MW00837108

BLACKWELL'S FIVE-MINUTE VETERINARY CONSULT

EQUINE

SECOND EDITION

BLACKWELL'S FIVE-MINUTE VETERINARY CONSULT

EQUINE

SECOND EDITION

Jean-Pierre Lavoie, DVM, Diplomate ACVIM
Professor
Department of Clinical Sciences
Faculte de Medecine Veterinaire
Universite de Montreal
St-Hyacinthe, Quebec, Canada

Kenneth William Hinchcliff, BVSc, PhD, Diplomate ACVIM
Professor and Dean
Faculty of Veterinary Science
The University of Melbourne
Melbourne, Australia

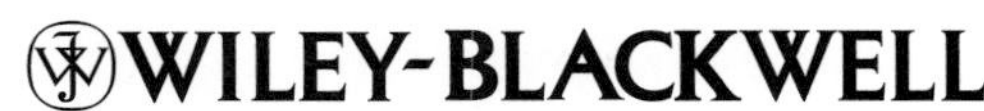

A John Wiley & Sons, Ltd., Publication

Blackwell Publishing was acquired by John Wiley and Sons in February 2007. Blackwell's publishing program has been merged with Wiley's global Scientific, Technical, and Medical business to form Wiley-Blackwell.

Editorial Office
2121 State Avenue, Ames, Iowa 50014-8300, USA

For details of our global editorial offices, for customer services, and for information about how to apply for permission to reuse the copyright material in this book, please see our website at www.wiley.com/wiley-blackwell.

Library of Congress Cataloging-in-Publication Data

Blackwell's five-minute veterinary consult : equine / [edited by] Jean-Pierre Lavoie, Kenneth William Hinchcliff. – 2nd ed.
p. ; cm.
Rev. ed. of: 5-minute veterinary consult : equine / Christopher M. Brown. c2002.
Includes bibliographical references and index.
ISBN 978-0-8138-1487-2 (alk. paper)
1. Horses–Diseases–Handbooks, manuals, etc. I. Lavoie, Jean-Pierre, 1957-. II. Hinchcliff, Kenneth W. (Kenneth William), 1956-. III. Brown, Christopher M. (Christopher Miles) 5-minute veterinary consult. IV. Title: Five-minute veterinary consult.
[DNLM: 1. Horse Diseases–Handbooks. 2. Veterinary Medicine–Methods–Handbooks.
SF 959 B632 2008
SF951.B867 2008
636.1′089–dc22 2008024700

A catalog record for this book is available from the U.S. Library of Congress.

Set in Adobe Garamond by Aptara
Printed in United States by Sheridan Books, Inc.
2 2011

PREFACE

One may ask what, in an era of widespread electronic availability of information, is the use of another textbook of equine medicine? The answer lies within the pages of this book in the form of a wealth of high-quality information presented in a compact format by topic experts. The result is a readily sourced body of information that does not need to boot up, never has a "blue screen" failure, and does not have a battery to go flat. Moreover, the book is readily browsed, allowing the reader to explore and find relevant information rapidly.

The purpose of this book is not to provide a detailed description of diseases of horses but rather to present a synopsis of the salient aspects of the important and common diseases with an emphasis on diagnosis and treatment. As such, this book, while useful for students, is intended for readers with a sound understanding of veterinary medicine who require a brief reminder of important aspects of disease.

This second edition of *Blackwell's Five-Minute Veterinary Consult: Equine* is built on the imposing body of work done on the first edition, supervised by Chris Brown and Joe Bertone. The quality of this second edition of the book is dependent on the hard work, knowledge, and attention to detail of the section editors and authors. The strength of this book is a tribute to their talents, whereas blame for any weaknesses can be laid at our feet.

J. P. Lavoie
K. W. Hinchcliff

CONSULTING EDITORS

JEAN-PIERRE LAVOIE, DVM,
Diplomate ACVIM
Professor
Department of Clinical Sciences
Faculte de Medecine Veterinaire
Universite de Montreal
St-Hyacinthe, Quebec, Canada
Volume Editor

KENNETH WILLIAM HINCHCLIFF,
BVSC, PhD,
Diplomate ACVIM
Professor and Dean
Faculty of Veterinary Science
University of Melbourne
Melbourne, Australia
Laboratory Tests, Volume Editor

ASHLEY BOYLE, DVM,
Diplomate ACVIM
Assistant Professor of Medicine
Section of Field Service
University of Pennsylvania
School of Veterinary Medicine
New Bolton Center
Kenneth Square, Pennsylvania, USA
Infectious Disease

DENNIS E. BROOKS, DVM, PhD,
Diplomate ACVO
Professor
Department of Large Animal Clinical
Sciences
University of Florida
Gainesville, Florida, USA
Ophthalmology

ELIZABETH J. DAVIDSON, DVM,
Diplomate ACVS
Assistant Professor in Sports Medicine
New Bolton Center
University of Pennsylvania School of
Veterinary Medicine
Kennett Square, Pennsylvania, USA
Musculoskeletal

DOMINIC DAWSON, DVM
Large Animal Medicine Resident
Department of Clinical Sciences
Cornell University Hospital for Animals
Cornell University College of Veterinary
Medicine
Ithaca, New York, USA
Urinary

DANIEL Q. ESTEP, PhD,
Certified Applied Animal Behaviorist
Co-Owner, Animal Behavior Associates
Littleton, Colorado, USA
Behavior

CAROLINE HAHN, DVM, MSc, PhD,
MRCVS,
Diplomate ECEIM, ECVN
Senior Lecturer
Veterinary Clinical Sciences
Royal (Dick) School of Veterinary
Studies
University of Edinburgh
Roslin, Midlothian, United Kingdom
Neurology

DAVID HODGSON, BVSC, PhD,
Diplomate ACVIM, FACSM
Head of Department
Large Animal Clinical Sciences
Virginia-Maryland Regional College of
Veterinary Medicine
Virginia Tech
Blacksburg, Virginia, USA
Hematopoietic

JENNIFER HODGSON, BVSC,
DIP VET PATH, PhD,
Diplomate ACVIM
Associate Professor
Biomedical Sciences and Pathobiology
Virginia-Maryland Regional College of
Veterinary Medicine
Virginia Tech
Blacksburg, Virginia, USA
Hematopoietic

DANIEL JEAN, DVM,
Diplomate ACVIM
Professor
Veterinary Clinical Sciences
Faculte de Medecine Veterinaire
Universite de Montreal
St-Hyacinthe, Quebec, Canada
Respiratory

MICHEL LEVY, DVM,
Diplomate ACVIM
Associate Professor, Large Animal
Medicine
Department of Veterinary Clinical
Sciences
School of Veterinary Medicine
Purdue University
West Lafayette, Indiana, USA
Endocrine/Metabolism

GWENDOLEN LORCH, DVM, MS,
Diplomate ACVD
Clinical Instructor of Dermatology
Department of Veterinary Clinical
Sciences
College of Veterinary Medicine
The Ohio State University
Columbus, Ohio, USA
Dermatology

CELIA M. MARR, PhD, MRCVS,
Diplomate ECEIM, EIM
Specialist in Internal Medicine
Rossdales Equine Hospital
Honorary Professor
Glasgow University Veterinary School
Newmarket, Suffolk, United Kingdom
Cardiology

MARGARET C. MUDGE, VMD,
Diplomate ACVS
Clinical Assistant Professor
Equine Emergency and Critical Care
Galbreath Equine Center
The Ohio State University
Columbus, Ohio, USA
Neonatology

OLIMPO OLIVER-ESPINOSA, DVM,
MSc, DVSc
Associate Professor, Salud Animal
Clinica de Grandes Animales
Salud Animal Facultad de Medicina
Veterinaria y de Zootecnia
Universidad Nacional de Colombia
Bogata DC, Cundinamarca, Colombia
Gastroenterology

GILLIAN A. PERKINS, DVM,
Diplomate ACVIM
Lecturer
Department of Clinical Sciences
College of Veterinary Medicine
Cornell University
Ithaca, New York, USA
Urinary

ROBERT H. POPPENGA, DVM, PhD,
Diplomate ABVT
Professor of Clinical Veterinary
Toxicology
California Animal Health and Food
Safety Laboratory
School of Veterinary Medicine
University of California–Davis
Davis, California, USA
Toxicology

VIRGINIA B. REEF, DVM,
Diplomate ACVIM
Professor of Medicine in the Widener Hospital
Director of Large Animal Cardiology and Ultrasonography
Chief, Section of Sports Medicine and Imaging
New Bolton Center
University of Pennsylvania School of Veterinary Medicine
Kennett Square, Pennsylvania, USA
Cardiology

HENRY STAMPFLI, DVM, PhD,
Diplomate ACVIM
Associate Professor Large Animal Medicine, Clinical Studies
Ontario Veterinary College
University of Guelph
Guelph, Ontario, Canada
Gastroenterology

CORINNE SWEENEY, DVM,
Diplomate ACVIM
Professor of Medicine
Associate Dean and Executive Hospital Director
The George D. Widener Hospital for Large Animals
New Bolton Center
University of Pennsylvania School of Veterinary Medicine
Kennett Square, Pennsylvania, USA
Infectious Disease

VICTORIA LEA VOITH, DVM, PhD,
Diplomate ACVB
Professor
College of Veterinary Medicine
Western University of Health Sciences
Pomona, California, USA
Behavior

CONTRIBUTORS

EMMA N. ADAM, BVetMed, Diplomate ACVIM, ACVS
Surgeon
Equine Sports Medicine and Surgery
Weatherford, Texas, USA

JENNIFER G. ADAMS, DVM, Diplomate ACVIM
Clinical Instructor, Anesthesiology
Department of Small Animal Medicine
College of Veterinary Medicine
University of Georgia
Athens, Georgia, USA

FRANCISCO JOSE ALVAREZ-BERGER DVM, DIPLOMATE ACVIM
Clinical Instructor
Veterinary Clinical Sciences
The Ohio State University
Columbus, Ohio, USA

VINCENT J. AMMANN, DVM, Diplomate ACVIM
Equine Practitioner
La Maison Cassou
Montagut, France

CLAIRE B. ANDREASEN, DVM, PhD, Diplomate ACVP
Professor and Chair
Department of Veterinary Pathology
College of Veterinary Medicine
Iowa State University
Ames, Iowa, USA

LUIS G. ARROYO, LicMedVet, DVSc
PhD Student
Department of Pathobiology
Ontario Veterinary College
University of Guelph
Guelph, Ontario, Canada

JANE E. AXON, BVSc, MACVSc, Diplomate ACVIM
Director
Clovelly Intensive Care Unit
Scone Veterinary Hospital
Scone, New South Wales, Australia

JOHN D. BAIRD, BVSc, PhD
Professor, Large Animal Medicine
Department of Clinical Studies
Ontario Veterinary College
University of Guelph
Guelph, Ontario, Canada

JANE A. BARBER, DVM, MS, Diplomate ACT
Clinical Theriogenologist
Veterinary Specialties at the Lake
Sherrils Ford, North Carolina, USA

RALPH E. BEADLE, DVM, PhD
Professor Emeritus
Veterinary Clinical Sciences
School of Veterinary Medicine
Louisiana State University
Baton Rouge, Louisiana, USA

KERRY BECKMAN, DVM
Owner
Gas Light Equine Veterinary Practice
Lanesville, Indiana, USA

DENNIS J. BLODGETT, DVM, PhD, Diplomate ABVT
Associate Professor
Biomedical Sciences and Pathobiology
Virginia Tech
Blacksburg, Virginia, USA

PAUL B. BLOOM, DVM, Diplomate ACVD and ABVP
Assistant Adjunct Professor
Small Animal Clinical Science
Michigan State University
Owner and Staff Dermatologist
Allergy, Skin and Ear Clinic for Pets
East Lansing, MI, USA

PATRICK JACQUES BOURDEAU, DVM, PhD, DIPLOMATE EVPC, ECVD,
Agregation in Parasitology,
Dipl Intitut Pasteur in Mycology
Full Professor,
Parasitology/Dermatology/Mycology,
Chairperson,
Department of Clinical Sciences
Unit
Dermatology/Parasitology/Mycology,
Exotic and Zoo Animals
National Veterinary School,
Centre Hospitalier Veterinaire
Nantes, France

LUDOVIC BOURE, Med Vet, MSc, DES, Diplomate ACVS, ECVS
Associate Professor
Department of Clinical Studies
Ontario Veterinary College
University of Guelph
Guelph, Ontario, Canada

ASHLEY BOYLE, DVM, Diplomate ACVIM
Assistant Professor of Medicine
Section of Field Service
University of Pennsylvania,
School of Veterinary Medicine
New Bolton Center
Kennett Square, Pennsylvania, USA

JOHAN BROJER, DVM, MSc, PhD, Diplomate ACVIM
Assistant Professor
Clinical Sciences, Equine Internal Medicine
Faculty of Veterinary Medicine
Swedish University of Agricultural Sciences
Uppsala, Sweden

DENNIS E. BROOKS, DVM, PhD, Diplomate ACVO
Professor
Department of Large Animal Clinical Sciences
University of Florida
Gainesville, Florida, USA

CHRISTOPHER M. BROWN, BVSc, PhD, Diplomate ACVIM
Dean, College of Veterinary Medicine
Michigan State University
East Lansing, Michigan, USA

TERESA A. BURNS, DVM
Resident, Equine Internal Medicine
Department of Veterinary Clinical Sciences
College of Veterinary Medicine
The Ohio State University
Columbus, OH, USA

MARIA E. CADARIO, DVM, Diplomate ACT
Equine Theriogenologist
Gainesville, Florida, USA

CARLA L. CARLETON, DVM, MS, Diplomate ACT
Associate Professor, Theriogenology
Large Animal Clinical Sciences
Equine Theriogenologist,
Veterinary Medical Center
Michigan State University,
College of Veterinary Medicine
East Lansing, Michigan, USA

STAN W. CASTEEL, DVM, PhD, Diplomate ABVT
Professor of Toxicology
Department of Veterinary Pathobiology
College of Veterinary Medicine
University of Missouri
Columbia, Missouri, USA

ALFRED CAUDLE, DVM, Diplomate ACT
Professor
Large Animal Medicine
Large Animal Department
University of Georgia
Athens, Georgia, USA

JOHN CHRISTIAN, DVM, PhD
Associate Professor of Clinical Pathology
Department of Comparative Pathobiology
Purdue University
West Lafayette, Indiana, USA

LAIS R. R. COSTA, MV, MS, PhD, Diplomate ACVIM, ABVP
Assistant Professor in Large Animal Medicine
Department of Clinical Sciences
Cummings School of Veterinary Medicine, Hospital of Large Animals
Tufts University
North Grafton, Massachusetts, USA

NATHALIE COTE, DVM, DVSc, Diplomate ACVS
Equine Surgeon
Milton Equine Hospital
Campbellville, Ontario, Canada

LAURENT COUETIL, DVM, PhD, Diplomate ACVIM
Director
Equine Research Program and Equine Sports Medicine Center
Professor, Veterinary Clinical Sciences, Purdue University School of Veterinary Medicine
Chief, Large Animal Medicine, Purdue University Teaching Hospital
West Lafayette, Indiana, USA

NICOLA C. CRIBB, MA, VetMB, DVSc, Diplomate ACVS
Staff Surgeon
Veterinary Teaching Hospital
Ontario Veterinary College
University of Guelph
Guelph, Ontario, Canada

MARK V. CRISMAN, DVM, MS, Diplomate ACVIM
Professor, Section Chief
Large Animal Clinical Science
Virginia-Maryland Regional College of Veterinary Medicine
Virginia Tech
Blacksburg, Virginia, USA

SHARON LYNN CROWELL-DAVIS, DVM, PhD, Diplomate ACVB
Professor
Anatomy and Radiology
Veterinary Teaching Hospital
College of Veterinary Medicine, University of Georgia
Athens, Georgia, USA

ANTONIO M. CRUZ, DVM, MVM, MSc, Dr. Vet Med, Diplomate ACVS, ECVS
Associate Professor
Department of Clinical Studies
University of Guelph
Ontario Veterinary College
Guelph, Ontario, Canada

ROBIN M. DABAREINER, DVM, PhD, Diplomate ACVS
Associate Professor of Lameness
Department of Large Animal Medicine
Texas A & M University
College Station, Texas, USA

MARTIN DAVID, DVM, MS, Diplomate ACVP
Clinical Pathologist
IDEXX Laboratories
Adjunct Professor, Veterinary Technology Program
Community College of Denver, Center for Health Sciences
Westminster, Colorado, USA

FLORENT DAVID, DVM, MSc, Diplomate ACVS, ECVS
Assistant Professor in Large Animal Surgery
Department of Veterinary Surgery
School of Agriculture, Food Science, and Veterinary Medicine
University College of Dublin
Beltfield, Dublin, Ireland

ELIZABETH J. DAVIDSON, DVM, Diplomate ACVS
Assistant Professor in Sports Medicine
University of Pennsylvania
School of Veterinary Medicine
New Bolton Center
Kennett Square, Pennsylvania, USA

HILDE E. V. DE COCK, DVM, PhD, Diplomate ACVP
Professor in Veterinary Pathology
Department of Veterinary Medicine
University of Antwerp
Antwerp, Belgium

THOMAS J. DIVERS, DVM, Diplomate ACVIM, ACVECC
Professor of Medicine
Department of Clinical Sciences
Cornell Hospital for Animals
Cornell University
Ithaca, New York, USA

PATRICIA M. DOWLING, DVM, MSc, Diplomate ACVIM and ACVCP
Professor, Veterinary Clinical Pharmacology
Department of Veterinary Biomedical Sciences
Western College of Veterinary Medicine
University of Saskatchewan
Saskatoon, Saskatchewan, Canada

NORM G. DUCHARME, DMV, MSc, Diplomate ACVS
James Law Professor of Surgery
Department of Clinical Sciences
Medical Director, Clinical Sciences, Equine and Farm Animal Hospital
College of Veterinary Medicine, Cornell University
Ithaca, New York, USA

WENDY MARLENE DUCKETT, DVM, MSc, Diplomate ACVIM
Associate Professor
Health Management
Atlantic Veterinary College
University of Prince Edward Island
Charlottetown, Prince Edward Island, Canada

DANIEL Q. ESTEP, PhD
Certified Applied Animal Behaviorist
Co-Owner
Animal Behavior Associates
Littleton, Colorado, USA

TIM J. EVANS, DVM, MS, PhD, Diplomate ACT, ABVT
Assistant Professor
Veterinary Pathology
Veterinary Medical Diagnostic Laboratory
University of Missouri-Columbia
Columbia, Missouri, USA

LAURA C. FENNELL, BVSc(Hons)
Resident in Equine Medicine
Equine Center
Department of Veterinary Clinic and Hospital
University of Melbourne
Werribee, Victoria, Australia

GREGORY L. FERRARO, DVM
Director, Center for Equine Health
School of Veterinary Medicine
University of California–Davis
Davis, California, USA

ANNA M. FIRSHMAN, BVSc, PhD, Diplomate ACVIM
Assistant Professor, Large Animal Medicine
Clinical Sciences
Lois Bates Acheson Veterinary Teaching Hospital
Oregon State University
Corvallis, Oregon, USA

GRACE FORBES, BVSc
Resident, Equine Medicine Department
Department of Veterinary Clinic and Hospital Equine Centre
The University of Melbourne
Werribee, Victoria, Australia

JENNIFER JACOBS FOWLER, DVM
Consulting Veterinarian
Princeton, New Jersey, USA

NICHOLAS FRANK, DVM, PhD, Diplomate ACVIM
Associate Professor
Department of Large Animal Clinical Sciences
University of Tennessee
University of Nottingham School of Veterinary Medicine and Science
Knoxville, Tennessee, USA, and Nottingham, United Kingdom

JOSE M. GARCIA-LOPEZ, VMD, Diplomate ACVS
Assistant Professor in Large Animal Surgery
Department of Clinical Sciences
Hospital for Large Animals
Tufts University Cummings School of Veterinary Medicine
North Grafton, Massachusetts, USA

TAM GARLAND, DVM, PhD, Diplomate ABVT
Branch Chief of Ag Security
Department of Homeland Security
Washington, District of Columbia, USA

TERRY C. GERROS, DVM, MS, Diplomate ACVIM
Equine Internal Medicine Consultant
IDEXX Laboratories, Inc.
Owner-Veterinarian
Santiam Equine Clinic
Salem, Oregon, USA

LIBERTY M. GETMAN, DVM,
Diplomate ACVS
Lecturer in Large Animal Surgery
Department of Clinical Studies
New Bolton Center
University of Pennsylvania School of Veterinary Medicine
Kennett Square, Pennsylvania, USA

SHANNON B. GRAHAM, DVM
Equine Field Service
Department of Clinical Sciences
New Bolton Center
University of Pennsylvania School of Veterinary Medicine
Kennett Square, Pennsylvania, USA

STEVEN T. GRUBBS, DVM, PhD,
Diplomate ACVIM
Senior Scientist
Clinical Development
Boehringer Ingelheim Vetmedica, Inc.
St. Joseph, Missouri, USA

BRIANNE GUSTAFSON
Student Intern
New York State Department of Agriculture and Markets
Iowa State University College of Veterinary Medicine, Class of 2009
Albany, New York, USA

RICHARD P. HACKETT, DVM, MS,
Diplomate ACVS
Professor of Surgery
Department of Clinical Sciences
Cornell University
Ithaca, New York, USA

CAROLINE HAHN, DVM, MSc, PhD,
Diplomate ECEIM, ECVN, MRCVs
Senior Lecturer
Veterinary Clinical Sciences
Royal (Dick) School of Veterinary Studies
University of Edinburgh
Roslin, Midlothian, United Kingdom

JEFFERY O. HALL, DVM, PhD,
Diplomate ABVT
Associate Professor
Head of Diagnostic Toxicology
Animal, Dairy, and Veterinary Sciences
Utah State University
Logan, Utah, USA

DIANA M. HASSEL, DVM, PhD,
Diplomate ACVS, ACVECC
Assistant Professor, Equine Emergency Surgery and Critical Care
Department of Clinical Sciences
Colorado State University
Fort Collins, Colorado, USA

HUGO HILTON, BVMandS, MRCVS,
Resident II: Large Animal Medicine
Veterinary Medical Teaching Hospital
University of California–Davis
Davis, California, USA

KENNETH WILLIAM HINCHCLIFF, BVSc, PhD, DIPLOMATE ACVIM
Professor and Dean
Faculty of Veterinary Science
University of Melbourne
Melbourne, Australia

LAURA JOHANNA MARIA HIRVINEN, DVM
Resident in Equine Surgery
Department of Veterinary Clinical Sciences
Galbreath Equine Center
The Ohio State University
Columbus, Ohio, USA

JENNIFER L. HODGSON, BVSc, DipVetPath, PhD,
Diplomate ACVM
Associate Professor
Biomedical Sciences and Pathobiology
Virginia Maryland Regional Collge of Veterinary Medicine
Virginia Tech
Blacksburg, Virginia, USA

STEPHEN HOOSER, DVM, PhD,
Diplomate ABVT
Professor, Toxicology
Department of Comparative Pathobiology
Head, Toxicology; Assistant Director Animal Disease Diagnostic Lab
School of Veterinary Medicine, Purdue University
West Lafayette, Indiana, USA

KATHERINE ALBRO HOUPT, VMD, PhD,
Diplomate ACVB
Professor
Clinical Sciences
Director, Behavior Clinic
College of Veterinary Medicine, Cornell University
Ithaca, New York, USA

JEREMY D. HUBERT, BVSc, MRCVS, MS,
Diplomate ACVS
Associate Professor, Equine Surgery
Department of Veterinary Clinical Sciences
Equine Health Studies Program
Louisiana State University
Baton Rouge, Louisiana, USA

KRISTOPHER J. HUGHES, BVSc, FACVSc,
Diplomate ECEIM, MRCVS
Senior Clinical Fellow in Equine Clinical Studies
Department of Companion Animal Sciences
University of Glasgow
Glasgow, Scotland, United Kingdom

SAMUEL HURCOMBE, BSc, BVMS, MS,
Diplomate ACVIM
Resident, Equine Internal Medicine
Department of Veterinary Clinical Sciences
College of Veterinary Medicine
The Ohio State University
Columbus, Ohio, USA

ARMANDO R. IRIZARRY-ROVIRA, DVM, PhD,
Diplomate ACVP
Research Advisor– Pathologist
Department of Toxicology and Drug Disposition, Eli Lilly and Company
Adjunct Associate Professor of Veterinary Anatomic and Clinical Pathology
Department of Comparative Pathobiology
Purdue University
Greenfield, Indiana, USA

DANIEL JEAN, DVM,
Diplomate ACVIM
Professor
Department of Clinical Sciences
Faculte de Medecine Veterinaire
Universite de Montreal
St-Hyacinthe, Quebec, Canada

IMOGEN JOHNS, BVSc,
Diplomate ACVIM
Lecturer in Equine Medicine
Department of Veterinary Clinical Sciences
Royal Veterinary College
University of London
North Mymms, Herts, United Kingdom

SORAYA V. JUARBE-DIAZ, DVM,
Diplomate ACVB
Certified Applied Animal Behaviorist
Tampa, Florida, USA

MARIA ELISABETH KALLBERG, DVM, PhD
Assistant Professor
Small Animal Clinical Sciences
University of Florida
Gainesville, Florida, USA

DANIEL G. KENNEY, VMD,
Diplomate ACVIM
Staff Veterinarian
Veterinary Teaching Hospital
Ontario Veterinary College
University of Guelph
Guelph, Ontario, Canada

BEVERLY A. KIDNEY, DVM, MVetSc, PhD,
Diplomate ACVP
Associate Professor
Department of Veterinary Pathology
Western College of Veterinary Medicine
University of Saskatchewan
Saskatoon, Saskatchewan, Canada

DONALD P. KNOWLES, DVM, PhD,
Diplomate ACVP
Research Leader
Animal Disease Research Unit, ADRU-ARS-USDA
Department of Veterinary Microbiology and Pathology
Washington State University
Pullman, Washington, USA

SANDRA NOGUEIRA KOCH, DVM, MS,
Diplomate ACVD
Assistant Clinical Professor
Veterinary Clinical Sciences
College of Veterinary Medicine
University of Minnesota
Saint Paul, Minnesota, USA

THOMAS GADEGAARD KOCH, DVM
PhD Candidate, Department of Biomedical Sciences
Staff Veterinarian, Large Animal Medicine, Department of Clinical Studies
Ontario Veterinary College
University of Guelph
Guelph, Ontario, Canada

JUDITH KOENIG, Dr.Med.Vet, DVSc,
Diplomate ACVS, ECVS
Assistant Professor
Clinical Studies
Ontario Veterinary College
University of Guelph
Guelph, Ontario, Canada

ANDRÁS M. KOMÁROMY, DrMedVet, PhD,
Diplomate ACVO and ECVO
Assistant Professor of Ophthalmology
Department of Clinical Studies
University of Pennsylvania
Philadelphia, Pennsylvania, USA

ANITA MAUREEN KORE, DVM, PhD,
Diplomate ABVT
Senior Toxicology Specialist
Toxicology Assessment and Compliance
Assurance, 3M
Saint Paul, Minnesota, USA

JEFFREY LAKRITZ, DVM, PhD,
Diplomate ACVIM
Associate Professor
Head, Food Animal Medicine and
Surgery
Veterinary Clinical Sciences
The Ohio State University
Columbus, Ohio, USA

ROLF E. LARSEN, DVM. PhD,
Diplomate ACT
Professor
Department of Clinical Studies
School of Veterinary Medicine
St. George's University
St. George's, Grenada

SHEILA LAVERTY, MVB,
Diplomate ACVS, ECVS
Professor
Department of Clinical Sciences
Faculte de Medecine Veterinaire
Universite de Montreal
St. Hyacinthe, Quebec, Canada

JEAN-PIERRE LAVOIE, DVM,
Diplomate ACVIM
Professor
Department of Clinical Sciences
Faculte de Medecine Veterinaire
Universite de Montreal
St-Hyacinthe, Quebec,
Canada

SONIA SARAH LE JEUNE, DVM,
Diplomate ACVS
Assistant Professor of Clinical Equine
Surgical Emergency and Critical Care
Department of Surgical and Radiological
Sciences
Large Animal Teaching Hospital
University of California–Davis
Davis, California, USA

MATHILDE LECLERE, DVM,
Diplomate ACVIM
PhD Student
Department of Clinical Sciences
Faculte de Medecine Veterinaire
Universite de Montreal
St-Hyacinthe, Quebec, Canada

LAURELINE LECOQ, DMV, DES,
Clinician
Department of Clinical Sciences
Veterinary Teaching Hospital
University of Montreal
St-Hyacinthe, Quebec, Canada

LAURA CARYN LEE, BVSc,
Large Animal Resident
Department of Large Animal Medicine
Virginia-Maryland Regional College of
Veterinary Medicine
Blacksburg, Virginia, USA

RENAUD LEGUILLETTE, DMV, MSc, PhD,
Diplomate ACVIM
Assistant Professor
Veterinary Clinical and Diagnostic
Sciences
Faculty of Veterinary Medicine
University of Calgary
Calgary, Alberta, Canada

MICHEL LEVY, DVM,
Diplomate ACVIM
Associate Professor, Large Animal
Medicine
Department of Veterinary Clinical
Sciences
School of Veterinary Medicine
Purdue University
West Lafayette, Indiana, USA

JEANNE LOFSTEDT, BVSc, MS,
Diplomate ACVIM
Professor, Large Animal Internal
Medicine
Department of Health Management
Atlantic Veterinary College
University of Prince Edward Island
Charlottetown, Prince Edward Island,
Canada

MAUREEN T. LONG, DVM, PhD,
Diplomate ACVIM
Associate Professor
Department of Infectious Diseases and
Pathology
College of Veterinary Medicine
University of Florida
Gainesville, Florida, USA

GWENDOLEN LORCH, DVM, MS,
Diplomate ACVD
Clinical Instructor of Dermatology
Department of Veterinary Clinical
Sciences
College of Veterinary Medicine
The Ohio State University
Columbus, Ohio, USA

MARGO LEE MACPHERSON, DVM, MS,
Diplomate ACT
Associate Professor
Large Animal Clinical Sciences
University of Florida
Gainesville, Florida, USA

JOHN E. MADIGAN, DVM, MS,
Diplomate ACVIM
Professor, Medicine and Epidemiology
School of Veterinary Medicine
University of California–Davis
Davis, California, USA

K. GARY MAGDESIAN, DVM,
Diplomate ACVIM, ACVECC, ACVCP
Associate Professor, Critical Care
Medicine and Epidemiology
University of California–Davis
Davis, California, USA

NICHOLAS MALIKIDES, BVSc, PhD,
FACVSc, MVCS, DVCS, MRCVS
Head, Pre-Clinical Development
Yarrandoo R and D Centre
Novartis Animal Health Australasia
Kemps Creek, New South Wales,
Australia

ERIN MALONE, DVM, PhD,
Diplomate ACVS
Associate Clinical Professor
Large Animal Surgery
Department of Veterinary Population
Medicine
University of Minnesota, College of
Veterinary Medicine
St. Paul, Minnesota, USA

RICHARD A. MANSMANN, VMD, PhD
Director, Equine Podiatry and
Rehabilitation Services
Director, Outreach Equine Health
Program
North Carolina State University College
of Veterinary Medicine
Veterinary Teaching Hospital
Raleigh, North Carolina, USA

CELIA M. MARR, PhD, MRCVS,
Diplomate ECEIM, EIM
Specialist in Internal Medicine
Rossdales Equine Hospital
Honorary Professor
Glasgow University Veterinary School
Newmarket, Suffolk, United Kingdom

BENSON B. MARTIN JR., VMD,
Diplomate ACVS
Associate Professor Sports Medicine
Department of Clinical Studies
New Bolton Center
University of Pennsylvania
Kennett Square, Pennsylvania, USA

CYNTHIA ANN McCALL, PhD, PAS,
Diplomate ACAABS
Professor
Extension Horse Specialist
Animal Sciences
Auburn University
Auburn, Alabama, USA

SUE M. McDONNELL, PhD,
Certified Applied Animal Behaviorist
Adjunct Professor in Behavior and
Reproduction
Clinical Studies
New Bolton Center
University of Pennsylvania School of
Veterinary Medicine
Kennett Square, Pennsylvania, USA

ERICA C. McKENZIE, BSc, BVMS, PhD,
Diplomate ACVIM
Assistant Professor, Large Animal
Medicine
Department of Clinical Sciences
Oregon State University
Corvallis, Oregon, USA

ROBERT H. MEALEY, DVM, PhD,
Diplomate ACVIM
Associate Professor
Department of Veterinary Microbiology
and Pathology
Washington State University
Pullman, Washington, USA

CARLOS EDUARDO MEDINA-TORRES, MV,
MSc
Resident: Large Animal Internal
Medicine, Veterinary Teaching Hospital
Doctor in Veterinary Science Candidate,
Department of Clinical Sciences
Ontario Veterinary College
University of Guelph
Guelph, Ontario, Canada

CAROLE C. MILLER, DVM, PhD,
Diplomate ACT
Program Chair, Veterinary Technology
Division of Life Sciences
Athens Technical College
Athens, Georgia, USA

CLIFF MONAHAN, DVM, PhD
Parasitologist
Department of Veterinary Preventive Medicine
College of Veterinary Medicine
The Ohio State University
Columbus, Ohio, USA

LUIS MONREAL, DVM, PhD,
Diplomate ECEIM
Associate Professor
Departament de Medicina I Cirurgia Animals, Facultat de Veterinaria
Head of the Equine Internal Medicine Service, Equine Teaching Hospital
Universitat Autonoma de Barcelona
Bellaterra, Barcelona, Spain

SANDRA E. MORGAN, DVM, MS,
Diplomate ABVT
Associate Professor
Physiological Sciences
College of Veterinary Medicine
Oklahoma State University
Stillwater, Oklahoma, USA

PETER R. MORRESEY, BVSc,
Diplomate ACT, ACVIM
Clinician, Medicine Department
Rood and Riddle Equine Hospital
Lexington, Kentucky,
USA

MARGARET C. MUDGE, VMD,
Diplomate ACVS, ACVECC
Clinical Assistant Professor
Equine Emergency and Critical Care
Galbreath Equine Center
The Ohio State University
Columbus, Ohio, USA

AMELIA S. MUNSTERMAN, DVM, MS,
Diplomate ACVS
Clinical Instructor
Equine Emergency and Critical Care
J. T. Vaughan Large Animal Teaching Hospital
Auburn University
Auburn, Alabama, USA

SHANNON J. MURRAY, DVM
Equine Surgery Resident
Veterinary Clinical Sciences
Galbreath Equine Center
The Ohio State University
Columbus, Ohio, USA

MATTHIAS A. MUURLINK, BVSc (Hons), MScVSc,
Registrar
Equine Centre
Veterinary Clinical Hospital
University of Melbourne
Melbourne, Australia

ROSE NOLEN-WALSTON, DVM,
Diplomate ACVIM
Assistant Professor
Clinical Sciences
New Bolton Center
University of Pennsylvania School of Veterinary Medicine
Kennett Square, Pennsylvania, USA

YVETTE S. NOUT, DVM, PhD,
Diplomate ACVIM, ACVECC
Postdoctoral Researcher
Neurological Surgery
University of California–San Francisco
San Francisco, California, USA

OLIMPO OLIVER-ESPINOSA, DVM, MSc, DVSc
Associate Professor
Clinica de Grandes Animales
Salud Animal
Facultad de Medicina Veterinaria y de Zootecnia
Universidad Nacional de Colombia
Bogata DC, Cundinamarca, Colombia

ERIC J. PARENTE, DVM
Associate Professor of Surgery
Department of Clinical Sciences
New Bolton Center
University of Pennsylvania School of Veterinary Medicine
Kennett Square, Pennsylvania, USA

DEBORAH A. PARSONS, DVM,
Diplomate ACVIM
Sole Proprietor, Veterinarian
Parsons Equine Internal Medicine Services
Langley, British Columbia, Canada

JOHN R. PASCOE, BVSc, PhD,
Diplomate ACVS
Professor of Surgery and Executive Associate Dean
School of Veterinary Medicine
University of California–Davis
Davis, California, USA

GILLIAN A. PERKINS, DVM,
Diplomate ACVIM
Lecturer
Department of Clinical Sciences
College of Veterinary Medicine
Cornell University
Ithaca, New York, USA

RICHARD J. PIERCY, MA VetMB, MS, PhD, MRCVS,
Diplomate ACVIM
Senior Lecturer in Equine Medicine and Neurology
Veterinary Clinical Sciences
Royal Veterinary College
Herts, United Kingdom

KONNIE H. PLUMLEE, DVM, MS,
Diplomate ABVT, ACVIM
Laboratory Director
Veterinary Diagnostic Laboratory
Arkansas Livestock and Poultry Commission
Little Rock, Arkansas, USA

CARYN E. PLUMMER, DVM,
Diplomate ACVO
Assistant Professor, Comparative Ophthalmology
Small and Large Animal Clinical Sciences
College of Veterinary Medicine,
Veterinary Medical Center
University of Florida
Gainesville, Florida, USA

ROBERT H. POPPENGA, DVM, PhD,
Diplomate ABVT
Professor of Clinical Veterinary Toxicology
California Animal Health and Food Safety Laboratory
School of Veterinary Medicine
University of California–Davis
Davis, California, USA

PHILIP EDWARD PRATER, DVM,
Diplomate ACT
Associate Professor
Agricultural Sciences
Veterinary Technology
Morehead State University
Morehead, Kentucky, USA

BIRGIT PUSCHNER, DVM, PhD,
Diplomate ABVT
Professor of Veterinary Clinical Toxicology
School of Veterinary Medicine
California Animal Health and Food Safety Laboratory
University of California–Davis
Davis, California, USA

MERL F. RAISBECK, DVM, MS, PhD,
Diplomate ABVT
Professor, Veterinary Toxicology
Department of Veterinary Sciences
University of Wyoming
Laramie, Wyoming, USA

VIRGINIA B. REEF, DVM,
Diplomate ACVIM
Mark Whittier and Lila Griswold Allam Professor of Medicine in the Widener Hospital
Chief, Section of Sports Medicine, Clinical Studies
Director of Large Animal Cardiology and Ultrasound, Sports Medicine and Imaging
New Bolton Center
University of Pennsylvania School of Veterinary Medicine
Kennett Square, Pennsylvania,
USA

LAURA K. REILLY, VMD,
Diplomate ACVIM
Adjunct Assistant Professor
Department of Clinical Studies
New Bolton Center
University of Pennsylvania School of Veterinary Medicine
Kennett Square, Pennsylvania, USA

N. EDWARD ROBINSON, BVetMed, PhD, MRCVS,
Hon Diplomate ACVIM;
Docteur Honoris Causa (Liege)
Matilda R. Wilson Professor
Large Animal Clinical Sciences
Michigan State University
East Lansing, Michigan, USA

JULIE ROSS, MA, VetMB, MRCVS,
Diplomate ACVIM
Veterinary Surgeon
Centre for Preventive Medicine
Animal Health Trust
Lanwades Park
Newmarket, Suffolk, United Kingdom

WILSON K. RUMBEIHA, BVM, PhD,
Diplomate ABT, ABVT
Associate Professor
Pathobiology and Diagnostic Investigation
Michigan State University
East Lansing, Michigan, USA

KAREN ELIZABETH RUSSELL, DVM, PhD,
Diplomate ACVP
Associate Professor
Department of Veterinary Pathobiology
College of Veterinary Medicine and Biomedical Sciences
Texas A & M University
College Station, Texas, USA

CHRISTOPHER T. RYAN, VMD
Lecturer, Department of Clinical Studies
Field Service
New Bolton Center
University of Pennsylvania School of Veterinary Medicine
Kennett Square, Pennsylvania, USA

SANDRA J. SARGENT, DVM,
Diplomate ACVD
Pittsburgh Veterinary Specialty and Emergency Center
Pittsburgh, Pennsylvania, USA

WILLIAM KENT SCARRATT, DVM,
Diplomate ACVIM
Associate Professor
Large Animal Clinical Sciences
Virginia-Maryland Regional College of Veterinary Medicine
Virginia Tech
Blacksburg, Virginia, USA

JENNIFER R. SCHISSLER, DVM
Resident
Veterinary Clinical Sciences, Dermatology
The Ohio State University
Columbus, Ohio, USA

HAROLD C. SCHOTT II, DVM, PhD,
Diplomate ACVIM
Professor
Large Animal Clinical Sciences
Michigan State University
East Lansing, Michigan, USA

JAMES SCHUMACHER, DVM, MS,
Diplomate ACVS
Professor
Large Animal Clinical Sciences
University of Tennessee
Knoxville, Tennessee, USA

BARBARA L. SHERMAN, MS, PhD, DVM,
Diplomate ACVB, CAAB
Clinical Associate Professor
Department of Clinical Sciences
North Carolina State University
College of Veterinary Medicine
Raleigh, North Carolina, USA

JO ANN SLACK, DVM,
Diplomate ACVIM
Assistant Professor of Ultrasound and Cardiology
Department of Clinical Studies
New Bolton Center
University of Pennsylvania School of Veterinary Medicine
Kenneth Square, Pennsylvania, USA

MARIANNE VAN SLOET OLDRUIBENBORGH.OOSTERBAAN, DVM, PdD,
Diplomate ECEIM
Spec KNMcD Equine Internal Medicine
Associate Professor, Equine Sciences
Faculty of Veterinary Medicine
Utrecht University
Utrecht, the Netherlands

KATIE J. SMITH, Bvet Med, MS,
Diplomate ACVS
Lecturer in Large Animal Surgery
Department of Surgery
New Bolton Center
University of Pennsylvania School of Veterinary Medicine
Kennett Square, Pennsylvania, USA

JANICE SOJKA, VMD, MS,
Diplomate ACVIM
Associate Professor
Veterinary Clinical Sciences and Large Animal Medicine
Purdue University
West Lafayette, Indiana, USA

WENDY S. SPRAGUE, DVM, PhD
Clinical Instructor
Department of Microbiology, Immunology and Pathology
Colorado State University
Fort Collins, Colorado, USA

GAIL ABELLS SUTTON, DVM, MSc,
Diplomate ACVIM
Clinical Instructor
Large Animal Department
University Veterinary Hospital,
Hebrew University of Jerusalem
Faculty of Agricultural, Food and Environmental Quality Sciences
Koret School of Veterinary Medicine
Rehovot, Israel

RAYMOND W. SWEENEY, VMD,
Diplomate ACVIM
Professor of Medicine
Chief Section of Medicine
Department of Clinical Studies
New Bolton Center
University of Pennsylvania School of Veterinary Medicine
Kennett Square, Pennsylvania, USA

CORINNE R. SWEENEY, DVM,
Diplomate ACVIM
Professor of Medicine
Associate Dean and Executive Hospital Director
The Gorge D. Widener Hospital for Large Animals
New Bolton Center
University of Pennsylvania, School of Veterinary Medicine
Kennett Square, Pennsylvania, USA

PATRICIA ANN TALCOTT, MS, DVM, PhD,
Diplomate ABVT
Associate Professor
VCAPP, Veterinary Diagnostic Toxicologist
Washington Animal Disease Diagnostic Laboratory
College of Veterinary Medicine
Washington State University
Pullman, Washington, USA

RACHEL HSING HSING TAN, BVSc (Hons), DVSc, MACVSc, MS ,
Dplomate, ACVIM
Chief Resident, Large Animal Internal Medicine
Large Animal Clinical Sciences
Virginia-Maryland Regional College of Veterinary Medicine
Virginia Tech
Blacksburg, Virginia, USA

DOUGLAS H. THAMM, VMD,
Diplomate ACVIM
Assistant Professor of Oncology
Department of Clinical Sciences
College of Veterinary Medicine and Biomedical Sciences
Colorado State University
Fort Collins, Colorado, USA

JENNIFER S. THOMAS, DVM, PhD,
Diplomate ACVP
Associate Professor
Department of Pathobiology and Diagnostic Investigation
Michigan State University
East Lansing, Michigan, USA

LARRY J. THOMPSON, DVM, PhD,
Diplomate ABVT
Senior Research Scientist
Quality and Food Safety
Product Technology Center
Nestle Purina PetCare
St. Louis, Missouri, USA

WALTER R. THRELFALL, DVM, MS, PhD,
Diplomate ACT
Professor and Head
Theriogenology Area
The Ohio State University
Columbus, Ohio, USA

PETER J. TIMONEY, MVD, PhD, MSc, FRCVS
Veterinary Science
University of Kentucky
Lexington, Kentucky, USA

ASHEESH K. TIWARY, DVM, MS,
Diplomate ABVT
Toxicologist
California Animal Health and Food Safety Laboratory System
School of Veterinary Medicine
University of California–Davis
Davis, California, USA

SUSAN J. TORNQUIST, DVM, PhD,
Diplomate ACVP
Associate Professor
Department of Biomedical Sciences
College of Veterinary Medicine
Oregon State University
Corvallis, Oregon, USA

JOSIE L. TRAUB-DARGATZ, DVM, MS,
Diplomate ACVIM
Professor
Clinical Sciences Department
Animal Population Health Institute
College of Veterinary Medicine and Biomedical Sciences
Fort Collins, Colorado, USA

SUSAN C. TROCK, DVM, MPH, ACPVM
Epidemiologist
Animal Health Diagnostic Laboratory
Cornell University
New York State Department of Agriculture and Markets
Ithaca, New York, USA

SANDRA C. VALDEZ-ALMADA, DVM, Diplomate ABVP, ACVS
Equine Surgeon
San Luis Rey Equine Hospital
Bonsall, California, USA

ANDREW W. VAN EPS, BVSc, MACVSc,
Resident, Large Animal Medicine
Department of Clinical Studies
New Bolton Center
University of Pennsylvania School of Veterinary Medicine
Kennett Square, Pennsylvania, USA

MODEST VENGUST, DVM, Diplomate ACVIM
Veterinary Faculty
University of Ljubljana
Ljubljana, Slovenia

LAURENT VIEL, DVM, MSc, PhD
Professor, Large Animal Internal Medicine
Department of Clinical Studies
Ontario Veterinary College, University of Guelph
Guelph, Ontario, Canada

VICTORIA LEA VOITH, DVM, PhD, Diplomate ACVB
Professor, Animal Behavior
College of Veterinary Medicine
Western University of Health Sciences
Pomona, California, USA

PETRA A. VOLMER, DVM, MS, Diplomate ABT and ABVT
Assistant Professor
Veterinary Biosciences
University of Illinois
Urbana, Illinois, USA

ELIZABETH ANNE WALMSLEY, BVSc, MRCVS
Resident in Surgery
Equine Department
University of Melbourne Equine Center
University of Melbourne
Werribee, Victoria, Australia

JOHANNA L. WATSON, DVM, PhD, Diplomate ACVIM
Associate Professor
Department of Medicine and Epidemiology
School of Veterinary Medicine
University of California, Davis
Davis, California, USA

J. SCOTT WEESE, DVM, DVSc, Diplomate ACVIM
Associate Professor
Department of Pathobiology
Ontario Veterinary College
University of Guelph
Guelph, Ontario, Canada

STEPHEN D. WHITE, DVM, Diplomate ACVD
Professor
Medicine and Epidemiology
School of Veterinary Medicine
University of California
Davis, California, USA

ROBERT H. WHITLOCK, DVM, PhD, Diplomate ACVIM
Associate Professor of Medicine
Director of Botulism Laboratory
Clinical Studies
New Bolton Center
University of Pennsylvania School of Veterinary Medicine
Kennett Square, Pennsylvania, USA

PAMELA A. WILKINS, DVM, PhD, Diplomate ACVIM, ACVECC
Associate Professor
Department of Clinical Studies and Chief, Emergency, Critical Care, and Anesthesia
George D. Widener Hospital for Large Animals
New Bolton Center
University of Pennsylvania School of Veterinary Medicine
Kennett Square, Pennsylvania, USA

W. DAVID WILSON, BVMS, MS
Professor, Department of Medicine and Epidemiology
Director, Veterinary Medical Teaching Hospital (VMTH)
School of Veterinary Medicine
University of California, Davis
Davis, California, USA

SHARON G. WITONSKY, DVM, PhD, Diplomate ACVIM
Associate Professor
Large Animal Clinical Sciences
Virginia-Maryland Regional College of Veterinary Medicine
Virginia Tech
Blacksburg, Virginia, USA

Contents

CONTENTS

BEHAVIOR

CARDIOLOGY

Dermatology

Endocrine/Metabolism

Gastroenterology

HEMATOPOIETIC

INFECTIOUS DISEASES

LABORATORY TESTS

Musculoskeletal

Neonatology

NEUROLOGY

OPHTHALMOLOGY

RESPIRATORY

THERIOGENOLOGY

TOXICOLOGY

URINARY

Blackwell's Five-Minute Veterinary Consult

Equine

Second Edition

ABDOMINAL DISTENTION IN THE ADULT HORSE

BASICS

DEFINITION

Process by which the abdomen becomes enlarged leading to a change in its normal contour and shape

PATHOPHYSIOLOGY

The accumulation of fluid, gas, or ingesta in the peritoneal GI tract and/or peritoneal cavity, presence of abdominal masses, increased size of abdominal organs, or abdominal wall abnormalities may result in the distention and/or change in shape of the abdominal contour.

SYSTEMS AFFECTED

• GI—Any condition, physical or functional, resulting in the vascular or nonvascular obstruction of the GI transit
• Cardiovascular—Fluid sequestration may lead to a decreased circulating volume and hypovolemic shock. Often compounded by the presence of vascular compromise of the GI tract leading to translocation of bacteria and/or toxins to the systemic circulation. Hemoperitoneum may occur from trauma or rupture of mesenteric vessels due to increased traction or trauma (e.g., during foaling), from any other abdominal viscera (e.g., rupture of the spleen or liver), or ascites secondary to heart failure.
• Behavioral—Flank watching, pawing, rolling or violent episodes of thrashing.
• Respiratory—Abdominal distention or herniated abdominal viscera (diaphragmatic hernia) may lead to hypoventilation.
• Musculoskeletal/nervous/ophthalmologic/skin—Due to self-inflicted trauma secondary to abdominal pain.
• Reproductive—Hydrops and ruptured of prepubic tendon is seen in pregnant mares and both conditions will manifest as change in the abdominal contour.

SIGNALMENT

• All horses are susceptible.
• Pregnant mares—hydrops (anytime during pregnancy), uterine torsion (mid-term), uroperitoneum (postpartum), rupture of the mesocolon (postpartum) leading to hemoperitoneum and large colon torsion (peripartum)
• Rupture of the prepubic tendon occurs in older, sedentary mares in late pregnancy.
• Miniature horses—predisposed to fecaliths, enteroliths, and small colon impactions
• Older horses—predisposed to pedunculating lipomas

SIGNS

Historical

The clinical progression should help the clinician differentiate between vascular and nonvascular GI obstructions and other non-GI causes of distention. Also, signalment and geographical location, time of year, and sex should provide clues toward a final diagnosis.

Physical

• Evaluate progression of clinical signs, historical facts, and cardiovascular system.
• Rectal examination is practical, inexpensive, and quick, but evaluates only the caudal abdomen.
• Abdominal ultrasound examination may help determining location, nature, and severity of the cause of colic.

CAUSES

Accumulation of Gas

• Functional obstruction—primary ileus due to increased sympathetic drive. Secondary ileus due to pain (visceral or musculoskeletal), ischemic necrosis (e.g., verminous arteritis), electrolyte abnormalities (e.g., endurance horses), dehydration, inflammation of the bowel (enteritis) or abdominal cavity (peritonitis), and drugs (e.g., α_2 agents, morphine)
• Physical obstruction—Either vascular (large colon volvulus, mesenteric root volvulus, strangulating lipoma) or nonvascular (impaction, enteroliths, nephrosplenic entrapment)
• Cecal tympany from abnormal cecal motility patterns
• Grain overload
• Free gas within the abdominal cavity may occur secondary to trauma or anaerobic infections
• Colitis

Accumulation of Fluid

• Hemoperitoneum—ruptured viscera or myenteric vessel
• Uroperitoneum—ruptured bladder secondary to obstructive urolithiasis or traumatic parturition
• Hydrops amnion or allantois
• Ascites—peritonitis, neoplasia, hypoproteinemia, right-sided heart failure
• Colitis or enteritis—secretory process leading to accumulation of fluid in lumen of large colon or small intestine
• Cecal impaction with fluid due to abnormal motility patterns
• Pyometra/mucometria

Solid Mass

• Abscess
• Neoplasia—lymphosarcoma, squamous cell carcinoma, mammary adenocarcinoma, mesothelioma, hemangiosarcoma, and hepatic neoplasia

Body Wall Abnormality

• Hernia
• Prepubic tendon rupture

RISK FACTORS

• Cribbing may predisposed to tympany of the colon and epiploic foramen entrapment.
• Gastric ulcers predispose to gastric rupture.
• Sudden exposure to large amounts of carbohydrate-rich feed or diets consisting of increased proportions of highly fermentable feedstuff (especially whole-grain corn) and decreased amounts of roughage can predispose to gastric tympany and large colon displacement or volvulus.
• Colonic impactions often occur in horses that are old or debilitated or that have poor dentition.
• Sudden change in physical activity or sudden stall rest imposed by another injury.
• Sudden change of diet, even hay batch, has been associated with colic and gas distention of the abdomen
• Enterolithiasis occurs frequently in the states of California, Florida, and Indiana.
• Sand impactions are seen frequently in the southern states, including Florida and Arizona, and the coastal states, including California and New Jersey.
• Ileal hypertrophy has been associated with ingestion of Bermuda grass hay.
• Periparturient mares are at increased risk of large colon volvulus, particularly if has happened in the past.
• Miniature horses are predisposed to small colon impactions.
• Overconditioned and old horses are predisposed to strangulating lipomas.

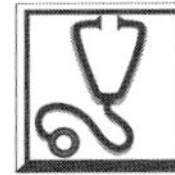

DIAGNOSIS

DIFFERENTIAL DIAGNOSIS

Differentiating Similar Signs

Other conditions also associated with abdominal distention:
• Marked subcutaneous edema along the ventral abdomen and thorax—hypoproteinemia, disturbed regional lymphatic drainage (e.g., pleuropneumonia), cardiac failure postoperative following abdominal celiotomy
• Pregnancy
• "Hay belly"—may be diagnosed on history (malnourished or severely parasitized horses, diets high in poor-quality roughage) and by fecal examination
• Pendulous abdomen secondary to Cushing's disease—usually accompanied by other distinctive signs, such as hirsutism
• Extreme obesity—ribs not palpable, fat deposits evident along crest of neck, over tailhead, etc.
• Subcutaneous emphysema from penetrating chest wound, ruptured trachea or subcutaneous anaerobic infection—characteristic crepitus noticed on palpation of the skin

Differentiating Causes

Signalment, history, physical examination, laboratory work, rectal palpation, and ultrasound examination findings often provide sufficient information to permit a tentative diagnosis. Some conditions are associated with characteristic findings:
• GI gas accumulation (bloat)—On auscultation of the abdomen, few to no GI sounds may be heard, and increased gaseous distention may be identified on percussion as a hyperresonant "ping"; depending on the inciting cause and the degree of distention present, various degrees of abdominal pain are usually present.
• Ascites from right-sided heart failure—Tricuspid insufficiency results in findings including heart murmur, exercise intolerance, jugular distention and pulse, and edema of the ventral abdomen, pectoral muscles, and distal limbs. Progression of the disease is slower than acute abdominal distention due to GI obstruction.
• Ascites from intra-abdominal mesothelioma—Because this tumor originates from the fluid-producing cells of the peritoneum, several liters of peritoneal fluid may be produced

within a 24-hr period; ascites may be more dramatic than is noted with other conditions.

- Body wall defect from prepubic tendon rupture—One of the only causes of unilateral abdominal distention in the horse; also results in cranioventral positioning of the mammary gland, cranial tilting of the pelvis, and severe ventral abdominal swelling.
- Presence of diarrhea may point toward the presence of colitis or enteritis.

CBC/BIOCHEMISTRY/URINALYSIS

Results are dependent on the cause. It is important to asses PCV, TP, and WBC and differential.

OTHER LABORATORY TESTS

- Abdominocentesis should be performed carefully in pregnant mares with intestinal distention, where the bowel may be torn easily by inadvertent penetration with a needle or teat cannula despite proper restraint.
- WBC count, TP level, and SG of the peritoneal fluid should be measured, and the fluid should be assessed cytologically for evidence of degenerate neutrophils, neoplastic cells, bacteria, or plant material. An increase in WBC count and TP levels and the appearance of degenerate neutrophils are indicative of increasing inflammation within the abdomen.
- Hemoperitoneum—free-flowing blood during the centesis procedure. Should be differentiated from puncture of the spleen during the procedure (PCV of the obtained sample higher than that of the circulating blood).
- Uroperitoneum—ratio of peritoneal fluid to serum Cr >2:1.

IMAGING

- Abdominal radiography may be of benefit in the diagnosis of gas accumulation within bowel segments in small horses and ponies. Enteroliths or sand impactions may be evident in adult horses in the mid- to ventral abdomen on the lateral view. Standing radiographs of these regions in a 500-kg horse require ≈450 mA and 100 kVp and therefore are mostly available at referral centers.
- Ultrasonography of the abdomen can be used to identify the location, amount, character, and echogenicity of peritoneal fluid and abdominal viscera, particularly thickness of the intestinal wall.

DIAGNOSTIC PROCEDURES

- Laparoscopy permits direct visualization of the abdominal cavity in the standing horse and can be used to provide a definitive diagnosis of the cause of abdominal distention. However, it must be used carefully in cases of abdominal distention to not damage accidentally any abdominal viscera upon entrance in the abdominal cavity. In the presence of GI distention, the ability of identifying the nature of the obstruction may be compromised.

Exploratory laparotomy through a flank incision in the standing horse is very limiting and should only be performed in selected cases as a therapeutic intervention if a confirmed diagnosis such as nephrosplenic entrapment or uterine torsion has been made. Exploratory laparotomy through a ventral midline incision in the anesthetized horse should not be delayed unnecessarily as it may be a life-saving diagnostic and therapeutic tool if used appropriately.

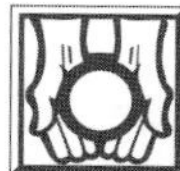

TREATMENT

- Treatment is dependent on the cause of abdominal distention.
- Cardiovascular stabilization through rehydration and correction of electrolyte and acid-base abnormalities should be initiated prior to treatment of the primary disease process.
- In horses with severe gaseous distention, trocharization of the cecum and/or large colon may be necessary to improve ventilation. Any horse that is trocharized should be treated preemptively with broad-spectrum antibiotic therapy to reduce and minimize the inherent risk of peritonitis. The site for trocharization is situated within the paralumbar fossa and can be delineated through auscultation and percussion of the distended viscus. The author prefers the highest point possible and on the right side this may coincide with the cecal attachment to the body wall, thereby decreasing the incidence of direct peritoneal contamination. The trocharization site should ideally be situated in the mid-proximal region of the most tympanitic area. A longer catheter may be used in this procedure to ensure that the viscus is entirely decompressed. Following clipping and aseptic preparation of the site, a small bleb of local anesthetic should be injected into the skin and muscle layers. A 5.25-in. (13.3-cm) 14-gauge stiff intravenous catheter with stylet should be used for trocharization. The catheter should be inserted through the skin, muscle layers, and distended viscus with a gentle thrust. The stylet could be removed once the viscus has been penetrated and maintained until no further escaping gas is heard or fluid is seen at the hub of the catheter. The audible escape of gas confirms correct placement within the lumen of the distended viscus. In order to prevent laceration of the bowel wall, the needle/catheter should be held carefully during the decompression phase and the hand should follow gently in the direction that GI motility dictates. As the bowel becomes decompressed, the catheter may require further advancement into the lumen of the viscus. In order to prevent leakage of intestinal contents from the tip of the catheter into the peritoneal cavity, the catheter should not be withdrawn until the decompression process is complete. The catheter is then withdrawn while injecting 10 mL of procaine penicillin or gentamicin. The trocarization site should be wiped clean with alcohol.
- Horses with abdominal distention should be confined to a stall and monitored continuously until a diagnosis has been made and appropriate treatment initiated. Feed should be withheld from horses showing any signs of abdominal discomfort. Prompt and adequate referral to a hospital facility may be required in cases requiring surgical intervention or prolonged nursing care.

MEDICATIONS

Drug therapy is dictated by the inciting cause.

FOLLOW-UP

Plans for monitoring are based on cause and treatment.

MISCELLANEOUS

PREGNANCY

- Termination of pregnancy may be indicated in mares with hydrops or nonresolving uterine torsion. In case of mares with hydrops if bred in the future, a different stallion should be selected.
- Induction of parturition may be necessary in mares close to term that have experienced rupture of the prepubic tendon. These mares should be monitored carefully and parturition attended as they may require assistance with delivery due to their inability to perform effective abdominal press for fetal expulsion.

SYNONYMS

Bloat

SEE ALSO

See Causes.

ABBREVIATIONS

- Cr = creatinine
- GI = gastrointestinal
- PCV = packed cell volume
- SG = specific gravity
- TP = total protein
- WBC = white blood cell

Suggested Reading

Foreman JH. Abdominal distention. In: Reed SM, Bayly WM (eds). Equine Internal Medicine. Philadelphia: WB Saunders, 1998.

Author Antonio M. Cruz

Consulting Editors Henry Stämpfli and Olimpo Oliver-Espinosa

ABDOMINAL HERNIA IN ADULT HORSES

BASICS

OVERVIEW

Abdominal hernia is an exteriorization of internal organs through a defect or an anatomic opening in the abdominal wall. In adult horses, abdominal herniae include ventral, incisional, and acquired inguinal/scrotal hernia.

SIGNALEMENT

Ventral Hernia

Most frequently seen in older, late-term pregnant mares. The draft breeds appear to be predisposed.

Incisional Hernia

It is a complication of ventral celiotomy in 10%–15% of horses. No breed or sex predilection. Incisional herniation can develop up to 3 mo after ventral celiotomy, but acute form develops within 8 days after surgery.

Acquired Inguinal/Scrotal Hernia

• Inguinal hernia refers to the passage of intestine and/or omentum through the vaginal ring into the inguinal canal. • Scrotal hernia describes presence of herniated contents in the scrotum. • Distal jejunum and ileum are most frequently involved, but omentum or small colon may also herniate.
• Acquired inguinal/scrotal hernia occurs exclusively in the intact male horse but isolated cases of inguinal herniation in geldings and mares have been reported.
• Standardbred, Tennessee Walking Horses, American Saddlebreds, and draft breeds seem to be predisposed.

SIGNS

Ventral Hernia

Mares with ventral hernia walk slowly and often lie down. Often, the herniae are painful and the horses have an increased heart and respiratory rates. A large swelling over the flank or caudal ventral abdomen is present. Orientation of the pelvis and the mammary gland is normal. Signs of colic may be present if the herniated content is compromised.

Incisional Hernia

Brown serosanguineous discharge from the incision and progressive increase in drainage of peritoneal fluid are commonly observed prior to dehiscence. Ventral swelling developing over the abdominal incision site is observed. Gaps in the abdominal wall between sutures may be palpated.

Acquired Inguinal/Scrotal Hernia

Scrotal swelling may be mild in inguinal hernia but marked in horses with scrotal hernia. The testis on the hernia side is usually firmer and cooler compared to the opposite testis. Abdominal pain may vary from mild to severe depending on degree of intestinal strangulation.

CAUSES AND RISK FACTORS

Ventral Hernia

In pregnant mares, old broodmares, and twin gestation. Often associated with degenerative changes in the body wall. It can also be associated with trauma and hydrallantois.

Incisional Hernia

Incisional infection and swelling, postoperative endotoxemia and pain, repeated surgeries, and use of chromic gut suture predispose hernia formation after celiotomy.

Acquired Inguinal/Scrotal Hernia

Inguinal/scrotal hernia often follows breeding activity or strenuous athletic exercise. Large vaginal rings may predispose to herniation, but it also occurs in horses with small to normal-size vaginal rings.

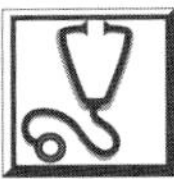

DIAGNOSIS

DIFFERENTIAL DIAGNOSES

Ventral Hernia

Prebubic tendon rupture. Clinical signs are similar; however, the pelvis becomes tilted cranioventrally. Cranioventral displacement of the udder can lead to rupture of blood supply and blood can be observed in the milk of such mares.

Incisional Hernia

Postoperative wound infection, severe peri-incisional edema, seroma, and sinus formation are easily differentiated from incisional herniae with the abdominal wall being intact on palpation and ultrasonographic examination.

Acquired Inguinal/Scrotal Hernia

Torsion of the spermatic cord, infectious epididymitis or orchitis, thrombosis of the testicular artery, hydrocele, hematocele, and testicular neoplasia

CBC/BIOCHEMISTRY/URINALYSIS

Unremarkable in absence of secondary intestinal obstruction

IMAGING

Abdominal Ultrasonography

Transcutaneous abdominal ultrasonographic examination with a 3.5- or 5-MHz transducer is used to rule in herniation, to evaluate the extent of the abdominal wall defect, and to identify hernia contents. May also reveal presence of herniated intestine in acquired inguinal/scrotal hernia or rule out hydrocele, hematocele, and testicular neoplasia

OTHER DIAGNOSTIC PROCEDURES

External Palpation

To define the hernia ring and hernia contents but is more difficult with extensive abdominal edema. Mares with ventral hernia resist deep palpation of affected area. Palpation of inguinal regions and scrota is mandatory in stallions with signs of colic.

Rectal Palpation

• Ruling out prepubic tendon rupture by rectal palpation can be difficult, depending on the defect's location and size of the fetus. Palpation of distended loops of intestine associated with abdominal pain warrants immediate exploratory laparotomy. • Rectal palpation of stallions with inguinal/scrotal herniae reveals presence of a loop of intestine entering the vaginal ring. Multiple loops of distended intestine are usually palpated with intestinal obstruction.

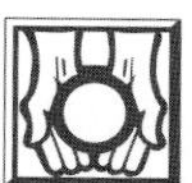

TREATMENT

Ventral Hernia and Incisional Hernia

Ventral or incisional herniae are treated initially conservatively by supporting the ventral abdominal wall, decreasing the amount of local inflammation and edema, and preventing worsening of the condition. Affected horses should be rested, fed with low-bulk feed, and monitored for signs of intestinal obstruction. Abdominal pressure bandage should be applied for 24 hr a day and removed twice daily for cold (initial phase) or warm (chronic phase) hydrotherapy for 20–30 min. Ventral or incisional hernia may resolve with conservative treatment, but for the surgical closure of the abdominal defect 8–12 weeks after its occurrence is usually required. Application of a mesh will be performed based on the size of the wall defect and the surgeon's preference. Horses with acute severe incisional dehiscence (eventration) are emergency surgical candidates.

Acquired Inguinal/Scrotal Hernia

Treatment of acute inguinal/scrotal hernia is surgical. During early phase, when intestinal strangulation has not yet occurred, it may be possible to reduce the hernia using external inguinal/scrotal massages under general anesthesia in dorsal recumbency.

MEDICATION

DRUG(S)

Ventral and Incisional Hernia

Pending surgical correction, the use of NSAIDs (phenylbutazone 2.2 mg/kg PO q12 h) is advocated to decrease abdominal edema. Parenteral broad-spectrum antibiotics are also required for incisional hernia. Resolution of incisional infection is mandatory prior to attempting surgical correction.

FOLLOW-UP

• The prognosis for ventral hernia is guarded. Incisional and inguinal/scrotal herniations warrant a favorable prognosis.
• From 3 to 5 mo of rest is required after surgical correction of both ventral and incisional herniae.

Suggested Reading

Kawcak CE, Stashak TS. Predisposing factors, diagnosis, and management of large abdominal wall defects in horses and cattle. JAVMA 1995;206:607–611.

Mair TS, Smith LJ. Survival and complication rates in 300 horses undergoing surgical treatment of colic. Part 2: Short-term complications. Equine Vet J 2005,37:303–309.

Author Ludovic Bouré
Consulting Editors Henry Stämpfli and Olimpo Oliver-Espinosa

ABDOMINOCENTESIS

BASICS

OVERVIEW

• Procedure for sampling peritoneal fluid by collection through the abdominal wall
• Fluid is collected into EDTA and into a sterile clot tube for bacterial culture or biochemical tests.
• Equine abdominal fluid normally appears clear and colorless to slightly yellow and does not clot.
• Total protein commonly is assessed by refractometer and normally is <2.5 g/dL.
• Nucleated cell count in fluid from normal horses is <10,000 cells/μL, with a predominance of nondegenerative neutrophils (22%–98%) and large mononuclear cells (1%–68%), which include mesothelial cells and macrophages. Small lymphocytes may comprise 0%–36% of the total and eosinophils up to 7%; mast cells and basophils rarely are seen. Normally, few erythrocytes are present.
• Biochemical measurements other than total protein may include lactate as an indicator of intestinal ischemia and creatinine and/or potassium to diagnosis uroabdomen.

PATHOPHYSIOLOGY

• Normal peritoneal fluid is a dialysate of plasma; many of the low-molecular-weight substances in blood are present in the peritoneal fluid at similar concentrations.
• High-molecular-weight molecules (e.g., proteins) normally are not present in abdominal fluid.
• Cells in normal peritoneal fluid include mesothelial cells and small numbers of cells from the blood and lymphatics.
• Fluid circulates constantly through the abdominal cavity and is drained via lymphatic vessels. When fluid production exceeds drainage, an effusion develops. This may occur with some systemic disorders (e.g., cardiovascular disease) or with local disorders of abdominal organs or mesothelium. Changes in peritoneal fluid protein, cell numbers and types may reflect those disorders.
• In the face of inadequate intestinal perfusion and ischemia, anaerobic glycolysis can result in increased peritoneal fluid lactate concentration.

SYSTEMS AFFECTED

• GI
• Hepatobiliary
• Hemic/lymphatic/immune
• Renal/urologic
• Cardiovascular
• Reproductive

SIGNALMENT

Any breed, age, or sex

SIGNS

• Colic
• Chronic weight loss
• Abdominal distention
• Diarrhea

CAUSES AND RISK FACTORS

• Peritonitis caused by compromised gut wall
• Hemorrhage
• Neoplasia
• Intestinal parasitism and secondary thromboembolism
• Inflammation of abdominal organs
• Breeding and foaling injuries
• Bile or urine leakage
• Postsurgical inflammation
• Abdominal abscess
• Decreased oncotic pressure
• Congestive heart failure

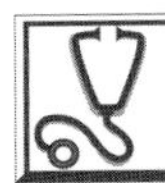

DIAGNOSIS

DIFFERENTIAL DIAGNOSIS

Peritonitis

• Fluid is an exudate with increased nucleated cell count and a predominance of neutrophils.
• Total protein usually is >2.5 g/dL because of inflammation.
• Bacteria are present in septic peritonitis and may be intracellular or extracellular.
• With gut rupture, cells often are degenerate and mixed bacterial types, ciliated protozoa and plant material may be seen.
• Postsurgical peritonitis also produces an exudate with increased cell numbers and total protein within 24 hr. Neutrophils generally are not degenerate and no bacteria are seen. Increased RBC numbers may be seen.

Hemorrhage

• With a splenic tap, PCV is higher in abdominal fluid than in blood, and small lymphocyte numbers may be increased.
• With hemorrhage into the abdomen, PCV of fluid is lower than that of blood. Platelets are absent, and erythrophagocytosis may be present.
• With blood contamination at the time of sampling, fluid initially may look clear, with bloody streaks appearing during sampling. Phagocytosis of RBCs is not seen, and platelets may be present.

Neoplasia

Diagnosis may be established on finding neoplastic cells in fluid but absence of neoplastic cells does not rule out neoplasia, because tumor cells may not exfoliate into fluid.

Parasitism

Migration of parasitic larvae may be associated with increased eosinophils, but this does not occur often and is not diagnostic for parasitism.

Uroabdomen

- Typically, peritoneal fluid creatinine and potassium are increased compared to serum concentrations.
- Hyperkalemia, marked hyponatremia, and hypochloremia are typical but are not present in all cases.

Ascites

- A transudate with low cell numbers and low protein content may be present with hypoalbuminemia or lymphatic or vascular obstruction or stasis.
- Serum biochemical profile and history contribute to this diagnosis.

Congestive Heart Failure

Increased hydrostatic pressure within vessels may result in a modified transudate with a higher cell count and protein level than a transudate, but these values may be normal for equine abdominal fluid.

CBC/BIOCHEMISTRY/URINALYSIS

- Inflammatory causes of abdominal effusion may be associated with leukocytosis or hyperfibrinogenemia if disease is systemic.
- Left shift or toxic changes in neutrophils indicate systemic inflammation.
- Serum biochemistries help to assess causes of transudates—panhypoproteinemia is consistent with GI protein loss; elevated liver enzymes suggest hepatic disease.
- Serum electrolytes and comparison of serum and fluid creatinine aid in diagnosis of uroperitoneum.

OTHER LABORATORY TESTS

Bacterial culture is helpful in some cases, such as abdominal abscess.

IMAGING

Ultrasonography

- May be used to look for intestinal entrapment, intussusception, masses, adhesions, enlarged liver, and enteroliths
- Ultrasonographic location of peritoneal fluid sometimes helps in performing abdominocentesis.

Abdominal Radiography

In adult horses, may aid in establishing the diagnosis of diaphragmatic hernia, sand, and enteroliths.

OTHER DIAGNOSTIC PROCEDURES

- Laparoscopy may be used to establish the diagnosis in cases of chronic colic or weight loss.
- Gastroscopy can be useful in establishing the diagnosis of gastric ulcers, impaction, and neoplasia.
- Exploratory laparotomy is necessary for definitive diagnosis in some cases.

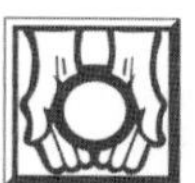

TREATMENT

Directed at the underlying cause

MEDICATIONS

None

FOLLOW-UP

POSSIBLE COMPLICATIONS

Accidental enterocentesis (rarely associated with clinical disease) causes increased nucleated cell count in abdominal fluid within 4 hours.

MISCELLANEOUS

AGE-RELATED FACTORS

Foals normally have protein levels similar to peritoneal fluid cell counts (<1500 cells/μL) but lower than adults.

PREGNANCY

No significant differences in fluid from mares that are pregnant or have recently foaled compared with fluid from nonperipartum mares.

ABBREVIATIONS

- GI = gastrointestinal
- PCV = packed cell volume

Suggested Reading

Latson KM, Nieto JE, Beldomenico PM, Snyder JR. Evaluation of peritoneal fluid lactate as a marker of intestinal ischaemia in equine colic. Equine Vet J 2005;37:342–346.

Parry BW, Brownlow MA. Peritoneal fluid. In: Cowell RL, Tyler RD, eds. Cytology and Hematology of the Horse. Goleta, CA: American Veterinary Publications, 1992:121–151.

Author Susan J. Tornquist

Consulting Editor Kenneth W. Hinchcliff

ABNORMAL ESTRUS INTERVALS

BASICS

DEFINITION/OVERVIEW

Estrus—period of sexual receptivity by the mare for the stallion.
• Abnormal—individual's overt display of sexual behavior for longer or shorter periods than normal. • Abnormal interestrus intervals result from short or long estrus or diestrus intervals.

ETIOLOGY/PATHOPHYSIOLOGY

• Mare—seasonally polyestrus in spring and summer months. • Average estrous cycle—21 days (range: 19–22); period of time between ovulations • Estrus coincides with P4 levels <1 ng/mL. • Estrus and estrous cycle lengths repeatable in individual mare from cycle to cycle.

Key Hormonal Events in the Equine Estrous Cycle

• FSH causes ovarian follicular growth.
• Estradiol (E2) stimulates increased GnRH pulse frequency to decreased LH secretion. • LH surge causes ovulation; E2 returns to basal levels 1–2 days post-ovulation. • Progesterone (P4) rises from basal levels (<1 ng/mL) at ovulation to >4 ng/mL by 4–7 days post-ovulation. • P4 causes decreased GnRH pulse frequency, allowing increased FSH secretion to stimulate a new wave of ovarian follicles to develop during diestrus. • $PGF_2\alpha$ (endometrial origin) is released 14–15 days post-ovulation, causing luteolysis and concurrent decline in P4 levels.

Estrus Length

In normal, cycling mares—average 5–7 days; range 2–12 days

Diestrus Length

Less variable than estrus in normal, cycling mares, averaging 15 +/− 2 days

Sexual Behavior

• Absence of P4 allows onset of estrus behavior even if E2 is present in small quantities.
• Conditions that eliminate P4 and/or >E2 concentrations are likely to induce estrus behavior. Persistence of these conditions results in abnormal estrus periods or interestrus intervals. The converse is also true.

SYSTEMS AFFECTED

• Reproductive • Behavioral • Endocrine

SIGNALMENT

• Any breed • Mares of age >20 years tend to have prolonged transition periods, >estrus duration, fewer estrous cycles per year • Ponies may have longer estrous cycles than horses (average 25 days).

SIGNS

Historical

• Chief complaints—infertility, failure to show estrus, prolonged estrus, split estrus, or frequent estrus behavior • Teasing records—Review methods, frequency, teaser type (pony, horse, gelding), stallion behavior (aggressive/passive, vocalization, proximity), and handler experience.
• Seasonal influence—Individual variation (onset/duration/termination of cyclicity) can be mistaken for estrus irregularity. • Mare's reproductive history—Can clinical abnormalities be linked to estrous cycle length, teasing, foaling, previous injuries, or genital infections?
• Pharmaceutical—Clinical abnormalities related to current and historical drug administration?

Physical Examination

• Body condition—Poor condition/malnutrition may add to/cause abnormal estrous cycles.
• Perineal conformation—Poor vulvar conformation can result in pneumovagina, ascending infection, urine pooling and may result in symptoms consistent with behavioral estrus. • Clitoral size—Enlargement may be related to prior treatment with anabolic or progestational steroids or intersex conditions.
• TRP—Essential to evaluate abnormal cycles; uterine size and tone; ovarian size, shape and location; cervical relaxation. Serial examinations, minimum 3 per week, may be needed (several weeks) to define her estrous cycle.
• U/S—Define uterine and ovarian features, normal and abnormal. • Vaginal examination—To identify inflammation, urine pooling, cervical competency or abnormal conformation. Also identify stage of estrous cycle (appearance, degree of external cervical os relaxation).

CAUSES

Shortened Estrus Duration

• Seasonality—Estrus duration decreases in height of breeding season; more efficient folliculogenesis. • Silent estrus—Normal cyclic ovarian activity but minimal or no overt sexual receptivity. Often behavior-based problem—nervousness, foal-at-side, maiden mare; possibly previous anabolic steroid use.

Lengthened Estrus Duration

• Seasonality—Erratic estrus behavior with transition periods is common. Vernal transition receptivity can be short or long; protracted estrus behavior most common. • Ovarian neoplasia (GCT, GTCT)—affected mare chronically, anestrus exhibits persistent or frequent estrus behavior or stallion-like behavior • Congenital disorders—Gonadal dysgenesis due to chromosomal defects (e.g., XO, XXX) may underlie anestrus, erratic estrus, or prolonged estrus. • Hormone imbalance—Older mares may fail to ovulate and exhibit prolonged estrus; may be ineffective LH release.

Shortened Interestrus Interval

• Uterine disease—Uterine inflammation may cause atypical endogenous $PGF_2\alpha$ release, luteolysis, and early return to estrus. • Systemic illness—Endotoxin-induced $PGF_2\alpha$ release can cause premature luteolysis and a shortened interestrus period. • Iatrogenic/pharmaceutical—$PGF_2\alpha$ administration, intrauterine infusions, uterine biopsy procedure can cause corpus luteum regression, early return to estrus.

Lengthened Interestrus Interval

• Prolonged corpus luteum (CL) activity:
  ○ A normal diestrus ovulation—if CL is immature, it fails to respond to endogenous $PGF_2\alpha$ release.
  ○ Severe uterine disease may prevent release of uterine $PGF_2\alpha$.
  ○ Early embryonic death after maternal recognition of pregnancy
  ○ Persistent CL
  ○ Luteinization of an ovarian hematoma
  ○ Persistent CLs also associated with consumption of fescue forages
• Pregnancy—CL persists if a conceptus is present. Estrus behavior during pregnancy can be normal.
• Iatrogenic/pharmaceutical:
  ○ Treatment with progestin compounds suppresses behavioral estrus.
  ○ NSAIDs—potential interference with endometrial $PGF_2\alpha$ release; result—prolonged CL activity
  ○ No evidence that chronic PGF_2 treatment (label dosing) inhibits spontaneous formation and release of endogenous $PGF_2\alpha$
• GnRH agonist (deslorelin) implants—stimulate ovulation, associated with prolonged interovulatory intervals; effect more profound if $PGF_2\alpha$ is used during the diestrus period to short-cycle the mare.

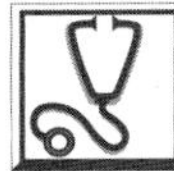

DIAGNOSIS

DIFFERENTIAL DIAGNOSIS

Differentiating Conditions with Similar Symptoms

• Frequent urination:
  ○ Cystitis/urethritis
  ○ Bladder atony
  ○ Urine pooling
  ○ Vaginitis or pneumovagina
  ○ May mimic submissive urination and be confused with behavioral estrus
• Defensive or aggressive behavior can be confused with anestrus—review or alter teasing methods.

Differentiating Causes

• Minimum database—Need full medical and reproductive history, teasing, physical examination, TRP, U/S, vaginal examination
• May be useful—uterine cytology, culture, and biopsy
• Silent estrus—often due to poor detection
  ○ *Diagnosis*—TRP minimum 3 per week with frequent serum P4 assays to detect a short or inapparent estrus period
• Transition period in the Northern Hemisphere extends from February to April; mare begins to develop follicles but not regular estrous cycles.
  ○ Characterized by persistent estrus behavior, irregular estrus periods, or irregular diestrus intervals
  ○ *Diagnosis*—Season, combined with serial TRP and U/S, confirms numerous small to large follicles on both ovaries that fail to progress to ovulatory size.
• GCT/GTCT—any age but more typical in middle-aged or older mares. Affected ovary enlarges; ovulation fossa often fills in; contralateral ovary—smaller, inactive
  ○ U/S–affected ovary—multilocular "honeycomb" appearance

- *Diagnosis*—TRP and U/S–endocrine assays

• Gonadal dysgenesis—usually ID when the mare enters the breeding herd and fails to have normal estrous cycles
- *Diagnosis*—TRP and U/S confirm absence of normal ovarian tissue and a juvenile reproductive tract. Karyotyping for a definitive diagnosis.

• Ovulation in diestrus—Corpus luteum formed from a diestrus ovulation may be insufficiently mature to be lysed by endogenous $PGF_{2}\alpha$ at the end of diestrus. Ovulations after day 10 of the estrous cycle result in persistent CL activity.
- *Diagnosis*—demonstration of a normal reproductive tract with failure of clinical estrus for >2 weeks post-ovulation; P4 levels of >4 ng/mL for >2 weeks

CBC/BIOCHEMISTRY/URINALYSIS
N/A

OTHER LABORATORY TESTS
• Serum P4 concentrations
- Basal levels of <1 ng/mL indicate no functional luteal tissue.
- Active CL function is associated with P4 levels of >4 ng/mL.

• Serum testosterone and inhibin concentrations
- Mare testosterone values typically <50–60 pg/mL and inhibin values <0.7 ng/mL
- Hormone levels suggestive of a GCT/GTCT (in a nonpregnant mare)—testosterone >50–100 pg/mL (if thecal cells are present), inhibin >0.7 ng/mL, with P4 <1 ng/mL

IMAGING
Transrectal U/S—routine to evaluate equine ovaries reproductive tract.

OTHER DIAGNOSTIC PROCEDURES
• Uterine endoscopy can help identify intrauterine adhesions, glandular or lymphatic cysts, and polyps.

• Uterine cytology, culture, and biopsy

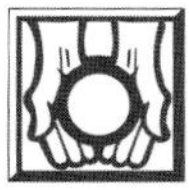

TREATMENT

• Vary teasing methods—Silent estrus may be a reflection of poor teasing management.

• Monitor the problem mare, including TRP and U/S, 3 times weekly to best define the reproductive cycle.

• Poor vulvar conformation—Control pneumovagina by vulvoplasty; a portion of the dorsal vulvar commissure is closed surgically.

• GCT/GTCT—ovariectomy

• Urine pooling, rectovaginal fistula and cervical tears—surgical correction

• Artificial lighting—management tool to initiate earlier ovarian activity
- Mares bred earlier in the season, foal earlier the next year; accommodate breed registries that use the January 1 universal birth date.
- Photostimulation does not eliminate vernal transition; merely shifts it to an earlier time of onset.
- Photostimulation should begin ≥90 days prior to the onset of early season breeding.

MEDICATIONS

DRUG(S) OF CHOICE
• $PGF_{2}\alpha$ (10 mg IM) or its analogs to lyse CL tissue.

• If follicle is ≥35 mm—deslorelin 2.1 mg implant SC or hCG (2500 IU IV) can stimulate ovulation.

• Altrenogest (0.044 mg/kg PO daily, minimum 15 days) can be used to shorten the duration of vernal transition, provided multiple follicles >20-mm diameter are present and the mare is demonstrating behavioral estrus.
- $PGF_{2}\alpha$ (10 mg IM) on day 15 of the altrenogest treatment increases the reliability of this transition management regimen.

CONTRAINDICATIONS
$PGF_{2}\alpha$ and its analogs—contraindicated in mares with heaves, or other bronchoconstrictive disease.

PRECAUTIONS
• Horses
- $PGF_{2}\alpha$ causes sweating and colic-like symptoms due to its stimulatory effect on smooth muscle cells. If cramping has not subsided within 1–2 h, symptomatic treatment should be instituted.
- Antibodies to hCG can develop after treatment; desirable to limit hCG use to no more than 2–3 times during one breeding season. The half-life of these antibodies ranges from 30 days to several months; typically do not persist from one breeding season to the next
- Deslorelin implants—associated with suppressed FSH secretion and decreased follicular development in the diestrus period immediately following use; results in a prolonged interovulatory period in nonpregnant mares. Implant removal post-ovulation is recommended. Injectable product still available in the United States
- Altrenogest, deslorelin, and $PGF_{2}\alpha$ should not be used in horses intended for food.

• Humans
- $PGF_{2}\alpha$ or its analogs should not be handled by pregnant women or persons with asthma or bronchial disease. Accidental exposure to skin—wash off immediately.
- Altrenogest should not be handled by pregnant women or persons with thrombophlebitis and/or thromboembolic disorders, cerebrovascular disease, coronary artery disease, breast cancer, estrogen-dependent neoplasia, undiagnosed vaginal bleeding, or tumors that developed during the use of oral contraceptives or estrogen-containing products. Accidental exposure to skin—wash off immediately.

POSSIBLE INTERACTIONS N/A

ALTERNATIVE DRUGS
• Cloprostenol sodium (250 μg/mL IM), a prostaglandin analog
- Product used similar to natural prostaglandin but fewer side effects
- While not currently approved for use in horses, it is in broad use in the absence of an alternative.

FOLLOW-UP

PATIENT MONITORING
Until normal cyclicity is established or pregnancy confirmed, regular TRP examinations are recommended.

POSSIBLE COMPLICATIONS
Unless corrected, abnormalities in estrus behavior frequently result in infertility.

MISCELLANEOUS

PREGNANCY
• Prostaglandin administration to pregnant mares can cause CL lysis and abortion, especially if <40 days pregnant.

• Carefully rule out pregnancy before using any prostaglandin product.

SYNONYMS
• Anestrus • Prolonged diestrus
• Pseudopregnancy • Short estrus

SEE ALSO
• Aggression • Anestrus • Clitoral enlargement
• Disorders of sexual development
• Early embryonic death • Endometritis
• Large ovary syndrome • Ovulation failure
• Pneumovagina/pneumouterus • Prolonged diestrus • Pseudopregnancy • Pyometra
• Urine pooling/urovagina • Vaginitis and vaginal discharge • Vulvar conformation

ABBREVIATIONS
• CL = corpus luteum
• E2 = estradiol
• FSH = follicle-stimulating hormone
• GCT = granulosa cell tumor
• GnRH = gonadotropin-releasing hormone
• GTCT = granulosa theca cell tumor
• hCG = human chorionic gonadotropin
• LH = luteinizing hormone
• P4 = progesterone
• $PGF_{2}\alpha$ = PGF, natural prostaglandin ($F_{2\alpha}$)
• TRP = transrectal palpation
• U/S = ultrasound, ultrasonography

Suggested Reading

Hinrichs K. Irregularities of the estrous cycle and ovulation in mares (including seasonal transition). In: Youngquist RS and Threlfall WR, eds. Current Therapy in Large Animal Theriogenology. St. Louis, MO: Saunders Elsevier, 2007;144–152.

McCue PM, Farquhar VJ, Carnevale EM, Squires EL. Removal of deslorelin (Ovuplant™) implant 48 h after administration results in normal interovulatory intervals in mares. Therio 2002;58:865–870.

Author Carole C. Miller

Consulting Editor Carla L. Carleton

ABNORMAL SCROTAL ENLARGEMENT

BASICS

DEFINITION/OVERVIEW

A condition causing the gross appearance of the scrotum to deviate from normal size and texture, e.g., scrotal enlargement and/or asymmetry.

ETIOLOGY/PATHOPHYSIOLOGY

- Equine scrotum and associated contents are positioned on a horizontal axis between the hind limbs of the animal and are relatively well protected from external insult.
- Scrotal skin is thin and pliable, and contents are freely movable within the scrotum.
- Blunt trauma (breeding accident, jumping) is the most common cause of scrotal abnormality.
- Trauma can result in scrotal hemorrhage, edema, rupture of the tunica albuginea, hematocoele, hydrocoele, and inflammation.
- Similar signs can occur with inguinal/scrotal herniation, torsion of the spermatic cord, or neoplasia.

SYSTEM AFFECTED

Reproductive

GENETICS

N/A

INCIDENCE/PREVALENCE

Dependent on cause—traumatic, vascular, infectious/noninfectious, neoplastic

SIGNALMENT

- Intact male horses
- Any age

SIGNS

Historical

- Gross changes in the size of the scrotum (usually acute)
- Pain (generally colic-like symptoms)
- Reluctance to breed, jump, or walk
- Extreme environmental temperatures (hot or cold)

Physical Examination

- Increased scrotal size (unilateral or bilateral)
- Abnormal testicular position
- Abnormal scrotal temperature (too warm or cold)
- Edema/engorgement of scrotum and/or contents
- Scrotal laceration
- Derangements in systemic parameters (elevated HR, RR, inappetence, CBC abnormalities)
- Any combination of abnormalities may be present and not all signs are present in every animal.

CAUSES

- Three most common:
  - Trauma, may include testicular hematoma/rupture
  - Inguinal/scrotal hernia
  - Torsion of the spermatic cord, also known as testicular torsion
- Inflammatory/infectious causes:
  - EIA
  - EVA/EAV
  - Orchitis/epididymitis
- Neoplasia
  - Primary scrotal—melanoma, sarcoid
  - Testicular neoplasia—seminoma, teratoma, interstitial cell tumor, Sertoli cell tumor
- Noninflammatory scrotal edema
- Hydrocele/hematocele
- Varicocele
- See also: Abnormal Testicular Size

RISK FACTORS

- Breeding activity
- Large internal inguinal rings
- Systemic illness
- Extremes of ambient temperature (hot or cold)

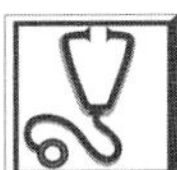

DIAGNOSIS

DIFFERENTIAL DIAGNOSIS

Differentiating Causes

- Duration of problem
  - Acute—traumatic injury, torsion of spermatic cord, herniation, infection
  - Chronic—neoplasia, temperature-induced hydrocele/edema, varicocele, infection
- History of recent breeding, semen collection, and/or trauma
- Palpation of the caudal ligament of the epididymis (attaches epididymal tail to caudal testis and aids in the determination of testicular orientation)
- Palpation of the inguinal rings
- U/S (see Imaging)

CBC/BIOCHEMISTRY/URINALYSIS

- Inflammatory or stress leukocyte response
- Increased fibrinogen
- Results of serum biochemistry profile and urinalysis are usually normal.

OTHER LABORATORY TESTS

- EVA
  - SN or CF
  - Acute and convalescent serum samples
  - If stallion is seropositive, carrier state is determined with virus isolation.
  - Virus isolation from serum and/or seminal plasma
  - Semen is best sample for diagnosis (freeze portion of ejaculate and send to approved lab with serum samples).
  - **Send samples to an approved laboratory.**
- EIA
- AGID or ELISA, the Coggins test

IMAGING—SCROTAL U/S

Examination of scrotal contents may reveal:

- Bowel with inguinal/scrotal herniation
- Rupture of the testis/tunica albuginea
  - Accumulation of hypoechoic fluid in scrotum with loss of discrete hyperechoic tunica albuginea around testicular parenchyma
  - Hypoechoic appearance of contents will gradually contain echogenic densities with the formation of fibrin clots.
- Engorgement of the pampiniform plexus and/or testicular congestion with torsion of the spermatic cord
  - Doppler can verify loss of blood flow to the testis.
- Hypoechoic dilation of venous plexus of spermatic cord with varicocele
- Hypoechoic accumulation of fluid within the vaginal cavity with hydrocele
- Loss of homogeneity in testicular parenchyma with neoplasia
  - May see areas of increased or decreased echogenicity or be variable throughout

OTHER DIAGNOSTIC PROCEDURES

- Needle aspirate and cytology—to differentiate hydrocele from recent hemorrhage
- Neoplasia—diagnosed using fine needle aspirate and/or biopsy

PATHOLOGICAL FINDINGS

Dependent on etiology

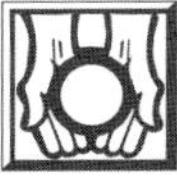

TREATMENT

Treatment is directed at the cause of scrotal enlargement.

- Management of inflammation is a primary concern with abnormal scrotal enlargement.
- Sexual rest is indicated for all causes of scrotal enlargement.

APPROPRIATE HEALTH CARE

Inpatient or Outpatient Treatment?

- Acute scrotal enlargement warrants hospitalization for treatment and care.
- Chronic scrotal enlargement may or may not warrant hospitalization; etiology dependent

NURSING CARE

• Cold therapy (cold packs, ice water baths, water hose) for acute scrotal trauma is implemented only in the absence of testicular rupture.
  ○ Testicular tunics *must* be intact.
• Cold therapy sessions should not exceed 20 min and can be repeated every 2 hr.
• Scrotal massage with emollient salve—useful to reduce scrotal edema and ischemic injury
• Fluid removal should be considered with hydrocele.
  ○ Use only an aseptically placed needle or an IV catheter.
  ○ Excess fluid accumulation may cause thermal damage to the testes.
• Administration of IV fluids is dependent on systemic status of the horse.

ACTIVITY

The need to restrict activity depends on etiology of scrotal enlargement.

DIET

Diet modification is necessary only with secondary ileus or as a preoperative consideration.

CLIENT EDUCATION

• Fertility may be irreversibly impaired with acute scrotal trauma.
• Semen evaluation should be performed 90 days after nonsurgical resolution of scrotal enlargement.
• Compensatory semen production may occur in the remaining testis of a horse undergoing hemicastration.
• Following removal of a neoplasia, examine carefully for evidence of metastatic tumor growth (serial examinations).

SURGICAL CONSIDERATIONS

• Hemicastration is the treatment of choice for:
  ○ Torsion of the spermatic cord, if the duration of vascular compromise has caused irreversible damage and/or gonadal necrosis
  ○ Unilateral inguinal/scrotal herniation
  ○ Testicular rupture
  ○ Unilateral neoplasia
  ○ Varicocele
  ○ Nonresponsive hydrocele/hematocele
• Primary repair of scrotal laceration is required to protect scrotal contents.
  ○ Repair generally fails due to extensive scrotal edema associated with traumatic injury.

MEDICATIONS

DRUG(S) OF CHOICE

• Anti-inflammatory therapy (phenylbutazone 2–4 mg/kg P/O or IV BID or flunixin meglumine 1 mg/kg IV BID) indicated in all cases
• Diuretics (furosemide 0.5–1 mg/kg IV) may be useful in managing scrotal edema.
• Antibiotic therapy should be considered in cases of scrotal laceration or scrotal hemorrhage.
• Tetanus toxoid should be administered for scrotal trauma or prior to surgery.

CONTRAINDICATIONS, PRECAUTIONS, POSSIBLE INTERACTIONS, ALTERNATIVE DRUGS

N/A

FOLLOW-UP

PATIENT MONITORING

Semen collection and evaluation 90 days after complete resolution of cause and/or surgery

PREVENTION/AVOIDANCE

N/A

POSSIBLE COMPLICATIONS

• Infertility
• Endotoxemia
• Laminitis
• Scrotal adhesions
• Death

EXPECTED COURSE AND PROGNOSIS

N/A

MISCELLANEOUS

ASSOCIATED CONDITIONS, AGE-RELATED FACTORS, ZOONOTIC POTENTIAL, PREGNANCY, SYNONYMS

N/A

SEE ALSO

• Abnormal testicular size

ABBREVIATIONS

• AGID = agar gel immunodiffusion
• CBC = complete blood count
• CF = complement fixation
• EIA = equine infectious anemia
• ELISA = enzyme-linked immunosorbent assay
• EVA = equine viral arteritis
• EAV = equine arteritis virus
• HR = heart rate
• RR = respiratory rate
• SN = serum neutralization
• TRP = transrectal palpation
• U/S = ultrasound, ultrasonography

Suggested Reading

Love CC. Ultrasonographic evaluation of the testis, epididymis and spermatic cord of the stallion. In: Blanchard TL, Varner DD, eds. The Veterinary Clinics of North America: Equine Practice. Stallion Management. 1992;8:167–182.

Varner DD, Schumacher J, Blanchard T, Johnson L. Diseases and Management of Breeding Stallions. Goleta: American Veterinary Publications, 1991.

Author Margo L. Macpherson
Consulting Editor Carla L. Carleton

ABNORMAL TESTICULAR SIZE

BASICS

DEFINITION/OVERVIEW

Any condition causing the gross appearance of a testis to deviate from normal size and texture, e.g., testicular enlargement, reduction, and/or asymmetry

ETIOLOGY/PATHOPHYSIOLOGY

- The testes and epididymides are positioned in a horizontal orientation between the hind limbs of the horse and are freely movable within the scrotum.
- The scrotum and contents, while relatively protected from external insult, are at increased risk for injury during breeding or athletic activity.
- *Acute enlargement* of a testis occurs after trauma, torsion of the spermatic cord, or orchitis/epididymitis.
  - May be of bacterial, viral, autoimmune, or parasitic origin
- *Testicular neoplasia* is uncommon in the horse.
  - Seminoma, teratoma, Sertoli cell tumor, interstitial cell tumor
  - Of these, seminoma is the most frequently reported testicular tumor of the stallion.
  - Most equine testicular tumors arise from germ cells, including seminomas and teratomas.
  - The effect of neoplasia on testicular size (increase or decrease) may be insidious.
- *Hypoplastic* and *degenerative testes* are smaller than normal.
- *Testicular degeneration* can be transient or permanent.
  - An acquired condition, degeneration may arise from thermal injury, infection, vascular insult, hormonal disturbances, toxins, and age.
- *Testicular hypoplasia* is an irreversible condition.
  - Hypoplastic testes are incompletely developed.
  - Condition is usually congenital.
  - Suspected causes include genetic aberrations, teratogens, cryptorchidism, and postnatal insult.

SYSTEMS AFFECTED

- Reproductive
- Other systems (respiratory, GI, lymphatic) may be affected subsequent to metastasis of primary testicular neoplasia.

GENETICS

Cryptorchism and testicular hypoplasia are subjected to having genetic components.

INCIDENCE/PREVALENCE

Dependent on etiology

SIGNALMENT

- Intact male horses
- Any age

SIGNS

Historical

- Recent history of breeding or semen collection
- Gross changes in the size of a testis
- Reduced fertility
- Pain (generally colic-like symptoms)
- Reluctance to breed, jump, or walk

Physical Examination

- Increased or decreased scrotal size
- Increased or decreased testicular size
- Abnormal testicular texture (too soft or firm)
- Abnormal testicular position
- Abnormal scrotal temperature (too warm or cold)
- Edema/engorged scrotum and/or contents
- Derangements in systemic parameters (elevated HR, RR, inappetence, CBC abnormalities)

CAUSES

- Three most common
  - Trauma
  - Cryptorchidism
  - Torsion of the spermatic cord
- Testicular degeneration
- Testicular hypoplasia
- Testicular hematoma/rupture
- Neoplasia
  - Seminoma
  - Teratoma
  - Interstitial cell tumor
  - Sertoli cell tumor
- Orchitis/epididymitis
  - Bacterial infection
  - EIA
  - EVA, EAV
  - *Strongylus edentatus* infection
  - Autoimmune

RISK FACTORS

- Breeding activity
- Systemic illness
- Temperature extremes
- Anabolic steroid use

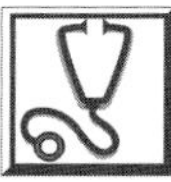

DIAGNOSIS

DIFFERENTIAL DIAGNOSIS

Differentiating Similar Signs

- Scrotal enlargement due to scrotal hydrocele/hematocele and scrotal or inguinal hernia may be confused with testicular enlargement.
- U/S examination and measurement of the testes is the best means of differentiating the pathologies.

Differentiating Causes

- Duration of problem:
  - *Acute*: traumatic injury, torsion of spermatic cord, infection
  - *Chronic*: cryptorchidism, neoplasia, infection, testicular degeneration/hypoplasia
- History of recent breeding and/or trauma
- Palpation of the caudal ligament of the epididymis (attaches epididymal tail to caudal testis and aids in the determination of testicular orientation).
- Testicular hypoplasia is usually congenital, while testicular degeneration is acquired.
- U/S (see Imaging).

CBC/BIOCHEMISTRY/URINALYSIS

- Inflammatory or stress leukocyte response.
- Eosinophilia may be an indicator of a parasitic infection.
- Increased fibrinogen in peripheral blood.
- Serum biochemistry profile and urinalysis are usually normal.

OTHER LABORATORY TESTS

- EVA:
  - SN or CF
  - Requires acute and convalescent serum samples
  - If stallion is seropositive, carrier state is determined with virus isolation.
  - Semen is best sample for diagnosis (freeze portion of ejaculate and send to approved lab with serum samples).
  - **Send samples to an approved laboratory.**
- EIA:
  - AGID or ELISA, the Coggins test.
- Testicular degeneration:
  - Endocrine profile (LH, FSH, testosterone, estrogens) from pooled samples obtained hourly for a minimum of four samples (due to pulsatile release of hormones)
  - Abnormal elevation of FSH and low total estrogen concentration are indicative of testicular degeneration.

IMAGING, SCROTAL/TESTICULAR U/S

Testicular parenchyma should appear uniformly echogenic. Aberrations that may be identified by U/S include:

- Rupture of the testis/tunica albuginea
  - Hypoechoic fluid accumulates in the scrotum with loss of discrete hyperechoic tunica albuginea around testicular parenchyma.
  - Hypoechoic appearance of contents will gradually be replaced with echogenic densities as fibrin clots form.
- Engorgement of the pampiniform plexus and/or testicular congestion with torsion of the spermatic cord
  - Doppler can verify loss of blood flow to the testis.
- Loss of homogeneity in testicular parenchyma with neoplasia
  - Neoplasia results in heterogeneity (usually a circumscribed area) in testicular parenchyma.
  - May see areas of increased or decreased echogenicity or be variable throughout

OTHER DIAGNOSTIC PROCEDURES

- Needle aspirate and cytology—diagnose and/or differentiate recent hemorrhage or neoplasia

- Testicular histopathology—diagnose and/or differentiate neoplasia and testicular degeneration/hypoplasia
- Semen evaluation is useful in the diagnosis of testicular degeneration or hypoplasia.
    - Oligospermia
    - Azoospermia
    - Premature release of spermatids

PATHOLOGICAL FINDINGS

N/A

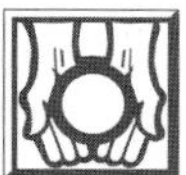

TREATMENT

Treatment is directed at the cause of testicular abnormality.

APPROPRIATE HEALTH CARE

Inpatient versus Outpatient

- Most causes of testicular enlargement require hospitalization for treatment/resolution.
- Horses with testicular degeneration that are not systemically ill may be managed on the farm.
- Horses with hypoplastic testes can be managed on an outpatient basis.

NURSING CARE

- Cold therapy (cold packs, ice water baths, water hose/hydrotherapy) is indicated for acute orchitis/epididymitis.
- Cold therapy sessions should not exceed 20 min and can be repeated every 2 hr.
- Sexual rest is indicated in most cases until resolution of the problem.
- Administration of IV fluids is dependent on systemic status of the horse.

ACTIVITY

Restriction depends on cause of the testicular aberration.

DIET

Modification is necessary only with cases of secondary ileus or as a preoperative consideration.

CLIENT EDUCATION

- Fertility may be permanently lowered.
- Testicular degeneration and subsequent reduction in semen quality can be transient or permanent, depending on the inciting cause.
- Testicular hypoplasia is a permanent condition.
- Horses with neoplasia should be examined carefully for evidence of metastatic tumor growth.
- Compensatory sperm production may occur in the remaining testis of a horse undergoing hemicastration.
- Serial semen evaluations are beneficial to monitor fertility status of horses following testicular insult and treatment.
    - Semen should be evaluated 75–90 days after complete resolution of testicular insult.

SURGICAL CONSIDERATIONS

- Hemicastration is the treatment of choice for:
    - Torsion of the spermatic cord, if the duration of vascular compromise has caused irreversible damage and/or gonadal necrosis
    - Testicular rupture
    - Unilateral neoplasia or any condition causing irreparable damage to testis/es

MEDICATIONS

DRUG(S) OF CHOICE

- Anti-inflammatory therapy (phenylbutazone 2–4 mg/kg PO or IV BID or flunixin meglumine 1 mg/kg IV BID) is indicated in most cases.
- Antibiotic therapy should be considered in cases of orchitis/epididymitis and testicular trauma.
- Tetanus toxoid should be administered after testicular trauma and/or prior to surgery.
- Antiparasitic therapy for *Strongylus edentatus* infection (ivermectin 0.2 mg/kg PO q30days until resolution of lesions)

CONTRAINDICATIONS PRECAUTIONS, POSSIBLE INTERACTIONS, ALTERNATIVE DRUGS

N/A

FOLLOW-UP

PATIENT MONITORING

Semen collection and evaluation 90 days after complete resolution of testicular problem and/or surgery

POSSIBLE COMPLICATIONS

- Infertility/subfertility
- Endotoxemia
- Laminitis
- Scrotal adhesions
- Death

EXPECTED COURSE AND PROGNOSIS

Dependent on etiology

MISCELLANEOUS

ASSOCIATED CONDITIONS

- Cryptorchidism is commonly associated with testicular hypoplasia.
- Male equine hybrids (mules or hinnies) often have hypoplastic testes.

AGE-RELATED FACTORS

- Prepubertal testes are small and can be misdiagnosed as pathologically hypoplastic.
- Testicular growth increases rapidly from 12 to 24 mo of age in horses.
- Testes may take 4–5 years to reach full size and maturity.

ZOONOTIC POTENTIAL

N/A

PREGNANCY

N/A

SYNONYMS

N/A

SEE ALSO

- Cryptorchidism
- Abnormal scrotal enlargement

ABBREVIATIONS

- AGID = agar-gel immunodiffusion
- CBC = complete blood count
- CF = complement fixation
- EAV = equine arteritis virus
- EIA = equine infectious anemia
- ELISA = enzyme-linked immunosorbent assay
- EVA = equine viral arteritis
- FSH = follicle-stimulating hormone
- GI = gastrointestinal
- HR = heart rate
- LH = luteinizing hormone
- RR = respiratory rate
- SN = serum neutralization
- U/S = ultrasound, ultrasonography

Suggested Reading

Brinsko SP. Neoplasia of the male reproductive tract. In: Savage CJ, ed. Veterinary Clinics of North America: Equine Practice. 1998;14:517–533.

Love CC. Ultrasonographic evaluation of the testis, epididymis and spermatic cord of the stallion. In: Blanchard TL and Varner DD, eds. Veterinary Clinics of North America: Equine Practice. Stallion Management. 1992;8:167–182.

Varner DD, Schumacher J, Blanchard T, Johnson L. Diseases and Management of Breeding Stallions. Goleta: American Veterinary Publications; 1991.

Author Margo L. Macpherson

Consulting Editor Carla L.Carleton

ABORTION, SPONTANEOUS, INFECTIOUS

BASICS

DEFINITION

Fetal loss >40 days; maternal, placental, or fetal invasion of microorganisms

PATHOPHYSIOLOGY

- Fetal death by microorganisms
- Fetal expulsion after placental infection, insufficiency, or separation
- Premature parturition by microbial toxins, fetal stress, combination mechanisms
- Result: fetal absorption, maceration, autolysis; live fetus incapable of extrauterine survival

SYSTEMS AFFECTED

- Reproductive
- Other organ systems if maternal systemic disease

INCIDENCE/PREVALENCE

- 5%–15% infectious abortion
- Abortion storm, especially EHV-1

SIGNALMENT

Nonspecific, associated specific risk factors

SIGNS

General Comments

- Early pregnancy loss unobserved often termed *asymptomatic*
- Unless complications occur, abortion may occur rapidly; sole sign is relatively normal, previously pregnant mare later found open
- Signs—none to multisystemic and life-threatening
- May be multiple animals
- Most *symptomatic* spontaneous infectious abortions are in second half of gestation

Historical

One or more:

- Vaginal discharge—mucoid, hemorrhagic, serosanguinous
- Premature udder development; dripping milk
- Anorexia or colic; GI disease
- Failure to deliver on expected due date
- Recent (1–16 weeks before presentation) systemic infectious disease
- Other mares, recent abortions
- Inadequate EHV-1 prophylaxis
- History of placentitis
- Previous endometrial biopsy with moderate/severe endometritis or fibrosis
- None/excessive abdominal distention consistent with gestation length
- Behavioral estrus, pregnant mare—may be normal depending on gestation length, time of year, gestation length at time of loss
- Climactic and environmental conditions favor increased ETC (*Malacosoma americanum*) populations and development of MRLS in early and late pregnant mares.
- Possibly geographical location if MRLS and nocardioform placentitits

Physical Examination

- Fetal parts/placental structures protruding through vulvar lips; abdominal straining or discomfort
- Vulvar discharge (variable appearance); premature udder development, dripping milk
- A previously documented pregnancy is inapparent at next examination; evidence of fetal death by palpation, transrectal or transabdominal U/S
- Anorexia, fever, signs of concurrent systemic disease, especially with endotoxemia, dystocia, RFM
- Evidence of placental separation with transrectal or transabdominal U/S

CAUSES

- *Viruses*
  - EHV-1 (1P and 1B strains); EHV-4–>7 mo of gestation; rarely EHV-2
  - EVA (>3 mo of gestation)
  - EIA—direct causal relationship not yet established
  - Vesivirus—recent correlation between antibodies of vesivirus and equine abortion
- *Bacteria*
  - Placentitis and possible, subsequent fetal infection by *Streptococcus* sp., *Actionobacillus* sp., *Escherichia coli, Pseudomonas* sp., *Klebsiella* sp., *Staphylococcus* sp., nocardioform actinomycetes (to include *Amycolatopsis* sp., *Cellulosimicrobium* sp., *Crossiella* sp., and *Rhodococcus* sp.), *Taylorella equigenitalis* (rare, reportable), and *Leptospira* serovars
  - Endotoxemia cause release of $PGF_{2\alpha}$ (especially <80 days of gestation [day 60 in many mares]; may be factor later in gestation, if repeated exposure)
  - Exposure to ETC setae in conjunction with MRLS theorized associated with microscopic bowel puncture and bacteremic spread to fetus and/or placenta
- Rickettsiae
- *Ehrlichia risticii*—PHF
- *Fungi*—placentitis caused by *Aspergillus* sp., *Candida* sp., or *Histoplasma capsulatum*
- Protozoa
- *Sarcocystis neurona* or, possibly, *Neospora* sp. in aborted fetuses from EPM affected mares
- MRLS
  - Early (≈40–150 days' gestation) and late (>269 days of gestation) abortion syndromes
  - Association with ETCs

RISK FACTORS

- Pregnant mares intermixed with young horses or horses-in-training are susceptible to EHV-1, EVA, or *Ehrlichia risticii.*
- Immunologically naïve mares brought to premises with enzootic EHV-1, EVA, *Ehrlichia risticii,* or *Leptospira* infections
- Pregnant mares traveling to horse shows or competitions
- Poor perineal conformation—predisposes mares to bacterial or fungal placentitis and, possibly, subsequent fetal infection
- Concurrent maternal GI disease or EPM
- Large numbers ETCs in pastures with pregnant mares
- Geographical location with respect to MRLS and nocardioform placentitis

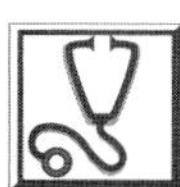

DIAGNOSIS

- Except for placentitis and abortion secondary to endotoxemia, most abortions are *asymptomatic;* expelled fetus and fetal membranes vary in condition—intact to autolytic
- Definitive causative diagnosis of equine abortion in ≅50%–60% of all cases
- Excluding twins and EHV-1, diagnostic rate may approach only 30% if limited samples are submitted and accompanied by moderate to severe fetal and placental autolysis.

DIFFERENTIAL DIAGNOSIS

Other Causes of Abortion

Abortion, spontaneous, noninfectious

- Twinning
- Fetal abnormalities—teratogenesis
- Umbilical cord abnormalities—excessive twisting; thrombosis
- Placental pathology
- Maternal malnutrition, other noninfectious systemic disease
- Old mare, history of EED or abortion
- Old mare, poor endometrial biopsy (inflammation, fibrosis)
- Endophyte-infected tall fescue pasture, exposure to ergotized grasses, small cereal grains during last month of gestation—no mammary development (agalactia, if term is reached); phytoestrogens; xenobiotics

Other Causes—Signs of Labor or Abdominal Discomfort

- Normal parturition
- Dystocia unassociated with abortion
- Prepartum uterine artery rupture
- Colic associated with uterine torsion
- Discomfort associated with hydrops of fetal membranes or prepubic tendon rupture
- Colic unassociated with reproductive disease

Other Causes—Vulvar Discharge

- Normal parturition
- Dystocia unassociated with abortion
- Normal estrus
- Endometritis
- Metritis or partial RFM
- Mucometra or pyometra

CBC/BIOCHEMISTRY/URINALYSIS

Determine inflammatory or stress leukocyte response, other organ system involvement

OTHER LABORATORY TESTS

Maternal Progesterone

- Indicated if pregnancy outcome is doubtful (prediagnosis of an infectious cause of impending abortion), with suspected endotoxemia
- ELISA or RIA for progesterone may be useful at <80 days of gestation (normal levels vary from >1 to >4 ng/mL, depending on reference lab).
- At >100 days, RIA detects both progesterone (very low >day 150) and cross-reacting 5α-pregnanes of uterofetoplacental origin. Acceptable levels of 5α-pregnanes vary with stage of gestation and laboratory used.

Other Maternal Hormones

See Abortions, noninfectious.

Maternal Serology

- Take serum samples in all cases of abortion in which cause is unknown. Paired sample (21 days later), may be indicated.
- Diagnostic for abortions by *Leptospira* serovars
- Confirms EVA abortion

IMAGING

Transrectal and Transabdominal U/S

- Evaluate fetal viability, placentitis, alterations in appearance of amniotic and/or allantoic fluids.
- Other gestational abnormalities

DIAGNOSTIC PROCEDURES

Pathology, Serology, Molecular Techniques, and Culture

If fetus and membranes are available, sample:

- Fresh/chilled fetal thoracic or abdominal fluid, serum from fetal heart or cord blood, if available
- Fetal stomach content
- 10% Formalin-fixed and chilled/frozen samples of fetal membranes (allantochorion; allantoamnion), fetal heart, lung, thymus, liver, kidney, lymph nodes, thymus, spleen, adrenal, skeletal muscle, and brain

Molecular Techniques

Specific PCR, other molecular analyses, various samples for selected viral infections

Maternal Uterine Swabs

May aid in establishing diagnosis of abortions caused by placentitis

ABORTION, SPONTANEOUS, INFECTIOUS

PATHOLOGICAL FINDINGS

Viruses

- EHV
  - Gross—pleural effusion, ascites, fetal icterus, pulmonary congestion and edema; 1-mm, yellowish-white spots on enlarged liver; fetus is fresh.
  - Histopath (EHV-1 and -4)—areas of necrosis; prominent, eosinophilic, intranuclear inclusion bodies in lymphoid tissue, liver, adrenal cortex, and lung as well as a hyperplastic, necrotizing bronchiolitis; FA staining of fetal tissues; virus isolation from aborted fetus
- EVA
  - Few gross lesions
  - Autolyzed fetus
  - Placental/fetal vascular lesions
- Vesivirus
  - Nonspecific lesions

Bacteria and Fungi

- Fetal infection and placentitis
  - Gross—pleural effusion, ascites; enlarged liver; rare plaques of mycotic dermatitis; placental edema and thickening with fibronecrotic exudate (chorionic surface), especially at cervical star (especially if fungal)
  - Histopath—inflammatory disease; autolysis may make interpretation difficult
- Leptospirosis
  - Gross—fetal icterus and autolysis
  - Histopath—nonspecific; mild, diffuse placentitis

Endotoxemia

Fetus minimally autolyzed

Rickettsiae

Ehrlichia risticii:

- Gross—placentitis
- Histopath—typical fetal lesions include colitis, periportal hepatitis, lymphoid hyperplasia, and necrosis

Protozoa

Sarcocystis neurona—anecdotal reports on histopath, aborted fetuses from EPM plus mares

MRLS

Path findings—similar to bacterial infections

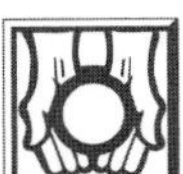

TREATMENT

APPROPRIATE HEALTH CARE

- Except late-gestational placentitis (>270 days) and endotoxemia, no therapy indicated to preserve fetal viability with spontaneous, infectious abortion
- Aborting mares—only prophylactic therapy for metritis or endometritis. Therapy limited to intrauterine, may include a systemic component
- Preexisting GI disease and complications may warrant hospitalization and intensive care

NURSING CARE

Most affected horses require limited nursing care, except for endotoxemia and gram-negative septicemia, dystocia, RFM, metritis, and laminitis.

ACTIVITY

Paddock exercise to permit observation

CLIENT EDUCATION

Inform owners of possible complications of abortion.

MEDICATIONS

DRUG(S) OF CHOICE

- Altrenogest 0.044–0.088 mg/kg PO daily—start later during gestation, continue longer, or use only short periods of time depending on serum progesterone levels during first 80 days of gestation, clinical circumstances, risk factors, clinician preference. Note—Serum levels reflect only endogenous progesterone, not exogenous/oral product.
- If near term, altrenogest frequently is discontinued 7–14 days before foaling date unless indicated otherwise by fetal maturity/viability, or actual gestational age is in question.

CONTRAINDICATIONS

Altrenogest only used to prevent abortion in cases of endotoxemia or placentitis (>270 days of gestation) if fetus is viable.

PRECAUTIONS

Altrenogest—absorbed through skin; wear gloves and wash hands.

ALTERNATIVE DRUGS

Injectable progesterone (150 to 500 mg oil base IM)

FOLLOW-UP

PATIENT MONITORING

- 7–10 days postabortion—TRP and U/S, monitor uterine involution
- Assess genital tract health—vaginal speculum, uterine culture and cytology, endometrial biopsy
- Base treatment on clinical results. Uterine culture <14 days postpartum or postabortion is affected by contaminants at parturition

PREVENTION/AVOIDANCE

Vaccines

- A killed-virus EHV-1 vaccine, 5, 7, and 9 mo of gestation; approved for abortion prevention in pregnant mares; 2-mo interval due to short-lived vaccinal immunity
- EVA vaccine; not specifically labeled for abortion prevention
  - MLV
  - Only open mares 3 weeks before anticipated exposure to infected semen or in enzootic conditions
  - Isolate first-time vaccinated mares, 3 weeks after exposure to infected semen.
  - Some countries forbid importation of horses with titers to EVA.

Additional Prophylactic Steps

- Segregate pregnant mares from horses susceptible/exposed to infections.
- Isolate immunologically naïve individuals until immunity to enzootic infections is established/enhanced. Depending on infectious agent, protection may only be accomplished postpartum.
- Limit transport of pregnant mares to exhibitions or competitions.
- Isolate aborting mares, proper disposal of contaminated fetal tissues
- Proper diagnostics to ID infectious cause
- Correct poor perineal conformation, prevent placentitis.
- Prevent pregnant mare exposure to ETCs until 7–8 weeks after ETC death.
- Insecticides to control ETCs; consider toxicity of insecticides.

POSSIBLE COMPLICATIONS

Future fertility and reproductive value impaired by dystocia, RFM, endometritis, laminitis, septicemia, trauma to genital tract

EXPECTED COURSE AND PROGNOSIS

- Most patients recover with appropriate treatment.
- Complications—significant impact on mare's survivability and future fertility
- Prognosis—guarded for pregnancy maintenance with endotoxemia and placentitis

MISCELLANEOUS

ASSOCIATED CONDITIONS

- Abortion, noninfectious
- Dystocia
- EHV-1
- Endometritis
- EPM
- EVA
- Metritis
- Pericarditis, MRLS
- Placental insufficiency
- Placentitis
- PHF
- Premature placental separation
- RFM

AGE-RELATED FACTORS

Immunologic status of young mares

SEE ALSO

- Abortion, noninfectious
- Dystocia
- Endometrial biopsy
- Endometritis
- Fetal stress/viability
- High-risk pregnancy
- Metritis
- Placental insufficiency
- Placentitis
- Premature placental separation
- RFM

ABBREVIATIONS

- EED = early embryonic death
- EHV = equine herpesvirus
- EIA = equine infectious anemia
- ELISA = enzyme-linked immunosorbent assay
- EPM = equine protozoal encephalomyelitis
- ETC = eastern tent caterpillar
- EVA = equine viral arteritis
- FA = fluorescent antibody
- MRLS = mare reproductive loss syndrome
- PCR = polymerase chain reaction
- PHF = Potomac horse fever
- RIA = radioimmunoassay
- RFM = retained fetal membranes/placenta
- TRP = transrectal palpation
- U/S = ultrasound, ultrasonography

Suggested Reading

Christensen BW, Roberts JF, Pozor MA, et al. Nocardioform placentitis with isolation of *Amycolatopsis* spp in Florida-bred mare. J Am Vet Med Assoc 2006;228:1234–1239.

Giles RC, Donahue JM, Hong CG, et al. Causes of abortion, stillbirth, and perinatal death in 3,527 cases (1986–1991). J Am Vet Med Assoc 1993;208: 1170–1175.

Kurth A, Skilling DE, Smith AW. Serologic evidence of vesivirus-specific antibodies associated with abortion in horses. Am J Vet Res 2006;67:1033–1039.

Webb BA, Barney WE, Dahlman DL, et al. Eastern tent caterpillars (*Malacosoma americanum*) cause mare reproductive loss syndrome. J Insect Physiol 2004;50:185–193.

Author Tim J. Evans

Consulting Editor Carla L. Carleton

ABORTION, SPONTANEOUS, NONINFECTIOUS

BASICS

DEFINITION

Fetal loss >40 days (term *stillbirth* may apply >300 days) associated with a variety of noninfectious conditions

PATHOPHYSIOLOGY

- Fetal death/premature parturition from some intrinsic structural or functional defect or exposure to xenobiotics
- Fetal expulsion <80 days of gestation after CL loss as a result of endometritis or other factors
- Fetal death/expulsion by placental insufficiency or separation
- Fetal stress, dead twin fetus, maternal stress, or combination
- Fetal reabsorption, maceration, mummification, autolysis, or live fetus incapable of extrauterine survival

SYSTEM AFFECTED

Reproductive

INCIDENCE/PREVALENCE

- 5%–15% spontaneous abortion, multiple risk factors
- Breed predisposition for twinning

SIGNALMENT

- Nonspecific
- Breeds—Thoroughbred, draft mares, Standardbreds, related breeds (twinning)
- Mares >15 years
- Maiden American Miniature Horse mares—anecdotal placental insufficiency

SIGNS

General Comments

- Depending on cause, time of fetal death, stage of gestation, duration of condition, and whether pregnancy ended in dystocia or with RFM, dam may show few signs or, in extreme cases, suffer life-threatening multiorgan system disease.
- Most in second half of gestation

Historical

- Signs consistent with labor at unexpected stage of gestation
- Dystocia, birth of nonviable foal
- Vaginal discharge—mucoid, hemorrhagic, or serosanguinous
- Premature udder development; dripping milk
- Anorexia or colic
- Recent systemic disease
- Moderate/severe endometritis or fibrosis
- Failure to deliver on expected due date
- None/excessive abdominal distention consistent with stage of gestation
- Behavioral estrus in pregnant mare—normal for stage of gestation; dependent on time of year and stage of pregnancy when lost
- Geographical location—endophyte-infected fescue pastures/hay and/or ergotized grasses or grains

Physical Examination

- Fetal/placental structures protruding through vulvar lips; abdominal straining or discomfort
- Vulvar discharge (variable appearance), premature udder development, dripping milk
- Previously diagnosed pregnancy absent at next examination; fetal death determined by palpation or transrectal/transabdominal U/S
- Twin fetuses identified by transrectal/transabdominal U/S
- Evidence of placental separation or hydrops of fetal membranes during transrectal/transabdominal U/S
- Signs of concurrent, systemic disease, dystocia, or RFM
- Note—Signs variable. Mares pregnant at early check can remain asymptomatic but abort; unobserved, early in gestation. Abortion may be rapid without signs.

CAUSES

Twins

- Twin pregnancies that persist >40 days—≅70% end in abortion/stillbirth.

Luteal Insufficiency/Early CL Regression

- Anecdotal, somewhat controversial
- Caused by increased levels of luteal progesterone at <80 days of gestation

Placental Abnormalities

- Umbilical cord torsion—cord twists are normal, must be evidence of vascular compromise, e.g., cord thrombus, to confirm diagnosis
- Long umbilical cord/cervical pole ischemia disorder
- Confirmed body pregnancy
- Placental separation
- Villous atrophy or hypoplasia
- Hydrops

Fetal Abnormalities

- Developmental abnormalities—hydrocephalus; anencephaly
- Fetal trauma
- Chromosomal abnormalities

Maternal Abnormalities

- Concurrent maternal disease, maternal stress
- Trauma
- Malnutrition—starvation; selenium deficiency
- Severe maternal anxiety—anecdotal
- Moderate to severe endometritis or fibrosis
- Maternal chromosomal abnormalities

Xenobiotics

- Ergopeptine alkaloids associated with fescue toxicosis or ergotism (prolonged gestation is more common)
- Phytoestrogens—anecdotal
- Xenobiotics causing maternal disease—cardiac glycosides, taxine alkaloids, carbamates, organophosphates
- Xenobiotics causing placental and/or fetal disease—originally suspected with respect to MRLS; considered less likely at present time
- Possible deleterious effects of medications on pregnancy—EPM therapies (anecdotal)
- Repeated large doses of corticosteroids during late gestation

Iatrogenic Causes

• $PGF_{2\alpha}$—may require repeated injections if >40 days of gestation
• Procedures mistakenly done on a pregnant mare—AI; intrauterine infusions; samples taken for cytology, culture, or biopsy

RISK FACTORS

• Family history of twinning or noninfectious, spontaneous abortion
• Systemic maternal disease
• Grazing endophyte-infected fescue, ergotized grasses, or plants producing phytoestrogens (anecdotal) late in gestation
• Exposure to xenobiotics

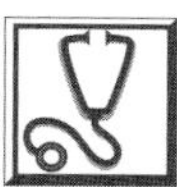

DIAGNOSIS

• Most mares asymptomatic before aborting
• Fetus(es)—variable condition, fresh to autolytic
• Definitive diagnosis possible ≅50%–60% of cases
• Excluding twins and EHV-1, diagnosis is only 30% if few samples are submitted and moderate/severe autolysis of fetal and placental tissues.

DIFFERENTIAL DIAGNOSIS

Other Causes of Abortion

• Infectious, spontaneous abortion
• Placentitis—by physical examination or by lab diagnostics

Other Causes of Signs of Labor or Abdominal Discomfort

• Normal parturition
• Dystocia unassociated with abortion
• Prepartum uterine artery rupture
• Colic associated with uterine torsion
• Discomfort associated with hydrops of fetal membranes or prepubic tendon rupture
• Colic unassociated with reproductive disease

Other Causes of Vulvar Discharge

• Normal parturition
• Dystocia unassociated with abortion
• Normal estrus
• Endometritis
• Metritis or RFM
• Mucometra or pyometra

CBC/BIOCHEMISTRY/URINALYSIS

Determine inflammatory/stress leukocyte response, other organ system involvement

OTHER LABORATORY TESTS

Maternal Progesterone

• Indicated with history of abortion or in an old mare, previous biopsy presence of endometritis or fibrosis
• ELISA or RIA <80 days of gestation; acceptable levels are >1 to >4 ng/mL, depending on reference lab
• >100 days of gestation, RIA detects progesterone (may be very low >150 days) and cross-reacting 5α-pregnanes of uterofetoplacental origin
• Decreased maternal levels of 5α-pregnanes with cases of equine fescue toxicosis

Maternal Estrogens

• Reflect fetal estrogen production and viability, especially conjugated estrogens, e.g., estrone sulfate

Maternal Relaxin

• Decreased maternal relaxin concentration—thought associated with abnormal placental function

Maternal Prolactin

• Decreased prolactin secretion, late gestation, associated with fescue toxicosis and ergotism

Maternal T_3/T_4

• Anecdotal reports of lower levels in mares with history of conception failure, EED, or abortion
• Significance of low T_4 levels is unknown.

Cytogenetic Studies

• If suspect maternal chromosomal abnormalities
• Difficult if fetus autolysis

Maternal and Fetal Assays for Xenobiotics

• Indicated in cases of specific intoxications
• Sample the dam's whole blood, plasma, or urine samples
• Sample fetal serum from heart blood, thoracic or abdominal fluid, liver, and kidney

Feed Analysis

Indicated for specific xenobiotics—ergopeptine alkaloids, phytoestrogens, heavy metals, or endophyte (*Neotyphodium coenophialum*)

IMAGING

Transrectal/transabdominal U/S to confirm pregnancy, diagnose twins, evaluate fetal viability and development, assess placental health, diagnose other gestational abnormalities, e.g., hydrops of fetal membranes

DIAGNOSTIC PROCEDURES

• If entire fetus and placenta are available, appropriate samples for pathology, histology, culture, and serology
• Fresh/chilled fetal thoracic or abdominal fluid or serum from fetal heart or cord blood (if available); fetal stomach contents; 10% formalin-fixed and chilled/frozen samples of fetal heart, lung, thymus, liver, kidney, lymph nodes, spleen, adrenal gland, skeletal muscle and brain; 10% formalin-fixed and chilled/frozen fetal membranes (i.e., allantochorion and allantoamnion)
• Uterine swabs from dam may be useful to establish placentitis diagnosis
• Unless cause is obvious, e.g., twins, iatrogenic, rule out infectious causes of abortion, especially if multiple mares are at risk.

ABORTION, SPONTANEOUS, NONINFECTIOUS

PATHOLOGICAL FINDINGS

Twins

- Two fetuses, often dissimilar in size, with one mummified or severely autolytic
- Avillous chorionic membrane at point of contact of two placentae

Placental Abnormalities

- Umbilical cord torsion—confirm with evidence of vascular compromise
- Villous atrophy or hypoplasia may suggest endometrial fibrosis.
- Placental edema, gross and histopathological, consistent with equine fescue toxicosis
- Hydrops allantois and amnion—a gross diagnosis if dam suffers prepartum death

Fetal Abnormalities

Developmental abnormalities—hydrocephalus; anencephaly; gross and histopath confirmation

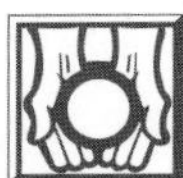

TREATMENT

APPROPRIATE HEALTH CARE

- Treatment only if early diagnosis of the pathologic process, before irreversible fetal or placental compromise occurs
- Main therapeutic approach to twinning—early selective reduction
- Late-gestation twin diagnosis—pregnancy may be maintained until term, in some instances, with progestin and antibiotic therapy.
- Mares with abortion history—evaluate and treat before rebreeding; progestin supplementation may be appropriate, especially with suspected luteal insufficiency (anecdotal) or early luteal regression, but this therapy is controversial and is contraindicated in some circumstances; ET may be indicated for mares with a history of repeated abortion.
- Signs of fescue toxicosis or ergotism can be treated with D_2-dopamine receptor antagonists; cases of abortion, i.e., stillbirth, frequently occur before therapy begins.
- Aborting mares generally only require prophylactic therapy for metritis or endometritis.
- Most patients managed on an ambulatory basis
- Systemic maternal disease may need hospitalization and intensive care.

NURSING CARE

Most noninfectious abortions require limited nursing care, unless systemic disease develops.

ACTIVITY

Limit to paddock exercise to allow observation.

CLIENT EDUCATION

Problem mares are likely to have future reproductive problems.

MEDICATIONS

DRUGS OF CHOICE

See specific topics.

History of Abortion, Endometritis, or Fibrosis

- Treat with altrenogest 0.044–0.088 mg/kg PO daily.
- Begin 2–3 days after ovulation or at diagnosis of pregnancy; continue to at least 100 days of gestation.
- Taper dose gradually during a 14-day period at end of treatment.

Altrenogest

- Start later in gestation, continue longer, or use for only short periods of time depending on serum progesterone levels during the first 80 days of gestation (>1 to >4 ng/mL), clinical circumstances, risk factors, and clinician preference.
- If used near term, altrenogest often discontinued 7–14 days before expected foaling date, unless otherwise indicated by assessment of fetal maturity/viability or questions arise regarding accurate gestational age

CONTRAINDICATIONS

- Uses of altrenogest—prevent abortion of viable fetus, for noninfectious placentitis, and endotoxemia
- Monitor fetal viability at least weekly to avoid retaining a dead fetus in utero or lead to development of pyometra.
- Altrenogest absorbed through skin; wear gloves and wash hands.
- Anecdotal success of supplemental progestin to maintain equine pregnancy

ALTERNATIVE DRUGS

- Progesterone 150–500 mg oil base IM daily
- T_4 supplementation—anecdotal success treating subfertile mares; use remains controversial, considered deleterious by some clinicians

ABORTION, SPONTANEOUS, NONINFECTIOUS

FOLLOW-UP

PATIENT MONITORING

- 7–10 days post-abortion—TRP, U/S, or both; evaluate uterine involution.
- Rate of involution depends on therapy used, presence of systemic disease, secondary complications.
- Further examination—vaginal speculum, uterine cytology/culture, endometrial biopsy

PREVENTION/AVOIDANCE

- Early recognition of at-risk mares
- Records of double ovulations
- Early twin diagnosis (<25 days, as early as day 14 or 15)
- Selective embryonic/fetal reduction
- Managing preexisting endometritis before next breeding
- Remove mares from fescue pasture during last third of gestation (minimum 30 days).
- Domperidone (1.1 mg/kg PO daily) at earliest signs of equine fescue toxicosis or 10–14 days prior to due date, continue until parturition and development of normal mammary gland
- Injection with fluphenazine (25 mg IM in pony mares) on day 320 of gestation has been suggested for prophylaxis of fescue toxicosis.
- Careful use of medications in pregnant mares
- Avoiding exposure to known toxicants.

POSSIBLE COMPLICATIONS

- Recovery uneventful after many asymptomatic abortions
- Dystocia, RFM, metritis, laminitis, septicemia, endometritis, reproductive tract trauma may impact the mare's future well-being and reproductive value.

EXPECTED COURSE AND PROGNOSIS

Uneventful recovery in most cases with appropriate treatment

MISCELLANEOUS

AGE-RELATED FACTORS

- Development of chronic endometritis and endometrial fibrosis
- Maiden American Miniature Horse mares

PREGNANCY

Pregnancy associated by definition

SEE ALSO

- Abortion, infectious
- Endometritis
- Fetal stress/distress/viability
- High-risk pregnancy
- Hydrops allantois/amnion
- Metritis, postpartum
- Multiple ovulations
- Placental insufficiency
- Placentitis
- Premature placental separation
- RFM
- Twin pregnancy

ABBREVIATIONS

- AI = artificial insemination
- CL = corpus luteum
- EED = early embryonic death
- EHV = equine herpesvirus
- ELISA = enzyme-linked immunosorbent assay
- EPM = equine protozoal encephalomyelitis
- ET = embryo transfer
- MRLS = mare reproductive loss syndrome
- RIA = radioimmunoassay
- RFM = retained fetal membranes/placenta
- U/S = ultrasound, ultrasonography

Suggested Reading

Evans TJ, Rottinghaus GE, Casteel SW. Ergopeptine alkaloid toxicoses in horses. In: Robinson NE, ed. Current Therapy in Equine Medicine, ed 5. Philadelphia: Saunders, 2003:796–798.

Giles RC, Donahue JM, Hong CG, et al. Causes of abortion, stillbirth, and perinatal death in 3,527 cases (1986–1991). J Am Vet Med Assoc 1993;208:1170–1175.

LeBlanc MM. Abortion. In: Colahan PT, Mayhew IG, Merritt AM, Moore JM, eds. Equine Medicine and Surgery, ed 5. St. Louis: Mosby, 1999:1202–1207.

Author Tim J. Evans

Consulting Editor Carla L. Carleton

ACER RUBRUM (RED MAPLE) TOXICOSIS

BASICS

OVERVIEW

• An equine disease that follows ingestion of wilted or dried *Acer rubrum* (red maple) leaves and is characterized by methemoglobinemia, hemolytic anemia, and Heinz-body formation
• Most frequently reported in the eastern half of North America, where trees are more prevalent
• The specific toxin has not been identified, but apparently is found only in wilted or dried leaves, because the disease has not been induced using fresh leaves.
• Clinical findings are consistent with oxidative injury to RBCs, resulting in the formation of methemoglobin (i.e., oxidation of iron in hemoglobin from ferrous to ferric form), Heinz bodies (i.e., precipitated oxidized hemoglobin), and hemolytic anemia.
• Affected organ systems include
  ○ Cardiovascular—tachycardia secondary to anemia
  ○ Hemic—methemoglobinemia, hemolytic anemia, and Heinz bodies
  ○ Renal—pigmenturia, hematuria, and proteinuria; renal failure secondary to hemoglobin deposition in the kidney
  ○ Reproductive—abortion secondary to fetal hypoxia
  ○ Respiratory—polypnea secondary to anemia

SIGNALMENT

• No breed predilections
• No gender predilections
• No age predilections
• No genetic basis

SIGNS

• Acute death can result from rapid formation of methemoglobin. Alternatively, hemolytic crisis can develop over several days as the hemolysis and methemoglobinemia progressively worsen.
• Historical findings include lethargy, weakness, anorexia, and perhaps colic or fever.
• Physical examination findings include yellow or brown mucous membranes, red or brown urine, tachycardia, polypnea, and dehydration.

CAUSES AND RISK FACTORS

It usually occurs during the summer and fall months after an event that results in leaf wilting such as tree pruning, fallen branches after a storm, or autumn leaves falling.

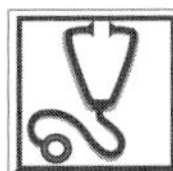

DIAGNOSIS

DIFFERENTIAL DIAGNOSIS

• Consider all causes of equine hemolytic anemia, which include oxidant poisons, EIA, immune-mediated hemolytic anemia, piroplasmosis, and liver failure.
• Hemolytic anemia accompanied by Heinz bodies and/or methemoglobinemia indicates oxidant toxicosis. The most common causes in horses are onions, red maple, and phenothiazine anthelmintics, which can only be differentiated by a history of ingestion.

CBC/BIOCHEMISTRY/URINALYSIS

• Interpretation of laboratory findings may be difficult because of the hemolysis, with resultant discoloration of the serum and urine.
• Decreased PCV, hemoglobin, and erythrocyte count confirm anemia, whereas increased MCHC and MCH support intravascular hemolysis with hemoglobinemia.
• Heinz bodies are not present in all cases. They may be seen on routinely-stained blood smears but are more apparent in new methylene blue–stained smears.
• Serum bilirubin, especially unconjugated bilirubin, is increased because of hemolytic anemia and inappetence.
• Urinalysis results include proteinuria and hemoglobinuria, with few or no intact erythrocytes.
• Increased albumin and total protein result from dehydration.
• BUN and creatinine increase if a pigment nephropathy develops and causes acute renal failure.
• Elevated liver enzymes and creatine phosphokinase may occur, probably secondary to cell damage caused by anemia-induced hypoxia.
• Eccentrocytes and ghost cells have been reported.

OTHER LABORATORY TESTS

The percentage of methemoglobin in the blood often is elevated.

IMAGING

N/A

OTHER DIAGNOSTIC PROCEDURES

N/A

PATHOLOGICAL FINDINGS

- Gross findings include generalized icterus, enlarged spleen, and discolored kidneys. Petechiae and ecchymoses may be present on serosal surfaces.
- Histopathologic findings include erythrophagocytosis by macrophages, renal pigment casts and sloughed epithelial cells, splenic and hepatic hemosiderin, and centrilobular hepatic lipidosis. Pulmonary thrombosis has been reported in one horse.

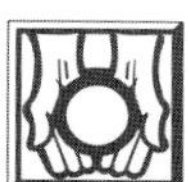

TREATMENT

- The decision regarding inpatient or outpatient treatment depends on severity of the clinical signs and ability of the owner to care for the animal. Frequently monitor progression of the methemoglobinemia and anemia.
- Give IV fluids to replace fluid deficits and to maintain adequate renal perfusion.
- Blood transfusion may be needed with severe anemia.
- Limit physical activity of anemic animals.
- Continuous nasal oxygen administration may be helpful.
- Offer a high-quality diet, especially because affected horses often lack an appetite.

MEDICATIONS

DRUG(S) OF CHOICE

- Ascorbic acid has been used for its antioxidant effects (30–50 mg/kg q12h added to IV fluids).
- It also can be given orally but may take several doses to achieve adequate tissue levels.

CONTRAINDICATIONS/POSSIBLE INTERACTIONS

- Do not treat methemoglobinemia with methylene blue because of its poor efficacy in horses and reports that it may increase Heinz-body formation.
- NSAIDs may be necessary to control pain but can compromise renal function.

FOLLOW-UP

PATIENT MONITORING

Monitor methemoglobinemia and anemia, and adjust therapy based on the severity and speed of progression.

PREVENTION/AVOIDANCE

- Instruct owners not to plant red maples.
- Prune or remove existing trees only when no leaves are on the trees.
- Owners should check for fallen branches immediately after storms.

EXPECTED COURSE AND PROGNOSIS

- Prognosis depends on the quantity of leaves ingested and how soon veterinary care is sought after ingestion.
- Death is attributed to severe methemoglobinemia or anemia or to renal failure secondary to pigment nephropathy.

MISCELLANEOUS

ASSOCIATED CONDITIONS

Laminitis can occur during or after the course of the disease.

PREGNANCY

Anemia and methemoglobinemia can result in fetal hypoxia, followed by abortion.

ABBREVIATIONS

- EIA = equine infectious anemia
- MCH = mean corpuscular hemoglobin
- MCHC = mean corpuscular hemoglobin concentration
- PCV = packed cell volume

Suggested Reading

Alward A, Corriher CA, Barton MH, et al. Red maple (*Acer rubrum*) leaf toxicosis in horses: a retrospective study of 32 cases. J Vet Intern Med 2006;20;1197–1201.

Merola V, Volmer PA. Red Maple. In: Plumlee KH, ed. Clinical Veterinary Toxicology. St. Louis: Mosby, 2004.

Author Konnie H. Plumlee
Consulting Editor Robert H. Poppenga

ACIDOSIS, METABOLIC

BASICS

DEFINITION

- A disruption of acid-base homeostasis producing increased H^+ concentration, which is reflected by acidemia—decreased blood pH and low plasma HCO_3^-
- Plasma bicarbonate level is ≅ 24 mEq/L.
- pH of arterial blood ranges from 7.35 to 7.45.

PATHOPHYSIOLOGY

- Fixed acid is produced via normal metabolic processes in large quantities daily.
- H^+ is regulated by intracellular and extracellular buffering, respiratory buffering (i.e., variation of CO_2 levels via changes in ventilation), and regulation of HCO_3^- via renal excretion of H^+.
- Renal H^+ excretion is accomplished by direct secretion of limited amounts of H^+, increased generation of ammonium ions, and titration to phosphates and urates (titratable acidity).
- Resorption of HCO_3^- occurs when H^+ is secreted—90% in the proximal tubule, the remainder in the distal nephron.
- The minimum pH (4.5) of the tubular fluid limits secretion of H^+.
- Titratable acidity increases minimally in acidotic patients.
- In most species, production of ammonia with subsequent excretion of ammonium ion is the major mechanism by which the kidney handles an acid load.
- Intracellular and extracellular buffering of H^+ occurs immediately or within minutes and is accomplished by proteins (primarily albumin and hemoglobin), phosphates, and bicarbonate.
- Carbonate storage in bone also is a significant site of intracellular buffering.
- The most important buffer is HCO_3^-, because it is present in high concentrations and the end product of its activity, CO_2, is readily eliminated by the lungs.
- Respiratory compensation responds within minutes and is effective for mild and moderate acidemia.
- Definitive regulation of H^+ and HCO_3^- levels is accomplished by the kidney.
- Renal processing of an acid load begins within hours but may take days to normalize pH.
- Inability to excrete H^+, loss of HCO_3^-, increased production of H^+ (i.e., lactic acidosis), and accumulation of acids are the major mechanisms producing metabolic acidosis.
- Hyperproteinemia (i.e., weak acids) and overhydration (i.e., dilutional acidosis) also produce metabolic acidosis via alteration of the balance between strong cations and anions in body fluids.

SYSTEMS AFFECTED

Respiratory

- Peripheral and central chemoreceptors sense low pH in blood or CSF and stimulate hyperventilation to increase elimination of CO_2 and increase pH.
- Decreased respiratory muscle strength can lead to muscle fatigue and worsening metabolic status, especially in neonates.

Cardiovascular

- Decreased cardiac contractility
- May predispose to arrhythmias
- Vasodilation of arterioles; constriction of veins
- Vascular effects may be offset by catecholamine effects.

Neuroendocrine

- Catecholamine release
- CNS depression
- CSF acidosis in acute situations
- Vasodilation of cerebral vessels leading to increased cerebral blood flow and CSF pressure

Renal

- The kidney responds to low arterial pH by increasing H^+ excretion and generating increased levels of HCO_3^- to bring the systemic pH back to normal.
- This response begins within hours, but it may take days to be effective.

Metabolic

- Inhibition of anaerobic glycolysis
- Insulin resistance
- Decreased affinity for oxygen–hemoglobin binding, enhancing release of oxygen to the tissues
- Increased protein catabolism
- Increased ionized calcium concentration

SIGNALMENT

Any equine

SIGNS

- Historical and physical examination findings vary primarily with the underlying cause.
- Weakness, depression, and tachypnea are clinical signs specific to acidosis.

CAUSES

- Many diseases result in metabolic acidosis via more than one mechanism.
- Loss of bicarbonate most commonly is seen in horses with colitis; RTA results in HCO_3^- loss both directly and indirectly, depending on the type of tubular dysfunction.
- Renal failure results in an inability to excrete H^+ and accumulation of uremic acids.
- Increased H^+ production (i.e., lactic acidosis) is seen with diseases producing decreased effective circulating blood volume—hypotension or hypovolemia caused by inadequate intake, hemorrhage, isotonic or hypotonic fluid loss or sequestration (e.g., uroperitoneum, peritonitis, pleuritis, ascites, nonstrangulating types of colic), strangulating lesions of the GI tract, endotoxemia, or cardiac failure.
- Chronic causes of hypoxemia produce lactic acidosis.
- Grain overload produces metabolic acidosis via production of lactic acid, fluid sequestration in the GI tract, secretion into the GI tract, and endotoxemia.
- High-intensity anaerobic exercise results in production of lactate, which can affect fluid balance/SID and result in metabolic acidosis, however, this is short-lived.
- Severe exertional rhabdomyolysis associated with anaerobic exercise produces lactic acidosis.
- Acute or end-stage hepatic failure may result in metabolic acidosis due to failure of the detoxification systems of the liver.
- Asphyxia at parturition may cause multiorgan damage or failure, which can result in metabolic acidosis in neonates.
- Accumulation of exogenous acids is uncommon, as this is usually caused by ingestion of toxic substances; it may be seen with salicylates, propylene or ethylene glycol, paraldehyde, and methanol.
- Malignant hyperthermia is uncommon but has occurred in anesthetized horses and results in severe lactic acidosis.
- Proteins are weak acids; conditions producing significant hyperproteinemia (e.g., chronic infection, immune-mediated disease, plasma cell myeloma, lymphoma) produce metabolic acidosis.
- Excessive or inappropriate fluid therapy, especially in neonates, produces free-water excess and dilutional acidosis.
- TPN can lead to metabolic acidosis when cationic (i.e., lysine, arginine) or sulfur containing amino acids are metabolized, as H^+ is formed.
- Endotoxemia produces acidosis via several mechanisms—hypotension, decreased cardiac contractility, tissue ischemia, fluid shifts, hypoxemia, hepatic damage, etc.

RISK FACTORS

- Patients with chronic renal failure or chronic hypoxemia (i.e., COPD) may be at greater risk for acidosis with progression of their primary problem or if acid load develops for other reasons.
- Horses on acetazolamide for HYPP may develop acidosis more readily, as acetazolamide is a carbonic anhydrase inhibitor that causes increased HCO_3^- excretion.
- Highly anionic diets have been suggested to induce metabolic acidosis in equine.

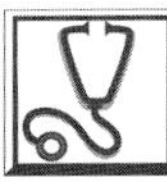

DIAGNOSIS

DIFFERENTIAL DIAGNOSIS

- Some causes of metabolic acidosis can be identified on physical examination (i.e., diarrhea, dehydration, colic with ischemic lesions).
- Decreased HCO_3^- levels are also seen in conditions with chronic respiratory alkalosis; Pco_2 is low if compensation is occuring, but pH will be normal or mildly increased.

LABORATORY FINDINGS

Drugs That May Alter Lab Results

- Excessive anticoagulant may falsely decrease results via dilution.
- Excessive sodium heparin may alter HCO_3^- levels, because it is an acidic compound.

Disorders That May Alter Lab Results

With poor peripheral perfusion or cardiovascular shunt, results of blood gas analysis on samples taken from peripheral vessels may differ from those taken elsewhere or not reflect the overall systemic condition.

Valid If Run in Human Lab and if sample submitted properly?

CBC/BIOCHEMISTRY/URINALYSIS

- Measurement of serum electrolytes and protein levels is important to determine the cause and to guide treatment.
- Calculation of the anion gap also may be useful, especially in mixed acid-base disorders.

- Proportionate changes in sodium and chloride levels occur with alterations of fluid balance.
- Normal sodium levels with hypochloremia or hyperchloremia indicate acid-base imbalance.
- Disproportionate changes in Na^+/Cl^- usually are associated with simultaneous acid-base imbalance and hydration abnormalities.
- Albumin/protein levels are not considered when calculating the anion gap; however, because proteins are weak acids, hyperproteinemia can produce the condition—dehydration, chronic infection, and neoplasia.
- Urinalysis and fractional excretion of electrolytes are useful in cases of renal failure and RTA.

Horses Affected with Hyperchloremia and Normal AG

- Loss of HCO_3^-—diarrhea, type II RTA, and primary respiratory alkalosis; however, severely affected colitis patients often are acidotic and low in Na^+, K^+, Cl^-, and HCO_3^- because of water intake after isotonic fluid loss.
- Addition of Cl^-—fluid therapy with Cl^--containing fluids (i.e., 0.9% NaCl, KCl), salt poisoning, TPN, NH_4Cl, or KCl supplementation
- Cl^- retention—renal failure, type I or IV RTA, and acetazolamide therapy

Horses Affected with Increased AG

Accumulation of unmeasured anions:

- Lactate—conditions with hypovolemia or hypotension (e.g., shock, sepsis, cardiac failure, ischemic/inflammatory types of colic); conditions with inflammation or fluid sequestration (e.g., pleuritis, peritonitis, uroperitoneum, grain overload); conditions utilizing anaerobic glycolysis (e.g., anaerobic exercise, severe exertional rhabdomyolysis, malignant hyperthermia)
- Phosphates, sulfates, and organic acids—renal failure, toxic ingestion

OTHER LABORATORY TESTS

Total CO_2

- Measured by many labs using the same sample submitted for electrolytes
- Closely approximates HCO_3^-, because most CO_2 is carried in the blood as bicarbonate
- Respiratory alkalosis also decreases Tco_2; differentiation can only be made with blood gas analysis.
- Analyze rapidly with minimal room-air exposure within the sample tube as CO_2 will decrease.

IMAGING

Diagnosis of cardiac, renal, and hepatic failure can be facilitated via ultrasonography.

DIAGNOSTIC PROCEDURES

Biopsy for suspected organ failure and cytology and microbiology of exudates or effusions may be useful with inflammation or infection.

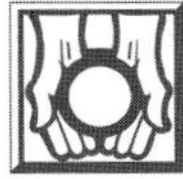

TREATMENT

- Directed at the primary cause. Alkalinizing therapy is described below.
- Replacement of fluid losses with balanced isotonic fluids may be all that is needed to restore acid-base status in mild cases.
- With hypovolemia caused by hemorrhage, hypertonic saline, colloids, or blood transfusion may be necessary to restore effective circulating volume in addition to crystalloid therapy.
- Specific electrolyte losses should be addressed, i.e., K^+, Ca^{2+}, in GI cases. Levels may change with alkalinizing therapy.

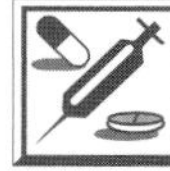

MEDICATIONS

DRUG(S) OF CHOICE

- Alkalinizing therapy is reserved for patients with a pH < 7.2 that persists following rehydration or volume replacement.
- Sodium bicarbonate is most frequently utilized.
- The bicarbonate deficit is calculated as follows: Base deficit × body weight (kg) × 0.3 (ECF space [0.5 in foals]) = HCO_3^- (mEq)
- A negative BE or 24 − (total CO_2 or HCO_3^-) can be used for the base deficit.
- In acute cases, $\frac{1}{2}$ the deficit can be given safely over 30 min, in fluids or as a 5% solution to adults.
- Isotonic bicarbonate (1.3%) is a good choice in neonates or severely affected adults with colitis.
- Correction to a pH >7.2 and BE ≥ -5 is usually adequate, especially with organic acidoses, because these are metabolized once the primary problem improves.

CONTRAINDICATIONS

Sodium bicarbonate cannot be mixed with calcium.

PRECAUTIONS

- Use bicarbonate therapy cautiously in patients with respiratory compromise, because the CO_2 that is generated may not be eliminated, causing a further decrease in pH.
- Hyperosmolar solutions may cause vascular irritation and affect tonicity of the CSF.
- Sodium load may affect blood volume in neonates and patients with compromised renal, neurologic, or cardiac function.
- Rebound alkalosis or cerebral acidosis is reported from overdose or too-rapid administration of bicarbonate since both CO_2 and H_2CO_3 cross the blood-brain barrier.

POSSIBLE INTERACTIONS

Alkalinizing therapies (i.e., HCO_3^-). Lactate can combine with Ca^{2+} in crystalloid solutions that form a harmful precipitate.

ALTERNATIVE DRUGS

- Replacement IV fluid solutions with other alkalinizing agents (e.g., lactate, citrate) are effective, because these are metabolized to HCO_3^-. Adequate hepatic function must be present, so these may not be useful in severely acidotic, hypoxemic, or septic patients.
- Oral rehydration solutions (1–2 gallons PO q2h in adults without ileus) have been used as primary therapy or an adjunct to IV fluid therapy in less severe cases.
- THAM, tromethamine, can be used as an alkalinizing agent. Its use does not increase CO_2 or sodium levels, and can be useful in patients with pneumonia or hypernatremia.

FOLLOW-UP

PATIENT MONITORING

Serial blood gas analysis to evaluate efficacy of therapy should be repeated within a few hours of initial treatment and thereafter according to patient response.

POSSIBLE COMPLICATONS

- Electrolyte abnormalities—hyperkalemia
- Cardiac arrhythmias, hypotension
- Severe, untreated metabolic acidosis with a pH <7.0 may result in death.

MISCELLANEOUS

ASSOCIATED CONDITIONS

- Hyperchloremia
- Hyperkalemia
- Respiratory alkalosis

AGE-RELATED CONDITIONS

- Asphyxia during parturition in neonates of any gestational age
- Conditions associated with premature neonates

ZOONOTIC POTENTIAL N/A

PREGNANCY

Metabolic acidosis may decrease uterine blood flow and result in placental insufficiency.

SYNONYMS

Nonrespiratory acidosis

SEE ALSO

- Causes of colitis • RTA

ABBREVIATIONS

- AG = anion gap
- BE = base excess
- COPD = chronic obstructive pulmonary disease
- CSF = cerebrospinal fluid
- ECF = extracellular fluid
- GI = gastrointestinal
- HYPP = hyperkalemic periodic paralysis
- RTA = renal tubular acidosis
- SID = strong ion difference
- TPN = total parenteral nutrition

Suggested Reading

Carlson GP. Fluid, electrolyte, and acid-base balance. In: Kaneko JJ, Harvey JW, Bruss ML, eds. Clinical Biochemistry of Domestic Animals, ed 5. San Diego: Academic Press, 1997:485–516.

Guyton AC, Hall JE, eds. Unit VII: Respiration. Textbook of Medical Physiology, 11th ed. Philadelphia: Elsevier Saunders, 2006:470–533.

McGinness GS, Mansmann RA, Breuhaus BA. Nasogastric electrolyte replacement in horses. Compend Cont Educ Pract Vet 1996;18:942–951.

Rose BD, Post TW, eds. Chapter 19: Metabolic Acidosis. In: Clinical Physiology of Acid-Base and Electrolyte Disorders, ed 5. New York: McGraw-Hill Professional, 2000, 2001:578–646.

Author Jennifer G. Adams

Consulting Editor Kenneth W. Hinchcliff

ACIDOSIS, RESPIRATORY

BASICS

DEFINITION

- Increase in blood Pco_2
- Homeostatic mechanisms maintain normal blood levels within a narrow range.
- Arterial levels range from 35–42 mm Hg.
- Venous levels range from 43–49 mm Hg.

PATHOPHYSIOLOGY

- CO_2 is formed in all tissues during metabolic energy production and diffuses passively out of cells and into the blood in gaseous form.
- Most of this CO_2 (65–70%) combines with water almost instantaneously to form carbonic acid, which then dissociates into bicarbonate ion and hydrogen.
- Most CO_2 is transported in the blood as bicarbonate. Some is bound to proteins, especially deoxygenated hemoglobin, and a small amount is dissolved directly into plasma.
- In the lungs, the reverse occurs, and CO_2 passively diffuses out of capillaries into the alveoli.
- The three forms of CO_2 exist in equilibrium in the blood, but the Pco_2 as measured by blood gases depends on the dissolved portion.
- The chemical components of the carbonic acid equilibrium are:

$$CO_2 + H_2O = H_2CO_3 = H^+ + HCO_3^-$$

- Alveolar CO_2 then is removed mechanically by ventilation as air moves in and out of the lungs.
- Hypercapnia is present only when tissue production exceeds the capacity of normal lungs to eliminate CO_2 or when components of the respiratory system are abnormal.
- Hypercapnia is uncommon in conscious patients, because the respiratory center responds to even minor abnormalities by increasing minute ventilation.
- Respiratory acidosis results from disease or alteration of the respiratory center in the medulla and peripheral chemoreceptors that control respiration, the mechanical components (i.e., chest wall, respiratory muscles), or the conducting airways, alveoli, and pulmonary vasculature, which are directly involved in gas exchange, by causing hypoventilation, barriers to diffusion, or V/Q mismatching.
- Because CO_2 diffuses very readily across the respiratory membrane in direct proportion to ventilation, hypoventilation usually has the most significant effect on blood levels.
- Hypermetabolism, as seen with malignant hyperthermia, may produce CO_2 in greater amounts than the lung can eliminate.
- Increased CO_2 also develops as a compensatory response of the lungs to metabolic alkalosis.

SYSTEM AFFECTED

Respiratory—See Pathophysiology.

SIGNALMENT

- Any horse
- Almost every anesthetized patient develops some degree of hypercapnia when breathing spontaneously.
- Because of their size, equines are especially predisposed to hypoventilation under anesthesia.

SIGNS

Historical Findings

- Respiratory noise may be heard, especially with exercise, in cases of upper airway obstruction.
- Exercise intolerance may be reported with many causes.

Physical Examination Findings

- None if minute ventilation is increased via increased tidal volume; if not, tachypnea may be present.
- Anesthetized animals with very high levels of CO_2 may have increased rate or depth of respiration.
- Decrease or absence of airway sounds may be found at auscultation in cases with damage or disease of the chest wall or thorax.
- Abnormal sounds may be present with pulmonary disease.

CAUSES

- Nasal edema, cysts, mass lesions, or infection of the paranasal sinuses; laryngeal or pharyngeal paralysis; soft-palate displacement; pharyngeal or epiglottal cysts; and tracheal masses or collapse all cause upper airway obstruction and impede airflow into the lungs.
- Injury or disease of the thorax, diaphragm, or pleura may restrict movement of the chest wall or respiratory muscles or lead to atelectasis because of fluid, blood, air, or intestinal organs in the pleural space.
- Uroperitoneum, diseases producing portal hypertension (e.g., cardiac or liver failure), and other diseases that result in large volumes of peritoneal fluid also may restrict diaphragmatic movement. Some may lead to pleural effusion as well.
- Displacement or distention of the intestine can restrict diaphragmatic movement.
- Weakness or paralysis of the respiratory muscles can be seen with neurologic dysfunction—encephalitis, botulism, tetanus, cranial or spinal trauma, and so on.
- Severe cases of pulmonary disease (e.g., viral, bacterial, or interstitial pneumonias), allergic small airway disease, and COPD affect gas exchange, ventilation, and diffusion.
- Hypoventilation caused by lung collapse, muscle relaxation, and decreased sensitivity of the respiratory centers to CO_2 occurs in all anesthetized horses. Heavy sedation also may produce temporary hypercapnia via muscle relaxation and respiratory center insensitivity.
- Exhaustion of the CO_2, absorbent, improper ventilator settings, or improper set up of the breathing system can lead to hypercapnia under anesthesia as well.
- Pregnant animals are more prone to hypoventilation under anesthesia because of abdominal distention from the pregnant uterus.
- Defective cellular metabolism of muscle is seen with malignant hyperthermia. This syndrome is very rare but has been seen in horses with inhalant anesthesia or succinyl choline administration. Abnormal metabolic processes in muscle cells are triggered, resulting in tremendous production of heat and CO_2, such that elimination mechanisms are overwhelmed and respiratory acidosis results.
- Anaerobic exercise produces temporary respiratory acidosis, because ventilation is limited when chest wall movement is linked to stride at high speeds.

RISK FACTORS

- General anesthesia; heavy sedation
- Pregnancy, which increases the volume of abdominal contents and may predispose to hypercapnia under anesthesia.
- Prolonged recumbency
- History of malignant hyperthermia in related individuals.
- Prematurity, dystocia, asphyxia or sepsis, persistent fetal circulation, or pulmonary hypertension in neonates.

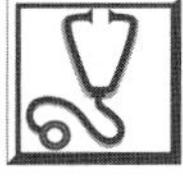

DIAGNOSIS

DIFFERENTIAL DIAGNOSIS

- Physiologic states or disease processes that present with tachypnea—fever, hyperthermia, excitement, anxiety, painful conditions, hypoxemia, metabolic acidosis, and CNS derangements.
- Under anesthesia, tachypnea also may result from a light plane of anesthesia, hypoxemia, metabolic acidosis, or faulty anesthetic rebreathing systems.
- Diseases resulting in metabolic alkalosis may have a compensatory hypercapnia—upper GI obstruction, early large colon impactions or simple obstructions, supplementation with bicarbonate or other alkalinizing agents. Measurements of pH in these cases often are still higher than normal, because compensatory hypoventilation is limited once hypoxemia develops.

LABORATORY FINDINGS

Drugs That May Alter Lab Results

N/A

Disorders That May Alter Lab Results

- With poor peripheral perfusion or cardiovascular shunt, results of blood gas analysis on samples taken from peripheral vessels may differ from those taken elsewhere or not reflect the overall systemic condition.
- Exposure to room air via air bubbles in the sample may change the Pco_2 level, because the sample equilibrates with the air.

• Cellular metabolism of RBCs continues after sampling; if not measured quickly, CO_2 levels may be falsely elevated.

Valid If Run in Human Lab?

Yes, if properly submitted.

CBC/BIOCHEMISTRY/URINALYSIS

N/A

OTHER LABORATORY TESTS

• Arterial blood gas analysis is necessary to evaluate adequacy of ventilation and gas exchange and to document hypercapnia.
• Handheld analyzers are available and easy to use, and some require only small amounts of whole blood. Otherwise, syringes should be heparinized before sampling.
• Perform sampling anaerobically. Immediately evacuate any air bubbles, and cap the needle with a rubber stopper.
• Perform analysis within 15–20 min. If not possible, samples can be stored on ice, and results will be valid for 3–4 hr.

IMAGING

N/A

DIAGNOSTIC PROCEDURES

• Capnography or capnometry to measure CO_2 indirectly from expired gases.
• Samples of end-tidal gases reflect arterial Pco_2 levels, because this gas is essentially alveolar gas.
• Continuous monitoring on anesthetized or ventilated patients.
• $\dot{V}/\dot{Q}$ mismatch is always present in anesthetized or recumbent patients, and end-tidal levels may underestimate arterial levels by $\cong$10–15 mm Hg.

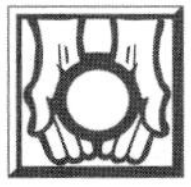

TREATMENT

• Emergency therapy occasionally may be necessary for upper airway obstructions—passage of a nasotracheal tube or tracheotomy.
• Definitive therapy for hypercapnia involves resolution of the primary disease process affecting ventilation, diffusion, or gas exchange; improvement of ventilation usually is most effective.
• Avoid excessive anesthetic depth. Lightening of anesthesia may improve ventilation and decrease Pco_2 levels. If depth is adequate, controlled ventilation is necessary when hypoventilation is severe (i.e., >60 mm Hg).
• In neonates, postural therapy and coupage may improve gas exchange. Improvement of overall status, especially cardiovascular and neurologic, may improve respiratory function dramatically.
• With severe lung disease, treat hypercapnia with controlled ventilation. This generally is not feasible in adults, but neonates respond well. Heavy sedation or muscle relaxant therapy may be necessary in some individuals; however, most relax once respiratory function improves.

MEDICATIONS

DRUGS OF CHOICE

Doxapram

• A respiratory stimulant that may be a useful adjunct (0.5–1 mg/kg IV or an infusion of 0.02–0.05 mg/kg per min) in emergency resuscitation and some patients, especially foals with neurologic or muscular weakness.
• Anesthetized patients who are breathing poorly may respond temporarily to its effects, but controlled ventilation, decreasing depth, and anesthetic reversal are more specific and appropriate therapies.
• Not indicated for healthy patients being weaned from controlled ventilation

Other Drugs

Anti-inflammatory therapy with corticosteroids or bronchodilator therapy with α_2-agonists or xanthine derivatives may be useful in patients with allergic airway disease and COPD once environmental factors are controlled.

CONTRAINDICATIONS

• Controlled ventilation may cause barotrauma in foals with meconium aspiration.
• Partial obstruction of the small airways may lead to air trapping in alveoli, which may rupture.

PRECAUTIONS

• Monitor ventilated patients continuously for airway obstruction caused by accumulation of secretions, kinking of tubing, hoses, and so on.
• Oxygen toxicity can develop with inspired Po_2 >50% or if Pao_2 >100 mm Hg is maintained for prolonged periods (10–12 hr).

POSSIBLE INTERACTIONS

N/A

ALTERNATIVE DRUGS

N/A

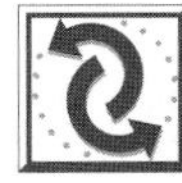

FOLLOW-UP

PATIENT MONITORING

• Decreased respiratory effort should be seen quickly after improvement of ventilation.
• Use serial arterial blood gas analysis or capnometry to assess adequacy of ventilation and monitor progress, especially during weaning.

POSSIBLE COMPLICATIONS

• Respiratory acidosis lowers systemic pH and may affect ionization of protein-bound drugs.
• Acidosis decreases heart contractility and may cause or contribute to CNS depression.
• Hypercapnia and the resultant acidosis predispose patients to cardiac arrhythmias, especially under anesthesia.
• The $Paco_2$ level greatly affects cerebral blood flow and CSF pressure.
• Severe or prolonged hypercapnia may contribute to brain damage or herniation in cases with head trauma.

MISCELLANEOUS

ASSOCIATED CONDITIONS

Disorders that result in metabolic alkalosis

AGE-RELATED FACTORS

Neonates, especially premature foals, may be more prone to hypercapnia because of decreased compliance of the lungs and lack of strength (i.e., immaturity) of the chest wall.

ZOONOTIC POTENTIAL

N/A

PREGNANCY

See Risk Factors.

SYNONYMS

• Hypercapnia
• Hypercarbia
• Hypoventilation

SEE ALSO

See specific diseases in Causes.

ABBREVIATIONS

• CNS = central nervous system
• COPD = chronic obstructive pulmonary disease
• CSF = cerebrospinal fluid
• GI = gastrointestinal
• $\dot{V}/\dot{Q}$ = ventilation/perfusion

Suggested Reading

Coons TJ, Kosch PC, Cudd TA. Respiratory care. In: Koterba AM, Drummond WA, Kosch PC, eds. Equine Clinical Neonatology. Philadelphia: Lea & Febiger, 1990:200–239.

Section VII: Respiration. In: Guyton AC, ed. Medical Physiology, 9th ed. Philadelphia: WB Saunders, 1992:465–526.

Palmer JE. Ventilatory support of the neonatal foal. Vet Clin North Am Equine Pract 1994;10:167–186.

Author Jennifer G. Adams

Consulting Editor Kenneth W. Hinchcliff

ACTINOBACILLOSIS

BASICS

OVERVIEW

• Acute rapidly progressive septicemia due to *Actinobacillus equuli* or *A. suis*–like organisms in neonatal foals.
• *A. equuli* is a gram-negative coccobacillary to rod-shaped pleomorphic organism that produces flat gray 1- to 3-mm colonies after 24-hr incubation on blood agar. *A. equuli* is a normal inhabitant of the mucous membranes of the alimentary tract.
• Fetal infection may follow transplacental infection. The kidneys are a frequent site of neonatal infection.
• In adults, infection is frequently endogenous and results from fecal contamination or spread from oral mucous membranes. Adults have soft tissue abscesses, respiratory infections, and rarely conjunctival, urinary tract, joint, guttural pouch, skin, and genital tract infections.

SIGNALMENT

• Foals <2 days of age
• Adults of any age and use

SIGNS

Foals

• Acute onset, depression, diarrhea, recumbency, distended painful joints, sudden death
• Fever may not be present and foals may be hypothermic. If left untreated, foals may progress rapidly to septic shock.
• Bone and joint infections in neonates may not be obvious for days to weeks and may be unaccompanied by signs of systemic disease.

Adults

• Signs are generally referable to the affected organ system.
• Primary peritonitis due to *Actinobacillus* has been reported in adult horses.

CAUSES AND RISK FACTORS

Foals

• Commonly seen associated with failure of passive transfer of immunoglobulins. Perinatal stress, prematurity, and/or unsanitary environmental conditions may predispose the foal.
• Portals of entry include respiratory tract, gastrointestinal tract, placenta, and umbilical remnant.

Adults

• Pneumonia and pleuropneumonia may develop secondary to viral infection or stressful events including but not limited to general anesthesia, athletic events, transport over prolonged distance, and other environmental stressors and concurrent illnesses.
• Trauma may predispose to abscess formation.

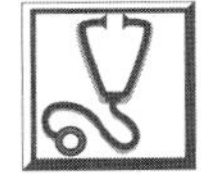

DIAGNOSIS

DIFFERENTIAL DIAGNOSIS

Foals

• Any other cause of neonatal sepsis including bacterial, viral, and fungal agents
• Gram-negative organisms are the most common bacterial agents isolated in cases of neonatal sepsis, although infections with only gram-positive pathogens have been reported.
• Foals with equine herpevirus type 1 and equine viral arteritis infections may appear identical to foals with bacterial infection.
• Foals with perinatal hypoxic-ischemic anoxic or inflammatory insults may present with nearly identical clinical signs, depending on severity.

Adults

• Any other cause of fever
• Any other cause of peritonitis
• Any other bacterial, viral, or fungal agent causing pneumonia or pleuropneumonia

Other causes of respiratory distress, fever, coughing, and nasal discharge should be considered, including:
• Sinusitis
• Guttural pouch empyema
• Heaves (recurrent airway obstruction)
• Inflammatory airway disease
• Interstitial pneumonia
• Mycoplasma infections
• Neoplasia
• Dysphagia

CBC/BIOCHEMISTRY/URINALYSIS

Foals

• Leukocytosis or leukopenia
• Hyperfibrinogenemia at birth is occasionally present with in utero infections. Hyperfibrinogenemia is common in postnatal infections.
• Increased creatinine and/or blood urea nitrogen with renal involvement
• Metabolic acidosis, hypoxemia, and hypercapnia may be observed with foals in septic shock.
• Hypoglycemia may be present.
• Frequent complete or partial failure of passive transfer (serum IgG <800 mg/dL)
• Urinalysis may be abnormal with renal involvement.

Adults

• Leukocytosis and hyperfibrinogenemia are possible.
• Low PCV in longstanding infection due to anemia of chronic disease
• Other abnormalities, depending on body system involved

OTHER LABORATORY TESTS

N/A

IMAGING

Foals

• Thoracic radiographs may demonstrate pulmonary involvement. Radiographs of affected joints may not show acute changes; bony involvement may take days to become radiographically apparent.

• Ultrasonographic examination of the umbilical remnant may demonstrate focal infection. Ultrasonographic examination of kidneys may be abnormal.

Adults

Radiographic and ultrasonographic evaluation of affected body system may be beneficial.

OTHER DIAGNOSTIC PROCEDURES

Foals

• Blood culture may be diagnostic.
• Bacterial culture of synovial fluid may be diagnostic and should be attempted in affected joints.
• Kidneys frequently have multifocal microabscesses at post-mortem examination.

Adults

• Culture of affected body system may be diagnostic.
• Culture of peritoneal fluid may be diagnostic.
• Culture and cytology of transtracheal aspirates and thoracocentesis fluids may be diagnostic. Because *A. equuli* is a normal inhabitant of equine gastrointestinal mucosa, results should be interpreted cautiously.

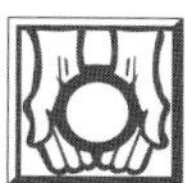

TREATMENT

Foals

Affected foals are quite ill and are best managed in a hospital. Administer intranasal oxygen supplementation as needed.

MEDICATIONS

DRUG(S) OF CHOICE

Foals

• Administer isotonic polyionic balanced fluids or 0.9% NaCl to maintain adequate hydration and fluid balance. Intravenous plasma as required based on serum or plasma IgG concentrations.
• Intravenous dextrose or parenteral nutrition as needed for nutritional management.
• Broad-spectrum antimicrobial therapy, gentamicin 12 mg/kg IV SID or amikacin 25–30 mg/kg IV SID and potassium penicillin 10,000 IV/kg IV QID or ceftiofur sodium 10 mg/kg IV QID. Monitor plasma creatinine concentration. Therapeutic drug monitoring desirable.
• Foals with systemic inflammatory response syndrome (SIRS) or multiple organ dysfunction syndrome (MODS) may require more intensive fluid management and inopressor therapy.
• Foals with severe respiratory disturbance may require assisted ventilation.
• Regional limb perfusion and/or direct instillation with antimicrobials of choice for septic joints

Adults

Antimicrobial therapy based on culture and sensitivity results

MISCELLANEOUS

Antimicrobial therapy should be modified based on response and culture/sensitivity results. Therapeutic monitoring of aminoglycoside levels should be performed. Continue treatment until clinical signs have resolved and white blood count, differential, and fibrinogen concentration are within normal limits for 48 hours.

Actinobacillus spp. were commonly isolated from foals lost to mare reproductive loss syndrome (MRLS) and adult horses affected by pericarditis during the same time period.

ABBREVIATIONS

• SIRS = systemic inflammatory response syndrome
• MODS = multiorgan dysfunction syndrome
• MRLS = mare reproductive loss syndrome

Suggested Reading

Stewart AJ, Hinchcliff KW, Saville WJ, et al. Actinobacillus sp. bacteremia in foals: Clinical signs and prognosis. J Vet Intern Med 2002;16:464–471.

Author Pamela A. Wilkins
Consulting Editor Ashley G. Boyle and Corinne R. Sweeney

ACUTE ADULT ABDOMINAL PAIN–ACUTE COLIC

BASICS

DEFINITION

Clinical signs associated with discomfort originating within the abdominal cavity. May develop acutely or progressively. Considered chronic when persist for >3–4 days.

PATHOPHYSIOLOGY

- It originates primarily from the gastrointestinal tract but may also arise from other abdominal structures such as liver, spleen, kidneys, uterus, bladder, or peritoneum.
- Intestinal pain may originate from increased intramural tension, tension on the mesentery, regional or generalized ischemia, mucosal inflammation, smooth muscle spasms associated with hypermotility, or a combination of any of these.
- Nonstrangulated lesions have no compromise to the local blood supply.
- Intraluminal lesions (impaction, foreign body, concretions), extraluminal lesions (adhesions, strictures), mural lesion (thickening), as well as spasmodic colic, intestinal displacement, ileus, and inflammatory bowel disease are usually considered nonstrangulated lesions.
- Strangulated lesions, such as torsion and incarceration, are usually associated with compromised local blood supply, intestinal necrosis and cardiovascular shock.

SYSTEMS AFFECTED

- Gastrointestinal—anywhere from the stomach to the small colon can be involved. The large colon and the distal part of the small intestine are most commonly involved.
- Cardiovascular system—dehydration and endotoxemia may lead to shock and result in organ failure.
- Other systems can be the source of abdominal pain.

SIGNALMENT

Nonspecific. There may be an age, breed, or sex predisposition for a specific problem (e.g., intussusception of the small intestine is more commonly seen in young horses; pedunculated lipomas are commoner on older horses; large colon torsion commonly seen around parturition in mares; pain from the reproductive tract is seen in pregnant or postpartum mares and in stallions of breeding age).

SIGNS

General Comments

Signs of abdominal pain may be subtle initially and are often easily missed and the source of pain may be difficult to identify.

Historical

Signs can appear acutely or following an episode of anorexia, depression, and/or decrease in fecal output. History of change in exercise regimen, diet, or availability of drinking water may also precede the signs of colic, which can be of different intensity:

- Mild—decrease in appetite, and fecal output, mild depression, yawning, extended neck and rolling of the upper lip in Flehmen-like response, teeth grinding
- Moderate—pawing at the ground, flank watching, groaning, posture for urinating but only a small quantity of urine is passed, leaning against the wall, kicking the abdomen with the hind legs, ears pinned backward, lying down more frequently, may attempt to roll
- Severe abdominal pain—walking in a tight circle, constantly getting up and down, rolling, traumatizing self and handlers, sweating, labored breathing

Physical Examination

Signs may vary, depending on stage of the disease:

- General findings—abdominal distention, sweating, increase in respiratory rate, elevated or subnormal body temperature, abnormal quality and quantity of feces
- Cardiovascular findings—congested mucous membrane, increase in capillary refill time and in heart rate, dehydration and cold extremities are suggestive of a strangulated lesion or to a severe inflammatory process such as colitis or peritonitis
- Gastrointestinal findings—increase, decrease or absence in gut motility, gas-filled resonant viscus on percussion. Gastric reflux on passage of the nasogastric tube is most commonly associated with lesions located at the level of the stomach or small intestine.
- Abnormalities on rectal examination—distention of a viscus by gas, liquid, or food; displacement of a viscus; thickening of the intestinal wall; uterine or renal abnormalities; findings will assist in the differentiation among problems involving the small intestine, large colon, cecum, small colon, or nongastrointestinal lesions

CAUSES

Gastrointestinal

- Gastric—gastric ulcers, gastric distention or impaction, gastric rupture, gastric tumor
- Small intestine—nonstrangulated obstructive lesion: duodenal ulcer, duodenojejunal enteritis, ascarid impaction, ileal impaction, ileal hypertrophy, stricture. Strangulated obstructive lesion: incarceration of a segment of the small intestine into the epiploic foramen, a space/rent in the mesentery/inguinal ring/gastrosplenic ligament, strangulation by a lipoma, volvulus, adhesions, etc.
- Large intestine—nonstrangulated obstructive lesion: ulceration, colitis, impaction, idiopathic gas distention, mild displacement, nephrosplenic entrapment, enterolith, adhesions, sand impactions. Strangulated obstructive lesion: volvulus, herniation, incarceration, thromboembolic infarction
- Cecum—nonstrangulated obstructive lesion: impaction, adhesions. Strangulated obstructive lesion: cecal-cecal or ceco-colic intussusception, thromboembolic infarction, torsion, incarceration
- Small colon—nonstrangulated obstructive lesion: impaction, enterolith. Strangulated obstructive lesion: incarceration, strangulating lipoma, submucosal hematoma, thromboembolic infarction
- Reproductive—uterine torsion, uterine laceration, abortion, parturition, testicular torsion, hematoma in the broad ligament, trauma
- Renal/urologic—renal/ureteral/bladder/urethral calculi, cystitis, renal inflammatory processes
- Hepatobiliary—hepatitis, hepatobiliary calculi
- Others—peritonitis, hemoperitoneum

RISK FACTORS

- No access to water
- Sudden change in diet
- Poor enteric parasite control
- Pregnancy
- Previous abdominal surgery
- Congenital abnormalities
- Certain medication

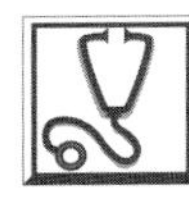

DIAGNOSIS

N/A

DIFFERENTIAL DIAGNOSIS

Other causes of pain that might mimic pain originating from the abdominal cavity include myositis, pleuropneumonia, neurologic diseases such as rabies, and musculoskeletal injuries.

CBC/BIOCHEMISTRY/URINALYSIS

Increase in PCV and TP in face of dehydration. Possible hypoproteinemia secondary to protein loss in the intestinal lumen and/or in the abdominal cavity. Leukopenia in acute inflammatory process and endotoxemia or leukocytosis in chronic inflammatory process. Possible metabolic acidosis related to cardiovascular shock and release of lactic acid and/or loss of bicarbonate and electrolytes (colitis) or metabolic alkalosis if a large amount of gastric reflux is present, resulting in loss of chloride. Hypokalemia and hypocalcemia can be present, especially if the horse has been anorexic or is a lactating mare. Hypochloremia and hyponatremia may be present in colitis. Alkaline phosphatase may be increased. Azotemia is found in horses with severe dehydration or urinary tract disease. The increase in some or all of the following is suggestive of liver disease: GLDH, AST, GGT, conjugated bilirubin and bile acids. A selective increase in serum GGT in a horse with colic is suggestive of a displacement of the right colon.

OTHER LABORATORY TESTS

Abdominal Paracentesis

- Normal fluid has a pale, clear yellow color.
- Turbidity of the sample indicates an elevation of WBCs, RBCs, or contamination with intestinal contents.
- Increase of the protein level and WBCs is indicative of primary peritonitis or secondary to morphologic change of the viscera.
- A sanguineous fluid is probably indicative of intra-abdominal bleeding or a strangulated obstructive lesion.
- A foul-smelling reddish-brown fluid with an increase in the RBC, WBC, and protein is indicative of presence of necrotic bowel.
- Presence of plant materials in the absence of an enterocentesis suggests intestinal rupture.
- Few leukocytes or cells should be present if an enterocentesis was performed.

Urinalysis

A change in specific gravity, increase in leukocyte content, RBC, and pH may be noticed in cases with renal disease.

IMAGING

Radiographs

May be useful in the identification of sand impactions or enteroliths in adults. In foals they help in the localization of gas, fluid, and impaction distention. May also help to identify congenital abnormality such as atresia coli.

Ultrasonography

Evaluate the amount, quality, and characteristics of abdominal fluid; motility, wall thickness and diameter of small intestine and its location; evaluation of the nephrosplenic space for presence of intestine; motility and wall thickness of the large intestine; other abnormal findings, such as intussusceptions, abscesses, or adhesions.

Endoscopy

- Gastroscopy—evaluation of the stomach for ulcers, impaction, or tumor. In small horses, the duodenum may also be observed.
- Cystoscopy—evaluation of the urethra, bladder, and opening of the ureters for inflammation or calculi.
- Laparoscopy—visualization of abdominal viscera

Nuclear scintigraphy

Can be used to assess motility, presence of inflammation and infection of the gastrointestinal tract, and the reticuloendothelial function

OTHER DIAGNOSTIC PROCEDURES

Exploratory laparotomy or laparoscopy.

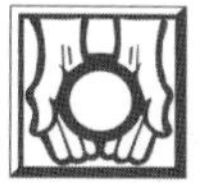

TREATMENT

- Horses should be taken off feed until diagnosis of the underlying problem.
- Indication for an exploratory laparotomy includes: signs of severe abdominal pain, unresponsiveness to medical treatment, moderate to severe abdominal distention, ileus or progressive reduction in gut motility, progressive increase in heart rate or heart rates above 60–70/min, cardiovascular compromise or deterioration, presence of moderate to severe gas distention or of a displacement of the large colon on rectal examination, gas distention of small intestine on rectal examination, gastric reflux, abnormal paracentesis findings, or presence of severe impaction of the large colon or the cecum. Animals presenting with these signs should be referred to a surgical facility.
- Supportive treatment for medical and surgical cases includes intravenous fluids, gastric decompression if necessary, electrolyte replenishment, and control of the abdominal pain.

MEDICATIONS

DRUG(S) OF CHOICE

- Analgesics—control the abdominal pain
- NSAIDs—dipyrone 10 mg/kg, flunixin meglumine 0.5–1.1 mg/kg IV, IM q8 h, phenylbutazone 2.2–4.4 mg/kg IV q12–24 h, ketoprofen 1.1–2.2 mg/kg, α_2-blockers such as xylazine 0.25–0.5 mg/kg IV, IM, detomidine 5–10 µg/kg IV, IM, or romifidine 0.02–0.05 mg/kg IV, IM can also be given if the pain is not controlled by NSAIDs.
- The narcotic analgesics such as butorphanol 0.02–0.075 mg/kg IV or meperidine (pethidine 2 mg/kg) can be given alone or in conjunction with xylazine. These two drugs potentiate each other.
- Any drugs should be used judiciously as they may mask clinical signs and may lead to postponement of surgery, thereby decreasing the chance of survival. Furthermore, most of these drugs have a detrimental effect on gastrointestinal motility.
- Spasmolytics (indicated in spasmodic colic)—hyoscine 20–30 mL IV and *N*-butylscopolammonium bromide 0.3 mg/kg
- Laxatives—for treatment of impactions
  - Mineral oil—10 mL/kg via nasogastric tube
  - Osmotic laxative—diluted disodium 0.5 g/kg or magnesium sulfate 0.5–1 g/kg in 4 L of warm water via nasogastric tube.
  - Dioctyl sodium succinate (DSS) 10–30 mg/kg of a 10% solution via nasogastric tube.
  - Fluids, via an indwelling nasogastric line (4–5 L/hr) or intravenously
- Parenteral fluid treatments—In cases of dehydration or moderate to severe impaction problems, intravenous fluid (100–200 mL/kg/day). If cardiovascular shock is present, hypertonic saline (2 L of 7% NaCl in an adult horse) prior to balanced electrolyte solutions. Electrolyte imbalances should be corrected, especially hypokalemia and hypocalcemia, which are important for intestinal motility. Moderate to severe bicarbonate deficit should be corrected as well as low plasma protein level (<45 g/L).
- Treatment of endotoxemia—flunixin meglumine 0.25 mg/kg q6 h. Other antiendotoxemic treatments include hyperimmune plasma (see Endotoxemia).
- Intestinal motility stimulants (see Ileus)—Postoperative ileus is the most common indication. Metoclopramide (0.1 mg/kg/hr in a constant drip infusion over several hours); lidocaine (1.3 mg/kg IV as a bolus followed by 0.05 mg/kg/min infusion); erythromycin lactobionate (1 g QID IV in 1 L saline).
- Antimicrobial therapy if peritonitis is suspected or if surgery is performed

CONTRAINDICATIONS

Acepromazine is contraindicated due to its peripheral vasodilatory effect.

PRECAUTIONS

Repeat use of α_2-blockers and butorphanol causes prolonged ileus. Repeat dose of NSAIDs, especially in presence of dehydration, can result in gastric or large colon ulceration as well as renal damage.

FOLLOW-UP

PATIENT MONITORING

The patient should be monitored closely for deterioration of clinical signs and cardiovascular status until resolution of the abdominal pain. Following resolution of these signs, reintroduction to feed should be done gradually.

POSSIBLE COMPLICATIONS

- Endotoxemia
- Laminitis
- Circulatory shock
- Adhesions
- Gastrointestinal rupture
- Peritonitis

AGE-RELATED FACTORS

Older horses are more predisposed to strangulated lipoma and epiploic foramen entrapment; pregnant mares are more predisposed to large colon torsion; and younger horses are more predisposed to ulcer problems, intussusception, and ascarid impactions.

PREGNANCY

Mares in late gestation or in the postpartum period are predisposed to large colon torsion. Parturition can present clinical signs similar to a gastrointestinal accident.

SYNONYM

Colic

ABBREVIATIONS

- PCV = packed cell volume
- TP = total protein

Suggested Reading

Mair T, Divers T, Ducharme N. Section 1. Diagnostic procedure in equine gastroenterology. In: Manual of Equine Gastoenterology. Philadelphia: WB Saunders, 2002:3–46.

Mair T, Divers T, Ducharme N. Section 4. Colic. In: Manual of Equine Gastoenterology. Philadelphia: WB Saunders, 2002:101–141.

Author Nathalie Coté

Consulting Editors Henry Stämpfli and Olimpo Oliver-Espinosa

ACUTE EPIGLOTTIDITIS

BASICS

OVERVIEW

Epiglottiditis is a nonspecific inflammatory disease of the epiglottis.

SIGNALMENT

- Primarily racehorses (2–10 years) in active race training or other horses undergoing repeated, strenuous exercise
- Occasionally seen in older horses (15–18 years) associated with neoplasia
- No known breed or sex predilection

SIGNS

- Chief complaints—variable amount of abnormal respiratory tract noise and exercise intolerance
- Coughing during eating is fairly common.
- Some horses act mildly pained when swallowing.

CAUSES AND RISK FACTORS

- Cause—unknown
- Repeated, strenuous exercise may induce inflammatory changes on the lingual (ventral) mucosal epiglottic surface between this tissue and the dorsal surface of the free edge of the soft palate.
- The role of inhaled particulate matter during galloping, abrasive feed or bedding material during swallowing, and bacterial or viral infections is unknown.

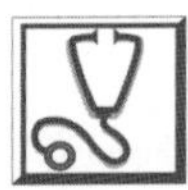

DIAGNOSIS

DIFFERENTIAL DIAGNOSIS

- The diagnosis is established based on endoscopy of the upper respiratory tract.
- Occasionally, the endoscopic appearance is misinterpreted as epiglottic entrapment by the aryepiglottic folds.
- May be associated with epiglottic abscess or chondritis

CBC/BIOCHEMISTRY/URINALYSIS

These tests are not typically performed.

OTHER LABORATORY TESTS

Additional laboratory tests are not typically performed.

IMAGING

Imaging is not usually performed.

DIAGNOSTIC PROCEDURES

- During routine endoscopy, the epiglottis may appear swollen and discolored (reddish-purplish), primarily along the lateral margins and ventral (lingual) mucosal surfaces. This swelling may obscure the normal, serrated margins and cause the epiglottis to appear more rounded and bulbous. The ventral mucosal surfaces often are ulcerated, and in more chronic, untreated cases, granulation tissue surrounded by fibrous connective tissue is seen. The epiglottis looks thicker and may be elevated a variable amount into an abnormal axis above the soft palate.
- If ulceration is seen at the rostral tip or dorsal surface of the epiglottic cartilage one should suspect associated epiglottic chondritis and abscessation.
- Horses with epiglottiditis often intermittently displace the soft palate dorsally and may experience difficulty replacing the soft palate into a normal position underneath the epiglottis.
- The caudal free margin of the soft palate may have a variable amount of inflammation, ulceration, or thickening. If the inflammatory insult is more diffuse, then inflammation of adjacent structures characterized by reddening, thickening, edema, and ulceration may occur in the corniculate processes of the arytenoids and adjacent nasal pharyngeal mucosa.

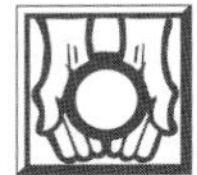

TREATMENT

- Outpatient (stall-side) basis
- Discontinue exercise for a minimum of 7–14 days, depending on the extent of the problem.
- If swallowing is difficult or stimulates coughing, hay may need to be eliminated from the diet or, at least, made wet until the inflammation resolves; a complete ration or gruel made from pellets may be easier to swallow.

MEDICATIONS

DRUG(S) OF CHOICE

- Epiglottiditis usually responds to medical therapy consisting of NSAIDs, parenteral corticosteroids, and topical pharyngeal sprays that contain anti-inflammatory and antimicrobial medication.
- With evidence of infection or a fever, antimicrobial therapy may be indicated—IM procaine penicillin G, PO trimethoprim sulfamethoxazole, or IM or IV ceftiofur at normal recommended dosages for 5–7 days.
- Horses are initially treated with phenylbutazone (4.4 mg/kg IV) or flunixin meglumine (1.1 mg/kg IV) and dexamethasone (0.044 mg/kg IV). Ten to 20 mL of a pharyngeal spray (750 mL of Furacin, 250 mL of DMSO, 1000 mL of glycerin, and 2.0 g of prednisolone) is sprayed slowly, while watching for swallowing, into the pharynx twice daily for 7–14 days through a 10-F catheter introduced into the nasal pharynx via the nasal passages. After the initial IV dose of either phenylbutazone or flunixin meglumine and dexamethasone, oral therapy is continued with phenylbutazone (2.2 mg/kg PO twice daily for 7–14 days) and prednisolone (2.2 mg/kg PO once daily for 7 days). The same dose is then administered orally every other day for three treatments. Subsequently, a dose of 0.45 mg/kg is given orally every other day for three treatments.

CONTRAINDICATIONS/POSSIBLE INTERACTIONS

No contraindications

FOLLOW-UP

PATIENT MONITORING

Substantial improvement in the overall appearance of the epiglottis and adjacent tissue and in pharyngeal function usually is seen at follow-up endoscopy after about 1 week of therapy with acute inflammation. Continue rest and therapy until healing is judged complete based on repeated endoscopy performed at about 1-week intervals.

PREVENTION/AVOIDANCE

Horses with more chronic-appearing inflammation or with associated epiglottic abscess and/or chondritis may require more protracted therapy (2–4 weeks), and complete resolution of thickening and cartilage deformity may not occur. Occasionally, epiglottic entrapment may develop, but this usually can be corrected using dorsal midline division or excision with a curved bistoury or a contact laser. Extremely bulbous or fibrotic-appearing entrapping membranes may need to be excised through a laryngotomy.

POSSIBLE COMPLICATIONS

Advise owners that healing may result in fibrosis or cicatrix on the lingual epiglottic surface sufficient to interfere with normal soft-palate function. Endoscopy may reveal intermittent or persistent dorsal displacement of the soft palate, which may need surgical treatment—laryngeal tie-forward, soft-palate trim, or excision of fibrous connective tissue on the subepiglottic surface.

EXPECTED COURSE AND PROGNOSIS

Epiglottiditis is a serious, potentially career-limiting or -ending problem in racehorses. Prognosis depends primarily on severity of the condition during the initial examination and the degree of involvement of the arytenoid cartilage. Resolution of acute inflammation results in complete return to normal exercise tolerance and elimination of abnormal respiratory tract noise. Horses with more chronic or extensive lesions may experience epiglottic deformity and suffer from intermittent to persistent dorsal displacement of the soft palate despite appropriate medical or surgical therapy.

SEE ALSO

- Dorsal displacement of the soft palate
- Inspiratory dyspnea

ABBREVIATION

- DMSO = dimethylsulfoxide

Suggested Reading

Hawkins JF, Tulleners EP. Epiglottitis in horses: 20 Cases (1988–1993). J Am Vet Med Assoc 1994;205:1577–1580.

Infernuso T, Watts AE, Ducharme NG. Septic epiglottic chondritis with abscessation in 2 young Thoroughbred racehorses. Can Vet J 2006;47:1007–1010.

Author Norm Ducharme; Eric Tulleners (First Edition)

Consulting Editor Daniel Jean

ACUTE HEPATITIS IN ADULT HORSES (THEILER'S DISEASE)

BASICS

OVERVIEW

• Many conditions can potentially lead to acute liver failure in adult horses, with the most common being a syndrome occurring 4–10 weeks after animals have received an equine biologic. This is usually tetanus antitoxin, but other agents have been implicated—equine serum and encephalitis vaccine. • Acute failure of liver functions leads to various biochemical derangements, with accumulation of some agents, lack of some, and imbalances in others. These biochemical imbalances are responsible for many of the clinical signs seen in this disease.

SIGNALMENT

Predominantly in adult horses

SIGNS

• Usually sudden in onset and rapidly progressive, with death occurring 2–6 days after onset of signs in some cases. • Horses are often very icteric and pass dark urine caused by the presence of bilirubin. • Many have signs of hepatic encephalopathy, which can manifest in various ways that may change during the course of the disease. • Initially, there may be subtle changes in behavior, progressing to excitement or depression with head pressing. • Some may wander aimlessly around the stall or paddock.
• Frequent yawning has been reported in some cases. • If animals live long enough and are outside in the sun, they may develop photosensitive dermatitis on white parts of the body. • Possible hemorrhagic diathesis or hemolysis terminally.

CAUSES AND RISK FACTORS

• Most commonly associated with administration of an equine biologic 4–6 weeks before the onset of signs; however, not all cases have been exposed to an equine biologic. • Some epidemiologic evidence suggests that some cases may result from an infectious agent, probably a virus. None has been isolated as yet, however, and attempts to reproduce the disease with material from affected horses have failed.
• Occasional cases caused by *Clostridium novyi* type B have been described.

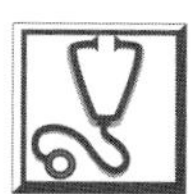

DIAGNOSIS

DIFFERENTIAL DIAGNOSIS

• Acute onset of icterus in adult horses has multiple causes—prehepatic, hepatic, or posthepatic; serum biochemistries and CBC assist in differentiating these causes.
• Prehepatic—red maple leaf toxicity, wild onion toxicity, phenothiazine toxicity, and nitrate poisoning • Hepatic—anorexia, Theiler's disease, *C. novyi,* bacterial cholangiohepatitis, EIA, EVA, *Strongyle* sp. migration, arsenic toxicity, and halogenated hydrocarbons.
• Posthepatic—cholelithiasis and other causes of biliary obstruction. • Signs of hepatic encephalopathy can be very similar to those of several acute neurologic diseases—rabies, EEE, WEE, and acute protozoal myeloencephalitis. Icterus and serum biochemical changes help in differentiating these problems. • Hematuria, hemoglobinuria, myoglobinuria, and bilirubinuria may cause pigmenturia; urinalysis and serum biochemistries aid in differentiation.

CBC/BIOCHEMISTRY/URINALYSIS

• Bilirubin—moderate increase in unconjugated and conjugated levels • Liver enzymes—increases in SDH (IDH), AST, GGT, and ALP
• Some may assay LDH, particularly isoenzyme 5. • Glucose—normal to low
• Urea—normal to low • Bilirubinuria
• CBC—usually normal

OTHER LABORATORY TESTS

Bromsulfalein clearance—2.2 mg/kg IV. Half-life is determined by sampling at 3, 6, and 9 min after injection; normal half-life is 2.8 +/− 0.5 min. Half-life is prolonged when >50% of liver function is lost. Archaic test.

IMAGING

Ultrasonography may suggest the liver is smaller than normal, with a loss of normal parenchymal structure.

DIAGNOSTIC PROCEDURES

• Liver biopsy is performed on the right side between the 12th and 14th intercostal spaces, where a line drawn from the tuber coxae to the elbow intersects the selected intercostal space. Ultrasound guidance may ensure accurate placement of the biopsy needle.
• Coagulation profile recommended by some before biopsy
• Histopathology defines the nature and severity of the lesions.

PATHOLOGIC FINDINGS

• The liver is usually smaller than normal, but it may be enlarged in peracute cases.
• Generalized icterus
• Histologically, centrolubular to midzonal hepatocellular necrosis, with mononuclear cell accumulation in the portal triads
• Possibly mild bile ductule proliferation in more chronic cases

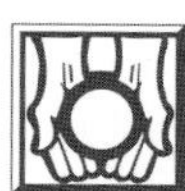

TREATMENT

• Restrict activity, and avoid sunlight.
• In cases with hepatic encephalopathy, house the horse in a quiet place, preferably padded to avoid injury.
• If the horse is still eating, a high-carbohydrate, low-protein diet is recommended. The protein should be high in BCAAs—two parts beet pulp with one part cracked corn and added molasses. Oat or grass hay is preferred over alfalfa, and the diet should be fed in small amounts five or six times daily.

MEDICATIONS

DRUG(S) OF CHOICE

• Xylazine (0.5–1.0 mg/kg) or detomidine (0.05–0.4 mg/kg) can be used to control the signs of hepatic encephalopathy.
• In hypoglycemic animals, 10% glucose solution at 0.2 mL/kg may be given, followed by continuous drip of 5% glucose solution at 2 mL/kg per hour, reducing after 24 hr to half this rate.
• If the animal is not drinking, administer IV polyionic fluids at maintenance rates.
• Reduced production and absorption of toxic metabolites can be achieved with mineral oil and neomycin (20–30 mg/kg QID), both via stomach tube.

CONTRAINDICATONS/POSSIBLE INTERACTIONS

• Neomycin should not be given for more than 24–36 hr, because it may induce severe diarrhea.
• Because the liver metabolizes many drugs, their duration of action may be increased in acute hepatic disease.

FOLLOW-UP

PATIENT MONITORING

Monitor liver enzymes and bilirubin every 2–3 days.

PREVENTION/AVOIDANCE

N/A

POSSIBLE COMPLICATIONS

N/A

EXPECTED COURSE AND PROGNOSIS

• Horses with severe hepatoencephalopathy have a poor prognosis, but if the animal survives for a week after the onset of clinical signs, recovery is possible.
• If the SDH (IDH) continues to fall, then the prognosis improves.

MISCELLANEOUS

ASSOCIATED CONDITIONS, AGE-RELATED FACTORS, ZOONOTIC POTENTIAL, PREGNANCY

N/A

ABBREVIATIONS

• ALP = alkaline phosphatase
• AST = aspartate aminotransferase
• BCAAs = branched-chain amino acids
• EEE = Eastern equine encephalomyelitis
• EIA = equine infectious anemia
• EVA = equine viral arteritis
• GGT = γ-glutamyltranspeptidase
• IDH = iditol dehydrogenase (SDH)
• LDH = lactate dehydrogenase
• SDH = sorbitol dehydrogenase (IDH)
• WEE = Western equine encephalitis

Suggested Reading

Divers TJ. Liver disease and liver failure in horses. Proc Am Assoc Equine Pract 1983;29:213–223.

Aleman M, Nieto JE, Carr EA etal. Serum hepatitis associated with commercial plasma transfusion in horses. J. Vet. Int. Med 2005;19:120–122.

Author Christopher M. Brown
Consulting Editor Michel Lévy

ACUTE RENAL FAILURE (ARF)

BASICS

DEFINITION

A consequence of an abrupt, sustained decrease in GFR, resulting in azotemia and disturbances in fluid, electrolyte, and acid-base homeostasis

PATHOPHYSIOLOGY

- Usually prerenal or renal; most commonly due to hemodynamic or nephrotoxic insults
- Except for neonatal bladder rupture and urolithiasis, postrenal failure is uncommon in horses (see Uroperitoneum and Urolithiasis).
- Perpetuated by decreased GFR in damaged glomeruli and tubular obstruction with desquamated tubular epithelial cells and debris

SYSTEMS AFFECTED

- Renal/urologic—failure • Endocrine/metabolic—disturbances in electrolyte and acid-base homeostasis • GI—inappetence, possible diarrhea, and increased risk of ulcers
- Nervous/neuromuscular—occasional ataxia or encephalopathy in severe cases • Hemic/lymphatic/immune—altered hemostasis and increased susceptibility to infection
- Musculoskeletal—acute laminitis in severe cases; often refractory to treatment

GENETICS N/A

INCIDENCE/PREVALENCE

Low

GEOGRAPHIC DISTRIBUTION NA

SIGNALMENT

Breed Predilections

N/A

Mean Age and Range

- Foals <30 days of age (especially when receiving nephrotoxic medications) may be at greater risk, but all ages can be affected.

Predominant Sex

None

SIGNS

General Comments

Clinical signs of ARF are vague and nonspecific.

Historical

- Often secondary to other problems leading to hypovolemia and renal ischemia—colic, diarrhea, prolonged exercise, rhabdomyolysis, or septicemia/endotoxemia • Previous administration of nephrotoxic drugs

Physical Examination

- Lethargy, anorexia, dehydration, edema, ulcers, or uremic odor in the oral cavity
- Severity of lethargy and anorexia often are greater than would be expected for the primary disease process. • Rectal examination may reveal an enlarged, painful left kidney. • Laminitis, often rapidly progressive • Markedly azotemic patients may have neurologic deficits—ataxia, hypermetria, and mental obtundation.

CAUSES

Prerenal Failure

- Hemorrhagic, hypovolemic, or endotoxic shock • Prolonged, exhaustive exercise • Severe rhabdomyolysis, vasculitis, or hemolytic diseases
- Disseminated intravascular coagulation

Intrinsic Renal Failure

- Prolonged duration of above disorders, lack of adequate fluid support, or concurrent use of normal dosages of nephrotoxic medications—aminoglycosides; NSAIDs
- Excessive doses of NSAIDs or prolonged use of gentamicin, particularly in dehydrated horses
- Other nephrotoxins include heavy metals (e. g., mercury [in counterirritants or blisters], lead, cadmium), endogenous pigments (e. g., hemoglobin, myoglobin), vitamins D and K_3, and high doses of oxytetracycline, especially when administered to neonates with flexural deformities. • In occasional cases, infectious agents—*Actinobacillus equuli* in neonates; *Leptospira* sp. in all age groups

RISK FACTORS

- Renal hypoperfusion • Exposure to nephrotoxins, particularly in patients with dehydration or primary renal disease

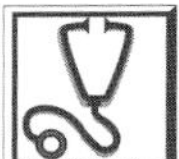

DIAGNOSIS

DIFFERENTIAL DIAGNOSIS

- All conditions leading to hemorrhagic, hypovolemic, or endotoxic shock; severe rhabdomyolysis; vasculitis and hemolytic diseases; or disseminated intravascular coagulation • Prerenal failure—oliguria with concentrated urine (specific gravity >1.035) and rapid correction of azotemia with rehydration
- Postrenal failure—stranguria, anuria, or uroperitoneum • Chronic renal failure—weight loss, poor body condition, ventral edema, PU/PD, hypercalcemia, and limited improvement of azotemia with fluid therapy

CBC/BIOCHEMISTRY/URINALYSIS

- Normal to high PCV, variable leukogram, CBC changes reflect underlying primary disease process. • Progressive (moderate to severe) increases in BUN (50–150 mg/dL) and Cr (2.0–20 mg/dL) • Variable hyponatremia, hypochloremia, hyperkalemia, hypocalcemia, and hyperphosphatemia—hyperkalemia and hyperphosphatemia more common with intrinsic ARF and uroperitoneum • Mild to moderate metabolic acidosis, severity varying with the underlying disease process; development of renal tubular acidosis may complicate recovery. • Mild to moderate hyperglycemia
- USG— high (>1.035) with prerenal failure, low (<1.020) with intrinsic ARF; specific gravity best assessed in urine collected during initial patient evaluation (before rehydration)
- Intrinsic cases may be accompanied by mild to moderate proteinuria, glucosuria, pigmenturia, and increased RBCs and casts on sediment examination. • Urine pH—normal to acidic, especially with concurrent depletion of body potassium stores • Myoglobinuria or hemoglobinuria/hematuria (see Pigmenturia)

OTHER LABORATORY TESTS

- Increased fractional clearances (i.e., excretions) of sodium and phosphorous; decreased clearance of potassium • Enzymuria—urinary GGT:Cr ratio >25 • Rising titers to *Leptospira* spp. may be found in horses with ARF attributable to leptospirosis.

IMAGING

Transabdominal/Transrectal Ultrasonography

- Kidneys may be enlarged (diameter, >8 cm; length, >15 cm), with increased echogenicity of renal cortices. • Rarely subcapsular/perirenal edema or hemorrhage • Variable dilation of renal pelves—may be marked in obstructive postrenal failure • Nephrolithiasis/ureterolithiasis would indicate underlying chronic renal failure and possible "acute-on-chronic" exacerbation of renal failure.

OTHER DIAGNOSTIC PROCEDURES

- Urine collection—Collect initial urine produced by all at-risk horses. • Percutaneous renal biopsy with routine histopathological, immunohistochemical, and electron microscopic evaluation of the sample may provide information regarding cause, severity, and prognosis. Pursued with caution, however, because life-threatening hemorrhage can be a complication. • Central venous pressure >8–10 mm Hg indicates fluid overload and assists with fluid therapy.

PATHOLOGICAL FINDINGS

- Gross—enlargement of kidneys due to nephrosis and subcapsular and interstitial edema, causing tissue to bulge onto cut surfaces
- Histopathological—Glomeruli may be congested and have a cellular infiltrate; tubules have denuded or flattened epithelium and varying amounts of accumulated debris.

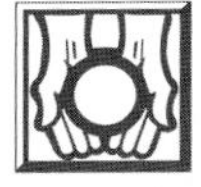

TREATMENT

AIMS OF TREATMENT

- Address underlying primary condition.
- Improve GFR with fluid therapy and medications aimed at restoring normal renal function.

APPROPRIATE HEALTH CARE

- Properly recognize and treat all underlying primary disease processes, usually on an inpatient basis for continuous fluid therapy.
- Reassess dosage schedule of, and possibly discontinue, potentially nephrotoxic medications.

NURSING CARE

Fluid Therapy

- After initial measurement of body weight, correct estimated dehydration with normal (0.9%) saline or another potassium—poor electrolyte solution over 6–12 hr. • Fluids may be supplemented with calcium gluconate or sodium bicarbonate if hyperkalemia or acidosis requires specific correction. • Monitor for subcutaneous and pulmonary edema—increased respiratory rate and effort as evidence of overhydration. • Monitor urine output. • CVP may be helpful in determining fluid replacement plan. • Use maintenance fluid therapy judiciously in animals not clinically dehydrated.

Oral Electrolyte Supplementation

• Sodium chloride (30 g) can be administered in concentrate feed or as an oral slurry/paste BID–QID to encourage increased drinking and urine output. • Potassium chloride can be supplemented in nonhyperkalemic patients with total body potassium depletion—common with anorexia of 2 days.

ACTIVITY

Stall rest, with limited hand-walking for grazing grass if appetite is poor

DIET

• Encourage intake by offering a variety of concentrate feeds, bran mash, and hay types.
• Hand-walking or short periods of turn-out to graze grass encourage feed intake.

CLIENT EDUCATION

• Prognosis is most dependent on progression of the underlying primary disease process.
• ARF may complicate recovery, prolong hospitalization and treatment, and increase cost.

SURGICAL CONSIDERATIONS N/A

MEDICATIONS

DRUG(S) OF CHOICE

• Judicious fluid therapy is the mainstay of treatment—see Nursing Care.
• Furosemide—For oliguria/anuria (i.e., lack of urination during first 6 hr of fluid therapy), this diuretic may be administered 2 times (1–2 mg/kg IV) at 1- to 2-hr intervals; if effective, urination should be observed within 1 hr after the second dose; if ineffective, discontinue treatment.
• Mannitol—has been used in the past as an osmotic diuretic agent for oliguria/anuria unresponsive to furosemide; however, recent evidence suggests that this treatment is not of benefit in critically ill human patients and ROUTINE USE OF MANNITOL IN PATIENTS WITH ARF IS NO LONGER RECOMMENDED.
• Dopamine—has been used in the past as a continuous rate infusion (3–5 μg/kg per minute IV in a 5% dextrose solution) for persistent oliguria/anuria; however, this drug can induce arrhythmias and recent evidence suggests that this treatment is not of benefit in critically ill human patients and ROUTINE USE OF DOPAMINE IN PATIENTS WITH ARF IS NO LONGER RECOMMENDED.
• Antiulcer drugs (e. g., omeprazole 2–4 mg/kg PO q24 h or cimetidine 5–10 mg/kg IV q8 h in anorexic horses) may be useful in decreasing the associated risk of gastric ulcer disease.

CONTRAINDICATIONS

• Furosemide—at repeated dosages can result in electrolyte derangements
• Avoid all nephrotoxic medications.

PRECAUTIONS

• Monitor response to fluid therapy (i.e., urine output)—as little as 40 mL/kg of IV fluids (20 L per 500-kg horse) may produce increases in CVP and significant pulmonary edema in oliguric/anuric patients.
• Reassess dosage schedule of drugs eliminated by urinary excretion; consider discontinuing all potentially nephrotoxic medications—gentamicin, tetracycline, and NSAIDs.

POSSIBLE INTERACTIONS

Use of multiple anti-inflammatory drugs (e. g., corticosteroids and one or more NSAIDs) will have additive negative effects on renal blood flow; avoid combined administration in azotemic patients.

ALTERNATIVE DRUGS

Consider peritoneal dialysis or hemodialysis (foals only) in refractory cases.

FOLLOW-UP

PATIENT MONITORING

• Assess clinical status (emphasizing hydration), urine output, and body weight at least twice daily during the initial 24 hr of treatment and at least daily thereafter.
• Assess magnitude of azotemia and electrolyte and acid–basis status at least daily for the initial 3 days of treatment.
• Consider placing a central venous line to maintain central venous pressure <8 cm H_2O in more critical patients and neonates.

PREVENTION/AVOIDANCE

• Anticipate compromised renal function in patients with other diseases or undergoing prolonged anesthesia and surgery; institute appropriate treatment to minimize dehydration and potential renal damage.
• Ensure adequate hydration status in patients receiving nephrotoxic medications.
• Avoid concurrent use of multiple anti-inflammatory drugs—NSAIDs.

POSSIBLE COMPLICATIONS

• Pulmonary and peripheral edema; conjunctival edema may be dramatic.
• Severe hyperkalemia accompanied by cardiac arrhythmias, cardiac arrest, and death
• Laminitis—often refractory to supportive care
• Signs of neurologic impairment—ataxia; mental obtundation
• GI ulceration or bleeding
• Coagulopathy
• Sepsis

EXPECTED COURSE AND PROGNOSIS

• Prognosis for recovery varies with the underlying primary disease process.
• Prognosis for recovery from prerenal failure and nonoliguric intrinsic ARF usually is favorable if azotemia decreases by 25%–50% after the initial 24 hr of treatment; extent of recovery of renal function in patients with intrinsic failure may require 3–6 weeks to fully assess.
• Guarded prognosis for patients with Cr >10 mg/dL at initial evaluation and when azotemia remains unchanged after the initial 24 hr of treatment.
• Poor prognosis for patients that have persistent anuria, increased magnitude of azotemia after the initial 24 hr of treatment, that rapidly develop edema, or that remain oliguric >72 hr.

MISCELLANEOUS

ASSOCIATED CONDITIONS

• Colic; enterocolitis
• Pleuritis; peritonitis; septicemia
• Laminitis
• Exhausted horse syndrome—multiorgan failure
• Rhabdomyolysis

AGE-RELATED FACTORS

• Neonates with hypoxic-ischemic multiorgan damage or septicemia may have increased risk of intrinsic ARF.
• Neonates, especially premature or dysmature foals, may have markedly elevated Cr concentrations (approaching 25 mg/dL) due to placental insufficiency; this azotemia typically resolves in 2–3 days and should not be confused with intrinsic ARF or uroperitoneum.

ZOONOTIC POTENTIAL

Leptospirosis has infectious and zoonotic potential; avoid direct contact with infective urine.

PREGNANCY

Postpartum mares are at risk of hemorrhagic shock and prerenal failure or intrinsic ARF consequent to rupture of a uterine artery.

SYNONYMS

• Acute nephrosis
• Acute tubular necrosis
• Vasomotor nephropathy

SEE ALSO

• Anuria/oliguria
• CRF

ABBREVIATIONS

• Cr = creatinine
• CVP = central venous pressure
• GGT = γ-glutamyltransferase
• GFR = glomerular filtration rate
• GI = gastrointestinal
• PU/PD = polyuria/polydipsia
• USG = urine specific gravity

Suggested Reading

Bayly WM. Acute renal failure. In: Reed SM, Bayly WM, Sellon DC, eds. Equine Internal Medicine, ed 2. Philadelphia: WB Saunders, 2004:1221–1230.
Divers TJ, Whitlock RH, Byars TD, Leitch M, Crowell WA. Acute renal failure in six horses resulting from hemodynamic causes. Equine Vet J 1987;19:178–184.
Geor RJ. Acute renal failure in horses. Vet Clin NA: Equine Pract 2007;23:563–576.
Schmitz DG. Toxins affecting the urinary system. Vet Clin North Am Equine Pract 2007;23:677–690.

Author Harold C. Schott II
Consulting Editor Gillian A. Perkins

ACUTE RESPIRATORY DISTRESS SYNDROME IN FOALS

BASICS

DEFINITION

Respiratory distress is defined as ventilatory efforts in excess of the metabolic demands. ARDS is defined as acute onset of respiratory distress.

PATHOPHYSIOLOGY

• Inflammatory stimuli may initiate events leading to clinical signs of respiratory failure—aspiration pneumonia; viral, bacterial, or fungal infections; thermal injury (i.e., heat stroke), systemic or pulmonary sepsis/endotoxemia, or inhalation of irritant gases, or smoke may be the initiating insult. • A manifestation of SIRS, leading to MODS, resulting in azotemia, liver dysfunction, ileus, or DIC and bleeding • Diffuse injury to pulmonary alveolar epithelium and capillary endothelium, leading to pulmonary edema • Immunosuppression may be a factor associated with development of ARDS/interstitial lung disease in foals infected with *Pneumocystis carinii.*

SYSTEMS AFFECTED

• Primarily respiratory • Often accompanied by dysfunction of the renal, hepatic, and cardiovascular systems and by clotting cascades as disease progresses—MODS

INCIDENCE/PREVALENCE

• Not established, but relatively uncommon • Worldwide, in areas with hot summer weather

GEOGRAPHIC DISTRIBUTION

Worldwide.

SIGNALMENT

• All ages, but foals 1–8 months of age are predisposed (mean age, 3.5 +/− 1.0 months). • No sex or breed predilections

SIGNS

• Acute or peracute depression, lethargy, fever, tachypnea, pronounced respiratory effort, nostril flaring, increased abdominal and intercostal effort (i.e., "double expiratory lift" or "heave line" or paradoxical breathing pattern), and cyanosis • Nasal discharge and cough are frequent but inconsistent findings. • Thoracic auscultation—loud bronchial sounds over central airways, with either increased or diminished peripheral airway sounds

CAUSES

• Likely the common end result of a variety of different intrapulmonary (inhaled) or systemic insults that initiate SIRS and lead to MODS • Heat stress may play a role. Foals with subclinical respiratory disease have limited ability to dissipate body heat. Use of erythromycin during hot weather is associated with increased susceptibility to environmental temperatures. • Viral and bacterial pneumonia can produce respiratory distress in foals with widespread infections throughout the lungs. *Rhodococcus equi* is cultured from approximately 25% of foals with respiratory distress, and opportunistic pathogens (e.g., β-hemolytic *Streptococcus* spp., enteric bacteria, *Actinobacillus* spp., *Pseudomonas aeruginosa, P. carinii*) may be involved in ARDS. • Lesions in affected foals are similar to those in ruminants with atypical interstitial pneumonia, suggesting that intoxication may contribute to this syndrome.

RISK FACTORS

• Unknown • Risk factors—preexisting subclinical to clinical respiratory tract disease; treatment with antimicrobial agents (particularly erythromycin) or bronchodilators, producing significant interactions in some patients; viral, bacterial, or fungal respiratory tract or systemic infection; heat stress; inhaled irritant gases and pneumotoxicants; and immunosuppression

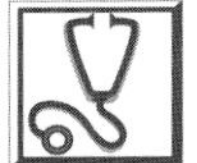

DIAGNOSIS

DIFFERENTIAL DIAGNOSIS

• Viral pneumonia—equine influenza, equine viral arteritis, equine herpesviruses 1 and 4, equine paramyxovirus, and equine adenovirus • Bacterial pneumonia • *P. carinii* infection • Pulmonary abscessation or granuloma • Upper airway dysfunction, with aspiration of oropharyngeal fluids • Ingestion or exposure to xenobiotics

CBC/BIOCHEMISTRY/URINALYSIS

Common abnormalities—neutrophilic leukocytosis, elevated fibrinogen, and anemia

OTHER LABORATORY TESTS

• Arterial blood gas—arterial hypoxemia, hypercapnia, and respiratory acidosis • Blood culture may help to identify bacteria. • Other laboratory abnormalities— dehydration, disseminated intravascular coagulation, and injury to other organs—may be seen.

IMAGING

Thoracic Radiography

• Findings vary, depending on the stage of injury. • Lesions include prominent interstitial patterns, coalescing to alveolar infiltrates, with superimposed, mixed bronchial patterns of varying severity throughout all lung fields. • A prominent miliary reticulonodular pattern is observed commonly in foals with *P. carinii* infection. • Other changes sometimes include consolidating anteroventral pneumonia or diffusely distributed pyogranuloma in foals with concurrent *R. equi* infection.

Transthoracic Ultrasonography

Consolidation, abscesses, or other lesions in some foals

OTHER DIAGNOSTIC PROCEDURES

• Because many foals are near death, ante-mortem culture of respiratory secretions before initiation of treatment may not be practical. • Routine culture of lower airway secretions should be accompanied by cytologic evaluation. • Examination of tracheal wash or bronchoalveolar fluid reveals acute inflammation, with large numbers of neutrophils some with phagocytized bacteria. • Recognition of *P. carinii* is difficult. • Transthoracic lung biopsy may be useful, but should not be performed in foals with severe respiratory distress or tendency to bleed.

PATHOLOGIC FINDINGS

Gross Findings

• Lungs are diffusely red, wet, heavy, firm, and fail to collapse when chest is opened. • In many instances, lungs have a lobulated appearance, with dark, reddened areas interspersed between areas of more normal appearing tissue. • A substantial number of foals also have other lung lesions (e.g., *R. equi* pyogranuloma) representing preexisting pulmonary disease. • Many foals demonstrate hypoxemia- or sepsis-induced lesions in other organs.

Histopathologic Findings

• Pulmonary lesions—diffuse, necrotizing bronchiolitis; alveolar septal necrosis; and filling of alveolar spaces with large numbers of mononuclear cells, pneumocytes, and epithelioid-like cells with hyaline membranes

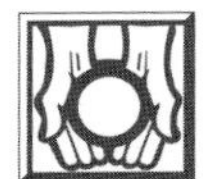

TREATMENT

AIMS OF TREATMENT

• Minimize ventilatory and metabolic demands • Reduce core body temperature (in hyperthermic foals) • Reduce lung edema and inflammation • Promote adequate oxygenation • Discontinue predisposing medications (e.g., erythromycin) • Eliminate infectious agents with broad-spectrum antimicrobial therapy • Support fluid and nutritional needs.

APPROPRIATE HEALTH CARE

• Avoid transporting these patients until temperature decreases. Transportation in extreme temperatures may result in their death. • On-farm examinations during high environmental temperatures should be conducted after moving the mare and foal to a controlled environment on the premises or awaiting stabilization and the cooler period of the day before transportation.

NURSING CARE

• These cases are respiratory emergencies and require immediate attention. • Reduce core body temperature using alcohol baths, fans, and/or misters or by carefully moving the mare and foal to a cooler area protected from direct sunlight or to an air-conditioned stall. • Cold-water enemas provide significant relief, especially when used in conjunction with the above treatments. • Judicious use of chilled IV fluids lowers core temperature; however, rapid infusion of large volumes may exacerbate pulmonary edema. Preferably, fluids should be selected to correct acid-base status and blood electrolyte abnormalities. Balanced electrolytes (e.g., lactated Ringer's solution) are appropriate initial therapy. • Insufflation of humidified oxygen (10–15

L/min) is facilitated by placement of a nasal or transtracheal catheter.

ACTIVITY

Reduce the patient's activity, by confinement to a clean, cool stall with appropriate environmental temperature and humidity control—fans, misters, or swamp coolers.

DIET

- Lowering body temperature may improve feed intake.
- Allow nursing foals adequate time with the mare, and provide high-quality feed.

CLIENT EDUCATION

- Education is aimed at prevention.
- Proper management of the neonate is imperative, because early handling and training of foals to accept physical examination and daily rectal temperature (preferably in the morning, when ambient environmental temperatures are low) allow early detection of subclinical cases.
- Clients should observe mares and foals carefully, on a daily basis, and consult a veterinarian when foals appear to be unthrifty or depressed.
- Removal of foals from extremes of heat and placement in well-maintained stalls providing shade or fans to lower temperature are beneficial.
- Minimize exposure to high environmental temperatures, providing cooler stalls for foals treated with antimicrobial agents (especially erythromycin).

SURGICAL CONSIDERATIONS

- Evaluate thorax for effusion or pneumothorax.
- Evaluate upper airway function to determine patency of the upper airway.
- In HYPP +/+ foals, hyperkalemic episodes may result in laryngeal paralysis.

MEDICATIONS

DRUG(S) OF CHOICE

- The treatment protocol should specifically address inflammation and hyperthermia.
- Use of corticosteroids in stressed foals demonstrating clinical signs of sepsis is controversial; however, single or multiple doses of short-acting corticosteroids (e.g., dexamethasone sodium phosphate [0.05–0.2 mg/kg IV q12–24h], prednisolone sodium succinate [0.5–1.0 mg/kg IV q8–12h]) provide potent, short-duration relief of pulmonary inflammation in many cases.
- NSAIDs (e.g., flunixin meglumine [0.25–1.0 mg/kg q12–24h]) may be useful in reducing body temperature, decreasing the systemic effects of sepsis or endotoxemia, and reducing discomfort.
- Appropriate antibiotic therapy should be guided by bacteriologic culture, if possible.

Use of oral antibiotics (e.g., trimethoprim-potentiated sulfonamides [30 mg/kg q12h]), parenteral antibiotics (e.g., procaine penicillin G [22,000 IU/kg IM q12h]), or cephalosporins (e.g., ceftiofur [2.2–5 mg/kg IM, IV, or SQ q12h]) may be substituted for antimicrobial agents used prior to onset of respiratory distress.

CONTRAINDICATIONS

Discontinue any medications (especially erythromycin/rifampin) and drugs with an effect that may be altered by concurrent therapy with drugs undergoing metabolism by the liver—theophylline, aminophylline.

PRECAUTIONS

- Because sepsis may represent the underlying cause in some foals, overuse of corticosteroids is discouraged.
- Use NSAIDs with caution, due to gastrointestinal and renal effects.

POSSIBLE INTERACTIONS

- Drugs such as erythromycin/rifampin that induce or inhibit hepatic drug metabolizing enzymes may alter the disposition of concurrently used medications (e.g., methylxanthines), leading to side effects.
- Septic animals are more likely to have multiorgan dysfunction, and hepatic and renal function should be monitored during therapy.
- NSAIDs may result in gastrointestinal or renal compromise in anorexic and dehydrated patients.

ALTERNATIVE DRUGS

- Aminoglycosides (amikacin sulfate, gentamicin sulfate) used in combination with β-lactams (penicillins and cephalosporins).
- Rifampin in combination with erythromycin, clarithromycin, or azithromycin may be indicated for *R. equi*.

FOLLOW-UP

PATIENT MONITORING

- Reduction in body temperature and respiratory rate and effort and improvement in mucous membrane color typically indicate clinical improvement.
- Frequent thoracic auscultation may reveal increased bronchovesicular sounds in foals with positive response to therapy.
- Arterial blood gas analysis is the most sensitive indicator function.
- Repeated thoracic radiography is useful; however, overall radiographic appearance may lag behind clinical appearance by days or weeks.

PREVENTION/AVOIDANCE

- Client education regarding prevention and early recognition of respiratory tract disease in foals is beneficial—minimizing heat stress, control of dust, manure dispersal, and plasma therapy on farms with endemic *R. equi*.
- Client education regarding use of anthelmintics and vaccination of mares and foals against respiratory pathogens
- Client education regarding potential adverse effects of use of drugs such as erythromycin during hot weather

POSSIBLE COMPLICATION

Chronic interstitial pneumonia

EXPECTED COURSE AND PROGNOSIS

- The initial prognosis is guarded to poor in most affected foals.
- The mortality rate is high.
- Long-term outcomes vary, but cases that are recognized and treated early respond well.
- In survivors, the diffuse alveolar pattern tends to resolve quickly, whereas increased interstitial pattern resolves over weeks or months.

MISCELLANEOUS

AGE-RELATED FACTORS

- Can occur at all ages
- In 1- to 8-month foals

SYNONYMS

- Bronchointerstitial pneumonia
- ALI
- Interstitial pneumonia
- Respiratory distress

SEE ALSO

- Inspiratory dyspnea
- Expiratory dyspnea

ABBREVIATIONS

- ALI = acute lung injury
- ARDS = acute respiratory distress syndrome
- DIC = disseminated intravascular coagulation
- HYPP = hyperkalemic periodic paralysis
- MODS = multiorgan dysfunction syndrome
- SIRS = systemic inflammatory response syndrome

Suggested Reading

Derksen FJ. Interstitial pneumonia in foals. In: Colahan PT, Mayhew IG, Merritt AM, Moore JN, eds. Equine Medicine and Surgery, ed 5.St. Louis: Mosby, 1999:552.

Dunkel B, et al. Acute lung injury/acute respiratory distress syndrome in 15 foals. Equine Vet J 2005;37:435–440.

Lakritz J, et al. Bronchointerstitial pneumonia and respiratory distress in young horses: Clinical, clinicopathologic, radiographic, and pathological findings in 23 cases (1984–1989).J Vet Int Med. 1993; 7:277–288.

Wilkins PA, Seahorn T. Acute respiratory distress syndrome. Vet Clin North Am Equine Pract 2004;20:253–273.

Wilson WD, Lakritz J. Bronchointerstitial pneumonia and acute respiratory distress. In: Robinson NE, ed. Current Therapy in Equine Medicine, ed 5.St. Louis: WB Saunders, 2003:674–677.

Authors Jeffrey Lakritz and W. David Wilson
Consulting Editor Daniel Jean

ADENOVIRUS

BASICS

OVERVIEW

- Causes fatal respiratory disease in Arabian foals with SCID
- May be a severe pathogen in Fell Pony foals affected by "Fell Pony syndrome"
- Other breeds may be affected as foals, but seldom succumb.
- Approximately 25% of affected foals also have diarrhea.
- A role for adenovirus in the development of respiratory disease in adult horses has been suggested.

SIGNALMENT

- Foals are usually older than 8–10 weeks when clinical signs become present.
- Adenovirus affects primarily Arabians, although other breeds are affected sporadically, in particular, Fell Ponies.
- SCID-affected foals are frequently clinically normal at birth.

SIGNS

- Signs are essentially identical to other causes of foal pneumonia and include fever, tachypnea, dyspnea, depression, and abnormalities on thoracic auscultation.
- Mild to moderate diarrhea may also be present.

CAUSES AND RISK FACTORS

Foals with SCID have a defect in lymphoid stem cells that may result from altered purine metabolism. The absence of an adaptive immune response causes these foals to be susceptible to even minor pathogens, such as adenovirus. Due to maternally derived immunity reaching a nadir at 1–2 months of age, these foals become unable to mount an appropriate immune response and deteriorate after 2 months of age. Foals that are immunosuppressed for other reasons, such as Fell Pony syndrome, are also susceptible. It has been suggested that adenovirus may predispose foals to bacterial pneumonia and may play a significant role in the pathogenesis of bacterial pneumonia in non-SCID foals. An antigenically distinct adenovirus has been identified in non-SCID foals with diarrhea, usually associated with concurrent rotavirus infection. The role of adenovirus in foal diarrhea is not clear.

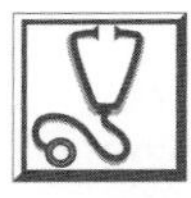

DIAGNOSIS

DIFFERENTIAL DIAGNOSIS

Other viral and bacterial causes of pneumonia in immunocompromised foals include, but are not limited to, the following:

- Equine herpesvirus type 1
- Equine influenza virus
- Equine arteritis virus
- *Streptococcus equi* var *zooepidemicus*
- *Actinobacillus equuli*
- *Pasteurella* spp.
- *Klebsiella pneumoniae*
- *Salmonella* spp.
- *Bordetella bronchiseptica*
- *Rhodococcus equi*

Other causes of diarrhea in foals include, but are not limited to, bacterial, viral, and parasitic causes.

CBC/BIOCHEMISTRY/URINALYSIS

Ante-mortem diagnosis of SCID is supported by finding appropriate clinical signs in an Arabian foal of the appropriate age with persistent severe lymphopenia ($\leq$500 cells/μL) and the absence of IgM on SRID (see below).

OTHER LABORATORY TESTS

- Antibody titers—SCID foals do not demonstrate a 4-fold rise in antibody titer to adenovirus, whereas non–SCID-affected foals develop a rise in antibody titer in 10 days.
- Virus isolation—Adenovirus may be isolated from normal and infected foals.
- Histopathology—Intranuclear inclusions can be detected in tissues. Ante-mortem testing may demonstrate intranuclear inclusions in conjunctival and nasal epithelial cells. At post-mortem examination there is gross and histologic evidence of lymphoid hypoplasia of the thymus, spleen, and lymph nodes.
- SRID—Precolostral testing of SCID foals also demonstrates an absence of IgM, but as IgM is absorbed by the foal from colostrum, foals with adequate transfer of maternal antibody cannot be tested until IgM levels have waned, usually at $\geq$3 weeks of age.
- Fell Pony syndrome—Measurement of IgM after 4 weeks of age (concentration will be decreased) and demonstration of B-cell lymphopenia will aid in diagnosis.

IMAGING

- Radiographs are consistent with pneumonia.
- Ultrasonographic imaging of lymphoid tissues may be suggestive of, but not diagnostic for, SCID.

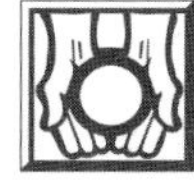

TREATMENT

- There currently is no treatment specifically for adenovirus.
- In non-SCID foals, treatment is primarily supportive, with broad-spectrum antimicrobial coverage provided.
- Foals with SCID and Fell Pony syndrome eventually die, and treatment is not productive. There has been some investigation into immunologic reconstitution of SCID patients by transplantation of bone marrow stem cells. This treatment remains experimental as of the time of this writing.

MEDICATIONS

DRUG(S) OF CHOICE

- Non-SCID foals should be treated for concurrent bacterial infection based on culture and sensitivity results.
- Foals with adenovirus associated with rotavirus should be treated with supportive therapy, including intravenous isotonic polyionic fluid replacement of deficits and nutritional support as warranted.

CONTRAINDICATIONS/POSSIBLE INTERACTIONS

N/A

FOLLOW-UP

CLIENT EDUCATION

- Prevention of SCID requires identification of carriers and removal of them from breeding programs.
- Approximately one of four foals from the mating of two heterozygotes results in an SCID foal.
- Arabian foals should be tested at birth for IgM levels (presuckle) and lymphocyte count. Those foals with an absolute lymphopenia should be closely monitored until 5 months of age. Alternatively, there are genetic tests available now to identify carriers of the genetic defect.
- Recommendations for client education regarding Fell Pony syndrome are not yet established.

MISCELLANEOUS

ABBREVIATIONS

- SCID = severe combined immunodeficiency syndrome
- SRID = serial radial immunodiffusion

Suggested Reading

Thomas GW, Bell SC, Carter SD. Immunoglobulin and peripheral B-lymphocyte concentrations in Fell pony foal syndrome. Equine Vet J 2005;37:48–52.

Author Pamela A. Wilkins

Consulting Editors Ashley G. Boyle and Corinne R. Sweeney

ADRENAL INSUFFICIENCY

BASICS

OVERVIEW

- Synonymous with hypoadrenocorticism and "steroid let-down syndrome"
- Characterized by glucocorticoid and mineralocorticoid deficiency caused by adrenal cortex destruction (i.e., primary AI or Addison's disease) or ACTH deficiency (i.e., secondary AI)
- Primary AI—Both glucocorticoid and mineralocorticoid are deficient.
- Secondary AI—Mineralocorticoid secretion usually is normal.

SYSTEMS AFFECTED

- Endocrine
- Cardiovascular
- Renal
- Musculoskeletal
- GI
- Behavioral

SIGNALMENT

Any age, sex, and breed

SIGNS

- Acute cases—muscular weakness, hypotension, anorexia, hemoconcentration, hypothermia, polyuria, cardiovascular collapse, and death
- Chronic cases—depression, anorexia, weight loss, poor hair coat, exercise intolerance, polyuria/polydipsia, mild abdominal pain, salt craving, and diarrhea

CAUSES AND RISK FACTORS

- Chronic administration of glucocorticoids, exogenous ACTH, or anabolic steroids
- Pituitary-adrenal axis immaturity attributable to prematurity in neonatal foals
- Adrenal hemorrhage and necrosis subsequent to septicemia or severe bouts of endotoxemia

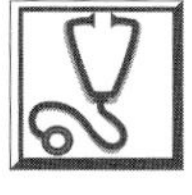

DIAGNOSIS

DIFFERENTIAL DIAGNOSIS

- Acute cases—endotoxemia, septicemia, renal failure, and colitis
- A normal ACTH stimulation test rules out adrenal insufficiency.

CBC/BIOCHEMISTRY/URINALYSIS

- Acute AI is characterized by hemoconcentration, hyponatremia, hypochloremia, hyperkalemia, decreased sodium:potassium ratio (reference range, >27), and hypoglycemia.
- Additional abnormalities—metabolic acidosis and azotemia
- Chronic cases, including secondary AI—mineralocorticoid secretion (i.e., aldosterone) is generally maintained. Therefore, serum electrolytes are within normal limits.

OTHER LABORATORY TESTS

- With insufficient aldosterone secretion, fractional excretion of sodium (reference range, <1%) is increased despite a normal or low serum sodium concentration.
- Administration of exogenous ACTH (1 U/kg IM) resulting in less than a doubling of the cortisol baseline 6–8 hr later is consistent with AI. Alternatively, synthetic ACTH (Cosyntropin 100 μg IV for a neonatal foal) may be used. Less than a doubling of the cortisol baseline 1 hr later is consistent with AI. Because acute AI is life-threatening, dexamethasone (0.044 mg/kg IV) should be administered simultaneously with exogenous ACTH. Serum cortisol is measured 2 hr later, and horses with AI exhibit a negligible increase in cortisol. This eliminates any delay in treatment while diagnostic tests are being performed.

IMAGING

N/A

DIAGNOSTIC PROCEDURES

N/A

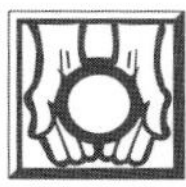

TREATMENT

- Complete rest and avoidance of stress, particularly surgery, infection, and trauma.
- Treat the underlying primary cause.
- Provide sodium supplementation (e.g., salt) to horses with increased sodium losses.

MEDICATIONS

DRUGS

- Glucocorticoid and, if necessary, mineralocorticoid replacement. The maintenance dose of prednisolone, which is equivalent to daily corticosteroid secretion in normal adult horses, is approximately 25 mg/day. However exposure to stress dramatically increases corticosteroid requirements. During periods of stress, increase the dose by 2- to 10-fold and divide into 2–3 daily doses.
- Acute AI—dexamethasone in conjunction with IV crystalloid solutions (i.e., normal saline) and dextrose in cases of hypoglycemia. Although dexamethasone has minimal mineralocorticoid activity, 20 mg administered daily is sufficient to maintain adrenalectomized horses alive.
- Mineralocorticoid replacement with fludrocortisone may be considered.

CONTRAINDICATIONS/POSSIBLE INTERACTIONS

N/A

FOLLOW-UP

PATIENT MONITORING

- Monitor electrolytes, renal function, acid-base balance, and hydration status.
- Once the animal is stable, adrenal recovery can be documented by repeating ACTH-stimulation tests.

PREVENTION/AVOIDANCE

Avoid excessive use of exogenous glucocorticoids, ACTH, and anabolic steroids.

POSSIBLE COMPLICATIONS

Excessive glucocorticoid administration, especially with long-acting forms (e.g., triamcinolone), increases susceptibility to infections and may result in laminitis.

EXPECTED COURSE AND PROGNOSIS

N/A

MISCELLANEOUS

ASSOCIATED CONDITIONS, AGE-RELATED FACTORS, ZOONOTIC POTENTIAL, PREGNANCY

N/A

ABBREVIATIONS

- ACTH = adrenocorticotropin hormone
- AI = adrenal insufficiency
- GI = gastrointestinal

Suggested Reading

Toribio RE. The adrenal glands. In: Reed SM, Bayly WM & Sellon DC, ed. Equine Internal Medicine, ed 2. St Louis: Saunders, 2004:1357–1361.

Author Laurent Couëtil
Consulting Editor Michel Lévy

AFLATOXICOSIS

BASICS

OVERVIEW

- Aflatoxicosis is the condition of intoxication by the *Aspergillus* fungal metabolite, aflatoxin.
- Diffuse liver disease is its hallmark with acute and chronic forms dictated by dose and duration of exposure.
- Aflatoxin-contaminated feed grains, especially corn, are the sources of toxin.
- Aflatoxin is usually produced on grain grown during drought conditions.

SIGNALMENT

Younger horses are more susceptible.

SIGNS

- Ponies given single lethal doses of aflatoxin (2 mg/kg) had increased temperatures, elevated heart and respiratory rates, tenemus, bloody feces, and tetanic convulsions.
- Some ponies died within 3 days while others lived for 32 days post-dosing. Ponies administered high oral doses (0.4 mg/kg for 5 days or the equivalent of several ppm in the feed) of aflatoxin were lethargic, anorectic and slightly icteric on the 5th day. Serum liver enzymes were elevated on the 4th day of dosing. Signs of hepatic encephalopathy such as belligerence, somnolence, circling, blindness, and head pressing may occur when serum ammonia levels are sufficiently elevated. Chronic low-level exposure may present as an ill-defined loss of condition.

CAUSES AND RISK FACTORS

The most likely contaminated diets are corn-based, while less likely exposure comes from diets containing peanut and cottonseed meals. Forage is an unproved source of aflatoxin.

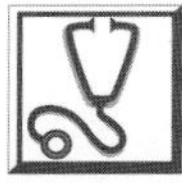

DIAGNOSIS

- Signs and lesions of aflatoxicosis reflect liver disease. None are pathognomonic for either acute or chronic aflatoxin poisoning.
- Feed concentrations of several hundred ppb aflatoxin in grain rations, together with appropriate clinical sings, are supportive of a diagnosis.
- Ill-thrift is associated with lower levels of aflatoxin intake.

DIFFERENTIAL DIAGNOSIS

Elevated serum hepatic enzyme levels can occur in association with many multisystemic diseases. Specific causes of hepatic disease include

- Fumonisin-induced mycotoxicosis—detection in feed
- Alsike clover or kleingrass toxicoses—evidence of exposure
- Hepatic neoplasia or abscessation—imaging or biopsy
- Biliary obstruction—serum chemistries and biopsy
- Theiler's disease—history, biopsy
- Pyrrolizidine alkaloid-containing plants such as *Amsinckia* spp., *Crotalaria* spp., and *Senecio* spp. cause chronic progressive liver disease—history of consumption, biopsy

CBC/BIOCHEMISTRY/URINALYSIS

- White blood cell counts, especially lymphocytes, are decreased and serum glucose is decreased. Total serum lipid and cholesterol are increased.
- Elevations of prothrombin time and serum AST, ALT, and GGT were consistent with the severe liver necrosis and biliary hyperplasia seen post-mortem.

OTHER LABORATORY TESTS

- Chemical analysis of feed samples is necessary to confirm the presence of aflatoxin. The inability to obtain samples at the time of exposure often precludes detection of aflatoxin levels consistent with acute intoxication.
- Feed concentrations necessary to induce acute intoxication typically approach the ppm range, while chronic exposure to several hundred ppb is sufficient to induce subclinical liver damage and associated ill-thrift.

IMAGING

N/A

OTHER DIAGNOSTIC PROCEDURES

- Necropsy findings include fatty liver, hemorrhagic enteritis and pale swollen kidneys.
- Histologic changes in the liver include fatty degeneration, centrilobular necrosis, periportal fibrosis, and bile duct hyperplasia.

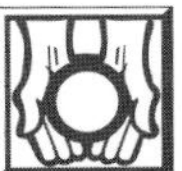

TREATMENT

Specific antidotes are unavailable. Horses suffering only moderate liver damage will benefit from supplementation with high-quality protein, fat-soluble vitamins, and selenium. Management for liver failure includes high-carbohydrate, low-protein diets.

MEDICATIONS

DRUG(S) AND FLUIDS

Dextrose 5% should be given slowly IV to hypoglycemic animals. Balanced electrolyte solutions are given for maintenance.

CONTRAINDICATIONS/POSSIBLE INTERACTIONS

Drugs subject to hepatic clearance should be given cautiously.

FOLLOW-UP

PATIENT MONITORING

Liver enzymes should be monitored to evaluate liver function.

PREVENTION/AVOIDANCE

Reliable feed sources are critical when grains are produced during drought conditions. Test grain before feeding.

EXPECTED COURSE AND PROGNOSIS

Survival of acute intoxication does not guarantee complete recovery. Ponies have died from liver failure up to 30 days following a single toxic dose of aflatoxin.

ABBREVIATION

- ppb = parts per billion

Suggested Reading

Raisbeck MF. Feed-associated poisoning. In: Robinson NE, ed. Current Therapy in Equine Medicine, ed. 3. Philadelphia: WB Saunders, 1992:366–372.

Author Stan W. Casteel
Consulting Editor Robert H. Poppenga

AFRICAN HORSE SICKNESS

BASICS

OVERVIEW

- Infectious disease affecting the cardiovascular and respiratory systems, characterized by fever and edema
- Not reported in the United States. Most commonly found on the African continent, with recent outbreaks investigated in South Africa, Zimbabwe, and Mozambique. India, Turkey, Iraq, Syria, Lebanon, Jordan, and Spain have reported outbreaks in the past.
- Geographic range of the disease is limited by that of its principal vector, *Culicoides* spp. The disease is most prevalent in low-lying, moist, warm areas.

SIGNALMENT

- All breeds of horses as well as other equids, such as donkeys and mules, are susceptible.
- There is no apparent breed, age, or sex predilection.
- Angora goats are also susceptible. Zebras and elephants may serve as natural reservoirs of the virus that causes AHS. Dogs fed uncooked infected horse meat have developed AHS.

SIGNS

- Fever (but not accompanied by inappetence)
- Pulmonary edema with coughing, frothy nasal discharge, dyspnea
- Subcutaneous edema of head and neck, edema of supraorbital fossa
- Colic

CAUSES AND RISK FACTORS

- Caused by the AHS virus, a viscerotropic RNA virus of the genus *Orbivirus*
- Transmitted by arthropod vectors, primarily *Culicoides* spp., but also mosquitoes and ticks
- Spread of the disease to uninfected countries can occur through travel of infected horses or movement of infected insect vectors in aircraft or heavy wind.
- Virus affects vascular endothelium, resulting in the clinical sign of edema that predominates.
- Disease occurs seasonally, during warm wet periods.

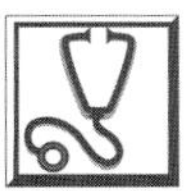

DIAGNOSIS

DIFFERENTIAL DIAGNOSIS

- Equine infectious anemia, equine viral arteritis, purpura hemorrhagica, equine anaplasmosis and equine piroplasmosis may have similar clinical presentation as AHS and may require laboratory testing to differentiate it.
- Index of suspicion for AHS should be raised when there is a history of travel to countries known to harbor the disease.
- Congestive heart failure may result in pulmonary and subcutaneous edema, but heart murmurs and/or venous distention should be present, and fever may not be present.

CBC/BIOCHEMISTRY/URINALYSIS

N/A

OTHER LABORATORY TESTS

- Definitive diagnosis depends on isolation of virus from whole blood or tissues, or antibodies to AHS virus in serum.
- In the United States, if AHS is suspected, the federal area veterinarian in charge should be notified immediately so that appropriate samples can be forwarded for testing.

IMAGING

- Thoracic radiography may reveal evidence of pulmonary edema.
- Thoracic ultrasound may reveal pleural effusion or pericardial effusion.

PATHOLOGIC FINDINGS

- Pulmonary edema, with frothy fluid in the bronchi and trachea
- Pleural effusion
- Pericardial effusion
- Yellow gelatinous edema fluid in the musculature of the neck and jugular groove
- Petechial hemorrhages on endocardium, epicardium, and oral mucous membranes and tongue

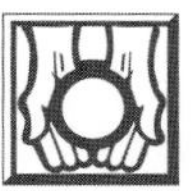

TREATMENT

There is no specific treatment for AHS. Supportive nursing care and symptomatic treatment may improve outcome in some cases, but usually the course of the disease is not altered by treatment.

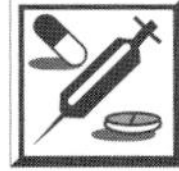

MEDICATIONS

DRUG(S) OF CHOICE

N/A

CONTRAINDICATIONS/POSSIBLE INTERACTIONS

N/A

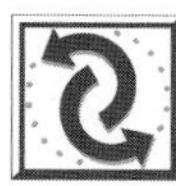

FOLLOW-UP

PREVENTION/AVOIDANCE

- Vaccination is effective. However, 42 antigenic strains of the virus exist, and vaccination with one strain does not result in immunity to heterologous strains, so polyvalent strains of vaccine should be used.
- Vaccination should be combined with other measures aimed at limiting exposure to insect vectors, such as fly-proof stabling, pasturing only during daylight, use of insect repellents, and keeping horses on high ground away from low-lying, swampy, insect-infested areas.
- Countries free of the disease restrict importation of horses from countries known to harbor the disease, or impose quarantine of at least 60 days in insect-proof housing.

EXPECTED COURSE AND PROGNOSIS

- Mortality in horses generally is high, up to 90%. In mules and donkeys, mortality may be lower (50%).
- The incubation period ranges from 7 to 21 days. Once clinical signs are observed, the clinical progression is rapid. Death usually occurs within 4–5 days after the onset of fever.
- Survivors do not harbor the virus.

MISCELLANEOUS

ZOONOTIC POTENTIAL

The disease does not affect humans.

ABBREVIATION

- AHS = African horse sickness

Suggested Reading

Committee on Foreign Animal Diseases of the US Animal Health Association, Foreign Animal Diseases "The Gray Book" online, 1998, http://www.vet.uga.edu/vpp/gray·book/FAD/AHS.htm

The African Horse Sickness Website, The African Horse Sickness Trust, 2005, http://www.africanhorsesickness.co.za/

Author Raymond W. Sweeney

Consulting Editors Ashley G. Boyle and Corinne R. Sweeney

AGALACTIA/HYPOGALACTIA

BASICS

DEFINITION

- Agalactia—postpartum lactation failure
- Hypogalactia—subnormal milk production

PATHOPHYSIOLOGY

- Estrogens (fetoplacental unit) in late gestation induce mammary duct development.
- P4 stimulates lobuloalveolar growth.
- Lactogenesis is triggered by the sharp decrease of P4 and sharp increase of prolactin just prior to parturition.
- The increased production of prolactin by the anterior pituitary gland results from suppression of a prolactin inhibitory factor (likely dopamine) and release of a hypothalamic prolactin-releasing factor (proposed to be serotonin).
- Agalactia/hypogalactia may be caused by alterations of hormonal events (endocrine disease), defects in mammary tissue itself (mammary disease), or as a result of systemic illness or disease.

SYSTEMS AFFECTED

- Reproductive
- Endocrine/metabolic

SIGNALMENT

Mores of any breed or age may be affected.

SIGNS

General Comments

- Tall fescue predominant in central and southeast United States; fescue syndrome
  - Grazing endophyte-infected fescue—most likely cause of lactation failure
  - Predominant finding—agalactia at parturition
- South America—fungus-infected feed, *Claviceps purpurea* (ergot) implicated in agalactia

Historical

- Grazing endophyte-infected tall fescue or ergot-infected feeds prepartum
- Prolonged gestation, dystocia, thickened fetal membranes, retained fetal membranes, and red bag
- Previous history—agalactia/hypogalactia or mammary gland disease
- Clinical evidence of systemic disease; known exposure to infectious disease

Physical Examination

- Weak, septicemic foal—FPT and/or inadequate nutrition
- Flaccid udder and secretion of a clear or thick, yellow-tinged fluid from the teats
- Mastitis—swollen, painful udder, warm to the touch, secretion of grossly or microscopically abnormal milk
- Distinct, palpable masses with mammary abscessation or neoplasia

CAUSES

Endocrinologic Disorders

- Ingestion of tall fescue grass—infected with *Neotyphodium coenophialum* (formerly *Acremonium coenophialum*) or feedstuffs infected with *Claviceps purpurea* sclerotia.
- Ergot alkaloids depress prolactin secretion (dopamine DA_2 receptor agonists and serotonin antagonists).
- Abortion/premature birth affects normal P4, estrogen, and prolactin fluctuations needed for lactation onset.

Mammary Gland Disease

- Inflammation and/or infection
- Abscessation or fibrosis
- Neoplasia
- Trauma

Systemic Disease

- Any debilitating systemic disease or stress-producing disorder
- Malnutrition/nutritional deficiency

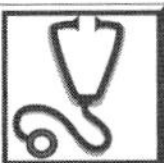

DIAGNOSIS

DIFFERENTIAL DIAGNOSIS

Differentiating Similar Signs

- Differentiate agalactia/hypogalactia from behavioral nursing problems.
  - Mare anxiety, pain, udder edema
  - Direct examination of udder and secretions
  - Observe interaction between mare and foal as its attempts to nurse.
- Failure of milk letdown can occur in mares.
  - Oxytocin stimulates milk letdown, NOT milk secretion.

DIFFERENTIATING CAUSES

- Indicators of fescue syndrome
  - History of fescue ingestion
  - Prolonged gestation
  - Dystocia
  - Retained fetal membranes, thickened fetal membranes
  - Weak, dysmature foal, mare with agalactia
- Full physical examination to differentiate—mastitis, mammary fibrosis, neoplasia, abscessation, traumatic injury, systemic illness

OTHER LABORATORY TESTS

Serum prolactin levels are decreased in fescue-induced agalactia.

OTHER DIAGNOSTIC PROCEDURES

- If mastitis is suspected
  - Cytology or culture of udder secretion
- If neoplasia is suspected
  - Fine-needle aspirate—cytology
  - Biopsy—histopathology

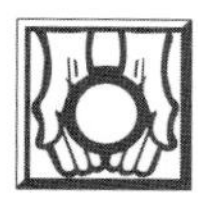

TREATMENT

- Mastitis
  - Lactating cow intramammary treatments
  - Systemic antibiotics based on culture/sensitivity
  - Frequent stripping of mammary gland
  - Hot-packs or hydrotherapy
  - Correct nutritional deficiencies.
- FPT foals
  - Nutritional supplementation during period of agalactia
  - Plasma transfusions

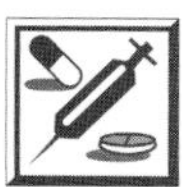

MEDICATIONS

DRUG(S) OF CHOICE FOR FESCUE TOXICITY

- Domperidone (1.1 mg/kg PO daily)
  - Selective DA_2 dopamine receptor antagonist; reverses effects of fescue ingestion.
  - Not approved by FDA; still experimental product.
  - No known side effects associated with treatment of pregnant mares.
  - Treat minimum15 days prepartum; discontinue when/if lactation is observed at foaling.
  - If agalactic at foaling and not treated prior to parturition, initiate treatment at foaling and continue for 5 days or until lactation ensues.
- TRH—2.0 mg, SQ, BID, 5 days, begin day 1 postpartum
  - Increases serum prolactin, due to its action as a prolactin releasing factor

CONTRAINDICATIONS

- Perphenazine, dopamine receptor antagonist—published, but:
  - Severe side effects in horses preclude its use.
  - Sweating, colic, hyperesthesia, ataxia, posterior paresis
- Metoclopramide used to treat agalactia of unknown origin
  - Significant risk for developing severe CNS side effects in horses
  - Its use is contraindicated.

PRECAUTIONS

- Remove pregnant mares from endophyte-infected fescue pastures/hay minimum 30 days, preferably 60–90 days, prepartum.
- If removal is not possible, treat with domperidone during last 2–4 weeks of gestation.

ALTERNATIVE DRUGS

- Acepromazine maleate (20 mg IM TID)
  - Some dopamine antagonistic properties, tried as agalactia treatment
    - At least one report of it having no effect on lactation
  - Sedation is the No. 1 primary side effect.
- Reserpine (0.5–2.0 mg IM q48h or 0.01 mg/kg PO q24h)
  - Depletes serotonin, dopamine, and norepinephrine in the brain and other tissues
  - GI motility greatly increased; can cause profuse diarrhea
  - Sedation—common side effect
  - Not Food and Drug Administration approved for agalactia
- Sulpiride (3.3 mg/kg PO daily)
  - Dopamine antagonist to treat agalactia; less effective than domperidone
  - Not FDA approved for agalactia

FOLLOW-UP

PATIENT MONITORING

- If effective, most treatments stimulate milk production in 2–5 days.
- In absence of other systemic signs, agalactia is not life-threatening.
- Foals need intensive medical and nutritional management with prolonged agalactia.

MISCELLANEOUS

ASSOCIATED CONDITIONS

Mare

Prolonged gestation, abortion, dystocia, uterine rupture, thickened placental membranes, red bag, retained fetal membranes, infertility, prolonged luteal function, early embryonic death, weak and dysmature foals

Neonate

- FPT
- Malnutrition
- Starvation

SEE ALSO

- Dystocia
- Fescue toxicosis
- Mastitis
- Prolonged pregnancy
- Retained fetal membranes
- FPT

ABBREVIATIONS

- FPT = failure of passive transfer
- P4 = progesterone
- TRH = thyrotropin-releasing hormone

Suggested Reading

Evans TJ, Youngquist RS, Loch WE, Cross DL. A comparison of the relative efficacies of domperidone and reserpine in treating equine "fescue toxicosis." Proc AAEP 1999;45:207–209.

Van Camp SD. Abnormalities of lactation. In: Youngquist RS, Threlfall WR, eds. Current Therapy in Large Animal Theriogenology. St. Louis, MO: Saunders Elsevier, 1997:131–134.

Author Carole C. Miller

Consulting Editor Carla L. Carleton

AGGRESSION

BASICS

DEFINITION

• Behaviors that do, or attempt to do, injury to another with the apparent motivation of causing harm. Predation is generally not considered aggression. • Agonistic behaviors include threats, offensive aggressive behaviors, defensive behaviors, and submissive behaviors. • Occurs in specific contexts or circumstances and is influenced by numerous variables, including internal states (e.g., hormones, hunger, fear), external stimuli (e.g., presence of offspring), learned experiences, etc. • Can be classified in overlapping categories—according to the target, e.g. people, predators, horses, other animals; according to function and motivation, e.g., establishing dominance status, maternal, defensive, redirected, etc.; whether offensive or defensive.

PATHOPHYSIOLOGY

• Not necessarily a pathological condition, but usually a normal, species-typical behavior
• When extreme in frequency or intensity, can be a sign of an underlying pathological condition
• Any pathophysiology that results in pain
• Hypothyroidism and acute liver failure have been associated with aggressiveness.
• Hypertestosteronism in mares—ovarian tumors such as arrhenoblastoma and granulosa-thecal cell; testicular feminization syndrome in mares • Retained testicles in males that may produce testosterone or e.g., estrogen
• Agents that affect the CNS—encephalopathies, rabies • Obsessive-compulsive self-mutilation; generally isolated stallions • Low blood serotonin levels have been associated with aggressive behavior. • Anabolic steroids may cause aggression.

SYSTEMS AFFECTED

• Several behavioral systems of the horse may be affected. • Musculoskeletal, skin, ophthalmic injuries as a consequent of aggression
• Reproductive behaviors may be interrupted; attachment behaviors may be severed between mare and foal, horse and person. • Frequent or prolonged states of aggression can result in chronic stress and result in changes in the hypothalamic-pituitary-cortical continuum. Chronic stress can affect immune function, body maintenance. Sympathetic arousal.
• Interference with learning and learned behaviors

GENETICS

Genetics has been shown to influence specific types of aggressive behaviors in many species, but the mechanisms are unknown.

INCIDENCE/PREVALENCE

Unknown

GEOGRAPHIC DISTRIBUTION

Unknown

SIGNALMENT

Breed Predilections

Maternal aggressive protection of foals is reported more often in Arabian mares.

Age

• Any age • Maternal aggression—more common among mares with unweaned foals
• Playful aggression—most common in young horses and colts • Intermale aggression—more common and intense in mature males

Predominant Sex

Intact males are more likely to show aggression to other horses and people.

SIGNS

General Comments

• Aggressive behaviors range from mild threats to intense injurious acts. • Mild forms include laying back of ears, lowering and extending head, nodding or swinging of head and neck, shifting of hindquarters toward another with the body or mild pushing. • Moderate aggression adds threats to bite, strike or kick, tail switching, sometimes slight hopping motions with rear quarters, head and body bumping, harsh vocal squeals. There is apparent restraint in intensity and effort. • High levels of aggression include serious efforts to bite, strike or kick, severe bites, and attempts to knock opponent off balance. Rearing and striking with forelegs (boxing).
• Play aggression includes components of above but of low intensity, usually not causing any or serious harm between unshod horses. • Defensive behaviors include moving away and/or shifting rear quarters toward aggressor. • Offensive behaviors usually involve head-on approach and threat. • Submissive behaviors include deferring to more dominant animal and "snapping" (jaw-waving, teeth-clamping, or *unterlegenheitsgebarde*). Sometimes a slight sucking sound occurs. The ears are usually in a somewhat horizontal position.

Historical

• Vary with the circumstances and kind of aggression shown
• Ask questions to identify exactly what behaviors are occurring. Determine when, where, how often they occur, when did they start and how did they progress, the targets of the aggression; the situations that tend to make it worse and situations when it does **not** occur; and what has been done thus far to deal with the problem. These answers form the basis for treatment and risk assessment. • Aggressiveness associated with endocrine abnormalities is generally of gradual onset. • Mares with elevated testosterone levels may show "stallion-like" behaviors, e.g. mounting other mares, vocalizing like a stallion, herding other mares, and aggression to other horses.

Physical Examinations

• Should be unremarkable, unless some underlying pathology is present • Examine carefully for pain. • Reproductive tract abnormalities • Retained testicles • Mares may have ovarian enlargements and cystic morphology, enlarged clitoris, blind vaginal sac, "cresty neck."

CAUSES

• Pain • Fear/defense • Play aggression usually is inhibited and causes no injuries among unshod horses of similar ages and weight. May cause serious injury to people.
• Protective—occurs in defense of other animals or people with whom the aggressor has a relationship and that are perceived to be under threat.
• Dominance—Dominance hierarchies exist in groups of horses and are usually initially established via aggression, threats, and reciprocal deference. Once hierarchies are established and there is sufficient opportunity for the subordinate horse to defer, high levels of aggression rarely occur. • Resource guarding—food, preferred pasture partners, water, shelter, etc. Usually directed toward other horses but can be directed toward people.
• Redirected—occurs during conflict situations in which a horse attacks another animal or person when access to the original target is blocked • Redirected aggression occurs when a horse is motivated to be aggressive but either is physically or psychologically prevented from aggressing the eliciting stimuli and, instead, redirects the aggression to another target.
• Infanticide—Stallions may kill foals that are not theirs or are not recognized as theirs.
• Sex related—occurs as part of courtship, copulation, or intrasexual competition. A mare may attack a stallion attempting to mate her, or a stallion may attack a mare that he is attempting to mate. Stallions may fight with each other in the presence or absence of mares. Mares may attack each other for access to stallions or to block access to a stallion. • Endocrine abnormalities

RISK FACTORS

• Inappropriate use of punishment • Horses reared in isolation from other horses may not develop adequate social skills and may develop inappropriately rough play aggression with people. • Small enclosures and poorly designed enclosures that prevent escape or deferral to threats • Inadequate designs of water and feeding sites that result in fighting over access to resources • Hand feeding treats can lead to "nipping." • Adjacent stabling of horses that exhibit aggression toward each other
• Sharp edges or protruding sharp wires on barriers between horses that engage in aggressive play with each other

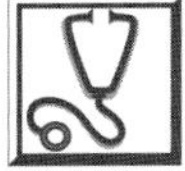

DIAGNOSIS

DIFFERENTIAL DIAGNOSIS

• Rule out pathological conditions, especially painful etiologies, before establishing a nonmedical behavioral diagnosis.
• Aberrant, intense, or steadily increasing aggressiveness warrants comprehensive medical workup.
• Nonmedical diagnoses are based on circumstances and behavioral signs exhibited and rule-outs of medical causes.

CBC/BIOCHEMISTRY/URINALYSIS

Dependent on clinical signs

OTHER LABORATORY TESTS

• Dependent on clinical signs
• Self-mutilating directed to right side warrants endoscopic examination for gastric ulcers.

• Aggression in mares, especially when accompanied by stallion-like behaviors, warrants testosterone, estrogen, and inhibin assays.
• Karyotyping of mares exhibiting stallion-like behaviors
• Thyroid panels

IMAGING

Transrectal ultrasonography of reproductive organs

OTHER DIAGNOSTIC PROCEDURES

• Rectal palpation
• Vaginal examination

PATHOLOGICAL FINDINGS

Dependent on etiology of aggression

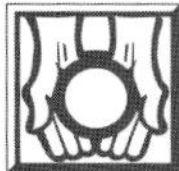

TREATMENT

AIMS OF TREATMENT

• Identify underlying reason for aggression and contributing factors.
• Correct medical causes.
• Specific treatments vary with the kind of aggression.
• Most treatments of nonmedical conditions involve changing the physical or social environment and/or using behavior modification techniques to change the motivational state of the animal.
• Behavior modification must be done precisely if it is to be safe and effective. Referral to an experienced and competent veterinary behaviorist, applied animal behaviorist, or trainer usually is necessary to help the client implement the plan.
• Assess the risks of treating and keeping a horse exhibiting aggression. Factors to consider are length of time the behaviors have been occurring, severity of aggression, number of situations in which the behaviors occur, predictability of the aggression, ease of stopping or preventing it, number of different targets, environment of the horse, and the people and other animals that may interact with the horse.

APPROPRIATE HEALTH CARE N/A

NURSING CARE N/A

ACTIVITY

• Prevent or control access to targets of aggression.
• Increase appropriate and safe types of exercise.

DIET

Reduction of energy and protein intake is reported to reduce activity level and aggressiveness. However, numerous interventions (generally increased exercise and changes in environment) are usually also implemented simultaneously and it is difficult to assess the effect of the diet.

CLIENT EDUCATION

• Advise owner of risks involved with keeping the animal when considering treatment. Aggressive animals can deliver serious injury or cause death, and keeping an aggressive animal may place the client at risk of criminal and civil legal actions.
• Advise owner that even if underlying medical reasons are alleviated, there may be residual behavior patterns that require behavior modification and/or training.

SURGICAL CONSIDERATIONS

• Removal of abnormal gonads in mares (ovarian tumors, aberrant testicular tissue) has a good prognosis.
• Castration of stallions and colts usually reduces, but does not always eliminate, aggressive behaviors directed towards other horses and people. Age and experience of horse prior to castration are reported to be unrelated to effectiveness of castration.
• Castration only cures self-mutilation that appears to be self-directed intermale aggression by stallions about 30% of the time. Seventy percent remain unaffected by castration.

MEDICATIONS

DRUGS OF CHOICE

• No drug is approved by the US Food and Drug Administration for use with aggressive problems in horses.
• Pain medications may help to reduce or eliminate pain-elicited aggression.
• Anxiolytics or antidepressants may help with fear-motivated aggression.

CONTRAINDICATIONS

Benzodiazepines may increase aggressive behaviors.

PRECAUTIONS

• Inform clients that use of psychoactive drugs for aggression problems constitutes off-label and experimental use.
• Inform clients regarding possible benefits, dangers, and side effects.
• Obtain written informed consent before prescribing off-label medication.

POSSIBLE INTERACTIONS

N/A

ALTERNATIVE DRUGS

N/A

FOLLOW-UP

PATIENT MONITORING

• Contact clients on a regular basis to check compliance with recommendations and to provide additional support.
• Behavioral problems generally require intensive follow-up.

PREVENTION/AVOIDANCE

• Rear young foals with other horses. Ideally should remain with mother for 6 mo and allowed access to other foals and (appropriate) horses as much as possible and for as long as possible.
• Sufficient exercise
• Adequate space to play and defer to dominant horses
• Ground work that results in the horse consistently and quickly yielding to the requests of the handler. Most easily accomplished with naïve and young horses
• Avoid inappropriate use of punishment.
• If the aggression is not pathophysiologic, at the first indication there might be an aggressive behavior problem; advise client to seek help from a qualified, accomplished professional who addresses such behaviors.

POSSIBLE COMPLICATIONS

See Client Education.

EXPECTED COURSE AND PROGNOSIS

• Resolution of aggressive and stallion-like behaviors of mases with ovariectomy is good.
• Removal of normal or retained testicles in males generally results in reduction of aggressive and typically masculine behaviors. Approximately one-third retain some aggressive behaviors to other horses and interested in mares. From 5% to 17% retain some aggressiveness toward people.
• Treatment of hypothyroidism with levothyroxine can effectively reduce aggressive behavior in horses.
• Successful treatment of nonmedical causes of aggression is dependent on many variables (see above).

MISCELLANEOUS

ASSOCIATED CONDITIONS, AGE-RELATED FACTORS, ZOONOTIC POTENTIAL, PREGNANCY, SYNONYMS

N/A

SEE ALSO

• Excessive maternal behavior/foal stealing
• Fears and phobias
• Maternal foal rejection
• Male sexual behavior problems
• Endocrine disorders
• Training and learning problems

Suggested Reading

Crowell-Davis SL. Normal behavior and behavior problems. In: Kobluk CN, Ames TR, Geor RJ, eds. The Horse: Diseases and Clinical Management. Philadelphia: WB Saunders, 1995:1–21.

Houpt KA. Domestic Animal Behavior for Veterinarians and Animal Scientists, ed 4. Ames, IA: Blackwell Publishing, 2005.

McGreevy P. Equine Behaviour: A Guide for Veterinarians and Equine Scientists. Philadelphia: WB Saunders, 2005.

Mills DS, McDonnell S. Domestic Horse: The Origins, Development, and Management of Its Behaviour. New York: Cambridge University Press, 2005.

Waring GH. Horse Behavior, ed 2. Norwich, NJ: Noyes Publications/William Andrew Publishing, 2003.

Authors Victoria L. Voith and Daniel Q. Estep

Consulting Editors Victoria L. Voith and Daniel Q. Estep

ALKALINE PHOSPHATASE (ALP)

BASICS

DEFINITION

• Serum ALP is mainly used as a marker for cholestasis. • Routine chemistry panels report total ALP, but nonhepatic tissues (especially bone) may contribute to total ALP. • Is infrequently used as a marker for changes in other tissues; requires isoenzyme separation techniques. • For routine interpretations, the potential contributions by nonhepatic tissues must be taken into account before interpreting increased ALP as evidence for cholestasis.
• Reference intervals vary depending on the assay substrate employed; thus, comparisons across labs may not be valid.

PATHOPHYSIOLOGY

• Two genes produce distinct ALP isoenzymes—intestinal ALP and tissue-unspecific ALP. • Generally, the intestinal ALP gene is expressed only in the intestine and the tissue-unspecific ALP gene elsewhere; however, the equine kidney expresses both.
• Posttranslational modification (especially glycosylation) produces additional tissue-specific isoforms of ALP (e.g., bone, liver) and affects circulating half-life. • Various ALP forms can be quantified, but only at specialized labs. • High tissue concentrations occur in kidney, intestine, liver, and bone; lower concentrations occur in placenta and other tissues. • Although intestine and kidney have much higher tissue concentrations than liver and bone, renal ALP usually is not released into blood, and intestinal ALP has a very short half-life of ≅8 min. Thus, serum concentrations normally consist mostly of liver and, to a lesser extent, bone ALP. • Liver ALP activity generally is greatest on the biliary canalicular membrane of hepatocytes. Increased blood activity results from increased synthesis (i.e., induction) or membrane release. The mechanism of release into the blood is proposed to involve membrane solubilization by bile salts, release of membrane fragments, or biliary regurgitation. A serum phospholipase contributes to cleavage of the enzyme from the membrane. • Cholestasis leads to increased serum ALP concentrations. Hepatocellular injury alone (e.g., carbon tetrachloride toxicity) has little effect. Bile duct ligation leads to nearly 3-fold elevations within 10 days. Presumably, much higher increases would require considerable chronicity. • Recent work suggests that ALP rises with biliary proliferation, as seen with GGT. • Because increased ALP involves enzyme induction, serum ALP increases in acute obstructive jaundice are preceded by other markers such as conjugated bilirubin and bile salts.

SYSTEMS AFFECTED

• Hepatobiliary—Increases are associated with cholestasis. • Musculoskeletal—Increases are associated with increased osteoblastic activity.
• GI—Severe GI disease can be associated with mild increases, the source of which (i.e., mucosal cells versus secondary liver changes) is often unclear. • Reproductive—Placental increases during pregnancy; impact on serum concentrations is equivocal. Semen ALP comes mainly from the epididymus and testes. High ALP and few/no sperm confirms decreased sperm production versus ejaculatory failure or blockage.

SIGNALMENT

• Neonates and foals—Activity at days 1–3 of age is up to 20-fold above that of adults. Values decrease to <5- to 10-fold by 2 weeks, and then taper to adult levels by 6 mo–1 year.
• Pregnancy—Equivocal impact on serum ALP; some diseases associated with cholestasis and increased ALP are more common in pregnant mares (e.g., hyperlipemia, Theiler's disease, etc.).
• Ponies and donkeys—particularly susceptible to hyperlipemia and hepatic lipidosis • Other factors—depend on the underlying cause

SIGNS

General Comments

Signs do not result directly from increased serum ALP activity but from the underlying disease process.

Historical Findings

• Owners may report icterus, dark yellow/orange urine, anorexia, weight loss, listlessness, and behavioral changes associated with hepatic failure in conditions associated with cholestasis.
• Abdominal pain (e.g., sweating, rolling) may occur with acute hepatopathies (i.e., capsular swelling) or biliary obstructions.

Physical Examination Findings

• Icterus is common. • Increased pulse and respiratory rates, fever, photosensitization, weight loss, or obesity vary with the type and severity of the underlying disease process.

CAUSES

Hepatobiliary System

• Metabolic—secondary to severe anemia (see Hematopoietic System), hyperlipemia, or fasting (<50% increase within 2–3 days, nonpathological) • Immune-mediated, infectious—chronic active hepatitis, Theiler's disease (i.e., serum hepatitis), amyloidosis, endotoxemia, viral (e.g., EIA, EVA, EHV in perinatal foals), bacterial (e.g., Tyzzer's disease, salmonellosis), fungal, protozoal (piroplasmosis), and parasitic (e.g., liver flukes, strongyle larval migrans) • Nutritional—hepatic lipidosis
• Degenerative—cirrhosis; cholelithiasis
• Toxic—pyrrolizidine alkaloid–containing plants (e.g., senecio, crotolaria), alsike clover, aflatoxin, rubratoxin; chemical toxins (e.g., arsenic, chlorinated hydrocarbons, phenol, paraquat) primarily cause hepatocellular injury; cholestasis secondary to hepatocellular swelling may increase ALP; some anesthetics (e.g., halothane) are associated with mild, transient increases. • Anomaly—biliary atresia; portovascular shunts • Neoplastic—primary liver tumors (rare); metastatic neoplasia (uncommon)

Musculoskeletal System

• Rapid bone growth—juveniles • Severe bony lesions

GI System

Severe GI disease—diarrhea

Reproductive System

Pregnancy increases placental ALP, with mild increases in total serum ALP.

Hematopoietic System

• Severe anemia (e.g., acute EIA, red maple leaf toxicity, onion toxicity, postparturient hemorrhage) leads to hypoxic injury and hepatocellular swelling, with subsequent cholestasis. • Hepatic lymphosarcoma, leukemias, and so on

RISK FACTORS

Those associated with any disease leading to cholestasis; exposure to serum products in periparturient mares (serum hepatitis); pregnant ponies (hepatic lipidosis), etc. See Causes.

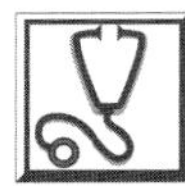

DIAGNOSIS

DIFFERENTIAL DIAGNOSIS

• Increases caused by bone ALP mostly are seen in growing animals. In adults, increased bone ALP likely involves lameness or obvious bony lesions. Increases from bone ALP are relatively mild. • Highest elevations generally are associated with long-standing conditions involving severe cholestasis—chronic active hepatitis, cirrhosis, cholelithiasis, and lipidosis.
• Concurrent obesity and high enzyme levels suggest hyperlipemia/lipidosis, whereas anorexia and weight loss are typical of most other differentials.

LABORATORY FINDINGS

Drugs That May Alter Lab Results

• Arsenate, beryllium, cyanide, fluoride, manganese, phosphate, sulfhydryl compounds, and zinc may cause falsely low values.
• Complexing anticoagulants (e.g., citrate, EDTA, oxalate) inhibit the enzyme and should not be used for sample collection.

Disorders That May Alter Lab Results

• Extreme icterus, severe lipemia, and marked hemolysis may affect values. • Activity tends to increase with storage.

Valid If Run in Human Lab?

• Valid, but concentrations vary with the methodology used. • Equine reference intervals should be generated in-house or based on literature values using the same methodology.

CBC/BIOCHEMISTRY/URINALYSIS

• No routine laboratory tests provide a causative or specific diagnosis for increases. • Most suggest a type of injury (e.g., process, cholestasis, insufficiency) rather than a cause. • Others, confirming the presence of cholestasis, support a suspected hepatic origin for the increase.

Erythrocytes

• Nonregenerative anemia may be seen with liver disease. • Microcytosis is associated with portosystemic shunts. • Acanthocytes, schistocytes (hepatic microvascular disease) are associated with decreased RBC survival and may contribute to mild hemolytic anemia. • Severe hemolytic anemia (regardless of mechanism) can cause hypoxic injury leading to hepatocellular swelling and secondary cholestasis.

Leukocytes

• Neutrophilia or neutropenia and monocytosis may occur with inflammatory liver disease—bacterial cholangiohepatitis. • Evidence of antigenic stimulation (e.g., lymphocytosis, reactive lymphoid cells) may be seen.

Glucose

• Postprandial hyperglycemia or fasting hypoglycemia may occur with hepatic insufficiency/shunts.
• Hypoglycemia with liver disease carries a guarded prognosis.

Albumin

• Decreased production with hepatic insufficiency may decrease serum levels; usually a late event.
• Albumin is a negative acute-phase reactant—Mild decreases may occur with inflammation.

BUN

Decreased levels (especially relative to creatinine) occur with hepatic insufficiency/shunts due to decreased conversion of ammonia to urea.

GGT

Increases with either injury or cholestasis

Bilirubin

• Conjugated—increases with cholestasis
• Unconjugated—increases with increased RBC destruction (i.e., hemolysis), or decreased hepatic uptake and with fasting

Cholesterol

• May decrease with hepatic insufficiency/shunts
• Sometimes increases with cholestasis and lipid metabolic disorders—hyperlipemia

Triglycerides

Increased with hyperlipemia

Urinalysis

• Bilirubinuria indicates cholestasis.
• Ammonia urates may be observed with hepatic insufficiency/shunt.

OTHER LABORATORY TESTS

Bile Acids

• Sensitive indicator of hepatic disease but not specific for the type of process—injury, cholestasis, or insufficiency.
• Assesses enterohepatic circulation, adequate hepatocellular perfusion, and hepatobiliary function.
• More sensitive than ALP for cholestasis

Ammonia

Serum concentrations are affected by hepatic uptake and correlate inversely with hepatic functional mass.

Clearance Tests (BSP, ICG)

• Prolonged clearance intervals with decreased functional mass or cholestasis
• Accelerated clearance (possibly masking insufficiency) with hypoalbuminemia

Serology

Depends on the degree of suspicion for specific diseases—viral, fungal, and so on

Coagulation Tests

May be prolonged with hepatic insufficiency/shunting—prothrombin time; activated partial thromboplastin time.

IMAGING

Ultrasonography—useful for assessing liver size, shape, position, and parenchymal texture; may help to detect focal parenchymal lesions (e.g., abscesses, neoplasms) and abnormalities in the biliary tree (e.g., dilatations, obstructions) or large vessels (e.g., shunts, thrombosis).

DIAGNOSTIC PROCEDURES

Aspiration cytology or biopsy for microbiologic testing, cytologic imprints, and histopathological evaluation may provide specific diagnostic information.

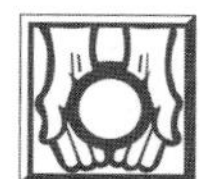

TREATMENT

• Decision regarding outpatient versus inpatient treatment depends on the severity of disease, intensity of supportive care required, need for isolation of infectious conditions, and so on.
• Fluid and nutritional support may be needed.
• Anorexic and hypoglycemic cases may benefit from IV 5% dextrose (2 mL/kg per hr); otherwise, fluid support depends on specific electrolyte and acid-base abnormalities.
• Avoid negative energy balance, especially in ponies and donkeys, to avoid/treat hyperlipemia and hepatic lipidosis.
• Toxicities or hepatic insufficiency may warrant efforts to reduce production/ absorption of toxins.
• Mineral oil by nasogastric tube helps to reduce toxin absorption.
• Lactulose (0.3 mL/kg q6h) by nasogastric tube is suggested to combat GI ammonia production/absorption but also causes diarrhea.
• A high-carbohydrate, low-protein diet reduces ammonia production.
• Specific therapy, including surgery, depends on the specific underlying cause.

MEDICATIONS

DRUG(S) OF CHOICE

Depend on the suspected cause and observed complications

CONTRAINDICATIONS

Depend on the suspected cause and observed complications

PRECAUTIONS

• Depend on the suspected cause
• With suspected hepatic insufficiency, assess coagulation profiles before invasive procedures.

POSSIBLE INTERACTIONS

Depend on the underlying cause

ALTERNATIVE DRUGS

Depend on the underlying cause

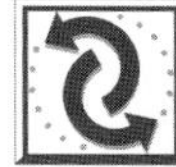

FOLLOW-UP

PATIENT MONITORING

Serial chemistries can help to establish a prognosis by characterizing disease progression and identifying evidence of improvement—Initial evaluation at 1- to 2-day intervals helps to establish the disease course; subsequent testing can be at increasing intervals, depending on signs and severity.

PREVENTION/AVOIDANCE

Depends on the underlying cause

POSSIBLE COMPLICATIONS

Depend on the underlying cause

EXPECTED COURSE AND PROGNOSIS

Depend on the underlying cause

MISCELLANEOUS

ASSOCIATED CONDITIONS

• Depend on the underlying cause
• One study showed ALP values >900 IU/L were associated with increased risk of nonsurvival (hazard ratio = 10.66).

AGE-RELATED FACTORS

• See Signalment.

ZOONOTIC POTENTIAL

Depends on the underlying cause

PREGNANCY

See Signalment.

SYNONYMS

N/A

SEE ALSO

• See Causes.

ABBREVIATIONS

• BSP = sulfobromophthalein
• EHV = equine herpesvirus
• EIA = equine infectious anemia
• EVA = equine viral arteritis
• GGT = γ-glutamyltransferase
• GI = gastrointestinal
• ICG = indocyanine green

Suggested Reading

Barton MH, Morris DD. Disorders of the liver. In: Reed S, Bayly W, Sellon D, eds. Equine Internal Medicine, ed 2. St. Louis: WB Saunders, 2004.

Durham AE, Newton JR, Smith KC, Hillyer MH, Hillyer LL, Smith MRW, Marr CM, Retrospective analysis of historical, clinical, ultrasonographic, serum biochemical and haematological data in prognostic evaluation of equine liver disease. Equine Vet J 2003;35:542–547.

Hoffmann W, Baker G, Rieser S, Dorner J. Alterations in selected biochemical constituents in equids after induced hepatic disease. Am J Vet Res 1987;48:1343–1347.

West HJ. Clinical and pathological studies in horses with hepatic disease. Equine Vet J 1996;28:146–156.

The author and editor wish to acknowledge the contribution to this chapter of Armando Irizarry-Rovira, author in the previous edition.

Author John A. Christian

Consulting Editor Kenneth W. Hinchcliff

ALKALOSIS, METABOLIC

BASICS

DEFINITION

- A disruption of acid-base homeostasis producing decreased H^+ concentration reflected by alkalemia—increased pH and high plasma HCO_3^-, Tco_2, or BE.
- Normal plasma bicarbonate level in horses is ≅24 mEq/L.
- Normal pH of arterial blood ranges from 7.35 to 7.45.
- Hypoventilation should increase CO_2 levels to lower pH; however, respiratory compensation is limited once hypoxemia develops.

PATHOPHYSIOLOGY

- The kidney normally is extremely capable of responding to a high pH, correcting metabolic alkalosis (MAK) via excretion of HCO_3^- into the urine. Even with daily administration of high bicarbonate levels, the alkalosis is short lived in normal horses. Therefore, MAK persists only when an initiating factor develops simultaneously with conditions in which renal excretion of HCO_3^- is impaired or reabsorption is enhanced.
- Excessive loss of H^+, retention of HCO_3^-, and contraction of ECF volume without loss of HCO_3^- (i.e., contraction alkalosis) are the common mechanisms thought to initiate MAK.

SYSTEMS AFFECTED

Respiratory

Peripheral and central chemoreceptors sense high pH in blood or CSF and depress ventilation to decrease removal of CO_2; hypercapnia and hypoxemia may follow.

Cardiovascular

- Cardiac arrhythmias
- Arteriolar vasoconstriction
- Decreased coronary blood flow

Neuroendocrine

- Decreased cerebral blood flow caused by vasoconstriction
- Neurologic signs (e.g., delirium, seizures, lethargy, stupor) are rare but can be seen with severe alkalemia.
- Neuromuscular excitability and tetany may occur.

Metabolic

- Increased affinity of oxygen-hemoglobin binding, which inhibits release of oxygen to the tissues
- Decreased ionized calcium concentration

Renal

The kidney responds to high pH by very effective HCO_3^- excretion under otherwise normal conditions. This response develops within hours, but it may take days to complete.

SIGNALMENT

- All breeds, ages, and sexes
- Horses used for endurance exercise may be more likely to be affected.

SIGNS

- Recent participation in endurance events or other exercise of long duration and moderate intensity may be included in the history.
- Physical examination findings vary with the primary cause.

CAUSES

- Some causes may include both an initiating factor(s) and condition(s) that encourage maintenance of alkalosis.
- GI loss of H^+ is seen with gastric reflux that occurs with anterior enteritis, ileus, or early small intestinal obstruction.
- Salivary loss of Cl^- occurs with dysphagia, esophageal trauma or obstruction, and esophagostomy.
- Cl^- loss is seen with gastric reflux, excessive sweating (especially in endurance horses), and diuretic therapy (especially with furosemide).
- K^+ depletion is associated with anorexia, restriction of GI intake, polyuric renal failure, and diuretic therapy (especially with acetazolamide).
- Endurance horses with exertional rhabdomyolysis present with MAK, likely associated with the loss of fluid and electrolytes via sweating.
- Equine sweat contains large amounts of chloride and potassium relative to serum levels. Fluid loss can be extreme with moderate-intensity exercise over long periods, especially in warm, humid conditions. Therefore, fluid and electrolyte losses can be very significant—even life-threatening—in sweating horses.
- Most of the mentioned conditions involve contraction alkalosis—fluid loss/shifts involving Na and Cl but not HCO_3^-.
- Bicarbonate therapy may result in MAK in race horses, especially if also given diuretics.
- Because proteins are weak acids, hypoproteinemia (especially albumin) produces MAK.

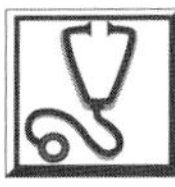

DIAGNOSIS

DIFFERENTIAL DIAGNOSIS

- Increased bicarbonate levels also are seen in conditions with respiratory acidosis. Pco_2 is high but the pH close to normal or high on blood gas analysis.
- Compensation may be very effective in chronic respiratory acidosis.

LABORATORY FINDINGS

Drugs That May Alter Lab Results

- Excessive anticoagulant may falsely decrease results via dilution.
- Excessive sodium heparin may alter HCO_3^- levels.

Valid If Run in Human Lab?

Yes, if properly submitted

CBC/BIOCHEMISTRY/URINALYSIS

- Measurements of serum electrolytes, protein levels, and serum chemistries are important to determine the cause and to guide treatment.
- Proportionate changes in sodium and chloride levels occur with alterations of fluid balance. Normal sodium levels with hypochloremia or hyperchloremia indicate acid-base imbalance, whereas disproportionate changes usually are associated with simultaneous acid-base imbalance and hydration abnormalities.
- Potassium and chloride are decreased in horses that sweat excessively. Potassium may be low because of the primary cause or as a response to the extracellular shift of H^+.
- Ionized calcium is decreased.
- Magnesium may be decreased, especially with sweat loss and colic.
- Urinalysis may reveal decreased urine pH.

OTHER LABORATORY TESTS

- Many labs measure Tco_2 using the same sample submitted for electrolytes.

• The T_{CO_2} closely approximates HCO_3^-, because most CO_2 is carried in the blood as bicarbonate.
• Like MAK, respiratory alkalosis also results in high T_{CO_2}. These conditions can be differentiated only by complete blood gas analysis.
• The T_{CO_2} must be analyzed rapidly and with minimal room-air exposure within the sample tube, because CO_2 can dissipate from the sample.

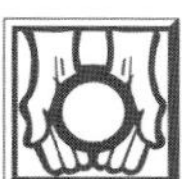

TREATMENT

• Treatment of the primary cause is essential.
• Replacement of fluid losses with isotonic fluids may be all that is needed to restore acid-base status in mild cases.
• Address specific electrolyte losses.
• Large volumes may be needed in some endurance athletes with excessive fluid losses from sweating or hyperthermia.

MEDICATIONS

DRUGS OF CHOICE

• With hypochloremia, give fluids containing chloride, or the alkalosis will not be corrected even if hydration is restored.
• Saline or Ringer's solution with added calcium and KCl is the fluid of choice.
• With excessive potassium loss, PO supplementation is necessary if the horse remains anorexic.

CONTRAINDICATIONS

Any alkalinizing therapy (i.e., LRS) can worsen the alkalosis. Check contents of oral electrolyte therapies closely.

PRECAUTIONS

• Give calcium-containing solutions slowly to avoid arrhythmias.
• Monitor cardiac rhythm during administration.

POSSIBLE INTERACTIONS

N/A

ALTERNATIVE DRUGS

Oral rehydration solutions have achieved good results in horses, being very effective in mild cases and an excellent adjunct to IV therapy. From 1–2 gallons can be given PO every few hours to adults without ileus.

FOLLOW-UP

PATIENT MONITORING

Serial blood gas analysis and measurement of electrolytes and calcium are very important in evaluating efficacy of therapy; repeat within a few hours of initial treatment and thereafter according to patient response.

POSSIBLE COMPLICATIONS

• Hypokalemia
• Hypocalcemia
• Other, rare complications—cardiac arrhythmias, colic, synchronous diaphragmatic flutter, tetany, and neurologic signs

MISCELLANEOUS

ASSOCIATED CONDITIONS

• Hypochloremia
• Hypokalemia
• Respiratory acidosis

SEE ALSO

• Exertional rhabdomyolysis
• Exhausted horse syndrome
• Heat exhaustion
• Hyperthermia

ABBREVIATIONS

• BE = base excess
• CSF = cerebrospinal fluid
• ECF = extracellular fluid
• GI = gastrointestinal
• LRS = lactated Ringer's solution
• MAK = metabolic alkalosis

Suggested Reading

Androgue HJ, Madias NE. Management of life-threatening acid-base disorders. Part 2. N Engl J Med 1998;338:107–111.

Carlson GP. Fluid, electrolyte, and acid-base balance. In: Kaneko JJ, Harvey JW, Bruss ML, eds. Clinical Biochemistry of Domestic Animals, ed 5. San Diego: Academic Press, 1997:485–516.

Hinchcliff KW, ed. Fluids and electrolytes in athletic horses. Vet Clin North Am Equine Pract 1998;14:1–225.

Sampieri F, Schott HC, et al. Effects of oral electrolyte supplementation on endurance horses competing in 80 km rides. Eq Vet Journal Suppl 2006 Aug(36): 19–26.

Author Jennifer G. Adams

Consulting Editor Kenneth W. Hinchcliff

ALKALOSIS, RESPIRATORY

BASICS

DEFINITION

- A decrease in blood P_{CO_2} and pH
- Arterial P_{CO_2} tensions of <35 mm Hg
- Venous P_{CO_2} tension <43 mm Hg

PATHOPHYSIOLOGY

- Most (65%–70%) CO_2 combines with water almost instantaneously to form carbonic acid, which then dissociates into bicarbonate ion and hydrogen. Therefore, most CO_2 is transported in the blood as bicarbonate, with some bound to proteins (especially deoxygenated hemoglobin) and a small amount dissolved directly into plasma.
- In the lungs, the reverse occurs, and CO_2 passively diffuses out of capillaries and into the alveoli.
- These three forms of CO_2 exist in equilibrium in the blood, but P_{CO_2} as measured by blood gases depends on the dissolved portion.
- Alveolar CO_2 then is removed mechanically by ventilation as inspired air displaces alveolar gas, which is expired.
- Respiratory alkalosis is present with hyperventilation or when tissue production of CO_2 drops but ventilation remains unchanged.

SYSTEMS AFFECTED

- The brain is most affected by CO_2 levels, because hypocapnia decreases cerebral blood flow.
- Low pH affects acid-base balance, protein binding, and electrolyte levels directly in the blood and via effects on the kidney.
- The kidney responds to low pH by generating more H^+ and excreting more HCO_3^-. It also reabsorbs Cl^- to maintain electroneutrality. Alkalosis decreases serum potassium and ionized calcium levels.
- Severe alkalemia can cause venoconstriction and predispose to arrhythmias, and it may result in hyperexcitability of muscle and nervous tissue.

SIGNALMENT

Any horse

SIGNS

Respiratory rate, volume, or both usually are increased.

CAUSES

Acute

- Usually is a temporary change in response to a stimulus causing hyperventilation
- Physiologic causes of hyperventilation—exercise, fever, and hyperthermia
- Psychological causes—pain, anxiety, excitement, and fear
- Stimulation of medullary respiratory centers by CNS disorders, early septicemia, acidosis, or endotoxemia may result in hyperventilation.
- Anemia, hypovolemia, and hypoxemia of any cause increase respiration in response to tissue hypoxia.

Chronic

- May result from chronic respiratory disease (e.g. pleuropneumonia) or chronic, painful conditions (e.g., laminitis, septic arthritis)
- Overventilation with mechanical ventilators produces low P_{CO_2} in anesthetized patients and sick neonates.
- Hypothermia or decreased metabolic rates seen with prolonged general anesthesia may lower tissue CO_2 production and produce respiratory alkalosis in patients ventilated at appropriate settings.
- Also seen as a compensatory response to primary metabolic acidosis

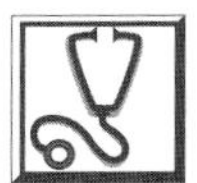

DIAGNOSIS

DIFFERENTIAL DIAGNOSIS

- Physiologic states or disease processes that present with tachypnea—fever, hyperthermia, excitement, anxiety, painful conditions, hypoxemia, metabolic acidosis, and CNS derangements; most of these can be differentiated with history and physical examination findings.
- Most acute problems have low pH and low P_{CO_2}.
- Chronic respiratory alkalosis results in compensatory metabolic acidosis, in which bicarbonate is low and pH should be normal, because compensation is very effective in this circumstance.
- Acute metabolic acidosis has low bicarbonate. Often, pH remains low in severe cases, because respiratory compensation rarely is complete.

LABORATORY FINDINGS

Disorders That May Alter Lab Results

- With poor peripheral perfusion or cardiovascular shunt, results of blood gas analysis on samples taken from peripheral arteries may differ from those taken elsewhere or may not reflect the patient's overall systemic condition.

• Prolonged exposure to air may alter CO_2 levels, because RBC metabolism continues and equilibration with room air may occur.

Valid If Run in Human Lab?
Yes, if properly submitted

OTHER LABORATORY TESTS
• Blood gas analysis is the definitive laboratory test.
• Venous samples may be adequate to identify the condition, but arterial samples are necessary to evaluate adequacy of pulmonary function as a cause.
• Handheld analyzers are now available and easy to use. Some require only small amounts of whole blood; otherwise, heparinize syringes before sampling.
• Perform sampling anaerobically. Immediately evacuate any air bubbles present, and cap the needle with a rubber stopper.
• Analysis should be performed within 15–20 min. If not, samples can be stored on ice, and results will be valid for 3–4 hr.

DIAGNOSTIC PROCEDURES
• Capnography is an indirect method of measuring CO_2 levels.
• Samples of ET gases reflect arterial Pco_2, because ET gas is essentially the same as alveolar gas.
• Continous monitoring can be performed on anesthetized or ventilated patients via a gas-sampling port incorporated into the endotracheal tube or attached to an adapter.
• Because some $\dot{V}/\dot{Q}$ mismatch usually is present, ET levels may underestimate arterial tension by 10–15 mm Hg.
• Periodically compare values obtained via capnography with those via blood gas analysis.

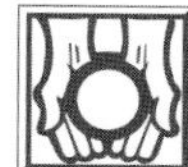

TREATMENT

• Most often, treatment of the primary problem resolves the need for hyperventilation, or metabolic rate will increase and normal Pco_2 levels return.
• Alteration of ventilator settings in anesthetized patients is necessary to return CO_2 and pH to normal; however, this may decrease oxygen levels.

MEDICATIONS

PRECAUTIONS
• Monitor ventilated patients continuously for airway obstruction caused by accumulation of secretions, movement of endotracheal tube, kinking of tubing or hoses, and so on.
• Inspiratory pressure should range from 20 to 30 cm H_2O in normal patients.
• Pressures of $\geq$40 cm H_2O may be utilized in patients with abdominal distention—those anesthetized for colic surgery.
• Pressures of >40 cm H_2O compromise venous return and cardiac output.

FOLLOW-UP

PATIENT MONITORING
• Decreased respiratory effort should be seen quickly after resolution of the primary problem.
• Evaluate repeat blood gases analyses soon after institution of mechanical ventilation to ensure appropriate settings have been selected. Further evaluation thereafter is dictated by the patient's condition.

POSSIBLE COMPLICATIONS
Severe alkalemia can result in neurologic signs from decreased cerebral blood flow, muscular excitability, and cardiac arrhythmias.

MISCELLANEOUS

ASSOCIATED CONDITIONS
• Hyperchloremia
• Hypokalemia
• Metabolic acidosis

PREGNANCY
Pregnant females often hyperventilate because of decreased lung volume caused by abdominal distention from the gravid uterus.

SYNONYMS
• Hypocapnia
• Hypocarbia

ABBREVIATIONS
• ET = end-tidal, refers to gas expired at the end of expiration, which should be the alveolar gas most recently involved in gas exchange
• $\dot{V}/\dot{Q}$ = ventilation-perfusion ratio

Suggested Reading

Adrogue JG, Madias NE. Management of life-threatening acid-base disorders. Second of two parts. N Engl J Med 1998;338:107–111.

Rose BD, Post TW, eds. Chapter 21: Respiratory Alkalosis. In: Clinical Physiology of Acid-Base and Electrolyte Disorders, ed 5. New York: McGraw Hill, 2001:673-681.

Author Jennifer G. Adams
Consulting Editor Kenneth W. Hinchcliff

ALOPECIA

BASICS

DEFINITION

• Alopecia is an absolute decrease in the number of hairs per given area of body surface or hairs that are shorter than normal even though their number is within normal limits. It is a loss or lack of the hair from skin areas where it is normally present.
• Alopecia is congenital or acquired.
• *Congenital* alopecia is rare in horses.
• *Acquired* alopecia can be subdivided into *infectious* and *noninfectious* causes. Common etiologies of acquired alopecia are adnexal destruction or atrophy secondary to infection, physical trauma, immune-mediated reactions, nutritional supplements and deficiencies, toxicities, physiologic stressors, hypersensitivities, neoplasia, and various miscellaneous causes.

PATHOPHYSIOLOGY

• *Acquired* alopecia represents a disruption in the growth of the hair follicle with or without damage to the hair bulb, follicular wall, hair shaft, or both. The animal is born with a normal hair coat, has or had normal hair follicles at one time, and is or was capable of producing structurally normal hairs.
• *Congenital* alopecia is the result of abnormal morphogenesis or lack of adnexa (therefore hair) in regions of the body where they normally are expected. Animals with congenital hypotrichosis may be born with varying degrees of hypotrichosis or a complete haircoat; however, if born with a complete haircoat, a rapid onset of progressive permanent alopecia within the first few months of life ensues.

SYSTEM AFFECTED

Skin/exocrine

GENETICS

Congenital alopecia does not necessarily imply a genetic basis, although in most cases the disease is based on genetic abnormalities and thus is hereditary. The exact mode of inheritance is unknown.

INCIDENCE/PREVALENCE

True incidence is unknown.

GEOGRAPHIC DISTRIBUTION

Presumably worldwide

SIGNALMENT

• Congenital hypotrichosis has been documented in certain Arabian lines and a blue roan Percheron.
• Appaloosas with foundation bloodlines have hair dystrophy/thinning of the long mane and tail hair.
• Acquired alopecia can occur in all breeds.
• Both sexes are affected equally.

SIGNS

General Comments

• May be an acute onset or slowly progressive

• Multifocal patches of circular alopecia are most commonly associated with bacterial folliculitis, dermatophytosis, or dermatophiliosis
• Large diffuse areas of alopecia may indicate an immune-mediated etiology or congenital abnormality.
• Congenital hypotrichosis may be regional, multifocal, or generalized. It might become clinically apparent only weeks after birth and usually does not continually progress with age.

CAUSES

• Noncicatricial alopecia (nonscarring causes)
  ○ Mild to moderate inflammation of the hair follicle (folliculitis and furunculosis)
  ○ Defects in the hair shaft
  ○ Hair follicle dystrophies
  ○ Altered hair follicle function
  ○ Trauma (self-induced from pruritus)
• Cicatricial alopecia (scarring causes)
  ○ Physical, chemical, or thermal injury
  ○ Severe furunculosis
  ○ Neoplasia
  ○ Severe inflammatory disease such as in cutaneous onchocerciasis

Congenital Causes

• Congenital hypothyroidism may be a cause of congenital hypotrichosis and alopecia.
• Trichorrhexis nodosa is a hair shaft defect that may be hereditary or acquired.
• Congenital hypotrichosis
• Epidermolysis bullosa
• Mane and tail dystrophy
• Follicular dysgenesis

Acquired Causes

Infectious

• Bacterial
  ○ The most common bacterial infection is dermatophiliosis. Folliculitis and furunculosis due to *Staphylococcus* spp. and *Corynebacterium pseudotuberculosis* are uncommon. Other bacterial causes are abscesses due to *Fusiformis* and *Streptococcus* spp.
• Fungal
  ○ Dermatophytosis due to *Microsporum gypseum, M. equinum* or *M. canis* or *Trichophyton equinum* var. *equinum* causes alopecia. Other fungal causes are mycetoma and the subcutaneous mycosis such as phycomycosis and pythiosis.
• Parasitic
  ○ Follicular parasitic infections of the follicle that result in alopecia are rare and include *Demodex equi* and *Pelodera strongyloides*. Other more common parasitic infections that cause alopecia are *Culicoides*, onchocerciasis, lice, ticks, oxyuriasis, and mites (*Sarcoptes* spp., *Chorioptes* spp., and *Trombiculid* spp.).
• Viral
  ○ Viral papillomas—congenital, cutaneous, or pinnal

Noninfectious

• Immune mediated
  ○ Cell-mediated autoimmune disease directed toward the hair follicle and adnexa
    • Alopecia areata • Hair follicle dystrophy—possible variant of alopecia areata • Sebaceous adenitis—rare anecdotal reports and one case report in 2006; however, diagnosis is questionable.
  ○ Drug eruptions • Pemphigus foliaceus
  • Systemic lupus erythematosus
  • Sarcoidosis
• Physical
  ○ Burns from chemicals, hot, cold, or ropes
  • Scalding from exudate, urine, or feces
  • Tail and mane rubbing as stable vice

• Neoplasia
 ○ Sarcoids • Squamous cell carcinoma
• Miscellaneous
 ○ Symmetrical atrophy of hair follicles secondary to endocrine disorders is extremely rare to nonexistent. • Anagen and telogen effluvium • Anhidrosis • Iodism • Selenium, mimosine, or mercury toxicities • Copper deficiency

RISK FACTORS

N/A

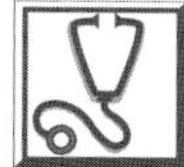

DIAGNOSIS

DIFFERENTIAL DIAGNOSIS

• Accurate diagnosis of alopecia requires a careful history and physical examination.
• Key points in the history include recognition of breed predispositions for congenital alopecia, the duration and progression of lesions, the presence or absence of pruritus, or evidence of contagion.
• The distribution of lesions should be noted (focal, multifocal, generalized, or symmetrical), and the hairs examined to determine if they are being shed from the hair follicle or broken off. Signs of secondary infections or ectoparasites should be noted. The degree of crusts, scale, and exudate helps prioritize the differentials.
• Patchy, localized to multifocal
 ○ Bacterial folliculitis and furunculosis
 ○ Dermatophytosis
 ○ Dermatophilosis
 ○ Linear alopecia
 ○ Alopecia areata—results from selective and reversible damage to anagen hair follicles. Initial lesions may be focal, multifocal well-circumscribed alopecia that progresses to diffuse alopecia. The mane and tail are often involved and hoof dystrophies can occur. The alopecic skin has minimal or no visible inflammation. Prognosis varies, some cases spontaneously resolve, some respond to immunosuppressive doses of steroids, while others have no hair regrowth.
• Generalized, symmetrical, and large patchy multifocal

a. Normal shed—"physiologic telogen effluvium"
 ○ Telogen effluvium—a reaction pattern characterized by widespread alopecia in response to severe metabolic stress. Serious illness, high fever, pregnancy, and adverse reaction to supplements are all potential inducers of telogen effluvium. Rapid premature cessation of anagen growth leads to abrupt synchronization of the follicular cycle such that hair follicles proceed in unison through catagen and telogen. This leads to hair loss of variable severity when old telogen hairs are forced out by new, synchronous anagen hairs. Hair loss usually occurs within 3–4 weeks after the insult but may occur up to 2 mo later. Alopecia resolves spontaneously if the initiating factor is no longer present, and new anagen hairs grow.

b. Anagen effluvium—a reaction pattern characterized by shedding during anagen arrest. Severe stresses such as high-dose cytotoxic therapy, infection, or metabolic disease halts anagen hair growth and results in hair loss within days to weeks of the insult. The hairs are lost due to structural weakness or dysplastic changes damaging the hair shaft.

CBC/BIOCHEMISTRY/URINALYSIS

Useful to rule out metabolic causes

OTHER LABORATORY TESTS N/A

IMAGING N/A

OTHER DIAGNOSTIC PROCEDURES

• Cytology should be obtained from pustules, papules, erosions, or ulcers. Neutrophilic exudate with intra-and/or extracellular cocci representative of a secondary folliculitis are easily identified if cytology is sampled from ruptured pustules or impression smears made from the underside of crusts or a fresh erosion or ulcer. Impression smears from the surface of lesions often do NOT show bacteria, but rather numbers of shed keratinocytes.
• Direct hair examination (trichography)–Hairs will either have anagen or telogen roots. Telogen hairs have uniform shaft diameters and slightly rough-surfaced tapered spear-shaped angular non-pigmented roots. Anagen hairs have rounded smooth pigmented bulbs that bend. Distal ends of hair shafts may appear fractured from self-induced trauma. No normal animal should have all of its hairs in telogen but rather should have an admixture of anagen and telogen. Anagen defluxion reveals fragmented hair shafts with the absence of roots.
• Perform skin scrapings to rule out ectoparasites.
• Perform bacterial and DTM cultures to determine bacterial species and susceptibility and/or dermatophyte infections.
• Perform skin biopsies if the tests listed above do not identify or suggest an underlying cause. A biopsy evaluates hair follicles, adnexal structures, inflammation, and anagen/telogen ratios. Biopsies may reveal evidence for bacterial, parasitic or fungal causes of alopecia but should NOT be considered as the definitive test for determination of alopecia caused by infectious agents. If cytologic identification reveals evidence of folliculitis, treat the patient with appropriate antimicrobials, parasiticides, or antifungals for a minimum of 3 weeks. If no improvement in the degree of alopecia is noted, obtain a biopsy for histopathology, preferably, while the patient is still receiving treatment. Often biopsies submitted from patients with moderate to severe bacterial folliculitis make it difficult to determine and may mask the primary cause of alopecia. Submit biopsies from affected and non-affected sites.
• Definitive diagnosis of alopecia areata requires histologic confirmation. Multiple biopsies need to be collected as pathognomonic lesions can be sparse. Biopsy from newly developed areas of alopecia, rather than older lesions.

PATHOLOGICAL FINDINGS

• Biopsies of telogen effluvium are misleading, as they will demonstrate most follicles in the active growing (anagen) phase. Often the hair cycle has returned to normal by the time the decision to biopsy has been made.
• Anagen effluvium findings include apoptosis and fragmented cell nuclei in the keratinocytes of the hair matrix of anagen follicles, as well as eosinophilic dysplastic hair shafts within the pilar canal.

ALOPECIA

• Alopecia areata has two major histologic features. The first is hair follicle miniaturization and the second feature is lymphocytic bulbitis. The lymphocytic bulbitis involves anagen follicles and is best found in recently developed areas of alopecia. A lymphocytic mural folliculitis affecting the follicular isthmus is possible. The bulbitis may be very difficult to demonstrate especially in chronic lesions where the inflammation may be nonexistent. Chronic lesions only exhibit small telogen follicles lacking hair shafts that may be somewhat atrophic.
• Histologic findings of alopecia secondary to infectious organisms are covered in the appropriate dermatology sections.

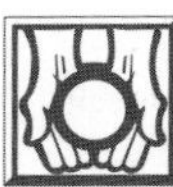

TREATMENT

AIMS OF TREATMENT
The clinical approach to alopecia is to identify the cause and, if the etiology is something that may benefit from pharmaceutical treatment, then therapy may resolve the clinical signs.

APPROPRIATE HEALTH CARE
Relevance equated to etiology; most require outpatient medical management.

NURSING CARE
Relevance equated to etiology

ACTIVITY
Patients with multifocal to generalized hypotrichosis may be more susceptible to hypothermia and solar dermatoses.

DIET
Telogen effluvium has been associated with the administration of a feed supplement.

CLIENT EDUCATION
Relevance equated to etiology

SURGICAL CONSIDERATIONS N/A

MEDICATIONS

DRUG(S)
• Varies with cause
• Dermatophytosis—lime sulfur or enilconazole, miconazole/chlorhexidine rinses; systemic griseofulvin
• Dermatophilosis—topical antimicrobial therapy
• Bacterial folliculitis—systemic and topical antimicrobial therapy
• Pemphigus foliaceus—immunosuppressive therapy
• There are no hair growth–promoting pharmaceuticals for horses.

CONTRAINDICATIONS N/A

PRECAUTIONS N/A

POSSIBLE INTERACTIONS
None

ALTERNATIVE DRUGS
None

FOLLOW-UP

PATIENT MONITORING
Varies with cause

PREVENTION/AVOIDANCE
• Varies with cause
• Patients with documented congenital alopecia and their parents should not be used for breeding.

POSSIBLE COMPLICATIONS N/A

EXPECTED COURSE AND PROGNOSIS
• Prognosis is based on whether the alopecia is classified as noncicatricial or cicatricial.
• *Cicatricial* alopecia is characterized by permanent destruction of the hair follicles and regrowth of hair will not occur.
• In *noncicatricial* alopecia, future hair growth will occur if the causative factors are eliminated or corrected.
• Telogen and post anagen effluvium resolve upon identification and elimination of cause.

MISCELLANEOUS

ASSOCIATED CONDITIONS N/A

AGE-RELATED FACTORS N/A

ZOONOTIC POTENTIAL
Dermatophytosis and dermatophiliosis are zoonotic.

PREGNANCY
• Post-partum telogen effluvium is thought to be due to the physiologic stress of pregnancy and lactation.
• Avoid the use of griseofulvin to treat dermatophytosis in pregnant mares.
• Mares that receive iodine-deficient diets give birth to weak or dead foals with no haircoat.

SYNONYMS
• Alopecia = hypotrichosis
• Telogen effluvium = telogen defluxion or defluvium
• Anagen effluvium = anagen defluxion or defluvium

SEE ALSO
• Dermatophytosis
• Pemphigus foliaceus
• Bacterial folliculitis
• Dermatophilosis
• Linear alopecia
• Sarcoids

ABBREVIATION
• DTM = dermatophyte test medium

Suggested Reading

Pascoe RRR, Knottenbelt DC. Manual of Equine Dermatology. London: WB Saunders, 1999:68.
von Tscharner C, Kunkle GA, Yager JA; Stannard's illustrated equine dermatology notes. Alopecia in the horse – an overview. Vet Dermatol 2000;11:191–203.

Author Gwendolen Lorch
Consulting Editor Gwendolen Lorch

AMITRAZ TOXICOSIS

BASICS

OVERVIEW

- Amitraz is a formamide acaricide widely used for the control of mites and ticks in veterinary medicine.
- While not approved for use in horses, it is sometimes used intentionally for ectoparasite control and accidental exposures may occur. Amitraz may be deliberately administered intravenously to alter performance in athletic horses.
- Amitraz has complex pharmacological and toxicological effects in animals. It acts on α_2-adrenergic receptors in the central nervous system and both α_1- and α_2-adrenergic receptors in the periphery. It is also believed to inhibit monaminoxidase, block prostaglandin E_2 synthesis, and cause a local anesthetic effect.
- Amitraz-induced central nervous system stimulation or depression appears to be dose dependent with high doses causing depression while low doses result in hyperreactivity to external stimuli, and in some cases, to aggressive behavior.
- Amitraz reduces smooth muscle activity in the gastrointestinal tract. Clinically and experimentally, this results in a reproducible and reversible impaction colic syndrome.
- Amitraz depresses respiratory rate centrally, probably by inhibiting respiratory neurons located in the ventral portion of the brain. α_2-Adrenergic agonists can reduce both sensitivity of the breathing center to increased P_{CO_2} and tidal volume, thus accentuating respiratory depression.
- Amitraz inhibits antidiuretic hormone and thus may promote diuresis.
- Amitraz and its active metabolite both induce hyperglycemia and hypoinsulinemia by inhibiting insulin secretion mediated by α_2-adrenergic receptors located within the pancreatic islets.
- Amitraz is more slowly metabolized in ponies than sheep, which may explain its toxicity in equines.
- Clinical signs of amitraz toxicosis are usually referable to the central nervous or gastrointestinal systems.

SIGNALMENT

N/A

SIGNS

- Affected horses display signs of tranquilization, depression, ataxia, muscular incoordination, and impaction colic, which may persist for days.
- The impaction colic syndrome is characterized by rapid cessation of gastrointestinal sounds, gastrointestinal stasis, extensive impaction, and tympany throughout the large colon.

CAUSES AND RISK FACTORS

- Amitraz toxicity after topical application is due either to deliberate exposure for parasite control or accidental exposure.
- Because of its known sedative/tranquilizing actions, amitraz may be deliberately administered intravenously to alter performance in athletic horses.
- Amitraz in stored solutions may break down to the highly toxic *N*-3,5-dimethylphenyl-*N*-methyl formadine derivative and more easily induce toxicosis.
- In a chronic low-dose toxicity study in horses, there were no demonstrable adverse effects from amitraz.

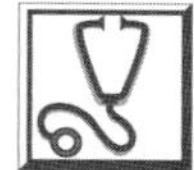

DIAGNOSIS

DIFFERENTIAL DIAGNOSIS

- Signs of colic can be due to many other disorders.
- Signs of depression and ataxia can be due to viral disease (e.g., rabies, equine encephalomyelitis, West Nile virus), hepatoencephalopathy, meningitis, and brain abscess or tumor.

CBC/BIOCHEMISTRY/URINALYSIS

- With acute intoxication, total protein and packed cell volume may increase due to dehydration and a mild acidosis may be seen.
- Hyperglycemia and hypoinsulinemia result from inhibition of insulin release.

OTHER LABORATORY TESTS

Drug-testing laboratories have methods for the detection of amitraz and its major metabolite in performance horses.

IMAGING

N/A

OTHER DIAGNOSTIC PROCEDURES

N/A

PATHOLOGICAL FINDINGS

In an experimental model, amitraz-treated horses had fecalith obstruction in the proximal small colon aboral to marked colonic impaction.

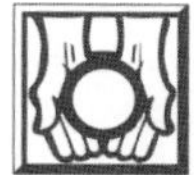

TREATMENT

- If dermal exposure to amitraz occurs, horses should be immediately bathed with soap and water to reduce absorption.
- If ingested, activated charcoal (1–4 g/kg PO in water slurry [1 g of AC in 5 mL of water]) can be administered via nasogastric tube to reduce absorption.
- Laxatives and/or a laxative diet may be used to manage the gastrointestinal effects.
- Oxygen and mechanical ventilation may be necessary if respiratory depression is severe.
- Fluid therapy may be beneficial.

MEDICATIONS

DRUG(S)

- The α_2-adrenergic antagonists yohimbine and atipamezole are used for treatment of amitraz intoxication in dogs and cats, but their use has not been documented for amitraz-intoxicated horses.
- Yohimbine is a α_2-adrenergic antagonist with high affinity for the α_2-adrenergic receptors α_2A, α_2B, and α_2C and a low affinity for the α_2D receptor. Yohimbine reverses amitraz-induced sedation in horses. A suggested dose for horses is 0.15 mg/kg IV slowly.
- Atipamezole is a potent and selective α_2-adrenergic antagonist approved to reverse sedative and analgesic effects of medetomidine in dogs. It is considered a new generation of α_2-adrenergic antagonists due to its high selectivity for α_2-adrenergic receptors, like α_2A, α_2B, and α_2C receptors, and has a 100-times higher affinity for the α_2D receptor than yohimbine. Atipamezole has a higher affinity for α_2-adrenergic receptors and is more efficacious in reversing amitraz toxicity in cats than yohimbine. A suggested dose for horses is 0.1mg/kg IV.

CONTRAINDICATIONS/POSSIBLE INTERACTIONS

- While used in humans to treat amitraz-induced bradycardia, atropine is contraindicated in horses due to the known sensitivity of horses to the anticholinergic effects on gastrointestinal motility.
- Adverse drug interactions are possible with heterocyclic antidepressants, xylazine, benzodiazepines, and macrocyclic lactones.

FOLLOW-UP

EXPECTED COURSE AND PROGNOSIS

The impaction colic effects of amitraz toxicosis may persist for days, but affected horses usually return to normal with treatment.

Suggested Reading

Queiroz-Neto A, Zamur G, Goncalves SC, et al. Characterization of the antinociceptive and sedative effect of amitraz in horses. J Vet Pharmacol Ther 1998;21:400–405.

Author Patricia M. Dowling
Consulting Editor Robert H. Poppenga

AMMONIA, HYPERAMMONEMIA

BASICS

DEFINITION

• Free ammonia (NH_3) is a nonprotein nitrogen compound that can permeate cells and result in hyperammonemia. At physiologic pH, almost all blood ammonia is the ammonium ion (NH_4^+), which is less permeable for cells. In order to eliminate waste nitrogen as ammonia, the mammalian body converts it to an excretable form, urea. To a lesser extent, ammonia is eliminated by conversion to glutamine.
• Reference intervals for plasma ammonia are 7.6–63.4 μmol/L, but are very dependent on the type of assay and reported units. Hyperammonemia is when concentrations exceed the established laboratory reference intervals.

PATHOPHYSIOLOGY

• Blood ammonia is derived primarily from dietary nitrogen with the gastrointestinal tract action of bacterial proteases, ureases, and amine oxidases resulting in the major source of blood ammonia.
• Ammonia is also derived from catabolism of glutamine and protein, and skeletal muscle exertion. Ammonia is delivered to the liver via the portal vein or hepatic artery, where functional hepatocytes remove ammonia to form urea by means of the Krebs-Henseleit urea cycle.
• If functional liver mass is inadequate, ammonia is not converted to urea, and plasma ammonia concentrations increase. Serum urea concentrations also rise when glomerular filtration is inadequate. Acid-base status affects the absorption of ammonia.
• As blood pH increases, free ammonia (NH_3) increases and can permeate cells via nonionic diffusion to produce toxicity. Ammonia is one of the compounds responsible for clinical signs of hepatic encephalopathy.
• Other described neurotoxins in hepatic encephalopathy are: alterations in monoamine neurotransmitters due to altered aromatic amino acids, alterations in γ-aminobutyric acid (GABA) and/or glutamate, and increased endogenous benzodiazepine-like substances.

SYSTEMS AFFECTED

• Nervous—Ammonia is neurotoxic and the brain is affected by high plasma concentrations.
• The degree of hyperammonemia does not necessarily correlate to the severity of hepatic encephalopathy signs because other compounds are involved. Ammonia interferes with the blood-brain barrier, cerebral blood flow, cellular excitability, neurotransmitter metabolism, and ratios of neurotransmitter precursor amino acids.
• Degenerative changes of the neurons and supporting cells have been observed in chronically affected animals (Alzheimer cells).

GENETICS

N/A

INCIDENCE/PREVALENCE

N/A

GEOGRAPHIC DISTRIBUTION

N/A

SIGNALMENT

• Portal-caval shunts have been reported in foals (rare).
• The presence of hyperammonemia is most often associated with diseases of the liver.

SIGNS

General Comments

• Clinical signs of hyperammonemia are primarily those of hepatic encephalopathy, although this is not the only substance responsible for all of the clinical signs.
• Signs may be sporadic and progressive and worsen after feeding.

Historical

Ptyalism, behavior changes, visual deficits (blindness), compulsive circling, pacing, anxiety, head pressing, stupor, coma, unusual positions/posture, sudden falling to the ground, violent thrashing

Physical Examination

Stunted growth, loss of body condition, poor hair coat, mentation changes and aberrant behavior. Similar findings as discussed in liver disease, e.g., icterus may be observed, especially in horses with acute hepatitis. In animals affected chronically, neuronal degeneration occurs and signs become persistent.

CAUSES

• Liver disease—Hepatic encephalopathy is a prominent clinical feature of hepatic failure in the horse, and is associated with acute hepatitis and hepatic cirrhosis. Abnormalities of the urea cycle, abnormal portal blood flow, or any disorder that results in markedly impaired liver function can cause hyperammonemia. Decreased functional hepatic mass can result from pyrrolizidine alkaloid toxicity, acute hepatitis, chronic active hepatitis, hepatotoxic drugs or chemicals, Tyzzer's disease in foals, and hyperlipidemia in ponies with associated hepatic dysfunction.
• Portosystemic shunts—acquired or congenital
• Toxicities—urea toxicity/poisoning, ammonium salt fertilizer toxicity

RISK FACTORS

• Horses in known areas with hepatotoxic plants would be prone to develop hepatopathies.
• Administration of equine-derived biologics may induce hepatopathies.
• Feedstuffs contaminated with high levels of urea, nitrogen, or ammonium salts

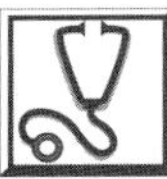

DIAGNOSIS

DIFFERENTIAL DIAGNOSIS

• Hepatic encephalopathy must be differentiated from primary neurologic diseases such as inflammatory, degenerative, infectious, or neoplastic CNS diseases. Rabies should be a differential diagnosis for abnormal behavior in the horse. Behavior-based alterations or problems should be ruled out.
• Differentiation consists of evaluating the history, signalment, and results of serum biochemistry, hematology, urinalysis, and hepatic biopsy.
• Possible intestinal bacterial overgrowth resulting in transient hyperammonemia (proposed)

CBC/BIOCHEMISTRY/URINALYSIS

Findings vary with the nature of the liver disease.
• CBC—microcytosis may occur in animals with portosystemic shunts, but may be difficult to determine in the horse; RBC histograms may be useful.
• Biochemistry—liver enzymes may be normal in animals with portosystemic shunts, but bile acid concentrations as well as ammonia concentrations will be elevated. Usually, other biochemical abnormalities are present, indicating hepatic dysfunction if the liver disease is severe enough to produce hepatic encephalopathy. Finding elevated liver enzymes (SDH, GDH, ALP, GGT, or AST) and hyperbilirubinemia, hypoglycemia (not common), hyper- or hypocholesterolemia, or late hepatic failure, and low BUN support a diagnosis of liver disease.
• Urinalysis—ammonia biurate crystals and low urine specific gravity due to underlying liver disease in some animals

OTHER LABORATORY TESTS

• Measurement of serum bile acid concentrations has largely replaced ammonia assays due to convenience of sampling.
• Coagulation factor production may be decreased in liver failure resulting in prolonged PT and PTT.

IMAGING

Ultrasound evaluation of the liver and portal vessels is advised.

OTHER DIAGNOSTIC PROCEDURES

Hepatic biopsy is often necessary.

PATHOLOGICAL FINDINGS

- Decreased functional hepatic mass; decreased liver size; microhepatica
- Portosystemic shunt
- Degenerative changes of the neurons and supporting cells have been observed in chronically affected animals.

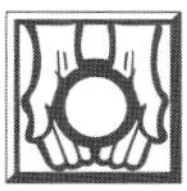

TREATMENT

AIMS OF TREATMENT

Prevent signs and adverse effects of hepatic encephalopathy.

APPROPRIATE HEALTH CARE

Fluid administration is needed to correct dehydration and maintain tissue perfusion. It is important to maintain normal plasma potassium concentrations because low plasma potassium may increase the intracellular movement of ammonia.

NURSING CARE

Given above

ACTIVITY

Restrict activity.

DIET

Feed a very low protein diet, or fast the patient initially, and then institute a protein-restricted diet when the patient is stable.

CLIENT EDUCATION

Discussion of the prognosis with a hepatopathy and related causes

SURGICAL CONSIDERATIONS

Correction of hepatic shunts

MEDICATIONS

DRUG(S) OF CHOICE

- Lactulose is an acidifying agent used to decrease ammonia absorption from the intestine and lower plasma ammonia concentration in equine hyperammonemia. Lactulose acts as a cathartic laxative and maintains ammonia in its nonabsorbable ammonium ion form.
- Antibiotics with a broad spectrum against intestinal flora have been used orally, such as a nonabsorbable aminoglycoside (e.g., neomycin). Metronidazole has been used in companion animals and in horses with acute colitis, but caution should be used with this drug because decreased hepatic clearance also can result in neurologic signs.

CONTRAINDICATIONS

Any drugs that affect the CNS must be used with caution because of the common association of hyperammonemia with hepatic encephalopathy and possibly impaired hepatic metabolism. Barbiturates and benzodiazepam-like drugs are of particular concern.

PRECAUTIONS

Sodium bicarbonate in fluids should be administered slowly, because rapid correction of acidosis may favor intracellular ammonia movement.

POSSIBLE INTERACTIONS

Because of impaired hepatic metabolism, any drugs that inhibit metabolism by the liver or are metabolized by the liver should be used with caution or the dosage should be adjusted.

ALTERNATIVE DRUGS

N/A

FOLLOW-UP

PATIENT MONITORING

Repeated assessment of plasma ammonia can be helpful. Monitoring of serum potassium and glucose is advised in critical patients.

PREVENTION/AVOIDANCE

N/A

POSSIBLE COMPLICATIONS

Inaccuracy is the biggest problem because of the labile nature of ammonia in blood samples. Delay in processing results in false readings of high ammonia concentration.

EXPECTED COURSE AND PROGNOSIS

Guarded prognosis for most causes of hyperammonemia

MISCELLANEOUS

ASSOCIATED CONDITIONS

N/A

AGE-RELATED FACTORS

Congenital hepatic shunts are found in young animals versus acquired shunts that may occur at various ages.

ZOONOTIC POTENTIAL

N/A

PREGNANCY

N/A

SYNONYMS

N/A

SEE ALSO

- Hepatic encephalopathy
- Liver/hepatic diseases
- Hepatic enzyme
- Bile acids

ABBREVIATIONS

- ALP = alkaline phosphatase
- BUN = blood urea nitrogen
- CNS = central nervous system
- GDH = glutamate dehydrogenase
- GGT = γ-glutamyltransferase
- PT = prothrombin time
- PTT = partial thromboplastin time
- SDH = sorbitol dehydrogenase

Suggested Reading

Barton MH, Morris DD. Diseases of the liver. In: Reed SM, Bayly WM, eds. Equine Internal Medicine. Philadelphia: WB Saunders, 1998:713–716.

McGorum BC, Murphy D, Love S, Milne EM. Clinicopathological features of equine primary hepatic disease: a review of 50 cases. Vet Rec 1999;145:134–139.

Peek SF, Divers TJ, Jackson CJ. Hyperammonaemia associated with encephalopathy and abdominal pain without evidence of liver disease in four mature horses. Equine Vet J 1997;29:70–74.

Tennent BC. Hepatic function. In: Kaneko JJ, Harvey JW, Bruss ML, eds. Clinical Biochemistry of Domestic Animals, ed 5. San Diego: Academic Press, 1997:332–334.

Author Claire B. Andreasen

Consulting Editor Kenneth W. Hinchcliff

AMYLASE, LIPASE, AND TRYPSIN

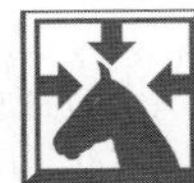

BASICS

DEFINITION

- Serum amylase or lipase concentrations above laboratory reference interval in horses are suggestive of pancreatic disease.
- Pancreatic disease is rare in horses.
- Reference range for serum activity of amylase and lipase are <35 IU/L and <87 IU/L, respectively.
- Amylase and lipase are rarely measured in routine equine serum biochemical profiles.
- Trypsin is released from damaged pancreatic cells.

PATHOPHYSIOLOGY

- Amylase in the blood comes from a number of sources, including the intestinal mucosa, liver, and pancreas.
- Amylase is cleared from the blood by the kidneys, so renal dysfunction could lead to higher concentrations remaining in the blood.
- Damage to pancreatic cells can cause leakage of amylase into the blood or peritoneal fluid, but this is not common in the horse.
- Lipase is derived from the pancreas, gastrointestinal mucosa, and other tissues. Clinical serum assays detect all forms of lipase.
- Although uncommon in the horse, damage to pancreatic cells can cause release of lipase into the blood or peritoneal cavity.
- Panniculitis can result in abnormally high serum activity of amylase and lipase. This disease is often associated with pancreatitis.
- Increased activity of trypsin in blood is a result of leakage from damaged pancreatic cells, usually in horses with colic.

Systems Affected

Pancreas, peritoneum, peripheral adipose tissue

SIGNALMENT

N/A

SIGNS

Varies with underlying cause:

- Pancreatitis—colic, gastric reflux, tachycardia, and signs of hypovolemic shock
- Hyperlipemia—depression, anorexia, and lipemia serum
- Other intestinal diseases—colic, gastric reflux, and tachycardia
- Panniculitis (inflammation of adipose tissue) sometimes evident as colic

CAUSES

- Proximal enteritis
- High intestinal obstructions
- Intestinal mucosal damage
- Hyperlipemia
- Cortisol administration
- Heparin-induced lipoprotein lipase activity
- Obstruction to common bile and pancreatic duct
- Renal disease with renal failure
- Pancreatitis
- Panniculitis

RISK FACTORS

Unknown other than risk factors for colic

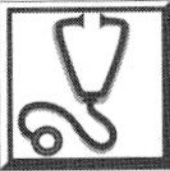

DIAGNOSIS

DIFFERENTIAL DIAGNOSIS

- Colic with small bowel distention should lead a clinician to suspect inflammation or obstruction of the small intestine rather than pancreatic inflammation, although colic and ileus can be caused by peritonitis secondary to pancreatitis.
- In a pony or miniature horse, hyperlipemia should be considered.

LABORATORY FINDINGS

Drugs That May Alter Lab Results

N/A

Disorders That May Alter Lab Results

- Hemolysis inhibits lipase activity.
- Lipemia falsely decreases serum lipase activity measured by kinetic assays.

Valid If Run in Human Lab?

Not unless horse reference intervals are available

CBC/BIOCHEMISTRY/URINALYSIS

- Peritoneal fluid amylase and lipase activities are usually less than those in blood except in pancreatitis.
- GGT is concentrated in the pancreas as well as the liver, so increased serum activity could mean pancreatitis as well as hepatitis or cholestasis, or elevations of GGT could be secondary to the proximity of the bile duct to an inflamed pancreatic duct.

OTHER LABORATORY TESTS

- Serum triglycerides above 500 mg/dL would mean hyperlipemia and expected increases in serum lipase or lipoprotein lipase activity.
- Nonesterified fatty acid (NEFA) concentrations >0.5 mEq/L could mean hyperlipemia due to fat mobilization and expected increases in serum lipase activity.
- Urine GGT:creatinine ratio above 25–50 would indicate renal tubular damage and possible impairment of renal excretion of amylase or lipase.
- Abdominocentesis has been used for cytology to define inflammation and for chemical comparisons of peritoneal amylase and lipase concentrations to serum concentrations. Finding peritoneal fluid concentrations above serum concentrations can be indicative of pancreatitis, but this also can be a nonspecific finding in peritonitis/serositis.

DIAGNOSTIC PROCEDURES

Exploratory celiotomy may be indicated in cases of colic with undiagnosed causes of continued pain or indications of small intestinal obstruction. Abdominal fluid analysis should precede this invasive procedure.

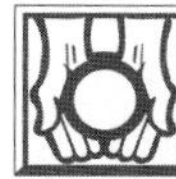

TREATMENT

Treatment varies with the underlying cause. There is no specific treatment for pancreatitis in horses.

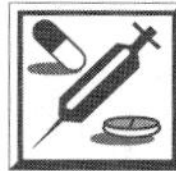

MEDICATIONS

As appropriate for underlying disease

FOLLOW-UP

PATIENT MONITORING

- Repeat blood and peritoneal fluid activity of amylase, lipase, and typsin.
- Observe every hour for signs of colic.

POSSIBLE COMPLICATIONS

- Small intestinal obstruction, pancreatitis, and hyperlipemia can cause death.
- Distention of the stomach may cause rupture and death due to peritonitis.
- Leakage of amylase and lipase into the peritoneal cavity can induce nonseptic peritonitis.

MISCELLANEOUS

SEE ALSO

- Colic
- Gastric reflux

ABBREVIATIONS

- GGT = γ-glutamyltransferase
- NEFA = nonesterified fatty acid

Suggested Reading

Grulke S, Gangl M, Deby-Dupont G, *et al.* Plasma trypsin level in horses suffering from acute intestinal obstruction. Vet J 2002:63;283–291.

Parry BW, Crisman MV. Serum and peritoneal fluid amylase and lipase reference values in horses. Equine Vet J 1991;23:390–391.

Waitt LH, Cebra CK, Tornquist SJ, *et al.* Panniculitis in a horse with pancreatitis and pancreatic fibrosis. J Vet. Diagn Invest 2003:18;405–408.

The author and editor wishe to acknowledge the contribution to this chapter of Erwin G. Pearson, author in the previous edition.

Author Kenneth W. Hinchcliff
Consulting Editor Kenneth W. Hinchcliff

ANAEROBIC BACTERIAL INFECTIONS

BASICS

DEFINITION

Anaerobic bacterial infections are caused by organisms that live and grow in the absence of molecular oxygen. Anaerobic bacteria are classified as either facultative or obligate, the former growing with or without oxygen. The anaerobic infections discussed here are caused by obligate anaerobic organisms.

PATHOPHYSIOLOGY

Dermal and mucosal surfaces serve as protective barriers to infection. Normal flora and commensal bacteria contribute to this protective barrier. A breach in this protective barrier allows normal flora or commensal bacteria to gain access and potentially allows pathogenic infection to become established. There is a delicate balance between normal flora and commensal bacteria. When this balance is upset, commensal bacteria may become pathogenic or allow normally sterile sites to become contaminated. In other cases, contamination of a wound or an injection site by environmental organisms may lead to infection. Infectious challenge is dependent on inoculum size, virulence of the organism, and microbial resistance. Anaerobic organisms establish invasion through virulence factors, and release of enzymes and toxins; these result in tissue destruction and provide protection from the host's defenses. Anaerobic infections develop primarily in body sites where there is low oxygen tension, a low redox potential, or both.

SYSTEMS AFFECTED

Upper Respiratory Tract

• Apical abscesses • Sinusitis • Pharyngeal abscesses

Lower Respiratory Tract

- Pneumonia
- Pulmonary abscesses
- Pleuropneumonia
- Pleuritis

Gastrointestinal System

- Peritonitis
- Abdominal abscesses
- Enteritis
- Colitis

Musculoskeletal System

- Soft-tissue abscesses
- Foot abscesses
- Thrush
- Canker
- Osteomyelitis
- Sequestrums
- Septic arthritis
- Tenosynovitis
- Clostridial myonecrosis

Neuromuscular System

- Botulism
- Tetanus

Vascular System

- Omphalophlebitis/Omphalitis
- Thrombophlebitis

Hematopoietic System

- Septicemia

Reproductive System

- Metritis

INCIDENCE/PREVALENCE

Dependent on the organism, body system infected, and how early the infection is noted and treatment is instituted

GEOGRAPHIC DISTRIBUTION

Worldwide distribution

SIGNALMENT

Any age, breed, and sex can be affected.

SIGNS

Signs are variable depending on what system is involved and which organism is involved.

Upper Respiratory Tract

- Nasal discharge
- Facial swelling and crepitation
- Malodorous exudates

Lower Respiratory Tract

- Cough
- Nasal discharge
- Malodorous breath, sputum, pleural fluid
- Fever
- Inappetance
- Abnormal lung sounds
- Lethargy

Gastrointestinal System

- Abdominal discomfort
- Fever
- Diarrhea
- Inappetance
- Reflux

Musculoskeletal System

- Swollen and painful muscles or joints
- Lameness
- Fever
- Crepitation over swollen muscles

Neuromuscular System

- Stiffness and rigid posture
- Flashing third eyelid
- Trismus (lockjaw)
- Convulsions
- Dysphagia
- Loss of muscle tone leading to recumbency
- Ataxia

Vascular System

- Swollen and painful umbilicus
- Fever
- Lethargy
- Inappetance
- Swollen, hard, painful veins

Hematopoietic System

- Fever
- Depression
- Tachycardia, +/− arrhythmias
- Tachypnea, +/− dyspnea
- Mucous membrane alterations
- Laminitis
- Abdominal discomfort

Reproductive System

- Vaginal discharge
- Fever
- Lethargy
- Endotoxemia

CAUSES *(most common)*

Upper Respiratory Tract

- *Bacteroides* spp.
- *Fusobacterium* spp.
- *Peptostreptococcus* spp.

Lower Respiratory Tract

- *Bacteroides* spp.
- *Clostridium* spp.
- *Eubacterium lentum*
- *Peptostreptococcus* spp.

Gastrointestinal System

- Peritonitis/abdominal abscesses—*Bacteroides* spp., *Fusobacterium* spp., *Peptostreptococcus* spp.
- Enteritis/colitis—*Clostridium* spp. and *Bacteroides* spp.

Musculoskeletal System

- Soft-tissue/foot abscesses and canker—*Bacteroides* spp. and *Fusobacterium necrophorum*
- Osteomyelitis/sequestrums—*Clostridium* spp.
- Septic arthritis/tenosynovitis—*Clostridium* and *Bacteroides* spp.
- Myonecrosis—*Clostridium* spp.

Neuromuscular System

- Botulism—*Clostridium botulinum*
- Tetanus—*Clostridium tetani*

Vascular System

- *Bacteroides fragilis, Propionibacterium acnes, Peptostreptococcus magnus,* and/or *Clostridium septicum*

Hematopoietic System

- *Clostridium septicum*

Reproductive System

- *Bacteroides fragilis, Peptococcus, Peptostreptococcus, and Fusobacterium* spp.

RISK FACTORS

Concurrent diseases, corticosteroid therapy, antibiotic therapy, immunosuppression, leukopenia, tissue anoxia, prior or concurrent aerobic infections, or the presence of a foreign body may also predispose the horse to anaerobic infections.

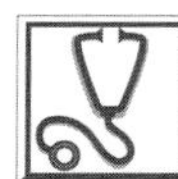

DIAGNOSIS

DIFFERENTIAL DIAGNOSIS

Upper Respiratory Tract

- Aerobic infection (*Streptococcus* spp., *Staphylococcus* spp.)
- Fungal infection (*Cryptococcus neoformans, Coccidioides immitis*)
- Granuloma
- Neoplasia (anaerobes may proliferate in necrotic neoplastic tissues)

Lower Respiratory Tract
• Aerobic infection (*Streptococcus* spp., *Staphylococcus* spp., *Escherichia coli, Klebsiella, Pasturella, Bordetella* spp.)
• Fungal infection (*Coccidioides, Cryptococcus, Histoplasma, Aspergillus, Candida* spp.)
• *Mycoplasma* infection
• Thoracic trauma
• Esophageal rupture
• Neoplasia—Primary (rare), metastatic (more common)

Gastrointestinal System
• Peritonitis—Aerobic infection (*Streptococcus* spp., *E. coli)*, neoplasia,
• Abdominal abscesses—Aerobic infection (*Streptococcus* spp., *Rhodococcus equi, Corynebacterium pseudotuberculosis)*, neoplasia, granuloma
• Enteritis/colitis—*Salmonella* spp., Potomac horse fever, idiopathic, parasitic, antibiotic-associated, NSAID drug toxicity, fungal infection

Musculoskeletal System
• Aerobic infection (*Staphylococcus aureus, Corynebacterium pseudotuberculosis)*
• Fungal infection
• Neoplasia

Neuromuscular System
• Botulism—Laminitis, myositis/myopathy, exertional rhabdomyolysis, EPM, tick paralysis
• Tetanus—Acute laminitis, hypocalcemic tetany, rabies, HYPP

Vascular System
• Aerobic infection (*Streptococcus* spp., *E. coli, Proteus* spp.)

Hematopoietic System
• Aerobic infection (*Streptococcus* spp., *Staphylococcus* spp., *E. coli, Actinobacillus* spp., *Salmonella* spp., *Klebsiella* spp.)

Reproductive System
• Aerobic infection (*Streptococcus zooepidemicus, E. coli, Klebsiella* spp., *Staphylococcus* spp., *Proteus* spp., *Pseudomonas* spp., *Corynebacterium* spp.)
• Fungal infection (*Candida* spp.)
• Neoplasia

CBC/CHEMISTRY/URINALYSIS
• Inflammatory leukogram
• Hyperfibrinogenemia
• Elevated total protein
• +/− Anemia of chronic disease
• Clinical chemistry is usually normal unless there is secondary systemic involvement or severe disease.

OTHER LABORATORY TESTS
• Direct cytology—All aspirated fluids should be gram stained.
• Anaerobic culture—Aspirates/tissue specimens must be placed in the appropriate anaerobic bacterial transport medium and stored at room temperature with minimal exposure to oxygen.
• Clotting profile
• Fluorescent antibody testing
• Direct immunofluorescence testing

IMAGING
• Radiographs of the affected anatomical region revealing abscessation, fluid line, areas of consolidation, or lytic bone changes
• Sonograms of the affected anatomic region revealing gas echos, fluid, abscessation, areas of consolidation, or masses

OTHER DIAGNOSTIC PROCEDURES
• Fecal cultures
• Bone biopsies
• Identification of toxins or spores in feed, gastrointestinal contents, or serum for botulism (extremely difficult)

PATHOLOGIC FINDINGS
Lesions are characterized by necrotic, edematous, emphysematous, and hyperemic tissues. Neutrophils, monocytes, and macrophages may accumulate in the tissue architecture, with bacteria interspersed.

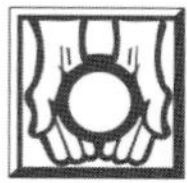

TREATMENT

AIMS OF TREATMENT
Elimination of infection with effective antimicrobial therapy and exposure to oxygen, drainage of purulent exudates, and debridement of necrotic tissue if possible

APPROPRIATE HEALTH CARE
Initial hospitalization for intensive therapy, antimicrobials, and debridement/drainage. Hyperbaric oxygen therapy can be utilized in areas with extensive tissue necrosis. Once stabilized, the patient may return home for continued care.

NURSING CARE
Dependent on severity/duration of infection, body system affected, and causative organism. Care may include staged debridement, frequent hot compress therapy, and/or bandaging. Intensive care of indwelling tubes for constant drainage of body cavities may be required. Supportive care includes intravenous fluids and/or total/partial parenteral nutrition.

ACTIVITY
Most likely decreased or restricted and will depend on the body system affected

DIET
The diet will most likely remain unchanged.

CLIENT EDUCATION
Some cases may be life-threatening depending on the extent of the illness and complications may arise. In cases with severe muscle necrosis requiring debridement or fasciotomies, a cosmetic appearance may not be likely.

SURGICAL CONSIDERATIONS
Surgery may be necessary to perform fasciotomies, to debride necrotic tissue, or to skin graft large areas that sloughed tissue during active infection. Surgery may also be required for the placement of an indwelling catheter to allow for lavage and flushing.

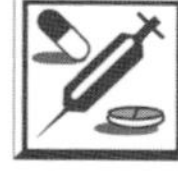

MEDICATIONS

DRUG(S) OF CHOICE

Penicillin
First line of defense against anaerobic infections. Excellent activity against most anaerobic infections, except beta-lactamase producing *Bacteroides*. Preferred drug for clostridial infections. Dose: 22,000–44,000 IU/kg QID IV (aqueous) or BID IM (procaine).

ANAEROBIC BACTERIAL INFECTIONS

Ampicillin

Comparable to penicillin in its spectrum, but it is expensive in some countries, limiting its use to foals. Dose: 25–100 mg/kg IV QID.

Cephalosporins

First-generation cephalosporins are generally less efficacious for anaerobic infections compared to penicillins. Cefoxitin (second generation) kills *Bacteriodes fragilis* but may be used less due to expense. Other cephalosporin activity for anaerobic infections is unpredictable.

Trimethoprim-Sulfonamides (TMS)

TMS is effective against some obligate anaerobes but activity is unpredictable. Dose: 15–30 mg/kg BID PO.

Metronidazole

Consistently effective against obligate anaerobes including *Bacteriodes fragilis,* not effective against facultative anaerobes or aerobes. It is rapidly absorbed after oral administration (bioavailability 75%–85%) and distributes well into synovial fluid, peritoneal fluid, cerebrospinal fluid, and urine, but has poor endometrial concentrations. It is used orally in cases of diarrhea caused by *Clostridium difficile.* It can also be given per rectum to horses that are anorexic or are refluxing; the bioavailability is about 30%. Dose: 15–25 mg/kg PO, IV, or per rectum QID–TID.

Chloramphenicol

All obligate anaerobes are susceptible. It has good tissue penetration into CNS, peritoneal, pleural, and synovial fluids. Absorption decreases with repeated oral administration; the result is lower concentrations with subsequent doses. Dose: 45–60 mg/kg PO TID–QID.

Rifampin

Usually not necessary in most anaerobic infections but it may be useful in polymicrobial infections in walled-off abscesses. Most strains of *Bacteroides* and *Clostridium* are sensitive to rifampin. Dose: 5 mg/kg PO BID.

Tetracyclines

Can be used for anaerobic infections but penicillin-resistant *Bacteroides* spp. are demonstrating tetracycline resistance. Dose: 5–7.5 mg/kg IV BID.

Aminoglycosides

Ineffective against anaerobes due to mechanism of action requiring oxygen activity

CONTRAINDICATIONS

Any drug causing diarrhea or enteritis. Static drugs like chloramphenicol are not recommended for immunocompromised patients.

PRECAUTIONS

Sustained high dose systemic penicillin therapy may have complications including secondary immune-mediated anemia, thrombocytopenia, and procaine reactions. Chloramphenicol can cause the development of aplastic anemia rarely in humans. Oral administration of metronidazole may cause anorexia but resolves when the drug is discontinued.

POSSIBLE INTERACTIONS

Chloramphenicol may affect the metabolism of other drugs. Concurrent administration of cimetidine with metronidazole may decrease the metabolism of metronidazole and increase the likelihood of dose-related side effects.

FOLLOW-UP

PATIENT MONITORING

Response to therapy can be noted by monitoring changes in clinical signs. Hematologic and sonographic evaluations also help to establish the patient's response to therapy.

PREVENTION/AVOIDANCE

Intramuscular injections have been reported to cause severe necrotizing myonecrosis; avoid giving IM injections if possible or monitor injection sites closely after administration. Provide proper and immediate treatment of wounds to help prevent anaerobic infections.

POSSIBLE COMPLICATIONS

The possibility of complications depends on the body system affected and the severity of the disease. Severe infections may result in severe tissue sloughing, laminitis, endotoxemia, or death.

EXPECTED COURSE AND PROGNOSIS

Depends on the body system affected and the severity of the disease

MISCELLANEOUS

ASSOCIATED CONDITIONS

Depends on the body system affected and the severity of the disease

PREGNANCY

Infection of the reproductive tract may result in breeding and conception problems.

ABBREVIATIONS

- EPM = equine protozoal myeloencephalitis
- HYPP = hyperkalemic periodic paralysis
- NSAID = nonsteroidal anti-inflammatory drug

Suggested Reading

Long MT. Mechanisms of establishment and spread of bacterial and fungal infections. In: Reed SM, Bayly WM, Sellon DC, eds. Equine Internal Medicine, ed 2. Philadelphia: WB Saunders, 2004:59–70.

Moore RM. Pathogenesis of obligate anaerobic bacterial infections in horses. Compend Contin Educ Pract Vet 1993;15(2):278–286.

Moore RM. Diagnosis and treatment of obligate anaerobic bacterial infections in horses. Compend Contin Educ Pract Vet 1993;15(7):989–994.

Peek SF, Semrad SD, Perkins GA. Clostridial myonecrosis in horses (37 cases 1985-2000). Equine Vet J 2003;35:86–92.

Wilson DA. Management of severely infected wounds. NAVC 2006;249–251.

Author Shannon B. Graham

Consulting Editors Ashley Boyle and Corinne R. Sweeney

ANAPHYLAXIS

BASICS

OVERVIEW

• An immediate hypersensitivity reaction (type I) where antigen-antibody reactions involve mast cells and basophils • IgE is most commonly involved. • Previous exposure to an antigen (allergen) is required to stimulate antigen-specific IgE synthesis. IgE molecules bind to and sensitize the mast cell/basophil. Subsequent exposure to allergen results in release of pharmacologically active substances that mediate anaphylaxis. • Sensitization occurs ≈10 days after first exposure to the allergen. It can persist for years. • Clinical signs usually occur within seconds-minutes of antigen reexposure. They range from mild inflammatory reactions to severe, life-threatening disorders (anaphylactic shock).

SIGNS

• Exposure to the allergen may occur by ingestion, inhalation, contact with skin, or systemic introduction (e.g., IV injection).
• Clinical signs are related to a species-specific tissue distribution of mast cells and smooth muscle. The lung and GIT are the primary target (shock) organs in the horse; involvement of skin and feet also may occur. • Signs are attributable to the inflammatory mediators, enzymes, and cytokines released from sensitized cells. These dilate blood vessels and increase vascular permeability (erythema, edema, and emphysema), stimulate smooth muscle constriction especially in the lungs and GIT (bronchospasm, dyspnea, diarrhea, and abdominal pain), and stimulate secretion of airway mucus and gastric acid. • Reactions may be localized or systemic. Additional signs include restlessness, excitement, urticaria, pruritus, piloerection, generalized sweating, salivation, lacrimation, tachycardia, laminitis, and cardiac arrhythmia. • Severe dyspnea, systemic hypotension, and anoxia may lead to recumbency, convulsions, and death from asphyxia, shock, or cardiac arrest. Death may occur within 5min but usually occurs in ≈1hr.
• Alternatively, signs may be transient and disappear spontaneously within a few hours.

CAUSES AND RISK FACTORS

• A wide range of antigens may induce anaphylaxis, but repeated parenteral administration of the same biological preparations at high doses increases the risk of inducing severe reactions. • Reactions can occur at any time in the course of administration including, rarely, after the first injection of a drug (e.g., penicillin). • Agents implicated include, but are not limited to, insect venom, vaccines, blood products, thiamine, vitamin E/selenium, anthelmintics, penicillin, trimethoprim-sulfa, chloramphenicol, aminoglycosides, tetracyclines, halothane, thiamylal, and guaifenesin. • Rarely reactions may occur during initial exposure to highly charged or osmotically active agents (e.g., iodinated radiocontrast media, dextran). These perturb mast cell membranes. • The sensitizing agent is frequently not identified.

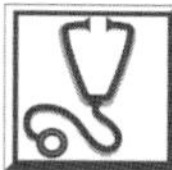

DIAGNOSIS

DIFFERENTIAL DIAGNOSIS

• Clinical signs within a few minutes to hours after injection or reexposure to a foreign antigen is a hallmark of anaphylaxis. Response to treatment may help confirm the diagnosis.
• Acute pneumonia can resemble anaphylaxis, but horses are usually more toxemic with lung changes prominent in ventral lobes compared to widespread involvement with anaphylaxis.
• An inappropriate dose or route of drug administration (such as intracarotid injection) may result in collapse associated with neurological deficits (e.g., blindness, seizures).

CBC/BIOCHEMISTRY/URINALYSIS

Hemoconcentration, leukopenia, thrombocytopenia, hyperkalemia, increases in hepatic and myocardial enzyme activities, and coagulation deficits are reported. Their diagnostic relevance is uncertain.

OTHER LABORATORY TESTS

Provocative intradermal/conjunctival challenge testing with the suspected antigen may help confirm diagnosis (response time ≈20min), but value is questionable due to high rate of false-negatives and risk of inducing anaphylaxis.

PATHOLOGICAL FINDINGS

• Severe, diffuse pulmonary emphysema, and peribronchiolar edema are common at necropsy.
• Widespread petechiation, edema, and extravasation of blood in the wall of the large bowel, subcutaneous edema, congestion of the kidney, spleen, and liver, and evidence of laminitis may be observed.

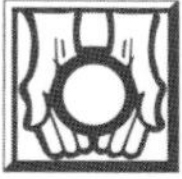

TREATMENT

• Therapeutic goals include reversal of the effects of mediators, prevention of their further release and maintenance of respiratory and cardiovascular function.
• Treatment, if required, should be administered immediately; a few minutes' delay may result in death.
• Identify and remove inciting antigen— if possible.
• Less severe reactions may only warrant monitoring.
• Signs suggestive of anaphylactic shock require aggressive therapy.
• Large-volume fluid therapy is indicated in hypotensive patients.

MEDICATIONS

DRUG(S)

• Epinephrine is the most effective treatment of systemic anaphylaxis/shock. Epinephrine can be given at 0.01–0.02 mg/kg of a 1:1000 dilution [1.0 mg/ml] IM or 0.01 mg/kg of 1:10,000 dilution [0.1 mg/ml] IV.
• Corticosteroids potentiate the effect of epinephrine. Rapid-acting glucocorticoids (prednisolone sodium succinate, 0.25–1.0 mg/kg IV) are recommended in cases of local and systemic anaphylaxis; longer-acting glucocorticoids (dexamethasone, 0.05–0.1 mg/kg IV) are less effective for systemic reactions.
• Antihistamines (tripelennamine hydrochloride 1 mg/kg IM) are in common use but provide variable results due to the presence of mediators other than histamine.
• Atropine is of little value.
• Hypotension refractory to IV fluid and epinephrine therapy may be treated with a dilute dobutamine solution (50 mg in 500mL of 5% dextrose). Administer 1–3 μg/kg/min to effect. Ideally, dobutamine administration requires blood pressure and ECG monitoring.

CONTRAINDICATIONS/POSSIBLE INTERACTIONS

• Epinephrine may cause profound excitement and potentiate myocardial ischemia, increasing the risk of arrhythmia.
• Dobutamine potentiates hypoxemia-induced cardiac arrhythmias.
• Glucocorticoid administration has been associated with laminitis.

FOLLOW-UP

PATIENT MONITORING

• Horses with less severe anaphylactic reactions should be monitored carefully.
• Horses with anaphylactic shock warrant intense therapy and monitoring.
• Continuous blood pressure and cardiac monitoring are recommended to determine efficacy of therapy or worsening of cardiac abnormalities.

PREVENTION/AVOIDANCE

Administration of drugs (especially antibiotics) may result in acute anaphylactic reactions and death. Therefore, caution must be used if there is any suspicion that a horse may be sensitized to these agents.

EXPECTED COURSE AND PROGNOSIS

Variable and will depend on the severity of the reaction, speed of diagnosis, and administration of treatment.

MISCELLANEOUS

SEE ALSO

• Eosinophilia and basophilia
• Blood transfusion reactions

Suggested Reading

Swiderski C. Hypersensitivity disorders in horses. Vet Clin North Am 2000;16:131–151.

Author Jennifer Hodgson
Consulting Editors David Hodgson and Jennifer Hodgson

ANEMIA

BASICS

DEFINITION

A decrease in the erythrocyte content or oxygen-carrying capacity of blood as a consequence of a decrease in PCV, RBC count, and, except in cases of intravascular hemolysis, a decrease in Hb concentration to less than the lower limit of the laboratory reference interval.

PATHOPHYSIOLOGY

- Anemia is not a disease but a hematologic clinical sign that develops when one or more of the following 3 basic pathophysiologic mechanisms is present:
  - Blood loss (internal/external hemorrhage)
  - Increased RBC destruction (intravascular or extravascular hemolysis)
  - Decreased or ineffective RBC production
- Characterization of anemia in horses as regenerative (due to hemorrhage or hemolysis) or nonregenerative (due to decreased/ineffective marrow production) is assessed most accurately by examination of bone marrow aspirates. Serial monitoring of PCV and plasma TP concentration also may be helpful. Evaluation of immature RBC and RBC indices in peripheral blood is unrewarding in horses as equine reticulocytes or nucleated RBCs are rarely released into circulation until mature, even during intense erythropoiesis.
- The circulating RBC mass is extremely labile due to the effects of breed, age, level of activity, and splenic contraction, which can increase the RBC by ≈50%.
- Nonregenerative anemia occurs when the rate of erythropoiesis is insufficient to replace aged RBCs removed by the mononuclear phagocyte system. Nonregenerative anemia usually develops slowly due to the long life span of equine RBCs (≈150 days).
- Mechanisms associated with nonregenerative anemia may include:
  - Diseases that interfere with erythropoiesis (e.g., by shortening erythrocyte life span or decreasing responsiveness to erythropoietin)
  - Deficiency or alterations in specific substances necessary for RBC production or
  - Diseases that damage or displace normal bone marrow elements and affect RBC precursors alone, or affect all marrow precursors (WBCs, RBCs, platelets)

SYSTEMS AFFECTED

- Although dependent on the severity and rate of development of anemia, the decreased oxygen-carrying capacity, the decreased circulating RBC mass, and reduced blood viscosity are the main consequences of anemia.
- Hemic/lymphatic/immune systems
- Cardiovascular and respiratory systems
- Hepatobiliary, renal, musculoskeletal, and GI systems

SIGNALMENT

There is no breed, sex, or age predilection for anemia, although some specific primary diseases that result in anemia are more likely in some types of horses.

SIGNS

General Comments

Anemia generally occurs secondary to another disease. Clinical signs relate to the compensatory mechanisms activated in response to anemia as well as the primary disease process, which often are more prominent.

Historical

- Vary depending on the primary disease process, although frequently are related to trauma with visible hemorrhage, and exposure to oxidant toxins, medications, parasites, or infectious agents.
- Most common presenting complaints are exercise intolerance, signs of depression, and inappetence.

Physical Examination

- May be subclinical in horses with chronic anemia, although exercise may induce exaggerated tachycardia, weakness and reduced performance.
- In acute or severe cases, tachycardia, tachypnea, and low-grade holosystolic heart murmur are present at rest.
- Pale mucous membranes
- Other signs depend on the primary disease process and may include:
  - Icterus, fever and pigmenturia in cases of hemolysis
  - Weight loss, polyuria, and polydipsia in chronic renal failure
  - Weight loss, fever, and lethargy in cases caused by chronic infectious, inflammatory, neoplastic, or immune-mediated processes

CAUSES

Hemorrhage

- External hemorrhage due to trauma, surgery, or external parasites
- Epistaxis due to guttural pouch mycosis, pulmonary abscess, severe pnuemonia, EIPH, ethmoid hematoma, fungal rhinitis, sinusitis, neoplasia, or trauma
- Hemothorax due to trauma, ruptured pulmonary abscess, ruptured great vessel, or aneurysm
- Hematuria due to pyelonephritis, erosive cystitis, urolithiasis, urogenital neoplasia, trauma, or urethral ulceration
- Hemoperitoneum due to trauma, ovarian hemorrhage, mesenteric vessel rupture, aneurysm, or abdominal abscess
- GI hemorrhage due to ulceration (e.g., gastric or duodenal ulcers in foals, NSAID toxicosis), parasites (particularly large strongyles), granulomatous inflammatory disease, neoplasia (e.g., gastric squamous cell carcinoma), or foreign bodies
- Coagulopathy

Hemolysis

- Immune-mediated disease—secondary immune-mediated anemia (e.g., bacterial, viral, or parasitic antigens, neoplasia, or drugs), autoimmune hemolytic anemia, and NI
- Infectious diseases—piroplasmosis (*Babesia caballi* and *Theirleria equi*), ehrlichiosis (*Anaplasma phagocytophila*), and EIA
- Oxidant-induced—wilted red maple leaf, phenothiazine anthelmintics, wild onions and familial methemoglobinemia
- Iatrogenic; hypotonic or hypertonic solutions administered IV
- Other toxicities—intravenous dimethyl sulfoxide, heavy metal toxicosis, bacterial toxins (*Clostridium* sp.), snake envenomation
- Miscellaneous—end-stage hepatic disease, hemolytic uremic syndrome, hemangiosarcoma, and disseminated intravascular coagulation

Nonregenerative Anemia

- Anemia of chronic disease associated with infectious, inflammatory, neoplastic, or endocrine disorders
- Iron deficiency due to chronic hemorrhage (especially GI) and nutritional deficiency (particularly foals)
- Bone marrow failure—myelophthisis, myeloproliferative disease, bone marrow toxins (e.g., phenylbutazone), radiation, immune-mediated, and idiopathic hypoplastic anemia
- Miscellaneous—chronic renal disease, chronic hepatic disease, and recent hemorrhage or hemolysis

RISK FACTORS

- Depends on risk factors for the primary disease process
- Age (e.g., neoplasia, middle uterine artery rupture) and sex (e.g., idiopathic urethral hemorrhage in geldings)
- Any infectious or inflammatory disease
- Foals consuming incompatible colostrum are at risk for NI.
- Inadequate preventative anthelmintic use or long-term high-dose phenylbutazone administration
- Geographical location for exposure to infectious agents or toxic plants

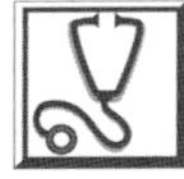

DIAGNOSIS

DIFFERENTIAL DIAGNOSIS

- Differentiation of the primary disease causing anemia should be the focus of investigations.
- Initial investigations should focus on identifying the basic mechanisms (see Causes) involved using historical, clinical, hematologic and biochemical findings.
- When onset of clinical signs is sudden, or if there is a history of trauma, severe external or internal hemorrhage or severe hemolysis should be suspected.
- Chronic nonregenerative anemia secondary to infectious, inflammatory, or neoplastic conditions usually is indicated when there is fever, weight loss, and dramatic increases in heart and respiratory rates if the horse is subjected to exercise or stress.
- Laboratory error due to insufficient mixing of samples, delay in analysis of samples. or samples left in hot conditions (hemolysis) may result in a falsely low PCV or RBC count and falsely high MCH and MCHC.

CBC/BIOCHEMISTRY/URINALYSIS

- PCV, total RBC count, and (except in cases of intravascular hemolysis) Hb concentrations below the lower limit of reference intervals.
- Reticulocytes, nucleated RBCs, Howell-Jolly bodies, polychromasia, and anisocytosis are

rarely observed in horses with regenerative anemia and RBC indices are less useful for diagnosis or classification of anemia.
- A moderate increase in MCV (hemolytic anemia) and RDW (hemorrhagic anemia) may occur 2–3 weeks after onset of regenerative anemia. Additionally, increased MCH values may indicate presence of free Hb and hemolysis and decreased MCH, MCHC, and MCV may indicate iron deficiency anemia.
- Heinz bodies may be observed near the cellular margins of RBCs stained with New Methylene Blue in horses with hemolytic anemia due to oxidative injury.
- Spherocytosis, indicative of immune-mediated hemolytic anemia, may be difficult to detect in equine blood smears due to the small size and lack of central pallor of normal RBCs. In addition, rouleaux formation of normal equine RBCs may complicate identication of autoagglutination in cases of immune-mediated hemolytic anemia.
- Neoplastic cells may be observed in blood smears of horses with myeloproliferative disorders.
- Severe neutropenia and thrombocytopenia may be observed in horses with myelophthisis.
- Horses with blood loss usually have a concomitant decrease in PCV and plasma TP, whereas horses with hemolytic anemia usually have decreased PCV, normal plasma TP and marked increases in serum total direct bilirubin concentration with normal liver enzymes.
- Horses with nonregenerative anemia due to inadequate erythropoiesis usually have decreased PCV, normal or increased TP (due to increased globulin and fibrinogen concentrations), and an inflammatory leukogram.
- Bilirubinuria or hemoglobinuria may occur with some hemolytic disorders.
- Isosthenuria in horses with chronic renal failure

OTHER LABORATORY TESTS

- Positive direct Coombs test is evidence for immune-mediated hemolytic anemia.
- Blood diluted with saline (1:4) aids in differentiating erythrocyte autoagglutination from normal rouleaux formation in horses with immune-mediated hemolytic anemia.
- Serum iron concentration usually is increased, total iron-binding capacity usually decreased and storage iron usually increased in horses with anemia of chronic disease.
- Serum iron concentration, percentage saturation of transferrin, and storage iron usually are decreased, while total iron-binding capacity usually is increased in iron deficiency anemia.
- Coggins test or C-ELISA test for diagnosis of EIA
- Serology for *Babesia, Theileria* or *A. phagocytophila.*
- Identification of organisms in blood smears

IMAGING

- As indicated to diagnose underlying disease processes
- Ultrasonography or radiography may assist in detecting thoracic or abdominal hemorrhage.

OTHER DIAGNOSTIC PROCEDURES

- Bone marrow aspiration or core biopsy may demonstrate increased erythropoiesis and a decreased myeloid-to-erythroid (M:E) ratio in horses with regenerative anemia or may reveal decreased erythropoiesis and an increased M:E ratio with nonregenerative anemia. Infiltration with abnormal cell types may be observed in myelodysplasia or myeloproliferative disorders.
- Abdominocentesis or thoracocentesis to detect internal hemorrhage
- Fecal occult blood to detect GI hemorrhage. However, this test lacks sensitivity and specificity.
- Endoscopy to assist in detecting respiratory or GI hemorrhage

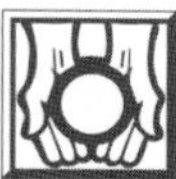

TREATMENT

AIMS OF TREATMENT

The major aims of therapy in horses with anemia are to identify and eliminate the primary cause, provide nursing care, ensure adequate tissue perfusion, and administer blood transfusions if indicated.

APPROPRIATE HEALTH CARE

- Inpatient medical management may be necessary depending on severity and rapidity of onset of anemia and underlying disease condition.
- Cross-matched whole blood or packed RBC transfusion is recommended if PCV decreases to <0.08–0.12 L/L (<8%–12%).
- Large-volume, isotonic (e.g., lactated Ringer's solution) or small-volume hypertonic saline (7% NaCl) fluid therapy if patient has signs of hemorrhagic shock

NURSING CARE

- Close monitoring of vital signs, serial determination of PCV and TP, and adjustment of rate are essential in horses receiving fluid therapy.
- Monitor horses for renal failure induced by hemoglobinuria or hypoxia and for laminitis.

DIET

- Ensure access to oxidative plant toxins is eliminated.
- Oral iron supplementation in horses with confirmed iron deficiency anemia. However, for horses with external blood loss, iron supplementation is rarely required because most diets are rich in this element.

SURGICAL CONSIDERATIONS

May be indicated in horses with significant uncontrolled internal hemorrhage, although these horses have a high anesthetic risk.

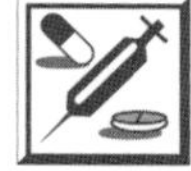

MEDICATIONS

DRUG(S) OF CHOICE

Specific therapy indicated for the primary underlying disease process

PRECAUTIONS

- Severe reactions to blood transfusions may occur and necessitate careful monitoring and prompt therapy (see Blood Transfusion Reactions).
- Hypertonic saline should be used with caution in horses with uncontrolled bleeding as it may cause increased blood loss.
- Corticosteroids should be used with caution in horses with suspected chronic infectious condition.
- Parenteral administration of iron formulations is not recommended because iron deficiency is extremely rare and there is the possibility of serious adverse reactions.

FOLLOW-UP

PATIENT MONITORING

Monitor PCV to assess regenerative responses. PCV should increase by an average of 0.5%–1% per day within 3–5 days of an acute hemorrhagic or hemolytic episode.

EXPECTED COURSE AND PROGNOSIS

Highly dependent upon the cause, severity, and rapidity of onset

MISCELLANEOUS

SEE ALSO

- Hemorrhage, acute
- Hemorrhage, chronic
- Myeloproliferative diseases
- Blood transfusion reactions

ABBREVIATIONS

- EIA = equine infectious anemia
- EIPH = exercise-induced pulmonary hemorrhage
- GI = gastrointestinal
- Hb = hemoglobin
- IV = intravenous
- MCH = mean cell hemoglobin
- MCHC = mean cell hemoglobin concentration
- MCV = mean cell volume
- NI = neonatal isoerythrolysis
- NSAID = non-steroidal anti-inflammatory drug
- PCV = packed cell volume
- RDW = red cell distribution width
- RBC = red blood cell
- TP = total protein
- WBC = white blood cell

Suggested Reading

Hurcombe SD, Mudge MC, Hinchcliff KW. Clinical and clinicopathologic variables in adult horses receiving blood transfusions: 31 cases (1999–2005). J Am Vet Med Assoc 2007;231;267–274.

Malikides N, Hodgson DH, Rose RJ. Hemolymphatic system. In: Rose RJ, Hodgson DR, eds. Manual of Equine Practice, ed 2. Philadelphia: WB Saunders, 2000:451–473.

Sellon DC. Disorders of the hematopoietic system. In: Reed SM, Bayly WM, Sellon DC, eds. Equine Internal Medicine. St Louis: WB Saunders, 2004:721–768.

Author Nicholas Malikides
Consulting Editors Jennifer Hodgson and David Hodgson

ANEMIA, PURE RED CELL APLASIA

BASICS

OVERVIEW

• Pure red cell aplasia is characterized by selective reduction or hypoplasia of erythroid precursors in the bone marrow resulting in development of a nonregenerative anemia. The white cell (granulocytic) and platelet (megakaryocytic) cell precursors are not affected (as they are in aplastic anemia/pancytopenia).
• In horses, pure red cell aplasia has been reported secondary to repeated doses of rhEPO.
• Primary pure red cell aplasia, described in a number of case reports in dogs and cats and considered to be an immune-mediated disorder responsive to treatment with corticosteroids and/or lymphocytotoxic drugs, has not been reported in horses.

SIGNALMENT

Most commonly this anemia is reported in performance horses such as racing Standardbreds and Thoroughbreds.

SIGNS

• Can occur in the absence of other systemic disease
• Signs depend on the severity and duration of anemia and may consist of poor performance, weight loss, signs of depression, inappetence, weakness, mucous membrane pallor, and tachycardia and polypnea (exaggerated when horses subjected to stress).
• Prolonged or severe nonregenerative anemia may cause tissue hypoxia resulting in cardiac, hepatic, and renal dysfunction and can be life-threatening.

CAUSES AND RISK FACTORS

• The strongest risk factor, and likely cause, of the disorder is repeated administration of rhEPO to race horses in order to increase total red cell mass and oxygen-carrying capacity with the aim of enhancing athletic performance.
• Although the mechanism for erythroid hypoplasia is unclear in this syndrome, the recombinant hormone may induce production of anti-rhEPO antibodies that bind endogenous equine erythropoietin, preventing the latter hormone from stimulating RBC differentiation and multiplication in bone marrow.
• Increased frequency of exposure may lead to an exaggerated immune response and more severe clinical signs.

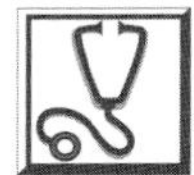

DIAGNOSIS

DIFFERENTIAL DIAGNOSIS

Other Causes of Inadequate Erythropoiesis

• Anemia of chronic disease associated with infectious, inflammatory, or neoplastic disorders. In general, these disorders also result in leukocytosis and elevated fibrinogen concentrations.
• Folate deficiency after treatment of EPM with antifolate drugs, which, paradoxically, occurs in horses administered oral folic acid while receiving antifolate drugs. Diagnosis of EPM and exposure to these drugs easily distinguishes this from pure red cell aplasia.
• Aplastic anemia. Granulocytic and megakaryocytic stem cell lines in bone marrow also fail to undergo differentiation resulting in generalized marrow hypoplasia and peripheral pancytopenia.
• Primary myelophthisic disease may cause anemia in the presence of leukopenia or thrombocytopenia. Because the life span of platelets and WBCs is shorter than that of RBCs, clinical signs of thrombocytopenic hemorrhage, infection, and fever typically precede those of anemia.
• Erythropoietin deficiency from chronic renal failure. Signs specifically referable to the renal system will also be present (e.g., polyuria, polydipsia, renal azotemia, reduced urine concentrating ability).

Other Causes of Anemia

• Chronic EIA may also cause significant bone marrow suppression. These horses are sero- or virus-positive for EIAV.
• Regenerative anemia caused by external or internal hemorrhage and infectious (e.g., low-grade equine piroplasmosis, ehrlichiosis), immune-mediated (e.g., immune-mediated hemolytic anemia and its various causes), or toxic (e.g., oxidant-induced) hemolysis may be differentiated from pure red cell aplasia by the presence of icterus, increased bilirubin concentrations, bilirubinuria, and decreased bone marrow M:E ratios.
• Iron deficiency anemia secondary to chronic hemorrhage. Measurement of decreased serum ferritin concentrations can be used to distinguish this condition from pure red cell aplasia.

CBC/BIOCHEMISTRY/URINALYSIS

• Anemia, with PCV 0.16 L/L (16%) or below
• Normal WBC count, platelet numbers and plasma fibrinogen concentrations
• Normal urinalysis

OTHER LABORATORY TESTS

- Reported cases have demonstrated increased serum iron and serum ferritin concentrations.
- Negative Coggins test for EIA and negative Coombs test for immune-mediated hemolytic anemia
- Bone marrow aspiration demonstrates an increased M:E ratio and erythroid hypoplasia, confirming nonregenerative anemia.
- Serum from affected horses may inhibit rhEPO-induced proliferation of erythroid progenitors in vitro.
- Other diagnostic tests appropriate to rule out other disorders on the differential diagnostic list

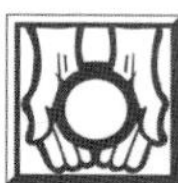

TREATMENT

- Avoid further rhEPO administration.
- Blood transfusion from a cross-matched donor is warranted if anemia is severe (< 8–12%) and there are clinical signs of tissue hypoxia (e.g. tachypnea, tachycardia, weak pulse pressure, weakness).

MEDICATIONS

DRUG(S) OF CHOICE

Dexamethasone (0.05 mg/kg once daily) has been used to treat horses with pure red cell aplasia, although efficacy is unproven. The dose should be adjusted or discontinued depending on a favorable or negative response, respectively.

CONTRAINDICATIONS/POSSIBLE INTERACTIONS

Avoid iron supplementation, because the iron binding-capacity of the serum may be exceeded, leading to hepatic necrosis.

FOLLOW-UP

PATIENT MONITORING

- Monitor the degree of anemia with serial PCV measurements over several weeks to months.
- Some horses are nonresponsive and die despite multiple transfusions and steroid administration, whereas others recover completely.

MISCELLANEOUS

SEE ALSO

- Anemia
- Pancytopenia

ABBREVIATIONS

- EIAV = equine infectious anemia virus
- EPM = equine protozoal myeloencephalitis
- M:E = myeloid:erythroid
- PCV = packed cell volume
- RBC = red blood cell
- rhEPO = recombinant human erythropoietin

Suggested Reading

Piercy RJ, Swardson CJ, Hinchcliff KW. Erythroid hypoplasia and anemia following administration of recombinant human erythropoietin to two horses. J Am Vet Med Assoc 1998;212:244–247.

Piercy RJ, Hinchcliff KW, Reed SM. Folate deficiency during treatment with orally administered folic acid, sulfadiazine and pyrimethamine in a horse with suspected equine protozoal myeloencephalopathy. Equine Vet J 2002:34;311–316.

Woods PR, Campbell G, Cowell RL. Nonregenerative anemia associated with administration of recombinant human erythropoietin to a thoroughbred racehorse. Equine Vet J 1997;29:326–328.

Author Nicholas Malikides

Consulting Editors Jennifer Hodgson and David Hodgson

ANEMIA, HEINZ BODY

BASICS

DEFINITION

• Acute or chronic hemolytic anemia following exposure to agents that oxidize and denature RBC hemoglobin.
• Heme-depleted hemoglobin aggregates onto RBC membranes to form Heinz bodies, resulting in cells more prone to lysis and removal from the circulation by intravascular hemolysis or via the RES (also called mononuclear phagocytic system).

PATHOPHYSIOLOGY

• Exposure of RBCs to oxidant toxins, drugs, or chemicals results in oxidation of sulfhydryl groups and formation of disulfide linkages in the protein component of the hemoglobin molecule.
• The denatured or heme-depleted hemoglobin precipitates to form Heinz bodies, which attach to the RBC membrane and cause increased cell fragility with resultant intravascular hemolysis, or cause deformability changes with subsequent premature RBC removal by the spleen (extravascular hemolysis).
• Many of these toxins also cause methemoglobin formation. This results from ferrous iron (Fe^{2+}) in the hemoglobin molecule being oxidized to the ferric form (Fe^{3+}). Methemoglobin cannot transport oxygen, resulting in tissue hypoxia.
• Heinz body hemolytic anemia and methemoglobinemia may occur solely, or in combination (the latter producing a more severe clinical syndrome) as a consequence of an oxidant insult.

SYSTEMS AFFECTED

• The systems affected by Heinz body anemia are dependent on the severity and rate of development of the hemolytic anemia.
• Hemic/lymphatic/immune system; regenerative anemia is observed and may result in marked RBC hyperplasia in the bone marrow and splenomegaly. Pyrexia may result from release of hemoglobin and other end products of RBC breakdown.
• Cardiovascular and respiratory systems may be involved resulting in increased heart and respiratory rates, a holosystolic heart murmur, and pallor of mucous membranes.
• Renal system involvement can occur when there is significant intravascular hemolysis with hemoglobinemia causing pigment nephropathy and acute renal failure.
• Hepatobiliary system; hemolytic anemia can result in hyperbilirubinemia and icterus, while hypoxia may result in hepatocellular damage.
• GIT involvement can occur due to hypoxic damage to intestines. This may result in motility disorders, colic or diarrhea.
• Musculoskeletal system involvement can occur due to hypoxic damage to laminae, and shock from severe acute hemorrhage may result in laminitis.

INCIDENCE/PREVALENCE

• No incidence or prevalence data currently is available for oxidant-induced hemolytic anemia in horses.
• Horses with red maple leaf toxicosis have a reported case fatality rate of 30 – 40%.

GEOGRAPHIC DISTRIBUTION

• *Acer rubrum* (red maple) is a common tree in the eastern United States.

SIGNALMENT

• Can occur in horses of any breed, age or sex.

SIGNS

Historical Findings

• Access to wilted or dried leaves or bark of red maple (*A. rubrum*) or other oxidative toxins (e.g. phenothiazine, wild onions). Dried red maple leaves may remain toxic for as long as 30 days.
• Sudden onset of lethargy, inappetence and signs of depression are common presenting signs.
• May result in acute, apparently unexplained death.

Physical Examination Findings

• Signs of anemia including exercise intolerance, weakness, pale or icteric mucous membranes, tachypnea, tachycardia, or holosystolic heart murmur.
• Brown coloration of mucous membranes, serum/plasma or urine in horses with significant methemoglobin formation (generally from wilted red maple leaf intoxication).
• Occasionally affected horses are febrile.
• Oliguria or polyuria due to acute, pigment-induced renal failure.
• Discolored urine from hemoglobinuria.
• Rectal examination may reveal an enlarged spleen.
• Severely affected horses may become debilitated and (sudden) death may occur.

CAUSES

• Ingestion of wilted or dried red maple leaves or bark.
• Ingestion of wild or domestic onions.
• Phenothiazine toxicity (usually through access to ruminant supplements or salt blocks that contain phenothiazine)

RISK FACTORS

• Exposure to toxins (e.g., wilted or dried [not fresh] red maple leaves, onions)
• Possibly higher risk with ingestion of wilted red maple leaves in autumn compared to spring
• Poorly conditioned horses may be at greater risk of phenothiazine toxicosis
• Horses are innately sensitive to oxidant toxins due to a poorly developed protective mechanism of equine RBC to reverse the natural processes of hemoglobin oxidation (due to the large oxygen load it carries).

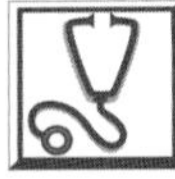

DIAGNOSIS

DIFFERENTIAL DIAGNOSIS

• Other diseases causing anemia must be differentiated from Heinz body hemolytic anemia.
• Hemorrhage is usually evident from history. Physical examination findings may indicate thoracic or abdominal disease.
• Horses with EIA will have a positive Coggins or C-ELISA test.
• Horses with piroplasmosis may have intracellular organisms on Giemsa or New Methylene Blue stained blood smears and/or be seropositive or seroconvert on convalescent titer.
• Horses with granulocytic ehrlichiosis may have granular inclusion bodies in the cytoplasm of neutrophils in Giems stained blood smears and/or be seropositive or seroconvert on convalescent titer.
• Horses with immune-mediated hemolytic anemia will have a positive Coombs test. This test gives a negative result in Heinz body anemia.
• Other causes of hemolytic anemia such as envenomation and heavy metal toxicosis (e.g. chronic consumption of lead, copper or selenium) must be differentiated based on history of exposure.
• Horses with chronic inflammatory, infectious or neoplastic disorders may have anemia, e.g. lymphosarcoma (usually a more chronic history, often including weight loss or organ-specific clinical signs) or purpura hemorrhagica (usually a history of exposure to antigens of *Streptococcus equi* or other respiratory pathogens).
• Familial methemoglobinemia is a hereditary disorder described in Standardbreds.
• Nitrate/nitrite toxicity resulting in methemoglobinemia and anemia can be differentiated based on history of exposure.

CBC/BIOCHEMISTRY/URINALYSIS

• Mild to severe anemia; PCV is often <0.20 L/L (<20%).
• Eccentrocytes, RBC fragments and anisocytosis may be observed on direct blood smears.
• Neutrophilic leukocytosis may be present.
• Increased MCH indicates hemoglobinemia and the presence of intravascular hemolysis.
• Serum chemistry abnormalities may include increased total and indirect bilirubin, increased BUN and creatinine concentrations (in horses with hemoglobinuric nephrosis) and increased serum hepatic enzyme activity (reflecting hepatic hypoxia).
• Results of urinalysis may include bilirubinuria, hemoglobinuria (no microscopic hematuria), methemogobinuria and proteinuria.

OTHER LABORATORY TESTS

• Heinz bodies can be visualized using a blood smear stained with New Methylene Blue. They appear as bluish-green, oval to serrated, refractile granules located near the RBC margin or protruding from the cell.
• Negative direct antiglobulin (Coombs) test.
• Increased RBC osmotic fragility.
• Bone marrow aspiration may reveal a regenerative response and increased erythropoiesis is indicated with an M:E ratio <0.5.
• Blood methemoglobin concentration if mucous membranes or urine are brown-tinged. The normal value is ≤1.77% of total hemoglobin. Affected horses may have methemoglobin concentrations >40% total hemoglobin.

IMAGING

• Splenic/hepatic ultrasonography may be used to detect splenic/hepatic enlargement, which may appear hyperechoic or hypoechoic. There may be some loss of architecture due to increased fluid component.

OTHER DIAGNOSTIC PROCEDURES

• A thorough diagnostic workup should be undertaken to rule out other causes of hemolytic anemia.

PATHOLOGICAL FINDINGS

• Pale or icteric tissues
• Enlarged liver and spleen and severe, diffuse congestion of the kidneys
• If chronic, possible signs of congestive heart failure include pulmonary embolism, pulmonary edema, cardiomegaly, or hepatic congestion.
• Histopathologic lesions might include renal tubular nephrosis with hemoglobin casts, centrilobular hepatic degeneration and necrosis, and phagocytized RBCs and hemosiderin in the spleen and liver.

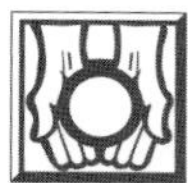

TREATMENT

AIMS OF TREATMENT

• Treatment of Heinz body hemolytic anemia involves identification and removal of the oxidant source and provision of supportive care.

APPROPRIATE HEALTH CARE

• Even if several days have elapsed since exposure to the oxidant, activated charcoal (8–24 mg/kg PO via nasogastric intubation) should be administered to reduce further absorption of toxin.
• In-hospital medical management may be necessary depending on severity and rapidity of onset of the anemia.
• Balanced IV fluid therapy with isotonic crystalloid solutions to prevent hemoglobin-induced nephropathy and promote diuresis.
• Cross-matched blood transfusion if PCV decreases to < 8–12%, or if there is persistent tachycardia, tachypnea, prolonged CRT, mucous membrane pallor and weak pulse pressure or a poor response to isotonic fluid therapy.
• Oxygen therapy may be useful but often is ineffective if hemoglobin oxygen-carrying capacity is too low.

NURSING CARE

• Close monitoring of catheter asepsis, vital signs, fluid rates (to avoid hemodilution) and blood hematology and clinical chemistry are indicated and likely aid recovery.
• Concomitant monitoring for renal failure induced by hemoglobinuria or hypoxia and for laminitis also is necessary.

ACTIVITY

• Minimize activity and stress.
• No forced exercise

DIET

• Provide the horse with a balanced diet, including good-quality hay and grain.
• Fresh water should be available *ad libitum*.

CLIENT EDUCATION

• The hazards of exposure to wilted red maple leaves (including red maple hybrids) should be explained and suggestions given concerning housing and removal of branches blown down in storms or cut down in areas where horses may have access to them.

MEDICATIONS

DRUG(S)

• There is no specific medicinal treatment for Heinz body anemia and treatment is mainly supportive.
• Along with administration of isotonic IV fluids for pigment-induced nephropathy, furosemide or dopamine may be indicated in cases with oliguria or anuria.
• Dexamethasone (0.05–0.1 mg/kg IV q12–24 h) may help to stabilize cellular membranes and decrease phagocytosis of damaged RBCs.

CONTRAINDICATIONS

• Use of Methylene Blue or other reductive therapy may be detrimental, because these agents may enhance Heinz body formation.

ALTERNATIVE DRUGS

• Vitamin C or ascorbic acid (30 mg/kg twice daily, diluted in IV fluids) may be used as antioxidant therapy in cases involving methemoglobin-associated conditions although there is no strong evidence of efficacy.

FOLLOW-UP

PATIENT MONITORING

• Serial determination of PCV should be performed to assess the bone marrow regeneration and response to treatment. The PCV should remain stable or slowly increase over time.
• Renal function should also be reassessed and signs reflective of laminitis monitored, particularly in horses also receiving corticosteroid therapy.

PREVENTION/AVOIDANCE

• Limiting access to excess phenothiazine, onions, or wilted red maple leaves.

POSSIBLE COMPLICATIONS

• Laminitis
• Nephropathy
• General debilitation
• Abortion, weak foals

EXPECTED COURSE AND PROGNOSIS

• Prognosis for recovery depends on the amount of oxidant ingested and whether or not methemoglobinemia also is present. If the inciting cause can be removed and methemoglobinemia is minimal or absent, the prognosis for recovery is fair to good. Several weeks may be required for full recovery.
• The prognosis is guarded in horses with red maple leaf toxicosis when methemoglobinemia is present.

MISCELLANEOUS

ASSOCIATED CONDITIONS

• Methemoglobinemia
• Pigment nephrosis

PREGNANCY

• Horses severely affected, and with general debilitation, may abort or deliver a weak foal.

SYNONYMS

• Methemoglobinemia
• Oxidative hemoglobinemia
• Oxidant-induced hemolysis

SEE ALSO

• Anemia
• Anemia, immune-mediated
• EIA
• Methemoglobinemia

ABBREVIATIONS

• BUN = blood urea nitrogen
• C-ELISA = competitive enzyme-linked immunosorbent assay
• CRT = capillary refill time
• EIA = equine infectious anemia
• GIT = gastrointestinal tract
• IV = intravenous
• MCH = mean corpuscular hemoglobin
• M:E = myeloid:erythroid
• PCV = packed cell volume
• PO = per os
• RBC = red blood cell
• RES = reticuloendothelial system

Suggested Reading

Alward A, Corriher CA, Barton MH, Sellon DC, Blikslager AT, Jones SL. Red maple (*Acer rubrum*) leaf toxicosis in horses: A retrospective study of 32 cases. J Vet Intern Med 2006; 20:1197–1201.

Corriher CA, Parvianen AKJ, Gibbons DS, Sellon DC. Equine red maple leaf toxicosis. Compend Contin Educ Pract Vet 1999; 21:74–80.

Davis E, Wilkerson MJ. Hemolytic anemia. In: Robinson NE, ed. Current Therapy in Equine Medicine 5ed. Philadelphia: WB Saunders, 2003: 344–348.

George LW, Divers TJ, Mahaffey EA, Suarez JH. Heinz body anemia and methemoglobinemia in ponies given red maple (*Acer rubrum*) leaves. Vet Pathol 1982;19:521–533.

Pierce KR, Joyce JR, England RB, Jones LP. Acute hemolytic anemia caused by wild onion poisoning in horses. J Am Vet Med Assoc 1972;160:323–327.

Author Nicholas Malikides
Consulting Editors Jennifer Hodgson and David Hodgson

ANEMIA, IMMUNE-MEDIATED

BASICS

DEFINITION

• IMHA is an acute or a chronic destruction of RBCs associated with immunoglobulin and/or complement attachment to either RBC antigens or foreign antigens coating the surface of RBCs.
• Affected RBCs are most commonly removed by the RES (also called mononuclear phagocyte system) after immunoglobulin-mediated opsonization (extravascular hemolysis).
• Less commonly, they may undergo intravascular, complement-mediated lysis.

PATHOPHYSIOLOGY

• IMHA most commonly occurs secondary to agents that:
  ○ Alter the RBC membrane, exposing antigens to which the host produces antibody (e.g., infectious agents, neoplasia);
  ○ Form immune complexes that adsorb to the RBC and fix complement (e.g., infectious agents);
  ○ Directly bind to the RBC and act as haptens that bind antibody (e.g., drugs); or
  ○ Stimulate the immune system resulting in production of antibodies with cross-reactivity to RBCs (e.g., infectious agents, neoplasia).
• Occasionally, the immune system produces specific autoantibodies to normal erythrocyte antigens (e.g., primary or idiopathic autoimmune hemolytic anemia, NI, or transfusion reaction).
• Antibody- and/or complement-coated RBCs are removed from the circulation by extravascular hemolysis (if removed by the RES) and/or intravascular hemolysis (if complement-mediated).

SYSTEMS AFFECTED

• The hemic/lymphatic/immune systems are involved due to intravascular and/or extravascular hemolysis. In cases where extravascular hemolysis predominates, splenomegaly may occur. Pyrexia may result from release of hemoglobin and other end products of red cell breakdown.
• Cardiovascular and respiratory systems may be involved with increased heart and respiratory rates, holosystolic heart murmur, and pallor of mucous membranes observed.
• Hepatobiliary system—Hemolytic anemia can result in hyperbilirubinemia and icterus while hypoxia may result in centrilobular degeneration.
• The renal system may be involved in cases where significant intravascular hemolysis and hemoglobinemia cause pigment nephropathy.
• The gastrointestinal tract may be involved due to hypoxic damage to intestines resulting in motility disorders, colic or diarrhea.

INCIDENCE/PREVALENCE

• No incidence or prevalence data are available for immune-mediated hemolytic anemia for specific horse populations. Weak evidence from in-practice experience suggests IMHA is a rare consequence of other disease states in adult horses. These forms of IMHA are reported to have a low case fatality rate.
• NI, which is a specific form of IMHA, is reported in foals in most countries, particularly horse studs where there are large numbers of breeding mares.

SIGNALMENT

Can occur in horses of any breed, age, or sex.

SIGNS

General Comments

IMHA often reflects a primary, underlying disease process such as infection or neoplasia.

Historical

• History generally reflects an underlying disease process and may include chronic weight loss (e.g., neoplastic diseases) or signs of depression and inappetence (e.g., infectious diseases).
• Exercise intolerance, weakness, and lethargy are common presenting signs.
• There may be a history of exposure to blood transfusion(s) or certain drugs.

Physical Examination

• Signs of anemia—Severity proportional to the degree of anemia.
• Exercise intolerance, weakness, pale or icteric mucous membranes, fever, tachypnea, tachycardia, holosystolic heart murmur, abdominal pain, and hemoglobinuria may be observed.
• Rectal examination may reveal an enlarged spleen.
• In foals with NI, there is usually an acute onset of intravascular hemolysis, with weakness and icterus during the first few days of life.
• Severe debilitation and death may occur in severe cases.

CAUSES

Primary Immune-Mediated

• NI
• Autoimmune hemolytic anemia
• Incompatible blood transfusion

Secondary Immune-Mediated

• Infectious—e.g., EIA, acute viral infections, infection with *Clostridium perfringens*, injection site abscess
• Neoplastic—e.g., lymphosarcoma and hemangiosarcoma
• Drug-associated—e.g., penicillins, cephalosporins, and trimethoprim-sulfamethoxazole
• Microangiopathic—disseminated intravascular coagulation
• Systemic lupus erythematosus

RISK FACTORS

• Foals born to multiparous dams that have previously had a blood transfusion(s), or the mare is known to be RBC antigen Aa or Qa negative, are at increased risk of developing NI.
• Exposure to incompatible blood transfusion and certain drugs

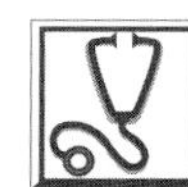

DIAGNOSIS

DIFFERENTIAL DIAGNOSIS

• Other diseases causing anemia must be differentiated from IMHA.
• Horses with hemorrhage (acute or chronic) often have a history of external blood loss or signs referable to thoracic or abdominal disease.
• Horses with Heinz-body anemia (e.g., wilted red maple leaf toxicosis, onion toxicosis, phenothiazine toxicosis) may have a history of exposure to oxidative toxins and presence of Heinz bodies or methemoglobinemia on routine blood analysis.
• Horses with purpura hemorrhagica often have a history of exposure to *Streptococcus equi* ss *equi* or other respiratory tract pathogens. In these cases edema of the legs, abdomen, and face and petechial hemorrhages of mucous membranes are common.

CBC/BIOCHEMISTRY/URINALYSIS

• PCV is often <0.20 L/L (<20%).
• May have neutrophilic leukocytosis
• RBC autoagglutination may be observed, but must be distinguished from rouleaux formation or RBC clumping due to other inflammatory disorders. Spherocytes may be observed in blood smears, but are more difficult to identify in horses due to the lack of central pallor in normal equine RBCs.
• Increased MCH suggests intravascular hemolysis, which may also result in discolored plasma.
• Increased serum total bilirubin concentration (indirect greater than direct)
• Bilirubinuria and hemoglobinuria may be observed in the rarer cases where intravascular hemolysis occurs.

OTHER LABORATORY TESTS

• Positive direct antiglobulin (Coombs) test, which detects presence of antibody on the surface of RBCs. False-negative results are possible, particularly if there has been prior corticosteroid therapy. False-positive results also can occur, emphasizing the need to use multiple methods to confirm the diagnosis of IMHA.
• Confirmation of true autoagglutination is performed by diluting EDTA-anticoagulated blood 1:4 with physiologic saline solution. RBCs should remain augglutinated with saline dilution.
• RBC osmotic fragility may be increased in IMHA, although this test can be positive with RBCs damaged by oxidant insults.
• Bone marrow aspiration reveals a diffuse, regenerative erythron (M:E ratio is <0.5).
• Infectious causes of IMHA may have positive serology and/or evidence of hematologic parasites on direct or special stained blood smears:
  ○ Horses with EIA will be seropositive for virus on Coggins or C-ELISA tests;
  ○ Horses with equine piroplasmosis may have organisms observed in Giemsa or New Methylene Blue stained blood smears, be seropositive or seroconvert on their convalescent titer;
  ○ Horses with equine granulocytic ehrlichiosis may have granular inclusion bodies observed in cytoplasm of neutrophils in Giemsa stained blood smears, be seropositive or seroconvert with acute and convalescent samples.

IMAGING

• Splenic/hepatic ultrasound determines splenic/hepatic enlargement and highlights hyperechoic or hypoechoic areas indicating loss of architecture.

- Radiography of the thorax is usually within normal limits unless a primary neoplasia is the underlying cause.

OTHER DIAGNOSTIC PROCEDURES
A thorough diagnostic workup should be performed to rule out neoplasia and infectious causes of secondary IMHA.

PATHOLOGICAL FINDINGS
- Necropsy findings may include an enlarged liver and spleen and pale or icteric tissues.
- If chronic, there may be signs of congestive heart failure (with pulmonary embolism, pulmonary edema, cardiomegaly), renal tubular nephrosis with hemoglobin casts, and centrilobular hepatic degeneration and necrosis.

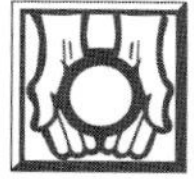

TREATMENT

AIMS OF TREATMENT
- Treatment of IMHA involves identification and resolution (if possible) of any underlying infection or disease, reduction of the immune response, and provision of supportive care.
- Administration of any drugs should be discontinued as IMHA could be caused by an adverse drug reaction. If antimicrobial therapy is required, a molecularly dissimilar antibiotic should be used.

APPROPRIATE HEALTH CARE
- Most cases of IMHA are treated in hospitals, especially if severe.
- Balanced polyionic IV fluid therapy may be indicated to expand vascular volume and induce diuresis.
- Emergency medical therapy with cross-matched blood transfusion is indicated if there is evidence of tissue hypoxia (PCV <8%–12%). In foals, washed RBCs from the dam or appropriate blood-typed blood is optimal.

NURSING CARE
- Serial analysis of PCV in order to monitor response to therapy should be performed.
- Close monitoring of vital signs and adjustment of fluid rate is essential in horses receiving fluid therapy.
- In foals with NI, provide adequate warmth and hydration, avoid stress and confine mare and foal to restrict activity.

ACTIVITY
Minimize or eliminate activity, but allow the animal access to fresh air and sunshine if possible.

DIET
- Make efforts to keep the horse eating a balanced diet, with good-quality hay and grain.
- Fresh water should be available *ad libitum*.

CLIENT EDUCATION
- Clients should be made aware that horses with primary (or autoimmune) IMHA often require long-term corticosteroid therapy and often are found to have incurable neoplastic disease.

Additionally, long-term administration of corticosteroids may increase the risk of laminitis, tendon laxity, and immunosuppression leading to secondary infections.

- Clients should be educated in preventative measures for NI.

SURGICAL CONSIDERATIONS
Consider splenectomy if the primary cause cannot be identified.

MEDICATIONS

DRUG(S)
- In adults, corticosteroids (dexamethasone, 0.05–0.2 mg/kg IV or IM q12–24h) are indicated until PCV ceases to decline. The dose may then be decreased by 0.01 mg/kg/day until the total dose is 20 mg/day (for a 500-kg horse), after which alternate-day oral prednisolone is recommended. Alternatively, oral prednisolone (2–3 mg/kg) may be used in place of dexamethasone at any time during therapy, although, anecdotally, dexamethasone is more efficacious.
- From 4 to 7 days often are needed for corticosteroids to have a therapeutic effect (with stabilization of PCV) and up to 10 weeks of treatment may be necessary.

CONTRAINDICATIONS
Corticosteroids may exacerbate underlying infectious diseases so should be used only in horses that are EIA (Coggins) negative and horses free of other infectious disorders.

PRECAUTIONS
- Cross-match blood before blood transfusion.
- Corticosteroid therapy may predispose horses to laminitis and exacerbate an undiagnosed infectious process. They also should be used with caution in pregnant mares.

ALTERNATIVE DRUGS
The immunosuppressive agents azathioprine (5 mg/kg PO once daily) and cyclophosphamide (300 mg/m^2 body surface area) have been used successfully in one horse that was nonresponsive to corticosteroids.

FOLLOW-UP

PATIENT MONITORING
The PCV should be carefully monitored during dexamethasone treatment. The frequency of dexamethasone administration can be increased to twice daily in horses initially commenced on once/day treatment if the PCV does not stabilize within 24–48hr.

PREVENTION/AVOIDANCE
Avoid drugs known to have caused secondary IMHA.

POSSIBLE COMPLICATIONS
- Pigment nephropathy may occur secondary to intravascular hemolysis.
- Laminitis

EXPECTED COURSE AND PROGNOSIS
- If the primary cause can be identified and successfully treated, the prognosis for IMHA is good.
- Red cell numbers replenish as the immune-mediated response resolves. This may take several weeks in some horses.
- Horses requiring constant corticosteroid treatment (if diagnosed with idiopathic autoimmune hemolytic anemia) may have an incurable underlying disease such as neoplasia (e.g., lymphosarcoma). The prognosis for survival in these horses is poor.

MISCELLANEOUS

ASSOCIATED CONDITIONS
- Pigment nephropathy with intravascular hemolysis
- Laminitis

PREGNANCY
Use corticosteroids cautiously in pregnant mares.

SYNONYMS
- Autoimmune hemolytic anemia
- Immune-mediated hemolytic disease

SEE ALSO
- Anemia
- Anemia, Heinz-body
- Babesiosis
- Equine infectious anemia
- Hemorrhage, acute

ABBREVIATIONS
- C-ELISA = competitive enzyme-linked immunosorbent assay
- IM = intramuscular
- IV = intravenous
- EIA = equine infectious anemia
- IMHA = immune-mediated hemolytic anemia
- MCH = mean corpuscular hemoglobin
- M:E = myeloid:erythroid ratio
- NI = neonatal isoerythrolysis
- PCV = packed cell volume
- PO = per os
- RBC = red blood cell
- RES = reticuloendothelial system

Suggested Reading
Mair TS, Taylor FGR, Hillyer MH. Autoimmune haemolytic anaemia in eight horses. Vet Rec 1990;126:51.

McConnico RS, Roberts MC, Tompkins M. Penicillin-induced immune-mediated hemolytic anemia in a horse. J Am Vet Med Assoc 1992;201:1402–1403.

Messer NT, Arnold K. Immune-mediated hemolytic anemia in a horse. J Am Vet Med Assoc 1991;198:1415–1416.

Sellon DC. Disorders of the hematopoietic system. In: Reed SM, Bayly WM, Sellon DC, eds. Equine Internal Medicine. St Louis: WB Saunders, 2004:721–768.

Author Nicholas Malikides
Consulting Editors Jennifer Hodgson and David Hodgson

ANEMIA, IRON DEFICIENCY

BASICS

OVERVIEW

• Iron is stored in horses as hemoglobin (65% of total iron stores), ferritin, and hemosiderin.
• Iron deficiency may arise from either chronic external loss of blood (most common in adult horses) or dietary deprivation (in young rapidly growing foals). Unless adult horses have inadequate access to soil, pasture or feed, inadequate iron intake is unlikely.
• Iron deficiency results in delayed hemoglobin synthesis, resulting in arrested and ineffective RBC maturation in bone marrow and anemia. The small hemoglobin deficient RBCs (i.e., hypochromic microcytes) produced have reduced deformability and life span.
• Nonregenerative anemia and reduced blood hemoglobin concentration may lead to compromised oxygen delivery to tissues.
• Nonheme, iron-containing enzymes may also be depleted and result in impairment of cell-mediated immunity and neutrophil killing of ingested bacteria.

SIGNALMENT

• No breed or sex predilections
• Rapid growth of foals is associated with high tissue demands for iron. Mare's milk has low iron concentrations (≈0.88 μg/g of milk by 2 weeks and ≈0.6 μg/g by 8 weeks postpartum) and therefore deficiency may occur in foals with limited access to pasture, iron-rich soils, or not consuming forage or grain.

SIGNS

• Initially, clinical signs may be absent or mild due to adequate physiologic compensation for the gradual reduction in oxygenation.
• Lethargy and exercise intolerance may be the first overt clinical signs noted.
• When PCV is <12%, tissue hypoxia can cause tachycardia, tachypnea, pale mucous membranes, systolic heart murmur, and signs of depression.

CAUSES AND RISK FACTORS

Risk factors for chronic hemorrhage may include inadequate preventative anthelmintic use, phenylbutazone administration, and exposure to toxins.

Chronic, Low Grade Hemorrhage

• Severe internal parasitism (*Strongylus vulgaris*, small strongyles) or external parasitism (e.g., heavy infestation of sucking lice—*Haematopinus asini*)
• Bleeding GI, respiratory, and urinary tract lesions (e.g., gastroduodenal ulcers, NSAID toxicosis, neoplasia [especially gastric squamous cell carcinoma], hemorrhagic or erosive cystitis, guttural pouch mycosis, and ethmoid hematoma)
• Coagulopathies leading to chronic blood loss (e.g., heritable coagulopathies, warfarin toxicosis, moldy sweet clover [dicumarol] toxicosis)

Diet

Inadequate dietary intake (foals)

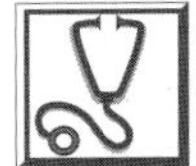

DIAGNOSIS

DIFFERENTIAL DIAGNOSIS

• Causes of low-grade, hemolytic anemia must be ruled out including immune-mediated hemolysis, oxidant-induced hemolysis, and parasite-induced hemolysis. Distinguishing features may include hemoglobinemia, hemoglobinuria, and a normal serum protein concentration. Serum iron concentrations may be increased.
• Causes of decreased erythrocyte production must be ruled out including anemia of chronic disease and aplastic anemia. Increased serum ferritin concentrations are typical in anemia of chronic disease and bone marrow morphology is diagnostic for aplastic anemia.

CBC/BIOCHEMISTRY/URINALYSIS

• Normochromic, normocytic anemia is initially observed, but usually develops into a microcytic, hypochromic, nonregenerative anemia in later stages. Microcytosis often precedes hypochromasia.
• Thrombocytosis may be observed.
• Decreased plasma protein and albumin concentrations

OTHER LABORATORY TESTS

Initial Stage

• Decreased stainable iron (Prussian Blue stain) in bone marrow macrophages
• Decreased serum ferritin concentrations (reference range 85–155 ng/mL) where serum ferritin <45 ng/mL is highly indicative of iron deficiency.

Later Stages

• Decreased SI concentration (reference range, 120–150 μg/dL)
• Normal or increased TIBC (reference range, 300–400 μg/dL)
• Decreased percentage transferrin saturation (= 100 × SI/TIBC). Reference range is 30%–50% (Arabian horses ≈68%) with values <16% reflecting insufficient iron available for erythropoiesis.
• Presence of microcytes (decreased MCV) with decreased hemoglobin concentration (hypochromia, decreased MCHC)
• SI, serum ferritin, and TIBC may be affected by conditions other than iron

deficiency including acute and chronic inflammation, renal disease, and corticosteroid therapy.

OTHER DIAGNOSTIC PROCEDURES

- Cytology of bone marrow aspirate may show a predominance of late rubricytes and metarubricytes, depletion of macrophage iron, and sideroblasts.
- A diagnostic workup of causes of chronic hemorrhage is required.

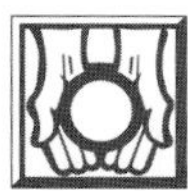

TREATMENT

- Horses with lethargy, intolerance to mild exercise, or a PCV <15% should be restricted to stall rest.
- Blood transfusion is rarely necessary unless PCV drops below 8% (0.08 L/L) or there are clinical and laboratory signs of tissue hypoxia.

MEDICATIONS

DRUG(S)

- Appropriate treatment of underlying disease process to resolve chronic blood loss
- Oral ferrous sulfate (1.0 g/450 kg body weight) is the safest means to administer iron. Iron requirements for a 450-kg horse are ≈800 mg/day for maintenance and ≈1100–1300 mg/day during pregnancy and lactation.
- Iron cacodylate (1 g/adult horse) may be given slowly IV, but must be used with caution due the possibility of an anaphylactic reaction.

CONTRAINDICATIONS/POSSIBLE INTERACTIONS

- Do not administer iron dextrans due to idiosyncratic reactions (anaphylaxis and sudden death).
- Iatrogenic iron overload has been reported in adult horses given unnecessary oral and/or parenteral iron supplementation.
- Do not give foals iron-containing products during the first 2 days of life as fatal toxic hepatopathies may result.

FOLLOW-UP

PATIENT MONITORING

- Monitor response to therapy of underlying disease and ensure no further hemorrhage.
- Monitor SI, TIBC, and percentage saturation at ≈2-week intervals.
- Discontinue iron supplementation when values for PCV, SI, TIBC, and percentage saturation return to within reference ranges.

PREVENTION AVOIDANCE

Ensure that sucking foals have access to pasture and, when of an appropriate age, forage and grain.

POSSIBLE COMPLICATIONS

May result in death if horses are left untreated

EXPECTED COURSE AND PROGNOSIS

- If the underlying disease is successfully treated, iron deficiency anemia is reversible.
- Weeks of iron supplementation may be required, depending on the severity of anemia and the degree of iron store depletion.

MISCELLANEOUS

SEE ALSO

- Anemia
- Anemia, aplastic (pure red cell aplasia)
- Anemia, Heinz body
- Anemia, immune-mediated
- Hemorrhage, chronic equine infectious anemia

ABBREVIATIONS

- GI = gastrointestinal
- PCV = packed cell volume
- SI = serum iron
- TIBC = total iron-binding capacity

Suggested Reading

Morris DD. Diseases of the hemolymphatic system. In: Reed SM, Bayly WM, eds. Equine Internal Medicine. Philadelphia: WB Saunders, 1998:558–602.

The author and editors wish to acknowledge the contributions of Catherine W. Kohn, author of this topic in the previous edition.

Author Nicholas Malikides

Consulting Editors Jennifer Hodgson and David Hodgson

ANESTRUS

BASICS

DEFINITION/OVERVIEW

Period of reproductive inactivity, ovaries small and static. Characterized by indifferent behavior of mare to stallion.

ETIOLOGY/PATHOPHYSIOLOGY

Seasonally polyestrus, estrous cycles (*ovulatory period*) in spring and summer; primarily regulated by photoperiod; light begins a cascade:
• Increasing day length decreases melatonin secretion (pineal gland).
• Decreasing melatonin allows increased production and release of GnRH.
• Increased GnRH stimulates gonadotropin release (FSH and LH).
• FSH promotes folliculogenesis and ultimately the onset of estrus behavior.
• When sufficient LH is present, ovulation occurs; end of vernal transition = onset of cyclicity

Average estrous cycle—21 days (range 19–22); time between 2 ovulations that coincides with progesterone levels of <1 ng/mL. Estrus, estrous cycle lengths—quite repeatable in individual mare, cycle to cycle. Key hormonal events of equine estrous cycle:
• FSH causes follicular growth.
• Estradiol (follicular) stimulates increased GnRH pulse frequency and secretion of LH.
• LH surge causes ovulation; estradiol returns to basal levels 1–2 days post-ovulation.
• Progesterone (CL origin) rises from basal levels (<1 ng/mL) at ovulation to >4 ng/mL by 4–5 days post-ovulation.
• Progesterone causes decreased GnRH pulse frequency and increased FSH secretion; it stimulates a new wave of follicular development beginning in diestrus.
• Endogenous $PGF_{2\alpha}$ (endometrial) is released 14–15 days post-ovulation causing luteolysis and concurrent decline in progesterone levels.

SYSTEMS AFFECTED

• Reproductive
• Endocrine

SIGNS

Historical

• Chief complaint—failure of mare to accept stallion. Rarely reported—stallion-like behavior.
• Teasing—Review methods used, records, frequency, teaser type (pony, horse, gelding), stallion behavior (aggressive/passive, vocalization, proximity), and handler experience.
• Seasonal influences—Evaluate normal individual variation of onset, duration, termination of cyclicity.
• Individual reproductive history—estrous cycle length, teasing response, foaling data, previous genital tract injuries/infections, and relationship to clinical abnormalities.
• Pharmaceuticals—Current and historical drug history may relate to clinical abnormalities.

Physical Examination

• Poor body condition/malnutrition may contribute to anestrus.
• Poor perineal conformation can result in pneumovagina, ascending infections and/or urine pooling, anestrus/infertility.
• Clitoral enlargement may relate to drug history—anabolic steroids, progestational steroids, or intersex conditions.
• TRP is essential to evaluate suspected anestrus mare. Assess uterine size and tone, ovarian size, shape and location, and cervical relaxation. Serial TRP 3 times a week over 1–3 weeks to completely define status.
• Transrectal U/S to define normal and abnormal features of uterus and ovaries
• Vaginal examination (digital and/or speculum) to identify inflammation, urine pooling, cervical competency, conformational abnormalities; determine stage of the estrous cycle.

CAUSES

Normal Physiologic

• *Winter anestrus*—≈20% of mares cycle through the winter (Northern Hemisphere—November to January); most enter a period of ovarian quiescence. Failure to cycle is normal during winter anestrus.
• *Two transitional phases* occur yearly—*autumnal* transition (ovulatory to anestrus) and *vernal* transition (anestrus to cyclicity/ovulatory). Behavioral patterns vary during transition periods. Individual variation in onset and length of transitional periods is normal.
• Behavioral anestrus (silent heat)—a normal estrous cycle as determined by serial TRP, failures to demonstrate estrus
• Pregnancy—After recognition of pregnancy, CL progesterone production continues; majority of pregnant mares exhibit anestrus behavior.
• Pseudopregnancy—Embryo dies after recognition of pregnancy or formation of endometrial cups, resulting in persistent CL activity and behavioral anestrus.
  ○ eCG (by endometrial cups, 35–150 days pregnancy) is luteotropic, role in maintaining primary CL and formation of secondary CLs of pregnancy.
• Postpartum anestrus—>95% of mares reestablish cyclic activity ≤20 days postpartum. Some fail to continue cycling after first postpartum ovulation, due to prolonged CL function or ovarian inactivity.
• Age-related conditions—Puberty occurs at 12–24 mo. Individual variation by age, weight, nutrition, and season. Aged mares can have protracted seasonal anestrus; >25 years may last for senescence, cycles cease.

Congenital Abnormalities

• Gonadal dysgenesis—no functional ovarian tissue; can result in anestrus, erratic estrus, or prolonged estrus
  ○ Behavioral estrus may be due to adrenal-origin steroid production and absence of progesterone.
  ○ Typically flaccid, infantile uterus, hypoplastic endometrium, small, nonfunctional ovaries
  ○ Most common chromosomal defect is XO monosomy (Turner's syndrome).
• Intersex conditions—XY sex reversal chromosomal abnormality

Endocrine Disorders

• Cushing's disease—Adenomatous hyperplasia of pars intermedius of pituitary leads to destruction of FSH- and LH-secreting cells and/or overproduction of glucocorticoids.
  ○ May be increased adrenal-origin androgens causing suppression of the normal hypothalamic-pituitary-ovarian axis
  ○ Primary hypothalamic-pituitary-ovarian axis interference is proposed as cause of anestrus.

Ovarian Abnormalities—See Large Ovary Syndrome

• Ovarian hematoma • Ovarian neoplasia

Uterine Abnormalities

Pyometra—Severe uterine infections can destroy the endometrium, prevents formation and release of $PGF_{2\alpha}$, needed for CL regression. Appears as prolonged diestrus or anestrus.

Iatrogenic/Pharmacologic

• Anabolic steroids—Affected mares behave as if in anestrus, silent estrus, or show increased aggression.
• Progesterone/progestin—Continued treatment inhibits estrus behavior.
• NSAIDs—Potential to interfere with endogenous $PGF_{2\alpha}$ release; result is prolonged CL activity. No evidence that exogenous treatment [recommended therapeutic dose] inhibits spontaneous formation and release of endogenous $PGF_{2\alpha}$

RISK FACTORS

Postpartum anestrus occurs more often in early foaling mares and mares in poor body condition at time of parturition.

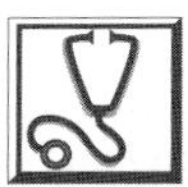

DIAGNOSIS

DIFFERENTIAL DIAGNOSIS

Differentiating Causes

• Critically review teasing records, general and reproductive history—foaling data, evidence of infections, injuries, medications that may affect reproductive health. • Serial TRP with/without U/S over 2–3 weeks is adequate to differentiate transitional and behavioral anestrus; fewer examinations for pregnancy, hypoplastic ovaries, large ovary syndrome/ovarian neoplasia, pyometra • EED after the formation of endometrial cups, may result in anestrus or pseudopregnancy. • Gonadal dysgenesis and intersex conditions—base on history (anestrus, irregular estrus), TRP and U/S (small ovaries, flaccid uterus and cervix), repeated low serum progesterone concentrations (<1 ng/mL q7days for 5 weeks) and karyotype.

OTHER LABORATORY TESTS

• Serum progesterone
  ○ Basal—<1 ng/mL—no functional CL present.
  ○ Active CL—>4 ng/mL
• Serum testosterone and inhibin
  ○ Mare—<50–60 pg/mL, inhibin <0.7 ng/mL.
  ○ Levels suggestive of GCT/GTCT (in a nonpregnant mare) are—testosterone >50–100 pg/mL (if thecal cells are significant

tumor component), inhibin >0.7 ng/mL, progesterone <1 ng/mL.
- Serum eCG—measured by ELISA
- GnRH stimulation test—to ID primary hypothalamic or pituitary dysfunction
- Karyotype—if suspect gonadal dysgenesis or intersex conditions

IMAGING

Transrectal U/S of reproductive tract. See related topics.

DIAGNOSTIC PROCEDURES

Uterine cytology, culture and biopsy—diagnosis, select treatment/monitor progress of pyometra and endometritis

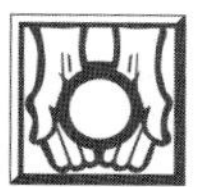

TREATMENT

- Combination—alter management techniques, vary teasing methods to elicit a response from a mare and/or base timing of AI on TRP and U/S.
- Artificial lighting—hasten onset of vernal transition, also known as manipulation of photoperiod. Duration of transition remains unchanged. Expose mare to 14.5–16 hr light/day or, alternatively, to additional 1–2 hr light at 10 hr after dusk (*flash lighting*). A minimum of 60 (some mares up to 90) days of supplemental light is needed to progress from anestrus to cyclicity. Added light typically starts December 1 (Northern Hemisphere).
- Mare due to foal early in the year—add supplemental lighting 2 mo prior to parturition, improve postpartum cyclicity and decrease potential for lactational anestrus.
- Treating a mare with progesterone while she is in anestrus/early vernal transition will suppress ovarian activity. Coupling artificial lighting as described above for 60 days, until minimal ovarian activity is achieved (multiple 15- to 20-mm follicles present), followed by progesterone therapy, can achieve earlier onset of regular estrous cycles.
- Ovarian tumors/ovariectomy
  - With removal of a GCT/GTCT, suppression (inhibin) of contralateral ovary is gone, allowing it to recover.
  - Latent period for return of ovarian activity is affected by when tumor is removed; e.g., best if OVX is done in autumn, then mare can respond to normal increase in day length as she transitions into the next season.

MEDICATIONS

DRUG(S) OF CHOICE

- $PGF_{2\alpha}$ (Lutalyse [Pfizer] 10 mg IM) or analogs—lyse persistent CL. Multiple injections may be needed with pseudopregnancy.
- Deslorelin injectable GnRH analog to induce ovulation within 48 hr if follicle(s) >30 mm
- hCG 2500 IU IV to induce ovulation in mares with follicle(s) >35 mm • Altrenogest (Regu-Mate [Intervet] 0.044 mg/kg PO daily minimum 15 days) to shorten vernal transition, providing follicles >20-mm diameter are present at onset of treatment and mare is exhibiting behavioral estrus • Its use in seasonally deep anestrus mares is not recommended. • $PGF_{2\alpha}$ (Lutalyse) on day 15 of altrenogest treatment increases the reliability of this transition management regimen.

CONTRAINDICATIONS

$PGF_{2\alpha}$ and its analogs—contraindicated in mares with heaves or other bronchoconstrictive disease

PRECAUTIONS

- Horses
  - $PGF_{2\alpha}$ causes sweating and colic-like symptoms due to its stimulatory effect on smooth muscle cells. If cramping has not subsided within 1–2 hr, symptomatic treatment should be instituted.
  - Antibodies to hCG can develop. Desirable to limit its use to no more than 2–3 times during one breeding season. Half-life of antibodies ranges from 30 days to several months; typically do not persist from one breeding season to the next
  - Deslorelin implants not currently sold in the United States; injectable product is available. Implants were associated with suppression of FSH and decreased follicular development in the diestrus period immediately following implant use; led to prolonged interovulatory period in nonpregnant mares. Implant removal post-ovulation helped some.
  - Progesterone supplementation—potential to decrease uterine clearance; its use may be contraindicated in mares with a history of uterine infection.
  - Altrenogest, deslorelin, and $PGF_{2\alpha}$ should not be used in horses intended for food.
- Humans—With either product below, accidental skin exposure should be washed off immediately.
  - $PGF_{2\alpha}$ or its analogs should not be handled by pregnant women or persons with asthma or bronchial disease.
  - Altrenogest should not be handled by pregnant women or persons with thrombophlebitis, thromboembolic disorders, cerebrovascular or coronary artery disease, breast cancer, estrogen-dependent neoplasia, undiagnosed vaginal bleeding, or tumors that developed with use of oral contraceptives or estrogen-containing products.

ALTERNATIVE DRUGS

Cloprostenol sodium (Estrumate [Schering-Plough Animal Health] 250 μg/mL IM), a prostaglandin analog. Used in similar fashion as natural prostaglandin, but fewer side effects. Not currently approved for use in horses, but is an analog in widespread use in absence of an alternative.

FOLLOW-UP

PATIENT MONITORING

- Serial TRP during the breeding season; establish diagnosis for etiology of anestrus behavior.
- Pseudopregnant mares return to normal cyclic activity upon regression of endometrial cups, as eCG decreases.
  - eCG can persist up to 150 days.
  - If embryonic death is confirmed, intervention up to 150 days may be ineffective.

POSSIBLE COMPLICATIONS

Infertility may result from intractable persistent anestrus.

AGE-RELATED FACTORS

Postpartum anestrus occurs more often in old mares.

MISCELLANEOUS

PREGNANCY

$PGF_{2\alpha}$ to pregnant mares can lyse CL, causing abortion, especially if <40 days pregnant. Rule out pregnancy before injecting this drug or its analogs.

SYNONYMS

- Gonadal dysgenesis • Gonadal hypoplasia
- Lactational anestrus • Postpartum anestrus

SEE ALSO

- Abnormal estrus intervals • Aggression
- Cushing's syndrome • Disorders of sexual development • EED • Endometritis
- Large ovary syndrome • Ovarian hypoplasia
- Ovulation failure • Prolonged diestrus
- Pyometra

ABBREVIATIONS

- AI = artificial insemination
- CL = corpus luteum
- eCG = equine chorionic gonadotropin
- EED = early embryonic death
- FSH = follicle-stimulating hormone
- GCT/GTCT = granulosa cell tumor/granulosa-theca cell tumor
- GnRH = gonadotropin-releasing hormone
- hCG = human chorionic gonadotropin
- LH = luteinizing hormone
- OVX = ovariectomy
- $PGF_2\alpha$ = natural prostaglandin
- TRP = transrectal palpation
- U/S = ultrasound, ultrasonography

Suggested Reading

Hinrichs K. Irregularities of the estrous cycle and ovulation in mares (including seasonal transition). In: Youngquist RS, Threlfall WR, eds. Current Therapy in Large Animal Theriogenology. St. Louis, MO: WB Saunders Elsevier, 2007:144–152.

McCue PM, Farquhar VJ, Carnevale EM, Squires EL. Removal of deslorelin (Ovuplant™) implant 48 h after administration results in normal interovulatory intervals in mares. Theriogenology 2002;58:865–870.

Sharp D, Robinson G, Cleaver B, Porter M. Clinical aspects of seasonality in mares. In: Youngquist RS, Threlfall WR, eds. Current Therapy in Large Animal Theriogenology. St. Louis, MO: WB Saunders Elsevier, 2007:68–73.

Author Carole C. Miller

Consulting Editor Carla L. Carleton

ANGULAR LIMB DEFORMITY

BASICS

DEFINITION

ALD is an abnormal rotation from the normal axis of the limb in the frontal plane. Valgus is the lateral deviation of the limb distal to the location of the deformity, while varus is the medial deviation of the limb to the location of the deformity. The deformity is named by the joint around which the deviation is centered (e.g., carpal valgus).

PATHOPHYSIOLOGY

There are two main categories associated with the etiology of ALD—perinatal factors and developmental factors.

Perinatal Factors

• Flaccidity of periarticular soft tissue structures and perinatal soft tissue trauma can lead to unstable joints, resulting in abnormal loading of the articular surfaces inducing ALD (manually correctable in the early stages). • Anything to jeopardize the intrauterine environment of the foal (i.e., placentitis, twin foal) and premature birth (<315 days) may result in incomplete ossification (carpus and tarsus) at birth. If the joints are unevenly loaded while the bones are not yet ossified, the uneven pressure may result in abnormal shape once ossification occurs, leading to permanent ALD.

Developmental Factors

• Unbalanced nutrition (i.e., "crib feeding" leading to excessive grain intake, unbalanced trace minerals) can result in disproportionate growth at the level of the physis, causing ALD. • Frequently observed in rapidly growing foals • Can occur days to months after birth • Excessive exercise and trauma can result in microfractures and crushing of the growth plate leading to early closure in severe cases (i.e., Salter-Harris type V fracture).

SYSTEM AFFECTED

Musculoskeletal—One or more joints may be involved in the front limbs and/or hindlimbs, including the fetlock, carpus, and tarsus. Most commonly, the angular limb deformity originates at the carpus. Carpal valgus deformity is the most commonly observed ALD, but tarsal valgus and fetlock varus are also seen commonly.

GENETICS

N/A

INCIDENCE/PREVALENCE

Most foals are born with some form of angular limb deformity; however, most cases resolve within 4 weeks without intervention.

GEOGRAPHIC DISTRIBUTION

N/A

SIGNALMENT

Most commonly encountered in neonatal foals

Breed Predilections

Observed in all breeds, most commonly Thoroughbreds, Quarter Horses, and Miniature Horses

Age and Range

May either be present at birth or develop days to months following birth

Predominant Sex

N/A

SIGNS

General Comments

• Natural growth of foals can lead to spontaneous correction of the ALD. However, foals with ALD must be monitored appropriately, as if they do not correct their conformation, there is a limited window during which time surgical intervention can occur prior to various physis closures. • Ideal conformation varies between breeds and type of work desired (i.e., pleasure versus racing).
• Each foal will respond differently to treatment.

Historical

• Prematurity/dysmaturity • Placentitis or twinning in the mare • Witnessed or suspected trauma at the physis • Crib-feeding practices on the farm

Physical Examination

• A valgus deformity results in what is termed "splay foot" due to the lateral deviation; outward rotation of the entire limb ("toed out") should not be mistaken for deviation of the limb at the level of the carpus or fetlock (carpal valgus or fetlock valgus). • A varus deformity results in what is termed "pigeon toed" due to medial/axial deviation.

CAUSES

Perinatal Factors

• Prematurity • Dysmaturity
• Hypothyroidism • Twin foal • Placentitis
• Ligamentous laxity • Perinatal soft tissue trauma • Intrauterine malpositioning

Developmental Factors

• Nutritional imbalances • External trauma to the physis • Overload of a limb • Excessive exercise

RISK FACTORS

N/A

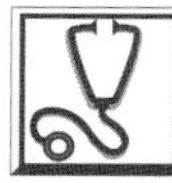

DIAGNOSIS

DIFFERENTIAL DIAGNOSIS

• Laxity of periarticular soft tissues
• Incomplete ossification/collapse of the cuboidal bones • Diaphyseal curvature (MCIII/MTIII)

CBC/BIOCHEMISTRY/URINALYSIS

N/A

OTHER LABORATORY TESTS

N/A

IMAGING

Radiography allows for determination of the location and the degree of the deformity, as well as concurrent physitis or physeal crushing, or cuboidal bone crushing. Radiographs should be centered over the joint of interest, including the mid-diaphysis of the bones proximal and distal to the deformity (long cassettes will allow for easier assessment of the deformity). Only two views are required for ALD (lateromedial and dorsopalmar/dorsoplantar). If there is evidence of joint problems, oblique images should be included.

OTHER DIAGNOSTIC PROCEDURES

• Examination of the limb in both a standing and a flexed position • Observation of the foal from several angles • Examination from a position perpendicular to a frontal plane through the limb—the toe should point in the same direction as the carpus.
• Observation of the foal at a walk
• Manipulation/palpation of the limb can help determine whether the deformity was caused by perinatal (manual correction) or developmental factors (permanent).

PATHOLOGICAL FINDINGS

• Asymmetric early closure of either the medial or lateral physis due to injuries or inflammation • Delayed ossification

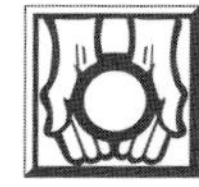

TREATMENT

AIMS OF TREATMENT

To manage ALD, either conservatively or by providing surgical intervention, if needed, in order to correct growth. A straighter limb will allow for more even load-bearing and should reduce the incidence of athletic injury.

APPROPRIATE HEALTH CARE

N/A

NURSING CARE

Splints and Casts

• The purpose is to maintain the limb in proper alignment and to facilitate adequate weight-bearing without adverse consequences.
• For foals with incomplete ossification of the cuboidal bones and deviation of the limbs
• Problems with casts and splints in foals include osteopenia and tendon/ligament laxity. Ending the cast/splint at the level of the fetlock can help prevent these problems.
• Splints should be changed every 3–4 days.
• Casts should be changed every 10–14 days.

Corrective Shoeing

• Application of glue-on/composite materials with an extension on the medial aspect (valgus deformities) or the lateral aspect (varus deformities) may assist in correction of the deformity. • Hoof trimming may also be performed—the outside of the hoof should be lowered for valgus deformity; the inside for varus deformity. It is important to not overtrim or create an abnormal hoof shape that will further alter normal weight-bearing.

ACTIVITY

Stall Rest

• Effective treatment for newborn foals, specifically for incomplete ossification and straight limbs. The maximum period of rest is 1 month. • Foals with ALD due to disproportionate growth at the level of the physis (>10 degrees) and diaphyseal deformities should be stall rested for 4–6 weeks. • Foals with laxity of the periarticular supporting structures require exercise in addition to stall rest. • It is important not to prolong stall rest beyond 4–6 weeks.

DIET

Balanced nutrition is very important.

CLIENT EDUCATION

• Early recognition and treatment are important. • The examination of a foal for ALD should begin shortly after birth, followed by examination once a week for 4 weeks, and once monthly for 6 months. This allows close monitoring to determine if the foal will self-correct or need surgical intervention.

SURGICAL CONSIDERATIONS

Growth Acceleration (Periosteal Transection and Elevation)

• Periosteal transection is performed on the concave aspect of the limb (e.g. lateral aspect of the distal radial physis for a carpal valgus deformity) in order to accelerate growth. Studies have indicated an 80% improvement in foals that have undergone a periosteal transection. The procedure is relatively inexpensive and easy, with the ability to be performed in the field. • Foals should have this surgery at 4 weeks (earlier if the deformity is severe) to 3 months of age (limited growth beyond this time). The timing of surgery also depends on the site of abnormal growth (below). • The maximum effect is observed within 2 months.
• Overcorrection of the deformity has not been observed. • A bandage should be maintained for 10–14 days following surgery.
• Keep the foal on stall rest for 2–3 weeks after surgery.

Growth Retardation (Transphyseal Bridging)

• Performed in foals <3 months with severe ALD or foals with significant ALD following the rapid growth phase (MClll/MTlll and proximal phalanx = 2 months, tibia = 4 months, and radius = 6 months). • The bridging is performed on the convex aspect of the affected limb. • The goal is to retard growth on the convex side of the limb, allowing the shorter side of the affected limb to keep growing. • Screws and cerclage wires are the most commonly used implants.
• Current techniques include two screws, one inserted in the center of the epiphysis and one into the proximal physis, with cerclage wire connecting the two in a figure-eight pattern. A more recent technique includes one transphyseal screw, which can be used across the physis of the distal MClll/MTlll, the distal radius and the distal tibia. Surgical staple techniques and small bone plates have also been described for use in transphyseal bridging. Periosteal transaction and elevation are often performed in combination with growth retardation techniques. • A bandage should be maintained for 10–14 days. • Stall rest the foal for 2–3 days following surgery.
• Evaluate radiographically every 2 weeks to assess. • Implants need to be removed as soon as the deformity has been corrected, as overcorrection can occur.

Corrective Osteotomy

• Osteotomies have been performed for correction of significant ALD in foals with closed growth plates. • Current techniques—closing wedge osteotomy, step osteotomy in the sagittal plane and step osteotomy in the frontal plane. • Most frequently performed on MClll/MTlll
• Maintain a bandage and splint or cast for several weeks following surgery.

MEDICATIONS

DRUG(S)

For surgical cases, NSAIDs (flunixin meglumine 1.1 mg/kg IV daily or q12h) and antibiotics (i.e., gentamicin 6.6 mg/kg IV daily or Amikacin 25–30 mg/kg IV daily and potassium penicillin 22,000 IU/kg IV q6h) can be given as needed perioperatively.

CONTRAINDICATIONS

N/A

PRECAUTIONS

NSAIDs can have an ulcerogenic effect on foals. Ulcer prophylaxis may include oral Gastrogard (omeprazole 1–2 mg/kg PO once daily) or ranitidine (10 mg/kg PO q8h or 1.5 mg/kg IV q8h in 250 mL saline) while the foal is in the hospital and receiving NSAIDs.

POSSIBLE INTERACTIONS

N/A

ALTERNATIVE DRUGS

N/A

FOLLOW-UP

PATIENT MONITORING

• Foals with splints and casts should be assisted to nurse if unable to on their own.
• Following transphyseal bridging, the horse should be monitored so that once the correction has taken place and radiographs have confirmed this, the implants are removed to prevent overcorrection. • Foals with incomplete ossification of the cuboidal bones should be evaluated at 2-week intervals to assess ossification progress.

PREVENTION/AVOIDANCE

Balanced nutrition is very important.

POSSIBLE COMPLICATIONS

• Nonsurgical management—pressure sores, osteopenia, and tendon/ligament laxity from cast/splint application • Surgical management—hematoma/seroma formation at surgery site, incisional infection, wound dehiscence • Overcorrection is possible if transphyseal bridging implants are not removed as soon as ALD has been corrected.
• Failure of passive transfer may result if foals are unable to nurse due to ALD following birth.

EXPECTED COURSE AND PROGNOSIS

• Studies have indicated an improvement in approximately 80% of foals that have undergone a periosteal transection. It has been reported that an athletic use was pursued for 80% of foals with ALD of the carpus and 27.3% of foals with ALD of the metacarpus/metatarsus after transphyseal bridging.

MISCELLANEOUS

ASSOCIATED CONDITIONS

N/A

AGE-RELATED FACTORS

Timing of intervention is important, as the greatest effects of surgical manipulation will occur during the rapid growth phases.

ZOONOTIC POTENTIAL

N/A

PREGNANCY

N/A

SYNONYMS

N/A

SEE ALSO

Flexural limb deformity

ABBREVIATIONS

• ALD = angular limb deformity
• MClll = third metacarpal bone
• MTlll = third metatarsal bone

Suggested Reading

Auer JA. Angular limb deformities. In: Auer JA, ed. Equine Surgery. Philadelphia: WB Saunders, 2006:1130–1149.

Bramlage LR. The science and art of angular limb deformity correction. Equine Vet J 1999;31:193–196.

Read EK, Read MR, Townsend HG, Clark CR, Pharr JW, Wilson DG. Effect of hemi-circumferential periosteal transection and elevation in foals with experimentally induced angular limb deformities. JAVMA 2002;221:536–540.

Trumble T. Orthopedic disorders in neonatal foals. Vet Clin North Am Equine Pract 2005;21:357–385.

Author Shannon J. Murray
Consulting Editor Margaret C. Mudge

ANHIDROSIS

BASICS

OVERVIEW

Anhidrosis (also known as dry coat disease or a nonsweater, or as "dry puffers") is the inability to sweat effectively in response to appropriate stimuli. The current theory is that overstimulation of sweat gland β_2-receptors causes diminished function or a period of unresponsiveness of the receptors.

SIGNALMENT

No coat color, age, sex, or breed predilections. Up to 20% of horses may be affected when exercising in a hot, humid climate.

SIGNS

- Extended tachypnea after exercise, later combined with a lack or reduction of sweating
- Horses recently introduced into a hot and humid climate may sweat excessively before showing signs of anhidrosis.
- With acute onset, horses may demonstrate partial or complete absence of sweating when exposed to appropriate stimuli.
- Horses with long-standing anhidrosis may exhibit dry and flaky skin with alopecia, lethargy, and decreased water intake. Body areas that may retain the ability to sweat include under the mane, saddle and halter regions, and the axillary, inguinal, and perineal regions.

CAUSES

- Systemic—Heat-stressed horses may have higher-than-normal levels of circulating catecholamines. Anhidrotic horses have significantly higher levels of epinephrine compared with normal horses at rest. These catecholamines act as β_2-agonists and may overstimulate the sweat gland receptors, which results in either desensitization of the receptor (i.e., the receptor is sequestered away from its normal site to another site within the cell) or down-regulation (i.e., decreased number of receptors). Down-regulation is a long-term mechanism that may involve altered synthesis or degradation of receptor proteins.
- Horses maintained in hot, humid climates are at risk, and exercise magnifies this risk.

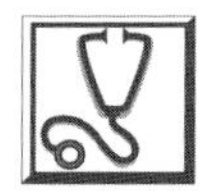

DIAGNOSIS

DIFFERENTIAL DIAGNOSIS

Respiratory diseases that cause an increase in the respiratory rate (both obstructive and restrictive diseases)

CBC/BIOCHEMISTRY/URINALYSIS

Dehydration, as evidenced by prerenal azotemia and, possibly, increased urinary specific gravity

DIAGNOSTIC PROCEDURES

Intradermal injections, in the neck area below the mane, of a specific β_2-agonist (e.g., terbutaline sulfate, salbutamol sulfate), serial dilutions (10^{-3} to 10^{-8} [w/v]), and a control injection of sterile saline— read the results at 30 min. Normal horses sweat in response to all dilutions, whereas anhidrotic horses show a diminished response to some or all.

PATHOLOGICAL FINDINGS/HISTOPATHOLOGY

Thickened basal lamina, evidence of poor myoepithelial contraction, thickened connective tissues, and marked reduction of vesicles in the secretory cells. Luminal microvilli often are absent and the lumen of the duct is obstructed with cellular debris.

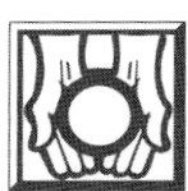

TREATMENT

- Advise clients that sound environmental management is the only reliable treatment option at present.
- Horses with acute anhidrosis who exhibit signs of heat stress should be immediately taken to a cooler environment, and attempts to reduce the body temperature should be made.
- Restrict to a stall with adequate air movement (i.e., a fan) during hot periods of the day.
- If exercise is necessary, do so during the cooler periods of the day. After exercise, make sure the horse is "cooled off" adequately by hosing it down with water.

- Concentrates should be fed in decreased amounts. Allow access to cool, fresh water as well as water with electrolyte supplementation.
- Inform clients that these horses will be prone to poor performance and will only improve once the capability to sweat effectively has returned.
- It may not occur again in a horse's lifetime but is usually is a lifelong problem. However, when it does occur attempts to provide a cool, dry environment must be made.
- If exogenous β_2-agonists such as clenbuterol for concurrent respiratory problems are being administered, consider this as a possible cause and cease administration.

MEDICATIONS

DRUG(S) OF CHOICE

- Supplemental electrolytes, especially potassium salts, can be added to the feed or water.
- Some anecdotal reports of success with iodinated casein (10–15 g/day for 4–8 days) and with 1000–3000 IU PO of vitamin E (i.e., natural α-tocopherol) daily for 1 mo.
- Amino acid supplements, especially those with tyrosine, are commercially available. (Tyrosine is necessary for the resensitization of sequestered β_2-receptors.)

PRECAUTIONS

Anaphylaxis has been reported when using injectable vitamin E.

ALTERNATIVE DRUGS

Drugs that either reduce down-regulation or decrease sympathetic drive are still in the investigative stages.

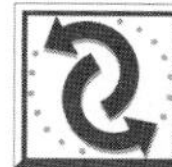

FOLLOW-UP

PATIENT MONITORING

Normal thermoregulatory abilities allow a horse to reduce its body temperature to within normal limits approximately 30 min after exercise. Monitor respiration and rectal temperature post-exercise.

PREVENTION/AVOIDANCE

- Do not expose anhidrotic horses, especially when exercising, to extreme ambient temperatures.
- Exercise during the cooler periods of the day and stall the horse in a cooler environment (e.g., an air-conditioned stall) during the hotter periods of the day.
- Relocating the horse to a more temperate climate may lead to resolution of the clinical signs.
- Avoid administration of exogenous β_2-agonists such as clenbuterol.

POSSIBLE COMPLICATIONS

Heat stroke may occur if horses are exercised during the hotter periods of the day.

EXPECTED COURSE AND PROGNOSIS

- Most horses respond to a change in environment and begin to sweat normally after a few weeks.
- Horses that have previously suffered from the disease will usually, but not necessarily, become anhidrotic if exposed to hot, humid conditions again.

MISCELLANEOUS

ASSOCIATED CONDITIONS

Skin lesions—dry, flaky skin and alopecia, especially around the eyes and shoulders

SEE ALSO

Skin diseases

Suggested Reading

Hubert JD, Norwood G, Beadle RM. Equine anhidrosis. Vet Clin North Am Equine Pract 2002;18:355–369.

Authors Jeremy D. Hubert and Ralph E. Beadle

Consulting Editor Michel Lévy

ANOREXIA AND DECREASED FOOD INTAKE

BASICS

DEFINITION

Anorexia is the loss of appetite or lack of desire for food. Some conditions that cause anorexia may not lead to complete loss of appetite, but merely reduced food intake.

PATHOPHYSIOLOGY

Appetite Suppression

• Anorexia in general appears to be the result of a modification of central regulation of feeding behavior in the hypothalamus. • Many factors and substances appear to be involved in regulating feed intake. • Anorexia associated with alterations of smell and taste has not been shown in the horse. • Decreased food intake has been associated with parasitic infections, but the mechanism is unknown. • Pain and depression appear to cause anorexia, as well as causing dehydration, electrolyte imbalances, acid-base disorders, micronutrient deficiencies, and changes in concentrations of neurotransmitters, hormones, or mediators. • Serotonin agonists decrease food intake, apparently via central histaminergic activity. • The neurotransmitter neuropeptide Y and various cytokines may cause CACS. Cytokines induce anorexia when administered peripherally or directly into the brain. Administration of specific cytokine antagonists mitigates cachexia in experimental animal models. • Other primary disease conditions, such as infection, inflammation, injury, toxins, immunologic reactions, and necrosis, may cause anorexia via cytokines as well. • In addition, a proteoglycan has been identified on the cell membranes of animals and has been named *satiomem.* It reduces food intake and may be a satiety or anorexigenic substance. • Reduced food intake can also be caused by various conditions affecting the lips, mouth, tongue, pharynx, esophagus, or stomach, and may include painful conditions, mechanical obstructions, or nervous or neuromuscular dysfunctions.

SIGNALMENT

Any signalment

SIGNS

May be a lack of interest in food or an interest only in certain types of food. May note difficulty or inability in prehension, chewing, or swallowing of food, and food may appear at the nostrils. Nasal discharge and cough can occur due to foreign material entering trachea, acquired aspiration pneumonia, or both. Some of the signs seen in horses with anorexia may include the following:
• Increased salivation (ptyalism) due to:
• Inability to swallow • Hypoesthesia of the face (CN-V) • Neurogenic atrophy of the masticatory muscles (CN-V, motor component)
• Bilateral paralysis of facial muscles (CN VII)
• May expel partially chewed food ("quidding")
• Oral lesions

CAUSES

Anorexia

Commonly due to gastrointestinal or abdominal disorders, including colic. May be secondary to one of the following primary disease processes in any organ system:
• Inflammation • Infections (bacterial, viral, fungal, or parasitic) • Injury • Toxins
• Immunologic reactions • Malignancy
• Necrosis • Dehydration • Electrolyte imbalances • Acid-base disorders • Severe respiratory distress • Neurologic disorders
• Uremia or renal tubular acidosis • Cardiac disease • Metabolic disorders • Side effects of medications • Pain

Food prehension problems may be due to:
• Pain in lips, tongue, or mouth (e.g., ulcers, lacerations, dental "points") • Mechanical obstructions (e.g., severe swelling of the lips)
• Nervous dysfunction of the lips or tongue

Mastication problems may be due to:
• Pain (in teeth, mandibles, maxilla, sinuses, muscles, or temporomandibular joint)
• Neurologic dysfunction

Swallowing problems may be due to:
• Pain (in pharynx or esophagus) • Mechanical obstructions in pharynx or esophagus
• Neurologic dysfunction (e.g., CN-IX although questioned lately) • Unpalatable food due to contamination or spoilage

RISK FACTORS

Choke, which is the layperson's term for feed impaction of the esophagus, occurs more commonly in animals that bolt their food or have defective teeth.

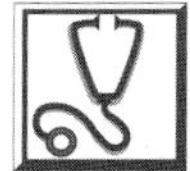

DIAGNOSIS

DIFFERENTIAL DIAGNOSIS

Anorexia

• Colic • Esophagitis • Gastrointestinal ileus
• Gastric ulcers and pyloric stenosis • Peritonitis

Secondary to a primary disease process in any organ system
• Renal failure (uremia)
• Renal tubular acidosis
• Cardiac amyloidosis
• Severe respiratory distress
• Depression of the nervous system—especially cerebral disorders
• Inflammation or endotoxemia
• Injury
• Toxins (e.g., monensin, lead)
• Immunologic reactions
• Malignancy
• Necrosis

Secondary to diseases leading to dehydration, electrolyte imbalances, or acid-base disorders
• Hypertriglyceridemia
• Side effect of metronidazole or toltrazuril or cyproheptadine

Dysphagia

Food prehension problems may be due to:
• Mucosal disease—oral erosions or ulcers, swellings, growths, or crusts
• Vesicular stomatitis
• Contact with chemical irritants
• Phenylbutazone toxicity
• Mechanical trauma; yellow bristle grass, foxtails
• Postsurgical complications
• Mechanical obstructions—severe swelling of the lips
• Snake bites
• Bee stings
• Nervous dysfunction of the lips
• Bilateral CN-VII damage
• Yellow star thistle (nigropallidal encephalomalacia) poisoning
• Rabies
• Equine protozoal myelitis
• Verminous encephalitis

Mastication problems may be due to:
• Musculoskeletal problems
• Postsurgical complications
• Pain (in teeth, mandibles, or maxilla (e.g., fractured mandible), sinuses (e.g., sinusitis), temporomandibular joint
• Pain or other problems of masticatory muscles (e.g. myodegeneration)
• Vitamin E/selenium deficiency causing masseteric myopathy
• Botulism or tick paralysis causing paresis of masticatory muscles and tongue
• Tetanus causing trismus
• Mechanical obstructions
• Premolar caps (deciduous teeth)
• Foreign body
• Neurologic problems
• CN-V bilaterally
• CN-XII damage
• Rabies
• Lead toxicity
• Equine protozoal myelitis
• Verminous encephalitis

Swallowing problems may be due to:
• Pain in pharynx or esophagus
• Esophagitis
• Pharyngitis or pharyngeal trauma
• Pharyngeal abscess
• Neoplasia
• Strangles
• Hyoid bone injury
• Mechanical obstructions or abnormalities in pharynx or esophagus
• Esophageal intraluminal occlusion; choke or foreign body
• Esophageal stricture, stenosis, or diverticulum
• Megaesophagus or esophageal ectasia
• Persistent right aortic arch
• Esophageal intramural inclusion cysts
• Rostral displacement of the palatopharyngeal arch
• Dorsal displacement of the soft palate in foals
• Ulcers of the soft palate secondary to dorsal displacement in adult horses
• Pharyngeal foreign body
• Cysts—epiglottic, dorsal pharyngeal, aryepiglottic, soft palate, guttural pouch, or laryngeal
• Strangles or other retropharyngeal abscess causing external compression
• Cleft palate
• Neoplasia of the tongue
• Nervous or neuromuscular problems
• Severe cerebrum or brain stem (forebrain) disease; hydrocephalus, trauma, leukoencephalomalacia, equine protozoal myelitis, verminous encephalitis
• Lead toxicity
• Senecio toxicity
• CN-IX damage

• Guttural pouch disease (CN-IX to CN-XI damage)
• White muscle disease–nutritional muscular dystrophy
• Hyperkalemic periodic paralysis
• Tetanus
• Botulism
• Tick paralysis
• Weak suckle reflex, poor pharyngeal tone
• Prematurity/dysmaturity, neonatal maladjustment syndrome, bacterial meningitis, viral encephalitis, hypoglycemia, or depression in foals
• Electrolyte disorders (hypokalemia and hypocalcemia)
• Post upper respiratory surgical complications
• Postanesthetic myasthenia
• Myotonia congenita
• Rabies
• Ruptured rectus capitus ventralis muscle
• Grass sickness
• Pharyngeal–cricopharyngeal incoordination

CBC/BIOCHEMISTRY/URINALYSIS

• Free (unconjugated or indirect) bilirubin elevations, unless cachexic, in which case bilirubin levels may be normal
• Laboratory findings (CBC, biochemistry, fibrinogen) consistent with the primary disease process (e.g., inflammation, internal organ damage)
• Laboratory findings (CBC, biochemistry, fibrinogen) consistent with a secondary disease (e.g., aspiration pneumonia)

OTHER LABORATORY TESTS

Based on primary disease processes

IMAGING

• Radiography of guttural pouches for swallowing problems
• Fluoroscopy or radiography of barium swallow for swallowing problems
• Radiography of mandible, temporo-mandibular joint and teeth for painful mastication
• Radiographs of thorax for aspiration pneumonia
• Ultrasound of the tongue
• Abdominal ultrasound for primary inflammatory or neoplastic problems

OTHER DIAGNOSTIC PROCEDURES

• Examination of the food supply for evidence of contamination or spoilage
• Careful observation of individual when offered food
• Oral examination for painful chewing
• Passage of a nasogastric tube (for difficulty swallowing) to rule out “choke”
• Neurologic examination for difficulty swallowing
• Endoscopy of guttural pouches for nervous cause of swallowing problems
• Endoscopy of pharynx, larynx, and esophagus for swallowing problems
• Rectal examination for internal organ disease

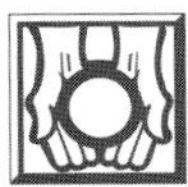

TREATMENT

Depends on the primary problem

DIET/ACTIVITY

Offer highly palatable and varied feed in cases of anorexia. Supply feed that is easy to chew and swallow in case of dysphagia. Force-feeding by nasogastric intubation or parenteral nutrition may be required. Activity should be limited to stall rest or hand-walking in most cases.

MEDICATIONS

DRUG(S) OF CHOICE

• Depends on primary disease process
• Oral administration of 40 g of KCl once or twice daily in anorectic patients

CONTRAINDICATIONS

KCl administration may be contraindicated in patients with abnormal renal function or those suspected of having hyperkalemic periodic paralysis.

FOLLOW-UP

PATIENT MONITORING

The patient should be monitored for dehydration, electrolyte imbalance, acid-base abnormalities, and weight loss, and, in cases of dysphagia, aspiration pneumonia.

POSSIBLE COMPLICATIONS

• Dehydration
• Hypokalemia
• Hypocalcemia
• Metabolic alkalosis with salivary loss
• Weight loss
• Aspiration pneumonia with dysphagia

EXPECTED COURSE AND PROGNOSIS

Depends on the underlying cause

MISCELLANEOUS

ASSOCIATED CONDITIONS

• Other primary disease conditions, such as infection, inflammation, injury, toxins, immunologic reactions, and necrosis
• Cancer-related anorexia/cachexia syndrome (CACS), a syndrome of anorexia and weight loss that occurs secondary to malignancy
• Guttural pouch disease can cause neurologic damage to CN-IX–CN-XI and impair chewing and swallowing as well as causing mechanical obstruction to swallowing.
• Tetanus
• Neonatal maladjustment syndrome may interfere with swallowing or the suckle reflex.
• Moderate jaundice may occur due to increased indirect bilirubin levels in the blood. This is an idiosyncratic finding in the horse that occurs with fasting or decreased intake of feed.
• Dehydration, electrolyte imbalances (hypokalemia, hypocalcemia), or acid-base disorders as a result of lack of intake of fluid and electrolytes may exacerbate the anorexia.
• Salivary loss of electrolytes leads to metabolic alkalosis and hypochloremia, primarily.
• Secondary or conditional PCM involves weight loss with prolonged anorexia.
• Aspiration pneumonia occurs secondary to dysphagia.

AGE-RELATED FACTORS

Cleft palate, hydrocephalus, and nutritional muscular dystrophy (white muscle disease) are noted most commonly in the neonatal period.

ZOONOTIC POTENTIAL

Rabies can cause anorexia or dysphagia. Precautions should be taken while examining and treating the patient.

SYNONYM

Decreased appetite

SEE ALSO

• Aspiration pneumonia
• Botulism
• Cerebral disorders of the central nervous system
• Choke
• Colic
• Dental disease
• Epiglottic cysts
• Esophagitis
• Fractured mandible
• Gastric ulcers
• Gastrointestinal ileus
• Guttural pouch disease
• Lead toxicity
• Monensin toxicity
• Organophosphate toxicity
• Peritonitis
• Pharyngeal abscess
• Phenylbutazone toxicity
• Rabies
• Renal failure (uremia)
• Ruptured rectus capitis ventralis muscle
• Sinusitis
• Snake bites
• Strangles
• Tetanus
• Tick paralysis
• Yellow star thistle poisoning
• Vesicular stomatitis
• Vitamin E/selenium deficiency causing swollen masseter muscles

ABBREVIATIONS

• CACS = cancer-related anorexia/cachexia syndrome
• CN = cranial nerve
• PCM = protein–calorie malnutrition

Suggested Reading

Amory H, Perron MF, Sandersen C, Delguste C, Grulke S, Cassart D, Godeau JM, Detilleux J. Prognostic value of clinical signs and blood parameters in equids suffering from hepatic disease. J Equine Vet Sci 2005;25:18–25.
Mayhew IG. Large Animal Neurology: A Handbook for Veterinary Clinicians. Philadelphia: Lea & Febiger, 1989.
Stratton-Phelps M. Assisted enteral feeding in adult horses. Compend Cont Educ Pract Vet 2004;26:46–49.

Author Gail Abells Sutton
Consulting Editors Henry Stämpfli and Olimpo Oliver-Espinosa

ANTHRAX

BASICS

OVERVIEW

Anthrax is a rapidly fatal septicemic disease of animals and human beings caused by *Bacillus anthracis,* which occurs in localized regions worldwide. In the horse, infection usually results from ingestion of soil, forage, or water contaminated with *B. anthracis* spores. In the animal, the organism germinates and produces exotoxins that impair phagocytosis and vascular integrity resulting in hemorrhage, edema, renal failure, shock, and almost invariably death. When *B. anthracis* is exposed to the environment, long-lasting spores are formed that are a potential source of infection for other animals.

SIGNALMENT

- Gender, age, or breed disposition have not been reported.
- In cattle, anthrax is reported to occur in adult animals, with males more frequently affected, probably due to differences in grazing habits.

SIGNS

- Fever, depression, and death in <4 days is characteristic of the acute form.
- Severe colic, bloody discharge from body orifices, and painful subcutaneous swellings may be noted.
- A chronic form resulting in pharyngeal edema has been described.
- The peracute form, in which death occurs with few clinical signs, appears to be less common in horses than in ruminants.

CAUSES AND RISK FACTORS

- The source of infection is usually soil contaminated by exudates from infected animals. *B. anthracis* forms spores that are very resistant to environmental conditions and most disinfectants, and these spores may persist in the soil for decades. Ingestion of contaminated soil, feed, or water is the most common route of infection, but the organisms may also be inhaled or inoculated by biting insects.
- Anthrax is most common in tropical and subtropical climates but is seen sporadically in temperate regions, usually in the summer. Anthrax usually occurs in regions with alkaline soils and with climatic cycles of heavy rain and drought.
- Overgrazing increases the risk of disease by increasing the ingestion of soil. Coarse forages may contribute to infection by causing breaks in the oral mucosa.

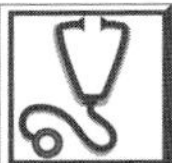

DIAGNOSIS

DIFFERENTIAL DIAGNOSIS

- Lightning strike can be differentiated on the basis of history of storms and absence of post-mortem findings typical of anthrax.
- Colic and enteritis can be differentiated by finding evidence of gastrointestinal disease at post mortem.
- Purpura hemorrhagica has similar signs but is not rapidly fatal.
- Toxicity can be differentiated based on history and lack of post-mortem findings typical of anthrax.
- Malignant edema may appear similar, but crepitation of swellings is not found with anthrax.

CBC/BIOCHEMISTRY/URINALYSIS

Routine laboratory findings have not been reported.

OTHER LABORATORY TESTS

Bacterial culture of blood or exudate is useful, although results may be negative early in disease or if antibiotics have been administered. Cultures should only be performed in a facility capable of containment to prevent infection of laboratory personnel.

IMAGING

N/A

OTHER DIAGNOSTIC PROCEDURES

- Organisms may be seen by microscopic examination of blood smear or edema fluid. Bacilli are gram-positive, have blunt ends, are encapsulated, and occur singly or in short chains.
- Fluorescent antibody of blood or tissue may be diagnostic.

PATHOLOGIC FINDINGS

- Due to human health risk and danger of environmental contamination, necropsy should not be performed if anthrax is strongly suspected. Diagnosis can be made without necropsy.
- Dark, nonclotting blood from orifices; absence of rigor mortis; splenomegaly; and lymphadenopathy are hallmarks of anthrax.
- Serosal and mucosal hemorrhage and edema of many organs are seen.

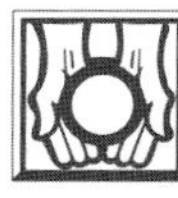

TREATMENT

- The high mortality and rapid course of disease usually limit opportunity for treatment. The prognosis is poor even with treatment.
- Isolate affected and in-contact animals.

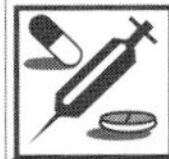

MEDICATIONS

DRUG(S) OF CHOICE

- Penicillin G (40,000 IU/kg IV q4–6 h) or oxytetracycline (5–11 mg/kg IV q12 h) is traditionally recommended. Enrofloxacin (7.5 mg/kg PO q24 h or 5 mg/kg IV q24 h) is potentially a good choice in adult horses. Continue treatment for at least 5 days.
- Anthrax antiserum may be useful but is not available in the United States.

CONTRAINDICATIONS/POSSIBLE INTERACTIONS

N/A

FOLLOW-UP

- Regulatory officials should be notified when anthrax is suspected and the premises placed under quarantine.
- Carcasses should not be opened, and may be disposed of by burning or deep (>6 ft) burial with lime. The area can be disinfected with 5% aqueous lye or 10% formaldehyde.
- Susceptible animals should be vaccinated. An avirulent live spore vaccine is administered subcutaneously and provides immunity in 1 week. Some authors recommend a second vaccination in 2–4 weeks. Annual boosters are required to maintain immunity. Severe adverse reactions have been reported; therefore, the vaccine is indicated only in endemic regions. No antibiotics should be administered within 5 days before or after vaccination, or the vaccine organism may be inactivated.

MISCELLANEOUS

ZOONOTIC POTENTIAL

Anthrax is a zoonosis; inhalation or ingestion of spores may lead to fatal disease. Gloves and mask should be worn if it is necessary to contact infected material or animals. Cutaneous anthrax is the most common form in human beings, resulting from inoculation of an open wound with spores.

SYNONYMS

- Woolsorters' disease
- Charbon
- Splenic fever

Suggested Reading

Pipkin AB. Anthrax. In: Smith BP, ed. Large Animal Internal Medicine. Philadelphia: Mosby, 2002:1074–1076.

Author Laura K. Reilly

Consulting Editors Ashley G. Boyle and Corinne R. Sweeney

ANTICOAGULANT RODENTICIDE TOXICOSIS

BASICS

OVERVIEW

- Ingestion of anticoagulant rodenticides interferes with normal blood clotting in horses.
- Anticoagulant rodenticides are the most commonly used class of rodenticides.
- First-generation anticoagulants (i.e., warfarin, pindone, coumafuryl, coumachlor) are short-acting coumarin derivatives requiring multiple feedings to result in toxicosis.
- Intermediate anticoagulants (i.e., chlorophacinone, diphacinone) require fewer feedings than first-generation chemicals and, thus, are more toxic to nontarget species.
- Second-generation anticoagulants (i.e., brodifacoum, bromadialone, difethialone) are highly toxic to nontarget species after a single feeding.
- Most anticoagulant rodenticides commonly used today are long-acting, second-generation anticoagulants, with activity in the body of ≅1 month.
- Coagulopathy has been reported in horses after a dose of brodifacoum of 0.125 mg/kg (equal to ingestion by an average-size horse of 1 kg of bait containing 0.005% brodifacoum).
- Warfarin has been used therapeutically (30–75 mg per 450 kg) in horses with navicular disease, laminitis, venous arteritis, DIC, and thrombophlebitis.

SIGNALMENT

- May affect all animals
- Poisoning can occur after accidental ingestion of bait packages or as a result of malicious intent.
- Poisoning is rare in horses because of the amount of bait needed to be ingested to cause signs.
- Iatrogenic warfarin toxicosis may result from overdosing, dietary vitamin K deficiency, or concurrent use of protein-bound drugs that increase the concentration of active, unbound warfarin.

SIGNS

- Bleeding diathesis ranging from mild to severe
- Hemorrhage—internal or external
- Signs generally manifest within 3–5 days after ingesting bait.
- Signs are similar to those seen with dicumarol toxicosis.

CAUSES AND RISK FACTORS

The mechanism of anticoagulant rodenticide toxicosis is the same as that for dicumarol toxicosis.

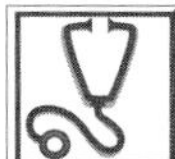

DIAGNOSIS

DIFFERENTIAL DIAGNOSIS

- Moldy sweet clover ingestion—history of ingesting plant, detection of dicumarol in forage or tissue samples
- DIC—reduced plasma concentrations of platelets and coagulant and anticoagulant proteins; increased concentrations of coagulant byproducts; petechial hemorrhages
- Severe liver disease—clinical pathology, liver biopsy

CBC/BIOCHEMISTRY/URINALYSIS

Blood loss anemia

OTHER LABORATORY TESTS

- Elevated PT and aPTT
- Chemical analysis of whole blood or liver tissue for specific anticoagulant

IMAGING

N/A

DIAGNOSTIC PROCEDURES

N/A

PATHOLOGICAL FINDINGS

Hemorrhages may occur in any part of the body.

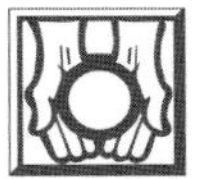

TREATMENT

- Blood or plasma transfusions may help.
- Handle horses with care to avoid stress and further hemorrhage.
- Attempt correction of organ dysfunction resulting from accumulation of extravascular blood (e.g., thoracocentesis) only if the situation is life-threatening and after normal blood coagulation is restored.
- Adding alfalfa hay to the diet may help to provide a source of increased dietary vitamin K_1.

MEDICATIONS

DRUG(S) OF CHOICE

- Vitamin K_1 (phytonadione 2.5 mg/kg q12h SQ initially then PO after ≅3 days and continuing for 3–5 weeks) effectively reverses the clotting defect.
- AC at 1–4 g/kg body weight in water slurry (1 g AC in 5 mL water) PO. One dose of cathartic PO with AC if no diarrhea or ileus (70% sorbitol at 3mL/kg or sodium or magnesium sulfate at 250–500 mg/kg).

CONTRAINDICATIONS/POSSIBLE INTERACTIONS

- Do not use vitamin K_3 (menadione) in horses. Vitamin K_3 is ineffective against anticoagulant rodenticide toxicosis and is nephrotoxic.
- Medications that are highly plasma protein bound may exacerbate toxicosis.
- Drugs generally contraindicated are NSAIDs, phenothiazine tranquilizers, local anesthetics, antihistamines, sulfonamide antibiotics, anabolic steroids, and epinephrine.

FOLLOW-UP

PATIENT MONITORING

- Continue monitoring for blood loss.
- Check PT 2–3 days after the last dose of vitamin K_1 to determine if additional treatment is necessary.

PREVENTION/AVOIDANCE

Prevent access to bait packages.

POSSIBLE COMPLICATIONS

N/A

EXPECTED COURSE AND PROGNOSIS

Prognosis is based on the severity of blood loss and damage to organ systems affected by hemorrhage.

MISCELLANEOUS

ASSOCIATED CONDITIONS, AGE-RELATED FACTORS, ZOONOTIC POTENTIAL

N/A

PREGNANCY

- Lactating mares may excrete anticoagulant rodenticides in their milk.
- Monitor foals for any coagulopathies, and treat with vitamin K_1 if PT rises.

SEE ALSO

Dicumarol (moldy sweet clover) toxicosis

ABBREVIATIONS

- AC = activated charcoal
- aPTT = activated partial thromboplastin time
- DIC = disseminated intravascular coagulation
- PT = prothrombin time

Suggested Reading

McConnico RS, Copedge K, Bischoff KL. Brodifacoum toxicosis in two horses. J Am Vet Med Assoc 1997;211:882–886.

Ayala I, Rodriguez MJ, Martos N, Zilberschtein J, Ruiz I, Motas M. Fatal brodifacoum poisoning in a pony. Can Vet J 2007;48:627–629.

Author Anita M. Kore

Consulting Editor Robert H. Poppenga

ANURIA/OLIGURIA

BASICS

- *Anuria*—lack of urine production
- *Oliguria*—decreased urine production (<0.25 mL/kg per hr, or <125 mL/hr in a 500-kg horse)
- Anuria or oliguria may be physiologic or pathological.
- This chapter will focus on intrinsic renal failure causing anuria and oliguria.

SYSTEM AFFECTED

Renal/urologic

SIGNALMENT

Breed Predilections

No age, sex, or bred predisposition documented

CAUSES AND RISK FACTORS

- Physiologic oliguria—hyperosmolality; any disease process leading to renal hypoperfusion (e. g., dehydration, hypotension, low cardiac output).
- Pathological anuria/oliguria—intrinsic ARF or birth trauma (e.g., dystocia) would increase the risk of urinary tract disruption and uroperitoneum in neonates and their dams; penile trauma is more common in breeding stallions.

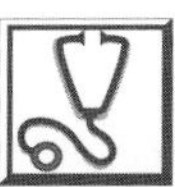

DIAGNOSIS

DIFFERENTIAL DIAGNOSIS

Pathologic Anuria/Oliguria

- Intrinsic ARF, terminal CRF, lower urinary tract disruption resulting in uroperitoneum, and urinary tract obstruction consequent to urolithiasis
- Bladder displacement
- Progressive abdominal distention should increase suspicion of uroperitoneum.
- Repeated posturing to urinate, with little urine passed, supports urinary tract obstruction.

CBC/BIOCHEMISTRY/URINALYSIS

- Normal to high PCV in most cases; mild to moderate anemia possible with terminal CRF.
- Moderate to severe increases in BUN (50–150 mg/dL) and Cr (2.0–20 mg/dL).
- Variable hyponatremia, hypochloremia, hyperkalemia, hypocalcemia, and hyperphosphatemia—hyperkalemia and hyperphosphatemia more common with intrinsic ARF; hyperkalemia most apparent with urinary tract disruption and development of uroperitoneum.
- Mild to moderate metabolic acidosis—depending on the underlying disease process.
- Mild to moderate hyperglycemia—attributed to stress.
- USG — high (>1.035) with physiologic oliguria, low (<1.020) with oliguria due to intrinsic ARF; specific gravity best assessed in urine collected during initial patient evaluation (before rehydration) or while the horse is not receiving fluids.
- Oliguria with intrinsic ARF may be accompanied by mild to moderate proteinuria, glucosuria, pigmenturia, and increased numbers of RBCs and casts on sediment examination.
- Urine pH—normal to acidic, especially with concurrent depletion of body potassium stores

IMAGING

Transabdominal and Ultrasonography

- Kidneys may be enlarged, with loss of detail of corticomedullary junction, in intrinsic ARF.
- Kidneys typically are reduced in size, with increased parenchymal echogenicity, in CRF.

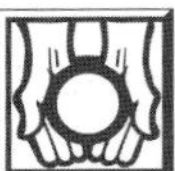

TREATMENT

- Treat anuria/oliguria as a medical emergency because persistent renal hypoperfusion may lead to ischemic ARF.
- If untreated, metabolic disturbances, most notably hyperkalemia, may lead to cardiac arrhythmias and death.
- Once the patient is stabilized (largely with supportive treatment in the form of IV fluid therapy), pursue further diagnostic evaluation to determine if surgical intervention (for correction of uroperitoneum or relief of obstruction) is needed.
- Proper recognition and treatment of all primary disease processes, usually on an inpatient basis for continuous fluid therapy, is warranted.
- Avoid nephrotoxic medications.

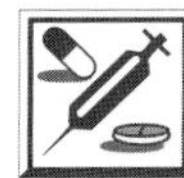

MEDICATIONS

DRUG(S) OF CHOICE

- Fluid therapy to correct renal hypoperfusion—after initial measurement of body weight, correct estimated dehydration with normal (0.9%) saline or another potassium-poor electrolyte solution over 6–12 hr; monitor closely for subcutaneous and pulmonary edema (i.e., increased respiratory rate and effort); conjunctival edema may develop rapidly in horses with intrinsic oliguric to anuric ARF; use maintenance fluid therapy judiciously in animals that are not clinically dehydrated; if hemorrhage is contributing to hypovolemia and renal hypoperfusion, initial treatment with hypertonic saline and/or a blood transfusion may have value.

• Severe hyperkalemia (>7.0 mEq/L) or cardiac arrhythmias—treat with agents that decrease serum potassium concentration (e.g., sodium bicarbonate [1–2 mEq/kg IV over 5–15 minutes]), or counteract the effects of hyperkalemia on cardiac conduction (e.g., calcium gluconate [0.5 mL/kg of a 10% solution by slow IV injection]).
• Furosemide—this diuretic may be administered two times (1–2 mg/kg IV) at 1–2-hr intervals; if effective, urination should be observed within 1 hour after administration of the second dose; if ineffective, discontinue.
• Based on recent evidences in critically ill human patients the ROUTINE USE OF MANNITOL or DOPAMINE IN EQUINE PATIENTS WITH ARF IS NO LONGER RECOMMENDED.

CONTRAINDICATIONS

Avoid all nephrotoxic medications unless specifically indicated for the underlying disease process, and then modify dosage accordingly.

PRECAUTIONS

• Monitor response to fluid therapy closely—as little as 40 mL/kg of IV fluids (20 L to a 500 kg horse) may produce significant pulmonary edema.
• Reassess dosage schedule of drugs eliminated by urinary excretion; consider discontinuing all nephrotoxic medications (especially gentamicin, tetracycline, and NSAIDs).

POSSIBLE INTERACTIONS

Use of multiple anti-inflammatory drugs (e.g., corticosteroids and one or more NSAIDs) will have additive negative effects on renal blood flow; avoid combined administration in azotemic patients.

FOLLOW-UP

PATIENT MONITORING

• Assess clinical status (emphasizing hydration), urine output, and body weight frequently for the first 3 days.
• Assess magnitude of azotemia and electrolyte and acid–basis status at least daily for the first 3 days of treatment.
• Consider placing a central venous line to maintain central venous pressure <8 cm H_2O in more critical patients and neonates.

POSSIBLE COMPLICATIONS

• Severe hyperkalemia accompanied by cardiac arrhythmias, cardiac arrest, and death
• Pulmonary and peripheral edema; conjunctival edema may be dramatic.

MISCELLANEOUS

ASSOCIATED CONDITIONS

• Colic; enterocolitis
• Pleuritis; peritonitis; septicemia
• Exhausted horse syndrome—multiorgan failure

AGE-RELATED FACTORS

Neonates afflicted with hypoxic-ischemic multiorgan damage or septicemia may be at increased risk of anuric/oliguric ARF.

ZOONOTIC POTENTIAL

Leptospirosis has infectious and zoonotic potential; avoid direct contact with infective urine.

SEE ALSO

• ARF
• CRF
• Urolithiasis
• Urinary tract obstruction
• Uroperitoneum

ABBREVIATIONS

• ARF = acute renal failure
• CRF = chronic renal failure
• GFR = glomerular filtration rate
• PCV = packed cell volume
• USG = urinary specific gravity
• UTI = urinary tract infection

Suggested Reading

Bayly WM. Acute renal failure. In: Reed SM, Bayly WM, eds. Equine Internal Medicine. Philadelphia: WB Saunders, 1998:848–856.

Geor RJ. Acute renal failure in horses. Vet Clin North Am Equine Pract 2007;23:563–576.

Schott HC. Chronic renal failure. In: Reed SM, Bayly WM, eds. Equine Internal Medicine. Philadelphia: WB Saunders, 1998:856–875.

Author Harold C. Schott II

Consulting Editor Gillian Perkins

AORTIC REGURGITATION

BASICS

DEFINITION

• Occurs when the aortic valve allows blood to leak into the left ventricular outflow tract during diastole, creating a holodiastolic decrescendo murmur with its PMI in the aortic valve area. • The murmur radiates toward the left cardiac apex and the right side.

PATHOPHYSIOLOGY

• The aortic leaflets do not form a complete seal between the aorta and left ventricle.
• During diastole, blood regurgitates into the left ventricular outflow tract, causing a left ventricular volume overload. As this volume overload becomes more severe, stretching of the mitral annulus occurs, and mitral regurgitation often develops. Mitral regurgitation compounds the severe left ventricular volume overload, and these horses often rapidly develop congestive heart failure.
• Severe regurgitation results in decreased coronary artery blood flow and decreased myocardial perfusion. • Ventricular arrhythmias may develop secondary to decreased myocardial perfusion.

SYSTEM AFFECTED

Cardiovascular

GENETICS

N/A

INCIDENCE/PREVALENCE

N/A

GEOGRAPHIC DISTRIBUTION

N/A

SIGNALMENT

Usually horses >10 years

SIGNS

General Comments

Often an incidental finding during routine auscultation

Historical

• Poor performance • Possibly congestive heart failure

Physical Examination

• Grade 1–6/6, decrescendo or musical holodiastolic murmur with PMI in the aortic valve area (left or right fourth intercostal space) radiating to the left apex and right side
• Other, less common findings—bounding arterial pulses, atrial fibrillation, ventricular premature depolarizations, accentuated third heart sounds, and congestive heart failure

CAUSES

• Degenerative changes of the aortic leaflets
• Fenestration of aortic leaflets
• Nonvegetative valvulitis • Flail aortic leaflet
• Infective endocarditis • Ventricular septal defect • Congenital malformation • Disease of the aortic root

RISK FACTORS

Old age

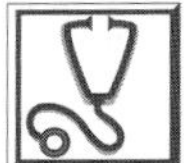

DIAGNOSIS

DIFFERENTIAL DIAGNOSIS

Pulmonic regurgitation—rare; murmurs usually are soft or not detectable and should have PMI in the pulmonic valve area; bounding arterial pulses are not present; differentiate echocardiographically.

CBC/BIOCHEMISTRY/URINALYSIS

May have neutrophilic leukocytosis and hyperfibrinogenemia with bacterial endocarditis

OTHER LABORATORY TESTS

• Elevated cardiac isoenzymes may be present (e.g., cardiac troponin I, CK-MB, HBDH, LDH-1 and LDH-2) with concurrent myocardial disease.
• Positive blood culture may be obtained from horses with bacterial endocarditis.

IMAGING

Electrocardiography

• Ventricular premature depolarizations may be present in horses with severe regurgitation and be caused by poor myocardial perfusion.
• Atrial fibrillation often develops in horses with marked left ventricular volume overload and subsequent left atrial enlargement.

Echocardiography

• Most affected horses have thickened aortic valve leaflets.
• An echogenic band parallel to and a nodular thickening of the left coronary leaflet free edge are the most common findings.
• Prolapse of an aortic leaflet (usually the noncoronary or right coronary leaflet) into the left ventricular outflow tract frequently is detected.
• Fenestration of the aortic leaflet, flail aortic leaflet, vegetations associated with infective endocarditis, or aortic root abnormalities infrequently are detected.
• Left ventricle—enlarged and dilated, with a rounded apex
• Thinning of the left ventricular free wall and interventricular septum
• Increased septal–to–E point separation may be present.
• Pattern of left ventricular volume overload
• Normal or decreased fractional shortening in a horse with left ventricular enlargement is consistent with myocardial dysfunction.
• Dilatation of the aortic root in horses with longstanding regurgitation
• High-frequency vibrations on the mitral valve septal leaflet usually are detected with M-mode echocardiography and are created by turbulence in the left ventricular outflow tract.
• In some horses, high-frequency vibrations may be visualized on the interventricular septum instead of, or in addition to, vibrations on the mitral valve septal leaflet.
• High-frequency vibrations on the aortic leaflets usually are visualized in horses with musical holodiastolic murmurs.
• Premature mitral valve closure may indicate more severe aortic insufficiency.
• Pulsed-wave or color-flow Doppler reveals a jet or jets of regurgitation in the left ventricular outflow tract. Size of the jet at its origin is a good indicator of severity. Size and extent of the regurgitation jet represent another means of semiquantitating its severity, as is strength of the regurgitation signal.
• Continuous-wave Doppler assessment of the spectral tracing of the regurgitation jet also provides an estimate for the severity of regurgitation—a steep slope and a short pressure half-time indicate more severe regurgitation.

Thoracic Radiography

• Left-sided cardiac enlargement may be detected in horses with moderate to severe regurgitation.
• Pulmonary edema may be present in affected horses with congestive heart failure.

DIAGNOSTIC PROCEDURES

Cardiac Catheterization

• Right-sided catheterization may reveal elevated pulmonary capillary wedge pressures and pulmonary arterial pressures in horses with severe regurgitation and concurrent mitral regurgitation.
• Right ventricular and atrial pressures may be elevated in affected horses with congestive heart failure.
• Oxygen saturation of blood obtained from the right atrium, right ventricle, and pulmonary artery should be normal.

Continuous 24-Hour Holter Monitoring

Use in the diagnosis of horses with suspected ventricular premature depolarizations.

PATHOLOGIC FINDINGS

• Focal or diffuse thickening or distortion of one or more aortic leaflets may be present.
• Nodules, bands, plaques, and fenestrations have been described on the aortic leaflets at postmortem examination.
• Flail aortic leaflets, infective endocarditis, or congenital malformations of the aortic valve infrequently are detected.
• Aortic root dilatation usually is present in horses with severe, long-standing regurgitation.
• Jet lesions usually are detected on the ventricular side of the mitral valve septal leaflet and, less frequently, on the interventricular septum.
• Left ventricular enlargement and thinning of the left ventricular free wall and interventricular septum in horses with significant regurgitation.
• Atrial myocardial thinning with atrial dilatation has been documented in horses with atrial fibrillation and enlargement.
• Inflammatory cell infiltrate has been detected in horses with myocarditis and aortic regurgitation; however, most affected horses do not have significant underlying myocardial disease.

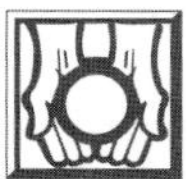

TREATMENT

AIMS OF TREATMENT

• Management by intermittent monitoring in horses with aortic regurgitation that is mild or moderate in severity • Palliative care in horses with severe aortic regurgitation

APPROPRIATE HEALTH CARE

• Most affected horses require no treatment and can be monitored on an outpatient basis.
• Horses with moderate to severe regurgitation may benefit from long-term vasodilator therapy, particularly with ACE inhibitors.
• Treat horses with severe regurgitation and congestive heart failure for the congestive heart failure with positive inotropic drugs, vasodilators, and diuretics on an inpatient basis, if possible, and monitor response to therapy.

NURSING CARE

N/A

ACTIVITY

• Affected horses are safe to continue in full athletic work until the regurgitation becomes severe or ventricular arrhythmias develop.
• Monitor horses with moderate to severe regurgitation by ECG during high-intensity exercise to ensure they are safe for ridden activities. These horses can be used for lower-level athletic activities until they begin to develop congestive heart failure.
• Horses with significant ventricular arrhythmias or pulmonary artery dilatation are no longer safe to ride.

DIET

N/A

CLIENT EDUCATION

• Regularly palpate the arterial pulses to monitor the progression of left ventricular volume overload. Bounding arterial pulses indicate significant left ventricular volume overload. Moderate to severe regurgitation usually is present in these horses.
• Regularly monitor cardiac rhythm; any irregularities other than second-degree AV block should prompt ECG.
• Carefully monitor for exercise intolerance, respiratory distress, prolonged recovery after exercise, increased resting respiratory rate or heart rate, or cough; if detected, seek a cardiac reexamination.

SURGICAL CONSIDERATIONS

N/A

MEDICATIONS

DRUGS

• Severe regurgitation—Administor enalapril (0.25–0.5 mg/kg PO q24h or q12h) or another ACE inhibitor.
• ACE inhibitors prolong the time to valve replacement in humans with moderate to severe regurgitation.
• The bioavailability of enalapril is poor but horses with moderate to severe regurgitation have experienced a decrease in left ventricular chamber size with ACE inhibitors.
• Treatment of affected horses in heart failure include digoxin, furosemide, and vasodilators.

CONTRAINDICATIONS

ACE inhibitors and other vasodilators must be withdrawn before competition to comply with the medication rules of the various governing bodies of equine sports.

PRECAUTIONS

ACE inhibitors can cause hypotension; thus, do not give a large dose without time to accommodate to this treatment.

POSSIBLE INTERACTIONS

N/A

ALTERNATIVE DRUGS

Most other vasodilatory drugs should have some beneficial effect in horses with moderate to severe regurgitation, but they may be less effective than the ACE inhibitors.

FOLLOW-UP

PATIENT MONITORING

• Frequently monitor arterial pulses and cardiac rhythm.
• Reexamine horses with mild to moderate regurgitation by ECG every year.
• Reexamine horses with severe regurgitation by echocardiography every 6 mo to monitor progression of valvular insufficiency and determine if the horse continues to be safe to ride or drive.

PREVENTION/AVOIDANCE

N/A

POSSIBLE COMPLICATIONS

Chronic regurgitation—ventricular arrhythmias; atrial fibrillation; mitral regurgitation; congestive heart failure

EXPECTED COURSE AND PROGNOSIS

• Most affected horses have a normal performance life and life expectancy.
• Progression of regurgitation associated with degenerative valve disease usually is slow. With the typical onset of regurgitation that occurs in old horses, other problems are more likely to end of horse's performance career or shorten life expectancy.
• Affected horses with congestive heart failure usually have severe underlying valvular heart disease and myocardial disease and a guarded to grave prognosis for life. Most affected horses being treated for congestive heart failure respond to the supportive therapy and improve. This improvement usually is short lived, however, and most are euthanized within 2–6 mo of initiating treatment.

MISCELLANEOUS

ASSOCIATED CONDITIONS

N/A

AGE-RELATED FACTORS

Old horses are more likely to be affected.

ZOONOTIC POTENTIAL

N/A

PREGNANCY

• Affected mares should not experience any problems with pregnancy unless the regurgitation is severe.
• Treat pregnant affected mares with congestive heart failure for the underlying cardiac disease with positive inotropic drugs and diuretics; ACE inhibitors are contraindicated because of potential adverse effects on the fetus.

SYNONYMS

Aortic insufficiency

SEE ALSO

• Infective endocarditis
• Ventricular septal defect

ABBREVIATIONS

• ACE = angiotensin-converting enzyme
• AV = atrioventricular
• CK-MB = MB isoenzyme of creatine kinase
• HBDH = α-hydroxybutyrate dehydrogenase
• LDH = lactate dehydrogenase
• PMI = point of maximal intensity

Suggested Reading

Else RW, Holmes JR. Cardiac pathology in the horse. I. Gross pathology. Equine Vet J 1972;4:1–8.

Gardner SY, Atkins CE, Sams RA, Schwabenton AB, Papich MG, Characterization of the pharmacokinetic and pharmacodynamic properties of the angiotensin-converting enzyme inhibitor, enalapril, in horses. J Vet Intern Med 2004:18;231–237.

Reef VB. Cardiovascular ultrasonography. In: Reef VB, ed. Equine Diagnostic Ultrasound. Philadelphia: WB Saunders, 1998:215–272.

Reef VB, Spencer P. Echocardiographic evaluation of equine aortic insufficiency. Am J Vet Res 1987;48:904–909.

Young L. Equine aortic valve regurgitation: a disease worthy of further consideration. Equine Vet Educ 2007:19;469–470.

Author Virginia B. Reef

Consulting Editor Celia M. Marr

AORTIC ROOT RUPTURE

BASICS

DEFINITION

A defect in the wall of the aorta at the aortic root, usually in the right sinus of Valsalva

PATHOPHYSIOLOGY

- Aortic rupture results in the exsanguination into the thoracic cavity, cardiac tamponade from hemopericardium, or a shunt between the aorta and heart.
- With an aortic rupture confined to the right sinus of Valsalva, an aorticocardiac fistula is created. Blood from the aorta shunts into the right side of the heart, at either the atrial or ventricular level, depending on the site of the rupture.
- Subendocardial dissection of blood into the interventricular septum is common, with subsequent rupture into the right or left ventricle (more commonly, the rupture is into the right ventricle).
- Often associated with a unifocal ventricular tachycardia that may be associated with dissection of blood into the interventricular septum

SYSTEM AFFECTED

Cardiovascular

INCIDENCE/PREVALENCE

More frequently occurs in old horses, particularly males

SIGNALMENT

Often occurs during or after breeding or other exercise

SIGNS

General Comments

Often interpreted by owners as colic, because the horse appears distressed, may be looking at its flanks, and acts uncomfortable

Historical

- Acute onset of colic or distress, usually after exercise or breeding
- Less commonly, exercise intolerance; syncope

Physical Examination

- Tachycardia
- Tachypnea
- Continuous machinery murmur—usually loudest on the right side
- Bounding arterial pulses
- Other, less common findings—jugular pulses and distention, ventricular tachycardia (unifocal), and congestive heart failure

CAUSES

- A congenital aneurysm in the wall of the aortic root, usually in the right sinus of Valsalva, predisposes to aortic root rupture.
- Necrosis and degeneration of the aortic media have been associated, especially in old breeding stallions.
- Aberrant parasite migration in the ascending aorta is unlikely.

RISK FACTORS

- Aortic aneurysm
- Aortitis

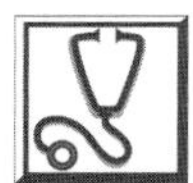

DIAGNOSIS

DIFFERENTIAL DIAGNOSIS

Ventricular Septal Defect with Aortic Regurgitation

- Murmurs are systolic (band shaped and pansystolic) and diastolic (holodiastolic and decrescendo), not continuous.
- Arterial pulses usually are not bounding, unless the associated aortic regurgitation is severe.
- No history of acute colic or distress
- Differentiate echocardiographically.

Patent Ductus Arteriosus

- No history of acute colic or distress
- No unifocal ventricular tachycardia
- Differentiate echocardiographically.

CBC/BIOCHEMISTRY/URINALYSIS

Elevated serum creatinine and BUN may occur because of impaired renal perfusion, which is associated with sustained ventricular tachycardia and blood loss.

OTHER LABORATORY TESTS

Serum cardiac troponin I and cardiac isoenzymes of creatine phosphokinase and lactate dehydrogenase can be elevated with significant myocardial cell injury.

IMAGING

ECG

Uniform ventricular tachycardia with a heart rate of >100 bpm may be present.

Echocardiography

- Two-dimensional echocardiography is diagnostic for a defect in the aortic root at the sinus of Valsalva or for a sinus of Valsalva aneurysm.
- The rupture may be a small, irregular defect in the aortic wall (usually associated with the right aortic leaflet) or be visualized flailing in the right atrium or ventricle.
- Anechoic to echoic fluid may be detected dissecting subendocardially into the interventricular septum, most frequently along the right ventricular side; however, dissection of blood subendocardially along the left side also occurs.
- Right atrial or ventricular enlargement if the aorta has ruptured into one of these chambers
- Paradoxical septal motion with severe right ventricular volume overload
- Ruptured tricuspid chordae tendineae or ruptured or flail tricuspid valve leaflet may be detected, particularly with rupture of an aneurysm of the sinus of Valsalva.
- Subendocardial dissection of blood along the left side of the interventricular septum may result in rupture into the left ventricle and left ventricular volume overload.
- Hyperdynamic interventricular septum and left ventricular free wall are associated with left ventricular volume overload, producing increased fractional shortening, until the myocardium starts to fail.
- Rupture of a mitral valve chordae tendineae and a flail mitral valve leaflet may occur, producing acute onset of severe mitral regurgitation.
- Significant left ventricular volume overload can lead to dilatation of the mitral annulus and mitral regurgitation.
- Use color-flow Doppler, pulsed-wave Doppler, or contrast echocardiography to localize the shunt associated with the aortic cardiac fistula.
- Continuous-wave Doppler can be used to determine peak velocity of the shunt flow.

Thoracic Radiography

- An enlarged cardiac silhouette should be present in horses with a large aorticocardiac shunt.
- Pulmonary overcirculation and edema may be detected.

DIAGNOSTIC PROCEDURES

Cardiac Catheterization

- Elevated right ventricular pressure, pulmonary arterial pressure, pulmonary capillary wedge pressure, and oxygen saturation of the blood are detected in horses with aorticocardiac fistula into the right ventricle.
- With a shunt into the right atrium, right atrial pressures and oxygen saturation also are elevated.

Arterial Blood Pressure

Demonstrates the wide difference between peak systolic pressure and end-diastolic pressure associated with continuous shunting of blood from the aorta into the heart

PATHOLOGIC FINDINGS

- Post-mortem examination confirms the site and extent of the rupture and the presence of aorticocardiac fistula.
- Path of the dissection can be traced and the rupture into the right atrium, tricuspid valve, right ventricle, or left ventricle confirmed.
- Dissecting tracts into the interventricular septum usually are lined with immature and mature fibrous tissue, and disruption of the conduction system has been detected.
- Degeneration and necrosis of the aortic media have been reported in some horses with aortic root rupture but not in other affected horses.
- An absence of media in the right sinus of Valsalva was reported in one horse with a sinus of Valsalva (i.e., aortic root) aneurysm.
- Fibrosis and scarring of the rupture site have been reported in old breeding stallions that died of unrelated causes.
- Biatrial and biventricular enlargement usually is detected, and hepatic congestion and pulmonary edema may be present.

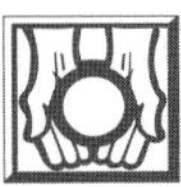

TREATMENT

AIMS OF TREATMENT

Palliative care

APPROPRIATE HEALTH CARE

- Closely monitor affected horses with ventricular tachycardia if the tachycardia is uniform, the heart rate is >120 bpm, no R-on-T complexes are detected, and no clinical signs of cardiovascular collapse are observed.
- If ventricular tachycardia is multiform, R-on-T complexes are detected, heart rate is >120 bpm, or with clinical signs of cardiovascular collapse, institute antiarrhythmic treatment on an inpatient basis.
- If congestive heart failure also is present, institute treatment for congestive heart failure as well. Consider humane destruction, however, because the horse is no longer safe to use for athletic work.

NURSING CARE

- Perform continuous ECG monitoring during the attempted conversion from ventricular tachycardia to sinus rhythm.
- Keep horses quiet and unmoving during antiarrhythmic treatment.

ACTIVITY

- Stall confinement until conversion to sinus rhythm has been successfully achieved
- Restrict athletic activity as much as possible once ventricular tachycardia has been converted.

CLIENT EDUCATION

- Affected horses are not safe to ride or use for any type of athletic work because of the risk of sudden death associated with further aortic rupture or development of fatal ventricular arrhythmia.
- If the horse is a breeding stallion and such continued use is desired, warn the stallion and mare handlers (and all other personnel involved) about the risk of sudden death.
- Develop an emergency plan in the event the stallion becomes unsteady or unsafe to handle.

SURGICAL CONSIDERATIONS

N/A

MEDICATIONS

DRUG(S) OF CHOICE

Antiarrhythmics

- Indicated with multiform ventricular tachycardia, R-on-T complexes, heart rate >120 bpm, or clinical signs of cardiovascular collapse
- Drug selection depends on severity of ventricular tachycardia and associated clinical signs.
- IV lidocaine is rapidly acting and has a very short duration of action. However, it also has CNS effects in horses and, thus, must be used carefully.
- IV procainamide and quinidine gluconate have been effective in converting sustained, uniform ventricular tachycardia but have a slower onset of action.
- IV magnesium sulfate has been successful in converting sustained ventricular tachycardia and is not arrhythmogenic.

ACE Inhibitors

- May be indicated in stallions to decrease resistance to forward flow once ventricular tachycardia has been converted.
- Enalapril (0.5mg/kg PO BID) has no effect on the stallion's libido, breeding performance, or fertility.
- Other vasodilators or antihypertensive drugs can be considered, but their effect on breeding stallions is unknown.

CONTRAINDICATIONS

Other vasodilators or antihypertensive drugs have the potential to adversely affect the stallion's libido, breeding performance, or fertility.

PRECAUTIONS

Affected horses could experience sudden death at any time; thus, everyone working around these horses must be aware of the safety issues involved.

POSSIBLE INTERACTIONS

Any antiarrhythmic drug has the potential to cause development of a more adverse arrhythmia as well as to convert to sinus rhythm.

ALTERNATIVE DRUGS

Propranolol

- The IV form is less likely to be effective but should be considered in affected horses with refractory ventricular tachycardia.
- Lowers systolic blood pressure

Propafenone

- Very effective in converting refractory ventricular tachycardia
- The IV form is not available in the United States (but is available abroad); only an oral form is available in this country.
- May have a synergistic effect with procainamide in horses with refractory ventricular tachycardia

FOLLOW-UP

PATIENT MONITORING

- Routine monitoring of heart rate and of respiratory rate and rhythm after conversion to sinus rhythm
- Persistent tachypnea, tachycardia, or new arrhythmias indicate deterioration in clinical status.

AORTIC ROOT RUPTURE

• Return of venous distention and jugular pulsations or development of ventral edema or coughing indicates the onset of congestive heart failure and worsening of ventricular volume overload.

PREVENTION/AVOIDANCE

• With congenital aneurysms of the sinus of Valsalva, control of systemic blood pressure may prolong the time until rupture occurs.
• With degenerative changes in the aortic media, antihypertensive drugs theoretically should have some benefit. However, identification of horses at risk has not yet been accomplished.
• Routine echocardiography of old breeding stallions and high-performance horses potentially at risk may help to identify these horses before development of a tear in the aortic root.

POSSIBLE COMPLICATIONS

• Deterioration of uniform ventricular tachycardia into fatal ventricular arrhythmia
• Severe, acute congestive heart failure from massive right atrial or ventricular, left atrial, and left ventricular volume overload
• Tricuspid valve rupture, leading to massive tricuspid regurgitation and congestive heart failure
• Rupture of a chordae tendineae of the tricuspid or mitral valve, leading to massive tricuspid or mitral regurgitation, respectively, and acute, right- or left-sided congestive heart failure
• Sudden death

EXPECTED COURSE AND PROGNOSIS

• Prognosis for life of affected horses is grave, with sudden death expected in those with extracardiac or intrapericardial rupture.
• Onset of congestive heart failure is likely after development of an intracardiac fistula, and the speed of its development depends on the location and size of the shunt.

MISCELLANEOUS

ASSOCIATED CONDITIONS

Aortic root aneurysm

AGE-RELATED FACTORS

Old horses are more likely to be affected, but horses as young as 4 years have been diagnosed.

PREGNANCY

• Rupture of a sinus of Valsalva aneurysm has been seen in one late-gestation pregnant mare. The volume expansion of late pregnancy may predispose pregnant mares to aortic rupture at this time.
• Aortic root rupture has been seen in one mare during early pregnancy. This mare experienced acute onset of ventricular tachycardia and subendocardial dissection of blood into the interventricular septum but survived to have the foal.

SYNONYMS

• Aortic cardiac fistula
• Aorticocardiac fistula

SEE ALSO

• Ventricular tachycardia

ABBREVIATIONS

• CNS = central nervous system

Suggested Reading

Lester GD, Lombard CW, Ackerman N. Echocardiographic detection of a dissecting aortic root aneurysm in a Thoroughbred stallion. Vet Radiol Ultrasound 1992;33:202–205.

Marr CM, Reef VB, Brazil T, Thomas W, Maxson AD, Reimer JM. Clinical and echocardiographic findings in horses with aortic root rupture. Vet Radiol Ultrasound 1998;39:22–31.

Reef VB, Klump S, Maxson AD, et al. Echocardiographic detection of an intact aneurysm in a horse. J Am Vet Med Assoc 1990;197:752–755.

Roby KA, Reef VB, Shaw DP, Sweeney CR. Rupture of an aortic sinus aneurysm in a 15-year-old broodmare. J Am Vet Med Assoc 1986;189:305–308.

Rooney JR, Prickett ME, Crowe MW. Aortic ring rupture in stallions. Pathol Vet 1967;4:268–274.

Author Virginia B. Reef
Consulting Editor Celia M. Marr

ARSENIC TOXICOSIS

BASICS

OVERVIEW

- Results from excessive exposure to arsenic-containing pesticides, arsenic-contaminated soils, burn piles, and water or feed
- Ashes from CCA-treated lumber are high in arsenic.
- Toxicity depends on the form of arsenic ingested.
- Trivalent inorganic forms (e.g., arsenic trioxide; sodium, potassium and calcium salts of arsenite) are 10-fold more toxic than inorganic pentavalent forms (e.g., sodium, potassium, and calcium salts of arsenate).
- Toxicity of organic pentavalent forms used as growth promoter in swine (e.g., arsanilic acid, roxarsone) has not been determined for horses.
- Trivalent inorganic arsenicals inhibit cellular respiration and damage capillaries.
- Pentavalent inorganic arsenicals uncouple oxidative phosphorylation, leading to deficits in cell energy.

SIGNALMENT

No breed or sex predilections

SIGNS

- Peracute or acute syndromes are most likely.
- Peracute—patient often found dead; death caused by cardiovascular collapse
- Acute—intense abdominal pain, hypersalivation, severe watery diarrhea, decreased abdominal sounds, muscle tremors, weak and rapid pulse with signs of circulatory shock, ataxia, depression, and recumbency; if the animal survives for several days, oliguria and proteinuria secondary to renal damage
- Chronic—not described in horses

CAUSES AND RISK FACTORS

Ingestion of arsenic-containing products or arsenic-contaminated soils, water, or feed

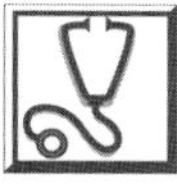

DIAGNOSIS

DIFFERENTIAL DIAGNOSIS

- Lead toxicosis—evidence of neurologic dysfunction is likely.
- Mercury toxicosis
- NSAID toxicosis—history of previous use
- Cantharidin toxicosis—evidence of cystitis
- Salmonellosis
- Colitis X
- Acute cyathastomiasis
- Clostridial colitis

CBC/BIOCHEMISTRY/URINALYSIS

- Reflect circulatory shock and possible liver and kidney damage
- Hemoconcentration—elevated PCV and plasma total protein
- Leukopenia with degenerative changes in PMNs
- Azotemia
- Electrolytes—hypokalemia; hyponatremia; hypochloremia
- Hyperglycemia
- Hyperbilirubinemia
- Elevated LDH and CK

OTHER LABORATORY TESTS

- Ante-mortem—measurement of arsenic in urine, whole blood, or GI contents
- Post-mortem—measurement of arsenic in liver or kidney
- Chronic exposures—arsenic can be measured in hair.
- Arsenic is rapidly excreted after exposure ceases.

IMAGING

N/A

DIAGNOSTIC PROCEDURES

N/A

PATHOLOGICAL FINDINGS

Gross

- GI hemorrhage, mucosal congestion, edema, and erosion are either localized or throughout the GI tract, which may be filled with watery, dark-green, black, or hemorrhagic ingesta, with necrotic material from mucosal sloughing.
- Pulmonary edema and epicardial and serosal hemorrhage

Histopathologic

Necrotizing, hemorrhagic typhlocolitis, with necrotizing vasculitis, renal tubular necrosis, and hepatic fatty degeneration

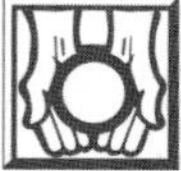

TREATMENT

- Urgent treatment is necessary.
- Remove animal from known or potential source of exposure.
- GI decontamination
- Treat circulatory shock and acidosis.
- Appropriate fluid therapy

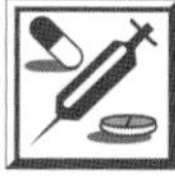

MEDICATIONS

DRUG(S)

- Hasten elimination of absorbed arsenic with chelators.
  - Dimercaprol (British anti-lewisite) is the classic arsenic chelator (loading dose of 4–5 mg/kg given by deep muscular injection, followed by 2–3 mg/kg q4h for 24 hr and then 1 mg/kg q4h for 2 days); adverse reactions include tremors, convulsions, and coma.
  - DMSA is a less toxic chelator (equine dose not established, but 10 mg/kg PO q8h is suggested).
- Control abdominal pain.
  - Flunixin meglumine (1.1 mg/kg IV or IM q24h for 5 days) or butorphanol tartrate (0.1 mg/kg IV q3–4h up to 48 hr)
  - Xylazine hydrochloride (0.5–1 mg/kg IV or IM) may be used in conjunction with butorphanol (0.02–0.03 mg/kg IV).
- Demulcents—mineral oil or kaolin-pectin

CONTRAINDICATIONS/POSSIBLE INTERACTIONS

Use NSAIDs cautiously because of possible adverse GI and renal effects.

FOLLOW-UP

- Monitor renal and hepatic function.
- Provide a bland diet, containing reduced amounts of high-quality protein.
- Identify source of exposure, and properly dispose of source.
- Expected course and prognosis depend on the severity of clinical signs.
- If the animal survives, recovery should be complete.

MISCELLANEOUS

ASSOCIATED CONDITIONS, AGE-RELATED FACTORS, ZOONOTIC POTENTIAL, PREGNANCY

N/A

ABBREVIATIONS

- CCA = chromated copper arsenate
- CK = creatine kinase
- DMSA = 2,3-dimercaptosuccinic acid, succimer
- GI = gastrointestinal
- LDH = lactate dehydrogenase
- PCV = packed cell volume
- PMN = polymorphonucleocytes

Suggested Reading

Casteel SW. Metal toxicosis in horses. Vet Clin North Am Equine Pract 2001;17:517–527.

Pace LW, Turnquist SE, Casteel SW, Johnson PJ, Frankeny RL. Acute arsenic toxicosis in five horses. Vet Pathol 1997;34:160–164.

Author Robert H. Poppenga

Consulting Editor Robert H. Poppenga

ARTIFICIAL INSEMINATION

BASICS

DEFINITION/OVERVIEW

- Extended fresh, cooled, frozen semen introduced into the mare's uterus using aseptic technique
- Standard AI—minimum 300–1000 × 10^6 PMS deposited into *uterine body*
- DHI or low-dose AI—1–25 × 10^6 PMS deposited into *tip of uterine horn* (ipsilateral to dominant follicle)

ETIOLOGY/PATHOPHYSIOLOGY

Advantages

- AI increases live cover.
- Efficient use of semen
- Ejaculate divided—several AI doses, greater number of mares bred in a season (120 by AI; 40–80 by live cover)
- Wider use of genetically superior stallions.
- Eliminate cost and risk of transport, mares with foals at side.
- Antibiotics in semen extenders prevent many genital infections.
- Fewer breeding injuries
- Continue using stallions with problems (musculoskeletal and behavioral).
- Protect mares with genital tract impairments or recent surgical repair from further breeding-related trauma.
- Semen quality assessed before AI
- Low-dose AI—stallions with limited availability or costly semen due to
  - Excessive size of book
  - Low sperm cell production or high percentage of dead sperm
  - Use of sex-sorted sperm
  - Epididymal spermatozoa collected at the time of castration or stallion's death

SYSTEM AFFECTED

Reproductive

SIGNALMENT

- Thoroughbreds allow only live cover.
- All other breed registries allow AI; may impose restrictions

SIGNS

Historical

Records of mare's prior cycles—help predict days in heat, time of ovulation

Teasing and Physical Examination

- Ovulation timing is critical.
  - Predict by her history, teasing response, results of genital tract TRP and U/S.
  - During estrus—tease daily; not less than every other day
  - On 2nd day of estrus, begin daily or every-other-day TRP.
  - Perform U/S, as needed, to determine optimal time to breed.
- TRP—record dominant follicle (35+ mm), uterine edema, relaxing cervix
- Follicle size and growth, increasing uterine estrual edema (cartwheel appearance) evident with U/S
- Preovulatory follicle may become irregular/pear-shaped 12–24 hr preovulation.
- Estrual edema peaks 72–96 hr, decreases to light or absent by 36 hr preovulation in young, normal mares.
- OVD, CH, CL—evidence of ovulation

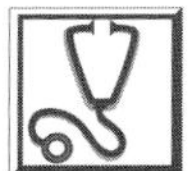

DIAGNOSIS

PROCEDURAL ISSUES

Timing and Frequency of Breeding

- Depends on semen longevity—affected by stallion idiosyncrasy, semen preservation method (fresh, cooled, frozen)
- Equine ova—short viability, 8–18 hr postovulation

Teasing and Examinations

- GnRH analog or hCG when preovulatory follicle is ≥35 mm to induce ovulation within 36–42 hr. AI as close to ovulation as possible.
- U/S 4–6 hr post-AI for presence of intrauterine fluid (especially new/DUC mare, or if bred with frozen semen) and for ovulation
- Evaluate normal, fertile mares 24–48 hr after AI for ovulation.

Fresh (raw or extended) Semen

- Routine breeding—every other day
  - Begin day 2–3 of estrus until they tease out, or
  - When a large preovulatory follicle is detected by TRP and U/S.
- Inseminate within 48 hr preovulation to achieve acceptable pregnancy rates.

Cooled Transported Semen

- More intense management; fertility of cooled semen from some stallions decreases markedly >24 hr.
- GnRH analog or hCG when preovulatory follicle is ≥35 mm to induce ovulation within 36–42 hr; order semen—overnight shipment
- Inseminate ≤12–24 hr preovulation for acceptable conception rates.
- Semen with poor post-cooling fertility should be sent *counter to counter* (i.e., airline transport).
  - Administer Deslorelin or hCG 24–36 hr before expected semen arrival; ensure ovulation is very close to time of AI.
  - No advantage to keeping a 2nd AI dose to rebreed next day. Mare's uterus is best incubator for sperm, not a chilled shipper.

Frozen Thawed Semen

- Precise timing of AI post-thaw longevity is reduced to ≤12–24 hr.
- Mare management—serial, daily teasing, TRP, and U/S
- Deslorelin or hCG when dominant follicle ≥35 mm
- TRP and U/S—TID–QID, ensure AI as close before ovulation as possible; most important, ≤6–8 hr postovulation
- New frozen semen strategy for AI if have multiple doses:
  - Deslorelin or hCG when dominant follicle ≥35 mm
  - AI at 24 hr and again at 40 hr after injection; ensures viable sperm are available during ovulatory period
  - Treat mare if intrauterine fluid is present 4–6 hr after first AI.
  - Pregnancy rate is equivalent to a one-time AI 6 hr postovulation, but minus the intensive labor and fewer veterinary examinations.

Low-Dose Insemination

- Allows use of a reduced dose of semen (fresh, cooled, frozen)
- Varies with semen quality
  - DHI dose has been decreased to as few as 14×10^6 motile, frozen-thawed sperm.
  - Average of 60–150 × 10^6 of PMS for DHI.
  - Semen is deposited at the UTJ, tip of uterine horn ipsilateral to dominant follicle.
- DHI can be either hysteroscopically guided or transrectally guided (with or without U/S).
- Mare management varies according to method of semen preservation.

General Comments

- If ovulation has not occurred within the recommended times for fresh (48 hr), cooled (24 hr), or frozen (6–12 hr) semen, rebreed the mare.
- Older ova or semen—due to poor timing, percentage of EED increases.

OTHER LABORATORY TESTS

Progesterone level of >1 ng/mL confirms ovulation.

IMAGING

U/S

DIAGNOSTIC PROCEDURES

Semen Analysis

- Minimum parameters—volume, motility, concentration
- Morphology—optional, but of particular use if a stallion has fertility problems
- Small sample of cooled or frozen semen should be saved and warmed (at 37° C) to evaluate immediately after AI.
- Slide, coverslip, and pip—prewarm, stallion semen very susceptible to cold shock
- The total number of sperm should be at least 300–1000 × 10^6 PMS (concentration [in millions of sperm per mL] × volume used).

Stallion's Disease Status

Should be negative for EIA, EVA, CEM, and venereal diseases

Mare Selection

- Her fertility takes on special significance if using frozen semen or its quality is less optimal.
- Include reproductive history +/− normal estrous cyclicity, results of uterine culture and cytology, presence of intrauterine fluid during estrus.
- Fertility alters by status—normal maiden > normal pluriparous > older maiden, pluriparous or barren mare

Prebreeding Uterine Culture and Cytology of Mare

- All, except young maiden mares, should have at least one negative uterine culture and cytology prebreeding.
  - Avoid transmitting infections to the stallion.
  - Early identification of possible mare problems
  - Maximize the likelihood of first-cycle conception.
- Pregnancy rates are lower and EED higher for mares treated for uterine infections during the same cycle as the AI.

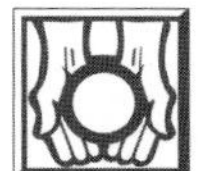

TREATMENT

Prebreeding

- Presence of ≥2-cm height of prebreeding uterine fluid, then LRS uterine lavage immediately before AI
- Does not affect fertility

AI Technique

- Sterile and disposable equipment. Mares are restrained and the perineal area is thoroughly cleansed with a mild detergent, antiseptic solution or soap; then completely remove any residue (minimum three rinses).
- Sterile sleeve on arm and nonspermicidal lubricant applied to dorsum of the gloved hand.
  - 250–56 cm (20–22 inch) AI pipet is carried in the gloved hand.
  - Index finger is first passed through the cervical lumen. It serves as a guide by which the pipet can readily be advanced (advanced to a position no more than 2.5 cm into the uterine body).
  - Syringe with a nonspermicidal plastic plunger (e.g., Air-tite) containing the extended semen is attached to the pipet, and the semen is slowly deposited into the uterus. The remaining semen in the pipet is delivered by using a small bolus of air (1 mL) in the syringe.

Fresh Extended Semen

- Perform AI immediately after collection.
- Semen can be mixed with an appropriate extender for immediate insemination, with semen-to-extender ratio of 1:1 or 1:2, if the ejaculate volume is small and of high concentration.

Cooled Transported Semen

- Semen is collected, diluted in semen extender, and cooled to 5°–6° C for 24–48 hr. With transport, there can be a modest decrease of fertilizing capacity (stallion fertility dependent).
- A semen-to-extender ratio of 1:3 or 1:4 is acceptable; may be as high as 1:19
- Semen longevity optimized by extending the ejaculate to a final sperm concentration of 25–50 × 10^6 sperm/mL.

Frozen Thawed Semen

- Frozen semen is packed in 0.5–5 mL straws and stored in liquid N_2.
- A 5-mL straw contains from 600–1000 × 10^6 sperm cells.
- Dependent on post-freeze viability of the spermatozoa, only one straw may be needed.
- A 0.5-mL straw contains 200–800 × 10^6 sperm cells.
  - Number of straws needed depends on post-thaw motility and method of AI.
  - Thawing protocols vary and are reported ideally to be paired with a particular freezing method. Seek specific information regarding thawing. In the absence of a recommended protocol, 37° C for 30–60 seconds may provide an acceptable alternative.

ARTIFICIAL INSEMINATION

• If details are not provided with frozen semen received, seek instructions regarding thawing before the day of AI to ensure proper handling.
• Post-thawing, semen should be in the mare within 5 min.
• Post-AI uterine treatment is strongly recommended. The high concentration of sperm cells in a thawed straw and absence of seminal plasma (provides a natural protective effect in the uterus) may induce an acute PMIE.

Low-Dose Insemination Procedures (LDI)

• Sedation of the mare is recommended. Procedure should be performed quickly ($\leq$10 min) and avoid inducing uterine trauma.
• *Hysteroscopic AI*—introduction of an endoscope into the mare's uterus:
  ○ Approach and visualize the UTJ ipsilateral to the dominant follicle.
  ○ Small catheter is passed through the endoscope's channel and semen deposited at/on the UTJ.
• *DHI*—Pass a flexible AI pipet through the cervix toward the tip of the uterine horn ipsilateral to the dominant follicle.
  ○ Pipet is guided by either TRP or U/S.
  ○ Semen is deposited close to or onto the UTJ.
  ○ *Manual TRP elevation of the tip of the uterine horn may help pass the pipet.*

Post-Breeding

• U/S examination 4–6 hr after AI for presence of intrauterine fluid.
  ○ If present, lavage uterus with sterile saline or LRS, followed by oxytocin beginning 4–6 hr after AI.
  ○ Repeat oxytocin at 2-hr intervals until 8–10 hr post-AI, and again at 12–24 hr until the inflammation resolves.

MEDICATIONS

DRUG(S) OF CHOICE

• Ovulation induction most effective if follicle is $\geq$35 mm
  ○ Within 36–42 hr with hCG (1500–3000 IU IV); response range is 12–72 hr.
  ○ Within 36–42 hr with GnRH analogue (Deslorelin 1.5 mg IM)
• Ecbolic drugs may be used to treat PMIE and DUC.
• Prostaglandins—Misoprostol for cervical relaxation or intrauterine $PGF_{2\alpha}$ (0.25 mg) 2 hr before deep AI (only with good-quality semen)

CONTRAINDICATIONS

See Endometritis.

PRECAUTIONS

See Endometritis.

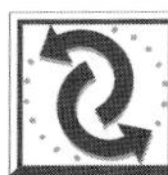

FOLLOW-UP

PATIENT MONITORING

• Begin teasing by 11 days post-ovulation.
  ○ Early detection of endometritis—indicated by a shortened cycle due to endogenous prostaglandin release
• U/S for pregnancy 14–15 days post-ovulation includes ruling out potential twins versus lymphatic cyst.
• Follow-up TRP and U/S—24–30 days; confirm heartbeat in the embryo.
• Serial TRP pregnancy examinations—45, 60, 90, and 120 days

POSSIBLE COMPLICATIONS

• AV preparation, handling, maintenance
• Semen evaluation at collection—ship adequate AI dose and/or send correct number of semen straws.
• Shipping methods—Equitainer, reusable box cooling containers, vapor tank
  ○ With cooled shipments, entire breeding program is at the mercy of airlines/couriers.
• Operator skill—to manipulate and place semen through the cervix, into the uterine lumen or to the tip of the horn, in a proper and timely manner
• Misidentification of stallions/mares

MISCELLANEOUS

PREGNANCY

Cooled Semen

Per cycle pregnancy rates are equivalent to on-farm AI with fresh semen (60%–75%) if semen quality remains good after cooling period of 24 hr at 5–6° C.

Frozen Semen

• Pregnancy rates decrease for most stallions.
• Spermatozoa suffer many stresses; anticipate attrition rate of $\cong$50% with freezing and thawing.
• First-cycle pregnancy rates—30%–40% (range—0%–70%); wide range between stallions
  ○ Intense breeding management and good quality of semen—positive impact on the pregnancy rate
• Candidate selection for frozen semen breeding
  ○ Most fertile—young, maiden and normal pluriparous mares
  ○ Least fertile—old, maiden or barren and abnormal pluriparous mares
• Older eggs or semen
  ○ Due to poor timing; pregnancy rate decreased by 30 days; increased EED

SYNONYMS

Artificial breeding

SEE ALSO

• Conception failure
• Delayed uterine clearance
• Early embryonic death
• Endometritis
• Semen evaluation, abnormal
• Semen evaluation, normal
• Venereal diseases

ABBREVIATIONS

• AI = artificial insemination
• AV = artificial vagina
• CEM = contagious equine metritis
• CH = corpus hemorrhagicum
• CL = corpus luteum
• DHI = deep horn insemination
• DUC = delayed uterine clearance
• EIA = equine infectious anemia
• EED = early embryonic death
• EVA = equine viral arteritis
• GnRH = gonadotropin-releasing hormone
• hCG = human chorionic gonadotropin
• LRS = lactated Ringer's solution
• OVD = ovulation depression
• PMIE = persistent mating-induced endometritis
• PMS = progressively motile sperm
• TRP = transrectal palpation
• U/S = ultrasound, ultrasonography
• UTJ= utero-tubal junction

Suggested Reading

Blanchard TL, Varner D, Schumacher J. Semen collection and artificial insemination. In: Manual of Equine Reproduction. St. Louis; Mosby–Year Book, 1998:111–125.
Brinsko SP. Insemination doses—how low can we go? Therio 2006;66:543–550.
Morris LH. Low dose insemination in the mare—an update. Anim Reprod Sci 2004;82–83:625–632.

Author Maria E. Cadario
Consulting Editor Carla L. Carleton

ARYTENOID CHONDROPATHY

BASICS

OVERVIEW

• A septic inflammatory process of one or both arytenoid cartilages, resulting in deformation with enlargement • This interferes with the ability of the affected arytenoid cartilage to fully abduct during forced inspiration and/or to resist collapsing airway pressure during inspiration.

SIGNALMENT

• Male and Thoroughbred racehorses are more commonly affected. • Incidence increases with age.

SIGNS

• Upper respiratory noise, exercise intolerance, or both • The disease usually worsens gradually, with progressive involvement of one or both arytenoid cartilages. • The condition leads to ventilation interference proportional to the loss of abductory function and the mechanical size of the affected arytenoid cartilages. The more intense the high-intensity exercise occurs, the more severe is the hypoventilation, so the horse does not "finish" or close well. • In show horses, loss of points during competition because of upper respiratory noise may be the main concern; this upper airway noise resembles that of horses with laryngeal hemiplegia.

CAUSES AND RISK FACTORS

• Physical trauma to the mucosa of the arytenoid cartilage caused by air turbulence or aspiration of track surface particles during exercise or severe coughing or intubation (e. g., endotracheal, nasogastric) procedures.
• Upper airway infection leading to cartilage sepsis
• In many cases, the inciting cause is never found.

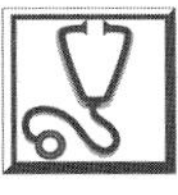

DIAGNOSIS

DIFFERENTIAL DIAGNOSIS

• Laryngeal hemiplegia • Congenital malformation of the laryngeal cartilages

CBC/BIOCHEMISTRY/URINALYSIS

Of no value.

OTHER LABORATORY TESTS

• Arterial blood gases during exercise
• Hypoventilation can be evaluated using arterial blood gases—typically at maximal exercise $PaCO_2$ can be >50 mm Hg; PaO_2 may be <65 mm Hg in affected horses.

IMAGING

• Lateral radiography of the larynx may reveal enlarged laryngeal cartilages, sometimes with associated osseous metaplasia. • Ultrasound examination of the larynx using the mid-ventral and caudoventral windows to evaluate for abscess and the caudolateral window to assess the presence of disease in the lateral aspect of the arytenoid cartilage.

OTHER DIAGNOSTIC PROCEDURES

• The diagnosis is established on the basis of videoendoscopic examination at rest:
 ○ The body of the arytenoid is irregular and thickened. ○ A mass of granulation tissue may protrude from the axial surface of the arytenoid cartilage into the airway. The size or location of the protruding mass has no correlation with the amount of abduction remaining. ○ The corniculate process may be deformed. ○ Contact (i.e., "kissing") lesions may be observed on the contralateral arytenoid cartilage.
• Eventually, the condition leads to decreased or total inability of the affected arytenoid cartilage to abduct during inspiration.

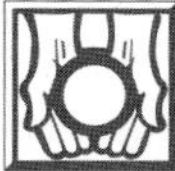

TREATMENT

• Medical treatment is indicated only in acute cases with mucosal ulceration and swellings.
• Consider laser-assisted excision of intralaryngeal granulations if the affected arytenoid cartilage retains abductory function. • Partial arytenoidectomy (excision of the body and corniculate process of affected arytenoid cartilage) is the treatment of choice to restore exercise capacity and to reduce upper airway noise. • Permanent tracheotomy can be used in countries where athletic competition is allowed with this procedure and to salvage the animal for breeding purposes.

MEDICATIONS

DRUG(S) OF CHOICE

• Acute case: broad-spectrum antibiotics and NSAIDs. • Chronic case: none, other than routine perioperative antimicrobial and anti-inflammatory agents. • Use of nasopharyngeal spray, consisting of various anti-inflammatory and antimicrobial agents (e. g., 250 mL of 90% DMSO, 500 mL of nitrofurazone, and 50 mL of prednisolone [25 mg/mL] mixed with 250 mL of glycerin) can be applied (20 mL BID) using a soft rubber feeding tube. • If the airway is significantly compromised, a temporary tracheotomy may be needed until the swelling resolves.

FOLLOW-UP

PATIENT MONITORING

• Videoendoscopy of the upper airway 6 weeks after surgery to monitor patient response • Final response to treatment or continuation of monitoring of affected horses is made on the basis of evaluating exercise tolerance and upper respiratory noise. • Laser resection of the unsupported ipsilateral aryepiglottic fold might be needed to improve airway patency.

POSSIBLE COMPLICATIONS

• Horses undergoing removal of the corniculate and body of the arytenoid cartilage have a slightly increased risk for tracheal aspiration of feed during deglutition. In addition, these procedures do not fully restore the airway diameter, so a mild degree of airway obstruction persists, which may interfere with performance or result in upper airway noise during exercise. • Bilateral arytenoidectomy increases the risk for tracheal aspiration of feed during deglutition and for glottic stenosis because of webbing at the resection site.

EXPECTED COURSE AND PROGNOSIS

• Horses with acute swelling of the arytenoid cartilage may respond favorably to NSAIDs, topical anti-inflammatory agents, and antibiotics. • Untreated horses exhibit a progressive increase in exercise intolerance and upper respiratory noise. • Horses with focal elevated granulations on the axial surface of the arytenoid cartilage that maintain abductory function may respond to simple "lumpectomy." • Horses with generalized involvement of an arytenoid cartilage and without surgical treatment often develop contralateral contact or "kissing" lesions.
• Horses with unilateral lesions treated surgically have a fair prognosis (60%) for elimination or significant reduction of exercise intolerance; however, the prognosis is guarded (20%) in horses with bilateral lesions.

MISCELLANEOUS

SEE ALSO

• Dynamic collapse of the upper airways
• Laryngeal hemiparesis/hemiplegia

ABBREVIATION

• DMSO = dimethylsulfoxide

Suggested Reading

Hay WP, Tulleners E. Excision of intralaryngeal granulation tissue in 25 horses using a neodymium: YAG laser (1986 to 1991). Vet Surg 1993;22:129–134.

Haynes PF, Snider TG, McLure JR, et al. Chronic chondritis of the equine arytenoid cartilage. J Am Vet Med Assoc 1980;177:1135–1142.

Lumsden JM, Derksen FJ, Stick JA, et al. Evaluation of partial arytenoidectomy as a treatment for equine laryngeal hemiplegia. Equine Vet J 1994;26:92–93.

Radcliffe CH, Woodie JB, Hackett RP, Ainsworth DM, Erb HN, Mitchell LM, Soderholm LV, Ducharme NG. A comparison of laryngoplasty and modified partial arytenoidectomy as treatments for laryngeal hemiplegia in exercising horses. Vet Surg 2006;35(7):643–652.

Tulleners EP, Harrison IW, Raker CW. Management of arytenoid chondropathy and failed laryngoplasty in horses: 75 Cases (1979–1985) J Am Vet Med Assoc 1988:192;670–675.

Authors Norm Ducharme and Richard P. Hackett

Consulting Editor Daniel Jean

ASCARID INFESTATION

BASICS

OVERVIEW

- Parasitic roundworm infection caused by *Parascaris equorum*.
- The infection prevalence may be up to 100% in tested farms and up to 80% in foals, with the highest incidence occurring between 100 and 180 days of age.
- The parasite has a direct life cycle that follows the oral-fecal route. Adults, in the small intestine of infected horses, produce large numbers of eggs, which are passed in the feces. The eggs become infective in 10 days to 6 weeks by developing into larvae (L_2). These highly resistant eggs accumulate in the environment, sticking to different surfaces, including the mare's mammary gland. When ingested, the larvae are released in the small intestine and migrate through the intestinal wall into the bloodstream, reaching the liver via the portal circulation. In the liver, they migrate to a hepatic vein, accessing the caudal vena cava and finally the pulmonary circulation. Molting of the larvae occurs in the lungs, followed by tracheal ascending migration and subsequent deglutition. Arrival to the small intestine completes the life cycle, and a final molting and maturation into the adult form take place.

SYSTEMS AFFECTED

- It affects primarily the GI system, causing enteritis, maldigestion, and malabsorption.
- The hepatobiliary and respiratory systems—An exaggerated inflammatory response to migrating larvae, resulting in temporary lung and liver damage in sensitized horses. Varying forms of tracheobronchitis have also been described.

SIGNALMENT

- Any ages, but primarily in foals and weanlings up to 9–12 mo of age
- Debilitated and immunocompromised adult horses can also be infected.

SIGNS

- Decreased growth rate, generalized weakness, a dull hair coat and dry skin, "pot-bellied" appearance, and decreased appetite
- In severe cases, colic due to obstruction can occur.
- Acute colic signs with peritonitis due to perforation of the intestine.
- Coughing and mucopurulent nasal discharge with or without systemic illness may be seen during periods of larval imigration through the lungs.

CAUSES AND RISK FACTORS

The disease is caused by *P. equorum*, the roundworm from the family Ascarididae. Animals at risk are susceptible foals and weanlings grazing on infested pastures.

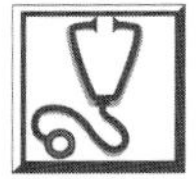

DIAGNOSIS

DIFFERENTIAL DIAGNOSIS

Any causes of colic, ill thrift, weakness, malabsorption, and malnutrition

CBC/BIOCHEMISTRY/URINALYSIS

- Eosinophilia may be seen during larval migration, 10–40 days postinfection.
- Leukopenia and mild anemia have been reported.
- In severe cases, hypoproteinemia can be detected.

OTHER LABORATORY TESTS

Coprology for detection of the eggs (see Other Diagnostic Procedures)

IMAGING

Adult ascaris may be seen on transabdominal ultrasound, within the intestinal lumen or in the peritoneal cavity after intestinal perforation.

OTHER DIAGNOSTIC PROCEDURES

The infestation is confirmed by fecal flotation techniques.

PATHOLOGIC FINDINGS

- Adult forms are found in the intestinal lumen or free in the abdominal cavity following intestinal perforation.
- Hemorrhagic and edematous lesions around necrotic areas in the lungs, liver, and associated lymph nodes are seen during larval migration.
- Microscopy after larval migration reveals multiple foci of white tracts within a fibrotic liver parenchyma.
- Lymphocytic nodules may develop in the lungs after multiple episodes of reinfection in a sensitized host.

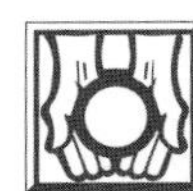

TREATMENT

Treatment is indicated for fecal egg counts greater than 100 eggs per gram. Following sudden and complete paralysis of all ascarids after anthelmintic therapy, small intestinal obstruction or impaction may occur. Emergency surgical intervention for removal of dead parasites and correction of secondary complications such as intussusceptions and intestinal volvulus are then required. Ascarid impaction should be suspected in colicky foals and weanlings with a recent history (24 hr) of deworming.

MEDICATIONS

The regular use of anthelmintics is the treatment of choice for patent infections with *P. equorum* and should be administered to foals and weanlings every 6–8 weeks, starting at 1.5–2 mo of age.

DRUG(S) OF CHOICE

- Anthelmintics available at present do not eliminate migrating larvae. Therefore, preventative therapy should be given until 1 year of age.

• Broodmares should be treated at monthly intervals in the last trimester of pregnancy to reduce environmental contamination.
Recommended anthelmintics:
• Fenbendazole 10 mg/kg PO given for 5 consecutive days (varies in effectiveness against ascarids)
• Pyrantel pamoate 6.6 mg/kg PO
• Levamisole 8 mg/kg PO
• Daily prophylactic administration of pyrantel tartrate (2.64 mg/kg) in the feed also prevents penetration of the intestinal wall by ascarid larvae.
• Moxidectin 0.4 mg/kg PO and ivermectin 0.2 mg/kg PO were advocated to be 100% efficient in eliminating ascarid infection in horses, but resistance to these and other macrocyclic lactone anthelmintics has been identified in Europe, Canada, and the United States in recent years.

CONTRAINDICATIONS/POSSIBLE INTERACTIONS

If severe parasite burdens are suspected, anthelmintics that result in paralysis of the parasites (e. g., pyrantel pamoate, piperazine, organophosphates, ivermectin) should be avoided because it may result in small intestinal obstruction or impaction and can lead to intestinal rupture and peritonitis. Therefore, anthelmintics with a slower action such as benzimidazoles are recommended.

FOLLOW-UP

PATIENT MONITORING

Fecal floatation should be conducted in 10% or more of the foals every 4–6 mo. If 10% of foals or more are positive, failure of the anthelmintic therapy and/or the prevention and control strategies should be suspected.

PREVENTION/AVOIDANCE

• Contaminated facilities should be disinfected with a 5% phenolic compound and sprayed with a high-pressure hose.
• Grazing of broodmares, foals, and weanlings on heavily contaminated pastures should be avoided.
• *P. equorum* eggs can remain viable in the environment for many years.
• Frequent removal of manure from stalls and pastures also reduces transmission between foals and reinfection following treatment.

POSSIBLE COMPLICATIONS

Overdose of anthelmintic can result in toxicity.

EXPECTED COURSE AND PROGNOSIS

• Prognosis is favorable in uncomplicated cases, but a delay in growth and development is common.
• Infection rates start to decline at 6 mo of age, and immunity is long lasting. Patent infections are rarely seen in adults except in immunocompromised animals.

MISCELLANEOUS

ASSOCIATED CONDITIONS

• Gastrointestinal obstruction
• Septic peritonitis

ZOONOTIC POTENTIAL

Human infection, although extremely rare, may occur after ingestion of a viable egg.

PREGNANCY

Transplacental infection with *P. equorum* is not known to occur, nor is the transfer of ascarid larvae in colostrum.

Suggested Reading

Bowman DD. Georgi's Parasitology for Veterinarians, ed 8. Philadelphia: WB Saunders, 2002.
Foreyt WJ. Veterinary Parasitology Reference Manual, ed 5. Ames, IA: Blackwell Publishing Professional, 2001.

Author Carlos Medina-Torres
Consulting Editors Henry Stämpfli and Olimpo Oliver-Espinosa

ASPARTATE AMINOTRANSFERASE (AST)

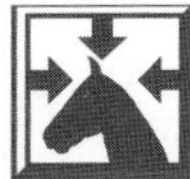

BASICS

DEFINITION

- Catalyzes transamination of 2-oxoglutarate and L-aspartate to glutamate and oxaloacetate
- Present in many tissues—liver, striated muscle, erythrocytes, and others
- Reported normal AST activity in horses varies from 48 to 456 IU/L.

PATHOPHYSIOLOGY

- Increases in AST activity are typically indicative of hepatocellular and/or striated muscle injury; however, increased AST activity will occur with hemolysis because of the high AST content in erythrocytes.
- Magnitude of the elevation generally is proportional to the number of hepatocytes affected, not to the severity of a particular insult.
- With skeletal muscle injury, magnitude of AST elevation is not necessarily proportional to the extent of tissue injury.
- Increases above the reference interval occur with intramuscular injections and in downer animals.
- AST is a sensitive indicator of hepatocellular and striated muscle injury; however, because it is present in many tissues, AST lacks specificity. Other biochemical tests need to be examined concurrently with AST to localize the source of the increase (i.e., SD for liver and CK for muscle).
- After tissue injury AST activity increases more slowly and remains increased longer than SD or CK.
- Increased SD, with normal or increased AST, indicates acute or ongoing hepatocellular injury. If serial serum chemistry analyses reveal continuously or progressively increased activities of both enzymes, ongoing hepatocellular injury is likely. During treatment of hepatic disease, the enzymes can be used to monitor cessation of the insult. If, after documenting recent hepatocellular injury, serial serum chemistry analyses reveal increased AST and progressively decreasing or normal SD activity, cessation of the original insult is likely. Because of its longer half-life, AST may increase even after cessation of the original insult, and the activity may remain increased for weeks.
- A similar interpretative approach is used when determining if muscle injury is present. Muscle and hepatocellular injury can occur concurrently, and increases in AST, CK, and SD may be seen together.

SYSTEMS AFFECTED

- Musculoskeletal
- Hepatobiliary
- Cardiovascular (myocardium)
- Hemic (erythrocytes)

GENETICS

N/A

INCIDENCE/PREVALENCE

N/A

GEOGRAPHIC DISTRIBUTION

N/A

SIGNALMENT

- Depends on the primary disease process and secondary complications

SIGNS

Historical

- Depend on the cause of the increases in AST activity
- Strenuous exercise or overtraining

Physical Examination

- Depends on the cause of the increases in AST activity
- Muscle disorders—reluctance or inability to move, stiffness, and recumbency
- Liver disorders—jaundice, neurologic deficits, discolored urine, anorexia, abdominal pain, weight loss, and fever
- Clinical signs due to hepatic failure generally do not appear until 75% of the hepatic functional mass is lost.

CAUSES

- Degenerative conditions—cirrhosis, rhabdomyolysis, and choleliths
- Anomaly, congenital diseases—polysaccharide storage myopathy; biliary atresia
- Metabolic diseases—shock, hypovolemia, hypoxia caused by severe anemia or during anesthesia, and severe GI disease
- Neoplastic or nutritional diseases—primary neoplasia, metastatic neoplasia, leukemia, hepatic lipidosis, and vitamin E/selenium deficiency
- Infectious and immune-mediated diseases—hepatitis of various causes (e.g., viral, bacterial, protozoal, fungal, parasitic), serum sickness, amyloidosis, endotoxemia, and chronic active hepatitis
- Toxic or trauma—pyrrolizidine alkaloid-containing plants, ferrous fumarate in newborn foals, cottonseed, castor bean, oaks, and alsike clover; fungal toxins, such as aflatoxins, cyclopiazonic acid, fumonisin, phalloidin (i.e., mushrooms), rubratoxins; blue-green algae; and chemical compounds/elements, such as ethanol, chlorinated hydrocarbons, carbon tetrachloride, monensin, copper, iron, and petroleum and its products

RISK FACTORS

- Risk factors vary according to the specific disease.
- Familial disease, exposure to infected animals, overweight and miniature ponies, poor nutrition, excessive exercise, exposure to toxic compound or plants, or excessive exercise
- Halothane anesthesia, particularly of prolonged duration, may result in hepatic injury in horses.

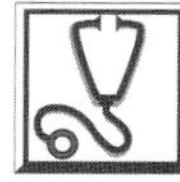

DIAGNOSIS

DIFFERENTIAL DIAGNOSIS

See Causes.

CBC/BIOCHEMISTRY/URINALYSIS

CBC

- Erythrocytes—liver disease may cause nonregenerative anemia and morphologic changes (e.g., acanthocytes, target cells, nonspecific poikilocytosis, normochromic microcytosis in portosystemic vascular shunts); severe anemia of any cause may produce cellular injury from tissue hypoxia.
- Leukocytes—leukocytosis or leukopenia may be seen with inflammatory diseases and leukemia; morphologic changes of the leukocytes (e.g., neutrophil toxicity in inflammation; neoplastic cells) also may be seen.
- Platelets—quantitative decreases and increases may be seen with a variety of systemic diseases that may affect the liver or striated muscle.

Serum/Plasma Biochemistry Profile

- Glucose—increased in diabetes mellitus, glucocorticoid influence (e.g., exogenous, endogenous); decreased in end-stage liver disease, sepsis/endotoxemia
- BUN—increased in severe rhabdomyolysis from secondary renal injury; decreased in liver insufficiency and end-stage liver disease from decreased conversion of ammonia to urea
- Albumin—decreased in end-stage liver disease from decreased production; minimally to mildly decreased in inflammation
- Globulins—generally increased in end-stage liver disease and with chronic antigenic stimulation
- SD—increased with acute and ongoing hepatocellular injury
- ALP—increased with concurrent cholestatic disease
- GGT—increased with cholestatic disease or hepatocellular injury
- CK—increased with acute or ongoing muscle injury
- Conjugated bilirubin—increased in cholestatic disease
- Unconjugated bilirubin—increased with anorexia and prehepatic cholestasis (i.e., massive in vivo hemolysis)
- Cholesterol—may be increased with cholestasis and lipid disorders, and decreased in hepatic insufficiency.
- Triglycerides—increases may be associated with hepatic lipidosis.
- Because of high AST activity in erythrocytes, hemolysis falsely elevates serum/plasma AST activity.
- Prolonged in vitro exposure of serum or plasma to erythrocytes falsely increases AST activity even before visible signs of hemolysis are present. To avoid this confounding factor, prompt separation of plasma/serum from the cellular components of blood is strongly recommended.
- If laboratory analysis will not occur within 1–2 days, freeze the plasma/serum.

Urinalysis

Bilirubinuria—Conjugated bilirubin, detected by the commonly used dipstick and diazo tablet methods, indicates cholestatic disease and should not be increased if only hepatocellular injury is present.

OTHER LABORATORY TESTS

SBA

- Sensitive test for hepatobiliary disease, but not specific for the type of hepatobiliary disease
- May be increased with cell injury, cholestasis, or hepatic insufficiency/decreased functional mass; specificity for the latter condition is greatly

increased when SBA are increased in cases with normal or minimally increased markers for hepatocellular injury (e.g., SD, AST, GGT) and cholestasis (e.g., ALP, GGT, conjugated bilirubin).

• Main advantage over plasma ammonia, a more specific test for hepatic insufficiency/ decreased functional mass, is that immediate sample analysis is not necessary.

Plasma Ammonia

• Hepatic insufficiency/decreased functional mass is indicated if fasting or challenge ammonia concentration is increased.
• A sensitive and specific test, because it is not affected by other factors (e.g., cholestasis). However, ammonia measurement requires special handling, which limits its general availability.
• Consult reference laboratory for specific sample submission requirements.

Coagulation Tests and Fibrinogen

• The liver manufactures many of the coagulation factors; significant decreases in liver function may lead to deficiencies in these factors and to coagulation abnormalities.
• APTT and PT—Decreased APTT and PT are seen when <30% of the activity of the factors is present.

Serologic Tests

Helpful in detecting infectious causes

Toxicology

• Analysis of tissue biopsy material, feed, ingesta, serum/plasma, or other body fluids may indicate presence of a toxin.
• Contact reference laboratory regarding sample selection and submission recommendations.

Bacterial, Fungal, or Viral Culture

• May establish a definitive diagnosis regarding the infectious agent involved and help to guide treatment.
• Request bacterial antibiotic sensitivity to determine appropriate antibiotic therapy.
• Contact reference laboratory regarding sample selection and submission recommendations.

Sulfobromophthalein and Indocyanine Green Dye—Clearance Tests for Evaluation of Hepatic Function

These tests have been replaced by plasma ammonia and SBA.

IMAGING

Ultrasonography for Liver Disease

• Limited by position and size of the liver
• Evaluate size, echogenicity, shape, and position.
• Useful for guidance when obtaining biopsy material for cytology, histopathology, and microbiology
• Helpful in the evaluation of muscle and tendon injuries
• Other diagnostic imaging modalities such as radionucleotide imaging are expensive and available only at select institutions.

OTHER DIAGNOSTIC PROCEDURES

• Aspiration cytology and histopathology of formalin-fixed tissue (particularly liver)
• Cytology has the advantages of simplicity, quicker turnaround, better individual cellular detail, and better recognition of individual infectious organisms.
• Histopathology has the advantage of allowing examination of the tissue architecture and lesion distribution.
• Success of these procedures depends on the quality of the sample, area sampled, and the disease process itself; some hepatic diseases do not have significant microscopic alterations.

PATHOLOGICAL FINDINGS

Pathological findings will depend on the primary disease process and complications.

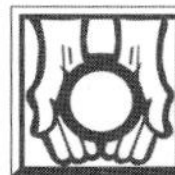

TREATMENT

AIMS OF TREATMENT

Depend on the primary disease process and secondary complications

APPROPRIATE HEALTH CARE

Depends on the primary disease process and secondary complications

NURSING CARE

Depends on the primary disease process and secondary complications

ACTIVITY

Depends on the primary disease process and secondary complications

DIET

Depends on the primary disease process and secondary complications

CLIENT EDUCATION

Depends on the primary disease process and secondary complications

SURGICAL CONSIDERATIONS

Depends on the primary disease process and secondary complications

MEDICATIONS

DRUG(S) OF CHOICE

Depends on the primary disease process and secondary complications

CONTRAINDICATIONS

With suspected hepatic insufficiency, assess the relative safety/risk of performing invasive procedures (e.g., fine-needle aspiration, tissue biopsy, laparoscopy, surgery) in light of the coagulation panel results.

PRECAUTIONS

Depends on the primary disease process and secondary complications

POSSIBLE INTERACTIONS

Depends on the primary disease process and secondary complications

ALTERNATIVE DRUGS

Depends on the primary disease process and secondary complications

FOLLOW-UP

PATIENT MONITORING

Serial serum biochemical analyses to monitor progression or improvement of the disease process (see Pathophysiology)

PREVENTION/AVOIDANCE

Depends on the primary disease process and secondary complications

POSSIBLE COMPLICATIONS

Depends on the primary disease process and secondary complications

EXPECTED COURSE AND PROGNOSIS

Depends on the primary disease process and secondary complications

MISCELLANEOUS

ASSOCIATED CONDITIONS

Depend on the primary disease process and secondary complications

AGE-RELATED FACTORS

See Signalment.

ZOONOTIC POTENTIAL

Infectious diseases such as salmonellosis

PREGNANCY

See Signalment.

SYNONYMS

Previously known as glutamate oxaloacetate transaminase (SGOT)

SEE ALSO See Causes.

ABBREVIATIONS

• GI = gastrointestinal
• ID = iditol dehydrogenase
• SBA = serum bile acids

Suggested Reading

Bain PJ. Liver. In: Latimer KS, Mahaffey EA, Prasse KW, eds. Duncan and Prasse's Veterinary Laboratory Medicine Clinical Pathology, ed 4. Ames, IA: Iowa State University Press, 2003.

Cardinett GH. Skeletal muscle function. In: Kaneko JJ, Harvey JW, Bruss ML, eds. Clinical Biochemistry of Domestic Animals, ed 5. San Diego: Academic Press, 1997.

Kramer JW, Hoffmann WE. In: Kaneko JJ, Harvey JW, Bruss ML, eds. Clinical Biochemistry of Domestic Animals, ed 5. San Diego: Academic Press, 1997.

Peek SF. Liver disease. In: Robinson NE. Current Therapy in Equine Medicine, ed 5. Philadelphia: Saunders, 2003.

Valberg SJ, Hodgson DR. Diseases of Muscle. In: Smith BP, ed. Large Animal Internal Medicine, ed 3. St. Louis, 2002.

The author and editor wish to acknowledge the contribution to this chapter of John A. Christian, co-author in the previous edition.

Author Armando R. Irizarry-Rovira
Consulting Editor Kenneth W. Hinchcliff

ASPIRATION PNEUMONIA

BASICS

OVERVIEW

• May develop after inhalation of foreign material and bacteria into the lower respiratory tract • Causes include dysphagia, obstructive esophageal disorders, GI reflux, and accidental inhalation of foreign material (e.g., administration of medication into the lung via a nasogastric tube). • Characterized by ventral consolidation of the lungs • Other organ systems may be involved depending on the primary cause.

SIGNALMENT

• No sex or breed predisposition has been observed.
• Foals appear more prone to GI reflux and subsequent AP.

SIGNS

Historical Findings

• Dysphagia, ptyalism, or discharge of food, water, or milk from the nostrils may have been observed before the onset of respiratory signs. • Recent history of drenching or nasogastric intubation should be investigated.

Physical Examination Findings

• Clinical signs—depression, anorexia, fever, tachypnea, dyspnea, nasal discharge, and coughing.
• Foul-smelling breath or nasal discharge suggests anaerobic infection. • Abnormal lung sounds are often heard on auscultation.

CAUSES AND RISK FACTORS

Dysphagia

• Neurologic diseases affecting cranial nerves IX and X—guttural pouch diseases, botulism, lead toxicity, and viral encephalitis • Primary myopathies of pharyngeal and laryngeal musculature—white muscle disease and hyperkalemic periodic paralysis • Diseases causing pharyngeal obstruction—strangles, pharyngeal abscess, neoplasia, foreign body, dorsal displacement of the soft palate, rostral displacement of the palatopharyngeal arch, and cysts • Congenital abnormalities—cleft palate and hypoplasia of the soft palate
• Iatrogenic causes—pharyngeal and laryngeal surgery

Esophageal Disorders

• Esophageal obstruction—foreign body, feed impaction, stricture, compression (e.g. abscess, neoplasia) • Megaesophagus • Esophageal diverticulum • Esophageal fistula

GI Reflux

Gastric outflow obstruction is usually secondary to ulcer disease in foals.

Accidental Inhalation of a Foreign Body

Administration of fluids by drenching or nasogastric tube

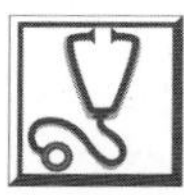

DIAGNOSIS

DIFFERENTIAL DIAGNOSIS

• Acute bronchopneumonia—often follows viral infection or stressful events (e.g., anesthesia, transportation, strenuous exercise)
• Pleuropneumonia—possible complication of AP, bronchopneumonia, pulmonary abscess, or secondary to thoracic trauma or esophageal rupture; auscultation, percussion, ultrasonography, radiography, or thoracocentesis helps confirm pleural effusion.
• Interstitial pneumonia—thoracic radiography most commonly reveals marked increase in overall lung opacity. • Respiratory distress syndrome—severe respiratory distress noted 24–48 hours after birth caused by surfactant deficiency; thoracic radiography typically shows diffuse, ground-glass appearance of the lungs with air bronchograms.

CBC/BIOCHEMISTRY/URINALYSIS

• Elevated WBC count with absolute neutrophilia is common. • Band neutrophils may be present.
• Hyperfibrinogenemia, hyperglobulinemia, and anemia are common findings with chronic pneumonia.

OTHER LABORATORY TESTS

• Increased blood and tissue concentrations of lead are diagnostic for lead toxicity. • Decreased whole-blood selenium concentration and glutathione peroxidase activity with increased serum creatinine kinase (CK) and aspartate amino-transferase (AST) are consistent with white muscle disease. • Hyperkalemic periodic paralysis may be diagnosed by genetic testing or by finding hyperkalemia during clinical episodes.

IMAGING

• Thoracic radiography commonly reveals ventral patchy opacity often obscuring the cardiac silhouette.
• Contrast radiography may help to diagnose causes of esophageal diseases. • Thoracic ultrasonography is a sensitive means of detecting pleural effusion.

OTHER DIAGNOSTIC PROCEDURES

• Tracheobronchial aspiration for cytology, gram stain, and culture (both aerobic and anaerobic); with pleural effusion, collect fluid sample by thoracocentesis for cytology and culture • Endoscopy of the respiratory and upper GI tracts may help to identify the primary cause.

PATHOLOGIC FINDINGS

• Consolidation of the ventral region of the lungs
• Acute cases—severely affected areas are hemorrhagic and edematous. • Chronic cases—affected lung may be necrotic and filled with purulent material. • Pleural space involvement—fibrinous exudate and adhesions

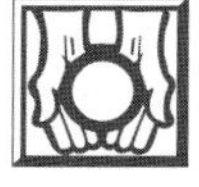

TREATMENT

• Treat severe dyspnea according to the cause—restore airway patency, drain pleural effusion, etc. • Nasal oxygen (6–10 L/min) if severe hypoxemia ($PaO_2 < 60$ mm Hg) • The primary disease must be treated. • Stall rest is imperative. • Dysphagic horses may be fed via an indwelling nasogastric tube. • With pleural effusion, thoracocentesis or placement of indwelling chest tubes can achieve drainage; a one-way valve attached to the tube prevents pneumothorax. • Administer fluid therapy as needed.

MEDICATIONS

DRUG(S) OF CHOICE

• Promptly initiate systemic administration of broad-spectrum antimicrobials while waiting for culture results. • Preferred combinations include sodium or potassium penicillin (22,000–40,000 IU/kg IV q6h), aminoglycoside (gentamicin [6.6–8.8 mg/kg IV q24h] or amikacin [15–20 mg/kg IV or IM q24h] for foals), and metronidazole (15–25 mg/kg IV or PO q6–8h). • Other antimicrobial choices include procaine penicillin G (22,000 IU/kg IM q12h), trimethoprim-sulfamethoxazole (30 mg/kg PO q12h), ceftiofur (1–5 mg/kg IV or IM q12h), or chloramphenicol (20–50 mg/kg PO q6–8h for adults and foals >1 week). • Administer antimicrobial drugs systemically until the horse's condition is stable and improving; treatment may then be switched to long-term oral antimicrobials. • NSAIDs—flunixin meglumine (1.1 mg/kg PO or IV q12–24h) or phenylbutazone (2.2–4.4 mg/kg PO or IV q12h)

CONTRAINDICATIONS/POSSIBLE INTERACTIONS

Use aminoglycosides and NSAIDs with caution in horses with compromised renal function or dehydration.

FOLLOW-UP

PATIENT MONITORING

• Monitor clinical signs, especially respiratory rate and efforts, and rectal temperature. • Follow progress of pulmonary lesions by radiography. • Ultrasonography helps to monitor pleural effusion.

PREVENTION/AVOIDANCE

• Prevent or avoid exposure to primary causes.
• Vitamin E and selenium supplementation for white muscle disease

POSSIBLE COMPLICATIONS

• Lung abscess • Pleuritis • Disseminated intravascular coagulation • Laminitis • Thrombophlebitis • Septicemia

EXPECTED COURSE AND PROGNOSIS

• Expect a long and protracted course of treatment.
• Prognosis is guarded.

MISCELLANEOUS

SEE ALSO

• Hemorrhagic nasal discharge
• Pleuropneumonia
• Acute respiratory distress syndrome

ABBREVIATIONS

• AP = aspiration pneumonia
• GI = gastrointestinal

Suggested Reading

Ainsworth DM, Hackett R. Bacterial pneumonia. In: Reed SM, Bayly WM, Sellon DC, eds. Equine Internal Medicine, ed 2. St. Louis: WB Saunders, 2004:321–323.

Author Laurent Couëtil
Consulting Editor Daniel Jean

ATHEROMA OF THE FALSE NOSTRIL

BASICS

OVERVIEW

- An epidermal inclusion cyst of the false nostril (nasal diverticulum)
- Also called false nostril cyst
- Present at birth and becomes apparent with age as the cyst enlarges
- Usually a cosmetic issue only
- The term "atheroma" is a misnomer as it implies a sebaceous cyst.
- The false nostril cysts in horses are not sebaceous cysts.

SIGNALMENT

- Any age
- Usually becomes apparent after weaning to 3 years of age. Most often at yearling age.
- No known sex or breed predilections

SIGNS

- Soft to firm, spherical swelling covered by normal skin in the caudal dorsal to lateral aspect of the false nostril at the area of the nasomaxillary notch
- Typically unilateral, but can be bilateral
- Not painful on palpation
- Size increases with age and can reach a size of up to 5cm
- Usually not associated with respiratory compromise unless very large

CAUSES AND RISK FACTORS

- Congenitally aberrant epithelial tissue between the skin and mucous membrane of the false nostril
- Can slowly enlarge due to progressive exfoliation of keratinized material within the cyst

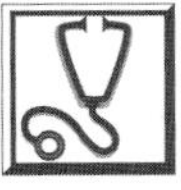

DIAGNOSIS

Characteristic location and physical features of the swelling

DIFFERENTIAL DIAGNOSIS

- An abscess can be ruled out as there is no heat or pain associated with the cyst.
- Cysts could become inflamed if keratinized material leaks into the surrounding tissue.

CBC/BIOCHEMISTRY/URINALYSIS

N/A

OTHER LABORATORY TESTS

- Aspirated fluid is white to gray, milky to creamy in appearance and odorless.
- Cytologically, the cyst fluid contains keratinized and nonkeratinized squamous epithelial cells.
- Trichrome staining reveals keratinized and nonkeratinized squamous epithelial cells and keratinous debris.
- Histologically, the cyst lining is comprised of varying thickness of stratified squamous epithelium.

IMAGING

- Ultrasonographic findings consistent with cystic structure, usually unilocular, mostly homogeneous echogenicity

OTHER DIAGNOSTIC PROCEDURES

- Palpation
- Ultrasonographic evaluation
- Centesis
- Histological evaluation

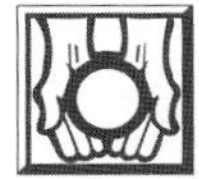

TREATMENT

- Do nothing. Usually not removed unless for cosmetic reasons or for airway noise or impairment from large swelling size.
- If removed surgically, it is imperative to remove the entire cyst lining to prevent recurrence.
- Total surgical removal can be done under general anesthesia or standing with sedation and local anesthesia of the infraorbital nerve.
- The cyst can be approached surgically through the skin over the dorsum of the swelling. The cyst then is dissected in its entirety, and the wound is closed.
- Another option is to open the cyst ventrally into the false nostril, drain the contents, and remove the lining using a burr instrument. In this technique, the wound is left open to heal by second intention.
- A technique has been reported using intralesional injection of neutral-buffered 10% formalin after aspirating the cyst contents. Injection of formalin until leakage around the needle is seen (2–4.5 mL). There is transient swelling within 24 hours of injecting the formalin. Desiccation of the cyst occurs after a few weeks.

MEDICATIONS

DRUGS

Draining and cauterizing or sclerosing the cyst has been done using tincture of iodine, silver nitrate, or both followed by packing; this requires daily treatment and carries a high risk of recurrence.

CONTRAINDICATIONS/POSSIBLE INTERACTIONS

Transient swelling if chemical ablation is used.

FOLLOW-UP

Usual precautions for tetanus prophylaxis and asepsis of the surgical site

POSSIBLE COMPLICATIONS

- A cyst may become abscessed if infection is introduced during centesis.
- Transient swelling after surgery
- Recurrence if lining not removed
- Infection at surgery site
- Scar formation
- White hair at surgery site

EXPECTED COURSE AND PROGNOSIS

Favorable prognosis for both leaving the atheroma untouched and for surgical removal if needed

MISCELLANEOUS

ASSOCIATED CONDITIONS

In addition to false nostril cysts, other congenital cutaneous cysts reported in horses are dentigerous cysts and, very rarely, dermoid cysts.

AGE-RELATED FACTORS

May increase in size with age

ZOONOTIC POTENTIAL

None

PREGNANCY

N/A

SEE ALSO

N/A

Suggested Reading

Frankeny RL. Intralesional administration of formalin for treatment of epidermal inclusion cysts in five horses. J Am Vet Med Assoc 2003;223:221–222.

Schumacher J, Dixon PM. Diseases of the nasal cavities. In: McGorum BC, Dixon PM, Robinson NE, Schumaker J, eds. Equine Respiratory Medicine and Surgery. Philadelphia: WB Saunders, 2007:372–373.

Author Wendy Duckett
Consulting Editor Daniel Jean

ATOPIC DERMATITIS

BASICS

DEFINITION

Chronically relapsing, inflammatory, pruritic skin disease resulting from a predispostion to develop IgE-mediated hypersensitivities to inhaled or cutaneously absorbed environmental allergens

PATHOPHYSIOLOGY

The complete pathomechanism of equine AD is unknown. Susceptible animal is sensitized to environmental allergens resulting in the production of allergen-specific IgE. Upon further exposure to percutaneously absorbed or inhaled allergens, an immediate type I hypersensitivity ensues. The reaction commences by binding of allergen-specific IgE to FcεRIα receptors on mast cells ultimately causing degranulation and liberation of inflammatory mediators such as histamine, cytokines, chemokines, and proteolytic enzymes. The culmination of these inflammatory processes is pruritus and/or urticaria.

SYSTEMS AFFECTED

• Skin • Respiratory

GENETICS

• Genetic predisposition and heritability of AD in horses are unknown. AD must have a genetic component due to the clinical observation that the disease appears more often within certain breeds. • One stallion with AD has five offspring with AD, each from a different mare—suggesting a dominant mode of inheritance.

INCIDENCE/PREVALENCE

True incidence is unknown; estimated at 2%–4% of the equine population; within the top 10 most common equine dermatoses

GEOGRAPHIC DISTRIBUTION

Recognized worldwide; local environmental factors (temperature, humidity, and flora) influence the seasonality, severity, and duration of signs.

SIGNALMENT

Breed Predilections

Arabians, Thoroughbred, Quarter Horses, and Warmbloods have been reported to be predisposed.

Mean Age and Range

Mean 5–6.5 years of age (2–12 years); signs may be mild the first year and usually progress each year.

Predominant Sex

• Both sexes affected equally • In a recent small regional study, males (geldings > stallions) were twice as likely as mares to develop AD.

SIGNS

General Comments

• Hallmark sign—chronic relapsing seasonal or nonseasonal pruritus and/or urticaria (rubbing, itching, biting themselves, stomping, tail flicking, rarely head shaking, and agitation)
• Primary lesions are wheals representing an urticarial reaction and/or papules. • Secondary lesions reflect self-induced trauma from intense pruritus at the affected body site and consists of alopecia, excoriations, erosions to ulcers, scale, lichenification, hypopigmentation, and mane and tail loss. Lesions may be symmetrical.
• Urticaria in AD may be pruritic or nonpruritic.

Historical

• Most commonly affected sites include face, pinnae, chest, ventral thorax and abdomen, extremity extensor and flexor surfaces • Other common sites include the mane, dorsolateral neck, croup, and tail base. • Clinical signs may begin in any season and progress from seasonal to nonseasonal. • Symptoms become progressively more severe with time.

Physical Examination

• Clinical signs of atopy-associated recurrent airway obstruction include head shaking, snorting, bilateral mucopurulent nasal discharge, conjunctivitis, dry unproductive coughs, labored breathing, stomping, and face rubbing on front legs or objects and exercise intolerance.
• Uncommon clinical signs are head shaking and laminitis.

CAUSES

• Airborne pollens (trees, grasses, weeds) • Mold spores (indoor and outdoor) • Animal danders (mouse, cat, cow, poultry, goat) • Possibly storage and house dust mites

RISK FACTORS

• Temperate environments with long allergy seasons, high pollen and mold spore levels
• Concurrent pruritic dermatoses, such as insect hypersensitivity or ectoparasitic disease (summation effect)

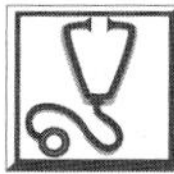

DIAGNOSIS

DIFFERENTIAL DIAGNOSIS

• Insect hypersensitivity—may occur concurrently with AD • Ectoparasites (pathogens and incidentals) • Cutaneous adverse food reaction—rare • Contact hypersensitivity
• For respiratory disease—respiratory infection (bacterial, fungal, viral), congestive heart failure, and bronchitis

CBC/BIOCHEMISTRY/URINALYSIS

Eosinophilia is rare.

OTHER LABORATORY TESTS

Serologic Allergy Tests

• Detects relative levels of allergen-specific IgE in the serum • Controversy exists as to the usefulness of serum allergy tests in horses; the author does not recommend the use of these tests. • A positive result does not always correlate with clinical manifestation of allergy; therefore, results of these tests must be interpreted cautiously. • The effects of antihistamines and corticosteroid administration on test results are unknown. • Many false-positive and -negative results occur with the currently available assays. Lack of repeatability of test results and sensitivity are common. • Do not use to diagnose cutaneous adverse reaction to food or supplements.

IMAGING

N/A

OTHER DIAGNOSTIC PROCEDURES

Intradermal Testing

• Detects levels of allergen-specific IgE in the skin directed to a panel of allergens that are region specific and thought to be clinically-relevant to the patient's disease. • IDT is the gold standard test for allergen hypersensitivity identification in horses.
• Performed for identification of allergens to include in ASIT, possible avoidance or decrease in exposure • Intradermal injection of allergens results in raised turgid wheals. The reaction is given a subjective score (usually 0–4+) based on its size and turgidity compared to the positive and negative controls. • Reactions are interpreted at 15–30 min for an immediate IgE-mediated type I hypersensitivity and 4 hr for the IgE-mediated late-phase reaction. • Normal horses have one or more positive intradermal reactions. • Interpret results in terms of the horse's environment, clinical signs, and history to determine allergens that should be avoided and included in ASIT. • Before performing IDT, a withdrawal period of 14 days is observed for oral and topical antihistamines as well as topical steroid preparations and 30 days for parenteral corticosteroids. • Cytology from erosions or ulcers shows a neutrophilic exudate with intra- and/or extracellular cocci representative of a secondary folliculitis. • Perform skin scrapings to rule out ectoparasites. • Perform bacterial and DTM cultures to determine bacterial species and susceptibility and/or dermatophyte infections.

PATHOLOGICAL FINDINGS

• Skin biopsy—will not rule out other differential diagnosis such as insect or food hypersensitivity • Histopathological changes—epidermal hyperplasia with superficial and deep, perivascular to interstitial dermatitis wherein the eosinophil is the predominant inflammatory cell. Concurrent focal eosinophilic infiltrative and/or necrotizing mural folliculitides and/or eosinophilic granulomas are possible.

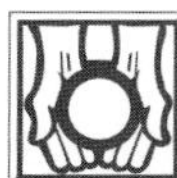

TREATMENT

AIMS OF TREATMENT

Reduce pruritus and secondary infections.

APPROPRIATE HEALTH CARE

Outpatient medical management

NURSING CARE

Frequent bathing using cool water (antimicrobial shampoos, sulfur/salicyclic acid, +/− colloidal oatmeal rinses or leave-on conditioners) helps to remove allergens, crusts, bacteria, and debris; control secondary infections; hydrate dry skin; and provide antipruritic effects.

ACTIVITY

Avoid offending allergens if possible by changing environment.

DIET

Essential fatty acid supplementation may be beneficial in some cases.

CLIENT EDUCATION

• Imperative to discuss the progressive nature of the disease • Advise disease is not curable, but rather manageable and life-long therapy may be needed. • Advise that commitment to proper management of horses with AD can lead to a horse that has a good quality of life and can continue to work. • Discuss that therapeutic modifications over the life of the horse are to be expected. • Due to the potential hereditary factor, owners should be advised to remove affected individual from breeding stock.

SURGICAL CONSIDERATIONS

N/A

MEDICATIONS

DRUG(S) OF CHOICE

Allergen-Specific Immunotherapy

• Subcutaneous administration of gradually increasing doses of causative allergens in an attempt to reduce sensitivity • Allergens for inclusion are based on correlation of history with positive intradermal results and knowledge of local flora. • A useful nonsteroidal long-term treatment alternative when signs last longer than 2 mo or when nonsteroidal forms of therapy are ineffective • Anticipated improvement may be seen as early as 2 mo; however, minimum treatment duration of 12–14 mo is necessary to determine efficacy. • Reports indicate 50%–75% of horses with AD show at least a 50%–100% improvement in clinical signs with ASIT.

Corticosteroids

• Best selection—prednisolone, greater bioavailability than prednisone, tablets or syrup (compounded) at 0.5–1.5 mg/kg q24h until control achieved; then reduce to lowest-dose alternate-day regimen, for example, 0.2–0.5 mg/kg q48h • For horses that do not respond to prednisolone, try dexamethasone powder or injectable. Initial loading oral or IV dose of 0.02–0.1 mg/kg q24h for 3–5 days; then taper to 0.01–0.02 mg/kg q48–72h for maintenance. • Repository injectable corticosteroids should be avoided as withdrawal upon an adverse reaction is not possible.

Antihistamines—A Nonsteroidal Alternative for Long-term Control

• Not useful when moderate to severe pruritus is present; rather use as a preventative either before the onset of severe pruritus or in a maintenance regimen to suppress pruritus once controlled. • Pharmacokinetic data for the use of antihistamines in horses are limited. Anecdotal reports suggest that H_1-receptor antagonist hydroxyzine hydrochloride/pamonate (0.5–1 mg/kg q8h), chlorpheniramine (0.25 mg/kg q12h), diphenhydramine (0.75–1.0 mg/kg q12h), or pyrilamine malate (1 mg/kg q12h) may decrease pruritus and provide a steroid-sparing effect. • Antihistamines should be given at least 10–14 days before efficacy is determined. If no response, select another class of antihistamine.

Tricyclic Antidepressants

Used to control hypersensitivity with a stress or psychogenic component. Horses may respond to doxepin HCl (0.5–0.75 mg/kg q12h PO) or amitriptyline (1–2 mg/kg q12h PO).

CONTRAINDICATIONS

• Due to the anticholinergic properties of antihistamines and tricyclic antidepressants, do not use in patients with a history of cardiac arrhythmias, colic, glaucoma, or urinary retention disorders. Antihistamines may thicken mucus in the respiratory tract. Extra caution should be used in horses with respiratory problems due to excess mucus. • Avoid corticosteroid use during pregnancy and lactation unless the benefits outweigh the risks. Risks are likely low.

PRECAUTIONS

• Corticosteroids—Use judiciously to avoid iatrogenic hyperglucocorticism, diabetes mellitus, polydipsia and polyuria, aggravation of bacterial folliculitis, decreased muscle mass, weight loss, poor wound healing, and behavior changes. • Antihistamines—can produce sedation and/or behavior changes, whole body or fine tremors or seizures. High doses of antihistamines cause birth defects in laboratory animals. Antihistamines should only be used in pregnant or lactating animals if the benefits outweigh the risks. Do not administer antihistamines intravenously in the horse due to potential CNS stimulation. • Note drug withdrawal times and regulations pertaining to horse show or racing associations.

POSSIBLE INTERACTIONS

• If diuretics such as furosemide are given with corticosteroids, an increased risk of electrolyte imbalances due to calcium and potassium losses exists. • Prednisolone interacts with phenytoin, phenobarbital, rifampin, erythromycin and the anticholinesterase drugs, neostigmine and pyridostigmine. • Antihistamines have an additive effect when combined with other CNS-depressant drugs, such as tranquilizers.

ALTERNATIVE DRUGS

Polyunsaturated omega 3 and 6 fatty acids—variable response in decreasing pruritus; provide support for epidermal barrier function and anti-inflammatory properties. Use as adjunctive therapy. Response noted within 2–8 weeks after starting therapy. Exact dosing for horse is lacking; the author uses 180 mg of EPA/10 lb q24h.

FOLLOW-UP

PATIENT MONITORING

• Examine patient every 2–6 weeks when a new course of therapy is commenced. • Monitor pruritus, self-trauma, secondary bacterial dermatitis, and possible adverse drug reactions. • Once an acceptable level of pruritus is achieved, examine patient every 4–12 mo. • CBC, serum biochemical profile, and fibrinogen are recommended within the first week of starting corticosteroid therapy and then every 1–4 mo thereafter if chronic corticosteroid therapy cannot be avoided.

PREVENTION/AVOIDANCE

• Avoidance of allergens is not always possible or practical, especially as many patients have multiple allergens contributing to their disease. • Prevention of the disease may be possible if patient is moved to another region of the country.

POSSIBLE COMPLICATIONS

• Secondary bacterial dermatitis • Secondary laminitis, colic, and iatrogenic hyperadrenocorticism due to chronic steroid administration

EXPECTED COURSE AND PROGNOSIS

• Not life-threatening unless intractable pruritus persists • No reports of spontaneous remission exist.

MISCELLANEOUS

ASSOCIATED CONDITIONS

• Insect hypersensitivity • Eosinophilic granulomas • Allergic conjunctivitis and rhinitis • Recurrent airway obstruction • Inflammatory airway disease • Summer pasture–associated obstructive pulmonary disease

AGE-RELATED FACTORS

Severity worsens with age.

ZOONOTIC POTENTIAL

N/A

PREGNANCY

• Corticosteroids—contraindicated during pregnancy • Antihistamines—no information on teratogenicity is available for horses; consider this before treating pregnant mares.

SYNONYMS

Equine atopy

SEE ALSO

• Insect hypersensitivity • Urticaria • Bacterial dermatitis • Ectoparasites

ABBREVIATIONS

• AD = atopic dermatitis • ASIT = allergen specific immunotherapy • IDT = intradermal test • DTM = dermatophyte test medium

Suggested Reading

Scott DW, Miller WH Jr. Equine Dermatology. St. Louis: Saunders, 2003: 480.

Author Gwendolen Lorch

Consulting Editor Gwendolen Lorch

ATRIAL FIBRILLATION

BASICS

DEFINITION

- An irregularly irregular cardiac rhythm, with variable-intensity heart sounds and pulses and inconsistent diastolic intervals
- Can be sustained or paroxysmal (resolving spontaneously within 48 hr of onset)

PATHOPHYSIOLOGY

- A critical atrial mass must be present for the condition to occur.
- Predisposing factors—large atrial mass, high vagal tone, shortened and nonhomogeneous effective refractory period, potassium depletion, atrial premature depolarizations, rapid atrial pacing
- Produces no change in cardiac output at rest without underlying cardiac disease
- During high-intensity exercise, produces a marked increase in the heart rate response and fall in cardiac output and exercise capacity
- Present in many horses with CHF but is not the cause of CHF

SYSTEM AFFECTED

Cardiovascular

SIGNALMENT

Higher incidence in Standardbreds, Draft, and Warmblood horses

SIGNS

General Comments

Causes exercise intolerance in performance animals, but often an incidental finding in sedentary horses

Historical

- Exercise intolerance
- Exercise-induced pulmonary hemorrhage—often profuse
- Weakness or collapse

Physical Examination

- Irregularly irregular heart rhythm
- Variable-intensity heart sounds and arterial pulses
- Absent fourth heart sound
- Cardiac murmurs with predisposing cardiac disease

CAUSES

- Normal horses have sufficient atrial mass and high vagal tone to develop AF without evident underlying heart disease.
- Diseases causing atrial enlargement further predispose horses to AF.

RISK FACTORS

- AV valve insufficiency
- CHF
- Electrolyte disturbances

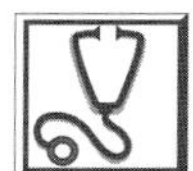

DIAGNOSIS

DIFFERENTIAL DIAGNOSIS

- Second-degree AV block—Regular rhythm is interrupted by pauses containing fourth heart sound.
- Atrial tachycardia with second-degree AV block—Rhythm usually is regularly irregular; fourth heart sounds are present.
- Sinus rhythm with multifocal ventricular premature depolarizations—Need ECG to differentiate.

CBC/BIOCHEMISTRY/URINALYSIS

Low plasma potassium or urinary fractional excretion of potassium may be present.

OTHER LABORATORY TESTS

- Elevated cardiac isoenzymes (e.g., CK-MB, HBDH, LDH-1 and LDH-2, cardiac troponin I) may be present but are usually within the normal range.
- RBC potassium concentrations may be decreased.

IMAGING

ECG

- No P waves, replaced by baseline "f" waves
- The "f" waves may be coarse or fine and may occur 300–500 times per minute.
- Irregular R-R interval
- Some variation in the amplitude of QRS and T complexes usually is present, but these complexes are normal in appearance.

Echocardiography

- Most have little or no discernible underlying cardiac disease; therefore, the echocardiogram is normal.
- Some have low shortening fraction (24%–32%). This should return to normal within several days of conversion to normal sinus rhythm.
- Mild left atrial enlargement with sustained AF
- Atrial enlargement due to congenital defects or AV valve insufficiency may be present.

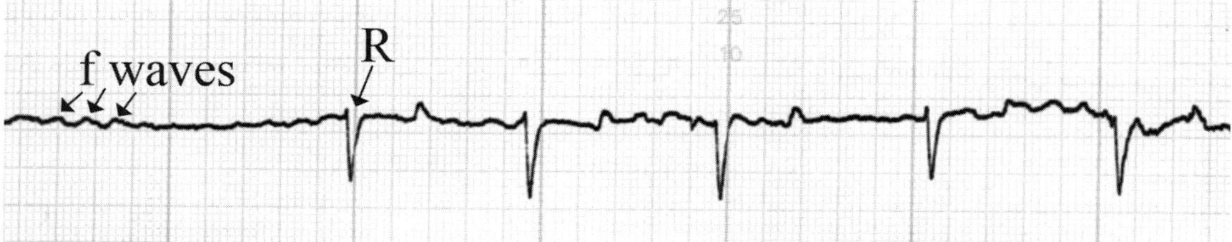

Figure 1.

Base-apex lead, 25 mm/sec, 5 mm = 1 mV.

DIAGNOSTIC PROCEDURES

Continuous 24-Hour Holter Monitoring

Use in horses with suspected paroxysmal AF to identify underlying arrhythmias.

Exercise Electrocardiography

- Useful to detect exercise-induced arrhythmias and to determine exercise limitations if the AF is not or cannot be converted

PATHOLOGIC FINDINGS

- Grossly and histopathologically normal heart in horses with no underlying cardiac disease
- Focal or diffuse atrial fibrosis may be present in horses with long-standing AF.
- Myocarditis, myocardial necrosis, and fatty infiltration have been documented in affected horses.
- Both atrial and ventricular enlargement in horses with significant AV valvular disease

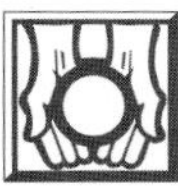

TREATMENT

AIMS OF TREATMENT

- Restoration of sinus rhythm and athletic performance in horses with exercise intolerance but no, or minimal, underlying heart disease
- Palliative care for horses with AF in conjunction with CHF

APPROPRIATE HEALTH CARE

- Monitor horses for 24–48 hr to determine if the condition will resolve without treatment (i.e., paroxysmal).
- In horses with AF and CHF, institute treatment for congestive heart failure—for example, using digoxin (0.0022 mg/kg IV) and furosemide (1–2 mg/kg IV, not PO).
- If AF is sustained, CHF is not present, and exercise intolerance is present, pharmacological or electrical cardioversion should be considered.

NURSING CARE

- Perform continuous ECG throughout attempted conversion to sinus rhythm.
- Keep horses quiet and unmoving during quinidine treatment.

ACTIVITY

- AF cases should not perform high-intensity exercise.
- AF cases usually can perform successfully as pleasure horses, in lower-level athletic competition, as broodmares, and as breeding stallions.

DIET

- Oral potassium supplementation may be indicated with low plasma potassium, low RBC potassium, or low urinary fractional excretion of potassium or with excessive sweating.
- Potassium chloride salt can be added to the feed (1 tbsp BID, gradually increasing to 1 oz BID).

CLIENT EDUCATION

- Discuss treatment-associated risks with owners—see Possible Complications.
- Discuss predisposing factors with owners to minimize the likelihood of future episodes.

SURGICAL CONSIDERATIONS

- Successful transvenous electrical conversion of horses under general anethesia has been described.
- This utilizes a biphasic current delivered between electrodes placed in the right atrium and left pulmonary artery using pressure waveforms, echocardiography, and radiography to guide and confirm electrode placement.
- Initial reports of success rates from one center are very encouraging.

MEDICATIONS

DRUG(S) OF CHOICE

The drug of choice for conversion is quinidine sulfate or gluconate.

Quinidine Gluconate

- Indicated with AF of duration ≤2 weeks and no underlying cardiac disease.
- Administered in boluses of 0.5–1 mg/kg every 5–10 min to a total dose of 10 mg/kg.

Quinidine Sulfate

- Indicated in horses with sustained AF
- Administered via nasogastric intubation at 22 mg/kg q2h to a total of four to six treatments, then q6h until the horse shows signs of toxicity or has converted to sinus rhythm.

CONTRAINDICATIONS

- Do not administer quinidine sulfate or gluconate to affected horses with CHF.
- Horses with a resting heart rate of >60 bpm and/or grade 3/6 or louder systolic murmurs are likely to have CHF.

PRECAUTIONS

Quinidine is associated with the following complications.

Cardiovascular

- Prolonged QRS duration—indicates quinidine toxicity.
- Rapid supraventricular tachycardia—treat aggressively with digoxin to slow heart rate.
  - Digoxin is recommended in conjunction with quinidine in horses with myocardial dysfunction or rapid heart rate during quinidine treatment.

ATRIAL FIBRILLATION

- ○ If heart rate exceeds 100 bpm, consider digoxin—0.011 mg/kg PO or 0.0022 mg/kg IV.
- ○ If a heart rate exceeds 150 bpm, consider digoxin (0.0022 mg/kg IV) and sodium bicarbonate (1 mEq/kg IV).
- ○ If the heart rate remains high, administer propranolol—0.03 mg/kg IV.
- ○ If a horse receiving quinidine only on day 1 does not convert, consider adding digoxin orally on day 2.
- ○ Base subsequent digoxin administration during quinidine treatment on serum digoxin concentration and need to control heart rate or to improve myocardial contractility.

- Ventricular arrhythmias require treatment unless ventricular rhythm is slow (<100 bpm), uniform, and no R-on-T is detected.
- Treat ventricular arrhythmias with magnesium sulfate—2–5 mg/kg bolus IV q5min to 50 mg/kg total or propranolol—0.03 mg/kg IV.
- Hypotension—monitor and treat, if severe, with intravenous fluids to effect and, if necessary, phenylephrine (0.1–0.2 μg/kg per minute IV to effect).
- Sudden death—Try to prevent with continuous ECG and treatment of any arrhythmias that occur.

GI

- Flatulence—resolves on return of quinidine plasma concentrations to negligible levels.
- Oral ulcerations—Prevent by not administering quinidine via nasogastric tube.
- Diarrhea—indicates quinidine toxicity, resolves on return of quinidine plasma concentrations to negligible levels.
- Colic—indicates quinidine toxicity; treat with analgesics as needed.

Respiratory

Upper respiratory tract obstruction—Treat with passage of a nasotracheal tube to relieve the upper airway obstruction; administer corticosteroids and antihistamines; emergency tracheotomy, if necessary

Dermatologic

Urticaria—Treat with corticosteroids and antihistamines.

Reproductive

Paraphimosis—resolves on return of plasma quinidine concentration to negligible levels

Musculoskeletal

Laminitis—If the horse is uncomfortable, administer analgesics.

Neurologic

- Indicates quinidine toxicity
- Ataxia—resolves on return of plasma quinidine concentration to negligible levels
- Convulsions—Administer anticonvulsants.
- Bizarre behavior—resolves on return of plasma quinidine concentration to negligible levels

POSSIBLE INTERACTIONS

Quinidine competes with digoxin for binding to plasma protein, causing potential digoxin toxicity.

ALTERNATIVE DRUGS

Oral, but not intravenous, flecanide and intravenous amiodarone have recently been proposed.

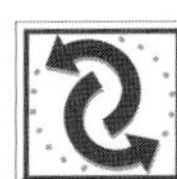

FOLLOW-UP

PATIENT MONITORING

- Perform continuous ECG during treatment, because antiarrhythmic drugs are also arrhythmogenic.
- Measure QRS duration before each dose; discontinue treatment if QRS duration ≥25% of the pretreatment value.
- Discontinue treatment if rapid supraventricular tachycardia, ventricular arrhythmia, diarrheal colic, ataxia, convulsions, bizarre behavior, urticaria, upper respiratory tract obstruction, or laminitis occurs.
- Following conversion, perform 24-hour Holter monitoring. If atrial ectopy is found, rest and corticosteroid therapy may be indicated.
- Riders should regularly monitor cardiac rhythm; any irregularities or poor performance should prompt reexamination.

PREVENTION AVOIDANCE

• Discontinue administration of furosemide and bicarbonate milkshakes.
• Administer potassium or other electrolyte supplementation, if indicated.
• See Supraventricular Arrhythmias.

POSSIBLE COMPLICATIONS

• If AF is not or cannot be treated, clinical signs will persist.
• Some horses with AF also have exercise-induced ventricular arrhythmias; this possibility should be explored if AF is not or cannot be treated and the horse is to continue to be used for ridden exercise—see Ventricular Arrhythmias.

EXPECTED COURSE AND PROGNOSIS

• Most horses with little or no underlying cardiac disease convert to sinus rhythm with quinidine therapy.
• Recurrences occur in ≅25% of horses with a suspected duration of atrial fibrillation of ≤4 mo.
• Recurrences occur in ≅60% of horses with a duration of atrial fibrillation of >4 mo.
• Recurrence is mostly likely during the first year after conversion but can occur at any time.
• Prognosis for return to the previous level of athletic performance is excellent in converted horses without significant underlying cardiovascular disease.
• Horses with sustained AF that do not convert to sinus rhythm with treatment or that are not candidates for conversion usually have a normal life expectancy and can be safely used for lower-level athletic performance.
• With significant valvular insufficiency, severity of the valvular heart disease and its progression determine the horse's useful performance life and life expectancy.
• Horses with CHF usually have severe underlying valvular heart or myocardial disease and have a guarded to grave prognosis for life.
• Most affected horses treated for congestive heart failure respond to the supportive therapy and improve for a short time but are euthanized within 2–6 mo of initiating treatment.

MISCELLANEOUS

ASSOCIATED CONDITIONS

Any cardiac disease resulting in atrial enlargement predisposes to atrial fibrillation.

AGE-RELATED FACTORS

• Old horses are more likely to have significant underlying cardiac disease with valvular insufficiency and atrial enlargement.
• These horses usually are not candidates for conversion because of significant underlying cardiac disease.

PREGNANCY

• Affected pregnant mares without underlying cardiac disease and congestive heart failure should not experience any problems.
• Affected pregnant mares with CHF can be treated for the underlying cardiac disease with positive inotropic drugs (e.g., digoxin) and diuretics (e.g., furosemide).

SYNONYMS

A fib

SEE ALSO

• Congestive heart failure
• Mitral regurgitation
• Tricuspid regurgitation
• Supraventricular arrhythmias
• Ventricular arrhythmias

ABBREVIATIONS

• AF = atrial fibrillation
• AV = atrioventricular
• CK-MB = MB isoenzyme of creatine kinase
• CHF = congestive heart failure
• GI = gastrointestinal
• HBDH = α-hydroxybutyrate dehydrogenase
• LDH = lactate dehydrogenase
• RBC = red blood cell

Suggested Reading

De Clercq D, van Loon G, Baert K, Tavernier R, Croubels S, De Backer P, Deprez P. Effects of an adapted intravenous amiodarone treatment protocol in horses with atrial fibrillation. Equine Vet J. 2007;39:344–349.

McGurrin MK, Physick-Sheard PW, Kenney DG, Kerr C, Hanna WJ. Transvenous electrical cardioversion of equine atrial fibrillation: technical considerations. J Vet Intern Med. 2005;19:695–702.

Reef VB, Levitan CW, Spencer PA. Factors affecting prognosis and conversion in equine atrial fibrillation. J Vet Intern Med 1988;2:1–6.

Reef VB, Reimer JM, Spencer PA. Treatment of equine atrial fibrillation: new perspectives. J Vet Intern Med 1995;9:57–67.

Risberg AI, McGuirk SM. Successful conversion of equine atrial fibrillation using oral flecainide. J Vet Intern Med. 2006;20:207–209.

Author Virginia B. Reef

Consulting Editor Celia M. Marr

ATRIAL SEPTAL DEFECT

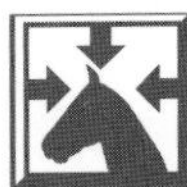

BASICS

DEFINITION

• A congenital defect (i.e., hole) in the interatrial septum that creates a communication between the right and left atria
• Can be located in the atrial septum immediately adjacent to the ventricular septum (i.e., atrium primum defect), in the area of the foramen ovale (i.e., atrium secundum defect), or in the most basilar portion of the interatrial septum (i.e., sinus venosus–type defect).
• ASD can occur in isolation or in conjunction with other cardiac anomalies in complex congenital cardiac disease.
• The atrial septum forms in the fetus from the septum primum and the septum secundum. The slit-like communication between these septa (i.e., the foramen ovale) allows passage of blood from right to the left atrium in the fetus.
• The foramen ovale is functionally closed in normal neonates within 24–48 hr of birth, but anatomic closure may not be complete until 9 weeks.

PATHOPHYSIOLOGY

• A patent foramen ovale occurs when the foramen ovale fails to close.
• Failed formation of one of the two septa results in the other forms of ASD.
• Blood shunts from the higher-pressure left atrium to the lower-pressure right atrium in foals with ASD, creating a left atrial, right atrial, and right ventricular volume overload.
• Size of the ASD determines severity of the volume overload. In horses with a large ASD, the right and left atrial and right ventricular volume overload is severe.
• Over time, stretching of the tricuspid annulus occurs, and tricuspid regurgitation develops. As the tricuspid regurgitation becomes more severe, increases in right atrial pressure result in increased hepatic venous pressure and development of clinical signs of right-sided congestive heart failure.

SYSTEM AFFECTED

Cardiovascular

GENETICS

• Not yet determined in horses
• Although heritable in other species, it is rare in horses.

INCIDENCE/PREVALENCE

These defects are uncommon as isolated congenital defects and more frequently occur in conjunction with complex congenital heart disease, particularly tricuspid and pulmonic atresia.

SIGNALMENT

Most frequently diagnosed in neonates, foals, and young horses, but may be diagnosed at any age

SIGNS

General

May be detected as an incidental finding, but usually is part of a more complex, congenital cardiac disorder

Historical

• Exercise intolerance—medium-size to large ASDs
• Congestive heart failure—large ASDs

Physical Examination

• No murmur may be present, or a coarse, band- or ejection-shaped, holosystolic murmur with PMI in pulmonic valve area may be detected.
• Premature beats or an irregularly irregular heart rhythm of atrial fibrillation may be present with larger ASDs.

CAUSES

• Failed closure of the foramen ovale
• Congenital malformation of the interatrial septum

RISK FACTORS

• Premature foal
• Neonatal pulmonary hypertension
• Neonatal respiratory distress syndrome

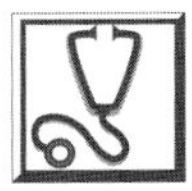

DIAGNOSIS

DIFFERENTIAL DIAGNOSIS

• Physiologic flow murmur—Differentiate echocardiographically.
• Pulmonic stenosis (rare)—murmur usually louder; differentiate echocardiographically.
• Aortic stenosis (rare)—murmur usually louder; weak arterial pulses; differentiate echocardiographically.
• Tricuspid atresia—murmur usually louder; foal is unthrifty, tachycardic, and hypoxemic; differentiate echocardiographically.
• Pulmonic atresia—murmur usually louder; may have a continuous machinery murmur; foal is unthrifty, tachycardic, and hypoxemic; differentiate echocardiographically.

CBC/BIOCHEMISTRY/URINALYSIS

N/A

OTHER LABORATORY TESTS

N/A

IMAGING

Electrocardiography

• Atrial premature depolarizations or atrial fibrillation may be present in horses with right and left atrial enlargement.
• Persistent atrial fibrillation has been reported in some affected foals and horses.

Echocardiography

• Can determine location of the ASD
• Atrial septal dropout is detected at the ASD location and should be confirmed by visualization in two mutually perpendicular planes.
• The left and right atria and right ventricle are enlarged, dilated, and have a rounded appearance.
• Paradoxical septal motion is detected with a severe right ventricular volume overload.
• Pulmonary artery dilatation is seen in horses with a large shunt.
• Interrogate the entire atrial septum with pulsed-wave or color-flow Doppler with suspected ASD.
• Contrast or color-flow Doppler reveals the shunt from the left to the right atrium through the ASD.
• A small amount of positive contrast may be seen in the left atrium in horses with normal pulmonary arterial pressures or with the Valsalva maneuver at contrast echocardiography.
• A jet of tricuspid regurgitation may be present in horses with a large ASD and marked right atrial and ventricular volume overload.

Thoracic Radiography

Increased pulmonary vascularity and cardiac enlargement may be detected in horses with large shunts.

DIAGNOSTIC PROCEDURES

Cardiac Catheterization

• Right-sided catheterization can be performed to directly measure right atrial, right ventricular, and pulmonary arterial pressures and to sample blood for oxygen content.
• Elevated right atrial, right ventricular, and pulmonary arterial pressures and increased oxygen saturation of right ventricular and pulmonary arterial blood have been seen in horses with larger ASDs.

Continuous 24-Hour Holter Monitoring

Use in identifying intermitent atrial premature depolarizations.

PATHOLOGIC FINDINGS

• Defect in the atrial septum
• Jet lesions along the defect margins and on the adjacent right atrial endocardium
• Left atrial, right atrial, and right ventricular enlargement and thinning of the left atrial, right atrial, and right ventricular free wall in horses with a significant shunt
• Pulmonary artery dilatation in horses with a large shunt or that have developed pulmonary hypertension
• With congestive heart failure, ventral and peripheral edema, pleural effusion, pericardial effusion, chronic hepatic congestion, and, occasionally, ascites may be detected.

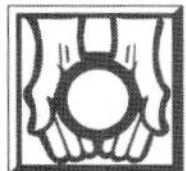

TREATMENT

AIMS OF TREATMENT

• Management by intermittent monitoring in horses with small ASDs
• Palliative care in horses with large ASDs and those with complex congenital cardiac defects

APPROPRIATE HEALTH CARE

• Most affected horses require no treatment and can be monitored on an outpatient basis.
• Monitor horses with large shunts on an annual basis.
• Affected horses with congestive heart failure can be treated for congestive heart failure with positive inotropic drugs, vasodilators, and diuretics. Consider humane destruction if congestive heart failure develops, however, because only short-term, symptomatic improvement can be expected.

NURSING CARE

N/A

ACTIVITY

• Affected horses are safe to continue in full athletic work until significant tricuspid regurgitation or atrial fibrillation develops.
• Horses with small defects can be in unrestricted activity and may be able to compete reasonably successfully in upper-level athletic competition.
• Monitor horses with hemodynamically significant defects echocardiographically on an annual basis to ensure they are safe to ride and compete. These horses can be used for lower-level athletic competition but are unlikely to compete at the upper levels of athletic performance.
• Affected horses that develop atrial fibrillation need a complete cardiovascular examination to determine if they are safe to use for lower-level athletic performance.
• Horses with significant pulmonary artery dilatation no longer are safe to ride.

DIET

N/A

CLIENT EDUCATION

• Regularly monitor cardiac rhythm; any irregularities of the rhythm, other than second-degree AV block, should prompt ECG.
• Carefully monitor for exercise intolerance, respiratory distress, prolonged recovery after exercise, increased resting respiratory or heart rate, cough, generalized venous distention, jugular pulses, or ventral edema; if detected, obtain a cardiac reexamination.

SURGICAL CONSIDERATIONS

• Closure of the ASD would be possible with a transvenous umbrella catheter if the diameter of the umbrella was large enough to close the defect.
• Surgical closure is not financially feasible or practical for obtaining equine athletes at this time.

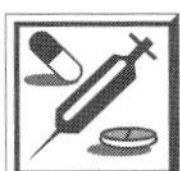

MEDICATIONS

DRUG(S) OF CHOICE, CONTRAINDICATIONS, PRECAUTIONS, POSSIBLE INTERACTIONS, ALTERNATIVE DRUGS

N/A

FOLLOW-UP

PATIENT MONITORING

Frequently monitor cardiac rate, rhythm, and respiratory rate and effort.

PREVENTION/AVOIDANCE

N/A

POSSIBLE COMPLICATIONS

Large ASD—atrial fibrillation; congestive heart failure

EXPECTED COURSE AND PROGNOSIS

• Horses with small defects should have a normal performance life and life expectancy.
• Horses with moderate defects also have a normal life expectancy. These horses usually perform successfully only at lower levels of athletic competition, and they may develop atrial fibrillation.
• Horses with large defects have a guarded prognosis, because they may have a shortened life expectancy and performance life, even at the lower levels of athletic competition.
• Affected horses with congestive heart failure usually have a guarded to grave prognosis for life. Most such horses being treated for congestive heart failure should respond to the supportive therapy and transiently improve; however, once congestive heart failure develops, euthanasia is recommended.

MISCELLANEOUS

ASSOCIATED CONDITIONS

• Complex congenital cardiac disease, particularly tricuspid and pulmonic atresia, is likely.
• Tricuspid regurgitation can develop in horses with significant left atrial, right atrial, and right ventricular volume overload secondary to stretching of the tricuspid annulus.
• Pulmonic regurgitation can develop in horses with isolated defects.
• Pulmonic valve leaflets may no longer coapt with stretching of the pulmonary artery from the volume overload.

AGE-RELATED FACTORS

Young horses are more likely to be diagnosed.

ZOONOTIC POTENTIAL

N/A

PREGNANCY

Breeding affected horses is discouraged. The condition is rare, however, and the heritable nature of this defect in horses is not known.

SYNONYMS

N/A

SEE ALSO

• Atrial fibrillation
• Supraventricular arrhythmias

ABBREVIATIONS

• ASD = atrial septal defect
• AV = atrioventricular
• PMI = point of maximal intensity

Suggested Reading

Reef VB. Cardiovascular disease in the equine neonate. Vet Clin North Am Equine Pract 1985;1:117–129.

Reef VB. Cardiovascular ultrasonography. In: Reef VB, ed. Equine Diagnostic Ultrasound. Philadelphia: WB Saunders, 1998:215–272.

Reef VB. Echocardiographic findings in horses with congenital cardiac disease. Compend Contin Educ Pract Vet 1991;13:109–117.

Reppas GP, Canfield PJ, Hartley WJ, Hutchins DR, Hoffmann KL. Multiple congenital cardiac anomalies and idiopathic thoracic aortitis in a horse. Vet Rec 1996;138:14–16.

Taylor FG, Wooton PR, Hillyer MH, Barr FJ, Luce VM. Atrial septal defect and atrial fibrillation in a foal. Vet Rec 1991;128:80–81.

Author Virginia B. Reef
Consulting Editor Celia M. Marr

AURAL PLAQUES

BASICS

OVERVIEW

• Aural plaques are whitish plaques on the inner surface of the pinna of horses.
• Likely related to papilloma virus infection
• May or may not be associated with varying degrees of ear sensitivity
• Lesions do not spontaneously regress.
• Treatment has been unsuccessful until recently.

SIGNALMENT

• Common in both sexes and all breeds.
• Not frequently observed in horses <1year of age.

SIGNS

• Depigmented, well-demarcated papules and plaques covered with keratin deposits located on the concave surface of the pinna. Lesions are single, multiple, or coalescing and may affect one or both pinna.
• Horses can be asymptomatic or may resent bridling or handling of the ears.
• Head shaking has been rarely reported.
• Symptoms may be aggravated by biting flies.

CAUSES AND RISK FACTORS

• Bovine papilloma virus is suspected.
• Abrasions and insect bites may be involved in transmission.

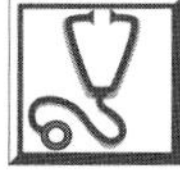

DIAGNOSIS

DIFFERENTIAL DIAGNOSIS

• Sarcoids—usually identified on the external surface of the pinna or at the margins of the ear. They may be coexistent with aural plaques.

CBC/BIOCHEMISTRY/URINALYSIS

N/A

OTHER LABORATORY TESTS

N/A

IMAGING

N/A

OTHER DIAGNOSTIC PROCEDURES

Diagnosis is based on classic appearance and can be confirmed by biopsy.

PATHOLOGICAL FINDINGS

Histologic features consistent with papilloma virus infection including papillated epidermal hyperplasia, koilocytosis, and increased numbers and size of keratohyalin granules.

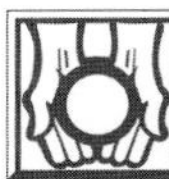

TREATMENT

• Multiple treatments are advocated but none have been shown consistently effective.
• CO_2 laser ablation, corticosteroids, tretinoin, and Eastern blood root in zinc chloride have all been tried with variable results and recurrence is common.
• Management of affected horses often involves minimizing resistance to ear handling and protecting ears from biting insects.

MEDICATIONS

DRUG(S) OF CHOICE

• Imiquimod (Aldara) has recently been evaluated in a clinical trial and is effective at removing the plaques. Recurrence rates are as yet undetermined.
• Imiquimod is applied topically as a thin layer 2–3×/week every other week until resolution (typically 3–4 mo of every other week treatment).

CONTRAINDICATIONS/POSSIBLE INTERACTIONS

A strong local inflammatory response is consistently observed with imiquimod due to its mechanism of action. This can make it difficult to clean the ears prior to the subsequent treatment. Sedation is often needed, particularly for the second or third treatments of the treatment weeks. Owners should be warned of the reaction and temporarily increased sensitivity due to local inflammation.

FOLLOW-UP

PATIENT MONITORING

• Monitoring for complete resolution is important. Imiquimod causes enough local reaction that it can be difficult to determine if the plaques are still present. One to 2 weeks without treatment allows better evaluation and recheck evaluation at 1 mo post-treatment is strongly recommended.
• Each lesion must be treated. No effect is observed on untreated lesions.

PREVENTION/AVOIDANCE

• *Generally* not possible
• Use of fly repellents with permethrin/pyrethrin (for quick insect knockdown) and piperonyl butoxide (as a pesticide synergist) in addition to fly masks that provide ear coverage may help prevent development of additional lesions.

POSSIBLE COMPLICATIONS

• Ear sensitivity and pain on cleaning
• Imiquimod can cause skin erosions or ulcers, particularly if applied in a thick layer. Erosions appear to be more common in the first month of treatment. The amount of reaction seems to decrease as the plaques resolve.

EXPECTED COURSE AND PROGNOSIS

• Aural plaques persist without treatment.
• Post-treatment skin depigmentation may occur.
• Initial results with imiquimod treatment suggest that after resolution of the plaques, horses are less sensitive to ear manipulation than prior to treatment.

MISCELLANEOUS

ASSOCIATED CONDITIONS

None known

AGE-RELATED FACTORS

None known

ZOONOTIC POTENTIAL

None

PREGNANCY

Does not affect disease or treatment

SEE ALSO

• Papillomatosis
• Sarcoid

Suggested Reading

Berman B, Hengge U, Barton S. Successful management of viral infections and other dermatoses with imiquimod 5% cream. Acta Dermatol Enereal 2003;suppl 214:12–17.

Fairley RA, Haines DM. The electron microscopic and immunohistochemical demonstration of a papillomavirus in equine aural plaques. Vet Pathol 1992;29:70–81.

Williams MA: Papillomatosis: warts and aural plaques. In: Robinson ME, ed. Current Therapy in Equine Medicine, ed 4. Philadelphia: WB Saunders, 1997.

Authors Erin Malone and Sheila Torres
Consulting Editor Gwendolen Lorch

AZOTEMIA AND UREMIA

BASICS

DEFINITION

• Azotemia—the accumulation of nitrogenous waste (e.g., urea, Cr, other nitrogenous substance) in blood, plasma, or serum.
• Uremia—the clinical manifestation of azotemia; a multisystem disorder resulting from the effects of uremic toxins on cellular metabolism and function. • Cr and SUN (serum urea nitrogen) typically are measured in serum and used as indices of azotemia.

PATHOPHYSIOLOGY

• Serum urea concentration is determined by rate of urea synthesis by hepatocytes and rate of clearance by the kidneys. • Increased protein catabolism results in elevated SUN. • Decreased GFR may result from decreased renal perfusion (i.e., prerenal azotemia); primary renal disease, either insufficiency or failure (i.e., renal azotemia); or urinary obstruction (i.e., postrenal azotemia). • Azotemia results from resorption of urine when urinary tract rupture (i.e., postrenal azotemia) results in accumulation of urine in the body cavities (abdomen) or subcutaneously.
• Creatinine is a result of muscle creatine metabolism; serum levels reflect the rate of synthesis and rate of excretion. • Rate of synthesis is relatively constant except in the face of rhabdomyolysis. • Renal excretion is dependent on GFR. • Creatinine is not resorbed by renal tubules. • Low serum urea levels may result after prolonged diuresis or as a result of impaired liver function. • There is no clinical significance to decreased creatinine levels.

SYSTEMS AFFECTED

• Generalized or systemic effects—depression, weakness, weight loss, edema, and dehydration
• Gastrointestinal—anorexia, uremic stomatitis, uriniferous breath, excessive dental tartar, gingivitis, oral/gastric ulceration, mild protein-losing enteropathy, diarrhea, and melena
• Neuromuscular—dullness, lethargy, gait imbalance, tremors, behavioral changes, seizures, and stupor • Endocrine/metabolic—renal secondary hyperparathyroidism, inadequate production of erythropoietin and 1,25-dihydrocholecalciferol, decreased hormone clearance that prolongs plasma half-life (e.g., parathormone, gastrin), decreased tissue sensitivity (e.g., insulin, parathormone), decreased hormone production (i.e., testosterone), and hypersecretion to reestablish homeostasis (i.e., parathormone)
• Cardiovascular—elevated blood pressure, heart murmur, and cardiac dysrhythmia
• Respiratory—dyspnea • Hemic/lymphatic/ immune— anemia and impaired immune function

GENETICS

No genetic predisposition

GEOGRAPHIC DISTRIBUTION

None

SIGNALMENT

All ages, breeds, and sexes

SIGNS

General Comments

• Azotemia does not always equate to clinical signs of disease described here. • Unless the animal is uremic, clinical findings are limited to the process causing azotemia—dehydration, urinary outflow tract obstruction, or rupture.

Historical

• Weight loss • Anorexia • Abnormal urination
• Depression • Lethargy • Dental tartar
• Uriniferous breath • Poor performance
• Lumbar pain • Colic • Abdominal distension
• Poor hair coat • Prolonged posturing to urinate • PU/PD

Physical Examination

• Fever • Anorexia • Depression • Oral pallor
• Poor body condition • Ventral edema • Oral ulceration • Excessive dental tartar • Scleral injection • Colic • Distended abdomen • Urine scalding • Dysuria • Hematuria • Halitosis

CAUSES

Prerenal Azotemia

• Renal hypoperfusion caused by decreased circulating volume or decreased blood pressure
• Protein catabolism associated with fever, infection, trauma, myositis, thermal injury, and corticosteroid therapy • General anesthesia
• Prolonged exercise

Renal Azotemia

Acute or chronic renal failure—primary renal dysfunction affecting glomeruli, renal tubules, renal interstitium, or renal vasculature and impairing 60%–75% of renal function

Postrenal Azotemia

• Obstruction of the urinary tract • Rupture of the urinary outflow tract

RISK FACTORS

Medical Conditions

• Renal disease • Diarrhea • Endotoxemia
• Acute blood loss • Septic shock • Prolonged exercise • Urolithiasis • Exposure to nephrotoxic chemicals or plants • Dehydration • Acidosis
• Hepatic disease • Neoplasia

Drugs

• Aminoglycosides
• NSAIDs
• Diuretics

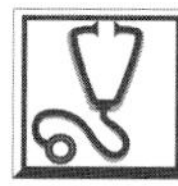

DIAGNOSIS

DIFFERENTIAL DIAGNOSIS

• Prerenal azotemia—dehydration, hypovolemia, acute blood loss, decreased cardiac output, exhaustive disease syndrome, some colic cases
• Renal azotemia
  ○ *Acute renal failure* with increased or decreased urine output is suggestive of vitamin K_3 toxicity, red maple leaf toxicosis, aminoglycoside toxicosis, other nephrotoxic chemicals, vasomotor nephropathy, abnormal kidney size, and rarely leptospirosis.
  ○ *Chronic renal failure* with progressive weight loss, PU/PD, pitting edema, other signs over several weeks or months suggests chronic glomerulohephritis or pyelonephritis, amyloidosis, polycystic kidney disease, renal hypoplasia, and nephrolithiasis.
• Postrenal azotemia—abrupt decrease in urine output and acute signs of uremia, abdominal distension, stranguria and signs of colic may suggest ruptured ureter, ruptured bladder, or obstructive urolithiasis.

CBC/BIOCHEMISTRY/URINALYSIS

CBC

Nonregenerative anemia caused by decreased erythropoietin production occurs with chronic renal failure.

Biochemistry

• Consider hydration status, presenting complaint and physical exam findings when interpreting SUN/Cr levels.
• In horses, the SUN:Cr ratio is unreliable in differentiating acute from chronic renal failure.
• Correcting dehydration deficits and restoring renal perfusion dramatically reduces SUN and Cr in patients with prerenal azotemia.
• Relieving outflow obstruction or correcting the rent in the excretory pathway rapidly decreases the degree of azotemia in patients with postrenal azotemia.
• Hyponatremia and hypochloremia are common in horses with renal disease and can occur with third-compartment spacing of fluid as in uroperitoneum.
• Hyperkalemia is a common finding in urinary tract disruption and uroperitoneum.
• Calcium and phosphorus levels vary in renal disease.
• Hypercalcemia and hypophosphatemia often are found with chronic renal failure; hypocalcemia and hyperphosphatemia are seen with acute renal failure.
• Hypercalcemia in renal failure depends on dietary content and intake of calcium.

Urinalysis

• Urine specific gravity >1.020 and urine osmolality >500 mOsm/kg are consistent with prerenal azotemia.
• Fluid therapy and some medications (e.g., furosemide, α_2-receptor agonists, steroids) may render the urine specific gravity value inconclusive.
• Dehydrated horses with primary renal disease usually lose the ability to concentrate urine;urine specific gravity and osmolality are <1.020 and <500 mOsm/kg, respectively.
• Urine specific gravity does not differentiate postrenal, prerenal or primary renal azotemia.

IMAGING

Radiography

Rarely is used to evaluate the urinary tract in adult horses but is useful in foals and miniature horses

Ultrasonography

• The urinary tract can be examined either transrectally or transabdominally.
• Bladder ultrasonography is best performed transrectally using a 5-MHz probe.
• Transcutaneous ultrasonography of the right or left kidney is best performed with a 2.5- or 3-MHz probe.
• Assess the size and shape of both kidneys and the architecture and echogenicity of the parenchyma.

AZOTEMIA AND UREMIA

• The renal medulla is more echolucent than the renal cortex. The renal pelvis varies in echogenicity.
• With acute renal failure, kidneys may be normal or enlarged, and parenchymal abnormalities often are not detected.
• With chronic renal failure, kidneys are smaller and more echogenic than normal.
• Cystic or mineralized areas more often are associated with chronic renal disease or congenital anomalies.
• Acoustic shadowing represents calculi formation.

Renal Scintigraphy

May be used to document renal function but commonly is not performed

OTHER DIAGNOSTIC PROCEDURES

Urine GGT:Cr Ratio

• Reflects GGT leakage from damaged renal tubular epithelium containing GGT compared to the constant excretion of Cr
• Calculated as (Urine GGT/Urine Cr) × 100
• A ratio of >25 suggests proximal tubular damage; this elevation may occur before azotemia develops.
• Finding an elevated ratio depends on having enough remaining tubules that can leak GGT—severe renal fibrosis may yield values in the normal range.

Fractional Excretion of Electrolytes

• Measurement of electrolytes in serum and urine can be compared to assess renal damage.
• Calculated as (Urine [electrolyte] × Serum Cr)/(Serum [electrolyte] × Urine Cr).
• Reported reference intervals for sodium fractional excretion range from 0.01–0.70 in healthy horses.
• Poor indicator of renal function

Rectal Examination

• Bladder—determine size, wall thickness, and presence of calculi or mural mass.
• Left kidney—determine size and texture.
• Ureter—usually not detectable; enlarged in association with pyelonephritis or ureterolithiasis

Ultrasound-Guided Renal Biopsy

Can be used to confirm the diagnosis of primary renal failure, to differentiate acute from chronic renal disease, and to identify a specific cause

Urethrocystoscopy

• Extremely useful diagnostic aid when evaluating abnormal urination, especially in geldings and stallions.
• In adult male horses, a flexible endoscope with an outside diameter of <12 mm and a length of ≥1 m is adequate to evaluate the urethra and urinary bladder.
• Normal urethral mucosa is pale pink, with longitudinal folds.
• If the urethra is dilated with air (e.g., to aid passage of the endoscope), the mucosa may appear reddened, and a prominent vascular pattern may appear.
• The ischial arch and colliculus seminalis are the most common sites of posturination or postbreeding hemorrhage in geldings and stallions.
• In the dorsal aspect of the trigone, the ureteral openings can be visualized to determine the source of hematuria or pyuria.
• Biopsy of a bladder mass or collection of a sterile urine sample can also be obtained.

Renal Scintigraphy

May be used to document renal function but is rarely performed

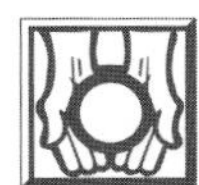

TREATMENT

PRERENAL AZOTEMIA

• Correct the underlying cause of renal hypoperfusion and/or correct the dehydration deficit.
• Fluid replacement is primary therapy.
• More aggressive treatment in conditions that can lead to primary renal damage or failure

PRIMARY RENAL AZOTEMIA

• Measures to stop or reverse the immediate cause
• Supportive care to alleviate clinical signs of uremia; to correct fluid, electrolyte, and acid–base abnormalities; and to resolve the problems associated with decreased renal hormones

POSTRENAL AZOTEMIA

• Eliminate the urinary obstruction or correct the cause of urine leakage.
• Surgical intervention often is required, but correction of any metabolic derangements is paramount.
• Solute diuresis can follow correction of postrenal azotemia; thus, additional fluid therapy may be required to prevent dehydration.

FLUIDS

• IV fluid therapy is indicated for most azotemic patients.
• Commonly used fluids—0.9% saline, Ringer's, and lactated Ringer's solution.
• Base the amount of fluid administered on the dehydration or volume deficit.
• Correction of the fluid deficit can occur during the first 6 hr without untoward effects, except in patients with hypoproteinemia/ hypoalbuminemia and with signs of cardiac disease.

MEDICATIONS

DRUGS OF CHOICE

Treat any patient exhibiting signs of shock appropriately.

CONTRAINDICATIONS

Use nephrotoxic drugs (e.g., aminoglycosides, NSAIDs) with caution in patients with azotemia.

PRECAUTIONS

• Use caution when administering fluids to horses with chronic renal failure, because they may develop significant peripheral and pulmonary edema.
• Use IV fluids cautiously in oliguric or anuric patients to minimize overhydration.
• Use NSAIDs and corticosteroids cautiously. Although they can limit intrarenal inflammation, they also nonselectively block vasodilatory mediators of renal blood flow under conditions of renal hypoperfusion and are not recommended for chronic renal failure.
• Use caution with drugs requiring renal excretion. Horses should be well hydrated when using aminoglycosides and NSAIDs.
• Be aware of adverse reactions and toxic effects that may require altering dosage schedules.

FOLLOW-UP

PATIENT MONITORING

• Serum urea nitrogen, Cr, and electrolyte concentrations 24 hr after initiating fluid therapy; hydration status; and urine outflow.
• In neonates, monitoring body weight may be helpful.
• With severe acid-base derangements, more frequent monitoring may be required.

POSSIBLE COMPLICATIONS

• Failure to promptly correct prerenal azotemia caused by renal hypoperfusion may result in ischemic renal failure.
• Failure to correct renal azotemia may result in uremia.
• Failure to correct postrenal azotemia (e.g., urinary tract obstruction, uroperitoneum) may result in renal damage or death caused by hyperkalemia and uremia.

MISCELLANEOUS

AGE-RELATED FACTORS

• Primary renal failure may occur at any age, but older horses may be at higher risk for azotemia regardless of the cause.
• Postrenal azotemia caused by ruptured bladder is more common in neonatal foals.

PREGNANCY

The ability of a mare to maintain a viable pregnancy decreases as renal function decreases.

SYNONYMS

N/A

SEE ALSO

• Renal failure, acute
• Renal failure, chronic
• Urinary tract obstruction

ABBREVIATIONS

• GFR = glomerular filtration rate
• GGT = γ-glutamyltransferase
• PU/PD = polyuria/polydipsia

Suggested Reading

Diseases of the urinary system. In: Radostits OM, Gay CC, Hinchcliff KW, Constable PD. Veterinary Medicine: A Text Book of the Diseases of Cattle, Horses, Sheep, Goats, and Pigs, ed 10. London: WB Saunders, 2006:543–552.

Author Terry C. Gerros
Consulting Editor Kenneth W. Hinchcliff

BABESIOSIS

BASICS

DEFINITION

A tick-borne, noncontagious disease caused by infection of erythrocytes by either of two distinct protozoan parasites, *Babesia caballi* and *B. equi.*

PATHOPHYSIOLOGY

- Infection with *B. caballi* or *B. equi* results in clinical signs referable to infection and lysis of erythrocytes; dual infections occur.
- The erythrocytic stage of *B. equi* can lyse erythrocytes in the absence of specific immune responses; however, the precise role of immune responses to parasite antigens of *B. equi* and *B. caballi* in anemia is not known.
- Occlusion of capillaries within the pulmonary, hepatic, and central nervous system occurs during acute infection with *B. caballi.*
- Those surviving acute infection are persistently infected and represent a problem for the international movement of horses, because several countries, including the United States, restrict the entry of horses based on their serologic status to *B. equi* and *B. caballi.*
- Intrauterine transmission appears to occur with *B. equi* but is rare with *B. caballi* infections; abortions due to fetal infections have been reported for both parasites.

SYSTEMS AFFECTED

- Hemic/lymphatic/immune—Lysis of infected erythrocytes leads to anemia and icterus.
- Nervous, hepatobiliary, respiratory—Occlusion of capillaries by *B. caballi* can lead to dysfunction within these organ systems.

GENETICS

N/A

INCIDENCE/PREVALENCE

- Infection and clinical disease occur when susceptible horses move into endemic areas or persistently infected horses move into a nonendemic area with tick vectors capable of transmission. Compounding concerns about movement of persistently infected horses is the lack of knowledge about the ability of tick species in nonendemic areas to transmit *B. equi* and *B. caballi.*
- Disease and persistent infection have been reported in southern Florida, the U.S. Virgin Islands, part of Asia, Russia, India, the Middle East, Europe, Africa, Australia, South America, Central America, Mexico, the Philippines, and numerous Caribbean islands.
- Tick vectors include species of *Dermacentor, Hyalomma,* and *Rhipicephalus.*

SIGNALMENT

- Horses, donkeys, their cross-breeds, and zebras are susceptible to babesiosis.
- No known breed, age, or sex predilections

SIGNS

General Comments

- Clinical signs depend on the immune status of the horse.
- Horses that survive acute infection are immune to clinical disease on reinfection; however, an exception may be those infected with *B. caballi* and treated by chemotherapy.
- Although chemotherapy with imidocarb reduces the parasitemia in both *B. equi* and *B. caballi* infections, its ability to clear persistence infection for either parasite is controversial.
- In endemic areas, clinical babesiosis seldom is seen, except when nonimmune (i.e., uninfected) horses are introduced.

Historical Findings

- Acute disease—lethargy, anorexia, fever, anemia, petechial hemorrhages of mucous membranes, and icterus
- Hemoglobinuria and subcutaneous edema can be observed during progression of *B. equi* infection.
- Exercise intolerance (related to the level of anemia) is common.

Physical Examination Findings

- Signs are common only during the acute phase of infection.
- During acute *B. caballi* infection, high fever, lethargy, hyperemia of mucous membranes with petechial hemorrhages, ventral edema, constipation, colic, dehydration, and icterus are seen.
- Acute *B. equi* infection is similar, with hemoglobinuria and a more pronounced icterus.

CAUSES

- Caused by infection of erythrocytes with the hemoprotozoan parasites *B. caballi* or *B. equi*
- Anemia—result of hemolysis caused by replication of the erythrocyte-stage parasites.
- *B. caballi* sequesters in the capillaries of organ systems, including the CNS, leading to occlusion of blood flow.

RISK FACTORS

The primary risk factor is movement of uninfected (i.e., nonimmune) horses into endemic areas.

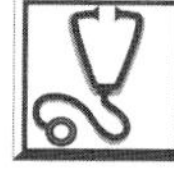

DIAGNOSIS

DIFFERENTIAL DIAGNOSIS

- EIA—Infected horses are seropositive.
- Purpura hemorrhagica—Petechial hemorrhages and ventral edema are common; often a history of previous exposure to *Streptococcus equi* or other respiratory pathogens; hemolysis is uncommon.
- Equine viral arteritis virus—Hemolysis is uncommon; diagnosis can be confirmed serologically or by viral isolation.
- Equine ehrlichiosis—Hemolysis is uncommon.
- Trypanosomiasis
- Leptospirosis
- Red maple-leaf poisoning—Heinz bodies and methemoglobinemia are common.

CBC/BIOCHEMISTRY/URINALYSIS

- Anemia
- Leukocytosis
- Hyperbilirubinemia
- Hemoglobinuria (*B. equi*)

OTHER LABORATORY TESTS

- Persistently infected horses have no indication of infection but for specific antiparasite antibody and, occasionally, a level of parasites in the peripheral blood, detection is possible by light microscopy. Definitive diagnosis currently depends on identification of *Babesia* organisms in Giemsa-stained blood smears or by transfusion of blood into a susceptible animal. PCR assays have been reported for detection of both parasites.
- Direct parasitologic verification of chronic *B. caballi* infection is almost impossible but occasionally is successful with *B. equi* infection. The USDA in 2005 adopted cELISA as the official serologic test for equine babesiosis; this test measures antibodies to an erythrocyte stage protein epitope of *B. equi* or *B. caballi.*
- Horses that test positive on cELISA are restricted from entry into the United States. Serum submitted to state diagnostic laboratories is forwarded to the National Veterinary Services Laboratory (Ames, IA) for testing.
- *B. equi* and *B. caballi* can now be routinely cultured.

IMAGING

N/A

DIAGNOSTIC PROCEDURES

N/A

PATHOLOGIC FINDINGS

- Horses that die of acute infection may demonstrate subcutaneous edema, serous exudates in the body cavities and pericardium, pronounced icterus, hepatomegaly, splenomegaly, glomerulonephropathy, and petechial hemorrhages of mucosal membranes.
- Histologically, the spleen contains macrophages with intracellular erythrocytes (erythrophagocytosis), the renal tubular epithelium often is degenerated, and hemoglobin is deposited in renal tubules.

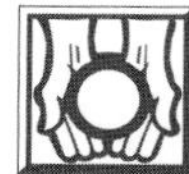

TREATMENT

APPROPRIATE HEALTH CARE

Inpatient or outpatient, depending on the severity of clinical signs

NURSING CARE

Routine care; intensive care usually not needed

ACTIVITY
Restrict activity.

DIET
Normal diet

CLIENT EDUCATION
Inform clients of the reportable nature of this infection and its significance regarding the international movement of horses.

SURGICAL CONSIDERATIONS
N/A

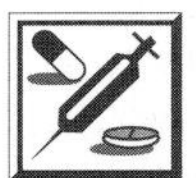

MEDICATIONS

DRUG(S) OF CHOICE
• Imidocarb is the most effective and safest chemotherapy to date, but its ability to clear *B. caballi* infections remains uncertain. Also, effective therapy for elimination of *B. equi* infection has not been found. Recommended doses are, for *B. equi,* 4 mg/kg every third day for a total of four treatments and, for *B. caballi,* 2 mg/kg for 2 consecutive days for a total of two treatments. A higher dosage used for *B. equi,* 4 mg/kg every third day for a total of four treatments, has also be used for *B. caballi*. Each dose is given IM and divided among at least four injection sites.
• Colic, transient salivation, and purgation are common after imidocarb treatment.
• Glycopyrrolate at 0.0025 mg/kg and/or atropine sulfate at 0.01 mg/kg administered intravenously has been recommended for colic associated with imidocarb treatment.
• Do not initiate retreatment after use of imidocarb for *B. equi* infection 30 days after the first treatment.

CONTRAINDICATIONS
• In endemic regions, antibabesial therapy may lead to susceptibility on reinfection. This is especially true for *B. caballi* infections, in which chemotherapy (imidocarb) may clear persistent infections.
• Donkeys appear very susceptible to the toxic side effects of imidocarb and should not be treated with this drug.

PRECAUTIONS
N/A

POSSIBLE INTERACTIONS
N/A

ALTERNATIVE DRUGS
• Several chemotherapies with antibabesial activity have been tested; these therapies include phenamidine, benenil, and diampron.
• For *B. equi,* parvaquone and buparvaquone have been tested.
• Imidocarb is the most effective and safest of all therapies tested to date.

FOLLOW-UP

PATIENT MONITORING
Monitor hydration status and percentage parasitemia in the peripheral blood.

PREVENTION/AVOIDANCE
Control in endemic areas is most effectively directed at tick vectors.

POSSIBLE COMPLICATIONS
N/A

EXPECTED COURSE AND PROGNOSIS
• Horses that survive acute infection usually, with appropriate supportive care, can return to normal activity. Owners should be advised that such animals are persistently infected and remain a potential source of parasite transmission to susceptible horses.
• Although chemotherapy eliminates *B. caballi* infection in most cases, chemotherapy has not been identified that eliminates *B. equi* infection.

MISCELLANEOUS

ASSOCIATED CONDITIONS
N/A

AGE-RELATED FACTORS
N/A

ZOONOTIC POTENTIAL
N/A

PREGNANCY
Abortion (especially with *B. equi* infection) is a possible outcome.

SYNONYMS
Piroplasmosis

ABBREVIATIONS
• CNS = central nervous system
• EIA = equine infectious anemia virus
• cELISA = competitive enzyme-linked immunosorbent assay
• USDA = U.S. Department of Agriculture

Suggested Reading

Friedhoff KT. The piroplasms of Equidae—Significance for international commerce. Berl Munch Tierarztl Wochenschr 1982;95:368–374.

Holman PJ, Chieves L, Frerichs WM, Olson D, Wagner GG. Culture confirmation of the carrier status of *Babesia caballi*—infected horses. J Clin Microbiol 1993;31:698–701.

Knowles DP. Control of *Babesia equi* parasitemia. Parasitol Today 1996;12:195–198.

Knowles DP. 1996. Equine babesiosis (Piroplasmosis): A problem in the international movement of horses [guest editorial]. Br Vet J 1996;152:123–126.

Knowles RC. Equine babesiosis: Epidemiology, control and chemotherapy. Equine Vet Sci 1988;8:61–64.

Author Don Knowles

Consulting Editors Ashley G. Boyle and Corinne R. Sweeney

BACK PAIN

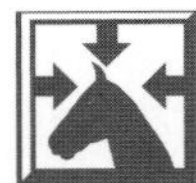

BASICS

OVERVIEW

- Back pain is either primary bone pain from the spine and its associated ligaments or pain from the epaxial muscles.
- There are 18 thoracic, 6 lumbar, and 5 fused sacral vertebrae. Cranial and caudal articular processes articulate by their facet joints. Joints are composed of a fibrous intervertebral disk. Supraspinous and interspinous ligaments provide stability of the vertebrae. Epaxial, iliopsoas, longissimus dorsi and iliocostalis muscles manipulate the spine.
- Abnormal stresses to these structures result in injury and back pain.
- Musculoskeletal system—back (thoracolumbar spine and associated soft tissue structures)

SIGNALMENT

- Middle-aged performance horses
- Jumping, racing, and dressage horses are particularly susceptible.

SIGNS

Historical

- Decrease or change in performance
- Previous trauma such as a fall or starting gate "incident"
- Ill-defined signs of discomfort (inappetence, crankiness, reluctance to lie down)
- Resentment to grooming or being saddled or mounted ("cold backed")
- Behavioral abnormalities (bolting, rearing, bucking, refusal to move forward, jump or break out of the starting gate)
- Stilted gait

Physical Examination

- Disuse atrophy of back musculature
- Kyphosis ("roached back")
- Lordosis
- Scolosis
- Resentment, tightening, spasm or fasciculation to back musculature palpation
- +/− Lack of flexibility
- Ill-defined gait alterations (lack of impulsion, general stiffness, gait deterioration when ridden, elevation of the head)

CAUSES AND RISK FACTORS

- Spinal malformations (kyphosis, lordosis, scolosis)
- Short-backed or long-backed conformation
- Poor or improper training methods
- Chronic coexisting hindlimb lameness
- Abnormal hindlimb conformation (straight hindlimb, sickle hock)
- Poorly fitting saddle
- Sports that require jumping
- Specific diseases that cause primary back pain
  - Impingement (overriding) of dorsal spinous processes ("kissing spines")
  - Fractured withers
  - Vertebral bone fractures
  - Vertebral spondylosis or discospondylosis
  - Osteoarthritis of vertebral body articular processes

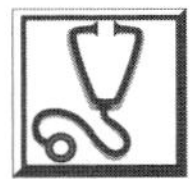

DIAGNOSIS

DIFFERENTIAL DIAGNOSIS

- Bilateral lameness (i.e., distal tarsitis, navicular syndrome)—Rule out with lameness examination and imaging.
- Exertional rhabdomyolosis—Rule out with muscle enzyme elevation, increased radiopharmaceutical uptake in affected muscles, muscle biopsy histology.
- PSSM—Rule out with muscle biopsy histology.
- EPM—Rule out with clinical signs of neurologic deficits, elevated titer in serology, or CSF analysis.
- HYPP—Rule out with hyperkalemia during clinical manifestation, DNA testing.
- Lyme disease—Rule out with significantly elevated titers in paired serum samples.

CBC/CHEMISTRY/URINALYSIS

Mild elevation in serum CK, AST, and/or LDH

OTHER LABORATORY TESTS

Serology (titer or Western blot) for EPM and Lyme disease—Elevation in paired serum titers may indicate active disease.

IMAGING

- Radiography—+/− normal, narrowing, or loss of interspinous space, sclerosis and/or osteolysis of spinous processes, ventral and/or lateral bony proliferation (spondylosis)
- Nuclear scintigraphy—increased radiopharmaceutical uptake in spinous processes and/or affected muscles, focal "hot spots" with vertebral fracture
- Ultrasonography—supraspinous desmitis, calcification, or acute tear in epaxial muscles

OTHER DIAGNOSTIC PROCEDURES

- Diagnostic analgesia—local infiltration between dorsal spinous processes, local infiltration of affected musculature, periarticular infiltration of sacroiliac joints
- Neurologic examination
- Sedation and riding—Horses with behavioral problems often improve.
- CSF analysis—Rule out meningitis, equine protozoal myelitis.
- Muscle biopsy—Rule out primary muscle disorders (exertional rhabdomyolosis, PSSM) with characteristic histologic abnormalities.
- DNA analysis—Rule out HYPP.

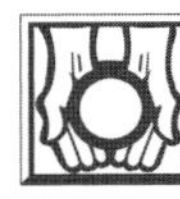

TREATMENT

- Appropriate treatment for primary lameness
- Training management—progressive warmup (lunge without saddle then lunge with saddle then walk with rider, etc.), lowering the neck (i.e., long and low exercises)
- Assess and replace poorly fitting saddle.
- Extracorporeal shock wave therapy—3 treatments at 3-week intervals at site of injury
- Surgical resection of dorsal spinous processes—may be successful in horses that do not respond to medical therapy. Six months of postop convalescence is generally required.
- Acupuncture—multiple intradermal treatments at the site of injury, usually 9 acupuncture points, weekly for 8 treatments

- For vertebral body fracture—stall rest for 2 mo followed by small paddock turnout for 2 mo
- Additional treatments:
  - Physical therapy (massage)
  - Therapeutic ultrasound
  - Low power laser therapy
  - Chiropractic therapy
  - Magnetic blanket

MEDICATIONS

DRUG(S)

- NSAIDs—phenylbutazone (2.2– 4.4 mg/kg daily to BID)
- Interspinous or perispinal injections—corticosteroids (40–60 mg of methylprednisolone acetate per site) +/– Sarapin
- Intra-articular methylprednisolone acetate (20–40 mg) in vertebral facet or sacroiliac joints. Ultrasound guidance ensures accurate placement.
- Methocarbamol (10 mg/kg IV or 40–60 mg/kg PO daily)
- Tiludronate (1 mg/kg IV, slow rate infusion)
- Multiple intramuscular injections of 2% iodine in oil within sore muscle followed by 4–6 weeks of mild exercise
- Mesotherapy—intradermal injections corresponding to the sites of the lesion. After treatment, exercise is restricted and gradually increased.

CONTRAINDICATIONS/POSSIBLE INTERACTIONS

Gastrointestinal sensitivity with phenylbutazone

FOLLOW-UP

PATIENT MONITORING

Periodic lameness and behavior evaluations

PREVENTION/AVOIDANCE

- Avoid poorly fitting tack.
- Institute proper training and treatment once diagnosed; frequent treatments are often necessary.

POSSIBLE COMPLICATIONS

- Failure of accurate diagnosis and treatment
- Infection after injection(s)

EXPECTED COURSE AND PROGNOSIS

- For acute epaxial muscle injury, early diagnosis and treatment can be successful.
- For most other back pain, accurate diagnosis is difficult. Timely and appropriate treatment is challenging. Prognosis is variable and determined by response to therapy.
- Vertebral body fracture can be successfully treated with early diagnosis and rest.

MISCELLANEOUS

ASSOCIATED CONDITIONS

Distal tarsitis

AGE-RELATED FACTORS

None

ZOONOTIC POTENTIALS

None

SEE ALSO

- Exertional rhabdomyolosis
- PSSM
- Distal tarsitis
- HYPP
- EPM

ABBREVIATIONS

- AST = aspartate aminotranferase
- CK = creatine phosphokinase
- LDH = lactate dehydrogenase
- CSF = cerebrospinal fluid
- PSSM = polysaccharide storage myopathy
- HYPP = hyperkalemic periodic paralysis
- EPM = equine protozoal myelitis

Suggested Reading

Denoix JM, Dyson SJ. Thoracolumbar spine. In: Ross MW, Dyson SJ, eds. Diagnosis and Management of Lameness in the Horse. St. Louis: Elsevier, 2003:509–521.

Author Benson B. Martin Jr.

Consulting Editor Elizabeth J. Davidson

BACTEREMIA/SEPTICEMIA

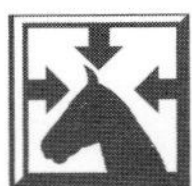

BASICS

DEFINITION

• *Bacteremia* refers to the presence of viable bacteria in the circulating blood. • *Septicemia* is defined as systemic disease caused by circulating microorganisms, including viral and fungal microorganisms, and their products. • *Endotoxemia* specifically refers to the presence of endotoxin (lipopolysaccharide) within the circulating blood and implies the presence of clinical signs associated with the circulating endotoxin.

PATHOPHYSIOLOGY

In cases of bacteremia, bacteria must gain access to the circulation, necessitating a breach of normal protective mechanisms. This occurs most commonly in the neonate, although adults may be affected, particularly if they are immunocompromised. Portals of entry commonly include the respiratory tract, gastrointestinal tract, placenta, umbilicus, and surgical and traumatic wounds. In a generally healthy animal, normal defense mechanisms rapidly clear circulating bacteria from the bloodstream.

In cases of septicemia, normal defense mechanisms are overwhelmed, allowing the establishment of localized or generalized infection. Passive acquisition of immunoglobulins from maternal colostrum provides for neutralizing and opsonizing activity in the neonate. The phagocytic and killing functions of polymorphonuclear neutrophils are crucial to the initial defense against invading pathogens. These functions, although present, appear to be impaired in the neonate. Other aspects of innate immunity appear to be less effective in the neonate than in the adult, increasing the risk of septicemia in the neonate. The large majority of pathogens associated with neonatal septicemia are gram-negative bacteria, predominantly *Escherichia coli,* although gram-positive bacteria are gaining recognition in some geographic areas as a major cause of neonatal septicemia. Viral, fungal, and protozoal pathogens are also recognized causes of septicemia. In adults, septicemia can be associated with enterocolitis (e.g., Salmonellosis) because loss of the mucosal gastrointestinal barrier provides a route for entry of bacteria and fungi.

Endotoxemia results from the elucidation of LPS from the bacteria cell wall of gram-negative pathogens. Endotoxemia is recognized as a sequela to gram-negative sepsis in the neonate. Endotoxemia in adults is frequently associated with enterocolitis and pleuropneumonia. Circulating LPS interacts with immune cells, macrophages, and lymphocytes to initiate production of a cascade of soluble immune mediators to produce a wide variety of systemic effects. Imbalance in the production of immune mediators (interleukins, prostaglandins, leukotrienes) can result in septic shock.

SYSTEMS AFFECTED

All body systems can be affected. The cardiovascular system undergoes hyperdynamic responses in early septic shock, systemic hypoperfusion, and cardiac depression in later stages.

SIGNALMENT

• Foals generally within the first 3 days of age, although may occur at almost any age
• Adult horses of any age, sex, or breed

SIGNS

General Comments

A large variety of clinical signs are associated with infection, and specific signs depend on the stage of the disease process and the organ systems involved.

Historical Findings

• Foals with septicemia may have a history of perinatal problems, dystocia, premature/dysmature/postmature birth, previous abnormal siblings, etc. Failure of passive transfer is commonly reported. Poor management and poor environmental conditions may be present. • Affected adults may have concurrent immunosuppression or other disease processes.

Physical Examination Findings

• Early signs—nonspecific, vague, or nonexistent. Easily attributable to other disease processes. Signs include lethargy, scleral injection, petechiation, mucous membrane injection, loss of suck reflex in foals, increased lethargy, or sleepiness. • Fever is present inconsistently. • Diarrhea may be the earliest localizing sign in septic foals. • Other signs—seizures, colic, respiratory distress, uveitis, subcutaneous abscesses, lameness, gait abnormality, joint distention, and periarticular edema • Early septicemia/sepsis—normal blood pressures and blood pressure gradient, variable fever, injected mucous membranes, normal to brisk capillary refill time, tachycardia, agitation, and depression • Late-stage septic shock is characterized by hypoperfusion and cool distal limbs and extremities, depression, unresponsiveness, hypotension, hypothermia, and gray mucous membranes with delayed capillary refill time.

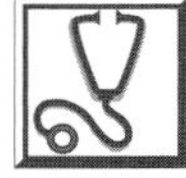

DIAGNOSIS

DIFFERENTIAL DIAGNOSIS

Foals

Hypoxic ischemic asphyxial or inflammatory perinatal insult, prematurity, and viral sepsis

Adults

Early sepsis can be confused with almost any disease process. Late-stage septic shock is difficult to misdiagnose. Major differentials at that point are hypovolemia (e.g., blood loss) and cardiogenic shock.

CBC/BIOCHEMISTRY/URINALYSIS

CBC

Leukocytosis or leukopenia may be present. Increased numbers of band neutrophils occur in some cases. Neutropenia is common. Platelet counts may be decreased with associated DIC. Fibrinogen may be normal, increased, or decreased (DIC), depending on stage of disease.

Biochemistry

Hypoglycemia is common in foals and some adult horses. There is metabolic acidosis with advancing hypoperfusion as well as increased lactate concentrations. Creatinine and serum urea nitrogen concentrations are increased, with dehydration and acute renal failure secondary to renal hypoperfusion in late stages. End-stage sepsis is associated with multisystem organ failure.

Urinalysis

With acute renal failure there are increased protein and cells, as well as altered fractional excretion of sodium and potassium. The animal shows a loss of the ability to concentrate. Urinary parameters may not be valid in animals on intravenous fluid therapy and may not reflect underlying pathology accurately.

OTHER LABORATORY TESTS

Arterial Blood Gas Analysis

Hypoxemia, hypercapnia, and/or acidosis (mixed respiratory and metabolic), particularly in animals with acute respiratory distress syndrome and/or PE.

DIAGNOSTIC PROCEDURES

• Blood culture required for definitive diagnosis • Culture from localized infection • Serial fecal cultures in cases of suspected salmonellosis, clostridiosis • Clostridial toxin determination from feces for suspected clostridiosis

PATHOLOGIC FINDINGS

• Pathology is associated with affected organ systems.• Pneumonia, focal abscess, pleuritis, peritonitis, enterocolitis, joint and/or physeal infection, meningitis, etc.
• Findings associated with DIC include jugular thrombosis, pulmonary thromboembolism, general or localized petechiae and ecchymoses, spontaneous hemorrhage, hemorrhage associated with venipuncture, and laminitis. Septic shock and end-stage multiorgan failure findings may include pulmonary edema, tubular and interstitial nephritis, hepatic lipidosis, hepatic necrosis, myocardial necrosis, and/or gastrointestinal mucosal abnormalities.

IMAGING

• Thoracic radiography may demonstrate pneumonia or PE. Radiographs of affected joints may be normal at early stages, or may demonstrate radiolucency or other changes associated with the physis or other bony areas

with advanced disease. • Thoracic ultrasound may demonstrate pleural fluid or areas of pleural/parenchymal consolidation.
• Abdominal ultrasound may demonstrate thickened areas of small and large intestine, abnormal gastrointestinal motility, and increased peritoneal fluid. • Cardiac ultrasonography demonstrates early increases in fractional shortening and decreased end-systolic volume, whereas later stages show decreased cardiac contractility and ejection fractions.

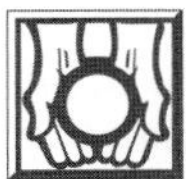

TREATMENT

APPROPRIATE HEALTH CARE

Septic neonates and adults without evidence of septic shock may be treated at home. Horses and foals with evidence of early or late septic shock will benefit from referral to a facility where advanced 24-hour care can be more readily provided.

NURSING CARE

Nursing care in cases of septic shock may be intensive. Continuous intravenous fluid therapy is generally necessary, and intranasal oxygen supplementation should be considered. Affected foals will be recumbent and require frequent turning to prevent decubital sores and lung atelectasis. Hypothermia is common and may require heat lamps and warming blankets.

ACTIVITY

Activity should be restricted.

DIET

Septic foals and adults are frequently anorexic. In addition, gastrointestinal function may be compromised and gastrointestinal rest may be required. Parenteral nutrition should be considered for all foals and in adults in cases in which finances are not a primary concern. Foals with evidence of gastrointestinal discomfort and/or bloat should not be fed until signs resolve. Foals and adults with hypothermia should not be fed enterally, even if they demonstrate an appetite, until they are normothermic.

CLIENT EDUCATION

Foals and adults that do not have serious additional disease beyond localized or mild sepsis frequently respond to treatment and survive. Survival decreases with the onset of severe sepsis, although rapid and aggressive intervention at this stage improves survival. Foals and adults with hypotensive septic shock have a guarded to grave prognosis, even with intensive care.

SURGICAL CONSIDERATIONS

• Localized abscesses that are readily accessible may be drained surgically.
• Infected umbilical remnants in foals may be removed surgically if the condition of the patient is stable enough to warrant general anesthesia.
• Lavage and/or arthroscopy for debridement of infected joints may be indicated.

MEDICATIONS

DRUG(S) AND FLUIDS

• Broad-spectrum antimicrobial therapy in cases where culture is pending or culture results are negative. Antimicrobial therapy should then be based on culture and sensitivity results.
• Equine plasma should be administered to foals with failure of passive transfer of maternal antibody. Plasma should be given until serum IgG is >800 mg/dL. Plasma therapy may need to be repeated, and IgG may be consumed or lost due to disease processes.
• Plasma and/or whole blood are ideal volume expander fluids, but may not be readily and rapidly available for resuscitation.
• Hyperimmune anti-endotoxin plasma (J-5) therapy may benefit affected foals and adults.
• Adults and foals with dehydration and either early or late septic shock require the administration of intravenous fluids.
• Crystalloids may initially be administered rapidly in shock boluses of 20 mL/kg over 20 min. The patient should then be reassessed and additional boluses given as necessary.
• Colloidal fluids (Hetastarch) given at a dose of 10 mg/kg may aid in resuscitation of early or late septic shock.
• Cases with hypotensive septic shock may require pressor agents. Vasopressin, norepinephrine, and dobutamine are commonly used and require administration at a constant rate of infusion. Use of these drugs requires that blood pressure and cardiac rate and rhythm be monitored constantly.
• Nonsteroidal anti-inflammatory agents may aid in combating endotoxemia. Flunixin meglumine at 0.25 mg/kg is commonly administered TID IV to adult horses; use of NSAIDs should be judicious in foals due to complications of gastrointestinal ulceration and renal dysfunction.
• Intravenous DMSO, although controversial, can be administered at 0.25–1.0 g/kg SID or BID as an anti-inflammatory agent and for diuresis.
• Short-acting corticosteroid therapy (dexamethasone 0.01–0.1 mg/kg IV SID; also controversial) may be used with septic shock.

CONTRAINDICATIONS/PRECAUTIONS/ POSSIBLE INTERACTIONS/ ALTERNATIVE DRUGS

• Corticosteroids have been associated with laminitis in the adult horse.
• Pressor agents may cause cardiac dysrhythmias or result in decreased renal perfusion at certain dosages.

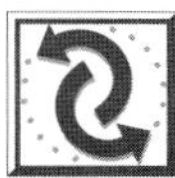

FOLLOW-UP

PATIENT MONITORING

• Animals with sepsis and septic shock are in delicate physiologic balance. All interventions should be monitored carefully for any change in the patient's condition.
• Electrolyte and creatinine values should be obtained daily if animals are on intravenous fluids; otherwise, they should be obtained every other day. Urinary output should be monitored. Any decrease is suggestive of poor renal perfusion and possible renal failure.
• Blood glucose should be monitored twice daily if possible, particularly in septic shock patients.
• Frequent arterial blood gas determinations are desirable in cases of septic shock.
• Aminoglycoside antimicrobials are nephrotoxic and ototoxic given at high dosages and dosage frequencies. Therapeutic drug monitoring should be performed.
• Arterial blood pressure should be monitored, along with heart rate and rhythm.
• Serial white blood cell counts and fibrinogen determinations aid in monitoring response to therapy. Antimicrobial treatment should continue until clinical signs are resolved and white blood count and fibrinogen concentration are within normal range.

PREVENTION/AVOIDANCE

Sepsis and septic shock are best treated by prevention. Clients should be educated as to the importance of early ingestion of good-quality colostrum by neonates and good management practices.

MISCELLANEOUS

ABBREVIATIONS

• DIC = disseminated intravascular coagulopathy
• DMSO = dimethylsulfoxide
• LPS = lipopolysaccharide
• PE = pulmonary edema

Suggested Reading

Keusis B, Spier SJ. Endotoxemia. In: Reed SM, Bayley WM, eds. Equine Internal Medicine. Philadelphia: WB Saunders, 1998:639–451.

Koterba AM, House JK. Neonatal infection. In: Smith BP, ed. Large Animal Internal Medicine. Philadelphia: Mosby, 1996:344–353.

Mackay RJ. Endotoxemia. In: Smith BP, ed. Large Animal Internal Medicine. Philadelphia: Mosby, 1996:733–742.

Wilkins PA. Disorders of foals. In: Reed SM, Bayley WM, Sellon DC, eds. Equine Internal Medicine, ed 2. St. Louis: WB Saunders, 2004:1381–1431.

Author Pamela A. Wilkins

Consulting Editors Ashley G. Boyle and Corinne R. Sweeney

BACTERIAL DERMATITIS—METHICILLIN-RESISTANT STAPHYLOCOCCI

BASICS

DEFINITION

• Staphylococci are gram-positive, opportunistic pathogens that can cause a variety of infections, including skin and soft tissue infections. Recently, MRS have emerged as important causes of disease. • Methicillin resistance is conferred by the *mecA* gene. This gene encodes for production of an altered penicillin binding protein with a low affinity for beta-lactam antimicrobials, thereby conferring resistance to all beta-lactam antimicrobials (penicillin, cephalosporins). MRS are often resistant to many other drug classes. • There is also concern about zoonotic transmission of certain MRS, particularly MRSA.

PATHOPHYSIOLOGY

• Staphylococci are commensal organisms and are often found in the nasal passages, in the gastrointestinal tract, and on the skin. Disease most often develops in response to compromised host barriers. • There are two main classifications of staphylococci—coagulase positive and coagulase negative.
 ○ Coagulase-positive staphylococci are the most common causes of disease. *S. aureus* is the main coagulase-positive *Staphylococcus* in horses. *S. intermedius* is less common but can cause disease, particularly pastern dermatitis. Disease caused by *S. hyicus* subsp. *hyicus* has also been reported in horses. The role of other species such as *S. schleiferi coagulans, S. pseudointermedius,* and *S. delphini* is unclear.
 ○ Coagulase-negative species are generally less pathogenic and most often affect compromised hosts.
• A variety of virulence factors may be involved in dermatologic disease, including proteases, hemolysins, leukocidins, dermonecrotoxins, exfoliative toxin, nucleases, and lipases. • The pathophysiology of disease is similar or identical to methicillin-susceptible staphylococcal infections.

SYSTEMS AFFECTED

Methicillin-resistant staphylococci cause infections at various body sites. Dermatitis may occur alone or associated with infections at other sites.

GENETICS

No genetic predisposition has been identified.

INCIDENCE/PREVALENCE

• The incidence of staphylococcal dermatitis is unclear. MRS dermatitis appears to be increasing based on published case reports and anecdotal information. Methicillin-resistant *S. aureus, S. intermedius,* and *S. schleiferi coagulans* are important emerging causes of dermatologic disease in dogs and cats. • There is minimal information regarding staphylococcal skin colonization. More information is available regarding nasal colonization of staphylococci. MRSA can be found in the nares of 0%–2% of healthy horses. MR-CoNS colonization is much more common, ranging from 30% to 60%, and high rates of skin carriage or colonization are likely. • Staphylococcal skin diseases are more common in the spring and summer in most regions, likely because of factors such as heavy riding/training, higher temperature, higher humidity, increased time outdoors and in rainy conditions, increased biting insect populations and shedding.

GEOGRAPHIC DISTRIBUTION

• MRSA infections have been reported in many countries in North America, Europe, and Asia. It is likely that MRSA is distributed in the horse population worldwide. MR-CoNS appear to be present worldwide.

SIGNALMENT

There are no breed, age, or sex predilections.

SIGNS

Clinical signs vary with the type of disease, and details are provided under specific topics. Diseases associated with staphylococci include folliculitis and furunculosis, pastern dermatitis, cellulitis, tail pyoderma, mucocutaneous pyoderma, and wound infections. There is no indication that infections caused by MRS are clinically discernable from those caused by susceptible strains.

CAUSES

Causes of specific staphylococcal dermatologic diseases are covered elsewhere. There should be no difference for MRS infections.

RISK FACTORS

Risk factors for MRS dermatitis have not been reported. A history of MRSA infection or colonization on the farm should increase suspicion. Prior antimicrobial therapy is associated with a higher risk of MRSA colonization and perhaps any MRS infection. Most MRS infections occur in the absence of identifiable risk factors.

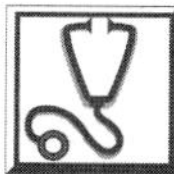

DIAGNOSIS

DIFFERENTIAL DIAGNOSIS

Differential diagnoses vary with the specific type of dermatologic disease and are covered elsewhere.

CBC/BIOCHEMISTRY/URINALYSIS

This type of testing is typically unnecessary. If recurrent disease is present, a comprehensive evaluation is indicated to identify underlying disease.

OTHER LABORATORY TESTS

• Cytologic examination—An abundance of neutrophils and clusters of intra- and extracellular cocci is suggestive of staphylococcal infection, but cannot differentiate methicillin-resistant from methicillin-susceptible. • Diagnosis is based on bacterial culture and susceptibility testing. Identification of MRS involves culture of the *Staphylococcus* spp. and identification of oxacillin resistance; oxacillin is used because it is more stable than methicillin in vitro. Oxacillin-resistant isolates are methicillin-resistant. Ideally, confirmation of methicillin resistance is done by detection of the *mecA* gene by PCR or PBP2a by latex agglutination test. Veterinarians should ensure that the laboratory they use tests staphylococci for oxacillin resistance. • Coagulase-positive staphylococci must be identified to the species level; "coagulase-positive *Staphylococcus*" is inadequate due to the additional concerns regarding MRSA versus other species. Speciation of coagulase-negative strains is less critical as there is currently no information suggesting that management or outcome varies between species. Interpretation of cultures of superficial skin surfaces can be difficult because staphylococci, particularly coagulase-negative species, are common on normal skin. Isolation of MRS, particularly MR-CoNS, from skin does not necessarily imply relevance.

IMAGING N/A

OTHER DIAGNOSTIC PROCEDURES

None

PATHOLOGICAL FINDINGS N/A

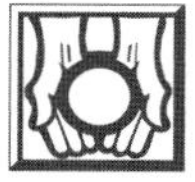

TREATMENT

AIMS OF TREATMENT

Aims of treatment are to eliminate the infection by prudent use of antimicrobials and to limit the risk of transmission to other horses or humans. Addressing underlying risk factors is critical.

APPROPRIATE HEALTH CARE

Most cases can be managed on the farm or as outpatients. The main reasons for hospitalization would be severe infection and an inability of the owner to properly treat the horse. Another possible reason is if the owner is immunocompromised, therefore at risk for developing zoonotic MRSA infection, and is the sole caretaker of the horse.

NURSING CARE

Nursing care is dependent on the specific staphylococcal disease. Infection control precautions should be instituted as described below.

ACTIVITY

Medically, there is no reason to limit activity. The main reason to limit activity is for infection control. MRSA is transmissible to other horses and humans, and infected horses should be isolated. There is less concern with other MRS; however, it is reasonable to restrict contact with these horses to prevent dissemination of these multi-drug–resistant organisms.

DIET

A good-quality diet should be provided, but there are no specific requirements.

CLIENT EDUCATION

• **MRSA is a zoonotic disease** and clients should be counseled on the risk of transmission. • Barrier precautions (gloves, protective outerwear) should be used when handling affected horses. • Hand hygiene (handwashing, use of alcohol-based hand rub) should be performed when in contact with the horse or its environment. The affected horse should be isolated from other horses until clinical signs have resolved and a negative nasal swab for MRSA culture has been obtained. The risk with other MRS is unclear and is probably lower.

SURGICAL CONSIDERATIONS N/A

MEDICATIONS

DRUG(S)

• There are two approaches to antimicrobial therapy—systemic and local. • Topical therapy is critical, particularly when there are few viable systemic antimicrobial options. Topical therapy can remove debris and affect the local bacterial population. The importance of the removal of organic debris is that it can inhibit some antimicrobials and antiseptics, and provide a more hospitable environment for bacterial growth. Antiseptics include chlorhexidine, dilute povidone-iodine, and acetic acid, which can be applied as antibacterial shampoos, with the added benefit of bathing removing organic debris, or as topical rinses. Topical antimicrobials include mupirocin and fusidic acid, although resistance to these drugs has emerged.
• Systemic therapy is thought to be superior to topical therapy in all but the most superficial infections and can be used alone or in combination with topical therapy. Select antimicrobials based on culture and susceptibility testing. Despite the degree of resistance, there is usually a reasonable antimicrobial option. MRS should be considered resistant to all beta-lactam antimicrobials, regardless of in vitro results. Fluoroquinolones should be avoided if possible because resistance can develop quickly. MRS may be susceptible to rifampin, but this drug should always be used with another antimicrobial to which the isolate is susceptible. Chloramphenicol is often useful based on susceptibility and the option of oral therapy; however, human exposure concerns should be taken into consideration.
• Duration of therapy is variable. In general, deeper infections need longer treatment. Duration of therapy is not necessarily longer for MRS, once the appropriate treatment is started. For deep infections, it is important that treatment duration is adequate; 10–12 weeks of therapy (or more) may be required in some cases.

CONTRAINDICATIONS

None

PRECAUTIONS

If topical antimicrobials are used, the horse should be prevented from licking the wound so antimicrobials are not removed or ingested. Ingestion of topical antimicrobials could pose a risk for antimicrobial-associated diarrhea.

POSSIBLE INTERACTIONS N/A

ALTERNATIVE DRUGS

There are ethical concerns about the use of drugs that are important in human medicine such as vancomycin, linezolid, and daptomycin, and there is minimal pharmacokinetic and safety information available for horses. Use of these drugs should be discouraged.

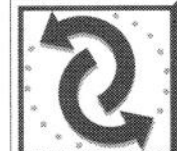

FOLLOW-UP

PATIENT MONITORING

• Reevaluation after initial therapy has been started is essential for severe and/or deep infections. For mild or superficial infections, the owner's monitoring may be adequate to evaluate response and further treatment plan.
• If there is poor initial response, the diagnosis should be reconsidered and testing repeated. Ideally, changes in antimicrobial therapy should be made after the culture is repeated and results reported.
• Relapses within 1–2 weeks of cessation of treatment usually occur because antimicrobial therapy was stopped too early. Relapses that develop later would suggest an underlying problem causing reinfection as opposed to treatment failure.
• With MRSA infections, it is important to consider infection and colonization independently. Horses can resolve the clinical infection and remain colonized in the nasal passages for a varying length of time (usually a few weeks). It is prudent to culture from the nares for MRSA after resolution of MRSA dermatitis to consider the horse noninfectious.

PREVENTION/AVOIDANCE

Prudent antimicrobial use is important to decrease the prevalence of MRSA in the population and to reduce that chance of a horse acquiring MRSA. The same probably applies to many other MRS, although it is likely that MR-CoNS are part of the normal microflora and there are no effective means of eliminating normal commensals. Application of general infection control practices may be useful for restricting the spread and impact of MRS infections.

POSSIBLE COMPLICATIONS

Systemic manifestations are unlikely. While it is possible for dissemination of infection to occur, this should be very uncommon, especially in an adult horse with no other significant comorbidities.

EXPECTED COURSE AND PROGNOSIS

The prognosis is more dependent on the type of disease than the pathogen involved and is good as long as an appropriate antimicrobial can be identified and administered.

MISCELLANEOUS

ASSOCIATED CONDITIONS

None

AGE-RELATED FACTORS

None

ZOONOTIC POTENTIAL

MRSA is a zoonotic pathogen, and transmission from colonized and infected horses to humans has been documented. Infection control precautions should be implemented to limit contact with infected horses. These include the use of barrier precautions (gloves, dedicated outerwear) whenever the horse or its environment is contacted, restricted contact, and careful attention to hand hygiene. People at higher risk for developing an MRSA infection, such as immunocompromised individuals, should not have contact with infected or colonized horses. The risk with other MRS is unclear and is likely minimal; however, it is sensible to implement the same precautions with any multidrug-resistant infection.

PREGNANCY

There are no additional concerns.

SYNONYMS N/A

SEE ALSO

• Bacterial dermatitis

ABBREVIATIONS

• MRSA = methicillin-resistant *Staphylococcus aureus*
• MRSI = methicillin-resistant *Staphylococcus intermedius*
• MR-CoNS = methicillin-resistant coagulase-negative staphylococci
• MRS = methicillin-resistant staphylococci
• PBP2 a = penicillin binding protein 2a

Suggested Reading

Baptiste KE, Williams K, Williams NJ, Clegg PD, Dawson S, Corkill JE, O'Neill T, Hart CA. Methicillin-resistant staphylococci in companion animals. Emerg Infect Dis 2005;11:1942–1944.

Scott DW, Miller WH Jr. Equine Dermatology. St. Louis, Saunders, 2003:207.

Weese JS, Archambault M, Willey BM, Hearn P, Kreiswirth BN, Said-Salim B, McGeer A, Likhoshvay Y, Prescott JF, Low DE. Methicillin-resistant *Staphylococcus aureus* in horses and horse personnel, 2000–2002. Emerg Infect Dis 2005;11:430–435.

Author J. Scott Weese
Consulting Editor Gwendolen Lorch

BACTERIAL DERMATITIS—SUPERFICIAL

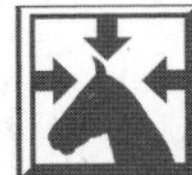

BASICS

DEFINITION

Bacterial skin infection confined to epidermis and the hair follicle.

PATHOPHYSIOLOGY

- Disruption of epidermal integrity results in skin infection.
- Moisture and minor frictional trauma in areas of tack contact result in maceration, allowing for opportunistic colonization.
- Coat changes, including shedding, clipping, as well as poor grooming, also contribute.
- Physiologic stress imparted by poor nutrition and underlying disease participates in bacterial dermatitis by impairing the cutaneous immune response.

SYSTEM AFFECTED

Skin/exocrine

GENETICS

Breeds with finer skin, such as Thoroughbreds, Quarter Horses, and Standardbreds, may be predisposed.

INCIDENCE/PREVALENCE

- Common although some clinicians report superficial bacterial dermatitis as rare in their patient populations
- Incidence is higher in spring and summer months secondary to increased grooming, shedding, and sweating, as well as more frequent riding and heavier work schedules.

GEOGRAPHIC DISTRIBUTION

Worldwide

SIGNALMENT

- Age is related to underlying cause and horses are of working and riding age.
- No sex predilection is evident.

SIGNS

- Areas most often involved include sites on the trunk and cervical areas where blankets and tack are in frequent contact. The distal limbs can also be involved (pastern dermatitis). Lesions can occur anywhere on the body and usually have a gradual onset.
- Rare clinical presentations are tail folliculitis or furunculosis and mucocutaneous staphylococcal pyoderma, which presents as uniform swelling, erosion, ulceration, fissuring, and heavy crusting of the lips or eyelids. Depigmentation of the lips or eyelids can occur with chronicity.
- Superficial dermatitis consists of papular and pustular lesions progressing to focal and coalescing ulceration, crusting, scale, and alopecia. Hair may initially stand erect before the lesions become readily visualized. Lesions can be remarkably painful. Pruritus is variable. With progression, furunculosis and deep pyoderma may ensue. Subsequent nodular, ulcerative disease with regional lymphangitis can result in scarring.

CAUSES

- *Staphylococcus aureus* is most frequently involved, followed by *Staphylococcus intermedius,* and, rarely, *Staphylococcus hyicus.*
- *Corynebacterium pseudotuberculosis* and *Streptococcus* sp. also cause superficial dermatitis.

RISK FACTORS

- Any category of skin disease can predispose to secondary bacterial infection; however, allergic, ectoparasitic, seborrheic, and follicular disorders are the most common causes.
- Constant exposure to inclement weather, filth, or trauma are all risk factors for secondary bacterial infections.

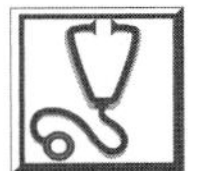

DIAGNOSIS

DIFFERENTIAL DIAGNOSIS

- Dermatophilosis
- Dermatophytosis
- Pemphigus foliaceus—a cause of pustular dermatitis disease that is not typically painful
- Onchocerciasis—pruritus is a consistent feature, rather than pain.
- Demodicosis—although rare

CBC/BIOCHEMISTRY/URINALYSIS

Not indicated unless suspect systemic disease

OTHER LABORATORY TESTS

N/A

IMAGING

N/A

OTHER DIAGNOSTIC PROCEDURES

- Cytologic examination should be performed. Neutrophils, intracellular and extracellar cocci indicate primary or secondary staphylococcal or streptococcal infection. Diphtheroid organisms indicate the presence of *Corynebacterium.* Lack of organisms on cytology does not rule out bacterial dermatitis.
- Culture and sensitivity provide the definitive diagnosis. Culture is best obtained from beneath a crust, or from a ruptured pustule. Punch biopsies of tissue can also be used if crusts and pustules are not present. Fungal culture is recommended to rule out dermatophytosis.
- Biopsies may show folliculitis and the presence of bacteria in crusts.
- Biopsies obtained for histopathology may require special stains to identify gram negative bacteria or acid fast organisms, or to rule out dermatophytosis.
- Perform skin scrapings to rule out ectoparasites and demodicosis.

PATHOLOGICAL FINDINGS

- Histopathologic findings vary with the type of infection.
- Classic folliculitis is characterized by suppurative luminal folliculitis or mural folliculitis, whereas *Staphylococcal* impetigo is characterized by large areas of suppurative epidermitis where cocci may be evident and/or discrete subcorneal or intragranular pustules composed of neutrophils. The dermis has a superficial to interstitial mixed inflammation with neutrophils predominating.
- Mucocutaneous pyoderma may have both epidermitis and luminal folliculitis. Variable, often neutrophilic serocellular crusting is observed in lesions complicated by self-trauma, erosion, and ulceration. The dermis contains a perivascular to lichenoid infiltrate. The infiltrate is composed predominantly of plasma cells, and there are mixtures of lymphocytes, neutrophils, and macrophages. Pigmentary incontinence may be mild to severe.

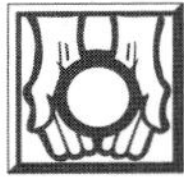

TREATMENT

AIMS OF TREATMENT

Treatment should be focused on eliminating infection and improving patient comfort. Physical, environmental, and physiologic factors predisposing the horse to bacterial dermatitis should be identified and eliminated, if possible.

APPROPRIATE HEALTH CARE

Outpatient treatment is appropriate. Severe, deep pyoderma may require hospitalization.

NURSING CARE

- Antiseptic shampoos containing chlorhexidine, chlorhexidine/miconazole, benzoyl peroxide, ethyl lactate, or povidone-iodine should be used. Products that contain sulfur, salicyclic acid, or selenium sulfide are antibacterial and help remove follicular secretions, crusts, and scale. Silvadene (silver sulfadiazine) cream or mupirocin ointment can be applied to focal lesions. When needed, a clean washable light cotton blanket or wrap can be used over topical treatments and changed daily.
- Allow a 10- to 15-min shampoo contact time. The timing of the bath depends on the severity of infection, the cause, and the response to antibiotic therapy.
- If bathing is not possible and the lesions are focal, 4% chlorhexidene spray or 2% chlorhexidene lotion may be used.
- Clip areas of matted hair.
- Disinfect tack and refrain from use during treatment.
- Proper husbandry and hygienic environment should be maintained during and after treatment.

ACTIVITY

The horse should be rested from riding and tack.

DIET

A good-quality nutritionally complete diet should be provided, but there are no specific requirements.

CLIENT EDUCATION

- If culture identifies a methicillin-resistant *Staphylococcus,* then education about potential zoonosis, appropriate hygiene, and barrier precautions is advised.
- Warn owners that recurrence is likely if an underlying cause is not found.

SURGICAL CONSIDERATIONS

Not necessary for superficial dermatitis; however, surgical excision may be curative for localized focal deep nodular bacterial disease.

MEDICATIONS

DRUG(S) OF CHOICE

- Analgesia with NSAIDs is indicated when painful.
- Systemic antimicrobial therapy is recommended with extensive involvement. Treatment should not be discontinued until lesions are resolved and preferably 2 weeks past clinical cure. If resolution plateaus or there is a relapse, then a repeat culture is indicated to assess for the development of resistance.
- Trimethroprim-sulfa—15–20 mg/kg q12h for 2 weeks or until resolution
- Procaine penicillin—20,000 IU/kg q12h IM for 10 days
- Oxytetracycline—5 mg/kg q24 h IV (not PO)
- Doxycycline—10 mg/kg PO q12h
- Ceftiofur—2 mg/kg q24h
- Enrofloxacin—5.0–7.5 mg/kg q24h

CONTRAINDICATIONS

- Because resistance can be rapid, fluoroquinolones are not recommended unless indicated by a culture and sensitivity result.
- Fluoroquinolones are not appropriate in horses <2 years of age.

PRECAUTIONS

- Doses and dosing schedule recommendations for horses may not be safe or efficacious for donkeys.
- Marbofloxacin at 2 mg/kg IV was found to be efficacious for gram-negative infections.
- Doses appropriate for gram-positive infections have not been established.
- Higher doses may result in neurologic side effects in this species.

POSSIBLE INTERACTIONS

NSAIDs are contraindicated when using systemic corticosteroids.

ALTERNATIVE DRUGS

Immunomodulatory agents may be considered in recurrent bacterial infections in which an underlying cause can not be identified after extensive investigation. Their use in horses are anecdotal, however, the use of autogenous bacterins, levamisole, EqStim (inactivated *Propionibacterium acne*; Neogen), Equimune (mycobacterial cell wall fraction; Bioniche Animal Health), or low-dose interferon-α 0.5 IU/kg PO may be helpful.

FOLLOW-UP

PATIENT MONITORING

Reevaluation to ensure that complete resolution is achieved is essential. For minor or less extensive manifestations, monitoring by the owner is adequate. If the initial response is poor, progression plateaus or relapse occurs, then repeat culture to identify resistance is necessary.

PREVENTION/AVOIDANCE

- Tack should be disinfected.
- Regular bathing or rinsing of the horse after strenuous work is recommended in tack-related cases.

POSSIBLE COMPLICATIONS

Disease is limited to the skin with no systemic involvement. Progressive, deep dermatitis, cellulitis, and scarring can occur.

EXPECTED COURSE AND PROGNOSIS

The prognosis for resolution is good.

MISCELLANEOUS

ASSOCIATED CONDITIONS

None

AGE-RELATED FACTORS

None

ZOONOTIC POTENTIAL

Methicillin-resistant *Staphylococcus aureus* transmission from horses to humans has been documented.

PREGNANCY

N/A

SYNONYMS

- Superficial pyoderma
- Acne
- Summer scab
- Summer rash
- Saddle scab
- Sweating eczema

SEE ALSO

- Bacterial dermatitis—methicillin-resistant staphylococci
- Pastern dermatitis
- Dermatophilosis
- Pemphigus foliaceus
- Dermatophytosis

ABBREVIATIONS

N/A

Suggested Reading

Scott DW, Miller WH Jr. Equine Dermatology. St. Louis: Saunders, 2003:207.

Author Jennifer R. Schissler

Consulting Editor Gwendolen Lorch

BACTERIAL MENINGITIS, NEONATE

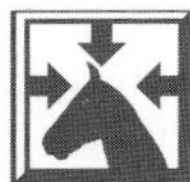

BASICS

OVERVIEW

Bacterial meningitis is an uncommon but potentially devastating sequel to septicemia in the equine neonate. An estimated 5%–10% of septic neonatal foals develop meningitis, resulting from hematogeneous spread of bacteria to the central nervous system. Bacterial meningitis can also result from penetrating trauma to the central nervous system; however, this is very uncommon in equine neonates. The rapidly progressive nature of the disease and the difficulties associated with drug penetration of the site of infection warrant a guarded to poor prognosis for affected foals. The disease is rapidly fatal if untreated.

SIGNALMENT

• Neonatal foals, usually less than 2 weeks of age • No breed or sex predisposition or genetic basis has been noted.

SIGNS

Clinical signs vary widely but usually include one or more of the following:
• Lethargy/depression • Decreased nursing
• Fever • Ataxia and weakness • Cervical stiffness/splinting of the neck • Hyperesthesia
• Opisthotonus • Cranial nerve deficits
• Anisocoria • Strabismus, nystagmus
• Recumbency • Seizures, coma (late findings; poor prognostic indicators) • Clinical signs are usually rapidly progressive (on the order of hours). Historical findings often include risk factors for septicemia (poor colostral intake, maternal illness, dystocia). Signs of other concurrent septic foci are frequently present (enteritis, arthritis, pneumonia, uveitis).

CAUSES AND RISK FACTORS

• Failure of transfer of passive colostral immunity is the single strongest risk factor for bacterial meningitis in the equine neonate. *Meningitis should not be ruled out in a patient with suspicious clinical signs based on a normal serum IgG concentration.* • The most common bacterial isolates from foals with septic meningitis are similar to those most commonly implicated in neonatal septicemia (especially gram-negative enteric bacteria).
• Infection may occur via the respiratory, gastrointestinal, or umbilical route.

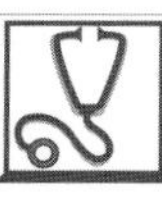

DIAGNOSIS

DIFFERENTIAL DIAGNOSIS

• Perinatal asphyxia syndrome—may also be concurrently septic; typically not rapidly progressive; normal CSF • Congenital anomaly—hydrocephalus, hydranencephaly, other brain anomalies
• Metabolic—hypoglycemia, hepatic encephalopathy, kernicterus, electrolyte and acid-base abnormalities
• Nutritional myodegeneration/white muscle disease—increased serum CK, AST values; neurologic deficits are not common, rather diffuse muscle stiffness or recumbency is seen. • Tetanus—normal CSF
• Trauma—external evidence typically present; imaging studies may be helpful.

CBC/BIOCHEMISTRY/URINALYSIS

• CBC—normal, increased, or decreased segmented neutrophils; toxic changes
• Biochemistry—hyperfibrinogenemia; hypogammaglobulinemia

OTHER LABORATORY TESTS

Serum IgG concentration—usually <400 mg/dL, often <200 mg/dL

IMAGING

Radiography of skull to rule out fracture, congenital anomaly

OTHER DIAGNOSTIC PROCEDURES

• CSF tap—*Analysis of cerebrospinal fluid is diagnostic.* Grossly, fluid usually discolored (yellow, orange) and turbid. Cytology reveals increased nucleated cell count (>6/μL, usually >100/μL), predominantly degenerate neutrophils; intracellular and extracellular bacteria often noted. Gram stain of CSF may identify the predominant bacterial population present, and may be used to guide empiric antimicrobial therapy.
• Bacterial culture and sensitivity testing performed on CSF is diagnostic and identifies pathogen(s). • Blood cultures may also be useful.

PATHOLOGIC FINDINGS

• Thickened, discolored, opaque meninges over cerebrum, cerebellum, brainstem
• Meningeal vascular congestion

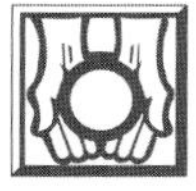

TREATMENT

Inpatient medical care and, often, emergency stabilization are required.
• Fluid therapy and nutrition if unable to nurse adequately from the mare. Fluids are especially needed in hypotensive septicemic foals as this will help maintain cerebral perfusion pressure. • Hyperimmune plasma IV if there is failure of transfer of passive immunity. • Padding to prevent self-trauma. A "foal sitter" or 24-hr nurse to stay with the foal can help with monitoring and prevention of self-trauma. • Nasal oxygen or mechanical ventilation for respiratory failure

MEDICATIONS

DRUG(S) OF CHOICE

Antimicrobials

• Broad-spectrum, rapidly bactericidal antimicrobial drugs that penetrate the blood-brain barrier are required for treatment. Should be started immediately, but guided by culture results and response to therapy
• Third-generation cephalosporins (cefotaxime 40 mg/kg IV q6h; ceftriaxone, 25 mg/kg IV q12h) are preferred; may be expensive. • Penicillin, tetracyclines, and aminoglycosides do not reliably penetrate CSF.
• Chloramphenicol—penetrates CSF well, but is bacteriostatic (not recommended)
• Trimethoprim-sulfonamide—penetrates CSF well, but organisms often resistant (not recommended)

Anti-inflammatory Medication

• Corticosteroids (dexamethasone 0.1 mg/kg IV or prednisolone 1–2 mg/kg IV)—decrease brain edema and intracranial pressure; should be given early in the course of the disease. No evidence of improved survival in horses
• DMSO (1 g/kg as a 5%–10% solution IV once daily)—free radical scavenging and lipid membrane stabilization. No strong evidence of clinical benefits
• NSAIDs (ketoprofen 1.1–2.2 mg/kg IV q12h or flunixin meglumine 0.5–1.1 mg/kg IV q12h) for analgesia

Seizure Control

• Diazepam (0.2–0.5 mg/kg IV as bolus, can be given every 15–20 min) • Midazolam (0.02–0.2 mg/kg/hr as CRI) • Phenobarbital (10–20 mg/kg IV over 20 min, then 5 mg/kg PO once daily)

CONTRAINDICATIONS/POSSIBLE INTERACTIONS

• Immunocompromise secondary to steroid administration is a concern in septicemic foals. • Avoid concurrent use of bacteriostatic and bacteriocidal antimicrobials.

FOLLOW-UP

PATIENT MONITORING

• Serial physical and neurologic examinations
• Recheck CBC, plasma fibrinogen concentration, +/− repeated CSF.

PREVENTION/AVOIDANCE

• Ensure adequate colostral intake and serum IgG >800 mg/dL within first 24 h of life. • Clean, hygienic environment for neonates

POSSIBLE COMPLICATIONS

Persistent neurologic deficits possible in recovered foals

EXPECTED COURSE AND PROGNOSIS

• Rapidly fatal without treatment • Guarded prognosis with treatment; poor if signs progress to seizures and/or coma • At least 4–6 weeks of antimicrobial treatment recommended

MISCELLANEOUS

ASSOCIATED CONDITIONS

Concurrent septic foci (pneumonia, arthritis, enteritis, uveitis, etc.)

AGE-RELATED FACTORS

Failure of transfer of passive immunity predisposes in the neonate.

ZOONOTIC POTENTIAL

Unlikely, but use caution if *Salmonella* sp. isolated from CSF, blood

SEE ALSO

• Septicemia/sepsis • Perinatal asphyxia syndrome

ABBREVIATIONS

• CSF = cerebrospinal fluid • DMSO = dimethylsulfoxide

Suggested Reading

MacKay RJ. Neurologic disorders of neonatal foals. Vet Clin North Am Equine Pract 2005;21:387–406.

Author Teresa A. Burns
Consulting Editor Margaret C. Mudge

BASISPHENOID/BASIOCCIPITAL BONE FRACTURE

BASICS

OVERVIEW
- Neurological disease caused by a fracture of the floor of the calvaria affecting petrous temporal bone and brainstem
- Due to trauma to the poll/nuchal crest

SIGNALMENT
- No breed or sex predilection
- Tends to occur in young untrained horses

SIGNS
- Many horses are unable to rise.
- Signs of changed mentation, with obtundation or coma due to damage to the reticular activating system
- May have hemorrhaging from nose or ears
- Poor pupillary light reflex and anisocoria are signs associated with cerebral edema, hemorrhage, and/or parenchymal laceration.
- With brainstem or cerebellar involvement, extensor rigidity and abnormal breathing patterns may be seen.
- Involvement of the vestibular systems in the cranial brainstem is indicated by a head tilt and nystagmus.
- Ophthalmic examination may show alterations of retinal vasculature patterns, blurring of the optic disc, and papilloedema due to increased intracranial pressure.

CAUSES AND RISK FACTORS
- Sharp trauma to the poll (nuchal crest) due to falling over backward.
- Most commonly associated with training of young horses.
- Can be seen in older horses with restrictive training methods such as sidelines or tying a rein around to the saddle to achieve bending.

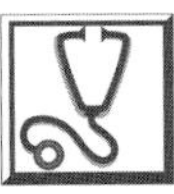

DIAGNOSIS

DIFFERENTIAL DIAGNOSIS
- Other forms of trauma to the brain—history, physical exam, skull radiographs
- Meningitis—CSF analysis
- Rabies and other encephalitis—CSF analysis/post-mortem rabies IFA of brain

CBC/BIOCHEMISTRY/URINALYSIS
Usually within normal limits

OTHER LABORATORY TESTS
- CSF analysis—Fluid obtained from the atlanto-occipital space is contraindicated if signs of increased intracranial pressure are seen, due to danger of herniation of the cerebrum under the tentorium cerebelli or herniation of the cerebellum through the foramen magnum. If fluid is obtained, it will likely have gross evidence of hemorrhage, including increased numbers of red blood cells, increased total protein content, as well as increased albumin. Platelets, increased immunoglobulins, white blood cells, erythrophagocytosis, and xanthochromia may also be seen.
- If the sample is obtained from the lumbosacral space acutely, it may well be within normal limits. If in the subacute period, it will show similar changes as seen with atlanto-occipital sample.

IMAGING
- Skull radiographs—essential but often unrewarding and difficult to obtain the diagnostic views.
- Adult horses will require a focused grid, high-energy x-ray machine and/or a fast film screen combination.
- Also, oblique views, if the horse will allow his head to be moved, may help highlight a fracture line.
- Fracture line in the basisphenoid or basioccipital bone, or separation of the suture line between these is diagnostic.
- Nonossified suture may appear in normal position.
- Look for fracture lines through occipital bones adjacent to the condyles.
- Advanced imaging techniques such as computed tomography may be useful.

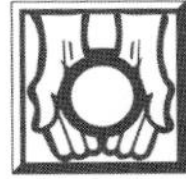

TREATMENT

- Keep horse in quiet, dark stable and minimize stimulation.
- Monitor support and breathing difficulties.
- Treat any lacerations or abrasions.
- Check for corneal abrasions and lacerations, treat appropriately.
- Turn horse frequently to minimize decubital ulcers.
- Do not overhydrate the patient, which could increase intracerebral pressure.

MEDICATIONS

DRUG(S) OF CHOICE
- Glucocorticoids in human head traumas are considered contraindicated, and their use should be judicious in horses with head trauma until studied further.
- DMSO not documented to be useful
- Sedation with α_2-agonist if patient is delirious and thrashing.
- Diuretics if horse remains in a coma or semicoma and recumbent for more than a few minutes: mannitol 0.25–2mg/kg IV over 20min
- If fracture of cranium is obvious, tetanus prophylaxis and systemic antibiotics such as penicillin should be considered.

FOLLOW-UP

- Patient monitoring—Serial neurological examinations are needed to access deterioration of condition.
- Expected course and outcome—If the horse can regain his feet in 4 hours or less, it will probably live. If not, the horse will either die or be euthanized.
- If the horse recovers, it will probably have residual neurological and proprioceptive deficits.

SEE ALSO
Head trauma

ABBREVIATIONS
- CSF = cerebrospinal fluid

Suggested Reading

Alderson P, Roberts I. Corticosteroids for acute traumatic brain injury. Cochrane Database Syst Rev 2005;(1):CD000196.

The author and editors wish to acknowledge the contribution of R. Jay Bickers, author of this chapter in the previous edition.

Author Caroline N. Hahn
Consulting Editor Caroline N. Hahn

BILE ACIDS

BASICS

OVERVIEW

- Bile acids are cholesterol derivatives synthesized by the liver and secreted via the biliary tree into the small intestine, where they function to emulsify dietary lipid and enhance its digestion by pancreatic lipases.
- The primary functions of bile acids are to:
  - Provide a route for cholesterol excretion
  - Stimulate hepatic bile flow
  - Enhance dietary lipid absorption
- During the course of the digestive process, primary bile acids are dehydroxylated by resident bacteria to secondary bile acids.
- Bile acids are reabsorbed from the gastrointestinal tract in the ileum; they are transported back to the liver via the portal circulation, where they are extracted by the liver, conjugated, and resecreted. Approximately 90% of the bile acid pool is concentrated in the enterohepatic circulation, and bile acids may be recycled up to 40 times per day.
- Under physiologic conditions, equilibrium exists between intestinal absorption, hepatic uptake from the portal circulation, and hepatic secretion of bile acids; this is represented and quantified as the serum bile acids (SBA). This value is relatively constant in healthy animals.
- In contrast to other domestic species, assessment of SBA in the horse can be performed at any time; relation to a meal is relatively unimportant, as the horse does not store bile acids in a gallbladder between meals. Further, SBA concentrations do not display diurnal variation in this species.
- Normal range depends somewhat on the laboratory performing the assay; however, most normal horses have concentrations lower than 10–12 μmol/L.
- Elevated SBA concentration is one of the more sensitive and specific clinicopathologic markers of hepatic disease; however, the exact nature of the lesion cannot be determined by this parameter alone, and further diagnostic testing is required.
- In the horse, the primary bile acids are taurocholic, taurochenodeoxycholic, glycochenodeoxycholic acid, and the majority of bile acids are conjugated with taurine. Conjugation is required for secretion.
- Three general mechanisms exist to cause increased SBA:
  - Failure of hepatocytes to extract bile acids from the portal blood
  - Biliary stasis/regurgitation
  - Portosystemic shunting
- Ileal disease in other species can cause decreased SBA due to decreased reabsorption (clinical significance, particularly in horses, unknown).

SIGNS

- Elevated SBA accumulation in the skin has been suggested to induce pruritus.
- Signs of hepatic dysfunction
  - Icterus
  - Anorexia, weight loss
  - Depression
  - Lethargy
  - Dependent edema
  - Hepatic encephalopathy (head pressing, wandering, mania, seizures, ataxia, yawning, inappropriate mentation, somnolence)
  - Photosensitization (erythema, exfoliation of nonpigmented skin)
  - Colic
  - Diarrhea
  - Hemolysis (rare, but grave finding)
  - Hemorrhagic diathesis (rare)

CAUSES AND RISK FACTORS

- Fasting for greater than 2–3 days will cause significant elevations in SBA in horses.
- Acute disease
  - Theiler's disease (serum hepatitis)
  - Hepatic lipidosis
  - Tyzzer's disease
  - Cholangiohepatitis
  - Acute biliary obstruction
    - Cholelithiasis/choledocholithiasis
    - Colon displacement
    - Hepatic torsion
- Arasitic hepatitis
- Toxic hepatopathy (iron, drugs, plants, mycotoxins)
- Viral hepatitis (EIA, EVA, EHV-1)
- Chronic disease
  - Pyrrolizidine alkaloid toxicity (*Crotolaria* spp., *Senecio* spp.)
  - Chronic active hepatitis
  - Cholelithiasis
  - Neoplastic disease
  - Hepatic abscess
- Congenital disease
  - Portosystemic shunt has been reported in a few foals but is rare.

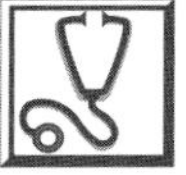

DIAGNOSIS

DIFFERENTIAL DIAGNOSIS

See differential diagnoses for liver disease.

CBC/BIOCHEMISTRY/URINALYSIS

- CBC—may suggest an inflammatory lesion as underlying cause of hepatic dysfunction (leukocytosis, neutrophilia; may show anemia of chronic disease)
- Biochemistry—other markers of hepatic dysfunction should be present (such as increased GGT, AST, SDH, ALP, bilirubin; decreased BUN, blood glucose may occur).

OTHER LABORATORY TESTS

- Blood ammonia concentration
- Plasma fibrinogen concentration (elevated with inflammatory disorders)

IMAGING

- Hepatic ultrasonography may be very helpful.
  - Hyperechogenicity noted in cases of hepatic fibrosis, hepatic lipidosis
  - Nodules
  - Biliary dilatation
  - Choleliths

OTHER DIAGNOSTIC PROCEDURES

- Hepatic biopsy is required to characterize hepatic lesions.
- Often helpful in formulating prognosis (acute hepatitis versus end-stage hepatic fibrosis)
- Assessment of coagulation profile should be performed prior to collecting biopsy (risk of hemorrhage in coagulopathic patients).

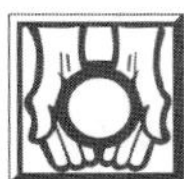

TREATMENT

• Definitive treatment of underlying cause is required, if possible.
• Treatment largely involves supportive care, as the initial insult inciting the hepatic disease may no longer be present in many cases (pyrrolizidine alkaloid hepatotoxicity, for example).
• Animals should be hospitalized, as many require intensive care.
• Fluid therapy
• Low-protein, high–soluble carbohydrate diet with a low aromatic amino acid–to–branched-chain amino acid ratio
• Padded stall, protective headgear and limb wraps for horses with neurologic complications

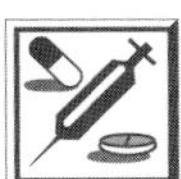

MEDICATIONS

DRUG(S) OF CHOICE

See treatment for hepatic dysfunction.

CONTRAINDICATIONS/POSSIBLE INTERACTIONS

See treatment for hepatic dysfunction.

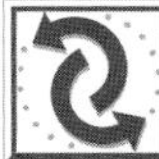

FOLLOW-UP

PATIENT MONITORING

• Serial monitoring of serum biochemical variables (esp. SDH, GGT, bilirubin, bile acids)
• Clinicopathologic parameters may remain abnormal in the face of clinical improvement.

PREVENTIOALN/AVOIDANCE

• Use caution in the administration of equine-origin biologics to adult horses.
• Avoid exposure to potentially hepatotoxic plants (*Senecio* sp., *Crotolaria* sp., etc.).

POSSIBLE COMPLICATIONS

• Coagulopathy and hemorrhagic diathesis with severe hepatic failure
• Self-trauma in patients with neurologic complications

EXPECTED COURSE AND PROGNOSIS

• Although the prognosis depends on the underlying cause of hepatic dysfunction, most etiologies carry a prognosis that is guarded (at best) to grave.
• SBA concentrations > 50 μmol/L have been associated with a grave prognosis in horses with pyrrolizidine alkaloid toxicosis.

MISCELLANEOUS

AGE-RELATED FACTORS

The SBA concentration of neonatal foals is substantially higher than that observed in adult horses. Age-matched controls should be used for interpretation purposes.

SEE ALSO

• Theiler's disease
• Tyzzer's disease
• Cholangiohepatitis
• Pyrrolizidine alkaloid toxicosis
• Cholelithiasis
• Photosensitization

ABBREVIATION

• SBA = serum bile acids

Suggested Reading

Barton MH and LeRoy BE. Serum bile acids concentrations in healthy and clinically ill neonatal foals. J Vet Intern Med 2007;21:508–513.

Engelking LR. Evaluation of equine bilirubin and bile acid metabolism. Compend Cont Educ Pract Vet 1989;11:328–336.

Author Teresa A. Burns

Consulting Editor Kenneth W. Hinchcliff

BILIRUBIN (HYPERBILIRUBINEMIA)

BASICS

DEFINITION

Hyperbilirubinemia is serum or plasma concentrations exceeding the reference interval.

PATHOPHYSIOLOGY

• Most bilirubin in the blood of healthy horses originates from the breakdown of hemoglobin by macrophages in the liver, spleen and bone marrow that have phagocytized senescent or damaged erythrocytes. • Macrophages release water-insoluble, unconjugated (indirect) bilirubin into the blood where it binds to albumin. This form of bilirubin does not normally pass through renal glomeruli into urine. • Unconjugated bilirubin enters hepatocytes by a carrier-mediated process. A small amount is refluxed back into the blood; however, most is conjugated to a water-soluble form that is excreted into the biliary system. Little conjugated (direct) bilirubin is regurgitated back into systemic circulation. • In the intestines, conjugated bilirubin is degraded into urobilinogen. A small amount of urobilinogen is passively absorbed into the portal circulation and excreted into urine. • Conjugated bilirubin is filtered by glomeruli and excreted in the urine. Bilirubinuria is associated with increased blood concentrations of conjugated bilirubin.
• Normal horses have higher blood concentrations of bilirubin (primarily unconjugated) when compared to many other species. • Hyperbilirubinemia occurs secondary to decreased food intake, hemolytic anemia, hepatocellular disease, and cholestatic disorders.

SYSTEM AFFECTED

Skin/Exocrine

• Icterus (yellow discoloration of the skin, sclera, or mucous membranes) is detected when plasma bilirubin concentrations exceed 2–3 mg/dL.
• A slight yellow discoloration of sclera or mucous membranes occurs in 10%–15% of normal horses.

Renal/Urologic

Dark-colored urine occurs with bilirubinuria.

GENETICS N/A

INCIDENCE/PREVALENCE N/A

GEOGRAPHIC DISTRIBUTION

N/A

SIGNALMENT

• All ages and breeds are affected. • Newborns are at risk for neonatal isoerythrolysis.

SIGNS

Historical

• Anorexia • Depression • Lethargy • Weakness
• Icterus

Physical Examination

• Hemolytic anemia—pale mucous membranes, tachycardia, and tachypnea • Hepatocellular disease or cholestatic disorders—weight loss, behavioral/neurologic changes, abdominal pain, fever, diarrhea, ascites, edema, hemorrhagic diathesis, photodermatitis, and pruritus

CAUSES

Prehepatic (Hemolytic) Hyperbilirubinemia

• Hemolytic disorders cause elevated total bilirubin (primarily unconjugated) when increased production overwhelms the ability of normal functioning hepatocytes to uptake, conjugate, and excrete bilirubin.
• Conjugated bilirubin may increase because of increased hepatic production and associated regurgitation or because of concurrent hepatobiliary disease.
• Causes for hemolytic disorders include immune-mediated disorders (e.g., neonatal isoerythrolysis, primary/idiopathic, or secondary to drug therapy, infectious agents, neoplasia), infectious diseases (e.g., babesiosis, equine infectious anemia), oxidant-induced damage (e.g., red maple leaf intoxication), fragmentation (e.g., DIC), and severe hepatic failure.

Fasting Hyperbilirubinemia

• The most common cause in horses.
• Unconjugated bilirubin predominates.
• Occurs secondary to many systemic diseases including intestinal disorders.
• Anorexia or decreased food intake is associated with elevated unconjugated bilirubin levels in the blood within 12 hr of onset.
• Bilirubinemia plateaus after 2–3 days and rarely exceeds 6–8 mg/dL.
• The mechanism likely involves impaired bilirubin uptake by hepatocytes.
• Values normalize once sufficient food intake resumes.

Hepatic Hyperbilirubinemia

• Hepatocellular disorders cause increased bilirubin because of impaired bilirubin uptake, conjugation, or excretion.
• Unconjugated bilirubin predominates.
• Suspect hepatocellular disease whenever conjugated bilirubin comprises greater than 25% of total bilirubin.
• Acute hepatocellular diseases more commonly are associated with hyperbilirubinemia than chronic diseases.

Cholestatic Hyperbilirubinemia

• Decreased bilirubin excretion occurs with hepatocyte swelling, periportal compression of bile ducts, or extrahepatic blockage of bile ducts.
• Endotoxemia/ sepsis may cause functional cholestasis.
• Both unconjugated and conjugated bilirubin increase; however, conjugated bilirubin rarely exceeds 30%–40% of total bilirubin.

RISK FACTORS

• Hyperbilirubinemia frequently occurs secondary to fasting or anorexia.
• Mild hyperbilirubinemia may occur for several days after prolonged exercise in healthy horses.

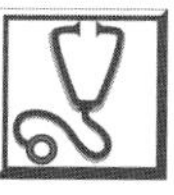

DIAGNOSIS

DIFFERENTIAL DIAGNOSIS

Prehepatic Hyperbilirubinemia

• Acute history of depression, weakness, or lethargy.
• Physical examination reveals pale mucous membranes and mild icterus.
• With severe anemia, heart murmurs may be auscultated, and heart and respiratory rates increase.

Fasting Hyperbilirubinemia

• History of anorexia of varying length.
• Physical examination reveals mild to moderate icterus.
• Clinical signs referable to the primary underlying disorder.

Hepatic or Cholestatic Hyperbilirubinemia

• Acute to chronic history of anorexia, depression, weight loss, or polydipsia.
• Physical examination may reveal moderate to severe icterus, abdominal pain, behavioral changes, ascites, edema, fever, diarrhea, steatorrhea, hemorrhagic diathesis, photodermatitis, or pruritus.

CBC/BIOCHEMISTRY/URINALYSIS

• Total and conjugated bilirubin usually are directly measured in serum or heparinized plasma. Unconjugated bilirubin is usually calculated.
• Exposure to sunlight or fluorescent lighting may decrease bilirubin concentration.
• Centrifuge blood within 4 hr of collection.
• Samples are stable up to 4 hr at room temperature, 7 days at 4° C, and 6 mo at –20° C or lower.
• Hemolysis, lipemia, or some drugs may cause artifactual changes in measured bilirubin concentrations, depending on the methodology used. Check with the laboratory performing the assay for possible interferences.

Prehepatic Hyperbilirubinemia

• Severe decreases in RBC count, hematocrit, and hemoglobin concentration.
• If hemolysis is intravascular, hemoglobinemia and hemoglobinuria are expected.
• Total protein and albumin concentrations are usually normal.
• Microscopy of a blood smear may reveal morphologic changes supporting a hemolytic process (e.g., agglutination, spherocytes, Heinz bodies, eccentrocytes, schistocytes, or erythroparasites).
• Neutrophilia with a left shift may be present.
• The activity of liver enzyme (e.g., AST, SDH) may be normal to slightly elevated due to hypoxia.

Fasting Hyperbilirubinemia

• RBC count, hematocrit, and hemoglobin concentration are normal to slightly decreased.
• Liver enzyme activities are normal to mildly elevated.
• Bile acid concentration may mildly increase.

Hepatic Hyperbilirubinemia

• RBC count, hematocrit, and hemoglobin concentration are normal to slightly decreased.
• Albumin concentration usually is normal in acute and decreased in chronic hepatocellular disease.
• Globulin concentrations are normal to increased.
• Liver enzyme (e.g., AST, SDH, ALP, GGT) activities are significantly increased, though the degree of elevation may lessen with chronicity.

BILIRUBIN (HYPERBILIRUBINEMIA)

- With significant impairment of hepatic function, BUN, glucose, and cholesterol may decrease.
- Concentrations of bile acids and ammonia increase.
- Elevated triglyceride concentration occurs with hyperlipemia and hepatic lipidosis.
- Bilirubinuria is detected.

Cholestatic Hyperbilirubinemia

- RBC count, hematocrit, and hemoglobin concentration are normal to slightly decreased.
- Total protein, albumin, BUN, glucose, and cholesterol concentrations usually are normal.
- Activities of enzymes indicative of hepatocellular damage (e.g., AST, SDH) are mildly increased; those indicative of cholestasis (e.g., ALP, GGT) are moderately to markedly increased.
- Serum bile acids concentration is elevated.
- Bilirubinuria is detected.

OTHER LABORATORY TESTS

- Prehepatic hyperbilirubinemia—consider Coggins test, direct Coombs test, antinuclear antibody test, osmotic fragility, or serology for babesiosis to determine cause of the anemia.
- Hepatic hyperbilirubinemia—measure clotting times (i.e., PT, aPTT) and FDP in horses with hemorrhagic diathesis or before surgery to assess risk of hemorrhage.

IMAGING

- Ultrasonography is useful to evaluate liver size, changes in hepatic parenchyma, and biliary patency.
- Radionucleotide imaging may detect altered blood flow or parenchymal changes.

OTHER DIAGNOSTIC PROCEDURES

Hepatic biopsy for histopathology and bacterial culture may identify the cause of hepatic or cholestatic hyperbilirubinemia.

PATHOLOGIC FINDINGS

- Hepatic disorders associated with hyperbilirubinemia include Theiler's disease, infectious hepatitis (e.g., bacteria, virus), toxic hepatopathies, chronic active hepatitis, neoplasia, and hepatic lipidosis.
- Cholestatic disorders associated with hyperbilirubinemia include cholangitis, cholelithiasis, hepatitis, neoplasia, fibrosis, and biliary hyperplasia.

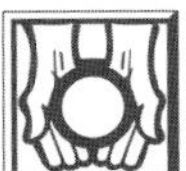

TREATMENT

AIMS OF TREATMENT

- Prehepatic hyperbilirubinemia: limit further erythrocyte destruction by eliminating the inciting cause.
- Fasting hyperbilirubinemia: no specific therapy for hyperbilirubinemia is required. Correct the underlying cause for decreased food intake.
- Hepatic or cholestatic hyperbilirubinemia: eliminate underlying cause and provide supportive care until liver regeneration occurs.

APPROPRIATE HEALTH CARE

- Medical management is appropriate for most horses.
- Surgery may be required in some cases of biliary obstruction.

NURSING CARE

- IV fluid therapy may be required to maintain hydration, cardiovascular function, renal perfusion, and electrolyte balance.
- Compatible whole-blood or packed RBC transfusions are required to restore erythrocyte mass in severely anemic horses.

ACTIVITY

Restrict activity until underlying abnormalities are corrected.

DIET

- Fasting hyperbilirubinemia: offer a high-quality diet; the icterus will resolve when food intake resumes.
- Decreased hepatic function: provide a balanced, high-quality diet (e.g., high carbohydrates, low protein)—a mixture of one-part cracked corn and two-parts beet pulp in molasses (2.5 kg of feed per 100 kg of body weight per day) can be divided into six feedings; oat or grass hay is recommended.

CLIENT EDUCATION N/A

SURGICAL CONSIDERATIONS N/A

MEDICATIONS

DRUG(S) OF CHOICE

Prehepatic Hyperbilirubinemia

- Discontinue any current drug therapy to rule out drug-induced IMHA.
- Treatment of IMHA includes immunosuppressive doses of corticosteroids—dexamethasone (0.05–0.2 mg/kg IM or IV SID, decreasing gradually once hematocrit stabilizes).

Hepatic or Cholestatic Hyperbilirubinemia

- Bacterial hepatitis or cholangitis are best treated with antibiotics determined by culture and sensitivity results.
- Chronic active hepatitis with a suspected immune-mediated origin may respond to corticosteroid therapy—dexamethasone (0.05–0.1 mg/kg IM or IV daily for 4–7 days, then gradually decreasing over several weeks).
- Hepatic encephalopathy—neomycin (10–100 mg/kg PO q6h for 1 day); lactulose (0.3 mL/kg via nasogastric tube q6h)

CONTRAINDICATIONS

Hepatic or cholestatic hyperbilirubinemia:

- Avoid drugs known to be hepatotoxic.
- Drugs associated with hepatocellular diseases include phenothiazine and erythromycin.
- Drugs associated with idiosyncratic hepatotoxicity include aspirin, diazepam, erythromycin, halothane, isoniazid, nitrofurantoin, phenobarbital, phenytoin, rifampin, and sulfonamides

PRECAUTIONS

Hepatic or cholestatic hyperbilirubinemia:

- Use drugs cautiously because many require biotransformation in the liver.
- Dosages of some drugs may need to be altered.
- Avoid analgesics, anesthetics, and barbiturates whenever possible.
- Avoid drugs that rely heavily on liver metabolism and excretion.

FOLLOW-UP

PATIENT MONITORING

- Hemolytic hyperbilirubinemia—serial CBCs as required by the underlying disease process.
- Hepatic or cholestatic hyperbilirubinemia—regular measurement of liver enzyme activities, albumin, and bilirubin as required by the underlying disease process.

EXPECTED COURSE AND PROGNOSIS

Depends on the underlying condition causing hyperbilirubinemia

MISCELLANEOUS

ASSOCIATED CONDITIONS

N/A

AGE-RELATED FACTORS

Bilirubin often is elevated in neonatal foals because of decreased hepatic uptake and conjugation and increased turnover of fetal hemoglobin; values decrease to adult levels within 2–4 weeks of birth.

ZOONOTIC POTENTIAL

N/A

PREGNANCY

N/A

SYNONYMS

- Icterus
- Jaundice

SEE ALSO

- Hemolytic anemia
- Hepatobiliary disease topics

ABBREVIATIONS

- ALP = alkaline phosphatase
- aPTT = activated partial thromboplastin time
- AST = aspartate aminotransferase
- DIC = disseminated intravascular coagulation
- FDP = fibrin degradation product
- GGT = γ-glutamyltransferase
- IMHA = immune-mediated hemolytic anemia
- PT = prothrombin time
- SDH = sorbitol dehydrogenase

Suggested Reading

Barton MH. Disorders of the liver. In: Reed SM, Bayly WM, Sellon DC, eds. Equine Internal Medicine, ed 2. Philadelphia: WB Saunders, 2004.

Sellon DC. Disorders of the hematopoietic system. In: Reed SM, Bayly WM, Sellon DC, eds. Equine Internal Medicine, ed 2. Philadelphia: WB Saunders, 2004.

Stockham SL, Scott MA. Fundamentals of Veterinary Clinical Pathology. Ames, IA: Iowa State University Press, 2002.

Author Jennifer S. Thomas

Consulting Editor Kenneth W. Hinchcliff

BLINDNESS ASSOCIATED WITH TRAUMA

BASICS

DEFINITION

Head injuries associated with ocular and optic nerve damage

PATHOPHYSIOLOGY

- Head trauma can result in periorbital and intraorbital injury as well as optic nerve and retinal damage as a result of shearing forces on the optic nerves.
- Deceleration forces such as falling over backward or hitting an obstacle can result in the brain accelerating backward in the calvaria; the eyes, however, are anchored by the bony orbits, resulting in stretching of the optic nerves.
- Retinal degeneration and optic nerve atrophy are evident on fundic examination, usually 2–6 weeks following the traumatic event.
- If there is trauma to the occipital lobes of the cerebrum, a degree of central blindness can also occur.

SYSTEMS AFFECTED

Central nervous system and other traumatized tissues

INCIDENCE/PREVALENCE

Unknown

GEOGRAPHIC DISTRIBUTION

No specific distribution

SIGNALMENT

No specific signalment

SIGNS

Historical

A recent history of trauma, especially when the horse rolled backward or received poll trauma

Physical Examination

- Lack of or sluggish pupillary light reflexes and menace response are indicative.
- Degrees of other central nervous system signs will depend on the extent of damage.
- Often, the pupils are widely dilated in bilateral optic nerve rupture.
- Within the next 2–6 weeks, there is generalized retinal degeneration and optic nerve atrophy in the affected eye(s).
- Central blindness due to trauma of the occipital lobe is characterized by normal pupillary light reflexes but an absent menace response.

CAUSES AND RISK FACTORS

- Trauma, most often to the back of the head
- Young animals, horses turned out together, and during competitive sports

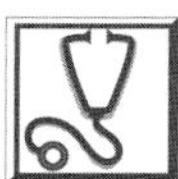

DIAGNOSIS

- Physical examination findings consistent with blindness and a recent history of trauma to, most commonly, the back of the head.
- Presence of concurrent neurological signs and lack of primary ocular lesions strongly suggest the diagnosis.

DIFFERENTIAL DIAGNOSIS

- Other causes for encephalopathies such as the equine encephalitides
- Simultaneous primary ocular trauma may complicate the diagnosis.

CBC/BIOCHEMISTRY/URINALYSIS

No specific abnormalities

OTHER LABORATORY TESTS

Electrolytes and glucose levels, particularly in foals

IMAGING

Skull radiography may indicate trauma, but if blindness is the only abnormality, it is likely that there will be no changes evident.

OTHER DIAGNOSTIC PROCEDURES

Computed tomography sensitive to bone lesions and hemorrhage; magnetic resonance imaging sensitive to soft tissue lesions

PATHOLOGIC FINDINGS

Hemorrhage, neuronal fiber degeneration, necrosis, and astrocytosis occur to varying degrees.

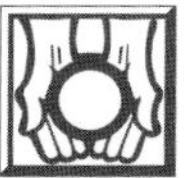

TREATMENT

AIMS OF TREATMENT

The optic nerve is part of the central nervous system and treatment options are as for traumatic brain injury. It is worth giving the horse a few weeks post injury before deciding to euthanize.

NURSING CARE

Activity

Adjust physical activity to the degree of vision.

Diet

N/A

Client education

N/A

SURGICAL CONSIDERATIONS

N/A

MEDICATIONS

DRUG(S) OF CHOICE

- Mannitol 0.25 g/kg slow IV if increased intracranial pressure is suspected (e. g., sudden deterioration in mentation)
- Phenobarbitone (loading 12–20 mg/kg IV, maintenance 6–12 mg/kg PO BID) if there is evidence of seizure activity
- Glucocorticoids in human head trauma are considered contraindicated, and their use should be judicious in horses with head trauma until further studied.

CONTRAINDICATIONS

N/A

PRECAUTIONS

N/A

POSSIBLE INTERACTIONS

N/A

ALTERNATIVE DRUGS

N/A

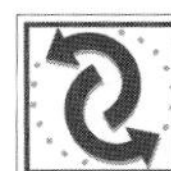

FOLLOW-UP

The horse may continue to improve for several weeks.

PATIENT MONITORING

Observe the animal over the course of several days to weeks; this is to allow cortical edema and retrobulbar hemorrhage to resolve.

PREVENTION/AVOIDANCE

If impaired vision, take care when turning out shod horses.

EXPECTED COURSE AND PROGNOSIS

Overall, prognosis is poor, but remarkable recoveries are occasionally observed.

SEE ALSO

Head trauma

Suggested Reading

Martin L, Kaswan R, Chapman W. Four cases of traumatic optic nerve blindness in the horse. Equine Vet J 1986;18:133–137.

Wang BH, Robertson BC, Girotto JA, Liem A, Miller NR, Iliff N, Manson PN. Traumatic optic neuropathy: A review of 61 patients. Plast Reconstr Surg 2001;107:1655–1664.

The author and editors wish to acknowledge the contribution of Joseph J. Bertone, author of this chapter in the previous edition.

Author Caroline N. Hahn

Consulting Editor Caroline N. Hahn

BLOOD CULTURE

BASICS

DEFINITION

• A diagnostic procedure used to identify pathogenic organisms of bacterial or fungal origin in the bloodstream.
• A positive blood culture is one in which pathogens have been grown, isolated and identified.
• A negative blood culture does not rule out microbial infection.
• Performing a blood culture involves collection of a 5–30 mL sample of blood with aseptic technique. Samples may be collected when the patient is febrile or on multiple occasions (1 hr apart) to increase the sensitivity of the test. Ideally, samples should be collected prior to institution of antimicrobial therapy. If antimicrobials have already been administered to the patient, discontinuation of antimicrobials for 24 hr before sampling and or addition of antimicrobial-inactivating enzymes to the culture broth may enhance bacterial recovery.

PATHOPHYSIOLOGY

A positive culture occurs when microorganisms are present in the systemic circulation due to a generalized infection or local infection not contained at the primary site.

SYSTEMS AFFECTED

• Hemic/lymphatic/immune—microorganisms, usually bacteria, must be present in the circulation for a blood culture to be positive; therefore the hemic system is always affected. Positive blood culture may be more likely to occur in immunosuppressed patients.
• Generalized infection may lead to localization at a primary site, therefore many different systems may be affected. In foals this commonly affects the gastrointestinal, respiratory, musculoskeletal (arthritis and osteomyelitis) and nervous systems. In adults, the cardiovascular (valvular endocarditis) system is commonly affected.
• Furthermore, generalized infection may develop subsequent to a severe local infection. In foals this may occur secondary to infection of the gastrointestinal (enterocolitis), respiratory (pneumonia) and cardiovascular (omphalophlebitis, venous thrombophlebitis) systems. In adults, generalized infection may arise subsequent to infection of the cardiovascular (venous thrombophlebitis), gastrointestinal or respiratory systems.

GENETICS

No genetic basis has been identified.

INCIDENCE/ PREVALENCE

• Positive blood culture in adult horses is uncommon.
• Positive blood culture has been reported to occur in 19% of patients admitted to a neonatal intensive care unit.
• Positive culture in neonatal foals has a case fatality rate of 15–45%.

GEOGRAPHIC DISTIBUTION

Positive blood cultures occur in patients from all geographic distributions, however the predominance of organisms cultured will vary between geographic areas.

SIGNALMENT

• Any age, breed or sex
• Positive cultures are most common in neonatal foals with septicemia.

SIGNS

Historical

• Adults may demonstrate inappetence, depression and lethargy.
• Historical findings may vary depending on whether there is a primary site of infection.
• Foals may demonstrate recumbency, poor suck reflex, weakness, diarrhea or colic.

Physical Examination

• Adults may demonstrate fever, anorexia, depression, tachycardia, tachypnea and mucous membrane hyperemia. Dehydration and shock may be present in some cases.
• Signs in foals vary widely. Foals may be standing, recumbent or comatose at presentation. Aberrations (elevated or decreased) in heart rate, respiratory rate and temperature are common. Absence of pyrexia does not rule out bacteremia.
• Signs may be referrable to a primary site of infection.
• Signs are difficult to differentiate from severe systemic inflammatory response syndrome with or without gram-positive or gram-negative toxemia.

CAUSES

Infectious Agents

Any condition that results in circulating microbes, usually bacteria

Adults

• Bacteremia involving *Streptococcus* sp., *Actinobacillus* sp., and *Pseudomonas aeruginosa*, among others, has been reported.

Neonatal Septicemia

Bacterial

• Gram-negative organisms more commonly isolated, these include: *Escherichia coli, Actinobacillus* sp., *Klebsiella* sp., *Salmonella* sp., *Enterobacter* sp.
• Gram-positive organisms include: *Enterococcus* sp., *Streptococcus* sp., *Staphlyococcus* sp. *Listeria monocytogenes.*
• Anaerobes include: *Clostridium* sp.

Mycotic

• *Candida* sp. is the most commonly identified fungal pathogen of foals. Prolonged antimicrobial therapy predisposes to fungal infections.

RISK FACTORS

Adults and Foals

• Leukopenia
• Severe underlying disease
• Venous thrombophlebitis
• Local infection or abscess, such as pulmonary infection, penetrating wound, castration, septic arthritis or synovitis
• Immunosuppression (endogenous or exogenous)

Neonates

• Maternal illness or placentitis
• Failure of transfer of passive immunity due to premature lactation, low immunoglobulin content of the colostrum, poor lactation, impaired nursing, insufficient intestinal absorption of immunoglobulins
• Neonatal immaturity/dysmaturity
• Heavy exposure to environmental pathogens
• Omphalophlebitis

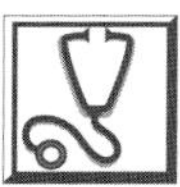

DIAGNOSIS

DIFFERENTIAL DIAGNOSIS

Differentiate from a false-positive culture caused by contamination. Contamination may result from poor aseptic technique, or errors in the collection, transfer or incubation of samples.

LABORATORY FINDINGS

Drugs That May Alter Lab Results

Antimicrobial administration prior to collection of sample for blood culture may impair microbial recovery.

Disorders That May Alter Lab Results

N/A

Valid If Run in Human Lab?

• Yes, however a veterinary laboratory could provide more useful interpretation of results.
• Knowledge of the likely organisms may influence culture techniques.
• Antimicrobials selected for sensitivity testing in human labs might not be appropriate for horses.

CBC/BIOCHEMISTRY/URINALYSIS

CBC

• Leukopenia or leukocytosis, left shift, toxic changes to neutrophils, elevated fibrinogen
• Hypoproteinemia may reflect failure of transfer of passive immunity in foals.
• Elevated PCV and TP with dehydration and shock

Biochemistry

• Abnormalities vary depending on organ system involved.
• Hyperproteinemia in adults
• Hypoalbuminemia and hyperglobulinemia in patients with abscesses at primary sites of infection
• Hypoglycemia is common in foals with bacteremia.

OTHER LABORATORY TESTS

• Abnormalities may be present in abdominal, pleural, synovial, or cerebrospinal fluid if these are sites of primary infection: increased protein, increased total nucleated cell count with degenerative changes in cell morphology and intracellular bacteria.
• Blood lactate concentration may be elevated. This is particularly useful in neonates.
• Serum immunoglobulin levels should be measured in neonates.
• Blood gas analysis may reveal metabolic acidosis and hypoxemia in neonates.

• Abnormalities in the clotting profile: increased prothrombin time, activated partial thromboplastin time, fibrin degradation products or D-dimer test; thrombocytopenia may occur in association with disseminated intravascular coagulation in severely affected patients.

IMAGING

Radiography, ultasonography, echocardiography, computed tomography, and leukocyte-labeled nuclear scintigraphy may be useful in identifying the primary focus of infection.

DIAGNOSTIC PROCEDURES

• If a focus of infection is identified, culture of a sample collected from that area is indicated.
• Endoscopy, thoracoscopy, laparoscopy may be indicated.
• Biopsies from suspected sites of primary infection may be indicated.

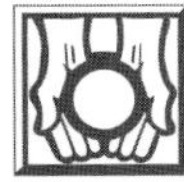

TREATMENT

ADULTS

• Hospitalization with inpatient medical management.
• Antimicrobial therapy: broad spectrum initially and then according to sensitivity results when they become available. NSAID therapy.
• Surgical drainage or resection of an infected focus should be performed if indicated.
• Specific therapy for venous thrombophlebitis or valvular endocarditis where these disease processes are also involved.

FOALS

• Hospitalization with inpatient medical management.
• Antimicrobial therapy: broad spectrum initially and then according to sensitivity results.
• Intravenous fluid therapy and administration of hyperimmune plasma.
• Surgical lavage and debridement of infected synovial structures or osteomyelitic lesions.
• Consider surgical excision with acquired patent urachus or umbilical remnant infection if not responding to medical therapy.

NURSING CARE

Keep patients in a clean, dry stall.

ACTIVITY

Rest adults for 6–8 weeks.

DIET

Anorexia occurs in many patients with positive blood cultures. Therefore, monitor nutritional intake and supplement with nasogastric feeding or total or partial parenteral nutrition where appropriate.

CLIENT EDUCATION

• Neonates with a positive blood culture carry a poor prognosis without intensive care.
• Endocarditis or primary abscessation may be difficult to treat successfully. Treatment may be prolonged and expensive.

MEDICATIONS

ANTIMICROBIALS

• Essential component of therapy
• Selection of agent is based on sensitivity results and in vivo activity.
• Broad-spectrum antimicrobials may be initiated following sample collection and prior to sensitivity results becoming available.
• Parenteral antimicrobials are preferred and should be continued for at least 7 days.
• Commonly used broad-spectrum antimicrobials include sodium or potassium penicillin G (10,000–50,000 IU IV q6h) in adults and neonates, in combination with an aminoglycoside (gentamicin 6.6–12 mg/kg IV q24h in neonates, 6.6 mg/kg IV q24h in adults or amikacin 25 mg/kg IV q24h in neonates). Third-generation cephalosporins present an alternative.
• Peak and trough concentration therapeutic drug monitoring recommended for aminoglycoside therapy

NSAIDs

• Flunixin meglumine (0.25 mg/kg IV q8 h to 1.1 mg/kg IV q12–24h)
• Phenylbutazone (2.2–4.4 mg/kg IV or PO q12–24h)
• NSAIDs should be used with caution in neonates due to increased risk of toxicity.

CONTRAINDICATIONS

Glucocorticoids are contraindicated in most situations in the face of infection due to immunosuppressive effects.

PRECAUTIONS

• Ensure pathogen is sensitive to selected antimicrobial and that the antimicrobial has suitable penetration and action in vivo.
• Reevaluate antimicrobials if inadequate response to therapy.

ALTERNATIVE DRUGS

N/A

FOLLOW-UP

PATIENT MONITORING

• Appropriate monitoring within intensive care facility
• Follow-up ultrasonography, radiography where appropriate
• Follow-up echocardiography in patients with valvular endocarditis
• Repeat sampling of primary sites of infection where appropriate

PREVENTION/AVOIDANCE

• Serum or plasma immunoglobulin concentration measured in neonates at 24 hr of age to detect failure of transfer of passive immunity
• Observed foaling
• Clean environment
• CBC at birth

POSSIBLE COMPLICATIONS

Relevant to underlying cause

MISCELLANEOUS

ASSOCIATED CONDITIONS

• Valvular endocarditis in adults
• Failure of transfer of passive immunity and septicemia in foals

AGE-RELATED FACTORS

Neonates more commonly affected

ZOONOTIC POTENTIAL

Organisms infecting horses have the potential to infect humans also although this is an unlikely scenario. *Salmonella* sp. is an example of this.

PREGNANCY

Organisms causing a generalized infection may localize to the placenta causing placentitis or fetal infection. This may result in abortion or neonatal septicemia.

SYNONYMS

N/A

SEE ALSO

• Fever
• Bacteremia
• Endocarditis
• Thrombophlebitis
• Enteritis/colitis/typhylitis
• Neonatal septicemia

ABBREVIATIONS

• PCV = packed cell volume
• TP = total protein

Suggested Reading

Corley KTT, Pearce G, Magdesian KG, Wilson WD: Bacteraemia in neonatal foals: clinicopathological differences between Gram-positive and Gram-negative infections, and single organism and mixed infections. Equine Vet J 2007;39:84–89.

Johns IC, Jesty SA, James FM. Pseudomonas aeruginosa sepsis in an adult horse with enteric salmonellosis. J Vet Emerg Crit Care 2006;16:219–223.

Marsh PS, Palmer JE. Bacterial isolates from blood and their susceptibility patterns critically ill foals: 543 cases (1991–1998). J Am Vet Med Assoc 2001;218:1608–1610.

Stewart AJ, Hinchcliff KW, Saville WJA, Jose-Cunilleras E, Hardy J, Kohn CW, Reed SM, Kowalski JJ. Actinobacillus sp. bacteremia in foals: clinical signs and prognosis. J Vet Intern Med 2002;16:464–471.

Weinstein MP. Current blood culture methods and systems: clinical concepts, technology, and interpretation of results. Clin Infect Dis 1996;23:40–46.

The author and editor wish to acknowledge the contribution to this chapter of Jill E. Parker, the author in the previous edition.

Author Laura C. Fennell
Consulting Editor Kenneth W. Hinchcliff

BLOOD TRANSFUSION REACTIONS

BASICS

OVERVIEW

• Indications for blood transfusions in horses include acute life-threatening hemorrhage, hemolytic anemia, or anemia due to erythropoietic failure. Potential complications include transfusion reactions and transmission of infectious diseases. • Transfusion reactions can be acute or delayed and are immune- or non–immune mediated. • They can vary in severity from mild urticarial reactions requiring no intervention, to worsening of hemolytic disease and/or anaphylactic shock requiring emergency resuscitative procedures. • Acute hemolytic reactions are most severe and are caused by antibodies binding to specific alloantigens on the surface of RBCs. These antigen–antibody complexes cause complement activation and subsequent lysis of RBCs with release of vasoactive substances. • Antibodies to RBC alloantigens can develop subsequent to blood transfusions or in multiparous mares exposed to fetal blood during pregnancy (see Neonatal Isoerythrolysis). • Antibodies develop within 3–10 days of original transfusion. Therefore blood transfusions given more than 3 days after an initial transfusion should be given with caution. • Incidence of adverse effects in response to blood transfusion is reported as 16%; fatal reactions are rare. • Differences in inherited blood types, WBC and platelet antigens, and protein polymorphisms contribute to incidence.

SIGNS

Historical

• Previous transfusion of blood or blood products • Transfusion of old, damaged, or hemolyzed blood • Improper or aseptic handling and storage of blood or transfusion supplies and equipment

Immune-Mediated Reactions

• Mild reactions include muscle fasciculations, piloerection, and urticaria with development of small wheals over the entire body, but most noticeable around the head. • Fever, hemoglobinemia, hemoglobinuria, and hypotension may occur in acute hemolytic reactions. • Poor response to RBC transfusion and mild icterus may be noted in delayed hemolytic reactions. • Systemic anaphylaxis is a serious reaction characterized by respiratory distress and hypotension.

Non–Immune-Mediated Reactions

• Signs associated with non–immune-mediated reactions may include fever, tachycardia, tachypnea, leukopenia, and hypotension (sepsis), hypertension and pulmonary edema (circulatory overload), muscle fasciculations with a decrease in ionized calcium concentration (citrate toxicity) and hemoglobinemia/hemoglobinuria (non–immune-mediated hemolysis). • Signs consistent with transmitted disease agents may be observed.

CAUSES AND RISK FACTORS

Immune-Mediated Reactions

• Acute hemolytic reactions are caused by recipient antibody reacting with infused donor RBC antigen. • Reactions also may occur when infused donor antibody reacts with recipient RBCs; these are usually milder. • Delayed hemolytic reactions occur when antibody to infused RBCs is formed by the recipient after transfusion. Hemolysis occurs in 3–14 days; it is usually mild. • Nonhemolytic febrile reactions can occur when there is an immune reaction to donor leukocytes, platelets, major histocompatibility antigens, or plasma proteins. • Urticaria and systemic anaphylaxis are mild and severe forms of type I hypersensitivity reactions, respectively, and occur in response to soluble proteins in donor plasma.

Non–Immune-Mediated Reactions

• Sepsis can result from contaminated blood due to poor collection or storage techniques.
• Circulatory overload occurs most commonly in neonates receiving large volumes of blood quickly. • Citrate toxicity is caused by rapid infusion of large volumes of citrated blood or plasma. • Transfusion of old, damaged, and hemolyzed RBCs due to excessive heating, freezing, or mechanical damage may result in non–immune-mediated hemolytic reactions.
• Infectious agents (e. g., equine infectious anemia virus, *Babesia spp.*) can be transmitted via blood transfusion.

RISK FACTORS

See Historical.

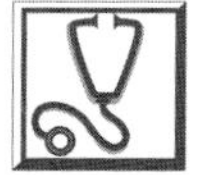

DIAGNOSIS

DIFFERENTIAL DIAGNOSIS

• If hemolysis is noted, rule out other causes of hemolytic disease. • If fever, respiratory distress, and hypotension occur, rule out other causes of infection or anaphylaxis.

CBC/BIOCHEMISTRY/URINALYSIS

• There may be hemoglobinemia, hemoglobinuria, bilirubinemia, and/or bilirubinuria. • Other changes may be present depending on underlying cause.

OTHER LABORATORY TESTS

Repeat cross-match to confirm incompatibility. However, even when both major and minor cross-matches are compatible, adverse reactions can still occur (mostly mild urticaria) indicating that cross-matching compatibilities are not 100% sensitive in identifying compatibility between donors and recipients.

OTHER DIAGNOSTIC PROCEDURES

Culture of transfused blood or blood culture from patient with suspected sepsis

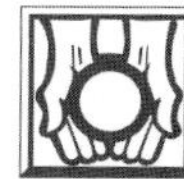

TREATMENT

• Emergency inpatient intensive care • Stop transfusion and maintain support (IV) with appropriate crystalloid or colloid solution.
• Monitor heart and respiratory rates and determine blood pressure. • If hypotension is observed, initiate infusion of fluids.

MEDICATIONS

DRUG(S)

• If severe anaphylaxis is observed, administer epinephrine (0.01 mg/kg of 1:1000 dilution [1.0 mg/ml] IM or 0.01 mg/kg of 1:10,000 dilution [0.1 mg/ml] IV) together with prednisolone sodium succinate (0.25–2.0 mg/kg IV) or dexamethasone (0.05–0.2 mg/kg IV).
• If reactions are less severe, dexamethasone (0.05–0.1 mg/kg IM or IV) or flunixin meglumine (0.25 mg/kg IV or IM) may be given.
• Appropriate IV antibiotics and fluid therapy should be given in cases of sepsis. • If volume overload with pulmonary edema is suspected, diuretics (furosemide 1 mg/kg IV) and intranasal oxygen (15 L/min) may be administered.

FOLLOW-UP

PATIENT MONITORING

Check vital signs, PCV, and plasma color before, during, and after transfusion.

PREVENTION/AVOIDANCE

• Use healthy donors; type or cross-match blood before transfusion. • Collect, store, and administer blood appropriately.

POSSIBLE COMPLICATIONS

• Hemolysis can lead to renal failure and DIC.
• Volume overload can lead to cardiac failure.

EXPECTED COURSE AND PROGNOSIS

• Most reactions follow an acute course.
• Prognosis is good if mild or moderate, but guarded if marked or occurs in a severely ill animal or when not recognized.

MISCELLANEOUS

PREGNANCY

An acute, severe reaction with resultant hypotension and organ ischemia in a pregnant mare may result in death/abortion of the foal.

SEE ALSO

- Anaphylaxis
- Anemia, immune-mediated
- Hemorrhage, acute
- Hemorrhage, chronic
- Neonatal isoerythrolysis
- Thrombocytopenia

Suggested Reading

Hurcombe SD, Mudge MC, Hinchcliff KW. Clinical and clinicopathological variables in adult horses receiving blood transfusions: 31 cases (1999–2005). J Am Vet Med Assoc 2007:231.

The author and editors wish to acknowledge the contributions of Jane Wardrop, author of this topic in the previous edition.

Author Jennifer Hodgson
Consulting Editors David Hodgson and Jennifer Hodgson

BLUE-GREEN ALGAE

BASICS

OVERVIEW

• Cyanobacterial proliferations occur in freshwater and saline ecosystems under certain environmental conditions leading to so-called algal blooms. • Blue-green algae exposure can lead to an acute intoxication affecting either the liver or the central nervous system. Reports of hepatotoxic blue-green algae poisoning are more frequent than that of neurotoxic algal intoxication. • Toxigenic blue-green algae include *Microcystis, Anabaena, Aphanizomenon, Oscillatoria, Lyngbya, and Planktothrix.*
• Microcystins are hepatotoxic blue-green algae toxins that have been found worldwide and are produced by *Microcystis, Anabaena, Planktothrix* and other genera. • Anatoxins, including anatoxin-a and anatoxin-a_s, are neurotoxic blue-green algae toxins that can be produced by *Anabaena, Plankothrix, Oscillatoria, Microcystis,* and other genera. • Cyanotoxin poisoning has occurred in animals and humans, but there are no documented cases in horses.

SIGNALMENT

N/A

SIGNS

Microcystin

• Acute hepatotoxicosis with clinical signs of diarrhea, weakness, pale mucous membranes and shock. • Progression of disease is rapid and death generally occurs within several hours of exposure.
• Animals that survive the acute intoxication may develop hepatogenous photosensitization.

Anatoxin-a

• Clinical signs include rapid onset of rigidity and muscle tremors, followed by paralysis, cyanosis and death as a result of potent nicotinic cholinergic stimulation. • Progression is very rapid and death usually occurs within minutes to a few hours of exposure.

Anatoxin-a_s

• Rapid onset of excessive salivation, lacrimation, diarrhea and urination is associated with muscarinic overstimulation. • Clinical signs of nicotinic overstimulation include tremors, incoordination and convulsions. • Respiratory arrest and recumbency may be seen prior to death. • Progression is very rapid and animals may die within 30 min of exposure.

CAUSES AND RISK FACTORS

• Algal bloom prevalence is increased with high water temperature and elevated nutrient concentrations. • Steady winds that propel toxic blooms to shore allow for ingestion by drinking animals. • Toxicity is strain specific and identification of potential toxin-producing strains should be followed up by toxicant detection to predict toxicity level. • Most microcystin-producing algal blooms are found in freshwater, but they also occur in saline environments. • Different algal species can be found in the benthic (e.g., on the sediment) or in the pelagic (water column) domains. Blooms of pelagic species are usually easily detected at the water surface of ponds, rivers or lakes. Blooms of benthic species cannot be easily detected as the algae are on the surface of sediment and stones in rivers or lakes.

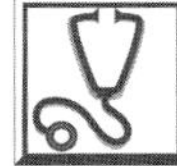

DIAGNOSIS

DIFFERENTIAL DIAGNOSIS

• Microcystin toxicosis—other causes of acute liver failure such as iron, amanitins, aflatoxins, cocklebur, alsike clover, Theiler's disease, and Tyzzer's disease—detection of toxicant, history
• Anatoxin-a—cyanide, yew, oleander, poison hemlock, insecticides, ionophore antibitiocs, intestinal compromise (e.g., torsion)— detection of toxicant, history, physical examination
• Anatoxin-a_s—organophosphorus and carbamate insecticides, slaframine—blood and brain acetylcholinesterase activity, detection of insecticide, history of feeding moldy clover

CBC/BIOCHEMISTRY/URINALYSIS

• Microcystins—increases in serum ALP, GGT, AST and bile acids, hyperkalemia, hypoglycemia
• Anatoxin-a and anatoxin-a_s—no significant findings

OTHER LABORATORY TESTS

Anatoxin-a_s—depressed blood cholinesterase activity

IMAGING

N/A

DIAGNOSTIC PROCEDURES

• Identification of the algae in the suspect water source or stomach content However, positive identification does not confirm intoxication because the toxicity of the cyanobacteria is strain specific, and morphological observations alone cannot predict the hazard level. • Detection of microcystins in gastric contents is confirmatory, but these tests are not routinely available at diagnostic laboratories. • Mouse bioassay (IP injection of algal bloom extract) was used in the past to determine the toxicity of algal blooms.

PATHOLOGICAL FINDINGS

Microcystin

• Detection of algal bloom material in GI tract and/or on legs or muzzle • Grossly evident liver enlargement; histologic lesions include progressive centrilobular hepatocyte rounding, dissociation, and necrosis, breakdown of the sinusoidal endothelium and intrahepatic hemorrhage.

Anatoxin-a and Anatoxin-a_s

• Detection of algal bloom material in GI tract and/or on legs • No lesions are found.

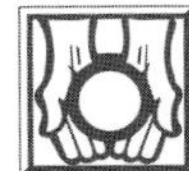

TREATMENT

• Often unsuccessful because of the rapid onset of clinical signs and death • GI decontamination with activated charcoal can be attempted but efficacy is questionable.
• Microcystin toxicosis—Provide supportive therapy to treat hypovolemia, electrolye imbalances; protect from sun exposure if hepatogenous photosensitization is present.
• Anatoxin-a toxicosis—general supportive care and specific measures to control seizures
• Anatoxin-a_s toxicosis—Atropine should be given at a test dose to determine its efficacy in animals with life-threatening clinical signs. After the test dose, atropine can be given repeatedly until cessation of salivation.

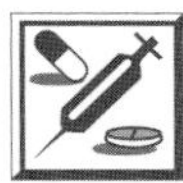

MEDICATIONS

DRUG(S) OF CHOICE

• AC (1–4 g/kg in water slurry [1 g of AC in 5 mL of water] PO) • Diazepam (adults: 25–50 mg IV, repeat in 30 min if necessary; foal: 0.05–0.4 mg/kg IV, repeat in 30 min if necessary) for seizure control • Atropine (given to effect, IV) in anatoxin-a_s intoxication

CONTRAINDICATIONS/POSSIBLE INTERACTIONS

N/A

FOLLOW-UP

PATIENT MONITORING

Microcystin toxicosis—monitor liver function, coagulation status, and risk of photosensitization.

PREVENTION/AVOIDANCE

• Horses should be denied access to water with visible algal blooms. • Reduce fertilizer application and run-off in fields surrounding ponds used for drinking water. • Use algicides for chemical control of algal blooms.

POSSIBLE COMPLICATIONS

Microcystin toxicosis—hepatic encephalopathy and hepatogenous photosensitization

EXPECTED COURSE AND PROGNOSIS

• Animals poisoned with blue-green algae toxins are often found dead. • Blue-green algae intoxications progress so rapidly that treatment is often too late. • Prognosis is poor. • Animals that survive acute microcystin poisoning may suffer from photosensitization.

ABBREVIATIONS

• AC = activated charcoal
• ALP = alkaline phosphatase
• AST = aspartate aminotrasferase
• GGT = γ-glutamyltransferase
• GI = gastrointestinal

Suggested Reading

Puschner B. In: Gupta RC, ed. Veterinary Toxicology—Basic and Clinical Principles. San Diego: Elesevier, 2007:714–724.
Puschner B, Galey FD, Johnson B, et al. Blue-green algae toxicosis in cattle. J Am Vet Med Assoc 1998;213:1605–1607.

Author Birgit Puschner
Consulting Editor Robert H. Poppenga

BORDETELLA BRONCHISEPTICA

BASICS

OVERVIEW

Bordetella bronchiseptica is a common respiratory pathogen in other animal species. Its role in equine respiratory disease is debated. It has been isolated from cultures of nasal and pharyngeal swabs from normal horses and was considered as a possible primary pathogen in horses with lower respiratory tract disease. It has also been cultured from a guttural pouch in one horse and has been associated with infertility in a mare.

SIGNALMENT

No breed, sex, or age predisposition.

SIGNS

Respiratory

Coughing, fever with associated inappetence, mucopurulent nasal discharge. Thoracic auscultation may reveal infrequent crackles and wheezes.

Reproductive

- Infertility
- Thickened uterine wall
- Hyperemic vaginal wall
- Uterine fluid

CAUSES AND RISK FACTORS

- *Bordetella* is a small, aerobic, gram-negative rod. The frequency of isolation from transtracheal aspirates varies with geographic location. Factors associated with the pathogenicity of *B. bronchiseptica* in equine respiratory disease are not known. In other animal species, *B. bronchiseptica* have attachment factors which adhere to respiratory cilia and produce toxins which inhibit phagocytic cells and damage respiratory epithelium. These result in an acute inflammation, altered mucociliary clearance, and increased mucus secretion.
- Factors compromising the normal airway defense mechanisms, such as transportation, confined close proximity, anesthesia, surgery, or recent viral infections, predispose horses to pneumonia in which *B. bronchiseptica* may be one of the pathogens.
- Recent antimicrobial therapies which eliminate competitive microorganism may predispose to *B. bronchiseptica* infection.

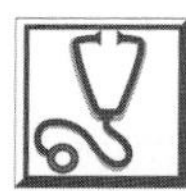

DIAGNOSIS

DIFFERENTIAL DIAGNOSIS

- Other infectious causes of lower respiratory tract disease can be differentiated with culture and cytology of transtracheal aspirates. Equine influenza, equine herpesviruses 1 and 4, and equine viral arteritis can be differentiated by viral isolation from acute-phase collection of nasopharyngeal secretions and a four-fold increase in antibody titers from serum samples collected 2 weeks apart.
- Noninfectious causes of coughing, such as allergic airway disease and upper airway disease, can be differentiated by lack of supportive laboratory data, endoscopic findings, transtracheal aspirate or bronchoalveolar lavage cytology, and lack of systemic illness.
- Other infectious causes of infertility can be differentiated with uterine culture and cytology.

CBC/BIOCHEMISTRY/URINALYSIS

Respiratory infection may be associated with elevated white cell count and fibrinogen.

OTHER LABORATORY TESTS

- Transtracheal aspirate cytology and culture. Cytologic examination reveals small gram-negative rods with a neutrophilic inflammation. This, however, does not differentiate *B. bronchiseptica* from other gram-negative infections.
- Uterine swab and lavage for culture and cytology.

IMAGING

- Thoracic radiography and ultrasonography are useful in evaluating the lower respiratory tract disease.
- Transrectal ultrasonography is useful in evaluation of the uterus.

DIAGNOSTIC PROCEDURES

Endoscopy

Assists in the evaluation of the upper respiratory tract and trachea and determining the origin of the nasal discharge and coughing.

Uterine Biopsy

Assists in the evaluation of uterine disease.

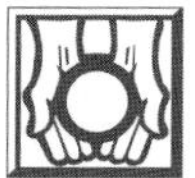

TREATMENT

The management and monitoring of the horse will depend on the extent of lung and pleural involvement. The horse should be rested until several weeks after clinical signs have resolved.

MEDICATIONS

DRUG(S) OF CHOICE

Antimicrobial therapy should be based on susceptibility results due to the variability of *B. bronchiseptica* susceptibility patterns. *B. bronchiseptica* is a potent β-lactamase inhibitor and in general is susceptible to aminoglycosides. Most reported isolates are sensitive to gentamicin (6.6–8.8mg q24h IV), oxytetracycline (6.6–11mg/kg q12h IV), trimethoprim-sulpha combination (30mg/kg q12h PO), and erythromycin (25mg/kg q12h PO). Therapy should continue until clinical signs resolve. Antimicrobial therapy should cover any other pathogenic bacteria that are isolated.

Intrauterine infusions for 5–7 days with antibiotics should be based on susceptibility tests.

FOLLOW-UP

PATIENT MONITORING

- Thoracic auscultation, rectal temperature, white blood cell count, plasma fibrinogen, thoracic radiographs and ultrasonographic findings should be used to monitor response to therapy.
- Uterine culture, cytology, and biopsy can be used to monitor response to therapy.

PREVENTION/AVOIDANCE

N/A

POSSIBLE COMPLICATIONS

- Chronic pneumonia, lung abscess formation, pleuritis, and adhesions may occur when other pathogens are involved.
- Antimicrobial induced colitis.

EXPECTED COURSE AND PROGNOSIS

Resolution of clinical signs usually occurs within 14 days with a primary *B. bronchiseptica* respiratory infection. Relapses have been reported to occur; however, further treatment with the same antibiotic regimen resulted in recovery. In small animals, unresponsiveness to antibiotics is related to the presence of *B. bronchiseptica* within the lumen of the respiratory tree rather than the lung parenchyma, thus medication is often accompanied with nebulization of an aminoglycoside. When other pathogens are involved with *B. bronchiseptica,* the treatment is for a longer period and complications associated with chronic pneumonia may occur. The reported *B. bronchiseptica* uterine infection resolved after 5 days of appropriate antibiotics.

MISCELLANEOUS

SEE ALSO

- Lower respiratory tract infection
- Pneumonia

Suggested Reading

Garcia-Cantu MC, Hartmann FA, Brown CM, et al. *Bordetella bronchiseptica* and equine respiratory infections: a review of 30 cases. Equine Vet Educ 2000;12:5–50.

Author Jane E. Axon

Consulting Editors Ashley G. Boyle and Corinne R. Sweeney

BASICS

DEFINITION

Borna disease causes sporadic cases of progressive, nonsuppurative polio encephalomyelomeningitis in sheep and horses in central Europe.

PATHOPHYSIOLOGY

- Borna disease virus is a single-stranded RNA virus that is now classified by itself in the Bornaviridae family.
- The clinical syndrome has been associated with virus-associated cell-mediated immunopathological reactions.
- Infection is believed to enter via the nasopharyngeal epithelium and trigeminal nerves and likely travels via axons to the brain.

SYSTEMS AFFECTED

Central nervous system

SIGNALMENT

Nonspecific

SIGNS

Historical

- Confirmed cases of clinical disease in horses so far are restricted to Germany, Switzerland, and Austria, but seropositive horses have been identified in the United States, Germany, the Netherlands, Poland, Israel, Iran, North Africa, and Japan.
- Furthermore, Borna disease virus–specific RNA has been detected in tissues from healthy horses in Japan and Germany, suggesting that these animals may represent potential virus reservoirs.

Physical Examination

- Subclinical encephalitis, peracute encephalitis through transient ataxia, and fever all occur.
- Typical clinical signs in sheep and horses are behavioral and mentation changes, ataxia, asymmetric vestibular signs, and various cranial nerve functional deficits.
- Circling, head pressing, constant yawning, aggressiveness, dysphagia, hyperesthesia, facial muscle fasciculations, stupor, and seizures all are described for horses and reflect the predominant forebrain and brainstem lesions; signs and lesions of cerebellar and spinal cord involvement are not common.
- Most prominently affected animals die.
- Abdominal discomfort may occur often in association with rectal impaction. Later, central nervous system signs become more pronounced.

CAUSES

Borna disease virus, a single-stranded RNA virus in the Bornaviridae family

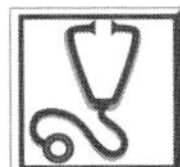

DIAGNOSIS

- Controversy still occurs over definitive diagnostic criteria for Borna disease.
- The high seroprevalence of the disease in horses in Europe probably results in overdiagnosis.
- Borna disease–specific antibodies can be recognized in cerebrospinal fluid with enzyme-linked immunosorbent assay. Virus isolation and in situ RT-PCR techniques are required to confirm the disease.

DIFFERENTIAL DIAGNOSIS

Other regionally associated viral encephalitides. More common diseases resulting in spinal cord or forebrain signs must be ruled out.

CBC/BIOCHEMISTRY/URINALYSIS

No consistent abnormalities other than stress and trauma-related changes

OTHER LABORATORY TESTS

A modest lymphocytic pleocytosis often is seen in cerebrospinal fluid during the early stages of the disease.

PATHOLOGICAL FINDINGS

There are often no gross pathology changes. On histopathological examination, the typical changes associated with viral encephalitides are present. These changes include nonpurulent encephalomyelitis and patchy discontinuous inflammatory lesions most prominent in the gray matter of the brainstem. The encephalitis is regarded as representing a cell-mediated immune response to the virus involving $CD4^+$ and $CD8^+$ cells. The identification of eosinophilic, neuronal, intranuclear Joest-Degen inclusion bodies, especially in the hippocampus, is almost pathognomonic for the disease.

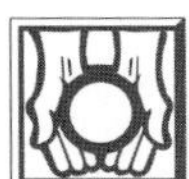

TREATMENT

Supportive care with no specific treatment

POSSIBLE COMPLICATIONS

Affected animals are usually euthanatized because the mortality rate is high and the virus can cause latent and persistent infection.

ZOONOTIC POTENTIAL

Some laboratory animals are susceptible to disease from exposure to homogenates of infected brain. The virus has been implicated in the pathogenesis of some neuropsychiatric diseases in humans.

Suggested Reading

Richt JA, Grabner A, Herzog S. Borna disease in horses. Vet Clin North Am Equine Pract 2000;16:579–596.

The author and editors wish to acknowledge the contribution of Brett Dolente and Joseph J. Bertone, authors of this chapter in the previous edition.

Author Caroline N. Hahn
Consulting Editor Caroline N. Hahn

BOTULISM

BASICS

DEFINITION

Gradually progressive, symmetric muscular weakness in horses characterized by dysphagia and eventual recumbency in most horses

PATHOPHYSIOLOGY

- Caused by systemic absorption of a potent neurotoxin elaborated by *Clostridium botulinum* that impairs transmission of electrical impulse from the nerve fiber to the adjacent muscle.
- After toxin absorption from the digestive tract or a wound previously infected with botulinum spores, botulinum toxin circulates in the bloodstream and, subsequently, is bound by specific endopeptidase receptors on motor end plates. Once attached to the receptor, the toxin is translocated within the cell and bound to acetylcholine vesicles, preventing electrical signals from reaching the myoneural junctions.
- The process of initial binding to the receptor, translocation within the cell, and final binding depends on the dose and requires several hours to a few days, depending on toxin dose. Thus, with relatively small doses of toxin (10^3 mouse lethal dose units), clinical signs may not become apparent for ≥ 10 days after ingestion. With massive doses (10^9 mouse lethal dose units), however, horses may become recumbent and die within 8 hours.
- Botulism spores are relatively ubiquitous in the environment. Ingestion rarely leads to clinical botulism, however, because the spores do not elaborate toxin unless present in an anaerobic environment with a high pH and appropriate nutrients.
- Botulism spores are pH sensitive and do not form toxin at a pH < 4.5. If forages are harvested too dry with inadequate fermentation toxin may be elaborated, if the pH is >4.5.
- Three forms of the disease are recognized in horses. The most common in adult horses is ingestion of the preformed toxin. Young foals develop toxicoinfectious botulism through ingestion of spores and subsequent sporulation with toxin formation in the gut. Toxin elaboration can also occur in wounds such as castration sites and deep penetrating wounds, including deep IM injections (wound botulism).

SYSTEMS AFFECTED

Neuromuscular

- Progressive muscular weakness over several hours to days frequently manifests as trembling of the larger muscle groups—triceps and large muscles of the rear limbs.
- As clinical signs progress, affected horses lie down more frequently than normal and, eventually, become so weak they are not able to stand. They may struggle to stand, get up and to stand for several minutes, then lie down, at first in sternal recumbency, then later lateral recumbency.
- Affected foals attempt to suckle the mare, but milk drools from the foal's mouth.

Gastrointestinal

- Some affected horses exhibit colic or abdominal pain as the primary sign prior to showing weakness.
- In addition to the systemic muscular weakness, most horses develop variable degrees of intestinal ileus, which may result in abdominal pain in some horses.

Musculoskeletal

- Progressive, symmetric muscle weakness
- Tetraparesis, not paraparesis

Respiratory

- Respiratory distress is evident only during the terminal phases of botulism.
- Horses with type C botulism may have an unusual type of respiratory effort, characterized by decreased respiratory rate (often 6–12/min) with an exaggerated abdominal lift during inspiration.

Ophthalmic

- Moderate mydriasis compared to other horses in the same light conditions
- Intact pupillary light reflex

Renal/Urologic

- Horses that remain standing can void the bladder, which helps to differentiate botulism from herpesvirus infections.
- Down horses will retain urine in the bladder, requiring periodic catheterization.

INCIDENCE/PREVALENCE

Type B

- Most frequently occurs in the mid-Atlantic region of the eastern United States, predominantly in central Kentucky, Virginia, Maryland, Delaware, and southeastern Pennsylvania.
- In most cases, occurs as an individual case
- In unusual circumstances, several cases may occur over a few days, suggesting a point source of toxin such as silage feeding to a group of horses or horses eating spoiled hay from large 750-lb hay bales, so-called "ag-bags," that has fostered growth of botulinum spores.
- More than 85% of equine botulism cases in the United States are type B.

Type A

Typically occurs in the western United States, especially in Idaho, Utah, and California

Type C

- May occur when a decomposing carcass, frequently a cat, contaminates feed materials
- More common in Arizona and New Mexico

SIGNALMENT

Age and Range

- Foals—peak occurrence between 6 days and 6 weeks of age
- Adults—any age

SIGNS

Historical

- Generalized muscle weakness or dysphagia typically is the first clinical sign detected.
- Astute owners also may detect mild depression, decreased exercise tolerance, and reluctance to eat hay or grain.

Physical Examination

- Moderately affected horses walk with a shuffling gait, occasionally dragging their toes, and show evidence of muscle weakness.
- Decreased tail tone with signs of muscle weakness is an early clinical sign.
- As the disease progresses, dysphagia becomes more obvious, and myasthenia leads to muscle tremors, difficulty in rising, and, finally, recumbency.
- Clinical signs are always symmetric, gradually progressive, and usually result in recumbency followed by death caused by respiratory paralysis or euthanasia (for humane considerations). Mildly affected horses may gradually progress over a few days, then stabilize at a certain point without recumbency and gradually recover over the next 5–14 days.

• Reduced tongue strength and slow tongue retraction are characteristic early signs. Assessment of tongue strength is best done by keeping the jaws closed with your left arm and hand over the bridge of the nose and gently pulling the tongue through the interdental space with your right hand ("tongue stress test"). Horses with normal strength retract the tongue with 1 or 2 contractions. If the tongue hangs over the mandible for even a few seconds, it is abnormal and suggestive of botulism.
• In advanced disease, before recumbency, affected horses retract the tongue very slowly, if at all. As the ability to retract the tongue diminishes, affected horses eat grain more slowly, and grain is mixed with more saliva than normal. The admixture of saliva and grain, with some grain falling out of the horse's lips during eating, is very characteristic and one of the earliest signs.
• Most normal horses consume an 8-oz cup of grain within 2 min (grain test). Accurate assessment of the time needed to consume a standard amount of grain (8 oz) and close observation of the horse eating the grain are essential in discerning early dysphagia. A delayed time to consume grain (>2 min) is one of the most sensitive clinical signs of botulism. The second most sensitive clinical index is delayed tongue retraction into the mouth. Both of these signs must be evaluated first in normal horses to appreciate the variation from horse to horse.
• Horses with early dysphagia may attempt to eat hay but have difficulty swallowing. Inability to swallow water usually occurs after inability to swallow hay. Horses seem to respond differently to the inability to drink water—many refuse even to attempt to drink; others immerse their muzzles under water.
• Recumbent horses are very difficult to assess clinically with regard to swallowing ability, because attempts in struggling to stand takes priority over eating and drinking.
• Vital signs are normal during the early stages of disease. Once the horse is recumbent, however, both the heart and respiratory rate increase in proportion to the intensity of the struggle to rise.
• Borborygmal sounds are typically reduced.

CAUSES

• The source of toxin in most cases of individual equine botulism is rarely determined but most likely is ingestion of a small amount of preformed toxin in roughage (typically hay). It is nearly impossible to subsequently identify toxin in roughage samples, because the offending material has been consumed.
• In herd outbreaks, the offending feed material usually is a point source, most often hay in plastic bags.
• Rarely has commercial grain been associated with equine botulism.
• Roughage contaminated with a carcass typically results in type C botulism.
• Wound botulism may develop secondary to infected castration sites, clamped umbilical hernias, and deep IM injections with counterirritants—iodine preparations.

RISK FACTORS

Never feed silage or fermented forages, because these may contain minute amounts of toxin.

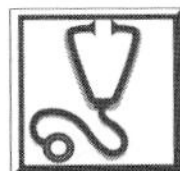

DIAGNOSIS

DIFFERENTIAL DIAGNOSIS

• Herpes myeloencephalopathy
• Ionophore toxicosis such as monensin or salinomycin
• Equine protozoal myelitis may result in similar signs but often is asymmetric, as is guttural pouch mycosis.

CBC/BIOCHEMISTRY/URINALYSIS

Until affected horses are recumbent, CBC and biochemistry profiles are within normal limits.

OTHER LABORATORY TESTS

Other routinely available diagnostic tests, including electrodiagnostic testing or nerve conduction studies, have little diagnostic value.

DIAGNOSTIC PROCEDURES

• Identification of toxin or spores in feed materials or GI contents has value only after the case is resolved, because these tests may take as long as 2–4 weeks to complete.
• Normal horses rarely, if ever, have detectable spores in their feces or GI contents.
• Laboratory identification of spores, together with compatible clinical signs, helps to confirm the diagnosis but is not definitive evidence.
• Detection of preformed toxin in serum or gut contents may be definitive but rarely is possible because of the exquisite sensitivity of horses to the toxin and the difficulty of identifying it in serum or gut contents.

PATHOLOGIC FINDINGS

Lack of gross and histologic lesions typifies horses with botulism.

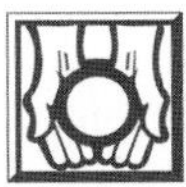

TREATMENT

APPROPRIATE HEALTH CARE

Confine affected horses to a box stall with no additional physical activity.

NURSING CARE

• Oral fluid therapy may be required in horses with complete dysphagia.
• Recumbent horses require an immense amount of nursing care to minimize decubital sores and other complications.
• Recumbent horses, especially males, also may need to have their bladder catheterized periodically to avoid necrosis of the bladder wall.

ACTIVITY

• Restriction of any muscular activity of affected horses is critical.
• Attempts to sling an affected horse are contraindicated and usually hasten the horse's death.
• Assistance to rise from recumbency should be <3 or 4 times/24 hr.
• Horses that struggle excessively when down have very poor prognosis for survival.

BOTULISM

CLIENT EDUCATION

- Once botulism has occurred on a farm, annual vaccination of all horses on the farm is strongly recommended every year.
- After the occurrence of botulism in one horse, owners should be very diligent for signs in other horses.

MEDICATIONS

DRUG(S) OF CHOICE

- Multivalent botulinum antitoxin (>100,000 IU) administered soon after the onset of clinical signs is *critical.* Only one dose is needed, since the half-life for equine origin antitoxin is ≅12 days in horses, thus providing circulating antitoxin for >50 days. Horses may be vaccinated concurrently.
- Antitoxin will not reverse clinical signs, but it should stop progression of the disease and allow patients to improve by growing more motor end plates at the myoneural junctions.
- One gallon of mineral oil is recommended for 1000-lb horses, since affected horses have ileus.

CONTRAINDICATIONS

- Aminoglycosides, which slow myoneural transmission and reduce survival in humans
- Metronidazole, which is ineffective and may predispose to toxicoinfectious botulism
- Neostigmine and 4-aminopyridine, which may provide transitory improvement but further deplete acetylcholine stores and exacerbate clinical signs

FOLLOW-UP

PATIENT MONITORING

- Monitor hydration status, and provide water with electrolytes PO with IV fluid therapy as indicated.
- During dysphagia, horses may be maintained with warm water (10–12 L) containing powdered alfalfa meal (2–3 kg) or an equivalent amount of pelleted feed that is readily soluble in water and should be administered twice daily via nasogastric tube.
- A marine bilge pump works much better than a traditional stomach pump.

PREVENTION/AVOIDANCE

- Three doses of monovalent type B botulinum toxoid ≅4 weeks apart are recommended to provide the most complete protection.
- Annual revaccination with a single dose of toxoid is adequate to maintain effective protection.
- Adequately vaccinated mares provide passive protection to newborn foals for several weeks if colostral ingestion is adequate.
- Foals are immunocompetent for botulism at birth, and the initial dose of toxoid should be given within the first 2–3 weeks of life.

POSSIBLE COMPLICATIONS

- Inhalation pneumonia secondary to dysphagia is a concern, but many horses recover without intensive antibiotic therapy.
- Massive decubital sores may result from recumbency in adults with botulism.

EXPECTED COURSE AND PROGNOSIS

- The more rapid the onset of clinical signs, the poorer is the prognosis for survival.
- In recumbent adults, the prognosis for survival is greatly reduced—usually <25%.
- Once given the antitoxin, horses remain stable for 2–4 days and then gradually improve during the next 5–10 days as they regain their ability to swallow both water and roughage. Muscle strength gradually returns during the next 30 days. Weak tongues may persist for several weeks, but affected horses seem to eat and swallow normally.

MISCELLANEOUS

SYNONYM

Forage poisoning in adults

ABBREVIATION

- GI = gastrointestinal

Suggested Reading

Schoenbaum MA, Hall SM, Glock RD, Grant K, Jenny AL, Schiefer TJ, Sciglibaglio P, Whitlock RH. An outbreak of type C botulism in 12 horses and a mule. J Am Vet Med Assoc 2000;217:365–368, 340.

Wilkins PA, Palmer JE. Botulism in foals less than 6 months of age: 30 cases (1989–2002). J Vet Intern Med 2003;17:702–707.

Author Margaret C. Mudge

Consulting Editors Ashley Boyle and Corinne Sweeney

BOTULISM, NEONATE

BASICS

OVERVIEW

• Botulism in foals (syn. "Shaker foal syndrome") is a syndrome of flaccid paralysis caused by neurotoxins produced by the anaerobic organism *Clostridium botulinum*.
• The disease results from production of the botulinum toxin in the intestinal tract ("toxicoinfectious" botulism). • Intoxication by type B toxin is most common in foals, although type A and C intoxications have also been reported in adult horses. • The toxin interferes with the release of acetylcholine from presynaptic vesicles at the neuromuscular junction.

SIGNALMENT

• No sex or breed predilection • Foals ranging from 1 week to 5 months are affected by the toxicoinfectious form of botulism.

SIGNS

• Weakness, muscle tremors, and dysphagia are characteristic. • Increased duration and frequency of recumbency, weak tongue, eyelid, and tail tone, and delayed PLR. • Respiratory distress and failure can occur secondary to diaphragmatic weakness or aspiration pneumonia. • Some foals may be found acutely dead.

CAUSES AND RISK FACTORS

• Toxicoinfectious form—most prevalent in foals; spores contaminating the soil are ingested by foals, proliferate within the intestinal tract, and release the toxin that causes disease.
• Wound botulism occurs when the bacteria proliferate under anaerobic conditions in a wound, injection site, or infected umbilicus.
• Foals born to mares that are not vaccinated against *C. botulinum* might be at higher risk, although vaccination of the mare does not confer complete protection to the foal. • Failure of transfer of passive immunity and lack of normal intestinal flora likely place foals at higher risk of toxicoinfectious botulism. • *C. botulinum* is found worldwide, but there are specific distributions of organisms that have distinct toxins. Type B organisms are most prevalent in the mid-Atlantic and Kentucky, usually found in the environment.

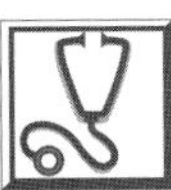

DIAGNOSIS

DIFFERENTIAL DIAGNOSIS

• Sepsis—Similar weakness can be seen, but septic foals will have neutropenia or leukocytosis, hyperfibrinogenemia, and may have focal sites of infection. • White muscle disease—Paralysis, if present, is not flaccid.
• Perinatal asphyxia syndrome—Signs of central neurologic deficits are more prominent.
• Prematurity/dysmaturity—may show weakness, but signs should be present from the time of birth • Hyperkalemic periodic paralysis—in horses of Quarter Horse (Impressive) lineage—muscle spasms or myotonia is present rather than muscle flaccidity.

CBC/BIOCHEMISTRY/URINALYSIS

• No specific changes on routine blood work, although changes compatible with dehydration (elevated PCV/TP, azotemia) and lack of milk intake (hypoglycemia) may be present. Mild neutrophilia may be present.
• Muscle enzymes (CK, AST) may be elevated due to prolonged recumbency.

OTHER LABORATORY TESTS

Blood gas—arterial blood gas may reveal hypercapnea and hypoxemia if there is hypoventilation due to respiratory weakness or prolonged lateral recumbency.

OTHER DIAGNOSTIC PROCEDURES

• Diagnosis is usually made on the basis of clinical signs and the exclusion of other differential diagnoses. • Identification of spores in feces or feed. • Demonstration of toxin in plasma, liver, gastrointestinal contents, or feed via mouse bioassay. • Serum antibiody titer to *C. botulinum*.

PATHOLOGIC FINDINGS (OPTIONAL)

No gross or microscopic findings specific to botulism, although other differentials may be ruled out.

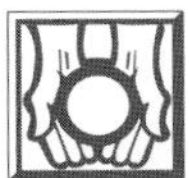

TREATMENT

• Neutralize botulism toxin—multivalent or polyvalent antitoxin. • Antimicrobial treatment of botulism infection—especially if continued production of toxin from *C. botulinum* in the gastrointestinal tract or liver, or from a wound is suspected. • Provide adequate nutrition via nasogastric tube or parenteral nutrition—If the foal is able to stand with assistance and hold itself sternal, it should be able to tolerate enteral feeding. Severely debilitated or weakened foals may initially need parenteral feeding with smaller trophic enteral feedings. • Intravenous fluids for rehydration and for maintenance requirements when enteral fluids are not tolerated.
• Respiratory support—oxygen supplementation; mechanical ventilation if needed. • Nursing care—turn every 2 hours; maintain in sternal recumbency, keep clean and dry.

MEDICATIONS

DRUG(S)

• Botulinum antitoxin—polyvalent (types A, B, C, D, and E) or monovalent (type B)
• Antimicrobial treatment—cephalosporins (ceftiofur 10 mg/kg IV QID), penicillin (22,000 IU/kg QID), metronidazole (15 mg/kg PO IV)

CONTRAINDICATIONS/POSSIBLE INTERACTIONS

• Aminoglycosides, procaine penicillin, and tetracycline are contraindicated due to their interference at the neuromuscular junction.
• Penicillins and metronidazole, although useful for treatment of the botulism organisms, may also contribute to a reduction in normal gastrointestinal flora and subsequent overgrowth of *C. botulinum*.

FOLLOW-UP

PATIENT MONITORING

• Monitor closely for signs of impending respiratory failure—significant abdominal effort, shallow breathing, decreasing Pa_{O_2}/increasing Pa_{CO_2}. • Although evaluations and monitoring should be frequent, efforts should be made to limit stress and exertion of the foal.

PREVENTION/AVOIDANCE

• Vaccinate mares against *C. botulinum* (type B toxoid is commercially available)—The mare should receive 3 doses 4 weeks apart, with an annual booster approximately 4–6 weeks prior to foaling. • Ensure adequate intake of good-quality colostrums.

POSSIBLE COMPLICATIONS

• Ventilatory failure • Aspiration pneumonia

EXPECTED COURSE AND PROGNOSIS

• Botulism toxin binds irreversibly at the neuromuscular junction, and this binding is not affected by administration of antitoxin. Weakness and respiratory difficulty may progress for 1–2 days after administration of the antitoxin, especially if there is a continued source of toxin production in the gastrointestinal tract.
• Recovery depends upon generation of new synapses. Signs of recovery are generally not seen for at least 3–5 days, and recovery may not be complete for at least 1 month. Foals have a good prognosis if treated early in the course of disease; however, treatment can be expensive and time-consuming.

MISCELLANEOUS

ASSOCIATED CONDITIONS

Aspiration pneumonia

AGE-RELATED FACTORS

Young foals (1 week to 5 months) can develop botulism via the toxicoinfecitous route. Older animals are more commonly affected by preformed toxin and occasionally by wound botulism.

SEE ALSO

Nutrition in foals

ABBREVIATIONS

• AST = aspartate aminotransferase • CK = creatinine kinase • PCV = packed cell volume
• PLR = pupillary light response
• TP = total protein

Suggested Reading

Wilkins PA, Palmer JE. Botulism in foals less than 6 months of age: 30 Cases (1989–2002). J Vet Intern Med 2003;17;702–707.

Author Margaret C. Mudge
Consulting Editor Margaret C. Mudge

BRADYARRHYTHMIAS

BASICS

OVERVIEW

• Bradyarrhythmia describes any cardiac arrhythmia that is associated with a slow heart rate.

• This includes the physiologic arrhythmias—first- and second-degree AV block, sinus arrhythmia, and sinus blocks and pauses—and the pathological arrhythmias—atrial standstill and advanced second- and third-degree AV block.

SIGNALMENT

All horses can be affected.

SIGNS

• Physiologic bradyarrhythmias produce no clinical signs and are usually easily abolished by exercising the horse to stimulate an increase in its heart rate. A slow heart rate is detected on cardiac auscultation, which is usually regularly irregular.

• During the pauses that occur with second-degree AV block, the fourth (atrial) heart sound can be auscultated.

• Pathological bradyarrhythmias lead to weakness and syncope.

CAUSES AND RISK FACTORS

• Physiologic arrhythmias are common and represent a normal mechanism to modify heart rate and blood pressure.

• Pathological arrhythmias are uncommon but can occur in association with potassium disturbances and myocardial pathology.

• Profound hyperkalemia in particular is associated with third-degree sinus bradycardia, atrial standstill, and AV block and can be seen in foals with uroperitoneum and foals or adult horses with renal failure.

• Advanced second-degree AV block can also occur in association with drugs such as the α_2-adrenergic sedative drugs and with the anesthetic inhalant agent halothane.

• Pathological bradyarrhythmias are also documented as a terminal event in horses dying of a variety of systemic diseases.

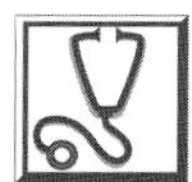

DIAGNOSIS

DIFFERENTIAL DIAGNOSIS

• Sinus bradycardia

• AV blocks

• Atrial fibrillation with a low normal heart rate

CBC/BIOCHEMISTRY/URINALYSIS

• Hyperkalemia may be present.

• Biomarkers of myocardial pathology such as cardiac troponin I may be increased with myocardial pathology.

IMAGING

• Electrocardiography is used to distinguish different forms of bradyarrhythmias and to identify atrial fibrillation.

• With AV block, there is prolongation of the PR interval (first degree), intermittent waves without a following QRS complex (second degree), or complete dissociation of the p and QRS complexes (third degree).

• With atrial standstill, p waves are absent.

• With sinus bradycardias, every P is followed by a QRS complex, but there is intermittent waxing and waning of the p-p interval and the R-R interval; with sinus pauses, there is a prolonged p-p interval; and with sinus blocks, the p-p interval is intermittently prolonged to more than two normal cardiac cycles.

• Echocardiography may be useful in identifying additional heart disease with pathologic bradyarrhythmias.

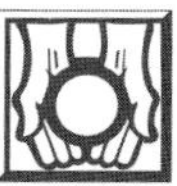

TREATMENT

• Physiologic bradyarrhythmias do not require treatment. It may be necessary to document that arrhythmias are not present during exercise by performing an exercising electrocardiogram.

• The aim of treatment in pathological bradyarrhythmias is first to identify predisposing causes such as drugs or hyperkalemia and then to remove these causes if possible.

• With uroperitoneum, abdominal drainage must be established, but the foal's electrolyte status must be stabilized before general anesthesia and surgery to repair the urinary defect are undertaken.

• With pathological bradyarrhythmias believed to be due to myocardial pathology, anti-inflammatory medications may be appropriate.

• Some cases of third-degree AV block have successfully been treated by placement of transvenous pacemakers.

MEDICATIONS

DRUG(S) OF CHOICE

- For treatment of hyperkalemia consider the following drugs:
- If symptomatic (bradycardia, muscle weakness) or serum potassium concentration >7.0 mmol/L
  - Calcium gluconate 40% 0.5 mL/kg IV over 10 min
  - Dextrose 0.5 g/kg with soluble insulin 0.1 unit/kg in 500 mL saline as IV infusion over 30–45 min
  - Sodium bicarbonate 1–2 mEq/kg IV over 15 min
- If not symptomatic and <7.0 mmol/L
  - Diuresis with at least 5 mL/kg/hr lactated Ringer's
  - Frusemide 1 mg/kg IV if horse well perfused
- For treatment of myocardial pathology, corticosteroids such as prednisolone 1 mg/kg PO every other day or dexamethasone 0.05–0.1 mg/kg IV or 0.1 mg/kg PO once a day for 3 or 4 days and then continued every 3–4 days in decreasing dosages are recommended.
- Where life-threatening bradyarrhythmias are observed during cardiopulmonary resuscitation, atropine or glycopyrrolate can be administered at 0.005–0.1 mg/kg IV.

CONTRAINDICATIONS/POSSIBLE INTERACTIONS

- Care should be taken that discontinuation of dextrose infusions does not lead to hypoglycemia, particularly when insulin has been administered concurrently.
- High-dose corticosteroid therapy has been associated with laminitis, particularly in cases in which other laminitis risk factors such as systemic illness and excessive body condition are present.

FOLLOW-UP

PATIENT MONITORING

Horses with pathological bradyarrhythmias should have their ECG monitored frequently until the arrhythmia resolves.

POSSIBLE COMPLICATIONS

- Physiologic bradyarrhythmias have no clinical consequences.
- Pathological bradyarrhythmias can be fatal.

EXPECTED COURSE AND PROGNOSIS

The clinical course and prognosis are generally determined by the underlying cause.

MISCELLANEOUS

ASSOCIATED CONDITIONS

- Uroperitoneum
- Renal failure
- Myocardial disease

AGE-RELATED FACTORS

Certain predisposing conditions, notably uroperitoneum, are more common in foals than in other age groups.

PREGNANCY

The presence of third-degree AV block will lead to a profound decrease in cardiac output and compromise blood supply to the fetus. Placement of a transvenous pacing device should be considered if this arrhythmia occurs in pregnant mares.

SEE ALSO

- Atrial fibrillation
- Myocardial disease

ABBREVIATION

- AV = atrioventricular

Suggested Reading

Reef VB. Arrhythmias. In: Marr CM, ed. Cardiology of the Horse. Philadelphia: WB Saunders, 1999:177.

Author Celia M. Marr

Consulting Editor Celia M. Marr

BROAD LIGAMENT HEMATOMA

BASICS

DEFINITION/OVERVIEW

• A rupture of the utero-ovarian, middle uterine, or external iliac arteries near the time of parturition
• Hemorrhage from the arteries can accumulate in the abdomen, in which case death is likely, or into the broad ligament, forming a hematoma. • Mares with a hematoma may appear to be in shock, with pale mucous membranes, but death rarely occurs if the broad ligament remains intact (does not rupture).

ETIOLOGY/PATHOPHYSIOLOGY

• With aging, the utero-ovarian and middle uterine artery walls undergo degenerative processes believed to result in loss of elasticity. • Secondary to the increased size or stretching, the arteries are more prone to rupture. • Preexisting damage to the intima and underlying media of the external iliac arteries (e.g., parasites) may result in necrosis and accumulation of material, predisposing them to thrombosis and rupture.

SYSTEMS AFFECTED

• Reproductive • Cardiovascular

GENETICS

Unknown

INCIDENCE/PREVALENCE

Can occur at any age, but most commonly reported in mares of >12 years of age

SIGNALMENT

• Pregnancy • Most common in mares >12 years of age • Any breed

SIGNS

General Comments

• Broad ligament hematoma (i.e., hemorrhage contained between separated layers of the broad ligament) usually is not fatal.
• Intraperitoneal hemorrhage (i.e., free blood into the abdomen) is a fatal sign.

Historical

• No cardinal, characteristic signs before artery rupture
• Pale mucous membranes, tachycardia • After rupture and with accumulation of hemorrhage, mares may show colic from pain associated with stretching of the mesometrium, the portion of the broad ligament attached to the uterus.

Physical Examination

• Mucous membranes may become pale from blood loss into the mesometrium. Clinical signs suggestive of hemorrhagic shock (tachycardia, delayed capillary refill time, sweating, etc.) • May appear anxious • TRP may reveal an enlarged broad ligament—unilateral is most common, but bilateral may occur.

CAUSES

• Degeneration of arterial vessel walls related to age
• With increased weight of the uterus and greater fetal movement, vessels break rather than stretch.

RISK FACTORS

• Pregnancy • Aging

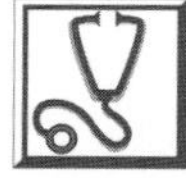

DIAGNOSIS

DIFFERENTIAL DIAGNOSIS

• Colic—TRP of the broad ligaments and surroundings structures is the best means of distinguishing broad ligament hematoma from a GI colic. • Old ilial fractures and pelvic abscesses may be present, but neither is associated with acute hemorrhage or pale mucous membranes.

CBC/BIOCHEMISTRY/URINALYSIS

Varying degrees of anemia after 24 hr of hematoma formation

IMAGING

U/S imaging is useful to differentiate hemorrhage from purulent material.

OTHER DIAGNOSTIC PROCEDURES

TRP is the preferred diagnostic method to confirm the condition.

PATHOLOGICAL FINDINGS

• Acute hemorrhagic enlargement in the broad ligaments/mesometrium during the peripartal period
• Free hemorrhage in the abdomen, at necropsy

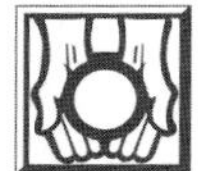

TREATMENT

APPROPRIATE HEALTH CARE

• Avoid moving the mare until she is medically stable, and the hematoma clots, contracts, and begins noticeably to reduce in size. • Prevent the mare from rolling, running, or becoming excited in any manner that might result in further bleeding from the weakened vessel or terminal rupture of the broad ligaments/mesometrium, permitting blood to escape into the abdomen.

NURSING CARE

• Restrict movement. • Maintain a quiet environment.

ACTIVITY

Restrict activity as much as possible, including hand walking, if necessary.

CLIENT EDUCATION

• Possibility of occurrence increases with age.
• Consider the possibility of arterial rupture before breeding an old mare.

SURGICAL CONSIDERATIONS

Attempts to ligate the damaged vessel may lead to further hemorrhage.

MEDICATIONS

CONTRAINDICATIONS

• Agents to enhance clotting have little or no value, because the primary mechanism to stem hemorrhage is not clot formation but the increased pressure within the broad ligament(s) that prevents further accumulation of blood. • Oxytocin administration is ill advised—The bleeding is occurring in the broad ligament; stimulation of uterine contractions may cause additional hemorrhage.

PRECAUTIONS

• Minimize movement of the mare. • If broad ligament hemorrhage began prepartum, be careful when extracting a fetus if the mare is in dystocia.
• Avoid transport to a veterinary hospital as it may be sufficient stimulus to rupture the damaged broad ligament, resulting in the mare bleeding to death internally.

FOLLOW-UP

PATIENT MONITORING

• Monitor PCV, total solids, CRT, and color of mucous membranes if broad ligament hematoma has been diagnosed. • Once a hematoma has been confirmed, subsequent serial TRPs should either be avoided, or be brief and gentle, to avoid iatrogenic rupture of a broad ligament that is stretched or under great pressure.

PREVENTION/AVOIDANCE

Avoid movement of the mare.

POSSIBLE COMPLICATIONS

• Death • Abscessation after clotting and hematogenous contamination of the hematoma with bacteria

EXPECTED COURSE AND PROGNOSIS

• Best outcome—slow regression of a hematoma, which is unlikely to return entirely to its prehematoma size and shape
• Once affected, mares are at increased risk of future rupture.

MISCELLANEOUS

ASSOCIATED CONDITIONS

• Abscess formation within the affected broad ligament/mesometrium • Death • Dystocia

AGE-RELATED FACTORS

All ages can be affected, but mares aged >12 years have a distinctly increased incidence.

PREGNANCY

Occurs either at or near term during an otherwise normal pregnancy

SYNONYM

Mesometrial hematoma

SEE ALSO

• Dystocia • Utero-ovarian, middle uterine, and iliac artery rupture

ABBREVIATIONS

• CRT = capillary refill time
• GI = gastrointestinal
• PCV = packed cell volume
• TRP = transrectal palpation
• U/S = ultrasound, ultrasonography

Suggested Reading

Asbury AC. Care of the mare after foaling. In: McKinnon AO, Voss JL. eds. Equine Reproduction. Philadelphia: Lea & Febiger 1993:979.

Pascoe RR. Rupture of the utero-ovarian or middle uterine artery in the mare at or near parturition. Vet Rec 1979;104:77–82.

Rooney JR. Internal hemorrhage related to gestation. In: Catcott EJ, Smithcors JF, eds. Progress in equine practice; Wheaton, IL: American Veterinary Publications, 1966:360–361.

Author Walter R. Threlfall
Consulting Editor Carla L. Carleton

BRUCELLOSIS

BASICS

OVERVIEW

Infection with *Brucella abortus,* a gram-negative coccobacillus, produces several outcomes in horses. The most common disease is supraspinous bursitis (fistulous withers), which results from the apparent predilection of the organism for synovial structures. Brucellosis, which is usually acquired from infected cattle, is difficult to treat and is a zoonosis. *Brucella suis,* transmitted from infected pigs, is a rare cause of bursitis or abortion in horses.

SIGNALMENT

No age, breed, or sex predilection has been reported.

SIGNS

• Most seropositive horses are asymptomatic.
• Supraspinous bursitis (fistulous withers) is the most common disease manifestation of *B. abortus* infection. This is marked by a painful swelling over the withers, which may open and drain purulent material. • Supraatlantal bursitis (poll evil) may also be caused by *B. abortus* infection. • Osteomyelitis and osteoarthritis have been reported.
• Generalized illness marked by fever, stiffness, and lethargy may be seen. • *B. abortus* infection is a rare cause of abortion in mares and infertility in the stallion. • Uveitis has been associated with *B. abortus* infection, but evidence for this is weak.

CAUSES AND RISK FACTORS

Most infections result from contact with *Brucella* -positive cattle, especially placental tissue and newborn calves. The organism can survive in the environment for weeks, so horses grazing pasture recently occupied by infected cattle are at risk. In *Brucella* -free areas, the prevalence of *Brucella* infections in horses is low. In areas where *B. suis* exists, contact with infected pigs would also pose a risk to horses. The route of infection is usually ingestion. *Brucella abortus* then travels to the lymphatics and enters phagocytic cells, leading to formation of granulomas.

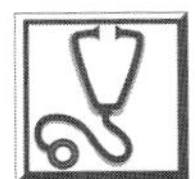

DIAGNOSIS

DIFFERENTIAL DIAGNOSIS

Fistulous withers may also result from infection of the supraspinous bursa by other agents, usually secondary to trauma or penetration of a foreign body. Failure to identify *Brucella* does not rule out infection because of the difficulty of isolating the organism and the common presence of secondary infection in cases that have developed fistulae. Radiographs or ultrasound may identify a foreign body or fracture of the spinous process.

Abortion in mares is usually a result of a noninfectious cause or an infection other than *Brucella.* History, culture, and histopathology of placental and fetal tissue may help identify the cause of abortion.

CBC/BIOCHEMISTRY/URINALYSIS

No consistent changes in CBC have been reported, but an elevated fibrinogen and neutrophilia may be detected.

OTHER LABORATORY TESTS

A rise in titer in paired serum samples 2 weeks apart is considered diagnostic. However, a high titer in conjunction with a history of exposure to infected cattle and typical clinical signs is usually sufficient for diagnosis of brucellosis in horses. Acute cases should be retested in 2 weeks before *Brucella* infection is ruled out.

IMAGING

• Radiographs of the dorsal spinous processes may help rule out fractures secondary to trauma. Also, infectious causes of fistulous withers frequently have radiographic evidence of osteomyelitis. • Contrast radiography of the fistulae may be used to determine the extent of the infection. • Ultrasonography is useful for determining location of fluid pockets and fistulous tracts. Irregularities in the surface of the bone are suggestive of osteomyelitis.

OTHER DIAGNOSTIC PROCEDURES

• Aspirate and culture of affected bursa or joint. *Brucella* is difficult to isolate and cultures should be performed in appropriate laboratories. If the withers has fistulated, secondary pathogens are usually isolated. If surgical excision is performed, a sample of material should be sent for culture.
• Intradermal testing is not considered reliable. • In cases of abortion, the organism may be cultured from placenta, fetal stomach, and vaginal discharge.

PATHOLOGIC FINDINGS

• Affected bursae have a thickened capsule and clear fluid unless fistulated, in which case the exudate is usually purulent.
• Osteomyelitis of the dorsal spinous processes may be present.

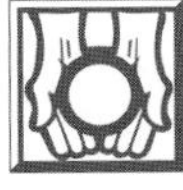

TREATMENT

• State regulatory authorities should be notified when brucellosis is suspected. In some states, treatment of *Brucella* -positive animals is prohibited. In all cases, animals should be isolated from other animals and precautions should be taken to prevent infection of people involved in the patient's care. • Lavage fistulous tracts with an antiseptic solution, such as 0.1% povidone iodine. Some authors recommend lavage with 10–50% DMSO solution. • Hydrotherapy of the swollen withers may be useful. • Horses with fistulous withers should not be ridden.
• Surgical curettage of the affected soft tissue and bone is indicated in cases that do not respond to antibiotic treatment. Patients may require more than one surgery to resolve the symptoms.

MEDICATIONS

DRUGS

• Recommended antibiotics include trimethoprim–sulfamethoxazole (30 mg/kg PO q12h), chloramphenicol, oxytetracycline, and rifampin. Many cases do not respond even after several weeks of therapy.
• Nonsteroidal anti-inflammatory drugs to reduce fever and inflammation, such as flunixin meglumine (1 mg/kg q12h) or phenylbutazone (2–4 mg/kg PO or IV q12h).
• Vaccination with strain 19 vaccine has been described. Three subcutaneous doses (5 mL) 10 days apart, or a single dose (25 mL) IV are the most commonly cited regimens. Although some authors report success with this treatment, serious adverse effects, including death, may result. This is an extra-label use of the vaccine, and the efficacy has not been determined. Use of RB51 vaccine in horses has not been reported.

CONTRAINDICATIONS/POSSIBLE INTERACTIONS

• Informed consent should be obtained before treatment with strain 19 vaccine. • Accidental injection of strain 19 vaccine may result in disease in humans. • Before administration of the *Brucella* vaccine, animals should be treated with dexamethasone (0.25 mg/kg IV) and aspirin (35 mg/kg PO) or flunixin meglumine (1.1 mg/kg).

FOLLOW-UP

• The prevalence of this disease is declining in areas where brucellosis has been eradicated.
• Cases of transmission from horses to cattle have been reported.

MISCELLANEOUS

ZOONOTIC POTENTIAL

Humans can contract brucellosis via direct contact with infected material, by ingestion or inhalation, or by inoculation with live vaccine. Gloves, mask, and protective eyewear should be worn when working with affected animals.

SYNONYMS

• Bangs disease • Undulant fever

Suggested Reading

Hawkins JF, Fessler JF. Treatment of supraspinous bursitis by use of debridement in standing horses: 10 cases (1968–1999). J Am Vet Med Assoc 2000; 217; 74–78.

Author Laura K. Reilly

Consulting Editors Ashley G. Boyle and Corinne R. Sweeney

BRUXISM

BASICS

DEFINITION

Bruxism is the medical term characterizing rhythmic or spasmodic grinding of the teeth, which is accompanied by a distinctive loud grinding sound. Bruxism may occur intermittently or, in more severe cases, may become incessant.

PATHOPHYSIOLOGY

Bruxism may be seen in a variety of clinical disorders:

• Foals—Bruxism is most commonly associated with gastroduodenal ulceration. This is especially true when gastric outflow is inhibited by stricture of the pylorus or duodenum and subsequent gastroesophageal reflux results in corrosive esophagitis. Intermittent bruxism may also occur with any painful condition.

• Adults—Bruxism in adults is often associated with pharyngeal pain or pain at the esophagus in the area of the palatopharyngeal arch. This area can be irritated by nasogastric intubation and indwelling nasogastric tubes. However, bruxism may occur in response to almost any painful condition. It is also observed with esophagitis and certain neurologic conditions such as Borna disease. Bruxism may infrequently be observed with gastric ulceration in adults.

SYSTEM AFFECTED

N/A

SIGNALMENT

No age, breed, or sex predisposition

SIGNS

Bruxism is a nonspecific clinical sign. It is usually a sign of discomfort or pain, or occasionally indicates frustration or neurological disease. Bruxism can therefore be present with a variety of clinical signs associated with the primary disease.

Historical

Historical findings are generally associated with primary disease. Health status of other horses on the premises should be checked. A history of recent nasogastric intubation or indwelling nasogastric may indicate traumatic causes for bruxism. Signs such as recent or ongoing colic, appetite, feces consistency, and attitude should be historically evaluated.

Physical Examination

When associated with pharyngeal pain, mild dysphagia is often present and is frequently characterized by salivation or by holding saliva in the mouth for prolonged periods. With gastric ulceration, foals may exhibit poor appetite, intermittent nursing (may nurse for short period and then act mildly uncomfortable), episodes of mild colic, diarrhea, pot-bellied appearance, salivation, or dorsal recumbency. Salivation and bruxism are usually indicative of severe glandular or duodenal ulcers with concurrent gastroesophageal reflux and delayed gastric emptying. Adults with gastric ulceration may exhibit poor appetite, lethargy, poor body condition, rough hair coat, and low-grade colic.

CAUSES

Trauma from nasogastric intubation, irritation from indwelling nasogastric tubes, gastroduodenal ulceration, reflux esophagitis, neurologic diseases such as Borna disease, any painful condition

RISK FACTORS

Passage of nasogastric tube, indwelling nasogastric tube, any painful illness

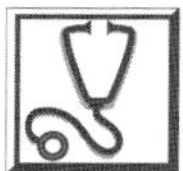

DIAGNOSIS

DIFFERENTIAL DIAGNOSIS

- Traumatic pharyngitis/esophagitis
- Gastritis/esophagitis
- Gastroduodenal ulceration
- Reflux esophagitis
- Gastric impaction
- Small intestine obstruction
- Borna disease
- Rabies
- Equine protozoal myeloencephalitis
- Head trauma
- Bacterial meningitis
- Foreign body or mass of the oral cavity, pharynx, esophagus, or stomach
- Severe inflammatory condition of the oral cavity, pharynx, esophagus, or stomach

CBC/BIOCHEMISTRY/URINALYSIS

These parameters are unlikely to assist in differentiating the cause of bruxism.

OTHER LABORATORY TESTS

N/A

DIAGNOSTIC PROCEDURES

Endoscopic Examination

Endoscopy is of value in determining if bruxism is a response to traumatic pharyngitis or esophagitis, reflux esophagitis, and/or gastroduodenal ulceration. Pharyngitis might be obvious; however, in some cases the lesion is in or behind the palatopharyngeal arch and difficult to visualize.

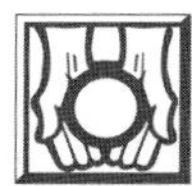

TREATMENT

• Bruxism may indicate serious medical conditions that require inpatient monitoring and care. If the patient is not drinking or is losing fluids through salivation, appropriate intravenous fluid therapy should be administered.

• Nasogastric intubation should be undertaken cautiously, and perhaps after the endoscopic examination had been undertaken should traumatic pharyngitis/esophagitis be considered the cause for bruxism.

• Exercise should be limited to hand-walking or paddock turnout. Horses with traumatic pharyngitis/esophagitis might benefit by eating a wet gruel rather than dry feed.

• Esophageal perforation may require extensive treatment, intensive care, and could have a poor prognosis.

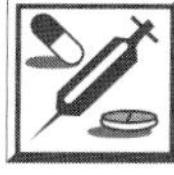

MEDICATIONS

DRUG(S) OF CHOICE

• Patients with painful conditions may benefit from administration of NSAIDs for pain control. In general, flunixin meglumine and ketoprofen are preferred for pain originating in the gastrointestinal tract and phenylbutazone is preferred for musculoskeletal pain. Flunixin is administered at 1.1 mg/kg, ketoprofen at 2.2 mg/kg, and phenylbutazone at 4.4 mg/kg.

• Gastric ulceration is treated with omeprazole or histamine H_2 receptor antagonists. Omeprazole is administered at 1–4 mg/kg PO once daily. Omeprazole has a time- and dose-related effect on healing of gastric ulcers. Therefore, higher doses result in more rapid and complete healing. However, lower doses are frequently effective in relieving clinical signs and promoting healing.

Omeprazole requires 3–5 days' treatment for maximum antisecretory effect to occur. Cimetidine is administered at 20–25 mg/kg PO or at 4–6 mg/kg IV q6–8 h. Ranitidine is administered at 6–8 mg/kg PO or 1.5–2.0 mg/kg IV q6–8 h.

CONTRAINDICATIONS

N/A

PRECAUTIONS

- NSAIDs may worsen gastroduodenal ulceration and can result in toxicosis if administered in excessive doses or if normal hydration is not maintained. NSAIDs also prolong mucosal healing. Between ketoprofen, flunixin meglumine, and phenylbutazone, the latter has the greatest potential for toxicity. When frequent dosing is necessary, ketoprofen has been shown to have less potential for toxicosis than flunixin meglumine or phenylbutazone.
- Signs of NSAID toxicosis are poor appetite, followed by loose feces, and, in some patients, oral ulceration. Serum total protein and especially albumin concentrations also decline.

POSSIBLE INTERACTIONS

Cimetidine and, to a lesser extent, omeprazole are hepatic cytochrome P450 inhibitors and might slow the metabolism of concurrently administered compounds that require this enzyme for metabolism and elimination. Drugs whose metabolism might be inhibited include phenylbutazone, diazepam, phenytoin, theophylline, and others.

ALTERNATIVE DRUGS

Butorphanol, xylazine, and detomidine may also be used for short-term relief of pain. For gastric ulceration, antacid compounds buffer gastric acid. They are impractical to use in most instances, and must be administered 4–6 times daily at approximately 250 mL/450 kg horse. Sucralfate is likely to be ineffective in the treatment of gastric stratified squamous lesions but could possibly be effective in glandular lesions. Sucralfate is administered as crushed tablets in syrup at 1 g/100 lb (1 g/45 kg) PO q6–8 h.

FOLLOW-UP

PATIENT MONITORING

Many patients exhibiting bruxism have serious medical problems and should be hospitalized for intensive monitoring. Foals exhibiting bruxism should be monitored carefully for development of gastroesophageal reflux and diminished gastric emptying.

POSSIBLE COMPLICATIONS

There are no significant complications associated with the bruxism itself. However, many complications may be associated with the primary disease process causing the patient to exhibit bruxism.

MISCELLANEOUS

ASSOCIATED CONDITIONS

Usually associated with primary disease

AGE-RELATED FACTORS

N/A

ZOONOTIC POTENTIAL

In endemic areas, rabies should be considered in patients showing neurologic signs of undetermined etiology.

PREGNANCY

N/A

SYNONYMS

- Odontoprisis
- Teeth grinding

SEE ALSO

- Gastric Ulcers and Erosions
- Regurgitation/Vomiting/Dysphagia

Suggested Reading

Bell RJW, Mogg TD, Kingston JK. Equine gastric ulcer syndrome in adult horses: a review. N Z Vet J 2007;55:1–12.

Bernard W. Colic in the foal. Equine Vet Educ 2004;6:409–413.

Doucet M, Vrins A. Les ulcères gastriques: physiopathologie, stratégies thérapeutiques et preventives. Pract Vet Equine 2004;144:35–41.

Hardy J, Stewart RH, Beard WL, *et al.* Complications of nasogastric intubation in horses: nine cases (1987–1989). JAVMA 1992;201:483–486.

Murray MJ. Gastroduodenal ulceration. In: Reed SM, Bayly WM, eds. Equine Internal Medicine. Philadelphia: WB Saunders, 1998.

Author Modest Vengust

Consulting Editors Henry Stämpfli and Olimpo Oliver-Espinosa

BURDOCK PAPPUS BRISTLE KERATOPATHY

BASICS

OVERVIEW
Burdock pappus (*Arctium* spp.) bristles are common conjunctival foreign bodies in the northeastern United States that can lead to chronic nonhealing lesions of the cornea. The ophthalmic system is affected.

SIGNALMENT
All ages and breeds affected

SIGNS
- History of unilateral ocular signs including photophobia, blepharospasm, lacrimation, ocular discharge characterized as either serous or mucopurulent, and a positive fluorescein dye uptake on the cornea.
- Most ulcers are near the nasal limbus, near the nictitans.
- The corneal erosions or ulcerations persist despite topical antibiotic medication.

CAUSES AND RISK FACTORS
Burdock pappus bristle are a common source of small conjunctival foreign bodies. The bristles may release irritating substances.

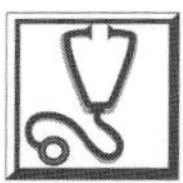

DIAGNOSIS

DIFFERENTIAL DIAGNOSIS
- Lid abnormalities such as distichiasis, trichiasis, and entropion; neuroparalytic and neurotrophic keratitis; keratoconjunctivitis sicca; corneal dystrophies; and corneal foreign bodies
- Inappropriate topical corticosteroid therapy causing delayed corneal healing
- Superficial nonhealing tumors with anterior stromol sequestration

CBC/BIOCHEMISTRY/URINALYSIS
N/A

OTHER LABORATORY TESTS
- Find the bristle.
- Rule out infectious causes (bacterial or fungal) with corneal scrapings for cytology and culture.

IMAGING
N/A

DIAGNOSTIC PROCEDURES
N/A

PATHOLOGIC FINDINGS
N/A

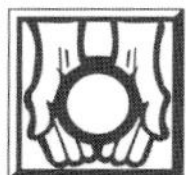

TREATMENT

- Conjunctivalectomy of the bristle foreign body and surrounding tissue under sedation and auriculopalpebral nerve block.
- Debridement of the conjunctiva behind the nictitans is often necessary.

MEDICATIONS

DRUG(S) OF CHOICE
After conjunctivalectomy—follow-up therapy with topical antibiotics 3–6 times daily (e. g., bacitracin-neomycin-polymyxin, chloramphenicol), topical 1% atropine SID to TID, and 1 to 2 g phenylbutazone BID PO

CONTRAINDICATIONS/POSSIBLE INTERACTIONS
Horses receiving topically administered atropine should be monitored for signs of colic.

FOLLOW-UP

EXPECTED COURSE AND PROGNOSIS
After removal of the bristle, healing of the corneal defect occurs within 3–14 days.

MISCELLANEOUS

ASSOCIATED CONDITIONS
Secondary bacterial infection

SEE ALSO
- Corneal ulceration
- Corneal/scleral lacerations
- Corneal stromal abscesses
- Recurrent uveitis
- Glaucoma
- Nonulcerative keratouveitis
- Eosinophilic keratitis
- Calcific band keratopathy
- Superficial nonhealing ulcers with anterior stromal sequestration

Suggested Reading

Brooks DE: Ophthalmology for the Equine Practitioner. Jackson, WY; Teton NewMedia, 2002.

Brooks DE, Matthews AG: Equine ophthalmology. In: Gelatt KN, ed. Veterinary Ophthalmology, ed 4. Philadelphia; Lippincott Williams and Wilkins, 2007.

Gilger BC, ed. Equine Ophthalmology. Philadelphia; WB Saunders, 2005.

Authors Andras M. Komaromy and Dennis E. Brooks

Consulting Editor Dennis E. Brooks

CALCIFIC BAND KERATOPATHY

BASICS

OVERVIEW

Calcific band keratopathy consists of depositions of calcium (hydroxyapatite) in or adjacent to the basement membrane of the corneal epithelium and anterior stroma and is a possible complication of chronic uveitis. The ophthalmic system is affected.

SIGNALMENT

All ages and breeds affected

SIGNS

- In addition to signs of chronic uveitis (e.g., synechiae, miosis, aqueous flare), variably dense, white, dystrophic bands or chalky plaques are noted in the interpalpebral region of the central cornea. These areas are often associated with scattered areas of fluorescein retention, usually the result of the lesions elevating the overlying epithelium.
- Calcium deposited at the level of corneal epithelial basement membrane may accumulate and disrupt the epithelium to result in painful ulcers and a secondary reflex uveitis.

CAUSES AND RISK FACTORS

The exact pathogenesis of calcium band keratopathy is unknown. It is an occasional complication of chronic cases of uveitis and has been noted following the chronic application of topical corticosteroids or phosphate-containing solutions (usually as a therapy for uveitis). Alterations of pH in the superficial cornea of the interpalpebral space and evaporation of tears in the same region have been postulated as contributing factors for the development of this condition.

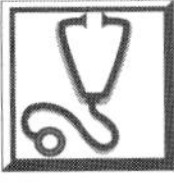

DIAGNOSIS

DIFFERENTIAL DIAGNOSIS

Lid abnormalities such as distichiasis, trichiasis, and entropion resulting in keratitis and corneal injury; bacterial or fungal keratitis; eosinophilic keratitis; corneal lipid degeneration; neuroparalytic and neurotrophic keratitis; keratoconjunctivitis sicca; corneal dystrophies; corneal foreign bodies; and chronic epithelial erosion (indolent ulceration).

CBC/BIOCHEMISTRY/URINALYSIS

N/A

OTHER LABORATORY TESTS

- Rule out infectious causes (bacterial or fungal) with corneal scrapings for cytology and culture. Scraping procedure causes audible and tactile evidence of mineralization.
- The dull, gritty appearance and character of corneal calcium are helpful in the diagnosis.
- Biopsy sample can be taken to histologically support the diagnosis of calcific band keratopathy. Von Kossa and alizarin red stains can detect the presence of calcium.

IMAGING

N/A

DIAGNOSTIC PROCEDURES

N/A

PATHOLOGIC FINDINGS

- Special stains (e.g., Kossa's method or alizarin red) confirm the presence of calcium deposits at level of lamina propria of epithelium and underlying superficial stroma.
- Vascularization is often noted, and an associated lymphocytic and neutrophilic cellular reaction is frequently present around the calcium deposits.

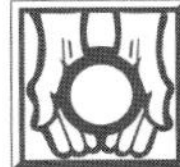

TREATMENT

- Superficial keratectomy is recommended. If calcific deposits are not removed, affected eyes remain painful despite medical treatment because of persistent or recurrent ulceration.
- Inappropriate topical corticosteroid therapy may cause delayed corneal healing.

MEDICATIONS

DRUG(S) OF CHOICE

- Topically administered calcium chelating drugs (dipotassium ethylene diamine tetraacetate 13.8%; Sequester-Sol) to dissolve the calcium deposits are usually only helpful if the corneal epithelium is absent or compromised.
- Topical antibiotic (e.g., chloramphenicol, bacitracin-neomycin-polymyxin), atropine (1%), and systemic nonsteroidal anti-inflammatory drugs (e.g., flunixin meglumine 0.25–1 mg/kg BID PO, IM, IV) should be used to protect any ulcerations and treat any resultant uveitis until the keratectomy site heals.

CONTRAINDICATIONS/POSSIBLE INTERACTIONS

- Risk of opportunistic infections due to topical corticosteroids for treatment of uveitis
- The rate of postkeratectomy infections can be high, usually due to a compromised cornea from chronic uveitis or prior use of topical corticosteroids.

FOLLOW-UP

EXPECTED COURSE AND PROGNOSIS

- Healing of keratectomy sites can occur with slight to severe scarring.
- Recurrence of calcium band keratopathy is possible with continued episodes of uveitis.
- The prognosis for vision is guarded because of subsequent corneal scarring and further uveitis episodes.
- Horses with dystrophic calcification due to severe corneal injury or infection in areas other than the interpalpebral fissure usually fare better than those with palpebral fissure lesions.

MISCELLANEOUS

ASSOCIATED CONDITIONS

Complication of uveitis

SEE ALSO

- Corneal ulceration
- Corneal/scleral lacerations
- Keratomycosis
- Corneal stromal abscesses
- Recurrent uveitis
- Glaucoma
- Nonulcerative keratouveitis
- Eosinophilic keratitis
- Herpes keratitis
- Burdock pappus bristle keratopathy
- Limbal keratopathy
- Superficial corneal erosions with anterior stromal sequestration

Suggested Reading

Brooks DE. Ophthalmology for the Equine Practitioner. Jackson, WY; Teton NewMedia, 2002.

Brooks DE, Matthews AG. Equine ophthalmology. In: Gelatt KN, ed. Veterinary Ophthalmology, ed 4. Philadelphia; Lippincott Williams and Wilkins, 2007.

Gilger BC, ed. Equine Ophthalmology. Philadelphia; WB Saunders, 2005.

Author Caryn E. Plummer

Consulting Editor Dennis E. Brooks

CALCIUM, HYPERCALCEMIA

BASICS

DEFINITION

Serum total calcium greater than the reference interval, or >13.5 mg/dL

PATHOPHYSIOLOGY

• PTH, calcitonin, and vitamin D act in conjunction with the intestine, bone, kidneys, and parathyroid glands to maintain calcium homeostasis. • Calcium absorption in the equine intestine, and hence serum calcium, is more dependent on the amount of dietary calcium and less dependent on vitamin D. • The equine kidney is important in calcium regulation; horses excrete a larger proportion of absorbed calcium in the urine than other mammals do.
• Disturbances in calcium homeostasis leading to hypercalcemia occur with organ dysfunction, abnormalities in hormonal balance and control, or production of a parathyroid hormone analog in certain malignancies. • Hypercalcemia of malignancy is associated with certain types of neoplasia. Tumor cells produce and secrete parathyroid-related hormone products, causing increased osteoclastic bone resorption and renal resorption of calcium. • Hypercalcemic states can lead to widespread soft-tissue mineralization.

SYSTEMS AFFECTED

Cardiovascular

• ECG changes associated with increased serum calcium progress from bradycardia to tachycardia (with or without extrasystoles/ ectopic beats) to ventricular fibrillation. • Hypervitaminosis D with secondary hypercalcemia and hyperphosphatemia can result in soft-tissue mineralization; lung, large vessels, endocardium are prone.

Endocrine/Metabolic

Hypercalcemia stimulates calcitonin release as a compensatory mechanism to decrease plasma calcium.

GI

Possible decreased contractility of GI smooth muscle

Neuromuscular

Decreased neuromuscular irritability can result from hypercalcemia and contribute to decreased performance.

Renal

Soft-tissue mineralization may occur with concurrent hypercalcemia and hyperphosphatemia.

SIGNALMENT

Renal Failure

• Horses with chronic renal failure usually are adult to old. • Suspect congenital abnormalities in young horses with renal failure.

Hypercalcemia of Malignancy

• Squamous cell carcinoma (e.g., cutaneous, GI, metastatic) generally occurs in adult and old animals. • Cutaneous squamous cell carcinoma more commonly occurs in animals with an area of white skin; common sites are nonpigmented, sparsely haired areas near mucocutaneous junctions. • Horses with lymphoma more often are young to middle-aged (2–9 years) but can be old as well.

SIGNS

General Comments

• Clinical signs in horses with hypercalcemia, regardless of cause, often are nonspecific.
• Weight loss, inappetence/anorexia, poor performance, and depression are most common.
• Clinical signs of hypervitaminosis D or hyperparathyroidism generally reflect the increased vitamin D or PTH activity causing increased renal and intestinal calcium reabsorption.

Historical

• With renal disease/failure, poor performance may be the presenting complaint. Less frequently, mild colic signs or abnormal frequency or volume of urination are noted. Confirmation of exposure to potential nephrotoxins requires an excellent history and investigation. • Depending on location of the alimentary tract squamous cell carcinoma, horses may exhibit signs of esophageal obstruction (e.g., dysphagia, ptyalism, choke), show a reluctance to eat or drink (despite interest in food and water), or have a prolonged history of anorexia and weight loss. • Horses with hypervitaminosis D may exhibit limb stiffness and painful flexor tendons and suspensory ligaments. • In a documented case of primary hyperparathyroidism in an old pony, intermittent weakness was the presenting complaint.

Physical Examination

Renal Failure

• Ventral edema—frequently seen with glomerulonephritis • Oral ulcerations
• Hematuria or PU/PD

Neoplasia

• Proliferative or erosive masses or nonhealing wounds in the periorbital region, genitalia, lips, nose, or anus suggest cutaneous squamous cell carcinoma. • During the late stages, metastasis to lymph nodes, lung, or bone can occur.
• Palpating abdominal masses or adhesions by rectal examination suggests GI tumors.
• Clinical findings in horses with lymphoma are nonspecific and relate to location of the tumor—cutaneous, alimentary, mediastinal, or multicentric.

CAUSES

Chronic Renal Disease/Failure

• Hypercalcemia secondary to decreased excretion of calcium carbonate occurs with chronic renal disease. • Hyper-, hypo-, or normocalcemia occurs with acute renal disease.
• Hypercalcemia in acute or chronic renal failure is more apt to develop in horses fed high-calcium rations. • Cause is difficult to determine, because many conditions or diseases may predispose to chronic progressive renal disease/failure—glomerulonephritis from immune complex deposition (e.g., streptococcal infection, equine infectious anemia), nephrotoxins (e.g., aminoglycoside antibiotics, NSAIDs, vitamin K_3, heavy metals [especially mercury], hemoglobin, myoglobin), chronic urinary tract obstruction, interstitial nephritis, amyloidosis, pyelonephritis, nephrolithiasis and ureterolithiasis, and congenital abnormalities (e.g., renal hypoplasia, or polycystic kidneys).

Neoplasia

• The most common paraneoplastic finding in horses is hypercalcemia.
• Tumors associated with hypercalcemia—lymphoma (common), squamous cell carcinoma (common), multiple myeloma (uncommon), adrenocortical carcinoma (uncommon), malignant mesenchymoma of the ovary (uncommon), and ameloblastoma (uncommon).

Hypervitaminosis D

Hypercalcemia from increased GI absorption and bone resorption is associated with ingestion of plants

Exercise

Calcium increases with exercise; however, because this ion is present in sweat, plasma concentrations may be reduced with large volumes of sweat loss.

Primary Hyperparathyroidism

• Potential causes—parathyroid adenoma, parathyroid hyperplasia, and carcinoma
• This condition is rare in horses but should be considered after ruling out all other causes of hypercalcemia.

Neonatal Hypecalcemia and Asphyxia

• Hypercalcemia with associated asphyxia has been seen in a number of newborn foals.
• Foals are severely hypotensive and exhibit somnolence.

Granulomatous Disease

Hypercalcemia, due to secretion of a parathyroid hormone-related protein, may be seen in horses with idiopathic systemic granulomatous disease.

RISK FACTORS

• Do not feed hypercalcemic horses legume hays (e.g., alfalfa, clover) or high-calcium rations.
• Fluid therapy for hypercalcemic horses should be devoid of calcium.

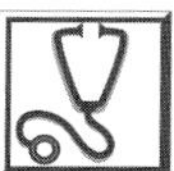

DIAGNOSIS

DIFFERENTIAL DIAGNOSIS

• Renal failure—azotemia, isosthenuria, and exposure to nephrotoxins
• Squamous cell carcinoma, lymphoma, and other neoplasia—clinical signs related to neoplasia, identification of tumor by cytology, and histopathology.
• Hypervitaminosis D—hypercalcemia with concurrent hyperphosphatemia occurs with overzealous supplementation; hyperphosphatemia may be absent with plant intoxication.
• Primary hyperparathyroidism—hypercalcemia, hypophosphatemia, increased serum PTH concentration, increased fractional excretion of phosphorus, and low to normal vitamin D_3 concentration.

LABORATORY FINDINGS

Drugs That May Alter Lab Results

Anticoagulants containing EDTA, citrate, oxalate, or fluoride chelate calcium can falsely decrease calcium measurements.

Disorders That May Alter Lab Results

- Of total calcium, ≅50% is bound to protein, predominantly albumin.
- Abnormalities in serum albumin or protein concentration directly affect total serum calcium concentration, but the correlation is not as strong in horses as in dogs. Correction formulas as determined for dogs have not been validated in horses.
- Total serum calcium may be falsely increased with hyperproteinemia if hyperalbuminemia is present; hypoalbuminemia or hypoproteinemia may obscure hypercalcemia.
- Acid–base status affects the amount of ionized and protein-bound calcium. Acidosis increases the ionized calcium fraction by decreasing the fraction bound to protein; alkalosis decreases ionized calcium by increasing the fraction bound to protein. Total calcium, however, usually remains within the reference interval.
- Lipemia and hemolysis may falsely elevate total calcium.

Valid If Run in Human Lab?

Yes

CBC/BIOCHEMISTRY/URINALYSIS

- Azotemia (increased serum creatinine and urea nitrogen) and isosthenuria (urine specific gravity, 1.008–1.015) support the diagnosis of renal failure, but other causes of azotemia with concurrent PU/PD must be ruled out.
- Hypophosphatemia, mild hyponatremia and hypochloridemia, and normo- or hyperkalemia can be present.
- Moderate to marked proteinuria is common with glomerulonephritis.
- Suspect urinary tract infection with moderate to many leukocytes in urine sediment.
- Hypercalcemia without concurrent azotemia or isosthenuria implies causes other than renal; suspect neoplasia.
- Consider vitaminosis D intoxication with concurrent hypercalcemia and hyperphosphatemia. Hyperphosphatemia is the earliest abnormality and may be more reliable for indicating hypervitaminosis D in oversupplementation than hypercalcemia. Hyperphosphatemia may be absent in plant intoxication. Urine specific gravity may be low.

OTHER LABORATORY TESTS

- Total serum calcium is reported during routine biochemical analysis.
- Measurement of ionized calcium concentration by ion-selective electrodes requires special sample handling and may not be readily available.
- With suspected primary hyperparathyroidism after ruling out all other diseases, measurement of PTH is indicated.

IMAGING

Ultrasonography of kidneys during chronic renal failure may reveal increased echogenicity (i.e., fibrosis) and is useful in assessing abnormalities (e.g., polycystic kidneys).

DIAGNOSTIC PROCEDURES

- Fine-needle aspiration or tissue biopsy of masses (endoscopic or ultrasound-guided) are indicated for establishing the diagnosis of neoplasia.
- Abdominal or thoracic fluid cytology may reveal neoplastic cells.
- Renal biopsy sometimes is useful in determining the morphological disorder and cause.

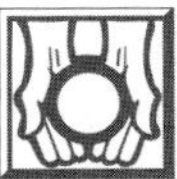

TREATMENT

- Unless cutaneous or localized, neoplasia carries a guarded to poor prognosis. Surgical excision, radiotherapy, cryosurgery, or hypertherapy are options with some localized tumors.
- Treatment of chronic renal disease/failure seldom is curative. Supportive treatment options include fluids to correct dehydration and acid-base disorders and antibiotics for concurrent infection or sepsis. Salt restriction is indicated if ventral edema develops, and a diet of high-quality carbohydrates (e.g., corn, oats), roughage (e.g., grass hay), and free access to fresh water is recommended. Avoid feeds high in protein or calcium.
- With severe hypercalcemia, administration of physiologic saline with loop diuretics (furosemide) will promote urinary calcium excretion.
- Because thiazide diuretics stimulate calcium resorption, use is contraindicated in hypercalcemia.
- Removal of vitamin D sources and time may result in recovery, but with soft-tissue mineralization in the heart or kidney, the prognosis is poor.

MEDICATIONS

DRUG(S) OF CHOICE

Chronic Renal Failure

- Good nutritional support and free access to fresh water, fluids and electrolytes, salt blocks if edema is absent (restrict if hypertension or edema develops), and vitamin B complex.
- Anabolic steroids may help to prevent muscle wasting.
- Supportive therapy may prolong life substantially in polyuric (urine output, >18 mL urine/kg per day), stabilized patients.

Hypervitaminosis D

- Removal of the source of vitamin D, fluid diuresis, corticosteroid administration, and low-calcium and -phosphorus feeds.
- In severe cases, treatment generally is unrewarding because of extensive soft-tissue mineralization.

CONTRAINDICATIONS

- Do not feed hypercalcemic horses legume hays (e.g., alfalfa, clover) or high-calcium rations.
- Fluid therapy for hypercalcemic horses should be devoid of calcium.
- Thiazide diuretics promote renal resorption of calcium.
- Avoid aminoglycoside antibiotics and NSAIDs, or use with extreme caution because of potential nephrotoxic effects.

PRECAUTIONS N/A

POSSIBLE INTERACTIONS N/A

ALTERNATIVE DRUGS N/A

FOLLOW-UP

PATIENT MONITORING

Chronic renal failure—frequent blood samples to monitor sodium, potassium, calcium, and bicarbonate status.

POSSIBLE COMPLICATIONS

- Soft-tissue mineralization
- See Contraindications.

MISCELLANEOUS

ASSOCIATED CONDITIONS N/A

AGE-RELATED FACTORS N/A

ZOONOTIC POTENTIAL N/A

PREGNANCY

- Increased calcium concentration in mammary secretions is a good indicator of impending parturition.
- Serum calcium remains within reference intervals unless an underlying disease process is present.

SYNONYMS

Hypercalcemia of malignancy—humoral hypercalcemia of malignancy; pseudohyperparathyroidism

SEE ALSO

- Hyperphosphatemia
- Hypocalcemia

ABBREVIATIONS

- GI = gastrointestinal
- PTH = parathyroid hormone
- PU/PD = Polyuria/polydipsia

Suggested Reading

Brewer BD. Disorders of equine calcium metabolism. Compend Cont Educ Pract Vet 1987;4:S244-S252.

Pringle J, Ortenburger A. Diseases of the kidneys and ureters. In: Kobluk CN, Ames TR, Geor RJ, eds. The Horse: Diseases and Clinical Management. Philadelphia: WB Saunders, 1995:583–596.

Schott HC. Chronic renal failure. In Robinson NE, ed. Current Therapy in Equine Medicine, ed 5. St. Louis: Saunders, 2003:845–848.

Toribio RE. Disorders of the endocrine system: Calcium disorders. In: Reed SM, Bayly WM, Sellon DC, eds. Equine Internal Medicine, ed 2. St. Louis: Saunders, 2004:1295–1327.

Turrel JM. Oncology. In: Kobluk CN, Ames TR, Geor RJ, eds. The Horse: Diseases and Clinical Management. Philadelphia: WB Saunders, 1995:1111–1136.

Author Karen E. Russell

Consulting Editor Kenneth W. Hinchcliff

CALCIUM, HYPOCALCEMIA

BASICS

DEFINITION

Total serum calcium less than the reference interval, or <10.0 mg/dL

PATHOPHYSIOLOGY

• Calcium, a major component of bone, also is necessary for blood coagulation, muscle contraction and neuromuscular excitability, hormone secretion, and enzyme activation.
• Fractions of total serum calcium occur as protein-bound (50%), ionized (40%), or complexed with other anions (10%).
• Ionized calcium is the physiologically active fraction. • Of the protein-bound fraction, ≅50% is complexed with albumin. • Serum albumin has a direct effect on total serum calcium concentration, but the correlation is not as strong in horses as in dogs. Ionized calcium usually is not affected by albumin concentrations. Acidosis increases the ionized calcium fraction by decreasing protein binding; alkalosis has the opposite effect. Total calcium usually remains within the reference interval.
• Hypocalcemia can be seen with dietary deficiency or imbalance, sepsis, GI disease, hypocalcemic tetany (e.g., lactation, transport, idiopathic, eclampsia), hypoalbuminemia or hypoproteinemia, toxicosis (cantharidin [blister beetle], oxalate), administration of certain drugs (tetracycline, furosemide, bicarbonate), excessive sweating, exertional rhabomyolysis, renal disease, or pancreatic disease.

SYSTEMS AFFECTED

Skeletal

• In response to hypocalcemia, calcium is mobilized from bone to maintain other metabolic functions. • Consequences include too little or abnormal bone formation, bone demineralization, and a skeleton more prone to injury.

Neuromuscular

• Most acute cases manifest by tetany rather than paresis. • Hypocalcemia may lead to increased neuroexcitability and seizures.

GI

Decreased contractility may lead to hypomotility and ileus, especially with decreased ionized calcium.

Reproductive

Retained placenta and acute endometritis are seen in mares with hypocalcemia and may occur due to decreased uterine tone and contractility, possibly resulting from a mechanism similar to that seen with ileus.

Cardiovascular

• SDF (i.e., contraction of one or both flanks coincident with heartbeat) is thought to result from altered membrane potential of the phrenic nerve and its discharge in response to electrical impulses generated during myocardial depolarization. • S_4–S_1 heart sounds may be obscured by thumping caused by contracture of the diaphragm. • Hypocalcemia is the most consistent electrolyte abnormality in this condition.

SIGNALMENT

• Depends on underlying disease or condition
• Lactation tetany most frequently occurs in mares ≅10 days post foaling or 1–2 days post weaning. • Draft breeds are more susceptible.

SIGNS

Historical

• History varies with the underlying cause.
• Owners may describe fatigue or exhaustion; abdominal pain, anorexia, or depression after ingestion of alfalfa; lameness, swollen painful joints, or poor growth; or diets of high-grain content and low-quality roughage or bran supplement added to grain (especially wheat or rice bran, which are high in phosphorus).

Physical Examination

General Clinical Signs

• Tetany, increased muscle tone or weakness, stiffness, muscle fasciculation, SDF, tachypnea, cardiac arrhythmias, trismus, ileus, colic, normal to high body temperature, sweating, and excitation. • In very severe cases, incoordination, recumbency, convulsions, and death.

Dietary Calcium Deficiency or Imbalance

• Clinical signs manifest in the skeletal system.
• Early signs include intermittent shifting-leg lameness, generalized joint tenderness, or stilted gait. • As the disease progresses, abnormal bone formation and enlarged facial bones (e.g., NHP, bighead) occurs.

Cantharidin Toxicosis

• Abdominal pain • GI or urinary tract irritation • Elevated respiratory and heart rates
• Watery feces • Fever • Sweating • Shock

Pancreatic Disease

• Weight loss • Diarrhea • Abdominal pain
• Gastric distention • Shock

CAUSES

Hypoalbuminemia or Hypoproteinemia

• The protein-bound fraction of calcium is directly affected by serum protein concentration; low serum protein concentrations may mask hypercalcemia. • Correction formulas determined for dogs have not been validated in horses.

Dietary Calcium Deficiency or Imbalance

• Occurs from lack of dietary calcium or factors limiting calcium utilization—excess phosphorus (in the form of inorganic phosphorus, phylate phosphate); oxalic acid. • Calcium deficiency may go undetected for many weeks or months; adults have large calcium reserves. • In young animals, skeletal mass does not keep up with increasing body size; the skeleton is more prone to injury. • NHP occurs from low calcium and excess phosphorus intake. • PTH secretion increases a compensatory mechanism to correct disturbance in mineral homeostasis induced by nutritional imbalance. • Rickets occurs from combined calcium and vitamin D deficiency.
• Young, growing animals with vitamin D deficiency may be hypocalcemic, hypophosphatemic, and have elevated ALP. The vitamin D deficiency causes defective mineralization of new bone, resulting in painful swelling of the physis and metaphysis of long bones and costochondral junctions, bowed limbs, and stiff gait. • Natural cases of rickets in foals are not well documented and probably are quite rare.

Cantharidin Toxicosis

Ingestion of alfalfa hay or alfalfa-containing products contaminated with blister beetles (*Epicauta* sp.).

Hypocalcemic Tetany (Lactation, Transport)

• Lactation tetany generally occurs ≅10 days post foaling or 2 days post weaning. • Draft mares, mares that produce large amounts of milk, and mares on pasture only or a marginal plane of nutrition are at greatest risk.
• Prolonged transportation or strenuous activity can predispose to hypocalcemia and tetany.
• Concurrent hypomagnesemia is common in hypocalcemic tetany.

Sepsis and GI Disease

• Sepsis and GI disease are common causes of hypocalcemia. • Endotoxemia may be the underlying stimulus that triggers several mechanisms leading to hypocalcemia. • Plasma calcium concentrations may decline during the postoperative period after abdominal surgery and while receiving IV fluid therapy. • Tendency to hypocalcemia may contribute to reduced GI smooth muscle activity, with gastric fluid accumulation and delayed fecal passage.

Excessive Sweating and Exertional Rhabdomyolysis

• Horses lose calcium, chloride, and potassium in sweat. • Endurance horses are especially prone to electrolyte imbalances and acid–base disturbances (e.g., alkalosis) after prolonged activity, and may develop SDF. • Hypocalcemia has been reported in neonatal foals with severe rhabdomyolysis. • The pathogenesis of hypocalcemia in exertional rhabdomyolysis is not understood.

Renal Disease

Horses with acute renal failure may be hypo-, hyper-, or normocalcemic.

Oxalate Toxicity

Several plant species contain oxalates, which, in excess, reduce calcium absorption.

Pancreatic Disease

• Pancreatic disease is rare in horses. • Acute pancreatitis is difficult to diagnose antemortem.
• Horses in which pancreatic atrophy was the only abnormality at necropsy presented with SDF, tetany, generalized muscle tremors, and hypocalcemia.

RISK FACTORS

See Causes.

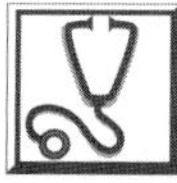

DIAGNOSIS

DIFFERENTIAL DIAGNOSIS

• Diet, reproductive, and exercise history aid in differentiating many of the causes of hypocalcemia. • Tetanus—normal serum calcium, history of wound, does not exhibit SDF, does not respond to treatment with calcium, hyperresponsive to sound, and show prolapse of the third eyelid. • Strychnine—normal serum calcium. • Exertional rhabdomyolysis, myositis–marked increases in CK and AST; myoglobinuria. • Colic—abdominal pain; other signs of GI disease. • Laminitis—extremely painful feet, bounding digital pulses, and characteristic stance.

LABORATORY FINDINGS

Drugs That May Alter Lab Results

EDTA, citrate, or oxalate-containing anticoagulants chelate calcium, causing a false decrease in calcium measurements.

Disorders That May Alter Lab Results

• Of total calcium, ≅50% is bound to protein, predominantly albumin. • Abnormalities in serum albumin or protein concentration directly affect total serum calcium concentration, but the correlation is not as strong in horses as in dogs. Correction formulas determined for dogs have not been validated in horses. • Total serum calcium may be falsely decreased in the face of hypoproteinemia; hyperalbuminemia or hyperproteinemia may obscure hypocalcemia.
• Acid–base status affects the amount of ionized and protein-bound calcium. Acidosis increases the ionized calcium fraction by decreasing the fraction bound to protein; alkalosis decreases ionized calcium by increasing the fraction bound to protein. Total calcium usually remains within the reference range. • Lipemia and hemolysis may falsely elevate total calcium.

Valid If Run in Human Lab?

Yes

CBC/BIOCHEMISTRY/URINALYSIS

• General—Concurrent hypomagnesemia commonly is seen during many conditions associated with hypocalcemia. • Cantharidin toxicosis—hypomagnesemia, hematuria, and normal to isosthenuric urine specific gravity
• Excessive exercise, endurance events, SDF—hypocalcemia, hypokalemia, hypochloremia, and alkalosis • NHP—normal renal function; depending on stage of disease, hypocalcemia, hyperphosphatemia, and elevated ALP • Pancreatic disease—increased amylase, lipase, GGT, and peritoneal amylase

OTHER LABORATORY TESTS

• Total serum calcium is reported with routine biochemical analysis.
• Measurement of ionized calcium concentration by ion-selective electrodes requires special sample handling and may not be readily available.
• Dietary deficiency or imbalance—review of dietary history, inspection of feed, and chemical analysis for calcium and phosphorus.
• NHP—increased urinary phosphorus and decreased urinary calcium concentrations.
• Cantharidin toxicosis—presence of blister beetles in hay; determination of cantharidin in urine or stomach contents is definitive; loss of activity of toxic principal in urine occurs ≅5 days after consumption; urine collected early is most diagnostic.

IMAGING

Conventional radiology has little benefit in detecting loss of skeletal mineralization until losses exceed 30%.

DIAGNOSTIC PROCEDURES N/A

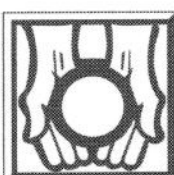

TREATMENT

• General—often symptomatic to control pain with analgesics; maintain hydration with fluids; broad-spectrum antibiotics with suspected bacterial infections; supplementation with high-calcium feeds (e.g., alfalfa, legume hays).
• NHP—correct dietary deficiency or imbalance by supplying the deficient nutrient.
• Cantharidin toxicosis—no antidote available; remove contaminated feed; supportive therapy (e.g., evacuate GI tract, maintain hydration, control pain, diuretics).
• Sources of calcium include alfalfa or legume hay, molasses, limestone, bonemeal, or dicalcium phosphate.
• Dietary calcium:phosphorus ratio should not exceed 1.5–2:1.

MEDICATIONS

DRUGS OF CHOICE

IV calcium solutions—20% calcium borogluconate diluted with saline, dextrose, or lactated Ringer's solution.

CONTRAINDICATIONS N/A

PRECAUTIONS

• Calcium is cardiotoxic.
• Administer solutions containing calcium slowly, with constant monitoring of heart rate and rhythm.
• Stop treatment at once if dysrhythmia or bradycardia develops.
• Rapid IV administration of tetracycline, which chelates calcium, can lead to cardiac arrhythmias, recumbency, sudden collapse and death.
• Furosemide administration promotes urinary calcium and magnesium excretion, which can lead to hypocalcemia.
• Excessive bicarbonate administration causes alkalosis, which decreases calcium.

POSSIBLE INTERACTIONS N/A

ALTERNATIVE DRUGS N/A

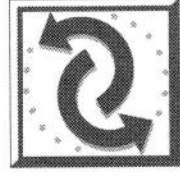

FOLLOW-UP

PATIENT MONITORING

With hypocalcemic tetany, recovery may take several days, and relapses can occur.

POSSIBLE COMPLICATIONS N/A

MISCELLANEOUS

ASSOCIATED CONDITIONS

SDF has been associated with many diseases and conditions—PO administration of large quantities of sodium bicarbonate to hypochloremic and volume-depleted horses, salmonellosis, severe diarrhea, laminitis, abdominal disorders, postoperative rhabdomyolysis, myositis, uterine torsion, lactation tetany, overexertion, cantharidin toxicosis, thoracic hematoma, and trauma.

AGE-RELATED FACTORS

Young animals may be more prone to skeletal abnormalities resulting from dietary deficiency or imbalance.

PREGNANCY

See Causes—hypocalcemic tetany; lactation tetany

SYNONYMS

• NHP—bighead disease, bran disease, osteodystrophia fibrosa, and Miller's disease
• SDF—thumps

SEE ALSO

• Hyperphosphatemia—NHP

ABBREVIATIONS

• ALP = alkaline phosphatase
• AST = aspartate aminotransferase
• CK = creatine kinase
• GGT = γ-glutamyltransferase
• GI = gastrointestinal
• NHP = nutritional secondary hyperparathyroidism
• PTH = parathyroid hormone
• SDF = synchronous diaphragmatic flutter

Suggested Reading

Bertone JJ. Nutritional secondary hyperparathyroidism. In Robinson NE, ed. Current Therapy in Equine Medicine, ed 3. Philadelphia: WB Saunders, 1992:119–122.
Brewer BD. Disorders of equine calcium metabolism. Compend Cont Educ Pract Vet 1987;4:S244-S252.
Capen CC. Nutritional secondary hyperparathyroidism. In: Robinson NE, ed. Current Therapy in Equine Medicine. Philadelphia: WB Saunders, 1983:160–163.
Dart AJ, Snyder JR, Spier SJ, Sullivan KE. Ionized calcium concentration in horses with surgically managed gastrointestinal disease: 147 cases (1988–1990). J Am Vet Med Assoc 1992;1244–1248.
Helman RG, Edwards WC. Clinical features of blister beetle poisoning in equids: 70 cases (1983–1996). J Am Vet Med Assoc 1997;211:1018–1021.
Freestone JF, Melrose PA. Endocrine diseases. In: Kobluk CN, Amers TR, Geor RJ, eds. The Horse: Diseases and Clinical Management. Philadelphia: WB Saunders, 1995:1137–1164.
Toribio RE. Disorders of the endocrine system: Calcium disorders. In: Reed SM, Bayly WM, Sellon DC, eds. Equine Internal Medicine, ed 2. St. Louis: Saunders, 2004:1295–1327.

Author Karen E. Russell
Consulting Editor Kenneth W. Hinchcliff

CANTHARIDIN TOXICOSIS

BASICS

OVERVIEW

- Cantharidin is the toxic compound found in blister beetles (primarily *Epicauta* spp. but also *Pyrota* spp.).
- Toxicosis results from ingestion of baled alfalfa hay, or other alfalfa feeds, containing dead beetles.
- Cantharidin is rapidly absorbed from the GI tract and excreted in the urine.
- The vesicant properties of cantharidin cause irritation, vesicle formation, ulceration, or erosions throughout the GI tract and bladder.
- Colic and/or sudden death
- Hypocalcemia, hypomagnesemia, renal failure, cardiac abnormalities
- Large swarms of blister beetles concentrate in alfalfa fields from the southern United States.

SIGNALMENT

- All ages affected
- No genetic or sex predisposition

SIGNS

- Typically several horses are affected within minutes to hours after feeding alfalfa.
- Severity depends on the amount of cantharidin ingested.
- High doses = sudden death within hours; lower doses = symptoms that last for days
- Restlessness, irritability
- Sweating, fever
- Colic, pawing the ground
- Muscle fasciculations
- Diaphragmatic flutter
- Anorexia, loose stools, oral lesions
- Playing in water without drinking
- Congested mucous membranes, increased capillary refill times
- Tachycardia, tachypnea
- Stranguria, hematuria
- Aggressive behavior
- Seizures before death

CAUSES AND RISK FACTORS

- Feeding of baled alfalfa that has been crimped or alfalfa cubes/pellets increases risk.
- Malicious poisoning has occurred.

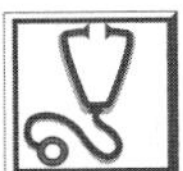

DIAGNOSIS

DIFFERENTIAL DIAGNOSIS

- Colic from a variety of other causes
- Ionophore toxicosis
- History of feeding alfalfa or alfalfa products, hypocalcemia with or without concurrent hypomagnesemia, and discovery of beetles in hay or GI contents

CBC/BIOCHEMISTRY/URINALYSIS

- Hypocalcemia, hypomagnesemia, hyposthenuria
- Hematuria

OTHER LABORATORY TESTS

N/A

IMAGING

N/A

OTHER DIAGNOSTIC PROCEDURES

- Any level of cantharidin detected is considered clinically significant.
- Urine (500 mL) is the specimen of choice for cantharidin analysis; intestinal contents (500 mL) can also be tested.
- Rapid renal clearance (3–4 days)
- Liver, kidney, and serum can be used but are not the specimens of choice.

PATHOLOGICAL FINDINGS

- Large doses can result in sudden death without gross lesions.
- Gross lesions may start in the lips and oral cavity but are most common in the terminal esophagus and stomach, less frequent in the intestines, and consist of areas of ulceration or erosion that may (or may not) be hemorrhagic.
- Reddening of the mucosal lining of the entire GI tract and urinary bladder has been noted.
- White streaks on the heart may be seen grossly.
- Microscopic lesions include acantholysis of mucosa of the GI tract, epithelium of the urinary tract, and endothelium of vessels. Myocarditis, renal tubular nephrosis, and degenerative changes in the kidneys and digestive tract can also be seen.

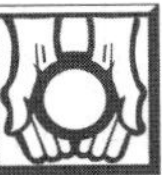

TREATMENT

- Cantharidin toxicosis is an emergency and requires in-hospital treatment.
- Focus treatment on enhancing fecal and urinary elimination of cantharidin, correcting dehydration, managing serum calcium and magnesium abnormalities, and controlling pain.
- Intensive supportive treatment may be required for 3–10 days, depending on the severity of illness.
- Initiate fluid therapy to adequately rehydrate the horse, decrease serum cantharidin levels, and aid in toxin excretion via the kidneys.
- Monitor serum calcium frequently.
- Stall rest for 5–10 days

MEDICATIONS

DRUG(S) OF CHOICE

- Administer AC (1–4 g/kg as an aqueous slurry) via nasogastric tube, then mineral oil (2–4 L) 2–3 hr later to prevent occupation of adsorptive sites on the AC.
- Repeated doses of mineral oil recommended
- Adult horses may receive 500 mL of a commercial calcium-containing fluid (not exceeding 23 g of calcium compound per 100 mL) if administered slowly. Dilute commercial calcium preparations in isotonic fluids to decrease the chance of adverse cardiac responses and to allow more rapid administration. Dilute calcium in a ratio of 1:4 with saline or dextrose if frequent administration is required to control synchronous diaphragmatic flutter or muscle fasciculations.
- Hypomagnesemia may require addition of magnesium as well as calcium to the isotonic fluids.
- Prednisolone sodium succinate (50–100 mg as an initial dose) may be administered IV over 1min for severe shock.

- Consider sucralfate (1 g per 45 kg PO q6–8h) in horses exhibiting clinical signs of gastritis— water playing.
- Commonly prescribed analgesics (e.g., flunixin meglumine) may not provide adequate pain relief. Therefore, administer α_2-adrenergic agonists (e.g., detomidine 20–40 μg/kg IV or butorphanol tartrate 0.02–0.1 mg/kg IV q3–4h, not to exceed 48hr). Detomidine at 40 μg/kg dose should provide analgesia for 45–75 min.
- Xylazine (1.1mg/kg IV) is also an α_2-adrenergic agonist and may be substituted for detomidine for analgesia.
- Use broad-spectrum antibiotic therapy if septic complications from GI mucosal ulceration are likely.

CONTRAINDICATIONS/POSSIBLE INTERACTIONS

- Do not include calcium in fluids containing sodium bicarbonate because of possible precipitation of calcium.
- Aminoglycoside antibiotics are potentially nephrotoxic and should be avoided.
- NSAIDs should be used with caution because of GI and renal complications.
- Diuretics—furosemide
- Acepromazine maleate—may potentiate shock
- Do not administer detomidine concurrently with potentiated sulfonamides (e.g., trimethoprim/sulfa) because fatal dysrhythmias can result.
- Use caution with corticosteroids—they are reported to cause laminitis.

FOLLOW-UP

PATIENT MONITORING

Monitor hydration status, electrolytes, and response to analgesics.

PREVENTION/AVOIDANCE

- Do not feed alfalfa.
- Owners should inspect individual flakes of hay for beetles when feeding.
- Cut hay before the bloom stage so plants do not attract adult blister beetles. First cutting and late cuttings are often safer because they are before and after peak beetle activity, respectively.

POSSIBLE COMPLICATIONS

- Complications are unusual, but laminitis has been reported.
- Any time the heart is damaged, there could be the possibility of sudden death.

EXPECTED COURSE AND PROGNOSIS

- Prognosis ranges from poor to excellent and depends on the amount of cantharidin ingested, early recognition of intoxication, and aggressiveness of therapy.
- A more favorable prognosis may be given if the animal survives for 2–3 days after toxin exposure.

MISCELLANEOUS

PREGNANCY

Use corticosteroids with caution in pregnant mares.

SYNONYMS

- Blister beetle poisoning
- Equine cantharidiasis

Suggested Reading

Gwaltney-Brant SH, Dunayer EK, Youssef HY. Terrestrial zootoxins. In: Gupta RC, ed. Veterinary Toxicology: Basic and Clinical Principles. New York: Elsevier, 2007:785–807.

Stair EL, Plumlee KH. Insects In: Plumlee KH. Clinical Veterinary Toxicology.St. Louis: Mosby, 2004:101–103.

Author Sandra E. Morgan

Consulting Editor Robert H. Poppenga

CARDIOTOXIC PLANTS

BASICS

DEFINITION

• Toxicosis caused by exposure to cardiotoxic plants
• Major toxins are cardiac glycosides, which are found in a number of unrelated plants, such as oleander (*Nerium oleander),* summer pheasant's eye (*Adonis aestivalis*), foxglove (*Digitalis purpurea*), lily-of-the-valley (*Convallaria majalis*), dogbane (*Apocynum* spp.), and some species of milkweed (*Asclepias* spp.).
• Oleander is cultivated widely in the southern United States and is most commonly associated with plant poisonings in horses. Therefore, oleander is discussed in detail as a representative of plants containing cardiac glycosides.
• Other cardiotoxic plants that have resulted in poisoning of horses include yew (*Taxus* spp.), grayanotoxin-containing plants (*Rhododendron* spp., *Kalmia* spp., and *Pieris japonica*), avocado (*Persea* spp.), and death camas (*Zigadenus* spp.).

PATHOPHYSIOLOGY

• Cardiotoxins present in plants cause acute intoxications and are believed to be rapidly absorbed from the gastrointestinal tract.
• Cardiac glycosides cause poisoning by inhibiting the cellular membrane Na^+/K^+-ATPase, which results in an indirect increase in intracellular Ca^{2+} concentrations and a subsequent positive inotropic effect. In addition, direct effects on the sympathetic nervous system are seen.
• Yews contain taxine alkaloids (major alkaloids are taxine A and taxine B) that are rapidly absorbed, metabolized, conjugated in the liver, and eliminated in urine as conjugated benzoic acid (hippuric acid). Taxine alkaloids can cause an increase in cytoplasmic calcium by interfering with both calcium and sodium ion channel conductance across myocardial cells. This results in the depression of cardiac depolarization and conduction. In addition, yews also contain nitriles (cyanogenic glycoside esters), ephedrine, and irritant oils that are likely to be responsible for the colic and diarrhea reported in animals exhibiting a subacute clinical syndrome.
• Grayanotoxins are diterpenes that exert their toxic effect by binding to sodium channels in excitable cell membranes. The resulting increase in membrane permeability to sodium ions maintains excitable cells in a state of depolarization. Accumulation of intracellular sodium results in an exchange with extracellular calcium and plays an important role in the control of transmitter release. The membrane effects caused by grayanotoxins account for the observed responses of skeletal and myocardial muscle, nerves, and the CNS.
• The toxic compound of avocado is called persin, but the exact mechanism of action remains unclear.
• Death camas contains steroidal alkaloids such as zygacine and zygadenine. The alkaloids decrease blood pressure, slow the heart rate, and lead to respiratory depression.

SYSTEMS AFFECTED

• Cardiovascular
• Gastrointestinal

GENETICS

N/A

INCIDENCE/PREVALENCE

• Oleander poisoning is relatively common in horses and is especially reported in California, Arizona, and Texas. Most cases of oleander poisoning are a result of ingestion of dried oleander clippings or oleander-contaminated hay.
• Yew, death camas, and avocado poisoning are relatively uncommon in horses. Poisonings should be suspected if plants are identified in the environment of the horses or found in hay.
• Grayanotoxin poisoning is uncommon in horses.

GEOGRAPHIC DISTRIBUTION

• Cardiotoxic plants have specific distributions in the United States.
• Oleander is commonly found across the southern United States, while summer pheasant's eye has been limited to some northern California counties.
• Grayanotoxins are found in several members of the Ericaceae (heath) family and are widely distributed in the United States. They are often found along the coastal regions as well as in the mountain areas.
• Avocado is extensively cultivated in California and Florida but can also be found as an ornamental in the Gulf Coast areas.
• Many species of death camas occur across the United States and are seasonal, with the greatest abundance being in the spring.

SIGNALMENT

No breed, age, or sex predilections

SIGNS

• Animals exposed to cardiotoxic plants are often found dead.
• Clinical signs of colic are often seen within hours of exposure.
• Progression is rapid and animals develop weakness, tremors, excessive salivation, incoordination, dyspnea, and sometimes convulsions.
• In cardiac glycoside poisonings, animals often have an irregular fast pulse with tachycardia, ventricular arrhythmias, or gallop rhythms.
• *Adonis* spp. poisoning in horses leads to gastrointestinal stasis, feed refusal, dyspnea, and cardiac arrhythmias.
• Horses exposed to avocado develop subcutaneous edema of the head and chest, submandibular edema, respiratory dyspnea, and cardiac arrhythmias.
• Clinical signs of *Taxus* poisoning in horses include incoordination, nervousness, difficulty in breathing, bradycardia, diarrhea, and convulsions, but sudden death is often all that is seen.
• Grayanotoxin poisoning can lead to depression, severe salivation, and abdominal pain. In severe cases, the animals may then become laterally recumbent and develop seizures, tachycardia, tachypnea, and pyrexia.

CAUSES

• Cardiotoxic plants most commonly associated with acute poisoning are oleander and yew.
• All parts of oleander are extremely toxic, whether the plant is fresh or dried. Ingestion of dried oleander clippings is a common source of poisoning. Five to 10 medium-sized oleander leaves can cause illness and death in an adult horse.
• All parts of the yew, green or dried with the exception of the red fleshy part surrounding the seed (aril portion) are toxic. Ingestion of yew clippings is most often the cause of poisonings. All species of *Taxus* are considered toxic.
• Grayanotoxin poisoning usually occurs when animals are offered plant trimmings or stray into wooded areas where little else is available to eat. The leaves of the plants are considered the greatest risk.
• Avocado leaves are especially toxic, but ingestion of fruit and seeds can also result in poisoning.
• Death camas leaves during the early stages of growth pose the greatest risk for poisoning. Seeds and fruits as well as the dried plant in hay are also toxic.

RISK FACTORS

• Fresh plant material is often considered to be of low palatability, so animals are most likely to ingest dried plant material.
• Plant trimmings present the most common source for oleander and yew poisoning.
• Contamination of hay or hay cubes with oleander is of great risk.
• The Guatemalan race of avocados and its hybrid ("Fuerte") are reportedly toxic, while the Mexican race has low toxicity.
• Many species of death camas occur across the United States and are seasonal with the greatest abundance being in the spring.

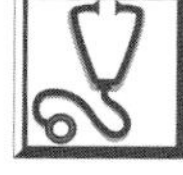

DIAGNOSIS

DIFFERENTIAL DIAGNOSIS

• Ionophore antibiotics—detection of toxic concentrations of ionophores in the feed, histologic lesions
• Cyanide poisoning—Mucous membranes are initially bright cherry red; evidence of exposure to cyanogenic plants, chemical analysis for cyanide in GI contents, liver, or muscle

• Organophosphorus or carbamate insecticide exposure—commonly associated with GI and neurologic signs, evaluation of cholinesterase activity, detection in GI contents
• Exposure to neurotoxic plants, such as poison hemlock, water hemlock, tree tobacco, lupine—chemical analysis for plant toxins in GI contents, history of presence of plants in the environment
• Exposure to star of bethlehem (*Ornithogalum* spp.)—mainly found in the Northeast and Midwest, severe diarrhea, history of presence of plants in the environment
• Myocarditis—Murmurs are usually present; differentiate echocardiographically.
• Endocarditis—fever; differentiate echocardiographically.
• Intestinal compromise (e.g., torsion, intussusception)—physical examination

CBC/BIOCHEMISTRY/URINALYSIS

• Serum chemistry changes are limited.
• Myocardial damage may result in hyperkalemia, elevated LDH, CK, and AST activities, and elevated cardiac troponin I.

OTHER LABORATORY TESTS

• Detection of cardiotoxins in serum, stomach, cecal, or colon contents, and liver
• Visual and microscopic examination of stomach or intestinal contents for plant fragments

IMAGING

N/A

DIAGNOSTIC PROCEDURES

ECG disturbances are supportive—atrioventricular conduction blocks and ventricular arrhythmias

PATHOLOGICAL FINDINGS

• In peracute cases, no lesions are found.
• Post-mortem lesions are generally nonspecific in animals that die. Lesions include reddening of the mucosa of the GI tract and congestion of organs.
• Horses with oleander poisoning have evidence of fluid in the pericardium and body cavities, endocardial hemorrhages, and multifocal myocardial degeneration and necrosis. Mural thrombi and subepicardial hemorrhage can be seen.
• *Taxus* poisoning is associated with mild to moderate endocardial hemorrhages in both ventricles. Histologically, acute multifocal contraction band necrosis of the ventricular wall and the papillary muscles and occasional neutrophilic and lymphocytic infiltrates in the interstitium of the myocardium are noted.
• There are no or very few lesions in cases of yew, grayanotoxin, or death camas poisoning.
• Avocado poisoning can result in fluid accumulation in the pericardial sac and in the thoracic and abdominal cavities. Edema of the gallbladder and perirenal tissues and a flabby, pale heart have been observed.

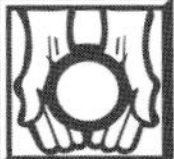

TREATMENT

AIMS OF TREATMENT

• Prevent further exposure to cardiotoxic plant.
• Decontamination
• Provide supportive therapy.

APPROPRIATE HEALTH CARE

• Immediate removal of the toxic plant material to prevent further exposure. Provide the animals with good-quality feed.
• Adsorption of toxins with AC has been suggested. Multidose AC is beneficial in oleander intoxications.
• Treatment of animals exposed to cardiotoxic plants is primarily supportive and symptomatic. Supportive therapy should include administration of IV fluids, antiarrhythmics, and antibiotics if indicated.
• Avoid stress.
• If edema is present in avocado poisoning, administration of diuretics is recommended.
• Atropine should be considered in cases of severe bradycardia.

NURSING CARE

• Decontamination procedures include administration of AC (1–4 g/kg PO in a watery slurry [1 g of AC in 5mL of water]) via stomach tube.
• Correct electrolyte losses according to clinical chemistry findings. Recommended IV fluid in oleander poisoning is 0.9% NaCl with 2.5% dextrose as a continuous rate infusion of 3 mg/kg/hr.

ACTIVITY

Keep the animal quiet.

DIET

Provide high-quality diet free of toxic plants.

CLIENT EDUCATION

• Recognize cardiotoxic plants of concern in the geographic location and prevent access by the horse.
• Provide adequate forage to limit ingestion of toxic plants.

SURGICAL CONSIDERATIONS N/A

MEDICATIONS

DRUG(S) OF CHOICE

• Antiarrhythmics (guided by ECG monitoring)
• Atropine (0.01–0.02 mg/kg IV) to treat bradyarrhythmias
• AC

CONTRAINDICATIONS

• Do not administer potassium in fluids if hyperkalemia is present.
• Avoid calcium-containing solutions and quinidine.

ALTERNATIVE DRUGS

Anticardiac glycoside Fab antibodies have been used in humans and small animals, but their efficacy is unknown in poisoned horses.

FOLLOW-UP

PATIENT MONITORING

Monitor progression of clinical signs and evaluate ECG.

PREVENTION/AVOIDANCE

• Horses should be denied access to landscaped yards and discarded clippings.
• Suspect forage should be inspected for the presence of cardiotoxic plants before allowing access.
• Hay should be inspected carefully for weeds, as many cardiotoxic plants remain toxic when dried (oleander, death camas, yew).

POSSIBLE COMPLICATIONS

N/A

EXPECTED COURSE AND PROGNOSIS

• Animals poisoned with cardiotoxic plants are often found dead.
• Cardiotoxic plant exposure progresses so rapidly that treatment is often too late. In oleander and yew intoxications, the prognosis is poor.
• If treatment is initiated promptly after the onset of clinical signs, the prognosis is fair.
• Animals that survive the acute poisoning may suffer from myocardial damage and may be more prone to stress.

MISCELLANEOUS

ASSOCIATED CONDITIONS

N/A

AGE-RELATED FACTORS, ZOONOTIC POTENTIAL, PREGNANCY

N/A

ABBREVIATION

• AC = activated charcoal

Suggested Reading

Casteel SW. Taxine alkaloids. In: Plumlee KH, ed. Clinical Veterinary Toxicology. St. Louis: Mosby, 2004:379–381.
Galey FG. Cardiac glycosides. In: Plumlee KH, ed. Clinical Veterinary Toxicology. St. Louis: Mosby, 2004:386–388.
Puschner B. Grayanotoxins. In: Plumlee KH, ed. Clinical Veterinary Toxicology. St. Louis: Mosby, 2004:412–415.
Tiwary AK, Puschner B, Kinde H, et al. Diagnosis of Taxus (yew) poisoning in a horse. J Vet Diagn Invest 2005;17:252–255.

Author Birgit Puschner
Consulting Editor Robert H. Poppenga

CASTRATION, HENDERSON CASTRATION INSTRUMENT

BASICS

DEFINITION/OVERVIEW
Surgical removal of the testes

ETIOLOGY/PATHOPHYSIOLOGY
The testes are removed to lessen stallion-like behavior and/or to remove testicular pathology.

SYSTEM AFFECTED
Reproductive

GENETICS
N/A

INCIDENCE/PREVALENCE
N/A

SIGNALMENT
Intact male horses of any age

SIGNS
Historical
Normal testis size, shape, and consistency

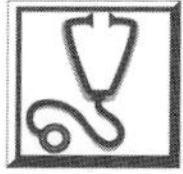

DIAGNOSIS

CAUSES, RISK FACTORS, DIAGNOSIS, DIFFERENTIAL DIAGNOSIS
N/A

CBC/BIOCHEMISTRY/URINALYSIS
Laboratory parameters should be normal prior to routine castration.

OTHER LABORATORY TESTS, IMAGING, DIAGNOSTIC PROCEDURES, PATHOLOGICAL FINDINGS
N/A

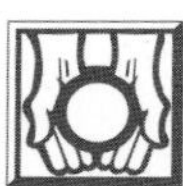

TREATMENT

N/A

APPROPRIATE HEALTH CARE
Routine castration is managed as an on-farm procedure.

NURSING CARE
- Stall confinement for complete recovery from anesthesia.
- Cold water therapy for 15–20 min daily for 3–5 days

ACTIVITY
- Normal activity in the pasture
- Forced exercise twice daily for 20 min for the first 10–12 days

DIET
N/A

CLIENT EDUCATION
- The Equine Henderson Castration Instrument is a relatively new, approved procedure.
- The procedure reduces hemorrhage, swelling, and surgical time.
- See Possible Complications.

SURGICAL CONSIDERATIONS
- The reader is referred to the article: *How to Use the Henderson Castration Instrument and Minimize Castration Complications.*
- Two testes must be present in the scrotum.
- The castration uses a closed technique under general anesthesia.

GENERAL ANESTHESIA
- Preoperative sedation with xylazine (1.0–1.1 mg/kg IV)
- Butorphanol (0.01–0.02 mg/kg IV) may be combined with xylazine to further sedation and analgesia.
- Induction with ketamine hydrochloride (2.2 mg/kg IV), which provides 15–20 min of surgical anesthesia.
- Patient in lateral recumbency with the upper rear limb pulled lateral to expose the testes.

SURGERY
- Three 30-second scrubs of the scrotal area using povidone-iodine (Betadine) and/or chlorhexidine scrub.
- After the second scrub, 2–5 mL of lidocaine is injected into each testis, for further analgesia.
- Two incisions are made over the testes, 1 cm from the midline of the scrotum, and a 3- to 4-cm strip of skin is removed to expose the testes.
- Stripe away the fascia from one exteriorized testicle exposing the spermatic cord to the inguinal ring.
- Insert and secure the Henderson Instrument into a 14.4v cordless hand-drill with a 0.375 removable chuck.
- Place the drill in a sterile shroud.
- Place the pliers of the Henderson on the spermatic cord proximal to the testicle (at the base of testis).
- Rotate (low torque setting) the Henderson in a clockwise direction slowly. Allow the tip of the Henderson Instrument to be drawn into the incision, approximately 2 cm, as it starts to rotate. As the spermatic cord twists, do not allow the instrument to go any farther into the incision. The rotation can be moderately increased, as the cord starts to elongate just before it fractures. Once the cord fatigues and fractures, more tension can be placed on the cord to complete separation and removal of the testis. A tightly coiled cord is left behind, which eliminates bleeding.
- The first testis is removed from the instrument and the other testis is removed in a similar manner. The incision site is inspected for bleeders. Excess fascia and/or fat is removed. The incision is left open and sprayed with a topical antiseptic/spray bandage. The horse is allowed to stand and is put into a stall to complete anesthetic recovery.

MEDICATIONS

DRUG(S) OF CHOICE
- Phenylbutazone (2–4 mg/kg PO or IV) is useful as an anti-inflammatory to help control swelling and pain postoperatively.
- Antibiotic therapy is not needed in a routine uncomplicated castration.
- Tetanus toxoid is a necessary and normal precautionary vaccination.

CONTRAINDICATIONS, PRECAUTIONS, POSSIBLE INTERACTIONS, ALTERNATIVE DRUGS
N/A

FOLLOW-UP

N/A

PATIENT MONITORING:
- The patient should be confined to the stall until the anesthesia has completely worn off, after which 20 min of moderate exercise twice daily should be provided.
- The surgical site should be monitored daily for hemorrhage, evisceration, excessive swelling, and/or infection.

PREVENTION/AVOIDANCE
N/A

POSSIBLE COMPLICATIONS
- Hemorrhage
  - Excessive hemorrhage may occur if too much tension is put on the spermatic cord before it fatigues and fractures.
- Minor hemorrhage occurs from the skin, but should stop within 30 min.
- Treatment for excessive hemorrhage should include identification and ligation of blood vessels.
- Excessive preputial/scrotal swelling results from poor drainage from the scrotum.
  - Tranquilization, surgical scrub, and manually opening the surgical site will allow drainage.
- Moderate forced exercise will help keep the surgical site open and draining.
- Excessive preputial/scrotal swelling may also result from infection. If infected—antibiotics, anti-inflammatory therapy, and drainage of the site are indicated.
- Evisceration of the abdominal contents is an uncommon occurrence, which can be fatal if not treated. The horse should be anesthetized, the intestinal contents cleaned, and viable intestine replaced. The superficial ring should be sutured closed.
- Masculine behavior following castration (with the standard or Henderson technique) is a learned behavior because all sources of testosterone have been removed (testis along with 4–5 cm of spermatic cord).

EXPECTED COURSE AND PROGNOSIS
N/A

MISCELLANEOUS

ASSOCIATED CONDITIONS, AGE-RELATED FACTORS, ZOONOTIC POTENTIAL, PREGNANCY
N/A

SYNONYMS
Gelding

Suggested Reading

Reilly MT, Cimetti LJ. How to use the Henderson Castration Instrument and minimize castration complications. Proc AAEP 2005;51.

Author Alfred B. Caudle
Consulting Editor Carla L. Carleton

CASTRATION, ROUTINE

BASICS

DEFINITION/OVERVIEW

Surgical removal of the testes

ETIOLOGY/PATHOPHYSIOLOGY

The testes are removed mainly to lessen stallion-like behavior.

SYSTEM AFFECTED

Reproductive

SIGNALMENT

Intact male horses of any age

SIGNS

Historical

• Normal testis size, shape, and consistency
• Reduced fertility • Pain (spermatic cord torsion, testicular torsion) • Failure to breed, walk, or jump without discomfort (performance affected)

PHYSICAL EXAMINATION

• Increased or decreased size, shape, and texture
• Abnormal testis position • Enlargement in scrotum and/or contents

CAUSES AND RISK FACTORS

• Diseased testis • Trauma to scrotum and/or testis • Cryptorchidism • Torsion of the testis
• Neoplasia • Hydrocele/hematocele
• Orchitis/epididymitis

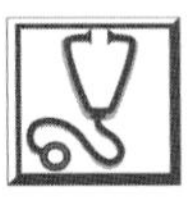

DIAGNOSIS

N/A

DIFFERENTIAL DIAGNOSIS

Normal testis

CBC/BIOCHEMISTRY/URINALYSIS

Laboratory parameters should be normal prior to routine castration.

OTHER LABORATORY TESTS, IMAGING, DIAGNOSTIC PROCEDURES, PATHOLOGICAL FINDINGS

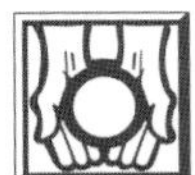

TREATMENT

APPROPRIATE HEALTH CARE

Routine castration is managed as an on-farm procedure.

NURSING CARE

• Stall confinement for complete recovery from anesthesia. • Cold water therapy for 15–20 min daily for 3–5 days.

ACTIVITY

• Normal activity in the pasture • Forced exercise BID for 20 min for the first 10–12 days.

CLIENT EDUCATION

• Six to 8 hr post-surgery, the horse needs moderate exercise (20 min BID), e.g., walking or at trot. • See Possible Complications.

SURGICAL CONSIDERATIONS

• Two testes must be present in the scrotum.
• Castration can be performed standing using local anesthesia or in lateral recumbency under general anesthesia. Standing castration has the advantage that recovery following surgery is faster and with less risk of injury during anesthetic recovery. Castration using general anesthesia, placing the animal in lateral recumbency, allows for greater safety for the surgeon, better exposure to the surgical site, and much better analgesia. • Closed technique (vaginal tunic is not incised) versus open technique (vaginal tunic is opened and the testes are completely exposed) can be standing or under general anesthesia.

General Anesthesia

• Preoperative sedation with xylazine (1.0–1.1 mg/kg IV) • Butorphenol (0.01–0.02 mg/kg IV) may be used combine with xylazine to achieve further sedation and analgesia. • Induction with ketamine hydrochloride (2.2 mg/kg IV), which provides 15–20 min of surgical anesthesia
• Patient in lateral recumbency with the upper rear limb pulled lateral, exposing the testes

Surgical Procedure

• Three 30-second scrubs of the scrotal area using povidine-iodine (Betadine) and/or chlorhexidine scrub • Following the second scrub, 2–3 mL of lidocaine is injected into each testis or spermatic cord, to achieve further analgesia. • Two incisions are made over the testes, 1 cm from the midline of the scrotum, and a 3- to 4-cm strip of skin is removed exposing the testes. • Strip away the fascia from one exteriorized testicle to expose the spermatic cord to the inguinal ring. • *Closed technique*—The emasculators are placed as close to the body wall as possible, removing as much of the cord as possible, and emasculated. • *Open technique*—The tunic over the testis is excised and the testis is exposed. The emasculators are placed closed to the body wall on the artery, vein, and nerve of the exposed cord and are emasculated followed by the exposed tunic, which is emasculated close to the body wall.
• The other testis is removed using either the closed or open technique.
  ○ In large stallions, the mesorchium should be separated above the epididymis and the cord separated into the neurovascular and musculofibrous (cremaster muscle, vaginal tunic, and ductus deferens) portions before emasculation.
• Following emasculation, maintain hold on one side of the stump to keep it in view and observe it for any bleeding. If there is no bleeding from the site, the incision is inspected to ensure that it is open and will drain readily (to avoid serum accumulation). • Remove any loose tags of fascia or fat that protrude from the incision. • Spray the area with an antiseptic solution and fly spray.

MEDICATIONS

DRUG(S) OF CHOICE

• Phenylbutazone (2–4 mg/kg PO or IV) is useful as an anti-inflammatory to help control swelling and pain postoperatively. • Antibiotic therapy is not needed for a routine, uncomplicated castration. • Tetanus toxoid +/− antitoxin depending on vaccination history

FOLLOW-UP

PATIENT MONITORING

• The patient should be confined to a stall until anesthetic recovery is complete, after which time 20 min of moderate, daily forced exercise BID should be provided. • The surgical site should be monitored daily for hemorrhage, evisceration, excessive swelling, and/or infection.

POSSIBLE COMPLICATIONS

• Minor hemorrhage occurs through the skin, which should stop within 30 min. • Treatment for excessive hemorrhage is identification and ligation of bleeding vessels. • Excessive preputial/scrotal swelling results from poor drainage from the scrotum.
  ○ Tranquilization, surgical scrub, and manually opening (stretching) the surgical site will facilitate drainage.
  ○ Moderate forced exercise is the best means to ensure the surgical site will remain open and draining.
  ○ Excessive preputial/scrotal swelling may also result from infection. If infected, antibiotics, anti-inflammatory therapy, and drainage of the site are indicated.
• Evisceration of the abdominal contents is an uncommon occurrence, which can be fatal if left untreated. The horse should be anesthetized and the intestinal contents cleaned and viable intestine replaced. The superficial inguinal ring should be sutured closed.
• Masculine behavior following castration is a reflection of learned behavior. Removal of the testes (verify by examining all tissues following emasculation) has eliminated the source of testosterone.

MISCELLANEOUS

SYNONYM

Gelding

Suggested Reading

McKinnon AO, Voss JL. Equine Reproduction. Philadelphia: Lea & Febiger, 1992.

Author Alfred B. Caudle
Consulting Editor Carla L. Carleton

CENTAUREA SPP. TOXICOSIS

BASICS

OVERVIEW

- *Centaurea solstitialis* (yellow star thistle) is an annual weed found commonly in the northwestern United States. The plant is about 1 m in height. The flower is yellow with a composite head and sharp thorns around the flower head.
- *Centaurea repens* (Russian knapweed) is a perennial weed found mainly in the western United States; it can appear in the eastern United States as well. The plant is about 1 m in height and has a cone-shaped flowering head that is pinkish-purple with spreading rhizomes, which make control difficult. In general, it is not readily grazed.
- Ingestion of either plant can result in ENE, or "chewing disease," characterized by the abrupt appearance of difficulties in eating and drinking. Typically, affected animals lose condition and die.

SIGNALMENT

There is no breed, age, or sex predilection.

SIGNS

- Drowsiness
- Difficulty eating and drinking
- Aimless walking with head low
- Hypertonicity of facial and lip muscles
- Tongue lolling
- Loss of body condition
- Dehydration
- Death

CAUSES AND RISK FACTORS

- Toxic principal is not conclusively identified, although it is suspected to be a sesquiterpene lactone.
- A lethal dose of fresh plant material has been given as 2.3–2.6 kg/100 kg body weight for *C. solstitialis* and 1.8–2.5 kg/100 kg body weight for *C. repens.*

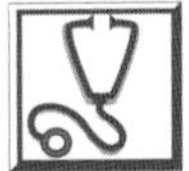

DIAGNOSIS

DIFFERENTIAL DIAGNOSIS

- Teeth or mouth abnormalities
- Other chronic disease processes

CBC/BIOCHEMISTRY/URINALYSIS

N/A

OTHER LABORATORY TESTS

N/A

IMAGING

MRI can be used to identify brain lesion.

DIAGNOSTIC PROCEDURES

- Positive identification of plants
- Evidence of consumption of *C. solstitialis* or *C. repens*

PATHOLOGICAL FINDINGS

Nigropallidal encephalomalacia—foci of necrotic tissue found in the brain, specifically in the globus pallidus and substantia nigra

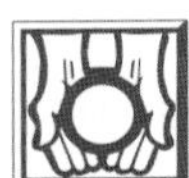

TREATMENT

- Removal from pasture or source of plants
- Supportive care

MEDICATIONS

DRUG(S) OF CHOICE

N/A

CONTRAINDICATIONS/POSSIBLE INTERACTIONS

N/A

FOLLOW-UP

Remove any nonaffected animals from suspect source.

MISCELLANEOUS

ABBREVIATION

- ENE = equine nigropallidal encephalomalacia

Suggested Reading

Burrows GE, Tyrl RJ. Toxic Plants of North America. Ames, IA: Iowa State University Press, 2001:156–160.

Author Larry J. Thompson
Consulting Editor Robert H. Poppenga

CEREBELLAR ABIOTROPHY

BASICS

DEFINITION

Disease associated with cerebellar dysfunction identified at birth or early in life

PATHOPHYSIOLOGY

Abiotrophy means "premature degeneration." Cerebellar abiotrophy may be an inherited metabolic defect of cortical cerebellar neurons in some breeds. The result is formation and then premature death of these neurons during late fetal or early postnatal life resulting in a cerebellum that may be normal at birth and degenerates thereafter. Degeneration can start in utero. The central nervous system is affected.

SIGNALMENT

• Foals may be affected at birth, but often disease is not evident until a few months of age.
• Cerebellar abiotrophy occurs in lines of Arabian horses and has been seen in Oldenburg, Gotland and Eriskay foals.

Historical

These clinical syndromes, for the most part, are not congenital. Affected animals have a normal gait for a period postnatally, then demonstrate a syndrome related to progressive cerebellar degeneration.

Physical Examination

The cerebellum processes peripheral proprioceptive input and coordinates the quality of motor activity through its efferent pathways; simplistically, it "tones down" somatic upper motor neurons in the brainstem. A basewide stance and hypermetric or hypometric ataxia may be prominent; some affected animals show hypometric gait at a walk, which becomes hypermetric at faster gaits. As with many neurologic diseases that result in abnormal gait in large animals, affected animals may pace. No weakness occurs. Severely affected animals may use their noses to assist in posturing. A head bob, intention tremor, and, in many cases, especially the Arabian horses, an absent menace response with intact vision and pupillary light reflexes are present.

CAUSES AND RISK FACTORS

The causes of these diseases are unknown, but there is a hereditary implication. Risk factors are unknown.

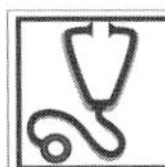

DIAGNOSIS

Signalment and clinical signs. Necropsy will be definitive.

DIFFERENTIAL DIAGNOSIS

• Cerebellar hypoplasia—i.e., cerebellum that is small at birth with no further signs of degeneration—is extremely rare in horses.
• Cerebellar dysfunction due to a structural lesion; rare.

CBC/BIOCHEMISTRY/URINALYSIS

No specific abnormalities

IMAGING

A small cerebellum may be evident on advanced (CT or MRI) imaging.

PATHOLOGIC FINDINGS

On gross post-mortem examination, the cerebellum weighs less than 10% of the whole brain weight. Histologically, evidence of degenerative Purkinje and granular cells and swollen Purkinje axons (torpedoes) may be prominent.

PROGNOSIS

Poor; this is a progressive condition.

Suggested Reading

deBowes RM, et al. Cerebellar abiotrophy. Vet Clin North Am 1987;3:345–352.

Hahn CN, Mayhew IG, MacKay RJ. The nervous system. In: Collahan PT, Mayhew IG, Merritt AM, Moore JN, eds. Equine Medicine and Surgery, ed 5. St. Louis: Mosby, 1999.

Palmer AC, Blakemore WF, Cook WR, Platt H, Whitwell KE. Cerebellar hypoplasia and degeneration in the young Arab horse: Clinical and neuropathological features. Vet Rec 1973;93:62–66.

Author Caroline N. Hahn
Consulting Editor Caroline N. Hahn

CERVICAL LESIONS

BASICS

DEFINITION/OVERVIEW

• Most common problems encountered—inflammation, lacerations and adhesions, and inability to dilate during estrus
• Congenital abnormalities and neoplasia of the cervix are rare.

ETIOLOGY/PATHOPHYSIOLOGY

• The thick circular muscular layer of the cervix, when normal, is responsible for expansion and contraction.
• Lesions may impair normal cervical function and competency, leading to infertility, repeated uterine infections, and possible pregnancy loss.

SYSTEM AFFECTED

Reproductive

GENETICS

N/A

INCIDENCE/PREVALENCE

More common in old and/or pluriparous mares

SIGNALMENT

• Old (mean age, 12–13 years), pluriparous mares (mean parity before surgery, 6.2 years) after either normal parturition or dystocia
• Old, pluriparous mares are more predisposed to cervicitis caused by pneumovagina, urovagina, or delayed uterine clearance.
• Young or old, nervous, maiden mares

SIGNS

Historical

• Infertility
• Recurrent uterine infections
• Pyometra
• Pregnancy loss

Physical Examination

• Vaginal examination—pneumovagina or urovagina; vaginal discharge; purulent material coming through the cervix; cervical and vaginal mucosal irritation; cervical lacerations or mucosal roughness; adhesions between the cervix and vaginal fornix or in the cervical lumen; intrauterine fluid accumulation, with or without cervical adhesions
• Intrauterine fluid accumulation after breeding

CAUSES

Infectious

• Associated with anatomic abnormalities (e.g., pneumovagina), vaginitis, and endometritis
• Severe acute cervicitis after inoculation/infection with *Taylorella equigenitalis* (CEM)
• See also Endometritis and Placentitis.

Noninfectious

Cervical Trauma
• Frequently occurs, resulting in full- or partial-thickness lacerations, during unassisted, prolonged parturition or dystocia (assisted, difficult foaling)
• Prolonged manipulation and traction, extended fetal pressure against the cervical walls, and use of a fetotome aggravate the outcome.
• Lacerations most frequently occur in the vaginal portion of the cervix but may extend toward the uterus, to and including the internal cervical os.
Two Types of Lacerations
• Overstretching or partial-thickness laceration of the muscular layer with intact mucosa
• Full-thickness laceration
Adhesions
• May be a sequel of cervical trauma during parturition or originate from use of irritating solutions for uterine therapy, pyometra, and, rarely, chronic endometritis
• May obliterate the cervical lumen and prevent it from opening and closing properly
Cervicitis
• May be iatrogenic (e.g., chemical substances) or secondary to trauma (e.g., parturition, dystocia, obstetric manipulation) or infection (e.g., vaginitis, endometritis)
• Individual sensitivity exists to use of diluted iodine, chlorhexidine, or acetic acid. These products may produce mucosal irritation, ulceration, and necrosis, even at low dilutions.
• May occur following the use of nonbuffered aminoglycosides, antibiotics, or antimycotics for endometritis
• Pneumovagina and urovagina result in vaginal, cervical, and uterine irritation.
Idiopathic
• Some maiden mares (young or old) show impaired cervical relaxation during estrus.
• No associated fibrosis or adhesions
• Affects ability to conceive by natural breeding and causes delayed uterine clearance
• Once affected mares conceive, the cervix dilates normally at parturition.
Neoplasia
• Very rare
• Uterocervical leiomyoma has been reported.
Developmental Abnormalities
Rare
Congenital Incompetency
Cervical aplasia, hypoplasia, and double cervix

RISK FACTORS

• Pluriparous and old mares
• Prolonged natural or assisted parturition
• >2 to 3 cuts with the fetotome
• Young or old maiden mares
• Aggressive uterine therapy
• Concurrent acute and chronic endometritis
• Pyometra

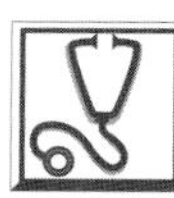

DIAGNOSIS

DIFFERENTIAL DIAGNOSIS

Other causes of vaginal discharge
• Endometritis
• Pyometra
• Placentitis

CBC/BIOCHEMISTRY/URINALYSIS

N/A

OTHER LABORATORY TESTS

N/A

IMAGING

U/S—fluid accumulation in the uterine lumen caused by a tight cervix (e.g., while still in estrus, after breeding) or adhesions

OTHER DIAGNOSTIC PROCEDURES

Cervical Examination

• The cervix is examined by TRP, direct visualization with a speculum, and direct vaginal/digital palpation. The latter is recommended over speculum examination.
• TRP—determines the size, tone, and degree of relaxation
• Vaginoscopy—provides information regarding cervical and vaginal color (e.g., hyperemia), presence of edema, secretions (e.g., pus, urine), cysts, varicose veins, or adhesions between the cervical os and vagina
• Digital palpation of the cervix is essential to evaluate lacerations or intraluminal adhesions. It is performed by placing the index finger into the cervical lumen and the thumb on the vaginal side of the cervix, then feeling carefully for defects around its full perimeter.
• To assess cervical patency, ability to relax, and the presence of intraluminal adhesions, perform cervical evaluation during estrus.
• To evaluate cervical closure and tone and for the presence and extent of lacerations, conduct the assessment during diestrus.
• During the noncycling phase of the year, mares can be placed on exogenous progesterone for 7 days to evaluate cervical tone, competency, and its ability to close.
• Only major defects can be detected in postpartum mares. Allow at least 7 days for substantial involution, reduction in size, and for normal postpartum inflammation to subside.

Timing of Repair in Postpartum Mares

• Postpartum mares may be evaluated for surgical readiness ≥30 days after foaling (i.e., after the 30-day heat) to allow for normal cervical involution.
  ○ Alternatively, if a mare has foaled normally, apart from its recurrent cervical tear, breeding earlier can readily be accomplished—skip foal heat, short-cycle, and AI on the next estrus, with daily or every-other-day serial TRP and US to determine the day of ovulation.
  ○ Surgical repair is ideally accomplished within 24–48 hr after ovulation.
  ○ It must occur ≤72 hr after ovulation, such that inflammation induced by the surgical procedure will have abated before entry of the embryo into the uterus by 5.5–6 days.
  ○ The use of progesterone supplementation, even double dose, is recommended during surgery and single dose, for a longer/prolonged period, if the mare is pregnant.
  ○ NSAIDs and antibiotics are also warranted in the perisurgical time period.
  ○ There is no need, nor should one attempt, to evaluate the repair before the mare's 14-day pregnancy check but not later than 30 days.
  ○ If the repair has been unsuccessful, considerations to terminate the pregnancy before endometrial cups develop may be appropriate.
  ○ If normal cervical tone and competency have been restored and the mare is found to be pregnant, further cervical examination is unnecessary at that time.

PATHOLOGICAL FINDINGS N/A

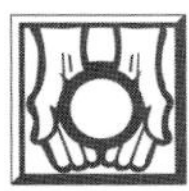

TREATMENT

APPROPRIATE HEALTH CARE

- Mucosal and submucosal lacerations are treated daily with antimicrobial/steroidal anti-inflammatory ointment to avoid cervical adhesions.
- Recently formed adhesions are manually debrided daily, and ointment is applied BID.
- Mature cervical adhesions may be bypassed by AI or reduced surgically, with guarded prognosis for fertility.
- Begin treatment of cervical lacerations immediately postpartum to prevent adhesions and infection.
- Infection—see Endometritis and Placentitis.
- Idiopathic—AI and treatment for delayed uterine clearance. If natural breeding is necessary, dilate the cervix manually or use prostaglandin E_1 (Misoprostol).

NURSING CARE

Treatment-induced inflammation—When using antiseptics or nonbuffered antibiotics, check for signs of acute mucosal irritation before administering subsequent treatments. If inflammation is present, it may be preferred to cease additional intrauterine therapy and change to systemic treatment.

ACTIVITY N/A

DIET N/A

CLIENT EDUCATION

- Routine postpartum evaluation of the reproductive tract of the mare, especially when there is a history of assisted, prolonged manipulation, or unassisted, traumatic parturition.
- Increase the likelihood of early identification of traumatic injuries and avoid loss of the breeding season.

SURGICAL CONSIDERATIONS

- Surgical repair may not be required when <50% of the vaginal portion of the cervix is affected (i.e., stretching, partial- or full-thickness lacerations not compromising the competency of the internal cervical os). Progesterone supplementation, beginning prior to the embryo's arrival and migration into the uterus, may provide sufficient benefit by increasing cervical tone, such that surgery is not required to overcome minor anatomic/functional damage.
- Cervical repair may be warranted for small cervical lacerations coupled with a history of infertility.
- Surgical repair is required for longitudinal, full- or partial-thickness lacerations within the cervical muscle, progressing cranially, that involve the junction of the external portion of the cervix with the vagina and therefore affect the ability of the cervix to close.
- With a successful surgical repair, prognosis is fair to good for delivering a term foal.
- Mild intraluminal adhesions are usually found after surgery. Apply ointment with antibiotics and steroids if not pregnant.
- Perform endometrial biopsy before surgery to evaluate the endometrium (biopsy category). Unnecessary repair and expense can be avoided if it is found that surgery cannot improve the mare's ability to carry a fetus to term.
- Anatomic defects resulting in cervicitis, such as pneumovagina and urovagina, should be surgically corrected.

MEDICATIONS

DRUG(S) OF CHOICE

- Progestin supplementation altrenogest
    - Double dose (0.088 mg/kg PO daily) during surgery
- Single dose (0.044 mg/kg PO daily) until 90–110 days gestation
- Systemic and oral antibiotics

See Endometritis.

- NSAIDs
    - Flunixin meglumine—anti-inflammatory dose, 1 mg/kg IV or IM BID
    - Phenylbutazone—2.2–4.4 mg/kg IV or PO BID
- Prostaglandin E_1 for cervical relaxation

Misoprostol 2000 μg/3 mL tube intracervically 4 hr before breeding. Cervix will be dilated for 8 hr. Less effective in older mares with previous cervical trauma. Frequent application produces irritation.

- Local therapy
    - Panalog ointment (anti-inflammatory, antibiotic, and antifungal). Frequency of application is based on severity of lesion or adhesions, from 3 times to once daily.

CONTRAINDICATIONS

See Endometritis.

PRECAUTIONS

- Be careful using antiseptics or nonbuffered antibiotics to treat infections of the vagina, cervix, or uterus.
- Minimize forced extraction during dystocia, use ample lubrication, and consider cesarean section in cases with intractable cervical induration, poor dilation of the birth canal, as well as with large, deformed, or contracted foals.

FOLLOW-UP

PATIENT MONITORING

- Do not examine the cervix for competency or patency until >2–4 weeks after surgical repair.
- Thirty days of sexual rest are recommended before AI or natural breeding. If live cover is necessary (i.e., Thoroughbreds), the use of a stallion roll is advised to limit full intromission by the stallion during cover.

PREVENTION/AVOIDANCE

- Unnecessary manipulation during parturition
- Use of irritants
- Check for normalcy of anatomic barriers that protect the genital tract (perineum, vulva, vestibulovaginal sphincter, and cervix), and repair any defects identified.

POSSIBLE COMPLICATIONS

- The scar/site of repair lacks the elasticity of normal cervical tissue. A high percentage will tear again at the next foaling and require annual surgical repair after foaling.
- The decision to perform subsequent surgeries is based on the degree of cervical damage after the most recent foaling, assessment of surgical cost, and breeding/treatment expenses versus the potential value of an additional foal.

EXPECTED COURSE AND PROGNOSIS

- Fair to good for maintenance of pregnancy after successful repair of cervical lacerations
- Guarded prognosis if repair was extensive or unsuccessful

MISCELLANEOUS

ASSOCIATED CONDITIONS

N/A

AGE-RELATED FACTORS

Most common in old, pluriparous mares and young or old maiden mares

ZOONOTIC POTENTIAL

N/A

PREGNANCY

See Expected Course and Prognosis.

SEE ALSO

- Artificial insemination
- Dystocia
- Endometritis
- Delayed uterine involution
- Pyometra

ABBREVIATIONS

- AI = artificial insemination
- CEM = contagious equine metritis
- TRP = transrectal palpation
- U/S = ultrasound/ultrasonography

Suggested Reading

Blanchard TL, Varner D, Schumacher J. Surgery of the mare reproductive tract. In: Manual of Equine Reproduction. St. Louis: Mosby–Year Book, 1998:165–167.

Sertich PL. Cervical problems in the mare. In: McKinnon AO, Voss JL, eds. Equine Reproduction. Philadelphia: Lea & Febiger, 1993:404–407.

Author Maria E. Cadario

Consulting Editor Carla L. Carleton

CERVICAL VERTEBRAL MALFORMATION

BASICS

OVERVIEW

CVM causes spinal cord compression. It is one of the most common causes of ataxia in horses in Europe and Australasia and is an important differential diagnosis in regions affected by inflammatory diseases such as equine protozoal myeloencephalitis and West Nile virus.

SIGNALMENT

- CVM is reported to be either due to developmental bone disease (type 1 CVM, more common in young lightbreed and Warmblood horses) or secondary to osteoarthritis of caudal cervical intervertebral joints (type 2 CVM, associated with somewhat older horses).There can be an overlap of these classifications. Affected horses are often large-frame, fast-growing horses that are usually described as large for their age.
- The genetic basis of this disease is still under debate. It is thought that there is at least a predisposition for the disease. Breeding trials involving both affected males and females have been unable to produce CVM cases; however, offspring did have a higher prevalence of OCD lesions in other joints.

SIGNS

- Neurological signs include progressive weakness and ataxia and can be acute in onset. Early in the course of the disease, it will only be evident in the pelvic limbs, but as the disease progresses, it will involve the thoracic limbs as well. The pelvic limbs appear more severely affected because pelvic limb proprioceptive tracts are more superficial in the spinal cord, and are compressed first.
- The neurological signs are due to proprioceptive and upper motor neuron deficits resulting in weakness and ataxia. These are characterized by knuckling of the fetlocks, toe dragging, a base wide stance, swaying of the body when moving, dysmetria, circumduction of the outside pelvic limb when tightly circled, and stepping on its own feet. These signs are usually bilaterally symmetrical.

CAUSES AND RISK FACTORS

- Osteochondrosis—commonly associated disease in affected horses. Can occur in multiple limbs and vertebral joints.
- Fast, excessive growth
- Overnutrition/nutritional imbalances—Predisposed foals have been shown to not develop clinical signs when put on near-starvation diets.

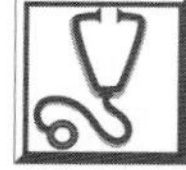

DIAGNOSIS

DIFFERENTIAL DIAGNOSIS

- Cervical fractures—History and/or evidence of trauma. Cervical radiographs.
- EPM: CSF and serum antibody titers
- EDM: young animals with history of low vitamin E status
- EHV-1—History of respiratory illness in other horses, cauda equina signs, viral identification using PCR or culture, CSF titers, CSF xanthochromia, rapidly progressive disease

IMAGING

Standing plain film lateral cervical radiographs—must be absolutely lateral

Type 1 CVM

- In some cases, the diagnosis can be made by the recognition of obvious vertebral malformation and malarticulation.
- To correct for magnification, measure the minimum width of vertebral canal and the width of the widest portion of the epiphysis of the cranial vertebral body. Divide the width of the canal by the width of the body. As a general guide, compression of the spinal cord is unlikely if the diameter of the vertebral canal is greater than half the diameter of the vertebral body.
- Myelography may contribute additional information and probably should be performed if the horse is going to surgery; however, it is rarely necessary in order to make the diagnosis.

Type 2 CVM

- The spinal cord in type 2 CVM is compressed secondary to arthritis of the caudal (C6-T1) cervical vertebrae. The diagnosis is made by finding enlarged and remodeled intervertebral joints of the caudal cervical vertebrae, although the specificity of the technique is low due to many normal older horses having similar radiographic changes.
- Myelography may be helpful; however, some of the compressions are in the lateral direction, while caudal cervical myelographs can only be evaluated in the lateral plane (lateral compressions are more evident on films taken in the dorsoventral plane).

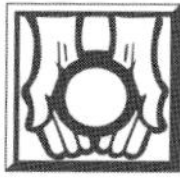

TREATMENT

- Conservative therapy—Horses that are overtly ataxic will never recover completely. Horses will become stronger with time but owners must be counseled of the risk of injury to the handler even if the horse is retired to pasture.
- Surgical—Ventral cervical vertebral stabilization. This procedure uses a stainless steel basket filled with cancellous bone graft to fuse the vertebrae. This has proved successful for both forms of CVM. The procedure is most successful in younger and mildly affected horses. Horses can take up to a full year to show improvement of neurological deficits; some never fully recover but still become athletes. Owners should be aware that this is a long-term commitment and there are still liability issues involved if the horse is put into training.

MEDICATIONS

None indicated; corticosteroids give no long-term benefit.

FOLLOW-UP

PATIENT MONITORING

Repeated assessment of ataxia and upper motor neuron weakness

PREVENTION/AVOIDANCE

Avoid overfeeding rapidly growing foals.

POSSIBLE COMPLICATIONS

Falling on rider and handler a serious risk

EXPECTED COURSE AND PROGNOSIS

Once clinical signs are seen, prognosis is hopeless unless surgery is undertaken.

MISCELLANEOUS

ASSOCIATED CONDITIONS

- Osteochondritis dissecans

AGE-RELATED FACTORS

- Often seen when first put to work (2–4 years old) or in horses >10 years old (type 2 CVM)

SEE ALSO

- EHV-1

ABBREVIATIONS

- CSF = cerebrospinal fluid
- CVM (some use CSM) = cervical vertebral malformation
- OCD = osteochondrosis
- EPM = equine protozoal myeloencephalitis
- EDM = equine degenerative myeloencephalopathy
- EHV-1 = equine herpesvirus 1

Suggested Reading

Hahn CN, Mayhew IG, MacKay RJ. The nervous system. In: Collahan PT, Mayhew IG, Merritt AM, Moore JN, eds. Equine Medicine and Surgery, ed 5. St Louis: Mosby, 1999.

van Biervliet J, Scrivani PV, Divers TJ, Erb HN, de Lahunta A, Nixon A. Evaluation of decision criteria for detection of spinal cord compression based on cervical myelography in horses: 38 Cases (1981–2001). Equine Vet J 2004;36:14–20.

The author and editor wish to acknowledge the contribution of R. Jay Bickers, author of this chapter in the previous edition.

Author Caroline N. Hahn
Consulting Editor Caroline N. Hahn

CESTRUM DIURNUM (DAY-BLOOMING JESSAMINE) TOXICOSIS

BASICS

OVERVIEW

- *Cestrum diurnum* L. (day-blooming jessamine) is a large shrub with alternate, simple leaves having smooth margins and lanceolate or elliptic in shape.
- The fragrant and showy blooms are ≅2.5 cm in length and are five-parted flowers that appear in axillary clusters. The flowers are white and sweet-scented in the day.
- The fruit is a small berry that is spheric and black when mature.
- The plant, introduced into the United States from the West Indies, prefers warmer areas, and is used as an ornamental in the South. It also may be found wild in the Florida Keys and in south Texas.
- The plant is a member of the Solanaceae family and contains several toxins. The unripe berry contains solanine, a GI irritant, and a cholinesterase-inhibiting glycoalkaloid. The ripe berry contains tropane alkaloids. Traces of saponins and nicotine are found as well.
- The agent of greatest concern is 1,25-dihydroxy vitamin D glucoside, which is found at high concentrations in the leaves; 1,25-dihydroxy vitamin D is the active metabolite of vitamin D.
- Ingestion of the plant results in hypercalcemia secondary to excessive calcium absorption and metastatic tissue calcification.

SIGNALMENT

N/A

SIGNS

- Progressive weight loss and lameness, increasing in severity during a 2- to 6-mo period
- Affected horses become stiff, are reluctant to move, and develop a short, choppy gait.
- Reluctance to move is especially evident when turning.
- Flexor and suspensory ligaments sensitive to palpation
- Slight to moderate kyphosis
- Elevated pulse and respiratory rates

CAUSES AND RISK FACTORS

N/A

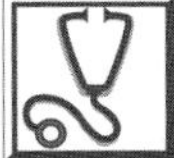

DIAGNOSIS

DIFFERENTIAL DIAGNOSIS

Vitamin D intoxication from other sources: historical or laboratory evidence of vitamin D oversupplementation; evidence of plant ingestion

CBC/BIOCHEMISTRY/URINALYSIS

- Hypercalcemia
- Serum phosphorus remains within normal limits.

OTHER LABORATORY TESTS

N/A

IMAGING

Evidence of tissue calcification

OTHER DIAGNOSTIC PROCEDURES

N/A

PATHOLOGICAL FINDINGS

Gross

- Hypervitaminosis D results in widespread soft-tissue mineralization (i.e., calcification), especially in arteries, ligaments, and tendons.
- Forelimb flexor tendons are more severely affected than those of the pelvic limb; however, all suspensory ligaments are calcified.
- Calcification occurs in the kidneys and lungs but is not a consistent finding.
- Cardiac calcification can occur, with the most severely calcified portion of the heart being the left atrium.
- Generalized osteoporosis and emaciation

Histopathologic

Hyperplasia of the parathyroid chief cells (i.e., C-cells)

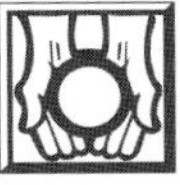

TREATMENT

- No documented efficacious treatment
- Promote diuresis and calciuresis with normal saline.

MEDICATIONS

DRUGS

- Promote diuresis and calciuresis with furosemide (1 mg/kg IV initial dose; if no increase in urine output is noted within 1 hr, the dose can be increased to 5 to 10 mg/kg IV; 1–3 mg/kg IV BID to QID). However, care should be taken to ensure that the horse does not become dehydrated. Preferable means of inducing diuresis is administration of isotonic, calcium-free fluids.
- Corticosteroids decrease bone release and intestinal absorption of calcium and promote calciuresis (prednisone at 0.02–4.4 mg/kg BID).
- Salmon calcitonin promotes bone deposition of calcium (dosage not well established).

CONTRAINDICATIONS/POSSIBLE INTERACTIONS

N/A

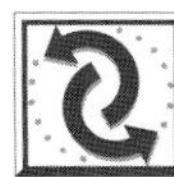

FOLLOW-UP

PATIENT MONITORING

Monitor serum calcium concentrations.

PREVENTION/AVOIDANCE

- Prevent access to the plant.
- When preventing access is impossible, remove the plant itself, because the dead leaves remain toxic.

POSSIBLE COMPLICATIONS

N/A

EXPECTED COURSE AND PROGNOSIS

N/A

MISCELLANEOUS

ASSOCIATED CONDITIONS, AGE-RELATED FACTORS, ZOONOTIC POTENTIAL, PREGNANCY

N/A

ABBREVIATION

- GI = gastrointestinal

Suggested Reading

Krook L, Wasserman RH, Shively JN, Tashjian AH Jr, Brokken TD, Morton JF. Hypercalcemia and calcinosis in Florida horses: implication of the shrub, *Cestrum diurnum*, as the causative agent. Cornell Vet 1975;65:26–56.

Author Tam Garland
Consulting Editor Robert H. Poppenga

CHLORIDE, HYPERCHLOREMIA

BASICS

OVERVIEW

Serum chloride concentration greater than the reference range—generally >111 mEq/L

PATHOPHYSIOLOGY

- Chloride is the major anion in the ECF.
- Serum chloride concentrations may increase and decrease in proportion to changes in serum sodium concentrations; these proportional increases and decreases relate to changes in body water and sodium homeostasis.
- Changes in serum chloride concentrations not proportional to those in serum sodium concentrations usually relate to acid-base abnormalities.
- Serum chloride concentrations tend to vary inversely with serum bicarbonate concentrations.
- Metabolic acidosis with a normal or low anion gap may be accompanied by hyperchloremia; in metabolic acidosis with a high anion gap, the serum chloride concentration is normal or low.
- Hyperchloremia may also occur when the serum bicarbonate concentration decreases in compensation for respiratory alkalosis.

SIGNS

- Depend on the underlying cause
- Neuromuscular—severe hypernatremia and hyperchloremia, resulting in marked hyperosmolality, may cause neurologic abnormalities because of water loss from neurons.
- See salt poisoning and water deprivation.

CAUSES AND RISK FACTORS

Chloride Increased Proportionately to Sodium

- High total body chloride—excessive NaCl intake (i.e., salt poisoning) with water restriction (rare).
- Iatrogenic causes—administration of excessive hypertonic NaCl.
- Normal total body chloride with excessive free water loss—inadequate water intake; early stages of diarrhea; central or nephrogenic diabetes insipidus; prolonged hyperventilation.

Chloride Increased Disproportionately to Sodium

- Suggests an acid-base abnormality.
- Metabolic acidosis with a low or normal anion gap—renal tubular acidosis, an uncommon disorder in horses, results in striking hyperchloremia, hypobicarbonatemia (especially proximal type II RTA) and metabolic acidosis.
- Compensated respiratory alkalosis–decreased bicarbonate as a compensatory response results in increased chloride.
- Acetazolamide treatment for hyperkalemic periodic paralysis

RISK FACTORS

- Inadequate water intake
- Psychogenic disorders leading to excessive consumption of salt/mineral block supplements

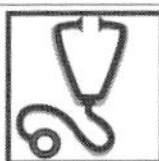

DIAGNOSIS

DIFFERENTIAL DIAGNOSIS

- History or physical examination to detect decreased water intake or excessive water loss resulting in dehydration
- Diseases resulting in metabolic acidosis with a normal or low anion gap—renal tubular acidosis (uncommon) or renal failure

CBC/BIOCHEMISTRY/URINALYSIS

Serum electrolyte analysis

Disorders That May Alter Lab Results

- Hemoglobin has a variable effect on serum chloride concentration; it may increase the concentrations with some methods.
- Bilirubin may falsely increase serum chloride concentrations.

OTHER LABORATORY TESTS

- Blood gas analysis is indicated where increases in chloride concentration are disproportionate to sodium concentration.
- Evaluate for primary metabolic (e.g., hypobicarbonatemia) or compensated respiratory alkalosis (decreased Pco_2).
- Urinalysis including pH determination, especially where RTA is suspected.
- Determine serum potassium and bicarbonate to calculate anion gap.

IMAGING

If neurologic signs are present, magnetic resonance imaging may show CNS edema formation.

OTHER DIAGNOSTIC PROCEDURES

N/A

PATHOLOGICAL FINDINGS

N/A

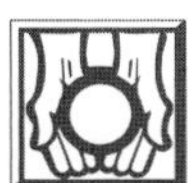

TREATMENT

- Treat the underlying cause.
- Change fluid therapy regimens in cases of iatrogenic causes of hyperosmolar fluid administration.

MEDICATIONS

DRUG(S) OF CHOICE

- Treat the primary cause.
- If sodium and chloride increases are proportional, ensure adequate water availability.
- If hypernatremia and hyperchloremia are long-standing, correction should be gradual to avoid neurologic damage.
- If chloride is increased disproportionately to sodium, evaluate and treat the acid–base imbalance.

CONTRAINDICATIONS/POSSIBLE INTERACTIONS

N/A

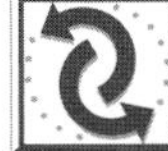

FOLLOW-UP

PATIENT MONITORING

Serum electrolyte concentrations and acid-base status to monitor response to fluid therapy

PREVENTION/AVOIDANCE

Ensure clean fresh water supply at all time in cases of water deprivation.

POSSIBLE COMPLICATIONS

- Depend on the underlying disorder
- Hypernatremia—seizures, convulsions, and permanent neurologic damage are possible in severe cases.
- Rapid replacement of fluid deficit with water in markedly hyperosmotic animals may result in cerebral edema and neurologic abnormalities. Reducing the hypertonicity of tissues with relatively hypotonic solutions should be performed slowly to prevent edema formation.

EXPECTED COURSE AND PROGNOSIS

- Depend on the primary disease process
- Poor if neurologic dysfunction is evident and worsens during treatment. This suggests cerebral edema.

MISCELLANEOUS

ASSOCIATED CONDITIONS

- Salt poisoning
- Renal tubular acidosis
- Water deprivation

AGE-RELATED FACTORS

N/A

ZOONOTIC POTENTIAL

N/A

PREGNANCY

N/A

ABBREVIATIONS

- CNS = central nervous system
- ECF = extracellular fluid
- P_{CO_2} = partial pressure of carbon dioxide
- RTA = renal tubular acidosis

Suggested Reading

Schmall LM. Fluid and electrolyte therapy. In: Robinson NE, ed. Current Therapy in Equine Medicine, ed 4. Philadelphia: WB Saunders, 1997.

The author and editor wish to acknowledge the contribution to this chapter by E. Duane Lassen, author in the previous edition.

Author Samuel D. A. Hurcombe

Consulting Editor Kenneth W. Hinchcliff

CHLORIDE, HYPOCHLOREMIA

BASICS

OVERVIEW

Serum chloride concentration less than the reference range—generally <99 mEq/L

PATHOPHYSIOLOGY

- Chloride is the major anion in the ECF.
- Serum chloride concentrations may increase and decrease in proportion to changes in serum sodium concentrations; these proportional increases and decreases relate to changes in body water and sodium balance.
- Alterations in serum chloride concentrations not proportional to changes in serum sodium concentrations usually relate to acid–base abnormalities, e.g., alterations in serum bicarbonate.
- Serum chloride concentrations tend to vary inversely with serum bicarbonate concentrations
- Metabolic alkalosis is usually accompanied by, and may result from, hypochloremia, which also may occur when serum bicarbonate concentrations increase in compensation for respiratory acidosis.
- Metabolic acidosis with an increased anion gap may result in serum chloride concentrations that are either normal or low.

SIGNS

- If accompanied by severe and acute hyponatremia, lethargy, central blindness, seizures, tremors, and abnormal gait are possible.
- If related to acid-base abnormality, respiratory rate may be increased or decreased. Other findings may be related to alkalemia such as ionized hypocalcemia and synchronous diaphragmatic flutter.
- Other signs depend on the underlying condition, e.g., diarrhea, colic, enterogastric reflux, etc.

CAUSES AND RISK FACTORS

Proportionate Decreases in Serum Chloride and Sodium Compared with Increased Total Body Water

- Third spacing—occurs when abnormal fluid volumes accumulate in body spaces (e.g., abdominal and thoracic cavities, GI tract; specific abnormalities resulting in equine third spacing include ruptured urinary bladder in foals, abdominal effusions associated with colic, colitis, and peritonitis from a variety of causes.
- Iatrogenic—Orally administered/provided hypotonic fluids or excessive IV administration of 5% dextrose solution (pseudo- hypochloremia/hyponatremia).
- Inappropriate water retention (rare) caused by congestive heart failure, hepatic fibrosis, severe hypoproteinemia, or syndrome of inappropriate ADH secretion.

Disproportionate Loss of Sodium and Chloride Compared with Loss of Total Body Water

- Renal disease
- Some forms of diarrhea and other diseases causing fluid sequestration in the GI tract.
- Prolonged diuresis secondary to psychogenic polydipsia, or hyperglycemia and glucosuria may result in medullary washout and subsequent hyponatremia, hypochloremia and metabolic alkalosis.
- Adrenal insufficiency or adrenal exhaustion
- Iatrogenic loss caused by GI fluid drainage via nasogastric intubation.
- Primary metabolic alkalosis—serum chloride decreases in compensation for increased serum bicarbonate. Metabolic alkalosis may result from excessive sweating in horses. Equine sweat contains a proportionally higher concentration of chloride than of sodium; excessive sweating can cause hypochloremia and metabolic alkalosis as a result of enhanced renal bicarbonate reabsorption in compensation for chloride loss.
- Compensatory response to a respiratory acidosis—serum bicarbonate concentration increases in compensation for the respiratory acidosis, and serum chloride concentration decreases to maintain electroneutrality.
- Metabolic acidosis with an increased anion gap is frequently associated with colic because of increased concentrations of other anions (e.g., lactate) provide the negative charges needed to maintain electroneutrality.
- Furosemide therapy—results in loss of chloride in the thick ascending loop of Henle.
- Sodium bicarbonate therapy—may lower serum chloride concentration in compensation for increased serum bicarbonate concentration.

RISK FACTORS

- Heavy sweating
- Colic and other GI disorders with voluminous enterogastric reflux and GI fluid sequestration
- Furosemide treatment promoting chloride wastage and metabolic alkalosis

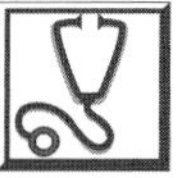

DIAGNOSIS

DIFFERENTIAL DIAGNOSIS

Proportional Decreases in Serum Chloride and Sodium Concentrations

- Ascites suggests third spacing. In foals, consider ruptured urinary bladder, and check BUN/creatinine in serum and fluid. In adults consider peritonitis, congestive heart failure, and other causes of ascites. Perform abdominal fluid analysis.
- Thoracic effusion suggests third spacing. Consider pleuritis, neoplasia, and other causes of thoracic effusions, and perform thoracic fluid analysis.
- Diarrhea suggests GI loss.
- Polyuria/polydipsia indicates the need for renal function assessment.

Disproportionate Decrease in Chloride Compared with Sodium

- Normal or low anion gap—consider excessive sweating as a cause of metabolic alkalosis; evaluate respiratory system for possible cause of respiratory acidosis.
- Increased anion gap—consider possible colic and other causes of increased lactate, phosphate, sulfate, ketone, or protein concentrations.

CBC/BIOCHEMISTRY/URINALYSIS

- Depends on the underlying disorder.
- Concurrent hyponatremia indicates need to consider diseases altering water balance or resulting in loss of sodium and chloride.
- Decreased serum potassium is more typical of GI fluid loss.
- Increased potassium is more typical of renal disease or uroperitoneum.
- Increased bicarbonate indicates metabolic alkalosis or compensation for respiratory acidosis.
- Decreased bicarbonate and increased anion gap indicate increased concentrations of ions other than bicarbonate or chloride.
- Increased BUN/creatinine may indicate renal failure or uroperitoneum.

Disorders That May Alter Lab Results

- Lipemia and hyperproteinemia may falsely lower chloride concentrations unless an ion-specific electrode is used.
- Marked hyperglycemia causes dilution of serum chloride via osmotic water movement.
- Hemoglobin has a variable effect on serum chloride concentrations.

OTHER LABORATORY TESTS

- Urinary fractional excretion ($[Na_u^+/Na_s^+]/[Cr_u/Cr_s]$)—increased fractional excretion accompanying hypochloremia suggests renal disease or furosemide treatment.
- Blood gas analysis if the decrease of chloride is disproportionate to that of sodium. Evaluate for primary metabolic alkalosis or compensated respiratory acidosis.
- Serum potassium and bicarbonate to calculate anion gap.
- Abdominal or thoracic fluid examination if these fluids are present in abnormal volumes. In foals, abdominal fluid urea nitrogen or creatinine concentrations are indicated if rupture of the urinary bladder is suspected.

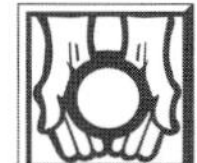

TREATMENT

Treat the underlying condition.

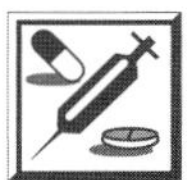

MEDICATIONS

DRUG(S)

- Treat the primary cause.
- If sodium and chloride decreases are proportional, see the discussion of treatment in Hyponatremia.
- If chloride is decreased disproportionately compared with sodium, evaluate and treat the acid–base imbalance.

FOLLOW-UP

PATIENT MONITORING

Serum electrolyte concentrations and acid–base status to monitor response to fluid therapy.

EXPECTED COURSE AND PROGNOSIS

- Variable, depending on the inciting cause.
- Hypochloremia secondary to gastrointestinal pathology has been associated with renal insuffiency and persistent azotemia in horses.

MISCELLANEOUS

ASSOCIATED CONDITIONS

- Other acid-base and electrolyte abnormalities
- See Hyponatremia.

SEE ALSO

- Hyponatremia
- Uroperitoneum

ABBREVIATIONS

- ADH = antidiuretic hormone
- ECF = extracellular fluid
- GI = gastrointestinal tract

Suggested Reading

Schmall LM. Fluid and electrolyte therapy. In: Robinson NE, ed. Current Therapy in Equine Medicine, ed 4. Philadelphia: WB Saunders, 1997.

The author and editor wish to acknowledge the contribution to this chapter by E. Duane Lassen, author in the previous edition.

Author Samuel D. A. Hurcombe
Consulting Editor Kenneth W. Hinchcliff

CHOLELITHIASIS

BASICS

OVERVIEW

- Refers to calculi in the biliary tree
- Relatively uncommon
- The pathogenesis is not fully understood but possibly involves conversion in the bile of conjugated bilirubin to unconjugated bilirubin by β-glucuronidase. The enzyme is present in the bile duct epithelium and in some bacteria.
- Most cases are associated with septic cholangitis, which suggests that bacterial enzymes may play a role.
- Unconjugated bilirubin combines with calcium in the bile to form calcium bilirubinate, which then precipitates to form the calculi, although many other compounds also are present—cholesterol, bile pigments, and sodium taurodeoxycholate.

SIGNALMENT

- Most affected horses are 5–15 years old; however, cases of cholelithiasis have been reported in horses as young as 3 years.
- No breed or sex predilections
- No reported geographic distribution

SIGNS

- Intermittent abdominal pain
- Icterus
- Fever
- Depression
- Weight loss
- Hepatic encephalopathy
- Photosensitization

CAUSES AND RISK FACTORS

- The condition is sporadic.
- No clearly established risk factors have been identified.

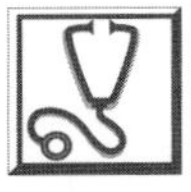

DIAGNOSIS

DIFFERENTIAL DIAGNOSIS

- Other causes of chronic liver disease (e.g., chronic active hepatitis, toxic hepatitis) can be differentiated with ultrasonography and liver biopsy.
- Mild, recurrent abdominal pain may more commonly be caused by GI problems—parasitism, abdominal abscesses and neoplasms, sand accumulation, and enteroliths; however, most of these conditions are not accompanied by changes in serum liver enzymes or icterus.
- Fever is common in many equine infectious conditions, but the chronic, recurrent causes include pleuropneumonia, abdominal abscesses, endocarditis, and EIA. Clinical pathology and physical examination will assist in differentiation.
- Weight loss is a feature in many of the chronic conditions listed above but also includes malnutrition, dental disease, chronic laminitis, chronic severe arthritis, and malabsorption. Again, clinical signs and laboratory data assist in differentiation.

CBC/BIOCHEMISTRY/URINALYSIS

- Liver enzymes may be elevated from time to time—AST, GGT, ALP, and SDH (IDH).
- Total bilirubin—Both conjugated and unconjugated levels may be elevated.
- CBC—neutrophilia
- Fibrinogen and globulin—elevated

OTHER LABORATORY TESTS

N/A

IMAGING

- Ultrasonography of affected livers usually reveals dilation of the bile ducts, which are thickened; normally, equine bile ducts are not readily visualized.
- The liver is usually enlarged and more echogenic than normal.
- Choleliths—most readily seen on the right side of the liver at the sixth or seventh intercostal space; may be hyperechoic and cast an acoustic shadow, although some may be sonolucent

DIAGNOSTIC PROCEDURES

Liver biopsy may be useful to define the nature of the pathology; a sample may be submitted for culture if septic cholangitis is suspected.

PATHOLOGIC FINDINGS

- In acute cases, the liver may be enlarged; in chronic cases, it may be smaller than normal.
- The liver surface may appear mottled, and the tissue appears firm.
- Possible icterus
- Bile ducts are often dilated and contain one or more calculi, which are usually greenish-brown.

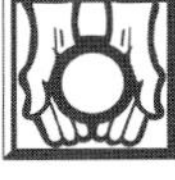

TREATMENT

- Both choledocholithotomy and choledocholithotripsy have been described as treatment of cholelithiasis in three horses; thus, these treatments have not been fully evaluated.
- Basic principles focus on the relief of obstruction, treatment of underlying hepatic disease, and therapy for infection.

MEDICATIONS

DRUG(S) OF CHOICE

- With suspected septic cholangitis, long-term antibiotic therapy is indicated.
- Gram-negative bacteria are the most frequently isolated; appropriate drugs include trimethoprim-sulfa combinations, chloramphenicol, ampicillin, and penicillin-gentamicin combinations.

CONTRAINDICATIONS/POSSIBLE INTERACTIONS

N/A

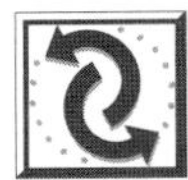

FOLLOW-UP

PATIENT MONITORING

N/A

PREVENTION/AVOIDANCE

N/A

POSSIBLE COMPLICATIONS

N/A

EXPECTED COURSE AND PROGNOSIS

- Prognosis depends on severity of the problem.
- Surgical intervention is not feasible in many cases because of limited access to the biliary tree and high risk of bile peritonitis.
- With antimicrobial therapy, sequential ultrasonography may assist with in monitoring whether progress is being made.

MISCELLANEOUS

ASSOCIATED CONDITIONS, AGE-RELATED FACTORS, ZOONOTIC POTENTIAL, PREGNANCY

N/A

ABBREVIATIONS

- ALP = alkaline phosphatase
- AST = aspartate aminotransferase
- EIA = equine infection anemia
- GGT = γ-glutamyltransferase
- GI = gastrointestinal
- IDH = iditol dehydrogenase (SDH)
- SDH = sorbitol dehydrogenase (IDH)

Suggested Reading

Peek SF, Divers TJ. Medical treatment of cholangiohepatitis and cholelithiasis in mature horses : 9 cases (1981–1998).Equine Vet J 2000;32:301–306.

Johnson JK, Divers TJ, Reef VB, *et al*. Cholelithiasis in horses: ten cases (1982–1986). J Am Vet Med Assoc 1989;194:405–409.

Author Christopher M. Brown

Consulting Editor Michel Lévy

BASICS

OVERVIEW

The choroid and retina are closely related anatomically and physiologically. The choroid is the primary supply of blood to the horse retina. Chorioretinitis is inflammation of the choroid and retina. The ophthalmic system is affected.

SIGNALMENT

N/A

SIGNS

Chorioretinitis is manifest in equine eyes as "bullet-hole" retinal lesions, diffuse chorioretinal lesions, horizontal band lesions of the nontapetal retina, and peripapillary chorioretinitis. Lesions near the optic disc are more likely to cause vision problems than peripheral retinal inflammatory disease.

• Focal chorioretinopathy or "bullet-hole" lesions are focal or multifocal circular scars of the peripapillary and nontapetal regions. They consist of a depigmented periphery and a hyperpigmented central area. Acute lesions, which are uncommon, appear as white or gray, exudative lesions. Vision is not impaired unless there are more than 10–20 bullet-hole lesions. EHV-1 may be associated with this type of lesion in horses. "Bullet-hole" lesions are nonprogressive, can be seen in all age groups, and are considered incidental findings.

• Diffuse chorioretinal lesions are vermiform, circular, or band-shaped lesions that are hyperreflective in the tapetal retina and large depigmented areas in the nontapetal retina that are associated with smaller areas of hyperpigmentation. These lesions are uncommon. They represent widespread prior inflammatory disease or infarctive lesions with subsequent retinal degeneration and scarring. Optic nerve atrophy may accompany these lesions. Vision is markedly reduced.

• Horizontal band lesions of the nontapetal zone are multifocal chorioretinal lesions appearing 1–2 disc diameters ventral to the optic disc. They radiate in a horizontal fashion around the posterior pole.

• Peripapillary chorioretinitis is commonly associated with anterior uveitis. Fluffy, raised exudates adjacent to the optic disc are found in the active stage. Vasculitis can be observed in some cases with white or pale exudates surrounding affected retinal vessels. In the chronic stage, scar tissue develops, often but not necessarily in a butterfly shape around the papilla. "Butterfly lesions" may be associated with ERU, especially with concurrent signs of anterior uveitis.

CAUSES AND RISK FACTORS

• Lesions can be caused by infectious agents (e. g., leptospirosis, EHV-1, *Onchocerca cervicalis* microfilaria), immune-mediated uveitis of unknown origin, trauma, or vascular disease.

• Foals born to mares with respiratory disease can have chorioretinitis.

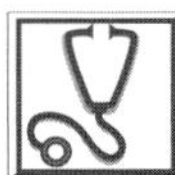

DIAGNOSIS

DIFFERENTIAL DIAGNOSIS

Chorioretinitis does usually not recur unless it is part of the ERU syndrome. Anterior uveitis is common in ERU but does not develop in many cases with chorioretinitis.

CBC/BIOCHEMISTRY/URINALYSIS

Possible signs of systemic disease, such as infection or immune-mediated disorder

OTHER LABORATORY TESTS

Rule out infectious causes of chorioretinitis by serologically testing for infectious agents.

IMAGING

N/A

DIAGNOSTIC PROCEDURES

Electroretinography will help to assess functionality of the retina.

PATHOLOGIC FINDINGS

Type of cellular reaction depends on underlying cause.

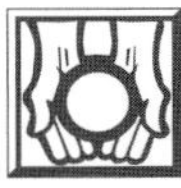

TREATMENT

• Remove underlying cause if known.
• Observed changes cannot be reversed.
• Goal of treatment is to stop the progression of the disease process.
• Chronic, inactive lesions do not require treatment.

MEDICATIONS

DRUG(S) OF CHOICE

• Systemic medication according to the underlying cause.
• In addition (if lesions appear active), nonsteroidal drugs such as flunixin meglumine (0.25–1.0 mg/kg BID PO), phenylbutazone (1 g BID IV or PO), or aspirin (15 mg/kg/day).
• Topical medication is only indicated if anterior uveitis is also present: prednisolone acetate (1%) or dexamethasone (0.1%) at least 4–6 times a day and atropine (1%) SID to TID.

CONTRAINDICATIONS/POSSIBLE INTERACTIONS

Horses receiving topically administered atropine should be monitored for signs of colic.

FOLLOW-UP

EXPECTED COURSE AND PROGNOSIS

The goal of the treatment for chorioretinitis is to preserve the present status, i.e., to prevent progression of the disease.

MISCELLANEOUS

ASSOCIATED CONDITIONS

Possible signs of systemic infection

AGE-RELATED FACTORS

N/A

PREGNANCY

Some infectious agents causing chorioretinitis can threaten pregnancy (e. g., *Leptospira*).

SEE ALSO

• Recurrent uveitis
• Stationary night blindness
• Ischemic optic neuropathy

ABREVIATIONS

• EHV-1 = equine herpesvirus 1
• ERU = equine recurrent uveitis

Suggested Reading

Brooks DE: Ophthalmology for the Equine Practitioner. Jackson, WY; Teton NewMedia, 2002.

Brooks DE, Matthews AG: Equine ophthalmology. In: Gelatt KN, ed. Veterinary Ophthalmology, ed 4. Philadelphia; Lippincott Williams and Wilkins, 2007.

Gilger BC, ed. Equine Ophthalmology. Philadelphia; WB Saunders, 2005.

Authors Andras M. Komaromy and Dennis E. Brooks

Consulting Editor Dennis E. Brooks

CHRONIC PROGRESSIVE LYMPHEDEMA

BASICS

OVERVIEW

- Chronic progressive disease characterized by progressive swelling of the lower limbs associated with the development of thick skin folds, dermal fibrosis, hard nodules, marked hyperkeratosis, and surface ulceration
- Caused by chronic lymphedema

SIGNALMENT

- Described in Shires, Clydesdales, and Belgian draft horses
- Probably affects many heavy draft horse breeds, especially with heavy feathering of the distal limbs
- Certain familial lines of draft horse breeds are more affected than others.
- May also exist in heavy breeds of cart horses such as Cobbs and Gypsy Vanners; however, this has yet to be investigated.

SIGNS

- Onset at young age, usually when 2–4 years old, rarely in older horses
- Progresses throughout life
- Both forelimbs and hindlimbs are affected, although the lesions tend to be milder on the forelimbs.
- Lesions most often start in the palmar/plantar region of the pastern and progress to encircle the limb. Over time, these lesions can spread up the legs to the tarsus or carpus.
- Initially, there is mild swelling with one or two thick skin folds and multiple small, well-demarcated ulcerations often only visible after clipping the long feathering.
- In the chronic stage, the lower limb enlargement becomes permanent, the swelling becomes extremely firm to palpation, ulcerations become large and coalesce, and hard dermal nodules that can measure several centimeters develop.
- Often, the hoof quality in these individuals is poor, characterized by flaky, brittle hoof walls that chip, split, and form deep cracks. Foot canker is also a frequent sequelae.
- Severe bacterial or fungal lymphangitis often occurs as the end stage of the long-term progression. Euthanasia is often the only recourse in these individuals.

CAUSES AND RISK FACTORS

- The underlying cause is poor function of the lymphatic system resulting in chronic lymphedema; reason for the malfunction is not known.
- Chronic stasis of lymph fluid induces diffuse and nodular fibrosis, ischemia of the skin and subcutaneaous tissues; followed by recalcitrant surface ulceration
- Irritation of the skin, by bacterial infections, mites, poor skin hygiene, and microtrauma, exacerbates the condition.

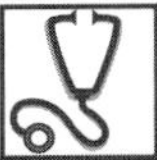

DIAGNOSIS

DIFFERENTIAL DIAGNOSIS

- In the initial stages, the pastern dermatitis complex commonly seen in light horse breeds is the usual differential diagnosis.
- In later stages, the disease is distinct especially in association with breed predilection.

CBC/BIOCHEMISTRY/URINALYSIS

None

OTHER LABORATORY TESTS

- Skin biopsies are usually nondiagnostic, suggestive of chronic hyperplastic dermatitis.
- Sometimes minimal signs of vasculitis are present; therefore often misdiagnosed as nonspecific leukocytic vasculitis or photosensitivity

IMAGING

- Isotopic lymphoscintigraphy proved valuable for diagnosis of CPL in draft horses. For this, a radioactive labeled colloid is injected subcutaneously at different sites proximal to the hoof. The particulate radiopharmaceutical is subsequently taken up by the lymphatics and its flow detected by a gamma camera. In limbs of affected horses, a profound delay and reduction in lymphatic clearance of the particulate radiopharmaceutical is seen when compared with clinically normal horses. End stage CPL may be characterized by complete lack of lymphatic flow.

• The reliability of lymphoscintigraphy for diagnosis of subclinical CPL is still unknown.

PATHOLOGICAL FINDINGS

• On necropsy, depending on the stage of the disease, the lesions are characterized by variable amounts of edema fluid and/or dense fibrous tissue in the deep dermis and subcutis.
• Thick-walled, dilated lymphatic vessels expand the deep soft tissues over the entire length of the distal limbs.
• The firm dermal nodules consist entirely of dense connective tissue.
• On histopathology there is marked epidermal hyperplasia, dermal fibrosis, prominent neovascularization and variable chronic inflammation.

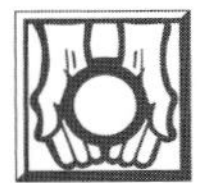

TREATMENT

• Currently, no curative treatment is known.
• All employed treatment modalities are palliative in nature and, at best, can only be expected to slow the progression of the disease.
• Early diagnosis is crucial for good clinical management.
• Supportive treatment is based on two principles: 1) reduction of skin inflammation through prompt treatment of secondary microbial infections, mite infestation and skin irritation, and 2) reduction of tissue edema through regular exercise.

MEDICATIONS

DRUG(S) OF CHOICE

None

CONTRAINDICATIONS/POSSIBLE INTERACTIONS

N/A

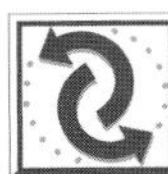

FOLLOW-UP

• CPL affected horses require a lifelong labor-intensive management.
• Good skin hygiene and avoiding excessive wetness or soiling of the skin
• It is essential to treat any type of infection/inflammation of the skin immediately.

MISCELLANEOUS

ABBREVIATION

• CPL = chronic progressive lymphedema

Suggested Reading

De Cock HEV, Affolter VK, Wisner ER, et al. Progressive swelling, hyperkeratosis and fibrosis of distal limbs in Clydesdales, Shires and Belgian draft horses suggestive of primary lymphedema. Lymphatic Res Biol 2003;1:191–199.

De Cock HEV, Affolter VK, Wisner ER, et al. Lymphoscintigraphy of draught horses with chronic progressive lymphoedema. Equine Vet J 2006;38:148–151.

Authors Hilde E. V. De Cock and Gregory L. Ferraro

Consulting Editor Gwendolen Lorch

CHRONIC RENAL FAILURE (CRF)

BASICS

DEFINITION

Results from a substantial and permanent decrease in GFR

PATHOPHYSIOLOGY

• Usually a consequence of GN or CIN • CIN encompasses all non-GN causes of CRF—permanent loss of renal function after a bout of hemodynamic/ischemic or toxic ARF, NSAID nephropathy, or pyelonephritis. • The hallmark of CIN is development of interstitial fibrosis. • Renal anomalies (e.g., hypoplasia, dysplasia) or polycystic kidney disease may cause CRF. • Impaired urine concentrating ability (i.e., isosthenuria) occurs when more than of two-thirds of nephron function is lost.
• Azotemia develops after loss of more than three-fourths of nephron function.
• Disturbances in fluid, electrolyte, and acid-base homeostasis are less severe than with ARF, but the loss of renal function is irreversible.

SYSTEMS AFFECTED

• Renal/urologic—failure • Endocrine/metabolic—disturbances in electrolyte and acid-base homeostasis; decreased erythropoietin production • GI—inappetence, possible diarrhea, and increased risk of ulcers
• Nervous/neuromuscular—Occasional ataxia or dementia in severe CRF; tremors or muscle fasciculations may accompany metabolic disturbances. • Hemic/lymphatic/immune—alterations in hemostasis (i.e., platelet dysfunction); increased susceptibility to infection, anemia (decreased erythropoietin)

GENETICS N/A

INCIDENCE/PREVALENCE

Reported to be 0.12%, increasing to 0.51% for stallions >15 years

SIGNALMENT

Breed Predilections

• May be more common in Clydesdales
• A heritable form of polycystic kidney disease may occur in some breeds (Arabians and Paints).

Mean Age and Range

Old horses (>15 years) are at greater risk.

Predominant Sex

Old stallions may be at greater risk; however, this may reflect more extensive diagnostic investigation of valuable breeding animals.

SIGNS

Historical

• Because CRF can be a long-term sequel to other underlying disease processes (e.g., colic, diarrhea, prolonged exercise, rhabdomyolysis, purpura hemorrhagica, or neonatal septicemia) that initially led to ischemic ARF or GN, historical questioning should pursue all previous medical and surgical problems. • May develop months to years after nephrotoxin-induced acute tubular necrosis or papillary necrosis (NSAIDs)
• Insidious-onset mild lethargy, partial anorexia, and weight loss • Astute owners may complain of ventral edema and mild polyuria and polydipsia (with clear-appearing urine). • If detected at an earlier stage, decreased performance may be the initial presenting complaint.

Physical Examination

• Weight loss and poor hair coat with mild lethargy, reduced appetite, edema, excessive dental tartar, and uremic odor in the oral cavity may be found. • Affected horses usually are not clinically dehydrated. • Voided urine usually is clear and pale yellow, unlike the cloudy urine of normal horses. • Rectal examination may reveal a small, firm left kidney with an irregular surface and, rarely, bilateral ureteral distension due to obstruction with uroliths. • With end-stage disease, anuria may develop with anorexia, and more marked lethargy may be accompanied by ataxia, hypermetria, and mental obtundation.

CAUSES

• Immune-mediated GN initiated by chronic infections (e.g., equine infectious anemia, streptococcal diseases) or autoimmune disease
• May be a sequel to ischemic or nephrotoxic ARF, leading to CIN • Less commonly, ascending infections may lead to bilateral pyelonephritis and nephrolithiasis and/or ureterolithiasis. • Long-term use of NSAIDs with papillary necrosis and nephrolithiasis
• Amyloidosis and renal neoplasia—rare • In horses <5 years and with no history of medical problems, anomalies of development—renal hypoplasia or dysplasia; polycystic kidney disease

RISK FACTORS

• Previous episodes of ARF or UTI likely are important risk factors. • Prior medical or surgical diseases, especially when treatment included aminoglycoside antibiotics and NSAIDs • Long-term use of NSAIDs

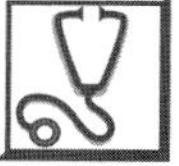

DIAGNOSIS

DIFFERENTIAL DIAGNOSIS

• A broad list of disorders that may lead to lethargy, partial anorexia, and weight loss
• Physical examination findings with CRF are nonspecific, but detection of azotemia, especially when accompanied by hypercalcemia, makes CRF rise to the top of the list. • Prerenal or intrinsic ARF—supported by another underlying disease process producing renal ischemia or recent/concurrent exposure to nephrotoxic agents • Postrenal ARF—supported by stranguria, anuria, or uroperitoneum

CBC/BIOCHEMISTRY/URINALYSIS

• Normal to low PCV (attributed to decreased serum erythropoietin concentration and shortened RBC life span), leukocyte count usually within normal ranges, and platelets normal to decreased
• Increased BUN (100–250 mg/dL) and Cr (2.0–20 mg/dL); BUN:Cr ratio usually >10; Cr usually >5.0 mg/dL with horses presented for chronic ill thrift
• Variable hyponatremia, hypochloremia, and hyperkalemia—not as severe as with ARF
• Hypercalcemia and hypophosphatemia with CRF are somewhat unique to horses; the former appears to result from decreased renal calcium excretion in the face of ongoing intestinal absorption, because elevated plasma parathormone concentrations have not been documented in these cases.
• Mild to moderate hypoalbuminemia
• Mild to moderate hypertriglyceridemia (i.e., hyperlipemia) and hypercholesterolemia
• Mild to moderate metabolic acidosis may accompany end-stage disease.
• USG—isosthenuria (1.008–1.014) is a hallmark feature.
• GN—moderate to marked proteinuria that may increase USG to 1.020
• Urine sediment is relatively devoid of crystals, but otherwise may be unremarkable. Increased RBCs support lithiasis or neoplasia, and increased leukocytes support UTI.

OTHER LABORATORY TESTS

• Increased fractional clearances (i.e., excretions) of sodium and chloride with advanced disease.
• Increased urine protein:creatinine ratio (>2:1) supports GN.
• Quantitative urine culture and antimicrobial sensitivity should always be performed because significant bacteriuria may occur without pyuria.
• Coagulation panel when performing renal biopsy or investigating GN (decreased anti-thrombin III)

IMAGING

Transabdominal and Transrectal Ultrasonography

• Kidneys may be small (diameter, <6 cm; length, <12 cm), with irregular surfaces.
• Parenchymal echogenicity typically increased (echogenicity of left kidney similar to that of the spleen), with loss of detail of corticomedullary junction
• Bilateral nephrolithiasis/ureterolithiasis and variable hydronephrosis may be detected.
• Multiple cystic structures may be found with polycystic kidney disease or pyelonephritis.

Urethroscopy/Cystoscopy

• Useful with suspected obstructive disease or pyelonephritis
• Urine samples may be collected from each ureter during cystoscopy by passing tubing through the biopsy channel of the endoscope.

DIAGNOSTIC PROCEDURES

GFR

• Measuring changes in GFR over time may be the most accurate way to follow the progressive decrease in renal function.
• A simple method to estimate decline in GFR is to plot the inverse of Cr over time; however, plasma disappearance of sodium sulfanilate, exogenous Cr, or radionuclides are more accurate.

Biopsy

• Percutaneous renal biopsy with routine histopathology, immunohistochemistry and electron microscopy of the sample may provide information regarding cause (i.e., GN versus CIN) but rarely affects prognosis or supportive treatment.
• Pursue biopsy with caution, because life-threatening hemorrhage can be a complication.

PATHOLOGICAL FINDINGS

Gross

• Characterized by firm, shrunken kidneys, with irregular surfaces • Renal capsule is often adhered to parenchyma. • Kidneys typically are pale, with narrowed cortices. • See Urolithiasis and Urinary Tract Infection. • Enlarged kidneys with multiple cysts are found with polycystic kidney disease.

Histopathological

• Variable glomerular, tubular, and interstitial changes • End-stage kidney disease may preclude histologic categorization of the initiating cause.

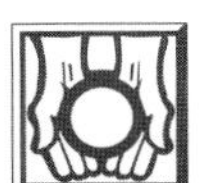

TREATMENT

APPROPRIATE HEALTH CARE

• Proper recognition and treatment of all underlying disease processes
• Fluid therapy, usually on an inpatient basis, to rule out ARF or acute-on-chronic disease
• Discontinue potentially nephrotoxic medications.

NURSING CARE

Fluid Therapy

• After initial measurement of body weight, monitor magnitude of azotemia, and USG, diuresis with 5% dextrose or normal (0.9%) saline at 2-fold the maintenance rate for 24–48 hr.
• Monitor closely, because significant pulmonary edema may develop after administering as little as 40 mL/kg of IV fluids.
• Increased urine output and decreased azotemia should occur in patients with ARF or acute-on-chronic disease.
• Horses with more severe CRF typically gain weight and develop edema, with little decrease in magnitude of azotemia.

Oral Electrolyte Supplementation

• With serum bicarbonate <20 mEq/L, 30 g of sodium bicarbonate may be administered once or twice daily.
• Electrolyte supplementation should be discontinued if it produces or exacerbates edema.

ACTIVITY

• When clinical signs are mild and the horse's attitude is good, light exercise (e.g., 30 min of walking and trotting) can be continued daily or a few days each week.
• Maintain on high-quality pasture with walk-in shelter or in a stall with frequent hand-walking for grazing grass if appetite is poor.

DIET

• Access to fresh water at all times
• The ideal diet for affected horses provides adequate caloric intake without excessive protein intake.
• Offering a variety of concentrate feeds, bran mash, and access to good-quality pasture is the recommended diet. Grass hay is preferred to alfalfa due to the higher protein and calcium content of the latter; however, if appetite for grass hay is poor, feed alfalfa.
• Supplementation with fat (rice bran or 12–16 oz. of oil added to concentrate feed) effectively increases caloric intake.
• Antioxidants—Vitamins C and E could be added to the diet. Feeding an omega-3 fatty acid–rich diet (fish oil and vegetable oil rich in linolenic acid) could decrease inflammation and slow the progression of the disease. However, this has not been investigated in the horse.

CLIENT EDUCATION

Inform clients that prognosis is poor for long-term survival but fair to guarded for short-term survival, especially when Cr <5.0 mg/dL.

SURGICAL CONSIDERATIONS

Surgery is only required for acute-on-chronic disease due to obstructive urolithiasis—ureteral, cystic, or urethral calculi.

MEDICATIONS

DRUG(S) OF CHOICE

• Judicious use of oral electrolytes—see earlier.
• Antioxidant supplements— see earlier.
• ACE inhibitors – (Enalapril 2 mg/kg PO q12 h) may be helpful in the patient with proteinuria and edema but is often cost prohibitive.
• Antiulcer drugs (e.g., omeprazole 2–4 mg/kg PO q24 h) may be useful in combating decreased feed intake in affected horses with accompanying gastric ulcers.

CONTRAINDICATIONS

• Corticosteroids and NSAIDs may exacerbate renal hypoperfusion and the decline in GFR.
• Avoid all nephrotoxic medications unless specifically indicated for a concurrent disease process, and then modify dosage accordingly.

PRECAUTIONS

• Monitor response to fluid therapy closely—as little as 40 mL/kg of IV fluids (20 L to a 500-kg horse) may produce significant pulmonary edema in oliguric/anuric patients.
• Discontinue oral electrolyte supplementation if it produces or exacerbates edema.

POSSIBLE INTERACTIONS N/A

ALTERNATIVE DRUGS N/A

FOLLOW-UP

PATIENT MONITORING

• Assess clinical status (emphasizing attitude and appetite), edema formation, body weight, and magnitude of azotemia at least monthly during the initial few months of supportive care and every 2–3 mo thereafter.
• Assess electrolyte and acid-basis status whenever changes in clinical status are noted.

PREVENTION/AVOIDANCE

• Anticipate compromised renal function in patients with other diseases or undergoing prolonged anesthesia and surgery; institute appropriate treatment to minimize dehydration and potential renal damage.
• Ensure adequate hydration status in patients receiving nephrotoxic medications.
• Avoid prolonged use of NSAIDs unless necessary.

POSSIBLE COMPLICATIONS

• Pulmonary and peripheral edema with fluid therapy
• Oral and GI ulceration or GI bleeding
• Signs of neurologic impairment—ataxia; mental obtundation

EXPECTED COURSE AND PROGNOSIS

• Issue a poor prognosis and consider euthanasia for horses that are emaciated, anuric, or have Cr >10 mg/dL at initial evaluation.
• Issue a guarded prognosis for short-term survival for patients with Cr of 5–10 mg/dL at initial evaluation.
• Issue a fair prognosis for short-term survival for patients with Cr <5 mg/dL that are in good body condition at initial evaluation.

MISCELLANEOUS

ASSOCIATED CONDITIONS

• UTI
• Urolithiasis

AGE-RELATED FACTORS

• Renal function decreases with age; old horses likely are at greater risk.
• In horses <5 years, likely due to a developmental anomaly—renal hypoplasia or dysplasia

PREGNANCY

Although not well documented, pregnant mares may be at increased risk of UTI. Mares with CRF have successfully carried foals to term but the prognosis for a viable foal is guarded.

SYNONYMS

• Kidney failure
• Chronic renal disease

SEE ALSO

• ARF
• Urolithiasis
• Urinary tract infection

ABBREVIATIONS

• ARF = acute renal failure
• CRF = chronic renal failure
• CIN = chronic interstitial nephritis
• GFR = glomerular filtration rate
• GI = gastrointestinal
• GN = glomerulonephritis
• PCV = packed cell volume
• UTI = urinary tract infection
• USG = urinary specific gravity

Suggested Reading

Schott HC. Chronic renal failure in horses. Vet Clinics North Amer: Eq Pract 2007;(23):593–612.

VanBiervliet J, Divers TJ, Porter B and Huxtable C. Glomerulonephritis in horses. Compend Contin Educ 2002;24(11):892–902.

Schott HC. Chronic renal failure. In: Reed SM, Bayly WM, Sellon DC, eds. Equine internal medicine, ed 2. Philadelphia: WB Saunders, 2004:1231–1253.

Author Harold C. Schott II

Consulting Editor Gillian A. Perkins

CHRONIC WEIGHT LOSS

BASICS

DEFINITION

Chronic weight loss is not a specific problem of the digestive system but it is a common clinical manifestation of gastrointestinal disease. It can be defined as loss of body weight over time (over 4–5 weeks) and may be due to decreased fat and muscle mass or loss of gastrointestinal content and total body water, or a combination of these factors.

PATHOPHYSIOLOGY

Weight loss can result from many different clinical conditions. Loss of weight in the horse can occur due to lack of adequate food and/or water, poor-quality food, inability to prehend or swallow, maldigestion or malabsorption of food, increased loss of nutrients once absorbed, and increased catabolism. Inadequate caloric intake is likely the most common cause of weight loss, with endoparasitism following suit, and may also be due to specific nutrient deficiencies, chronic liver disease, neoplasia, and malabsorption. The pathophysiologic events leading to weight loss are multifold and depend on underlying causes. For details, see specific problems.

SYSTEM AFFECTED

Gastrointestinal

• Dental diseases • Oral ulcerations • Tongue paralysis • Pharyngeal paresis or paralysis • Retropharyngeal masses • Esophageal strictures • Gastric ulceration • Duodenal and jejunal malabsorption • Maldigestion • Intestinal infections and noninfectious infiltrative and neoplastic disorders • Chronic diarrhea • Intestinal motility disturbances • Intra-abdominal abscesses • Parasitism • Chronic grass sickness

Endocrine/Metabolic

• Pituitary adenoma of the pars intermedia in the horse due to increased metabolic rate, including muscle wasting induced by hyperadrenocorticism
• Diabetes mellitus due to endocrine pancreatic insufficiency

Hemic/Lymphatic/Immune

• Lymphoma leading to cancer cachexia
• Inflammatory bowel disease leading to malabsorption • EIA

Hepatobiliary

Chronic hepatic failure

Cardiovascular

• Congestive heart failure, leading to decreased liver and gastrointestinal function • Valvular endocarditis due to occult infections

Renal/Urologic

Chronic renal failure

Neuromuscular

Equine motor neuron disease and associated muscle wasting

Behavioral

• Cribbing • Oral stereotypy

Respiratory

• Heaves
• Chronic pleuropneumonia

Skin/Exocrine

Pemphigus foliaceus

Musculoskeletal

Chronic painful lameness (e.g., severe laminitis)

Nervous

Neurologic conditions that impair prehension, chewing, and swallowing

SIGNALMENT

Age is important, especially in cases where parasitism is suspected (young horses), various bacterial diseases (*Rhodococcus equi, Lawsonia intracellularis*), or neoplasia, which is more commonly observed in older horses.

SIGNS

Signs vary according to the primary condition, but commonly, decrease in body condition and reduced appetite are observed.

CAUSES

A search of weight loss on Consultant® (Maurice White Cornell, 2007) listed 303 possible causes of weight loss in the horse. The causes include occult infections, such as abdominal abscesses, pulmonary abscesses, pleuropneumonia, sinusitis, valvular endocarditis, and tooth problems; the whole group of malabsorption syndromes, including IBD and neoplasia; chronic renal failure; chronic hepatic failure; chronic parasitism; chronic viral infections (EIA); and endocrinopathies.

RISK FACTORS

Any condition leading to catabolic situations

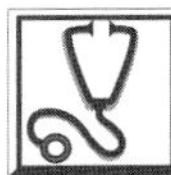

DIAGNOSIS

CBC/BIOCHEMISTRY/URINALYSIS

To work up a chronic weight loss case, a minimal database should include CBC, serum biochemical profile, and fibrinogen. CBC findings may be nonspecific, but total protein might be increased (e.g., due to hyperglobulinemia in occult infections) or decreased (e.g., due to protein-losing enteropathies). Anemia of chronic disease might be present with a hematocrit of <0.3L/L (<30%). There might be leukocytosis. Biochemistry should help to differentiate between specific organ failure problems such as hepatic or renal diseases. Serum electrophoresis might assist in characterizing dysproteinemias and in separating conditions such as occult infections from neoplasia or parasitism.

OTHER LABORATORY TESTS

Hyperfibrinogenemia in inflammatory or neoplastic disease

DIAGNOSTIC PROCEDURES

• Abdominocentesis can be useful in identifying the abdomen to be the site of occult infections.
• Ultrasonography is used to detect abscesses (abdominal, pleural, etc).
• In individual cases, exploratory laparatomy might be required.
• Glucose and xylose absorption tests where small intestine malabsorption is suspected.
• When stomach ulcers are suspected, gastroscopy should be performed.

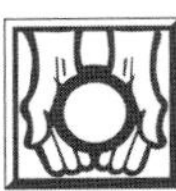

TREATMENT

See specific conditions.

MEDICATIONS

DRUG(S) OF CHOICE

See specific conditions.

FOLLOW-UP

PATIENT MONITORING

Monitoring feed intake and body weight of animal

POSSIBLE COMPLICATIONS

Secondary infections due to debilitated immune system of the horse

MISCELLANEOUS

AGE-RELATED FACTORS

Poor dentition might be a major factor in weight loss in older horses.

ZOONOTIC POTENTIAL

Chronic salmonellosis

ABBREVIATIONS

• CBC = complete blood count
• COPD = chronic obstructive pulmonary disease
• EIA = equine infectious anemia
• IBD = inflammatory bowel disease

Suggested Reading

Brown CM. Chronic weight loss. In: Brown CM, ed. Problems in Equine Medicine. Philadelphia: Lea & Febiger, 1989:6–21.
Roberts MC. Malabsorption syndromes in the horse. Compend Cont Educ Pract Vet 1985:7:S637–S647.
McClure JJ. Chronic weight loss without diarrhea, pain, or icterus. In: Anderson NV: Chapter 27, Veterinary Gastroenterology, ed 2. Philadelphia: Lea & Febiger, 1992.
Stämpfli H, Oliver OE. Chronic diarrhea and weight loss in three horses. Vet Clin North Am Equine Pract 2006;22:e27-e35

Authors Olimpo Oliver-Espinosa and Henry Stämpfli
Consulting Editors Henry Stämpfli and Olimpo Oliver-Espinosa

CLEFT PALATE

BASICS

• Cleft palate (palatoschisis) is a rare defect of the secondary (hard and soft) palates.
• Congenital clefts result from an interruption of the midline closure of the embryonic palatine folds. Closure of the palate proceeds from rostral to caudal, so either the soft palate or both soft and hard palate may be affected. Unlike in humans, defects of the nares and lips have not been reported. • Acquired clefts result from trauma during surgery and may involve the hard or soft palate.

PATHOPHYSIOLOGY

• The soft and hard palate provide a strict separation of the respiratory and digestive tract.
• The palate also provides stability to the nasopharynx and nasal passages to reduce airway resistance during exercise. • Clefts extending rostral to the levator veli palatini muscle result in contamination of the respiratory tract. • Clefts caudal to the levator veli palatini muscle may not cause significant contamination. • Cleft soft palate will permit dorsal displacement of the palate, resulting in exercise intolerance due to an expiratory obstruction.

SIGNALMENT

• Congenital cleft palate is seen in foals of any breed and sex, with a reported frequency of 4% of all reported congenital abnormalities. Age of presentation will depend on severity of the cleft.
• Acquired clefts occur in horses of any age that have a history of recent surgery.

SIGNS

• Milk draining from a foal's nose after nursing
• Water or food-stained discharge from the nares of adult horses • Coughing after eating or drinking • Signs of aspiration pneumonia—fever, lethargy, increased respiratory rate, harsh lung sounds • Chronic clefts—present stunted and in poor condition due to lack of adequate nutritional intake and persistent respiratory disease

CAUSES AND RISK FACTORS

• The cause of congenital cleft palate has not been determined. Risk factors may include toxins, nutritional deficiencies, infection, radiation exposure, hormonal and environmental factors, and metabolic abnormalities at the time of palate fusion (around the 47th day of gestation). • Causes of acquired cleft palate include iatrogenic trauma to the palate during pharyngeal or oral surgery, such as aggressive staphlectomy (palate trim) and treatment of epiglottic entrapment via a nasal approach. Iatrogenic hard palate clefts or oronasal fistula is common secondary to trauma from a dental punch during tooth repulsion.

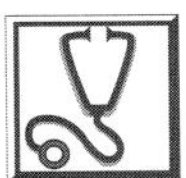

DIAGNOSIS

DIFFERENTIAL DIAGNOSIS

• Esophageal obstruction • Dysphagia

CBC/BIOCHEMISTRY/URINALYSIS

• CBC and fibrinogen—leukocytosis and hyperfibrinogenemia will usually be seen with secondary aspiration pneumonia.

OTHER LABORATORY TESTS

• IgG is assessed in all neonatal foals—ensures adequate transfer of passive immunity due to the possibility of inadequate colostrum intake caused by the cleft. • Blood cultures are indicated in foals with pneumonia or failure of transfer of passive immunity to rule out septicemia.

IMAGING

• Thoracic radiographs are necessary to determine the extent of aspiration pneumonia.
• Thoracic ultrasound will provide information regarding the pleural surface.

OTHER DIAGNOSTIC PROCEDURES

Endoscopy (nasal or oral) is essential to determine the extent and prognosis. Diagnosis is made based on lack of continuity of the palate, or abnormal visibility of oral structures from the nasopharynx.

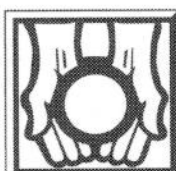

TREATMENT

• Primary, one-stage, surgical closure of the cleft is indicated—transhyoid pharyngotomy for caudal clefts of the soft palate or a mandibular symphysiectomy for extensive soft palate defects or hard palate clefts (may be combined with a transhyoid pharyngotomy). • Extensive nursing care is required after surgery. • Severity of aspiration pneumonia may increase the anesthetic risk. • The chronicity and severity of the cleft will affect the severity of the pneumonia.
• The size of the head of younger foals may reduce surgical access, but delaying surgery may increase the severity of pneumonia.

MEDICATIONS

DRUG(S) OF CHOICE

• Prompt administration of broad spectrum antibiotics is indicated. Antibiotics are continued for approximately 5 days postoperatively, but continued treatment with antibiotics is often required for treatment of secondary aspiration pneumonia.
• Antimicrobial combinations include sodium or potassium penicillin (22,000–44,000 U/kg IV q6h), an aminoglycoside (gentamicin in adults [6.6 mg/kg IV q24h] or amikacin in foals [25 mg/kg IV q24h]), and metronidazole (15–25 mg/kg PO q8h). • Procaine penicillin can be substituted (22,000–44,000 units/kg IM q12h). • Other antimicrobial choices include trimethoprim-sulfamethoxazole (20–30 mg/kg PO q12h) and chloramphenicol (44 mg/kg PO q8h). • NSAIDs—for endotoxemia and inflammation—flunixin meglumine (1.1 mg/kg IV/PO q12h) or ketoprofen (1.1–2.2 IV q12h). • Tetanus antitoxin and/or tetanus toxoid should be administered to all surgical patients.

CONTRAINDICATIONS/POSSIBLE INTERACTIONS

• Enrofloxacin should not be used in foals.
• Aminoglycosides and NSAIDs have nephrotoxic and negative gastrointestinal side effects, especially in dehydrated patients.
• Chloramphenicol has human health risks.

FOLLOW-UP

PATIENT MONITORING

• Evaluate the suture line by endoscopy no earlier than 1 week after surgery to prevent dehiscence. • Monitor clinical signs of pneumonia, including temperature, respiratory rate, and effort. • Follow progress of pneumonia by radiography for pulmonary lesions or ultrasonography for pleural lesions. • Patients with extensive repairs, especially those involving the hard palate, should be fed via nasogastric tube to reduce the risk of dehiscence of the suture line.

PREVENTION/AVOIDANCE

Owners are recommended not to breed animals with cleft palates, although inheritance is unknown.

POSSIBLE COMPLICATIONS

• Dehiscence—suspected if there is a recurrence of feed/milk from nostrils, generally in the first 7–14 days postoperatively • Incisional infection
• Osteomyelitis of the mandible • Nonunion of the mandibular symphysis • Persistent soft palate displacement • Oronasal fistula • Pneumonia

EXPECTED COURSE AND PROGNOSIS

• Successful repair occurs in 50%–60% of patients with midline clefts and minimal tissue loss.
• Clefts involving both hard and soft palate, >20% of the soft palate alone, or asymmetric clefts have a poor prognosis.
• Prognosis is reduced by concurrent respiratory disease.
• Poor prognosis for future athleticism—often stunted due to malnutrition and may have persistent respiratory insufficiency after resolution of pneumonia

MISCELLANEOUS

ASSOCIATED CONDITIONS

• Aspiration pneumonia
• Poor growth and development
• Exercise intolerance

SEE ALSO

• Pneumonia, neonatal

Suggested Reading

Semevolos S, Ducharme NG. Cleft palate. In: Mair TS, Divers TJ, Ducharme NG eds. Manual of Equine Gastroenterology. Philadelphia: WB Saunders, 2002:79–88.

Author Amelia S. Munsterman
Consulting Editor Margaret C. Mudge

CLITORAL ENLARGEMENT

BASICS

DEFINITION/OVERVIEW

- The clitoris appears larger than normal and may appear to protrude through the vulvar lips at the ventral commissure.
- It develops from the embryonic genital tubercle in the absence of testicular testosterone production, or testosterone's conversion by 5α-reductase to the active form, dihydrotestosterone.
- The clitoris is the female homologue of the penis.
- Corpus cavernosum clitoris—erectile tissue
- Corpus clitoris (body of the clitoris)—5 cm in length
- Crura—attached to the ischial arch
- Glans clitoris—2.5 cm in diameter; situated in the fossa at the ventral commissure of the vulva; well-developed median sinus and lateral sinuses may be present.

ETIOLOGY/PATHOPHYSIOLOGY

See Causes and Risk Factors.

SYSTEM AFFECTED

Reproductive

GENETICS

N/A

SIGNALMENT

- Females
- Congenital
- Concurrent ovarian neoplasia—GTCT.
- Iatrogenic drug administration—anabolic steroid, progestin
- Intersex condition

SIGNS

- Historical—known drug administration; female offspring of treated mare
- Enlargement of the glans clitoris beyond the expected norm
- May be visible externally as swelling of the ventral vulval commissure
- May protrude from the clitoral sinus between labia
- May be associated with abnormal cyclicity
- May be associated with other structural genital anomalies—internal and/or external
- May be associated with other signs of virilism—stallion-like behavior and conformation

CAUSES AND RISK FACTORS

- Administration of anabolic steroids
- Progestin (Altrenogest) usage for estrus control, behavior modification, and pregnancy maintenance—female progeny have associated altered gonadotropin secretion and increased clitoral size to 21 mo of age; no effect on reproductive function
- Aberrant endogenous sex-steroid production—GCT in dam during gestation alters fetal development.
- Hormonally active ovarian neoplasm in post-pubertal female—GTCT

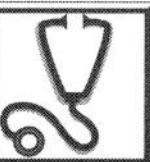

DIAGNOSIS

DIFFERENTIAL DIAGNOSIS

- Intersex conditions
- Pseudohermaphrodite is associated with clitoral enlargement.
- Hypospadia penis
- Hypoplastic penis with incomplete closure of embryonic urethral folds.
- Associated with prominent perineal median raphe, ventrally displaced vulva, and caudad direction of penis
- Most common presentation—64, XX male

CBC/BIOCHEMISTRY/URINALYSIS

N/A

OTHER LABORATORY TESTS

Hormonal Assay

- Testosterone/hCG challenge—baseline blood sample; administer 3000 IU hCG IV, with additional blood samples collected at 3 and 24 hr; increased testosterone indicates testicular tissue is present (i.e., Leydig cell production).
- Estrone sulfate—produced by Sertoli cells in the testicle; couple with hCG challenge to improve diagnostic accuracy
- Investigate (rule out presence of) a GTCT by measurement of inhibin (raised in 87%) and testosterone (raised in 54%).

Immunology

- Test for presence of 5α-reductase or cytosolic receptor.
- Use labial skin only as the receptors are site specific.

IMAGING

- U/S—coupled with TRP of internal genitalia for ovarian pathology or internal genital anomaly
- Note there is no pathognomonic appearance of a GTCT.

DIAGNOSTIC PROCEDURES N/A

PATHOLOGICAL FINDINGS N/A

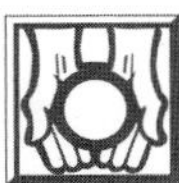

TREATMENT

APPROPRIATE HEALTH CARE, NURSING CARE, ACTIVITY, DIET, CLIENT EDUCATION, SURGICAL CONSIDERATIONS

N/A

MEDICATIONS

DRUG(S) OF CHOICE, CONTRAINDICATIONS, PRECAUTIONS, POSSIBLE INTERACTIONS

N/A

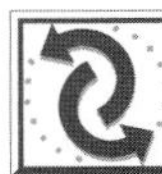

FOLLOW-UP

For control/prevention:

- Rational causative drug use
- If genetic, analysis of pedigree
- If heritable, elimination of parent stock from breeding pool

PATIENT MONITORING, PREVENTION/AVOIDANCE, POSSIBLE COMPLICATIONS, EXPECTED COURSE AND PROGNOSIS

N/A

MISCELLANEOUS

ASSOCIATED CONDITIONS

Intersex conditions

AGE-RELATED FACTORS

Congenital

ZOONOTIC POTENTIAL

N/A

PREGNANCY

Associated abnormalities may preclude fertility.

SEE ALSO

Disorders of sexual development

ABBREVIATIONS

- GCT = granulosa cell tumor
- GTCT = granulosa theca cell tumor
- hCG = human chorionic gonadotropin
- TRP = transrectal palpation
- U/S = ultrasonographic examination

Suggested Reading

Hughes JP. Developmental anomalies of the female reproductive tract. In: McKinnon AO, Voss JL, eds. Equine Reproduction. Philadelphia: Lea & Febiger, 1993:409–410.

McCue PM. Equine granulosa cell tumors. Proceedings of the 38th annual convention of the American Association of Equine Practitioners, Orlando, FL, 1992:587–593.

Noden J, Squires EL, Nett TM. Effect of maternal treatment with altrenogest on age at puberty, hormone concentrations, pituitary response to exogenous GnRH, oestrous cycle characteristics and fertility of fillies. J Reprod Fertil 1990;88:185–195.

Skelton KV, Dowsett KF, McMeniman NP. Ovarian activity in fillies treated with anabolic steroids prior to the onset of puberty. J Reprod Fertil Suppl 1991;44:351–356.

Author Peter R. Morresey

Consulting Editor Carla L. Carleton

CLOSTRIDIAL MYOSITIS

BASICS

DEFINITION

Clostridial myositis is an infection of muscle by *Clostridium* spp. most frequently associated with intramuscular injection. The infection may remain localized and form a focal abscess or migrate along fascial planes, resulting in diffuse cellulitis.

PATHOPHYSIOLOGY

The frequent temporal association between intramuscular injections and clostridial myositis suggests entry of the organism at the time of injection. However, injection of irritating substances may produce local tissue necrosis and an anaerobic environment ideal for proliferation of spores already present in muscle. In cattle, *Clostridium* spp. are thought to be absorbed from the gastrointestinal tract and remain dormant in tissue until conditions exist for proliferation. Due to the ubiquitous nature of clostridial organisms, they may contaminate wounds and surgical sites. Clostridial organisms are also common in subsolar abscesses. Regardless of the origin, the release of potent clostridial exotoxins leads to local tissue necrosis, systemic toxemia, and organ dysfunction. In this most severe form, the term "*malignant edema*" is used to reflect the systemic involvement and high mortality.

SYSTEM AFFECTED

Musculoskeletal

This is the primary system affected. Necrotizing toxins released by the organism lead to local tissue necrosis.

Cardiovascular, Respiratory, Renal, and Hemic

Exotoxins absorbed from the site of infection cause damage to cell membranes, leading to hemolysis, increased capillary permeability, and multiple organ dysfunction.

GENETICS

N/A

INCIDENCE/PREVALENCE

Some geographic areas may have a greater incidence due to higher environmental contamination by clostridial organisms.

SIGNALMENT

Clostridial myositis occurs in horses of any breed or age. Horses on a high plane of nutrition may be predisposed due to proliferation of clostridial organisms in the alimentary tract.

SIGNS

Historical Findings

Intramuscular injection with a non-antibiotic medication is the most common cause of clostridial myositis, and thus owners should be questioned about recent medications, treatments, or illnesses. The most commonly implicated medication is flunixin meglumine. Depending on the site of infection, horses may be stiff and reluctant to walk, lame, or unwilling to raise or lower the head to eat. Pain and systemic toxemia may lead to anorexia and tachypnea. Vague signs of discomfort are easily mistaken for colic.

Physical Examination Findings

If myonecrosis is related to intramuscular injection, common sites of injection should be palpated for heat, pain, swelling, and crepitus. Small puncture wounds are occasionally only visible once the hair over the affected area is clipped. Swellings are initially warm and painful and later become cool, firm, and necrotic. Muscle pain may cause a lame or stiff gait, reluctance to walk, depression, anorexia, tachypnea, and tachycardia. Dehydration, depression, delayed capillary refill time, poor peripheral pulses, and cool extremities suggest systemic toxemia and inadequate peripheral perfusion and shock. Oral mucous membranes may be dark red to blue. Fever is common.

CAUSES

Clostridial myositis is most often associated with *C. perfringens* (type A) and *C. septicum,* but *C. chauvoei, C. novyi, and C. fallax* have also been reported.

RISK FACTORS

Although any intramuscular injection could potentially result in a clostridial infection, medications that are irritating and result in tissue necrosis (such as nonsteroidal anti-inflammatory drugs and vitamin solutions) are frequently associated with this syndrome.

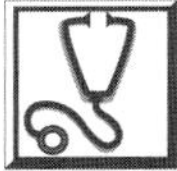

DIAGNOSIS

DIFFERENTIAL DIAGNOSIS

When clostridial myositis is secondary to an injection, the diagnosis can be complicated by previous medical problems. Pain associated with myonecrosis may be confused with colic, exertional myopathy, laminitis, or abscesses from other causes. Severe pain, fever, toxemia, and shock rarely result from an abscess due to other less virulent organisms.

CBC/BIOCHEMISTRY

If clostridial infection is localized into an abscess, a CBC may reveal only a modest leukocytosis with left shift and neutrophilia. Hyperfibrinogenemia may be present if infection is present for more than a few days. When severe systemic toxemia develops, leucopenia, thrombocytopenia, and hemolysis can occur. Increases in muscle enzymes CK and AST may be mild compared to the apparent severity of toxemia perhaps due to the focal nature of the disease, destruction of enzyme, or lack of enzyme absorption into systemic circulation. Dehydration and shock may result in azotemia and hemoconcentration.

OTHER LABORATORY TESTS

Clostridial toxins may result in disseminated intravascular coagulation and alterations in platelet count, PT, PTT, and antithrombin-III.

IMAGING

Ultrasonography may reveal an encapsulated abscess or diffuse tissue edema, necrosis, cellulitis, and echogenic foci of emphysema. Differentiation between focal abscesses and diffuse cellulitis aids in defining areas for treatment. Abscesses should be lanced and lavaged. Fasciotomy / myotomy is appropriate if diffuse cellulitis and myonecrosis are present.

DIAGNOSTIC PROCEDURES

A tentative diagnosis can be made based on a history of intramuscular injection or wound and a rapid onset of severe heat, pain, crepitus, and swelling of affected tissues. Diagnosis can be confirmed by aspiration of purulent or serosanguinous material for anaerobic culture, cytology, or fluorescent antibody identification. Care should be taken to properly prepare sites for aspiration to avoid contamination with surface organisms. Samples should be collected and placed in media designed for transportation of anaerobic specimens and submitted to a laboratory as soon as possible. Muscle biopsies frequently reveal characteristic gram-positive rods.

PATHOLOGIC FINDINGS

Systemic toxemia results in the degeneration of parenchymatous tissues. Malodorous serosanguinous fluid and emphysema are present in dark-colored necrotic muscle.

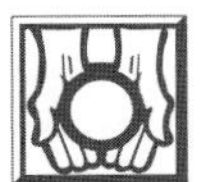

TREATMENT

APPROPRIATE HEALTH CARE

Treatment options are dictated by the severity of the disease. Focal encapsulated abscesses may be managed in the field; however, referral should be considered for horses with signs of systemic toxemia (tachycardia, increased capillary refill time, abnormal mucous membrane color, poor peripheral pulses, or cool extremities).

NURSING CARE

Oral or parenteral fluids are indicated if dehydration is present and balanced polyionic fluids (lactated or acetated Ringer's solution) should be administered intravenously if there are signs of shock. Hot-packing may aid in drainage of abscesses, whereas later in the course of the disease cold hydrotherapy may decrease the activity of inflammatory mediators. Feed should be provided at head level for horses with neck pain associated with infection of cervical musculature.

ACTIVITY

Activity should be limited to decrease movement of bacteria along fascial planes.

DIET

N/A

CLIENT EDUCATION

Clients should be educated about proper intramuscular injection techniques.

SURGICAL CONSIDERATIONS

Focal abscesses may be drained by incision, lavage, and placement of a drain. Diffuse cellulitis and tissue edema are important to identify sonographically because medical management may be more appropriate for this type of infection. Depending on the severity of the disease, fenestration of infected tissue with vertical incisions is helpful in reducing an anaerobic environment. Incisions are made through skin and necrotic muscle so as to aerate tissues and reduce pressure associated with severe edema. Minimal sedation and hemostasis are frequently necessary due to the necrotic nature of the tissue incised.

MEDICATIONS

DRUG(S) OF CHOICE

Horses with severe systemic signs are initially given potassium or sodium penicillin (44,000 IU/kg IV) every 2 to 4 hr until stabilized and then four times daily. Focal abscesses can be managed with drainage and penicillin (22,000 IU/kg IM q12h). Metronidazole (15–25 mg/kg PO q6h) is also effective against *Clostridium* spp. and can be given orally. Analgesics and anti-inflammatory medications (flunixin meglumine 1.1 mg/kg IV q12h) are indicated.

CONTRAINDICATIONS

N/A

PRECAUTIONS

Hydration and renal function should be monitored when using nonsteroidal anti-inflammatory medications in horses with severe systemic disease.

POSSIBLE INTERACTIONS

N/A

ALTERNATIVE DRUGS

Chloramphenicol (50 mg/kg PO q6h) also has activity against anaerobic bacteria; however, due to the potential for irreversible aplastic anemia in people, its use should be avoided if possible. Trimethoprim-potentiated sulfonamides are efficacious *in-vitro* but have questionable *in-vivo* efficacy. Rifampin is effective against most *Clostridium* spp.; however, it is generally used in combination with other antimicrobials due to the development of resistance.

FOLLOW-UP

PATIENT MONITORING

N/A

PREVENTION/AVOIDANCE

Clostridial myonecrosis may result from intramuscular injections even when proper technique is followed. Avoiding intramuscular injection of irritating substances may reduce the incidence of this disease.

POSSIBLE COMPLICATIONS

Severe toxemia may lead to shock, renal insufficiency, laminitis, intravascular hemolysis, disseminated intravascular coagulation, or death.

EXPECTED COURSE AND PROGNOSIS

Small, focal abscesses may respond well to drainage and systemic antimicrobials. Horses with diffuse myositis, toxemia, and shock have a guarded to poor prognosis in spite of aggressive therapy. *Clostridium septicum* and *C. chauvoei* infections are usually fatal; however, *C. perfringens* infections have a better prognosis.

MISCELLANEOUS

ASSOCIATED CONDITIONS

N/A

AGE-RELATED FACTORS

N/A

ZOONOTIC POTENTIAL

Clostridium perfringens is the most common cause of malignant edema in people.

PREGNANCY

N/A

SYNONYMS

- Malignant edema
- Clostridial myonecrosis
- Clostridial cellulitis

SEE ALSO

- Botulism, neonate
- Tetanus
- Tyzzer's disease
- Enteric clostridiosis

ABBREVIATIONS

- AST = asparate aminotransferase
- CK = creatinine kinase
- PT = prothrombin time
- PTT = partial thromboplastin time

Suggested Reading

Rebhun WC, Shin SJ, King JM, et al Malignant edema in horses. J Am Vet Med Assoc. 1985,187;732–736.

Peek SF, Semrad AD, Perkins GA. Clostridial myonecrosis in horses (37 cases 1985–2000). Eq Vet J. 2003, 35(1):86–92.

Author Kerry E. Beckman

Consulting Editors Ashley G. Boyle and Corinne R. Sweeney

CLOSTRIDIUM DIFFICILE ENTEROCOLITIS

BASICS

DEFINITION

Clostridium difficile enterocolitis is an inflammation of the small intestine and large colon commonly resulting in diarrhea and varying degrees of toxemia. It is caused by strains that produce toxin (s).

PATHOPHYSIOLOGY

C. difficile is acquired through ingestion or may be present in low numbers in the gastrointestinal tract (GI). In either case, it is not known why proliferation of this organism occurs, but it is hypothesized to be due to a disruption of the normal, protective gastrointestinal microflora and in some cases follows the use of antibiotics. This organism produces two major toxins (toxin A and B), a cytotoxin and an enterotoxin, that work synergistically. However, strains that only produce toxin B are capable of inducing disease. These toxins cause clinical signs both by their direct toxic effects on the colon and through proinflammatory effects on neutrophils. The net result is varying degrees of fluid secretion, mucosal damage, and intestinal inflammation. Some strains of *C. difficile* also produce a binary toxin (CDT), but its role in equine enterocolitis is unknown.

SYSTEMS AFFECTED

Gastrointestinal

C. difficile can cause diarrhea ranging in severity from cow-pie consistency feces to profuse and watery feces. Borborygmi are variable in intensity, but typically have a fluid sound. Mild to severe colic may be present.

Cardiovascular

Dehydration and cardiovascular shock can ensue. Venous thrombosis at injection or catheter sites can occur.

Musculoskeletal

Peripheral edema may occur due to hypoproteinemia. Laminitis is another common sequel.

INCIDENCE/PREVALENCE

It is usually a sporadic condition, but outbreaks have been reported. It is more commonly reported in certain geographic areas, but this may be partly because the diagnosis of this condition is not done in all regions.

SIGNALMENT

There is no reported breed, age, or sex predilection.

SIGNS

Historical Findings

There is occasionally a history of depression, anorexia, colic and/or pyrexia. Diarrhea is not always the initial complaint. There may be a history of recent antibiotic use, however not all cases are associated with antibiotic therapy.

Physical Examination Findings

Diarrhea is present in most cases. Dehydration may be present, suggested by decreased skin turgor, tacky oral mucous membranes, and increased capillary refill time. Rectal temperature may be subnormal, normal, or increased. Tachycardia is often present. Intestines are hypermotile or hypomotile but fluid-sounding gastrointestinal sounds may be present. Signs of endotoxemia and peripheral edema may be present. Colic may result from fluid and gas distension of the GI tract.

CAUSES

Infectious

The proliferation of the toxigenic strains of the anaerobic gram-positive *C. difficile* and the production of its exotoxin

RISK FACTORS

Risk factors for *C. difficile* enterocolitis have not been clearly established in the horse. However, it is presumed that any condition altering the normal intestinal microflora could allow proliferation of toxigenic *C. difficile.* Antibiotic use is a well-documented risk factor in humans for developing *C. difficile* colitis and is presumed to be a significant risk factor in the horse as well. *C. difficile* colitis has also been reported in mares whose foals were being treated with erythromycin succinate, presumably through low-dose antibiotic exposure. This syndrome has recently been reproduced experimentally. This organism is also a major nosocomial pathogen in human medicine, so hospitalization may be a risk factor as well. Other stressors, such as surgery and transportation, may play a role.

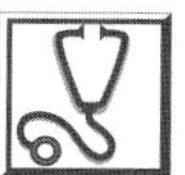

DIAGNOSIS

DIFFERENTIAL DIAGNOSIS

- Salmonellosis
- Potomac horse fever
- *Clostridium perfringens* enterocolitis
- Cyathostomiasis
- NSAID-induced colitis
- Cantharidin toxicosis
- Chronic sand impaction
- Idiopathic colitis

CBC/BIOCHEMISTRY/URINALYSIS

CBC

The packed cell volume is often elevated, depending on the degree of dehydration. Total protein levels are variable and may be increased due to hemoconcentration or decreased due to protein loss into the intestinal tract. Leukopenia with neutropenia is often present, frequently with a left shift. Neutrophils may be degenerate. A leukocytosis develops at later stages of the disease.

Biochemistry

Hyponatremia and hypochloremia are characteristic. Hypokalemia is sometimes present, but hyperkalemia in response to a metabolic acidosis is common. Hypocalcemia and hypoalbuminemia are also common. Prerenal azotemia is common in dehydrated animals.

OTHER LABORATORY TESTS

Culture of this organism is difficult, requires specialized equipment for anaerobic culture and, by itself, is not diagnostic. Testing of isolates to determine whether they are able to produce toxins supports a diagnosis, but is not considered to be confirmatory. The clinical standard for diagnosis is detection of *C. difficile* toxins A or B in feces using ELISA. Tests that only detect toxin A should not be used as the sole test because strains that do not produce toxin A but produce toxin B can cause disease in horses. Antigen testing of feces can be used as a screening test. Antigen negative results have a high negative predictive value, but antigen positive samples should be tested further to determine whether toxins are present. Polymerize chain reaction (PCR) has been used to detect toxin genes in fecal samples of human patients and is also under investigation in horses. The clinical utility of this technique is currently unclear.

Bacterial culture for *Salmonella* spp. should also be performed because it is a major differential diagnosis, and co-infection can occur.

IMAGING

Abdominal ultrasonography may be performed, and the large colon may appear hypoechoic with increased motility.

DIAGNOSTIC PROCEDURES

Palpation per rectum may be required in cases of colitis to rule out another gastrointestinal lesion.

PATHOLOGIC FINDINGS

The pathologic lesions in *C. difficile* colitis are not well described in horses. The large intestine, including the cecum, is the main site affected in adult horses. The only gross abnormality may be fluid intestinal contents. More severe cases may have marked intestinal edema and hemorrhage, with petechiae and ecchymoses throughout. Histologically, there is mild to severe inflammation, and edema and hemorrhagic necrotizing enterocolitis may be present.

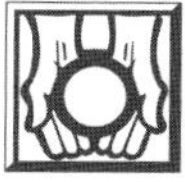

TREATMENT

APPROPRIATE HEALTH CARE

This condition is best managed intensively due to the frequent need for aggressive fluid therapy and the high risk of secondary problems. If the diarrhea is not severe and adequate hydration can be maintained, treatment on the farm could be attempted.

NURSING CARE

Intravenous (IV) fluid therapy is the most important treatment of this condition. A balanced polyionic electrolyte solution should be administered. The rate of fluid administration depends on the degree of dehydration and the amount of fluid content of the diarrhea. Mild to moderate cases of metabolic acidosis resolve with fluid therapy. Sodium bicarbonate may be required in certain cases to correct a severe metabolic acidosis. In severely hypokalemic horses, 20–40 mEq/L of potassium chloride can be added to the IV fluids. Intravenous administration of KCl should not exceed 0.5 mEq/kg/hr.

An oral electrolyte solution containing 35 g KCl and 70 g of NaCl in 10 L of water should be provided, along with clean, fresh drinking water. Hypertonic saline (4–6 mL/kg IV of 5–7.5% NaCl) may be indicated in severely dehydrated animals. This provides rapid volume expansion and also appears to increase myocardial contractility, vasodilation, and peripheral perfusion. It is essential that isotonic fluid therapy follow the use of hypertonic saline. Due to the high incidence of venous thrombosis in colitis cases, the catheter site should be monitored frequently. If distal limb edema develops, leg wraps should be applied and changed daily. Deep bedding should be provided if there are signs of laminitis. Ditrioctahedral smectite (Biosponge™)that has been shown to bind to *C. difficile* toxins *in vitro* and has been used with anecdotal success in horses.

ACTIVITY

Activity is restricted due to the need for IV fluid therapy and the potential for disease transmission. Horses that display signs of colic may benefit from short walks to stimulate progressive motility and help pass diarrhea. Because all diarrheic horses should be considered infectious, animals should be handled accordingly and an isolated area should be used and disinfected appropriately. While uncommon, outbreaks of *C. difficile* diarrhea have been reported and co-infection with *Salmonella* can occur, so close adherence to infection control practices is essential.

DIET

Horses should be provided with free choice hay. This may help stabilize the disrupted GI flora, provide electrolytes such as potassium and calcium, and decrease weight loss as affected animals can become very catabolic. It is recommended to feed hay in a hay net because hypoproteinemic horses eating off the ground may develop severe facial edema. Higher energy feeds can also be offered. Large amounts of grain should be avoided due to the risk of further GI flora disruption.

Due to the severe catabolic state that occurs in colitis, forced enteral feeding or partial or total parenteral nutrition may be required. The cost of parenteral nutrition is often prohibitive.

CLIENT EDUCATION

Clients should be made aware of the potential for mortality and the serious risk of secondary problems such as laminitis and jugular vein thrombosis. They should also be warned that the horse should be considered infectious, and appropriate sanitation of contaminated areas should be recommended.

SURGICAL CONSIDERATION

N/A

MEDICATIONS

DRUG (S) OF CHOICE

- Metronidazole—15–25 mg/kg PO q6–8-hr.
- Flunixin meglumine: 0.25–0.5 mg/kg q8-hr IV can be used for its purported anti-endotoxic effects, 1.1 mg/kg can be used for analgesia.
- Fresh-frozen plasma is beneficial in severely hypoproteinemic animals (<40 g/L) (4.0 g/dL). Although not proved to be of added benefit in cases of colitis, some clinicians believe that the use of serum from horses hyperimmunized to *Escherichia coli* J5 strain helps moderate the effects of endotoxemia.
- KCL—25–50 g PO q12–24 h. If the horse is eating but remains hypokalemic, oral administration of KCl once or twice a day is an easy and cost-effective route of supplementation.
- Lamitinis treatment—See the appropriate chapter in this text.

CONTRAINDICATIONS

Metronidazole may be teratogenic and is therefore contraindicated in pregnant mares.

PRECAUTIONS

The 1.1 mg/kg dose of flunixin meglumine may be nephrotoxic in dehydrated animals. It may mask severe pain that indicates a surgical lesion, and should be used judiciously when the diagnosis is still in question.

POSSIBLE INTERACTIONS

Cimetidine should not be used concurrently with metronidazole because there is interaction through hepatic inhibition.

ALTERNATIVE DRUGS

N/A

FOLLOW-UP

PATIENT MONITORING

Affected animals should be monitored frequently to evaluate hydration status, character and volume of diarrhea, presence of edema, and to observe for signs of colic. Packed cell volume and total protein levels should be evaluated at least daily during the initial course of disease. Increases in urea and creatinine seen on presentation should be reevaluated after rehydration to ensure it was due to prerenal azotemia and not to renal failure. Serum or plasma electrolyte levels should be monitored to determine whether electrolyte supplementation, especially potassium and calcium, is required. The IV catheter site should be monitored frequently. The feet should be checked frequently for any sign indicative of laminitis.

PREVENTION/AVOIDANCE

Antibiotics should be used judiciously to decrease the risk of disruption of the GI microflora.

POSSIBLE COMPLICATIONS

- Endotoxemia
- Laminitis
- Jugular vein thrombosis
- Renal failure

EXPECTED COURSE AND PROGNOSIS

Reported mortality rates for *C. difficile* enterocolitis range from 10% to 40%, however referral hospital-based studies are a biased population and the overall mortality rate is likely lower. Death can occur from the primary gastrointestinal disease; however, euthanasia is often opted for due to expense of treatment, poor response to initial treatment, or development of severe laminitis. The prognosis is good when the diarrhea resolves shortly after presentation and no signs of laminitis occur.

MISCELLANEOUS

ASSOCIATED CONDITIONS

- Laminitis
- Venous thrombosis

AGE-RELATED FACTORS

N/A

ZOONOTIC POTENTIAL

As the causative organism of colitis in humans and some *C. difficile* strain (s) affecting horses are the same, it is advisable to treat all affected horses as zoonotic risks.

PREGNANCY

Metronidazole should not be administered to pregnant mares. An increased risk of abortion may be present due to endotoxemia and hypovolemic shock.

SYNONYMS

N/A

SEE ALSO

Laminitis

ABBREVIATIONS

N/A

Suggested Reading

Weese JS, Toxopeus L, Arroyo L. *Clostridium difficile* associated diarrhoea in horses within the community: predictors, clinical presentation and outcome. Equine Vet J. 2006; 38:185–188.

Baverud V, Gustafsson A, Franklin A, Lindholm A, Gunnersson A. *Clostridium difficile* associated with acute colitis in mature horses treated with antibiotics. Eq Vet J 1997;29:279–284.

Jones RL, Shideler RK, Cockerell GL. Association of *Clostridium difficile* with foal diarrhea. In: Equine Infectious Diseases V. Lexington: University of Kentucky Press. 1988;5:236–240.

Knoop FC, Owens M, Crocker IC. *Clostridium difficile:* Clinical disease and diagnosis. Clin Microbiol Rev. 1993;6:251–265.

Weese JS, Parsons DA, Stämpfli HR. Association of *Clostridium difficile* with enterocolitis and lactose intolerance in a foal. J Am Vet Med Assoc. 1999;214:229–232.

Authors Luis G. Arroyo and J. Scott Weese
Consulting Editors Henry Stämpfli and Olimpo Oliver-Espinosa

COAGULATION DEFECTS, ACQUIRED

BASICS

DEFINITION

- Several acquired disorders can affect the coagulation system resulting in deficient hemostatic function and subsequent bleeding tendencies.
- They may be classified as:
  - Disorders that cause a deficient fibrin clot formation, known as coagulation defects.
  - Disorders that cause a deficient platelet plug formation due to platelet function deficiencies (e.g., idiopathic thrombocytopenia, thrombasthenia, antiplatelet drug administration) or endothelial damage (e.g., vasculitis). These are discussed elsewhere.
  - Disorders in which primary hemostasis and coagulation factor pathways are inadequate due to a consumptive coagulopathy (e.g., DIC). DIC is discussed in detail elsewhere.
- Acquired coagulation defects are characterized by an inability to form fibrin and a fibrin clot, resulting in hemorrhage. Causes of acquired coagulation defects include vitamin K deficiency, drug-induced coagulation deficiency, hepatic failure, and DIC.

PATHOPHYSIOLOGY

- The pathogenesis of sweet clover, rodenticide, and warfarin toxicosis is identical in that they inhibit vitamin K, which is essential for hepatic synthesis of several coagulation factors (II, VII, IX, and X) and protein C.
- Vitamin K deficiency results in a gradual decrease of coagulation factors in circulating blood, which causes progressive clinical signs of coagulation defect and unexpected bleeding.
- The gradual decrease of coagulation factor concentrations in plasma depends on the half-life of these factors. Factor VII is the vitamin K–dependent factor with the shortest half-life (<6–7hr); therefore, its concentration decreases rapidly. This affects the extrinsic coagulation pathway and subsequently prolongs the PT value. As the condition progresses, plasma concentrations of other coagulation factors decrease, affecting also the intrinsic pathway and subsequently prolonging the aPTT value.
- Sweet clover hay may contain dicumarol, a well-known vitamin K antagonist.
- First- (warfarin, dicumarol) and second-generation (brodifacoum, bromodiolone) rodenticides are vitamin K antagonists.
- Warfarin has been used as an oral anticoagulant in horses and has been recommended to treat navicular disease and thrombophlebitis. When warfarin is given in combination with other protein-bound drugs such as phenylbutazone, warfarin toxicosis is likely. Phenylbutazone competes with warfarin for plasma albumin binding, increasing the concentration of free warfarin in the circulation. Simultaneous administration of both drugs is therefore not recommended.
- Warfarin toxicosis can similarly result in horses with hypoalbuminemia.
- Heparin is a non–vitamin K–dependent anticoagulant that acts by potentiating the activity of the main plasma coagulation inhibitor (antithrombin). In cases of heparin overdosage, coagulation function is markedly inhibited and it may result in a hemorrhagic tendency.
- In cases of hepatic failure, a coagulation defect occurs due to a decrease in coagulation factor synthesis, especially fibrinogen and the vitamin K–dependent factors.

SYSTEMS AFFECTED

- Hemic/lymphatic/immune—Coagulation deficiencies are associated with prolonged bleeding after wounds/trauma or spontaneous hemorrhages.
- Other systems may be affected, depending on the sites of hemorrhage. The most frequently affected system is the musculoskeletal (i.e., hematomas in joints, muscle groups) and spontaneous bleeding into the respiratory and gastrointestinal tracts.

INCIDENCE/PREVALENCE

- Vitamin K deficiency in horses is very rare. However, toxicosis caused by ingestion of moldy sweet clover hay has been reported in all herbivores.
- Anticoagulant toxicosis is rare now because warfarin administration is currently not recommended in horses, and heparin administration is restricted to patients receiving critical care, in which low doses of heparin are given to prevent hypercoagulation and DIC.
- Many horses (up to 50% in some reports) with hepatic disease may have abnormal coagulation parameters.

SIGNS

General Comments

- Historical findings depend on the cause of the coagulation defect.
- Clinical signs of acquired coagulation defects are similar to those of the hemorrhagic form of DIC, but these must be differentiated in order to institute appropriate therapy.

Historical

- Excessive hemorrhage after minor trauma or surgery
- Unexplained epistaxis or other mucosal bleeding
- Previous exposure to moldy sweet clover hay or rodenticides
- Previous anticoagulant administration
- Preexisting chronic inflammatory intestinal disorder consistent with lipid malabsorption condition or a chronic cholestatic disorder

Physical Examination

- The clinical signs are characterized by spontaneous bleeding from body orifices or into body cavities and hematoma formation.
- The most common signs associated with spontaneous hemorrhage include subcutaneous or intramuscular hematomas, hemarthrosis, epistaxis, hematuria, melena, and ecchymoses in mucous membranes.
- Prolonged bleeding from wounds or after minor surgical procedures may also be observed.
- Normally, there are no petechial hemorrhages in mucous membranes. This finding can be used to distinguish this condition from a primary hemostatic deficiency (e.g., platelet disorder) and DIC. In cases of DIC, other clinical signs associated with the underlying disease are also observed.

CAUSES

- The most common causes of vitamin K deficiency are:
  - Ingestion of moldy sweet clover (*Melilotus* spp.); fresh or contained in hay or silage
  - Accidental ingestion of rodenticides containing first- or second-generation anticoagulants
  - Chronic intestinal malabsorption problems that decrease vitamin K absorption
- The anticoagulants most frequently used in equine medicine that may cause a coagulation deficiency disorder are:
  - Warfarin, which has previously been advocated as an oral anticoagulant for use in horses (no longer recommended)
  - Heparin (unfractioned and LMWH), which is recommended for treatment of endotoxemia
- Hepatic failure

RISK FACTORS

Administration of warfarin together with other albumin-binding drugs, such as phenylbutazone, or any condition that causes hypoalbuminemia may increase the risk of warfarin toxicosis.

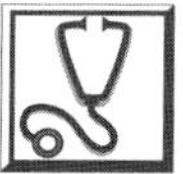

DIAGNOSIS

DIFFERENTIAL DIAGNOSIS

- Hemorrhagic diatheses caused by acquired coagulation defects must be differentiated from other causes of spontaneous hemorrhage and/or ecchymotic hermorrhages.
- DIC (hemorrhagic form) can be difficult to distinguish from an acquired coagulation defect. However, differentiation is required as different treatments are indicated. Clinical signs, identification of an underlying disease consistent with DIC and plasma D-dimer concentrations may assist differentiation.
- Inherited coagulation deficiencies (e.g., hemophilia A) can also be difficult to distinguish from an acquired coagulation defect, but both disorders are treated similarly.
- Platelet disorders (i.e., thrombocytopenia) can be differentiated by platelet counts or tests of platelet function.
- Vasculitis can be differentiated by histopathology and identification of the underlying cause of the vasculitis, e.g., purpura hemorrhagica.

CBC/BIOCHEMISTRY/URINALYSIS

- The platelet count usually remains within the normal range. Thrombocytopenia is rarely observed, in contrast to DIC.
- Urinalysis may show hematuria.
- In cases of hepatic failure, liver enzymes (i.e., SDH, GLDH, GGT) are markedly elevated.

OTHER LABORATORY TESTS

- PT and aPTT are typically prolonged (>15 and 65 seconds, respectively). In the initial stages of vitamin K deficiency, regardless of its cause (e.g., warfarin or sweet clover toxicosis), PT values are prolonged first and aPTT may remain within normal limits. However, in more chronic cases, PT and aPTT are markedly prolonged. Ongoing monitoring is recommended to assess clinical progression.

- ACT (a simple variation of aPTT) is also prolonged. Some clinicians prefer this test as it can be performed using portable devices. However, PT and aPTT are usually more reliable.
- Plasma D-dimer concentration is commonly within normal limits (0–500 ng/mL), although body cavity hemorrhages and hematomas may produce a mild increase (normally <1000 ng/mL). Higher increases in D-dimer concentration (>2000 ng/mL) is commonly observed in horses with DIC but is rare in vitamin K deficiency. This laboratory finding and the diagnosis of an underlying disease known to be associated with DIC are the key factors used to diagnose and treat a bleeding episode caused by a consumption coagulopathy (hypercoagulation and DIC).
- TT and aPTT are specifically recommended to detect overdoses of unfractioned heparin as these times are markedly prolonged in cases of heparin toxicosis. On the other hand, an overdose of LMWH has to be confirmed by measuring plasma anti–factor Xa activity and aPTT, which are above therapeutic limits and markedly prolonged, respectively.

IMAGING

Ultrasound and radiography may be used to diagnose and monitor the progression of body cavity hemorrhages and other sites of hemorrhage (e.g., within muscles).

OTHER DIAGNOSTIC PROCEDURES

Cytology of collected fluid (usually by ultrasound-guided centesis) can confirm the presence of body cavity hemorrhages, hemarthroses, or hematomas.

PATHOLOGICAL FINDINGS

Hemorrhages and hematomas in a variety of tissues, especially the respiratory and gastrointestinal tracts

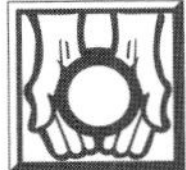

TREATMENT

AIMS OF TREATMENT

- In cases of vitamin K deficiency (i.e., rodenticide toxicosis), treatment consists of removal of the source of the toxin, vitamin K administration, and restoration of coagulation factor synthesis.
- The aim of this treatment differs significantly from the aims of treatment for the hemorrhagic form of DIC, and therefore it is important to differentiate if the coagulation defect is due to vitamin K deficiency or DIC before treatment is initiated.
- In cases of hepatic failure, the aim of treatment is to replace the deficient coagulation factors and to identify and treat the underlying cause of liver failure, and thus allow liver function to improve.

APPROPRIATE HEALTH CARE

- Horses with acquired coagulation defects should, ideally, be managed as inpatients due to the need for close monitoring of clotting times and for control of bleeding complications.
- Patients with profuse bleeding should be managed as a life-threatening emergency (see Hemorrhage, Acute).

NURSING CARE

- Fresh (frozen) plasma transfusion may be necessary in cases of severe bleeding in order to replace plasma clotting factors.
- Minimize trauma and venipunctures in these patients.

ACTIVITY

Minimize exercise and trauma while clotting times (PT and aPTT) remain prolonged.

DIET

All green leafy feeds, including hay and fresh pasture, contain high concentrations of vitamin K_1. Thus, good-quality alfalfa hay is recommended.

MEDICATIONS

DRUG(S)

- In cases with identified vitamin K deficiency, horses should be treated with vitamin K_1 (0.5–1mg/kg SC q6h) until PT values return to normal (usually within 24 hr in warfarin toxicosis). In horses intoxicated with brodifacoum, several weeks of vitamin K_1 administration (2.5 mg/kg SC or PO q12h) may be required due to the long half-life of this toxin.
- Antifibrinolytic drugs, such as aminocaproic acid (20–40 mg/kg IV diluted in saline solution and given over 30–60 min), may be used in order to reduce bleeding until hepatic synthesis of coagulation factors is restored.
- In cases of heparin toxicosis, a heparin antagonist such as protamine sulfate (1mg for every 100 U of heparin administered) has been recommended, but may have significant side/deleterious effects.

CONTRAINDICATIONS

- Administration of other anticoagulants and/or antiplatelet drugs may worsen the coagulation defect.
- Parenteral administration of vitamin K_3, which is nephrotoxic to horses and may produce signs of colic and acute renal failure.

POSSIBLE INTERACTIONS

- A number of drugs may interfere with vitamin K_1 binding including phenylbutazone, heparin, phenytoin, salicylates, quinidine, potentiated sulfas, and steroid hormones.
- These drugs should be avoided during treatment.

FOLLOW-UP

PATIENT MONITORING

- Continuously monitor clotting times (PT and aPTT) until normalization.
- Other coagulation parameters, such as plasma D-dimer concentration and platelet count, may also be monitored.

PREVENTION/AVOIDANCE

Warfarin administration is not currently recommended in horses due to complications.

POSSIBLE COMPLICATIONS

Tissue hemorrhages may be complicated by secondary infections.

EXPECTED COURSE AND PROGNOSIS

- Vitamin K deficiencies have a good prognosis and rapid resolution when diagnosed early and treated appropriately.
- Prognosis of coagulation defects due to hepatic failure is usually guarded.

MISCELLANEOUS

PREGNANCY

Rodenticides may cross the placenta and cause coagulation defects in the fetus.

SYNONYMS

Hypocoagulable disorders

SEE ALSO

- DIC
- Coagulation defects, inherited
- Thrombocytopenia
- Petechiae ecchymoses, and hematomas
- Purpura hemorrhagica
- Hemorrhage, acute
- Dicumarol (moldy sweet clover) toxicosis
- Anticoagulant rodenticide toxicosis

ABBREVIATIONS

- ACT = activated clotting time
- aPTT = activated partial thromboplastin time
- DIC = disseminated intravascular coagulation
- LMWH = low-molecular-weight heparin
- PT = prothrombin time
- TT = thrombin time

Suggested Reading

Monreal L. Monitoring the coagulation. In: Corley K, Stephan J eds. The Equine Hospital Manual. Oxford: Blackwell Publishing, 2008.

Schmitz DG. Toxicologic problems. In: Reed SM, Bayly WM, Sellon DC, eds. Equine Internal Medicine, ed 2. St Louis: Saunders, 2004.

Sellon DC. Disorders of the hematopoietic system. In: Reed SM, Bayly WM, Sellon DC, eds. Equine Internal Medicine, ed 2. St Louis: Saunders, 2004.

Author Luis Monreal
Consulting Editors Jennifer Hodgson and David Hodgson

COAGULATION DEFECTS, INHERITED

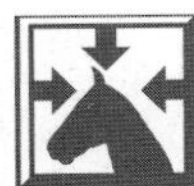

BASICS

OVERVIEW

- Several inherited coagulation deficiencies have been diagnosed in horses; all are rare.
- Reported inherited deficiencies affecting horses include:
  - von Willebrand's disease (vWF deficiency). vWF is involved in platelet adhesion to subendothelial collagen at sites of vascular injury and platelet adhesion to other platelets. The defect results in abnormal platelet adhesion and platelet plug formation, and consequently prolongation of bleeding time after wounding, trauma, or minor surgical procedure.
  - Glanzmann thrombasthenia is a deficiency/dysfunction of the platelet glycoprotein IIb/IIIa complex, which is responsible for platelet adhesion to endothelial collagen, vWF, and/or fibrinogen during platelet adhesion and subsequent aggregation. This defect also leads to bleeding.
  - A heritable Glanzmann-thrombasthenia-like platelet function defect has been recently reported in a Thoroughbred mare and its offspring.
  - Hemophilia A (factor VIII deficiency) results in a defect in the intrinsic coagulation pathway, with deficient clot formation. The severity of clinical signs is inversely related to the plasma factor VIII activity. Consequently, affected horses may show a bleeding tendency after minor trauma/surgical procedures, spontaneous bleeding episodes, or hemorrhage into body cavities, joints, etc. Intramuscular and subcutaneous hematomas also occur.
  - Prekallikrein deficiency leads to a defective initiation of the intrinsic coagulation pathway as this glycoprotein stimulates activation of factor XII. Subsequently, there is an increased bleeding tendency after trauma, but this deficiency does not result in spontaneous hemorrhage.
  - Protein C deficiency results in a hypercoagulable state and a higher frequency of thrombotic events as this protein is an important plasma coagulation inhibitor (together with antithrombin III).

SIGNALMENT

- Most of these inherited disorders occur in young purebred horses and are inherited in an autosomal recessive pattern. Thus both parents must be carriers of the genetic defect.
- Hemophilia A is the most frequently diagnosed inherited coagulation disorder of horses. It affects only males and has been diagnosed in Thoroughbred, Standardbred, Quarter Horse, and Arabian colts. It is an X-linked–recessive chromosomal abnormality that is usually evident in colts <6 mo of age, although a few cases have been diagnosed in older horses (up to 3 years).
- Prekallikrein deficiency has been reported in families of American Miniature and Belgian horses, affecting males and females. Horses with severe signs are homozygous for this genetic defect, although heterozygous horses are asymptomatic.
- vWF deficiency has been reported in young Quarter Horses and Thoroughbreds.
- Glanzmann thrombasthenia has only been reported in 2 adult horses (Thoroughbred cross; Quarter Horse).
- Protein C deficiency has been diagnosed in a Thoroughbred colt.

SIGNS

There are 3 clinical forms depending on the coagulation defect.

- When the specific deficiency affects platelet function or primary hemostasis (e.g., vWF deficiency, Glanzmann thrombasthenia), the main clinical signs are spontaneous epistaxis or bleeding involving mucosal surfaces (e.g., gingival), and prolonged bleeding after any trauma. Petechiae may also be observed.
- When the defect affects clot formation or secondary hemostasis (e.g., hemophilia A), the main clinical signs are a bleeding tendency with spontaneous hemorrhages or prolonged bleeding after trauma/surgery. Bleeding into body cavities and joints, as well as intramuscularly and subcutaneously is common. Petechiae are not reported.
- When the deficiency is related to a coagulation inhibitor defect (e.g., protein C deficiency), signs are related to the subsequent hypercoagulable state, and are consistent with a thrombotic disorder.

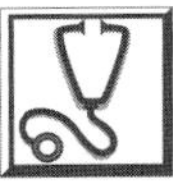

DIAGNOSIS

DIFFERENTIAL DIAGNOSIS

- DIC (hemorrhagic form)—clinical signs and plasma D-dimer concentrations may assist differentiation.
- Acquired coagulation defects can be difficult to distinguish from inherited defects, but both disorders are treated similarly.
- Platelet disorders (e.g., thrombocytopenia) can be differentiated by platelet counts or tests of platelet function.

CBC/BIOCHEMISTRY/URINALYSIS

- Few or no changes in hemogram, serum biochemistry, and urinalysis
- Most affected animals have a normal platelet counts, although mild thrombocytopenia may be noted if profuse bleeding has occurred.

OTHER LABORATORY TESTS

- von Willebrand's disease—abnormally prolonged template bleeding time, normal to abnormally prolonged aPTT, and decreased plasma vWF antigen concentration
- Glanzmann thrombasthenia—abnormally prolonged template bleeding time but normal platelet count, clotting times and vWF antigen concentration. Platelet aggregation responses to main agonists are markedly impaired. The number of fibrinogen receptors present on platelets is markedly reduced.
- Hemophilia A—abnormally prolonged aPTT, normal PT, and reduced plasma factor VIII activity support the diagnosis.
- Prekallikrein deficiency—abnormally prolonged aPTT, normal PT, and reduced plasma prekallikrein activity support the diagnosis.
- Protein C deficiency—reduced plasma protein C activity and/or antigen concentration.

IMAGING

Ultrasonography can be used for suspected hematomas, hemothorax, or hemoperitoneum, and may assist in ultrasound-guided centesis.

OTHER DIAGNOSTIC PROCEDURES

Cytology can confirm the presence of hemorrhage into body cavities, hemarthrosis, or hematomas.

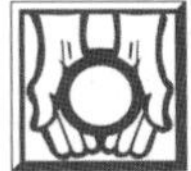

TREATMENT

Potential treatments are based on resupply of the deficient factor by means of whole blood or plasma transfusions. Owners should be informed that these diseases have no cure.

MEDICATIONS

CONTRAINDICATIONS/POSSIBLE INTERACTIONS

Other treatments that can affect platelet function (e.g., colloids) or coagulation system function (e.g., anticoagulants such as heparin) may exacerbate the bleeding tendency.

FOLLOW-UP

PATIENT MONITORING

Patients with platelet or coagulation deficiencies require continuous monitoring due to the risk of recurrent hemorrhagic episodes.

PREVENTION/AVOIDANCE

- Affected animals and their parents should not be used for breeding.
- Blood transfusions before surgical procedures may be necessary to reduce intrasurgical and postsurgical risk of bleeding.

EXPECTED COURSE AND PROGNOSIS

There is no cure.

MISCELLANEOUS

PREGNANCY

Do not breed affected horses.

SEE ALSO

- Coagulation defects, acquired
- Hemorrhage, acute
- Hemorrhage, chronic

ABBREVIATIONS

- aPTT = activated partial thromboplastin time
- DIC = disseminated intravascular coagulation
- PT = prothrombin time
- vWF = von Willebrand factor

Suggested Reading

Zimmel DN. Hemostatic disorders. In: Robinson NE, ed. Current Therapy in Equine Medicine, ed 5. Philadelphia: Saunders, 2003.

Author Luis Monreal

Consulting Editors Jennifer Hodgson and David Hodgson

COCCIDIOIDOMYCOSIS

BASICS

OVERVIEW

Coccidioidomycosis is a systemic fungal infection of animals and humans caused by the dimorphic fungus, *Coccidioides immitis*, which grows in soil of arid or semi-arid regions of the southwestern United States and South America. Disease results from inhalation of arthrospores, although rarely disease may result from ingestion or cutaneous inoculation of the organism. Infection most commonly produces granulomatous lesions in the respiratory system and associated lymph nodes. Osteomyelitis, abortion, mastitis and nasal granuloma have also been reported. The incubation period is not known.

SIGNALMENT

The influence of age, gender, and pregnancy status has not been determined. Arabian horses may be overrepresented in the case population.

SIGNS

Weight loss and respiratory symptoms (cough, nasal discharge, tachypnea) are the most common findings. Thoracic auscultation frequently reveals wheezes and/or areas of dullness corresponding with a pleural effusion or a pulmonary mass. Other signs include:

- Fever
- Lameness
- Intermittent colic
- Vaginal discharge, abortion
- Cutaneous abscesses
- Ventral edema

CAUSES AND RISK FACTORS

Coccidioides immitis is endemic in localized areas of California, Arizona, New Mexico, Texas, Nevada, and Utah.

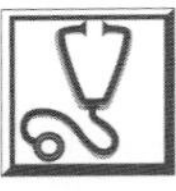

DIAGNOSIS

DIFFERENTIAL DIAGNOSIS

- Bacterial pneumonia may appear similar, but bacteria are usually identified by culture or cytology of tracheal aspirate.
- Recurrent airway obstruction (heaves) patients usually are not febrile and have normal hematology and fibrinogen concentrations.
- Neoplasia, such as lymphosarcoma, could appear similar but often has abnormal cells and a negative culture of tracheal aspirate or pleural effusion.
- Infectious and noninfectious causes of abortion may be diagnosed by history, culture, and histopathology of placental and fetal tissues.

CBC/BIOCHEMISTRY/URINALYSIS

- Hyperfibrinogenemia
- Hyperproteinemia
- Leukocytosis
- Neutrophilia
- Anemia

OTHER LABORATORY TESTS

Serologic testing is indicated when coccidioidomycosis is suspected. A positive titer is considered diagnostic of infection in a patient with clinical signs. Correlation between high titer and fatal disease has been noted.

IMAGING

- Thoracic radiography may show an increased interstitial pattern in the lung and evidence of enlarged mediastinal lymph nodes. Pleural effusion may also be detected. Osteomyelitis of vertebrae has been reported. These findings are not specific for coccidioidomycosis.
- Thoracic ultrasonography may reveal pleural effusion or abscess, although these findings are not pathognomonic for coccidioidomycosis.

DIAGNOSTIC PROCEDURES

- Culture of pleural fluid, peritoneal fluid, or transtracheal aspirate may yield *C. immitis* but the organism is difficult to isolate.
- Pleural and peritoneal fluids may be tested for *C. immitis* antibodies.
- Pleural and peritoneal fluids may have an elevated protein and white blood cell count, but these changes are not diagnostic for coccidioidomycosis.
- Intradermal testing with coccidioidin is nonspecific.
- In cases of abortion, the organism may be cultured from vaginal discharge or placental or fetal tissue.

PATHOLOGIC FINDINGS

Histopathology reveals granulomas or pyogranulomas in pulmonary parenchyma, thoracic lymph nodes, and often other sites, such as liver, bone, and peritoneum. The organism may be observed microscopically.

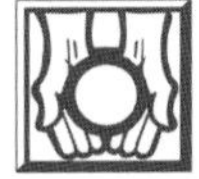

TREATMENT

- Treatment of coccidioidomycosis is difficult and costly. Most reported cases have not responded to treatment.
- If treatment is elected, many patients may be managed as outpatients. Others, however, require intensive support, including intravenous fluids and nutritional supplementation, and may be best managed in a hospital.
- If infection is limited to the nasal cavity, surgical excision may be beneficial, although recurrence is possible.

MEDICATIONS

DRUG(S) OF CHOICE

A recent report describes successful treatment with fluconazole at a loading dose of 14 mg/kg PO and 5 mg/kg daily thereafter. Itraconazole (2.6 mg/kg PO q12h) was successful in one case after several months of treatment.

FOLLOW-UP

- Clinical signs and hematology should improve if treatment is effective.
- There is no vaccine for this disease and the organism cannot be eliminated from the soil. If possible, control dust in endemic areas.
- Prognosis is grave. Most reported cases died or were euthanized. Treatment of generalized cases is likely to be expensive and ineffective, although itraconazole may prove useful. In other species, some cases resolve without treatment. It is not known if this is the case in horses.

MISCELLANEOUS

ZOONOTIC POTENTIAL

This disease is not considered contagious, but care should be taken to avoid aerosolization of infected fluids or tissue.

Suggested Reading

Higgins JC, Pusterla N, Pappagianis D. Comparison of *Coccidioides immitis* serological antibody titres between forms of clinical coccidioidomycosis in horses. J Am Vet Med Assoc 2005; 226: 1888–1892.

Author Laura K. Reilly

Consulting Editors Ashley G. Boyle and Corinne R. Sweeney

COCCIDIOSIS

BASICS

OVERVIEW

Equine coccidiosis is a protozoal infection of the intestinal tract of equids. The pathogenic capacity of equine coccidiosis has not been clearly demonstrated. Oocysts of *Eimeria leukarti* have been identified in the feces of normal horses and horses with diarrhea. The prepatent period is normally between 16 and 36 days. The meronts (schizonts) develop in the jejunum and ileum, mainly in the lacteal of these intestinal sections. This infestation has a worldwide distribution and has been reported on five continents. International reports indicated a prevalence of 0.6%–2.6% in horses but mainly in foals. However, recent studies in Kentucky have shown prevalences of *Eimeria leuckarti* oocysts between 28% and 41.6% in foals and between 86% and 100% of the farms studied.

SIGNALMENT

Detection of the causative organism is more prevalent in foals but it also occurs in adult horses. The organism is also a parasite of donkeys.

SIGNS

Because there are so many doubts of the pathogenic properties of the etiologic agent of equine coccidiosis, its presence is recorded as an incidental finding. Signs associated with this infestation are profuse diarrhea, massive intestinal hemorrhage, chronic diarrhea, catarrhal inflammation of the jejunum, and cecocolic intussusception.

CAUSES AND RISK FACTORS

The causative organism of equine coccidiosis is *E. leuckarti.*

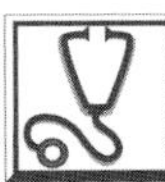

DIAGNOSIS

DIFFERENTIAL DIAGNOSIS

The finding of oocysts in the feces of any horse with diarrhea should not be taken as evidence of cause and effect. A thorough investigation for other causes (e.g., salmonellosis, Potomac horse fever, cyathastomiasis) should be undertaken.

CBC/BIOCHEMISTRY/URINALYSIS

N/A

OTHER LABORATORY TESTS

Fecal flotation is the main diagnostic method. Saturated sodium nitrate gives better concentration of oocysts of *E. leuckarti.*

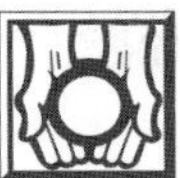

TREATMENT

There is no therapeutic regimen reported for equine cocccidial infestation.

Suggested Reading

Lyons ET, Drudge JH, Tolliver SC. Natural infection with *Eimeria leuckarti* : prevalence of oocysts in feces of horse foals on several farms in Kentucky during 1986. Am J Vet Res 1988;49:96–98.

Lyons ET, Tolliver SC. Prevalence of parasite eggs (Strongyloides westeri, Parascaris equorum, and strongyles) and oocysts (Emeria leuckarti) in the feces of Thoroughbred foals on 14 farms in central Kentucky in 2003. Parasitol Res 2004:94:400–404.

Lyons ET, Tolliveer SC, Collin SS. Field studies on endoparasites of Thoroughbred foals on seven farms in central Kentucky in 2004. Parasitol Res 2006;98:496–500.

Author Olimpo Oliver-Espinosa
Consulting Editors Henry Stämpfli and Olimpo Oliver-Espinosa

COLIC–CHRONIC / RECURRENT

BASICS

DEFINITION

Chronic abdominal pain–discomfort (colic) originating usually, but not exclusively, from the gastrointestinal tract and that has been present constantly or intermittently for > 3 days. It may also originate from other abdominal organs such as liver, spleen, kidney, uterus, and peritoneum.

PATHOPHYSIOLOGY

Pain from within the intestinal tract may result from intramural tension, tension on a mesentery, inflammation, spasm associated with hypermotility, or a combination of these. Most cases of chronic colic usually exclude strangulating obstructive events.

SYSTEMS AFFECTED

Gastrointestinal

The cardiovascular system may be affected due to progressive dehydration, toxemia, or shock secondary to gastrointestinal events.

Other Systems Affected

Other systems such as urinary, reproductive, or hepatic may also be involved.

SIGNALMENT

Nonspecific; for example, small intestinal intussusceptions are more commonly seen in young animals. Previous abdominal surgery results in a risk of adhesions leading to chronic colic.

SIGNS

General Comments

Signs of chronic/recurrent abdominal pain are usually mild to moderate in nature.

Historical

- There may be a recent history of change in diet or exercise regimen, lack of access to drinking water, deworming, weight loss, previous infection, or abdominal surgery. Furthermore, a change in attitude (depression), appetite, and fecal output may be noticed.
- *Chronic abdominal pain* refers to continuous or intermittent signs of abdominal pain of more than 3 days' duration.
- *Recurrent abdominal pain* refers to several episodes of transient or prolonged abdominal pain separated by a period of a few days or weeks in which the horse is usually normal.
- The signs of abdominal pain are usually of mild to moderate intensity and may include extended neck and rolling of the upper lip (Flehmen-like response), teeth grinding, pawing at the ground, flank watching, kicking of the abdomen with the hind legs, ears pinned back, lying down more frequently, and attempting to roll.

Physical Examination

Vital signs are usually normal to moderately elevated. The following signs might be observed:

- General findings—none to moderate abdominal distention
- Cardiovascular findings—normal to mild changes in color of the mucous membrane, normal or mild increase in capillary refill time, normal to moderate increase in heart rate, and dehydration may occur with time. May have signs of endotoxemia such as hyperemic mucous membranes and increase in heart rate if the problem is related to a septic process or enteritis/colitis.
- Gastrointestinal findings—normal, decrease, or increase in gut motility; abnormal sounds may be heard in sand impactions; may have a gas-filled viscus on percussion; may have presence of gastric reflux on passage of the nasogastric tube. If gastric reflux is present, lesion most likely located at the level of the stomach or small intestine. The pH of the gastric reflux may also be helpful in identifying the origin of the reflux. Feces are normal, reduced, or absent, or there may be diarrhea.
- Abnormalities on rectal examination—distension of a viscus by gas, liquid, or food; displacement of a viscus; uterine or renal abnormalities. May have a painful response on palpation of a specific area.

CAUSES

The most common cause of chronic colic located at the gastrointestinal level is impaction of the large colon, but there are a variety of other causes, such as chronic peritonitis, enteritis/colitis, colonic displacement, ulceration (colonic and gastric), and intussusception. For recurrent abdominal pain, the most common cause is spasmodic colic but also includes inflammatory processes such as chronic ulceration, partial disturbance of the intestinal lumen due to adhesions, intussusception, enteroliths, intra-abdominal masses such as abscesses and neoplasms, and sand impactions. Many of these conditions are related to altered motility, and intestinal parasitism probably has a significant role in the etiology of this.

Gastrointestinal

- Gastric—gastric ulcer, gastric neoplasia
- Small intestine—duodenal ulcer, duodenojejunal enteritis, adhesions, stricture, intussusception, neoplasia, impaction, etc.
- Large intestine, cecum, and small colon—impaction, ulceration, spasmodic colic, enteroliths, sand impaction, neoplasia, displacement

Reproductive

- Uterine torsion
- Late stage of pregnancy

Renal/Urologic

- Renal/ureteral/bladder/urethral calculi
- Pyelonephritis
- Cystitis
- Renal inflammatory process

Hepatobiliary

- Hepatitis
- Hepatobiliary calculi
- Abscesses

Other Systems Affected

- Peritonitis
- Mesenteric abscesses
- Abdominal neoplasia (e.g., lymphosarcoma)

RISK FACTORS

Previous surgery, diet (feeding coastal grass hay), environment, excessive use of NSAIDs, *Anoplocephala* infestation, no access to water, sudden change in exercise, history of deworming, pregnancy. Horses with severe dental disease may fail to masticate coarse herbage and be prone to impactions.

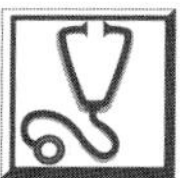

DIAGNOSIS

N/A

DIFFERENTIAL DIAGNOSIS

Other causes of pain that might resemble pain originating from the abdominal cavity include myositis, pleuropneumonia, neurologic, and musculoskeletal injury.

CBC/BIOCHEMISTRY/URINALYSIS

- Increase in PCV and plasma proteins might be present due to dehydration.
- Hypoproteinemia secondary to intestinal loss is seen in conditions such as chronic ulceration, intussusception, neoplasia, and inflammatory bowel disease.
- Leukocytosis in chronic inflammatory process may be present.
- Anemia may result from chronic inflammatory processes or chronic bleeding (ulceration, neoplasia).
- Hypochloremia, hyponatremia, and low bicarbonate concentrations are seen in colitis.
- In cases of abdominal pain related to renal problems, an increase in leukocyte count, red blood cells, and pH may be observed in the urine.
- Presence of azotemia occurs in severely dehydrated horses or in cases of renal disease.
- Liver enzymes may also be increased if hepatic disease is present.

OTHER LABORATORY TESTS

- Abdominal paracentesis—Cytology of the abdominal fluid may be normal or may reveal presence of an inflammatory process. This is indicated by an elevation of the protein level and leukocyte count. The presence of abnormal or mitotic cells may suggest lymphosarcoma. Bacteriology of abdominal fluid in cases of peritonitis may be helpful in isolating an agent and appropriately choosing the antibiotic therapy.

- Melena in feces—Ulcerative disease, intussusception of the small intestine
- Fecal analysis for the presence of parasitic eggs and sand
- Fecal bacteriology might help identifying the cause of inflammatory abdominal pain (*Salmonella* spp., *Clostridia* spp.). Culture and sensitivity of abdominal fluid if peritonitis is present
- Urinalysis—A change in specific gravity or an increase in leukocyte content, red blood cell, and pH may be noticed if renal disease is present.

IMAGING

- Radiographs—May be useful in identification of sand impaction or enteroliths
- Ultrasonography—Evaluation of the amount, quality, and characteristics of abdominal fluids; evaluation of wall thickness and diameter of small intestine; evaluation of the nephrosplenic space; and abnormal findings such as intussusception, abscess, or adhesions. Also useful in evaluating the kidneys, liver, spleen, and uterus.
- Endoscopy/gastroscopy—Evaluation of the glandular and nonglandular part of the stomach for ulcer or impaction. The duodenum may be also observed in small horses.
- Cystoscopy—Evaluation of the urethra, bladder, and opening of the ureters for inflammation urolithiasis
- Laparoscopy—visualization of abdominal viscera

DIAGNOSTIC PROCEDURES

- Histology—Biopsy of kidney or liver if these are suspected to be the origin of the problem; intestinal biopsy (requires an exploratory laparotomy or laparoscopy).
- Exploratory laparotomy or laparoscopy—To identify the origin of the problem if has not been determined by other tests

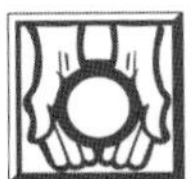

TREATMENT

The treatment depends on the source of the problem. The treatment may be supportive or curative, medical, or surgical. Moderate or severe cases of cecal impaction are an indication to perform exploratory laparotomy to prevent cecal rupture.

MEDICATIONS

DRUG(S) OF CHOICE

Analgesics

Analgesics control the abdominal pain and include:

- NSAIDs—flunixin meglumine 0.5–1.1 mg/kg q8–12 h
- α_2-agonists, such as xylazine 0.25–0.5 mg/kg IV, IM or romifidine 0.02–0.05 mg/kg IV, IM can also be given in more severe cases.
- Although usually not needed unless signs of pain are severe, the narcotic analgesics such as butorphanol or meperidine (pethidine) can be given alone or in conjunction to xylazine.

Spasmolytic

Hyoscine 20–30 mL IV

Laxative

To soften ingesta; mainly use for impaction.

- Mineral oil–10 mL/kg via nasogastric tube
- Osmotic laxative–diluted magnesium sulfate 0.5–1 g/kg in 4 L warm water via nasogastric tube
- DSS 10–30 mg/kg of a 30% solution
- Intravenous fluid of balanced electrolyte solution 100–200 mL/kg/day

Fluids

- Parenteral—In case of dehydration or moderate to severe impaction, intravenous fluid therapy should be initiated with a balanced electrolyte solution (lactated Ringer's). Unbalanced electrolytes should be corrected, especially hypokalemia and hypocalcemia, which are important for intestinal motility.
- Orally—impaction with normal gastrointestinal motility, 5 L of water every 2 hr can be given per nasogastric tube (check for gastric reflux prior to giving water).

Antibiotic Therapy

Antibiotic therapy should be started if peritonitis is suspected or surgery is performed. Usually, broad-spectrum antibiotics such as a combination of penicillin 20,000 UI/kg IV QID and gentamicin 6.6 mg/kg IV daily or trimethoprim-sulfa 30 mg/kg IV BID are given. Surgical exploration may be necessary to determine the cause of chronic or recurrent signs of abdominal discomfort. Other treatments are specific according to diagnosis, such as sand impaction, enteroliths, and parasitism.

PRECAUTIONS

Repeated use of α_2-agonists and butorphanol causes prolonged ileus. Repeat doses of NSAIDs, especially in cases of dehydration, can result in gastric or large colon ulceration as well as renal damage.

POSSIBLE INTERACTIONS

N/A

ALTERNATIVE DRUGS

N/A

FOLLOW-UP

PATIENT MONITORING

The heart rate and cardiovascular status of the horse should be monitored closely to detect any deterioration.

POSSIBLE COMPLICATIONS

Chronic signs of pain nonresponsive to medical treatment, intestinal rupture secondary to intestinal necrosis due to an enterolith, and severe impaction are indications for an exploratory laparotomy.

ZOONOTIC POTENTIAL

N/A

PREGNANCY

Late stage of pregnancy can result in intermittent mild signs of abdominal discomfort.

SYNONYM

Chronic/recurrent colic

ABBREVIATION

- DDS = dioctyl sodium succinate

Suggested Reading

Hillyer MH, Mair TS. Recurrent colic in the mature horse: a retrospective reviews of 58 cases. Equine Vet J 1997:29;421–424.

Hotwagner K, Iben C. Evacuation of sand from the equine intestine with mineral oil, with and without psyllium. J Anim Physiol Anim Nutr 2008;92:86–91.

Huskamp B, Scheidemann W. Diagnosis and treatment of chronic recurrent caecal impaction. Equine Vet J Supple 2000;32:65–68.

Mair TS, Hillyer MH. Chronic colic in the mature horse: a retrospective review of 106 cases. Equine Vet J 1997:29;415–420.

Schramme M. Investigation and management of recurrent colic in the horse. Practice 1995;17:303–314.

White NA. Epidemiology and etiology of colic. In: White NA, ed. The Equine Acute Abdomen. Philadelphia: Lea & Febiger, 1990.

Author Nathalie Coté

Consulting Editors Henry Stämpfli and Olimpo Oliver-Espinosa

COLIC IN FOALS

BASICS

DEFINITION

Colic refers to abdominal pain, most commonly due to a gastrointestinal disorder.

PATHOPHYSIOLOGY

- Obstructive conditions, such as meconium impaction, cause gas and fluid distention proximal to the obstruction, and subsequent abdominal distention and pain. Prolonged/severe distention or direct compression by an intraluminal mass (e.g., impaction) can lead to reduced intestinal wall perfusion.
- Enteritis and enterocolitis (see Diarrhea, neonatal) can be caused by a variety of bacterial and viral organisms. Small intestine and colon can become distended with fluid and gas and may also have spasmodic contractions, leading to colic pain.
- Strangulating lesions of the small or large intestine (such as small intestinal volvulus) generally cause acute, severe pain, and rapid hemodynamic deterioration. Strangulations occlude the intestinal lumen and the blood supply. Hemorrhagic strangulations are seen when venous return is occluded, but arterial supply continues. Ischemic strangulation occurs when venous and arterial blood supplies are occluded simultaneously. Production of free radicals during reperfusion can lead to further intestinal damage.
- Duodenal stricture or obstruction can occur secondary to gastroduodenal ulceration, usually in foals 1–4 mo of age.
- Damage to the intestinal wall secondary to enterocolitis, obstruction, or strangulation can lead to bacterial translocation and subsequent endotoxemia. Endotoxin is responsible for many of the clinical signs (fever, tachycardia, leukopenia, injected mucous membranes).
- Adhesions are a relatively common complication of abdominal surgery in neonatal foals. They form as fibrin adheres to areas of serosal injury.

SYSTEMS AFFECTED

- GI
- Cardiovascular—Decreased fluid intake, third-spacing of fluid in the intestinal lumen, and losses via reflux or diarrhea can lead to hypovolemic shock. Endotoxemia will compound the effects on the cardiovascular system and may lead to decompensated shock.

GENETICS

- Generalized abdominal pain or colic does not have a genetic predisposition.
- Specific causes of colic, such as lethal white syndrome, do have a genetic basis.

INCIDENCE/PREVALENCE

Incidence of colic in foals appears to be lower than that in adult horses; however, there are causes of colic that are specific to or more common in foals.

GEOGRAPHIC DISTRIBUTION

No specific geographic distribution, although sand colic is more prevalent in coastal areas (CA, FL, NJ).

SIGNALMENT

- Miniature horses have a higher incidence of fecalith formation.
- Overo-overo cross Paint foals are at risk of intestinal aganlionosis (LWFS).
- Foals 24–48 hr of age are most commonly affected by meconium impaction and enterocolitis. Less commonly, atresia coli, lethal white syndrome, GI ulceration, and congenital inguinal hernias are causes of neonatal colic.
- Foals 2–5 days of age—enterocolitis, ruptured bladder, atresia coli, ulcers
- Older foals—enterocolitis, ulcers, duodenal stenosis, small intestinal volvulus, intussusception, hernias
- Colts are at risk of inguinal hernias and appear to be at higher risk of ruptured bladder and meconium impaction.

SIGNS

Signs of colic in neonatal foals can be inconsistent, and may be complicated by concurrent disease states (e.g., septicemia). Foals may be depressed and anorexic rather than displaying "classic" colic signs such as pawing or rolling.

Historical

- Not nursing well—Foal may have dried milk on its head, and mare's udder will be full.
- Decreased fecal passage
- Previous gastric ulceration can predispose to gastric outflow obstruction in older foals.

Physical Examination

- Depression, lethargy
- Abdominal distention
- Tachycardia, tachypnea
- Tail flagging, straining/tenesmus
- Decreased or increased borborygmi
- Rolling, lying on back, persistent recumbency
- Mucous membranes vary from pink to injected to congested/ cyanotic.
- Signs of self-trauma (e.g., abrasions over the eyes) indicate colic pain prior to presentation.

CAUSES

- Bacterial—Septicemia can lead to enterocolitis. Other common causes of entercolitis in foals include *Clostridium difficile* and *C. perfringens*.
- Congenital—Intestinal atresia, LWFS, and hernia are congenital problems in foals.
- Intussusceptions are associated with tapeworm infestations in older foals and adults; this is not a common cause of colic in neonates, but may be related to altered peristalsis.
- Small intestinal volvulus can occur secondary to enteritis or may be idiopathic—Progressive fluid distention and altered motility may contribute to volvulus at the base of the mesentery.
- Diaphragmatic hernias are uncommon in neonatal foals but may be congenital or traumatic in origin.

RISK FACTORS

- Failure of transfer of passive immunity places foals at higher risk of septicemia (and therefore enterocolitis) and might predispose to meconium retention.
- NSAIDs and stress contribute to formation of gastric and duodenal ulcers in foals.

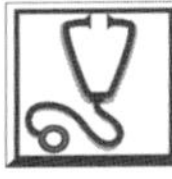

DIAGNOSIS

DIFFERENTIAL DIAGNOSIS

- Simple obstruction—should not have significant metabolic deterioration in the acute stages; if foal is <48 hr of age, suspect meconium impaction.
- Strangulating obstruction—small intestinal volvulus, large intestinal volvulus, strangulating hernia—rapid deterioration, pain refractory to analgesics, usually have pronounced abdominal distention
- Enterocolitis—reflux or diarrhea present; fluid-filled bowel on ultrasound; suspect in leukopenic or septicemic foals
- Uroperitoneum—Abdominal fluid and serum electrolytes and creatinine are usually diagnostic.
- Diaphragmatic hernia—Thoracic/ abdominal radiography and ultrasonography are most useful.

CBC/BIOCHEMISTRY/URINALYSIS

- Dehydration and hypoglycemia are common in neonatal foals that have not been nursing.
- Leukopenia (especially with enterocolitis) and leukocytosis are commonly seen with gastrointestinal inflammation.
- Electrolyte disturbances are seen with uroperitoneum (hyperkalemia, hyponatremia, hypochloremia).
- Azotemia (prerenal or postrenal) with dehydration or uroabdomen

OTHER LABORATORY TESTS

IgG—will be low (<800 mg/dL) if there is failure of transfer of passive immunity

IMAGING

- Abdominal radiography
  - Gas dilation of large and small intestine is visible. Radiodense fecaliths or impactions may be visualized. Standing or lateral views are usually adequate, although a dorsoventral view can be obtained, if needed.
  - Contrast radiography (upper GI) is useful for identifying gastric outflow obstruction; barium enemas can help in diagnosis of meconium impaction and atresia coli.
- Abdominal ultrasound—Evaluation of the small intestine is best performed with ultrasonography—distention, wall thickness, and motility can be assessed. Free abdominal fluid may be seen on ultrasound, and integrity of the bladder can also be assessed.

OTHER DIAGNOSTIC PROCEDURES

- Abdominocentesis—indicated if there is excessive free fluid, or if information from abdominal fluid will change the treatment or surgical decision. Use 20-gauge needle or teat cannula. Normal values: WBC <5000/µL, TP <2.5 g/dL. TP can increase with enteritis; WBCs, TP, and lactate may increase with ischemic lesions. Caution should be used when there is significant abdominal distention—bowel in foals is very friable, and there is risk of intestinal perforation.
- Measure abdominal circumference to monitor for increasing abdominal distention.
- Digital rectal examination—Use a well-lubricated finger; may detect firm meconium.
- Nasogastric reflux—>500 mL (usually >2 L) net reflux may indicate small intestinal ileus, enteritis, or pyloric outflow obstruction. Normal gastric emptying time for liquids is approximately 30 min. Relief of pain after refluxing is suggestive of enteritis or a gastric outflow obstruction.
- Gastroduodenal endoscopy—Identify gastric ulcers and duodenal ulceration/stricture.

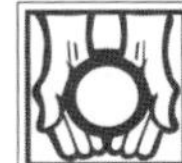

TREATMENT

AIMS OF TREATMENT

- Pain management—may be needed for short-term management of acute colic. Repeated administration of analgesics or sedation should always be accompanied by reassessment of the foal's status (possible need for changes in treatment or a decision for surgery).
- Treat underlying conditions—septicemia, perinatal asphyxia syndrome.
- Antimicrobials for perioperative coverage or for treatment of enterocolitis
- Supportive care—rehydration, treatment of hypotension and acidosis; correct electrolyte imbalances.
- Decision for surgery is based on the severity of pain, lack of response to analgesics, increasing abdominal distention, evidence of strangulation, or deterioration of condition despite medical treatment.
- Ulcer prophylaxis or treatment of existing ulcers. Septicemic neonates usually have alkaline gastric pH, and treatment with proton pump inhibitors or H_2 blockers may be contraindicated in this group.

APPROPRIATE HEALTH CARE

If colic is persistent (unresponsive to initial medications), the foal should be referred for inpatient medical treatment, and possibly for emergency medical stabilization, and if required, for emergency surgery.

NURSING CARE

- Fluid therapy—BES replacement fluids (Plasmalyte 148 or lactated Ringer's) for rehydration, unless hyperkalemia is present
- Gastric decompression (reflux) via nasogastric tube for cases of enteritis or gastric outflow obstruction

ACTIVITY

- The foal may be confined to a stall or small pen/cage while intravenous fluids are administered and the foal is observed closely for changes in clinical condition.
- If abdominal surgery is performed, the foal should be restricted to a stall for 3–4 weeks, and a small paddock for an additional 4 weeks to allow for healing of the ventral midline incision.

DIET

Parenteral nutrition is indicated if enteral feeding cannot be tolerated (due to obstruction, ileus, or enterocolitis).

CLIENT EDUCATION

- Discuss importance of adequate colostrum intake if failure of transfer of passive immunity is an underlying risk factor.
- If there is a congenital problem (LWFS), discourage rebreeding same mare and stallion and recommend genetic testing.

SURGICAL CONSIDERATIONS

- Surgery may be indicated if the foal is persistently painful and refractory to analgesics, has progressive abdominal distention, has evidence of sepsis or ischemia on abdominocentesis, or has evidence of complete obstruction on abdominal radiographs or ultrasound.
- The foal must be stabilized prior to surgery, especially if there are significant electrolyte or acid-base derangements, as these metabolic abnormalities increase the risk of anesthetic complications.
- Abdominal adhesions are a frequent and serious consequence of abdominal surgery in foals. Precautions such as gentle tissue handling, administration of NSAIDs and broad-spectrum antimicrobial drugs, lubrication of serosal surfaces with sodium carboxymethylcellulose, and omentectomy should be taken to help reduce the chance of significant postoperative adhesions.

COLIC IN FOALS

MEDICATIONS

DRUG(S)

Pain Management

- α_2-Agonist, e.g., xylazine (0.4–1.0 mg/kg IV)
- Butorphanol (0.04–0.1 mg/kg IV)
- NSAIDs, e.g., flunixin meglumine (0.5–1.1 mg/kg IV q12h)

Antimicrobials

- Penicillin (22,000 IU/kg IV q6h)
- Amikacin (25 mg/kg IV q24h)

Ulcer Prophylaxis

See Gastric ulcers, neonate

CONTRAINDICATIONS

Enrofloxacin should not be used in foals.

PRECAUTIONS

- NSAIDs increase the risk of gastric ulceration and can also mask a more serious underlying condition.
- Aminoglycosides should not be used in dehydrated or azotemic foals.

ALTERNATIVE DRUGS

Cephalosporins can be used as a broad spectrum antimicrobial (Ceftiofur 10 mg/kg IV q6h).

FOLLOW-UP

PATIENT MONITORING

- The neonatal foal with colic should be monitored closely for dehydration, hypoglycemia, and changes in cardiovascular status.
- Measure abdominal circumference and monitor for fecal passage to assess for resolution of impaction and gas distention.

PREVENTION/AVOIDANCE

Adequate colostrum intake should reduce the risk of meconium impaction and may reduce the risk of infectious enterocolitis.

POSSIBLE COMPLICATIONS

- In foals <7 days of age, concurrent diseases such as septicemia, perinatal asphyxia syndrome, and prematurity are common (colic is usually secondary).
- Recurrence of colic is possible in cases of enterocolitis.
- Adhesions are a common complication of colic surgery in foals, with as many as 30% developing clinically significant intestinal adhesions.

EXPECTED COURSE AND PROGNOSIS

- Simple obstruction, such as meconium impaction. has an excellent prognosis. Other medical colic will often resolve within 24–48 hr of treatment, although colic complicated by debilitating diseases such as sepsis have a more guarded prognosis.
- Short-term survival has been reported to be 61%–65% for foals with colic surgery.
- Long-term survival in surgically treated foals is approximately 35%–45%, with poorer prognosis for foals <14 days of age and for foals with strangulating GI lesions.
- Atresia coli, LWFS, and gastroduodenal rupture have a grave prognosis.

MISCELLANEOUS

ASSOCIATED CONDITIONS

Septicemia

AGE-RELATED FACTORS

Specific types of colic (e.g., meconium impaction, ruptured bladder) in foals are age related.

SEE ALSO

- Meconium impaction
- Lethal white foal syndrome (Ileocecocolic aganglionosis)
- Diarrhea, neonate

ABBREVIATIONS

- BES = balanced electrolyte solution
- GI = gastrointestinal
- LWFS = lethal white foal syndrome
- TP = total protein
- WBC = white blood cell

Suggested Reading

Bernard W. Colic in the foal. Equine Vet Educ 2004;6:409–413.

Bryant JE, Gaughan EM. Abdominal surgery in neonatal foals. Vet Clin North Am Equine Pract 2005;21:511–535.

Vatistas NJ, Snyder JR, Wilson WD, Drake C, Hildebrand S. Surgical treatment for colic in the foal (67 cases): 1980–1992. Equine Vet J 1996;28:139–145.

Author Margaret C. Mudge

Consulting Editor Margaret C. Mudge

CONCEPTION FAILURE

BASICS

DEFINITION OVERVIEW

Maternal structural or functional defects that prevent:

- The fertilized ovum from normal embryonic development.
- Transport of the embryo into the uterus on day 6 after ovulation.
- Embryonic survival until pregnancy is diagnosed by transrectal U/S ≥14 days after ovulation

ETIOLOGY/PATHOPHYSIOLOGY

- Defective embryo
- Unsuitable oviductal or uterine environment
- Early CL regression
- Failure of "maternal recognition of pregnancy"
- Luteal insufficiency — anecdotal
- Oviductal blockage or impaired function

SYSTEMS AFFECTED

Reproductive

INCIDENCE/PREVALENCE

The "normal" rate of conception failure is ≅ 30% but approaches 50% to 70% in old, subfertile mares.

SIGNALMENT

- Old (>15 years) mares
- Certain heterospecific matings: stallion × jenny

SIGNS

Historical Findings

- Diagnosis of failure of pregnancy by transrectal U/S at >14 days after ovulation following appropriately timed breeding with semen of normal fertility.
- Diagnosis of failure of pregnancy by TRP at >25 days after ovulation following appropriately timed breeding with semen of normal fertility
- Return (possibly early) to estrus after appropriately timed breeding with semen of normal fertility.
- Previous exposure to endophyte-infected fescue or ergotized grasses and grains.

Physical Examination Findings

- Nonpregnant uterus, possibly with edema of endometrial folds or accumulation of intrauterine (luminal) fluid.
- Absence of a CL
- Mucoid or mucopurulent vulvar discharge

CAUSES

Defective Embryos

- Old mares
- Seasonal effects

Endometritis

- Early CL regression
- Unsuitable/hostile uterine environment

Unsuitable Uterine Environment

- Endometritis
- Endometrial lymphatic cysts of sufficient size to impede embryonic mobility, resulting in failure of "maternal recognition of pregnancy."
- Inadequate secretion of histotrophs

Xenobiotics

- Equine fescue toxicosis and ergotism
- Phytoestrogens — anecdotal

Oviductal Disease

- Unsuitable/hostile environment for embryonic development
- Oviductal blockage

Endocrine Disorders

- Hypothyroidism — anecdotal
- Luteal insufficiency — anecdotal

Maternal Disease

- Fever
- Pain — anecdotal

RISK FACTORS

- Age of >15 years.
- Anatomic defects predisposing the genital tract to endometritis
- Seasonal effects
- Foal heat breeding — anecdotal
- Inadequate nutrition
- Exposure to xenobiotics — fescue toxicosis and ergotism
- Some heterospecific matings — stallion x jenny
- Mating-induced endometritis

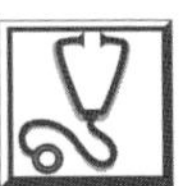

DIAGNOSIS

DIFFERENTIAL DIAGNOSIS

Mistiming of Insemination or Breeding

- Monitor follicular development and ovulation by TRP or U/S.
- Appropriate timing of insemination or breeding.
- Ovulation induction to complement timing of insemination or breeding.

EED

Transrectal U/S to detect pregnancy at >14 days, but that is absent on subsequent examination at <40 days of gestation.

Pregnancy Undetected by Transrectal U/S

- Careful, systematic visualization of the entire uterus — horns, body, and region near cervix.
- A slow sweep, twice per examination, over the entire tract will reduce "misses."

Ovulation Failure

- TRP or U/S (preferred) to confirm ovulation and formation of a CL.
- Serum progesterone level 6 to 7 days after ovulation or at end of estrus.

Poor Semen Quality

Monitoring/examination of ejaculate for adequate number of spermatozoa and evaluation of progressive motility and normal morphology.

Ejaculation Failure

- Observation of "flagging" of stallion's tail.
- Palpation of ventral penile surface during live cover or collection of semen in an AV to confirm ejaculation was complete: 6 to 10 pulses of the urethra.
- Examination of dismount semen sample for motile spermatozoa.

Mishandling of Semen

Systematic review of all procedures and examination of semen collection equipment, extenders, incubator temperature, and any containers coming into contact with semen that may be causing death of spermatozoa.

Impaired Spermatozoal Transport

- Transrectal U/S to ensure absence of intrauterine fluid at insemination or breeding.
- Vaginal speculum and digital cervical examination to assess cervical patency and to rule out urovagina.

CBC/BIOCHEMISTRY/URINALYSIS

Not indicated, unless signs of concurrent systemic disease are present.

OTHER LABORATORY TESTS

Maternal Progesterone

- May be indicated at >6 days after ovulation to evaluate CL function.
- ELISA or RIA for progesterone — acceptable levels vary from >1 to >4 ng/mL, depending on the reference lab.

Maternal T_3 /T_4 Levels

- Anecdotal reports of lower levels in mares with history of conception failure, EED, or abortion.
- Significance of low T_4 levels is not clear at present.

Cytogenetic Studies

- May be indicated with suspected maternal chromosomal abnormalities.

Feed Analysis

- May be indicated for specific xenobiotics (e.g., ergopeptine alkaloids, phytoestrogens, heavy metals) or endophyte (*Neotyphodium coenophialum*).

IMAGING

Transrectal U/S is essential to confirm ovulation and early pregnancy and to detect intrauterine fluid and endometrial cysts.

OTHER DIAGNOSTIC PROCEDURES

Thorough Reproductive Evaluation

- Indicated prebreeding for individuals predisposed to conception failure (e.g., barren, old mares with history of conception failure and/or endometritis).
- Transrectal U/S, vaginal speculum, endometrial cytology/culture, and endometrial biopsy to detect anatomic defects, endometritis, or fibrosis.

CONCEPTION FAILURE

Transrectal U/S

If performed earlier than normal, at 10 days, to determine presence of embryo; confusion with endometrial cysts often results.

Embryo Recovery

- Same procedure as for ET.
- Performed to detect embryonic transport – into uterus (6 to 8 days after ovulation) or oviduct (2 to 4 days after ovulation).
- Flush may be therapeutic as well.

Hysteroscopy

Endoscopy of uterine lumen and uterotubal junctions.

Oviductal Patency

- Starch granules or microspheres are deposited on the ovarian surface.
- Uterine lavage is then performed.
- Recovery of starch granules/microspheres in the lavage fluid is evaluated.

Laparoscopy

To evaluate normal structure and function of ovarian-uterine tubal interaction.

PATHOLOGIC FINDINGS

Endometrial biopsy – presence of moderate to severe, chronic endometritis or fibrosis.

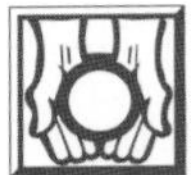

TREATMENT

APPROPRIATE HEALTH CARE

- Treat pre-existing endometritis before insemination or breeding of mares during physiologic breeding season when they have adequate body condition.
- Inseminate or breed foal heat mares if ovulation occurs >10 days postpartum and no intrauterine fluid is present.
- Uterine lavage 4 to 8 hours post-mating and administration of oxytocin and cloprostenol (see below) to treat PMIE.
- Progestin supplementation.
- Anecdotal reports of oviductal flushing to resolve oviductal occlusion.
- Various forms of advanced reproductive technologies (e.g., embryo, zygote) to retrieve embryos from the uterus (days 6 to 8 after ovulation) or oviduct (≅days 2 to 4 after ovulation); successful IVF is in the early stages of development.
- Primary, age-related (most are from aged mares) embryonic defects are refractory to treatment.
- Most cases of conception failure can be handled in an ambulatory situation.
- Increased frequency of U/S monitoring of follicular development and ovulation, or to permit insemination closer to ovulation, as well as more technical diagnostic procedures, may need to be performed in a hospital setting.
- Adequate restraint and optimal lighting (usually the problem is an excess of light) may not be available in the field to permit quality U/S examination.

NURSING CARE

- Generally requires none.
- Minimal nursing care after more invasive diagnostic and therapeutic procedures.

ACTIVITY

- Generally no restriction of broodmare activity, unless contraindicated by concurrent maternal disease or diagnostic or therapeutic procedures.
- Preference may be to restrict activity of mares in competition because of the impact of stress on cyclicity and ovulation.

DIET

Generally no restriction, unless indicated by concurrent maternal disease.

CLIENT EDUCATION

- Emphasize the effects of aging, i.e. the aged mare's conception failure and her refractoriness to treatment.
- Inform regarding the cause, diagnosis, and treatment of endometritis.
- Inform regarding the seasonal aspects and nutritional requirements of conception.
- Inform regarding the role that endophyte-infected fescue and certain heterospecific breedings might play in conception failure.

SURGICAL CONSIDERATIONS

- Indicated for repair of anatomic defects predisposing mares to endometritis.
- Certain diagnostic and therapeutic procedures.

MEDICATIONS

DRUG(S) OF CHOICE

- See specific sections for drug recommendations.

Altrenogest

- Mares with a history of conception failure or moderate to severe endometritis (i.e., no active, infectious component) or fibrosis: altrenogest (Regu-Mate, Hoechst-Roussel Agri-Vet; 0.044 to 0.088 mg/kg PO, SID; begin 2 to 3 days after ovulation or at diagnosis of pregnancy and continue until at least day 100 of gestation; taper daily dose over a 14-day period at the end of treatment).
- Altrenogest administration may be started later during gestation, continued longer, or used for only short periods of time, depending on serum progesterone levels during the first 80 days of gestation (>1 to >4 ng/mL, depending on the reference lab), clinical circumstances, risk factors, and clinician preference.
- If used near term, altrenogest frequently is discontinued 7 to 14 days before the expected foaling date, depending on the case, unless otherwise indicated by assessment of fetal maturity/viability or by questions regarding the accuracy of gestational length.

Oxytocin

- IM administration of 10 to 20 IU, 4 to 8 hours post-mating for PMIE.

Cloprostenol

- IM administration of 250 µgm 12 to 24 hours post-mating for PMIE.

CONTRAINDICATIONS

- Use altrenogest only to prevent conception failure of noninfectious endometritis.
- Iatrogenic administration of oxytocin and cloprostenol to pregnant mares (adverse effects are dependent on stage of pregnancy).

PRECAUTIONS

- Use transrectal U/S to diagnose pregnancy at ≥14 to 16 days after ovulation to identify intrauterine fluid or pyometra early in the disease course for appropriate treatment.
- If pregnancy is diagnosed, frequent monitoring (weekly initially) may be indicated to detect EED.
- Altrenogest is absorbed through the skin, so persons handling this preparation should wear gloves and wash their hands.
- Cloprostenol can be absorbed through the skin, so persons handling this preparation should wear gloves and wash their hands after treating mares.
- Although supplemental progestins are used widely to treat cases of conception failure, any reported success is purely anecdotal.
- Primary, age-related embryonic defects do not respond to supplemental progestins.

ALTERNATIVE DRUGS

- Injectable progesterone (150 to 500 mg/day, oil base) can be administered IM, SID instead of the oral formulation. Variations, contraindications, and precautions are similar to those associated with altrenogest.
- Other injectable and implantable progestin preparations are available commercially for use in other species. Any use in horses of these products is off-label, and no scientific data are available regarding their efficacy.
- Thyroxine supplementation has been successful (anecdotally) for treating mares with histories of subfertility. Its use remains controversial, however, and it is considered deleterious by some clinicians.

FOLLOW-UP

PATIENT MONITORING

- Accurate teasing records.
- Reexamination of mares treated for endometritis before breeding.
- Early examination for pregnancy by transrectal U/S.
- Monitor embryonic and fetal development with transrectal or transabdominal U/S.

PREVENTION/AVOIDANCE

- Recognition of at-risk mares.
- Management of endometritis before breeding.

• Removal of mares from fescue-infected pasture and ergotized grasses and grains after breeding and during early gestation.
• Prudent use of medications in bred mares.
• Avoiding exposure to known toxicants.

POSSIBLE COMPLICATIONS

• Later EED
• High-risk pregnancy
• Abortion

EXPECTED COURSE AND PROGNOSIS

• Young mares with resolved cases of endometritis may have a fair to good prognosis for conception and completion of pregnancy.
• Old mares (>15 years) with a history of conception failure or chronic, moderate to severe endometritis or fibrosis have a guarded to poor prognosis for conception and completion of pregnancy.

MISCELLANEOUS

ASSOCIATED CONDITIONS

• Abortion
• Conception failure – stallions
• EED
• ET
• Endometritis
• Metritis

AGE-RELATED FACTORS

• Development of chronic endometritis and endometrial fibrosis
• Age-related embryonic defects

PREGNANCY

• Condition is pregnancy—associated by definition
• Increased risk of EED or abortion

SEE ALSO

• Abortion
• Early embryonic death
• Embryo transfer
• Endometrial biopsy
• Endometritis
• Metritis
• Ovulation failure
• Pregnancy diagnosis

ABBREVIATIONS

• AV = artificial vagina
• CL = corpus luteum
• EED = early embryonic death
• ELISA = enzyme-linked immunosorbent assay
• ET = embryo transfer
• IVF = in vitro fertilization
• PMIE = post-mating induced endometritis
• RIA = radioimmunoassay
• T_3 = triiodothyronine
• T_4 = thyroxine
• TRP = transrectal palpation
• U/S = ultrasound, ultrasonography

Suggested Reading

Evans TJ, Rottinghaus GE, Casteel SW. Ergopeptine alkaloid toxicoses in horses. In: Robinson NE, ed. Current Therapy in Equine Medicine 5. Philadelphia: Saunders, 2003;796–798.

LeBlanc MM. Persistent mating-induced endometritis. In: Robinson NE, ed. Current Therapy in Equine Medicine 5. Philadelphia: Saunders, 2003;234–237.

Paccamonti D. Endometrial cysts. In: Robinson NE, ed. Current Therapy in Equine Medicine 5. Philadelphia: Saunders, 2003;231–234.

Author Tim J. Evans
Consulting Editor Carla L. Carleton

CONGENITAL CARDIAC ABNORMALITIES

BASICS

OVERVIEW

- Congenital cardiac abnormalities include any structural cardiac malformation present from birth, usually due to either a failure in embryologic development or a persistence of fetal circulation.
- VSD occurs when there is incomplete development of the ventricular septum during embryonic development.
- High (paramembranous) defect in the ventricular septum is most common; subpulmonic defect (less common) communicates below the pulmonary valve.
- ASDs—can involve various portions of the atrial septum
- PDA—ductus arteriosus shunts blood from the pulmonary artery to the descending aorta in the fetal circulation; it can remain patent as a single defect or, more commonly, as part of a complex congenital cardiac abnormality. The ductus arteriosus normally closes in response to changes in pressure gradients at birth and to inhibition of prostaglandins.
- Patent foramen ovale—The foramen ovale shunts blood from the right atrium to the left atrium to bypass the lungs in the fetal circulation. The foramen ovale normally closes when the lungs expand (pulmonary vascular resistance falls). This opening can remain patent if pulmonary hypertension is present. In normal foals functional closure occurs in the first 24–48 hours of life.
- Truncus arteriosis—normally partitions into aorta and pulmonary artery in the fetus. If there is failure to partition, communication occurs across a large VSD.
- Tricuspid atresia—prevents flow of blood from right atrium to right ventricle. Blood must be shunted across an ASD or patent foramen ovale.
- Tetralogy of Fallot includes VSD, right ventricular outflow obstruction, overriding aorta, and right ventricular hypertrophy.
- VSD is the most commonly recognized. Other forms of congenital cardiac abnormality are very rare. Reportedly 3.5% incidence in causes of neonatal death or euthanasia
- Left-to-right shunting occurs with ASD, VSD, and PDA. Blood shunted from the left ventricle to the right heart will increase volume in the pulmonary artery, and will therefore increase venous return to the left atrium and left ventricle, eventually causing left ventricular hypertrophy and dilation. Larger shunts will result in left-sided heart failure. VSDs that allow pressures to equilibrate between left and right ventricles can lead to biventricular hypertrophy.

SIGNALMENT

- There is thought to be a genetic predisposition to congenital cardiac abnormalities, although the specific genetic factors are unknown at this time. VSD appears to have a genetic link in the Arabian breed. Standardbred and Quarter Horse breeds may also be more commonly affected with VSD.
- Defects are present from birth; however, the time to recognition of the problem will vary depending on severity of clinical signs. Cardiac anomalies are most often recognized in the first weeks to months after birth.
- No sex predilection

SIGNS

Commonly, left-to-right shunts secondary to congenital cardiac anomalies will result in left-sided or biventricular heart failure, leading to signs of exercise intolerance, respiratory distress, and jugular venous distention.

Historical

- Premature foals may be at higher risk of left-to-right shunts at the foramen ovale.
- Exercise intolerance
- Stunted growth

Physical Examination

- Heart murmur—usually grade 3/6 or higher, but absence of a murmur does not rule out congenital cardiac anomaly
  - VSD—holosystolic, auscultated on both sides, but PMI usually on right; louder murmur generally correlates with smaller defect.
  - PDA—continuous machinery murmur, usually loudest on left; heard in most foals for the first 15 min of life; can be heard in normal foals for up to the first 3 days of life
  - Tetralogy of Fallot—loud, left-sided systolic murmur; may have a palpable thrill
- Lethargy, weakness
- Cyanotic mucous membranes at rest or with exercise (most common with right-to-left shunting)
- Tachypnea/dyspnea; may have harsh lung sounds
- Jugular venous distention
- Bounding pulses

CAUSES AND RISK FACTORS

- Teratogenic exposure, viral infection, or hypoxic damage early in pregnancy are suspected causes of congenital cardiac abnormalities.
- Breed is likely a risk factor.
- Prematurity may also be associated with failure to revert from fetal circulation.

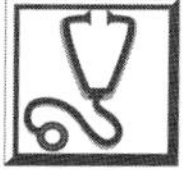

DIAGNOSIS

DIFFERENTIAL DIAGNOSIS

- Pneumonia—thoracic radiographs and 2D echocardiography should elucidate the cause of respiratory compromise.
- Physiologic cardiac murmur—usually left-sided, systolic; no echocardiography abnormalities, and foal should not show clinical signs of cardiac disease
- Anemia—lethargy and weakness

CBC/BIOCHEMISTRY/URINALYSIS

Polycythemia may be seen in response to chronic hypoxemia.

OTHER LABORATORY TESTS

Blood gas analysis—arterial hypoxemia, usually minimally responsive to oxygen supplementation, especially with right-to-left shunts. Arterial CO_2 is normal or reduced.

IMAGING

- Echocardiography—2D views can often confirm the defect, although Doppler studies are often needed to find VSDs in atypical locations and to estimate the pressure difference across the ventricles. Echocardiography is also useful for determining ventricular hypertrophy.
- Radiography—cardiomegaly and pulmonary edema

OTHER DIAGNOSTIC PROCEDURES

Cardiac catheterization can be performed to measure pulmonary artery and pulmonary capillary wedge pressures.

PATHOLOGIC FINDINGS

Cardiac malformations are detected on gross examination at necropsy.

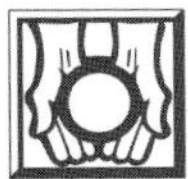

TREATMENT

- Supportive care with optimization of perfusion and appropriate exercise restriction constitute care for congenital cardiac abnormalities. There are no current surgical recommendations for horses with cardiac defects.
- Foals with significant shunts or complex cardiac defects are usually exercise intolerant and can become cyanotic when exercised.
- Breeding of affected animals should be discouraged.
- Medical management may be used for horses with CHF or acute decompensation.
- Although PDA and VSD have been successfully treated surgically in dogs, there are no surgical procedures currently described for use in foals.

MEDICATIONS

DRUG(S)

- Digoxin (0.01–0.02 mg/kg PO q12h) to improve myocardial function. Digoxin levels should be monitored to avoid toxic levels.
- Furosemide (1–2 mg/kg IV PRN) to treat pulmonary edema.

CONTRAINDICATIONS/POSSIBLE INTERACTIONS

Digoxin and furosemide should not be used in dehydrated patients.

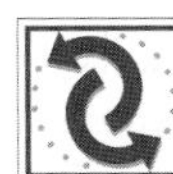

FOLLOW-UP

PATIENT MONITORING

- Horses with small VSDs can have successful athletic careers but should be monitored for development of CHF and atrial fibrillation (exercise intolerance, coughing, dyspnea, lethargy).
- Repeat echocardiography (recommended yearly) is useful for evaluating development of ventricular enlargement or hypertrophy as well as valvular insufficiency.

PREVENTION/AVOIDANCE

Horses with congenital cardiac anomalies should not be used for breeding, as the defects may be heritable.

POSSIBLE COMPLICATIONS

CHF

EXPECTED COURSE AND PROGNOSIS

- The prognosis with a VSD is dependent on the size of the defect. Horses with membranous VSDs that measure <2.5 cm at the largest diameter (and that have a higher peak velocity of shunt flow) tend to have a good athletic prognosis.
- Horses with large VSDs or with multiple congenital cardiac defects (e.g., tetralogy of Fallot) may be small and stunted and are likely to develop signs of CHF.

MISCELLANEOUS

ASSOCIATED CONDITIONS

N/A

AGE-RELATED FACTORS

N/A

ZOONOTIC POTENTIAL

N/A

PREGNANCY

Mares with significant shunting of blood due to congenital cardiac defects may develop signs of CHF during late-term pregnancy due to increased demand for cardiac output.

SEE ALSO

Congestive heart failure

ABBREVIATIONS

- ASD = atrial septal defect
- CHF = congestive heart failure
- 2D = two-dimensional
- PDA = patent ductus arteriosus
- PMI = point of maximal intensity
- VSD = ventricular septal defect

Suggested Reading

Bonagura JD, Reef VB. Disorders of the cardiovascular system. In: Reed SM, Bayly WM, Sellon DC, eds. Equine Internal Medicine, ed 2. St. Louis, Elsevier, 2004:355–459.

Chope K. Cardiac disorders. In: Paradis MR, ed. Equine Neonatal Medicine: A Case-Based Approach. Philadelphia: Saunders, 2006.

Reef VB. Evaluation of ventricular septal defects in horses using two-dimensional and Doppler echocardiography. Equine Vet J Suppl 1995;19:86–95.

Author Margaret C. Mudge
Consulting Editor Margaret C. Mudge

CONIUM MACULATUM (POISON HEMLOCK) TOXICOSIS

BASICS

OVERVIEW

- A potent toxic plant causing neurotoxicity and rapid death in horses
- *Conium maculatum* (poison hemlock) also is known as spotted hemlock, European hemlock, and Nebraska or California fern.
- The plant is a biennial herb with a fern-like appearance growing up to 10 feet in height, with a smooth, hollow, purple-spotted stem and a stout, white to pale yellow taproot.
- The lacy, triangular leaves resemble those of a carrot and have a musky odor, like that of a parsnip, when crushed.
- Small, white flowers cluster in flat-topped umbels 4–6 cm across.
- Grayish, round, tiny fruit with flattened ridges are produced during the second year.
- The plant commonly grows in disturbed soil along roadsides, field edges, railroad tracks, and stream banks throughout the United States.
- The whole green plant is toxic at doses of $\cong$1% of body weight; 4–5 pounds of fresh leaves are lethal for horses.
- The plant contains numerous piperidine alkaloids, with the most toxic being *N*-methyl coniine and γ-coniceine; coniine acts similarly to nicotine, first causing stimulation and then depression of the CNS.

SIGNALMENT

- All animals
- Horses readily eat the plant even if other forage is present.

SIGNS

- The clinical course is rapid, and horses may be found dead or die within a few hours.
- Initial signs include mydriasis, salivation, hypotension, colic, and diarrhea.
- Neurologic signs develop rapidly and include apprehension, muscle tremors, muscular weakness, incoordination, recumbency, paralysis, and coma.
- Death results from respiratory failure.

CAUSES AND RISK FACTORS

- The plant appears during the early spring, and most toxicoses occur at this time, when the plant is most palatable.
- The level of *N*-methyl coniine increases as the plant matures; the root becomes toxic only later in the year.
- The highest alkaloid concentration is in the seeds.
- Drying seems to reduce, but not eliminate, the toxicity.

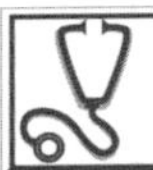

DIAGNOSIS

DIFFERENTIAL DIAGNOSIS

Other causes of sudden death in horses

CBC/BIOCHEMISTRY/URINALYSIS

N/A

OTHER LABORATORY TESTS

- Evidence of plant consumption
- Chemical analysis for coniine in the stomach contents and urine is available.

IMAGING

N/A

DIAGNOSTIC PROCEDURES

N/A

PATHOLOGICAL FINDINGS

- No diagnostic postmortem findings, but the toxin is eliminated via the kidneys and lungs, giving the urine and exhaled air a characteristic mousy odor.
- Nonspecific necropsy findings include diffuse congestion of the lungs, liver, and myocardium.

Conium maculatum (Poison Hemlock) Toxicosis

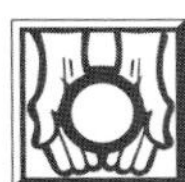

TREATMENT

- No specific treatment
- Early GI decontamination may be useful.
- Maintain body fluid and electrolyte balance.
- Respiratory support by mechanical ventilation may be helpful.
- Adequate nursing care of recumbent animals

MEDICATIONS

DRUGS

- AC (1–4 g/kg PO in water slurry [1 g of AC in 5 mL of water])
- One dose of a cathartic PO with AC if no diarrhea or ileus—70% sorbitol (3 mL/kg) or sodium or magnesium sulfate (250–500 mg/kg)

CONTRAINDICATIONS/POSSIBLE INTERACTIONS

N/A

FOLLOW-UP

PATIENT MONITORING

N/A

PREVENTION/AVOIDANCE

- Remove poison hemlock from all areas accessible by horses. Treatment with herbicides may be attempted. Ensure that all plants are dead before reintroducing horses, however, because herbicide-treated plants may be more palatable.
- Feed little or no hay that contains poison hemlock. Seeds may contaminate grains, making these feeds unsafe for consumption.

POSSIBLE COMPLICATIONS

N/A

EXPECTED COURSE AND PROGNOSIS

- Very guarded early prognosis
- Clinical course may last several hours to a day or two.
- Onset of signs occurs within ≅2 hr of ingestion.
- In severe cases, death occurs within 5–10 hr of the onset of signs.
- Because both the quantity of alkaloid in the plant and the quantity of plant consumed vary, not all horses that eat poison hemlock die.

MISCELLANEOUS

ASSOCIATED CONDITIONS

N/A

AGE-RELATED FACTORS

N/A

ZOONOTIC POTENTIAL

N/A

PREGNANCY

Poison hemlock has teratogenic effects in cattle and pigs; however, teratogenicity has not been reported in horses.

SEE ALSO

N/A

ABBREVIATIONS

- AC = activated charcoal
- GI = gastrointestinal

Suggested Reading

Burrows GM, Tyrl RJ. Toxic Plants of North America. Ames, IA: Blackwell Publishing, 2001:54–57.

Vetter J. Poison hemlock (*Conium maculatum* L.). Food Chem Toxicol 2004; 42:1373–1382.

Lopez TA, Cid MS, Bianchini ML. Biochemistry of hemlock (*Conium maculatum* L.) alkaloids and their acute and chronic toxicity in livestock. A review. Toxicon 1999; 37:841–865.

Author Anita M. Kore

Consulting Editor Robert H. Poppenga

CONJUNCTIVAL DISEASES

BASICS

OVERVIEW

Definition

Conjunctivitis is inflammation of the mucous membrane which covers the posterior aspects of the eyelids and nictitating membrane (palpebral conjunctiva) and the superficial surface of the sclera (bulbar conjunctiva). It may be infectious or noninfectious.

Pathophysiology

- Conjunctivitis is a nonspecific finding that indicates ocular inflammation and may also be seen in systemic disease. Infectious and noninfectious diseases of the lids, cornea, sclera, anterior uvea, nasolacrimal system, and orbit can result in conjunctivitis. The conjunctiva is a mucous membrane that can reflect systemic dysfunction through changes in color and in vascular appearance, as in anemia and jaundice.
- Environmental allergies or irritants may cause conjunctivitis.
- Habronemiasis is a parasitic conjunctivitis caused by aberrant migration of *Habronema* larvae. Habronemiasis may occur concurrently with SCC, which makes histologic examination of affected tissues crucial.
- Onchocerciasis can cause conjunctivitis, keratitis, and keratouveitis. The causative agent is *Onchocerca cervicalis* and the insect vector is the female *Culicoides*. Migrating larvae may invade the conjunctiva, cornea, and anterior uvea resulting in inflammation.
- The development of SCC has been associated with cell damage caused by the UV component of solar radiation. Animals with higher levels of exposure to sunlight or that live in high altitudes are more prone.

Systems Affected

Ophthalmic

SIGNALMENT

Breed Predilections

There are no breed predilections for noninfectious conjunctivitis.

Mean Age and Range

- Neonates—Conjunctivitis may be associated with neonatal maladjustment syndrome, septicemia, uveitis immune-mediated hemolytic anemia, and environmental irritants; dermoids are congenital; subconjunctival or episcleral hemorrhages may occur secondary to birth trauma or neonatal maladjustment syndrome. Conjunctivitis secondary to pneumonia is seen most commonly in 1- to 6-month-old foals.
- Adults—Ocular SCC prevalence increases with age.

Genetics

No proven genetic basis for conjunctiviti.

Predominant Sex

None proven

SIGNS

- Conjunctivitis—Conjunctival hyperemia, chemosis, and ocular discharge vary with type of disease.
- Onchocerciasis—Limbal conjunctival thickening and depigmentation, corneal edema, vascularization, stromal cellular infiltrate.
- Squamous cell carcinoma has two characteristic appearances—Proliferative mass which may or may not be ulcerated, or diffuse thickening and ulceration of tissue. May resemble granulation tissue or just an area of increased redness in the conjunctiva.
- Habronemiasis—Appearance ranges from granulomas, nodules, to small raised caseated plaques on the conjunctiva.
- Dermoid—Pigmented mass involving the limbus and varying degrees of the cornea.

CAUSES OF CONJUNCTIVITIS

- Infectious
  - Parasitic—*Habronema megastoma,* H. muscae,* Draschia megastoma, Onchocerca cervicalis, Thelazia lacrimalis, Trypanosoma* spp.
  - Viral—adenovirus, equine herpesvirus types 1 and 2, equine infectious anemia, equine viral arteritis, influenza type A2
  - Bacterial—*Moraxella equi, Streptococcus equi* subspecies *equi, Rhodococcus equi*, *Actinobacillus* spp. leptospirosis
  - Mycotic—*Aspergillus* spp., *Fusarium*
  - Protozoal—equine protozoal myeloencephalitis
- Neoplastic—SCC,* lymphoma, papilloma, hemangioma, hemangiosarcoma, mastocytoma, melanoma, multiple myeloma, etc.
- Secondary to other ocular/adnexal disease—ulcerative keratitis,* corneal stromal abscess,* anterior uveitis,* equine recurrent uveitis,* obstructed nasolacrimal duct
- Secondary to environmental causes—foreign bodies and debris,* trauma,* allergic reactions to dust and environmental pollutants
- Secondary to systemic disease—polyneuritis equi, vestibular disease syndrome, African horse sickness, epizootic lymphangitis, neonatal maladjustment syndrome

RISK FACTORS

- Recumbent foals are at risk for conjunctivitis secondary to environmental irritants.
- White, gray-white, and palomino hair color predisposes to ocular SCC.
- Lightly pigmented animals and those residing in areas with high UV indices are at the greatest risk.
- Warm weather and climates with heavy fly populations are risk factors for habronemiasis and other parasitic infections.

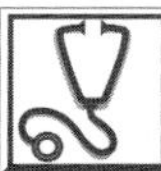

DIAGNOSIS

DIFFERENTIAL DIAGNOSIS

- Conjunctivitis is a nonspecific sign, reflecting the eye's limited mechanisms of response to injury. It is critical to differentiate primary conjunctivitis from conjunctivitis associated with ocular or systemic disease.
- Nodular/mass lesions of conjunctiva—habronemiasis, SCC, mastocytoma, hemangioma, hemangiosarcoma, papilloma and other neoplastic infiltrates, fungal granulomas, nodular necrobiosis, pseudotumors, dermoids, foreign body reaction

CBC/BIOCHEMISTRY/URINALYSIS

N/A

OTHER LABORATORY TESTS

- Cytology to identify mycotic, bacterial causes of conjunctivitis.
- Culture and sensitivity of mucopurulent discharge may be considered if a primary bacterial cause is suspected.
- Habronemiasis—conjunctival scraping reveals eosinophils, mast cells, neutrophils, plasma cells, rarely larvae.
- Biopsy and histopathology should be performed for mass lesions.

IMAGING

N/A

OTHER DIAGNOSTIC PROCEDURES

Complete ophthalmic examination is indicated to identify adnexal and ocular causes of conjunctivitis, including a thorough adnexal examination, fluorescein staining, and examination for signs of anterior uveitis.

GROSS AND HISTOPATHOLOGIC FINDINGS

Conjunctival Biopsy

- Onchocerciasis—microfilariae, eosinophils, lymphocytes
- Habronemiasis—eosinophils, mast cells, neutrophils, plasma cells, rarely larvae
- SCC—epithelial cells with neoplastic characteristics
- Lymphoma—large population monomorphic lymphocytes with neoplastic characteristics

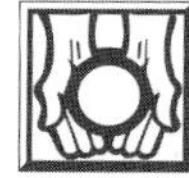

TREATMENT

INPATIENT VERSUS OUTPATIENT

Most horses with simple conjunctivitis associated with parasitic, bacterial, viral, and environmental causes can be treated on an outpatient basis. Treatment of some systemic and ocular diseases associated with complicated conjunctivitis may require hospitalization.

ACTIVITY

Restriction of activity may be required in cases where conjunctival disease is associated with systemic illness. If environmental irritation is suspected, then exposure to the inciting substance should be restricted or eliminated. Animals with ocular involvement/disease should not be ridden if visual status is compromised.

DIET

No change in diet is necessary. Hay should be fed at ground level rather than elevated hayracks or bags to avoid further irritation of the conjunctiva by dust and debris.

CLIENT EDUCATION

If there is evidence of self-trauma, a protective hood covering the affected eye should be placed on the horse. The client should be instructed to contact the veterinarian if the condition worsens in any way or shows little to no signs of improvement.

SURGICAL CONSIDERATIONS

- Treatment of conjunctival neoplasia may involve local resection, with adjunctive beta-irradiation, brachytherapy, cryotherapy, radiofrequency hyperthermia, or intralesional chemotherapy.
- Small lacerations of the conjunctiva will heal without primary closure. Large lacerations should be sutured with fine absorbable suture.
- Conjunctival foreign bodies and debris can usually be removed with topical anesthesia and liberal flushing of conjunctival fornices.

MEDICATIONS

DRUGS AND FLUIDS

- Parasitic conjunctivitis:
Habronemiasis—topical 0.03% echothiophate iodide (phospholine iodide) and ophthalmic neomycin/polymixin B with dexamethasone (Maxitrol) q12h. Multifocal lesions will require oral ivermectin (200 μg/kg). Intralesional triamcinolone may reduce size of granulomas, but this long-acting steroid must be used with extreme caution and not at all if the cornea is compromised in any way.
Onchocerciasis—systemic ivermectin with topical anti-inflammatories. Thelazia—topical phospholine iodide, flush conjunctival fornix
- Bacterial conjunctivitis—topical broad-spectrum antibiotic initially (triple antibiotic usually appropriate), may change after results of bacterial culture and sensitivity. Treat every 6–12 hours depending on severity of disease.
- Conjunctival lacerations—Treat with prophylactic broad-spectrum antibiotic topically.
- Allergic conjunctivitis—topical corticosteroid, reduce/eliminate exposure to inciting cause if possible.
- SCC—See Ocular/adnexal Squamous Cell Carcinoma.
- Ocular diseases inciting conjunctivitis—See appropriate section.
- Other systemic medication as indicated by concurrent systemic disease

CONTRAINDICATIONS

N/A

PRECAUTIONS

N/A

POSSIBLE INTERACTIONS

N/A

ALTERNATE DRUGS

Depends upon the primary condition and causative agents

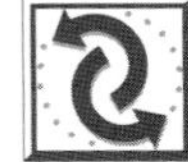

FOLLOW-UP

PATIENT MONITORING

The patient should be rechecked soon after beginning therapy (3–4 days), with specific time frame determined by disease and severity. Subsequent rechecks are dictated by the specific diagnosis, the severity of disease, and its response to treatment.

PREVENTION/AVOIDANCE

- Fly control in barns and pastures, fly hoods, and frequent periocular administration of insect repellent can help prevent the development of habronemiasis.
- A preventative health program including regular deworming with ivermectin will help prevent habronemiasis and onchocerciasis.
- The incidence of allergic/environmental conjunctivitis can be reduced/prevented by avoidance of the inciting agent.
- Treat any underlying ocular or systemic disease that may promote the conjunctival disease.
- Limit solar exposure in lightly pigmented animals to decrease the incidence of SCC.

POSSIBLE COMPLICATIONS

- Potential complications of conjunctival neoplasia and its treatment vary with the specific type of tumor.
- Possible complications of treatment include depigmentation in region of treatment, recurrence of the neoplasia, and metastatic spread.

EXPECTED COURSE AND PROGNOSIS

- Infectious conjunctivitis usually responds to appropriate treatment.
- Primary conjunctival infections respond well to topical therapy, usually within 5–7 days.
- Failure to respond or recurrence suggests an unidentified underlying cause (i.e., recurrent bacterial conjunctivitis associated with an unrecognized foreign body).
- Course and prognosis of conjunctival neoplasia depend on the specific type of neoplasia and the extent of invasion of surrounding tissues.
- Viral conjunctivitis may be recurrent.
- Allergic conjunctivitis is often difficult to eliminate completely due to the nature of the horse's environment.
- Prognosis associated with conjunctivitis secondary to systemic or ocular disease varies with the specific disease.
- Many systemic diseases that have conjunctivitis as a clinical sign can have serious and life-threatening consequences.

MISCELLANEOUS

ASSOCIATED CONDITIONS

N/A

AGE-RELATED FACTORS

N/A

ZOONOTIC POTENTIAL

N/A

PREGNANCY

Systemic absorption of topically applied medication is possible. Benefits of treatment should be considered against any risks posed to the fetus.

SYNONYMS

N/A

SEE ALSO

- Occular/adnexal SCC
- Ocular problems in the neonate
- Eyelid diseases
- Corneal ulceration
- Ulcerative keratomycosis
- Corneal stromal abscesses
- Recurrent uveitis
- Glaucoma

ABBREVIATION

- SCC = squamous cell carcinoma

Suggested Reading

Brooks DE: Ophthalmology for the Equine Practitioner. Jackson, WY; Teton NewMedia, 2002.

Brooks DE, Matthews AG: Equine ophthalmology. In: Gelatt KN, ed. Veterinary Ophthalmology, ed 4. Philadelphia; Lippincott Williams and Wilkins, 2007.

Gilger BC, ed. Equine Ophthalmology. Philadelphia; WB Saunders, 2005.

Author Caryn E. Plummer

Consulting Editor Dennis E. Brooks

CONTAGIOUS EQUINE METRITIS (CEM)

BASICS

DEFINITION/OVERVIEW

- Genital infection of stallions and mares caused by *Taylorella equigenitalis.*
- A reportable, highly contagious disease transmitted primarily by coitus.
- Transmission also may occur by contaminated equipment.
- Stallions are asymptomatic carriers.
- Organism is harbored in fossa glandis, urethral sinus, and smegma.
- It is also recoverable from the terminal urethra, preputial surface, and pre-ejaculatory fluid.
- Clinical signs only occur in mares; range from none to acute endometritis.
- The organism can persist in the clitoral sinuses and fossa.
    - Mares may be mechanical carriers via smegma of the clitoral fossa.

ETIOLOGY/PATHOPHYSIOLOGY

Stallions

The organism is harbored in various external regions of the genital tract and is transmitted primarily by coitus.

Mares

- 30 to 40% of mares bred by an infected stallion develop disease.
- Clinical signs range from none to acute endometritis.
- The organism initially is found in the endometrium and cervix.
- The organism less frequently is found in the vagina, vulva, clitoris, and oviducts.
- From 3 weeks to 4 months following exposure, the organism occasionally can be recovered from the ovarian surface, oviduct, uterus, cervix, and vagina.
- The organism is more reliably isolated from clitoral fossa and sinuses.
- Local IgA, IgM, and systemic IgG response.
- The organism also is recoverable from placentae of positive mares and genitalia of colts and fillies.
    - Acquired *in utero* or at parturition.

SYSTEMS AFFECTED

Reproductive

GENETICS

N/A

INCIDENCE/PREVALENCE

Transmission is dependent on carrier stallion or contaminated equipment.

SIGNALMENT

Breeding-age mares and stallions from countries identified as CEM-affected.

SIGNS

Stallions

Inapparent infection

Mares

- Within 2 to 7 days of infection, mares develop varying amount of odorless, grayish, mucopurulent discharge.
- Diffuse endometritis and cervicitis: severe and plasmacytic by 14 days; declines and persists as mild, diffuse, and multifocal for as long as 2 weeks.
- Shortened diestrus because of premature luteolysis.
- Temporary infertility
- No systemic involvement

CAUSES

- Two strains of *T. equigenitalis*
    - Streptomycin resistant
    - Streptomycin sensitive
- Contaminated equipment (e.g., specula, AI) and handling personnel (e.g., gloves).
- *T. asinigenitalis* resembles *T. equigenitalis.*
    - Has been isolated from donkey jacks at routine testing for CEM.
    - There is cross-reactivity with the CF utilized to identify mares recently infected with *T. equigenitalis*.

RISK FACTORS

- Carrier stallion
- Contaminated equipment
- No lifelong immunity
- Previous exposure does not afford absolute protection against subsequent challenge.

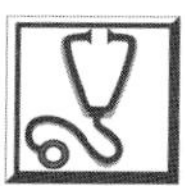

DIAGNOSIS

DIFFERENTIAL DIAGNOSIS

- Bacterial or fungal endometritis
- Pyometra
- Vaginitis
- Urinary tract infection
- Urine pooling
- Neoplasia of the uterus or vagina
- Persistent hymen

CBC/BIOCHEMISTRY/URINALYSIS

Unremarkable

OTHER TESTS

- Speculum examination
- Collection of cervical discharge
- Isolation of organism

IMAGING

U/S: intrauterine fluid suggestive of endometritis

OTHER DIAGNOSTIC PROCEDURES

Serology

- Detectable antibody in acute cases
    - Mares only CF positive 15 to 45 days post-infection.
- No value in stallions, because contamination is surface only.

Bacterial Cultures

- Stallions: urethral fossa and urethral sinus, distal urethra, penile skin, and preputial folds.
- Mares: clitoral sinus and fossa; endometrium, vaginal fluid, and cervix of estrus mare.
- Exacting culture requirements for *T. equigenitalis*
    - Immediately place swabs in Amies charcoal medium.
    - Keep at 4 °C for transport.
- Plate samples within 24 hours of collection in chocolate agar at 5% CO_2.
- Colonies usually form in 2 to 3 days; a recent streptomycin-sensitive strain may take as long as 6 days.
- Reportable disease that requires a federally approved laboratory for identification.

Cytology (Mares)

- Presence of PMNs, indicative of endometritis.
- Presence of morphologically suggestive bacteria.
    - Free or phagocytized gram-negative coccobacilli seen individually or in pairs, arranged end-to-end.

Test Breeding (Stallions)

- Breed to known CEM-negative mares. Does not consistently lead to colonization and seroconversion of test mares.

PCR

- Developed, but not yet sufficiently validated.
- Experimentally can discriminate between *T. equigenitalis* and *T. asinigenitalis*.
- Used in conjunction with culture, more effective technique than culture alone.

PATHOLOGIC FINDINGS

N/A

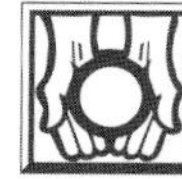

TREATMENT

APPROPRIATE HEALTH CARE

Under federal supervision at approved quarantine station.

Mares

- Intrauterine antibiotics: crystalline penicillin (5 to 10 million IU for 5 to 7 days).
- Cleansing of the clitoral fossa and sinuses with chlorhexidine scrub to remove all smegma.
- Pack with nitrofurazone ointment.

Stallions

- Completely extrude and wash penis in chlorhexidine scrub.
- Remove all smegma, especially from the urethral fossa and skin folds of prepuce.
- Nitrofurazone dressing for 5 days.

NURSING CARE

N/A

ACTIVITY

N/A

DIET

N/A

CLIENT EDUCATION

N/A

SURGICAL CONSIDERATIONS

Mares: clitoral sinusectomy or clitorectomy for intractable cases.

MEDICATIONS

DRUGS OF CHOICE

- Chlorhexidine (2% to 4%); higher concentrations can lead to penile irritation.
- Nitrofurazone (0.2% ointment)

CONTRAINDICATIONS

N/A

PRECAUTIONS

Mucosal irritation from drugs

POSSIBLE INTERACTIONS

N/A

ALTERNATIVE DRUGS

N/A

FOLLOW-UP

PATIENT MONITORING

Culture (Timing)

- Swabs 7 days after the last day of treatment for three consecutive sets of negatives.
- Stallions: every 2 days for three sets.
- Mares: three consecutive estrus periods.

Culture (Locations)

- Mares: swab the clitoris and endometrium at estrus before breeding; swab during abnormal estrous intervals.
- Stallions: swabs from teaser and breeding stallions before season begins.

Culture (Equipment)

- Disposable gloves, sleeves, and speculum
- Use AI when feasible or permitted by breed-society regulations.

PREVENTION/AVOIDANCE

- All horses older than 2 years entering the United States from CEM-affected countries must follow treatment and testing protocol.
- Mares: test three times in 7 days, then treat for 5 days; if three negative cultures are obtained, the mare is released.
- Stallions require negative culture and negative test-breeding to two known CEM-negative mares; if positive, repeat cycle until three consecutive, negative culture results are obtained.

POSSIBLE COMPLICATIONS

N/A

EXPECTED COURSE AND PROGNOSIS

Recovery with treatment, as described.

MISCELLANEOUS

ASSOCIATED CONDITIONS, AGE-RELATED FACTORS, ZOONOTIC POTENTIAL, PREGNANCY

N/A

SYNONYMS

Formerly *Haemophilus equigenitalis*

SEE ALSO

Venereal diseases

ABBREVIATION

- AI = artificial insemination
- CEM = contagious equine metritis
- CF = complement fixation test
- CO_2 = carbon dioxide
- IgA = immunoglobulin A
- IgG = immunoglobulin G
- IgM = immunoglobulin M
- IU = international units
- PCR = polymerase chain reaction
- PMN = polymorphonuclear cell
- U/S = ultrasound, ultrasonography

Suggested Reading

Baverud V, Nystrom C, Johansson KE. Isolation and identification of *Taylorella asinigenitalis* from the genital tract of a stallion, first case of a natural infection. Vet Microbiol. 2006;116;294–300.

Blanchard TL, Kenney RM, Timoney PJ. Venereal disease. Vet Clin North Am Equine Pract 1992;8:193–195.

Kristula MA, Smith BI. Diagnosis and treatment of four stallions, carriers of the contagious metritis organism – case report. Therio. 2004;61:595–601.

Timoney PJ. Aspects of the occurrence, diagnosis and control of selected venereal diseases of the stallion. In: Proceedings of the Stallion Symposium, Sponsored by the ACT/SFT, Hastings, Nebraska, December 1998 76–78.

Wakeley PR, Errington J, Hannon S, Roest HI, Carson T, Hunt B, Sawyer J, Heath P. Development of a real time PCR for the detection of *Taylorella equigenitalis* directly from genital swabs and discrimination from *Taylorella asinigenitalis*. Vet Microbiol. 2006;118:247–254.

Watson ED. Swabbing protocols in screening for contagious equine metritis. Vet Rec 1997;140:268–271.

Wood JL, Kelly L, Cardwell JM, Park AW. Quantitative assessment of the risks of reducing the routine swabbing requirements for the detection of *Taylorella equigenitalis*. Vet Rec. 2005;157:41–46.

Author Peter R. Morresey

Consulting Editor Carla L. Carleton

CORNEAL/SCLERAL LACERATIONS

BASICS

OVERVIEW

• Ocular trauma is the result of a redistribution of kinetic energy. It knows no boundaries with possible effects on any ocular structure such that ocular injury can have a variety of manifestations.
• Blunt injuries carry a worse prognosis than injury from sharp objects or missiles as blunt forces are transmitted throughout the eye. Sharp, penetrating injuries have the forces localized to the site of impact.

SIGNALMENT

Any age and breed of horse may suffer corneal laceration.

SIGNS

• The eye may be cloudy, red, and painful. Blepharospasm and lacrimation are present with focal or generalized corneal edema. Slight droopiness of the eyelashes of the upper eyelid may be a subtle sign of corneal ulceration.
• Full-thickness corneal/scleral perforations are usually associated with iris prolapse, shallow anterior chamber, and hyphema. If the corneal lesion extends to the limbus, the sclera should also be carefully checked for perforation because the scleral wound can be obscured by conjunctival chemosis and hemorrhage.

CAUSES AND RISK FACTORS

Trauma from nails, buckets, light fixtures, vegetative material, and tree branches can result in corneal/scleral lacerations.

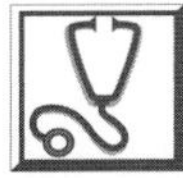

DIAGNOSIS

DIFFERENTIAL DIAGNOSIS

Ocular pain may also be found with corneal ulcers, uveitis, conjunctivitis, glaucoma, blepharitis, and dacryocystitis.

CBC/BIOCHEMISTRY/URINALYSIS

N/A

OTHER LABORATORY TESTS

N/A

IMAGING

N/A

DIAGNOSTIC PROCEDURES

Fluorescein dye staining of the cornea will reveal the laceration. Fluorescein dye may enter the anterior chamber.

PATHOLOGIC FINDINGS

N/A

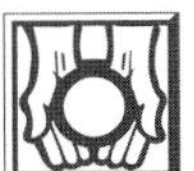

TREATMENT

• Medical therapy should be sufficient for superficial, nonperforating lacerations. Deep or irregular corneal lacerations require surgical support of the cornea and more aggressive therapy for iridocyclitis. Direct corneal suturing and conjunctival flaps are indicated to more rapidly restore corneal integrity.
• Both small and large full-thickness corneal perforations should be surgically repaired. Complications include infection, iris prolapse, anterior synechiae, cataract formation, and persistent iridocyclitis. Both small and large corneal or scleral full-thickness defects can result in phthisis bulbi if left untreated.
• A horse with a traumatic corneal perforation that defies repair, extensive extrusion of intraocular contents, severe intraocular hemorrhage, or evidence of bacterial infection should have the affected globe enucleated.

MEDICATIONS

DRUG(S) OF CHOICE

Medical therapy alone should be sufficient for superficial, nonperforating lacerations. Topically applied antibiotics (chloramphenicol, bacitracin-neomycin-polymyxin B, gentamicin; QID), atropine (1%; QID), and serum (QID) are recommended. Systemic NSAIDs (phenylbutazone 2 mg/kg BID PO; flunixin meglumine 1 mg/kg BID, PO, IM, IV) and broad-spectrum parenteral antibiotics are also indicated for full-thickness lesions.

CONTRAINDICATIONS/POSSIBLE INTERACTIONS

Horses receiving topically administered atropine should be monitored for signs of colic.

FOLLOW-UP

PATIENT MONITORING

• Horses with corneal lacerations should be monitored for continued blepharospasm and colic.
• The horse should be protected from self trauma with hard- or soft-cup hoods.
• Horses with corneal lacerations and secondary uveitis should be stall-rested till the condition is healed. Intraocular hemorrhage and increased severity of uveitis are sequelae to overexertion.
• Diet should be consistent with the training level of the horse.

PREVENTION/AVOIDANCE

N/A

POSSIBLE COMPLICATIONS

• Failure to detect a scleral tear will result in chronic hypotony and globe atrophy (phthisis bulbi).
• The eye of the horse does not tolerate much damage to its vasculature. Severe intraocular hemorrhage usually results in phthisis bulbi.
• Injury to the lens, iris, and retina can accompany blunt or sharp corneal/scleral trauma.
• Septic intrusion into the globe results in painful endophthalmitis. Such infection can spread to surrounding soft tissues and necessitates enucleation.

EXPECTED COURSE AND PROGNOSIS

• Small corneal lacerations can heal quickly if surgical and medical therapy is prompt. Larger lesions are associated with more uveitis and will be slower to heal.
• If the horse has a dazzle reflex in the damaged eye and a consensual pupillary light reflex in the good eye, then repair should be attempted.

MISCELLANEOUS

ASSOCIATED CONDITIONS

Corneal lacerations in the horse are always accompanied by varying degrees of iridocyclitis.

AGE-RELATED FACTORS

N/A

ZOONOTIC POTENTIAL

N/A

PREGNANCY

N/A

SEE ALSO

Iris prolapse

Suggested Reading

Brooks DE. Ophthalmology for the Equine Practitioner. Jackson, WY; Teton NewMedia, 2002.
Brooks DE, Matthews AG. Equine ophthalmology. In: Gelatt KN, ed. Veterinary Ophthalmology, ed 4. Philadelphia; Lippincott Williams and Wilkins, 2007.
Gilger BC, ed. Equine Ophthalmology. Philadelphia; WB Saunders, 2005.

Author Dennis E. Brooks
Consulting Editor Dennis E. Brooks

CORNEAL STROMAL ABSCESSES

BASICS

OVERVIEW

• A corneal abscess may develop after epithelial cells adjacent to a small epithelial puncture defect divide and migrate over the wound to seal infectious agents or foreign bodies in the stroma. This reepithelialization forms a barrier that protects the bacteria or fungi from topically administered antimicrobial medications.
• Stromal abscesses may also occur from endothelial invasion in iridocyclitis or a systemic disease.

SIGNALMENT

All ages and breeds of horses in all types of environments are at risk.

SIGNS

• The eye may be cloudy, red, and painful. Blepharospasm and tearing are present. Slight droopiness of the eyelashes of the upper eyelid may be a subtle sign of corneal abscessation.
• The diagnosis of stromal abscessation is based on the presence of a focal, yellow-white, stromal infiltrate with associated corneal edema. Single or multiple abscesses may be present. A mild to fulminating iridocyclitis occurs secondary to what appears initially to be a relatively benign corneal disease, causing severe pain and possible blindness. Corneal vascularization is variable at presentation, and may not reach the abscess site.
• Some cases have initial clinical signs suggestive of minor corneal trauma. Fluorescein dye retention is either negative, or positive over an area much smaller than the diameter of the corneal lesion.

CAUSES AND RISK FACTORS

Corneal stromal abscesses can be sterile or be infected by bacteria or fungi.

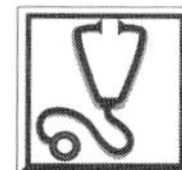

DIAGNOSIS

DIFFERENTIAL DIAGNOSIS

• Ocular pain may be associated with corneal ulcers, ERU, glaucoma, conjunctivitis, blepharitis, and dacryocystitis. • It may be difficult to differentiate a chronic stromal abscess with secondary uveitis from the NKU keratopathy noticed in horses in the southern United States. • A history of previous trauma, evidence of corneal ulceration, a yellow-white stromal infiltrate, and the varying corneal position of stromal abscesses help make the distinction. Nonulcerative keratouveitis cases have a pink, fleshy, stromal lesion located at the limbus with very painful anterior uveitis.
• Although melting and infected ulcers of horses are also associated with severe anterior uveitis, each is distinct in general appearance from a stromal abscess, with ulcers invariably retaining fluorescein stain over the majority of the lesion, and the stromal abscesses only retaining stain over a small area of the lesion in the acute stages, if at all.

DIAGNOSTIC PROCEDURES

• A large number of cytologic, microbiologic, and histologic specimens may fail to yield diagnostic results. It may be that the bacteria and/or fungi are killed by the initial medical treatment regimen, and the toxins subsequently released by the dying bacteria and fungi and degenerating leukocytes continue the stimulus for this interstitial keratitis, and prolong the anterior uveitis. • The keratectomy specimens may also be the only way to obtain a definitive etiologic diagnosis in order to institute proper antimicrobial therapy.

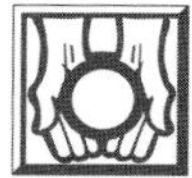

TREATMENT

• Many superficial stromal abscesses will initially respond positively with less uveitis to topical mydriatics/cycloplegics and to topical and systemic antibiotic and NSAID therapy but gradually worsen clinically, requiring surgical intervention. • Scraping over the stromal abscess may aid drug penetration and abscess healing in the early stages. • If significant improvement in the signs associated with a stromal abscess does not occur within the first 48–72 hours with intense and appropriate medical therapy, surgery can improve results and reduce the duration of medical therapy. • The use of systemic NSAID should be carefully adjusted, if medical therapy alone is used, to allow the control of anterior uveitis without significantly inhibiting the corneal vascularization necessary to heal corneal stromal abscesses. • Deep corneal abscesses do respond poorly to medical therapy. Most stromal abscesses involving Descemet's membrane are fungal infections, in my experience. Deep lamellar and penetrating keratoplasties are utilized in eyes with abscesses near Descemet's membrane, and eyes with rupture of the abscess into the anterior chamber. This aggressive surgical therapy can be very successful and is done to eliminate antigenic stimulation from the sequestered organisms and to remove the necrotic debris, metabolites and toxins from the degenerating leukocytes and microbes in the abscess. • Horses that undergo early surgery in the course of this disease tend to have a more rapid recovery than those in which surgery is delayed. If a positive response to medical therapy is not seen quickly, especially when the stromal abscesses are deep or severe uveitis is present, surgery should be considered. • The decision to perform surgery is based on continued progression of anterior uveitis despite intense medical therapy, imminent or preexistent rupture of the abscess into the anterior chamber, severe and unrelenting endophthalmitis, or anticipated poor visual outcome due to lack of vascularization of the stromal abscess.
• Penetrating keratoplasty, or corneal transplantation for the treatment of deep corneal stromal abscesses, with or without conjunctival pedicle grafts, is an effective treatment for this condition.

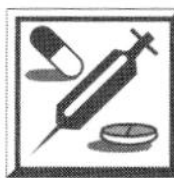

MEDICATIONS

DRUG(S) OF CHOICE

• Doxycycline (3 mg/kg BID PO), or gentamicin (2 mg/kg BID IV, IM)/penicillin K (10,000 IU/kg BID IM, IV) should be instituted initially. Topically applied antibiotics (chloramphenicol, bacitracin-neomycin-polymyxin B, gentamicin; QID), atropine (1%; QID), and serum (QID) are recommended. Systemic NSAIDs (phenylbutazone 2 mg/kg BID PO; flunixin meglumine 1 mg/kg BID PO, IM, IV) are also indicated. Topical natamycin or other antifungals are strongly recommended for deeper abscesses. • The intraocular injection of miconazole and fluconazole (0.1 mg/0.1mL solution), which can be performed at the time of surgery, has been effective adjunctive treatment in deep fungal stromal abscesses.

FOLLOW-UP

PATIENT MONITORING

• Ocular pain should be monitored and should diminish with resolution of the abscess. Self-trauma can be minimized with hard- or soft-cup face-masks or hoods. • The horse should be protected from self-trauma with hard- or soft-cup hoods. • Topically administered atropine is associated with colic. • Horses with stromal abscesses should be stall-rested until the condition is healed. Intraocular hemorrhage and increased severity of uveitis are sequelae to overexertion. • Diet should be consistent with the training level of the horse.

POSSIBLE COMPLICATIONS

Endophthalmitis, persistent uveitis, iris prolapse, ERU, and corneal ulcers are complications of stromal abscesses.

EXPECTED COURSE AND PROGNOSIS

• Stromal abscesses do not completely heal until they become vascularized, either directly from a conjunctival graft or from centripetal corneal vascular ingrowth. Deep and superficial corneal vascularization must occur in deep stromal abscesses for the lesion to resolve. Although some degree of corneal vascularization is generally present, it appears to grow much more slowly than the 1–2 mm/day described for the horse.
• Reepithelialization following corneal scrapings of medically treated horses is rapid and quite dramatic. Scraping over the stromal abscess may aid drug penetration and abscess healing in the early stages. Less benefit may be attained with scraping in the chronic stages. • Enucleation of painful blind eyes is necessary in a few cases.

MISCELLANEOUS

SEE ALSO

NKU

ABBREVIATIONS

• ERU = equine recurrent uveitis
• NKU = nonulcerative keratouveitis

Suggested Reading

Brooks DE: Ophthalmology for the Equine Practitioner. Jackson, WY; Teton NewMedia, 2002.

Brooks DE, Matthews AG: Equine ophthalmology. In: Gelatt KN, ed. Veterinary Ophthalmology, ed 4. Philadelphia; Lippincott Williams and Wilkins, 2007.

Gilger BC, ed. Equine Ophthalmology. Philadelphia; WB Saunders, 2005.

Author Dennis E. Brooks
Consulting Editor Dennis E. Brooks

CORNEAL ULCERATION

BASICS

DEFINITION

• Equine corneal ulceration is a sight-threatening disease requiring early clinical diagnosis, laboratory confirmation, and appropriate medical and surgical therapy.
• Both bacterial and fungal keratitis may present with a mild, early clinical course, but require prompt therapy if serious ocular complications are to be avoided.
• Ulcers can range from simple, superficial breaks or abrasions in the corneal epithelium, to full-thickness corneal perforations with iris prolapse.

PATHOPHYSIOLOGY

• The thickness of the equine cornea is 1.0–1.5 mm.
• The normal equine corneal epithelium is 8–10 cell layers thick but increases to 10–15 cell layers thick with hypertrophy of the basal epithelial cells following corneal injury. The epithelial basement membrane is not completely formed 6 weeks following corneal injury in the horse, in spite of the epithelium completely covering the ulcer site. Healing time of a 7-mm-diameter, midstromal depth, corneal trephine wound was nearly 12 days in noninfected wounds in horses.
• The environment of the horse is such that the conjunctiva and cornea are constantly exposed to bacteria and fungi. The conjunctival microbial flora of the horse varies, depending on the season and geographical area. Many bacterial and fungal organisms normally found in the horse conjunctival flora are potential ocular pathogens. *Staphylococcus, Streptococcus, Pseudomonas, Aspergillus*, and *Fusarium* spp. are common causes of corneal ulceration in the horse.
• The corneal epithelium of the horse is a formidable barrier to the invasion of bacteria or fungi. A defect in the tear film or corneal epithelium allows bacteria or fungi to adhere to the cornea and to initiate infection. Epithelial defects need not be full thickness, as corneas with partial-thickness epithelial defects are more susceptible to adherence by *Pseudomonas* than are corneas with a fully intact epithelium.
• Tear film neutrophils and some bacteria and fungi are associated with highly destructive protease and collagenase enzymes that can result in rapid corneal stromal thinning and perforation in the horse. Excessive protease activity is termed "melting" and results in a gelatinous appearance of the stroma. Total corneal ulceration ultimately requires the degradation of collagen, which forms the framework of the corneal stroma.
• Horse corneas demonstrate a strong fibrovascular healing response.

SYSTEM AFFECTED

Ophthalmic

GENETICS

There is no proven genetic predisposition to corneal ulceration in the horse, but the unique corneal healing properties of the horse in regard to excessive corneal vascularization and fibrosis appear to be strongly species specific.

INCIDENCE/PREVALENCE

Corneal ulceration is a common cause of ophthalmic disease in the horse and may be associated with bacterial and fungal infection.

SIGNALMENT

All ages and breeds of horses in all types of environments are at risk.

SIGNS

• The eye may be cloudy, red, and painful.
• Blepharospasm and tearing are present.
• Slight droopiness of the eyelashes of the upper eyelid may be a subtle sign of corneal ulceration.
• Corneal edema may surround the ulcer or involve the entire cornea.
• Signs of anterior uveitis are found with every corneal ulcer in the horse and include miosis and fibrin, hyphema, or hypopyon.

CAUSES

• Trauma is the most common cause of ulceration in the horse.
• Infection should be considered likely in every corneal ulcer in the horse. Infectious keratitis in horses develops in eyes with traumatic corneal abrasions, and eyes with epithelial defects due to chronic edema, keratoconjunctivitis sicca, exposure keratitis, neurotrophic keratitis, and neuroparalytic keratitis. Fungal involvement should be suspected if there is a history of corneal injury with vegetative material, or if a corneal ulcer has received prolonged antibiotic and/or corticosteroid therapy with slight or no improvement.
• Foreign bodies, chemical burns, and immune mechanisms may also cause corneal ulceration in horses.
• Persistent superficial ulcers may become indolent due to hyaline membrane formation on the ulcer bed.

RISK FACTORS

• The prominent eye of the horse may predispose to injury.
• Tear film proteases are elevated in both eyes of a horse with an ulcer in one eye.
• Healing of ulcers does not occur until tear film proteases are reduced to baseline levels.

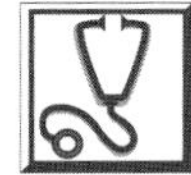

DIAGNOSIS

DIFFERENTIAL DIAGNOSIS

• Fluorescein dye retention is diagnostic of a corneal ulcer. The fluorescein should not be diluted but used at full strength.
• Uveitis, blepharitis, conjunctivitis, glaucoma, and dacryocystitis must be considered in the differential for the horse with a painful eye.

CBC/BIOCHEMISTRY/URINALYSIS

N/A

OTHER LABORATORY TESTS

• Microbial culture and sensitivity for bacteria and fungi are recommended for horses with rapidly progressive and deep corneal ulcers.
• Corneal cultures should be obtained first, followed by corneal scrapings for cytology.
• Mixed bacterial and fungal infections can be present.
• Vigorous corneal scrapings, at the edge and base of the lesion, to detect bacteria and deep hyphal elements can be obtained with the handle end of a sterile scalpel blade and topical anesthesia. Superficial swabbing cannot be expected to yield the organisms in a high percentage of cases. Stain cytologic specimens with Gram, Giemsa, or Wright's stain.

IMAGING

N/A

DIAGNOSTIC PROCEDURES

• All corneal injuries should be fluorescein stained to detect corneal ulcers. Small corneal abrasions are detected through the use of oblique transillumination and fluorescein dye retention.
• A "crater-like" defect that retains fluorescein dye at its periphery and is clear in the center is a descemetocele, and indicates the globe is at high risk of rupture. Descemet's membrane in the horse is 21 μm thick.

PATHOLOGIC FINDINGS

• Many early cases of equine ulcerative keratitis present, initially, as minor corneal epithelial ulcers or infiltrates, with slight pain, blepharospasm, epiphora, and photophobia.
• At first, anterior uveitis and corneal vascularization may not be clinically pronounced.
• Superficial and deep corneal vascularization and painful uveitis may occur.
• Extensive intrastromal lesions, vascularization, conjunctival injection, and corneal edema may then become evident.
• Corneal collagen breakdown or "melting" appears as a gelatinous, gray opacity to the margins and/or central regions of an ulcer.
• Cellular infiltration occurs rapidly and appears as white-to-yellow corneal lesions.
• A descemetocele can be recognized as a clearing at the bottom of a deep ulcer. It does not retain fluorescein dye, whereas deep ulcers retain fluorescein.
• Deep penetration of the stroma to Descemet's membrane with perforation of the cornea is a possible sequela to all corneal ulcers in horses.

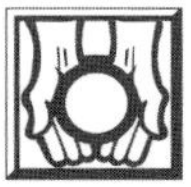

TREATMENT

APPROPRIATE HEALTH CARE

• Corneal ulceration should always be considered an emergency.

• The horse cornea can rapidly deteriorate if ulcerated and is prone to infection.
• Subpalpebral or nasolacrimal lavage treatment systems are used to treat a fractious horse or one with a painful eye that needs frequent therapy.

NURSING CARE

N/A

ACTIVITY

• Horses with corneal ulcers and secondary uveitis should be stall-rested until the condition is healed.
• Intraocular hemorrhage and increased severity of uveitis are sequelae to overexertion.

DIET

Diet should be consistent with the training level of the horse.

CLIENT EDUCATION

• A slowly progressive, indolent course often belies the seriousness of the ulcer.
• Corneal ulcers in horses may rapidly progress to descemetoceles.
• Corneal ulcers in horses are often very slow to heal.
• Anterior uveitis may be difficult to control.
• Scarring and vascularization of the cornea are common to the horse following ulceration.

SURGICAL CONSIDERATIONS

• Surgical placement of a conjunctival flap, corneoconjunctival transposition, or corneal transplantation may be indicated for rapidly progressive and deep corneal ulcers.
• Removing necrotic tissue by keratectomy speeds healing, minimizes scarring, and decreases the stimulus for iridocyclitis.
• Conjunctival grafts or flaps are used frequently in equine ophthalmology for the clinical management of deep, melting, and large corneal ulcers, descemetoceles, and for perforated corneal ulcers with and without iris prolapse.
• Nictitating membrane flaps are used for superficial corneal diseases including corneal erosions, neuroparalytic and neurotropic keratitis, temporary exposure keratitis, superficial corneal ulcers, and to reinforce a bulbar conjunctival graft.
• Panophthalmitis following perforation through a corneal stromal ulcer has a grave prognosis. To spare the unfortunate horse this chronic discomfort, enucleation is the humane alternative.
• Persistent ulcers may need surgical debridement and grid keratotomy to remove the hyaline membrane slowing healing.

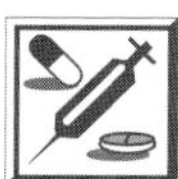

MEDICATIONS

DRUG(S) OF CHOICE

• Topically applied antibiotics, such as cefazolin, gentamicin, ciprofloxacin, or tobramycin ophthalmic solutions, may be used to treat bacterial ulcers. Amikacin (10 mg/mL) may also be used topically. Frequency of medication varies from q2h to q8h.
• Topically applied 1%–2% atropine is effective in stabilizing the blood-aqueous barrier, minimizing pain from ciliary muscle spasm, and causes pupillary dilatation. Atropine may be used as often as q4h, with the frequency of administration reduced as soon as the pupil dilates.
• Topically administered autogenous serum is used in ulcers with evidence of collagenolysis, infection, or chronicity. The serum can be administered topically as often as possible. Ten percent acetylcysteine or sodium EDTA can also be administered until stromal liquefaction diminishes. Both acetylcysteine and serum may be needed to arrest melting in some horse eyes.
• Systemic and topically administered NSAIDs such as phenylbutazone (1 g BID PO) or flunixin meglumine (1 mg/kg BID IV, IM, or PO) can be used orally or parenterally and are effective in reducing uveal exudation and relieving ocular discomfort from the anterior uveitis in horses with ulcers.

CONTRAINDICATIONS

Topical corticosteroids may encourage growth of bacterial and fungal opportunists by interfering with nonspecific inflammatory reactions and cellular immunity.

PRECAUTIONS

• Horses receiving topically administered atropine should be monitored for signs of colic.
• Hypomotility of the intestines can be induced with topical atropine in a small percentage of horses.

POSSIBLE INTERACTIONS

N/A

ALTERNATIVE DRUGS

Autogenous serum administered topically can reduce tear film and corneal protease activity in corneal ulcers in horses. The activity of serum against corneal proteases lasts at least 8 days. The serum can be stored at room temperature with little risk of contamination. Replace the serum with new serum every 5 days.

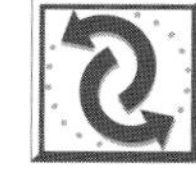

FOLLOW-UP

PATIENT MONITORING

• The clarity of the cornea, the depth and size of the ulcer, the degree of corneal vascularization, the amount of tearing, the pupil size, and intensity of the anterior uveitis should be monitored. Serial fluorescein staining of the ulcer is indicated to assess healing.
• As the cornea heals, the stimulus for the uveitis will diminish, and the pupil will dilate with minimal atropine therapy.
• Self-trauma should be reduced with hard- or soft-cup hoods.

PREVENTION/AVOIDANCE

Corneal ulcers in horses should be aggressively treated no matter how small or superficial they may be.

POSSIBLE COMPLICATIONS

Globe rupture, phthisis bulbi, and blindness are possible sequelae to corneal ulceration in horses.

EXPECTED COURSE AND PROGNOSIS

• The typical corneal ulcer in the horse heals slowly and with scarring. There is a strong tendency to vascularize.
• If the replication and spread of bacteria are not halted by the host response or the instillation of antibiotics, the process of stromal degradation and "melting" ultimately leads to total loss of stromal tissue and corneal perforation.
• Conjunctival flaps are necessary to save the globe and vision but are associated with scarring of the ulcer site. They are generally left in place 4–6 weeks.

MISCELLANEOUS

ASSOCIATED CONDITIONS

• Corneal infection and iridocyclitis are always major concerns for even the slightest corneal ulcerations.
• Iridocyclitis or uveitis is present in all types of corneal ulcers and must be treated in order to preserve vision.

AGE-RELATED FACTORS

N/A

ZOONOTIC POTENTIAL

N/A

PREGNANCY

N/A

SYNONYMS

N/A

SEE ALSO

N/A

Suggested Reading

Brooks DE. Ophthalmology for the Equine Practitioner. Jackson, WY; Teton NewMedia, 2002.

Brooks DE, Matthews AG. Equine ophthalmology. In: Gelatt KN, ed. Veterinary Ophthalmology, ed 4. Philadelphia; Lippincott Williams and Wilkins, 2007.

Gilger BC, ed. Equine Ophthalmology. Philadelphia; WB Saunders, 2005.

Author Dennis E. Brooks
Consulting Editor Dennis E. Brooks

CORYNEBACTERIUM PSEUDOTUBERCULOSIS

BASICS

DEFINITION

Corynebacterium pseudotuberculosis biovar *equi* causes three syndromes in horses, the most common form being external abscesses of the pectoral, ventral abdomen, axillary, or inguinal area. In less than 1 of 10 cases, the organism will spread internally, causing chronic internal infections associated with systemic illness. Ulcerative lymphangitis represents only a small percentage of the cases. The disease is seasonal, with most cases diagnosed between August and December with a peak in October and November in the Southwest. Occasional cases occur all year around.

PATHOPHYSIOLOGY

C. pseudotuberculosis is a soil-borne, facultative intracellular, facultative anaerobic bacterium than can survive for weeks to months in the environment. The disease is likely transmitted by mechanical vectors (house flies, horn flies, stable flies) and the bacterium penetrates the skin or mucosa where abrasions are present. Ventral midline dermatitis, caused by feeding habits of *Culicoides* and horn flies, seems to be a frequent route of entry. Incubation time ranges between 1 and 4 weeks. The high lipid content of the bacteria walls makes them resistant to phagocytosis, and a phospholipase D exotoxin is responsible for the increase in vascular permeability, causing edema and facilitating spread into the surrounding tissue and the regional lymph nodes. Typical abscesses have a thick capsule and contain copious amount of tan, odorless exudate. Pectoral abscesses give a pigeon breast appearance to affected horses (hence "pigeon fever"). Occasionally, the organism reaches one or more internal organs through lymphatic and/or hematogenous spread. Most affected horses mount a strong cellular and humoral immunity, the latter being apparently passively transmitted to foals.

SYSTEMS AFFECTED

- External abscesses
  - Skin and lymphatic
- Internal infection
  - Hepatobiliary
  - Respiratory
  - Renal
  - Occasionally other systems are involved
- Ulcerative lymphangitis
  - Musculoskeletal
  - Lymphatic

INCIDENCE/PREVALENCE

- In farms where the disease is considered endemic, cases are usually sporadic. In naïve populations, infection can take epidemic proportion.
- The case-fatality rate for external abscesses is less than 1%, but it ranges from 30% to 40% for internal infections, including euthanasia for economical reasons.

GEOGRAPHIC DISTRIBUTION

External abscess formation is usually restricted to the southwestern United States but has been seen in Wyoming, Utah, Colorado, and Kentucky in certain years. Ulcerative lymphangitis is not geographically restricted.

SIGNALMENT

Mean Age and Range

Horses of 1–5 years of age are more susceptible, but adult horses of any ages can be affected. The disease is uncommon in foals but has been reported occasionally between 3 and 6 months of age.

Predominant Sex

Mares may be slightly overrepresented.

SIGNS

General Comments

- External abscesses are often characteristic, but deeply located abscesses can be more difficult to recognize. Infection of the ventral abdomen often results in multiple small abscesses. Signs of systemic illness can be present, although less commonly than with internal infection.
- Atypical infection sites include septic arthritis, osteomyelitis, guttural pouch infection, abortion, metritis, and sinusitis.

Historical Findings

- Previous cases on the farm
- Internal infection—Concurrent external abscess is present or recently resolved in more than half of the cases.

Physical Examination Findings

- External abscesses
  - Painful swelling of the pectoral, ventral abdomen, axillary, sheath, or mammary gland area
  - Draining lesion with odorless exudate
  - Lameness and limb edema (with axillary and inguinal abscesses)
  - Fever/depression
- Internal infection
  - Anorexia
  - Fever
  - Lethargy
  - Weight loss
  - Ventral or limb edema
  - Tachycardia/tachypnea
  - Abdominal pain
  - Respiratory signs
  - Urinary infection
- Ulcerative lymphangitis
  - Cellulitis/lymphangitis in one or more limb
  - Multiple draining ulcerative lesions
  - Lameness
  - Fever

CAUSES

Seven genotypes of *C. pseudotuberculosis* biovar *equi* have been associated with the disease in horses. There is no known natural cross-species infection from small ruminants to horses.

RISK FACTORS

Geographic location (see earlier), age, the presence of other cases on the premises, and possibly being on pasture with other horses. Horses are more at risk in the months following a heavy rainfall winter, which favors breeding and survival of insects, and ventral midline dermatitis predisposes to the infection by providing a site of entry to the bacteria. In theory, immunocompromised horses are more at risk, but it has not been critically evaluated.

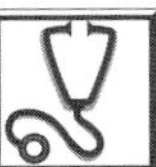

DIAGNOSIS

DIFFERENTIAL DIAGNOSIS

- External abscesses
  - Foreign body, trauma, neoplasia
  - Other causes of lameness for axillary and inguinal area abscesses
  - Other causes of ventral edema for ventral abscesses
  - *Streptococcus equi* (subsp. *zooepidemicus* or *equi*) and other bacterial infections should be considered, especially when the location is not typical.
- Internal infection
  - *Streptococcus equi* internal abscess, other internal abscesses
  - Pneumonia and pleuropneumonia of different etiology
  - Cholangiohepatitis, liver abscess, pyrrolizidine alkaloid toxicity, other liver diseases
  - Other causes of pyelonephritis
  - Neoplasia
- Ulcerative lymphangitis
  - Bacterial lymphangitis/cellulitis—staphylococcal and streptococcal infections, *Pseudomonas* sp., other bacterial infections
  - Fungal/protozoal lymphangitis/cellulitis—*Sporothrix schenckii*, *Pythium insidiosum* (phytiosis or swamp cancer).
  - Outside United States—*Burkholderia mallei* (cutaneous glanders) and *Histoplasma capsulatum* var. *farciminosum* (epizootic lymphangitis)

CBC/BIOCHEMISTRY/URINALYSIS

More frequently seen in internal infection than external abscesses (60% of the cases versus 30–40%):

- Neutrophilia, leucocytosis, anemia, hyperglobulinemia, increased fibrinogen concentration

Also with internal infection:

- Increased liver-associated enzymes with liver infection
- Pyuria, proteinuria, hematuria with kidney infection
- Rarely signs of intravascular disseminated coagulation with severe internal infection

OTHER LABORATORY TESTS

- Gram stain: gram-positive pleomorphic rod
- Bacterial culture: *C. pseudotuberculosis* grows well in 24–48 hours on blood agar plates. Small whitish opaque colonies. Can be isolated from draining lesions, needle aspiration or biopsy from internal organs, urine, tracheal wash, peritoneal or pleural fluid.
- Synergistic hemolysin inhibition (SHI) test measures serum IgG concentration directed to a *C. pseudotuberculosis* exotoxin: titers greater than 256 suggest an active infection and the vast majority of horses with internal infection have titers $\geq$512. Horses with external abscesses can have low titers and rarely horses with internal infection will fail to mount a serologic response. Titers can remain high for months (>1 year) after resolution of clinical signs.

CORYNEBACTERIUM PSEUDOTUBERCULOSIS

IMAGING

- External abscesses—Ultrasonography is useful to determine the depth of the abscess or the thickness of the capsule, especially when drainage is performed in a difficult location.
- Internal infection—Abdominal ultrasonography is useful in identifying the organ involved, for ultrasound-guided aspiration or biopsy, as well as for monitoring the progression of a lesion. Thoracic radiography and ultrasonography provide information on the extent of pneumonia. Internal infections often present as multiple hypoechoic lesions, as opposed to a single large encapsulated abscess as seen with external abscess.
- Ulcerative lymphangitis—Ultrasonography can be used to visualize distended lymphatics and find a site for needle aspiration. Radiographic exam can help to rule out other causes of lameness.

OTHER DIAGNOSTIC PROCEDURES

- Abdominocentesis (mild to severe peritonitis in most cases of liver, kidney, spleen, or mesenteric infection)
- Transtracheal wash, pleural fluid aspiration
- Hemoculture (only occasionally positive)

PATHOLOGIC FINDINGS

External abscesses are usually well encapsulated, while internal infection can be multifocal poorly encapsulated suppurative lesions containing gram-positive pleomorphic rods.

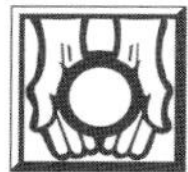

TREATMENT

AIMS OF TREATMENT

- External abscesses—Establish drainage and provide adequate analgesia if required during the maturation phase. Consider antimicrobial treatment in certain circumstances (systemic illness, recurrent or persistent infection, immunocompromised animal, pregnant mare).
- Internal infection—Eradicate the infection to prevent spreading to other organs.
- Ulcerative lymphangitis—Local treatment, systemic antimicrobials and adequate analgesia.

APPROPRIATE HEALTH CARE

- Most patients with external abscesses are treated at the farm. Repeated visits may be needed.
- Patients with internal infection can benefit from hospital setting for a precise diagnosis and initiation of antimicrobial therapy.
- Occasionally, a debilitated animal will benefit from emergency referral for immediate stabilization.

NURSING CARE

- External abscesses—hotpacking, poultice compound application, hydrotherapy. Abscesses should be lanced in a declive position, or a drain placed in deep abscesses, then lavaged daily with saline or diluted antiseptic. Exudate, including contaminated bedding, should be disposed of properly (to limit fly access).
- Internal infection—fluid therapy if dehydration present
- Ulcerative lymphangitis—hydrotherapy, bandaging

ACTIVITY

Limited during the time of infection, depending on the degree of systemic illness

CLIENT EDUCATION

To date, there is no evidence to support placing affected horses on a farm in quarantine; however, general hygiene, removal of contaminated bedding and fomites, and fly control should be emphasized. Topical insect repellent should be applied around draining abscesses, and on skin wounds and ventral abdomen of noninfected horses.

SURGICAL CONSIDERATIONS

Marsupialization or abscess removal has been reported.

MEDICATIONS

DRUG(S) OF CHOICE

- *Note:* To the author's knowledge, none of the drug combinations have been critically evaluated and compared.
- Isolates are susceptible to most antimicrobials in vitro. In vivo effectiveness is limited by the intracellular localization and the thick capsule surrounding external abscesses. Cost and route of administration will also guide the antimicrobial choice in most internal infection cases.
- Horses with external abscesses requiring antimicrobial administration can be treated with procaine penicillin (22,000 U/kg IM BID) or trimethoprim-sulfadiazine (30 mg/kg PO BID).
- Internal infection may have a better clinical outcome with a combination of ceftiofur (2–4 mg/kg IV, IM BID) and rifampin (5 mg/kg PO BID), but some horses will respond to penicillin or trimethoprim-sulfadiazine. Enrofloxacin (7.5mg/kg/day PO), chloramphenicol (50mg/kg PO TID), aminoglycoside-penicillin combination, and erythromycin estolate have been used with various success rates. The same recommendations could be made for ulcerative lymphangitis, but there are even less objective data available.
- Nonsteroidal anti-inflammatory drugs may be necessary to alleviate pain and control fever.

FOLLOW-UP

PATIENT MONITORING

For internal infection, the decision to discontinue therapy is based on resolution of clinical signs, normalization of clinicopathologic changes, and ultrasound or radiographic improvement. Titers should decrease as the infection is controlled but high titers can persist in some cases.

PREVENTION/AVOIDANCE

- See also "Client Education."
- No commercial vaccine is available for horses at the moment.

POSSIBLE COMPLICATIONS

- Recurrent or persistent infection
- Residual preputial swelling and fibrosis
- Antibiotic-associated diarrhea
- Purpura hemorrhagica (rare)
- Pregnant mares may abort, especially with internal infection. The risk for pregnant mares with external abscesses has not been evaluated, and it is not known if antibiotic treatment is of benefit.

EXPECTED COURSE AND PROGNOSIS

- External abscesses—The condition resolves within 2–3 weeks. The prognosis is excellent in most cases.
- Internal infection—Guarded prognosis (see Incidence/Prevalence) and prolonged antimicrobial treatment (1–2 months on average, sometimes more). In a small number of reported cases, all horses with confirmed internal infection that were not treated with antimicrobials did not survive. Horses that survive usually return to their previous use.
- Ulcerative lymphangitis—Should resolve within 1 month. Chronic edema and lameness can persist.

MISCELLANEOUS

ZOONOTIC POTENTIAL

C. pseudotuberculosis occasionally causes lymphadenitis in people in contact with farm animals, but there are no reports of a horse–to-human transmission.

PREGNANCY

See "Possible Complications."

SYNONYMS

- Pigeon fever
- Dryland or false distemper
- False strangles

Suggested Reading

Aleman M, Spier SJ, Wilson WD, Doherr MG. *Corynebacterium pseudotuberculosis*: 538 Cases (1982–1993). JAVMA 1996;209:804–809.

Doherr MG, Carpenter TE, Hanson KMP, Wilson WD, Gardner IA. Risk factors associated with *Corynebacterium pseudotuberculosis* infection in California horses. Prev Vet Med 1998;38:229–239.

Pratt SM, Spier SJ, Carroll SP, Vaughan B, Whitcomb MB, Wilson WD. Evaluation of clinical characteristics, diagnostic test results, and outcome in horses with internal infection caused by *Corynebacterium pseudotuberculosis*: 30 Cases (1995–2003). JAVMA 2005;227:441–448.

Spier SJ, Whitcomb MB. *Corynebacterium pseudotuberculosis*. In: Sellon DC, Long MT, eds. Equine Infectious Diseases St. Louis: Saunders, 2007:263–269.

Author Mathilde Leclère

Consulting Editors Ashley Boyle and Corinne Sweeney

COUGH

BASICS

DEFINITION

A sudden, forceful, noisy expulsion of air through the glottis to clear mucus, particles, and other material from the tracheobronchial tree and glottis

PATHOPHYSIOLOGY

- This reflex is a protective respiratory defense mechanism that, together with the mucociliary escalator, clears undesired material from the tracheobronchial tree proximal to the level of segmental bronchi.
- Initiated by stimulation of irritant receptors that ramify between epithelial cells from the level of the larynx down to the distal bronchioles and by receptors located in the lung parenchyma and pleura
- Receptors are stimulated by mechanical deformation, chemically inert dust particles, foreign bodies, pollutant gases, exposure to cold or hot air, inflammatory conditions, excessive mucus or exudates, and chemical mediators—histamine.
- Most of the afferent impulses travel in the vagus nerve, but also in the glossopharyngeal, trigeminal, and phrenic nerves, to cough centers in the medulla oblongata.

SYSTEMS AFFECTED

- Respiratory
- Musculoskeletal
- Cardiovascular
- Nervous

INCIDENCE/PREVALENCE

Unknown

GEOGRAPHIC INCIDENCE

Worldwide

SIGNALMENT

- All ages, breeds, and sexes
- Particular causes have a specific or general age predilection.
- Pneumonia caused by *Rhodococcus equi* and other bacteria is most common in foals aged from 4 weeks to 6 months.
- Viral infection is most common in weanlings, yearlings, and young adult performance horses.
- Heaves is most common in mature horses.

SIGNS

Historical

- Season and activity
  - Cough associated with heaves typically has a higher incidence when horses are confined indoors.
  - Summer pasture—associated obstructive airway disease and bacterial pneumonia in foals typically occur during late spring and summer.
- Housing and feeding practices
  - Cough associated with heaves occurs primarily in stabled horses fed hay and bedded on straw in poorly ventilated buildings.
  - Silicosis typically occurs in horses fed on the ground or grazed in bare, dusty paddocks in areas such as the Monterey Peninsula of California, which have exposed cristobalite silica shale.
- Speed of onset, contagiousness, duration, and characteristics
  - May suggest the underlying cause
  - Sudden onset and rapid spread are characteristics of viral infection, particularly influenza and EHV.
  - Cough-associated aspiration of food or a foreign body into the tracheobronchial tree is sudden in onset but does not spread to affect other horses.
  - Gradual onset and chronic course are typical for lower airway inflammatory disease, heaves, interstitial pneumonia, fungal pneumonia, and thoracic neoplasia.
  - Cough associated with lungworm infection typically has a sudden onset and chronic course, and may affect multiple horses.
  - Harsh, persistent cough suggests involvement of the major airways or exudate in the large airways secondary to pulmonary disease or aspiration.
  - Soft, infrequent cough often reflects inflammatory airway disease (IAD), heaves, interstitial lung disease, or pulmonary edema secondary to cardiac failure.
  - Productive cough frequently is reflected by swallowing movements afterward or by nasal discharge.
  - Exercise or activity frequently precipitates cough caused by many conditions, particularly those associated with airway irritation or fluid accumulation in airways. Cough associated only with exercise, however, often is a feature of EIPH or various other lower airway inflammatory diseases, including IAD.

Physical Examination

- Fever—usually indicates a primary infectious cause or secondary infection superimposed on a noninfectious cause
- No fever—typically found in heaves, IAD, abnormalities of the larynx or pharynx (other than retropharyngeal abscess), parasitic pneumonia, EIPH, tracheobronchial foreign body, tracheal collapse, and airway-oriented neoplasia (e. g., bronchial carcinoma)
- Food return via the nose—typically indicates esophageal obstruction, aspiration of food secondary to anatomic or neurologic derangement in the upper airway, severe pharyngeal inflammation, or cleft palate
- Pleurodynia—typically occurs with pleuropneumonia and other less common pleural inflammatory diseases
- Nasal discharge—reflects disease characterized by exudation or drainage of mucus or purulent exudate into the lower airways or, less commonly, aspiration of exudate draining into the pharynx or nasal passages secondary to guttural pouch or sinus disease

CAUSES

Most coughs are initiated by stimulation of receptors in the trachea and bronchi; therefore, cough is more likely to originate from diseases involving the lower than upper respiratory tract.

Upper Respiratory Tract Diseases

- Nasopharyngeal—rhinitis; sinusitis; pharyngitis; nasopharyngeal foreign body, cyst, hematoma, or tumor; strangles; cleft palate; dorsal or rostral displacement of the soft palate; guttural pouch empyema, tympany, or mycosis
- Laryngeal—hemiplegia, inflammation, epiglottic entrapment, epiglottic ulcer, foreign body, injuries, chondritis of the arytenoid cartilages, tumors, previous laryngeal or pharyngeal surgery
- Tracheal—inflammation, foreign body, smoke or chemical irritation, collapse, and tumor

Lower Respiratory Tract Diseases

- Bronchial—inflammation, infection, allergy/hypersensitivity, foreign body, and tumor
- Pulmonary—inflammation, infection, aspiration pneumonia, pulmonary edema, tumor, acute bronchointerstitial pneumonia, pneumoconiosis, and granulomatous pneumonia
- Pulmonary vascular—thrombosis/embolism, congestive cardiac failure, and pulmonary hypertension
- Pleural—inflammation, infection, hernia, and tumor

Other Diseases

Esophageal—obstruction, ulceration, inflammation, and tumor

RISK FACTORS

- Prolonged transportation predisposes to pleuropneumonia.
- Indoor housing in dusty environments, feeding of dusty hay, and use of dusty bedding may predispose to heaves.
- Viral respiratory infection predisposes to bacterial pneumonia and pleuropneumonia.
- Hot, dry, dusty outdoor conditions predispose foals to *R. equi* pneumonia.
- Mixing with other horses at shows, sales, and events predisposes to viral infections and strangles.
- Cograzing with donkeys or mules predisposes to lungworm infection.
- High ambient temperature or transportation of foals during hot weather predisposes to acute bronchointerstitial pneumonia.
- Poor parasite-control regimens predispose to parasitic pneumonitis resulting from ascarid migration.
- Congenital or acquired pharyngeal, palatal, and esophageal disorders, corrective upper airway surgery, and neurologic disorders that predispose to aspiration pneumonia

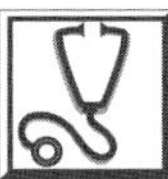

DIAGNOSIS

DIFFERENTIAL DIAGNOSIS

Differentiating Similar Signs

Because horses do not sneeze or vomit like humans or small animals, cough is not easily confused with other signs.

Differentiating Causes

See the sections on historical findings, physical examination findings, and risk factors.

CBC/BIOCHEMISTRY/URINALYSIS

- CBC typically is normal in noninflammatory diseases, whereas neutrophilia, with or without a left shift, and hyperfibrinogenemia are common in inflammatory diseases, particularly those caused by infection.
- Eosinophilia is a common finding in lungworm infection and some horses with granulomatous interstitial lung disease.

• Serum globulin concentration frequently is elevated in chronic inflammatory disease.

OTHER LABORATORY TESTS

• Serologic tests—for equine influenza, EHV-4, EHV-1, or equine viral arteritis
• Arterial blood gases in patients with signs of respiratory distress or cyanosis

IMAGING

• Thoracic ultrasonography in patients with suspected pulmonary consolidation, pulmonary abscesses or other masses, inflammatory pleural disease, pleural effusion, primary cardiac disease, and right heart disease secondary to a pulmonary condition
• Thoracic radiography (i.e., lateral projections) for differentiating types of lower respiratory tract disorders (consolidation, mass lesions, infiltrative interstitial disease, and pleural effusion)
• Radiography of the nasal passages, pharynx, larynx, guttural pouches, retropharyngeal structures, proximal esophagus, and trachea also may provide useful information.

OTHER DIAGNOSTIC PROCEDURES

• Endoscopy of the upper airway, guttural pouches, trachea, and bronchi detects anatomic, physiologic, and pathologic lesions and the source and nature of discharges.
• Bronchoalveolar lavage and collection of biopsy specimens of lesions or airway walls can be performed via the endoscope.
• Collection of nasal or nasopharyngeal swabs from horses with acute-onset cough and fever help to establish the diagnosis of acute viral infection and strangles. Diagnostic tests such as antigen-capture ELISA for influenza and PCR for herpesviruses, influenza, EVA, and other viruses, supplemented in some circumstances by viral isolation and serology and PCR testing of buffy coat samples (EHV-1 and EVA), facilitate rapid diagnosis of viral infection.
• Transtracheal aspiration with cytology and culture for evaluation of lower respiratory tract disorders
• Bronchoalveolar lavage with cytology for evaluation of lower respiratory tract disorders (heaves, inflammatory airway disease, silicosis, and granulomatous lung disease)
• Thoracocentesis with cytologic evaluation, determination of pH, glucose, lactate, and culture of aspirated fluid help to differentiate septic from nonseptic effusions.
• Direct and flotation fecal tests (e. g., Baermann) to detect ova or larvae of respiratory parasites and ascarids. Testing of donkeys or mules cograzed with affected horses may document asymptomatic infestation and shedding of lungworm ova.
• Lung biopsy and histologic examination are indicated for horses with suspected or confirmed diffuse, nonseptic lung disease (tumors or granulomas that can be visualized ultrasonographically).
• Echocardiography and electrocardiography in patients with suspected cardiac disease

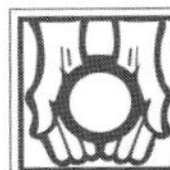

TREATMENT

AIMS OF TREATMENT

• Eliminate underlying infection
• Manage heaves through environmental modification, corticosteroids, and bronchodilators

APPROPRIATE HEALTH CARE

• Horses presented with cough usually are evaluated and managed as outpatients, unless respiratory distress, profound hypoxemia, cyanosis, serious choke, pleural effusion, pulmonary infarction, or congestive cardiac failure also are features of the disease process.
• Housing in a dust-free environment

NURSING CARE

Horses with suspected viral respiratory disease and contacts in the same airspace should be isolated as a group, either in the location currently occupied by the sick horses or in a separate isolation facility. Do not allow other horses to enter the same airspace occupied by sick horses.

ACTIVITY

Exercise restriction is best until a cause for the cough is established and corrected, especially when activity aggravates the cough.

DIET

• Appropriate for change in activity
• Cubed or pelleted food or haylage is preferred if pasture is not available.

CLIENT EDUCATION

Inform owners that a wide variety of conditions can be responsible for the cough and that an extensive workup may be required to define and treat the underlying cause.

SURGICAL CONSIDERATIONS

See the individual conditions causing cough.

MEDICATIONS

DRUG(S) OF CHOICE

Treatment is directed at the suspected or confirmed underlying cause rather than at attempting symptomatic relief by using cough suppressants (see relevant sections on individual diseases).

CONTRAINDICATIONS

• Do not use corticosteroids, except in foals with acute respiratory distress syndrome (i.e., acute bronchointerstitial pneumonia), unless allergic disease, hyperreactive airway disease, or anaphylaxis is suspected or confirmed and evidence of infection, parasitic infestation, or cardiac disease is lacking.
• Do not use cough suppressants in any patient in which a respiratory infection or clinically significant heart disease is suspected.

PRECAUTIONS

• Cough suppressants—indiscriminate use may obscure warning signs of serious pulmonary or cardiac disorders and predispose to life-threatening complications.
• Bronchodilator therapy may exacerbate hypoxemia in patients with $\dot{V}/\dot{Q}$ mismatch.
• NSAIDs may mask pleurodynia and fever in horses that are developing pleuropneumonia.

FOLLOW-UP

PATIENT MONITORING

• Cough may persist for several weeks after resolution of other signs in horses with infectious respiratory disease, because restoration of normal structure and function in the respiratory mucosa take several weeks.
• Continue exercise restriction until the cough disappears.

PREVENTION/AVOIDANCE

Contingent on diagnosis

POSSIBLE COMPLICATIONS

Some diseases that cause cough also can induce prolonged or permanent respiratory dysfunction and even death.

EXPECTED COURSE AND PROGNOSIS

Depend on cause of the cough

MISCELLANEOUS

AGE-RELATED FACTORS

See discussion of historical findings.

SEE ALSO

• See Causes.
• Purulent nasal discharge
• Acute respiratory distress

ABBREVIATIONS

• IAD = inflammatory airway disease
• EHV = equine herpesvirus
• EIPH = exercise-induced pulmonary hemorrhage
• ELISA = enzyme-linked immunoadsorbent assay
• EVA = equine viral anteritis
• PCR = polymerase chain reaction
• $\dot{V}/\dot{Q}$ = ventilation-perfusion ratio

Suggested Reading

Kohn CW, Cough. In: Reed SM, Bayly WM, Sellon DC, eds. Equine Internal Medicine, ed 2. St. Louis: Saunders, 2004:142–148.
Korpas J, Tomori Z. Cough and other respiratory reflexes. Progr Respir Rec 1979;12:15–18.
Korpas J, Widdicombe JG. Aspects of the cough reflex. Respir Med 1991;85(suppl A):3–5.
Wilson WD, Lofstedt J. Cough. In: Smith BP, ed. Large Animal Internal Medicine, ed 3. St. Louis: Mosby, 2002:46–54.

Author W. David Wilson
Consulting Editors Daniel Jean

CREATINE KINASE (CK)

BASICS

DEFINITION

The enzyme responsible for breakdown of creatine phosphate to creatine and phosphate. Releases energy for contraction and provides the sole source for energy in muscle at the initiation of exercise.

PATHOPHYSIOLOGY

• Skeletal muscle, myocardium and brain isoenzymes, with virtually no exchange between CSF and plasma.
• Therefore, significant increases in CK values are attributed to skeletal or cardiac muscle damage.
• Analysis of individual isoenzymes is generally not performed in the clinical setting. Use of CK to detect cardiac disease is problematic in horses and not recommended.
• Plasma half-life of CK is <2 hr in horses.
• After injury, serum activity typically peaks within 12 hr and returns to normal in 2–3 days (or, sometimes, as long as 7 days), provided the damage is not active and persistent.

SYSTEMS AFFECTED

• Increased serum activity is a result of a pathological condition, not a cause of disease.
• Systems affected in a given horse depend on the cause of the increased CK, not on the increased CK per se.

SIGNALMENT

• Depends on the specific cause. Muscle injury or exertion versus muscle disease.
• With polysaccharide storage disease, onset occurs at an early age, and there is said to be a familial pattern in some Quarter Horses and Belgian Draft Horses.
• Hyperkalemic periodic paralysis generally is seen in Quarter Horses.
• Otherwise, no convincing predilections for age, breed, or sex.

SIGNS

• History of muscular excertion, such as vigorous exercise, surgery (recumbency), seizures
• Palpably hard painful muscles, stiff gait, reluctant to move (exertional rhabdomyolysis)
• Discolored urine (myoglobinuria secondary to myonecrosis)
• Exercise intolerance—cardiac or muscle origin

COMMON CAUSES

Musculoskeletal

• *Exertional rhabdomyolysis—azoturia, myositis, tying-up; chronic or acute
• *Prolonged recumbency
• *Exercise/endurance event
• Trauma
• Clostridial myositis
• Hyperkalemic periodic paralysis
• Polysaccharide storage disease
• Vitamin E/selenium deficiency

Cardiovascular

• Monensin toxicity
• Acute cardiomyopathy (uncommon)

Nervous

• Disorders resulting in seizures, excessive muscular activity, or prolonged recumbency.
• *Note:* The serum CK is of muscular origin.

RISK FACTORS

• Improper conditioning
• Heavy training after prolonged rest
• Prolonged recumbency from any cause
• Monensin administration
• Trauma
• Medications administered by IM injection
• Seizures
• Poor nutrition

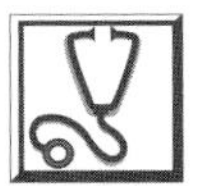

DIAGNOSIS

DIFFERENTIAL DIAGNOSIS

• History and physical examination (e.g., firm, swollen muscles; sweating; increased heart rate, body temperature, or respiratory rate) and degree of CK increase may suggest exertional rhabdomyolysis or capture myopathy and rule out other causes for gait abnormalities or discomfort.
• History and physical examination may indicate trauma, recent injections, or prolonged recumbency.
• Systemic signs and CBC, comprehensive chemistry profile, and urinalysis may suggest metabolic or infectious causes for recumbency, myositis, or endocarditis.
• A thorough history may elucidate recent IM injections, recent surgery, traumatic myocarditis, monensin toxicosis, cardiac causes (e.g., exercise intolerance), and seizures.
• Signalment is helpful in identifying polysaccharide storage disease.
• Signalment plus serum potassium determinations during an episode or induction of an episode by oral potassium challenge may suggest hyperkalemic periodic paralysis (*Note:* CK will be normal to moderately increased).
• If multiple farm animals are affected and feed quality is poor, suspect vitamin E/selenium deficiency.

LABORATORY FINDINGS

Drugs That May Alter Lab Results

N/A

Disorders or Problems That May Alter Lab Results

• Improper sample handling (consult with laboratory); gross hemolysis.
• Very high serum activity itself can alter reported values, because serum contains inhibitors of CK activity. Sample dilution may be necessary to bring extremely high values into the range of linearity for the instrument, but the resultant reduction in serum volume fraction reduces the inhibitor concentrations, resulting in higher CK values. This becomes important when CK values are monitored over time, because the actual value obtained from a diluted sample may not be accurate.

Valid If Run in Human Lab?

Yes

CBC/BIOCHEMISTRY/URINALYSIS

• Increased fibrinogen (with or without inflammatory leukogram) may be present with infectious causes, and physiologic leukocytosis may be present in horses that are excited, nervous, or in pain from myonecrosis.
• Increased AST often is seen with increased CK, depending on the time course.
• Initially, CK increases (peaks in 5–12 hr), and if muscle damage is not continuous, CK returns to baseline (usually by 2–3 days).
• AST may take several days to peak, has a more modest increase, and takes longer to return to baseline (may take several weeks).
• Samples should be taken over time, because increases in CK and AST indicate recent/active muscle damage.
• If CK remains increased, myonecrosis is ongoing; if AST remains increased but CK is falling, myonecrosis is not likely to be progressing.
• The degree of increase in CK may be helpful.
• Modest increases (<1000 IU/L), usually in the absence of increased AST, occur in normal horses from training, transport, or exercise.

- Endurance events may increase CK to >1000 IU/L, but activities generally return to baseline within 24–48 hr.
- IM injections result in relatively mild to moderate increases, but values in more extensive myonecrosis (e.g., vitamin E/selenium deficiency, exertional rhabdomyolysis) generally are well into the thousands and may exceed 100,000 IU/L.
- In milder forms of chronic exertional rhabdomyolysis, CK may be <1500–10,000 IU/L.
- Hyperkalemic periodic paralysis results in normal to moderately increased serum activity, even during an episode.
- Acid–base status is variable, depending on the cause and progression of myopathy.
- Moderate to severe myonecrosis results in myoglobinuria, regardless of the cause, but the absence of myoglobinuria does not rule out mild forms of chronic exertional rhabdomyolysis.

OTHER LABORATORY TESTS

Vitamin E/selenium determinations when indicated

IMAGING

Scintigraphy can be useful in localizing muscle pathology. Characteristic "tiger stripes" are seen in bone phase images.

DIAGNOSTIC PROCEDURES

- Biopsy for histopathology or muscle function tests to identify subtle cases of chronic exertional rhabdomyolysis or polysaccharide storage disease. The laboratory must specialize in muscle evaluation and be consulted before sample collection.
- Electromyography to rule out neuromuscular disease; also helpful in hyperkalemic periodic paralysis

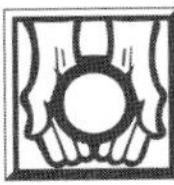

TREATMENT

- Supportive care includes minimizing movement, diminishing pain and anxiety, and maintaining fluid and electrolyte balance.
- IV fluid therapy with balanced electrolytes is indicated with moderate to severe cases, especially if myoglobinuria or sweating is present.
- Continue IV fluids at least until hydration is restored and urine is clear.

MEDICATIONS

DRUG(S) OF CHOICE

- No drug therapy is needed to specifically reduce CK, because increased serum activity is not harmful per se.
- With acute, severe myonecrosis, medications that reduce pain and anxiety may be of benefit—flunixin meglumine (1 mg/kg IV), ketoprofen (0.5 mg/kg), or phenylbutazone.
- Acepromazine at low doses for vasodilation and anxiety relief.
- With extreme pain, opiates, combined with xylazine (0.3–0.6 mg/kg) or detomidine (0.005–0.020 mg/kg).
- Recumbent, violent horses may be treated with phenobarbital by slow IV infusion to effect.
- Dantrolene sodium (recommended dosage varies by author: 2 or 10 mg/kg as a loading dose; alternatively, 2.5 mg/kg q1h) diluted in normal saline and administered by stomach tube to reduce calcium release from sarcoplasmic reticulum.

CONTRAINDICATIONS

Diuretics in muscle necrosis

PRECAUTIONS

- Avoid phenylbutazone in cases of myoglobinuria because of potential renal toxicity.
- Do not treat for acid–base abnormalities without blood gas data, because patients could be acidotic or alkalotic.
- Acepromazine at high doses is not recommended overall and is contraindicated at any dose in dehydration.
- If phenobarbital is used, titrate the dose to the patient.

FOLLOW-UP

PATIENT MONITORING

- CK and AST determinations over several days—during the initial episode, 24–48 hr later, and several days to a week after that. Reassess if parameters have not normalized.
- BUN, creatinine, and electrolyte determinations at similar timepoints to monitor renal and electrolyte status and response to therapy in cases of moderate to severe myonecrosis.

POSSIBLE COMPLICATIONS

- None solely caused by increased serum activity
- Myoglobin released from damaged muscles can cause irreversible renal failure without aggressive supportive care.

MISCELLANEOUS

AGE-RELATED FACTORS

None known

ZOONOTIC POTENTIAL

None known

PREGNANCY

N/A

SYNONYMS

Creatinine phosphokinase

SEE ALSO

- Myoglobin
- See Causes.

ABBREVIATION

- AST = aspartate aminotransferase

Suggested Reading

Beech J. Chronic exertional rhabdomyolysis. Vet Clin North Am Equine Pract 1997;13:145–168.

Cardinet GH. Skeletal muscle function. In: Kaneko JJ, Harvey JW, Bruss ML, eds. Clinical Biochemistry of Domestic Animals, ed 5. San Diego: Academic Press, 1997.

Duncan JR, Prasse KW, Mahaffey EA. Muscle. In: Veterinary Laboratory Medicine, ed 3. Ames, IA: Iowa State University Press, 1994.

The author and editor wish to acknowledge the contribution to this chapter of Ellen W. Evans, the author in the previous edition.

Author Elizabeth A. Walmsley

Consulting Editor Kenneth W. Hinchcliff

CRYPTORCHIDISM

BASICS

DEFINITION/OVERVIEW

- Failure of one or both testes to descend completely into its associated scrotal sac.
- Affected males are referred to as rigs, ridglings, originals or, if the testis is located in the inguinal canal, high flankers.
- False rig — a true castrate that retains some degree of stallion-like behavior.
- Complete abdominal cryptorchid – when the testis and entire epididymis are contained within the abdomen.
- Incomplete abdominal cryptorchid – when the testis and most of the epididymis are intra-abdominal but the ductus deferens and cauda epididymis (i.e., tail) are located in the inguinal canal.
- Inguinal cryptorchid – when the testis is located in the inguinal canal.
- Ectopic cryptorchid – when testis is subcutaneous and cannot be displaced manually into the scrotum.

ETIOLOGY/PATHOPHYSIOLOGY

- Embryologically, testes develop adjacent to the kidneys and are situated in the dorsal abdomen.
- Normal descent – both testes descend ventrally through the abdominal cavity and inguinal canals into the scrotum sometime during the last 30 days of gestation or first 10 days after birth.
- Abnormal descent – failure to descend may result from faults in development of the gubernaculum, vaginal process, vaginal ring, inguinal canal, or testis, or from persistence of the testicular suspensory ligament.
- Cryptorchidism – unilateral is more common, but may be bilateral.
- Spermatogenesis of abdominal testes is thermally suppressed with development arrested at the spermatogonia stage.
- Unilateral cryptorchids have normal fertility.
- Bilateral cryptorchidism results in sterility.
- If testes are retained in the inguinal canal, development may proceed to the primary spermatocyte stage.
- TRP of a retained testis – if inguinal, the testis often is palpable; if abdominal, the testis is difficult to locate by palpation (i.e., small and soft) but may be visualized at U/S.

SYSTEM AFFECTED

Reproductive

GENETICS

There appears to be some genetic link/heritability, but this doesn't explain the entire population of individuals affected by cryptorchidism.

INCIDENCE/PREVALENCE

- Higher incidence/risk – Quarter Horse, Percheron, Saddlebred, and pony breeds.
- Lower incidence/risk – Thoroughbreds, Standardbreds, Morgans, and Tennessee Walking Horses.
- Cryptorchidism is relatively common in horses, with a higher prevalence compared with that in dogs and cats.

SIGNALMENT

- All breeds
- Absence of a palpable testis in the scrotal sac by one month of age is presumptive evidence of cryptorchidism. After 12 months, inguinal retained testes rarely enter the scrotum but, reportedly, have entered in horses as old as 2 to 3 years of age.
- Unilateral is ≅10-fold more prevalent than bilateral.
- The left testis is retained slightly more often than the right in horses, which contrasts with dogs and cats, in which the right testis is twice as likely as the left to be retained.
- Left testes more often are intra-abdominal; right testes are equally likely to be inguinal or abdominal.

SIGNS

Historical Findings

- Stallion-like behavior in presumed geldings.
- Testes produce androgens regardless of location; even bilaterally affected individuals develop normal secondary sex characteristics and sexual behavior.
- Rarely associated with pain or other signs of disease.
- Isolated reports of torsion of the retained testis and of intestinal strangulation in association with a retained testis.

Physical Examination Findings

- Undescended testes are smaller and softer than scrotal testes.

CAUSES AND RISK FACTORS

- Cause unknown.
- Genetic research suggests a complex mechanism of inheritance involving several genes. The decreasing incidence of cryptorchidism in certain lines of horses suggests that *selective breeding influences the incidence.*
- Both autosomal dominant and autosomal recessive modes of inheritance have been proposed.
- In addition to genetics, other factors implicated in abnormal testicular descent include inadequate gonadotropic stimulation, intrinsically defective testes, and mechanical impediment of descent, all of which may, in turn, have a genetic basis.
- Cryptorchidism has been associated with intersexuality and abnormal karyotypes.

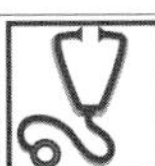

DIAGNOSIS

- Complete history
- Behavioral observation
- Often diagnostic to conduct a thorough visual examination and to palpate the scrotum and external inguinal region.
- External deep inguinal palpation and TRP often require tranquilization or sedation.

DIFFERENTIAL DIAGNOSIS

- Bilateral cryptorchid stallion
- Cryptorchid hemicastrate
- Gelding
- True anorchidism, in which neither testis develops, is extremely rare.
- Monorchid animals, having failed to develop a second testis, have been described in isolated reports.

CBC/BIOCHEMISTRY/URINALYSIS

N/A

OTHER LABORATORY TESTS

hCG Stimulation Test

- Administer hCG (10,000 IU IV), and collect blood samples as follows: baseline (pre-administration), 1-hour, and 2-hours.
- Stallions and cryptorchids show a 2- to 3-fold increase in serum testosterone levels.
- Geldings show no change in testosterone levels.

Serum Conjugated Estrogen Concentration

- Estrone sulfate
- Stallions and cryptorchids, >400 pg/mL.
- Geldings, <50 pg/mL.
- Not reliable in horses of <3 years and in donkeys of any age – donkeys have no detectable conjugated estrogens.

Fecal Conjugated Estrogen Concentration

- Noninvasive technique
- Estrogens are stable in feces for at least 1 week.

Serum Testosterone Concentration

- Stallion and cryptorchids, >100 pg/mL.
- Geldings, <40 pg/mL.
- Unreliable in horses less than 18 months of age.
- Less reliable than hCG stimulation test and conjugated estrogen determination because of wide seasonal variation in basal concentrations.

Serum Inhibin Concentration

- Stallions, 1 to 3 ng/mL
- Gelding, negligible

IMAGING

- Parenchyma of a cryptorchid testis is less echogenic and smaller than that of a normal descended testis.
- Percutaneous U/S may help to identify an inguinal testis.
- Transrectal U/S may help to identify an abdominal testis.

DIAGNOSTIC PROCEDURES

- Laparoscopy to identify an abdominal testis
- Less invasive procedures usually are sufficient to diagnose the problem and often are used in conjunction with laparoscopic cryptorchidectomy.

PATHOLOGIC FINDINGS

- Thermally-induced arrest of spermatogenesis in abdominal testis.
- Spermatocytogenic development may reach the primary spermatocyte stage if the testis is inguinal.
- Seminiferous tubule development is impeded.
- Elevated body temperature may induce interstitial cell hyperplasia.

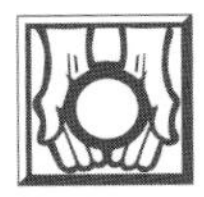

TREATMENT

No effective medical treatment available.

APPROPRIATE HEALTH CARE

Surgical removal of the retained testis.

NURSING CARE

N/A

ACTIVITY

N/A

DIET

N/A

CLIENT EDUCATION

Recommend castration of the cryptorchid individual.

SURGICAL CONSIDERATIONS

- Cryptorchidectomy via standard or laparoscopic approaches.
- Standard approaches: inguinal, parainguinal, paramedian, suprapubic, and flank; choice is dictated by the location of the testis.
- Laparoscopy can be performed with the horse standing or in dorsal recumbency. Remove the retained testis before the descended testis.
- Another, less reliable technique involves laparoscopic cautery and transection of the spermatic cord to induce avascular necrosis of the testis. Revascularization can occur, with subsequent production of testosterone.
- Orchiopexy (i.e., surgical placement of a retained testis into the scrotum) is considered unethical.

MEDICATIONS

DRUGS OF CHOICE

N/A

CONTRAINDICATIONS

N/A

PRECAUTIONS

N/A

POSSIBLE INTERACTIONS

N/A

ALTERNATIVE DRUGS

N/A

FOLLOW-UP

PATIENT MONITORING

- Cessation of stallion-like behavior occurs concomitant with decreasing androgen levels and may require 6 to 8 weeks.
- Some stallions castrated at an older age or, after having bred mares, retain stallion-like behavior even after removal of all testicular tissue.

POSSIBLE COMPLICATIONS

- Complications are uncommon, usually those associated with cryptorchidectomy.
- Possible sequelae – infection, hemorrhage, adhesion formation, eventration, and incomplete castration.

MISCELLANEOUS

ASSOCIATED CONDITIONS

Testicular cysts and neoplasia (e.g., teratoma, interstitial cell tumor, seminoma, Sertoli cell tumor) have been reported.

AGE-RELATED FACTORS

Endocrine assay is not reliable as a diagnostic tool in prepubertal males.

ZOONOTIC POTENTIAL

N/A

PREGNANCY

N/A

SYNONYMS

Lay terms include rigs, ridglings, originals or, if the retained testis is inguinal, high flanker.

SEE ALSO

- Scrotal evaluation
- Semen evaluation – abnormal
- Semen evaluation – normal
- Testicular enlargement
- Testicular tumors

ABBREVIATION

- hCG = human chorionic gonadotropin
- IU = international units
- IV = intravenous
- TRP = transrectal palpation
- U/S = ultrasound, ultrasonography

Suggested Reading

Mueller POE, Parks H. Cryptorchidism in horses. Equine Vet Educ 1999;11:77–86.

Rodgerson DH, Hanson RR. Cryptorchidism in horses. Part I. Anatomy, causes and diagnosis. Compend Contin Educ Pract Vet 1997;19:1280–1288.

Rodgerson DH, Hanson RR. Cryptorchidism in horses. Part II. Treatment. Compend Contin Educ Pract Vet 1997;19:1372–1379.

Authors Jane A. Barber and Philip Prater
Consulting Editor Carla L. Carleton

CYANIDE TOXICOSIS

BASICS

OVERVIEW

- The ingestion of plants containing cyanogenic glycosides can result in cyanide toxicosis. Although 55 cyanogenic glycosides have been reported (amygdalin, prunasin, and dhurrin, among others) in over 1000 different species of plants, the most important sources for animals have been the following genera: *Prunus, Sorghum, Triglochin, Pyrus, Suckleya,* and *Amelanchier*. Damage to the plant (including wilting and mastication) results in enzymatic degradation of the glycoside and release of cyanide.
- Cyanide ion has great affinity for the iron of cytochrome oxidase and will inhibit electron transport and cellular respiration.
- The blood can carry oxygen but it cannot be utilized by the cells, resulting in tissue anoxia.

SIGNALMENT

- No breed, size, sex or age predilection

SIGNS

- Onset usually rapid (20–120 min) after large ingestion
- Tachypnea
- Dyspnea
- Weakness
- Tachycardia
- Bright red mucous membranes
- Recumbency
- Terminal seizure-like activity
- Death

CAUSES AND RISK FACTORS

- Ingestion of large amounts of (usually wilted) plant material containing high concentrations of cyanogenic glycosides.
- Typical scenario is ingestion of fresh but wilted cherry leaves from branches broken off during storms.
- Reports indicate 100 g of wild black cherry leaves can be fatal to a 100-lb animal.
- Cyanide is volatile and dried cherry leaves or hay made from sorghum species are generally safe.

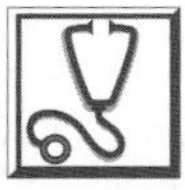

DIAGNOSIS

DIFFERENTIAL DIAGNOSIS

Carbon monoxide poisoning—measurement of carboxyhemoglobin in blood, CO measurement in environment, identified source for CO production

CBC/BIOCHEMISTRY/ URINALYSIS

N/A

OTHER LABORATORY TESTS

- Cyanide analysis of suspect material or stomach contents
- Place samples in airtight container and freeze immediately.
- Identification of suspect plant material in ingesta

IMAGING

N/A

DIAGNOSTIC PROCEDURES

N/A

PATHOLOGICAL FINDINGS

- Blood is bright red.
- Tracheal or pulmonary congestion or hemorrhage
- Other nonspecific agonal changes may be present.

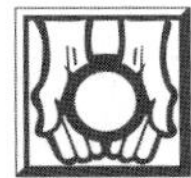

TREATMENT

- Supportive care
- Supplemental oxygen administration

MEDICATIONS

DRUGS

- Treatment must be administered soon after clinical signs are exhibited to be effective.
- Sodium nitrite is used to induce a methemoglobinemia, causing cyanide to dissociate from cytochrome oxidase and react with methemoglobin to form cyanmethemoglobin. Sodium thiosulfate will convert cyanide (by the enzyme rhodanese) to thiocyanate, which is excreted.
- Sodium nitrite 10–20 mg/kg as a 20% solution
- Sodium thiosulfate 30–40 mg/kg as a 20% solution
- Can be administered IV as a mixture of 1 mL of 20% sodium nitrite and 3 mL of 20% sodium thiosulfate at 4 mL per 45 kg of body weight. AC may help bind cyanide remaining in GI tract.
- Oral sodium thiosulfate (up to 20 g in solution) might detoxify cyanide in GI tract.

CONTRAINDICATIONS/ POSSIBLE INTERACTIONS

N/A

FOLLOW-UP

PATIENT MONITORING

N/A

PREVENTION/AVOIDANCE

Avoid additional exposure to cyanide-containing plants.

POSSIBLE COMPLICATIONS

N/A

EXPECTED COURSE AND PROGNOSIS

Death or recovery occurs rapidly.

MISCELLANEOUS

ASSOCIATED CONDITIONS

- Sorghum cystitis ataxia syndrome has been reported in horses following exclusive, long-term grazing on sorghum pastures.
- Syndrome is characterized by hindlimb ataxia, urinary incontinence, and subsequent skin irritation or scalding and cystitis.
- The lumbar and sacral segments of the spinal cord may have focal axonal degeneration and demyelination.
- Probably caused by thiocyanates formed from high, sublethal cyanide ingestion

AGE-RELATED FACTORS

N/A

ZOONOTIC POTENTIAL

N/A

PREGNANCY

N/A

ABBREVIATION

- AC = activated charcoal

Suggested Reading

Cheeke PR. Natural toxicants in feeds, forages, and poisonous plants. Danville, IL: Interstate Publishers, Inc., 1998.

Author Larry J. Thompson
Consulting Editor Robert H. Poppenga

CYTOLOGY OF BRONCHOALVEOLAR LAVAGE (BAL) FLUID

BASICS

OVERVIEW

• Material is collected from the small airways and alveoli by flushing with sterile saline and suctioning back through an endoscope, which has been placed in a bronchus. • Fluid is collected into EDTA for cytology and, for bacterial culture, into a sterile clot tube. • Direct smears, sediment preparations, or cytocentrifuged slides of fluid may be made. • Cytologic assessment and differential cell counts usually are made from smears stained with Wright's or Diff-Quick.
• Total nucleated cells may be counted on a hemacytometer. This is not routine, however, because standardizing the amount of saline recovered is difficult; thus, the value of total cell counts is questionable. • Total protein of a wash fluid is low, so protein content also is not routinely measured. • BAL fluid from normal horses contains predominantly macrophages, with small numbers of lymphocytes, columnar epithelial cells, and nondegenerative neutrophils. Mast cells and eosinophils are seen rarely. • Most samples contain a small amount of mucus, which appears as fibrillar strands of purple material. • Presence of squamous epithelial cells, often with adherent bacteria, indicates contamination from the oropharynx.

PATHOPHYSIOLOGY

• Material present in fluid from bronchoalveolar flushes represents the region of lung being sampled. • Detected abnormalities can include inflammatory cells; organisms, including bacteria, fungi, and rarely, lungworm larvae; evidence of hemorrhage; increased mucus and goblet cells; and material (e.g., pollens, particulates) that passes the mucociliary clearance apparatus. • Chronic inflammation or irritation of any type causes increased mucus production by epithelial cells of the airways.
• Neoplastic cells from metastatic or primary lung tumors typically are not found in BAL samples. • This technique may not be diagnostic for focal lung lesions, mild diffuse disease, or severe, chronic small airway disease that prevents lavage fluid from reaching affected alveoli.

SYSTEMS AFFECTED

• Respiratory • Hemic/lymphatic/immune

SIGNALMENT

Any breed, sex, or age

SIGNS

• Coughing • Dyspnea • Exercise intolerance
• Nasal discharge • Fever

CAUSES AND RISK FACTORS

• Acute or chronic inflammation • IAD • RAO
• EIPH • Parasitic inflammation
• Hypersensitivity • Neoplasia

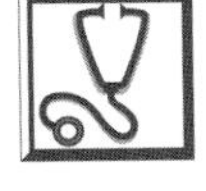

DIAGNOSIS

DIFFERENTIAL DIAGNOSIS

Acute or Chronic Inflammation

• Acute pulmonary inflammation is associated with increased neutrophil numbers, which may appear degenerative if bacteria are present.
• Bacteria may be intra- or extracellular. If primarily extracellular, examine cytologic samples for oropharyngeal contamination, which may lead to a false diagnosis of sepsis. • As inflammation becomes more chronic, the macrophage numbers typically increase, and neutrophils may seem relatively fewer but are, in fact, still present in increased numbers.
• Fungal elements may be observed, usually in association with increased macrophage and neutrophil numbers. • Viral infection of the lungs does not produce a typical inflammatory pattern in equine BAL fluid. • *Pneumocystis carinii* may be observed during pneumonias in immunosuppressed horses.

Inflammatory Airway Disease (IAD)

• This subset of inflammatory disease is characterized by nonseptic, neutrophilic inflammation and increased presence of mucus in airways. Increased percentages of eosinophils, and mast cells

Recurrent Airway Obstruction Heaves

• Typical findings—increased numbers/percentage of nondegenerative neutrophils (>20%) and increased mucus production, as evidenced by amount of mucus, Curschmann's spirals (i.e., casts of inspissated mucus from small airways), or increased goblet cells (i.e., columnar epithelial cells with distinct, round, purple granules of mucus in the cytoplasm). • Eosinophil and mast cell numbers may increase mildly in BAL fluid from horses with RAO. • Severity of chronic small airway disease may not correlate well with cytologic findings in many cases. Horses in remission often have BAL findings like those of normal horses.

EIPH

• Varied numbers of erythrocytes may be seen in BAL fluid from normal horses if mild trauma occurs during sampling. • Phagocytized RBCs or macrophages containing breakdown products of hemoglobin (e.g., hemosiderin) are most typical of pulmonary hemorrhage before sampling. These hemosiderophages may be present for up to 3 weeks following intrapulmonary bleeding.

Parasitic Inflammation

• Infection with the lungworm *Dictyocaulus arnfeldi* is associated with large numbers of eosinophils and macrophages in BAL fluid.
• Larvae typically are not seen.

Hypersensitivity

• Respiratory allergic reactions typically are associated with increased numbers of eosinophils. • Increased numbers of mast cells, neutrophils, and lymphocytes also may be seen.

Neoplasia

BAL is not usually considered a useful technique in the diagnosis of equine pulmonary neoplasia.

CBC/BIOCHEMISTRY/URINALYSIS

Inflammatory respiratory disease may be associated with neutrophilia, left shift, and hyperfibrinogenemia; however, these changes are neither consistent nor specific for respiratory disease.

OTHER LABORATORY TESTS

• Bacterial or fungal culture of BAL fluid when indicated; contamination often occurs while obtaining a sample and must be considered when interpreting culture results. • Blood gas analysis to evaluate gas exchange • Baermann funnel fecal examination to detect lungworms

IMAGING

Radiology and ultrasonography may be useful in localizing and characterizing lung lesions.

OTHER DIAGNOSTIC PROCEDURES

• Bronchoscopy • Lung biopsy

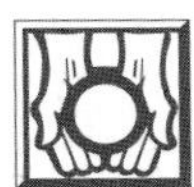

TREATMENT

Directed at the underlying cause

FOLLOW-UP

PATIENT MONITORING

Within 48 hours of BAL with sterile saline, a significant influx of neutrophils occurs into the lavaged region of the lung; recognize this effect if repeated BALs are performed.

MISCELLANEOUS

SEE ALSO

• Tracheal aspiration

ABBREVIATIONS

• BAL = bronchoalveolar lavage • EIPH = exercise-induced pulmonary hemorrhage • IAD = inflammatory airway disease • RAO = recurrent airway obstruction

Suggested Reading

Couetil LL, Hoffman AM, Hodgson J, Buchner-Maxwell VB, Viel L, Wood JLN, Lavoie J. Inflammatory airway disease of horses. J Vet Intern Med 2007;21:356–361.

Robinson NE, Berney C, Erberhart S, deFeijter-Rupp HL, et al. Coughing, mucus accumulation, airway obstruction, and airway inflammation in control horses and horses affected with recurrent airway obstruction. Am J Vet Res 2003;64:550–557.

Zinkl JG. The lower respiratory tract. In: Cowell RL, Tyler RD, eds. Cytology and Hematology of the Horse. Goleta, CA: American Veterinary Publications, 1992:77–87.

Author Susan J. Tornquist
Consulting Editor Kenneth W. Hinchcliff

CYTOLOGY OF TRACHEAL ASPIRATION (TA) FLUID

BASICS

OVERVIEW

- Transtracheal aspiration of fluid from the tracheal lumen is performed using a sterile, polyethylene catheter inserted between the tracheal rings.
- Another method for obtaining samples is via passage of an endoscope through the nostrils and pharynx into the trachea. A catheter is then advanced through the endoscope biopsy channel, beyond the tip of the endoscope, and into the trachea.
- Sterile saline (10–60 mL) is instilled and recovered by applying suction with a syringe.
- Retrieved fluid that appears cloudy or flocculent indicates a good sample has been obtained.
- The sample is aliquoted into a sterile tube for culture and into a tube containing EDTA for cytology.
- Direct smears, sediment preparations, or cytocentrifuged slides may be made.
- Most commonly, air-dried slides are stained with Wright's or Diff-Quik. Diff-Quik stain may fail to stain mast cell granules, making identification of mast cells problematic.
- Cell counts rarely are performed, because the amount of fluid infused and recovered is variable and the presence of mucus can lead to irregular distribution of cells.
- Protein content is also not commonly determined, because wash fluids usually are low in protein.
- In aspirates from normal horses, columnar epithelial cells, which may appear ciliated or nonciliated, are most common. Macrophages also are present in moderate numbers, along with small numbers of nondegenerate neutrophils and occasional eosinophils and lymphocytes. Multinucleated macrophages may be seen in low numbers.
- Mucus is present in many samples and appears as strands of purple fibrillar material.
- Squamous epithelial cells, organisms, and debris from the oropharynx or skin may be present and indicate contamination.

PATHOPHYSIOLOGY

- Samples from normal horses have a wide range of cell types and generally do not contain the same cell types as those obtained using BAL. This reflects differences in cell populations in the trachea and those lining alveolar spaces.
- Acute inflammation, especially bacterial, of the respiratory tract most often causes migration of inflammatory cells to the trachea.
- Other conditions (e.g., RAO) may not be diagnosed as readily by TA compared with BAL.
- With suspected septic conditions, sterile collection of material by TA is preferred over BAL; however, bacteria in the trachea without cytologic evidence of neutrophilic inflammation suggests nonpathogenic colonization of the trachea.
- Chronic inflammation or irritation of any type causes increased mucus production by epithelial cells of the airways.

SYSTEMS AFFECTED

- Respiratory
- Hemic/lymphatic/immune

SIGNALMENT

Any breed, sex, or age

SIGNS

- Coughing
- Dyspnea
- Exercise intolerance
- Nasal discharge
- Fever

CAUSES AND RISK FACTORS

- Acute or chronic inflammation—bacterial, fungal, or viral
- RAO
- EIPH
- Parasitic inflammation
- Hypersensitivity
- Neoplasia

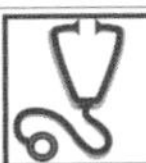

DIAGNOSIS

DIFFERENTIAL DIAGNOSIS

Acute or Chronic Inflammation

- Acute pulmonary inflammation is characterized by increased neutrophil numbers (generally >20%). This is most often associated with increased mucus.
- Bacterial infection often causes neutrophil degeneration.
- Bacteria may be present intracellularly or extracellularly. If primarily extracellular and increased numbers of degenerate neutrophils are not seen, examine cytologic samples for signs of oropharyngeal contamination, which may lead to a false diagnosis of sepsis.
- As inflammation becomes more chronic, macrophage numbers typically increase, and neutrophils may appear relatively fewer but, in fact, are still present in increased numbers.
- Fungal elements may be observed, usually in association with increased macrophage and neutrophil numbers.
- Viral infection of the lungs does not produce a typical inflammatory pattern.
- *Pneumocystis carinii* may be observed during pneumonias in immunosuppressed horses.

Recurrent Airway Obstruction (Heaves, Formerly Chronic Obstructive Pulmonary Disease)

- In chronic small airway inflammation, increased numbers of nondegenerate neutrophils and macrophages are seen, with no evidence of causative agents.
- Evidence of increased mucus, Curschmann's spirals (i.e., casts of inspissated mucus from small airways), or increased goblet cells (i.e., columnar epithelial cells with distinct, round, purple granules of mucus in the cytoplasm) are usually present.
- Numbers of eosinophils and mast cells may increase mildly in horses with RAO.
- Severity of chronic small airway disease may not correlate well with cytologic findings in many cases.

EIPH

• Few to moderate numbers of intact RBCs because of mild hemorrhage during TA are common.
• Phagocytized RBCs or macrophages containing the breakdown products of hemoglobin (e.g., hemosiderin) are consistent with pulmonary hemorrhage before sampling.

Parasitic Inflammation

• Infection with the lungworm *Dictyocaulus arnfeldi* most often results in large numbers of eosinophils and macrophages in the sample.
• Larvae have been found in unfixed, unstained sediment of tracheal fluid.

Hypersensitivity

• Respiratory allergic reactions typically are associated with increased numbers of eosinophils.
• Mast cells, neutrophils, and lymphocytes also may be present.

Neoplasia

TA is not usually considered a useful technique for the diagnosis of equine pulmonary neoplasia.

CBC/BIOCHEMISTRY/URINALYSIS

Inflammatory respiratory disease may be associated with neutrophilia, left shift, and hyperfibrinogenemia; however, these findings are neither consistent nor specific for respiratory disease.

OTHER LABORATORY TESTS

• Bacterial or fungal culture of aspirated fluid.
• Baermann funnel technique to detect lungworm larvae in feces may be indicated with marked eosinophilic inflammation and appropriate history.

IMAGING

Radiology and ultrasonography may be useful in localizing and characterizing lung lesions.

OTHER DIAGNOSTIC PROCEDURES

• Bronchoscopy
• Lung biopsy

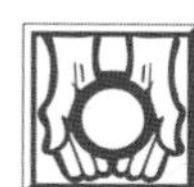

TREATMENT

Directed at the underlying cause

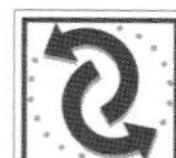

FOLLOW-UP

POSSIBLE COMPLICATIONS

Uncommon complications—infection, hemorrhage, or emphysema at the site

MISCELLANEOUS

AGE-RELATED FACTORS

Foals normally may have increased neutrophil numbers.

SEE ALSO

• Bronchoalveolar lavage

ABBREVIATIONS

• BAL = bronchoalveolar lavage
• EIPH = exercise-induced pulmonary hemorrhage
• RAO = recurrent airway obstruction
• TA = Tracheal aspiration

Suggested Reading

Holcombe SJ, Robinson NE, Derksen FJ, *et al.* Effect of tracheal mucus and tracheal cytology on racing performance in Thoroughbred racehorses. Equine Vet J 2006;38:300–304.

Author Susan J. Tornquist
Consulting Editor Kenneth W. Hinchcliff

DACRYOCYSTITIS

BASICS

OVERVIEW

Definition

The nasolacrimal system has both secretory and drainage components. Drainage of ocular secretions occurs through the puncta of the upper and lower eyelids into the nasolacrimal canaliculi, and subsequently the small nasolacrimal "sac." The "sac" drains to the nasolacrimal duct in the lacrimal canal of the lacrimal and maxillary bones, then opens into the ventrolateral nasal cavity. Dacryocystitis is inflammation of the lacrimal sac and/or NLD. It is seen frequently in horses.

Pathophysiology

- Dacryocystitis may develop as a primary problem or secondary to duct obstruction.
- Eyelid punctal atresia, nasolacrimal duct agenesis or incomplete formation of the duct, nasal punctal atresia and imperforate nasal puncta are congenital abnormalities which can result in severe dacryocystitis.
- There are many potential causes of acquired obstruction of the nasolacrimal system (fractures and other traumatic insults, inflammation, strictures, accumulation of environmental debris or foreign bodies, neoplasia, granulomas, sinusitis, upper arcade dental disease), although often an underlying cause cannot be determined.
- Usually dacryocystitis occurs as the result of obstruction of the NLD, followed by secondary retention of tears in the duct and bacterial proliferation in the stagnant tears.

SYSTEMS AFFECTED

Ophthalmic

SIGNALMENT

Breed Predilections

There are no breed predilections for dacryocystitis.

Mean Age and Range

- Dacryocystitis associated with a congenital abnormality of the nasolacrimal system is usually seen within the first 2–6 months of life, but occasionally not until 1 to 2 years of age, especially if the animal has been turned out after weaning.
- Acquired obstruction may occur at any point during an animal's life, however, for those induced by neoplastic causes, the incidence increases with age.

Genetics

No known genetic influence on development of dacryocystitis

Predominant Sex

No proven sex predilection

SIGNS

- Thick mucopurulent discharge at medial canthus, reflux exudation upon manipulation of the medial eyelid, mild conjunctival hyperemia.
- May be unilateral or bilateral when associated with congenital causes, acquired obstructions are usually unilateral.
- Atresia of the nasal puncta is most commonly unilateral.
- Globe and conjunctiva are usually not involved, unless chronic dacryocystitis has resulted in blepharoconjunctivitis.

CAUSES

Congenital Obstruction

- Nasal puncta atresia*
- Nasolacrimal duct agenesis
- Eyelid puncta atresia

Acquired Obstruction

- Traumatic disruption*
- Foreign body*
- Neoplasia (especially squamous cell carcinoma)
- Granuloma (habronemiasis)
- Sinusitis, rhinitis
- Periodontitis
- Fibrosis secondary to chronic inflammation
- *Thelazia lacrymalis*

RISK FACTORS

- White, grey-white, and palomino hair color and light periocular skin pigmentation predispose to ocular squamous cell carcinoma.
- Warm weather and climates with heavy fly population are a risk factor for habronemiasis and other parasitic causes.

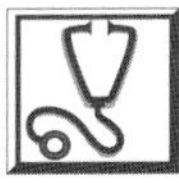

DIAGNOSIS

DIFFERENTIAL DIAGNOSIS

One must differentiate dacryocystitis from other causes of mucopurulent ocular discharge, including bacterial or parasitic conjunctivitis, neoplasia of eyelid or conjunctiva, secondary infection following ocular or eyelid injury, ocular foreign body.

CBC/BIOCHEMISTRY/URINALYSIS

Results usually normal

OTHER LABORATORY TESTS

- Aerobic and anaerobic bacterial culture and sensitivity of material flushed from puncta
- Habronemiasis—Scraping of the granuloma reveals eosinophils, mast cells, neutrophils, plasma cells, occasionally larvae.
- Biopsy and histopathology of mass lesions are necessary for proper diagnosis.

IMAGING

- Skull radiographs if fracture suspected from history or physical examination.
- Contrast dacryocystorhinography assists in identifying cause and location of obstruction. It involves instillation of 4–6 mL of radiopaque solution into puncta, followed by radiography or computed tomography. General anesthesia is necessary for this latter diagnostic technique.
- Rhinoscopy is indicated if sinusitis/rhinitis suspected.
- Microvideoendoscopy may be used to directly visualize NLD lesions.

OTHER DIAGNOSTIC PROCEDURES

- Complete ophthalmic examination is indicated to identify any primary ocular problem causing mucopurulent discharge or secondary ocular involvement.
- Patency of duct may be assessed initially by Jones dye test. Fluorescein dye is instilled into the eye, and the nasal puncta is observed for appearance of fluorescein within 5 minutes. Attempt should be made to flush duct with saline or irrigating solution from patent puncta. Topical anesthetic should be applied to both nasal mucosa and conjunctiva.
- Cannulation of nasolacrimal duct is performed using a 5 French urinary catheter or polyethylene tubing (size 160), inserted through nasal or eyelid puncta. Catheter may hit blind end several centimeters from nasal punctal opening where the duct is pressed laterally by a cartilaginous plate in the alar fold, and should be directed laterally.
- Dental and oral examination, and potentially dental radiography, should be performed if dental disease is suspected as inciting cause of dacryocystitis.

GROSS AND HISTOPATHOLOGIC FINDINGS

- Habronemiasis—eosinophils, mast cells, neutrophils, plasma cells, rarely larvae.
- Squamous cell carcinoma—epithelial cells with neoplastic characteristics.
- Other histopathologic findings possible depending on the type of neoplasia present.

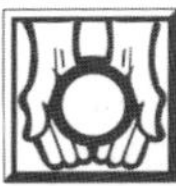

TREATMENT

INPATIENT VERSUS OUTPATIENT

Patients that require surgical intervention to reestablish patency of duct would be hospitalized for a short term basis. Those in which patency is reestablished with simple irrigation or cannulation can be treated on an outpatient basis.

ACTIVITY

Restriction of activity may be required for a short time following surgical procedures.

DIET

No change in diet is necessary. Hay should be fed at ground level rather than from elevated hayracks or bags if ocular disease is present.

CLIENT EDUCATION

The client should be informed of potential for recurrence, especially in cases of acquired obstruction or when a cause is unidentified.

SURGICAL CONSIDERATIONS

- Uncomplicated obstructions may be relieved by simply flushing the NLD and then applying topical broad-spectrum antibiotics and possibly anti-inflammatory agents.
- Nasolacrimal duct agenesis accompanied by nasal or eyelid punctal atresia necessitates surgical creation of a proximal or distal opening. If the duct is present, flushing of nasolacrimal system results in dilation of tissue overlying the site of the atretic or imperforate puncta. An incision through overlying tissue will establish patency, and a 5 French catheter placed in the nasolacrimal duct will allow epithelialization of the new puncta. Severe hemorrhage may occur following incision over the atretic nasal puncta. Ends of catheter/stent are sutured to skin of muzzle and near medial canthus, and the catheter/stent is left in place for 2–3 weeks and sometimes longer.
- Acquired obstructions are treated by removal of inciting cause when possible, irrigating duct, and catheterization of duct for 2–3 weeks. The indwelling stent is sutured to skin as described for congenital lesions.
- Conjunctivorhinostomy involves creation of mucous membrane-lined fistula between the ventromedial conjunctival surface and nasal cavity. This procedure is indicated for nasolacrimal duct obstruction that cannot be relieved with flushing or cannulation. Alternatively, canaliculorhinostomy involves creating a pathway from the canaliculi to the nasal cavity. Conjunctivosinostomy creates a connection between the conjunctiva and the maxillary sinus. All of these procedures must be performed under general anesthesia and involve drilling a hole through the lacrimal bone into the nasal cavity or the sinus and placing a stent until the connection is permanent and the incisions heal.

MEDICATIONS

DRUGS AND FLUIDS

- Topical triple antibiotic solution placed in eye 3–4 times daily until catheter is removed or until culture results specify the need to change antimicrobial agents.
- Topical corticosteroids (1% prednisolone acetate or 0.1% dexamethasone) are recommended to decrease swelling in the NLD as long as there are no ocular surface problems (corneal ulceration) that would make their use contraindicated.
- Systemic antibiotics are absolutely critical for 7–10 days if surgical establishment of the NDL has been performed. Appropriate antibiotic solution should be flushed through indwelling stent on a daily or every other day basis.

CONTRAINDICATIONS

N/A

PRECAUTIONS

N/A

POSSIBLE INTERACTIONS

N/A

ALTERNATE DRUGS

N/A

FOLLOW-UP

PATIENT MONITORING

The patient should be rechecked soon after the initial procedure to establish patency (7–10 days), with specific time frame determined by severity. Subsequent rechecks are dictated by severity of disease and response to treatment.

PREVENTION/AVOIDANCE

Fly control in barns and pastures, fly hoods, frequent periocular administration of insect repellent, and regular deworming with ivermectin, decreasing environmental dust, debris and other material that may accumulate in the NLD, and decreasing the amount or exposure to allergens may prevent the development of or decrease the incidence or severity of NLD obstructions and dacryocystitis.

POSSIBLE COMPLICATIONS

Potential complications vary with the inciting cause. They include recurrence of the dacryocystitis and failure to maintain patency of duct.

EXPECTED COURSE AND PROGNOSIS

- The prognosis for NLD obstructions and dacryocystitis is good, but depends upon the location, extent, and cause of the obstruction.
- Acquired obstructions resulting in dacryocystitis are more difficult to treat than congenital abnormalities.
- Foreign body and periodontal causes have the best response to therapy of acquired obstructions.
- Cannulation of the duct may be impossible in cases of neoplasia and maxillary fractures, and permanent correction of the obstruction and subsequent dacryocystitis may not be possible.

MISCELLANEOUS

ASSOCIATED CONDITIONS

N/A

AGE-RELATED FACTORS

N/A

ZOONOTIC POTENTIAL

N/A

PREGNANCY

Systemic absorption of topically applied medication is possible. Benefits of treatment should be considered against any risks posed to the fetus.

SEE ALSO

- Ocular problems in the neonate
- Ocular/adnexal squamous cell carcinoma

ABBREVIATION

- NLD = nasolacrimal duct

Suggested Reading

Brooks DE. Ophthalmology for the Equine Practitioner. Jackson, WY; Teton NewMedia, 2002.

Brooks DE, Matthews AG. Equine ophthalmology. In: Gelatt KN, ed. Veterinary Ophthalmology, ed 4. Philadelphia; Lippincott Williams and Wilkins, 2007.

Gilger BC, ed. Equine Ophthalmology. Philadelphia; WB Saunders, 2005.

Author Caryn E. Plummer

Consulting Editor Dennis E. Brooks

DEGENERATIVE MYELOENCEPHALOPATHY

BASICS

DEFINITION

EDM is a neuroaxonal dystrophy of young growing horses that affects all equids resulting in a diffuse degenerative disease of select areas of the brainstem and spinal cord.

PATHOPHYSIOLOGY

The exact pathogenesis of EDM remains speculative, but it is associated with vitamin E deficiency. Histopathologic findings include degrees of neuroaxonal dystrophy affecting spinal cord and brainstem nuclei with neuronal fiber degeneration within ascending and descending spinal cord pathways.

Risk factors associated with EDM include the exposure of foals to insecticides and wood preservatives but is most convincingly related to foals with poor access to vitamin E, such as spending time on dirt lots, and use of feeds with very low vitamin E levels. Foals that have access to green pastures appear to have a protective effect against development of EDM.

Vitamin E concentrations below control values of 1–4 mg/L have been shown to have a causative role in the pathogenesis and ensuing development of EDM. Prophylactic administration of vitamin E (2000 IU/day) to foals from sires known to produce EDM has resulted in a decreased incidence of the disease. Vitamin E acts as an intracellular antioxidant that protects lipid membranes from free radicals generated by normal oxidative processes of metabolism and inflammation. Inadequate amounts of vitamin E results in lipid peroxidation of cellular membranes, especially in the central nervous system. Current evidence supports the hypothesis that EDM is due to a vitamin E deficiency with a genetic predisposition.

GENETICS

It has been suggested the condition may be inherited in a polygenic mode or as a dominant disorder with variable expression.

GEOGRAPHIC DISTRIBUTION

The disease commonly reported in North America but has occurred in Great Britain and Continental Europe.

SIGNALMENT

- Species and breed—Domestic horses, Przewalski's horse, and zebras. Most commonly reported in Arabians, Quarter Horses, Appaloosas, Thoroughbreds, Standardbreds, and Paso Fino Horses. The neuroaxonal dystrophy reported in Morgan horses is likely to be an expression of the same disease.
- Mean age and range—Most affected animals exhibit clinical signs of ataxia during the first year of life. The onset of clinical signs has been reported as early as birth and as late as 12 years of age but rarely after 2 years of age. Most frequently, signs are first seen in suckling and weanling foals.

SIGNS

Clinical signs tend to have an insidious onset and be slowly progressive, but can have an apparent acute onset.

Historical

Many cases have involved horses that tended to be clumsy in the first few months of life and progressed slowly to visible ataxia in six months to two years. Owners have reported lameness of one limb that progressed to ataxia and often described by owners as an acute onset after the horse had a traumatic fall or injury. The fall may have been caused by a neurological dysfunction that was unnoticed.

Physical Examination

EDM can have very similar clinical signs to a focal cervical compressive disease. Animals show bilaterally symmetric ataxia, weakness, and dysmetria usually affecting all four limbs. Pelvic limbs are usually one to three grades more severely affected than the thoracic limbs. Severe cases can show hyporeflexia over the neck and trunk (local cervical, thoracolaryngeal and cutaneous trunci responses). There has been no evidence of cranial nerve deficits or muscle atrophy in horse with EDM.

PATHOLOGY

There are no gross lesions. Ascending and descending fibers are affected by a neuroaxonal dystrophy with prominent spheroid formation. Most severe in thoracic spinal cord, nucleus thoracicus and lateral cuneate nuclei of the rostral medulla oblongata.

CAUSES AND RISK FACTORS

Deficiencies of vitamins E [intrauterine to 1 year old appear to be critical] eg foals frequently spending time on dirt lots with no grass. There appears to be a familial predisposition to the disease.

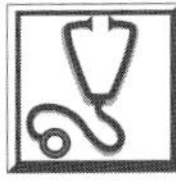

DIAGNOSIS

DIFFERENTIAL DIAGNOSIS: OTHER CAUSES OF ATAXIA IN HORSES <2 YEARS OF AGE

- Trauma: diagnosed by radiography if fractures of the vertebrae occur. Trauma may only cause injury to the spinal cord without bone involvement resulting in unobservable radiographic lesions.

• Cervical vertebral malformation (CVM) and occipital-atlanto-axial malformation (young Arabian foals): can be diagnosed by radiography. Horses with CVM do not have diffuse hyporeflexia of the neck and trunk.
• Equine protozoal myelopathy (EPM): an important differential diagnosis in parts of the Americas and should be ruled out. A negative serum titer has a strong negative predictive value.
• Equine herpesvirus 1 is usually associated with older horses and outbreaks of respiratory disease or abortion. The onset of disease is usually rapid with affected horses possibly showing signs of ataxia and lower motor neuron signs of incontinence with a flaccid anal sphincter and decreased tail tone. Horses with EHV-1 usually show the greatest deterioration in the first 24 hours and then begin to recover. A definitive diagnosis can be made in horses with a rising serum titer and/or CSF titer to EHV-1. A xanthochromic CSF tap and an increased total protein with a normal cell count are common with EHV-1.

OTHER LABORATORY TESTS

There is currently no definitive antemortem diagnostic test available to diagnose EDM. Serum α-tocopherol values tend to be low (<1.0 mg/l) and lower than unaffected herd mates.

IMAGING

Radiographs may be helpful in differentiating other etiologies of neurologic disease.

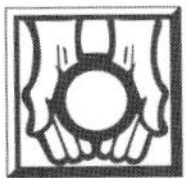

TREATMENT

Allow access to ample pasture and properly cured hay containing high amounts of vitamin E. Improper curing of hay results in hay with low levels of vitamin E, therefore properly cured hay should be fed.

MEDICATIONS

There are no therapeutic agents available to quickly return a horse with EDM to normal. Vitamin E has shown promise in prophylaxis on affected farms and as a treatment after signs appear.

Prophylaxis—supplement at least 2000 IU/day of α-tocopherol.

Therapeutic administration of 6000 IU/day of α-tocopherol mixed in grain daily has improved neurologic scores of affected horses. Improvement may be evident in affected horses during the first three to four weeks with slower improvements observed over the next year. The earlier gait deficits are recognized and treatment is started, the better the response to therapy.

CONTRAINDICATIONS

Toxic levels of vitamin E in horses have not been documented.

FOLLOW-UP

Horses placed on vitamin E therapy should be monitored for α-tocopherol levels in plasma and serum to ensure adequate absorption. If levels have not increased in 30 days a vitamin E absorption test should be run to rule out malabsorption of the fat-soluble vitamin. Each patient should have follow-up neurological examinations to enable continued assessment of the horse's condition.

MISCELLANEOUS

ABBREVIATIONS

• CVM = cervical vertebral malformation
• EDM = equine degenerative myeloencephalopathy
• EPM = equine protozoal myelopathy

Suggested Reading

Dill SJ, Correa MT, Erb HN, et al. Factors associated with the development of equine degenerative myeloencephalopathy. Am J Vet Res 1990;51:1300–1305.

Hahn CN, Mayhew IG, and MacKay RJ, The nervous system. In Collahan PT, Mayhew, IG, Merritt, AM, and Moore, JN, eds. Equine Medicine and Surgery, 5th ed. St Louis: Mosby, 1999.

Mayhew IG, Brown CM, Stowe HD, et al. Equine degenerative myeloencephalopathy: a vitamin E deficiency that may be familial. J Vet Intern Med 1987;1:45–50.

The author and editors wish to acknowledge the contribution of Steven T. Grubbs, author of this chapter in the previous edition.

Author Caroline N. Hahn
Consulting Editor Caroline N. Hahn

DELAYED UTERINE INVOLUTION

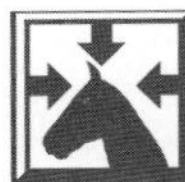

BASICS

DEFINITION/OVERVIEW

- Any delay in return of the uterus to its prepartum state.
- Delays may be of size, tone, endometrial regeneration, or elimination of bacteria from the uterine lumen.
- In normal mares, endometrial involution is complete by 13 to 25 days, with the exception of normal size, which may require as long as 35 days.

ETIOLOGY/PATHOPHYSIOLOGY

- DUC origin can be:
  - Mechanical, e.g., decreased muscular contractions.
  - Inflammatory, e.g., neutrophil influx.
  - Immunologic.
- DUC may follow dystocia or RFM and is characterized by compromised ability to eliminate postpartum debris and bacteria from the uterus.

SYSTEMS AFFECTED

Reproductive

SIGNALMENT

- All breeds
- Any mare of breeding age.
- More prevalent in old mares.

SIGNS

General Comments

- Because foal heat and rebreeding can occur within 5 to 18 days postpartum, it is extremely important for the uterus to return rapidly to normal postpartum.

Historical Findings

- A history of postpartum delayed involution may be suspected because of failure to conceive when bred during an early foal heat (ovulation less than 9 days postpartum).

Physical Examination Findings

- Evaluate uterine size and tone, and record if fluid is present.
- Note any abnormal discharge from the vulva.
- Any of the above may indicate delayed uterine involution.

CAUSES

- Individual predisposition to slower involution.
- Hormonal
- Immunologic
- Mechanical: reduced myometrial contractions
- Management: greater contamination at parturition may increase the time needed for involution.

RISK FACTORS

Increased incidence in:

- Old mares
- Post-dystocia
- Contaminated uterus at parturition
- Decreased oxytocin release, endogenous
- Failure of the uterus to respond to oxytocin, endogenous or exogenous

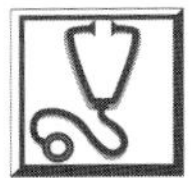

DIAGNOSIS

DIFFERENTIAL DIAGNOSIS

- Important to distinguish metritis from delayed uterine involution.
- Delayed uterine involution may accompany infection or inflammation of the uterus, but these are not necessarily co-dependent.

CBC/BIOCHEMISTRY/URINALYSIS

N/A

OTHER LABORATORY TESTS

Endometrial cytology to determine characteristics of any accumulated uterine fluid.

IMAGING

U/S

- Fluid within the postpartum uterine lumen
- Presence or absence of other findings (e.g., decreased uterine tone, increased uterine size) that are linked with delayed involution.

OTHER DIAGNOSTIC PROCEDURES

Endometrial cytology: presence of neutrophils

PATHOLOGIC FINDINGS

Indicators of delayed uterine involution, between 12- to 15-days postpartum

Uterus

- Intraluminal fluid
- Enlarged relative to days postpartum
- Decreased tone
- Endometrial cytology, increased number of leukocytes

Vulva/Vulvar

Discharge persists, abnormal by this time postpartum.

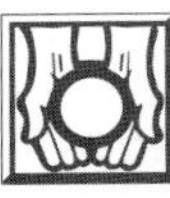

TREATMENT

APPROPRIATE HEALTH CARE

- DUC may accompany uterine infections or inflammation and should be differentiated from a combination of delayed involution with metritis.
- Delayed involution does not have an effect systemically, so systemic antibiotics are not needed, unless infection of the uterus is present and this is determined to be the desired method of uterine therapy.
- Local, intrauterine instillation of antibiotics may be contraindicated.
- Uterine flushes or use of hormonal stimulants (e.g., oxytocin, $PGF_2\alpha$) may be more appropriate therapy.

ACTIVITY

Normal activity

CLIENT EDUCATION

- Not all mares are ready to be bred at foal heat.
- Serial TRPs to determine the degree of uterine involution are advisable to select mares with the highest probability of conceiving if bred on a postpartum estrus.

MEDICATIONS

DRUG(S) OF CHOICE

- Oxytocin (20 IU IV or 20 IU IM, q 2 hours for the first 24 hours postpartum) and $PGF_2\alpha$ (10 mg IM) or prostaglandin analogue (cloprostenol, 250 μg IM), are the hormones of choice for aiding involution of the uterus.
- Uterine flushes (i.e., sterile saline or water), when indicated, may aid involution.
- Instillation of irritants or antiseptics (e.g., Lugol's solution) sometimes has value to further stimulate uterine involution.
- Antibiotics: *only* if a bacterial pathogen is confirmed present.

DELAYED UTERINE INVOLUTION

PRECAUTIONS

Do not over treat delayed uterine involution with unnecessary antibiotics or other local or systemic medications. Such treatments may further retard return of the uterus to normal and cost the owner additional expense without providing any measurable benefit.

FOLLOW-UP

PATIENT MONITORING

Examination of the uterus to determine return to normal is essential after therapy: TRP; U/S.

PREVENTION/AVOIDANCE

- Light exercise during late gestation and postpartum can aid uterine involution.
- Barn hygiene: mare's stall should be bedded with clean straw for foaling; especially maximize stall hygiene for the health of the mare and foal during the first several days postpartum; expense of bedding and labor is offset by improved reproductive health.

POSSIBLE COMPLICATIONS

- Failure to conceive.
- EED

EXPECTED COURSE AND PROGNOSIS

- Majority of mares return to normal without treatment, but for the extended time necessary for complete uterine involution to occur.
- In some cases, involution remains incomplete and may prevent conception or pregnancy maintenance.

MISCELLANEOUS

ASSOCIATED CONDITIONS

May or may not be coupled with a uterine infection.

AGE-RELATED FACTORS

Increased occurrence in old mares.

SEE ALSO

- Dystocia
- Postpartum problems
- Retained fetal membranes
- Uterine infection
- Vaginitis
- Vulvar discharge

ABBREVIATIONS

- DUC = delayed uterine clearance
- EED = early embryonic death
- RFM = retained fetal membranes
- TRP = transrectal palpation
- U/S = ultrasound, ultrasonography

Suggested Reading

McKinnon AO, et al. Ultrasonographic studies on the reproductive tract of mares after parturition: effect of involution and uterine fluid on pregnancy rates in mares with normal and delayed first postpartum ovulatory cycles. J AM Vet Med Assoc 1988;192:350–353.

Roberts SJ. Veterinary obstetrics and genital diseases (theriogenology). 3rd ed. Woodstock, VT: published by the author, 1986:584.

Stewart DR, et al. Concentrations of 15-keto-13,14-dihydroprostaglandin $PGF_2\alpha$ in the mare during spontaneous and oxytocin induced foaling. Eq Vet J 1984;16:270–274.

Vandeplassche M, et al. Observations on involution and puerperal endometritis in mares. Ir Vet J 1983;37:126–132.

Author Walter R. Threlfall

Consulting Editor Carla L. Carleton

DERMATOMYCOSES, SUBCUTANEOUS

BASICS

DEFINITION

Subcutaneous fungal infections are generally secondary to wound inoculations and are subdivided into the following categories:

1. Phaeohyphomycoses and eumycotic mycetomas—Nodular, slowly extensive, mycoses due to dematiaceous pigmented fungi (melanin pigments). With mycetomas, the lesions contain fungal grains and the disease is rarely invasive.
2. Sporotrichosis—Slowly extensive subcutaneous infection due to the yeast phase of *Sporothrix schenckii*, slowly invasive
3. Pythiosis—Subcutaneous and extensive infection due to *Pythium insidiosum*, rapidly invasive
4. Zygomycoses—Deep and progressive infections due to Zygomycetes (*Mucorales* and *Entomophtorales*), rapidly invasive

PATHOPHYSIOLOGY

• Phaeohyphomycoses and eumycotic mycetomas—Most dematiaceous fungi develop on soil and plants. After inoculating a wound, the fungus induces chronic inflammation.
• Sporotrichosis—Infection from wounds. The mold form is normally present in soil, plants, wood and water. After inoculation, the fungus changes to a yeast phase that slowly proliferates and extends to lymphatic vessels and lymph nodes. • Pythiosis—*Pythium insidiosum* develops on aquatic plants. Motile spores in water are attracted by damaged skin tissue and germinate on the surface of the skin. The invasion of skin (subcutis) results in proliferative necrotic extensive lesions. • Zygomycoses—After inoculation, the fungi develop in the dermis resulting in a pyogranulomatous inflammation with tropism for blood vessels.

SYSTEMS AFFECTED

Skin—all
• Phaeohyphomycoses and eumycotic mycetomas—skin only • Sporotrichosis—Lymphatics and rarely systemic • Pythiosis—Secondarily systemic • Zygomycoses—Occasionally nasal

INCIDENCE/PREVALENCE

• Dependent on geographic distribution
• Phaeohyphomycoses—Rare in the United States • Eumycotic mycetomas—Rare in the United States and Europe, with the most commonly reported fungus in the United States being *Pseudallescheria boydii* • Sporotrichosis—Sporadic cases mainly in rural areas
• Pythiosis—Most cases are seen during the summer and fall. The environmental factors of water, decaying vegetation and temperatures between 30°C and 40°C are the most influential factors governing the occurrence.
• Zygomycoses—Found in soil and decaying vegetation. Cases occur throughout the year.

GEOGRAPHIC DISTRIBUTION

• Eumycotic mycetomas—Found most frequently near the Tropic of Cancer, including Africa, South and Central America, India, and southern Asia
• Sporotrichosis—A worldwide disease most common in warm countries.
• Pythiosis—In tropical and subtropical areas of the world (e. g., Thailand, Japan, Indonesia, Burma, New Guinea, Colombia, Costa Rica, Brazil, and Australia). In the United States, cases are mainly seen in the Gulf Coast region and other southern states, however, it has also been documented in Oklahoma, Arkansas, Missouri, Kentucky, Tennessee, North and South Carolina, Virginia, New Jersey, and southern Indiana.
• Zygomycoses—*Rhizopus, Mucor, Absidia* (Mucorales) have a worldwide distribution. The two major species of *Entomophtorales* are *Basidiobolus ranarum* (Americas, Australia, Asia, and tropical Africa) and *Conidiobolus coronatus* (tropical Africa and southeast Asia). In the United States, states along the Gulf of Mexico

SIGNALMENT

• No apparent age, breed, or sex predilections
• Pythiosis—Commonly affected horses have had prolonged contact with water in lakes, ponds, swamps, and flooded areas. The horse is the most susceptible species.

SIGNS

Phaeohyphomycoses

• Firm single or multiple well-circumscribed dermal nodules (1–3 cm) on the face and legs but can be widely scattered. • Lesions initially haired but become alopecic, eroded, ulcerated, and drain • Papular satellites possible • Grossly pigmented, nonpruritic, and nonpainful

Eumycotic Mycetomas

• Lesions occur anywhere; however, single lesions on the distal extremities and face (muzzle) are the most common.
• As lesions progress, they become firm, alopecic, ulcerative plaques or nodules that may drain serous, purulent, or hemorrhagic discharge.
• On cut surface, suppurative exudate contains generally brown to black (rarely white to yellow) tissue grains (1–2 mm in size).
• Mycetomas discharge tissue grains in contrast to phaeohyphomycoses, which do not.

Sporotrichosis

• Cutaneolymphatic form most common. Nodules common on the distal extremity but can be found on the chest, proximal foreleg, shoulder, and perineal region.
• Firm dermal nodules linearly disposed along lymphatics and lymph nodes draining the area of the lesion
• Lymphangitis with enlarged thickened "corded" vessels
• Possible secondary fistulization with hemorrhagic rust to brown serosanguineous discharge
• Usually nonpruritic, nonpainful
• Primary cutaneous form occurs but is uncommon
• Rarely systemic infection

Pythiosis

• Disease affects ventral part of the body including the legs, chest, and ventrum. Occasionally nasal
• Progressive development of a tumor-like, ulcerative lesion; thick, sticky material exudes from the wound.
• May reach 50 cm in diameter
• Pruritus frequent, sometimes intense
• Visible hard, gritty, white coral–like masses named "kunkers" (2–10 mm) which are composed of fungal hyphae, host exudates, and protein
• Possible extension (bones, joints, lungs, digestive tract)

Zygomycoses

• *Basidiobolus* infects the lateral aspects of the head, neck, and body; lesions are usually single nodular eroded to ulcerative granulomas that may demonstrate moderate to severe pruritus.
• Fistulous tracts discharge a serosanguineous exudate from the lesions, which are frequently traumatized.
• *Conidobolus* affects almost exclusively the mucosa of the nose and mouth.
• Ulcerative pyogranulomas may cause mechanical blockage, resulting in dyspnea and nasal discharge.
• Vascular invasion and hematogenous spread more common with mucormycosis than entomophthoromycosis.

CAUSES

• Phaeohyphomycoses—*Bipolaris sphiciferum, Alternaria alternata, Exserohilum rostratum, Cladosporium* sp.
• Eumycotic mycetomas—*Curvularia geniculata* (black grained mycetoma), *Pseudoallescheria boydii* and *Aspergillus versicolor* (white grained mycetomas), *Altenaria*
• Sporotrichosis—*Sporothrix schenckii*
• Pythiosis—*Pythium insidiosum*
• Zygomycoses—two orders:
  1. *Mucorales* (genera include *Rhizopus, Mucor, Absidia,* and *Mortierella*)
  2. *Entomophthorales* (genera include *Conidiobolus* and *Basidiobolus*)

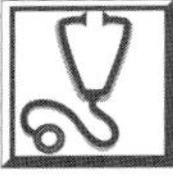

DIAGNOSIS

DIFFERENTIAL DIAGNOSIS

• Phaeohyphomycoses and eumycotic mycetomas—neoplasia (sarcoid, cutaneous lymphoma, melanoma), granulomas (foreign bodies, eosinophilic, bacterial), sporotrichosis, insect bite reactions, histoplasma infection, and molluscum contagiosum
• Sporotrichosis—cutaneous habronemiasis, foreign body and infectious granulomas, sarcoids, neoplasia, ulcerative and epizootic lymphangitis
• Pythiosis and zygomycoses—as for sporotrichosis

CBC/BIOCHEMISTRY/URINALYSIS

Pythiosis—anemia and hypoproteinemia

OTHER LABORATORY TESTS

• Sporotrichosis—Mold phase growth at 27°C or yeast growth on blood agar CO_2 enriched at 37°C
• Direct fluorescent antibody tests on biopsy specimen are performed at specialized laboratories like the Centers for Disease Control and Prevention, Atlanta, GA.
• PCR from skin biopsy for identification of *chitin synthase 1* gene

• Pythiosis—serology—A sensitive and specific ELISA is available through the Pythium Laboratory at Louisiana State University.
• Zygomycoses—A serum agar gel immunoprecipitation test is useful for the diagnosis of conidiobolomycosis.

OTHER DIAGNOSTIC PROCEDURES

• Definitive diagnosis for all subcutaneous mycoses is by demonstration of the organism via cytologic examination of exudate, culture of tissue or exudates, and/or histopathology.
• Pythiosis—Tissue samples should be submitted via overnight shipping at room temperature. An immunohistochemical stain can be used to identify *P. insidiosum* hyphae in histologic sections. Nested PCR assay is used for definitive identification of cultured isolates or organisms in tissue samples.

PATHOLOGICAL FINDINGS

• Phaeohyphomycoses and eumycotic mycetomas—Granulomatous dermatitis with septate, thick-walled, pigmented or not hyphae or yeast-like elements (organized in grains in mycetomas)
• Sporotrichosis—Special stains are required (periodic acid–Schiff or Gomori methenamine silver) as yeast are difficult to detect.
• Typically elongated yeasts in a granulomatous reaction with multinucleated giant cells
• Pythiosis—Pyogranulomatous dermatitis and panniculitis with eosinophils. Wide and irregular hyphae (special stains), frequently surrounded by eosinophilic Splendore-Hoeppli reaction and kunkers
• Zygomycoses—In excised tissues, a thickened fibrotic dermis has scattered, red to creamy white areas with a central core of necrotic tissue, which often contains hyphal forms surrounded by eosinophilic infiltrate of the Splendore-Hoeppli phenomenon. Tissue sections stained with GMS reveal large, branching sometimes septate, 4- to 20-μm hyphae.

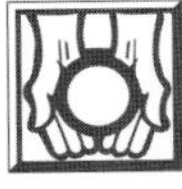

TREATMENT

AIMS OF TREATMENT

Attempt to reduce fungal burden via both medical and surgical management.

APPROPRIATE HEALTH CARE

• The treatment of choice is aggressive surgical excision of all infected tissue (at least 2–3 cm of apparent healthy margins).
• Chronic disease may not allow complete surgical excision.
• Medical management may reduce nonresectable lesions to the point that they become resectable.

CLIENT EDUCATION

• All subcutaneous dermatomycoses carry a fair to guarded prognosis if complete surgical excision cannot be achieved.
• Treatment duration is a least 3 weeks but often much longer.
• Treatment is expensive.

SURGICAL CONSIDERATIONS

• Wide surgical excision should be performed for all subcutaneous mycoses.
• Phaeohyphomycoses—the only effective treatment
• Eumycotic Mycetomas—recurrence is common
• Sporotrichosis—effective in limiting the disease
• Pythiosis—only possible in early cases
• Zygomycoses—early removal effective

MEDICATIONS

DRUG(S) OF CHOICE

• Phaeohyphomycoses—itraconazole—3 mg/kg orally q12 h for 1 mo beyond clinical cure; when complete surgical excision is not an option
• Eumycotic mycetomas, sporotrichosis, and zygomycoses—voriconazole at 3 mg/kg PO q12 h would maintain a plasma concentration of 2 μg/mL, which inhibits >95% *Aspergillus* spp., 50% of *Rhizopus* and *Mucor* spp., and *Sporotrichosis* in vitro.
• Sporotrichosis—ethylene diamine dihydroiodide (EDDI), drug of choice administered as a feed additive at a dosage of 1–2 mg/kg q12–24 h × 1 week; then reduce to 0.5–1.0 mg/kg q24 h for the remainder of the treatment. Continue treatment at least 1 mo past clinical cure.
• Zygomycoses and pythiosis—Amphotericin B given systemically after surgical excision must be dissolved in 5% dextrose and water. Initial daily dose is 0.3 mg/kg. Every third day the dose is increased by 0.1 mg/kg until a maximum dose of 0.8–0.9 mg/kg/day is reached.

CONTRAINDICATIONS

Use of azoles in horses with compromised hepatic function warrants careful monitoring of liver function during treatment or avoiding use of the drug if further hepatic compromise is considered to have serious clinical consequences.

PRECAUTIONS

• Tolerance to iodides is variable and some horses show signs of iodism. Stop treatment at least 1 week; then reinstitute at 75% of dosage responsible for toxic signs.
• Baseline biochemical profile should be performed to evaluate liver enzymes before administration of azoles.
• Ketoconazole is not recommended in the horse due to poor bioavailability.

ALTERNATIVE DRUGS

Pythiosis—Immunotherapy with *P. insidiosum* vaccine may be effective in early disease, but not chronic cases. The vaccine is not commercially available but may be obtained from Dr. Alberto L. Mendoza at the Medical Technology Program, Department of Microbiology and Molecular Genetics, 322 N. Kedzie Laboratory, Michigan State University, East Lansing, MI 48824-1031, USA. e-mail—mendoza9@msu.edu; fax ordering (517)-432–2006

FOLLOW-UP

PATIENT MONITORING

• Revaluate every 2–3 weeks for clinical signs and side effects associated with treatments.
• Pythiosis—ELISA serology can be used to monitor response to therapy; serology should be checked 2–3 mo after surgery or every 3 mo during medical therapy.

POSSIBLE COMPLICATIONS

• Phaeohyphomycoses and eumycotic mycetomas—osteomyelitits, arthritis, myositis
• Pythiosis—acute abdomen and death from gastrointestinal thrombosis and perforation

EXPECTED COURSE AND PROGNOSIS

• Unresponsive to therapy—not unexpected; consider alternative treatment or combined treatment regimens (supersaturated potassium iodide and itraconazole).
• Phaeohyphomycoses—Wide surgical excision may be curative, horses with multiple lesions may heal spontaneously within 3 mo after the diagnosis.
• Eumycotic mycetomas—Some response to aggressive surgical removal of affected nodules, but recurrence in common.
• Pythiosis—Prognosis is guarded to poor unless complete resection is possible.
• Zygomycoses—Chronic lesions have a poorer prognosis.

ZOONOTIC POTENTIAL

• Phaeohyphomycoses and eumycotic mycetomas and zygomycoses —No transmission directly between hosts
• Sporotrichosis—Humans are susceptible to sporotrichosis; however, there are no reports of transmission from an infected horse.
• Pythiosis—No evidence suggests transmission between hosts.

PREGNANCY

• Systemic iodides may cause abortion.
• Azoles antifungals are tetratogenic and should not be used in pregnant mares.

SYNONYMS

• Phaeohyphomycoses and mycetomas—chromomycosis, pseudomycetoma (dermatophytic mycetoma)
• Pythiosis—Swamp cancer, phycomycosis, hyphomycosis, Florida horse leeches,
• Zygomycoses—mucormycosis, entomophoromycosis, conodiobolosis, basidiobolosis

ABBREVIATIONS

• ELISA = enzyme-linked immunosorbent assay
• GMS = Gomori methenamine silver stain
• PCR = polymerase chain reaction

Suggested Reading

Chaffin MK, Schumacher J, McMullan WC. Cutaneous pythiosis in the horse. Vet Clin North Am Equine Pract 1995;11:91–103.

Author Patrick Bourdeau
Consulting Editor Gwendolen Lorch

DERMATOMYCOSES, SUPERFICIAL

BASICS

Skin fungal infections in horses are divided into four classes:

• Superficial (i.e., development on epidermis)—dermatophytoses and yeast dermatoses (*Candida* and *Malassezia*)

• Subcutaneous—In general, secondary to wound inoculations.
1. Rarely invasive—*Phaeohyphomycoses* and mycetomas
2. Slowly invasive—*Sporotrichosis*
3. Rapidly invasive—*Zygomycoses* and *Pythiosis*

• Systemic—Contamination is mainly respiratory or digestive, occasionally traumatic. Many signs other than cutaneous
1. *Cryptococcosis*
2. Yeast phases of dimorphic fungi—*Histoplasmosis farciminosi, Blastomycosis*, and *Coccidioidomycosis*

• Pseudomycoses—organisms related to fungi (*Protothecosis* and *Rhinosporidiosis*)

Only superficial mycoses are mentioned here.

DEFINITION

• Dermatophytoses—generally highly contagious dermatoses due to keratinophylic fungi—*Microsporum* sp. and *Trichophyton* sp.
• Yeast—Superficial fungal dermatoses. Most important yeasts are *Malassezia* and *Candida albicans*.

PATHOPHYSIOLOGY

Dermatophytoses—Two species specifically in horses—*Trichophyton equinum, Microsporum equinum*.

• Other zoophilic dermatophytes—*T. mentagrophytes* (rodents, ruminants, dogs, cats), *M. canis* (cats and dogs), *T. verrucosum* (cattle and sheep). Occasionally *M. gypseum* (soil) or *M. persicolor* (rodents) are involved. • Transmission by contact with infected horses or contaminated material • Dermatophyte spores have a very long resistance in environment (months to years).
• The spores remain quiescent until local conditions stimulate germination with invasion of stratum corneum and hair follicles. The hyphae in hairshafts produce arthroconidia that are released on surface and responsible for extension. Hairshafts are broken and lesions of alopecia and crusts with variable inflammation are seen.

Yeast—*Malassezia pachydermatis* (possibly another species) is a lipophilic yeast present on most of horses. Proliferation may induce inflammation. *Candida albicans* belongs to the digestive flora. In specific conditions, it may develop on skin.

SYSTEMS AFFECTED

• Skin/exocrine • Skin and possibly digestive and/or genital (*Candida albicans*)

GENETICS N/A

INCIDENCE/PREVALENCE

Dermatophytoses—One of the ten most frequent skin conditions in horses. Often misdiagnosed

GEOGRAPHIC DISTRIBUTION

• Dermatophytoses—Worldwide although relative frequency of species of dermatophytes may vary. • Yeast—Presumably worldwide

SIGNALMENT

• Dermatophytes—Any age. More frequent in young horses. • Yeast—No breed predilection. More frequent in mares? *Malassezia* (udder area). Nonseasonal

SIGNS

Dermatophytes

• Evolution influenced by host (age, immune status), fungus, and time • More inflammation is frequent with *Trichophyton* sp. • Papules, tufted hairs or urticaria-like lesions at early stage
• Annular alopecia (1–10 cm in diameter) and scaling • Become polycyclic by coalescence
• Moderate erythema (visible on white horses)
• Crusts occasionally thick • Occasionally multiple papular forms (miliary) • Pruritus usually minimal • Subcutaneous forms (mycetomas) are rare in horses.

Physical Examination

• Frequently starts from head, saddle, or axillae.
• More or less rapidly extensive • Individual lesions spontaneously cure with regrowth of hair from the center (occasionally darker in color).
• Mane and tail generally spared

Yeast

• *Malassezia*—intertrigo (axillae, groin, mammary gland, prepuce); odor; greasiness and sticky brownish material • *Candida*—acute inflammation, erythema, pustular, erosion, exudates (occasionally whitish) mainly periorificial, vulvovaginal, perineal or intertriginous areas, occasionally pruritic (even painful if *Candida*). Nodular cutaneous *candidiasis* represented as firm painful nodules covered by a normal haircoat has been reported.
• Oral candidiasis (white, pseudomembranous plaques and ulcers on the tongue and gingiva) occurs in immunodeficient foals.

CAUSES

• Yeast—Immunosuppressive diseases (viral infections, neoplasia) or immunosuppressive drug therapy may predispose to candidiasis. • Vulvovaginal candidiasis was reported in Thoroughbred mares following oral administration of a synthetic progestogen.

Defects in cornification and seborrheas

RISK FACTORS

Dermatophytes

• Collectivises of horses, contaminated barns, winter (controversial)
• Recent introduction of new horses or other animals

Yeast

• Candidosis precipitated by antibiotic treatments.
• Possible simultaneous digestive or genital candidosis • Increased humidity.

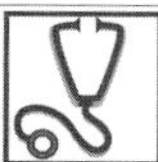

DIAGNOSIS

DIFFERENTIAL DIAGNOSIS

Dermatophytoses

• Bacterial folliculitis (mainly staphylococcal)—similar to identical annular lesions; same predisposed body locations, more frequent during hot periods; pseudocontagious
• Dermatophilosis (folliculitis with thick crusts and alopecia) • Urticaria (atopy, food, drug intolerances), frequent pruritus, rapid onset, alopecia is rare. • Alopecia areata (minimal reaction of skin) • Pemphigus foliaceus (crusts, frequently perioral) • Eosinophilic folliculitis
• Any nodular lesions (bacterial, fungal, or foreign-body granulomas, neoplasms) in cases of dermatophytic mycetoma

Yeast

• Other causes of greasiness, intertrigo, or periorificial inflammation • Other rare fungal superficial dermatoses (*Alternaria, Geotrichum*)
• Mucocutaneous candidiasis differentials include systemic lupus erythematosus, pemphigus vulgaris, erythema multiforme, drug eruptions, and vasculitis. • Nodular forms of candidiasis include infectious and sterile granulomatous disorders.

CBC/BIOCHEMISTRY/URINALYSIS

• Not indicated unless suspect systemic disease that is causing immunosuppression • If considering the use of oral azoles, a baseline biochemical profile should be performed to evaluate liver enzymes.

OTHER LABORATORY TESTS

Dermatophytes—Fungal Culture

• Identify the dermatophyte and possible origin.
• Growth difficult due to the abundance of contaminants
• Washing the skin surface before sampling could help.
• Dermatophyte test medium poorly reliable
• May need to include inoculation of crusts

Yeast—Fungal Culture

• Necessary to identify *C. albicans*. Pathogenic when isolated from skin.
• *Malassezia pachydermatis* is the only species that develops on routine medium agar at 30°C (others need Dixon medium).

IMAGING N/A

OTHER DIAGNOSTIC PROCEDURES

Dermatophytoses—Scrapings and Trichoscopy

Infected hairs broken, embedded in crusts, thickened and fibrous, containing hyphae, with surrounding arthrospores.

Yeast—Cytology on Direct Smears

Abundance of narrow (*Candida*) or wide (*Malassezia*) based budding yeasts. Occasionally hyphae (*Candida albicans*)

Cytology

• Abundant neutrophils, acantholytic cells (confusion with pemphigus); occasionally arthrospores (confusion with yeasts)
• Rarely concurrent bacterial folliculitis

DERMATOMYCOSES, SUPERFICIAL

PATHOLOGICAL FINDINGS

Dermatophytoses

- Follicular involvement with hyphae and arthrospores on histopathology
- Spores in the surface scales and crusts
- Folliculitis (intraluminal and mural)
- Perivascular and superficial neutrophilic and lymphocytic infiltrate, intraepidermal pustular dermatitis, hyperkeratotic epidermis
- Possibly furunculosis with fragments of infected hairs
- With mycetomas, a pyogranulomatous panniculitis containing (whitish 1–2 mm) granules of hyphae may be present.
- Observation easier with periodic acid–Schiff stain

Yeast

- *Malassezia*—Superficial mild infiltrate with hyperkeratosis and recognizable yeasts on and within the stratum corneum
- *Candida*—Erosive to ulcerative inflammation with yeasts, pseudo or septate hyphae

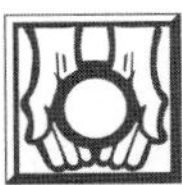

TREATMENT

AIMS OF TREATMENT

Dermatophytoses

- Although considered self-limiting, the infection may last for months and horses remain carriers and sources.
- The aim is to shorten the evolution, reduce lesions, and limit the risk of contamination.
- Topical therapy applied to the entire body is mandatory. Other mandatory therapy includes clipping and destruction of infected hairs.
- Due to the limited efficacy of systemic treatment, topical application is of primary importance.

Yeast

- Correction of the predisposing causes is fundamental.
- Excessive moisture must be avoided.

APPROPRIATE HEALTH CARE

Outpatient medical management is appropriate for dermatophytosis and yeast dermatitis.

NURSING CARE

N/A

ACTIVITY

Dermatophytes—Identification and isolation of infected horses are important to limit the contagion.

DIET

N/A

CLIENT EDUCATION

Dermatophytoses

- Inform that the disease is contagious to other horses and eventually humans. Other hosts may be of concern.
- The disinfection of all materials and housing is imperative for clinical success.
- The appropriate application of topical treatment is crucial for cure.

SURGICAL CONSIDERATIONS

N/A except for mycetomas (wide excision)

MEDICATIONS

DRUG(S)

Dermatophytoses

Topical

- Lotions or rinses are preferred to creams.
- Lime sulfur 2% (Lym Dip) or enilconazole 0.2% (Imaverol) if available. Applied twice weekly for at least 3–4 weeks

Systemic

- Griseofulvin (Fulvicin). Labeled for use in horses in many countries.
- Proposed dosages highly variable. Equivalent to 5 mg/kg 10–20 days or 10 mg/kg for 10 days mentioned active although the real efficacy or benefit remains controversial. Literature suggests that griseofulvin in other species used at much higher dosages and longer treatments are necessary for a better activity.

Yeast

Topical

Apply 2–3 times a week for at least 3 weeks.

Shampoos

- Chlorhexidine (2%–4%) or preferably miconazole (2%)
- If skin is particularly greasy (*Malassezia*), use a keratolytic shampoo.
- Selenium sulfide 1% or lime sulfur 2%

For localized dermatitis, consider clipping and applying topical chlorhexidine/miconazole or azole creams or ointments q12 h for 3–4 weeks.

CONTRAINDICATIONS

See Pregnancy.

PRECAUTIONS

Selenium sulfide can be irritating (rinse thoroughly).

POSSIBLE INTERACTIONS

Not reported in horses

ALTERNATIVE DRUGS

Dermatophytosis

Shampoos

- Their use is controversial. They allow the elimination of debris and infected hairs; but could increase the extension of infective spores.
- Chlorhexidine is only slightly active at high concentrations (4%) and could help for localized spot treatment.

Oral Azoles (ketoconazole, itraconazole)

- Have a limited indication due to the cost, limited information on bioavailability in horses, and possible need of administration intragastrically • Dosage of 10 mg/kg PO q24 h has been suggested for horses.

Vaccines

- Have been developed in different species, including horses, in some countries. • The preventive effect is not complete. • They could reduce duration and the extension of the infection in a group of horses.

Yeast

- Treatment with systemic azoles—a possible alternative but prohibitive cost • For refractory cases, consider the use of leave-on 2% lime sulfur or enilconazole rinses applied after twice-weekly medicated shampoos.

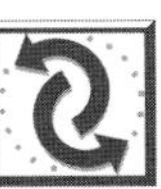

FOLLOW-UP

PATIENT MONITORING

Control at 7- to 10-day intervals and verify the clinical recovery.

PREVENTION/AVOIDANCE

The owner has to look carefully at other animals to detect new cases.

POSSIBLE COMPLICATIONS

N/A

EXPECTED COURSE AND PROGNOSIS

Dermatophytoses—With appropriate therapy, the extension is rapidly stopped and hair regrowth is noted. Complete cure in 3 to 6 weeks.

MISCELLANEOUS

ASSOCIATED CONDITIONS

Yeast—Possible allergic dermatitis

AGE-RELATED FACTORS

Any age although young horses frequently concerned.

ZOONOTIC POTENTIAL

Dermatophytosis

- Human contamination is not rare—mainly from *T. mentagrophytes, T. verrucosum* or *M. canis;* occasionally from *M. equinum;* rarely from *T. equinum.* • Lesions on neck, arms, legs—annular papulopustular and pruritic lesions, onychomycosis

Yeast

A minor concern, easily prevented by simple handwashing

PREGNANCY

The use of griseofulvin and oral azoles is contraindicated in pregnant animals.

SYNONYMS

Dermatophytosis

- Ringworm
- Microsporosis
- Trichophytosis

Yeast

- Candidosis
- Moniliasis
- Thrush

SEE ALSO

- Dematomycoses subcutaneous
- Superficial bacterial dermatitis
- Pemphigus foliaceus
- Dermatophilosis
- Alopecia

Suggested Reading

Scott DW,Miller WH Jr. Equine Dermatology. St. Louis: Saunders, 2003:261–313.

White SD. Equine bacterial and fungal diseases: a diagnostic and therapeutic update. Clin Tech Equine Pract 2005;4:302–310.

Author Patrick Bourdeau

Consulting Editor Gwendolen Lorch

DERMATOPHILOSIS

BASICS

OVERVIEW

Dermatophilosis is a common crusting dermatitis of horses that may affect multiple horses in a barn but not necessarily all of them. It typically occurs during periods of heavy rain. Tightly adherent crusts most commonly affect the dorsum of the trunk, especially the saddle region or the dorsal surface of both hind cannon bones. It is a cause of pastern dermatitis (grease heal, scratches). The face and neck occasionally are affected. This infection is easily resolved with topical and/or systemic antimicrobial therapy.

SIGNALMENT

No age, breed, or sex predilection has been recognized. Horses that are debilitated (e. g., poor nutrition, heavy parasite infestation) may develop a chronic infection. If a horse is kept in a wet stall or pen, chronic pastern dermatitis may ensue.

SIGNS

Clinical lesions vary with the stage of disease. Initially, follicular and nonfollicular papules and pustules form tightly adherent crusts. These progress to crusts that may cluster to form large coalescing crusted plaques associated with a thick yellow to light green suppurative exudate. When adherent crusts are removed, moist erosive erythematosus alopecic lesions are present. Alopecia is variable and can be mild or extensive dependent upon the stage and severity of disease. If lesions are palpated or are under a saddle, pain may be elicited. Pastern or fetlock involvement may cause lameness and localized swelling.

CAUSES AND RISK FACTORS

- Dermatophilosis is caused by a gram-positive, non–acid-fast facultative anaerobic actinomycete—*Dermatophilus congolensis.*
- Skin damage (from flies, allergies, brush) and moisture seem to be the two most important factors required for an infection to occur. Skin damage allows colonization while moisture is important to promote growth of the organism.
- Biting flies and ticks may spread the disease as well as fomites. Crusts, whether on the horse or in the environment, are infectious.

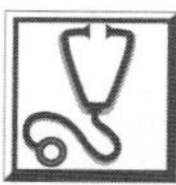

DIAGNOSIS

DIFFERENTIAL DIAGNOSIS

- Formulation of differential diagnoses depends on the distribution of the lesions. If the lesions are truncal, consider dermatophytosis, pemphigus foliaceus, demodicosis, staphylococcal folliculitis, and drug reactions.
- If only pastern involvement, then staphylococcal folliculitis/furunculosis, dermatophytosis, *Chorioptes* infestation, trombiculosis, irritant or allergic contact dermatitis, photosensitization, and vasculitis need to be ruled out.
- If limited to the white areas of the body, consider photosensitization due to liver disease, plant poisoning, or sunburn.

CBC/BIOCHEMISTRY/URINALYSIS

Generally, not of value; however, consider if photosensitization, malnutrition, heavy parasite burden, or chronic debilitating diseases (i.e., neoplasia) are considerations.

OTHER DIAGNOSTIC PROCEDURES

The distribution and types of lesions present are used to establish the diagnosis. Cytology of exudate and/or crust should be stained with a modified Wright's stain (Diff-Quik). Cytology collected by impression smears from a lesion in which the crust has been removed, as well as from the underside of a moist crust, is most rewarding. Dermatophilus are cocci that form parallel rows within branching filaments ("railroad tracks"). A skin culture is generally not imperative.

PATHOLOGICAL FINDINGS

- Histopathology may be necessary if cytologic examination fails to reveal the organism. The morphologic description from the submitted biopsy, as may be the cytology, may be pathognomic. Histopathological changes consistent with dermatophilosis include alternating layers of orthokeratotic and pararkeratotic hyperkeratosis. Inflammatory cells and the organism may be seen within the crusts.
- Upon submission, give location, morphologic appearance of lesions, and differential list and include crusts. Do not surgically prepare lesion for biopsy.

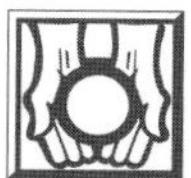

TREATMENT

- Be cognizant of the infectious and zoonotic potential of the crusts. Wear gloves when bathing the horse and especially when handling the crusts. The crusts should be disposed of in a trash bag, NOT discarded into the environment.
- There are two ESSENTIAL components to treatment.
  1. Keep the horse and its environment clean and dry.
  2. Gentle removal of the crusts after soaking
- Many cases will resolve when these two factors are instituted.

MEDICATIONS

DRUG(S)

- Topical therapy and establishing good management practices may be all that are needed. Bathe with a shampoo that has antimicrobial properties every day to every other day until the lesions are healed (typically 10–14 days). Allow a shampoo contact time of 10–15 min before rinsing. If bathing is not possible and the lesions are focal, 4% chlorhexidene spray or 2% chlorhexidene lotion may be used.
- Systemic treatment may be used in cases where topical therapy is not possible or has failed to be effective. Procaine penicillin G at 10,000 IU/lb q12h IM is very effective. Continue systemic therapy until the lesions are resolved. The author has had cases where only one dose of penicillin was required to resolve the lesions; in all probability, these cases were responding to management changes and topical therapy rather than a single dose of penicillin.

CONTRAINDICATIONS/POSSIBLE INTERACTIONS

None

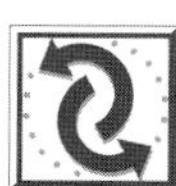

FOLLOW-UP

PATIENT MONITORING

Clinical appearance

PREVENTION/AVOIDANCE

- Management changes—control flies, keep the environment dry.
- If the horse is kept at a boarding stable, tell stable manager of the diagnosis so appropriate recommendations and modifications are made.
- The bacteria can survive in the environment for several years.

POSSIBLE COMPLICATIONS

None

EXPECTED COURSE AND PROGNOSIS

- Many cases are self-limiting once environmental factors are corrected.
- Excellent prognosis

MISCELLANEOUS

ASSOCIATED CONDITIONS

- Chronic infections may be associated with poor nutrition, heavy parasite infestation, viral diseases, or neoplasia.
- In some cases, white haired areas are more severely affected. Postulation exists that the infection with *Dermatophilus* results in a secondary photodermatitis.

AGE-RELATED FACTORS

None

ZOONOTIC POTENTIAL

Dermatophilus congolensis is a zoonotic disease; therefore, great care and precaution are needed when handling and discarding crusts.

PREGNANCY

No significance

SEE ALSO

- Superficial bacterial dermatitis
- Pemphigus foliaceus
- Pastern dermatitis
- Dermatophytosis

Suggested Reading

Pascoe RR, Knottenbelt DC. Manual of Equine Dermatology. London: Saunders, 1999:102.

Scott DW, Miller WH Jr. Equine Dermatology. St. Louis: Saunders, 2003:234.

Author Paul B. Bloom

Consulting Editor Gwendolen Lorch

DIAPHRAGMATIC HERNIA

BASICS

OVERVIEW

• Herniation of abdominal viscera into the thoracic cavity through a diaphragmatic defect. • Diaphragmatic hernia generally results in simple or strangulated obstruction of the herniated gastrointestinal viscera and in hypoventilation.

SIGNALEMENT

• No sex or breed predilection • Most frequently observed in adult horses

SIGNS

• Abdominal pain, which may vary from mild, intermittent episodes of colic to severe, intractable pain • Alteration in respiration, which may vary from exercise intolerance, to tachypnea, to respiratory distress depending on the degree of decrease in thoracic volume • Clinical signs suggestive of hypovolemic shock, such as blanched mucous membranes, tachycardia, and collapse, may be observed when severe hemorrhage occurs in the abdominal or thoracic cavity.

CAUSES AND RISK FACTORS

• Diaphragmatic defects may be either congenital or acquired. • Congenital defect results from incomplete fusion of the pleuroperitoneal folds, causing an enlarged esophageal hiatus. • Acquired defects result from sudden increases in intrathoracic or intra-abdominal pressure. Acquired defects are usually observed after external trauma, strenuous exercise, gastrointestinal distention, or pregnancy.

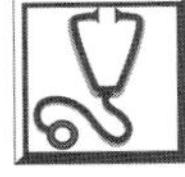

DIAGNOSIS

DIFFERENTIAL DIAGNOSIS

• All disorders resulting in acute abdominal pain in the horse should be included in the differential diagnosis. Intestinal conditions requiring surgical correction and severe medical conditions of the gastrointestinal tract, such as salmonellosis, colitis X, and Potomac horse fever, should therefore be included. Making a definitive diagnosis depends on a complete physical examination and appropriate auxiliary testing. • Pneumonia and pleuritis must be included in the differential diagnosis. Horses with diaphragmatic hernias usually are not pyrexic, depressed, or have inflammatory leukograms. • Horses with diaphragmatic hernia may be exercise intolerant. Any disorder of the respiratory, circulatory and musculoskeletal systems that result in exercise intolerance must be included in the differential diagnosis.

CBC/BIOCHEMISTRY/URINALYSIS

Not of diagnostic value

OTHER LABORATORY TESTS

Blood gas analysis reveals hypercapnia. Respiratory acidosis or uncompensated metabolic acidosis is usually observed in horses with diaphragmatic hernia, whereas the most common acid-base derangement in horses with colic is metabolic acidosis with respiratory compensation. The hypercapnia observed in horses with diaphragmatic hernia is associated with hypoventilation due to either thoracic pain or reduction of thoracic volume.

IMAGING

• Thoracic radiography—Standing lateral thoracic radiography is used to confirm a diagnosis of diaphragmatic hernia. Radiographic signs include gas-filled loops of intestines in the thoracic cavity, increased ventral thoracic density, and absence of the cardiac shadow. The most consistent radiographic sign is loss of the diaphragmatic shadow in the area of the hernia. • Thoracic ultrasonography—Thoracic ultrasonography reveals the presence of pleural fluid and of abdominal viscera in the thoracic cavity. Thoracic cavity and diaphragm are imaged using a 5.0- or 7.5-Mhz transducer. Ultrasonographic findings consistent with herniation of intestines in the thoracic cavity are presence of curved hyperechoic interfaces with reverberation artifact, attenuation of the ultrasound beam and slow peristaltic contractions.

OTHER DIAGNOSTIC PROCEDURES

• Auscultation of the thorax of horses with diaphragmatic hernia reveals regions of thoracic dullness or reduced cardiac sounds on the involved side of the thorax. Referred gastrointestinal sounds are frequently heard over the caudoventral thorax in normal horses and thus cannot be considered as definitive diagnosis. • Abdominal palpation per rectum may reveal an empty caudal abdomen, but this sign is not a consistent finding. • Abdominal paracentesis yields usually to a normal abdominal fluid; however, in the case of acute acquired diaphragm defect, abundant hemorrhagic fluid may be obtained. • Electrocardiography may reveal decreased amplitudes of the QRS complex caused by the herniated abdominal viscera that surround the heart and impair conduction of electrical impulses to the skin to form surface potentials.

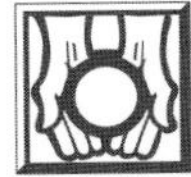

TREATMENT

• Emergency exploratory celiotomy is performed under general anesthesia with assisted positive-pressure ventilator. Surgical treatment consists of reduction of the herniated viscera, resection of devitalized intestine, and intestinal anastomosis. Repair of the diaphragmatic defect is not always possible and may require a second procedure. Meshes may have to be used to repair large diaphragmatic defects. • In horses with acute diaphragmatic defects secondary to trauma, surgery may be delayed if the animal's condition is stable. Delay allows development of fibrosis of the edges of the defect and easier surgical closure. • Preoperative fluid volume replacement therapy is accomplished with administration of lactated Ringer's solution at a rate of 6 to 12 mL/kg/hr. This solution is also used for maintenance fluid therapy postoperatively.

MEDICATIONS

DRUG(S) OF CHOICE

Preoperative and postoperative medication consist of the administration of systemic antibiotics (sodium penicillin G 20,000 IU/kg IV q6h and gentamicin sulfate 6.6 mg/kg IV q24h) and NSAIDs (flunixin meglumine 1 mg/kg IV BID).

CONTRAINDICATIONS/POSSIBLE INTERACTIONS

α_2-Agonist agents, such as xylazine, detomidine, and romifidine, should be used with caution in horses with diaphragmatic hernia because these drugs have depressive effects in both the cardiovascular and respiratory functions.

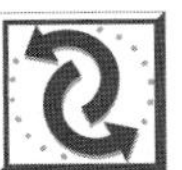

FOLLOW-UP

• Postsurgical monitoring for the development of pneumothorax or pleural effusion. • Restrict exercise for 90 days after the surgical correction of the hernia. • Prognosis for survival of horses with diaphragmatic hernia is poor to guarded.

MISCELLANEOUS

SEE ALSO

• Expiratory dyspnea • Inspiratory dyspnea • Pleuropneumonia • Thoracic trauma

Suggested Reading

Bristol DG. Diaphragmatic hernias in horses and cattle. Comp Contin Educ Pract Vet 1986;8:S407–S412.

Bryant JE, Sanchez LC, Rameriz S, Bleyaert H. What is your diagnosis? Herniation of the intestines into the caudal region of the thorax. J Am Vet Med Assoc 2002;15:1461–1462.

Malone ED, Farnsworth K, Lennox T, et al. Thoracoscopic-assisted diaphragmatic hernia repair using a thoracic rib resection. Vet Surg 2001;30:175–178.

Author Ludovic Bouré
Consulting Editor Daniel Jean

DIARRHEA, NEONATAL

BASICS

DEFINITION

• Diarrhea—increased volume and fluid content of feces, usually associated with abnormally frequent defecation • Neonatal foal—a foal <28 days of age

PATHOPHYSIOLOGY

• Varies with etiology of diarrhea, but a final common event is abnormal loss of water and electrolytes in feces. • Can result from abnormal secretion, increased luminal osmolality, and altered GI transit time. Loss of disaccharidase activity (lactase) secondary to destruction of enterocytes causes maldigestion of milk sugars and subsequent osmotic diarrhea. • Small intestinal disease (enteritis), colonic disease (colitis), or a combination of both can cause diarrhea in foals. • Loss of large volumes of electrolyte-rich fluid can result in electrolyte, fluid, and acid-base derangements. • Loss of enteric barrier function can allow absorption of enteric toxins (endotoxin) or translocation of enteric bacteria with subsequent toxemia, septicemia, and multiple organ dysfunction associated with hypovolemic or septic shock. • Translocation of enteric bacteria can result in disseminated disease such as septic arthritis or pneumonia.

SYSTEMS AFFECTED

• GI—as described earlier • Cardiovascular—With severe fluid loss from the vascular space to the intestinal lumen, hypovolemic shock can occur. • Renal—Hypovolemic shock and toxemia can cause prerenal or renal azotemia.

GENETICS

No genetic predisposition is recognized with the exception of Arabian foals with SCID.

INCIDENCE/PREVALENCE

• Common disease of foals • 25% of foals 0–7 days of age, 40% at 8–31 days of age, and 8% at 32–180 days of age have diarrhea at some point. • Case-fatality rate is low (≈3%).

GEOGRAPHIC DISTRIBUTION

N/A

SIGNALMENT

Breed Predilections

N/A

Age and Range

Sepsis-related diarrhea is most often seen in foals <2 weeks of age. Diarrhea due to viral infection or other causes is most commonly seen in foals <1 month of age.

Predominant Sex

None

CLINICAL SIGNS

Historical

• Often acute in onset but can be chronic. Some foals have mild diarrhea but are otherwise well. • More than one foal may be affected. • It is important to determine dietary history, deworming history, housing and other management practices, and medications administered.

Physical Examination

• Foals are often bright, alert, and responsive with normal vital signs. Presence of abnormal vital signs, depressed mentation, and/or dehydration is cause for concern.
• Consistency of diarrhea can vary from pasty to watery, and color of feces can vary from yellow to red, with the latter color resulting from hematochezia. • Severely ill foals often show signs of colic, abdominal distention, and/or tenesmus, often before onset of diarrhea.

CAUSES

Infectious

• Most foals with diarrhea do not have a definitive diagnosis. It is important to rule out infectious disease in situations in which there is more than one foal at risk. • Bacterial—septicemia, *Salmonella* sp., other gram-negative sepsis/endotoxemia, *Clostridium* (*difficile, perfringens* type C), *Rhodococcus equi* (usually >3 weeks of age); rare: *Escherichia coli*, *Lawsonia intracellularis* (older foals), *Bacteroides* sp., *Aeromonas* sp., *Yersinia pseudotuberculosis* • Viral—common: rotavirus; rare: adenovirus, coronavirus
• Protozoal—common: *Cryptosporidium* sp.; rare: *Giardia* sp. and *Eimeria leukarti*
• Parasitic—uncommon to rare: *Strongyloides westeri, Strongylus vulgaris*, and *Parascaris equorum*

Noninfectious Causes

• Foal heat diarrhea is a self-limiting diarrhea in foals during the first 2 weeks of life.
• Antibiotic induced (i.e., potentiated sulfonamides) • Lactose intolerance—secondary to infectious diarrhea
• Cathartics—overdosing of $MgSO_4$, DSS, castor oil • High stocking density • Housing on dirt or dry lots • Presence of other foals with diarrhea • Salmonellosis—carrier state in mare

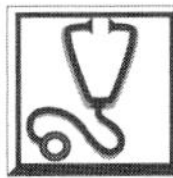

DIAGNOSIS

DIFFERENTIAL DIAGNOSIS

• Colic can be attributable to GI disease other than enteritis, or non-GI abdominal disease—Abdominal ultrasound, abdominal radiographs, and degree/severity of pain will help to differentiate diarrhea from other causes of colic. • Peritonitis—definitive diagnosis is by analysis of peritoneal fluid.
• Uroperitoneum—large amount of free fluid on ultrasound; abdominocentesis is diagnostic.

CBC/BIOCHEMISTRY/URINALYSIS

• Mildly affected, clinically stable foals rarely have abnormal hemogram or serum biochemical profile. • Sick foals are often leukopenic with neutropenia.
• Hypoproteinemia, depending on the cause. It can be attenuated by dehydration and caution should be used in assessing serum protein concentration as it can decline rapidly as the foal is rehydrated. • Acidemia (decreased pH, lowered Tco_2), hyponatremia, and hypochloremia are common in symptomatic foals.
• Hypoglycemia—not nursing or not digesting milk sugars • Azotemia—prerenal or renal origin • Some foals with diarrhea have inadequate serum concentrations of IgG.

OTHER LABORATORY TESTS

Infectious Causes

• Frank blood or hematochezia in neonates is consistent with clostridial diarrhea. • Culture feces or blood for bacteria (*Salmonella* sp., *E. coli, Actinobacillus* sp.) • Immunoassays for clostridial toxins—*C. difficile* toxins A or B, and *C. perfringens* toxins • IFA for *Cryptosporidium* sp. and *Giardia* sp.
• Immunoassay or electron microscopy for rotavirus • Fecal floatation for nematode parasites • Look for other clinical evidence of disease caused by *R. equi,* including disease in other foals, such as pneumonia, aseptic arthritis, uveitis, or intra-abdominal abscesses.
• Measure serum IgG concentration.

Noninfectious Causes

• Lactose absorption test (to detect lactose deficiency)—rarely necessary • Test feeding of lactose-free cow's milk results in resolution of diarrhea in 24 hr in lactose-intolerant foals.

IMAGING

Ultrasonography

• Use in foals with enteritis that do not (yet) have diarrhea. • Visualize distended, thickened, fluid-filled small intestines and fluid-filled large intestines. • Rule out other abdominal disease such as uroperitoneum, intussusception, and intestinal accidents.

OTHER DIAGNOSTIC PROCEDURES

• Measure abdominal circumference in a systematic fashion to monitor progression of distention. • Pass nasogastric tube for evidence of reflux/ileus in colicky foals.

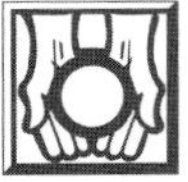

TREATMENT

AIMS OF TREATMENT

• Restore circulatory volume and correct electrolyte and metabolic derangement by administration of balanced, polyionic crystalloid fluids. • The principles of treatment of foals with diarrhea are to achieve normal hydration, acid-base status, and serum electrolyte concentrations; prevent systemic disease associated with translocation of enteric bacteria or toxins; and ensure adequate energy intake. Failure of transfer of passive immunity should be corrected. • Most foals with mild diarrhea that are otherwise asymptomatic do not require any treatment. Such foals are often administered oral products that contain antimotility agents, antimicrobials, and intestinal protectants (such as activated charcoal). The efficacy of these preparations is doubtful given that most foals with mild diarrhea recover if not treated. • Broad-spectrum antimicrobials are indicated in foals with abnormal vital signs suggestive of toxemia or bacteremia or at high risk of developing such. Foals with adequate serum IgG concentration and no abnormal clinical signs other than mild diarrhea should not be administered antibiotics.

APPROPRIATE HEALTH CARE

• Foals with severe diarrhea and hypovolemia require emergency inpatient intensive care management. • Less severe cases may be treated in the field, although it should be kept in mind that neonatal foals have minimal fluid and energy reserves.

NURSING CARE

• Depending on the degree of dehydration, fluid may be administered IV or PO. • IV administration of lactated Ringer's solution often is sufficient. • Alternatively, a 2.5% dextrose and 0.45% saline solution can be used initially. • With severe acidosis, isotonic sodium bicarbonate (1.3%; 13 g of sodium bicarbonate per 1 L of distilled water) can be used, but only if acidosis does not resolve with correction of volume and electrolyte deficits. • Dextrose solutions (2.5%–5.0%) to correct hypoglycemia • With less severe derangement of fluid and electrolyte balance, oral solutions formulated for treatment of diarrhea in calves can be used. • Administration of plasma to correct abnormally low serum IgG concentration • Important for prevention of secondary infection • Vaseline or zinc oxide around the perineum and back of hind legs helps to prevent hair loss and scalding of the skin. • Ophthalmic ointment may be useful in lubricating eyes if the foal is recumbent.

DIET

• GI rest in foals with severe diarrhea causing acid-base and electrolyte deficits refractory to fluid therapy. Provide nutrition parenterally or as lactose-free cow's milk. • Return foal to nursing the mare as soon as the foal can tolerate ingestion of milk. • Some foals continue to be lactose intolerant after resolution of infectious cause of the diarrhea. Some of these foals have resolution of diarrhea when fed lactose-free cow's milk.

MEDICATIONS

DRUGS

Broad-Spectrum Antimicrobial Therapy

• Penicillin or a first-generation cephalosporin and an aminoglycoside (e.g., amikacin [20–25 mg/kg q24h]) may be indicated in foals with suspected primary or secondary bacterial enteritis, primary or secondary peritonitis, or primary or secondary bacteremia. • With suspected clostridial enteritis, metronidazole (10–15 mg/kg PO or IV q8h) is recommended.

Intestinal Protectants

Uncertain efficacy. Products containing activated charcoal, smectite, or bismuth subsalicylate are often administered to foals with diarrhea. There is no objective evidence of efficacy.

Antispasmodic Drugs

Use motility-altering agents with caution.

Probiotics

Probiotics are available for use in foals. Their efficacy is unproved, and in fact routine administration might be associated with increased risk of diarrhea.

CONTRAINDICATIONS

• Avoid oral antimicrobials, particularly those associated with inducing diarrhea (e.g., erythromycin). • Avoid enteral nutrition in foals with severe diarrhea exacerbated by feeding (usually clostridial colitis, rotaviral diarrhea).

FOLLOW-UP

PATIENT MONITORING

• Foals can deteriorate rapidly and require intensive care. • Monitor attitude, appetite, fecal color and consistency, hydration status, and abdominal distention several times daily. Use laboratory data as clinically indicated, especially indicators of acid-base status, renal function, and serum electrolyte concentrations. • Monitor other foals for signs of diarrhea or colic.

PREVENTION/AVOIDANCE

• Implement isolation measures to control/prevent the spread of possible infectious agents. • If there is an outbreak of diarrhea due to *Salmonella* sp., institute a program of strict hygiene including washing the udder and perineum of prepartum mares immediately. • There are no vaccinations available for the common pathogens causing diarrhea in foals. • On farms that experience outbreaks of clostridial enteritis in foals, prophylaxis with metronidazole (10 mg/kg q12h for the first 4 days of life) and/or oral administration of 50–100 mL of bovine antitoxin to *C. perfringens* C, D, and E might provide some protection against disease.

POSSIBLE COMPLICATIONS

• Sepsis • Intussusception • Hypovolemic shock • Septic peritonitis • Septic arthritis • Peripheral arterial or venous thrombosis—distal limbs; jugular veins • Cerebral edema • Gastric ulceration

EXPECTED COURSE AND PROGNOSIS

• Uncomplicated osmotic diarrhea resolves rapidly when alternative nutrition (lactose-free milk or parenteral nutrition) is provided. Prognosis for foals with rotavirus diarrhea is excellent. • Diarrhea complicated by sepsis (enterocolitis) has a more guarded prognosis.

MISCELLANEOUS

ASSOCIATED CONDITIONS

• Septicemia • SCID • Peritonitis • Gastric ulceration

AGE-RELATED FACTORS

• Foals commonly develop a non–life-threatening diarrhea at 5–10 days of age (foal heat diarrhea). • High index of suspicion for clostridial enterocolitis in foals with hemorrhagic diarrhea <1 week of age

ZOONOTIC POTENTIAL

• *Salmonella* sp. • *Cryptosporidium* sp.

SYNONYMS

Scours

SEE ALSO

• Colic in foals • Gastric ulcers, neonate
• Fluid therapy, neonate

ABBREVIATIONS

• GI = gastrointestinal
• IFA = immunofluorescence assay
• SCID = severe combined immunodeficiency disease

Suggested Reading

Acute diarrhea of suckling foals. In: Radostits OM, Gay CC, Hinchcliff KW, Constable PD, eds. Veterinary Medicine: A Textbook of the Diseases of Cattle, Horses, Sheep, Goats and Pigs, ed 10. London: WB Saunders, 2004:274–277.

The author & editor acknowledge the contribution of Dr. N. Cohen to this topic in the first edition.

Author Kenneth W. Hinchcliff
Consulting Editor Margaret C. Mudge

DICUMAROL (MOLDY SWEET CLOVER) TOXICOSIS

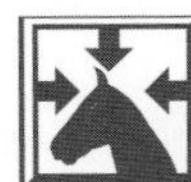

BASICS

OVERVIEW

- Sweet clover has erect stems and leaves divided into three segments and spikes of flowers, white or yellow, that give off a sweet odor when crushed.
- The white variety can grow as tall as 8 feet; the yellow variety grows to ≅6 feet.
- The plant grows in moist soils throughout the United States and Canada.
- In some areas, sweet clover is grown for hay and compares favorably with alfalfa in nutrient value; it also may become a weed invading pastures and growing along roadsides.
- Ingestion of moldy sweet clover hay interferes with normal blood clotting in horses.
- Sweet clovers (*Melilotus alba, M. officinalis*) and sweet vernal (*Anthoxanthum odoratum*) contain the nontoxic compound coumarin. When cut and baled for hay under high-moisture conditions, various molds metabolize coumarin to form dicumarol, which inhibits vitamin K epoxide reductase, in turn decreasing vitamin K_1 formation and leading to decreased prothrombin formation and bleeding.
- Dicumarol levels in hay >20 ppm suggest potential toxicity problems; most toxicoses in livestock are reported at levels >30 ppm.

SIGNALMENT

- All animals
- Poisoning occurs more commonly in cattle than in horses, because horses rarely eat moldy sweet clover hay.

SIGNS

- Bleeding diathesis, ranging from mild to severe
- Generally, horses show symptoms within 3–8 weeks after initial ingestion.
- Hemorrhage may be internal or external—epistaxis; fecal blood
- Swellings may appear over bony protuberances of the body because of bruising and hematoma formation.
- Lameness can result from hemorrhage into joint capsules and soreness may result from muscle hematomas.
- Profuse hemorrhage can occur during minor surgical procedures.
- Symptoms include anemia, pale mucous membranes, weakness, abnormal heartbeat, and death.
- Sudden death often is marked by massive hemorrhage into the thorax or abdominal cavity or around the brain.

CAUSES AND RISK FACTORS

Dicumarol interferes with normal blood clotting because of reduction in the concentrations of the active forms of clotting factors II (i.e., prothrombin), VII, IX, and X. This results from competitive inhibition between vitamin K epoxide and dicumarol for the enzyme vitamin K epoxide reductase, which converts inactive vitamin K epoxide back to its active vitamin K form in the body. Thus, dicumarol causes vitamin K deficiency by inhibiting regeneration of the active form of vitamin K.

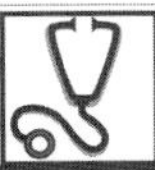

DIAGNOSIS

DIFFERENTIAL DIAGNOSIS

- DIC—reduced plasma concentrations of platelets and coagulant and anticoagulant proteins; increased concentrations of coagulant byproducts; petechial hemorrhages
- Severe liver disease—altered liver function tests
- Inherited deficiencies of coagulation factors—measurement of specific coagulation factors
- IMTP—thrombocytopenia; petechial hemorrhages

CBC/BIOCHEMISTRY/URINALYSIS

Blood loss anemia

OTHER LABORATORY TESTS

- Elevated PT and aPTT
- Chemical analysis of suspect hay for dicumarol content
- Liver tissue also may be analyzed.

IMAGING

N/A

DIAGNOSTIC PROCEDURES

N/A

PATHOLOGICAL FINDINGS

Hemorrhages may occur in any part of the body.

DICUMAROL (MOLDY SWEET CLOVER) TOXICOSIS

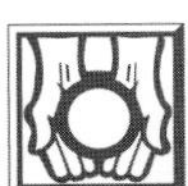

TREATMENT

• Massive blood or plasma transfusions may be helpful.
• Handle horses with care to avoid stress and further hemorrhaging.
• Attempt correction of organ dysfunction resulting from accumulation of extravascular blood (e.g., thoracocentesis) only if life-threatening and after normal blood coagulation has been restored.
• Adding alfalfa hay to the diet may help to provide a source of increased dietary vitamin K_1.

MEDICATIONS

DRUG(S) OF CHOICE

• Vitamin K_1 (i.e., phytonadione; 1.5 mg/kg SC or IM q12h for up to 3 days) effectively reverses the clotting defect.
• Improvement in PT after vitamin K_1 therapy usually is observed within 24 hr.

CONTRAINDICATIONS/POSSIBLE INTERACTIONS

Do not use vitamin K_3 (i.e., menadione), which is ineffective against dicumarol toxicosis and is nephrotoxic in horses.

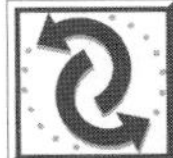

FOLLOW-UP

PATIENT MONITORING

Monitor for blood loss.

PREVENTION/AVOIDANCE

• Remove all moldy sweet clover hay from diet.
• Grazing sweet clover in a pasture has not been associated with coagulopathy.

POSSIBLE COMPLICATIONS

N/A

EXPECTED COURSE AND PROGNOSIS

• The time required to exhibit observable clinical signs in healthy horses fed contaminated hay depends on the dicumarol concentrations in that hay; onset of toxicosis is more delayed with lower dicumarol concentrations in the hay.
• Prognosis is based on the severity of blood loss and damage to organ systems affected by hemorrhage.

MISCELLANEOUS

ASSOCIATED CONDITIONS

N/A

AGE-RELATED FACTORS

N/A

ZOONOTIC POTENTIAL

N/A

PREGNANCY

Late-term abortions have been reported in cattle after moldy sweet clover intoxication, but this effect has not been specifically reported in horses.

SEE ALSO

Anticoagulant rodenticides

ABBREVIATIONS

• DIC = disseminated intravascular coagulation
• IMTP = immune-mediated thrombocytopenia
• PT = one-stage prothrombin time
• aPTT = activated partial thromboplastin time

Suggested Reading

Burrows GM, Tyrl RJ. Toxic Plants of North America. Ames: Blackwell Publishing, 2001:590–594.
Hintz HF. Molds, mycotoxins, and mycotoxicosis. Vet Clin North Am Equine Pract 1990;6:419–431.

Author Anita M. Kore
Consulting Editor Robert H. Poppenga

DISEASES OF THE EQUINE NICTITANS

BASICS

OVERVIEW

Definition

The nictitating membrane consists of a T-shaped cartilage with a seromucoid gland located at its base. This gland secretes a significant portion of the aqueous tear film. The nictitans is covered on both the palpebral and bulbar surfaces with conjunctiva, and diseases affecting the conjunctiva can also involve the nictitans. Movement of the nictitans distributes the tear film and protects the cornea. Protrusion of the nictitating membrane is passive and occurs secondary to retraction of the globe into the orbit. Sympathetic innervation functions to retract the nictitans. Horner's syndrome refers to sympathetic denervation.

Pathophysiology

- Protrusion of the nictitating membrane is usually a nonspecific sign of pain. Ocular diseases often result in ocular pain and secondary nictitans protrusion. Systemic disease can also cause nictitans protrusion.
- Horner's syndrome can be a result of central, preganglionic, or postganglionic lesions of the sympathetic innervation of the eye. The subsequent oculosympathetic paralysis is reflected in the loss of sympathetically mediated functions.
- Tetanus may be a complication of elective surgery or accidental wounds. Contamination of wounds by *Clostridium tetani* and the subsequent production of a neurotoxin results in the classic "sawhorse stance."

SYSTEMS AFFECTED

Ophthalmic

SIGNALMENT

Breed predilections

- There are no breed predilections for Horner's syndrome.
- Hyperkalemic periodic paralysis can cause protrusion of the nictitans and is seen most commonly in Quarter Horses.
- Squamous cell carcinoma, the most common neoplasm affecting the equine nictitans, has a high prevalence in draft horses, Appaloosas, and Paints.

Mean Age and Range

No detected age distribution of Horner's syndrome or protrusion of the nictitans. Ocular squamous cell carcinoma prevalence increases with age.

Genetics

Breed predilection for ocular squamous cell carcinoma suggests genetic influence.

Predominant Sex

No proven sex predilection

SIGNS

- Protrusion of the nictitating membrane, conjunctival hyperemia, chemosis, follicle development, ocular discharge
- Horner's syndrome—ptosis, nictitans protrusion, slight miosis, hyperemia of nasal and conjunctival mucosa, increased temperature, and sweating of base of ear, side of face, and neck of affected side
- Squamous cell carcinoma may have different appearances—proliferative/ulcerated or thickening/ulceration of tissue. May be complicated by habronemiasis.
- Habronemiasis—granulomas, nodules, often have yellow caseous exudate and necrotic mineralized tissue. May be nonhealing, ulcerated.
- Tetanus causes bilateral protrusion of the nictitans, spasms of the masseter muscles, stiff gait, and increased sensitivity to external stimulation.

CAUSES

Protrusion

- Ocular pain*
- Neoplasia*—squamous cell carcinoma most common
- Secondary to environmental causes*—foreign bodies and debris, trauma
- Horner's syndrome
- Tetanus
- Inflammation—bacterial, parasitic (habronemiasis), trauma
- Enophthalmos
- Space-occupying mass in orbit
- Loss of orbital mass—starvation, dehydration
- Decreased ocular mass—microphthalmos, phthisis bulbi
- Secondary to systemic disease—hyperkalemic periodic paralysis
- Congenital lack of pigmentation on leading edge—optical illusion of protrusion

RISK FACTORS

- White, gray-white, and palomino hair color predisposes to ocular squamous cell carcinoma.
- Warm weather, climates with heavy fly population are a risk factor for habronemiasis. Deficit vaccination programs increase the risk of tetanus.

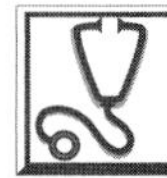

DIAGNOSIS

DIFFERENTIAL DIAGNOSIS

- Ocular pain—ulcerative keratitis, corneal stromal abscess, anterior uveitis, keratomycosis, corneal laceration, conjunctivitis
- Horner's syndrome—jugular vein and carotid artery injections, cervical abscesses, guttural pouch infections, neoplasia of neck and thoracic inlet, trauma to neck and thorax, mediastinal and thoracic masses
- Nodular/mass lesions of nictitans—squamous cell carcinoma, habronemiasis, mastocytoma, hemangioma, hemangiosarcoma, papilloma, fungal granulomas, nodular necrobiosis, foreign body reaction
- Space-occupying mass in orbit—neoplasia, abscess, hematoma, arteriovenous fistula

CBC/BIOCHEMISTRY/URINALYSIS

Results usually normal unless nictitans disease associated with systemic disease.

OTHER LABORATORY TESTS

- Habronemiasis—conjunctival scraping reveals eosinophils, mast cells, neutrophils, plasma cells, rarely larvae. Biopsy and histopathology for mass lesions.
- Consider bacterial culture and sensitivity if suspect bacterial inflammation.
- Other specific tests as indicated when systemic disease suspected.

IMAGING

N/A

OTHER DIAGNOSTIC PROCEDURES

- Complete ophthalmic examination is indicated to identify ocular causes of nictitans disease. Fluorescein stain and examination for signs of anterior uveitis (aqueous flare, miosis, hypotony). Examination behind nictitans may reveal foreign body, debris.
- Pharmacological testing to differentiate between central/preganglionic and postganglionic lesions in Horner's syndrome has not been evaluated in horses. Topical application of 1% phenylephrine or 0.1% epinephrine: rapid mydriasis within 20 minutes indicates postganglionic lesion, slow mydriasis within 30–40 minutes indicates preganglionic lesion. Topical application of 0.1% pilocarpine: rapid miosis within 20 minutes indicates postganglionic lesion, no miosis indicates preganglionic lesion.

GROSS AND HISTOPATHOLOGIC FINDINGS

- Nictitans/conjunctival biopsy—Habronemiasis: eosinophils, mast cells, neutrophils, plasma cells, rarely larvae. Squamous cell carcinoma: epithelial cells with neoplastic characteristics. Lymphoma: large population monomorphic lymphocytes with neoplastic characteristics. Multiple myeloma: large population neoplastic plasma cells. Other histopathologic findings possible depending on type of neoplasia present.

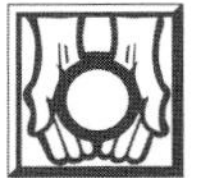

TREATMENT

INPATIENT VERSUS OUTPATIENT

- Most horses with nictitans protrusion or Horner's syndrome can be treated on an outpatient basis.

• Treatment of some ocular (severe ulcerative keratitis, corneal stromal abscess, keratomycosis, squamous cell carcinoma) and systemic (tetanus, severe hyperkalemic periodic paralysis) diseases associated with secondary nictitans involvement may require hospitalization.

ACTIVITY

• If environmental irritation is suspected, then exposure to the inciting substance should be restricted or eliminated.
• Animals with ocular involvement/disease should not be ridden if visual status is compromised.
• Animals affected with tetanus should be kept in quiet, dark environment.

DIET

No change in diet is necessary. Hay should be fed at ground level rather than elevated hayracks or bags if ocular disease is present.

CLIENT EDUCATION

• If there is evidence of self trauma when ocular disease is present, a protective hood covering the affected eye should be placed on the horse. The client should be instructed to contact the veterinarian if the condition worsens in any way. The problem may not be responding appropriately to treatment, may be progressing, or the patient may be having an adverse response to the medication. If hyperkalemic periodic paralysis is identified, the client should be informed of genetic basis of disease and advised against breeding the affected animal.

SURGICAL CONSIDERATIONS

• Squamous cell carcinoma is treated by surgical resection of the nictitans with adjunctive cryotherapy or chemotherapy. Enucleation or exenteration may be necessary depending on the type of neoplasia and extent of invasion of surrounding tissue.
• Foreign bodies and debris of the nictitating membrane can usually be removed with topical anesthesia and liberal flushing of conjunctival fornices.
• Surgical management of ocular diseases causing protrusion of nictitating membrane is addressed in appropriate chapters. Treatment of corneal stromal abscessation and keratomycosis may require conjunctival flap procedures, lamellar keratectomy, or penetrating keratoplasty.
• Thorough wound lavage and debridement is necessary in cases of tetanus.

MEDICATIONS

DRUGS AND FLUIDS

• Habronemiasis: topical 0.03% echothiophate iodide (phospholine iodide) and ophthalmic neomycin/polymixin B with dexamethasone q 12 hours. Multifocal lesions: oral ivermectin (200 microg/kg). Intralesional triamcinolone, 10–40 mg/lesion, may reduce size of granulomas.
• Bacterial inflammation: topical broad spectrum antibiotic initially (triple antibiotic usually appropriate), may change after results of bacterial culture and sensitivity. Treat every 6 hours to every 12 hours depending on severity of disease.
• Squamous cell carcinoma: See Ocular/adnexal Squamous Cell Carcinoma section.
• Ocular diseases inciting nictitans protrusion: See appropriate section.
• Other systemic medication as indicated by concurrent systemic disease.

CONTRAINDICATIONS

N/A

PRECAUTIONS

N/A

POSSIBLE INTERACTIONS

N/A

ALTERNATE DRUGS

N/A

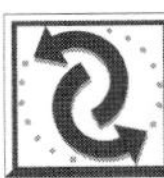

FOLLOW-UP

PATIENT MONITORING

The patient should be rechecked soon after beginning therapy (3–4 days), with specific time frame determined by disease and severity. Subsequent rechecks are dictated by severity of disease and response to treatment.

PREVENTION/AVOIDANCE

• Fly control in barns and pastures, fly hoods, frequent periocular administration of insect repellant, and regular deworming with ivermectin can help prevent the development of habronemiasis.
• Treat any underlying ocular or systemic disease which may be inciting the nictitans disease.

POSSIBLE COMPLICATIONS

• Potential complications of neoplasia of the nictitans and its treatment vary with the specific type of tumor.
• Possibilities include recurrence of the neoplasia and metastatic disease.

EXPECTED COURSE AND PROGNOSIS

• Course and prognosis of nictitating membrane neoplasia depend on the specific type of neoplasia and the extent of invasion of surrounding tissues.
• Horner's syndrome may be reversible depending on the cause. Resolution of cervical abscesses and guttural pouch disease may resolve associated Horner's syndrome. Neoplastic and traumatic causes are less likely to be correctable.
• Prognosis associated with nictitans protrusion secondary to systemic or ocular disease varies with the specific disease.
• Tetanus is a life-threatening disease with a prolonged recovery phase and intensive supportive care.

MISCELLANEOUS

ASSOCIATED CONDITIONS

N/A

AGE RELATED FACTORS

N/A

ZOONOTIC POTENTIAL

N/A

PREGNANCY

Systemic absorption of topically applied medication is possible. Benefits of treatment should be considered against any risks posed to the fetus.

SYNONYMS

N/A

SEE ALSO

• Conjunctival diseases
• Ocular/adnexal squamous cell carcinoma
• Corneal ulceration
• Ulcerative keratomycosis
• Corneal stromal abscesses
• Tetanus
• Hyperkalemic periodic paralysis

Suggested Reading

Brooks DE. Ophthalmology for the Equine Practitioner. Jackson, WY; Teton NewMedia, 2002.
Brooks DE, Matthews AG. Equine ophthalmology. In: Gelatt KN, ed. Veterinary Ophthalmology, ed 4. Philadelphia; Lippincott Williams and Wilkins, 2007.
Gilger BC, ed. Equine Ophthalmology. Philadelphia; WB Saunders, 2005.

Authors Heidi M. Denis and Dennis E. Brooks
Consulting Editor Dennis E. Brooks

DISORDERS OF SEXUAL DEVELOPMENT

BASICS

DEFINITION/OVERVIEW

- Sexual differentiation occurs sequentially at three levels:
  - Genetic
  - Gonadal
  - Phenotypic
- Errors at any level lead to varying degrees of genital ambiguity and aberrant reproductive function.
- Affected animals are known as intersexes or as particular classes of hermaphrodites.
  - True hermaphrodites or pseudohermaphrodites
  - The latter is further divided into male and female pseudohermaphrodites.

ETIOLOGY/PATHOPHYSIOLOGY

- Genetic sex is established at fertilization.
- Gonadal sex is controlled by genetic sex determination.
- Phenotypic sex is governed by gonadal function and target-organ sensitivity.

Disorders of Genetic Sex

- *Sex chromosomes*:
  - Abnormal number (aneuploidy)
  - Abnormal structure (deletion, duplication/insertion, reciprocal exchange, fusion, inversion)
- *Chimeras*—individual with coexisting, genetically distinct cell populations admixed *in utero* from different genetic sources
- *Mosaics*—individual with coexisting, genetically distinct cell populations caused by errors in chromosomal segregation during division of a single genetic source
- Normality of genetic sex development depends on normality of sex chromosomal pairings during gametogenesis and fertilization.
- Spontaneous errors affecting gonadal development may occur early during embryonic life.
- *Sry* gene initiates testicular development:
  - If present, the animal develops testicular tissue regardless of the number of X chromosomes present.
- 63, XO (most common)—ovarian dysgenesis, infantile tubular genitalia, small stature, phenotypic female; similar to Turner's syndrome in humans
- 65, XXY—hypoplastic testes, genitalia normal to hypoplastic, phenotypic male; similar to Klinefelter's syndrome in humans
- Numerous possible combinations (mixoploidies) are reported.

Disorders of Gonadal Sex

- *Sex reversal syndromes*—gonadal and genetic sex may disagree because of autosomal recessive genes or translocation of TDF to X chromosomes.
- XY with no testes—hypoplastic ovary/streak gonad; acyclic, sterile; female phenotype, but is XY female
- XX with varying degrees of testicular development—extreme form is XX male; otherwise, a true hermaphrodite forms.
- True hermaphrodite with ovotestes—ambiguous genitalia; named by genetic makeup, either XX or XY

Disorders of Phenotypic Sex

- Genetic and gonadal sex are in agreement; ambiguous external genitalia are present.
- Phenotypic sex development involves differentiation of tubular genitalia. (mesonephric and paramesonephric ducts) and external genitalia under direction of the gonad.
- Degree of masculinization of external genitalia relates to the proportion of testicular tissue and hence testosterone production of the intersex gonad.
- Male reproductive tract—gonad must produce testosterone (Leydig cells) and Müllerian-inhibitory substance (Sertoli cells) at correct time.
- Target organ (duct system) must have cytosolic receptors for testosterone and enzyme 5α-reductase to produce dihydrotestosterone, the androgen responsible for tubular and external genitalia differentiation.
- Hypospadia—Urethra opens ventrally on penis.
- Epispadia—Urethra opens dorsally on penis.
- Pseudohermaphrodite—named by the gonadal tissue present; male, testes; female, ovary
- Testicular feminization—genetic and gonadal male (XY chimera, testicle) but external genitalia female; target-organ insensitivity

SYSTEMS AFFECTED

- Reproductive
- Urinary

GENETICS

See Etiology/Pathophysiology.

INCIDENCE/PREVALENCE

N/A

SIGNALMENT

- Congenital disorder, by definition, means present at birth.
- Normal external genitalia may delay detection of problem until the affected individual enters a breeding program.

SIGNS

Historical

- Infertility; sterility
- Failure to display appropriate reproductive behavior with opposite sex; attraction to same sex

Physical Examination

External

- Female—normal or hypoplastic vulva; enlarged clitoris; presence of os clitoris; purulent vulvar discharge
- Male—penis, prepuce normal or hypoplastic; testes, scrotal or cryptorchid; hypospadia, epispadia (abnormal position of urinary orifice, closure of urethra)

Internal

- Abnormal gonadal position (cryptorchid), form (hypoplastic, fibrous) or type (ovotestis)
- Aberrant ductal derivatives—aplasia, hypoplasia, or cysts

CAUSES

- Congenital—heritable or spontaneous
- Genetic abnormalities—zygote fusion, abnormal sex chromosome number or structure. Transfer of TDF to autosomal chromosome
- Placental admixture not reported in equines
- Exogenous—steroid hormone use during pregnancy
- Progestins, androgens—masculinize females
- Estrogens, antiandrogens—feminize males

RISK FACTORS

N/A

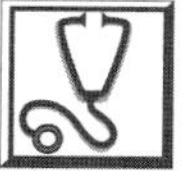

DIAGNOSIS

DIFFERENTIAL DIAGNOSIS

If phenotypically normal:

- Infectious infertility
- Noninfectious infertility—female, ovarian degeneration, endometrial degeneration; male, testicular hypoplasia or degeneration

CBC/BIOCHEMISTRY/URINALYSIS

Unremarkable, unless cystitis or infection results from aberrant genital structure

OTHER LABORATORY TESTS

Hormonal Assays

Testosterone

- Testosterone in XY mares correlates with phenotype and behavior.
- hCG challenge—baseline blood sample; administer 3000 IU hCG; additional blood samples at 3 and 24 hr.
- An increase in testosterone indicates testicular tissue is present, Leydig cell production

Estrone Sulfate

- Source in male is the testicles, Sertoli cells.
- Couple estrone sulfate test with testosterone levels (from an hCG challenge test) to improve diagnostic accuracy.

Immunology

- Test for 5alpha reductase or cytosolic receptor
- Use labial skin only; receptors are site-specific.

IMAGING

- U/S coupled with TRP; discovery of mass (neoplastic) or cyst (segmental aplasia with fluid dilations)
- Laparoscopy, laparotomy

OTHER DIAGNOSTIC PROCEDURES

PATHOLOGICAL FINDINGS

- Disorders are characterized by histopathology of gonad, morphology of tubular genitalia (duct derivatives), accessory glands (male), and external genitalia (increased anogenital distance, vulval folds, blind ended vagina).
- Karyotyping—culture of peripheral blood leukocytes and examination of metaphase spreads:
    - Collect whole blood in heparin or ACD.
    - Send samples unrefrigerated, by rapid courier.
    - Cultures require 48–72 hr.
- PCR
- Detection of *Sry*—whole blood in EDTA

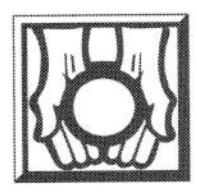

TREATMENT

APPROPRIATE HEALTH CARE

N/A, unless resulting pathology or physical/behavioral problems develop that require gonadectomy or hysterectomy to modify behavior

NURSING CARE

N/A

ACTIVITY

N/A

DIET

N/A

CLIENT EDUCATION

Some conditions are heritable and pedigree analysis is warranted in these cases.

SURGICAL CONSIDERATIONS

See Appropriate Health Care.

MEDICATIONS

DRUG(S) OF CHOICE, CONTRAINDICATIONS, PRECAUTIONS, POSSIBLE INTERACTIONS, ALTERNATIVE DRUGS

N/A

FOLLOW-UP

PATIENT MONITORING

Only if physical or behavioral complications develop

PREVENTION/AVOIDANCE

Remove carrier animals from the breeding population; gonadectomy

POSSIBLE COMPLICATIONS

N/A

EXPECTED COURSE AND PROGNOSIS

N/A

MISCELLANEOUS

ASSOCIATED CONDITIONS

If not detected early—

- Pyometra
- Cystitis
- Hematuria
- Gonadal neoplasia (intra-abdominal testis)

AGE-RELATED FACTORS

Congenital

ZOONOTIC POTENTIAL

N/A

PREGNANCY

Fertility is rare in affected animals.

SYNONYMS

- Hermaphrodite
- Intersex
- Klinefelter's syndrome, trisomy
- Mesonephric, wolffian
- Paramesonephric, müllerian
- Pseudohermaphrodite
- Turner's syndrome, monosomy X

ABBREVIATIONS

- ACD = acid citrate dextrose
- hCG = human chorionic gonadotropin
- *Sry* = sex-determining region of the Y chromosome
- TDF = testis-determining factor
- TRP = transrectal palpation
- U/S = ultrasound, ultrasonography

Suggested Reading

Bannasch D, Rinaldo C, Millon L, Latson K, Spangler T, Hubberty S, Galuppo L, Lowenstine L. SRY negative 64, XX intersex phenotype in an American saddlebred horse. Equine Vet J 2007;173:437–439.

Bowling AT, Hughes JP. Cytogenetic abnormalities. In: McKinnon AO, Voss JL, eds. Equine reproduction. Malvern: Lea & Febiger, 1993:258–265.

Chandley AC, Fletcher J, Rossdale PD, Peace CK, Ricketts SW, McEnery RJ, Thorne JP, Short RV, Allen WR. Chromosome abnormalities as a cause of infertility in mares. J Reprod Fertil Suppl 1975;23:377–383.

Halnan CR. Equine cytogenetics—role in equine veterinary practice. Equine Vet J 1985;17:173–177.

Kent MG, Schneller HE, Hegsted RL, Johnston SD, Wachtel SS. Concentration of serum testosterone in XY sex reversed horses. J Endocrinol Invest 1988;11:609–613.

Meyers-Wallen VN. Normal sexual development and intersex conditions in domestic animals. In: Proc Reprod Pathol Symp ACT/SFT 1997;18–28.

Meyers-Wallen VN, Hurtgen J, Schlafer D, et al. *Sry* XX true hermaphroditism in asa Fino horse. Equine Vet J 1997; 29:404–408.

Milliken JE, Paccamonti DL, Shoemaker S, Green WH. XX male pseudohermaphroditism in a horse. J Am Vet Med Assoc 1995;207:77–79.

Author Peter R. Morresey
Consulting Editor Carla L. Carleton

DISORDERS OF THE THYROID: HYPO- AND HYPERTHYROIDISM

BASICS

PATHOPHYSIOLOGY

• The thyroid gland is responsible for the synthesis of the thyroid hormones thyroxine (T_4) and triiodothyronine (T_3). These hormones are carried into target cells and result in a vast number of effects. The final result is regulation of resting metabolic rate in adult animals. In growing animals, thyroid hormones are essential for proper growth and maturation of the skeleton, respiratory tract, and other body systems.
• The net effect of hypothyroidism is decreased basal metabolic rate and decreased ability to respond to metabolic demands.
• Animals with systemic disease can exhibit the "euthyroid sick" syndrome—circulating thyroid hormone concentrations are reduced despite the presence of a normal thyroid axis. In these instances, the decreased thyroid concentrations are a response by the diseased animal that decreases the resting metabolic rate and thus conserves energy.
• In utero, thyroid hormones are necessary for proper bone, pulmonary, and nervous system development. Foals born with congenital hypothyroidism often have limb deformities caused by incomplete development of the carpal and tarsal bones, other skeletal deformities. They are often weak, with respiratory insufficiency.
• Hyperthyroidism caused by either an overdose of exogenous hormone or a secreting thyroid tumor produces an increased metabolic rate that manifests as weight loss and behavioral changes.

DEFINITION

• T_3 and T_4 are the hormones produced by the thyroid gland.
• Once excreted into the circulation, >99% is bound to circulating proteins (primarily albumin).
• Protein-bound thyroxine acts as a reservoir to maintain a steady supply of free T_4, which diffuses into cells, where it is deiodinated to form T_3. Similarly, the majority of circulating T_3 is protein bound, and the free T_3 is the biologically active form.
• Increased amounts of T_3 and T_4 in the circulation lead to hyperthyroidism, whereas decreased amounts results in hypothyroidism. Both are pathological conditions.
• Goiter is defined as an increase in thyroid size to twice its normal volume.

SYSTEM AFFECTED

Endocrine/Metabolic

• The endocrine system is primarily affected by abnormal T_3 and T_4; however, because thyroid hormones have such widespread effects, many other body systems are affected as well.
• Energy metabolism is altered by hypothyroidism, and affected horses have increased serum cholesterol and metabolize lipid poorly.

Musculoskeletal

• In foals with congenital hypothyroidism, the musculoskeletal system is dramatically affected.
• Affected foals are born with underdeveloped tarsal and carpal bones, prognathism, ruptured common digital extensor tendons, and forelimb contracture.
• Affected foals are often weak and need assistance to stand.
• Adult horses have an increased incidence of myositis and muscle abnormalities.

Behavioral

• Horses with abnormal thyroid levels may have altered behavior.
• Increased aggression and lethargy have been attributed to hypothyroidism.
• Nervousness and pacing have been attributed to hyperthyroidism.

Cardiovascular

• Thyroidectomized horses have bradycardia and decreased cardiac output, which results in exercise intolerance.
• Immature respiratory tract and respiratory insufficiency have been reported in hypothyroid foals.

SIGNALMENT

• No sex or breed predilections for abnormal T_3/T_4 levels.
• Hypothyroidism can occur at any age and exist in utero, with the foal showing characteristic signs at birth.
• Iatrogenic hyperthyroidism generally occurs in adults.
• Disease caused by thyroid tumors occurs in old horses (>10 years).

SIGNS

• Common clinical signs in foals born with congenital hypothyroidism—prognathism, ruptured common digital extensor tendon, forelimb contracture, retarded ossification and crushing of the carpal and tarsal bones, weakness, and poor suckle reflex.
• Less common clinical signs in foals born with congenital hypothyroidism—goiter, angular limb deformities, respiratory distress, abdominal hernia, poor muscle development, and osteoporosis.
• Hypothermia and bradycardia are consistent findings in adults with hypothyroidism.
• Other signs in adults associated with hypothyroidism include myositis, anhydrosis, laminitis, infertility, agalactia, poor hair coat, and poor growth.
• Horses with experimentally induced hypothyroidism develop edema of the distal limbs and coarsened features.
• The horse described with hyperthyroidism exhibited a thyroid tumor, weight loss, pacing, and nervousness.

CAUSES

• Many factors can lead to decreased blood thyroid hormone levels.
• Certain drugs, including phenylbutazone, iodine-containing compounds, corticosteroids, and sulfa drugs, may cause low serum levels.
• Ingestion of endophyte-containing fescue, high or low iodine levels, or high-carbohydrate diets can decrease circulating hormone levels.
• In most instances of hypothyroidism in adults, the cause is unknown.
• Iodine deficiency can cause hypothyroidism in horses, but this is extremely rare.
• Iodine deficiency or excess in the diets of broodmares can cause hypothyroidism in their foals; ingestion of endophyte-infected fescue also can result in congenital hypothyroidism.
• Training can decrease thyroid hormone levels. Some racehorses even have no detectable T_4 in their blood yet exhibit no signs of thyroid deficiency.
• Rarely, thyroid tumors cause hypothyroidism or hyperthyroidism in adults. In most instances, thyroid tumors are clinically silent. Debilitated horses or those with other severe diseases often have T_4 and T_3 levels < the reference ranges, which is termed *euthyroid sick syndrome*.
• Foals have increased thyroid hormone levels compared to old horses.
• Very cold weather also can lead to higher thyroid hormone levels.

RISK FACTORS

• Primarily dietary
• Excess or inadequate iodine or ingestion of other goitrogens can lead to hypothyroidism.
• In old horse populations, thyroid tumor is a risk factor for thyroid abnormalities.

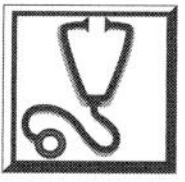

DIAGNOSIS

DIFFERENTIAL DIAGNOSIS

• The primary differential diagnosis for adults with suspected hypothyroidism is a pituitary tumor (i.e., equine Cushing's disease) or insulin resistance (equine metabolic syndrome); these horses, however, may have euthyroid sick syndrome. The "classic" presentation of hypothyroidism in adult horses—weight gain, laminitis, "cresty neck," and abnormal fat deposits—is now recognized as manifestations of idiopathic insulin resistance. Circulating thyroid hormone concentrations are normal in the vast majority of instances in these cases.
• Hypothyroidism can be ruled out by provocative testing with either TSH or TRH. A history of administration of a drug that decreases thyroid hormone values can explain abnormally low T_3 and T_4 levels not caused by true disease. A history of over administration of an exogenous thyroid supplement can explain abnormally high T_3 and T_4 levels.
• Differentials for foals with congenital hypothyroidism include fescue toxicosis, prematurity, angular limb deformities, and sepsis. Dietary history rules out abnormal iodine in the dam's diet. Physical examination and CBC should rule in sepsis or prematurity/dysmaturity without hypothyroidism.

LABORATORY FINDINGS

Drugs That May Alter Laboratory Results

N/A

Disorders That May Alter Laboratory Results

N/A

Valid If Run in Human Lab?

Laboratory determination of T_3, free T_3, T_4, and free T_4 is valid. Human thyroid values are commonly higher than equine; therefore use equine reference ranges to interpret results. Free T_3 and T_4 should be determined using the

DISORDERS OF THE THYROID: HYPO- AND HYPERTHYROIDISM

equilibrium dialysis method for most accurate results.

CBC/BIOCHEMISTRY URINALYSIS

Hypothyroid horses may exhibit anemia, leukopenia, and hypercholesterolemia.

OTHER LABORATORY TESTS

To confirm the diagnosis of hypothyroidism, consider provocative testing with a TRH or TSH response test. TSH is currently not readily available, but for a TRH stimulation test, give 1 mg TRH IV. Collect blood for T_3 and T_4 determination 0, 2, and 4 hr later. One expects to see baseline T_3 and T_4 in the reference range, the T_3 double at 2 hr, and T_4 to double at 4 hr.

IMAGING

Ultrasonography

- Imaging rarely is useful in diagnosing hypothyroidism.
- An enlarged thyroid gland caused by tumor or goiter could be seen via ultrasound.

Radiography

An enlarged thyroid gland caused by tumor or goiter might be seen as increased soft-tissue density on radiographs of the throat-latch area.

DIAGNOSTIC PROCEDURES

A fine-needle aspiration or biopsy may assist with assessing the thyroid gland.

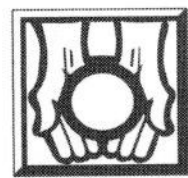

TREATMENT

APPROPRIATE HEALTH CARE

- Foals with congenital hypothyroidism may require inpatient medical management if the disease is severe.
- All other horses with abnormal T_3 and T_4 levels can be treated on an outpatient basis.

NURSING CARE

- Foals may need assistance standing and milk administered via nasogastric tube if they are too weak to suckle.
- Foals may need mechanical ventilation if they cannot ventilate on their own.
- Animals with poor hair coat may need blanketing, and cold temperatures should be avoided.

ACTIVITY

Limit activity in foals with musculoskeletal deformities—incomplete ossification of the carpal or tarsal bones.

DIET

- Examine the diet of any horse with hypothyroidism and the dams of foals born with hypothyroidism to ensure the proper amount of iodine is being fed.
- Pregnant mares should not receive endophyte-infected fescue hay, particularly during their last months of gestation or iodine supplementation.

CLIENT EDUCATION

- Prognosis for soundness is poor in most foals suffering from congenital hypothyroidism and should be discussed with owners before initiating expensive treatments.
- Adult horses with hypothyroidism respond well to exogenous replacement hormone, and their prognosis is generally good.
- Horses with hyperthyroidism should have their dose of thyroid supplement decreased.
- Animals that are euthyroid despite low blood T_3 and T_4 levels should have their primary disease treated, but do not require hormone supplementation.

SURGICAL CONSIDERATIONS

If the cause of increased or decreased T_3 and T_4 concentrations is a tumor of the thyroid gland, surgical removal of the affected thyroid lobe should be curative.

MEDICATIONS

DRUG(S) OF CHOICE

For decreased T_3 and T_4 levels caused by hypothyroidism, replacement therapy with thyroxine 20 μg/kg maintains T_4 and T_3 levels in the normal range for 24 hr; this constitutes a dose of 10 mg in a 1000-lb horse.

CONTRAINDICATIONS

When low resting T_3 and T_4 values exist because of some other severe disease (e.g., euthyroid sick syndrome), thyroid replacement therapies may cause further deterioration of the horse's condition. Thus, perform provocative testing to establish the diagnosis of hypothyroidism.

PRECAUTIONS

Exogenous thyroid hormones causes downregulation and, potentially, atrophy of the thyroid gland; gradually discontinue the hormone supplement over the course of several weeks.

POSSIBLE INTERACTIONS

N/A

ALTERNATIVE DRUGS

Other sources of thyroid hormone replacement—iodinated casein (5.0 g/day) and concentrated bovine thyroid extract (10 g/day)

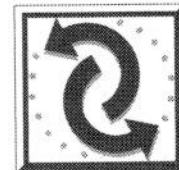

FOLLOW-UP

PATIENT MONITORING

- Monitor horses on thyroid supplement by measuring serum T_4 and T_3 levels every 30–60 days. If the serum levels are low, increase the dose of supplemetation until serum levels reach normal range; if the serum levels are too high or in the higher end of the normal range, decrease the dosage and retested in 30–60 days.
- Reconsider the original diagnosis if the patient fails to respond clinically after 6 weeks of therapy.

POSSIBLE COMPLICATIONS

N/A

MISCELLANEOUS

ASSOCIATED CONDITIONS

- Angular limb deformities, hypognathism, weakness, and respiratory distress often are associated with congenital hypothyroidism.
- Infertility and myositis have been associated with hypothyroidism in adults.
- Phenylbutazone is associated with low T_3 and T_4 levels.
- Euthyroid sick syndrome is associated with debilitating diseases including equine Cushing's disease.

AGE-RELATED FACTORS

- Higher T_3 and T_4 levels are normal in neonatal foals. Levels are highest at birth (10 adult levels), then decrease rapidly in the first weeks of life to adult levels.
- Resting T_3 and T_4 levels decline gradually over the life of a horse, and levels in old horses may be lower than those in younger animals.

ZOONOTIC POTENTIAL

N/A

PREGNANCY

N/A

SEE ALSO

- TRH and TSH stimulation tests

ABBREVIATIONS

- TRH = thyroid-releasing hormone
- TSH = thyroid-stimulating hormone

Suggested Reading

Allen AL, Doige CE, Fretz PB, *et al.* Congenital hypothyroidism, dysmaturity, and musculoskeletal lesions in Western Canadian foals. Proc AAEP 1993;39:207–208.

Breuhaus BA, Refsal KR, Beyerlein SL. Measurement of free thyroxine concentration in horses by equilibrium dialysis. J. Vet. Int. Med. 2006:20;371–6.

Frank N, Sojka J., Equine thyroid dysfunction, Vet Clin. North America, 2002:18:305–319.

Author Janice Sojka

Consulting Editor Michel Lévy

DISSEMINATED INTRAVASCULAR COAGULATION

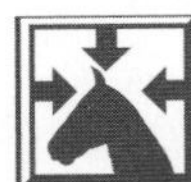

BASICS

DEFINITION

- Disseminated intravascular coagulation (DIC) is an acquired coagulation dysfunction characterized by a marked activation of the blood coagulation system that causes excessive thrombin activation, fibrin formation, and widespread intravascular fibrin deposition.
- The exaggerated activation of coagulation and subsequent deposition of microthrombi can lead to:
  - Ischemic lesions in organs and development of multiorgan failure
  - A depletion of platelets and coagulation factors (consumption coagulopathy), which may cause secondary profuse bleeding
- DIC is a syndrome that is always secondary to a severe underlying disorder, such as endotoxemia.

PATHOPHYSIOLOGY

- The underlying diseases induce platelet activation and an excessive formation of thrombin, but also may induce endothelial damage, inhibition of coagulation inhibitors, and defective fibrinolysis. These simultaneously occurring mechanisms ultimately produce the uncontrolled fibrin deposition and consumptive coagulation.
- Depending on the severity and duration of the underlying disorder and coagulation activation, 2 clinical forms of DIC can be observed:
  - The multiorgan failure form of DIC occurs when activation of coagulation is severe and fibrinolytic activity is inhibited. The widespread fibrin formation and microthrombi deposition in the microcirculation produce ischemic damage to tissues, which may contribute to MODS and MOFS.
  - The hemorrhagic form of DIC occurs when activation of coagulation is not as severe and the excessive formation of fibrin can be arrested by the fibrinolytic system. However when the above process is prolonged, the increased consumption of coagulation factors and platelet depletion may produce a consumptive coagulopathy and a subsequent hypocoagulable state, in which bleeding diatheses are the most evident clinical sign.
- Although there is debate regarding the contribution of the marked intravascular fibrin deposition to organ failure and mortality, there is ample evidence to indicate that DIC contributes to multiple organ failure. Histological studies, using specific stains for fibrin, demonstrate the presence of marked fibrin deposition in most capillaries of various organs.

SYSTEMS AFFECTED

- Hemic/lymphatic/immune; excessive fibrin formation and deposition occurs in blood vessels. Hypercoagulation may also induce vessel thrombosis after continuous endothelial damage associated with venipunctures or catheters (i.e., jugular thrombosis).
- Other systems may be affected depending on the organ affected by deposition of microthrombi, and/or the sites of hemorrhage. The most frequently affected organs are: cardiovascular (shock, cardiac arrhythmias), respiratory (pulmonary thromboembolism and hypoxemia), renal/urologic (azotemia), GIT (colic), hepatobiliary (increase in plasma hepatic enzymes and liver dysfunction).

INCIDENCE/PREVALENCE

- DIC is the most frequent hemostatic disorder of the horse. It has been reported in 55% of the ischemic and 36% of the severe inflammatory GIT disorders.
- DIC is also diagnosed in many septic newborn foals (>50%).

SIGNALMENT

Any sex, breed, and age may be affected.

SIGNS

General Comments

Clinical signs include those of the underlying disease and those of DIC.

Historical

They depend on the underlying disease.

Physical Examination

- In the MOFS form of DIC, horses may demonstrate clinical signs referable to the affected organ including hypotension, dyspnea, tachypnea, olyguria, colic, cardiac arrhythmias, etc.
- In cases of the hemorrhagic form of DIC, horses may have hemorrhagic diatheses, with excessive bleeding after wound or minor trauma, petechiations, or spontaneous bleeding from mucous membranes (i.e., epistaxis, melena).
- Catheter- and venipuncture-site thrombosis is common.

CAUSES

- Ischemic GIT disorders (e.g., small intestinal volvulus, large colon torsion)
- Inflammatory GIT disorders (e.g., colitis, anterior enteritis)
- Endotoxemia
- Neonatal septicemia
- Heat stroke
- Less commonly associated conditions include severe hemolysis, disseminated neoplasia, and other systemic inflammatory conditions (e.g., snake bite).

RISK FACTORS

Any disease or treatment that severely activates platelets and/or coagulation pathways, inhibits the fibrinolytic system, or causes significant endothelial damage

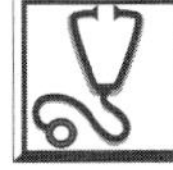

DIAGNOSIS

DIFFERENTIAL DIAGNOSIS

- The MOFS form of DIC requires differentiation from other causes of hypotension, renal failure, hypoxemia, etc.
- The hemorrhagic form of DIC requires differentiation from other coagulation deficiencies (acquired or inherited).

CBC/BIOCHEMISTRY/URINALYSIS

- Thrombocytopenia (<100,000 platelets/μL) due to platelet consumption
- Decrease in mean platelet component, which is consistent with platelet activation
- Other alterations in the CBC may be found associated with the underlying disease (e.g., neutropenia due to endotoxemia).
- In cases of MODS or MOFS, plasma biochemistry abnormalities may be detected depending on organ dysfunction (e.g., increase in creatinine, BUN, liver enzymes, etc).

OTHER LABORATORY TESTS

- Diagnosis of DIC may be achieved by demonstrating activation of the coagulation system.
- Laboratory evidence may include:
  - Procoagulant activation can be demonstrated using markers of thrombin generation, such as thrombin-antithrombin complexes (TAT). Elevations of their plasma concentrations are considered very sensitive indicators of DIC. However, their usefulness is limited because their testing is not widely available in veterinary diagnostic laboratories.
  - A consumptive coagulopathy, consistent with hypercoagulation, may be detected by evaluation of clotting times (PT and aPTT). Prolongation of clotting times sensitively detects consumptive coagulation, but it is not specific for DIC. A decrease in fibrinogen concentration is also consistent with clotting factor consumption.
  - Fibrinolytic activation results in increased plasma D-dimer concentration and is consistent with hyperfibrinolysis secondary to hypercoagulation. In DIC patients, plasma D-dimer concentration may be >2000 ng/mL. This test is considered a sensitive marker for DIC, although it has low specificity. Fibrin(ogen) degradation products (FDPs) have also been used to assess fibrinolysis, but this test is less reliable than evaluation of D-dimer concentration. Therefore, their use in clinical settings is being reduced.
  - Coagulation inhibitor consumption may be measured through a decrease in plasma concentrations of antithrombin activity and protein C. This consumption of inhibitors is consistent with severe hypercoagulation.
- No single laboratory test, that is routinely available, is sufficiently sensitive or specific to enable a diagnosis of DIC. Therefore, a diagnosis of DIC requires a combination of these laboratory findings (e.g., thrombocytopenia, prolonged clotting times, increased D-dimers, and reduced antithrombin and fibrinogen) in conjunction with appropriate clinical signs.

PATHOLOGICAL FINDINGS

- Serosal petechiations and ecchymoses may be evident on post-mortem examination.
- Thrombosis may be observed (infrequently) in gross examination, but microthrombosis is commonly misdiagnosed on histological examinations when using routine stains.
- Specific histochemical (PTAH) or immunohistochemical stains are required to accurately detect fibrin deposition in capillaries of different organs. The tissues most commonly reported to contain fibrin depositions are lungs, kidneys, and liver.

DISSEMINATED INTRAVASCULAR COAGULATION

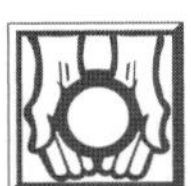

TREATMENT

AIMS OF TREATMENT

- The keystone for treatment of DIC is to control the underlying disease causing the severe, hypercoagulable state.
- The second aim is to control the hypercoagulable state (and subsequent consumptive coagulopathy).
- The mortality rate of DIC is low if patients are diagnosed and treated during the early stages of disease, but becomes high when multiorgan failure and/or bleeding diatheses are present. Thus, a primary objective for management of DIC is to treat patients at risk of DIC in order to reduce hypercoagulation from developing.
- Supportive therapy is also required for horses with DIC to reduce microthrombi deposition and secondary organ dysfunction and/or failure.

APPROPRIATE HEALTH CARE

DIC always requires emergency hospitalization and intensive care management.

NURSING CARE

- Fresh plasma (or fresh frozen plasma) transfusion (15–30 mL/kg) is only required in cases with severe consumptive coagulopathy and bleeding diatheses. This treatment slows progression of DIC and may help improve metabolic derangements caused by some primary diseases (e.g., the hypoalbuminemia in colitis).
- Low dose heparin therapy has also been given to patients with DIC added to the transfusion bags. However, the high cost of plasma transfusions and the poor prognosis of the hemorrhagic form of DIC makes this treatment difficult and impractical in horses. Horses with DIC may require intensive fluid therapy to control shock, improve tissue blood supply and reduce multiorgan failure. Crystalloid solutions (e.g., lactated Ringer's solution) are commonly used, but colloidal solutions (e.g., hetastarch) may also be indicated.

ACTIVITY

Totally limited as required for patients in intensive care

DIET

According to restrictions/prescriptions associated with the underlying disease (e.g., inflammatory or ischemic GIT disorders affecting small or large intestine)

SURGICAL CONSIDERATIONS

Only if the underlying disorder requires surgery (i.e., ischemic GIT problems)

MEDICATIONS

DRUG(S) OF CHOICE

- Drug treatment will include those required for the underlying disease, such as low-dose flunixin meglumine therapy for cases of endotoxemia or antibiotics in cases of neonatal septicemia.
- Antithrombotics (e.g., heparin) are administered during the early stages of DIC to reduce the excessive coagulation activation during the early stages of DIC. They are the most effective treatment for control of this disorder, although their administration has been considered controversial.
- LMWH (e.g., dalteparin, enoxaparin) are preferred as they do not produce many of the detrimental effects associated with unfractioned heparin (e.g., sodium heparin) such as erythrocyte agglutination. The safest dose of LMWH is 50 IU/kg of dalteparin SC q24h (or 0.5mg/kg of enoxaparin) over 3–4 days. If no LMWH is available, unfractioned heparin is recommended (40–100 IU/kg q12h). Sodium heparin may be administered SC or IV, but calcium heparin requires SC administration.
- The use of antiplatelet (e.g., aspirin) to reduce the hypercoagulable state has not been shown to be effective in horses (unlike humans or small animals). Differences in equine platelet function may explain this lower efficacy.

CONTRAINDICATIONS

- Antifibrinolytic drugs (e.g., aminocaproic acid) should not be used to reduce bleeding diatheses in patients with hemorrhagic episodes, as it reduces the main coagulation inhibitory system (fibrinolysis) and subsequently worsens hypercoagulation, microthrombi deposition and DIC.
- Hypertonic saline solution (7.5% NaCl) should not be used to control hypotension associated with an underlying disease (e.g., severe GIT disorders) as it may cause hemodilution of coagulation factors and thus increase the risk of bleeding.

POSSIBLE INTERACTIONS

Colloidal solutions may be administered to patients with DIC to treat the hypoalbuminemia caused by the underlying disease (e.g., colitis). Colloidal administration may reduce platelet function and may prolong hemorrhage. However, this effect might be considered beneficial to reduce excessive platelet activation.

FOLLOW-UP

PATIENT MONITORING

- Repeated physical examinations, with particular attention to evidence of MODS, MOFS, bleeding or venous thrombosis, should be performed.
- PT, aPTT, D-dimer concentration, and platelet counts should be closely monitored to assess clinical progression and effectiveness of treatment.
- In cases of MODS/MOFS, plasma biochemical parameters indicative of tissue dysfunction should be monitored (e.g., creatinine, BUN in case of renal failure, liver enzymes, etc).
- In cases where significant hemorrhage is observed, patients require similar monitoring to horses with acute hemorrhage.

POSSIBLE COMPLICATIONS

- MODS
- MOFS
- Shock
- Hypoxemia
- Acute renal failure
- Acute hepatic failure
- Cardiac arrhythmias
- Colic
- Laminitis
- Thrombophlebitis
- Fatal bleeding
- Death

EXPECTED COURSE AND PROGNOSIS

- In patients with clinical signs of DIC, prognosis is usually guarded to poor. Mortality rates are high due to the combination of DIC and the severity of the underlying disease.
- Prognosis is better if:
  - DIC is diagnosed at early stages of the disease.
  - Preventive treatment is effectively introduced.

MISCELLANEOUS

ASSOCIATED CONDITIONS

- Ischemic GIT disorders
- Colitis, proximal enteritis
- Septicemia in neonates
- Other systemic inflammatory disorders
- Heat stroke
- Others; severe hemolysis, disseminated neoplasia (i.e., melanosarcoma), etc.

SYNONYMS

Consumptive coagulopathy

SEE ALSO

- Coagulation defects, acquired
- Endotoxemia
- Septicemia, neonatal
- Thrombocytopenia
- Petechiae, ecchymoses, and hematomas

ABBREVIATIONS

- GIT = gastrointestinal tract
- LMWH = low-molecular weight heparin
- MODS = multiorgan dysfunction syndrome
- MOFS = multiorgan failure syndrome

Suggested Reading

Cotovio M, Monreal L, Navarro M, et al. Detection of fibrin deposits in tissues from horses with severe gastrointestinal disorders. J Vet Intern Med 2007;21:308–313.

Monreal L. Monitoring the coagulation disorder system. In: Corley K, Stephen J, eds. The Equine Hospital Manual. Oxford: Blackwell Publishing, 2008.

Monreal L, Aguilera E. Management of coagulation disorder in horses with coagulopathies. In: Corley K, Stephen J, eds. The Equine Hospital Manual. Oxford: Blackwell Publishing, 2008.

Author Luis Monreal

Consulting Editors Jennifer Hodgson and David Hodgson

DISTAL AND PROXIMAL INTERPHALANGEAL JOINT DISEASE

BASICS

OVERVIEW

- Any disease localized to the DIP or PIP
- The distal limb of the horse undergoes high stresses during locomotion.
- The DIP is a high-motion joint supported by collateral ligaments. During forward movement on flat ground, the joint flexes and extends. Circling, uneven ground, and/or an unbalanced foot results in sliding and rotation of the DIP. Any excessive or repetitive stress of the joint increases the occurrence of disease.
- The PIP is a low-motion joint supported by collateral ligaments, palmar ligaments, and the distal sesamoidean ligaments. Sliding and rotational forces are main contributing factors to joint disease.
- Any diseases involving the articular surface of the DIP or PIP (osteochondrosis, fractures, joint luxation) may result in osteoarthritis.
- Osteoarthritis of the DIP and PIP are commonly referred to as low ringbone and high ringbone, respectively.
- Musculoskeletal—foot (DIP) and pastern (PIP)

SIGNALMENT

- All breeds and types of horses
- Any age, although more common in middle-aged to older horses

SIGNS

- Lameness of variable degrees, often chronic, frequently progressive
- Lameness, frequently bilateral, although predominates in one limb
- Lameness may occur in any limb, but forelimbs are more common.
- Lameness is worse in circles or on hard ground.
- Resentment of distal limb flexion
- Dorsal proximal joint distension of the DIP, ballottement of joint fluid from medial to lateral midline
- Buttress foot (distortion of the dorsal distal pastern and dorsal hoof wall) in chronic DIP disease
- Firm periarticular outward swelling of the PIP in chronic disease

CAUSES AND RISK FACTORS

- Poor conformation
- Hoof imbalance
- Sports that require repetitive quick turns and abrupt stops, e.g., Western performance, polo, jumping
- Osteochondrosis of the DIP or PIP
- Articular fractures of first, second, or third phalanx

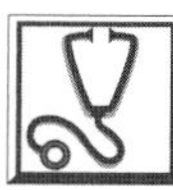

DIAGNOSIS

DIFFERENTIAL DIAGNOSIS

- Laminitis—Rule out with radiography.
- Other causes of forelimb lameness alleviated by DIP analgesia. The palmar pouch of the DIP is in close proximity to the palmar digital nerves. Analgesia of the DIP may diffuse to the nerves effectively anesthetizing their innervated structures. Differential include:
    - Navicular syndrome—Rule out with comprehensive imaging and additional selective nerve blocks (palmar digital analgesia and intra-articular analgesia of the navicular bursa)
    - Solar pain—Rule out with comprehensive imaging. Lameness may improve with application of foot pad.

CBC/CHEMISTRY/URINALYSIS

- None

OTHER LABORATORY TESTS

- None

IMAGING

- Radiography—In early or acute disease, radiographic evaluation may be normal. Periarticular osteophyte formation, loss of joint space, and subchondral bone sclerosis are signs of chronic disease.
- Ultrasonography—Desmitis of the collateral ligaments of the DIP can be a contributing factor for DIP disease. Desmitis of the collateral ligaments of the PIP, distal sesamoidean, or palmar pastern ligaments can be contributing factors for PIP disease.
- Nuclear scintigraphy—Generalized increased radiopharmaceutical uptake of the DIP or PIP may be apparent with advanced disease.
- MRI—Excellent imaging modality for assessment of subchondral bone, articular cartilage, and surrounding soft tissue structures of the foot.

OTHER DIAGNOSTIC PROCEDURES

- Diagnostic analgesia—Pain from the DIP will improve with palmar digital analgesia, abaxial analgesia, and intra-articular DIP analgesia. Pain from the PIP will improve with abaxial analgesia, palmar digital analgesia plus pastern ring block, and intra-articular PIP analgesia.
- Diagnostic arthroscopy—Limited visualization of the PIP and DIP. The dorsal and palmar pouches are accessible but challenging for osteochondral fragment removal.
- Synovial fluid analysis to rule out infectious arthritis

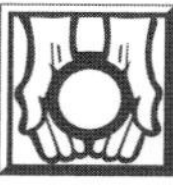

TREATMENT

- Rest periods from weeks to several months
- Restore hoof balance, shorten toe, and ease breakover of the foot.
- Intra-articular anti-inflammatory medication(s) of the DIP or PIP

DISTAL AND PROXIMAL INTERPHALANGEAL JOINT DISEASE

- Reduction in workload and expectations for the horse
- Arthroscopic removal of osteochondral fragmentation(s) when appropriate
- Surgical arthrodesis of the PIP joint is indicated in advanced disease. Three parallel screws placed in lag fashion, dorsal bone plate(s), or both have been used.
- Surgical arthrodesis of the DIP using lag screw fixation has been performed on a very limited basis for advanced disease.

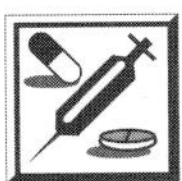

MEDICATIONS

DRUG(S)

- NSAIDs—phenylbutazone (2.2 mg/kg daily to BID for 7–10 days)
- Intra-articular corticosteroids—methylprednisolone acetate (20–40 mg) or triamcinolone (3–6 mg)
- Intra-articular sodium hyaluronate (10–20 mg)
- Combination of intra-articular corticosteroids and sodium hyaluronate
- Systemic chondroprotective drugs—polysulfated glycosaminoglycan (500 mg IM q4days for 7 treatments) or sodium hyaluronate (40 mg IV q7days for 3 treatments)
- Oral chondroprotective medications—glucosamine/chondrotin sulfate powder (1 scoop [3.3 grams] BID)

CONTRAINDICATIONS/POSSIBLE INTERACTIONS

- Intra-articular corticosteroid use is *not* recommended in horses with a previous history of laminitis.

FOLLOW-UP

PATIENT MONITORING

- Periodic lameness evaluation and radiographic assessment are recommended. In general, osteoarthritis of the DIP and PIP is progressive.

PREVENTION/AVOIDANCE

- Reduction in workload or alterative sport may slow the progression of disease.

POSSIBLE COMPLICATIONS

- Inability to perform expected sport due to chronic lameness

EXPECTED COURSE AND PROGNOSIS

- For PIP or DIP disease, early recognition and response to treatment may prolong the intended use of the horse.
- Osteoarthritis of the DIP or PIP is progressive and reduction in athletic soundness is expected.
- In chronic or advanced PIP disease, surgical arthrodesis is indicated. After arthrodesis, most horses with hindlimb and many horses with forelimb disease will return to athletic soundness.
- Horses with advanced DIP disease are candidates for retirement with or without surgical arthrodesis.

MISCELLANEOUS

ASSOCIATED CONDITIONS

- Older horses may have concurrent DIP disease and navicular syndrome.
- Horses may have a combination of osteoarthritis of the DIP and PIP.

AGE-RELATED FACTORS

- Most common in middle-aged horse

ZOONOTIC POTENTIALS

- None

SEE ALSO

- Osteoarthritis
- Osteochondrosis
- Navicular syndrome

ABBREVIATIONS

- DIP = distal interphalangeal joint
- PIP = proximal interphalangeal joint

Suggested Reading

Dyson SJ. The distal phalanx and distal interphalangeal joint. In: Ross MW, Dyson SJ, eds. Diagnosis and Management of Lameness in the Horse. St. Louis: Saunders, 2003:310–316.

Ruggles AJ. The proximal and middle phalanges and proximal interphalangeal joint. In: Ross MW, Dyson SJ, eds. Diagnosis and Management of Lameness in the Horse. St. Louis: Saunders, 2003:342–348.

Author Elizabeth J. Davidson
Consulting Editor Elizabeth J. Davidson

DISTAL TARSITIS

BASICS

OVERVIEW

- Lameness originating from pain from inflammation or osteochondral damage in the lower hock joints (DIT, TMT).
- Lay term for osteoarthritis of the distal tarsal joints is "bone spavin."
- The distal hock joints are low-motion joints and are prone to forces of compression and rotation. Excessive or repetitive forces result in inflammation and potentially osteoarthritis.
- Premature or dysmature neonates with delayed ossification of the small tarsal bones may develop "juvenile bone spavin."
- Musculoskeletal—hock (tarsus)

SIGNALMENT

- Any age horses but most common in middle-aged horses
- Horses used for athletic performance
- Rare in ponies, donkeys, mules, and draft breeds

SIGNS

Historical

- Intermittent and slowly progressive hindlimb lameness
- Usually bilateral but can be unilateral hindlimb lameness
- Warm out of the lameness during work
- Reduced performance such as increased time in speed events, resistance to stopping or turning correctly, reluctance to jump or collected work, difficulty maintaining/obtaining correct canter lead
- Dragging hind toes

Physical Examination

- Bony exostosis and/or heat on medial aspect of distal tarsal joints
- Lateral aspect of toe on hindlimb shoe is worn.
- "Stabbing" or "stabby" hindlimb gait
- Swing affected limb toward midline when walking or trotting
- Lameness worse after upper hindlimb flexion
- Painful to "Churchill test" (applying digital pressure to medial aspect of second metatarsal bone while the horse abducts the limb)

CAUSES AND RISK FACTORS

- Poor conformation: sickle or cow hocks, straight hindlimb, long toe-low heel hindlimb hoof conformation, height disparity between withers and croup
- Horses performing athletic activities that require jumping, abrupt stops, or excessive use of hindlimbs
- Delayed ossification of small tarsal bones
- Excessive exercise at a young age

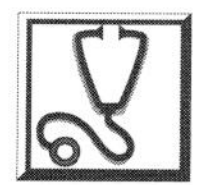

DIAGNOSIS

DIFFERENTIAL DIAGNOSIS

- Hindlimb proximal suspensory desmitis—Rule out with diagnostic analgesia and/or imaging.
- Stifle lameness—Rule out with diagnostic analgesia and/or imaging.
- Tarsocrural joint pain—Rule out with diagnostic analgesia and/or imaging.

IMAGING

Radiography

- Bony lesions can be subtle or absent in early disease.
- Periarticular osteophytes at the dorsal aspect of the joint(s), joint narrowing, subchondral sclerosis, and/or lysis
- Enthesiophye formation at the dorsal aspect of proximal third metatarsal bone
- In severe cases, extensive bone exostosis and ankylosis of the joints

Ultrasound

- Desmitis of the medial and lateral collateral ligaments
- Hindlimb suspensory desmitis should be ruled out.

Nuclear Scintigraphy

Generalized increased radiopharmaceutical uptake in the TMT and/or DIT

MRI

Tarsal bone edema and other subchondral bone injury

OTHER DIAGNOSTIC PROCEDURES

Diagnostic analgesia—intra-articular TMT and DIT or regional (peroneal/tibial) analgesia

PATHOLOGICAL FINDINGS

Ankylosis, bony lysis, and/or erosive cartilage lesions of DIT and/or TMT

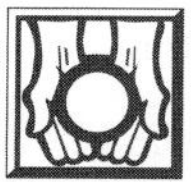

TREATMENTS

- Rest
- Restore hoof balance, shorten hind toes
- Intra-articular DIT and/or TMT anti-inflammatories
- Extracorporeal shockwave treatment
- Chemical arthrodesis of the distal tarsal joints in horses not responding to NSAIDs and intra-articular medications. Contrast arthrography prior to injection is required to ensure accurate intra-articular needle placement and assess proximal intertarsal joint communication. This method has fallen out

of favor due to severe pain and significant complications post injection.
- Surgical arthrodesis of the distal tarsal joints using subchondral forage and drilling across the distal tarsal joints. Stabilization of the joints with screws placed in lag fashion and cartilage ablation using Nd:YAG laser may facilitate ankylosis.
- Cunean tenectomy

MEDICATIONS

DRUG(S)
- NSAIDs—phenylbutazone (2.2 mg/kg daily to BID)
- Intra-articular corticosteroids—methylprednisolone acetate (20–40 mg) or triamcinolone (3–6 mg)
- Intra-articular sodium hyaluronate (10–20 mg)
- Combination of intra-articular corticosteroids and sodium hyaluronate
- Systemic chondroprotective drugs—polysulfated glycosaminoglycan (500 mg IM q4days for 7 treatments) or sodium hyaluronate (40 mg IV q7days for 3 treatments)
- Oral chondroprotective medications—glucosamine/chondrotin sulfate powder (1 scoop [3.3 g] BID)
- Intra-articular sodium monoiodoacetate (100 mg diluted in sterile saline)
- Chemical arthrodesis with ethyl alcohol has been used experimentally.

CONTRAINDICATIONS/POSSIBLE INTERACTIONS
- Intra-articular corticosteroids are not recommended in horses with previous history of laminitis.
- Chemical arthrodesis is contraindicated if the proximal intertarsal joint communicates with distal tarsal joints or tarsal sheath.
- Chemical arthrodesis may cause excessive edema and swelling or necrosis, joint sepsis, and severe post injection pain.

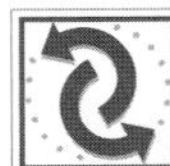

FOLLOW-UP

PATIENT MONITORING
- Lameness evaluation after intra-articular medications
- Periodic lameness evaluation for duration of athletic career
- Therapeutic trimming and shoeing every 6 weeks
- Radiographic assessment of tarsus 3–4 mo post chemical or surgical arthrodesis

PREVENTION/AVOIDANCE
Reduction or alterative workload

POSSIBLE COMPLICATIONS
- Laminitis can occur secondary to intra-articular medication with corticosteroids.
- Gastric ulceration, right dorsal colon inflammation or kidney damage secondary to chronic NSAIDs use
- Joint sepsis secondary to intra-articular medication
- Incomplete ankylosis and continued lameness
- Persistent soft tissue swelling, skin necrosis, and persistent lameness after chemical arthrodesis

EXPECTED COURSE AND PROGNOSIS
- Distal tarsitis is usually progressive but manageable with NSAIDs and/or periodic intra-articular medication(s). Many horses can return to previous athletic use with continued therapy.
- Distal intertarsal bone lysis carries a poor prognosis for returning to athletic use with medical therapy.
- After surgical arthrodesis by drilling and subchondral forage, 66% of horses return to their intended use but require 6–12 mo for ankylosis.
- Chemical arthrodesis should be used with caution due to possible postinjection complications.

MISCELLANEOUS

ASSOCIATED CONDITIONS
- Cunean bursitis
- Stifle disease (horses with straight hindlimb conformation)

AGE-RELATED CONDITIONS
- Middle-aged athletic horses
- +/− Young horses worked excessively

ABBREVIATIONS
- DIT = distal intertarsal joint
- Nd:YAG = neodymium:yttrium aluminum garnet laser
- TMT = tarsometatarsal joint

Suggested Reading

Jackman BA. Review of equine distal hock inflammation and arthritis. Int Am Assoc Equine Pract 2006;52:5–12.

Author Robin M. Dabareiner

Consulting Editor Elizabeth J. Davidson

DORSAL DISPLACEMENT OF THE SOFT PALATE

BASICS

OVERVIEW

• Horses are obligate nasal breathers, perhaps to allow maintenance of the olfactory senses during deglutition. The normal epiglottis is dorsal to the soft palate and contacts the caudal free margin, forming a tight seal around the base of the soft palate. The pillars of the soft palate converge dorsally, forming the palatopharyngeal arch. When the soft palate displaces dorsally, the epiglottis cannot be seen within the nasopharynx and is within the oropharynx, and the caudal free margin of the soft palate billows across the rima glottis during exhalation, creating airway obstruction.
• Results in a resistance to airflow during exhalation.
• Is a performance-limiting upper airway condition identified in 1.3% of 479 racehorses examined at rest. The true prevalence probably is higher, because palate displacement is a dynamic condition that most frequently occurs during intense exercise, making diagnosis at rest difficult. The prevalence of DDSP has been estimated to affect 10% of racehorses.
• This condition may be intermittent at exercise or permanent where the epiglottic cartilage is never seen dorsal to the soft palate.

SIGNALMENT

• This most common presentation is intermittent and is seen predominantly in racehorses and to a lesser degree in sport horses.
• The permanent form of this condition can affect all horse populations.

SIGNS

• Intermittent DDSP occurs in athletic horses during intense exercise.
• Usually associated with an abnormal upper respiratory noise during exhalation often referred to as gurgling.
• Approximately 10%–20% of horses with DDSP do not make a noise and are referred to as "silent displacers."
• Horses with intermittent DDSP generally have a history of exercise intolerance and may make a loud noise during exhalation; concurrent with these signs is open-mouth breathing.

CAUSES AND RISK FACTORS

The causes can be classified into two groups—(1) Intrinsic causes associated with structural abnormality of the nasopharynx such as subepiglottic cyst, subepiglottic masses, epiglottic cartilage deformity, epiglottitis, and palatal cyst or inflammation. It can also be due to decrease muscular activity of the palatinus and palatopharyngeus muscles as seen in horses with marked upper airway inflammation, guttural pouch disease and equine protozoal myelitis. (2) Extrinsic causes are those associated with factors affecting neuromuscular control of the position of the basihyoid bone and/or larynx such as caudal retraction of the larynx and dysfunction of the thyrohyoideus muscles.

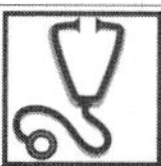

DIAGNOSIS

DIFFERENTIAL DIAGNOSIS

• When a noise is present it should be differentiated from with other expiratory upper airway obstruction such as epiglottic entrapment.
• Abnormal noise might not be present and because it is difficult to correlate the abnormal upper respiratory noise with the phase of respiration, any dynamic upper airway obstructions may need to be rule out such as laryngeal hemiplegia, arytenoid chondritis, vocal cord collapse, and aryepiglottic fold collapse. Endoscopy of the upper airway both at rest and while exercising on a treadmill may be required to differentiate these conditions from DDSP.
• Complete physical examination to rule out other causes of exercise intolerance–pulmonary disease, cardiac abnormalities, lameness, and neurologic disease

IMAGING

Lateral radiographs of the larynx/pharynx allow identification of soft palate displacement, the length of the epiglottic cartilage, and presence of subepiglottic and palatal cysts/mass. However these findings are more easily assessed by endoscopy.

DIAGNOSTIC PROCEDURES

• The diagnosis of intermittent DDSP is based on a history of sudden decrease in performance in the second half of the exercise intensity or competition and generally is associated with expiratory respiratory noise.

- Endoscopy of the upper airway at rest usually is normal. One can induce DDSP by inserting the endoscope in the proximal trachea and inciting the reflex of ventral displacement of the larynx or by a nasal occlusion test to mimic intense breathing efforts that occur during exercise. When the soft palate displaces dorsally, the epiglottis cannot be seen within the nasopharynx. The induction of DDSP is not an indicator of DDSP at exercise. Rather the difficulty in replacing the soft palate and the presence of an ulcer on the caudal edge of the soft palate are supportive of the condition.
- There is poor correlation with the observation of DDSP at rest and during exercise.
- To date, the best diagnostic test is treadmill endoscopy, in which the horse completes an incremental exercise test with the endoscope placed in the nasopharynx.

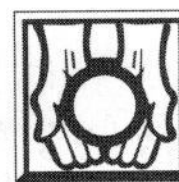

TREATMENT

- Treatment initially is directed at modifying or eliminating factors associated with the occurrence of DDSP.
- Condition and reevaluate unfit horses before considering surgery.
- If upper respiratory tract inflammation was diagnosed during the examination, treatment should include judicious use of systemic anti-inflammatory medication.
- Several surgical therapies and combination surgical therapies currently are performed as treatment—sternothyrohyoid myectomy, staphylectomy, procedures stiffening the soft palate (laser or cautery assisted or surgical imbrication), and combinations of these techniques. The most recent treatment introduced is a surgical repositioning of the larynx in a dorsal and forward position (laryngeal tie-forward) with transaction of the tendon of the muscles that apply caudal traction on the larynx (i.e., the sternothyroid muscles).

MEDICATIONS

DRUG(S) OF CHOICE

If upper airway inflammation is present a systemic course of anti-inflammatory agent may be indicated. For the average 450-kg horse, consider prednisolone (0.6 mg/kg PO BID for 14 days, 0.6 mg/kg PO daily for 14 days, and 0.6 mg/kg PO every other day for 14 days). Alternatively one may prescribe dexamethasone (PO or IV) 30 mg daily for 3 days, followed by 20 mg daily for 3 days, then 10 mg daily for 3 days, and 10 mg every other day for 3 treatments

CONTRAINDICATIONS/POSSIBLE INTERACTIONS

Previous episode of laminitis or equine protozoal myelitis

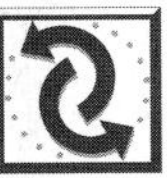

FOLLOW-UP

PATIENT MONITORING

Endoscopy 14–30 days after institution of medical treatment or 2–3 weeks after surgery.

POSSIBLE COMPLICATIONS

Tracheal aspiration of feed material is a possible complication after staphylectomy

EXPECTED COURSE AND PROGNOSIS

Prognosis after surgery is approximately 60%–80%.

MISCELLANEOUS

ASSOCIATED CONDITIONS

Pharyngitis

AGE-RELATED FACTORS

Higher prevalence in 2- to 3-year-olds

SEE ALSO

Dynamic collapse of the upper airway

Suggested Reading

Ducharme NG. Pharynx. In: Auer JA, Stick JA J, eds. Equine Surgery, ed 3. St. Louis: Saunders Elsevier, 2006:544–565.

Author Norm G. Ducharme
Consulting Editor Daniel Jean

DORSAL METACARPAL BONE DISEASE

BASICS

OVERVIEW

• Dorsal metacarpal bone disease, also known as "bucked shin complex," is stress related bone injury to the dorsal aspect of MCIII and occasionally MTIII. Two components of the disease are dorsal metacarpal periostitis ("bucked shins") and dorsal cortical stress fracture ("saucer fracture").
• High-strain cyclic fatigue causes decreased bone stiffness and the bone responds by adding new bone. "Bucked shin" is periosteal new bone formation along the dorsal aspect of MCIII. An MCIII with considerable periosteal new bone is less stiff and vulnerable to fatigue fracture. "Saucer fracture" is a fatigue fracture of the dorsal mid aspect of MCIII.
• Common racehorse disease in the United States and Australia and uncommon in the United Kingdom
• Musculoskeletal—dorsal MCIII, occasionally MTIII

SIGNALMENT

• Young (2- and 3-year-olds) healthy horses undergoing intense race training
• Thoroughbreds, Quarter Horses, Arabians, and uncommonly Standardbreds

SIGNS

• Sudden soreness, tenderness, or swelling of dorsal left or both MCIII following a high-speed workout ("breeze") or race
• Associated lameness, bilateral stiff or short, choppy forelimb gait
• Distinct dorsal convexity of MCIII when viewed from the lateral side
• "Saucer fractures" most commonly occur in left forelimb; focal swelling or bony knot along the dorsal or dorsolateral aspect of the mid MCIII

CAUSES AND RISK FACTORS

• Flat racing and race training
• Classically trained racehorses
• Race and training tracks with dirt surfaces
• Counterclockwise racing
• In Standardbreds, low incidence attributed to differences in speed and gait
• Most racehorses with a "saucer fracture" had previous episode of "bucked shins."

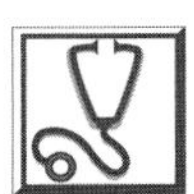

DIAGNOSIS

DIFFERENTIAL DIAGNOSIS

• Incomplete, longitudinal palmar MCIII cortical fracture—Rule out with radiography.
• Stress remodeling and stress fracture (avulsion fracture) of MCIII at the origin of the suspensory ligament—Rule out with radiography, nuclear scintigraphy, and ultrasonography.
• Periostitis due to direct trauma—Rule out with history of trauma.

IMAGING

Radiography

• "Bucked shins": periosteal roughening and/or thickening along dorsal and dorsomedial mid MCIII diaphysis
• "Saucer fracture": Short, oblique unicortical fracture in dorsal or dorsolateral MCIII cortex. Most fractures are diaphyseal and oriented dorsodistal to palmaroproximal, 30°–45° to the dorsal cortex.

Nuclear Scintigraphy

• "Bucked shins"—moderate to intense increased radiopharmaceutical uptake along the dorsal MCIII diaphysis
• "Saucer fracture"—focal increased radiopharmaceutical uptake ("hot spot") in dorsal MCIII diaphysis

THERMOGRAPHY

• Obvious change in thermal pattern due to marked temperature increase in dorsal MCIII

OTHER DIAGNOSTIC PROCEDURES

• Diagnostic analgesia—generally not necessary; high palmar analgesia with dorsal ring block in the proximal MCIII will confirm the location of pain.

PATHOLOGICAL FINDINGS

• Microradiographic evaluation of bone sections reveals appositional new bone formation on the dorsomedial periosteal surface of MCIII.

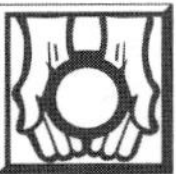

TREATMENT

• Anti-inflammatory therapy such as cold water hosing or icing, poultice, or antiphlogistic dressing for several days
• "Bucked shins"—Stall confinement until soft tissue swelling and pain subsides. For acute mild cases, 2 weeks of stall rest and hand walking are sufficient. Horses with marked periosteal reaction may require a more extended period of rest such as 4 weeks of stall

rest and hand walking followed by an additional 4–8 weeks of small paddock turn-out or "shed row" exercise.
• "Saucer fracture": Stall confinement and handwalked for 4–6 weeks followed by controlled exercise (small paddock or very light jogging) for an additional 6–8 weeks
• "Saucer fractures" are notorious for being slow to heal or failing to heal. Surgical management involves osteostixis (fenestration), screw fixation, or a combination of both.
• Additional therapies:
  ○ Thermocautery ("pin firing")
  ○ Cryotherapy ("freeze firing")
  ○ Periosteal picking—percutaneous irritation of the periosteum with a hypodermic needle
  ○ Extracorporeal shockwave therapy

MEDICATIONS

DRUG(S)

• NSAIDs (phenylbutazone 2.2–4.4 mg/kg daily to BID) for a few days
• Counterirritants ("paints" and "blisters")—topical medications applied to the dorsal MCIII to create hyperemia that facilitates healing

CONTRAINDICATIONS/POSSIBLE INTERACTIONS

• Long-term NSAID use is contraindicated due to their ability to impair bone healing and risk of catastrophic fracture in horses with a "saucer fracture."

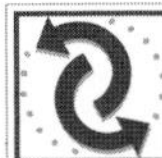

FOLLOW-UP

PATIENT MONITORING

• For acute mild disease, the dorsal MCIII should not be painful or hot and the horse should be sound within several days to weeks.
• For severe disease, follow-up scintigraphic evaluation of horses with "bucked shins" in several months will reveal a marked reduction or absence of increased radiopharmaceutical uptake.
• Radiographic evaluation is recommended to evaluate bony remodeling at monthly intervals for the duration of symptoms. Smooth, inactive periosteal thickening along the dorsal MCIII is desired.
• Radiographic evaluation in 3–4 months for bony healing of "saucer fractures."

PREVENTION/AVOIDANCE

• The most effective way of preventing "bucked shin complex" is by modifying the classic training protocols of racehorses. Revised training regimens are designed to stimulate cyclic loads under conditions that are similar to those experienced during a race, i.e., train at racing speeds. Horses are worked at or near racing speeds at least two times a week, initially at very short distances and increased gradually. As the horse is asked to go faster, the distance is decreased so the cycle repeats itself.
• Slow jogging and long gallops should be avoided.

POSSIBLE COMPLICATIONS

• Variable proportion of horses experience repeated or chronic episodes.
• Prolonged or incomplete bony healing of a "saucer fracture" with conservative treatment
• Catastrophic fracture in unrecognized "saucer fracture"

EXPECTED COURSE AND PROGNOSIS

• Prognosis for most horses with "bucked shins" is very good after early recognition and strict adherence to revised training protocol.
• The majority of horses with "saucer fractures" treated with osteostixis, screw fixation, or both will return to racing.

MISCELLANEOUS

ASSOCIATED CONDITIONS

Most horses with "saucer fractures" had previous episode of "bucked shins."

AGE-RELATED FACTORS

Young (<4 years of age) racehorses

ZOONOTIC POTENTIALS

None

SEE ALSO

Stress fractures

ABBREVIATIONS

• MCIII = third metacarpal bone
• MTIII = third metatarsal bone

Suggested Reading

Nunamaker DM. The bucked shin complex: etiology, pathogenesis, and conservative management. In: Ross MW, Dyson SJ, eds. Diagnosis and Management of Lameness in the Horse. St. Louis: Saunders, 2003:847–853.

Author Elizabeth J. Davidson
Consulting Editor Elizabeth J. Davidson

DOURINE

BASICS

DEFINITION/OVERVIEW

- Disease of equidae
- Natural infections reported only in horses and donkeys
- Causative agent—classically thought to be *Trypanosoma equiperdum*; however, position with the trypanozoon group is uncertain, with overlap noted between this and *T. evansi* and *T. brucei brucei*.
- Only a small number of laboratory strains of uncertain origin exist from the early 20th century. No recent isolates have been obtained.
- Venereal—only transmission; transmissible by direct contact
- Tropism for genital mucosa; cannot survive outside host
- Mortality high; debilitation; predisposition to other diseases

ETIOLOGY/PATHOPHYSIOLOGY

- Limited to venereal transmission
- Requires no vector host; low numbers of organisms in peripheral blood make biting insect transmission unlikely.
- The organism has a predilection for genital mucosa.
- Acute disease after incubation is characterized by pyrexia, debility, and multisystemic disease.

SYSTEMS AFFECTED

- GI—weight loss; emaciation
- Cardiovascular—intense anemia, dependent edema, and urticaria
- Lymphatic—peripheral lymphadenopathy
- Nervous—meningoencephalitis, progressive weakness, paresis, and paralysis
- Musculoskeletal—progressive weakness
- Reproductive—abortion
- Ophthalmic—keratoconjunctivitis

INCIDENCE/PREVALENCE

- Enzootic; endemic in Africa, Asia, Central and South America
- Eradicated in North America
- Low prevalence in parts of Europe

SIGNALMENT

Breeding mares and stallions

SIGNS

- Depend on strain and general health of the horse population
- Three phases of disease recognized:
  - Genital edema and tumefaction
  - Pathognomonic widespread raised cutaneous plaques 1–10 cm in diameter
  - Anemia, neurological compromise (hindquarter weakness; ataxia, hyperesthesia and hyperalgia), emaciation, death
- Approximately 50% of affected animals die of acute disease in 6–8 weeks.

Females

- Severe, edematous vulval and perineal swelling
- Mucopurulent vulval discharge
- Frequent, painful attempts at urination because of vaginal mucosal irritation
- Chronic cases develop urticarial subcutaneous plaques in vulva and surrounding tissues, as well as neck and ventral abdomen. These may regress within hours or days to areas of depigmentation.
- Abortion, if pregnant

Males

- Edema of prepuce, urethral process, penis, testes, and scrotum
- Paraphimosis may ensue.
- Purulent urethral discharge
- Inguinal LN enlargement
- Plaques and depigmented lesions, as in females

CAUSES

- Exposure to *T. equiperdum*
- Infection occurs across intact genital mucosal barriers.

RISK FACTORS

- Presence of asymptomatic carriers
- The organism periodically may be unrecoverable from the urethra or vagina.
- Transmission is not certain, even from matings with known-infected animals.
- Transport of horses from known-infected areas
- Urethral discharge from intact male
- Males may serve as noninfected mechanical carriers after breeding of infected females.

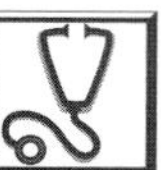

DIAGNOSIS

DIFFERENTIAL DIAGNOSIS

- EHV-3
- EIA
- EVA
- Endometritis

CBC/BIOCHEMISTRY/URINALYSIS

- Acute infection—leukocytosis; other inflammatory changes
- Chronic, debilitating infection results in anemia and extensive multisystemic disease.

OTHER LABORATORY TESTS

Cytology/Histopathology

- Causative organism in smears of body fluid or LN aspirates may yield organism—appears as flagellated protozoan. Mount as a wet film, appears motile with flagellar movement.
- Seminal fluid, mucus from prepuce, and vaginal discharges

Serology

- No definitive diagnosis at serological or molecular level. Neither serological nor DNA-based tests can provide subspecies trypanozoon identification.
- CF test is the most widely used and only internationally recognized test, however, developed in 1915.
- Also available—AGID, IFA, and ELISA tests

DIAGNOSTIC PROCEDURES

In the nervous form, the organism can be recovered from the lumbar and sacral spinal cord, sciatic and obturator nerves, and CSF.

PATHOLOGICAL FINDINGS

Primarily emaciation with enlargement of LNs, spleen, liver; periportal infiltrations in liver; and petechial hemorrhages in kidney

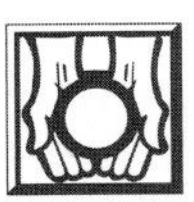

TREATMENT

APPROPRIATE HEALTH CARE

- International regulations impose slaughter of CF-positive horses.
- May be successful if treated early in the course of disease
- Chronic cases in particular are unresponsive to treatment.

CLIENT EDUCATION

Recovered treated animals may become asymptomatic carriers.

MEDICATIONS

DRUGS OF CHOICE

Quinapyramine sulfate—5 mg/kg divided doses SC

ALTERNATIVE DRUGS

- Diminazene—7 mg/kg as 5% solution injected SC; repeat at half-dose 24 hr later
- Suramin—10 mg/kg IV 2–3 times at weekly intervals

FOLLOW-UP

PATIENT MONITORING

- Body weight and condition
- CBC
- Neurologic examination

PREVENTION/AVOIDANCE

- Prohibit movement of horses from infected areas.
- Control breeding practices.
- Eradication—serological testing with slaughter of infected animals
- Consecutive negative tests at least 1 mo apart indicate freedom from disease.

POSSIBLE COMPLICATIONS

Multisystemic nature of the disease predisposes to multisystem failure.

EXPECTED COURSE AND PROGNOSIS

- Incubation period—1 week to 3 mo
- Approximately 50% of affected animals die of acute disease in 6–8 weeks.
- Course of disease—usually 1–2 mo but may last from 2–4 years

MISCELLANEOUS

PREGNANCY

Abortion

SEE ALSO

Venereal diseases

ABBREVIATIONS

- AGID = agar gel immunodiffusion
- CF = complement fixation
- CSF = cerebrospinal fluid
- EAV = equine arteritis virus
- EHV-3 = equine herpesvirus 3
- EIA = equine infectious anemia
- ELISA = enzyme-linked immunosorbent assay
- EVA = equine viral arteritis
- GI = gastrointestinal
- IFA = immunofluorescent assay
- LN = lymph node

Suggested Reading

Barrowman PR. Observations on the transmission, immunology, clinical signs and chemotherapy of dourine (*Trypanosoma equiperdum* infection) in horses, with special reference to cerebrospinal fluid. Onderstepoort Res 1976;43:55–66.

Claes F, Buscher P, Touratier L, Goddeeris BM. Trypanosoma equiperdum—master of disguise or historical mistake? Trends Parasitol 2005;21:316–321.

Clausen PH, Chuluun S, Sodnomdarjaa R, Greiner M, Noeckler K, Staak C, Zessin KH, Schein E. A field study to estimate the prevalence of Trypanosoma equiperdum in Mongolian horses. Vet Parasitol 2003;115:9–18.

Hagebock JM, Chieves L, Frerichs WM, Miller CD. Evaluation of agar gel immunodiffusion and indirect fluorescent antibody assays as supplemental tests for dourine in equids. Am J Vet Res 1993;54:1201–208.

Radositis OM, Blood DC, Gay CC. Veterinary Medicine, ed 8. London: Balliere Tindall, 1994:1220–1222.

Author Peter R. Morresey

Consulting Editor Carla L. Carleton

DUODENITIS–PROXIMAL JEJUNITIS (ANTERIOR ENTERITIS, PROXIMAL ENTERITIS)

BASICS

DEFINITION

DPJ is an inflammation of the proximal small intestine. It causes excessive fluid and electrolyte secretion, resulting in a functional ileus with small intestinal distention and gastric reflux.

PATHOPHYSIOLOGY

• Idiopathic condition • Lesions tend to be restricted to the duodenum and proximal jejunum, but pylorus and stomach can be affected. • Whatever the inciting factor, fluid and electrolyte accumulation occurs in the small intestine proximal to the site of disease. • As the intestine distends, signs of abdominal pain are displayed; with further distention, the intestine becomes compromised, resulting in increased secretion, decreased absorption, and poor perfusion. • Ileus may result from direct damage, distention, pain, toxemia or hypokalemia, and other electrolyte disturbances. • Net fluid movement into the small intestine combined with lack of aboral movement eventually results in gastric distention, which can develop to the point of rupture if the stomach is not decompressed.

SYSTEMS AFFECTED

GI

• Increased fluid secretion, decreased fluid absorption, and lack of aboral movement cause small intestinal distention, mainly in the duodenum and proximal jejunum. • Fluid accumulation in the small intestine progresses to gastric distention. • Signs of abdominal pain result from intestinal and gastric distention. • Some horses may also develop diarrhea. • Liver enzymes can be increased, but the mechanism involved is currently unknown.

Cardiovascular

As large volumes of fluid are sequestered in the proximal GI tract or removed through gastric decompression, dehydration can ensue. Cardiac arrhythmias may occur.

Musculoskeletal

• Laminitis is a relatively common secondary problem. • Marked muscle loss can result from the severe catabolic state and restricted food intake.

GENETICS

No known genetic basis

INCIDENCE/PREVALENCE

• Anecdotal reports indicate a greater prevalence in the southern United States; however, cases can occur in any region. • May occur throughout the year; however, is reported more often during the summer months in some areas

SIGNALMENT

• Horses >1 year are primarily affected, with a high proportion in those >9 years. • No sex predisposition

SIGNS

Historical

• Affected horses usually are presented with acute onset of colic, and signs can progress rapidly. • Occasionally, a history of recent introduction of a higher-energy diet or a too-lush pasture

Physical Examination

• Tachycardia, with the heart rate usually within 40–80 bpm, is typical. • Dehydration, depending on the severity and duration of disease. • Animals tend to be more depressed than painful, especially after gastric decompression; however some horses may be severely painful. • Initial volumes of gastric reflux are variable but may reach several liters. • Reflux fluid has a variable appearance, from green to brownish-red, and with or without a fetid odor. • Many horses also are pyrexic. • Distended small intestine is usually, but not always, palpable per rectum. • Clinical signs are very similar to those of an obstructive small intestinal lesion. Differentiation is critical because medical treatment of horses with obstructive lesions requiring surgery may affect the prognosis if surgical intervention is delayed. In general, horses with DPJ tend to be more depressed and to have a lower heart rate after gastric decompression, significantly more reflux, a less palpable distended small intestine, more GI sounds, and lower peritoneal WBC counts (with elevated peritoneal protein levels) compared to horses with surgical small intestinal lesions. None of these signs alone are diagnostic, however, and a definitive diagnosis could be confirmed only during surgical exploration or necropsy.

CAUSES

• Unknown, but an infectious agent is suspected. • *Clostridium difficile* was consistently recovered from the reflux and in some cases also from the feces of affected horses in a recent report. • *Salmonella* and other *Clostridium* spp. such as *C. perfringens* have been inconsistently recovered from reflux or feces of clinical cases. • Mycotoxins have been explored but not proven. • A diet high in concentrate, or a recent dietary change, may be a predisposing factor, perhaps because of development of an intestinal dysbacteriosis.

RISK FACTORS

A recent dietary change, with introduction of a higher level or concentrates or into a lush pasture, may predispose patients to this condition.

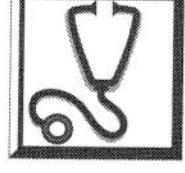

DIAGNOSIS

DIFFERENTIAL DIAGNOSIS

• Any condition causing colic and gastric reflux • Strangulating or nonstrangulating obstructive small intestinal lesions • Ileus • Large colon impaction, causing small intestinal compression

CBC/BIOCHEMISTRY/URINALYSIS

A leukocytosis may be present but is not diagnostic.

OTHER LABORATORY TESTS

A metabolic alkalosis may occur as a result of gastric HCl losses, but many animals may be acidotic because of hypovolemia, decreased tissue perfusion and electrolyte imbalance.

IMAGING

Abdominal ultrasonography—small intestinal distention not palpable per rectum may be visualized, but DPJ cannot be differentiated at imaging from other conditions causing small intestinal distension.

DIAGNOSTIC PROCEDURES

• Surgery—A definitive diagnosis usually is arrived at only by exploratory laparotomy, laparoscopy, or necropsy. • Abdominocentesis—A high peritoneal fluid protein level (>30g/L, and possibly >45g/L) with normal WBC numbers (<5–10 × 10^9 cells/L) is suggestive but is not diagnostic.

PATHOLOGICAL FINDINGS

Gross

• Lesions are present invariably in the duodenum, often in the jejunum, and occasionally in the pyloric region of the stomach. • The serosal surface typically contains petechial and ecchymotic hemorrhages. • The intestinal wall may be thickened from edema and inflammation. • The mucosa tends to be hyperemic.

Histopathological

• Lesions include fibrinopurulent exudation on the serosal surface, intramural hemorrhage, and hyperemia and edema of the mucosa and submucosa. • Depending on severity, there may be villous epithelial degeneration, epithelial cell sloughing, and neutrophilic infiltration. • In some cases, no gross or histologic lesions may be present.

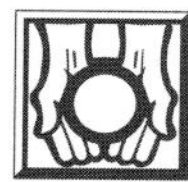

TREATMENT

APPROPRIATE HEALTH CARE

• Because of the difficulty in differentiating this condition from that of a surgical lesion and the intensive treatment and monitoring that are required, affected horses should be managed on an emergency inpatient basis. • Hyperimmune serum directed against the gram-negative core antigens (i.e., "anti-endotoxin" serum) can be administered in horses with signs of toxemia.

NURSING CARE

• Frequent monitoring is essential, especially early in the course of treatment, when the presence of a surgical lesion remains unclear. • Signs of colic and tachycardia indicate the need for gastric decompression. • Deep bedding may be beneficial considering the risk for development of laminitis.

IV Fluid Therapy

• Invariably indicated, with a balanced electrolyte solution • Administer daily maintenance (30–50mL/kg per day) plus correction of fluid deficits from dehydration and replacement of the fluid volume lost during refluxing. Initially, 50–100L/day may be required (average 450- to 500-kg horse). • IV fluid therapy initially may increase the volume of reflux obtained because of reduced intravascular oncotic pressure and increased capillary perfusion pressure. • Monitor serum electrolyte levels. • Approach IV supplementation of potassium with caution—20–40 mEq/L of KCl can be added to lactated Ringer's solution or saline in hypokalemic animals, but the rate of infusion should not exceed 0.5 mEq/kg per hr. • Hypocalcemia also is frequently encountered and can be treated with slow IV infusion (500mL of 23% calcium borogluconate).

Gastric Decompression

• A crucial component of treatment to relieve pain and prevent gastric rupture • Initially, nasogastric intubation may be needed every 1–2hr. A siphon must be established each time, because passage of a nasogastric tube does not always result in reflux, even with a distended stomach. • If <5L of fluid are obtained, the interval between refluxing can be increased. • If signs of colic or an elevated heart rate are observed, the stomach should be refluxed. • Leave the tube in place until refluxing has either ceased or decreased to 1–2L every 4hr.

ACTIVITY

If no signs of laminitis are present, it may be beneficial to walk the horse frequently for short periods of time to stimulate GI motility.

DIET

• Nothing should be given orally until the nasogastric tube is removed, after which a slow reintroduction of feed can begin. No concentrates should be fed initially. • Because there may be no food intake for a prolonged period in some cases, partial or total parenteral nutrition may be indicated.

CLIENT EDUCATION

• This condition can be frustrating and expensive to treat. • Owners should be aware that the affected horses may reflux for >1 week, and that expensive therapy (e.g., total or partial parenteral nutrition) may be indicated. • Laminitis is a common secondary problem, especially in larger horses. • Reported survival rate is generally good, and the majority of cases respond to medical therapy. • Death most often occurs from complications (e.g., laminitis, adhesions), or horses are euthanized because of economic concerns.

SURGICAL CONSIDERATIONS

• Surgical intervention is common during the early stages of this condition, because differentiation from a surgical small intestinal lesion is very difficult. • Surgery may be beneficial in the short term by confirming the diagnosis and decompressing the small intestine, but the possibility for secondary problems from the stress of anesthesia and risk of adhesion formation increases.

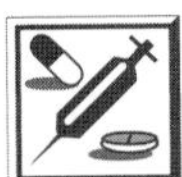

MEDICATIONS

DRUGS OF CHOICE

• Intestinal clostridiosis has been suggested as a cause; thus, penicillin may be administered—sodium penicillin (20,000–40,000 IU/kg IV q6h) or metronidazole (15–25mg/kg per rectum q8h). • Broad-spectrum antibiotics may be indicated with signs of toxemia or bacteremia. Options include a penicillin-aminoglycoside combination (sodium penicillin 20,000–40,000 IU/kg IV q6h/gentamicin 6.6mg/kg IV q24h), trimethoprim-sulfamethoxazole 24mg/kg IV q12h, or ceftiofur sodium 2mg/kg IV q12h. • Low-dose flunixin meglumine 0.25–0.5mg/kg IV q8h can be administered for its purported antiendotoxin effects. • If the stomach is decompressed, there usually is little need for analgesics. • Analgesics should be administered judiciously, because they may mask the progression of clinical signs that might indicate a surgical lesion. If analgesia is required, flunixin meglumine 1.1mg/kg IV q12h can be administered. • H_2-receptor antagonists (e.g., ranitidine 6.6mg/kg PO q8h or omeprazole [4mg/kg PO q24h) may be indicated after refluxing has ceased because of gastric irritation from distention, the primary disease process, and prolonged nasogastric intubation. • Heparin 40–100 IU/kg SC q8–12h has been suggested to reduce the incidence of intestinal adhesions and laminitis; monitor the PCV concurrently if this treatment is used. • Various prokinetics agents have been used. Some clinicians claim some success, however, no definitive results are available regarding the efficacy of these agents.

CONTRAINDICATIONS

Prokinetic agents are contraindicated if an obstructive small intestinal lesion is suspected. Reserve their use for the later stages in medical treatment, once an obstructive lesion has been ruled out or when DPJ has been confirmed via exploratory laparotomy or laparoscopy.

PRECAUTIONS

• Aminoglycosides and NSAIDs are potentially nephrotoxic and should not be administered until the patient's hydration status is normal. • Antibiotics have been implicated in the development of colitis.

FOLLOW-UP

PATIENT MONITORING

During the recovery period, monitor for signs of recrudescence of disease.

PREVENTION/AVOIDANCE

Because an intestinal dysbacteriosis may be involved in pathogenesis, institute feeding changes gradually.

POSSIBLE COMPLICATIONS

• Laminitis is the most common complication. • Intestinal adhesions are uncommon, unless surgical exploration was undertaken. • Other less common complications—peritonitis, aspiration pneumonia, and myocardial or renal infarcts.

EXPECTED COURSE AND PROGNOSIS

• Duration of reflux may be as short as 24 hr but typically lasts for 3–7 days (and may be even longer). • Reported survival rates range from 25–94%. • Prognosis is good for horses that stop refluxing within 72 hr. • Death most often results from economic concerns or complications, such as, laminitis or adhesions.

MISCELLANEOUS

ASSOCIATED CONDITIONS

• Aspiration pneumonia • Intestinal adhesions • Laminitis • Peritonitis

PREGNANCY

Pregnant mares may be at greater risk for abortion because of endotoxemia, systemic compromise from dehydration, and severe loss of body condition.

SYNONYMS

• Anterior enteritis • Proximal enteritis • Gastroduodenojejunitis

SEE ALSO

• Intestinal adhesions • Laminitis • Peritonitis

ABBREVIATIONS

• DPJ = duodenitis–proximal jejunitis • GI = gastrointestinal • PCV = packed cell volume

Suggested Reading

Arroyo LG, Stampfli HR, Weese JS. Potential role of *Clostridium difficile* as a cause of duodenitis-proximal jejunitis in horses. J Med Microbiol 2006;55:605–608.

Cohen ND, Toby E, Roussel AJ, Murphey EL, Wang N. Are feeding practices associated with duodenitis-proximal jejunitis? Equine Vet J 2006;38:526–531.

Freeman DE. Duodenitis-proximal jenunitis. Equine Vet Educ 2000;12:322–332.

White NA II, Tyler DE, Blackwell RB, Allen D. Hemorrhagic fibrinonecrotic duodenitis-proximal jejunitis in horses: 20 cases (1977–1984). JAVMA 1987;190:311–315.

Authors Luis G. Arroyo and J. Scott Weese
Consulting Editors Henry R. Stämpfli and Olimpo Oliver-Espinosa

DYNAMIC COLLAPSE OF THE UPPER AIRWAY

BASICS

DEFINITION

- This is a group of disorders that cause a transient obstruction to respiration within the pharynx, larynx, or both.
- Often cyclic and synchronous with inspiration.
- Results from fatigue of the musculature that normally maintains luminal patency of the pharynx and larynx.

PATHOPHYSIOLOGY

- The pathophysiologies for many of the abnormalities resulting in this condition have not yet been specifically characterized. All appear to be different forms of neuromuscular dysfunction or fatigue; however, most occur during the inspiratory phase of respiration, under the pull of high negative inspiratory pressures.
- With increased respiratory effort and muscular fatigue, the condition worsens, the obstruction becomes more severe, and a vicious cycle ensues.
- Airway turbulence may result in abnormal respiratory noise but is not always present.

SYSTEMS AFFECTED

- Upper respiratory tract
- With severe, more chronic conditions, the cardiopulmonary system may undergo secondary changes from repeated, high negative intrathoracic pressures and hypoxia.

SIGNALMENT

- Any age or breed
- More commonly diagnosed in racehorses because of the high negative inspiratory pressures created during strenuous exercise.
- Thoroughbreds (2–3 years) are the largest group affected.
- To date, axial deviation of the aryepiglottic folds has been identified only in racehorses.
- Quarter Horses with hyperkalemic periodic paralysis can have paroxysmal spasms of the pharynx and larynx during "paralytic episodes" that result in severe upper respiratory obstruction.

SIGNS

- Exercise intolerance or poor performance
- Abnormal upper respiratory noise during inspiration may occur depending on the degree and type of obstruction.
- Only dorsal displacement of the soft palate results in expiratory noise.
- Coughing
- Dysphagia

CAUSES

- Laryngeal hemiplegia most commonly affects the left arytenoid cartilage, results from idiopathic degeneration of the left recurrent laryngeal nerve, and causes a paresis of the primary abductor of the left arytenoid, the cricoarytenoideus dorsalis muscle.
- Infrequently, trauma to either the left or right recurrent laryngeal nerve associated with jugular thrombophlebitis can result in laryngeal hemiplegia.
- Epiglottic retroversion is presumed to be a dysfunction of the hypoepiglotticus muscle on the basis of experimental reproduction of the disorder after anesthetic blockade of the nerve (i.e., the hypoglossal) that supplies the hypoepiglotticus.
- Dorsal pharyngeal collapse can be reproduced experimentally with anesthetically induced dysfunction of the stylopharyngeus muscles.
- Other forms of collapse are thought to represent either specific muscle dysfunction within the pharynx or disproportionate force between the muscle groups.

RISK FACTORS

- High-speed exercise
- Hyperkalemic periodic paralysis in Quarter Horses

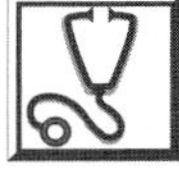

DIAGNOSIS

DIFFERENTIAL DIAGNOSIS

- Laryngeal hemiplegia
- Vocal cord collapse
- Intermittent dorsal displacement of the soft palate
- Pharyngeal collapse
- Epiglottic retroversion
- Axial deviation of the aryepiglottic folds
- Combinations of any of the above-mentioned distinct disorders

OTHER DIAGNOSTIC PROCEDURES

Resting Endoscopy

- Helps to evaluate any structural abnormalities predisposing to dynamic obstruction during exercise but rarely is definitive for a dynamic abnormality.
- More difficult to speculate on pharyngeal than on laryngeal forms of dynamic collapse.
- Assess laryngeal and pharyngeal function during normal breathing, nasal occlusion, and swallowing.
- Horses normally demonstrate some dorsal roof collapse of the pharynx and have air pass between the aryepiglottic folds and pharyngeal ostium during nasal occlusion. This is not an indication of a pharyngeal abnormality during exercise.
- With prolonged nasal occlusion, 60% of horses can be made to displace their palates, but they do not experience dynamic collapse during exercise.
- Horses that very readily displace their soft palate are more likely to displace it during a race.
- Horses that leave their palates displaced for an extended period of time or have difficulty replacing their palates with a swallow are more likely to have a pharyngeal abnormality during high-speed exercise. This may be a crude indication of some pharyngeal weakness.
- Horses commonly demonstrate asynchrony to their arytenoid movement yet achieve full abduction of both arytenoids during nasal occlusion or after swallowing (grade 2 on a scale of 1–4). These horses do not experience dynamic collapse during exercise. Horses that cannot fully and symmetrically abduct both arytenoids after swallowing or nasal occlusion (grade 3) are considered to be impaired.
- The degree of dynamic collapse depends on the degree of paresis and on the intensity of exercise. Racehorses likely undergo significant respiratory compromise with grade 3 laryngeal hemiplegia; show horses are more likely asymptomatic.

High-Speed Treadmill Endoscopy

- Often required to see the cause of upper respiratory collapse.

- Minimum requirements to ensure a valid test—Holter monitor to record heart rate during exercise, to determine heart rate relative to the horse's speed, and to guarantee the horse is maximally exerting itself by achieving a heart rate of ≅220 bpm or greater; videoendoscope linked to a video recorder to visualize the abnormality and play back the video in slow motion if the obstruction occurs too quickly to see in real time; and a physiologically fit horse exercised in tack (harness for Standardbreds) to minimize spurious results.
- Typical racehorse protocol—phase 1: warm up, 2 m/s for 4 min, 4.5 m/s for 1min, 7 m/s for 2 min; phase 2: walk until heart rate <90 bpm, stop and insert endoscope; phase 3: gradually accelerate to 9 m/s, incline treadmill to 3° (for Thoroughbreds); accelerate to 11 m/s, continue for 400 m; accelerate to 12 m/s, continue for 400 m; accelerate to 14 m/sec, continue for 1600 m; then decelerate to 12 m/s, continue for 400 m.
- Horses are unlikely to be capable of completing these steps as described; therefore, they are exercised as close to the desired speed as possible for the predetermined distances. Most horses require at least one schooling episode to become familiar enough with the treadmill to exercise at an adequate speed.
- Measurements of upper respiratory pressures and use of flow-volume loops during treadmill exercise can document respiratory obstruction but cannot discriminate between the many different abnormalities.

Analysis of Upper Respiratory Sounds

Spectrogram analysis can be used to some degree to determine if an abnormality is present and which abnormality exists.

PATHOLOGIC FINDINGS

N/A

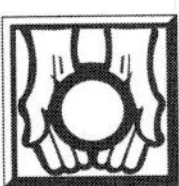

TREATMENT

AIMS OF TREATMENT

To create a stable open airway, resistant to high negative pressures.

SURGICAL CONSIDERATIONS

- Laryngeal hemiplegia is treated with surgical laryngoplasty (i.e., tieback procedure). The affected arytenoid is held in a fixed, partially abducted position with a nonabsorbable suture simulating the contracted cricoarytenoideus muscle. An adjunctive procedure (i.e., ventriculocordectomy) also can be performed to minimize obstruction at the ventral aspect of the glottis after a tieback.
- Axial deviation of the aryepiglottic folds has been treated effectively both with rest and with laser resection of the offending soft tissue; however, surgery affords a quicker return to training.
- There are multiple surgical procedures to consider for intermittent dorsal displacement of the soft palate, which demonstrates our inability to define the exact cause in each patient.
- Rest and oral anti-inflammatory treatment has been the only mode of therapy for other forms of dynamic collapse.

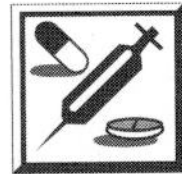

MEDICATIONS

DRUG(S) OF CHOICE

A 3–4-week course of an anti-inflammatory drug may be indicated during the period of rest to resolve any presumed inflammatory component causing the dysfunction. Prednisolone can be given at a tapering dose (0.8 mg/kg PO once daily for 7 days, then 0.8 mg/kg PO every other day for 3 treatments, then 0.4 mg/kg PO every other day for 3 treatments).

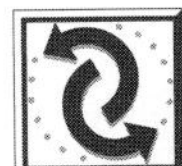

FOLLOW-UP

PATIENT MONITORING

- Resting endoscopy is necessary several weeks after any surgical intervention, and though it will not be definitive for determining the success of the surgery, it will determine the capability of the horse to resume training.
- An increase in performance or diminution of noise often is the criterion used to determine a successful treatment.
- Repeat high-speed treadmill endoscopy is the best method to determine a successful outcome from any treatment, but only after the horse has regained fitness.

POSSIBLE COMPLICATIONS

- Most common is failure to achieve primary goal.
- Increasing the risk of aspiration, or dysphagia is the second most common complication.

EXPECTED COURSE AND PROGNOSIS

Depending on the specific cause of collapse, the prognosis ranges from guarded to good.

MISCELLANEOUS

SEE ALSO

- Arytenoid chondritis
- Epiglottic entrapment
- Laryngeal hemiplegia
- Dorsal displacement of the soft palate

Suggested Reading

Derksen FJ. Evaluation of upper respiratory tract sounds. In: McGorum BC, Dixon PM, Robinson NE, Schumacher J, eds. Equine Respiratory Medicine and Surgery. Philadelphia: Elsevier, 2007:249–254.

Holcombe SJ, Ducharme NG. Disorders of the nasopharynx and soft palate. In: McGorum BC, Dixon PM, Robinson NE, Schumacher J, eds. Equine Respiratory Medicine and Surgery. Philadelphia: Elsevier, 2007: 437–458.

Parente EJ. Treadmill endoscopy. Equine Vet Educ 2004:15;250–254.

Author Eric J. Parente

Consulting Editor Daniel Jean

DYSTOCIA

BASICS

DEFINITION/OVERVIEW

Any difficult delivery with or without assistance

ETIOLOGY/PATHOPHYSIOLOGY

Attributed to—hereditary, nutritional, management, infectious, traumatic, and miscellaneous

- *Hereditary*—abnormalities of the genital tract, twinning, size of fetus' head, ankylosis of joints, hydrocephalus • *Nutrition and management*—dam's pelvic size (nutritional stunting), pelvic cavity fat, failure to observe animals near term (uterine inertia), close confinement of mares during entire gestation, etc. • *Infectious conditions of the placenta or fetus*—can result in uterine inertia, incomplete cervical dilatation, postural abnormalities due to fetal death, loss of placental attachment sites, etc.
- *Traumatic*—damage of abdominal wall, inhibits normal abdominal contractions; torsion of uterus, pelvic fracture, etc.
- *Miscellaneous*—postural changes occur for no apparent reason—posterior presentation, transverse presentation

Primary Uterine Inertia

- Uterine overstretching (i.e., hydrops, twins), increases in older, debilitated animals. • Uterine infections may predispose to inertia.
- Oxytocin—failure of its release or failure to affect a uterine response, etc.

Secondary Uterine Inertia

- Dystocia, uterine muscle is exhausted. • Failure of labor due to pain to the dam • Following prolonged dystocia with strong circular contractions in a fatigued uterus • Uterus may rupture if forced extraction is attempted.

Immediate Causes of Dystocia

- Causes relieved at the time of delivery can be divided into maternal and fetal. Most immediate causes are of fetal origin. • *Maternal causes*—stenosis of the birth canal, small pelvis, hypoplastic genital tract, lacerations and scars of the genital tract, pelvic tumors, persistent hymen, failure of cervical dilatation, uterine inertia, abortions, twinning, etc. • *Fetal causes*—abnormal presentation, position, and/or posture; excessive fetal size, fetal anasarca, fetal ascites, fetal tumors, ankylosed joints, hydrocephalus, fetal monsters, posterior presentation, wryneck, and transverse presentation

SYSTEMS AFFECTED

- Reproductive • Others possibly affected as condition progresses, with development of systemic illness

GENETICS

See Etiology/Pathophysiology.

INCIDENCE/PREVALENCE

- Dystocia rates—1% • Higher incidence—miniature horse breeds
- Geographic distribution—wherever pregnant mares are housed

SIGNALMENT

- Any breed • All ages affected

SIGNS

General Comments

Dystocia is always an emergency.

- Complete history • Do routine physical examination of the reproductive tract and fetal examination *before* deciding how to handle a dystocia.

Historical

- Stage 2 labor > 70 min or an abnormal presentation, position, and/or posture • May include premature placental detachment with the fetus remaining within the uterus
- Important—complete history includes
  - Mare's due date
  - Any previous dystocia or abnormal gestations
  - Recent systemic disease during gestation
  - Length of active labor (stages 1 and 2)
  - Rupture of allantoic membrane
  - Rupture of amniotic membrane
  - Any assistance given (potential for contamination)
  - Status of mare's mobility

Physical Examination

- If the mare is down and unable to rise, determine:
  - Cause
  - Hydration status
  - Whether she may be in shock or could go into shock before procedure is complete
  - CRT +/− toxic mucous membranes present
- TRP of genital tract should be performed to determine possible lacerations, uterine tone, presentation, position, and posture of fetus before entering the vagina.
- Genital tract examination following tail wrap and meticulous perineal wash
  - Use liberal amounts of lubricant.
  - Examine vulva, vagina, cervix, and uterus for possible lacerations.
  - Any lacerations—inform owner prior to palpation of the fetus or OB manipulation.
- Determine if fetus is viable by:
  - Gentle pressure over eyes (stimulate blink reflex).
  - Place fingers in fetal mouth (presence suckle reflex).
  - Pull on fetal limb (test—retraction by fetus).
  - Maximally flex limb (stimulate fetal motion, it *pulls away*).
  - Place finger in anus (test—sphincter contraction).
  - U/S examination to determine presence of heart beat or blood flow
- Evaluate fetal presentation, position, and posture.
- Determine if birth canal size will permit fetal passage.
- If fetus is dead, determine how long (may not be possible until after delivery).
  - TOD/time of death classification—corneas cloudy (dead 6–12 hr prior to delivery); emphysema and sloughing of hair of fetus (dead minimum 18 hr prior to delivery)

CAUSES

- All posterior presentations • All deviations from normal position (dorsosacral)
  - Dorsoilial
  - Dorsopubic
- Postural defects, flexion of the extremities (head and neck, limbs)
  - Most common cause of dystocia
  - Carpal, shoulder, hip flexion; lateral flexion of the head and neck
  - Ankylosis of joints
  - Hydrocephalic fetus, anasarca

RISK FACTORS

- Major causes involve fetal malposture. Therefore, it is impossible to state precisely why the fetus moves from normal delivery presentation, position, and posture (anterior presentation, dorsosacral position, with extended head and neck and both forelimbs [aka posture]), to an abnormality of any of these. • Older mares and mares with insufficient exercise have an increase of dystocia for unknown reasons.

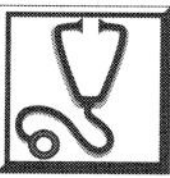

DIAGNOSIS

DIFFERENTIAL DIAGNOSIS

- The primary differential diagnosis for dystocia is prepartum colic.
  - Signs can be very similar, especially in early stages of dystocia.
  - In the case of colic, signs of abdominal distress continue to worsen, while with dystocia, it becomes obvious that the mare is not only uncomfortable but is straining.
- In the case of true breech delivery (fetus in posterior presentation, both rear legs flexed), the mare may not go into stage 2 labor, so straining may be absent.
- Examination of the reproductive tract (TRP and vaginal) will be extremely helpful to differentiate dystocia from colic.

CBC/BIOCHEMISTRY/URINALYSIS

CBC and blood chemistries may be indicated if the animal is hospitalized and the results are rapidly available.

IMAGING

Depending on the experience of the obstetrician, U/S may be used to determine fetal viability.

OTHER DIAGNOSTIC PROCEDURES

- Determine mare's mucous membrane color (normal, injected, muddy) and CRT. • Mare hydration status • Ability of the mare to move (ambulatory or down) • Determine if sufficiently stable to administer local anesthetics, epidurals, general anesthesia or sedation, if necessary.

It is always indicated to perform a TRP of the mare to determine—

- If lacerations exist within the uterus prior to vaginal examination • Fetal viability • Amount of uterine contracture around the fetus

A vaginal examination is performed to determine—

- Presence or absence of uterine tears • Degree of uterine contracture • Fetal viability • Fetal presentation, position, and posture • Amount of space between the fetus and the maternal pelvis
- Degree of cervical relaxation—

If cesarean section is not an option (and the mare's straining prevents adequate room to accomplish mutation), it is an additional means for field resolution.

- Heavy sedation or *light general anesthesia* of the mare, followed by:
  - Elevation of the mare's rear quarters (suspending by her hocks; *care must be taken* to protect the hocks with padding or towels before attaching chains or straps). May accomplish by using a lift, front-end loader, overhead beam, etc.
  - Mare placed in lateral recumbency, hocks elevated no more than 18–24 inches, usually sufficient
  - Allows the weight of the fetus and fluids in the relaxed uterus to fall deeper into the abdomen
  - Creates additional space for mutation and subsequent extraction
  - Whether the fetus is live or dead, this is an option, especially when cesarean section is not feasible or cost-prohibitive for the client.

PATHOLOGICAL FINDINGS

Depends on the cause of dystocia

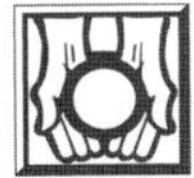

TREATMENT

APPROPRIATE HEALTH CARE

• Dystocia is generally best handled on the farm. Uterine size and room within which to accomplish mutation and extraction decrease with time and uterine contraction. • Vaginal deliveries can best be accomplished shortly after a dystocia is diagnosed, whether mutation and forced extraction or fetotomy is to be performed.

NURSING CARE

• Follow-up care consists of thorough examination of the uterus, cervix, vagina, vestibule, and vulva following the delivery.
• Broad-spectrum antibiotics should be placed into the uterus to reduce the number of organisms introduced during mutation and extraction of the fetus. • Uterine stimulants such as oxytocin can be beneficial and enhance uterine contractions (involution), and hasten return to normal size postpartum. • Systemic antibiotics may be necessary if indications of systemic involvement develop. • Uterine flushes or infusions may be indicated to enhance uterine contractility. • Other supportive therapy may be indicated for mares undergoing cesarean section.

ACTIVITY

• The mare's activity need not be restricted if a vaginal delivery was accomplished. • Mares undergoing cesarean section should be stall rested.

DIET

• Maintain the mare's regular diet, possible reduction of quantity fed, if indicated. Intent is to avoid intestinal displacement. • Changing the diet at the time of parturition further adds to the mare's stress and should be avoided.

CLIENT EDUCATION

• Emphasize that mares should not be permitted to be in prolonged labor, as it will reduce the probability of neonatal survival. • The position of the fetal extremities should be examined closely during delivery in order to determine if the fetus is in an abnormal delivery presentation, position, or posture at the earliest possible time.
- If the soles of the fetus are pointed down:
  - Anterior presentation with dorsosacral position or
  - Posterior presentation with dorsosacral position.
- Essential to determine if the head of the fetus is resting on its metacarpi (normal presentation, position, and posture).

SURGICAL CONSIDERATIONS

• Decide early in the intervention if a cesarean section is the best approach. • If the fetus is alive and no other correction (mutation, extraction) possible:
  - If the surgical approach can be made in a short enough period of time to maintain fetal viability, that decision must be reached quickly.

• If the fetus cannot be delivered alive, consideration must be given to fetotomy, especially if this procedure can be accomplished with one or two cuts on the farm. • If a cesarean section is to be performed, timing is critical.

MEDICATIONS

DRUGS OF CHOICE

• Epidural anesthesia can be used to assist in the delivery process; reduces contractions during an assisted delivery. Approximate dosage—1 mL of 2% carbocaine per 40 kg of body weight.
• Xylazine (0.5–1.0 mg/kg) can be used for sedation alone or combined with acepromazine (0.04 mg/kg). • General anesthetic agents can be used to induce anesthesia for cesarean section or to accomplish further corrective procedures.
• Following delivery the administration of oxytocin at a dosage of 10–20 IU per 500 kg IM will hasten uterine contractions and involution of the postpartum uterus.

CONTRAINDICATIONS

• Oxytocin should never be administered prepartum due to its potential to induce further uterine contracture, reducing further the space for fetal manipulation. • Exceeding recommended doses, especially early post-delivery, may result in uterine eversion (prolapse).

PRECAUTIONS

Regardless of the approach selected, care must be taken when manipulating the fetus during delivery.

ALTERNATIVE DRUGS

• Butorphenol • Dormosedan • Morphine

FOLLOW-UP

PATIENT MONITORING

• TRP is indicated daily or every other day depending on the findings to determine the size and tone of the uterus. • U/S examination + TRP—determine the presence or absence of uterine luminal fluid.

PREVENTION/AVOIDANCE

• Close observation of near-term mare will aid in early diagnosis of dystocia. • There is no method to prevent dystocia without doing an elective cesarean section or not breeding a mare.

POSSIBLE COMPLICATIONS

• Following dystocia, there may be lacerations of the cervix, vagina, vestibule, or vulva. • Uterine lacerations are also possible with resultant peritonitis. • Uterine inflammation or infection may result from the dystocia or the corrective methods used.

EXPECTED COURSE AND PROGNOSIS

- Prognosis decreases with:
  - Duration of dystocia
  - Inexperienced interference
  - Cause of dystocia
  - Other contributing factors
- Mares have a grave prognosis if >24 hr from onset of stage 2.
- Fetuses have a guarded prognosis >70 min from onset of stage 2.
- After initial examination of mare—discuss with owner the prognosis, fees, and best approach to resolve dystocia.
- Choices of approach include:
  - Mare standing, in lateral recumbency, or rear-quarters elevated—assisted forced extraction, manipulation (mutation) of fetus; fetotomy • Cesarean section • Euthanasia of dam
- Always give the owner a realistic prognosis and permit him/her to make the decision.

MISCELLANEOUS

AGE-RELATED FACTORS

Slight increased in dystocia in aged mares, possibly related to decreased uterine contractions

PREGNANCY

Condition limited to pregnant mares

SYNONYMS

• Difficult foaling • Difficult labor • Difficult delivery • Difficult parturition

ABBREVIATIONS

- CBC = complete blood count
- CRT = capillary refill time
- OB = obstetric
- TOD = time of death
- TRP = transrectal palpation
- U/S = ultrasound, ultrasonography

Suggested Reading

Asbury AC—Care of the mare after foaling. In: McKinnon AO and Voss JL, eds. Equine Reproduction. Philadelphia, Lea & Febiger, 1993:578–587.

Roberts SJ—Veterinary Obstetrics and Genital Diseases (Theriogenology), ed 3. Woodstock, VT: published by the author, 1986:326–351.

Author Walter R. Threlfall
Consulting Editor Carla L. Carleton

EARLY EMBRYONIC DEATH (EED)

BASICS

DEFINITION/OVERVIEW

Maternal structural or functional defects preventing normal embryonic development from early pregnancy diagnosis at 14–15 days to the beginning of the fetal stage at 40 days of gestation

ETIOLOGY/PATHOPHYSIOLOGY

• Defective embryo • Unsuitable uterine environment • Early regression of CL
• Luteal insufficiency—anecdotal

SYSTEM AFFECTED

Reproductive

GENETICS

N/A

INCIDENCE/PREVALENCE

• Normal rate is ≅5%–10%.
• Incidence may be much higher in old, subfertile mares.

SIGNALMENT

• Usually mares of >15 years, but not so with EED due to MRLS (all ages affected equally).
• Certain heterospecific matings: stallion × jenny

SIGNS

Historical

Return to estrus after previous diagnosis of pregnancy

Physical Examination

• At ≥40 days after ovulation, no evidence by transrectal U/S of a previously diagnosed pregnancy • At ≥40 days after ovulation, evidence by transrectal U/S of a previously diagnosed pregnancy undergoing EED (e.g., decreasing size, change in appearance of fluid, absence of heartbeat); a nonpregnant uterus (possibly with endometrial folds or intrauterine fluid); possible absence of CL; none or mucoid or mucopurulent vulvar discharge

CAUSES

• Defective embryos—old mares; seasonal effects • Endometritis—early CL regression; unsuitable uterine environment • Unsuitable uterine environment: endometritis; occurrence of endometrial cysts large enough to impede embryonic mobility (during transuterine migration) and failure of maternal recognition of pregnancy (more likely conception failure); inadequate secretion of histotrophs
• Xenobiotics: fescue toxicosis or ergotism; phytoestrogens (anecdotal); eastern tent caterpillar (MRLS) • Endocrine disorders: hypothyroidism (anecdotal); luteal insufficiency (anecdotal) • Maternal disease: fever; pain (anecdotal)

RISK FACTORS

• Age of >15 years
• Anatomic defects predisposing to endometritis
• Seasonal effects
• Foal heat breedings: anecdotal
• Inadequate nutrition
• Exposure to xenobiotics: fescue toxicosis or ergotism
• Some heterospecific matings: stallion × jenny
• Eastern tent caterpillars

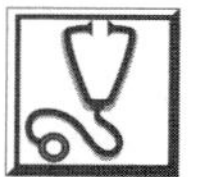

DIAGNOSIS

DIFFERENTIAL DIAGNOSIS

• Conception failure: failure to detect a 14-day pregnancy by transrectal U/S
• Previous misdiagnosis of pregnancy by transrectal U/S: endometrial cysts, intrauterine fluid, paraovarian cystic structures, and small ovarian follicles are distinguished from pregnancies based on shape, size, location, and reexamination.
• Pregnancies move at <16 days after ovulation (transuterine migration), grow, and develop/exhibit heartbeats.

CBC/BIOCHEMISTRY/URINALYSIS

Not indicated, unless signs of concurrent systemic disease are present

OTHER LABORATORY TESTS

Maternal Progesterone

• May be indicated at initial pregnancy examination to check for functional CL.
• ELISA or RIA for progesterone—acceptable levels vary from >1 to >4 ng/mL, depending on the reference lab.

Maternal T_3/T_4 Levels

• Anecdotal reports of lower levels in mares with history of failure of conception, early embryonic loss, or abortion.
• Significance of low T_4 levels is not clear at present.

Cytogenetic Studies

May be indicated with suspected maternal chromosomal abnormalities.

Feed Analysis

May be indicated for specific xenobiotics (e.g., ergopeptine alkaloids, phytoestrogens, heavy metals) or endophyte (*Neotyphodium coenophialum*).

IMAGING

Transrectal U/S is essential to confirm early pregnancy and normal embryonic development and to detect embryonic death, intrauterine fluid, and endometrial cysts.

OTHER DIAGNOSTIC PROCEDURES

Reproductive Evaluation of Mares

• In predisposed individuals (i.e., barren, old mares, or mares with history of EED), evaluation before breeding is indicated.
• Transrectal U/S, vaginal examination (speculum and manual digital), endometrial cytology/culture, and endometrial biopsy should detect anatomic defects and endometrial inflammation or fibrosis that may predispose a mare to conception failure (see Endometritis and Endometrial Biopsy).

Transrectal U/S

• Performed at weekly intervals in mares with history of EED
• Biweekly in normal mares to detect EED
• Follow embryonic growth and development, and distinguish the conceptus from cysts.

PATHOLOGICAL FINDINGS

Endometrial biopsy; for presence of moderate to severe, chronic endometrial inflammation and/or fibrosis (see Endometrial Biopsy).

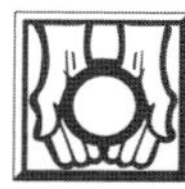

TREATMENT

APPROPRIATE HEALTH CARE

• Treatment of preexisting endometritis
• Insemination or breeding of mares during physiologic breeding season when they have adequate body condition.
• Insemination or breeding of foal heat mares when ovulation occurs at ≥10 days postpartum and no intrauterine fluid is present.
• Progestin supplementation.
• Various forms of embryo transfer to retrieve embryos from the uterus (6–8 days after ovulation) or oviduct (≅2–4 days after ovulation).
• Successful in vitro fertilization is in the early stages of development.
• Primary, age-related, embryonic defects are refractory to treatment (see Endometritis, ET, Ovulation Failure).
• Most cases can be handled in an ambulatory situation.
• Careful monitoring of embryonic development may require adequate restraint and optimal lighting in a hospital setting if such are not available in the field.

NURSING CARE

• Generally requires none
• Minimal nursing care after more invasive diagnostic and therapeutic procedures.

ACTIVITY

• Generally no restriction of broodmare activity, unless contraindicated by concurrent maternal disease or diagnostic or therapeutic procedures.
• Preference may be to restrict activity of mares in competition.

DIET

Mare can be fed a normal diet, unless contraindicated by concurrent maternal disease.

CLIENT EDUCATION

• Emphasize age-related aspects and their refractoriness to treatment.
• Educate regarding the cause, diagnosis, and treatment of endometritis.
• Inform regarding seasonal aspects and nutritional requirements of embryonic development.

• Clients should understand the role that endophyte-infected fescue and certain heterospecific breedings might play in conception failure.

SURGICAL CONSIDERATIONS

Surgery may be indicated in the repair of anatomic defects predisposing mares to endometritis or in certain therapeutic procedures.

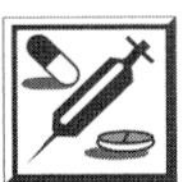

MEDICATIONS

DRUG(S) OF CHOICE

• See Endometritis and Metritis for specific drug recommendations.
• Mares with a history of EED or moderate to severe endometrial inflammation (i.e., no active, infectious component) and/or fibrosis—altrenogest (Regu-mate; Hoechst-Roussel Agri-Vet; 0.044–0.088 mg/kg PO q24h commencing 2–3 days after ovulation or at diagnosis of pregnancy, continued until at least day 100 of gestation [some clinicians prefer day 120], then gradually declining in daily dose over a 14-day period at the end of its administration).
• Altrenogest administration may be started later in gestation, continued longer, or used for only short periods of time depending on serum progesterone levels during the first 80 days of gestation (>1 to >4 ng/mL, depending on the reference), clinical circumstances, risk factors, and clinician preference.
• If used near term, altrenogest frequently is discontinued 7–14 days before the expected foaling date, depending on the case, unless otherwise indicated by assessment of fetal maturity/viability or questions exist regarding the correct gestational age.

CONTRAINDICATIONS

Use altrenogest only to prevent EED when infectious endometritis is not present concurrently.

PRECAUTIONS

Transrectal U/S

• Used to diagnose pregnancy at 14–16 days after ovulation
• To identify retention of intrauterine fluid or development of pyometra
• If pregnancy is diagnosed, frequent monitoring (weekly at first) may be indicated to detect EED.

Altrenogest

Because altrenogest is absorbed through the skin, those handling this preparation should wear nitrile gloves and wash their hands.

Progestins

• Widespread use of supplemental progestins in cases of EED is supported mainly by anecdotal reports of success.
• Primary, age-related, embryonic defects do not respond to supplemental progestins.

POSSIBLE INTERACTIONS N/A

ALTERNATIVE DRUGS

Progesterone

• Injectable progesterone (100–150 mg/day IM q24 h in an oil base) can be administered instead of altrenogest.
• Variations, contraindications, and precautions in administration are similar to those associated with altrenogest.
• Other injectable and implantable progestin preparations are available commercially for use in other species, but reports of their efficacy in mares are anecdotal.

T_4

• Supplementation has been successful anecdotally in mares with histories of subfertility.
• Its use remains controversial, and is considered deleterious by some clinicians.

FOLLOW-UP

PATIENT MONITORING

• Accurate teasing records
• Reexamination of mares diagnosed and treated for endometritis before breeding
• Early examination for pregnancy with transrectal U/S
• Monitoring of embryonic and fetal development with transrectal and/or transabdominal U/S

PREVENTION/AVOIDANCE

• Recognition of at-risk mares
• Management of preexisting endometritis before breeding
• Removal of mares from fescue pasture after breeding and during early gestation.
• Prudent use of medications in bred mares
• Avoiding exposure to known toxicants

POSSIBLE COMPLICATIONS

Later, high-risk pregnancy or abortion

EXPECTED COURSE AND PROGNOSIS

• Young mares with resolved cases of endometritis may have a fair to good prognosis for conception and completion of pregnancy.
• Mares of >15 years with a history of EED or chronic, moderate to severe endometrial inflammation and/or fibrosis have a guarded to poor prognosis for conception and completion of pregnancy.

MISCELLANEOUS

ASSOCIATED CONDITIONS

• Abortion
• Conception failure
• Endometritis
• Metritis

AGE-RELATED FACTORS

• Development of chronic endometritis and endometrial fibrosis
• Age-related embryonic defects

ZOONOTIC POTENTIAL

N/A

PREGNANCY

• By definition, EED is associated with pregnancy.
• Increased risk of abortion

SEE ALSO

• Abortion
• Conception failure
• Embryo transfer
• Endometritis
• Endometrial biopsy
• Metritis
• Pregnancy diagnosis

ABBREVIATIONS

• CL = corpus luteum
• EED = early embryonic death
• ELISA = enzyme-linked immunosorbent assay
• ET = embryo transfer
• MRLS = mare reproductive loss syndrome
• RIA = radioimmunoassay
• T_3 = triiodothyronine
• T_4 = thyroxine
• U/S = ultrasound, ultrasonography

Suggested Reading

Ball BA, Daels PF. Early pregnancy loss in mares: application for progestin therapy. In: Robinson NE, ed. Current Therapy in Equine Medicine, ed 4. Philadelphia: WB Saunders, 1997;531–533.

Dwyer RM, Garber LP, Traub-Dargatz JL, et al. Case-control study of factors associated with excessive proportions of early fetal losses associated with mare reproductive loss syndrome in central Kentucky during 2001. J Am Vet Med Assoc 2003; 222:613–619.

Evans TJ, Carleton CL. Conception failure. In: Brown CM, Bertone JJ, eds. The 5-Minute Veterinary Consult Equine. Philadelphia: Lippincott Williams and Wilkins, 2002:354–355.

Evans TJ, Rottinghaus GE, Casteel SW. Ergopeptine alkaloid toxicoses in horses. In: Robinson NE, ed. Current Therapy in Equine Medicine, ed 5. Philadelphia: Saunders, 2003:796–798.

Ginther OJ. Reproductive Biology of the Mare: Basic and Applied Aspects, ed 2. Cross Plains, WI: Equiservices, 1992:499–562.

Paccamonti D. Endometrial cysts. In: Robinson NE, ed. Current Therapy in Equine Medicine, ed 5. Philadelphia: WB Saunders, 2003:231–234.

Vanderwall DK, Squires EL, Brinsko SP, et al. Diagnosis and management of abnormal embryonic development characterized by formation of an embryonic vesicle without an embryo in mares. J Am Vet Med Assoc 2000;217:58–63.

Author Tim J. Evans

Consulting Editor Carla L. Carleton

EASTERN, WESTERN, AND VENEZUELAN ENCEPHALITIDES

BASICS

DEFINITION

EEE, WEE and VEE are encephalomyelitides of North and South America that spread from wild (sylvatic) reservoirs to horses and humans and other mammals, most often by mosquito species.

PATHOPHYSIOLOGY

Varying degrees of destructive encephalomyelitis associated with intraneuronal viral replication

SYSTEMS AFFECTED

Central nervous system, especially the cerebral cortex

INCIDENCE/PREVALENCE

Highly variable

GEOGRAPHIC DISTRIBUTION

North and South America only

SIGNALMENT

- There is no associated breed, sex, and age predisposition.
- Old and young horses may be at greater risk.

SIGNS

Historical

- Unvaccinated horses in endemic areas are at high risk.
- A recent history of cases in nearby areas and seasons with high vector numbers should increase suspicion.
- Cases may occur year round in southern latitudes.
- Cases of WEE occur in the western and mid-western United States, EEE cases tend to occur in the eastern and mid-western United States, and VEE cases have been reported in southern Texas and South America and occasionally in nearby locales.

Physical Examination

May be febrile and may show signs of colic

Neurologic

- Clinical signs, which vary in severity with each virus, usually are referable to diffuse cerebral disease, but sometimes signs of spinal cord disease predominate.
- Fever, prodromal malaise, colic, and anorexia may initially be evident; then there is a progressive, but often abrupt, onset of somnolence and peracute to acute diffuse brain signs.
- Dementia, head pressing, ataxia, blindness, circling, and seizures often become evident.
- Signs of spinal cord or brainstem involvement may occur first, occasionally with focal sensory, reflex and lower motor neuron signs, particularly in the brainstem.
- Cases of VEE may have similar or different clinical presentations compared with WEE and EEE. This is most likely due to the difference in strain pathogenicity.
- Diarrhea, severe obtundation, recumbency, and death may be noted before neurologic deficits are evident.
- Other associated signs include abortion, oral ulceration, pulmonary hemorrhage, and epistaxis.

CAUSES

Etiologic Agent

EEE, WEE, and VEE viruses are single-stranded, enveloped RNA viruses in the family Togaviridae, genus *Alphavirus.* They are vector borne and were classified as arboviruses.

RISK FACTORS

Poor vaccination programs and the presence of dense populations of insects (most often mosquitoes) spreading viral particles from the sylvatic reservoirs, which often include birds, rodents, and reptiles.

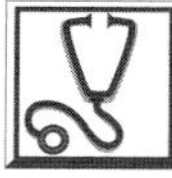

DIAGNOSIS

- Complement fixation, hemagglutination inhibition, and neutralizing antibodies are present early in the disease.
- A 4-fold rise in titer between acute and convalescent (7–10 days later) serum samples is considered positive for the diseases.
- An increased single sample titer in an unvaccinated animal is probably sufficient to establish a diagnosis.
- A single sample analysis must be interpreted cautiously if there is a history of vaccination against the viruses.
- Vaccinal versus wild virus–induced titers can be distinguished using serum hemagglutination-inhibition titers to EEE and WEE. EEE-to-WEE titer ratios of 4 or more are suspicious for EEE infection. A ratio of 8 or more is highly indicative of EEE. An ELISA can distinguish between vaccinal (IgG only) and virulent virus–induced (IgG and IgM) titers.

DIFFERENTIAL DIAGNOSIS

West Nile virus, rabies, leukoencephalomalacia, and hepatic encephalopathy—West Nile virus encephalomyelitis in the United States tends to result in less severe cerebral and more prominent spinal cord signs than in EEE and WEE.

CBC/BIOCHEMISTRY/URINALYSIS

No pathognomonic abnormalities

PATHOLOGIC FINDINGS

Gross necropsy findings are nonspecific. A gray discoloration with petechial hemorrhages of the brain and spinal cord is evident. There is often brain swelling and evidence of occipital-subtentorial herniation and brainstem compression. Histologic changes are characteristically strongly definitive. Diffuse gray matter predominant meningoencephalomyelitis with neuronal degeneration, gliosis, perivascular and neuroparenchymal infiltrates, and meningitis are highly suggestive for this disease group.

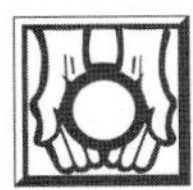

TREATMENT

AIMS OF TREATMENT

Treatment is supportive and should be aimed at metabolic maintenance and care and prophylaxis of self-induced trauma. No specific treatment will reduce morbidity and mortality.

NURSING CARE

Many horses, if they survive, have residual neurologic deficits: the ethics of nursing these cases should be discussed with owners.

CLIENT EDUCATION

Appropriate vaccination and vector control

MEDICATIONS

DRUG(S) OF CHOICE

Fluid and metabolic support can be useful. No specific drug treatment is likely to alter morbidity or mortality.

FOLLOW-UP

PATIENT MONITORING

Regular detailed neurologic examinations

PREVENTION/AVOIDANCE

Strict mosquito control and vaccination can prevent both human and equine cases. All equine cases should be reported to state health officials.

EXPECTED COURSE AND PROGNOSIS

Complete recoveries from the neurologic deficits associated with these viruses are reported, but they are rare. Animals that have recovered from EEE often have residual neurologic deficits that commonly include clumsiness, depression, and abnormal behavior. Neurologic sequelae are similar but less common in horses that recover from WEE. For horses that develop neurologic disease, the mortality rate for EEE is 75%–100%; for WEE, 20%–50%, and for VEE, 40%–80%. Reinfection is possible and survivors should be vaccinated.

POSSIBLE COMPLICATIONS

Self-induced trauma may be severe.

MISCELLANEOUS

ZOONOTIC POTENTIAL

- There is essentially no amplification of virus from horses afflicted with EEE and WEE. Hence, they are dead-end hosts.
- Horses with VEE have sufficient circulating viral concentrations that they act as amplifiers of disease.
- Ocular and nasal secretions from infected horses contain high concentrations of VEE.
- Infection via entry through the respiratory tract may occur by direct contact with infected animals.
- Equine and human survivors of VEE infection and clinical disease may develop chronic relapsing viremias and serve as chronic disease amplifiers.

ABBREVIATIONS

- EEE = Eastern equine encephalomyelitis
- VEE = Venezuelan equine encephalomyelitis
- WEE = Western equine encephalomyelitis

Suggested Reading

Del Piero F, Wilkins PA, Dubovi EJ, Biolatti B, Cantile C. Immunohistochemical, and virologic findings of Eastern equine encephalomyelitis in two horses. Vet Pathol 2001;38:451–456.

International Veterinary Information Service. Website. Available at: http://www.ivis.org/advances/Carter/toc.asp.

The author and editors wish to acknowledge the contribution of Joseph J. Bertone, author of this chapter in the previous edition.

Author Caroline N. Hahn
Consulting Editor Caroline N. Hahn

ECLAMPSIA

BASICS

Also known as puerperal tetany or lactation tetany

DEFINITION/OVERVIEW

• A rare metabolic condition resulting when serum calcium levels drop below 8 mg/dL in heavily lactating mares • Clinical signs are progressive and directly related to the level of serum calcium. • The mare develops muscle fasciculations beginning with the temporal, masseter and triceps muscles, demonstrates a stiff, stilted gait and rear limb ataxia, becomes anxious, and experiences tachycardia with dysrhythmias. • It usually occurs around 2 weeks after foaling and is associated with lactation and stress.

ETIOLOGY/PATHOPHYSIOLOGY

• The etiology is related to loss of calcium in the milk, particularly in those mares that are heavy milkers, especially when they are on lush pasture. • The condition is also seen most often in draft mares and heavy, well-muscled mares, Quarter Horse halter-type mares, that are working while lactating, or lactating mares that are transported over long distances. • The condition is also recognized in the heavily milking mare 1 to 2 days post-weaning.

SYSTEMS AFFECTED

• Mammary • Musculoskeletal • Cardiovascular • Neurologic

GENETICS

Draft breeds, but not exclusively

INCIDENCE/PREVALENCE

Rare

SIGNALMENT

Based primarily on clinical signs in conjunction with the appropriate historical information:
• Lactating mare 10 days postpartum or 1–2 days post-weaning or in late gestation
• Prolonged exercise or transport • On lush pasture • Serum calcium values in the 5–8 mg/dL range, coupled with associated clinical signs, confirm the diagnosis. • Draft mares—Belgian, Percheron, Clydesdale • No age predisposition • Unlikely occurrence in primiparous mares

SIGNS

- Signs of eclampsia vary and include:
  - Muscle fasciculations involving the temporal, masseter and triceps.
  - Generalized increased muscle tone; stiff, stilted gait; rear limb ataxia.
  - Trismus (tonic contraction of the muscles of mastication); dysphagia; salivation.
  - Profuse sweating; elevated temperature; anxiety, tachycardia with dysrhythmias.
  - Synchronous diaphragmatic flutter, convulsions, coma, and death.
  - If untreated, the condition is progressive over a 24- to 48-hr period and some of these mares die.
- The clinical signs are directly related to the level of serum calcium.
  - Increased excitability with calcium levels that are below normal (range 11–13 mg/dL) but >8 mg/dL
  - Calcium levels of 5–8 mg/dL usually produce signs of tetanic spasms and incoordination.
  - Serum calcium levels <5 mg/dL—often become stuporous and are recumbent

CAUSES

• Lactation • Exercise + lactation • Transport + lactation • Heavily lactating mare after foal has been weaned

RISK FACTORS

Lactation, postpartum, heavier milking mares

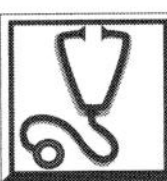

DIAGNOSIS

DIFFERENTIAL DIAGNOSIS

• Colic • Laminitis • Myositis • Tetanus
• Other neuromuscular disorders

CBC/BIOCHEMISTRY/URINALYSIS

Parameters should be within normal limits, except for possibly elevated muscle enzymes.

OTHER LABORATORY TESTS

• Normal laboratory ranges reported for serum calcium vary, e. g., (1) from 8.5 to 10.5 and (2) from 11 to 13 mg/dL. The majority of normal mares will be within 11–13 mg/dL. • It is best to know the normal range for serum calcium generated by *the laboratory that you regularly use*. • In addition to abnormally low levels of serum calcium, many affected mares have been reported to have abnormalities in serum levels of magnesium and phosphorus. • Hypocalcemia in the mare has been associated with hyper/hypophosphatemia and hyper/hypomagnesemia. • Reports suggest that hypomagnesemia/hypocalcemia is most commonly associated with transport of heavily lactating mares.

OTHER DIAGNOSTIC PROCEDURES

• Evaluate serum calcium, preferably ionized calcium, if available. • Evaluate serum protein. Normal ionized calcium possible despite hypocalcemia if severe hypoproteinemia. No clinical signs if ionized calcium is within normal range • There may be excess protein in the mare's urine.

PATHOLOGICAL FINDINGS

N/A

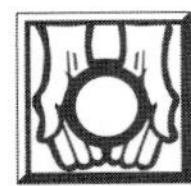

TREATMENT

APPROPRIATE HEALTH CARE

• Because of the progressive nature of this condition, therapy is recommended in nearly all cases. • A few mildly affected cases will recover without treatment.

NURSING CARE

• None • Occasional mare may require a second treatment, if relapse occurs.

ACTIVITY

Restrict transit of heavily lactating mares during the susceptible period, the first 10–12 days postpartum.

DIET

• Restrict access of heavily lactating mares to lush pasture if they have a history of eclampsia. • Feed high-protein, high-calcium diets post-foaling for mares previously prone to eclampsia.

CLIENT EDUCATION

• In addition to restricting access to lush pasture with a history of the eclampsia, reduce nutritional intake (quality) in heavily lactating mares for 1–2 weeks prior to weaning to reduce milk production.

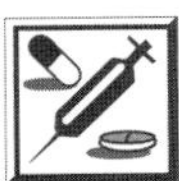

MEDICATIONS

DRUG(S) OF CHOICE

• IV calcium, in the form of 20% calcium borogluconate or 23% calcium gluconate
• Rate—250–500 mL per 500 kg body weight • Calcium solutions should be diluted 1:4 with saline or dextrose.

PRECAUTIONS

• Use caution when administering calcium solutions due to potential cardiotoxic effects.
• Imperative to monitor the heart for any alterations in rate or rhythm • If alterations occur, the treatment should be stopped immediately. • Dilution of the calcium with saline or dextrose reduces the potential for cardiotoxic effects.

FOLLOW-UP

PATIENT MONITORING

• A reduction in the clinical signs and a positive inotropic effect indicate treatment is effective. • If no response is evident after the initial treatment, a second treatment may be necessary in 30 minutes.

PREVENTION/AVOIDANCE

• Decreasing high-protein feeds in the mare's diet late in gestation may decrease incidence in susceptible mares. • In previously affected mares, decrease intake of calcium 2–5 weeks pre-foaling. • High-protein, high-calcium diets post-foaling for mares prone to eclampsia • See Client Education and Diet for susceptible mares.

POSSIBLE COMPLICATIONS

Cardiovascular effects

EXPECTED COURSE AND PROGNOSIS

• Most mares respond to treatment with a full recovery; however, relapses can occur, necessitating additional therapy. • Recurrence in the future if mares are foaling and maintained under the same management conditions

MISCELLANEOUS

PREGNANCY

This condition occurs either late in gestation or the peripartal period.

SYNONYMS

• Hypocalcemia • Lactation tetany • Transit tetany

SEE ALSO

• Dystocia

Suggested Reading

Fenger CK. Disorders of calcium metabolism. In: Reed SM, Bayly WM, eds. Equine Internal Medicine. Toronto: WB Saunders, 1998:930–931.

Valberg SJ, Hodgson DR. Diseases of muscle. In: Smith BP, ed. Large Animal Internal Medicine, ed 2. St. Louis, Mosby, 1996:1498–1499.

Author Carla L. Carleton
Consulting Editor Carla L. Carleton

ECTOPARASITES

BASICS

DEFINITION

Chorioptes equi, Psoroptes equi, and lice (*Damalinia equi* and *Haematopinus asini)* complete their life cycle on the horse and are transmitted to other horses by direct or indirect contact, such as via shared combs or brushes, saddle blankets, or rubbing on stalls or fences.

PATHOPHYSIOLOGY

The major manifestation with lice is the irritation, but blood loss to the level of clinical anemia is possible with sucking lice (*Haematopinus asini*). Multiplication of mites on the host is theoretically exponential until the nonspecific and specific immune reactions of the host limit the number of mites.

SYSTEM AFFECTED

Skin

GENETICS

No predisposition

INCIDENCE/PREVALENCE

- Sporadic and secondary to contact with another infested horse or the immediate environment containing scabs or hair shafts with eggs or larvae present.
- More common in barns with horses that are hauled frequently and return with subclinical infestations.

GEOGRAPHIC DISTRIBUTION

Worldwide

SIGNALMENT

Breed Predilections

- None, however, chorioptic acariosis is more common on breeds with feathered fetlocks, such as draft breeds.

Mean Age and Range

- Frequent in animals of an age to travel to events where exposure occurs

Predominant Sex

- None

SIGNS

General Comments

Mite and lice infections are more severe in colder months when hair coat length can mask their presence. Weight loss can be seen due to the chronic irritation rather than a direct interference with other systems. Infestations may produce typical clinical signs in some animals whereas others may exhibit few clinical signs or may be asymptomatic carriers.

Historical

Often involves travel to an equestrian event where exposure had occurred. Low level exposure may require months to develop into a noticeable infestation.

Physical Examination

Lice Infestation

- Common in sick, old, or otherwise debilitated animals
- Affected animals often have a long hair coat, making lice difficult to find.
- During warm months, lice will congregate in the longer hair of the mane and tail.
- Secondary seborrhea can camouflage the lice from detection. As the louse hangs onto the hair shaft when feeding, do not expect to find lice in alopecic areas.
- The hair coat is of poor quality represented by multifocal areas of alopecia and scale.
- Pruritus can vary from absent to severe, and predominately affects the neck, shoulders, mane, tail, and less often the legs.
- Lice glue their nits to hair shafts which are more numerous and noticeable than the adults. Examination of the tail and mane can identify the presence of *H. asini* nits. Adults also feed on the fetlocks and upper and inner thighs.
- *Damalinia equi*, the chewing louse of equids, prefers sites on the body such as the forehead, neck, and dorsolateral trunk rather than the neck and tail. When exercised, the increased body temperature tends to make the lice climb out toward the tip of the hairs and thus more easily identified.

Chorioptes (leg and tail mange)

- Live on the surface of the skin, do not penetrate the epidermis, and do not bite. These infections are generally less severe and less pruritic than psoroptic acariosis.
- Chorioptic acariosis commences with pruritus, irritation and restlessness represented by foot stamping and biting at the legs. The affected seeks every opportunity to rub or chew at its legs. Pruritus may be mild or absent in some cases.
- A mildly erythematous papular to crusted dermatitis involving the distal extremities is the initial clinical sign. Hind legs are always initially more severely affected, progressing into patchy alopecia with broken hair, prominent scaling, excoriations and hyperplasia of the affected regions. Exudation of serum with matting of leg hair and thick adherent crusts may develop over limited or extensive areas. Although lesions are generally localized to the lower limb, extension to involve the entire leg and ventrum may occur. Subtle lesions such as mild scale present on the ventral midline are described. Self-trauma results in secondary bacterial dermatitis. Generalized infestations result in a moth-eaten appearance with weight loss, irritability and exercise intolerance.

Psoroptes (mane and tail mange)

- *Psoroptes equis* is rare but highly contagious. Psoroptic mites do not burrow and feeding results in exudation of serum which hardens to form scabs.
- Lesions are found on regions such as under the forelock, base of the mane and tail and the axillary region. Lesions may slowly extend over the body. The mites prefer areas with thick hair such as the ears, mane, tail, and intermandibular areas.
- Intense pruritus is the hallmark clinical sign and results in head shaking and tail rubbing. Tail and mane hairs are often broken and distorted. Papules, vesicles, crusts, scaling, alopecia, excoriations, and exudation on the skin and ear margins are common. Lichenification of the ears, mane, and tail-head may be seen. Dorsal erythematous lesions that bleed easily when traumatized may develop.
- The species *P. hippotis* and *P. cuniculi* cause otoacariosis, which results in aural discharge, head-rubbing, head shaking, and carrying the ears in a downward droopy flat position.

Trombiculidiasis (harvest mite, chiggers)

Trombicula autumnalis infestation leads to seasonal pruritus of the sides of the face (perocular, perioral, and muzzle), feathers of the fetlocks, mane and tail, and sometimes the ventrum in pasture-grazed horses. Orange or brown sticky patches of serum are present on the legs forming matted erect hair tufts. Pruritus can be intense, resulting in stamping, head shaking, chewing at the legs and self-inflicted trauma. Secondary infections can produce boggy fetlocks.

CAUSES

Opportunistic infestations secondary to contact with another infested horse

RISK FACTORS

- Travel to equestrian events or trail rides
- Asymptomatic carriers of *C. equi* serve to perpetuate the infection from season to season.
- Horses with long, thick, and unclean coats may be more susceptible to psoroptic acariosis.
- Horses put out to pasture with tall grass in the late spring to late summer are a risk for development of trombiculidiasis.

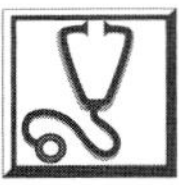

DIAGNOSIS

DIFFERENTIAL DIAGNOSIS

Differentials for lice infestation include the following:

- Chorioptic and psoroptic mange
- Trombiculidiasis
- *Culicoides* spp. hypersensitivity
- *Oxyuris equi* infestation
- *Dermanyssus gallinae*/*Tyroglyphus* spp. poultry mite infestation
- Stickfast fleas, spinose ear tick
- Insect hypersensitivities
- Dermatophilosis
- Microsporosis (ringworm)

Differentials for chorioptic and psoroptic infestations include the following:

- Trombiculidiasis
- Sarcoptic mange
- *Culicoides* hypersensitivity
- Pediculosis
- Dermatophilosis
- Dermatophytosis
- *Strongyloides westerni* dermatitis
- Pastern dermatitis
- Atopic dermatitis

Differentials for *Trombicula* infestations include all pruritic diseases of the distal extremities.

CBC/BIOCHEMISTRY/URINALYSIS

- Anemia with heavy *H. asini* infestations
- Nonspecific eosinophilia with mange infestations

OTHER LABORATORY TESTS

N/A

IMAGING

- Microscopy for differentiating the causative arthropod
- *D. equi* are 1–2 mm in size, have a relatively broad body with transverse strips on the abdomen and a square head, while *H. asini* are 3–3.5 mm in size, have a longer narrower body

with a sharp conical head and piercing mouth parts.

• *Chorioptes* can be easily seen with a magnifying lens or on low power of the microscope. This mite is 0.3–0.5 mm and has an oval body, a small head with blunt mouthparts, and long legs with suckers directly fixed to the extremity.
• *Psoroptes* are 0.4–0.8 mm in size with an oval body and elongated mouthparts and long legs with triarticulate sucker-bearing peduncles.
• Trombiculid larvae are orange to red and 0.25–1.0 mm, have six long legs and an oval body, and can sometimes be seen by the naked eye.

OTHER DIAGNOSTIC PROCEDURES

• Proper sampling technique improves the chances to demonstrate the mites. Clipping of the affected area is essential; otherwise, much of the specimen will stick to the surrounding hairs. Use a No. 10 blade coated with mineral oil to help collect the mites when performing superficial skin scrapes.
• Multiple superficial skin scrapings from the edge of fresh lesions are needed to recover superficial mites such as *Chorioptes* and *Psoroptes* mites as they often abandon alopecia and crusty lesions. Skin scrapings can be negative in asymptomatic carriers or in chronic disease. *Trombicula* are found in crusts of dried serum. Soften crusts in 10% KOH before examination under the microscope. The orange-colored larval stages are seen under low power.
• Other collection methods include acetate tape preparations or a firm toothbrush used to brush material downward onto a glass slide or Petri dish.
• An otoscope provides both a magnifying lens and good light in one tool and is useful for ectoparasite identification among the hairs.

PATHOLOGICAL FINDINGS

Skin biopsies from mange infestations are usually nonspecific unless fragments or entire parasites are present in the sections. The prominent findings are varying degrees of superficial perivascular dermatitis with numerous eosinophils and possible deep lymphoid nodules, a description compatible with both ectoparasites and hypersensitivities.

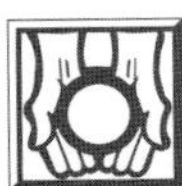

TREATMENT

AIMS OF TREATMENT

Prevent reinfestations with use of long-acting insecticides or acaricides. Treat all horses on the premises to prevent a single reservoir supplying the mites or lice for reinfestation.

APPROPRIATE HEALTH CARE

Outpatient medical management is appropriate for most cases.

NURSING CARE

Repeat treatments as needed.

ACTIVITY

As additional dispersal is by host mobility and transportation of infested hosts, limit the horse's contact with others in pastures, barns and transportaion vehicles.

DIET

Poor nutrition predisposes to many illnesses beyond lice and mites.

CLIENT EDUCATION

Prevention of infestations is achieved by the use of pyrethroid sprays or wipes during periods off premises and will aid in avoiding infestations when the horse returns to the barn.

SURGICAL CONSIDERATIONS

N/A

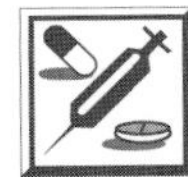

MEDICATIONS

DRUG(S)

• Shampooing the mane and tail with pyrethrin, pyrethroids, lime sulfur, or selenium sulfide products is an initial step in removal of adult lice, or washing the fetlocks in the case of a chorioptic mange infestation. This in itself is insufficient due to eggs that will hatch after shampooing. Removal of the nits from the mane and tail is beneficial. Long-acting pyrethroid, cypermethrin, or resmethrin sprays or wipes must then be applied to kill hatching larval stages of the arthropod. Fly wipes or sprays with pyrethroid compounds may require weekly application to achieve success.
• Fipronil spray (Frontline for dogs) is not approved for use on horses. Fipronil is highly effective against related arthropods, thus pharmacologically a worthy consideration. Application of the spray at 3-week intervals for 3 treatments should be completely effective.
• Ivermectin 200 μg/kg PO given twice at a 14-day interval is effective against *H. asini* but not *D. equi*.
• For chorioptic mange, clipping is advised before applying the antiparasitic agents. Ivermectin reduces mite numbers but is less effective. Treat the entire body as the mites can migrate to the neck, trunk, and face.
• For psoroptic acariosis, ivermectin at 200 μg/kg PO given twice at 14-day intervals is effective.
• For control of mange, a combination of a systemic macrocyclic lactone with the application of a topical acaricidal is the best treatment.
• Trombiculidosis is self-limiting if the horse is removed from the pasture; however, using topical acaracides effectively kills the larvae and corticosteroid treatment may be necessary to provide interim relief from the pruritus.

CONTRAINDICATIONS

• Amitraz use is contraindicated in horses.

PRECAUTIONS

• Feline susceptibility to pyrethroid compounds is dose dependent and the formulations for use on horses (0.05%–0.10%) are rarely of a level to achieve this toxicity, but some topical formulations for dogs and horses reach >50% permethrin, which cause neurological problems if applied directly to a cat. After applying a pyrethroid product directly to horses, a 2-hr drying time generally limits any toxic transfer from the horse to a cat. The use of environmental sprays with pyrethroids for fly control should be considered carefully for the effects on barn cats.
• Injectable ivermectin can cause serious side effects in some horses.

POSSIBLE INTERACTIONS

Not known

ALTERNATIVE DRUGS

Herbal remedies are available, but their effect is probably due more to daily grooming and application. Pyrethrins are plant derivatives.

FOLLOW-UP

PATIENT MONITORING

Observe for clinical signs of reinfestation.

PREVENTION/AVOIDANCE

Treat all horses on the premises to prevent a reservoir from initiating a second wave of infestations. For horses traveling to or returning from equestrian events consider topical treatments if contact with other infested horses is suspected. Parasiticidal treatments must be combined with other methods—isolation of all contaminated horses, avoidance of infested areas, and disinfection of barns and material.

POSSIBLE COMPLICATIONS

Reinfection can occur when using short-acting insecticides or acaricides.

EXPECTED COURSE AND PROGNOSIS

Excellent prognosis if all horses on a farm are treated.

MISCELLANEOUS

AGE-RELATED FACTORS

Exposure is required, thus more common in juveniles or adults rather than foals or weanlings, but infestation is possible if present on the breeding farm.

ZOONOTIC POTENTIAL

Infestations are species specific. Transient infestations on humans are possible for a matter of hours, but no establishment is possible.

PREGNANCY

No known complications

SEE ALSO

• Insect hypersensitivity
• Pastern dermatitis
• Atopic dermatitis

Suggested Reading

Lloyd DH, Littlewood JD, Craig JM, Thomsett LR. Practical Equine Dermatology. Oxford: Blackwell, 2003; 27.

Scott DW, Miller WH Jr. Equine Dermatology. St. Louis: Saunders, 2003; 27.

Author Cliff Monahan

Consulting Editor Gwendolen Lorch

EHRLICHIOSIS, EQUINE GRANULOCYTIC

BASICS

DEFINITION

This is a seasonal, tick-borne disease caused by a granulocytotropic rickettsial organism, *Anaplasma phagocytophilum* (previously *Ehrlichia equi).*

PATHOPHYSIOLOGY

- *Ixodes pacificus* (the Western black-legged tick) is a vector for *A. phagocytophilum* on the Pacific coast.
- *Ixodes scapularis* (the black-legged tick or deer tick) is the likely primary vector for the disease in the eastern and midwestern United States.
- Existence of a maintenance or sylvatic host is unknown but likely represents a wild reservoir; horses are considered dead-end hosts and are not directly contagious.
- Incubation period—8–25 days after experimental infection using ticks as vectors
- The agent affects granulocytes (both neutrophils and eosinophils) and causes a vasculitis and interstitial inflammation, leading to edema, petechial hemorrhages, ataxia, and hemolytic anemia.

SYSTEMS AFFECTED

- Behavioral—mentation alteration (i.e., lethargy) of varying degrees
- Hemic/lymphatic/immune—vasculitis, leading to edema and mucosal hemorrhages; hemolytic anemia
- Musculoskeletal—reluctance to move, limb edema
- Nervous—vasculitis in the CNS, leading to ataxia and recumbency
- Cardiac—Arrhythmias have been associated with myocarditis secondary to vasculitis within the myocardium.
- Myopathy—rare, but observed in one case

GENETICS

N/A

INCIDENCE/PREVALENCE

- There is a high prevalence in the Sierra Nevada foothills and northern coastal range of California and many areas of New England, as well as New York, Connecticut, New Jersey, and the Midwest including Illinois, Minnesota and other adjacent states. Anywhere the tick vector is present is at risk for the disease.
- Seroprevalence studies in northern California show a prevalence of 3.1–10.3%, depending on geographic location, and >50% seropositivity among horses on premises known to be enzootic for the disease.
- The disease is seasonal, having its highest occurrence during the late fall, winter, and spring and its peak during March in California.

SIGNALMENT

- Primarily affects horses, but donkeys have been experimentally infected
- No breed or sex predilections
- Horses ≥4 years are most severely affected.
- The disease has been reported in a foal as young as 2.5 months.

SIGNS

Historical Findings

- Lethargy
- High fever
- Anorexia
- Limb edema
- Tick exposure

Physical Examination Findings

- Pyrexia
- Anorexia
- Depressed mentation
- Limb edema (absent in young animals)
- Mild petechiae and ecchymoses on mucous membranes and sclerae
- Icterus
- Ataxia
- Reluctance to move
- Arrhythmias (rare)
- Recumbency (rare)

CAUSES

- *Anaplasma phagocytophilum*, a granulocytotropic rickettsia, spread by *Ixodes* ticks
- Close antigenic and genetic similarity to the agent of HGE and to European tick-borne fever affecting ruminants

RISK FACTORS

- Geography
- Exposure to *I. ricinus* complex ticks
- Age—Horses ≥4 years are most severely affected.
- Immune status

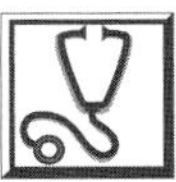

DIAGNOSIS

DIFFERENTIAL DIAGNOSIS

- Viral encephalitis—rapid progression of disease with high mortality
- Liver disease with hepatic encephalopathy—increased serum hepatic enzyme activities and bilirubin and bile acid concentrations
- Purpura hemorrhagica—history of exposure to antigens of *Streptococcus equi* or other respiratory pathogens; usually not thrombocytopenic
- EIA—seropositive on Coggins or ELISA tests
- Equine viral arteritis—respiratory signs; seropositive to virus.

CBC/BIOCHEMISTRY/URINALYSIS

- Leukopenia with neutropenia
- Thrombocytopenia
- Increased icteric index
- Anemia
- Hyperbilirubinemia (high unconjugated bilirubin)

OTHER LABORATORY TESTS

- Giemsa-, new methylene blue–, or Wright-stained peripheral blood smears show inclusion bodies (i.e., morula) within the cytoplasm of neutrophils and eosinophils. Inclusions are pleomorphic and blue-gray to dark blue in color, have a spoke-wheel appearance, and occur in 30–75% of circulating granulocytes within 3–6 days of the onset of fever.
- Buffy coat smears concentrate granulocytes and, therefore, increase the sensitivity of identifying inclusion bodies.
- Coagulopathies consistent with disseminated intravascular coagulation (DIC) may be present.
- Indirect fluorescent antibody tests are available for serology. A titer ≥1:10 suggests exposure which may not be acute. An increasing titer documents active infection but requires an acute and convalescent sample. A single sample with a cut off value of 1:40 can be seen from prior subclinical infection and is not diagnostic for acute infection.
- PCR amplification of DNA from buffy coats of infected horses is a very sensitive diagnostic tool when using real time TaqMan PCR. PCR is positive before inclusion bodies are first observed in neutrophils and persists while the animal is febrile.
- Immunohistochemistry of tissues from post mortem examination can be used for diagnosis.

IMAGING

N/A

DIAGNOSTIC PROCEDURES

N/A

PATHOLOGIC FINDINGS

- Mortality is rare, except for reasons of secondary complications. There is one recent report of mortality from the primary infection itself, thought to be due to severe vasculitis and DIC.
- Inflammation of small arteries and veins (vasculitis), hemorrhage, edema
- Mild inflammatory vascular or interstitial lesions in the heart, CNS, kidneys, and lung.

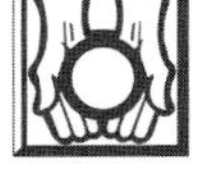

TREATMENT

APPROPRIATE HEALTH CARE

Hospitalize horses with severe ataxia or secondary complications; otherwise, uncomplicated cases can be managed in the field. The infection is often self-limiting, with horses recovering fully within 1–2 weeks.

NURSING CARE

- Supportive limb bandages for edema
- NSAIDs for antipyretic purposes
- Debilitated cases may benefit from IV fluid or electrolyte therapy.
- Corticosteroids may benefit horses with severe ataxia by reducing the severity of vasculitis.

EHRLICHIOSIS, EQUINE GRANULOCYTIC

ACTIVITY

Stall confinement for ataxic animals; otherwise, hand-walking may help to reduce edema.

DIET

N/A

CLIENT EDUCATION

When entering known *Ixodes* tick–infested areas, use tick repellents, and check horses closely for ticks upon return from these areas.

SURGICAL CONSIDERATIONS

N/A

MEDICATIONS

DRUG(S) OF CHOICE

Oxytetracycline (7 mg/kg IV q24h for 3–7 days diluted in 5% dextrose in water)–with this treatment, a marked decrease in rectal temperature and improvement in appetite and attitude should be observed in 12–24 hours. Doxycycline (10 mg/kg PO q12 h for 3–7 days) is an alternative used with success in field cases.

CONTRAINDICATIONS

N/A

PRECAUTIONS

- Tetracyclines can retard fetal skeletal development and discolor deciduous teeth; therefore, use with caution and only for a short duration during the first half of gestation, then only when the benefits outweigh the fetal risks.
- Monitor horses for signs of enterocolitis or diarrhea while on tetracycline therapy; the risk of diarrhea is greater with the oral route of administration of oxytetracycline, and may be less with doxycycline.
- Tetracyclines have been associated with photosensitivity and nephrotoxicity.
- NSAIDs have been associated with GI ulceration and nephrotoxicity.
- α_2-Agonist drugs (e.g., xylazine, detomidine) may induce tachypnea and respiratory distress in horses with pyrexia.

POSSIBLE INTERACTIONS

N/A

ALTERNATIVE DRUGS

N/A

FOLLOW-UP

PATIENT MONITORING

- Monitor temperature, attitude, and appetite for significant improvement within 12–24 hours of treatment.
- Evaluate serial buffy coat smear for inclusion bodies.
- Monitor hydration status and renal function while on oxytetracycline.

PREVENTION/AVOIDANCE

- Minimize exposure to *Ixodes* ticks through application of topical tick repellents when entering infested areas, and carefully examine horses for ticks on their return from such areas.
- Prevention is impractical in endemic areas, and many horses may experience subclinical infections and develop subsequent immunity.

POSSIBLE COMPLICATIONS

- Secondary bacterial infections, especially bronchopneumonia.
- Horses with severe ataxia may suffer traumatic injury (e.g., fractures).
- Cardiac arrhythmias, including ventricular tachycardia, may be associated with myocarditis; treatment of myocarditis consists of corticosteroids and antiarrhythmic drugs (e.g., quinidine) along with tetracycline therapy.
- Disseminated intravascular coagulation
- Recumbency

EXPECTED COURSE AND PROGNOSIS

- Excellent prognosis in uncomplicated cases.
- Horses are immune to reinfection for at least 2 years; no carrier or latent state has been documented.
- With therapy, horses show rapid improvement—a decrease in rectal temperature, increase in appetite, and improvement in overall demeanor should be noted in 12–24 hours; the ataxia should resolve within 2–3 days and the edema within several days.
- Left untreated, the disease is self-limiting in 2–3 weeks; however, affected horses exhibit more severe weight loss, edema, and ataxia and are at greater risk for secondary complications than horses treated with tetracycline. Laminitis is not associated with infection.
- Only one report of a confirmed death of a horse due solely to acute infection with *A. phagocytophilum*.

MISCELLANEOUS

ASSOCIATED CONDITIONS

N/A

AGE-RELATED FACTORS

Severity of clinical signs is associated with age—animals <1 year generally do not show signs of infection or at worst exhibit only slight lethargy and fever; animals 1–3 years of age show mild to moderate signs; and animals ≥4 years are affected most severely, with ataxia, icterus, edema, and petechial hemorrhages.

ZOONOTIC POTENTIAL

- The agent of HGE may represent one or more strains of the equine pathogen; however, horses are considered dead-end hosts and do not act as a source of human infection directly.
- Ticks are required as intermediate hosts.

PREGNANCY

- Two pregnant mares are reported to have been naturally infected with *A. phagocytophilum* during gestation and to have subsequently delivered live foals at full term.
- No abortions or congenital abnormalities have been described.
- Passive immunity is transferred to suckling foals but is short-lived in duration.

SYNONYMS

Equine ehrlichiosis

SEE ALSO

- Infectious anemia (IA)
- Thrombocytopenia

ABBREVIATIONS

- DIC = disseminated intravascular coagulopathy
- cELISA = competitive enzyme-linked immunosorbent assay
- EIA = equine infectious anemia
- GI = gastrointestinal
- HGE = human granulocytic ehrlichiosis
- PCR = polymerase chain reaction

Suggested Reading

Franzen P, Berg A-L, Aspan A, Gunnarsson A, Pringle J. Death of a horse infected experimentally with *Anaplasma phagocytophilum*. Vet Rec 2007;160:122–125.

Madigan JE, Gribble D. Equine ehrlichiosis in northern California: 49 Cases (1968—1981). J Am Vet Med Assoc 1987;190:445–448.

Madigan JE, Nietela S, Chalmers S, DeRock E. Seroepidemiologic survey of antibodies to *Ehrlichia equi* in horses of northern California. J Am Vet Med Assoc 1990;196:1962–1964.

Madigan JE, Richter PJ Jr, Kimsey RB, Barlough JE, Bakken JS, Dumler JS. Transmission and passage in horses of the agent of human granulocytic ehrlichiosis. J Infect Dis 1995;172:1141-1144.

Nolen-Walston RD, D'Oench SM, Hanelt LM, Sharkey LC, Paradis MR. Acute recumbency associated with *Anaplasma phagocytophilum* infection in a horse. J Am Vet Med Assoc 2004;224:1964–1966.

Reubel GH, Kimsey RB, Barlough JE, Madigan JE. Experimental transmission of *Ehrlichia equi* to horses through naturally infected ticks (*Ixodes pacificus*) from northern California. J Clin Microbiol 1998;36:2131–2134.

Richter PJ Jr, Kimsey RB, Madigan JE, Barlough JE, Dumler JS, Brooks DL. *Ixodes pacificus* (Acari: Ixodidae) as a vector of *Ehrlichia equi* (Rickettsiales: Ehrlichieae). J Med Entomol 1996;33:1–5.

Authors K. Gary Magdesian and John E. Madigan

Consulting Editors Ashley G. Boyle and Corrine R. Sweeney

EMBRYO TRANSFER (ET)

BASICS

DEFINITION/OVERVIEW

Removal of an embryo from the uterus or oviduct of one mare (the donor) and placement into the uterus or oviduct of another (the recipient)

SYSTEM AFFECTED

Reproductive

SIGNALMENT

- Mares of >15 years with a history of conception failure, EED, or abortion
- Young mares in competition
- Certain extraspecific matings—zebra into a horse

CBC/BIOCHEMISTRY/URINALYSIS

N/A

OTHER LABORATORY TESTS

- Dosing maternal progesterone may be indicated at recipient's initial pregnancy examination to check for functional CL.
- ELISA or RIA for progesterone—acceptable levels vary from >1 to >4 ng/mL, depending on the reference lab.
- Maternal T_3/T_4 levels—anecdotal reports of lower levels in mares with a history of conception failure, EED, or abortion; significance of low T_4 levels not clear at present

IMAGING

Transrectal U/S

- Indicated for donor and recipient at the time of flushing and transfer, respectively, to determine the absence of intrauterine fluid and the presence of CL
- Also used in one technique as a guide for the aspiration of oocytes

OTHER DIAGNOSTIC PROCEDURES

Prebreeding Reproductive Evaluation

- Indicated in individuals with a history of conception failure, EED, or abortion
- Indicated in mares being screened as potential ET recipients
- Transrectal U/S, vaginal examination (both by digital manual and speculum), endometrial cytology/culture, and endometrial biopsy should detect evidence of anatomic defects, endometritis, and fibrosis, which may predispose to conception failure.

Transrectal U/S

- To monitor follicular development and more precisely monitor ovulation in both the donor and recipient
- To time artificial, insemination or breeding
- To schedule ET for optimal success
- To confirm pregnancy in the recipient mare

Embryo Collection

May be used as a diagnostic procedure to determine if embryos can enter the oviduct or uterus

PATHOLOGICAL FINDINGS

Endometrial biopsy—moderate to severe, chronic endometritis or fibrosis may be indications for ET.

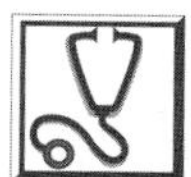

DIAGNOSIS

N/A

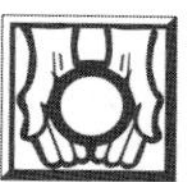

TREATMENT

APPROPRIATE HEALTH CARE

Most ETs are best handled in a hospital setting with adequate facilities and personnel.

Indications

- Mares with a history of conception failure, EED, repeated abortion, or high-risk pregnancy
- Mares with chronic, moderate to severe endometritis or fibrosis
- Mares in competition

Embryo Recovery Procedures

- Nonsurgical uterine flushing 6–8 days after ovulation
- Surgical oviductal flushing 2–4 days after ovulation
- Laparoscopic or transvaginal U/S-guided recovery of oocytes

Embryo Transfer Procedures

- Nonsurgical intrauterine transfer
- Surgical intrauterine transfer
- Pre–embryo stage procedures
- Laparoscopic or surgical oviductal transfer of zygotes—ZIFT
- In vitro fertilization
- Laparoscopic or surgical oviductal transfer of gametes—GIFT
- Cryopreservation of embryos and unfertilized oocytes
- See Cloning.

NURSING CARE

Generally required after more invasive procedures in donor and recipient mares

ACTIVITY

Generally restricted after more invasive procedures in donor and recipient mares

DIET

Normal diet, unless contraindicated by concurrent maternal disease or exercise restriction

CLIENT EDUCATION

- ET procedures are not approved by all breed registries.

- Recipient mares generally need to be fairly closely synchronized with donor mares—depending on the procedure, every 0–2 days.
- If the number of normal, synchronized recipients is limited, embryos can be transported to commercial facilities with large numbers of recipient mares.
- Embryo-freezing procedures are improving.

SURGICAL CONSIDERATIONS

- May be indicated to repair anatomic defects predisposing to endometritis.
- Surgical oviductal recovery and implantation

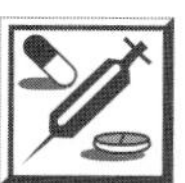

MEDICATIONS

DRUG(S) OF CHOICE

Progestins, antibiotics, anti-inflammatory medications, and intrauterine therapy may or may not be used depending on the case, procedures involved, and clinician preference.

FOLLOW-UP

PATIENT MONITORING

- Accurate teasing records
- Reexamination of donors diagnosed and treated for endometritis before ET
- Early transrectal U/S of recipient mare for pregnancy
- Transrectal U/S to monitor for embryonic and fetal development

PREVENTION/AVOIDANCE

N/A

POSSIBLE COMPLICATIONS

- Recipient conception failure or EED
- Endometritis in donor mares after the uterine flushing procedure
- Pregnancy in donor mare following an "unsuccessful flush," i.e., no embryo retrieved and follow-up prostaglandin injection not administered post-flush to the donor

EXPECTED COURSE AND PROGNOSIS

- Prognosis for successful pregnancy depends on the quality of the embryo (i.e., oocyte) and recipient mare.
- Prognosis for successful recovery of intrauterine embryo at 6–8 days after ovulation is ≅70% in normal mares (less in subfertile mares).
- Prognosis for successful surgical, intrauterine transfer of embryos is ≅70%–75% for embryos from normal mares (less from subfertile mares).
- Nonsurgical, intrauterine transfer of embryos has potential to be less successful (wide individual and facility variation) than surgical transfer but is becoming more widespread.
- Other embryo and early zygote procedures may have lower success rates and are still in development.
- Embryo cryopreservation techniques have been developed.
- Oocyte cryopreservation techniques are still being refined.

MISCELLANEOUS

ASSOCIATED CONDITIONS

- Abortion
- Conception failure
- EED
- Endometritis
- High-risk pregnancy

AGE-RELATED FACTORS

- Development of chronic endometritis and endometrial fibrosis
- Age-related embryonic defects, especially with old mares

PREGNANCY

By definition, the condition is associated with pregnancy.

SEE ALSO

- Abortion
- Conception failure
- EED
- Endometritis
- Endometrial biopsy
- High-risk pregnancy
- Pregnancy diagnosis

ABBREVIATIONS

- CL = corpus luteum
- EED = early embryonic death
- ET = embryo transfer
- ELISA = enzyme-linked immunosorbent assay
- GIFT = gamete intrafallopian transfer
- RIA = radioimmunoassay
- T_3 = triiodothyronine
- T_4 = thyroxine
- U/S = ultrasound
- ZIFT = zygote intrafallopian transfer

Suggested Reading

Carnevale EM. Oocyte transfer. In: Robinson NE, ed. Current Therapy in Equine Medicine, ed 5. Philadelphia: Saunders, 2003:285–287.

Squires EL. Management of the embryo donor and recipient mare. In: Robinson NE, ed. Current Therapy in Equine Medicine, ed 5. Philadelphia: Saunders, 2003:277–279.

Vanderwall DK. Embryo collection, storage, and transfer. In: Robinson NE, ed. Current Therapy in Equine Medicine, ed 5. Philadelphia: Saunders, 2003:280–285.

Author Tim J. Evans

Consulting Editor Carla L. Carleton

ENDOMETRIAL BIOPSY

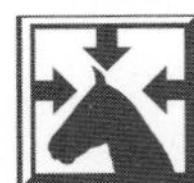

BASICS

DEFINITION

Histopathological evaluation of the endometrium to predict a mare's ability to carry a foal to term

PATHOPHYSIOLOGY

Seasonal Variation

• Normal histopathological endometrial changes driven by cyclic rise and fall of ovarian estrogen and progesterone. Variations reflect stage of estrous cycle and season. • Winter anestrus—endometrial atrophy; luminal and glandular epithelium becomes cuboidal, glands straight, low in density, secretions accumulate from myometrial hypotonia • Vernal transition—Increasing estrogen stimulates endometrial activity, increasing luminal, glandular epithelial activity, and gland density.
• Variations in luminal epithelium in spring breeding season; height—tall columnar in early diestrus; low/moderately columnar and cuboidal through diestrus; tall columnar in estrus
• Other springtime changes
  ◦ *Early estrus*—stromal edema develops, causing *physiologic nesting* of individual gland branches.
  ◦ *Estrus*—PMNs marginate on sides of venules and capillaries, without migrating into the stroma. Glands—straight, some degree of edema
  ◦ *Diestrus*—gland tortuosity increases and edema decreases.
• No seasonal effect on degree or distribution of histologic changes

Assessment of Inflammation and Degenerative Changes

• Degree and extent of inflammation and degenerative changes of endometrium—alterations due to age, natural challenges (coitus, pregnancy), contamination by bacteria, pneumovagina, urovagina, DUC, and other unknown causes • Nature of change—inflammatory cell infiltration, periglandular fibrosis, cystic glandular distention and lymphangiectasia, with/without periglandular fibrosis • High correlation between degree of changes and ability of endometrium to carry fetus to term. As duration and degree of endometrial damage and insult increase, probability of term pregnancy decreases. • Inflammation is associated with repeated natural challenges.
• Degenerative changes usually are progressive, associated with aging, clearly exacerbated by parity, chronic inflammation.

SYSTEM AFFECTED

Reproductive

SIGNALMENT

• Degenerative changes and chronic inflammatory cellular infiltration increase with age and parity.
• Abnormal anatomy, uterine insult, history of aggressive/prolonged treatment predispose to contamination and irritation independent of age or parity

SIGNS

Historical

Infertility of variable degrees
• Mare barren from previous/current breeding season, despite being bred ≤48 hr pre-ovulation with proven semen • Anestrus mare during breeding season • Mare with reproductive tract abnormalities
• History—EED, abortion • Mare with inconclusive cytologic/uterine culture findings for diagnosis of clinical endometritis

Physical Examination

• Biopsy—essential for prepurchase examination of broodmare prospect

CAUSES

Inflammation

• Most common endometrial abnormality
• Neutrophils predominate in acute; lymphocytes, plasma cells and macrophages in chronic endometritis • Chronic/active is less common; PMNs, lymphocytes, and plasma cells may be present concurrently—chronic change superimposed by acute result of persistent antigenic stimulation [contamination because of genital abnormalities (poor VC, RVF)]; semen in DUC mare also results in fluid accumulation and inflammatory cells. • Degree and cell type depend on severity of insult, length of exposure and infection. • Described by distribution (focal, diffuse), frequency (moderate, severe), cell type present (acute, chronic, chronic/active)
• Inflammatory cells may be in foci, scattered, diffuse distribution in *stratum compactum* (including capillaries and venules) and luminal epithelium.
• Chronic inflammation also may affect the *stratum spongiosum.* • Other types of cells occur less often—macrophages, siderophages, eosinophils. • Macrophages linked to irritating or poorly absorbed foreign matter
• Siderophages (macrophage contains hemoglobin pigment from digestion of blood) indicate previous foaling, abortion, hemorrhagic event—may have been as long as 2–3 years previously • Eosinophils often indicate acute irritation due to pneumovagina, urovagina, and, less often, fungal endometritis.

Fibrosis

• Irreversible • Increased variation in distribution than degree of fibrosis. Widespread distribution, any degree, correlates with low foaling rates. • Stromal cells deposit collagen in response to repeated acute/chronic inflammation, aging, other stimuli. • Most collagen deposition is periglandular. • *Nests* are clusters/branches of glands surrounded by collagen. • Periglandular fibrosis exerts pressure within the gland and decreases blood flow to the gland, leads to cystic glandular distention, epithelial atrophy, decrease in uterine secretions
• Calculi, mineral/organic substances, may be in lumen of endometrial glands • With periglandular fibrosis, can usually conceive, but pregnancy is lost <90 days due to impaired secretion of gland *uterine milk*, secretion critical for conceptus' nutrition • Prognosis indirectly correlates with number of collagen layers and frequency of nests per LPF, i.e., more layers = poorer prognosis.

Cystic Glandular Distention and Uterine Hypotonia

• If unassociated with fibrosis, may be due to impaired flow of secretions • Normal during anestrus and transition (seasonal variation)
• During breeding season—old, pluriparous mares with pendulous uteri; history of repeat breeding. Presents as clusters of cystic glands not surrounded by collagen, i.e., not fibrotic nests.
• Cystic glands may have inspissated material and exhibit epithelial hypertrophy. • Cystic glandular distention has been suggested to precede periglandular fibrosis. • In normal mares, glands are uniformly dilated after a recent abortion or pregnancy.

Lymphatic Stasis

• Characterized by dilated, dysfunctional lymphatic vessels • Histology—Dilated lymphatics are differentiated from widespread edema by endothelial cells lining a fluid-filled space. • Common in mares with pendulous uterus and DUC • TRP may reveal thickened but soft uterus, poor tone in diestrus.
• Widespread—associated with low foaling rates
• Coalescing lymphatic lacunae may become lymphatic cysts, 1–15 cm diameter • Lymphatic cysts identified by U/S, endoscopy, and, less frequently, TRP

Angiosis

• Angiosclerotic changes of uterine vessels associated primarily with parity, secondarily with aging. • Younger maiden mares—intact vessels. Older maiden mares—mild sclerosis in the intima and adventitia. Pluriparous mares—all layers affected; exhibit fraying and disruption of the intima with medial and adventitial elastosis and fibrosis • Incidence increases with parity independent of mare's age. • Severe angiosis—with phlebectasia and lymphangiectasia decreasing endometrial perfusion and drainage, results in edema formation • Consider in prognosis for classification, as it affects pregnancy outcome.

Nonseasonal Glandular Atrophy or Hypoplasia

• Decreased gland density during breeding season is abnormal; associated with ovarian dysgenesis or secretory tumors (ranulose cell tumor) • Focal glandular atrophy can develop in old, pluriparous mares.

Prognostic Categories

Category I—
• Endometrium optimal, expect ≥80% of mares to conceive and carry to term • Histologic changes—slight, focal, and irregularly distributed (scattered)
Category IIA—
• 50%–80% foaling rate with proper management • Conception and pregnancy maintenance slightly decreased • Histologic changes—slight to moderate, may improve with proper treatment, may include:
  ◦ Slight to moderate, diffuse cellular infiltration of superficial layers
  ◦ Scattered, frequent inflammatory or fibrotic foci
  ◦ Scattered, frequent periglandular fibrosis of individual branches, 1–3 collagen layers, or ≤2 fibrotic gland nests/LPF, at least 5 fields

ENDOMETRIAL BIOPSY

- Widespread lymphatic stasis without palpable changes

Category IIB—

• 10%–50% foaling rate with proper management • Histologic changes—more extensive and severe than IIA, still may be reversible, may include

- Diffuse, widespread, moderately severe cellular infiltration of superficial layers
- Widespread periglandular fibrosis of individual branches
- ≥4 collagen layers or 2–4 fibrotic gland nests/LPF in 5 fields
- Widespread lymphatic stasis, palpable changes in the uterus, usually noted as decreased uterine tone in diestrus

Category III—

• Foaling rate, even with optimal management and treatment, ≤10% • Greatly decreased chances of conception and pregnancy maintenance; difficult-to-treat conditions or severe, irreversible changes in endometrium
• Histologic changes

- Widespread, severe cellular infiltration
- Glandular fibrosis (≥5 fibrotic nests/LPF)
- Severe lymphatic stasis

• Endometrial hypoplasia with gonadal dysgenesis and pyometra with severe, widespread cellular infiltration and palpable endometrial atrophy. • Electron microscopy doesn't reveal major differences between categories I and II. Category III—increased cells with degenerative structures, fewer organelles and cilia on surface

RISK FACTORS

• Age • Parity • Anatomical abnormality—pneumovagina, urovagina, DUC
• Repeated inflammation by/resulting from coitus, DUC, infectious endometritis

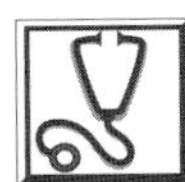

DIAGNOSIS

DIFFERENTIAL DIAGNOSIS

• History, physical, behavioral findings play important role in infertility. • Endometrial gland distention—*seasonal* (atrophy expected during anestrus, transition) and *nonseasonal* (endometrial atrophy linked with ovarian dysgenesis, recent abortion or pregnancy, pluriparous DUC mare, fibrosis) • Differentiate cystic glands (distention is ≤1 mm in diameter) from lymphatic cysts by origin and size. • Gland *nest* associated with proestrus edema = normal physiologic alteration; *nest* secondary to irreversible, periglandular fibrosis is abnormal.

IMAGING

U/S—method of choice to assess lymphatic cysts—location, number, and size

DIAGNOSTIC PROCEDURES

BSE

• Routine BSE or suspected endometritis—culture and cytology must precede biopsy to avoid contaminating swab.
• Perform biopsy with a sterile endometrial biopsy forcep, preferably when the mare is cycling and, if convenient, during estrus.
• Forcep is carried through cervix into uterine body; sample taken from caudal portion of the horn or at the junction of horn and body (i.e., approximate area of endometrial cups of pregnancy). Unless a gross abnormality is present, one sample is adequate to represent the entire endometrium; otherwise, take additional samples as needed. • Fix sample in Bouin's for 4–24 hr, then transfer into 70% ethanol/10% formalin until slides are prepared. Bouin's exposure >24 hr will make the sample brittle and difficult to section. • H&E is routine stain, may request others • If sample sent to lab for slide prep and interpretation, include complete history, stage of cycle and TRP findings on day of examination.

Endoscopy

To diagnosis intraluminal adhesions, endometrial cysts

PATHOLOGIC FINDINGS

• See category descriptions. • Culture and cytology from biopsy sample provide more accurate results compared to an endometrial swab.

EPICRISIS

• Clinical evaluation of the biopsy requires interpretation in concert with patient history, physical examination findings, bacteriology results, and previous treatments. • Include recommendations for treatment/management/prognosis.

CATEGORY I

A *normal* endometrium—if difficulties are encountered with conceiving or carrying to term and mare is not infected, focus on semen quality, estrus detection, timing of breeding and insemination with respect to ovulation, anatomic or behavioral abnormalities.

CATEGORIES IIA AND IIB

• Appropriate therapy to improve category
• Inflammation decreases if source of irritation is removed and contamination is decreased at breeding. • Pneumovagina and urovagina—surgical correction • Treat acute and chronic bacterial/fungal infections with appropriate local/systemic antibiotic/antifungal.
• Treat DUC—uterine lavage and oxytocin
• Lymphatic circulation—enhanced by cloprostenol ($PGF_{2\alpha}$ analog) 12–24 hr before and after breeding • Fibrosis and angiosis—irreversible • Uterine edema—if due to impaired perfusion/drainage, improve by increasing uterine tone with P+E.

CATEGORY III

• Often become pregnant, but lost at 40–90 days' gestation • Histologic changes either difficult to affect or irreversible • Therapy to decrease inflammation, lymphangiectasia + MCT at breeding • Extensive fibrosis decreases likelihood that category may improve with treatment. • If allowed by breed registry, consider category III as ET donor. • If improvement is impossible, cull mare.

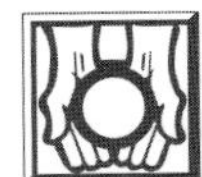

MEDICATIONS

DRUGS OF CHOICE

• Antibiotic based on culture and sensitivity
• P+E

- 3 mL of combined P (150 mg) + E (5–10 mg) daily, IM × 10 days or 10 mL once, Bio-release P + E
- Day 10 administer $PGF_{2\alpha}$ 10 mg IM
- Day 5 after breeding, if no fluid is in the uterus, resume treatment
- If pregnant at 14 days, continue to day 45

CONTRAINDICATIONS

Do not treat with P + E if mare is infected; she may develop pyometra.

FOLLOW-UP

PATIENT MONITORING

A repeat endometrial biopsy ≅2 weeks after treatment ends—means to determine effectiveness of therapy

POSSIBLE COMPLICATIONS

• Biopsy—relatively safe • Possible complications—uterine perforation, excessive hemorrhage (rare)

MISCELLANEOUS

AGE-RELATED FACTORS

• Direct correlation category to age • Category I—primarily young, maiden mares • Category II—old, pluriparous mares; high incidence of poor VC, pneumovagina, urovagina, DUC, periglandular fibrosis

PREGNANCY

Contraindication to biopsy

SYNONYMS

Uterine biopsy

SEE ALSO

• Endometritis • Metritis

ABBREVIATIONS

• BSE = breeding soundness examination
• DUC = delayed uterine clearance • EED = early embryonic death • ET = embryo transfer
• LPF = low-power field • MCT = minimum contamination technique • P = progesterone
• P+E = progesterone + estradiol-17β • PMN = polymorphonuclear leukocyte • RVF = rectovaginal fistula • U/S = ultrasound • VC = vulvar conformation

Suggested Reading

Gruninger B, Schoon HA, Schoon D, Menger S, Klug E. Incidence and morphology of endometrial angiopathies in relationship to age and parity. J Comp Pathol 1998;119:293–309.

Kenney RM, Doig PA. Equine endometrial biopsy. In: Morrow DA, ed. Current Therapy in Theriogenology. Philadelphia: WB Saunders, 1986:723–729.

Author Maria E. Cadario
Consulting Editor Carla L. Carleton

ENDOMETRITIS

BASICS

DEFINITION/OVERVIEW

- Infectious/noninfectious endometrial inflammation
- Major cause of mare infertility
- Multifactorial disease classified in one of four groups:
  - Infectious (active/acute, active/chronic, or subclinical) endometritis
  - PMIE
  - Endometritis due to an STD and,
  - Degenerative endometritis due to aging (angiosis, periglandular fibrosis)
- May involve more than one group/origin

ETIOLOGY/PATHOPHYSIOLOGY

Infectious Endometritis

- Uterus repeatedly exposed to contamination at breeding, parturition, and gynecological examinations.
- Uterine defense mechanisms to clear contamination, combination of:
  - Anatomic (physical) barriers
  - Cellular phagocytosis
  - Physical evacuation of uterine contents
- Anatomic integrity—loss of the vulvar seal, vestibular sphincter and cervical integrity caused by aging, parity and associated perineal accidents, or breed predisposition
  - Decreased function results in recurring aspiration of air (pneumovagina), urine (urine pooling), fecal material, and/or bacteria into the cranial vagina.
  - Contamination may increase during estrus, subsequent to vulvar and cervical relaxation.

PMIE

- Increased parity in aged mares and incomplete cervical dilation in maiden mares (old maiden mares, mares >12 years old) predisposes them to intrauterine fluid accumulation.
- Breeding (semen + bacterial contamination) induces a normal, transient, endometritis.
- Byproducts of inflammation normally are removed by uterine contractions through an open estrual cervix. Following ovulation, the cervix closes; fluids within the uterine lumen are cleared by the lymphatics.
- Intrauterine fluid is cleared (absent) by 12 hr post-mating in normal mares.
- The likelihood of fluid accumulation and lymphatic stasis increases if the uterus is suspended below the pelvic brim, uterine contractions are impaired, or normal contractions are incomplete, but coupled with negligible cervical dilation during estrus.
- Supportive structures of the genital tract stretch with each pregnancy.

Low Pregnancy Rate

- Direct—causes interference with embryo survival on its arrival into the uterus
- Indirect— by premature luteolysis; inflammation induces endometrial prostaglandin release.

SEXUALLY TRANSMITTED (VENEREAL) ENDOMETRITIS

- Mode of transmission is coitus or AI with infected semen.
- Most common bacteria are *Pseudomona aeruginosa*, *Klebsiella pneumonia,* and *Streptococcus zooepidemicus*.
  - All opportunistic organisms on the penile surface
  - Can become overwhelming if the normal penile bacterial flora is disturbed/altered

SYSTEM AFFECTED

Reproductive

GENETICS

N/A

INCIDENCE/PREVALENCE

Frequent

SIGNALMENT

Infectious Endometritis

Predisposition to contamination is caused by an inherent or acquired anatomical defect of the vulva, vestibular sphincter, or cervix.

PMIE

- Pluriparous mares—usually >12–14 years with pendulous uterus.
- Nulliparous mares—young or old, having incomplete cervical dilation during estrus

SIGNS

Historical

- Infertility
- Accumulation of uterine fluid (luminal) before and/or after breeding
- Failure to conceive after repeated breeding to a stallion of known fertility
- Early embryonic loss
- Hyperemia of the cervix/vagina
- Vaginal discharge

Physical Examination

- Can be inconclusive. Key diagnostic tools are patient history, cytology/culture, and U/S.
- Guarded swab to obtain samples for endometrial cytology and uterine culture
- Endometrial biopsy is indicated only in specific cases.

Infectious Endometritis

- Abnormal VC
- TRP is not very diagnostic.
- U/S usually reveals accumulation of echogenic fluid in the uterine lumen.
- Hyperemia of vaginal and cervical mucosa; discharge may be observed at the cervix.
- Endometrial cytology and uterine culture reveal neutrophils (>5 PMNs/hpf).
- Usually isolate a pure bacterial growth, single organism

PMIE

- External genitalia not always abnormal
- TRP, U/S, and cytology/culture results may be inconclusive in the spring, prior to onset of the breeding season.
- Signs of persistent inflammation usually appear post-breeding.
- May be hyperemia of the vaginal and cervical mucosa
- Pendulous, edematous uterus in older mares
- Presence of >2 cm (height, determined by U/S) of intrauterine fluid during estrus is diagnostic/predictive of PMIE.
- Post-breeding U/S reveals luminal fluid that persists for 12–24+ hr without treatment.
- Endometrial cytology reveals significant inflammation (>5 PMNs/hpf).
- Bacterial culture—usually negative

CAUSES

See Etiology/Pathophysiology.

RISK FACTORS

- Age >14 years old
- Multiparous and nulliparous mares that are >12–14 years
- Abnormal VC
- Excessive breeding (live covers or AI) during one or consecutive estrus periods
- Pendulous uterine suspension
- Cervix that fails to relax during estrus

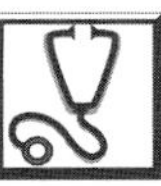

DIAGNOSIS

DIFFERENTIAL DIAGNOSIS

For Vaginal Discharge

- Pneumovagina—mucosal irritation by air, a foamy-appearing exudate accumulates on the vaginal floor
- Treatment-induced vaginitis and/or necrosis—may result from antiseptics used for uterine lavage. Individual mares vary in their response to a similar treatment.

- Bacterial vaginitis secondary to pneumovagina
- Necrotizing vaginitis—secondary to excessive manipulation and inadequate lubrication during dystocia, or contamination during the delivery of a dead, necrotic fetus
- Urine pooling—usually affects a population of mares with characteristics similar to those affected by endometritis
  - Diagnosis (by vaginal speculum)—presence of urine during estrus
  - Transrectal U/S reveals nonechogenic intrauterine fluid present before and variably after ovulation.
- Varicosities in the region of the vaginovestibular sphincter
  - May rupture and bleed during late pregnancy or during breeding
  - Diagnosis by vaginal speculum
- Lochia—normal finding up to 6 days postpartum
- Postpartum metritis
- Pyometra
- During pregnancy, vaginal discharge may be a sign of placentitis.
- Purulent cervical discharge—associated with ascending, infectious placentitis
- Serosanguinous cervical discharge with a negative bacterial swab indicates premature placental separation.
- Premature mammary development may develop with placental insufficiency of any origin.

CBC/BIOCHEMISTRY/URINALYSIS

N/A

OTHER LABORATORY TESTS

Microbiology

Aerobes

- Most common isolates—*S. zooepidemicus* and *E. coli*
- Guarded swab to sample the endometrial surface. Two different agar plates are used:
  - McConkey for gram-negative and blood agar for gram-positive and yeast
  - Incubate plates at 37° C, examine at 24 and 48 hr
- For subclinical endometrial infections, recommend culture be taken from endometrial biopsy sample or from the return solution of a low-volume lavage.
- *E. coli*, a fecal contaminant, results from poor VC.
- *P. aeruginosa* and *K. pneumoniae* usually are a venereal transmission.
  - Overgrowth may occur secondary to excessive use of intrauterine antibiotics.
- Other bacteria—*Staphylococcus, Corynebacterium, Enterobacter, Proteus* and *Pasteurella* spp.

Anaerobes

- *Bacteroides fragilis*
- May be recovered in some cases of postpartum metritis

Yeasts

- *Candida* spp.
- Usually follow(s) excessive antibiotic uterine therapy
- Use cytology slides and the blood agar plates for presence of *Candida* and *Aspergillus* spp.
- For a specific fungal culture, incubate in Sabouraud agar for 4 days.

Cytology

- Sample is of endometrial cells and intraluminal content.
- Scrape the endometrial surface with the swab tip or cap (if using a Kalayjian swab); gently roll the sample onto a slide and stain with Diff-Quick.
- Neutrophils indicate active inflammation. Recent breeding or gynecologic examination results in a transient, positive cytology.
- Persistent, positive cytology without bacterial growth most often suggests a recurrent, noninfectious cause, e.g., pneumovagina, urine pooling, or early stages of DUC. If treatment or surgical correction fails to improve fertility, do not rule out an infectious cause, e.g., subclinical endometritis.
- Positive culture with positive cytology—diagnostic for uterine infection
- Positive culture with negative cytology—indicates contamination during uterine sampling in 70% of the cases.
- May have negative cytology results in 30% of subsequently confirmed endometrial infections, due to the inability to reach the PMNs in the pendulous areas of the uterus (physically out of reach)

IMAGING

U/S

- Normal mares retain small amounts of intrauterine fluid up to 12 hr post-breeding.
- Mares with DUC often have luminal fluid present pre-breeding and always retain fluid for 12–24 hr post-breeding.

OTHER DIAGNOSTIC PROCEDURES

Endoscopy

- When other modalities fail to define the cause of infertility
- Better method is to visualize intrauterine adhesions affecting uterine drainage, luminal tumors, or uterine abscess (rare) that may not be palpable or visible by U/S.

Small-Volume Uterine Lavage

- For gross and bacteriologic evaluation of uterine content when subclinical endometritis is suspected
- Flush uterus with 60 mL of sterile saline, evaluate effluent, centrifuge, and culture the pellet.

Endometrial Biopsy

- To determine the presence or absence of endometritis when clinical and bacteriological findings are inconclusive
- Culture and cytology taken from endometrial biopsy sample yield accurate results.
- Inflammatory cells (neutrophils) are diagnostic, if present, of active endometritis.
- Low numbers of lymphocytes and plasma cells (indicative of chronic endometritis) are not always associated with infertility.
- Periglandular fibrosis—associated with early abortions—gestational age, 70–90 days
- Lymphatic stasis is common in mares with a pendulous uterus and DUC.

PATHOLOGICAL FINDINGS

Endometritis

- Cannot predict a mare's endometrial biopsy category, ranges from IIA to III (rarely)
- Category relates to the length of sexual rest, conformational abnormalities, and age.
- Histopathology associated with endometritis—mild, diffuse lymphocytic or neutrophilic infiltration; focally moderate fibrosis (1–4 nests); lymphangiectasia

PMIE

- Biopsy score at the beginning of the breeding season is not diagnostic.
- Category may be IIA or IIB, with mild inflammation and moderate fibrosis.
- After breeding, interstitial edema, lymphatic stasis, and diffuse, acute or subacute inflammation (PMN) usually develop.
- Serial sampling may be useful.

ENDOMETRITIS

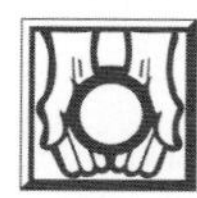

TREATMENT

APPROPRIATE HEALTH CARE

Minimize contamination during breeding:

• Wash mare's perineum and stallion's penis with clean water; dry the stallion's penis prior to mating or semen collection for AI.
• Limit to one breeding (live cover or AI) per estrus.
• Breed as close to ovulation as possible.
• Immediately prior to natural breeding (live cover), infuse semen extender (60–120 mL) with nonspermicidal antibiotic (antibiotic concentration compatible with sperm viability); MCT

NURSING CARE, ACTIVITY, DIET, CLIENT EDUCATION N/A

SURGICAL CONSIDERATIONS

• Consider feasibility of surgical correction of predisposing causes before treating a uterine infection—Caslick's vulvoplasty (pneumovagina); vaginoplasty; urethral extension (urine pooling); repair of cervical tears
• RVF and extensive cervical tears (foaling trauma)—prudent to wait for results of endometrial biopsy before surgery if the broodmare has been barren for >1 year. Chronic endometritis may have seriously diminished the mare's biopsy category in the interim.

MEDICATIONS

DRUGS OF CHOICE

General Principles

• Administer treatments during estrus, when the cervix is open; however, this issue remains a topic of some controversy.
• Organism is eliminated chemically (antibiotics, antiseptics) or mechanically (uterine lavage, ecbolic drugs).
• Local placement of antibiotics is preferred to systemic treatment; higher concentrations are achieved in the endometrium.
• Cost of systemic treatment is more than local administration.
• Most uterine infections in mares are luminal/endometrial.
• Systemic treatment is optional when access to the mare is limited (e.g., unsafe or unsanitary conditions) or when attempting to avoid further uterine contamination.
• Uterine lavage is the treatment of choice for mares with DUC and to evacuate debris from the uterus before antibiotic instillation.
  ○ Also enhances local uterine defenses by local irritation and stimulates PMN migration to the lumen
• Uterine lavage with LRS can be performed immediately prior to insemination when a mare has intrauterine fluid (e.g., rebreeding or multiple inseminations in a 24hr period).
• If oxytocin is used during/after the lavage, wait for 45–60 min before inseminating the mare.

Endometritis

• *Active/acute endometritis*—uterine lavage and oxytocin (daily or alternate days) followed by intrauterine infusion of chosen antibiotics
• Antibiotics are chosen based on culture and sensitivity and should be diluted in 60–120 mL of sterile saline (maximum volume infused).
• *Chronic inflammation*—Do not breed mare until 45–60 days after treatment.
• *Chronic active endometritis*—surgical correction of defective anatomic barriers before intrauterine treatment; uterine lavage and oxytocin if intrauterine fluid is present
• *Subclinical endometritis*—positive or negative cytology, no bacteria identified:
  ○ Uterine lavage with diluted antiseptics or antibiotics
  ○ If history warrants, consider post-breeding treatment.
• *Yeast infection*—uterine lavage and oxytocin, followed by intrauterine infusion with antifungal drugs (Nystatin, Clotrimazole, etc.); alternatively, uterine lavage with diluted 1% povidone-iodine solution (to the approximate color of light iced tea) or acetic acid (vinegar).
• One or two treatments of intrauterine infusion with 540 mg of Lufenuron (Program, oral suspension for flea control in cats) diluted in 60 mL of saline appears to be effective in some cases of fungal endometritis.
• Correct anatomic defects and culture and treat reservoirs of infection, e.g., vagina and clitoral fossa.

PMIE

• Manual cervical dilation pre-breeding, and systemic or local medication, may help intrauterine semen deposition and uterine clearance. Foaling, at least once, is highly recommended to improve cervical relaxation and drainage in old maiden mares.
• Promote uterine clearance by lavage and ecbolic drugs (oxytocin).
• Mare with no history or characteristics of DUC:
  ○ Begin her evaluation and treatment, if necessary, 12-hr post-breeding to let the normal mechanisms of clearance occur.
• If the mare has been diagnosed with PMIE:
  ○ 4–8 hr post-breeding treat to promote uterine clearance.
  ○ 4-hr interval ensures spermatozoa are in the oviduct, bacteria have not yet adhered or multiplied in the uterus.
• Oxytocin immediately before or immediately after lavage stimulates strong uterine contractions, clears the remaining uterine contents and promotes lymphatic drainage.
• Administer oxytocin every 2–4 hr in refractory cases, e.g., older maiden mares.
• $PGF_{2\alpha}$ and analogs (cloprostenol):
  ○ Sustains smoother uterine contractions longer than oxytocin (4–5 hr versus 45–60 min).
  ○ Successful in reducing persistent uterine edema by stimulating lymphatic drainage
  ○ Treat after each mating or suggested protocol.

U/S

• 4–8 hr post-AI or breeding (not ovulation), check for uterine fluid.
  ○ If fluid is present at a height of >2 cm free fluid, lavage uterus with1–3 L of sterile saline or LRS.
  ○ Administer oxytocin immediately before or after lavage.
  ○ If only a small amount of free fluid, administer oxytocin only.
• If possible, 12 hr after breeding—use cloprostenol if history includes dilated uterine lymphatics and poor drainage.
• 24 hr after breeding, if mare has free intraluminal fluid, use lavage and oxytocin.
  ○ Small amounts of fluid require only the use of oxytocin.
  ○ If free fluid and persistent edema in the walls—lavage the uterus/oxytocin and add a regimen of IM oxytocin alternating with IM cloprostenol every 4–6 hr.
  ○ If only edema is present, cloprostenol every 4–12 hr, up to 36 hr post-ovulation.
• 48-hr post-breeding—If the mare has not ovulated, rebreed and oxytocin/cloprostenol sequence begins anew. Prebreeding uterine lavage may be indicated.
• Treatment should continue, if necessary, no more than 3–4 days post-ovulation.
  ○ Embryo enters the uterus day 5 + 20 hr; allows treatment-induced uterine inflammatory response to subside.

Drugs and Fluids

Antibiotics

- Amikacin (0.5–2 g)—gram-negative; *Pseudomonas* and *Klebsiella* spp. An intrauterine infusion of Tris-EDTA increases the permeability of the *Pseudomonas* capsule to the antibiotic.
- Ampicillin (1–3 g)—gram-positive; streptococci
- Carbenicillin (2–6 g)—broad spectrum; persistent *Pseudomonas* spp.
- Gentamicin (0.5–2 g)—primarily gram-negative; streptococci
- Neomycin (3–4 g)—*E. coli* and *Klebsiella* spp.
- K-penicillin (5×10^6 U)—gram-positive; streptococci
- Ticarcillin (3–6 g)—broad spectrum
- Ceftiofur (1 g)—broad spectrum
- Aminoglycosides must be buffered before infusion. Mix the antibiotic with an equal volume of sodium bicarbonate, e.g., 1 mL of $NaHCO_3$ (7.5%) for every 50 mg of gentamicin or amikacin, then dilute in sterile saline.

Systemic Antibiotics

- K-penicillin
- Procaine penicillin G
- Gentamicin
- Amikacin
- Ampicillin
- Trimethoprim-sulfamethoxazole

Antimycotics

- Nystatin ($0.5–2.5 \times 10^6$ U)—*Candida* spp.
- Clotrimazole (500–700 mg)—*Candida* spp.
- Amphotericin B (100–200 mg)—*Aspergillus, Candida* and *Mucor* spp.; tablets must be crushed and well suspended in 60–120 mL of sterile saline.
- Lufenuron (540 mg); Program (270 mg oral suspension for cats), may inhibit fungal growth by disrupting the cell walls

Others

- DMSO may remove excessive endometrial mucus to allow better access to the bacteria by the antibiotic. At 5%–10%, bacteriostatic; >10%, bacteriocidal; 10%–20%, decreased growth of *Candida albicans* in vitro
- Intrauterine infusion with DMSO at >25% produces endometrial ulceration.

Uterotonic/Ecbolic Drugs

- Oxytocin (10 IU IV or 20 IU IM)
- Cloprostenol (250–500 g IM), prostaglandin of choice because of its effectiveness; fewer adverse effects

Cervical Dilation

- Prostaglandins, Misoprostol ointment (see Cervical Lesions)

CONTRAINDICATIONS

- Do not administer prostaglandin or its analogs >36 hr post-ovulation; affects progesterone production by the CL; it may result in EED.
- Intrauterine infusion of Enrofloxacin (Baytril) is contraindicated; not labeled for horses; highly irritating for endometrium.

PRECAUTIONS

Adverse reactions may occur with natural or synthetic prostaglandin—transient sweating, ataxia, and increased GI motility

POSSIBLE INTERACTIONS N/A

ALTERNATIVE DRUGS N/A

FOLLOW-UP

PATIENT MONITORING

- Complete the gynecologic evaluation with special attention to uterine culture/cytology on day 1 or 2 of the estrus after treatment.
- If no conception after several attempts, repeat the complete evaluation at 45–60 days after treatment.

PREVENTION AVOIDANCE N/A

POSSIBLE COMPLICATIONS

- Secondary bacterial/yeast overgrowth due to excessive use of antibiotics
- Uterine adhesions
- Pyometra

EXPECTED COURSE AND PROGNOSIS

N/A

MISCELLANEOUS

ASSOCIATED CONDITIONS N/A

AGE RELATED FACTORS

See Risk Factors.

ZOONOTIC POTENTIAL N/A

PREGNANCY N/A

SEE ALSO

- Cervical lesions
- Endometrial biopsy
- Postpartum metritis
- Pyometra
- Urine pooling

ABBREVIATIONS

- AI = artificial insemination
- CL = corpus luteum
- DUC = delayed uterine clearance
- EED = early embryonic death
- GI = gastrointestinal
- hpf = high-powered field (microscopy)
- LRS = lactated Ringer's solution
- MCT = minimum contamination technique
- PMIE = persistent mating-induced endometritis
- PMN = polymorphonuclear cell
- RVF = rectovaginal fistula
- STD = sexually transmitted disease
- TRP = transrectal palpation
- U/S = ultrasound, ultrasonography
- VC = vulvar conformation

Suggested Reading

Asbury AC, Lyle SK. Infectious causes of infertility. In: McKinnon AO, Voss JL, eds. Equine Reproduction. Philadelphia: Lea & Febiger, 1993:381–391.

Blanchard TL, Varner DD, Schumacher J. Uterine defense mechanisms in the mare. In: Manual of Equine Reproduction. St. Louis: Mosby, 1998:47–58.

Brinsko S, Rigby SL, Varner DD, Blanchard TL: A practical method for recognizing mares susceptible to post-breeding endometritis. Proc AAEP 2003;363–365.

Hess MB, Parker NA, Purswell BJ, Dascanio JD. Use of Lufenuron as a treatment for fungal endometritis in four mares. J Am Vet Med Assoc 2002; 221:266–267.

LeBlanc MM. Breakdown in uterine defense mechanisms in the mare. Is a delay in physical clearance the culprit? Proc Soc Therio 1994;121–129.

Vanderwall DK, Woods GL. Effect on fertility of uterine lavage performed immediately prior to insemination in mares. J Am Vet Med Assoc 2003;222:1108–1110.

Author Maria E. Cadario

Consulting Editor Carla L. Carleton

ENDOTOXEMIA

BASICS

DEFINITION

• Endotoxemia is a clinical syndrome characterized by the presence of endotoxin in the blood, generalized inflammatory response and systemic effects. Endotoxin (LPS) is a heat-stable toxin associated with the lipid portion of the outer layer of cell membranes in gram-negative bacteria. Endotoxemia occurs when either gram-negative bacteria or the LPS gain access to the systemic circulation. • The term *systemic inflammatory response syndrome* (SIRS) has been used to describe the clinical manifestation of overshooting inflammatory response caused by endotoxemia, gram-positive bacteria, viral and fungal infection, and severe trauma.

PATHOPHYSIOLOGY

• Endotoxin is released with gram-negative bacterial cell wall disruption by rapid multiplication, cell death, or bacterial killing from antimicrobial treatment. It is composed of complex LPS molecules, with the phospholipid moiety (lipid A) as the source of the toxicity, while the hydrophilic O-specific chain is responsible for most of the antigenic properties of the LPS and core oligosaccharide.
• Endotoxemia occurs through a series of events. First, LPS is absorbed from severe localized or disseminated gram-negative bacterial infection or as free LPS through hypoperfused or inflamed damaged epithelial surfaces; LPS spreads systemically. The GI tract normally contains a relatively large quantity of LPS, but the mucosa must be compromised by inflammation or ischemia for it to gain access to the systemic circulation. Any GI disorder that leads to severe mucosal inflammation and necrosis (*Salmonella* or *Clostridium* infection, strangulating and nonstrangulating obstructions, and toxin ingestion) can result in LPS absorption. Once in the systemic circulation, LPSs interact with blood constituents or can be removed by macrophages in liver, spleen, or pulmonary vasculature. Due to the hydrodrophobic nature of lipid A, endotoxins form aggregates in plasma. These aggregates are dispersed into monomers and are bound to an LPS-binding protein, inducing a severe inflammatory response. This occurs when LPS binding protein transfers endotoxin monomers to a cell surface receptor complex composed of a Toll-like receptor (*TLR4*), called cluster differentiation antigen 14 (CD14) and myeloid differentiation factor 2 (MD-2). This complex is present in inflammatory cells. LPS is a potent stimulus of the host inflammation, leading to activation of defense mechanisms that initiate overzealous inflammatory processes that cause the clinical manifestations seen in endotoxemia. These clinical manifestations are determined primarily by effects of inflammatory mediators, many of which are released after inflammatory cell stimulation (TNF, IL-1, IL-6, IL-8, IL-10, TXA_2, PGE_2, PAF, LTB_4, kinins, oxygen-derived free radicals, etc.). • The main effects are endothelial dysfunction, hemodynamic changes, neutrophil activation, coagulopathy, complement activation, acute phase response, shock, and organ failure. Clinical manifestations include fever, tachycardia, hypotension, coagulopathy, vascular damage, perfusion defects leading to vital organ damage and ultimately multiple organ system failure, and death.

SYSTEMS AFFECTED

Cardiovascular

• Reduced myocardial contractility
• Differential vasoconstriction and vasodilation in capillary beds • Vascular endothelial damage resulting in permeability changes, fluid leakage, and DIC • Compensatory responses involve increased heart rate and contractility and peripheral vasoconstriction in attempts to raise systemic blood pressure.

GI

Impaired mucosal perfusion may cause mucosal sloughing, allowing bacterial translocation and further LPS absorption

Hepatobiliary

Hepatic ischemia may cause hepatocellular enzyme increases and alter hepatic function, including impaired removal of bacteria from the portal circulation.

Renal

Acute renal failure may result from reduced renal blood flow and ischemic tubular damage.

Respiratory

Pulmonary edema and pulmonary thromboembolisms may occur.

SIGNS

Early

• Pyrexia • Depression • Tachycardia • Normal or high arterial blood pressure • Pale mucous membranes • Rapid capillary refill time
• Tachypnea and/or labored respiration

Late

• Tachycardia or bradycardia • Poor peripheral pulses • Arterial hypotension • Dark mucous membranes • Prolonged capillary refill time
• Cool extremities • Hypothermia • Peripheral edema • Abdominal pain • Diarrhea • Ileus
• Laminitis • Abortion • Petechial and ecchymotic hemorrhages • Death

Neonates

Neonates can show all of the above plus decreased suckling and weakness.

CAUSES

GI Disorders

Within the GI tract, LPS normally gains access to the blood through compromised mucosa that may also allow translocation of gram-negative bacteria.

Neonatal Septicemia

• Gram-negative bacteria proliferate in the tissues and gain access to the blood. • Localized or disseminated infectious focus causing gram-negative bacteremia or release of LPS into the circulation

RISK FACTORS

• The equine is particularly susceptible to gram-negative sepsis secondary to GI disease, metritis, pneumonia and pleuropneumonia, and neonatal septicemia. • Failure of passive transfer and high-risk pregnancies increase the risk of development of neonatal septicemia.

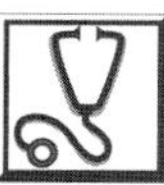

DIAGNOSIS

The diagnosis of endotoxemia is usually made based on appreciation of the primary disease process with a high risk of endotoxemia and the presence of the above mentioned clinical signs in combination with clinicopathologic laboratory findings. Although plasma endotoxin concentration can be measured by the *Limulus amebocyte* assay, use of it has been limited to research.

DIFFERENTIAL DIAGNOSIS

• Hypovolemic shock • Cardiogenic shock

CBC/BIOCHEMISTRY/URINALYSIS

• Initially, there is a neutropenia due to vascular margination (may be $<1000/\mu L$; 10^9 cells/L). This is followed by a neutrophilic leukocytosis with a left shift, due to induction of myeloid proliferation in the bone marrow. Toxic changes are usually present in the neutrophils.
• Hemoconcentration (increased PCV and total plasma protein) • Hyperproteinemia initially due to hemoconcentration, but may decrease significantly with GI losses • High hepatocellular enzymes and bilirubin due to ischemic hepatic injury • Azotemia may be due to renal or prerenal azotemia associated with blood volume depletion. • Initial hyperglycemia followed by hypoglycemia

OTHER LABORATORY TESTS

Coagulation Profile

• Prolongation of the aPTT and PTT
• Increased FDPs • Thrombocytopenia
• Decreased plasma fibrinogen • Decreased AT-III

Blood Gas Analysis

• Hypoxemia • Acid-base disturbances; metabolic acidosis due to decreased peripheral perfusion and hypoxemia

DIAGNOSTIC PROCEDURES

Aerobic and anaerobic blood cultures

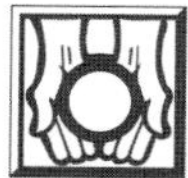

TREATMENT

Given the inflammatory mechanisms involved in endotoxemia and the deleterious effects on the life of the horse, the ideal treatment for endotoxemia is prevention. Close monitoring to prevent the development of the cascade of events should be instituted. Treatment should be initiated quickly and should be aimed at stabilization with aggressive symptomatic therapy, resolving the source of the gram-negative sepsis (inhibition of endotoxin release into circulation), controlling the inflammatory response (inhibition of cellular activation by LPS, inhibition of mediator synthesis), and providing supportive care while establishing tissue perfusion (fluid therapy and cardiovascular support), scavenging of LPS and management of coagulopathy. If the source of sepsis can be identified, it should be addressed.

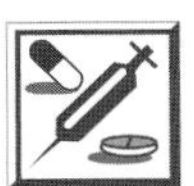

MEDICATIONS

DRUG(S) OF CHOICE

Fluid Therapy and Cardiovascular Support

• Fluid therapy—restoration of the circulating blood volume is the most important factor in restoring peripheral perfusion. • Balanced electrolyte solutions such as lactated Ringer's solution or 0.9% sodium chloride; in foals, dextrose should be added to the fluid therapy. • Rates of 10–20 mL/kg/hr to severely compromised horses • Use caution not to overhydrate and cause pulmonary edema because microvascular alterations may be present. Foals and adults with low plasma protein levels are particularly susceptible to edema formation. • Colloidal solutions (whole blood, plasma, hetastarch, dextrans) can be used to maintain the fluid in the vascular space. They should be initiated when plasma proteins are <4g/dL, 40g/L. • Colloids should be from a commercial source or from appropriate donors (Aa and Qa isoantibody negative). • 7.5% Hypertonic saline solution 4 mL/kg for rapid volume expansion • Sodium bicarbonate to treat severe metabolic acidosis that does not correct with volume expansion. Adult—0.5 mEq body weight (kg) (base deficit); give half the dose slowly intravenously over 20 min. Give the rest of the dose in crystalloid fluids over 4hr if necessary. Foals—0.7 mEq body weight (kg) (base deficit); then follow the same regimen as above. • Inotropic agents can be given to increase systemic blood pressure when it drops to <60mm Hg. • Dopamine hydrochloride—1–5 μg/kg/min by continuous IV administration • Dobutamine—2–5 μg/kg/min by continuous IV administration • Oxygen therapy if hypoxia and respiratory distress are present

Inhibition of Endotoxin Release

• Antimicrobials should be initiated soon after samples for culture have been obtained. Initially, broad-spectrum antimicrobials should be selected pending the results of the culture and susceptibility. Commonly used drugs include aminoglycosides, third-generation cephalosporins, potentiated sulfonamides, and expanded-spectrum penicillins. • Removal of infected tissues or fluids may be helpful.

Inhibition of Mediator Synthesis

Corticosteroids

The use of corticosteroids is controversial in this condition, but their use has been suggested because of their anti-inflammatory effects (decreasing TNF synthesis, decreasing the production of arachidonic acid–derived eicosanoids, stabilizing lysosomal membranes, and decreasing vascular permeability), thereby protecting against some of the effects of endotoxin. Lately, the use of cosrticosteroids in human medicine has been reevaluated. Low-dose cortcosteroids are now used in the treatment of septic shock with an increase in survival rate without increasing adverse events, while administration of high-dose corticosteroids is now totally discouraged. Whether corticosteroids will provide similar benefit in horses remains to be determined.

NSAIDs

NSAIDs are used for attenuation of the inflammatory cascade by inhibiting cyclooxygenase.

• Flunixin meglumine appears to have the most potent anti-endotoxic effects. • 0.5mg/kg q8–12h or 0.25mg/kg q6–8h • Aspirin to prevent thrombus formation • NSAIDs inhibit vasodilator prostaglandins; therefore, care must be taken with regard to renal damage.

Scavenger of LPS

Immunotherapy (Hyperimmune Antisera or Plamsa)

• O-chain specific antisera is not clinically useful due to the antigenic diversity in this region. • Different gram-negative bacteria share common core antigens; therefore, antibodies are aimed at the LPS core. • J5 hyperimmune plasma 4.4 mL/kg.

Polymixin B

• Cationic plypeptide antibiotic used to bind the lipid A portion of LPS • It is nephrotoxic and neurotoxic; caution is advised. • Reduced toxicity is achieved if the drug is administered as a conjugate with Dextran-70. • Current recomendatios is IV administration of 1000–6000 U/kg q8–12h.

CONTRAINDICATIONS

Glucocorticoids may be contraindicated in horse with severe bacterial infection or exhibiting signs of laminitis.

PRECAUTIONS

NSAID toxicity may result in GI ulceration and renal ischemia; therefore, careful patient monitoring is required along with adequate hydration of the patient and using the lowest effective dose possible.

POSSIBLE INTERACTIONS

Sodium bicarbonate and dopamine cannot be administered in the same intravenous line.

ALTERNATIVE DRUGS

• Pentoxyphylline • DMSO

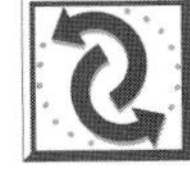

FOLLOW-UP

PATIENT MONITORING

• Vital parameters should be closely monitored in aggressive fluid therapy (heart rate, pulse intensity, mucous membrane color, respirations, lung sounds, urine output, mentation, rectal temperature). • Blood gas analysis and pulse oximetry to measure oxygenation and acid-base balance • PCV, serum total protein, serum electrolytes, hepatocellular enzymes, BUN, and serum creatinine should be monitored.

POSSIBLE COMPLICATIONS

• Laminitis • Electrolyte and acid-base disturbances • Pulmonary edema • Pulmonary thromboembolism • DIC • Renal dysfunction • Hepatic dysfunction • GI ischemia and bacterial translocation • Vasculitis and peripheral edema • Cardiac arrest

MISCELLANEOUS

ASSOCIATED CONDITIONS, AGE-RELATED FACTORS, ZOONOTIC POTENTIAL, PREGNANCY

N/A

SYNONYMS

• Endotoxic shock • Gram-negative sepsis

SEE ALSO

• DIC • Hypoxemia • Bacteremia • Septicemia

ABBREVIATIONS

• aPTT = activated partial thromboplastin time • AT-III = antithrombin III • BUN = blood urea nitrogen • DIC = disseminated intravascular coagulation • FDP = fibrinogen degradation products • GI = gastrointestinal • IL = interleukin • LPS = lipopolysaccharide • PAF = platelet-activating factor • PCV = packed cell volume • PG = prostaglandin • PTT = prothrombin time • TNF = tumor necrosis factor

Suggested Reading

Annane D, Sebille V, Charpentier C, Bollaert PE, Francois B, Korach JM, Capellier G, Cohen Y, Azoulay E, Troché G, Chaument-Riffaut P, Bellisant E. Effect of treatment with low dose of hydrocortisone and fludrocortisone on mortality of patients with septic shock. JAMA 2002;288:862–871.

Lohman KL, Barton MH. Endotoxemia. In Sellon DC, Long MT, eds. Equine Infectious Diseases. St. Louis: Saunders Elsevier, 2007:317–331.

Moore JM, Barton MH. Treatment of endotoxemia. Vet Clin North Am Equine Pract 2003;19:681–695.

Authors Olimpo Oliver-Espinosa and Deborah A. Parsons

Consulting Editors Henry Stämpfli and Olimpo Oliver-Espinosa

ENTEROLITHIASIS

BASICS

DEFINITION

Calculi composed of struvite (magnesium ammonium phosphate hexahydrate) that form in the ampulla of the right dorsal colon and subsequently cause partial or complete obstruction of the right dorsal, transverse, or descending colon

PATHOPHYSIOLOGY

- Enteroliths form and enlarge over a period of ≥1 years by deposition of concentric rings of struvite around a central nidus.
- Enterolith formation appears to be facilitated by the relative hypomotility of the right dorsal colon, a pH of colonic contents that is more alkaline than normal, and a high dietary intake of magnesium and protein (typical of alfalfa-rich diets).
- The valve-like effect of the enlarging enterolith at the junction of the right dorsal and transverse colon may intermittently cause partial colonic obstruction and colic.
- Complete colonic obstruction and persistent colic occur when large enteroliths lodge in the narrower distal portion of the right dorsal colon, or when enteroliths migrate aborally and become lodged in the smaller diameter transverse or descending colon.
- Pressure from the lodged enterolith may cause necrosis and rupture of the bowel wall, or the colon may rupture secondary to distension by gas and fluid that accumulate proximal to the obstructing enterolith.

SYSTEM AFFECTED

The gastrointestinal system is the only system affected.

GENETICS

There is no known genetic basis for this disease, although breed predilections do exist (see below).

INCIDENCE/PREVALENCE

Enterolithiasis has a worldwide distribution but is much more common in certain geographic areas, particularly parts of California and Florida. At the University of California, enteroliths were responsible for 15% of patients admitted for treatment of colic and almost 30% of patients undergoing celiotomy for treatment of colic between 1973 and 1996.

SIGNALMENT

- Enteroliths occur in all breeds, but Arabian and Arabian crosses, Morgans, American Miniatures. American Saddlebreds, and donkeys appear to be overrepresented. In endemic areas, Thoroughbreds, Standardbreds, and warmblooded horses are underrepresented, likely because they are predominantly younger horses in active training being fed higher levels of grain.
- There is no apparent sex predilection, although stallions are underrepresented.
- Middle-age adult horses >2 years of age are at greatest risk in endemic areas. The mean age for affected horses in a recent retrospective study was approximately 11.5 years, and the age range was 1–36 years.

SIGNS

Historical

Historical feeding of a diet containing >50% alfalfa is common to almost all cases. In about one-third of cases, recurrent colic of mild to moderate severity over a period of a few weeks to as long as a year is observed. Some horses develop severe colic signs acutely without any history of recurrent colic signs. Passage of small enteroliths in the feces is a feature of the history of about 15% of affected horses. Other horses show more nonspecific signs, such as attitude changes, intermittent anorexia, lethargy, weight loss, intermittent loose manure, resentment of tightening the girth, reluctance to exercise, or reluctance to travel down hills, before signs of colic appear.

Physical Examination

- Typical signs reflect mild to moderate abdominal discomfort and include pawing, looking at the flank, rolling, repeatedly lying down and getting up, sweating, and kicking at the abdomen.
- Other signs include tachycardia, anorexia, depression, intestinal hypomotility, lack of progressive peristalsis, bilateral abdominal distention, "dog-sitting" posture, prolonged capillary refill time, and tachypnea.
- Horses with multiple small, nonobstructing enteroliths may have progressive borborygmi resulting in a characteristic gravelly sound heard on auscultation of the colon.
- Signs reflecting endotoxemia may develop, particularly when the integrity of the bowel wall is compromised.

CAUSES

Enteroliths are caused by the deposition of concentric rings of struvite around a central nidus, which is usually a flintlike pebble (silicon dioxide), a piece of metal, or, less commonly, fibrous material, such as nylon baling twine, rubber fencing, or hair.

RISK FACTORS

- Proven risk factors include residing in an endemic area, feeding alfalfa as the predominant or sole forage, and lack of pasture grazing.
- In addition, consumption of hard water, residing predominantly in a stall or paddock, limited exercise, and feeding of diets low in grain may increase risk.
- The high magnesium content (3–6 times the daily requirement) and high protein content of alfalfa appear to provide magnesium and nitrogen for formation of struvite as well as promoting a high colonic buffering capacity and the alkaline colonic pH necessary for precipitation of struvite.
- Historically, the feeding of diets high in wheat bran and low in grass-based forages contributed to a problem with enterolith formation in millers' horses.

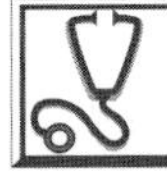

DIAGNOSIS

DIFFERENTIAL DIAGNOSIS

All other causes of colic (see relevant section), but particularly those that cause chronic or recurrent colic, including sand colic, internal abdominal abscess, gastric ulcer, thromboembolic colic, peritonitis, abdominal neoplasia, cholelithiasis, and nephrolithiasis should be included.

CBC/BIOCHEMISTRY/URINALYSIS

Changes are nonspecific for enterolithiasis. Increased hematocrit and hyperproteinemia are common secondary changes reflecting hemoconcentration and/or stress-associated splenic contraction.

OTHER LABORATORY TESTS

- In uncomplicated cases, peritoneal fluid is usually of normal to increased volume, has a normal appearance, and has laboratory parameters within normal limits.
- Secondary bowel wall compromise leads to amber discoloration, increased turbidity, increased protein concentration, and increased cell count changes compatible with a modified transudate.
- In cases of rupture, evidence of peritoneal contamination is observed (plant material, protozoa).

IMAGING

Abdominal radiography, preferably after fasting for ≥24hr, is useful diagnostically in many but not all horses. The technique is most successful in smaller horses and is more sensitive for detecting enteroliths in the large colon than enteroliths that have migrated to the small colon. Enteroliths are recognized by their spherical or tetrahedral shape, homogeneously increased density, sharp borders silhouetted against gas caps in the intestinal lumen, or the presence of a metallic nidus. Equivocal radiographic findings can often be resolved by one or more repeat examinations performed after continued fasting if permitted by the clinical condition of the patient. Abdominal ultrasound is of limited utility, except to help rule out other conditions.

DIAGNOSTIC PROCEDURES

Rectal examination findings may be within normal limits in up to 25% of horses with enterolithiasis; however, rectal examination frequently reveals distention of the large colon and, less often, tight mesenteric bands. Enteroliths are palpable on rectal examination in about 5% of cases. Placing the horse on a ramp to elevate the front end may enable palpation of enteroliths rectally.

PATHOLOGICAL FINDINGS

N/A

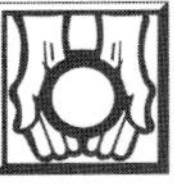

TREATMENT

Surgical intervention is the only treatment documented to be effective to eliminate formed enteroliths and is best performed via ventral celiotomy within a few hours of the onset of signs or, preferably, before signs of complete colonic obstruction are present. The preferred approach is to evacuate the colon via an enterotomy created at the pelvic flexure, after which the enterolith is gently manipulated to this site or to a second enterotomy site for removal.

APPROPRIATE HEALTH CARE

Initial evaluation and treatment of horses with enterolithiasis are handled appropriately on an outpatient basis. Horses that do not have a complete colonic obstruction frequently respond favorably to medical approaches commonly used to treat colic (i.e., withholding feed; administration of flunixin meglumine or similar NSAID; passage of a nasogastric tube; administration of fluids, laxatives, or lubricants such as mineral oil by nasogastric tube; or IV administration of polyionic fluids).
Transportation to a referral center is usually necessary for radiographic confirmation of the diagnosis and surgical management.

NURSING CARE

Prevention of rolling and self-induced trauma, provision of analgesia, maintenance of an indwelling nasogastric tube and fluid therapy are indicated before referral and during transportation. Intravenous fluid therapy is often indicated before, during, and after surgery.

ACTIVITY

As with any horse undergoing ventral celiotomy, stall rest with hand-walking is recommended for the first 4 weeks postsurgery, and the horse should not be returned to work or used for breeding for at least 2–3 months.

DIET

Feed should be withheld before and immediately after surgery. Feeding of small amounts is reintroduced 4–6 hr after surgery and increased to full intake over the next 5 days, unless precluded by complications such as ileus or enteritis. Alfalfa should be eliminated from the diet of horses that have had enteroliths removed surgically.

CLIENT EDUCATION

Restriction of exercise in the immediate postoperative period must be implemented. There is a high likelihood of recurrence unless diet and management are not changed (see Risk Factors).

SURGICAL CONSIDERATION

If the patient shows evidence of complete colonic obstruction or has a large, nonobstructing enterolith in the large colon, surgical removal of the enterolith is the only effective treatment.

MEDICATIONS

DRUG(S) OF CHOICE

See Appropriate Health Care.

CONTRAINDICATIONS

The use of neostigmine, bethanechol, or other potent prokinetics is contraindicated. Acepromazine is contraindicated in affected horses showing evidence of shock.

PRECAUTIONS

Repeated use of potent analgesics such as flunixin meglumine or ketoprofen to control colic pain should be avoided unless appropriate diagnostic and therapeutic intervention is also pursued.

POSSIBLE INTERACTIONS

N/A

ALTERNATIVE DRUGS

N/A

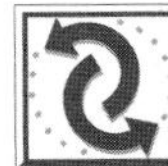

FOLLOW-UP

PATIENT MONITORING

Observation for signs of colic or inappetence. Follow-up annual abdominal radiographs may be helpful in detecting recurrence.

PREVENTION/AVOIDANCE

- Replace alfalfa hay in the diet with good-quality grass or oat hay. Alfalfa should make up <50%, and preferably 0%, of the diet.
- Supplement hay with 8fl oz (250mL/450kg) of apple cider vinegar daily, and/or mixed grain, to help acidify colonic contents.
- Provide regular exercise.
- Eliminate hard drinking water if possible.
- Minimize ingestion of nidi, such as pebbles and metallic objects, by not feeding horses on the ground and by carefully screening the feed and manger for foreign material.
- Intermittent administration of psyllium at a dose of 16oz (0.5 kg) orally once daily for the first 5 consecutive days of each month may help remove sand and other nidi from the large colon.
- Serious colic resulting from acute colonic obstruction can be avoided if large enteroliths recognized by radiographic examination or rectal examination are removed with elective surgery while horses are asymptomatic.

POSSIBLE COMPLICATIONS

Postoperative complications are uncommon. Apart from postoperative complications encountered after colic surgery (diarrhea, incisional infection, incisional hernia, laminitis, septic peritonitis, adhesions, impaction at the enterotomy site), the major complication is recurrence of enteroliths if dietary modification is not instituted.

EXPECTED COURSE AND PROGNOSIS

- Horses with small enteroliths in their large colon likely remain asymptomatic for months or years and often pass the enteroliths in their manure.
- Prognosis for horses with small nonobstructing enteroliths is good, provided appropriate dietary modification is initiated.
- Prognosis for horses with large nonobstructing enteroliths in the large colon is guarded without surgical removal because there is a high likelihood that these will eventually pass aborally and cause a complete colonic obstruction.
- Prognosis for recovery for horses with a complete colonic obstruction detected before bowel compromise has occurred is good following surgical removal of the stone. Complete recovery can be anticipated in >90% of cases in which surgery is performed before the bowel ruptures. Without surgery, the prognosis for horses with obstructing enteroliths is virtually hopeless.

MISCELLANEOUS

ASSOCIATED CONDITIONS

Colonic rupture, colonic displacement, septic peritonitis, endotoxemia, and the postoperative complications listed previously have been recognized in association with enterolithiasis.

AGE-RELATED FACTORS

Enterolithiasis is rarely a clinical problem in horses younger than 2 years. Peak incidence is in horses between 5 and 15 years of age.

ZOONOTIC POTENTIAL

N/A

PREGNANCY

Pregnant mares are likely at increased risk for abortion, as is the case for other causes of colic requiring surgery. Prophylactic use of NSAIDs (flunixin meglumine) and progestagens such as altrenogest is indicated in pregnant mares.

SYNONYMS

- Intestinal stones
- Intestinal calculi
- Intestinal bezoars
- Stones
- Rocks

SEE ALSO

Colic

Suggested Reading

Blue MG, Wittkopp RW. Clinical and structural features of equine enteroliths. JAVMA 1988;179:79–82.

Hassel DM, Langer DL, Snyder JR, Drake CM, Goodell ML, Wyle A. Evaluation of enterolithiasis in horses: 900 cases (1973–1996). JAVMA 1999;214:233–237.

Hassel DM, Rakestraw PC, Gardner IA, Spier SJ, Snyder JR. Dietary risk factors and colonic pH and mineral concentrations in horses with enterolithiasis. J Vet Intern Med 2004;18:346–349.

Hintz HF, Lowe JE, Livesay-Wilkins P, *et al*. Studies on equine enterolithiasis. Proc AAEP 1988;24:53–59.

Lloyd K, Hintz HF, Wheat JD, Schryver HF. Enteroliths in horses. Cornell Vet 1987;77:172–186.

Murray RC, Constantinescu GM, Green EM. Equine enteroliths. Compend Contin Educ Pract Vet 1992;14:1104–1113.

Authors W. David Wilson and Diana M. Hassel
Consulting Editors Henry Stämpfli and Olimpo Oliver-Espinosa

EOSINOPHILIA AND BASOPHILIA

BASICS

OVERVIEW

Eosinophilia

• Eosinophil count in peripheral blood > upper limit of the laboratory reference range; usually >800 cells/μL [$>0.8 \times 10^9$ cells/L]
• Eosinophilopoiesis is stimulated by T-cell–derived lymphokines (IL-3, IL-5, GM-CSF, and eosinophilopoietin). IL-5 also promotes eosinophil differentiation, maturation, survival and function.
• Eosinophils are normally found in subepithelial locations of tissues at the sites of entry of foreign particles such as the skin, respiratory, genitourinary, and GI tracts.
• Eosinophils have diverse functions including parasiticidal activity, regulation of allergic and inflammatory processes, and regulation of coagulation and fibrinolysis. • During recruitment, eosinophils in blood are primed by lymphokines, migrate to tissues under the influence of chemoattractants and are activated by cytokines, lipid mediators, complement, and immunoglobulins. • Recruitment is often associated with specific immune responses to parasites or allergens through release of histamine and other constituents of mast cells, basophils, and/or lymphokines. • Parasites may be destroyed or immune responses dampened. However, protracted eosinophilic inflammation can result in tissue damage and organ dysfunction. • Extensive tissue eosinophilia can occur without concurrent blood eosinophilia.
• Blood eosinophilia may arise from increased production, increased release from bone marrow reserve pool, redistribution from the marginated to circulating pool or prolonged vascular survival.

Basophilia

• Basophil count in peripheral blood >300 cells/μL [$>0.3 \times 10^9$ cells/L]. • Basophils are the least numerous and least understood WBC. • Production is antigen-specific and is regulated primarily by IL-3 and to a lesser degree by IL-5 and GM-CSF. • Basophils have morphologic and functional similarities with mast cells; both elicit immediate (type I) hypersensitivity reactions by release of stored mediators upon cross-linking of surface-bound IgE by specific antigens.
• Other functions include regulation of coagulation and fibrinolysis, lipolysis and parasite rejection.
• Basophilia and eosinophilia may exist concurrently as histamine released by basophils is chemotactic for eosinophils.

SIGNS

• Dependent on the underlying disease. • If weight loss, lethargy, diarrhea, colic. or ventral edema is observed, consider parasites or idiopathic hypereosinophilic syndrome.

CAUSES AND RISK FACTORS

Eosinophilia

• Eosinophilia most commonly occurs in diseases involving tissues with high concentrations of mast cells (e.g., skin and GI, respiratory, and urogenital tracts) and after an interaction between specific antigen, IgE, and mast cells/basophils. • In these diseases tissue eosinophilia is common; however, blood eosinophilia is not a consistent finding.

Parasitism

More common with parasites that exhibit tissue migration (e.g., *Parascaris equorum*, *Strongylus* spp., and *Dictylocaulus arnfeldi*).

Fungal infection

• Zycomycosis (*Conidiobolus* spp. or *Basidiobolus* spp.). • Pythiasis (*Pythium insidiosum*)

Idiopathic

Idiopathic hypereosinophilic syndromes, i.e., MEED, EE, eosinophilic granulomas

Neoplasia.

Eosinophilic leukemia or as a paraneoplastic condition with lymphoma (production of IL-5 by neoplastic T cells)

Immune

Type I hypersensitivity reactions—eosinophilia is rare in horses.

Basophilia

• Hypersensitivity reactions—rare
• Parasitism—rare • Basophilic leukemia in the horse has not been reported.

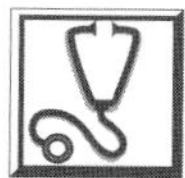

DIAGNOSIS

CBC/BIOCHEMISTRY/URINALYSIS

• Eosinophil and/or basophil count > the laboratory reference intervals. • Biochemical analysis may reveal evidence of specific organ dysfunction.

OTHER LABORATORY TESTS

Serologic antigen testing for diagnosis of atopic dermatitis; however, false-positives are common.

IMAGING

• Thoracic radiography may reveal space-occupying lesions of lymphoma or MEED. • Thoracic and abdominal ultrasonography may reveal lesions of lymphoma, MEED, or EE.

OTHER DIAGNOSTIC PROCEDURES

• Fecal flotation techniques detect nematode parasite ova or larvae if patent infection is present.
• Baermann technique detects *D. arnfeldi* larvae in feces.
• Abdominocentesis—eosinophils suggest parasitism, MEED or EE; abnormal lymphocytes may suggest lymphoma.
• Thoracocentesis—eosinophils suggest MEED; atypical lymphocytes suggest lymphoma. • Oral glucose absorption test—evidence of malabsorption may suggest lymphoma, MEED, or EE. • Rectal biopsy to detect lymphoma, MEED, or EE
• Endoscopy of the airways may reveal masses in cases of MEED or mucoid exudate associated with parasitic or allergic lung disease. • Tracheal aspirate and/or brochoalveolar lavage to detect eosinophilic inflammation and possibly parasite ova or larvae.
• Skin biopsy in cases of zygomycosis, pythiasis, MEED or eosinophilic granulomas. • Bone marrow aspirate/biopsy to detect myeloproliferative disease

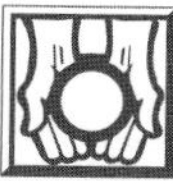

TREATMENT

• Treatment should be directed at underlying disease.
• Fluid therapy in animals with dehydration (e.g., from diarrhea)
• Environmental management in cases of suspected allergic disease • Aggressive surgical resection is required in cases of pythiasis.

MEDICATIONS

DRUG(S)

• Immunosuppressive treatment with corticosteroids—e.g., dexamethasone (0.2 mg/kg IV or IM once daily for 5 days) followed by prednisolone (1mg/kg PO once daily for 14 days, then 1mg/kg PO every second day).
• Appropriate anthelminitics for parasitism (e.g., ivermectin at 0.2 mg/kg PO)

CONTRAINDICATIONS/POSSIBLE INTERACTIONS

Corticosteroids should be avoided in horses with laminitis or infectious disease.

FOLLOW-UP

PATIENT MONITORING

Periodic CBC to monitor eosinophil and basophil counts

POSSIBLE COMPLICATIONS

Tissue eosinophil infiltration can cause organ dysfunction.

EXPECTED COURSE AND PROGNOSIS

• Depends on underlying condition • MEED and lymphoma have a poor to grave prognosis.
• Parasitism and EE have a guarded prognosis.
• Course of allergic diseases depends on ongoing antigen exposure.

MISCELLANEOUS

AGE-RELATED FACTORS

Eosinophils are absent at birth, then eosinophil counts increase to a mean of 353 cells/μL (0.353×10^9 cells/L) at 4 mo.

PREGNANCY

Corticosteroids should be avoided in the last trimester.

SEE ALSO

Anaphylaxis

ABBREVIATIONS

• EE = eosinophilic enterocolitis • GI = gastrointestinal • GM-CSF = granulocyte-macrophage colony stimulating factor • IgE = immunoglobulin E
• IL-3 = interleukin 3 • IL-5 = interleukin 5
• MEED = multisystemic eosinophilic epitheliotrophic disease

Suggested Reading

Latimer KS. Diseases affecting leukocytes. In: Colahan PT, el al., eds. Equine Medicine and Surgery, ed 5. St Louis: Mosby, 1999;1992–2001, 2025–2034.

Author Kristopher Hughes
Consulting Editors Jennifer Hodgson and David Hodgson

EOSINOPHILIC KERATITIS

BASICS

OVERVIEW

- EK is a relatively common disease of horses with an unknown etiology.
- An accumulation of mainly eosinophils and a few mast cells in the affected cornea is characteristic.

SYSTEM AFFECTED

Ophthalmic

SIGNALMENT

All ages and breeds affected

SIGNS

- The clinical appearance of EK in horses can be highly variable.
- Mild to severe blepharospasm, epiphora, chemosis, conjunctival hyperemia, mucoid discharge, corneal ulcers covered by raised, white, necrotic plaques
- A subset of horses with minimal discomfort and more chronic, nonulcerated, proliferative lesions of the cornea has been observed.

CAUSES AND RISK FACTORS

- The true etiology of this condition is yet to be illuminated.
- Possibly allergic or parasitic
- May be an immune-mediated or inflammatory manifestation of chronic ivermectin administration for parasite control

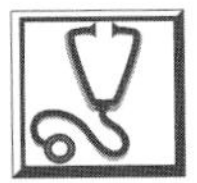

DIAGNOSIS

DIFFERENTIAL DIAGNOSIS

Allergic or hypersensitivity keratitis/ keratoconjunctivitis; eosinophilic granuloma; bacterial, mycotic, or viral keratitis; foreign body reaction; onchocerciasis; habronemiasis; corneal neoplasia such as squamous cell carcinoma or mastocytoma; traumatic keratitis with scarring; calcium or lipid degeneration

CBC/BIOCHEMISTRY/URINALYSIS

N/A

OTHER LABORATORY TESTS

- Rule out infectious causes (bacterial or fungal) with corneal scrapings for cytology and culture.
- Corneal scrapings of EK typically contain degenerate collagen, numerous eosinophils, and a few neutrophils, macrophages, lymphocytes, and mast cells.
- Cytology is usually diagnostic; however, biopsy for histology will help to confirm the diagnosis if corneal scrapings are not conclusive.
- In cases with an associated conjunctivitis, the distribution of inflammatory cells in a sample from the conjunctiva resembles that from the cornea.

IMAGING

N/A

DIAGNOSTIC PROCEDURES

N/A

PATHOLOGIC FINDINGS

Histologic examination finds eosinophilic, acellular granular material, and subepithelial fragmented degenerate collagen infiltrated by eosinophils, lymphocytes, plasma cells, and macrophages.

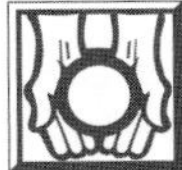

TREATMENT

- Medical therapy is aimed at decreasing the inflammatory response within the cornea.
- Often combination therapy is necessary.
- Superficial lamellar keratectomy to remove plaques speeds healing.

MEDICATIONS

DRUG(S) OF CHOICE

- Topical corticosteroids (1% prednisolone acetate or 0.1% dexamethasone) 3–4 times a day in early stages (despite corneal ulcerations)
- Topical mast cell stabilizers such as 4% cromolyn sodium and 0.01% iodoxamide or olopatadine can be necessary in some cases 3–4 times a day.
- Topical antibiotics (e.g., bacitracin-neomyxin-polymyxin, chloramphenicol), 1% atropine, and 0.03% phospholine iodide BID in combination with systemic nonsteroidal anti-inflammatory drugs (e.g., flunixin meglumine 0.25–1 mg/kg BID PO, IM, IV) to protect the corneal wounds from secondary infection and treat any associated uveitis
- Once improvement is noted, medical therapy should be tapered slowly.

CONTRAINDICATIONS/POSSIBLE INTERACTIONS

- Phospholine iodide is an acetylcholinesterase inhibitor which may be larvacidal for parasites. Its use is controversial.
- The use of topical NSAIDs may increase the severity of clinical signs in the horse, since they do not inhibit and may potentiate leukotrienes.
- Horses receiving topically administered atropine should be monitored for signs of colic.

FOLLOW-UP

EXPECTED COURSE AND PROGNOSIS

- Although therapy is often prolonged and these lesions are often slow to heal, the prognosis for resolution with diligent treatment is good.
- Scarring of the cornea may occur.
- May recur

MISCELLANEOUS

ASSOCIATED CONDITIONS

Uveitis

ABBREVIATION

- EK = eosinophilic keratitis/keratoconjunctivitis

SEE ALSO

- Corneal ulceration
- Corneal/scleral lacerations
- Corneal stromal abscesses
- Nonulcerative keratouveitis
- Burdock pappus bristle keratopathy
- Superficial nonhealing ulcers with anterior stromal sequestration
- Recurrent uveitis
- Glaucoma

Suggested Reading

Brooks DE. Ophthalmology for the Equine Practitioner. Jackson, WY; Teton NewMedia, 2002.

Brooks DE, Matthews AG., Equine ophthalmology. In: Gelatt KN, ed. Veterinary Ophthalmology, ed 4. Philadelphia; Lippincott Williams and Wilkins, 2007.

Gilger BC, ed. Equine Ophthalmology. Philadelphia; WB Saunders, 2005.

Authors Caryn E. Plummer

Consulting Editor Dennis E. Brooks

EPIGLOTTIC ENTRAPMENT

BASICS

OVERVIEW

• A result of the loose, aryepiglottic mucosa, which normally is on the ventral surface of the epiglottis, enveloping part or all of the dorsal surface of the epiglottis.
• Usually, the epiglottis remains in its normal, horizontal position dorsal to the soft palate, but the condition can occur concurrently with dorsal displacement of the soft palate (DDSP).
• Leads to varying degrees of respiratory compromise and exercise intolerance.
• Most often diagnosed during resting endoscopy because the entrapment is persistent.
• Also can occur intermittently.

SIGNALMENT

• Affects horses participating in intensive exercise primarily—Thoroughbred and Standardbred racehorses.
• Other breeds or horses engaged in other activities rarely are affected.
• Can occur at any age while in training
• No sex predilection.
• Rarely seen in older noncompetitive horses associated with a cough.

SIGNS

• Exercise intolerance is the most frequent chief complaint.
• Abnormal respiratory noise also may be present during exercise.
• Other signs—coughing, dysphagia, or nasal discharge.

CAUSES AND RISK FACTORS

• The cause is unknown.
• Racing is the most significant risk factor.
• Horses with a short or small epiglottis are predisposed.
• An obscure association exists between epiglottic entrapment and DDSP.

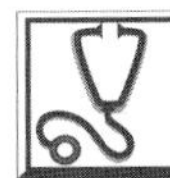

DIAGNOSIS

DIFFERENTIAL DIAGNOSIS

• Epiglottiditis – swelling of the epiglottis smooths out the normal scalloped edges and distorts the vascular pattern, but there is no edge of membrane over the top of the epiglottis as there is with an entrapment.
• Epiglottic deformity/hypoplasia – while there may be varying epiglottic deformity, there is no edge of membrane over the top of the epiglottis as there is with an entrapment.
• DDSP – Not even the outline of the shape of the epiglottis is visible above the palate since the epiglottis is below the palate (within the oropharynx) with a displacement.

CBC/BIOCHEMISTRY/URINALYSIS

N/A

OTHER LABORATORY TEST

• Arterial blood gases during exercise are typically normal without concurrent abnormalities (PaO_2 approximately 70 mmHg or greater).

IMAGING

• Upper airway endoscopy at rest—the most common diagnostic technique. The triangular-shaped epiglottis above the palate remains visible, but the entrapping membrane obscures the visualization of the normal serrated edge of the epiglottis and the vascular pattern. The normal vasculature on the dorsal surface of the epiglottis consists of two longitudinal vessels that extend from the base toward the apex and that arborize into smaller vessels extending toward the edge of the epiglottis. With chronicity, the entrapping membrane becomes very thickened and, sometimes, ulcerated at the apex of the epiglottis.
• With concurrent DDSP, it is difficult to see if the epiglottis is entrapped. Close inspection over the free edge of the palate may reveal another edge of membrane, representing the epiglottic entrapment, before the dorsal surface of the epiglottis is apparent. Sometimes there will be a bulge into the palate from the epiglottic entrapment below it.
• Skull radiography—when the epiglottis is entrapped, the normal, convex shape of the epiglottis above the palate is obscured on lateral skull radiographs.

OTHER DIAGNOSTIC PROCEDURES

- Initiating swallowing during resting endoscopy may induce an intermittent entrapment.
- High-speed treadmill endoscopy may be required to establish the diagnosis of intermittent entrapment.
- Local anesthetic and intravenous sedation may allow the clinician to elevate the epiglottis under videoendoscopic guidance with bronchoesophageal graspers to evaluate under the epiglottis. The presence of ulceration of the subepiglottic membrane may indicate previous intermittent entrapment.

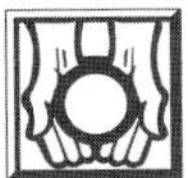

TREATMENT

- Surgical correction of the simple, nonulcerated entrapment entails axial division of the entrapping membrane in the standing horse with sedation and topical anesthetic. The division is performed with direct visualization, employing a laser fiber through the instrument portal of a videoendoscope. Axial division also can be performed with a hooked bistoury in the standing or anesthetized horse. With the hooked bistoury, general anesthesia is preferred to minimize the risk of inadvertent trauma to the pharynx or palate.
- Very thickened, ulcerated entrapping membranes often require surgical resection of the tissue. This can be approached through a laryngotomy under general anesthesia, or via transendoscopic laser surgery in the sedated horse.

MEDICATIONS

DRUGS

- Anti-inflammatory drugs (dexamethasone [10 mg IV SID], phenylbutazone [2.2mg/kg PO BID]) and throat sprays (10 mL of a furacin-based solution with 2 mg of prednisolone in a 1 mL-solution BID) for several days postoperatively.
- Antimicrobials (doxycycline 10 mg/kg PO BID for 7 days) are advised in cases of thickened membranes or ulceration, but may not be necessary in an uncomplicated entrapment without any ulceration or thickening of the entrapping membrane.

CONTRAINDICATIONS/POSSIBLE INTERACTIONS

- N/A

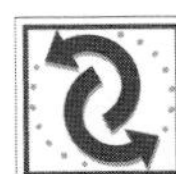

FOLLOW-UP

- Perform endoscopy postoperatively and before resuming training; further examinations depend on any change in performance.
- Epiglottic entrapment has a very low recurrence rate.

MISCELLANEOUS

ASSOCIATED CONDITIONS

- N/A

AGE-RELATED FACTORS

- N/A

ZOONOTIC POTENTIAL

- N/A

PREGNANCY

- N/A

SEE ALSO

- Acute epiglottiditis
- Dynamic collapse of the upper airway

ABBREVIATION

- DDSP = dorsal displacement of the soft palate

Suggested Reading

Epstein KL, Parente EJ. Epiglottic Fold Entrapment. In: McGorum BC, Dixon PM, Robinson NE, Schumacher J, eds. Equine Respiratory Medicine and Surgery. Philadelphia: Elsevier, 2007:459–466.

Author Eric J. Parente
Consulting Editor Daniel Jean

EQUINE CUSHING'S DISEASE

BASICS

DEFINITION

A slowly progressive disorder with a characteristic clinical picture. It is associated with functional adenomas or adenomatous hyperplasia of the pars intermedia of the pituitary gland.

PATHOPHYSIOLOGY

• The pars distalis and pars intermedia of the pituitary gland secrete the same precursor molecule, POMC, but they process it into different hormones. • The corticotroph cells of the pars distalis cleave POMC into ACTH and β-endorphin–related peptides. • The melanotroph cells of the pars intermedia cleave POMC mainly into MSH and β-endorphin–related peptides, with relatively small amounts of ACTH. • In health, glucocorticoid levels are maintained by ACTH secretion from the corticotroph cells. • Control of the pars intermedia appears to be via tonic inhibition of melanotrophs by dopamine secreted from hypothalamic neurons. Horses with ECD show oxidant-induced injury and degeneration of dopaminergic neurons of the hypothalamus and, consequently, decreased inhibition of the melanotrophs. This results in hyperplasia of the melanotrophs, significantly increasing POMC-related peptide synthesis and secretion (including ACTH).

SYSTEMS AFFECTED

Skin/Exocrine

Clinical signs most often include hirsutism, abnormal hair coat–shedding pattern, and hyperhidrosis.

Endocrine/Metabolic

Polyuria/polydipsia—this may be multifactorial:
• Excess cortisol can increase the GFR and antagonize the effect of ADH on water reabsorption in the renal tubules.
• Hyperglycemia can lead to an osmotic diuresis, although polyuria/polydipsia is also observed in euglycemic horses. • Compression or destruction of the pars nervosa by enlargement of the pars intermedia can decrease ADH secretion.

Musculoskeletal

Laminitis, particularly in ponies

Behavioral

It has been suggested that the more docile behavior of some patients is the result of increased β-endorphins.

GENETICS

N/A

INCIDENCE/PREVALENCE

The reported prevalence varies from 0.1% to 0.5% of equine hospital caseloads but probably is an underestimation since most cases are treated by private practitioners.

SIGNALMENT

• All breeds, but appears to be more prevalent in ponies and Morgans • Old horses—range, 10–35 years; mean, 20 years • No sex predilection

SIGNS

Historical

Affected horses may have various problems that do not necessarily appear directly related to a disease of the pituitary gland, e.g., weight loss, recurrent laminitis, infertility, or chronic infections.

Physical Examination

• Hirsutism is the most common sign and is characterized by a long, wavy hair coat. • In some, shedding of the winter coat is delayed; in others, hair grows earlier and faster during the fall months. • Excessive sweating, primarily in horses with hirsutism. • Polyuria and polydipsia in >50% of cases; however, this may not be noticed if the horse is on pasture for prolonged periods. • Weight loss is common and may be associated with parasitism, poor dentition, or concurrent infection. • Horses with ECD but without concurrent infections maintain normal body weight but may show decreased muscle mass, particularly over the back, and a pot-bellied appearance. • Less frequent signs—chronic laminitis, tachycardia, sinusitis, gingivitis, pneumonia, skin infections, delayed wound healing, infertility, lethargy, blindness, seizures, and abnormal bulging of supraorbital fat pads.

CAUSES

The pituitary lesion has been described as pituitary basophil, chromophobe adenomas, or a diffuse hyperplasia of the melanotroph cells.

RISK FACTORS

None known

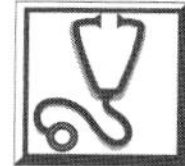

DIAGNOSIS

DIFFERENTIAL DIAGNOSIS

• Hirsutism is pathognomonic, except in breeds with a long hair coat—Missouri Foxtrotter or Bashkin. • Chronic weight loss—poor management, parasitism, poor dentition, hypothyroidism, other chronic systemic diseases, or neoplasia • Polyuria/polydipsia can be a sign of chronic renal failure, diabetes insipidus, or diabetes mellitus, although the latter two diseases are rare in horses. • Pheochromocytoma may cause episodes of hyperthermia, hyperhidrosis, tachypnea, and weight loss.

CBC/CHEMISTRY/URINALYSIS

• No consistent changes in laboratory values, although ≅60% show hyperglycemia
• Hyperlipidemia is noted frequently in ponies.
• Serum liver enzyme activity may be elevated.
• CBC—may show a stress leukogram

OTHER LABORATORY TESTS

Endocrinologic testing of the pituitary adrenal axis most often confirms the diagnosis.

Resting Plasma Cortisol Concentration

• Wide range of normal values—horses with pars intermedia dysfunction are often within the normal limits. • Physiologic elevation of cortisol can occur secondary to exercise, hypoglycemia, or stress. • Equine plasma cortisol levels have a diurnal rhythm with morning values higher than evening values. Affected horses appear to lose the diurnal variation. However, this cannot be used for a definitive diagnosis because the rhythm also may be absent in normal horses. • If a horse does have a marked diurnal variation, it probably does not have ECD.

Dexamethasone Suppression Test

• This is the most commonly used test for pituitary adrenocortical function and, in the author's experience, the test of choice in most cases, taking into account the effect of the season (fall versus winter and spring). • Plasma cortisol concentration is measured in samples collected immediately before and 19 hr after administration of dexamethasone (40 μg/kg IM). • Normal horses—administration in the late afternoon depresses cortisol production to less than 1 μg/dL by the following morning. However, in the fall, serum cortisol concentration of healthy horses may be >1 μg/dL after dexamethasone administration.
• Affected horses—administration produces a small degree of suppression, but not to the extent of normal horses; affected horses also rebound more quickly.

ACTH Stimulation Test

• Measurement of plasma or serum cortisol levels before and 8 hr after administration of ACTH gel (1 IU/kg IM) or 2 hr after synthetic ACTH gel (100 IU IV). • Normal horses—2- to 3-fold increase in plasma cortisol within 4–8 hr.
• Affected horses—exaggerated response with cortisol levels sometimes rising at least 4-fold.
• Because of the variable responsiveness of affected horses and the overlap in values with those of normal horses, this test fails to consistently differentiate affected and non-affected animals.

Resting Plasma ACTH Level

• Measurement of plasma endogenous ACTH concentration is valuable in establishing the diagnosis. • Normal values may vary between laboratories. • In one study, resting plasma ACTH levels were markedly higher in September than in January and May. • The sample requires special handling—blood must be collected in cold disodium EDTA tubes, kept at 4° C, promptly centrifuged, and the plasma stored at 70° C until assayed. • Values in stressed normal horses and those with early ECD can overlap.

TRH Response Test

• Affected horses will respond uniquely to administration of TRH (1 mg IV); in addition to the expected elevations in T_3 and T_4, plasma cortisol production increases significantly by 15–30 min and lasts for up to 90 min. • Normal horses—cortisol level decreases slightly. • This test has been used in horses with clinical signs of ECD and ambiguous dexamethasone suppression test results. • Recommended for use when dexamethasone is contraindicated—laminitis. • This test has been recently reviewed and its specificity has been questioned.

Combined Dexamethasone/TRH Stimulation Test

• Collect a baseline blood sample and administer dexamethasone (40 μg/kg IV). • Collect a second blood sample 3 hr later and then administer TRH (1.1 mg/kg IV). • Collect a third blood sample 30 min after TRH administration. • Normal horses—Cortisol levels decrease, as expected after dexamethasone administration, and remain low after TRH administration. • Affected horses—Plasma cortisol concentration decreases somewhat after dexamethasone administration but return to normal after TRH administration.

Glucose Tolerance Test, Insulin Levels, and Insulin Tolerance Test

• Affected horses have a deranged glucoregulatory mechanism and are often insulin resistant. • Normal horses challenged with glucose (0.5 g/kg IV as a 50% solution) show an immediate rise in plasma glucose concentration and return to baseline level in 1.5 hr. • Affected horses show a delayed return of plasma glucose concentration to baseline; basal insulin levels also are persistently increased, with or without hyperglycemia. • When subjected to an exogenous insulin tolerance test (0.4 IU/kg IV), affected horses show no significant decline in blood glucose.

Urinary Corticoid: Creatinine Ratio

• The urinary corticoid:creatinine ratio was determined in eight horses with ECD and found to be significantly greater than in control horses. Urine was collected in the morning, but values of affected and nonaffected horses overlapped.
• Do not use as the sole test to confirm the diagnosis.

IMAGING

• Computed tomography has been used to evaluate the pituitary gland. • Ventrodorsal radiography with contrast venography has been described.

DIAGNOSTIC PROCEDURES N/A

PATHOLOGICAL FINDINGS

• Necropsy usually reveals an enlarged pituitary gland (3- to 4-fold normal weight). • Tumors are composed of large columnar or polyhedral cells with hyperchromatic nuclei. • No metastases
• Enlargement of the adrenals and multiple sites of infections often are present.

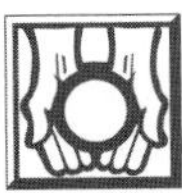

TREATMENT

APPROPRIATE HEALTH CARE

Pay particular attention to regular deworming, vaccination, dental care, and foot trimming.

NURSING CARE

Body clipping and appropriate blanketing are recommended for horses with heavy hair coat.

ACTIVITY

No need to decrease activity unless infections or laminitis are present.

DIET

Increase the energy content of the ration of horses showing signs of weight loss.

CLIENT EDUCATION

• Remind owners about the importance of husbandry.
• Owners need to be vigilant for complications (e.g., sinusitis, gingivitis, laminitis, nonhealing wounds) to readily recognize signs of disease and seek veterinary help early.

SURGICAL CONSIDERATIONS

Bilateral adrenalectomy has not been successful in the long term.

MEDICATIONS

DRUGS OF CHOICE

• Dopamine agonists (e.g., bromocriptine, pergolide) or serotonin antagonists (e.g., cyproheptadine).
• Pergolide mesylate is an expensive, long-acting, type 2 dopaminergic agonist that provides dopamine replacement therapy. Treatment recommendations are based on information extrapolated from human literature and anecdotal clinical accounts. The recommended starting dose is 0.001 mg/kg (0.5 mg for an average-size horse) PO once a day. Some ponies can be successfully maintained on 0.25 mg/day. Clinical improvement should be noted within a few weeks. If horses show no improvement at lower doses, the dose can be increased by 0.25–0.5 mg/day to a maximum of 0.011 mg/kg. If anorexia, colic, diarrhea, worsening of signs of laminitis, or other undesirable effects develop, decrease the dose.
• Bromocriptine can be given orally but apparently has poor bioavailability. It can be prepared in an injectable solution for intramuscular administration. Reported effective oral doses range from 0.03–0.09 mg/kg BID or 0.04 mg/kg PO in the morning and 0.02 mg/kg PO in the evening.
• Information regarding the basic pharmacokinetic behavior and metabolism of cyproheptadine in horses has not been collected. Reports of clinical efficacy vary from 35% to 75%. Initial recommended dose is 0.25 mg/kg PO once a day for 1 mo. If no clinical response occurs, the dose can be increased to 0.3–0.5 mg/kg.
• Cyproheptadine is less expensive than pergolide. Cases in which cyproheptadine is unsuccessful often respond to pergolide treatment.
• A complete treatment plan should include symptomatic therapy such as NSAIDs for laminitis and/or antibiotics for focal bacterial infections.

CONTRAINDICATIONS N/A

PRECAUTIONS N/A

POSSIBLE INTERACTIONS

Unknown

ALTERNATIVE DRUGS

There is one report of insulin used to treat the hyperglycemia associated with ECD. Even though improvement was noted, it was temporary because of the development of anti-insulin antibodies.

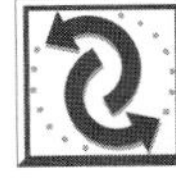

FOLLOW-UP

PATIENT MONITORING

• Clinical improvement manifests by decreased water consumption in polyuric/polydipsic horses, disappearance of pain associated with laminitis, increased weight, or shedding of the long hair (replaced by a shinier coat).
• Improvement also may be marked by a return to normal blood glucose levels in hyperglycemic horses.
• Objectively evaluate the efficacy of treatment by repeating a dexamethasone suppression test or reevaluating endogenous ACTH levels.

PREVENTION/AVOIDANCE

N/A

POSSIBLE COMPLICATIONS

N/A

EXPECTED COURSE AND PROGNOSIS

Prognosis varies, depending on the severity of clinical signs.

MISCELLANEOUS

ASSOCIATED CONDITIONS

In the lay literature, ECD often is associated with hypothyroidism. In more than 30 affected horses that were tested, the response of the thyroid to TRH stimulation was normal.

AGE-RELATED FACTORS

N/A

ZOONOTIC POTENTIAL

N/A

PREGNANCY

Abortion is possible in pregnant, affected mares.

SYNONYMS

• Hyperadrenocorticism
• Pituitary adenoma
• Pituitary-dependent hyperadrenocorticism
• Pituitary pars intermedia dysfunction

SEE ALSO

• Glucose, hyperglycemia
• TRH and TSH stimulation tests

ABBREVIATIONS

• ACTH = adrenocorticotropin hormone
• ADH = antidiuretic hormone
• ECD = equine cushing's disease
• GFR = glomerular filtration rate
• MSH = melanotropin
• POMC = pro-opiomelanocortin
• TRH = thyroid-releasing hormone

Suggested Reading

Donaldson MT, McDonnell SM, Schanbacher BJ *et al.* Variation in plasma adrenocorticotropic hormone concentration and dexamethasone suppression test results with season, age, and sex in healthy ponies and horses. J Vet Intern Med 2005;19:217–222.

Dybdal NO. Equine Cushing's disease. In: Smith BP, ed. Large Animal Medicine, ed 3. St. Louis: Mosby, 2002:1233–1236.

Schott II HC. Pituitary pars intermedia dysfunction: equine Cushing's disease. Vet Clin Equine 2002;18:237–270.

Author Michel Lévy
Consulting Editor Michel Lévy

EQUINE METABOLIC SYNDROME (EMS)/INSULIN RESISTANCE (IR)

BASICS

DEFINITION

• EMS is currently defined by (1) obesity and/or regional adiposity, (2) prior or current laminitis, and (3) IR.
• Clinical signs of EMS have been attributed to hypothyroidism in the past, but it is now known that low serum thyroid hormone concentrations are a consequence rather than a cause of obesity and IR.
• Insulin resistance can be broadly defined as a decrease in tissue responses to circulating insulin, which slows insulin-mediated glucose uptake into skeletal muscle, adipose, and liver tissues.
• Insulin resistance can also be associated with PPID and pregnancy.

PATHOPHYSIOLOGY

• Accumulation of body fat predisposes horses to IR.
• Obesity can lead to IR when myocytes and adipocytes expand with lipid, which interferes with insulin signaling. Accumulation of intracellular lipid also causes adipocytes to release more adipokines, which act locally and enter the circulation.
• Laminitis and IR are potentially related through three mechanisms: (1) impaired glucose delivery to hoof keratinocytes, (2) altered blood flow or endothelial cell function within the hoof vessels, and (3) proinflammatory or prooxidative states associated with chronic IR and/or obesity.
• In horses, NSC within pasture grass play an important role in IR. NSC include simple sugars, starch, and fructans (polymers of fructose), and levels of these components vary within the grass according to geographical location, soil type, weather conditions, and time of day.
• Excessive sugar consumption is likely to exacerbate IR and large quantities of NSC arriving in the hindgut can disrupt the intestinal flora.
• Insulin resistance could be a factor that increases the risk of pasture-associated laminitis.

SYSTEMS AFFECTED

• Skeletal muscle
• Adipose tissues
• Hoof laminae

GENETICS

• There is evidence from a closed herd of ponies within Virginia that IR follows a genetic pattern, but more extensive studies are required.
• Old-line Morgan horses are particularly susceptible to EMS.

INCIDENCE/PREVALENCE

• Pasture-associated laminitis accounts for approximately 45% of laminitis cases occurring on United States farms.
• Laminitis episodes occur more frequently in the spring as pastures turn green. Episodes also occur when the grass is challenged by dry conditions, growing quickly after summer rains, or adapting to the cooler temperatures of the fall season.

GEOGRAPHIC DISTRIBUTION

Horses with EMS are found throughout the United States, but the condition may be more common in regions with heavier rainfall and greener pastures. Epidemiological studies must be performed to determine the geographical distribution of EMS.

SIGNALMENT

• Morgan horse, Paso Fino, Arabian, and pony breeds are most affected.
• Also detected in Quarter Horse, Saddlebred, Tennessee Walking Horse, Thoroughbred, and Warmblood breeds of horse
• Obesity may develop when the horse matures (3 years of age), but most horses are between 5 and 15 years of age when laminitis first occurs.
• There does not appear to be a sex predilection.

SIGNS

• Generalized obesity and/or regional adiposity
• Regional adiposity refers to the presence of a "cresty neck" and fat deposits next to the tailhead, in the sheath, within the supraorbital fossae, or randomly distributed throughout the trunk region as subcutaneous masses.
• Divergent growth rings that are wider at the heel than the toe (founder lines) are also detected in some horses. These divergent growth rings are thought to indicate the occurrence of laminitis and may be detected in horses that do not have a history of lameness.

CAUSES

• Horses described as "easy keepers" are at greater risk.
• Environmental factors include the sugar content of the grass on pasture, the amount of grass and its rate of growth, feeding of concentrates, and the amount of exercise.
• Laminitis episodes are likely to be triggered by a combination of exacerbated IR and a gastrointestinal disturbance. Both of these challenges occur as the pasture grows rapidly in the spring or responding to other changes in weather and season.

RISK FACTORS

• Offspring of a mare or stallion with EMS
• "Easy keeper" metabolic status
• Lack of exercise
• Grazing on lush pasture
• Feeding of concentrates to an obese animal

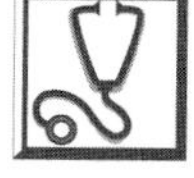

DIAGNOSIS

DIFFERENTIAL DIAGNOSIS

PPID (also called equine Cushing's disease) can develop as horses get older and can be recognized by loss of muscle mass, increase in caloric needs, and delayed haircoat shedding. Horses with EMS appear to develop the condition at a younger age (10–20 years of age).

CBC/BIOCHEMISTRY/URINALYSIS

• No CBC changes have been identified.
• Blood glucose concentrations may approach the high end of reference range.
• Glucosuria is not detected.

OTHER LABORATORY TESTS

• Serum insulin concentrations — the horse should be kept off pasture overnight and fed only hay for 12 hr prior to blood collection. Use the reference range for the laboratory, but a serum insulin concentration >30 μU/mL (also written as mU/L) is often used to define hyperinsulinemia and, therefore, compensated IR. Concentrations may be reported in pmol/L and the conversion factor is approximately 7. This test does not detect uncompensated IR.
• Serum glucose-to-insulin (G:I) ratio — this value can be calculated by dividing the glucose concentration (in mg/dL) by the insulin concentration (in μU/mL). For example, a horse with a serum glucose concentration of 80 mg/dL and serum insulin concentration of 5 μU/mL has a G:I ratio of 16. It has been proposed that a G:I ratio <10 supports the diagnosis of compensated IR, whereas a value <4.5 indicates decompensated IR. This term is used when there is an acute exacerbation in IR and serum insulin concentrations increase markedly, which causes the G:I ratio to decrease. This is not the same as uncompensated IR, which is characterized by pancreatic failure and insulin concentrations that are lower than expected. It should be noted that some laboratories report glucose concentrations in mmol/L, so these values must be multiplied by 18 to convert units to mg/dL.
• Serum or plasma triglyceride (TG) concentrations — elevated serum TG concentrations have been detected in ponies with IR and it has been suggested that this measure serves as an indicator of whole-body metabolic status. However, horses with EMS vary widely with respect to serum TG concentrations, so the presence or absence of hypertriglyceridemia cannot be used to diagnose IR.

IMAGING

Horses with EMS often show radiographic evidence of laminitis, including rotation and bony remodeling of the third phalanx. These abnormalities may be detected in the absence of any discernable lameness and provide evidence of prior subclinical laminitis events.

OTHER DIAGNOSTIC PROCEDURES

• Combined glucose-insulin test (CGIT)—used to confirm IR when blood glucose and insulin concentrations are within reference range. Horses should be kept off pasture and fed hay the night before and during the test. An intravenous catheter should be placed the night before. A preinfusion sample is collected and then 150 mg/kg body weight 50% dextrose solution is infused, immediately followed by 0.10 unit/kg body weight regular insulin. Blood samples are collected at 5, 15, 25, 35, 45, 60, 75, 90, 105, 120, 135, and 150 min post-infusion. Insulin resistance is defined as maintenance of blood glucose concentrations (measured with a glucometer) above the baseline value for 45 min or longer. There is a small risk of hypoglycemia when performing this test so two 60-mL syringes containing 50% dextrose should be kept on hand and administered if sweating, muscle fasciculations, or weakness is observed.

EQUINE METABOLIC SYNDROME (EMS)/INSULIN RESISTANCE (IR)

PATHOLOGICAL FINDINGS

- Affected horses can show evidence of regional adiposity, including enlarged adipose tissue deposits in the neck region or distributed throughout the subcutaneous tissues as masses.
- Gross or histopathologic evidence of laminitis is often present.

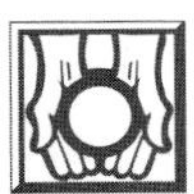

TREATMENT

AIMS OF TREATMENT

- Induce weight loss in horses with generalized obesity.
- Improve insulin sensitivity through weight loss, diet, and exercise.
- Avoid dietary triggers for laminitis.

NURSING CARE

See Laminitis.

DIET

- Individual horses should be fed according to their metabolic needs. Obese horses that are easy keepers can be placed on a simple diet of hay and a vitamin/mineral supplement.
- Obese horses can be fed hay in amounts equivalent to 1.5% of ideal body weight until weight loss is achieved.
- Hay fed to obese horses should have a lower (<12%) NSC content and samples can be tested by commercial laboratories. If the NSC content of the hay exceeds 12%, it should be soaked in cold water for 30 min to lower the sugar content.
- Horses with EMS should receive an additional 1000 IU vitamin E in their diet each day from supplements.
- Avoid feeds that exacerbate IR. Access to pasture must often be restricted or eliminated when managing horses and ponies with EMS. Horses with EMS can be managed by limiting grazing time to 1–2 hr per day (within the period from late night until mid-morning), housing in a grass paddock, strip grazing using an electric fence, or use of a grazing muzzle.
- Thinner insulin-resistant horses can usually be safely fed concentrates, but care must be taken to provide calories without exacerbating IR. Feeds that contain less starch and sugar are appropriate in these situations.

CLIENT EDUCATION

- Obesity is likely to be an important risk factor for EMS, so owners should alter feeding practices, increase exercise, and limit pasture access.
- Grazing should be limited or eliminated at high-risk times of the year.
- Owners and veterinarians should include body condition scoring in their routine heath care.
- Development of regional adiposity (e.g., cresty neck) should prompt measurement of blood glucose and insulin concentrations.

SURGICAL CONSIDERATIONS

None, with the exception of procedures used in some cases of chronic laminitis, including dorsal hoof wall resection and deep digital tenotomy.

MEDICATIONS

DRUG(S) OF CHOICE

- Levothyroxine sodium (Thyro-L; Vet-A-Mix, Lloyd, Inc., Shenandoah, IA) 12 mg per teaspoon
- Previously it was administered as a supplement in cases of suspected hypothyroidism, but now used as a pharmacologic agent to induce weight loss and improve insulin sensitivity in obese insulin resistant horses.
- Used when rapid weight loss is required in a horse that has suffered from laminitis and is threatened by subsequent episodes, and in horses that remain obese despite stringent diet and exercise interventions
- Administered at a dosage of 48 mg (equivalent to 4 teaspoons) for a 500-kg horse (total dose) once daily by mouth or in the feed for 3–6 mo. This total dose of 48 mg/day is not exceeded in larger horses, but lower dosages are selected for ponies, Miniature Horses, and donkeys.
- Serum thyroxine concentrations are usually between 60 and 100 ng/mL in treated horses. This range can be targeted when lower dosages are selected for smaller patients.
- At the completion of the treatment period, the dosage should be lowered to 24 mg (2 teaspoons)/day for 2 weeks and then 12 mg (1 teaspoon)/day for 2 weeks in order to allow endogenous thyroid hormone production to resume.

CONTRAINDICATIONS

- The dosages recommended above are not appropriate for thin horses with IR because weight loss will be induced.
- This treatment has not been evaluated in pregnant mares.

PRECAUTIONS

Cardiac hypertrophy and bone resorption have been associated with levothyroxine sodium use in humans, but not horses.

POSSIBLE INTERACTIONS

No known interactions

ALTERNATIVE DRUGS

Supplements that are thought to improve insulin sensitivity are also available to horse owners.

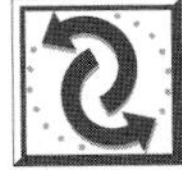

FOLLOW-UP

PATIENT MONITORING

- Blood glucose and insulin concentrations (plus the G:I ratio) should be rechecked after diet, exercise, or treatment interventions.
- Patients should be reevaluated at different times of the year because seasonal and dietary influences vary.
- If a CGIT was performed, repeat it after management practices have been instituted.

PREVENTION/AVOIDANCE

- Owners should avoid overfeeding their horses.
- Exercise is likely to prevent obesity and IR.
- Currently, it is only possible to recognize that the offspring of affected horses may be predisposed to EMS.

POSSIBLE COMPLICATIONS

Chronic damage to the hoof laminae and structures of the foot

EXPECTED COURSE AND PROGNOSIS

EMS is a manageable condition if recognized.

MISCELLANEOUS

ASSOCIATED CONDITIONS, AGE-RELATED FACTORS, ZOONOTIC POTENTIAL, PREGNANCY

N/A

SYNONYMS

- Insulin resistance syndrome
- Peripheral Cushing's syndrome

SEE ALSO

- Hyperlipidemia/hyperlipemia
- Laminitis
- Pituitary pars intermedia dysfunction (PPID)

ABBREVIATIONS

- EMS = equine metabolic syndrome
- IR = insulin resistance
- NSC = nonstructural carbohydrates
- PPID = pituitary pars intermedia dysfunction
- TG = triglyceride

Suggested Reading

BaileySR, Habershon-Butcher JL, Ransom KJ, *et al*. Hypertension and insulin resistance in a mixed-breed population of ponies predisposed to laminitis. Am J Vet Res 2008;69:122–129.

Johnson PJ, Messer NT, Kellon E. Treatment of equine metabolic syndrome. Compend Cont Educ Pract 2004;26:122–130.

Treiber KH, Kronfeld DS, Hess TM, *et al*. Evaluation of genetic and metabolic predispositions and nutritional risk factors for pasture-associated laminitis in ponies. J Am Vet Med Assoc 2006;228:1538–1545.

Treiber KH, Kronfeld DS, Geor RJ. Insulin resistance in equids: possible role in laminitis. J Nutr 2006;136:2094S–2098S.

Author Nicholas Frank

Consulting Editor Michel Lévy

ESOPHAGEAL OBSTRUCTION (CHOKE)

BASICS

DEFINITION

Choke, esophageal obstruction, refers to an inability to swallow as a sequela to partial or complete obstruction of the esophageal lumen by feed or foreign body. The disorder may occur as a single acute episode or as a chronic, intermittent problem.

PATHOPHYSIOLOGY

- Esophageal obstruction occurs with higher frequency at sites with naturally decreased esophageal distensibility. These areas are the mid-cervical region, the thoracic inlet, and the terminal esophagus.
- The most common type of obstruction is impaction with feed material such as beet pulp, pelleted feed, corncobs, grain, hay, and pieces of fruit or vegetable. Wood shavings and various foreign bodies can also cause obstruction of the esophagus.
- A frequent predisposing factor is improper mastication by older or younger horses caused by defective and erupting teeth, respectively. Improper mastication can also occur in gluttonous, sedated, or exhausted horses or in horses recovering from general anesthesia.
- Horses with preexisting lesions such as external esophageal compression, megaesophagus, and esophageal diverticulum or stricture experience recurrent obstructions at the affected site.
- Choke can also occur secondarily to neurologic disorders (botulism, rabies, leukoencephalomalacia, and yellow star thistle poisoning).

SYSTEMS AFFECTED

Gastrointestinal

Choke causes dysphagia. Sequelae to choke include esophageal perforation or stricture formation and megaesophagus.

Respiratory

Aspiration of feed material and saliva frequently occurs in horses with esophageal obstruction. This can lead to aspiration pneumonia. Other less common sequelae to choke are pleuritis and mediastinitis secondary to esophageal perforation.

Cardiovascular

The inability to drink water may result in dehydration.

Skin/Exocrine

Esophageal perforation can result in cervical cellulitis and fistula formation.

SIGNALMENT

Age Predisposition

Younger and older horses

SIGNS

General Comments

Ptyalism and feed-containing nasal discharge are the most common clinical signs of choke. Other clinical signs vary with the duration and the degree of the obstruction. Partial obstruction might cause intermittent clinical signs depending on the diet.

Historical

- Frequent, ineffectual attempts to swallow
- Retching
- Repeated extension of the head and neck
- Coughing during swallowing
- Nasal discharge of saliva mixed with feed
- Restlessness
- Sweating
- Anxiety

Physical Examination

- Dysphagia, coughing, ptyalism, and regurgitation of saliva and feed material through the mouth and nostrils
- Sweating and halitosis
- If the obstruction is located in the cervical esophagus, focal swelling may be palpated or visible.
- Patients with recurrent or chronic esophageal obstruction may demonstrate nonspecific clinical signs such as weight loss, depression, and hypovolemia.
- The presence of subcutaneous emphysema and/or cellulitis over the cervical region may indicate esophageal rupture.
- In cases of aspiration pneumonia, abnormal lung sounds such as crackles and wheezes can be present.

CAUSES

- Obstruction of the esophagus is most frequently caused by intraluminal impaction of feed material or, less commonly, by foreign bodies. Improper mastication due to erupting or defective teeth, sedation, exhaustion, and fracture of the hyoid bone are potential predisposing factors to intraluminal feed obstruction. Dry feeds (e.g., beet pulp, pelleted feeds, oats) are most often associated with the condition.
- Defects in the esophageal wall (intramural lesions) such as strictures, intramural abscesses or cysts, esophageal diverticula, and neoplasia (especially squamous cell carcinoma) usually result in recurrent esophageal obstructions.
- Acquired lesions causing external esophageal compression are relatively rare and include abscesses, tumors, regionally enlarged lymph nodes, cervical cellulitis, and diaphragmatic hernia.
- Congenital disorders such as megaesophagus, achalasia, vascular ring anomalies, and right aortic arch are rare causes of esophageal obstruction. Clinical signs of dysphagia may be present from birth, but this depends on the degree of obstruction. Esophageal motility disorders can result in esophageal obstruction and megaesophagus.

RISK FACTORS

- Poor dental care
- Rapid ingestion of feed
- Poor-quality feed; pelleted or dry feeds such as beet pulp and oats
- Inadequate water intake
- Previous episode of choke

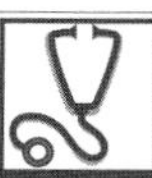

DIAGNOSIS

DIFFERENTIAL DIAGNOSIS

Bilateral nasal discharge caused by pharyngeal abscessation, guttural pouch empyema, strangles, or lung edema may be mistaken for esophageal obstruction. Neurologic disorders such as rabies, botulism, leukoencephalomalacia, and yellow star thistle poisoning can cause dysphagia. Guttural pouch mycosis may cause pharyngeal dysphagia by affecting the cranial nerves IX, X, and XII. Foreign bodies in the pharynx or oral cavity may produce similar clinical signs as esophageal obstruction. In those countries where it is recognized, acute grass sickness (equine dysautonomia) should be included in the differential list.

CBC/BIOCHEMISTRY/URINALYSIS

Packed cell volume and total serum protein evaluation provide additional information on the hydration status. Leukogram and fibrinogen may give more information about inflammatory reactions and should be obtained if aspiration pneumonia is suspected as a complication. Prolonged excessive salivary loss may cause hyponatremia, hypochloremia, and metabolic alkalosis.

IMAGING

Radiography

Radiographic evaluation of the esophagus supplies information concerning the nature and degree of the obstruction. Single- or double-contrast esophagraphy is useful to identify sites of partial or complete obstructions. Esophageal perforation, diverticulum formation, strictures, and esophageal ulcers and erosions may be diagnosed by contrast esophagraphy. Motility disorders can be diagnosed by positive contrast studies.

Fluoroscopy

It is particularly useful for dynamic studies of esophageal motility disorders.

DIAGNOSTIC PROCEDURES

Passage of a nasogastric tube is an important diagnostic tool. This procedure can confirm a tentative diagnosis of choke and determine the approximate location of the obstruction. Endoscopic evaluation of the esophagus gives further information about the nature of the obstruction. Predisposing factors such as strictures and diverticulum formation may also be identified by esophagoscopy.

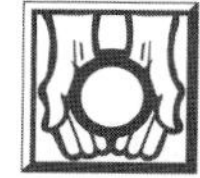

TREATMENT

Conservative Management

- Although some cases of esophageal obstruction resolve spontaneously, they should be treated as emergencies. The owner should be instructed to remove feed and water from the stall while waiting for the veterinarian to arrive. Most cases of esophageal obstruction can be successfully treated on the farm. Only a few cases require referral to an animal hospital.

- The basic approaches to treatment of esophageal obstruction are gentle esophageal lavage in conjunction with administration of drugs that result in relaxation of esophageal musculature and reduced level of anxiety. In cases of mild obstruction, administration of these drugs alone may result in muscular relaxation to allow the obstruction to pass. Gentle passage of a stomach tube may also be required, but this should be attempted with great care.
- If these procedures are unsuccessful, lavage of the esophagus can be done with warm water. A nasogastric tube is advanced to the level of the obstruction and warm water instilled into the tube, which allows water and ingesta to flow out of the tube. During the procedure, the patient's head should be kept at a low level to facilitate the exit of fluid and prevent aspiration. Numerous modifications of the lavage technique exist. A cuffed nasogastric tube may be used to decrease the risk of aspiration. Continuous lavage can be performed by passing a smaller tube through the larger cuffed esophageal tube. The procedures require patience and gentleness. If the impaction is not relieved, the lavages can be performed intermittently with the horse placed in a stall without access to feed, water, and bedding between the attempts.
- In most cases, the procedures described above relieve the esophageal obstruction. Refractory cases can be anesthetized, intubated with an endotracheal tube, and placed in lateral recumbency with the head lowered.

Dietary Management

- Dietary management after the esophageal obstruction has resolved relates to the degree of esophageal injury.
- Esophageal dilatation post obstruction increases the likelihood of reimpaction for at least 48 hr.
- If the impaction was transient and there is minimal or no superficial esophageal mucosal damage with no functional alteration, the horse can be fed small amounts of a pellet gruel after 12– 24 hr. The amount can be increased as the condition improves.
- Small amounts of hay presoaked in water can be gradually introduced after a couple of days.
- In horses with more complicated and/or prolonged esophageal impactions with moderate mucosal damage, feed should not be provided for at least 48–72 hr, depending on the extent of esophageal injury. If the esophageal damage is severe, the esophagus remains dilated, or if the esophageal transit time is prolonged, feed should be withheld for at least 72 hr.
- Ideally, mucosal healing should be monitored by endoscopic examinations to asses when feeding of the horse can begin. Hay should not be fed until 7–10 days depending on the lesions. Severe esophageal damage may require parenteral feeding.

Maintenance of Homeostasis

Intravenous isotonic fluids should be given if the horse is dehydrated or water consumption is restricted. The type of intravenous fluids used is based on acid-base and electrolyte derangements. Patients with hypochloremic metabolic alkalosis should be treated intravenously with 0.9% sodium chloride. However, most cases of esophageal obstruction do not require intravenous fluid therapy.

Surgical Management

- If all attempts to resolve the esophageal obstruction fail, surgical intervention is indicated.
- Prophylactic treatment with antibiotics should be administered before surgery and continued for several days postsurgery.
- Tetanus prophylaxis is necessary
- Before anesthetic induction, a nasogastric tube should be placed to the level of the obstruction.
- Depending on the location of the obstruction, different surgical approaches are used. Thoracic esophageal surgery requires rib resection and positive pressure ventilation. Detailed descriptions of esophageal surgery are found elsewhere.
- Complications following esophageal surgery are a major concern and include dehydration, dehiscence of the esophageal incision, laryngeal hemiplegia, chronic esophageal obstruction due to strictures, aspiration pneumonia, pleuritis, laminitis, and Horner's syndrome.

MEDICATIONS

DRUG(S) OF CHOICE

- Administration of xylazine, detomidine, or acepromazine provides sedation and muscle relaxation of the esophagus.
- The use of α_2-adrenergic agonists has the advantage of causing lowering of the head, thereby facilitating the lavage and decreasing the likelihood of aspiration.
- Anti-inflammatory drugs, such as flunixine meglumine and phenylbutazone, are used to control pain and treat inflammation.
- Broad-spectrum antibiotics are indicated if esophageal perforation or aspiration pneumonia is suspected or has occurred.
- The antibacterial spectrum should be targeted against gram-negative and gram-positive bacteria including anaerobic bacteria.
- Detailed descriptions of the treatment of aspiration pneumonia are found elsewhere.

CONTRAINDICATIONS

Administration of lubricating agents, such as mineral oil, or softening agents, such as DSS, in order to facilitate the removal of an esophageal obstruction are contraindicated because they might be aspirated.

PRECAUTIONS

NSAIDs should be administered cautiously to dehydrated animals due to their potentially nephrotoxic effects.

POSSIBLE INTERACTIONS

N/A

ALTERNATIVE DRUGS

A recent study indicates that oxytocin is capable of relaxing the proximal equine esophagus and may be valuable in the treatment of choke. However, the value of this approach has yet to be determined.

FOLLOW-UP

PATIENT MONITORING

- Endoscopy of the esophagus should be performed after the obstruction has been relieved in order to determine the presence and extent of esophageal lesions, establish the prognosis, and make recommendations for additional treatments and feeding regimen. Repeated esophagoscopies are indicated if mucosal damage has occurred. Strictures most often occur 15–30 days after mucosal damage. Surgery is required in some cases of esophageal strictures.
- Thoracic auscultation and monitoring of body temperature might identify aspiration pneumonia. Thoracic radiographs are indicated if aspiration pneumonia is suspected.

POSSIBLE COMPLICATIONS

- Recurrent esophageal obstructions
- Esophageal diverticulum
- Esophageal stricture
- Esophageal perforation
- Cellulitis
- Esophageal dilation
- Mediastinitis
- Aspiration pneumonia
- Pleuritis

MISCELLANEOUS

ASSOCIATED CONDITIONS

Aspiration pneumonia

AGE-RELATED FACTORS

Younger and older horses are most commonly affected.

PREGNANCY

α_2-Adrenergic agonists (detomidine and xylazine) may induce premature parturition if used during the last trimester of pregnancy.

SYNONYM

Choke

ABBREVIATION

- DSS = dioctyl sodium succinate

Suggested Reading

Jones SJ, Blikslager AT. In: Reed SM, Bayly WM, Sellon D, eds. Equine Internal Medicine, ed 2. St. Louis: Saunders, 2004.

Whithair KJ, Cox JH, Coyne CP, DeBowes RM. Esophageal obstruction in the horse. Compen Contin Educ Vet Pract 1990;1:91–96.

Author Johan T. Bröjer

Consulting Editors Henry Stämpfli and Olimpo Oliver-Espinosa

EXCESSIVE MATERNAL BEHAVIOR/FOAL STEALING

BASICS

OVERVIEW

- Uncommon
- Mares may show maternal behavior for a foal that is not her own without preventing care by the foal's biological mother. Such mares may stay closer to the foal than other herd members (except for the mother) and may stand for the foal to suckle.
- Mares that are not pregnant and currently have no foals of their own occasionally produce milk for a foal they have spontaneously adopted, but this phenomenon is rare.
- Some mares may prevent the foal's biological mother from caring for it.
- Endocrine changes that prepare prepartum mares to care for their own foals may prompt them to steal the foals of subordinate mares. Maternal behavior is under neural and hormonal control, with estrogen, progesterone, and oxytocin being most significant; however, the exact neuroendocrine mechanism for mismothering is unknown.

SIGNALMENT

Mares that are dominant to most other mares in the herd are the most likely to be successful in stealing foals of subordinate mares.

SIGNS

- A mare other than the mother remaining near a foal and standing for the foal to suckle
- In cases of true foal stealing, a mare remains between the foal and its biological mother and shows aggressive behavior (e. g., biting and kicking, or threatening such) toward the mother and may chase the mother away from the vicinity of the foal.

CAUSES AND RISK FACTORS

- Neuroendocrine mechanisms that prepare a prepartum mare to care for her own foal
- Parturition by a low-ranking mare within 48 hr of parturition by a high-ranking mare provides the stimulus of a neonatal foal to the higher-ranking mare.
- Very timid, nonaggressive, low-ranking biological mothers are most likely to have their foals stolen.
- Very aggressive nonmothers that are hormonally ready to care for a neonate are most likely to steal foals.

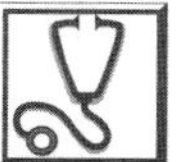

DIAGNOSIS

DIFFERENTIAL DIAGNOSIS, CBC/BIOCHEMISTRY/URINALYSIS, OTHER LABORATORY TESTS, IMAGING

N/A

OTHER DIAGNOSTIC PROCEDURES

In herds that are surveyed only periodically and for which the actual birth was not observed, it may be superficially unclear which of two mares fighting over a foal is the biological mother. Examine both mares to determine which has recently given birth and which is still pregnant. DNA analyses can be done later to positively identify the mother.

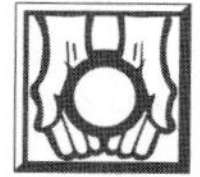

TREATMENT

- Isolate the foal and its biological mother from the mare attempting to steal the foal. Isolating the mother and foal from herd members not attempting to steal the foal may not be necessary, unless the foal requires medical attention.
- Colostrum for the foal that was stolen and the foal of the stealing mare if the history suggests that either may be unable to get colostrum from its mother
- Fluid therapy if dehydrated

MEDICATIONS

DRUGS OF CHOICE

N/A

CONTRAINDICATIONS/ POSSIBLE INTERACTIONS

N/A

PRECAUTIONS

Daily monitoring of herds of pregnant and nursing mares. Watch for signs suggestive of possible foal stealing.

FOLLOW-UP

PATIENT MONITORING

Once the stealing mare has her own foal, she is unlikely to attempt to steal a foal again; nevertheless, both mares should be observed carefully once returned to the herd to ensure no resumption of conflict.

POSSIBLE COMPLICATIONS

If a foal has been suckling a prepartum mare, it may have consumed her colostrum. Alternatively, its mother may have lost her colostrum during several hours of conflict with the foal-stealing mare, during which time the foal may have been unable to suckle. Be prepared to assess foals for dehydration and exhaustion. Provide stored colostrum, if available.

PRECAUTIONS

Daily monitoring of herds of pregnant and nursing mares. Watch for signs suggestive of possible foal stealing.

MISCELLANEOUS

ASSOCIATED CONDITIONS

Mares that steal foals may be more likely to engage in excessive aggression toward other herd members, regardless of the presence or absence of foals.

AGE-RELATED FACTORS

N/A

ZOONOTIC POTENTIAL

N/A

PREGNANCY

Mares in late pregnancy have the greatest risk of this behavior.

SYNONYMS

- Misdirected maternal behavior
- Mismothering

SEE ALSO

- Aggression

Suggested Reading

Crowell-Davis SL. Normal behavior and behavior problems. In: Kobluk CN, Ames TR, Geor RJ, eds. The Horse: Diseases and Clinical Management. Philadelphia: WB Saunders, 1995:1–21.

Crowell-Davis SL, Houpt KA. Maternal behavior. Vet Clin North Am Equine Pract 1986;2:557–571.

Author Sharon L. Crowell-Davis

Consulting Editors Victoria L. Voith and Daniel Q. Estep

ENDOCARDITIS, INFECTIVE

BASICS

DEFINITION

• Infective endocarditis usually is a bacterial infection of the valvular or mural endocardium. • A platelet fibrin thrombus is attached to the endocardium and is colonized by bacteria during periods of bacteremia. The platelet fibrin thrombus forms in response to collagen exposure on a denuded endothelial surface. Proliferation of a mass of fibrin and platelets containing bacteria occurs, resulting in a vegetative mass. • Bacterial infection is most likely to localize on a previously damaged valve. This accounts for the most common site of equine infection being the mitral valve, closely followed by the aortic valve. • The tricuspid valve most frequently is affected in horses with septic jugular vein thrombophlebitis.

PATHOPHYSIOLOGY

• Clinical signs depend on site and severity of the intracardiac infection, embolization of vegetations to any organ, constant bacteremia, and development of immune-complex disease. • Initially, the vegetative lesion, if large, may obstruct the outflow of blood from the chamber, resulting in a murmur of valvular stenosis. • As vegetative lesions grow or heal, valvular damage occurs. • Valvular incompetence and a murmur of valvular insufficiency usually develop. • There may also be concurrent myocarditis.

SYSTEMS AFFECTED

• Cardiovascular—primary • Respiratory—secondary • Neurologic—secondary • Renal—secondary • Splenic—secondary • Hepatic—secondary • GI—secondary • Musculoskeletal—secondary

GENETICS

N/A

INCIDENCE/PREVALENCE

No breed predilection

SIGNALMENT

• All ages, but horses <3 years constitute the majority of cases. • Males may have a slightly higher risk than females.

SIGNS

General Comments

Usually associated with fever of unknown origin

Historical

• Fever • Shifting leg lameness • Joint or tendon sheath distention • Jugular thrombosis

Physical Examination

• Fever • Tachycardia • Cardiac murmur; note this is not present in around 30% of horses with right-sided infective endocarditis. • Other, less common findings—arrhythmias, anorexia, depression, weight loss, coughing, and congestive heart failure

CAUSES

Bacterial infection of the valvular or mural endocardium most frequently involve streptococci, *Pasturella/Actinobacillus,* and *Pseudomonas* sp. But a wide range of bacterial species have been implicated, and fungal endocarditis has been reported rarely.

RISK FACTORS

• Preexisting endocardial damage • Septic jugular vein thrombophlebitis

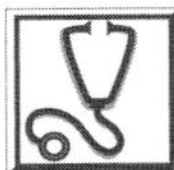

DIAGNOSIS

DIFFERENTIAL DIAGNOSIS

• Pericarditis—Heart sounds usually are muffled; friction rubs may be present; differentiate echocardiographically.
• Myocarditis—can occur concurrently; differentiate echocardiographically.
• Degenerative valve disease—Fever and depression are not present; differentiate echocardiographically. • Other diseases causing fever of unknown origin (e.g., peritonitis, pleuropneumonia, abscesses, neoplasia)—murmurs and shifting leg lameness usually are not present; differentiate echocardiographically and with clinicopathology, abdominocentesis or thoracocentesis, and abdominal or thoracic ultrasonography.

CBC/BIOCHEMISTRY/URINALYSIS

• Often, neutrophilic leukocytosis with hyperfibrinogenemia and anemia of chronic disease • BUN and creatinine may be elevated in horses with infective endocarditis.
• Azotemia may be detected in horses with renal emboli or may be prerenal in horses with low cardiac output.

OTHER LABORATORY TESTS

• Obtain three serial blood cultures at 1-hr intervals before treatment with antimicrobials, if possible. Positive bacterial growth will be obtained in ≅50% of cases. • Previous or concurrent antimicrobial therapy reduces likelihood of a positive blood culture.
• Elevated cardiac isoenzymes (e. g., cardiac troponin I, CK-MB, HBDH, LDH-1, and LDH-2) may be present with concurrent myocardial disease.

IMAGING

Electrocardiography

• Ventricular premature depolarizations or ventricular tachycardia most frequently is detected in horses with left-sided infective endocarditis. • Atrial fibrillation is most common in horses with marked atrial enlargement associated with AV valvular insufficiency.

Echocardiography

• Definitive diagnosis of infective endocarditis is established by identifying irregular, hypoechoic to echoic masses associated with the valve leaflet, chordae tendineae, or mural endocardium. • Determine the number of valve leaflets affected and size of the lesions.
• Doppler examination documents valvular insufficiency. • Small vegetative lesions and lesions in the atria may be difficult to detect with transthoracic echocardiography.

Thoracic Radiography

• Cardiac enlargement may be detected with severe valvular insufficiency. • Pulmonary edema may be detected in horses with congestive heart failure. • Pneumonia may be present in horses with right-sided endocarditis.

DIAGNOSTIC PROCEDURES

Continuous 24-hour Holter monitoring is used to identify concurrent arrhythmias.

PATHOLOGIC FINDINGS

• Focal or diffuse thickening or distortion of one or more affected valve leaflets with vegetative masses on the leaflet, chordae tendineae, or less frequently, mural endocardium. • Ruptured chordae tendineae and flail valve leaflets are infrequently detected. • Jet lesions usually are detected in the preceding chamber. • Enlargement of the respective atria and thinning of the atrial myocardium in horses with significant mitral or tricuspid regurgitation. • Ventricular enlargement and thinning of the ventricular free wall and interventricular septum in horses with significant regurgitation. • Pulmonary vein dilatation in horses with severe mitral regurgitation; pulmonary artery dilatation in horses with pulmonary hypertension. • Pale areas may be seen in the atrial myocardium with areas of inflammatory cell infiltrate, necrosis, and fibrosis detected histopathologically. • Infarcts and abscesses secondary to septic embolization of other organs, particularly the lung, kidneys, spleen, myocardium, and brain

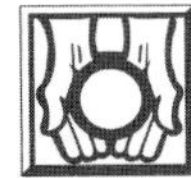

TREATMENT

AIMS OF TREATMENT

The goals of treatment are sterilization of the vegetations and provision of cardiovascular support.

APPROPRIATE HEALTH CARE

• Hospitalize horses with infective endocarditis, and treat with systemic, bacteriocidal, broad-spectrum antimicrobials that are initially empirical and subsequently based on results of blood culture and sensitivity. • Horses with moderate to severe mitral or aortic regurgitation may benefit from long- term vasodilator therapy. • Treat horses with severe mitral, aortic, or tricuspid regurgitation and congestive heart failure for congestive heart failure with positive inotropic drugs, vasodilators, and diuretics. • Closely monitor response to therapy with clinical, clinicopathologic, and echocardiographic reevaluations.

ENDOCARDITIS, INFECTIVE

NURSING CARE
N/A

ACTIVITY
• Stall rest and hand walking only while being treated for infective endocarditis. • Once a bacteriologic cure is achieved, rest with small paddock turnout for an additional month before being returned to work. • Ability of the horse to return to work successfully depends on severity of the residual valvular damage.
• Horses with significant ventricular arrhythmias or pulmonary artery dilatation are no longer safe to ride.

CLIENT EDUCATION
• Monitor the horse's temperature daily, preferably during the late afternoon or evening, during treatment of infective endocarditis and after discontinuation of antimicrobials. • Regularly monitor cardiac rhythm; any irregularities other than second-degree AV block should prompt ECG.
• Carefully monitor for exercise intolerance, respiratory distress, prolonged recovery after exercise, increased resting respiratory or heart rate, cough, or edema; if detected, see Patient Monitoring.

MEDICATIONS

DRUGS OF CHOICE

Infective Endocarditis
• To cure endocarditis requires sterilization of the vegetation. • Bacteriocidal antimicrobials can be administered IV for 4–6 weeks.
• Empirically, until blood culture and sensitivity results are available, potassium penicillin and gentocin are a good combination. Enrofloxacin is likely to penetrate vegetations and rifampin may be added to improve penetration of the antimicrobial into the lesion. • Administer aspirin to decrease platelet adhesiveness.
• With life-threatening ventricular arrhythmias, institute appropriate antiarrhythmic drugs.

Valvular Insufficiency
• With severe mitral or aortic regurgitation, use enalapril or other ACE inhibitor.
• During heart failure with mitral, aortic, or tricuspid regurgitation, use digoxin, furosemide, and vasodilators.

PRECAUTIONS
• Evaluate creatinine and BUN before starting aminoglycoside antimicrobials and use therapeutic drug monitoring to individualize dosage regimens. • ACE inhibitors can cause hypotension; thus, do not give as a large dose without time to accommodate to this treatment.

ALTERNATIVE DRUGS
Most other vasodilatory drugs should have some beneficial effect in horses with moderate to severe mitral and/or aortic regurgitation but may be less effective than ACE inhibitors.

FOLLOW-UP

PATIENT MONITORING
• Assess CBC and in particular serum creatinine and fibrinogen concentrations.
• Frequently monitor lesions echocardiographically during treatment with antimicrobials to assess the efficacy of treatment. • Once antimicrobials have been discontinued, monitor lesions echocardiographically 2 and 4 weeks later and periodically thereafter, depending on the valve affected and the severity of the valvular regurgitation that has developed.
• With severe valvular insufficiency, echocardiographic reevaluations are recommended at 3-mo intervals.

PREVENTION/AVOIDANCE
Institute aggressive treatment of septic jugular vein thrombophlebitis to minimize seeding of the tricuspid valve from septic emboli associated with the infected jugular vein.

POSSIBLE COMPLICATIONS
• Immune-mediated synovitis or tenosynovitis • Right-sided infective endocarditis—pulmonary thromboembolism, pulmonary abscess, and pneumonia
• Left-sided infective endocarditis—hepatic, splenic, and renal abscess; myocardial and cerebral infarction

EXPECTED COURSE AND PROGNOSIS
• Prognosis for horses is primarily determined by the valve(s) affected and severity of valvular damage that develops, and is also likely to be influenced by the organism(s) involved, and the response to antimicrobial treatment.
• Prognosis for horses with right-sided infective endocarditis is guarded and for left-sided infective endocarditis is grave.
• Achieving bacteriologic cure can be difficult. • Even when bacteriologic cure is achieved, continued damage to the affected valve occurs. This usually results in worsening of the valvular insufficiency already present. These horses may develop clinical signs associated with the worsening valvular insufficiency that shorten both useful performance life and life expectancy.

MISCELLANEOUS

ASSOCIATED CONDITIONS
• Septic jugular vein thrombophlebitis
• Preexisting valve damage • Congenital cardiac disease

AGE-RELATED FACTORS
Infective endocarditis is more frequent in horses <3 years of age.

ZOONOTIC POTENTIAL
N/A

PREGNANCY
• Pregnant mares are at risk for development of placentitis, and the fetus may become septic. • Treating pregnant mares with IV broad-spectrum bacteriocidal antimicrobials is important. Base the antimicrobial therapy on blood culture and sensitivity, if available, and choose antimicrobials that are safe for the developing fetus. • The volume expansion of late pregnancy places an additional load on the already volume-loaded heart and may precipitate congestive heart failure in mares with severe valvular insufficiency. • In pregnant mares with congestive heart failure, treat for the underlying cardiac disease with positive inotropic drugs and diuretics. ACE inhibitors are contraindicated because of potential adverse effects on the fetus.

SYNONYMS
• Vegetative endocarditis • Infective endocarditis

SEE ALSO
• Aortic regurgitation • Mitral regurgitation
• Tricuspid regurgitation

ABBREVIATIONS
• ACE = angiotensin-converting enzyme
• AV = atrioventricular • BUN = blood urea nitrogen • CK-MB = MB isoenzyme of creatine kinase • GI = gastrointestinal
• HBDH = α-hydroxybutyrate dehydrogenase
• LDH = lactate dehydrogenase

Suggested Reading

Buergelt CD, Cooley AJ, Hines SA, Pipers FS. Endocarditis in 6 horses. Vet Pathol 1985;22:333–337.

Kasari TR, Roussel AJ. Bacterial endocarditis. Part I. Pathophysiologic, diagnostic and therapeutic considerations. Compend Contin Educ Pract Vet 1989;11:655–671.

Marr CM. Cardiovascular Infections. In Sellon DC, Long MT, eds. Equine Infectious Disease, Philadelphia: WB Saunders, 2007: 21.

Maxson ADM, Reef VB. Bacterial endocarditis in horses: a review of 10 cases (1984–1995). Equine Vet J 1997;29:394–399.

Roussel AJ, Kasari TR. Bacterial endocarditis in large animals. Part II. Incidence, causes, clinical signs and pathologic findings. Compend Contin Educ Pract Vet 1989;11:769–773.

Author Virginia B. Reef
Consulting Editor Celia M. Marr

EXERCISE-ASSOCIATED ARRHYTHMIAS

BASICS

OVERVIEW

EAAs are common in athletic horses occurring most often as the heart rate speeds up or slows down following a period of intense exercise. Arrhythmias occurring during strenuous exercise are of greatest significance. It is difficult to be definitive when making an assessment of the significance of arrhythmias in individual cases as more data on their prevalence and prognostic significance are needed.

SIGNALMENT

• EAAs tend to be detected most often in performance animals, in part because this is the group that most often undergoes ECG evaluation during intense exercise. • EAAs are also occasionally identified in horses engaged in lower-level athletic performance.

SIGNS

• EAAs can be detected in association with signs of poor athletic performance or as incidental findings. • Some individuals with the more severe arrhythmias such as ventricular tachycardia or paradoxical atrial fibrillation present with signs of marked exercise intolerance, distress, or collapse at exercise.
• Cardiac arrhythmias are often assumed to account for sudden death at exercise, although this is extremely difficult to prove.

CAUSES AND RISK FACTORS

• Some EAAs, particularly those occurring in the pre- and post-exercise periods, represent normal (elsewhere) physiologic variants, occurring as the heart rate speeds up and slows down. • Dynamic airway obstruction and arterial hypoxemia can predispose to arrhythmias. • Electrolyte disturbances, particularly depletion of total body magnesium and potassium, are potential risk factors for paroxysmal atrial fibrillation. Hypocalcemia can also be important in some cases. Some horses with hyperkalemic periodic paralysis develop ventricular arrhythmias at exercise and these horses may also have dynamic airway obstruction. • Myocardial fibrosis, necrosis, and myocarditis can be associated with arrhythmias present at rest and exercise.

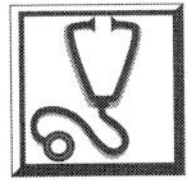

DIAGNOSIS

DIFFERENTIAL DIAGNOSIS

Other causes of poor performance and distress associated with exercise include upper airway disorders, exercise-induced pulmonary hemorrhage, lameness, and myopathy.

CBC/BIOCHEMISTRY/URINALYSIS

• Biomarkers of myocardial disease such as cardiac troponin I may be increased if there is myocardial necrosis present. • Arterial oxygen measurements, taken during exercise on a high-speed treadmill, may reveal hypoxemia.
• Assessment of electrolyte status using both serum electrolyte concentrations and fractional excretion of electrolytes can identify electrolyte disturbances.

IMAGING

• Electrocardiography during exercise is mandatory to identify the specific form of arrhythmia. • Radiotelemetric ECG can be used while horses exercise overground or on a high-speed treadmill and has the advantage that the operator can review the ECG in real-time.
• Holter monitor (ambulatory ECG) techniques can also be used to monitor the ECG while horses exercise overground. A recording of the ECG is subsequently downloaded and reviewed later. The lack of real-time data may be offset by the convenience of this method, particularly in horses whose normal workload cannot easily be emulated on a high-speed treadmill, such as long-distance endurance racehorses. Once EAAs have been identified, 24-hour continuous ECG is used to determine whether the arrhythmia is also present at rest.

OTHER DIAGNOSTIC PROCEDURES

Upper airway endoscopy during high-speed exercise can identify predisposing respiratory disorders.

PATHOLOGIC FINDINGS

Focal or diffuse myocardial necrosis, fibrosis, or inflammation may be identified in a small proportion of cases. Gross and histologic examination of the heart is often unremarkable in cases that die suddenly during exercise, but this does not preclude the possibility that a fatal arrhythmia may have been the cause.

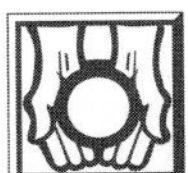

TREATMENT

• In horses with arrhythmias confined to the warm-up and post-exercise periods, no treatment may be necessary. • Horses that have more than one or two premature depolarizations during maximal exercise can potentially have clinical signs associated with these arrhythmias; if the arrhythmia is ventricular in origin, the possibility of collapse during exercise and consequent risk to a rider must be considered.
• Treatment should be aimed predisposing diseases such as dynamic airway obstruction.
• In the absence of obvious causes, a period of rest and corticosteroids are recommended with around a 40% chance that the arrhythmia will resolve.

MEDICATIONS

DRUG(S)

For treatment of myocardial pathology, corticosteroids such as prednisolone 1 mg/kg PO every other day or dexamethasone 0.05–0.1 mg/kg IV, or 0.1 mg/kg PO once a day for 3 or 4 days and then continued every 3–4 days in decreasing dosages are recommended.

CONTRAINDICATIONS/POSSIBLE INTERACTIONS

High-dose corticosteroid therapy has been associated with laminitis, particularly in cases in which other laminitis risk factors such as systemic illness and excessive body condition are present.

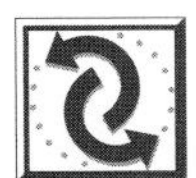

FOLLOW-UP

PATIENT MONITORING

Exercising ECGs following treatment are used to assess efficacy.

POSSIBLE COMPLICATIONS

• Ventricular arrhythmias at exercise can lead to collapse or sudden death with consequent risk to a rider. • Frequent supraventricular arrhythmias may predispose the horse to the development of atrial fibrillation and more severe exercise intolerance.

EXPECTED COURSE AND PROGNOSIS

• Many apparently healthy horses have EAAs consisting of atrioventricular block, usually immediately after strenuous exercise, sinus arrhythmia in the warm-up and post-exercise phases, or isolated supraventricular or ventricular premature depolarizations at any stage, providing there is no more than two at strenuous exercise. • Horses with frequent premature depolarizations during strenuous exercise or with paroxysmal atrial fibrillation will show more severe signs. Paroxysmal atrial fibrillation often occurs only once but frequent premature depolarizations tend to persist and will cause ongoing performance problems if they cannot be treated successfully.

MISCELLANEOUS

SEE ALSO

• Supraventricular arrhythmias • Ventricular arrhythmias • Myocardial disease • Atrial fibrillation • Dynamic airway obstruction

ABBREVIATIONS

• EAA = exercise-associated arrhythmia
• ECG = electrocardiography

Suggested Reading

Reef VB. Electrocardiography and echocardiography in the exercising horse. In Marr CM, ed. Cardiology of the Horse. Philadelphia: WB Saunders, 1999:150.

Author Celia M. Marr
Consulting Editor Celia M. Marr

EXERTIONAL RHABDOMYOLYSIS SYNDROME

BASICS

DEFINITION

Exercise-induced muscle necrosis

PATHOPHYSIOLOGY

• Exercise induces muscle necrosis resulting in the release of CK and myoglobin into circulation. • Myoglobinuria may cause renal tubular damage and acute renal failure.
• Both acquired and inherited forms of exertional rhabdomyolysis exist. • It may be a single (sporadic exertional rhabdomyolysis) or recurring (recurrent exertional rhabdomyolysis, PSSM) event.

SYSTEMS AFFECTED

• Musculoskeletal—muscle • Renal

GENETICS

• In Thoroughbreds, recurrent exertional rhabdomyolysis is an autosomal dominant trait resulting in disturbed intracellular calcium regulation. • In Quarter Horses, PSSM is an autosomal dominant trait (incomplete penetrance) resulting in abnormal glycogen synthesis and storage.

INCIDENCE/PREVALENCE

• 5%–7% of racing Thoroughbreds • 6% of Quarter Horses have PSSM, but it may be higher in specific subpopulations. • In Belgians, PSSM exceeds 30%. • Fatality rate is low, but mortality can occur with severe episodes.

GEOGRAPHIC DISTRIBUTION

Worldwide

SIGNALMENT

Breed Predilections

• Thoroughbreds, Quarter Horses, Drafts (particularly Belgians), Arabians, and Standardbred horses • Specific disciplines—polo, endurance, racing

Mean Age and Range

• Mean age of onset of signs in Quarter Horses (PSSM) is ~5 years, ranging from 1 day old to late maturity. • In Thoroughbred racehorses, 2-year-olds are most frequently affected.

Predominant Sex

In Thoroughbred racehorses, 2- to 3-year-old females are 3 times as likely to be affected. Gender bias resolves with increasing age.

SIGNS

General Comments

• The frequency and severity of episodes can be very variable. • Occurs any time from the onset of exercise until after exercise • Horses without active muscle necrosis or with subclinical disease (elevated CK/AST only) have few abnormalities. Muscle atrophy can indicate previous severe rhabdomyolysis.

Historical

• Training or management alterations
• Period of rest prior to episode • Variable signs from mild stilted gait to severe sweating, stiffness, and recumbency • Recurrent episodes of exertional rhabdomyolysis

Physical Examination

• Exercise intolerance • Stiffness, stilted gait
• Sweating • Reluctance to move • Swollen, and/or fasciculating muscles
• Tachycardia • Tachypnea • Distress
• Recumbency • Pawing, stretching, discomfort • Discolored (red/brown) urine
• Muscle atrophy • Usually normal between episodes

CAUSES

Acquired Causes

• Exercise exceeding level of training
• Exhaustive exercise • Dietary electrolyte and mineral imbalance • Electrolyte depletion during exercise • Vitamin E and/or selenium deficiency

Inherited Causes

• In Thoroughbreds, defective calcium regulation resulting in a low threshold for muscle contraction • PSSM is a defect of glycogen metabolism recognized in Quarter Horses, Paints, Drafts, and related breeds.

RISK FACTORS

• High starch (grain) diet • >24 hours of stall rest in horses with underlying muscle disease
• Sudden interruption of exercise routine
• Infectious respiratory disease
• Nervous temperament (Thoroughbreds, polo horses) • Lameness (Thoroughbreds)
• Genetic predisposition

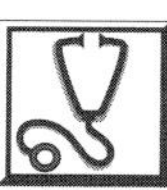

DIAGNOSIS

DIFFERENTIAL DIAGNOSIS

• The association between exercise and onset of signs in addition to physical examination and laboratory findings facilitates differentiation from other conditions.
• Conditions causing reluctance to move, acute recumbency and/or discolored urine, include:
  - Lameness/laminitis
  - Colic
  - Pleuropneumonia
  - Tetanus
  - Lactation tetany
  - Diseases causing intravascular hemolysis or bilirubinuria
  - Neurologic disease
  - Aortoiliac thrombosis
  - HYPP

CBC/BIOCHEMISTRY/URINALYSIS

• Elevated serum CK (<1000 U/L in subclinical disease to >50,000 U/L in severe cases) • Elevated serum AST and LDH
• Myoglobinuria • +/− Hypochloremia, hypocalcemia, metabolic alkalosis, hyponatremia, hyperkalemia (severe disease)
• +/− Elevated BUN and serum creatinine

OTHER LABORATORY TESTS

• Urinary fractional excretion of electrolytes
• Measurement of blood selenium and serum vitamin E

IMAGING

Nuclear scintigraphy—increased radiopharmaceutical uptake in damaged muscles; commonly gluteal, semitendinosus, and semimembranosus

OTHER DIAGNOSTIC PROCEDURES

• Muscle biopsy
  - Semimembranosus biopsy: Performed 4–5 inches below the tuber ischii after desensitizing the skin only with local anesthetic. The fascia can be undermined and a 3-cm^3 cube of muscle removed with minimal handling of the sample. The sample is wrapped in saline moistened gauze and shipped with ice packs within 24 hr to a specialized laboratory for analysis.
  - Gluteal and epaxial muscle biopsy—performed with Bergstrom or Tru-Cut needle at institutions that can process frozen sections (samples are too small to ship). Needle biopsy is quick and less prone to complications and permits a rapid return to exercise.
  - Frozen sections are superior to formalin sections for microscopic examination, but require processing at laboratories with the equipment and expertise.

• Submaximal exercise testing—Measure serum CK activity before 15 min of walk and trot and 4–6 hr after exercise. Abnormal response is indicated by >2- to 3-fold increase in CK. The test should be immediately terminated and CK measured in 4–6 hr if sweating, stiffness, or reluctance to continue is seen.

PATHOLOGICAL FINDINGS

• Muscle histologic abnormalities with recurrent exertional rhabdomyolysis—increased number of centrally located nuclei, myocyte degeneration and regeneration; abnormal sensitivity to caffeine or halothane of intact external intercostal muscle strips
• Muscle histologic abnormalities with PSSM—detection of abnormal polysaccharide inclusions

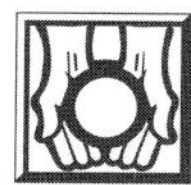

TREATMENT

AIMS OF TREATMENT

• Reduce discomfort and anxiety, prevent further damage. • Normalize hydration, acid-base and electrolyte status. • Restore or protect renal function.

APPROPRIATE HEALTH CARE

Severe rhabdomyolysis is an emergency. Inpatient management is preferable to facilitate fluid therapy but further muscle damage may occur with transport. Mildly to moderately affected horses can be managed as outpatients.

NURSING CARE

• IV or oral fluid therapy with balanced electrolyte solutions until myoglobinuria resolves • Provide deep bedding, particularly for recumbent patients. Slinging may be indicated to prevent prolonged recumbency and further muscle trauma.

ACTIVITY

• Horses recovering from mild exertional rhabdomyolysis can commence gentle exercise (at reduced intensity and duration than prior to the episode) in 24–48 hr if clinical signs of stiffness have resolved. • Horses should remain stall confined during recovery from severe exertional rhabdomyolysis and gentle exercise (hand walking) can commence as clinical appearance and serial CK measurements improve.

DIET

• Feed a palatable low-starch diet (grass hay) according to caloric requirements. • Avoid feeding susceptible horses >5 lb of grain per day. • Fat supplements (rice bran, vegetable oil) can be added if higher caloric requirements exist. • Eliminate high-starch supplements (molasses).

CLIENT EDUCATION

• Susceptible horses should not be stall rested for >24 hr at a time. • Daily turnout or forced daily exercise (riding or lunging) is ideal. Instruct owners that interruption of the exercise routine is a prominent risk factor. • Dietary starch should be restricted and high caloric requirements met with supplemental fat sources. • Breeding management should be discussed where an underlying hereditary muscle disorder is suspected.

SURGICAL CONSIDERATIONS

• Horses with underlying muscle disorders, particularly Thoroughbreds, may be at increased risk of rhabdomyolysis with inhalant anesthesia. Premedication with dantrolene (4–6 mg/kg PO to a fasted horse) may be considered for horses with a history of exertional rhabdomyolysis or adverse anesthetic reactions.

MEDICATIONS

DRUG(S) OF CHOICE

• Acepromazine (0.03–0.07 mg/kg IM or IV q8–12 hr) • For significant distress and pain, xylazine (0.2–0.4 mg/kg) or detomidine (0.01–0.02 mg/kg IM or IV) • Butorphanol (0.01–0.04 mg/kg IM or IV) may provide additional relief and can be administered to effect as an infusion by adding 0.08 mg/kg (40 mg for a mature horse) into a minimum of 10 L of IV fluids • NSAIDs—flunixin meglumine (1.1 mg/kg IV or PO) or phenylbutazone (2.2–4.4 mg/kg IV or PO) • Dimethylsulfoxide (1 g/kg IV or PO as a 10% solution) • +/− Methocarbamol (5–22 mg/kg IV slowly) • Dantrolene (4–6 mg/kg PO 90 min before exercise) prevents exertional rhabdomyolysis in Thoroughbreds with recurrent exertional rhabdomyolysis, but absorption may be negligible in nonfasted horses.

CONTRAINDICATIONS

Avoid acepromazine in dehydrated or shocky horses.

PRECAUTIONS

Avoid or minimize NSAID use in horses with myoglobinuria or high serum creatinine, and correct dehydration prior to use.

POSSIBLE INTERACTIONS

None

ALTERNATIVE DRUGS

Diazepam (0.05–0.5 mg/kg slow IV) for muscle relaxation

FOLLOW-UP

PATIENT MONITORING

• Horses recovering from mild to moderate exertional rhabdomyolysis can recommence exercise once clinical signs of stiffness resolve. • Horses with severe exertional rhabdomyolysis require longer recuperation and serial monitoring of serum CK and AST to help determine resolution of muscle damage and appropriate return to exercise (after muscle enzymes normalize). • Serum CK and AST can remain persistently mildly elevated in resting horses with PSSM so exercise can resume when clinical signs resolve.

PREVENTION/AVOIDANCE

• Daily exercise and avoidance of stall rest are critically important in preventing recurrent episodes in susceptible horses. • Eliminate/reduce high starch feeds. Grass hay should be fed (1.5%–2.0% body weight) with supplemental fat sources (rice bran, oil, commercial high fat feeds) to meet higher caloric needs. Susceptible horses should not consume more than 5 lb of grain/day. • Young Thoroughbreds with anxious temperaments may benefit from stress reducing management changes, such as feeding and exercising them before others and low dose sedatives (acepromazine) before training. • Horses with sporadic exertional rhabdomyolysis should respond to appropriate training regimes that prepare them for their intended athletic use.

POSSIBLE COMPLICATIONS

• Acute or chronic renal failure from myoglobinuria • Atrophy of affected muscles may develop weeks to months after severe rhabdomyolysis.

EXPECTED COURSE AND PROGNOSIS

• Horses with sporadic exertional rhabdomyolysis unrelated to hereditary muscle dysfunction have a good prognosis with appropriate management. • Horses with mild to moderate signs of PSSM or recurrent exertional rhabdomyolysis usually respond to a disciplined routine of daily exercise and appropriate dietary changes. • PSSM horses with late onset of signs have a good prognosis if the triggering management change can be identified and addressed. • PSSM horses developing signs early (<1 year of age) may have a less-favorable prognosis for athletic function. • Horses with repeated and severe episodes of muscle necrosis have a poor prognosis for athletic function if they display limited response to appropriate dietary and training changes. • Horses with acute or chronic renal failure as a result of rhabdomyolysis may have a good to guarded prognosis depending on the severity and response to treatment.

MISCELLANEOUS

ASSOCIATED CONDITIONS

A malignant hyperthermia–type reaction has been described in a low number of horses susceptible to exertional rhabdomyolysis during procedures using inhalant anesthetic agents. Thoroughbreds appear particularly predisposed. Premedication with dantrolene sodium (4–6 mg/kg PO to a fasted horse) may be an effective prevention strategy.

ZOONOTIC POTENTIAL

None

PREGNANCY

None

SYNONYMS

• Tying up • Monday morning disease
• Azoturia • Paralytic myoglobinuria
• Exertional myopathy

SEE ALSO

Polysaccharide storage myopathy

ABBREVIATIONS

• CK = creatine kinase
• PSSM = polysaccharide storage myopathy
• HYPP = hyperkalemic periodic paralysis
• LDH = lactate dehydrogenase
• AST = aspartate aminotransferase

Suggested Reading

MacLeay JM. Diseases of the musculoskeletal system. In: Reed SM, Bayly WM, Sellon DC, eds. Equine Internal Medicine, ed 2. St. Louis: Saunders, 2004:461–531.

McKenzie EC, Valberg SJ, Pagan JD. Nutritional management of exertional rhabdomyolysis. In: Robinson NE, ed. Current Therapy in Equine Medicine, ed 5. St. Louis: Saunders, 2003:727–734.

Valberg SJ, Hodgson DR. Diseases of muscle. In: Smith BP, ed. Large Animal Internal Medicine, ed 3. St. Louis: Mosby, 2002:1266–1291.

Author Erica C. McKenzie
Consulting Editor Elizabeth J. Davidson

EXERCISE-INDUCED PULMONARY HEMORRHAGE

BASICS

OVERVIEW

• Hemorrhage from the lung parenchyma associated with exertion and characterized by blood in the airways and, occasionally, by epistaxis.
• Precise mechanism unknown
• Current speculation—initial bleeding associated with pulmonary capillary stress failure. Exercising horses have high cardiac outputs and vascular pressures. High left atrial pressures (likely associated with low left ventricular compliance and, possibly, mitral valve resistance) contribute to high capillary pressures. If high transmural pressure (difference between intravascular [capillary] pressure and alveolar pressure) exceeds the tensile strength of the capillary wall, disruption occurs with hemorrhage into interstitial and alveolar spaces. Bleeding into airspaces is either sufficient to cause overt pulmonary hemorrhage or is cleared by the mucociliary blanket and visible in the tracheobronchial airways. Blood in the interstitium or alveoli elicits an inflammatory reaction and contributes to small airway disease and bronchial arterial neovascularization, which may also be a source of hemorrhage during subsequent exercise.
• Other factors—inhaled particles, viral respiratory disease, and air pollutants are considered to exacerbate inflammation. Changes in blood viscosity, hemostasis, and fibrinolysis occur with exercise but there is no known causal association with EIPH.
• Reported frequency—(1) based on airway endoscopic examination after exercise: 62% racing Quarter Horses, 35%–87% Standardbreds, >80% racing Thoroughbreds; (2) based on airway fluid aspirate or BAL—most (~100%) horses after strenuous exercise
• Reported for most strenuous activities—flat racing, pacing and trotting races, jumping, barrel racing, roping, steeple chase, 3-day eventing, draft-pulling competitions, polo, and endurance races
• Worldwide distribution

SIGNALMENT

• Occurs with onset of strenuous exercise and training, thus from 2 years of age
• Males, gelding, and females are equally affected.

SIGNS

• Occasionally, coughing and increased swallowing activity are found
• Occasionally, performance is impaired
• Rarely, abnormal airway sounds
• Commonly, no external clinical signs
• Typically <5% of affected horses have epistaxis

CAUSES AND RISK FACTORS

• Strenuous exercise
• Less commonly, underlying parenchymal disease

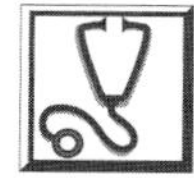

DIAGNOSIS

DIFFERENTIAL DIAGNOSIS

• Epistaxis—ethmoid hematoma, guttural pouch mycosis, sinonasal trauma, coagulopathy
• Airway blood—pulmonary abscess, pneumonia, foreign body, and neoplasia

CBC/BIOCHEMISTRY/URINALYSIS

Changes in CBC or biochemical panel indicate a concurrent disease process

OTHER LABORATORY TESTS

Cytologic examination of airway or BAL lavage fluid

IMAGING

• Thoracic radiography—increased homogeneous parenchymal density in dorsal caudal lung fields (not a consistent finding but, if present, usually clears in 3–5 days); increased interstitial density in the same lung region indicative of chronic EIPH.
• Endoscopy—airway endoscopy 30–90 minutes after strenuous exercise with identification of airway blood is the definitive diagnostic method. Blood usually clears from airways by 4–6 hours.
• Scintigraphy—perfusion deficit in caudodorsal lung field; ventilation scan is often normal.

OTHER DIAGNOSTIC PROCEDURES

• Cytology of airway contents (transtracheal or endoscopic aspiration, or BAL lavage)—presence of hemosiderophages (macrophages with intracytoplasmic hemosiderin) considered evidence of bleeding into the airways.
• Lung biopsy of the caudodorsal fields—hemosiderophages in alveolar or interstitial spaces

PATHOLOGIC FINDINGS

Gross

• Characteristic patchy to multifocal, symmetric, blue-brown to brown staining of the pulmonary parenchyma on the dorsal and diaphragmatic surfaces of the caudodorsal regions of the caudal lung lobe.
• Foci of subpleural scarring within discolored lung regions in association with enhanced subpleural vasculature.

Histopathologic

• Small airway disease—intraluminal debris, hypertrophy of lining cells, or fibrosis
• Pleural and interlobular septa fibrosis
• Interstitial fibrosis
• Hemosiderophage sequestration in airways, airspaces, and interstitium
• Obliteration of small airways

Exercise-Induced Pulmonary Hemorrhage

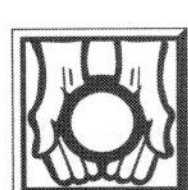

TREATMENT

- No known treatment
- Treat small airway disease if present
- Unless performance impaired, continue athletic activity
- Rest (30 days to 1 year) helps parenchymal repair but does not prevent EIPH

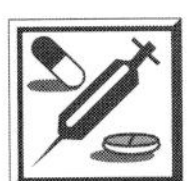

MEDICATIONS

DRUG(S) OF CHOICE

- Most commonly used—furosemide (0.25–1 mg/kg). Administration usually limited to 4 hours prerace; in some areas, other regulations guide administration. Dose occasionally split between IV and IM administration. Efficacy uncertain.
- Conjugated estrogen is administered occasionally in the belief that it counters capillary fragility; no evidence of efficacy.
- Aspirin—no evidence of efficacy for EIPH prevention.
- Nasal dilator strips—decrease airway (nasal resistance) during treadmill exercise and erythrocyte count in BAL fluid but efficacy in EIPH prevention unproven.
- Small airway disease—see the Inflammatory Airway Disease section

CONTRAINDICATIONS/POSSIBLE INTERACTIONS

Chronic furosemide administration, especially if the horse is dehydrated, may predispose electrolyte disorders

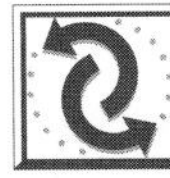

FOLLOW-UP

PATIENT MONITORING

- Repeat endoscopy examination after subsequent strenuous activities (e.g., training, racing, jumping) provides information on the frequency and severity of the condition.
- If severe bleeding, repeat examination in 24–48 hours to make sure bleeding has stopped; may indicate intercurrent disease.

EXPECTED COURSE AND PROGNOSIS

Resolution of lung pathology especially with continued strenuous exercise unlikely. Aged horses with a history of EIPH have parenchymal lesions years after retirement. Horses with reduced performance attributable to EIPH rarely improve after rest or palliative treatment.

MISCELLANEOUS

AGE-RELATED FACTORS

Increase prevalence with increasing age in actively competing horses

SEE ALSO

- Progressive ethmoidal hematoma
- Guttural pouch mycosis
- Hemorrhagic nasal discharge
- Inflammatory airway disease
- Pleuropneumonia

ABBREVIATION

- BAL = bronchoalveolar lavage
- EIPH = exercise-induced pulmonary hemorrhage

Suggested Reading

Hinchcliff KW. Exercise-induced pulmonary hemorrhage. In Smith BP, ed. Large Animal Internal Medicine. 4th ed. St. Louis: Mosby, 2007 (in press)

Marlin DJ. Exercise-induced pulmonary hemorrhage. In: Robinson NE, ed. Current Therapy in Equine Medicine. 5th ed. Philadelphia: WB Saunders, 2003:429–433.

Pascoe JR. Exercise-induced pulmonary hemorrhage: a unifying concept. Proc Am Assoc Equine Pract 1996;42:220–226.

Author John R. Pascoe
Consulting Editor Daniel Jean

EXPIRATORY DYSPNEA

BASICS

DEFINITION

• A sensation of difficult breathing.
• In animals, dyspnea is used to describe clinical signs associated with respiratory distress, which can be present throughout the respiratory cycle or be primarily associated with either inhalation (i.e., inspiratory dyspnea) or exhalation (i.e., expiratory dyspnea).
• The lay term for expiratory dyspnea (i.e., heaves) describes the abdominal push at end expiration.

PATHOPHYSIOLOGY

• As a primary clinical sign, usually associated with obstruction of the intrathoracic airways by mucus and bronchospasm; to move air from the lung through partially obstructed airways, the horse recruits its abdominal muscles and makes a noticeable, forced abdominal exhalation.
• Can also accompany inspiratory dyspnea in any animal with severe impairment of gas exchange

SYSTEMS AFFECTED

• Respiratory
• Cardiovascular
• Hemic/lymphatic/immune

GENETICS

In heaves, there is increasing evidence of a genetic susceptibility.

INCIDENCE/PREVALENCE

Unknown

GEOGRAPHIC DISTRIBUTION

Worldwide

SIGNALMENT

Depends on the underlying cause, but usually occurs in mature to old animals

SIGNS

Expiratory dyspnea is a sign, but associated signs can indicate the source of dyspnea.

Historical

• Accompanying inspiratory dyspnea and loud respiratory noises are indicative of a fixed airway obstruction – mass encroaching into the pharynx
• A preceding or accompanying cough indicates inflammation of the tracheobronchial tree.
• Inflammation of the lower airway can result in bilateral mucopurulent nasal discharge.
• Unilateral or bilateral nasal discharge, either purulent or hemorrhagic, can be a sign of a nasal or pharyngeal mass causing severe airway obstruction.

PHYSICAL EXAMINATION

• The condition is indicated by flared nostrils, increased excursions of the thorax during breathing, and a forced abdominal component to expiration, which becomes particularly obvious at end exhalation.
• The horse may rock forward during the abdominal effort.
• Careful observation reveals that the rib cage collapses rapidly at the start of exhalation and that the abdominal component is more prolonged.
• The abdominal effort raises intra-abdominal pressure and this leads to bulging of the anus.
• Fixed airway obstruction—nasal discharge, sometimes foul breath, and both inspiratory and expiratory dyspnea.
• Bronchitis/bronchiolitis—cough, wheezing audible at the nares, increased breath sounds on both inhalation and exhalation, and expiratory wheezes may be particularly evident; however, fever is unusual without a viral or bacterial cause.

CAUSES

Respiratory

• Extrathoracic causes are usually accompanied by inspiratory dyspnea–congestion of the nasal mucosa (e.g., Horner's syndrome, inflammatory disease), deviation of the nasal septum, space-occupying lesion affecting the nasal cavity (e.g., foreign body, intraluminal mass, ethmoid hematoma, extraluminal mass or swelling), congenital pharyngeal cysts, space-occupying masses encroaching on the pharynx (e.g., enlarged lymph nodes, guttural pouch enlargement (usually by tympanites), deformity of the larynx (e.g., edema, epiglottiditis, chondritis), and tracheal obstruction caused by trauma, masses or foreign body.
• Lower respiratory tract—severe bronchiolitis or heaves; infiltrative disease of the alveolar interstitium

Nonrespiratory

See Inspiratory dyspnea.

RISK FACTORS

See the individual conditions causing expiratory dyspnea.

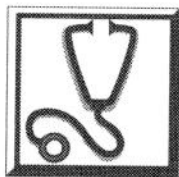

DIAGNOSIS

DIFFERENTIAL DIAGNOSIS

Differential Similar Signs

• Inspiratory dyspnea is characterized by an enhanced thoracic component to inhalation.
• Tachypnea (i.e., a rapid breathing in response to severe heat stress) is not accompanied by prolonged exhalation.
• Deep breathing after strenuous exercise has a marked inspiratory and expiratory component.

Differential Causes

• Fixed upper airway obstructions produce severe respiratory distress on both inhalation and exhalation and are accompanied by loud respiratory noise.
• Fever, malaise, and inappetence indicate infectious inflammatory disease.
• Expiratory dyspnea of gradual onset, precipitated by an environmental cause and accompanied by cough in an afebrile mature horse, is indicative of heaves (also known as recurrent airway obstruction).
• Expiratory dyspnea of sudden onset in a febrile young horse is indicative of infectious bronchiolitis.
• Once a fixed upper airway obstruction is ruled out, heaves is the most likely cause of expiratory dyspnea.

CBC/BIOCHEMISTRY/URINALYSIS

Depends on causes

OTHER LABORATORY TESTS

• With fixed airway obstruction, arterial blood gas analysis identifies hypoventilation (i.e., increased $PaCO_2$) and hypoxemia (i.e., low PaO_2), with the increase in $PaCO_2$ being almost equal to the decrease in PaO_2.
• Bronchitis/bronchiolitis usually is accompanied by obvious hypoxemia (i.e., $PaO_2 < 80$ mm Hg), with only a slightly elevated $PaCO_2$ (i.e., 45–50 mm Hg).

IMAGING

Radiography

• May identify a mass causing a fixed obstruction in the nose, pharynx, larynx, or trachea
• Bronchitis/bronchiolitis may not produce diagnostic radiographic signs.
• Diffuse interstitial alveolar disease may be observed as a diffuse increase in density, with or without a miliary pattern.

Endoscopy

• Essential for diagnosing a fixed airway obstruction.
• Can be used to assess the presence of mucopurulent exudate in the trachea, which is a sign of inflammation of the lower airways and lung.

OTHER DIAGNOSTIC PROCEDURES

• Cytology of the lower airways, preferably by bronchoalveolar lavage, can be used to determine the presence of lower airway inflammation.
• Bacterial culture of tracheal mucus or tracheal lavage revealing a relatively pure culture of a known pathogen is suggestive of infection.

PATHOLOGIC FINDINGS

Depend on cause of the dyspnea

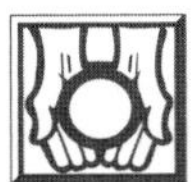

TREATMENT

AIMS OF TREATMENT

Maintain ventilation and gas exchange

APPROPRIATE HEALTH CARE

In- or outpatient medical management

NURSING CARE

- Supplemental oxygenation via a nasotracheal or nasopharyngeal catheter relieves hypoxemia and accompanying distress when dyspnea results from lung disease.
- With fixed airway obstruction, oxygen can be life-saving until the problem is surgically corrected.
- Heaves—move horse to a low-dust environment.

ACTIVITY

N/A

DIET

Heaves—use low-dust diet such as pasture, complete pelleted feed, or haylage.

CLIENT EDUCATION

If the cause of expiratory dyspnea is heaves, emphasis the importance of eliminating contact with dust, which can be coming from feed and bedding in stable or from dusty paddocks.

SURGICAL CONSIDERATIONS

- Relieve a fixed upper airway obstruction sufficient to cause panic or life-threatening hypoxemia (indicated by cyanosis) by tracheotomy.
- Nasotracheal intubation also can be used to bypass the obstruction, especially when it is to be corrected surgically within a short time.
- Tracheotomy is not useful for relief of expiratory dyspnea originating in the lower airway.

MEDICATIONS

DRUGS OF CHOICE

- Depend on cause of the dyspnea.
- Heaves—dilate airway with a bronchodilator, and relieve inflammation with corticosteroids (see Heaves). Atropine (0.02 mg/kg IV) provides almost immediate relief from dyspnea; other bronchodilators, either oral (e.g., clenbuterol 0.8–3.2 mg/kg BID) or inhaled (e.g., ipratropium bromide 2–3 μg/kg, albuterol 1–2 μg/kg, feneterol 2–3 μg/kg) should be used for maintenance.

CONTRAINDICATIONS

N/A

PRECAUTIONS

N/A

POSSIBLE INTERACTIONS

N/A

ALTERNATIVE DRUGS

N/A

FOLLOW-UP

PATIENT MONITORING

Heaves is a chronic problem that recurs whenever horses are exposed to the dusts and antigens that initiate the hypersensitivity response.

PREVENTION/AVOIDANCE

N/A

POSSIBLE COMPLICATIONS

Atropine may cause ileus and colic signs.

EXPECTED COURSE AND PROGNOSIS

N/A

MISCELLANEOUS

ASSOCIATED CONDITIONS

N/A

AGE-RELATED FACTORS

N/A

ZOONOTIC POTENTIAL

N/A

PREGNANCY

Fetal growth retardation and fetal death may be observed in mares with severely compromised respiratory function.

SEE ALSO

- Aspiration pneumonia
- Diaphragmatic hernia
- Fungal pneumonia
- Heaves
- Inspiratory dyspnea
- Pleuropneumonia
- Pneumothorax
- Acute respiratory distress syndrome

Suggested Reading

Hannas CM, Derksen FJ. Principles of emergency respiratory therapy. In : Colahan PT, Mayhew IG, Merritt AM, Moore JM, eds. Equine medicine and surgery. 4th ed. Goleta: American Veterinary Publications, 1991; 1:372–374.

Lavoie J-P, Recurrent airway obstruction (heaves) and summer-pasture-associated obstructive pulmonary disease. In: McGorum BC, Dixon PM, Robinson NE, Schumacher J, eds. Equine respiratory medicine and surgery. Oxford: Saunders, 2007: 565–589.

McGorum BC, Dixon PM. Clinical examination of the respiratory tract. In: McGorum BC, Dixon PM, Robinson NE, Schumacher J, eds. Equine respiratory medicine and surgery. Oxford: Saunders, 2007: 103–117.

Author N. Edward Robinson

Consulting Editor Daniel Jean

EXUDATIVE OPTIC NEURITIS

BASICS

OVERVIEW

• The optic discs are swollen with large, whitish, raised nodular masses spread across the surface of the optic disc.
• Retinal and optic disc hemorrhages may also be present.

SIGNALMENT

Older horses (>15 years); rare

SIGNS

Sudden onset of total blindness in bilateral cases; dilated pupils

CAUSES AND RISK FACTORS

Trauma; acute, massive hemorrhage

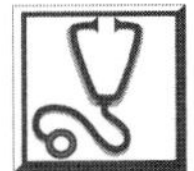

DIAGNOSIS

DIFFERENTIAL DIAGNOSIS

• Blindness due to cataracts, glaucoma, ERU, retinal detachment, central nervous system disease
• Must be distinguished from benign exudative/proliferative optic neuropathy in aged horses with otherwise normal findings in a visual eye

CBC/BIOCHEMISTRY/URINALYSIS

N/A

OTHER LABORATORY TESTS

N/A

IMAGING

N/A

DIAGNOSTIC PROCEDURES

Diagnosed by characteristic funduscopic appearance

EXUDATIVE OPTIC NEURITIS

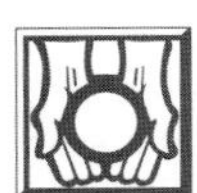

TREATMENT

N/A

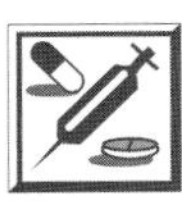

MEDICATIONS

No known therapy

CONTRAINDICATIONS/POSSIBLE INTERACTIONS

N/A

FOLLOW-UP

EXPECTED COURSE AND PROGNOSIS

Poor prognosis

MISCELLANEOUS

ASSOCIATED CONDITIONS

Dependent on cause

AGE-RELATED FACTORS

Older horses

SEE ALSO

- Traumatic optic neuropathy
- Ischemic optic neuropathy
- Retinal detachment
- Recurrent uveitis
- Acute cataract formation

ABBREVIATION

- ERU = equine recurrent uveitis

Suggested Reading

Brooks DE. Ophthalmology for the Equine Practitioner. Jackson, WY; Teton NewMedia, 2002.

Brooks DE, Matthews AG. Equine ophthalmology. In: Gelatt KN, ed. Veterinary Ophthalmology, ed 4. Philadelphia; Lippincott Williams and Wilkins, 2007.

Gilger BC, ed. Equine Ophthalmology. Philadelphia; WB Saunders, 2005.

Author Maria Källberg

Consulting Editor Dennis E. Brooks

EYELID DISEASES

BASICS

OVERVIEW

• A variety of conditions lead to abnormal function of the upper and lower eyelids predisposing the globe to secondary diseases such as conjunctivitis and keratitis. • Major categories of eyelid disease include congenital, inflammatory, neoplastic, and traumatic. Manifestation of each type of disease depends on age, environment, duration and progression of problem, and prior treatment. • Regardless of the etiology, all eyelid diseases disrupt the normal function of the equine eyelids—to provide the lipid part of the tear film, to distribute the tear film across the cornea, to protect the globe from excessive exposure to ultraviolet light, and to serve as an external barrier to foreign material from the external orbit. • Blinking in the horse should occur at about 5–25 times per minute. Keratitis may be secondary to a primary blinking disorder. • Systems affected are the eye and skin. • Squamous cell carcinoma and sarcoids have separate topics devoted to each of them and are not discussed here.

SIGNALMENT

• Eyelid melanomas are found in gray horses, with Arabians and Percherons at increased risk. Entropion is predominantly found in young foals. • Equine papillomas are common in immature horses. • Median age in one report of ocular lymphoma was 11 years with a range of 4 months to 21 years.jArabians may inherit juvenile Arabian leukoderma (unknown mechanism). Andalusians and Saddlebreds are also affected.

SIGNS (variable according to disease process)

• Eyelid disease may be acute or chronic. The owner may not notice a change in the eyelids until the disease is advanced. Trauma, however, is usually acutely recognized. • Blepharospasm • Epiphora • Conjunctivitis • Keratitis can be of two types: (1) acutely ulcerative and edematous and (2) chronic, pigmentary, and vascularized, possibly due to sicca.A mixed form is also recognized. • Rubbing at eye • Blepharedema • Periocular discharge ranging from frank blood if traumatic to purulent or serosanguinous if inflammatory or neoplastic. • Asymmetry of eyelids (comparing right eye to the left eye and upper to lower lids) can be due to raised firm or soft masses, erosive blepharitis, or overt trauma. • Lack of palpebral reflex may stem from a neurogenic disorder or trauma.

CAUSES AND RISK FACTORS

• Entropion* is an inward rolling of the eyelid margin. It can be a primary problem in foals or secondary to dehydration or emaciation as in perinatal asphyxia syndrome. Prior eyelid damage that leaves scarring may lead to a cicatricial entropion. Acquired or blepharospastic entropion is a secondary condition due to chronic irritation and pain, causing spasms of the orbicularis oculi muscle. One may see entropion with multiple causes, and therefore the pathophysiologies of each clinical presentation must be identified. • Some foals have eyelid abnormalities identified at birth. Microphthalmos causes a related macropalpebral fissure and often secondary entropion requiring intervention. Dermoids (choristomas) are aggregates of skin tissue aberrantly located within adnexal tissue, conjunctiva, and cornea and have been reported in the eyelids of foals. Eyelid colobomas are focal to diffuse areas of eyelid agenesis leading to exposure keratitis. Faulty induction of the surface ectoderm by defective or absent neuroectoderm is most likely to blame for some of these congenital anomalies. • Traumatic blepharitis* can develop into eyelid abscesses and may be associated with orbital fractures, penetrating and lacerating trauma, subpalpebral lavage system irritation, and bony sequestra. • *Trichophyton* or *Microsporum* spp. are known to cause blepharitis, as are *Histoplasma farciminosum* and *Cryptococcus mirandi.* • Equine papillomas from a papovavirus causes a focal eyelid inflammation in immature horses. • Demodex infestation may lead to lid alopecia, meibomianitis, and papulopustular blepharitis. • *Thelazia lacrimalis* is a spirurid nematode and a commensal parasite of the equine conjunctival fomices and nasolacrimal ducts. This parasite can cause diffuse blepharitis. • Habronemiasis,* a common cause of granulomatous blepharitis, occurs mainly in the summer months when house and stable flies serve as vectors. Dying microfilariae in the eyelids, conjunctiva, lacrimal caruncle, medial canthus, and nictitans are thought to incite a immune-mediated hypersensitivity. • Fly-bite blepharitis, dermatophilus, and staphylococcal folliculitis are other causes of blepharitis, especially in young foals. • Juvenile Arabian leukoderma, or "pinky" syndrome, is a cutaneous depigmentation condition affecting 6- to 24-month-old Arabians. This disease may present as several cycles of depigmentation and repigmentation. • Allergic blepharitis, eosinophilic granuloma with collagen degeneration, pemphigus foliaceous and bullous pemphigoid, solar blepharitis of nonpigmented skin, and St. John's wort photosensitization of the lids are also reported. • Topical chemical toxicities can also cause a caustic blepharitis. • Eyelid lacerations* are common in the horse. Upper eyelid damage is more significant because the upper lid moves 75% more to cover the cornea than the lower lid. Medial canthal lid trauma can involve the nasolacrimal system. • Tumors of the eyelids other than squamous cell carcinoma and sarcoids include but are not limited to melanoma, mast cell tumor and lymphoma.

* Blepharitis, or inflammation of the eyelids, has multiple causes including viral, fungal, parasitic, allergic, and immune-mediated.

DIAGNOSES

DIFFERENTIAL DIAGNOSES

• Many of the conformational eyelid diseases are confirmed on clinical presentation and successful outcome of medical or surgical intervention. Careful examination of the eyelids and the eye are essential to proper management of diseases such as entropion and microphthalmos. • Inflammation and neoplasia can look very similar on presentation; therefore, documenting an accurate history and performing other diagnostics (see later) will provide information and direct therapeutic efforts. • Quite often, blepharitis is nonspecific and may indeed mask a specific infection, parasitism, or neoplasia. • Habronemiasis may mimic mastocytomas, nodular necrobiosis, or fungal granulomas.

CBC/BIOCHEMISTRY/URINALYSIS

These tests are usually normal for eyelid diseases unless there is systemic involvement.

OTHER LABORATORY TESTS

• Cytology of tissue aspirates or impressions • Microbial culture and sensitivity if fungal or bacterial infection is suspect • Biopsy if neoplasia is a primary differential

IMAGING

N/A

CONTRAINDICATIONS

As in all cases involving ulcerative keratitis, all steroid preparations are contraindicated.

PRECAUTIONS

• Antifungal drugs, antiparasitic drugs, and chemotherapy may all be irritating to the local tissues. If a drug hypersensitivity is suspected, it should be temporarily discontinued and restarted with caution if necessary. • Many topical skin antibiotic preparations used in eyelid trauma can be highly irritating to the cornea: preventing ocular exposure to these drugs is advised.

POSSIBLE INTERACTIONS

N/A

ALTERNATE DRUGS

A current formulary should be consulted for alternatives to all types of topical medications.

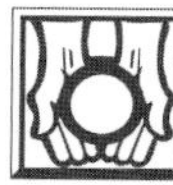

FOLLOW-UP

• Careful monitoring of the response to therapy is critical in managing eyelid diseases, as the correct diagnosis may not be evident initially and ocular health is dependent on normal eyelid function. A clean, dust-free environment eliminates the likelihood of irritant or allergic blepharitis. However, allergies to common barn items such as wood shavings and certain types of hay are not uncommon. • Loss of eyelid tissue or extreme post surgical scarring can be extremely detrimental to corneal health and without correction may lead to severe keratitis and loss of vision. • Eyelids have a tremendous blood supply and heal readily when treated appropriately. Because this tissue is also highly mobile, sutures in the eyelids may be left for 3–4 weeks to ensure proper wound healing. • Most eyelid tumors are locally invasive and will not metastasize if treated appropriately. • Certain types of tumors if left unchecked will be invasive and destroy adnexal tissue and the globe.

MISCELLANEOUS

ASSOCIATED CONDITIONS

Conjunctivitis, nasolacrimal disease, nictitans disease

AGE RELATED FACTORS

Horses known to have a difficult temperament or who are untrained (i.e., foals and yearlings) may be more likely to present for eyelid trauma.

PREGNANCY

• Systemic absorption of topical medication is possible. • General anesthesia versus sedation and local akinesia must always be contemplated in cases of eyelid surgery in pregnant mares.

SEE ALSO

• Ocular/adnexal squamous cell carcinoma
• Periocular sarcoids • Conjunctival diseases
• Ocular problems in the neonate
• Keratopathies • Dacryocystitis disease

DIAGNOSTIC PROCEDURES

• Complete ophthalmic examination for suspected congenital lesions • Instillation of topical anesthesia (proparicaine) differentiates blepharospastic entropion from other causes. • Look under nictitans and in conjunctival fornices for signs of tumor, parasites, or foreign bodies. • Flush nasolacrimal duct if obstruction is suspected. • Fluorescein stain for any painful eye.

PATHOLOGIC FINDINGS

Findings may range from simple blepharitis with neutrophilic (septic or non-septic), lymphocytic/plasmacytic, or eosinophilic infiltrates, to specific descriptions of differentiated tumors.

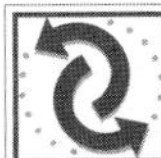

TREATMENT

• Most eyelid diseases are treated on an outpatient basis. More severe infections may require more intensive topical or systemic therapy, but could be managed by most horse owners and trainers. Periodic rechecks every few weeks initially are advised when tumors and severe eyelid malformations are being treated.
• If the pathology of the eyelids impairs vision or if a protective eye covering must be worn, activity should be restricted to the horse's ability to navigate safely until the visual impairment resolves. • No specific change in diet is necessary. Dust and debris should be kept to a minimum by feeding the hay at ground level. • Fly repellants or insecticide strips reduce the incidence of fly-strike blepharitis. • If caught early, most eyelid diseases are amenable to treatment. Medication may be 2 to 4 times per day for inflammatory causes. During treatment, a protective eye covering may be worn to keep dirt out and prevent further self-trauma induced by rubbing, and to protect any sutures that may be present. • Young foals with entropion can have temporary tacking sutures placed in a vertical mattress pattern (4–0 silk) 2–3 mm from the eyelid margin at the affected areas. They also can receive surgical staples in the affected areas until the causative mechanism has resolved. Older foals and adult horses with entropion can receive permanent reconstructive surgeries such as the Hotz-Celsus procedure.
• Blepharoplastic measures may be necessary in horses with primary anatomic entropion, eyelid colobomas, or severe eyelid trauma. • Lid trauma needs to be corrected as soon as possible to prevent undesirable scarring and secondary corneal desiccation and ulceration. • Papillomas may regress spontaneously, require surgery, cryotherapy, or autogenous vaccination.

MEDICATIONS

DRUGS AND FLUIDS

• In cases of exposure keratitis or conjunctivitis, supplemental lubrication in the form of artificial tears or ophthalmic antibiotic ointment is recommended until the eyelid problem is corrected. • For eyelid swelling due to acute trauma, ophthalmic antibiotic/steroid combinations may be indicated. Therapy for severe, chronic, or aggressive bacterial blepharitis should be directed by results of culture and sensitivity. • Intralesional steroid injections (triamcinolone 1–10 mg) may be effective against granulomatous diseases stemming from habronemiasis. Systemic ivermectin (200 g/kg PO once) is indicated for demodex and habronemiasis. • Topical therapy for solitary, focal habronema lesions consists of a topical mixture of 135 g of nitrofurazone ointment, 30 mL of 90% dimethylsulfoxide, 30 mL of 0.2% dexamethasone, and 30mL of a 12.3% oral trichiorphon solution. This is applied 2–3 times daily to the affected areas. • Topical 2% miconazole or thiabendazole is effective against eyelid ringworm, whereas systemic antifungals are effective against *Histoplasma* and *Cryptococcus*.

Suggested Reading

Brooks DE. Ophthalmology for the Equine Practitioner. Jackson, WY; Teton NewMedia, 2002.

Brooks DE, Matthews AG. Equine ophthalmology. In: Gelatt KN, ed. Veterinary Ophthalmology, ed 4. Philadelphia; Lippincott Williams and Wilkins, 2007.

Gilger BC, ed. Equine Ophthalmology. Philadelphia; WB Saunders, 2005.

Author Dennis E. Brooks
Consulting Editor Dennis E. Brooks

FAILURE OF TRANSFER OF PASSIVE IMMUNITY (FTPI)

BASICS

DEFINITION

• Inadequate passive immunity in neonates evidenced by abnormally low concentrations of immunoglobulins in serum at >18 hr of age. Foals that ingest an adequate volume of high-quality colostrum and absorb the immunoglobulins have serum IgG > 1500 mg/dL and often >2000 mg/dL. • IgG concentrations in serum of <800 mg/dL (8 g/L) are considered to place the foal at increased risk of infectious disease and have been termed "partial failure of transfer of passive immunity." It is important to note that some foals with IgG concentrations <800 mg/dL remain healthy. • IgG concentrations in serum <200 mg/dL are considered to represent complete failure of transfer of passive immunity (FTPI) and to place the foal at high risk of infectious disease in the neonatal period. • It is important to realize that these cutoff values are to some extent arbitrary and that the risk of a foal developing infectious disease in the neonatal period is a function of the amount of passive immunity it acquires and the size of the infectious challenge to the foal. The risk of infectious disease presumably increases relative to the lower the serum IgG concentration and the higher the challenge dose of an infectious organism. Other factors, such as concurrent illness, environmental stress, and malnutrition, can also contribute to the risk of infectious disease in the neonatal period.

PATHOPHYSIOLOGY

• Because of diffuse epithelial chorial placentation in mares, immunoglobulins do not cross the placenta during gestation.
• Foals are born immunologically competent but without immunologically significant concentrations of immunoglobulins in the blood. Humoral immunity of these foals during the neonatal period is dependent on absorption of adequate amounts of colostral immunoglobulin. • Immunoglobulins are concentrated by selective secretion in the mare's udder during the last 2 weeks of gestation. • Specialized epithelial cells in the foal's small intestine pass macromolecules via pinocytosis into local lacteals and, subsequently, into the blood. • Specialized epithelial cells are present at birth and are sloughed and replaced by nonspecialized intestinal epithelial cells; thus, the absorption process is both time and use dependent.
• Maximal absorption occurs after birth, decreases in efficiency by 12 hr, and is gone by 24 hr. • Immunoglobulin composition of colostrum is primarily IgGb and IgG(T), with smaller amounts of IgA and IgM; colostrum also contains factors such as cytokines, complement, and lactoferrin, which are important in upregulation of the foal's immune system and which provide local protection to the gastrointestinal tract. • Foals require approximately 2 g/kg of IgG to achieve a serum IgG concentration of 2000 mg/dL. • Good-quality colostrum (SG > 1.060) contains >3000 mg/dL (30 g/L) of IgG, and the average colostral IgG is about 10,000 mg/dL. • Foals (45 kg) need to ingest >1.5 L of acceptable-quality colostrum to have a reasonable expectation of serum IgG >800 mg/dL.

SYSTEMS AFFECTED

Systemic illness is associated with infectious, usually bacterial disease, with localization in the lungs (pneumonia) or joints (septic arthritis).

GENETICS N/A

INCIDENCE/PREVALENCE

FTPI has been reported to occur in 3%–24% of otherwise normal Thoroughbreds, Standardbreds, and Arabians in the United States, United Kingdom, and Australia.

GEOGRAPHIC DISTRIBUTION N/A

SIGNALMENT

• Breed predilections—No breed predilection is recorded. • Mean age and range—Affected foals are neonates, although signs of disease secondary to FTPI might not develop for days to weeks. • Predominant sex—No sex predilection is recorded.

SIGNS

General Comments

• There are no clinical signs pathognomonic of FTPI. • Foals with FTPI are at increased risk of developing sepsis, pneumonia, or septic arthritis, among other infectious diseases. The signs are typical of these diseases.

Historical Findings

• Foals born to mares >15 years are at increased risk. • Because colostrum is produced only once, premature lactation diminishes the quantity of colostrum in the udder, thereby reducing the amount available to the foal. • Mares kept on endophyte-infected tall fescue pasture or hay often fail to produce colostrum and milk.
• Foals must ingest an adequate amount of colostrum within 12–18 hr of birth, and preferably within 3 hr, in order to absorb sufficient IgG. Foals that are slow to stand and nurse, or that are unable to stand and nurse, are unable to ingest colostrum.

Physical Examination Findings

• Affected foals are clinically normal unless they develop infectious disease. • Many foals with partial FTPI that are kept in optimal conditions do not become sick.

CAUSES

• Ingestion of an inadequate amount of immunoglobulin can be due to production of an insufficient volume of colostrum, loss of colostrum through premature lactation, or colostrum that contains insufficient amounts of immunoglobulins. • Colostrum with a specific gravity <1.060 (as measured with a colostrometer; Equine Colostrometer, Jorgensen Laboratories, Loveland, CO; Gamma-Check-C, Veterinary Dynamics, San Luis Obispo, CA) has IgG concentration <3000 mg/dL and is associated with an increased risk of FTPI. • Failure of the foal to nurse by 3–6 hr after birth is associated with complete or partial FTPI; foals that fail to nurse by 12 hr usually have complete FTPI.

RISK FACTORS

• Illness or chronic debilitating disease in the mare during gestation, mares >15 years, and mares with poor mothering behavior have an increased incidence of affected foals. • Foals born in cold, overcast climates have an increased incidence compared to foals born in climates with more total solar radiation.
• Premature foals and foals with prolonged gestation (especially when associated with endophyte-infected fescue grass or hay) are at increased risk. • Any foal that is weak or otherwise poorly adapted to extrauterine life, such that the time to first suckle is >3 hr, is more likely to be affected.

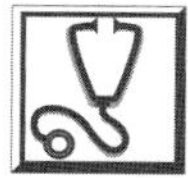

DIAGNOSIS

DIFFERENTIAL DIAGNOSIS

• Affected foals are clinically normal until they develop infectious disease. • Foals with sepsis or other medical conditions should have serum IgG concentrations measured.

CBC/BIOCHEMISTRY/URINALYSIS

Foals with serum total protein concentrations <4.0 g/dL are 2.5 times more likely to have FTPI. However, unlike the situation in calves, this is not a good screening test for FTPI in foals.

OTHER LABORATORY TESTS

• Serum IgG is detectable at 6 hr of age in foals that nursed by 2 hr and is almost maximal at 12–16 hr of age in these foals.
• The gold standard for measurement of serum IgG concentrations is the single radial immunodiffusion test. However, this test requires up to 24 hr to complete and is therefore of minimal clinical utility. • Other methodologies have been developed that provide a more rapid result. However, most of the more rapid tests have a high sensitivity (>80%) but low to moderate specificity (50%–70%). The result is that few foals with FTPI are missed by these tests but that many foals that have adequate serum IgG concentrations are classified as deficient. • An ELISA kit (CITE Foal IgG Test Kit; IDEXX Laboratories, Westbrook, ME) uses serum, plasma, or whole blood and provides semiquantitative measurement of IgG. The test has approximate sensitivity and specificity of 53% and 100%, respectively. The test methodology is modified by the manufacturer occasionally and the above characteristics can vary. • The zinc sulfate turbidity test (Equi-Z;

VMRD, Pullman, WA) measures total immunoglobulins based on formation of a precipitate of zinc ions and immunoglobulins. The test takes 1 hr and in the presence of hemolysis overestimates the concentration of immunoglobulins. The test has sensitivity and specificity of 97% and 57%, making it a good screening test. • The glutaraldehyde clot test (Gamma-Check-E; Veterinary Dynamics) is based on formation of a clot from interaction of the glutaraldehyde with immunoglobulin. The test has sensitivity and specificity of 100% and 59%, making it also a good screening test. • The latex agglutination test (Foalcheck; Centaur, Overland Park, KS) estimates the amount of IgG from the degree of agglutination of serum or blood with latex beads coated with anti-equine IgG antibody. The test has sensitivity and specificity of 72% and 79%, making it not a recommended test for testing foals for FTPI.

IMAGING N/A

OTHER DIAGNOSTIC PROCEDURES
N/A

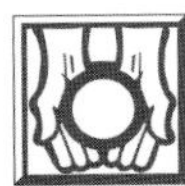

TREATMENT

TREATMENT GOALS
• Raise the serum IgG concentration to at least 800 mg/dL for a foal that has any risk factors for sepsis. • Foals with serum IgG 400–800 mg/dL may not require plasma transfusion if they are on a well-managed farm and are at low risk of sepsis.

APPROPRIATE HEALTH CARE
Colostrum and plasma can be given in the field, but if signs of septicemia or other systemic illness are apparent, referral is recommended.

NURSING CARE
• Foals <12 hr of age—Oral administration of colostrum with a specific gravity >1.060 is the preferred treatment. From 2 to 4 L of colostrum administered in 500-mL increments every 1–2 hr during the first 6–8 hr of life is desirable. Administration of bovine colostrum results in equine-specific passive immunity that is less than optimal and is not recommended. • In foals >12 hr—Adequate absorption for optimal IgG concentrations is unlikely and serum or plasma should be administered intravenously.
• Concentrated equine serum and lyophilized or other concentrated equine immunoglobulins are available. However, administration of the label dose results in suboptimal serum IgG concentrations and use of these products is not recommended.
• Plasma—Use of commercial frozen plasma is preferred because the donor horses should have been immunized against common equine pathogens, have tested negative for equine infectious anemia, have no clinically significant alloantibodies, and be Aa and Qa red cell antigen negative. Fresh plasma can be harvested from the mare or another horse with neither lysins nor agglutinins to equine RBC antigens. • Plasma should be transfused at a rate of 40 mL/kg to foals with serum IgG <400 mg/dL and at a rate of 20 mL/kg to foals with serum IgG of 400–800 mg/dL. Generally, a 45-kg well foal with IgG <400 mg/dL will require 2 L of plasma, and a foal with serum IgG of >400 mg/dL but <800 mg/dL will require 1 L of plasma.
• Measurement of serum IgG should be performed after transfusion to confirm that adequate IgG concentrations have been achieved. • Administer IV plasma through an in-line filter. Thaw frozen plasma slowly in a water bath at 39°–45°C (102°–113° F), and warm to at least 20° C before administration. The initial plasma or serum infusion should be slow and the foal observed for adverse reactions. Subsequently, the infusion may be given at 20–30 mL/kg/hr.

ACTIVITY N/A

DIET N/A

CLIENT EDUCATION N/A

SURGICAL CONSIDERATIONS N/A

MEDICATIONS

DRUG(S) OF CHOICE N/A

CONTRAINDICATIONS
• No contraindications to commercially available, fresh-frozen plasma • Use of fresh plasma from horses with agglutinins or lysins to equine RBC carries a risk for neonatal isoerythrolysis.

PRECAUTIONS
• Frozen plasma thawed at too high a temperature or in a microwave oven contains denatured proteins that subsequently can cause vasomotor reactions during administration, characterized by tachypnea, tachycardia, pyrexia, muscle fasciculations, blanching of the mucous membranes, and, in severe cases, marked hypotension. • If adverse reactions occur during administration of plasma or serum products, discontinue the infusion until signs abate, and then continue the infusion at a slower rate. If adverse reactions continue, terminate the infusion.
• Pretreatment of foals with flunixin (0.5–1.1 mg/kg) before infusion can decrease adverse reactions; however, this strategy should not be a substitute for proper handling of frozen plasma.

POSSIBLE INTERACTIONS
N/A

ALTERNATIVE DRUGS
N/A

FOLLOW-UP

PATIENT MONITORING
Foals with sepsis appear to have a reduced half-life of exogenous IgG and, thus, can need multiple transfusions to maintain serum concentrations above 800 mg/dL, and perhaps higher. Serum IgG concentrations should be measured every 48–72 hr in foals with sepsis.

PREVENTION/AVOIDANCE
• Ensure that newborn foals are able to stand and nurse within 3 hr of birth. If unable to nurse on their own, supplement with at least 1.5 L of good-quality colostrum via bottle or nasogastric tube (in 500-mL increments). • If the mare has dripped milk prior to delivery or has been exposed to fescue, the foal should receive good-quality colostrum or plasma transfusion shortly after birth.

POSSIBLE COMPLICATIONS
• Exogenous IgG may be redistributed to extravascular sites and cause complement activation with subsequent anaphylaxis-like reactions. • Complexes can be formed with preexisting antigens resulting in immune-mediated disease. • Catabolism of IgG can occur, particularly in foals that are sick or receiving inadequate nutrition.

EXPECTED COURSE AND PROGNOSIS
• Foals with uncomplicated FTPI have an excellent prognosis with appropriate treatment. • Complications with sepsis will lower the prognosis.

MISCELLANEOUS

ASSOCIATED DISEASES
Neonatal sepsis

AGE-RELATED FACTORS
N/A

ZOONOTIC POTENTIAL
N/A

PREGNANCY
N/A

SEE ALSO
Septicemia, neonatal

ABBREVIATIONS
• ELISA = enzyme-linked immunosorbent assay
• FTPI = failure of transfer of passive immunity

Suggested Reading

Radostits OM, Gay CC, Hinchcliff KW, Constable PD, eds. Veterinary Medicine: A Textbook of the Diseases of Cattle, Horses, Sheep, Goats and Pigs, ed 10. London: WB Saunders, 2004:164–168, 149–158.

Author Kenneth W. Hinchcliff
Consulting Editor Margaret C. Mudge

FEARS AND PHOBIAS

BASICS

DEFINITION

• *Fear*—an emotion of alarm and agitation caused by real or perceived danger and manifested by physiologic responses (e.g., tachycardia, trembling, elimination) and by behavioral responses (e.g., postural changes, ranging from ear flicks to charging, escape, immobility, and defensiveness including aggression)
• *Phobia*—a marked, persistent, and excessive fear of clearly discernible circumscribed objects or situations. Exposure to a phobic stimulus almost invariably provokes an immediate fear response, which may be expressed as heightened arousal or agitation, escape behavior, or defensive aggression, and subsequent avoidance of the phobic stimulus.

PATHOPHYSIOLOGY

• When evaluating an individual animal, medical explanations of fearful behavior must be considered, particularly in horses showing an acute change in their behavior or those that exhibit concomitant neurological abnormalities. Pain, toxin exposure, infectious conditions (e.g., rabies, tetanus, equine protozoal myelitis), and some ophthalmic conditions can cause animals to exhibit hyper-reactive responses that may mimic fear.
• Chronic conditions, such as pain, may affect responses to stimuli as horses attempt to avoid conditions previously associated with pain. Acute pain, such as a needle stick, may become associated with fear, leading to a conditioned response.
• There are learned and genetic (see later) etiologies to fearful and phobic responses.

SYSTEMS AFFECTED

• Nervous—motor restlessness, trembling, pacing, attempts to escape restraint or confinement, inattentiveness during training, inadequate performance, or aggression to handlers
• Neuromuscular—Trembling may occur.
• Gastrointestinal—inappetence or altered eating habits and increased defecation rate when fearful/reactive; gastric ulceration may be associated with chronic fearful states, including shipping/show stress and suboptimal housing.
• Cardiovascular—horses rated as reactive (fearful) in behavioral tests exhibited high mean heart rate and low heart rate variability.
• Respiratory—tachypnea or frequent snorting when exposed to fearful stimulus
• Endocrine/metabolic—Chronic fear may increase metabolic rates and elevate endogenous cortisol levels.
• Hemic/lymphatic/immune—Conditions of chronic fear may reduce immune competence.
• Musculoskeletal—Traumatic injuries may occur during escape attempts or restraint.
• Ophthalmic—Rule out abnormalities in cases of adult-onset fear responses.
• Skin/exocrine—Sweating may occur due to autonomic arousal.
• Reproductive—Fear may affect breeding performance and tractability by stallions and mares; cryptorchids and mares with granulosa cell tumors may be excessively reactive; chronic fear may be associated with abortion.
• Hepatobiliary—none
• Renal/urologic—none

GENETICS

• There is a strong genetic component to fear/phobic responses. Among horses that evolved as prey in open habitat, detection of unusual features in the environment that might represent a danger, followed by an avoidance reaction, such as running away, has been an effective strategy to ensure survival and reproductive success. When escape is not possible, defensive responses, such as kicking or biting, have been favored by natural selection. Although selective breeding of individuals with attenuated fear responses has been part of the process of domestication of the horse, some ancestral characteristics remain, including heritable (i.e., genetic) tendencies to monitor the environment and react to novel stimuli by exhibiting fears and phobias.
• Artificial selection by humans for certain traits, such as racing speed and showy performance, may favor horses that exhibit escape responses and are reactive. Genetic factors (breed, sire) appear to play a role in neophobic reactions. The mode of inheritance is not known.

INCIDENCE/PREVALENCE

• Common
• Aversion to veterinary and handling procedures may be a manifestation of fear.

GEOGRAPHIC DISTRIBUTION

Not limited geographically, although regional conventions for horse handling may affect the prevalence of fearful responses

SIGNALMENT

Breed Predilections

May be breed-specific differences in reactivity to novel stimuli and attempts to flee, especially breeds used for racing or for show in which activated movement is favored by selective breeding or training. Overt fear responses may be less commonly expressed in individuals of "cold-blooded" breeds.

Mean Age and Range

Any age; especially common in young animals lacking positive experiences with humans and novel situations

Predominant Sex

Any sex

SIGNS

Historical

• Vary according to temperament and prior experience; horses raised without exposure to humans may have a large flight distance compared with handled horses.
• Lack of systematic, positive training is associated with more reactive responses, especially in novel environments.
• Affected horses described as "spooky" or "flighty"

Physical Examination

• Usually unremarkable, may sweat, defecate excessively
• Acute—orientation toward the stimulus, head-up alert/immobility stance, spin, retreat. Aggression may be expressed if escape is prevented.
• Chronic—poor body condition, postural effects, often the opposite of acute reactions, such as droopy head position
• Signs of trauma may be evident secondary to attempts to escape fearful situations.
• Very fearful horses may be difficult to examine, attempting escape or reactive/defensive/aggressive behavior when approached or restrained.

CAUSES

• Fear responses are part of normal equine behavior; strongly influenced by individual temperament (e.g., hypersensitive individual), handling experience, and experience of handler.
• Although rare, phobic behavior may be a manifestation of an organic condition; medical causes of fears and phobias should be ruled out before seeking a behavioral explanation.
• Neonatal handling has not been shown to reduce adult reactions to novel situations any more than systemic, positive training.

RISK FACTORS

• Horses with minimal exposure to humans and their activities
• Excessive arousal or frustration
• Previous or current mismanagement, abuse, and/or inadequate or incompetent training
• Risk analysis consists of historical information, observation of the animal, and supporting medical and legal data. The goals are to prevent human injury, to reduce the client's and veterinarian's liability risk, and to establish a rational management/ rehabilitation plan.
• The situation is considered high risk if the horse has had a history or displays fear aggression (e.g., kicking, biting, lunging) when approached or handled. "Flighty" horses that unpredictably exhibit fearful behavior (e.g., bolting) and horses that exhibit fear-motivated aggression are dangerous, can cause death and therefore should be handled only by experienced personnel.

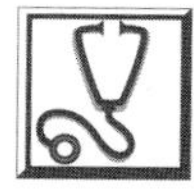

DIAGNOSIS

DIFFERENTIAL DIAGNOSIS

Identify pathological conditions associated with fears and phobias, including pain and sleep deprivation, before seeking a purely behavioral diagnosis.

CBC/BIOCHEMISTRY/URINALYSIS

- Usually normal; possible stress leukogram
- Abnormalities may suggest metabolic or endocrine explanations.

OTHER LABORATORY TESTS

May be indicated to rule out medical explanations

IMAGING

- May be indicated to identify sources of pain
- CT or MR imaging if congenital abnormalities or cerebral neoplasia are suspected

OTHER DIAGNOSTIC PROCEDURES

Postmortem fluorescent antibody test for any fearfully aggressive horse in which rabies is a differential diagnosis

PATHOLOGICAL FINDINGS

Uncommon, see above

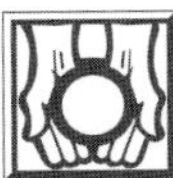

TREATMENT

AIMS OF TREATMENT

- The overall objective of treatment is to reduce fear and phobic responses in horses in order to manage them safely and improve their usefulness and welfare.
- Positive handling and progressive training by experienced handlers reduce fear responses and reactivity in novel environments.

Environmental Management

- Use adequate barriers and sufficient restraint to prevent human, self-induced injury, and escape.
- Use well-fitting, sturdy halters with leads and other necessary restraint devices; experience, patient handler.
- Establish safe, quiet environment to practice behavior modification techniques. Start in a familiar environment; then with success progress to unfamiliar environments.

Behavior Modification

- Positive reinforcement is used to reward acceptable behavior, starting with a simple task, then progressing to a more complex task. Rewards can be in the form of praise, petting, or food. Rewards may be preceded by a clicker or other conditioned reinforcer.
- Negative reinforcement is used to increase a desired behavior. A mildly aversive "pressure" is applied, such as pulling on a lead or tapping on the rump with a plastic bag on the end of a whip, until the horse responds, then the pressure is released. The horse learns when pressure is applied and it moves forward; it is rewarded by the removal of pressure. The "pressure" should not induce fear.
- Punishment may worsen fearful reactions, since the horse may associate the fearful stimulus with pain or distress, worsening the condition in the future. Punishment may also lead to increased situational fears, such as fear of the punisher (see chapter Training and Learning Problems).
- Desensitization/counterconditioning—Based on history and observations, list all situations in which the horse appears fearful or phobic. Align these situations along a continuum from least to most fearful. Initially, avoid all these situations. Teach the horse basic obedience commands from the ground (e.g., "whoa," "come along") using adequate equipment, such as halter and lead under nonfearful, familiar conditions. Reward the horse for being calm and obedient with praise, favored tactile contact, or food treats, or the release of constant pressure (e.g., from a halter or rein). Then, practice these control exercises in a range of environmental conditions so the horse generalizes the learning to different locations and situations. Escape behavior must be avoided since it is strongly reinforced by the diminished fear that results from greater distance from the stimulus.
- Next, when practicing control exercises, expose the horse to the least fearful stimulus on the fear continuum. The goal is to expose the horse to mildly fearful situations while in a nonfearful state under obedience control. Reward the horse for calm, tractable behavior. It may be necessary to reduce the intensity of the fearful stimulus by moving it farther away and only gradually moving it closer as the horse habituates to the stimulus. Eventually, a "good habit" can replace a "bad response," a process called counterconditioning.
- A "target," such as a tennis ball or pool buoy affixed to a wooden dowel, may be used in the counterconditioning process. Initially, the target needs to be "loaded," i.e., given positive value to the horse. This is accomplished by positioning the target so that the horse voluntarily approaches and touches the target. Immediately, this approach response should be marked with a praise word or the sound of a hand-held clicker. Then, the horse is given a suitable reward, such as a small food treat. This sequence should be repeated until the horse learns that, when it touches the target with its nose, a single reward is delivered. With time, the target can be used to distract the horse from fearful stimuli and to teach the horse to move forward under potentially fear-inducing conditions, such as walking into a transport trailer.

Other Factors

Recent techniques popularized by professional horse trainers, dubbed *horse whisperers*, use their keen observation of the horse, patience, and knowledge of equine communication to "tame" fearful horses. Such techniques avoid the confrontational and often abusive techniques previously used to "break" horses. These trainers are adept at shaping behavior using subtle positive and negative reinforcement as well as "learned helplessness" to produce calm, tractable horses with reduced fearful or phobic behavior. Practitioners of these techniques usually work with individual horses in social isolation, and they commonly use a high-fenced pen to prevent the horse's escape and to focus its attention on the trainer. Often these immediate training successes do not persist when the horse is managed by a less-experienced client in another, more complex environment.

APPROPRIATE HEALTH CARE

To avoid fears and phobias, positive-based, species-appropriate handling should be part of routine health care of all horses.

NURSING CARE

N/A

ACTIVITY

Regular exercise

DIET

- Dietary adjustment with vitamin B complex, thiamine, and/or vitamin B6 and magnesium may be helpful; maintain physiological range for calcium:magnesium ratio (1.5:1 to 2:1).
- Avoid excessive high-energy concentrates that may promote reactive behavior.

CLIENT EDUCATION

- Recommend handling of the affected horse by experienced persons.
- Recommend safe, quiet housing. Extreme fear reactions or phobic behavior can cause self trauma during an escape attempt.
- Chronic fear/phobic responses constitute a welfare issue. Horses in a chronic, high-fear state may eat or drink poorly, exhibit stereotypic behaviors such as cribbing, or develop gastric ulcers. Wild mustangs transported for long distances have died from the acidosis and dehydration associated with such a state. Thus, fears and phobias need to be addressed as a welfare issue.

SURGICAL CONSIDERATIONS

Because of the heritable nature of these behaviors, fearful/phobic stallions should be castrated.

MEDICATIONS

DRUGS OF CHOICE

Generally, drugs are not used for treatment. However, medication, when used with a systematic behavioral management program, may decrease arousal or anxiety and, thus, facilitate learning and safe handling.

CONTRAINDICATIONS

Racing, showing; for ethical and safety reasons, the drugs listed below are not recommended for use in performance animals.

FEARS AND PHOBIAS

PRECAUTIONS

No drugs are approved by the US Food and Drug Administration for treatment of fearful or phobic behavior in horses. No clinical trials have been performed on these extra-label drugs; our knowledge is based on evidence from other species and anecdotal information from a few, individual cases. Inform the client regarding the experimental nature of these treatments and the risk involved; document the discussion in the medical record.

ALTERNATIVE DRUGS

- Acepromazine, a phenothiazine tranquilizer, is used widely, and is valuable to reduce the effect of environmental stimuli, if acute fear-inducing situations can be anticipated. Side effects include priapism and paraphimosis in stallions.
- Fluoxetine, a selective serotonin reuptake inhibitor with anxiolytic and anticompulsive effects, may require 1–4 weeks to effect. Fluoxetine may decrease libido in breeding animals; higher doses of fluoxetine or imipramine may result in serotonin effects in the GIT.
- Fluphenazine decanoate, a phenothiazine dopamine antagonist, has been used to reduce reactivity. Serious extrapyramidal side effects (motor restlessness, altered mentation) have been reported. Diphenhydramine has been used successfully as an antidote.
- Reserpine, a *Rauwolfia* alkaloid used to enhance behavioral calming; side effects can include erratic behavior, colic signs; it should not be used if surgery is anticipated due to serious anesthetic risk.
- Synthetic hormones have been used, including the synthetic progestin altrenogest to suppress behavioral cycling in mares.
- Tricyclic antidepressants, such as amitriptyline or imipramine, have serotonin and norepinephrine reuptake inhibitor effects; may enhance behavioral calming; side effects can include mild sedation and anticholinergic effects. Imipramine is used to reduce anxiety in breeding males and is associated with masturbation and erection in males in sexual context. At high doses, imipramine (2–4 mg/kg PO q24h) can cause muscle fasciculations, tachycardia, and hyperresponsiveness to sound, likely due to norepinephrine effects.
- Oral tryptophan, a serotonin precursor, is purported to have calming effects, but one controlled study showed no such clinical response.
- A synthetic equine appeasing pheromone (Modipher EQ, VPL), commercially available and administered via intranasal spray, prior to exposure to an anxiety-producing situation, has been reported to reduce fear responses and tachypnea in a test situation.
- NSAIDs may be used for two weeks to rule out pain as an etiological factor.

FOLLOW-UP

PATIENT MONITORING

- Weekly to biweekly contact during the initial phases
- Clients frequently need feedback and assistance with behavior modification plans and medication management.

PREVENTION/AVOIDANCE

Helpful examination strategies:

- Rapid recognition of fearful/phobic behavior by the examiner
- Suitable restraint equipment
- A familiar, tractable horse within visual range
- A familiar, experienced handler utilizing rewards (praise, touch, food) in response to acceptable responses
- A familiar location that does not allow escape or injury, with nonslippery footing
- By the veterinarian—slow, nonjerky movements, monotone speech, allow the horse visual and olfactory inspection
- Chemical restraint, if necessary, to prevent injury and avoid a negative association with the veterinarian

POSSIBLE COMPLICATIONS

- Human injury caused by a horse exhibiting fear-motivated or phobic behavior
- To prevent human injury and extensive self-inflicted trauma of the horse, consider euthanasia for high-risk cases in which all other treatment options have failed.

EXPECTED COURSE AND PROGNOSIS

- Systematic behavior modification can reduce fear and phobic responses.
- The knowledge and patience of the handler greatly influence treatment success.
- Temperament differences between horses may limit treatment success.

MISCELLANEOUS

ASSOCIATED CONDITIONS

Pain may exacerbate fear responses. For example, a horse with foot pain may become fearful and resistant when shod due to anticipation of pain or punishment for not standing well; resistance to the protocol may result.

AGE-RELATED FACTORS

- Fear-motivated behavior problems are common in young horses with little training.
- Adult- or acute-onset fear-motivated behavior, particularly in previously well-handled animals, suggests a medical cause.

ZOONOTIC POTENTIAL

Rabies is a potential cause of fearful behavior or fear-motivated aggression.

PREGNANCY

Chronic use of behavioral medications is not recommended in pregnant animals.

SYNONYMS

N/A

SEE ALSO

- Trailer loading problems
- Training and learning problems

ABBREVIATION

- GIT = gastrointestinal tract

Suggested Reading

Falewee C, Gaultier E, Lafont C, Bougrat L, Pageat P. Effect of a synthetic equine maternal pheromone during a controlled fear-eliciting situation. Appl Anim Behav Sci 2006;101:144–153.

Karrasch S, Karrasch V, Newman A. You Can Train Your Horse to Do Anything: Target Training, Clicker Training, and Beyond. North Pomfret, VT: Trafalgar Square Publishing, 2000.

McDonnell SA. Oral imipramine and intravenous xylazine for pharmacologically-induced ex copula ejaculation in stallions. Anim Reprod Sci 2001;68(3–4):153–159.

McGreevy P. Equine Behaviour: A Guide for Veterinarians and Equine Scientists. Philadelphia: WB Saunders, 2005.

Mills DS, McDonnell S. Domestic horse: the origins, development, and management of its behaviour. New York: Cambridge University Press, 2005.

Momozawa Y, Ono T, Sata F, Kikusuui T, Takeuchi Y, Mori Y, Kusunose R. Assessment of equine temperament by a questionnaire survey to caretakers and evaluation of its reliability by simultaneous behavior test. Appl Anim Behav Sci 2003;84:127–138.

Voith VL. Fears and phobias. In: Voith V, Borchelt P (eds). Readings in Companion Animal Behavior. Trenton, NJ: Veterinary Learning Systems, 1996.

Waring GH. Horse Behavior, ed 2. Norwich, NJ: Noyes Publications/William Andrew Publishing, 2003.

Authors Barbara Lynn Sherman and Richard A. Mansmann

Consulting Editors Victoria L Voith and Daniel Q. Estep

FELL PONY SYNDROME

BASICS

OVERVIEW

• Familial disease of Fell Ponies that is characterized by immunodeficiency, progressive anemia, peripheral ganglionopathy, secondary opportunistic infection, and death usually by 3 months of age. • It was first described in the late 1990 s in England.

SIGNALMENT

• Fell Pony breed • Colts and fillies equally affected

SIGNS

• Nonspecific signs usually begin at approximately 2–3 weeks of age, including weight loss, depression, ill thrift, and lethargy. • Pale membranes • Fever secondary to opportunistic infection such as enteritis (diarrhea) and pneumonia is very common. • Glossal hyperkeratosis is a described finding. • Tachycardia and tachypnea are common findings often as a result of severe anemia and/or concurrent illness. • Concurrent infectious disease often with pathogens commonly observed in immunosuppressed individuals are common including cryptosporidial enteritis, adenoviral bronchopneumonia and/or pancreatitis, or disease states uncommon to immunocompetent animals.

CAUSES AND RISK FACTORS

• Genetically acquired disease is suspected, where an autosomal recessive mode of inheritance has been postulated although not proved. • This disease has been described in the United Kingdom, the United States, and the Netherlands. • Low morbidity and high (100%) mortality • Despite normal serum IgG concentrations, affected foals still develop severe opportunistic infection, suggesting that other segments of the immune system (e.g., cell-mediated immunity) are defective and essential for protection.

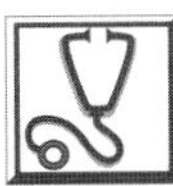

DIAGNOSIS

• No definitive genetic test exists.
• Immunologic testing:
  ○ Lymphocyte function tests are typically normal.
  ○ Normal distribution of $CD4^+$ and $CD8^+$ lymphocyte populations
  ○ Low serum immunoglobulin M and immunoglobulin A concentrations when measured at >3–4 weeks of age
  ○ Immunoglobulin G concentration may be normal and be maternally derived in origin.

DIFFERENTIAL DIAGNOSIS

• Sepsis—usually in neonatal foals (<2 weeks of age); typical gram-negative and gram-positive organisms • Infectious enteritis—generally responds to appropriate treatment; no anemia seen with typical infectious enteritis • Other immune deficiency syndromes (see Associated Conditions)

CBC/BIOCHEMISTRY/URINALYSIS

• Severe nonregenerative anemia with PCV often <15% and lymphopenia are common. • Thrombocytopenia is common. • Plasma protein concentrations and blood lymphocyte counts may be normal or low.

OTHER LABORATORY TESTS

• Bone marrow biopsy reveals marked erythroid hypoplasia with myeloid to erythroid ratios (M:E) 21–62:1. • Flow cytometry on peripheral blood leukocytes reveals severe B-cell lymphopenia (≤10% of normal counts) with normal to increased T-lymphocyte concentrations.
• T-lymphocytes have a decreased expression of major histocompatibility complex (MHC) class II.

IMAGING N/A

OTHER DIAGNOSTIC PROCEDURES

N/A

PATHOLOGICAL FINDINGS

• Necropsy findings reveal hypoplasia of lymphoid tissue including the thymus and an absence of secondary lymph node follicles and plasma cells. • Low numbers of plasma cells are evident in the spleen. • Peripheral ganglionopathy is characterized by neuronal chromatolysis in the cranial mesenteric, dorsal root, and trigeminal ganglia. • Bone marrow examination shows a paucity of erythroid precursor cell lines.

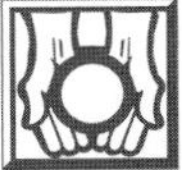

TREATMENT

• This condition is uniformly fatal; most foals die by 3 months of age. • Supportive care with intravenous fluids and parenteral nutrition
• Treat secondary infections with appropriate antimicrobials. • Blood transfusion with packed red blood cells may prolong survival temporarily. • Affected foals often respond initially to targeted supportive therapy but soon succumb to severe anemia and immunodeficiency. • Humane euthanasia should be considered in Fell Pony foals with clinical evidence of Fell Pony syndrome.

MEDICATIONS

DRUG(S) OF CHOICE

• Broad-spectrum antimicrobials: penicillin (22,000 IU/kg q6 h) and amikacin (25 mg/kg IV q24h) or ceftiofur (10 mg/kg IV q6h)
• Gastroprotectants may also be used if gastric ulceration is a concern (ranitidine 1.5 mg/kg IV q8h, sucralfate 10–20 mg/kg PO q6–8h).

CONTRAINDICATIONS/POSSIBLE INTERACTIONS

N/A

FOLLOW-UP

PATIENT MONITORING

• Repeat bloodwork to assess for worsening of anemia or efficacy of transfusions. • Monitor for development of opportunistic infections.
• Diagnosis of Fell Pony syndrome should be pursued, as further treatment is likely futile, and humane euthanasia is recommended.

PREVENTION/AVOIDANCE

If Fell Pony syndrome is presumed to be autosomal recessive, then the dam and sire of affected foals should be considered heterozygous for the condition. Genetic counseling might be important when considering future breeding of such animals. To avoid having affected foals, heterozygotes should not be bred together.

POSSIBLE COMPLICATIONS

N/A

EXPECTED COURSE AND PROGNOSIS

• Severe nonregenerative anemia, immunodeficiency, and overwhelming secondary infection occur rapidly in early life, ultimately causing death. • Many foals will die from disseminated intravascular coagulation related to severe septic shock.

MISCELLANEOUS

ASSOCIATED CONDITIONS

• No reports exist of a similar condition in humans or other species. • Other humoral immunity deficiencies exist in horses, including failure of transfer of passive immunity, transient hypogammaglobulinemia of young horses, severe combined immunodeficiency syndrome of Arabian foals, primary agammaglobulinemia, selective IgM deficiency, and common variable immunodeficiency.

AGE-RELATED FACTORS

Foals begin showing signs as maternally derived immunity begins to wane. The clinical course is typically rapid thereafter.

ZOONOTIC POTENTIAL

N/A

PREGNANCY

N/A

Suggested Reading

Gardner RB, Hart KA, Stokol T, Divers TJ, Flaminio MJ. Fell pony syndrome in a pony in North America. J Vet Intern Med 2006;20:198–203.

Scholes SF, Holliman A, May PD, Holmes MA. A syndrome of anaemia, immunodeficiency and peripheral ganglionopathy in Fell pony foals. Vet Rec 1998;142:128–134.

Author Samuel D. A. Hurcombe
Consulting Editor Margaret C. Mudge

FESCUE TOXICOSIS

BASICS

DEFINITION

• Toxicosis in pregnant mares associated with ingestion of endophyte-infected tall fescue (*Festuca arundinacea* Schreb.) during late gestation (i.e., post gestation day 300)
• The endophyte is a fungus (*Neotyphodium coenophialum*) that lives in a mutualistic relationship within the intercellular spaces of the plant. Previous names for the fungus include *Acremonium coenophialum* and *Epichloe typhina.*
• The endophyte produces ergot peptide alkaloids, the most prominent being ergovaline.
• The ergot peptide alkaloids produced by the endophyte are mycotoxins—secondary metabolites of a fungus.

PATHOPHYSIOLOGY

• Ergot peptides act as dopamine agonists, binding D2-dopamine receptors and suppressing prolactin secretion.
• Prolactin affects not only mammary development and milk production but also lipogenesis, immunity, and reproductive hormones.

SYSTEMS AFFECTED

Reproductive system and mammary gland

GENETICS

N/A

INCIDENCE/PREVALENCE

• Tall fescue occupies >35 million acres in the United States and is especially prominent in the Southeast.
• Most tall fescue pastures derive from a Kentucky 31 variety released in 1943 that was contaminated by an endophyte; >95% of tall fescue pastures are estimated to contain this endophyte.
• An estimated 688,000 horses are maintained on tall fescue pastures.
• One survey indicated that 53% of pregnant mares maintained on fescue pastures were agalactic, 38% had prolonged gestation, and 18% had stillborn or weak foals that died.

GEOGRAPHIC DISTRIBUTION

Tall fescue is most prominent in the southeastern United States, but it can be found over much of the eastern United States and is grown for grass seed in the Pacific Northwest.

SIGNALMENT

Pregnant mares during late gestation, with the last 30 days of pregnancy (i.e., post gestation day 300) being the most critical

SIGNS

Historical

• Lack of udder development in mare
• Mare is past her due date.
• "Red bag presentation" with premature placental separation of chorioallantois preceding foal through birth canal
• Mare is having foaling problem.
• Weak foal with "dummy-like" behavior
• Lower ADG is possible in yearlings not supplemented with concentrates.

Physical Examination Findings

• Typically, mares are 3–4 weeks past their due date.
• Agalactia in mares; milk appears brown or straw-colored rather than white.
• Larger-than-normal foal or inadequate preparation of the reproductive tract may cause dystocia; foal may be turned 90°in the pelvis.
• Placenta may be thickened enough that the foal has trouble breaking through, and the mare may retain the placenta.
• Foals are weak or stillborn.
• Foals are large and gangly, with long and fine hair coats, poor muscle mass, overgrown hooves, and nonerupted incisor teeth (i.e., dysmature).
• Foals may be hypothyroid, with signs of incoordination and poor suckling reflex.
• Foals may suffer from failure of passive transfer of colostral antibodies due to mare agalactia; septicemia problems in foals are common.

CAUSES

• Any tall fescue should be considered infected by the endophyte unless the owner has purposely planted an endophyte-free variety.
• Lower percentages of fescue in mixed pastures decrease the severity or likelihood of problems; however, minimal toxic concentrations of ergovaline in endophyte-infected tall fescue have not been determined for horses; any tall fescue exposure should be considered potentially toxic for mares.

RISK FACTORS

• Ergovaline concentrations are highest in seed heads during summer months; concentrations are increased by drought, excessive rain, and fertilization.
• Fescue hay retains its toxicity.
• Non–endophyte-infected fescue cannot become infected; however, endophyte-infected fescue will outcompete non–endopyte-infected fescue and will eventually take over a pasture.

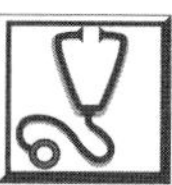

DIAGNOSIS

DIFFERENTIAL DIAGNOSIS

• Other causes of dystocia, placentitis, and dysmature foals
• Ergot alkaloids associated with ergot sclerotia from *Claviceps purpurea* in small grains or hay can mimic fescue toxicosis.

CBC/BIOCHEMISTRY/URINALYSIS

No major changes are likely, unless a stress leukogram caused by prolonged parturition is present.

OTHER LABORATORY TESTS

• Mares—decreased serum prolactin and progesterone concentrations; increased serum estradiol-17β
• Foals—decreased serum T_3 and plasma ACTH and cortisol concentrations

IMAGING

Ultrasonography may show a thickened placenta and large foal.

DIAGNOSTIC PROCEDURES

• Pasture or hay concentrations of ergovaline likely are >200 ppb dry weight.
• Endophyte contamination can be checked qualitatively by staining plant tillers at plant pathology laboratories or by ELISA testing.

PATHOLOGICAL FINDINGS

• Thickened, congested, and edematous placenta, with no significant bacterial cultures
• Edema is most severe in allantochorion at the area of the cervical star.
• The amnion is edematous throughout and the umbilical cord also may be edematous.
• Placenta may be ruptured in the uterine body rather than the typical location at the cervical star.

- Foals may have overgrown hooves and nonerupted incisor teeth.
- An enlarged thyroid in a foal is not apparent grossly, but large, distended thyroid follicles lined by flat, cuboidal epithelial cells can be seen histopathologically.
- If a mare dies from dystocia, uterine rupture may be present and the mammary gland undeveloped.

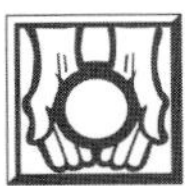

TREATMENT

APPROPRIATE HEALTH CARE, NURSING CARE, ACTIVITY, DIET, CLIENT EDUCATION, SURGICAL CONSIDERATIONS

N/A

MEDICATIONS

DRUG(S) OF CHOICE

- Oxytocin, uterine infusion of fluids, and possibly antibiotics/anti-inflammatory drugs for retained placentas
- Stored colostrum, antiserum, or plasma as immunoglobulin sources for foals not receiving enough colostrum; antibiotics for septicemia problems in foals
- Domperidone, a D2-dopamine antagonist, is marketed as an oral gel for mares; it is given at 1.1 mg/kg once a day for 7–10 days before anticipated parturition if the mare exhibits no signs of milk production; domperidone may be continued 5–10 days after foaling at the same dosage; agalactia in a mare that has already foaled can be treated twice a day at 1.1 mg/kg for 2 days and then once a day at 1.1 mg/kg for at least 3 more days.

CONTRAINDICATIONS

Domperidone stimulates GI motility; avoid use in mares with GI blockage or perforation.

PRECAUTIONS

- Domperidone treatment may cause leaking of milk and loss of colostrum prior to foaling; if this occurs, administer one-half the regular dose twice a day; if milk loss continues with the split dose, administer one-third or less of the regular dose twice a day; collect and save colostrum; if significant colostrum is lost, monitor serum IgG levels in the foal.
- Domperidone may cause a false-positive for the milk calcium test that is used to predict foaling date.

POSSIBLE INTERACTIONS

N/A

ALTERNATIVE DRUGS

N/A

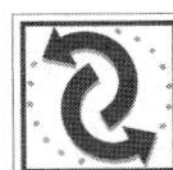

FOLLOW-UP

PATIENT MONITORING

- Monitor serum IgG concentration in foals to assess adequate passive transfer.
- Keep mares away from fescue for ≅1 week until lactating well.
- Bottle feeding of milk replacers or a nurse mare may be needed for foals.
- Mares may have rebreeding problems.

PREVENTION/AVOIDANCE

- Prevention is much more feasible than treatment.
- Remove mares from fescue pastures and fescue hay a minimum of 3–4 weeks before their foaling date; some practitioners recommend 6–8 weeks before foaling; mares should not be exposed to tall fescue beyond day 300 of gestation.
- If removal from fescue pasture is not possible, domperidone can be administered orally at 1.1 mg/kg per day during the last 10–14 days of gestation.
- Endophyte-infected tall fescue pastures can be replanted with other grasses or new novel varieties of endophyte-infected fescue, which do not produce ergovaline; new novel varieties of endophyte-infected fescue retain their resistance to overgrazing, insect damage, and drought stress without causing adverse effects in animals; non-endophyte-infected tall fescue is not very hardy or persistent.
- A glucomannan product produced from yeast cell walls is marketed as a binder of ergovaline in the GI tract.

POSSIBLE COMPLICATIONS

Dystocia or uterine rupture in mares

EXPECTED COURSE AND PROGNOSIS

Guarded prognosis for dysmature foals

MISCELLANEOUS

ASSOCIATED CONDITIONS, AGE-RELATED FACTORS, ZOONOTIC POTENTIAL

N/A

PREGNANCY

See above.

SEE ALSO

- Agalactia
- Dysmaturity
- Ergot alkaloids
- Failure of passive transfer
- Retained placenta

ABBREVIATIONS

- ACTH = adrenocorticotrophin hormone
- ADG = average daily gain
- ELISA = enzyme-linked immunosorbent assay
- ppb = parts per billion
- T_3 = triiodothyronine

Suggested Reading

Blodgett DJ. Fescue toxicosis. In: Galey FD, ed. The Veterinary Clinics of North America; Equine Practice; Toxicology. Philadelphia: WB Saunders, 2001:17(3).

Boosinger TR, Brendemuehl JP, Bransby DL, et al. Prolonged gestation, decreased triiodothyronine concentration, and thyroid gland histomorphologic features in newborn foals of mares grazing *Acremonium coenophialum*–infected fescue. Am J Vet Res 1995;56:66–69.

Cross DL. Fescue toxicosis in horses. In: Bacon CW, Hill NS, eds. Neotyphodium/Grass Interactions. New York, Plenum Press, 1997.

Author Dennis J. Blodgett

Consulting Editor Robert H. Poppenga

FETAL STRESS/DISTRESS/VIABILITY

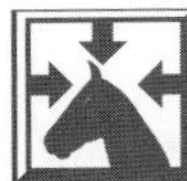

BASICS

DEFINITION

Parameters indicate less-than-ideal conditions for fetal survival (often impaired placental function) that, if they progress, will lead to fetal compromise and its eventual demise

PATHOPHYSIOLOGY

• Maternal systemic disease, fetal abnormalities and/or placental infection, insufficiency, and separation impede efficient fetal gas exchange and nutrient transfer. • The fetus responds physiologically or pathologically to these alterations in oxygenation and nutrient supply and dies if the impairment is not resolved.
• In some cases, acute fetal stress may cause premature birth of a nonviable foal.

SYSTEM AFFECTED

• Maternal—reproductive • Fetal—all organ systems

INCIDENCE/PREVALENCE

Sporadic

SIGNALMENT

• May be nonspecific • Thoroughbreds, draft mares, and related breeds—twins • Mares > 15 years • American Miniature Horse mares

SIGNS

Historical

• Maternal disease during gestation—colic, hyperlipemia, prepubic tendon rupture, uterine torsion, etc. • Mucoid, hemorrhagic, serosanguinous, or purulent vulvar discharge
• Premature udder development and dripping of milk • Previous examination indicating placentitis or fetal compromise • Previous abortion, high-risk pregnancy, or dystocia
• History of delivering a small, dysmature, septicemic, and/or congenitally malformed foal
• Preexisting maternal disease at conception—laminitis, equine Cushing's-like disease, endometrial inflammation, and/or fibrosis • Previous exposure to abortigenic xenobiotics or infections

Physical Examination

Maternal and Placental Signs

• Anorexia, fever, or other signs of concurrent, systemic disease • Abdominal discomfort
• Mucoid, hemorrhagic, serosanguinous, or purulent vulvar discharge • Premature udder development and dripping of milk • Placentitis, placental separation, or hydrops of fetal membranes by transrectal or transabdominal U/S • Excessive swelling along the ventral midline and evidence of ventral body wall weakening by palpation or transabdominal U/S
• Excessive abdominal distention • Maternal circulating levels of progestins, estrogens, and relaxin reflect fetal well-being and/or normal placental function.

Fetal Signs

• Fetal hyperactivity or inactivity (concurrent with maternal or placental abnormalities) may suggest a less-than-ideal fetal environment or fetal compromise. • Can be assessed by visual inspection or TRP of the mare • Transrectal or transabdominal U/S to measure directly some parameters (see Imaging)

CAUSES AND RISK FACTORS

Preexisting Maternal Disease

• Equine Cushing's-like disease • Chronic, moderate to severe endometrial inflammation and/or fibrosis • Laminitis

Gestational Maternal Conditions

• Malnutrition • Colic • Endotoxemia
• Hyperlipemia • Prepubic tendon rupture
• Uterine torsion • Ovarian granulosa cell tumor • Laminitis • Musculoskeletal disease
• Equine fescue toxicosis or ergotism • Exposure to other xenobiotics • Exposure to abortigenic infections, especially EHV and ETCs

Fetal Conditions

• Twins • Fetal abnormalities—hydrocephalus
• Delayed fetal development—small for gestational age; IUGR • Fetal trauma

Placental Conditions

• Placentitis
• Placental insufficiency
• Placental separation
• Hydrops of fetal membranes
• MRLS

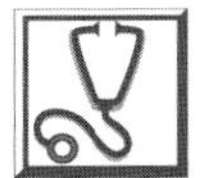

DIAGNOSIS

DIFFERENTIAL DIAGNOSIS

• Normal, uncomplicated, pregnancy—an active, normal fetus as assessed by TRP, transrectal or transabdominal U/S and various laboratory tests
• See sections for specific maternal, fetal and placental conditions.
  ○ Historical and physical examination findings suggesting maternal, fetal, or placental disease
  ○ Laboratory tests, imaging and other diagnostic procedures indicating maternal, fetal or placental disease

CBC/BIOCHEMISTRY/URINALYSIS

• CBC and a serum biochemistry profile may be indicated based on physical examination findings to determine a maternal inflammatory, stress, or left shift, e.g., degenerative or regenerative, leukocyte response.
• Other maternal organ-system involvement that may reflect primary maternal and/or fetal disease

OTHER LABORATORY TESTS

Maternal Progesterone

• May be indicated when uterofetoplacental unit function is in question
• After day 100 of gestation, RIA will detect both progesterone (may be very low after day 150) and cross-reacting 5a -pregnanes of uterofetoplacental origin.
• Decreased maternal 5a -pregnanes are seen in cases of equine fescue toxicosis.
• Normal ranges for levels of 5a -pregnanes may vary with gestational stage and by laboratory.

Maternal Estrogens

• Reflection of fetal estrogen production and viability, especially conjugated estrogens—estrone sulfate
• Normal levels vary by laboratory.

Maternal Relaxin

• Decreases with placental abnormalities

Allantoic/Amniotic Fluid Analysis

• May become a future means to assess fetal karyotype, pulmonary maturity, and to measure fetal proteins
• Samples may reveal bacteria, meconium, or inflammatory cells.
• A higher-risk technique in horses than in humans, and its utility is not yet established.

IMAGING

General Comments

• Transrectal and transabdominal U/S can be useful in diagnosing twins, assessing fetal stress/distress/viability, monitoring fetal development, evaluating placental health and diagnosing other gestational abnormalities, e.g., hydrops of fetal membranes.
• Confirmation of pregnancy and diagnosis of twins should be performed any time serious, maternal disease occurs or surgical intervention is considered for a mare bred within the last 11 mo.
• Twin pregnancy can be confirmed by identifying two fetuses (easier by transrectal U/S when the mare is <90 days pregnant) or ruled out by a nonpregnant uterine horn (by transabdominal U/S during late gestation).
• Fetal stress/distress/viability can be determined best by transabdominal U/S during late gestation. View fetus in both active and resting states for at least 30 min. Note abnormal fetal presentation and position.
• Abnormally high FHR after activity >100 bpm; >40 bpm difference between resting and active rates reflects fetal stress rather than distress.
• Abnormal fetal heart rhythm by echocardiography—may occur immediately before, after and during foaling; also may indicate distress from acute hypoxia.
• Abnormally low FHR—resting, <60 bpm; <50 bpm after day 330 of gestation
• Bradycardia and absence of heart rate variation with activity indicate CNS depression, probably from acute hypoxia.
• Persistent bradycardia correlates well with poor prognosis for survival.
• Absence of fetal heartbeat is a reliable sign of fetal death.
• Absence of fetal breathing movements correlates well with fetal distress.
• Alterations in fetal fluid amounts—
  ○ Normal range for maximal allantoic fluid depth, 4.7– 22.1 cm
  ○ Normal range for maximal amniotic fluid depth, 0.8–14.9 cm; increased amounts reflect hydrops; low amounts indicate fetal distress and longstanding, chronic hypoxia.
• Increased echogenicity of fetal fluids may reflect distress earlier during pregnancy; may be normal during later gestation.

DIAGNOSTIC PROCEDURES

• Fetal ECG has been used to detect twins and to assess fetal viability and distress, but largely has been replaced by transabdominal U/S with ECG capabilities.
• U/S-guided amniocentesis or allantocentesis—poses some risk to the pregnancy; utility not yet established; some interesting possible future applications
• After 2001 outbreak, MRLS research is under way to develop fetal catheterization techniques and other methods of prepartum evaluation.

FETAL STRESS/DISTRESS/VIABILITY

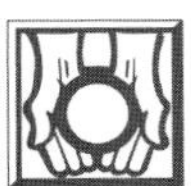

TREATMENT

GENERAL COMMENTS

- Early diagnosis of at-risk pregnancies is essential for successful treatment. The impact of maternal disease on fetal and placental health cannot be underestimated.
- With fetal distress, maintenance of pregnancy (while attempting to treat the cause of fetal compromise) must be balanced with the need to induce parturition (with or without cesarean section) if that becomes necessary to stabilize the mare's health.
- Parturition requires close supervision in cases of fetal stress and distress. The neonatal foal will very likely require intensive treatment.
- Individual circumstances and their sequelae require consideration to determine nature and timing of treatment.
    - PE findings
    - CBC and biochemistry profile results
    - Stage of gestation
    - Nature of maternal disease
    - Hydrops of fetal membranes
    - Evidence of fetal stress, distress or impending demise
    - Occurrence of complications such as dystocia or RFM
- Refer to individual topics for treatment recommendations.

APPROPRIATE HEALTH CARE

Monitoring/managing fetal stress/distress, including the prolonged examination times required for complete serial transabdominal fetal assessments, is best performed at a facility prepared to manage high-risk pregnancies, especially if distress is severe and parturition (induction or cesarean section) is imminent.

NURSING CARE

Depending on the nature of the maternal disease, fetal distress, and necessity of surgical intervention, intensive nursing care very likely will be required for the neonatal foal and mare.

ACTIVITY

- For most cases, exercise will be somewhat limited and supervised.
- Prepubic tendon rupture, laminitis and/or fetal hydrops may necessitate complete restriction of exercise.

DIET

Feed the mare an adequate, late-gestational diet with proper levels of energy, protein, vitamins, and minerals, unless contraindicated by concurrent maternal disease.

CLIENT EDUCATION

- Clients should be aware that early diagnosis is essential for fetal survival.
- Predisposing conditions compromising fetal well-being must be corrected and/or managed for a successful outcome.
- Induction of parturition and cesarean section are not without risk to the mare and foal.

SURGICAL CONSIDERATIONS

Cesarean section may be indicated when vaginal delivery is not possible or in dystocias not amenable to resolution by manipulation alone.

MEDICATIONS

DRUG(S) OF CHOICE

See recommendations in sections for specific conditions—dystocia, fescue toxicosis, high-risk pregnancy, induction of parturition, prepubic tendon rupture, RFM, hydrops, etc.

FOLLOW-UP

PATIENT MONITORING

- Mare and fetus need frequent monitoring until termination of pregnancy.
- Specific monitoring depends on the therapy undertaken, nature of the maternal and/or fetal disease, and complications that may develop.
- Vaginal speculum examination and uterine cytology and culture (as indicated) may be performed 7–10 days postpartum.
- Endometrial biopsy may be indicated as part of the postpartum examination as a prognostic tool for future reproduction.
- Appropriate therapeutic steps should be taken based on these findings.

PREVENTION/AVOIDANCE

- Early monitoring of mares with a history of fetal stress/distress/viability • Correction of perineal conformation to prevent placentitis
- Complete breeding records, especially for recognition of double ovulations, early diagnosis of twins (<25 days; ideally, days 14–15) and selective embryonic or fetal reduction
- Management of preexisting endometritis before breeding • Careful monitoring of pregnant mares for vaginal discharges and premature mammary secretions • Removing mares from fescue pasture or ergotized grasses or grains during last trimester (minimum of 30 days prepartum) • Avoid breeding or using ET procedures in mares predisposed to producing stressed, distressed, or dead foals due to congenital conditions. • Prudent use of medications in pregnant mares • Avoid exposure to known toxicants. • Management of ETCs for prevention of MRLS

POSSIBLE COMPLICATIONS

- Abortion, dystocia, RFM, endometritis, metritis, laminitis, septicemia, reproductive tract trauma, and impaired fertility affect the mare's well-being and reproductive value.
- Neonatal foals that have been compromised during pregnancy are more likely to be dysmature, septicemic, and subject to angular limb deformities than foals from normal pregnancies.

EXPECTED COURSE AND PROGNOSIS

- Pregnancies in which fetal stress has been diagnosed have a guarded prognosis for successful completion, if the predisposing conditions can be treated or managed.
- If evidence of fetal distress continues in the face of treating the mare and fetal viability is a concern, the prognosis for successful completion of gestation is guarded to poor.

MISCELLANEOUS

ASSOCIATED CONDITIONS

- Abortion, spontaneous, infectious • Abortion, spontaneous, noninfectious • Dystocia
- Endometritis • High risk pregnancy, neonate
- High risk pregnancy • Hydrops allantois and amnion • Metritis • Placental insufficiency
- Placentitis • Premature placental separation
- Prepubic tendon rupture • RFM

AGE-RELATED FACTORS

Generally, a greater concern in old mares

PREGNANCY

By definition, the condition is associated with pregnancy.

SYNONYMS

- Premature placental passage/separation • Red bag • RFM • Retained placenta

SEE ALSO

- Abortion, spontaneous, infectious • Abortion, spontaneous, noninfectious • Dystocia
- Embryo transfer • Endometrial biopsy
- Endometritis • High-risk pregnancy, neonate
- High-risk pregnancy • Hydrops allantois/amnion • Induction of parturition
- Metritis • Placental insufficiency • Placentitis
- Premature placental separation • Prepubic tendon rupture • RFM • Twin pregnancy

ABBREVIATIONS

- EHV = equine herpesvirus
- ET = embryo transfer
- ETC = Eastern tent caterpillar
- FHR = fetal heart rate
- IUGR = intrauterine growth retardation
- MRLS = mare reproductive loss syndrome
- PE = physical examination
- RIA = radioimmunoassay
- RFM = retained fetal membranes, retained placenta
- TRP = transrectal palpation
- U/S = ultrasound, ultrasonography

Suggested Reading

Evans TJ, Rottinghaus GE, Casteel SW. Ergopeptine alkaloid toxicoses in horses. In: Robinson NE, ed. Current Therapy in Equine Medicine, ed 5. Philadelphia: Saunders, 2003:796–798.

MacPherson ML. Induction of parturition. In: Robinson NE, ed. Current Therapy in Equine Medicine, ed 5. Philadelphia: Saunders, 2003:315–317.

Author Tim J. Evans

Consulting Editor Carla L. Carleton

FEVER

BASICS

DEFINITION

Fever is defined as a regulated elevation in the thermal set point. Body temperature is actively maintained at this new set point by the body's thermoregulatory mechanisms. Hyperthermia is differentiated from fever as it involves a loss of thermoregulation, resulting in an unregulated rise in body temperature.
• Adult—Normal rectal temperature 100.5° F (38.0° C) • Foal—normal rectal temperature 100°–102° F (37.8°–38.9° C)

PATHOPHYSIOLOGY

The febrile response is a physiologic reaction involving communication between the periphery and the central nervous system. This response involves complex interactions between cytokines, acute phase reactants and the neuroendocrine system. Fever can be induced by endogenous or exogenous pyrogens. Endogenous pyrogens are cytokines (i.e., IL-1β, TNF-α, IL-6, IFN-γ) that are released from cells of the immune system (most commonly, monocytes and macrophages) in response to infectious, inflammatory, neoplastic, traumatic, or immunologic stimuli. Exogenous pyrogens (bacterial products, foreign antigens) can stimulate the release of endogenous pyrogens or can directly stimulate a febrile response. Endogenous pyrogens act on the OVLT (cluster of neurons surrounded by the anterior hypothalamus and preoptic nucleus) to stimulate the production of prostaglandins (especially PGE_2) within the CNS. PGE_2 initiates a cascade that results in an increase in the set point for thermoregulation (in the hypothalamic regulatory center). It is unlikely that the cytokines involved cross the BBB, and their mechanism of communication with the CNS is incompletely understood. It is currently thought that cytokines activate receptors on the systemic side of the neuronal vasculature, resulting in intracellular changes that initiate the production of prostaglandins within the CNS. Toll-like receptors in the area of the OVLT bind exogenous pyrogens resulting in a similar intracellular cascade. Other mechanisms of fever production also exist involving the peripheral vagus nerve, opiate receptors, etc.
• Elevation of the thermoregulatory set point in fever results in the induction of heat conservation mechanisms (i.e., vasoconstriction, piloerection, behavioral changes, increased muscle activity). The duration and magnitude of the febrile response are controlled by endogenous antipyretics (IL-10, arginine vasopressin, α-melanocyte stimulating hormone). TNF-α can act as both an endogenous pyrogen and antipyretic hormone. Cytokine patterns in fever are complex, and vary depending on whether local or systemic inflammation is occurring.

SYSTEMS AFFECTED

All body systems can be affected by a fever-inducing disease process and can be the source of a febrile response.

GENETICS

Certain breeds are predisposed to disorders associated with fever—Fell Ponies (Fell Pony syndrome), Arabians (severe combined immunodeficiency).

INCIDENCE/PREVALENCE

The incidence/prevalence of fever-inducing diseases should be assessed on an individual disease basis.

SIGNALMENT

Nonspecific—different etiologies of fever are more common with animals of certain signalment.

HISTORY

Investigate recent exposure to new animals, recent travel, vaccination history, health of in-contact animals, diet, housing, previous medical history, medication administration, and course of fever.

CLINICAL SIGNS

It is essential that a complete, thorough physical examination is carried out. Horses with fever may show nonspecific signs such as lethargy, anorexia, and weight loss, or physical examination may identify a suspected source of the fever. Physical examination should include oral examination, rebreathing examination, rectal examination, lymph node palpation, and analysis of gait and neurologic status.

CAUSES

Infectious

Respiratory
• Upper respiratory tract—EHV-1, EHV-4, equine influenza virus, *Streptococcus equi*
• Guttural pouch empyema—secondary to upper respiratory tract infection or retropharyngeal lymph node abscessation, *S. equi, Streptococcus zooepidemicus*
• Retropharyngeal lymph node abcessation—*S. equi, S. zooepidemicus, Corynebacterium pseudotuberculosis, Actinobacillus, Mycobacterium avium*
• Sinusitis—primary; secondary to dental disease, trauma, neoplasia, etc.; *Streptococcus* spp., fungi, mixed bacterial infection
• Lower respiratory tract—*S. zooepidemicus, S. equi, Streptococcus pneumoniae, Pasteurella, Escherichia coli, Klebsiella, Pseudomonas, Bacteroides fragillis, Bacteroides melaninogenicus, Mycoplasma, Aspergillus,* phycomycetes, *Pneumocystis carinii, Coccidiodes immitis, Histoplasma capsulatum, Cryptococcus neoformans,* African horse sickness, *M. avium, Mycobacterium bovis, Mycobacterium tuberculosis, Nocardia asteroides,* adenovirus, hendra virus
• Pleuropneumonia—*S. zooepidemicus, Pasteurella, Actinobacillus, E. coli, Klebsiella, Bacteroides* • Foals—*Rhodococcus equi, S. zooepidemicus, S. equi, Staphylococcus epidermidis, Pasteurella, Pneumocystis carinii*
Gastrointestinal
• Peritonitis—primary—*Actinobacillus equuili;* secondary—bowel trauma, ischemia or vascular compromise; abdominal abscess rupture (*R. equi, S. equi*); secondary to immunodeficiency • Colitis—*Salmonella spp., Clostridium difficile, Clostridium perfringens, Ehrlichia risticii* (Potomac horse fever), Cyathastomiasis • Foals—*Salmonella* spp., *Clostridium perfringens, Clostridium difficile,* Rotavirus, Cryptosporidium, *Rhodococcus equi*
• Duodenitis—proximal jejunitis—possible association with *Clostridium perfringens*
• Abdominal abcessation—*Streptococcus equi, Rhodococcus equi, Corynebacterium pseudotuberculosis* • Gastric abscess—foreign body penetration, *Rhodococcus equi,* peritonitis • Vesicular *stomatitis*
Neurologic
• Cerebrum/brainstem—EEE, WEE, VEE, rabies, meningitis (*Streptococcus* spp., *Actinomyces, Klebsiella pneumoniae, E. coli, Salmonella* spp.), brain abscess, mycotic encephalitis, listeriosis, West Nile virus
• Spinal cord disease—EHV-1, vertebral osteomyelitis (*Rhodococcus equi, Streptococcus* spp., *Staphylococcus* spp., *Actinobacillus, Aspergillus, Brucella abortus*)
• Otitis media/interna—*Actinobacillus, Salmonella* spp., *Enterobacter, Pseudomonas, Streptococcus* spp., *Staphylococcus* spp., *Aspergillus*
Hepatic
• Cholelithiasis—associated with *Salmonella* spp., *E. coli, Aeromonas, Citrobacter,* group D *Streptococcus* • Cholangiohepatitis—Gram-negative enteric bacteria (*Salmonella* spp., *E. coli, Citrobacter), Aeromonas, Acinetobacter*
• Infectious necrotic hepatitis—*Clostridium novyii type B* • Tyzzer's disease—*Bacillus piliformis* • Chronic active hepatitis—unknown etiology—possibly bacterial or immune mediated • Liver abscess—adults—extension of bacteria from common bile duct or mesenteric lymph nodes; neonates—secondary to omphalophlebitis, bacteremia
Musculoskeletal
• Clostridial myonecrosis—*Clostridial* spp. (*C. perfringens* most common)
• *Streptococcus*-associated rhabdomyolysis—associated with *S. equi*
• Osteomyelitis/septic arthritis—Many different organisms can be involved, i.e. *E. coli, R. equi, Salmonella* spp., *Bacteroides* spp., *Enterobacteriaceae, Streptococcus* spp., *Staphylococcus* spp., fungi
• Fistulous withers—primary—*Brucella abortus, Actinomyces bovis;* secondary—*Streptococcus* spp., *E. coli, Pseudomonas*

Integument
• Cellulitis—*Staphylococcus* spp. (coagulase positive), *Streptococcus* spp., *Clostridial* spp.
• Dermatophilosis—*Dermatophilus congolensis*
• Subcutaneous abscess—*C. pseudotuberculosis*, foreign body, *S. equi*
• Urticaria—equine Getah virus

Hematologic
Anemia—Equine infectious anemia, piroplasmosis

Cardiovascular
• Vasculitis—equine viral arteritis, equine infectious anemia, *Anaplasma phagocytophilia*
• Phlebitis—Thrombophlebitis (*Streptococcus* spp., *Staphylococcus* spp., *Pasteurella, Actinobacillus, E. coli, K. pneumoniae*)
• Omphalophlebitis—Many organisms can be involved, i.e., *E. coli, Proteus, Streptococcus* spp. • Endocarditis—*Streptococcus* spp., *A. equuili, R. equi, Pasteurella* spp., *Candida parapsilosis, Erysipelothrix rhusiopathiae, S. aureus* • Pericarditis—Idiopathic • Septic—*A. equuili, Enterococcus fecalis, Streptococcus fecalis, C. pseudotuberculosis* • African horse sickness

Renal
Pyelonephritis—gram-negative infections common

Reproductive
Abortion—*Leptospirosis pomona*, EHV-1,

Systemic
Septicemia—neonates and adults (often secondary to immunodeficiency)

Inflammatory

Respiratory
• Smoke inhalation • Acute respiratory distress syndrome—possible association with *E. coli, R. equi, S. zooepidemicus*

Gastrointestinal
• Ulcerative duodenitis—foals • NSAID toxicity • Right dorsal colitis—associated with NSAID toxicity • Sterile peritonitis—uroperitoneum

Hepatic
• Chronic active hepatitis—etiology unknown, possibly immune mediated
• Theiler's disease—acute hepatic necrosis

Cardiovascular
Myocarditis—inflammation secondary to viral, bacterial, or parasitic disease

Integument
• Purpura hemorrhagica—secondary to viral disease, bacterial disease, drug administration, or toxin exposure. Most commonly associated with *S. equi.* • Thermal burns—pyrexia secondary to systemic inflammatory response syndrome and hypermetabolism
• Generalized granulomatous disease—unknown etiology • Pemphigous foliaceus—autoantibody formation against a desmosomal glycoprotein • Bullous pemphigoid—autoantibody formation against epithelial basement membrane • Systemic lupus erythematous—immediate-type hypersensitivity reaction associated with systemic immune complex formation
• Panniculitis—inflammation of subcutaneous adipose tissue precipitated by trauma, infection, autoimmune disease, vasculitis

Systemic
Systemic inflammatory response syndrome—can occur secondary to any process that causes injury or inflammation, i.e., trauma, bacterial infection, burns, endotoxin

Hematologic
• Immune-mediated hemolytic anemia—primary; secondary (associated with drugs, infection, neoplasia) • Neonatal isoerythrolysis—systemic immune complex reaction targeted against red blood cell antigens inherited from sire • Transfusion reaction—immunologic reaction—immediate-type hypersensitivity reaction due to presence of recipient antibodies to donor red blood cells, white blood cells, or plasma proteins • Nonimmunologic—due to contamination of donor product during collection, storage, or administration

Nutritional

• Nutritional myodegeneration—vitamin E and selenium deficiency—cardiac and skeletal forms • Hyperlipemia

Neoplasia

Fever can occur with any form of neoplasia.

Iatrogenic

• Myelogram—transient febrile response reported post myelogram (using Iohexol)
• Transport—depressed alveolar macrophage function and increased bacterial colonization of airways • Transfusion reactions • Adverse drug reaction • Antibiotic-associated colitis—associated with *C. difficile*

Trauma

Traumatic inflammation

Immunodeficiency

• Fever occurs as a result of increased susceptibility to infection. • Severe combined immunodeficiency—prevention of maturation of B cells and T cells • Selective IgM deficiency • Transient hypogammaglobulinemia—delayed onset of immunoglobulin synthesis by neonate
• Agammaglobulinemia—complete B-cell dysfunction • Fell Pony syndrome—anemia, peripheral ganglionopathy, B-cell lymphopenia, decreased IgM • Common variable immunodeficiency

Toxins

• Fescue toxicosis • Blister beetle toxicosis (Cantharidin) • Snake bite • Selenium
• Tetanus—fever due to tonic musculature activity • Castor bean toxicity *(Ricinus communis)* • Arsenic • Mercury • Chlorinated hydrocarbons • Dinotrophenol
• Trichloroethylene extracted feed • Propylene glycol • Algae • Pyrrolizidine alkaloid • Water hemlock *(Cicuta* spp.*)* • Jimson weed
• Mycotoxicosis

RISK FACTORS

• Exposure to infected animals • Poor hygiene
• Transportation • Immunodeficiency
• Intense exercise, showing, racing

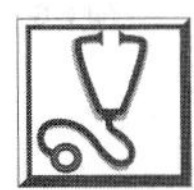

DIAGNOSIS

DIFFERENTIAL DIAGNOSIS

Initial history and physical exam must be thorough and detailed as described earlier. One retrospective study of fever of unknown origin in the horse identified the cause of fever to be of infectious origin in 43% of cases, neoplastic in 22%, immune mediated in 6.5%, and miscellaneous in 19%. In 9.5% of cases, a definitive etiology for fever could not be identified. This suggests that the majority of cases of fever of unknown origin are due to atypical manifestations of common disease rather than more unusual conditions. Thorough investigation can often be rewarding.

FURTHER DIAGNOSTICS

Depending on the abnormalities identified on initial clinical evaluation, ancillary testing will likely be required.

CBC/Chemistry/Urinalysis

• Hematology—fibrinogen—increased during active inflammation • Serum amyloid A—acute-phase protein; marker of the inflammatory response • White blood cell count/differential—Differential can be a useful marker of progression of disease process. • Blood smear—Check for red blood cell parasites and assess cell morphology.
• Packed cell volume and total protein—Assess for evidence of hemoconcentration, anemia, or hypoproteinemia. • Chemistry—Serum chemistry results can indicate specific organ compromise. • Urinalysis—Useful for identifying renal protein loss, urinary tract infection, and hematuria/hemoglobinuria. Urine can be tested for cantharidin toxin and leptospirosis (fluorescent antibody testing).

Other Laboratory Tests

• Blood culture—in any case where bacteremia is suspected • Immunoglobulin levels (neonates) • Coggins test—equine infectious anemia • Direct Coombs test—Use in cases of suspected hemolytic anemia.
• Antinuclear antibody test • Virus isolation (from blood, nasopharynx)—EHV-1, EHV-4, EIV • Serology—paired titers most useful EVA, EHV-1, EHV-4, EEE, WEE, VEE, *Anaplasma phagocytophilium, Brucella*
• Fungal serology • PCR—*Ehrlichia risticii, A. phagocytophilium*, piroplasmosis • Vitamin E level—Assess whole blood levels in cases of suspected nutritional myodegeneration.

Imaging

Ultrasonography
• Thorax—Assess effusion, consolidation, pleural masses.

FEVER

• Abdomen—Assess internal organs, intestinal wall thickness, peritoneal fluid.
• Jugular veins—If thrombosed, assess presence of infection, extent of thrombosis.
• Heart—Assess valves (for development of endocarditis), pericardium.
• Abscess/mass—useful to assess nature and extent of unidentified masses

Radiography

• Thorax—useful in cases of pneumonia, neoplasia, pleural effusion, masses
• Abdomen—limited usefulness, especially in adults—can do contrast studies to assess swallowing and gastric emptying
• Skull—useful in cases of sinusitis, guttural pouch empyema
• Musculoskeletal—Assess physitis, osteomyelitis, osteosarcoma, vertebral body abcessation.

Endoscopy

• Upper respiratory tract—Assess guttural pouches, pharyngeal region, nasomaxillary opening.
• Lower respiratory tract—Identify tracheitis, abnormalities in distal airways.
• Gastroscopy—Assess esophageal and gastric mucosa for ulceration, masses.
• Can also use to assess urethra, bladder, uterus, rectum, and sinuses

Nuclear Scintigraphy

• Identify regions of active inflammation.
• Can perform with radiolabeled white cells or radiolabeled albumin

MRI/CT

Perform studies of head in cases of suspected intracranial or brainstem disease or in cases of otitis interna/media or sinusitis.

Diagnostic Procedures

• Transtracheal wash—culture, cytology, Gram stain—Perform when lower respiratory tract disease is suspected. • Bronchoalveolar lavage—cytology, Gram stain—Perform when diffuse lower airway disease is suspected.
• Guttural pouch lavage—culture, cytology
• Abdominocentesis—culture, cytology, Gram stain—perform if suspect peritonitis or bowel compromise. • Thoracocentesis—culture (including *Mycoplasma* spp. culture), cytology, Gram stain • Sinucentesis—culture, Gram stain, cytology • Cerebrospinal fluid tap—Assess nucleated cell count and protein.
• Lymph node aspiration—culture, Gram stain, cytology • Abscess aspiration—culture, Gram stain, cytology • Fecal assessment—*Salmonella* culture, *Clostridium perfringens* toxin assay, *C. difficile* toxin assay, Rotavirus ELISA/latex agglutination, fecal egg count • Perform similar cultures and toxin assays on gastric reflux. • Biopsy—lung (if suspect parenchymal disease), liver, skin (biopsy area of developing lesions), muscle (immunofluorescent stain for *S. equi*), bone
• Synoviocentesis—cytology, cell count, total protein level, culture (if indicated)
• Pericardiocentesis—Sample pericardial fluid and perform cytology and culture. • Bone marrow aspirate/biopsy—Assess progenitor cells in selected cases of anemia, thrombocytopenia, or leukogram abnormalities.

PATHOLOGIC FINDINGS

Biopsy and necropsy findings vary depending on the cause of fever.

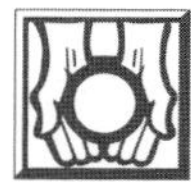

TREATMENT

Treatment should ideally be targeted at a known source of fever. Supportive nursing care should be provided with rest, temperature controlled environment and freely available food and water. Intravenous fluid therapy may be indicated in some cases and enteral or parenteral nutritional support may also be necessary. Pyrexia is a catabolic state and weight loss should be closely monitored.

CLIENT EDUCATION

Ensure client understands the clinical signs to look for in contact horses and encourage client to check horses' temperature daily. If quarantine is indicated, ensure the client understands the importance of this procedure.

SURGICAL CONSIDERATIONS

Exploratory laparotomy may be indicated in cases where an abdominal lesion is suspected but has not been identified by noninvasive means. Surgery may be necessary as an adjunct to medical therapy in some disease processes, i.e., sinusitis secondary to tooth root abscessation, septic arthritis.

MEDICATIONS

There is some debate as to whether treatment of fever is beneficial. Beneficial effects of fever include enhancement of host defenses and inhibition of certain neoplastic cells. Several animal studies looking at serious infection have shown an inverse correlation between mortality and temperature. In addition, the side effects of the commonly used antipyretic drugs (NSAIDs) must be taken into consideration (nephrotoxicity, gastric ulceration, colonic inflammation). Detrimental effects of fever include muscle atrophy and weakness due to increased catabolism, increased metabolic rate, and anorexia. These factors are used as arguments for the use of antipyretics. In addition, pyrexia can result in seizures (unlikely at temperatures below 108° F in most species) and prolonged fever can result in cardiovascular collapse. Reducing fever is often thought to improve patient comfort, but it is difficult to discern if this effect is due to reducing fever or secondary to the analgesic effects of most antipyretic medications. External cooling has been shown in humans to increase discomfort. This should be considered prior to administering alcohol baths.

DRUG(S) OF CHOICE

NSAIDs

NSAIDs are the traditional therapy to reduce fever. Benefits, disadvantages, and potential side effects of such treatments must be carefully weighed before such treatment is instituted. Commonly used NSAIDs include flunixin meglumine, phenylbutazone, and ketoprofen.

Corticosteroids

• Corticosteroids act as anti-inflammatory agents, and at higher doses as immunosuppressive agents. These drugs can be useful in the treatment of selected nonseptic inflammatory and immune mediated diseases. It is essential to ensure that no infectious causes of fever are present at the onset of corticosteroid use and to ensure that the patient is being appropriately treated for any ongoing infectious process. Corticosteroid treatment should be gradually tapered off after treatment due to induced suppression of the hypothalamic-pituitary-adrenal system. Commonly used corticosteroids include dexamethasone, prednisolone, and prednisolone sodium succinate.
• Other anti-inflammatory drugs that are in use include azathioprine, cyclophosphamide, aurothioglucose, and pentoxifylline.

Antimicrobials

• Ideally, the source of fever and etiologic agent should be identified before antimicrobial therapy is initiated. Bacterial sources of fever should be treated with antibiotics based on culture and sensitivity results. The location of infection must be taken into consideration with appropriate antimicrobials chosen to target this location (i.e., consider the ability of drugs to penetrate the blood-brain barrier in cases of meningitis). It is also important to consider any potential side effects. In circumstances where empirical treatment must be initiated without the benefit of culture and sensitivity results, broad spectrum antimicrobial cover should be initiated, bearing in mind the most likely organisms to be involved.
• Potential side effects must be taken into consideration and nonessential use of antibiotics should be avoided to prevent increased development of resistance and to avoid antibiotic-induced colitis. In some cases, local therapy is more appropriate than systemic therapy, and undesirable side effects are decreased with local therapy (i.e., intra-articular and regional administration in septic joints/osteomyelitis).
• Fungal disease can be difficult to treat in the horse due to the lack of availability of antifungal agents and the expense of treatment. Therapy should ideally be initiated based on culture and sensitivity results. Available antifungal agents include amphotericin B and itraconazole.
• Parasitism should be treated with institution of a comprehensive deworming program

based on the needs and facilities of the individual horse and property. It is important to monitor for development of resistance and to treat for encysted cyathastomes and tapeworms.

• Viral disease rarely has directed therapeutic options and care normally involves supportive therapy. Acyclovir has been used in treatment of the neurologic form of EHV-1, and interferon therapy has been tried in the treatment of West Nile virus. Other therapies may become available in the future.

Miscellaneous Treatment

Depending on the disease process, further therapy may be indicated (i.e., antiendotoxic treatment, red blood cell transfusion, plasma transfusion, intranasal oxygen, etc.).

PRECAUTIONS

NSAIDS

Can result in nephrotoxicity, gastric ulceration, or ulcerative colitis. Side effects are more common in dehydrated animals.

Corticosteroids

• Can induce hypothalamic-pituitary-adrenal system suppression or immunosuppression.
• Corticosteroids have been associated with development or worsening of laminitis in isolated cases.

Antimicrobials

• The use of any antibiotic can result in antibiotic-induced colitis. Aminoglycosides are nephrotoxic, and monitoring of renal parameters should be conducted along with therapeutic drug monitoring. Antibiotic use has the potential to increase resistance within a bacterial population; thus, indiscriminate antibiotic use must be avoided.
• Amphotericin B is potentially nephrotoxic; thus, careful monitoring must be implemented. Itraconazole should be used with care in cases with hepatic impairment.

POSSIBLE INTERACTIONS

Care should be taken in using multiple drugs that are potentially nephrotoxic in patients who are dehydrated or hypovolemic.

FOLLOW-UP

PATIENT MONITORING

Patients should be closely monitored for signs of disease progression or resolution. Therapeutic efficacy should be monitored by assessing clinical abnormalities on a regular basis (i.e., fibrinogen concentration, ultrasonographic or radiographic findings) and closely monitoring temperature, appetite, and attitude. While the patient is receiving medications, monitoring should be used to assess for side effects; i.e. monitor total protein, albumin, and creatinine while undergoing NSAID treatment, and monitor fecal consistency while receiving antimicrobials.

PREVENTION/AVOIDANCE

• Minimize transport of horses between farms and keep resident and transient populations separate.
• Follow simple biosecurity rules when working with horses, i.e., washing hands between animals, isolating animals with signs of disease.
• Maintain current vaccination status on all horses.

POSSIBLE COMPLICATIONS

• Many disease processes that cause fever have been associated with a risk for the development of laminitis.
• Many horses with severe infectious disease such as colitis or pleuropneumonia have subclinical coagulopathies and are at risk for jugular thrombophlebitis and disseminated intravascular coagulopathy.
• Anorexia can predispose horses and ponies and donkeys to hyperlipemia.

EXPECTED COURSE AND PROGNOSIS

Variable depending on cause of fever

MISCELLANEOUS

AGE-RELATED FACTORS

• Neonates—Neonates are immunodeficient prior to receiving colostrum; thus, they are at risk for a variety of infectious agents within the environment that can localize to various body tissues.
• Foals
  ○ Foals have an increased susceptibility to disease when maternal immunity wanes.
  ○ Stressful situations during the early period of life contribute to increased risk of infections.
  ○ *Rhodococcus equi*—Exact timing of infection and course of disease are still not fully understood. Signs of disease are seen between 1 and 6 months of age.
• Racehorses
  ○ Transportation and exercise can both contribute to compromised immune function and increased susceptibility to disease. Racehorse populations are often transient, with constant exposure to new horses occurring, thus increasing the risk of exposure to infectious agents.
  ○ Pleuropneumonia
  ○ Viral respiratory disease
• Older horses—neoplasia

ZOONOTIC POTENTIAL

• Rabies
• *Salmonella* spp.
• Brucellosis
• Leptospirosis
• EEE, WEE, VEE
• Anthrax
• Cryptosporidium
• *Clostridium difficile*
• *Rhodococcus equi* (immunocompromised individuals)
• Hendra virus

PREGNANCY

Fever and the associated inflammatory response can be detrimental to pregnancy; thus, fetal evaluations should be performed in febrile pregnant mares. Foaling should be attended and the foal carefully assessed for signs of in utero compromise. Drug therapy should be carefully considered in the late term mare to ensure there are no contraindications to the drugs chosen.

SYNONYM

Pyrexia

ABBREVIATIONS

• PCR = polymerase chain reaction
• BBB = blood-brain barrier
• CNS = central nervous system
• DIC = disseminated intravascular coagulopathy
• EEE – Eastern equine encephalitis
• EHV = equine herpesvirus
• EIV = equine influenza virus
• EVA = equine viral arteritis
• IFN = interferon
• IL = interleukin
• NSAID = nonsteroidal anti-inflammatory drug
• OVLT = organum vasculosum laminae terminalis
• PG = prostaglandin
• TNF = tumor necrosis factor
• VEE = Venezuelan equine encephalitis
• WEE = Western equine encephalitis

Suggested Reading

Dinarello CA. Infection, fever, and exogenous and endogenous pyrogens: Some concepts have changed. J Endotox Res 2004;10:201–222.

Greisman LA, Mackowiak PA. Fever: Beneficial and detrimental effects of antipyretics. Curr Opin Infect Dis 2002;15:241–245.

Hines MT. Changes in body temperature In: Reed SM, Bayly WM, Sellon DC, eds. Equine Internal Medicine, ed 2. St. Louis: Saunders, 2004:148–155.

Mair TS, Taylor FGR, Pinsent PJN. Fever of unknown origin in the horse: A review of 63 cases. Equine Vet J 1989;21:260–265.

Author Julie Ross

Consulting Editors Ashley G. Boyle and Corinne R. Sweeney

FLEXURAL LIMB DEFORMITY

BASICS

DEFINITION

Flexural limb deformity is ultimately the inability to fully extend a limb. Specifically, it is a conformational limb abnormality that can be defined as a deviation of the limb in the sagittal plane, described as either persistent hyperflexion or hyperextension of the joint region. The flexural deformity is named according to the joint involved. Joints commonly involved include: distal interphalangeal, metacarpophalangeal/metatarsophalangeal, and carpus. Flexural limb deformities may be congenital or acquired.

PATHOPHYSIOLOGY

There are two main categories associated with the etiology of FLD: congenital and acquired.

Congenital

• Present at birth • Pathophysiology is not completely understood but thought to involve genetic predisposition, intrauterine malpositioning and teratogens (i.e., ingestion of locoweed and hybrid Sudan grass by the mare, maternal influenza infection, collagen cross-linking, and equine goiter).
• Commonly—digital hyperextension deformities, and contractural deformities
• FLD is a common cause of dystocia in the mare.

Acquired

• Several factors are thought to contribute to the development of acquired flexural deformities, including nutrition, infectious polyarthritis. and trauma. • Nutrition— Excessive intake and abrupt changes in quality and quantity of feed can lead to accelerated growth in foals. It is believed that during the rapid growth phase, the longitudinal growth rate of the bone exceeds the ability of the tendons to lengthen passively, pulling the respective joint into flexion.
• Polyarthritis and trauma—Both are painful conditions that result in the "flexion result reflex," leading to an acquired contractural deformity.

SYSTEM AFFECTED

• Musculoskeletal: FLD is commonly found in the distal interphalangeal joint, metacarpophalangeal joint, metatarsophalangeal joint, and carpus.

GENETICS

Congenital FLD is thought to have a genetic predisposition.

INCIDENCE/PREVALENCE N/A

GEOGRAPHIC DISTRIBUTION

Worldwide

SIGNALMENT

Breed Predilections N/A

Mean Age and Range

• Congenital deformity—present at birth
• Acquired deformity—Flexural deformities at the distal interphalangeal joint usually occur at 1–4 mo of age; deformities at the metacarpophalangeal joint usually occur at 12–14 mo of age.

Predominant Sex N/A

SIGNS

General Comments

Flexural limb deformity is a common orthopedic problem in foals.

Historical

• Dystocia in the mare may occur secondary to flexural deformity in the foal. • The foal may have difficulty rising or ambulating. There is sometimes a history of failure to stand and nurse.

Physical Examination

- Congenital
    - Present at birth
    - Digital hyperextension—Toes lift off of the ground due to flaccidity of the flexor tendons and the foot may rock back on the heel. More severe cases result with the foal walking on the palmar/plantar surface of the phalanges, which can result in skin abrasions of the pastern and fetlock; occurs mainly in the hind limbs.
    - Contractural deformities—Foals with contracture usually have no voluntary extension of the affected limb. Often occurs bilaterally. If the deformity is located at the distal interphalangeal joint, the foals walk on their toes, and the dorsal hoof wall is often concave (dish-like) in appearance with increased heel length ("club foot") observed. If the metacarpophalangeal joint is involved, the foal will often have difficulty standing and knuckle over at the fetlock. If the carpus is affected, the foals can be observed to buckle forward.
- Acquired
    - Contractural deformity of the distal interphalangeal joint—short toe and steep dorsal hoof wall angle. Over time, a "boxy" appearance is observed as the heel increases in length relative to the toe. Stage I—Angle of the dorsal hoof wall is less than 90°. Stage II—angle of the dorsal hoof wall is >90°.
    - Contractural deformity of the metacarpophalangeal/metatarsophalangeal joint: Characterized from a straight angle to "knuckled-over" appearance at the fetlock. More common in the front limbs but can occur in the hind limbs.
    - Contractural deformity of the proximal interphalangeal joint: Commonly occurs bilaterally. Dorsal subluxation with audible click heard as the foal walks.

CAUSES

Congenital

• Genetic predisposition • Uterine malpositioning • Teratogens • Multifactorial
• Prematurity/dysmaturity (hyperextension/laxity)

Acquired

• Pain • High plane of nutrition • Rapidly growing foals • Infectious polyarthritis
• General disuse of limbs; thick bandages or casts (hyperextension/laxity) • Genetics
• Inability to bear weight of affected limb
• Overload of unaffected limb • Trauma

RISK FACTORS

• Multifactorial • Nutrition offering high energy and protein

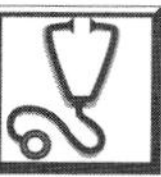

DIAGNOSIS

DIFFERENTIAL DIAGNOSIS

• Rupture of the common digital extensor or lateral digital extensor—swelling over the dorsolateral carpus—ends of the extensor tendon can be palpated within the tendon sheath.
• Rupture of the SDFT or DDFT could mimic digital hyperextension—palpation and ultrasound of the flexor tendons should differentiate.

CBC/BIOCHEMISTRY/URINALYSIS

Complete CBC/biochemistry workup prior to administration of oxytetracycline

OTHER LABORATORY TESTS N/A

IMAGING

Radiography and ultrasonography commonly show no abnormal findings. Radiographs may be helpful in detection of bony abnormalities such as osteochondrosis and degenerative joint disease. Premature foals with significant tendon/ligament laxity should have radiographs of the carpus and tarsus to assess for ossification of the cuboidal bones.

OTHER DIAGNOSTIC PROCEDURES

• Observation of the foal standing and walking
• Manipulation/palpation of the limb, in both weight-bearing and non–weight-bearing positions (difficulty in manipulating the limb into a normal position aids in determining prognosis). Palpation of the flexor tendons while attempting to straighten a limb with contracture can help to determine which tendon is involved (becomes taught).

PATHOLOGICAL FINDINGS N/A

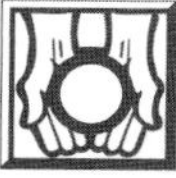

TREATMENT

AIMS OF TREATMENT

• Progress toward normal limb position
• Pain management to encourage weight bearing for contractural deformities
• Bandages/splints/casts/oxytetracycline to induce laxity and straighten the limb for contractural deformities • Strengthening of the musculotendinous unit for hyperextension deformities

APPROPRIATE HEALTH CARE N/A

NURSING CARE: CONSERVATIVE TREATMENT

Congenital Deformities

Digital Hyperextension Deformity

• Moderate exercise • Light bandages (protection of the palmar/plantar aspect of the phalanges) • Corrective shoeing, application of glue-on shoes with heel extensions

Contractural Deformity

• Encourage weight-bearing exercise (use NSAIDs if needed); physical therapy manipulation of the limbs in recumbent foals is also possible. • Oxytetracycline 3 g IV in 250 or

500 mL saline, by binding calcium ions thought to aid in tendon relaxation • Correct nutrition • Corrective shoeing, toe-extensions • Splints and casts, used to relax the muscle-tendon unit

Acquired Deformities

Distal Interphalangeal Joint

• Balanced nutrition • Exercise • NSAIDs will help keep the foal exercising during the painful passive stretching of the tendons.
• Toe-extensions increase tension in the DDFT resulting in stretching of the tendon unit.
• Casts also have been used to aid correction of the deformity.

Metacarpophalangeal Joint

• Balanced nutrition • Physical therapy
• NSAIDs, alleviate pain associated with stretching of the tendons. • Corrective shoeing—wedge pads used to raise the heel, alleviating the DDFT while bringing the fetlock into a more normal position

Carpal Joint

• Physical therapy and splints have been used to manage carpal region deformities.

Proximal Interphalangeal Joint

• Trimming of the hoof

ACTIVITY

See Nursing Care.

DIET

• Balanced nutrition is very important. Early weaning may be necessary for foals with acquired flexural deformities (lower plane of nutrition), especially if accompanied by angular limb deformity, physitis, or osteochrondrosis. Attention to the calcium-phosphorus balance may be important for flexural deformities.

CLIENT EDUCATION

• Creep feeding of young foals and high-energy diets in weanlings may contribute to the development of ALD.

SURGICAL CONSIDERATIONS

Congenital

• Digital hyperextension deformity—Historically, tenoplasty as surgical management for small or miniature foal patients has been described.
Contractural deformity—See Acquired Deformities.

Acquired Contractural Deformities

• Distal interphalangeal joint
  ○ Desmotomy of the accessory check ligament of the DDFT indicated for stage l contractural deformities. Correction observed immediately up to a few days following surgery.
  ○ Tenotomy of the DDFT recommended for stage ll contractural deformities, used as a salvage procedure.
• Metacarpophalangeal joint
  ○ Desmotomy of the accessory ligament of the DDFT or the SDFT, depending on which tendon palpates tighter, in order to allow for release. Transection of both accessory ligaments as well as the suspensory ligament may be required in severe cases; however, the prognosis for athletic soundness is poor.
• Carpal joint
  ○ Tenotomy of the ulnaris lateralis and flexor carpi ulnaris tendons. Transection of the palmar carpal ligament and palmar joint capsules has also been described, but with limited success. These procedures can also be used for refractory congenital carpal contracture.
• Proximal interphalangeal joint
  ○ Transection of the accessory ligament of the DDFT and the medial head of the DDFM has been described. Doral subluxation of the pastern that is not reducible may require realignment and surgical arthrodesis to achieve soundness.

MEDICATIONS

DRUG(S) OF CHOICE

• For surgical cases, NSAIDs (flunixin meglumine 1.1 mg/kg) and antibiotics (i.e., gentamicin 6.6 mg/kg IV daily or amikacin 25–30 mg/kg IV daily and potassium penicillin 22,000 IU/kg IV QID) can be given as needed perioperatively. • Oxytetracycline (for a 50-kg foal, 3 g in 250 or 500 mL saline IV, may be repeated 2–3 times given 24 hr apart). • NSAIDs to relieve pain associated with stretching of the tendons—flunixin meglumine (1.1 mg/kg IV or PO daily to BID), phenylbutazone (2–4 mg/kg IV or PO daily to BID), or ketoprofen (2.2 mg/kg IV daily)

CONTRAINDICATIONS N/A

PRECAUTIONS

• NSAIDs can have an ulcerogenic effect on foals—can administer oral GastroGard (omeprazole 1–2 mg/kg PO once daily) or ranitidine (10 mg/kg PO TID or 1.5 mg/kg IV TID in 250 mL saline) while the foal is in the hospital and receiving NSAIDs.
• Monitor renal values in foals prior to use of oxytetracycline. Renal failure has been reported in foals following administration for FLD.

POSSIBLE INTERACTIONS N/A

ALTERNATIVE DRUGS N/A

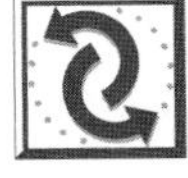

FOLLOW-UP

PATIENT MONITORING

• Monitor foals in splints and casts closely in order to avoid pressure sores. • Evaluation of standing and ambulating without splints is often needed to determine whether continued splinting is necessary, • Monitor renal values in foals receiving oxytetracycline (specifically creatinine and BUN).

PREVENTION/AVOIDANCE

Balanced nutrition (avoid high-energy and excessive protein diets)

POSSIBLE COMPLICATIONS

• Renal failure from oxytetracycline given to a neonate • Rupture of the common digital extensor tendon secondary to flexor tendon contracture • Nonsurgical management—pressure sores • Surgical management—hematoma/seroma formation at surgery site, incisional infection, wound dehiscence

EXPECTED COURSE AND PROGNOSIS

• Mild cases of congenital FLD respond within several days. If the deformity is corrected easily with manual reduction, the prognosis with medical treatment is generally good. • If medical management does not result in improvement of FLD, surgery intervention should be considered.
• Reasonable prognosis for desmotomy of the inferior check ligament with contracture at the distal interphalangeal joint • Poor athletic prognosis for moderate to severe FLD (especially for nonreducible carpal contracture and stage II contractural deformity at the distal interphalangeal joint)

MISCELLANEOUS

ASSOCIATED CONDITIONS, AGE-RELATED FACTORS, ZOONOTIC POTENTIAL, PREGNANCY

N/A

SYNONYM

Contracted tendons

SEE ALSO

Angular limb deformity

ABBREVIATIONS

• DDFM = deep digital flexor muscle
• DDFT = deep digital flexor tendon
• FLD = flexural limb deformity
• SDFT = superficial digital flexor tendon

Suggested Reading

Adams SB, Santschi ES: Management of congenital and acquired flexural limb deformities. Proc Am Assoc Equine Pract 2000;46:117.

Auer JA. Flexural limb deformities. In: Auer JA, ed. Equine Surgery. Philadelphia: WB Saunders, 2006:1150–1165.

Trumble T. Orthopedic disorders in neonatal foals. Vet Clin North Am Equine Pract 2005;21:357–385.

Author Shannon J. Murray
Consulting Editor Margaret C. Mudge

FLUID THERAPY, NEONATE

BASICS

DEFINITION

• Fluid therapy consists of oral or intravenous fluids administered for treatment of shock, fluid replacement, or fluid maintenance. • This topic will focus on intravenous fluid therapy in the foal, although in less debilitated foals, fluid requirements should be supplied by nursing or enteral feeding of mare's milk.

PATHOPHYSIOLOGY

• Neonates distribute fluids to the interstitial space rapidly due to a high capillary filtration coefficient. Because of this filtration as well as limited renal function, neonates do not handle large fluid loads as well as adults. Sepsis and hypoxia may exacerbate leakage of fluids into the interstitial space. • Neonatal foals have low urinary fractional excretion of sodium, and this sodium conservation is well-suited to the low sodium milk diet. However, the sodium in isotonic intravenous fluids may cause sodium overload. • Hemorrhagic shock results from loss of whole blood. The systemic effects of hypovolemia are compounded by the loss of oxygen-carrying capacity. • Hypovolemia—A decrease in circulating blood volume will lead to decreased perfusion of tissues, including vital organs. If perfusion impairment is severe or prolonged, organ failure may result. • Septic shock results from poor systemic vascular tone, reduced myocardial contractility, and maldistribution of blood flow. Fluid resuscitation is required, but inotropic and vasopressor therapy might also be required.

SYSTEMS AFFECTED

• Cardiovascular—Hypovolemia can reduce cardiac output and tissue perfusion.
• Renal/urologic—Hypovolemia and poor systemic perfusion will decrease renal blood flow and renal perfusion, leading to azotemia, and if the insult is severe enough, to renal failure (tubular necrosis). • Gastrointestinal— Poor perfusion can result in loss of mucosal barrier function, and secondary bacterial translocation.

GENETICS

N/A

INCIDENCE/PREVALENCE

N/A

GEOGRAPHIC DISTRIBUTION

N/A

SIGNALMENT

N/A

SIGNS

Historical

• Decreased nursing or lack of nursing for 4 hours or longer. Mare will have a full udder and may be streaming milk. • Fluids losses though diarrhea or third-spacing in the intestinal tract

Physical Examination

• Signs of dehydration include prolonged skin tent, sunken eyes, tacky mucous membranes, and prolonged capillary refill time. • Signs of hypovolemia include tachycardia, cold extremities, decreased urine production, depressed mentation, and poor pulse pressure.

CAUSES

Indications for Fluid Therapy

• Correct dehydration • Increase perfusion, treat hypovolemia • Sepsis/septic shock • Diarrhea or other gastrointestinal fluid losses
• Gastrointestinal disease preventing enteral intake • Volume replacement after acute blood loss (e.g., umbilical bleeding)

RISK FACTORS

N/A

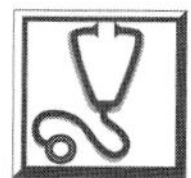

DIAGNOSIS

DIFFERENTIAL DIAGNOSIS

N/A

CBC/BIOCHEMISTRY/URINALYSIS

• Hemoconcentration (elevated PCV and TP) is common with dehydration. • Blood lactate concentration—If elevated it may indicate poor perfusion or tissue hypoxia, although this is not specific for the need for fluid therapy since sepsis, hepatic dysfunction, and respiratory compromise can also contribute to hyperlactatemia. • Urine specific gravity in normal foals is usually <1.008. Urine concentration will increase with dehydration and hypovolemia, provided renal function is normal. • Serum electrolytes should be monitored before and during fluid therapy.

OTHER LABORATORY TESTS

• Blood gas—Lactic acidosis occurs with significant hypovolemia or sepsis. • IgG should be checked in the neonatal foal—If plasma transfusion is required, this will need to be factored into the fluid therapy plan.

IMAGING

Vessel appearance on thoracic radiographs

OTHER DIAGNOSTIC PROCEDURES

• Central venous pressure—provides an estimate of right atrial pressure; single measurements are not very useful, but trends can be followed to help assess changes in preload and possible volume overload or end-points for fluid therapy.
• Blood pressure—Indirect or direct measurements can be used. Oscillometric indirect measurements using the cuff over the coccygeal artery are the most practical method.
• Urine output measurements— Urine can be obtained via urinary catheter in a closed collection system. Useful in the determination of renal blood flow and fluid balance • Cardiac output—Measurements are limited to referral centers; they may be useful in guiding fluid and vasopressor therapy in foals with septic shock.

PATHOLOGICAL FINDINGS

N/A

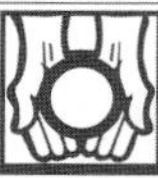

TREATMENT

AIMS OF TREATMENT

Shock Reversal

• Boluses up to 80 mL/kg crystalloid fluid may be needed. Fluids can be administered as boluses of 20 mL/kg (≈1 L in a 50-kg foal), with reassessment after each bolus.
• Rehydration—Volume needed can be estimated by the formula (% dehydration × weight [kg]). • Hemorrhagic shock—Volume replacement with crystalloid fluid is estimated at 3 times the volume of blood lost; however, blood transfusion is recommended with significant blood loss, and volume overload is a concern if the volume is replaced by both crystalloids and whole blood. More conservative resuscitation is recommended while blood is obtained for transfusion.

Correction of Electrolyte Abnormalities

• For conditions such as uroabdomen in which hyponatremia and hyperkalemia are present, fluid therapy can be used to correct these imbalances (e.g., by giving 0.9% saline) • As perfusion is improved and lactic acidosis is resolved, serum potassium concentration may fall; therefore, additional potassium supplementation may be needed.

Maintenance Fluids

• Fluids with lower sodium and higher potassium than that of plasma (e.g., Plasma-lyte 56 or Normasol-M) are more appropriate for maintenance requirements of neonatal foals.
• Daily requirements for maintenance fluid administration can be calculated using the Holliday-Segar formula:
  ○ 100 mg/kg/day for the first 10 kg body weight
  ○ 50 mL/kg for the second 10 kg body weight, and
  ○ 25 mL/kg for body weight above 20 kg
  ○ A 50-kg foal would therefore require 2250 mL/day. The use of this formula results in substantially lower volume delivered than with a more traditional estimate of 60–80 mL/kg/day.
• Fluids can be administered as a CRI or as boluses given every 1–4 hr. Although constant rate may be preferred, bolus administration may be easier for ambulatory foals that are housed with the mare.
• Additional fluid losses (diarrhea, reflux) should also be considered when determining fluid rates.
• Enteral and parenteral nutrition should be considered—Increasing volumes of nutrition will lower the intravenous fluid requirements.

APPROPRIATE HEALTH CARE

Intravenous fluids are generally administered as inpatient medical management. Foals with severe systemic disease or hypovolemic shock will require emergency inpatient intensive care management.

NURSING CARE

• Intravenous catheter care—Over-the-wire flexible 14- or 16-gauge catheters placed in sterile fashion are preferred for long-term fluid and medication administration. Over-the-needle catheters can be placed for emergency administration of fluids. • Catheter should be flushed with heparinized saline q6 h if fluids are not being administered continuously. • IV fluids containing dextrose should be discarded after 24 hr to reduce the risk of contamination.

ACTIVITY

• Foals requiring intravenous fluids must be restricted to a stall or small pen in order to maintain the IV catheter and deliver fluids. Foals may need to be separated from the mare (at least by a divider or in a pen) if they are receiving continuous IV fluids.

DIET

See Nutrition in Foals.

CLIENT EDUCATION N/A

SURGICAL CONSIDERATIONS

N/A

MEDICATIONS

DRUG(S) OF CHOICE

Intravenous Fluids

- Crystalloids
  - Lactated Ringer's, 0.9% saline, Plasmalyte 148, and Normosol-R are isotonic crystalloid solutions that can be used for fluid replacement. Normal saline is acidifying due to the high chloride concentration (154 mEq/L), and is generally preferred only if a potassium-free crystalloid is needed for resuscitation (as with uroperitoneum).
  - Plasmalyte 56 and Normosol-M are crystalloid maintenance solutions that are more appropriate for long-term fluid therapy. These solutions may not be readily available, but maintenance solutions low in sodium (40–80 mEq/L) and high in potassium (13 mEq/L) can be made using 0.45% saline or a combination with 5% dextrose in water.
- Colloids
  - Hetastarch 6% (10 mL/kg) is an example of a synthetic colloid that will remain in the vasculature for a longer period of time due to the large molecule size. There is no evidence of superiority of colloid fluids for resuscitation, but colloids are indicated when colloid oncotic pressure is low and volume resuscitation is needed.
- Plasma
  - Plasma is a natural colloid and is the most commonly used colloid in neonatal foals due to the frequent need for immunoglobulin supplementation.
- Whole blood
  - It should not be a first-line fluid for resuscitation unless hemorrhagic shock is present.

Fluid Supplementation

• Glucose—Start with a rate of 4–8 mg/kg/min (in a 50-kg foal, ≈250 mL/hr of a 5% dextrose solution) if enteral or parenteral feedings have not been initiated. Dextrose solution should not exceed 10%. Blood glucose should ideally be <150 mg/dL and >80 mg/dL. If hyperglycemia persists, treatment with insulin may be needed. • Potassium—Since this electrolyte is mainly intracellular, accurate estimates for supplementation are difficult to make. Supplementation of maintenance fluid may range from 10 to 40 mEq/L. The rate of potassium administration should not exceed 0.5 mEq/kg/hr. • Bicarbonate—Should not be used routinely to correct metabolic acidosis since lactic acidosis may resolve readily with fluid resuscitation. If pH <7.2 or there is significant loss of bicarbonate, a combination of intravenous and oral supplementation may be needed. The amount of bicarbonate required can be determined by the formula: Base deficit × 0.3 × Body weight kg), with half the calculated amount given initially, then blood gas reassessed. Bicarbonate is contraindicated with hypoventilation/abnormal respiratory function because the CO_2 produced cannot be eliminated. • Calcium and magnesium supplementation should be guided by ionized values. SIRS appears to produce hypocalcemia and hypomagnesemia; therefore, septic neonates may require supplementation.

CONTRAINDICATIONS

Hypertonic saline is generally not recommended for use in neonatal foals, since it causes rapid changes in osmolarity and foals have less ability to handle large sodium loads.

PRECAUTIONS

• Transfusion reactions are a risk with administration of plasma and other blood products. Any transfusions should be given slowly for the first 10 min, monitoring the foal for any reactions (tachycardia, fever, urticaria, tachypnea, sweating). • HBOCs can be used instead of whole blood or packed red cells if increased oxygen-carrying capacity is needed. The use of HBOCs is limited by expense and availability. • Hetastarch can prolong clotting times at does ≥20 mL/kg. Once Hetastarch has been administered, TP is no longer a good estimate of oncotic pressure, so COP should be directly measured with a colloid osmometer.

POSSIBLE INTERACTIONS

Bicarbonate- and calcium-containing solutions are incompatible.

ALTERNATIVE DRUGS

Dextran is an alternative to Hetastarch, although the risk of anaphylactic reaction limits its use in the horse.

FOLLOW-UP

PATIENT MONITORING

• Volume and perfusion status—The initial response to fluid therapy can be judged by an improvement in mentation, return of peripheral pulse and warmer extremities, urine production, and improvement in mucous membrane color and CRT. Recheck blood work should generally be monitored every 4–24 hr, and fluid composition and rate adjusted accordingly.
• Catheter complications—The IV catheter site should be examined at least daily for any heat, swelling, pain, discharge, or kinking/pulling out of the catheter. • Body weight q24h to estimate fluid balance and adequate nutrition

PREVENTION/AVOIDANCE

Frequent nursing is imperative for maintenance of normal hydration in neonatal foals. Any foal that has not been seen to nurse during a period of 4hr is at high risk of dehydration. Careful monitoring of nursing behavior and fluid losses (e.g., diarrhea) may help to prevent life-threatening hypovolemia.

POSSIBLE COMPLICATIONS

• Fluid overload—Pulmonary and cerebral edema are possible sequelae.
• Hypernatremia—Fluids that are high in sodium (replacement fluids) tend to result in hypernatremia if used for maintenance.
• Thrombophlebitis—Signs include heat, pain, and swelling at the site of catheter insertion, jugular vein thickening, and unexplained fever. The catheter should be removed immediately if thrombophelebitis is noted.

EXPECTED COURSE AND PROGNOSIS

• Foals with uncomplicated dehydration should respond rapidly to fluid therapy, although they may require continued fluid replacement if there are ongoing fluid losses or reduced intake.
• Prognosis depends on the underlying disease.

MISCELLANEOUS

AGE-RELATED FACTORS

Neonatal foals (<2 weeks old) have a large ISF reserve and altered handling of sodium loads compared to adults.

ZOONOTIC POTENTIAL

N/A

PREGNANCY

N/A

SYNONYMS

• Rehydration • Fluid resuscitation

SEE ALSO

• Nutrition in foals • Septicemia, neonatal
• Uroperitoneum

ABBREVIATIONS

- COP = colloid oncotic pressure
- CVP = central venous pressure
- HBOC = hemoglobin-based oxygen carrier
- ISF = interstitial fluid
- PCV = packed cell volume
- SIRS = systemic inflammatory response syndrome
- TP = total protein

Suggested Reading

Buchanan BR, Sommardahl CS, Rohrback BW, Andrews FM. Effect of a 24-hour infusion of an isotonic replacement fluid on the renal clearance of electrolytes in healthy neonatal foals. J Am Vet Assoc 2005; 227:1123–1129.

Palmer JE. Fluid therapy in the neonate: not your mother's fluid space. Vet Clin North Am Equine Pract 2004;20:63–75.

Author Margaret C. Mudge
Consulting Editor Margaret C. Mudge

FUMONISINS

BASICS

OVERVIEW

Fumonisins are a group of mycotoxins produced by the fungus *Fusarium verticillioides* (formerly *F. moniliforme*), which are responsible for the disease ELEM, also referred to as moldy corn disease. The most important of these is fumonisin B_1. ELEM is a fatal disease characterized by rapidly progressing neurologic impairment in horses and other equids. Distinctive lesions include softening and necrosis of cerebral white matter, as well as swollen and discolored livers.

PATHOPHYSIOLOGY

- Fumonisins are structurally similar to the sphingolipids sphingosine and sphinganine, which are necessary for cellular membrane function and cellular regulation. Fumonisins inhibit ceramide synthase, a sphingolipid metabolizing enzyme, resulting in accumulations of sphingosine and sphinganine and disruption of sphingolipid-dependent processes. Clinical and pathological effects are thought to be due to sphingolipid alterations on the vasculature of the brain, cardiovascular dysfunction, and, in some individuals, hepatocellular necrosis.
- For most species, fumonisins are poorly absorbed following oral administration and are rapidly eliminated. Fumonisin tissue concentrations are undetectable in most species studied. The toxicokinetics of fumonisins in horses have not been evaluated.

SYSTEMS AFFECTED

- Nervous
- Hepatobiliary

GENETICS

N/A

INCIDENCE/PREVALENCE

- Fumonisin outbreaks occur sporadically throughout regions of the world, including North America.
- Insect damage and adverse weather conditions are associated with increased fumonisin production. Conditions favoring fumonisin production include a period of drought during the growing season, followed by cool and moist conditions during pollination and kernel formation. Clinical outbreaks occur seasonally, generally from late fall to early spring. Numbers affected can be variable, with as many as 15%–25% of animals within a group being affected.
- ELEM outbreaks occur from time to time under environmental conditions favoring mold production in corn crops, as well as from contaminated corn shipped to other locations.

SIGNALMENT

- Horses, ponies, donkeys, and mules can be affected.
- Any age horse can be affected, but mature horses may be more susceptible.

SIGNS

- Both neurotoxic and hepatotoxic syndromes have been described, but generally some aspects of both syndromes are noted. The predominance of each syndrome is related to the concentration of fumonisin in the feed, the duration of toxin consumption, and the sensitivity of the particular horse.
- The neurologic syndrome is considered the most common. Signs of a fumonisin toxicosis are usually first noticeable following several weeks of daily ingestion of contaminated feed. Once initiated, clinical signs often have a sudden onset and are rapidly progressive.
- Depression, anorexia, blindness, ataxia, aimless wandering, lowered head and/or head pressing, circling, hyperexcitability, facial paralysis, paresis, recumbency, coma, and death
- Severely affected animals may die by 2–3 days; others may survive a week or more after onset of signs.
- Horses may be found dead without the owner noticing any unusual clinical signs.
- Body temperature usually remains normal.
- Depressed horses are usually unresponsive. However, some may become hyperexcitable and unpredictable when disturbed.
- Icterus, hemorrhages, and edema are possible with liver failure.

CAUSES AND RISK FACTORS

- Ingestion of corn and corn products contaminated with fumonisins, or foraging on damaged or moldy corn.
- Much less commonly, fumonisins have been reported in "black oats" feed from Brazil and in New Zealand forage grasses.
- Horses are the most sensitive species to fumonisins.
- The highest concentrations of fumonisins can be found in broken kernels and screenings.
- The minimum dietary concentration associated with induction of ELEM is about 8–10 ppm ingested for a period of approximately 30 days. Higher dosages result in signs as early as 7–10 days. High dosages seem to cause predominantly ELEM and lower exposures for longer periods favor the development of hepatotoxicosis.
- Fumonisins are water soluble, heat stable, and resistant to alkali treatments that render many other mycotoxins inactive during feed processing.

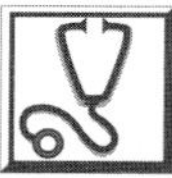

DIAGNOSIS

DIFFERENTIAL DIAGNOSIS

- Rabies—brain positive for rabies virus antigen using fluorescent antibody techniques, histpathology.
- Encephalitis—rapid progression of febrile syndrome with CNS inflammation, high serum antibody titers (especially if acute and convalescent serum samples are available), no history of appropriate vaccination, CSF analysis, pathologic changes in CNS
- Botulism—paralytic syndrome, detection of botulinum toxin via mouse bioassay or ELISA in feed, GI contents or liver.
- Head trauma—history of trauma, physical examination, imaging.
- Hepatic encephalopathy—underlying liver dysfunction, clinical pathology.
- Aflatoxicosis—clinical pathology compatible with liver disease, liver pathology, detection of aflatoxins in feed or liver.
- PA hepatotoxicosis—history of exposure to PA-containing plants, signs related to chronic wasting, clinical pathology compatible with liver disease, liver pathology, detection of PAs in feed.

CBC/BIOCHEMISTRY/URINALYSIS

- Serum biochemistry results are reflective of hepatic disease. Increases in serum lactate dehydrogenase, alkaline phosphatase, aspartate aminotransferase, γ-glutamyl transpeptidase, and bilirubin may be seen.
- Urinalysis is often normal.

OTHER LABORATORY TESTS

- Elevations in serum sphinganine to sphingosine ratios are often pronounced. This assay is performed by only a few diagnostic laboratories.
- Detection of fumonisins in feed specimens can be performed at many veterinary diagnostic laboratories. Representative feed samples can be difficult to obtain because of the long duration from consumption until clinical manifestations occur.
- To date reliable assays for detection of fumonisins in blood or tissues are not available.

• Culturing of the feed samples for the *Fusarium* fungus does not correlate to fumonisin concentrations, because high fumonisin concentrations have been found without the presence of the fungus while other samples have demonstrated large amounts of fungus without concomitant toxin production. Therefore, testing for the toxin is required to diagnose intoxication.
• When testing feed, it is important to obtain representative samples of the entire batch, at various locations and depths within the batch, in order to catch potential "hot spots."

IMAGING

N/A

OTHER DIAGNOSTIC PROCEDURES

Cerebral spinal fluid findings may include elevated protein concentrations, albumin, and IgG concentrations.

PATHOLOGIC FINDINGS

• Evaluation of the brain can reveal massive softening and liquefaction of subcortical cerebral white matter. Lesion size may range from a few millimeters to involving large portions of the white matter of either or both sides of the cerebral hemispheres. Areas surrounding the necrosis are usually edematous and hemorrhagic.
• The liver can appear swollen and brownish on gross examination.
• Histologic examination may reveal fatty change of hepatocytes, loss of hepatic architecture, scattered liver cell necrosis, portal fibrosis, bile stasis, and bile duct proliferation.

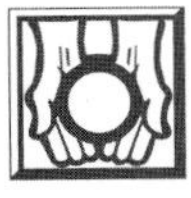

TREATMENT

• There is currently no successful treatment for horses with ELEM. Most horses die or are euthanized.
• Treatment is aimed at providing supportive care for animals with neurologic and/or hepatic disease and reducing further exposure to the source of contamination.
• Outpatient medical management.
• Because of the long latent period involved, gastrointestinal decontamination is of limited value.
• Horses with hepatic dysfunction should be treated with fluids and hepatoprotectants.
• Activity should be decreased to prevent injury in those horses exhibiting neurologic signs. Excitable horses should be sedated to prevent injury to the horse or handler.
• Contaminated feed should be replaced with mycotoxin-free feed.

MEDICATIONS

DRUG(S)

There is no antidote for fumonisins.

CONTRAINDICATIONS, PRECAUTIONS, POSSIBLE INTERACTIONS, ALTERNATIVE DRUGS

N/A

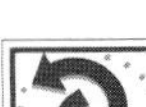

FOLLOW-UP

PATIENT MONITORING

• Neurologic function and hepatic enzymes should be monitored following removal from contaminated feed.
• Animal handlers should take caution around affected horses because their behavior may be unpredictable and serious injury may result.

PREVENTION/AVOIDANCE

• Animal owners should be informed about the conditions favoring toxin production, and the risks involved in feeding corn or corn-based products.
• Corn intended to be fed to horses should be periodically tested so that fumonisin concentrations are below FDA recommended guidelines. Currently, equine feeds should contain no more than 5 ppm dietary fumonisins, which, in turn, should constitute no more than 20% of the total diet.
• No binding agents are currently available to decrease fumonisin absorption following ingestion.
• Contaminated feeds should be either diluted with clean feed and retested prior to feeding or fed to a less sensitive species, such as ruminants.

POSSIBLE COMPLICATIONS

N/A

EXPECTED COURSE AND PROGNOSIS

Horses with ELEM have a poor prognosis and are not likely to recover despite treatment.

MISCELLANEOUS

ASSOCIATED CONDITIONS

N/A

AGE-RELATED FACTORS

N/A

ZOONOTIC POTENTIAL

N/A

PREGNANCY

Ingestion of fumonisin-contaminated corn has been associated with neural tube defects in humans. The significance of these findings to the pregnant mare and fetus has yet to be determined.

SYNONYMS

• Moldy corn disease
• ELEM
• Cornstalk disease

SEE ALSO

N/A

ABBREVIATION

• CNS = central nervous system
• ELEM = equine leukoencepalomalacia
• ELISA = enzyme-linked immunosorbent assay
• PA = pyrrolizidine alkaloid
• ppm = parts per million

Suggested Reading

Cheeke PR. Natural Toxicants in Feeds, Forages, and Poisonous Plants, ed 2. Danville: Interstate Publishers, 1998:122.
Marasas WFO, Riley RT, Hendricks KA, et al. Fumonisins disrupt sphingolipid metabolism, folate transport, and neural tube development in embryo culture and in vivo: a potential risk factor for human neural tube defects among populations consuming fumonisin-contaminated maize. J Nutr 2004;134:711–716.
Osweiler GD. Mycotoxins. Vet Clin North Am Equine Pract Toxicol 2001;17:547–566.
Smith GW, Constable PD. Fumonisins. In: Plumlee KH, ed. Clinical Veterinary Toxicology. St. Louis: Mosby, 2004.
Smith GW. Fumonisins. In: Gupta RC, ed. Veterinary Toxicology, Basic and Clinical Principles. New York: Elsevier, 2007.

Author Petra A. Volmer
Consulting Editor Robert H. Poppenga

FUNGAL PNEUMONIA

BASICS

OVERVIEW

Fungal pneumonia affects the respiratory tract. Two categories of fungal pneumonia have been described in the horse. The first is caused by primary fungal pathogens with discrete geographical restrictions, and caution should be taken diagnosing them outside of their endemic areas if no travel to these areas has occurred. The second form of fungal pneumonia is caused by opportunistic agents such as *Aspergillus* and other environmental species.

SIGNALMENT

Horses with fungal pneumonia may be any age but generally have significant immune impairment or comorbidity such as severe enteric disease. Geographic location is an important consideration for primary fungal pneumonia. *Pneumocystis jiroveci* (previously *Pneumocystis carinii*) has only been reported in foals 1.5–4 months of age.

SIGNS

• Primary fungal pneumonia does not always show dramatic respiratory signs, although weight loss, exercise intolerance, and cough are common. Secondary fungal pneumonias show signs that are generally typical of lower respiratory tract infection, including cough, fever, tachypnea, adventitial lung sounds, and nasal discharge. • Foals with *P. jiroveci* pneumonia typically present with severe respiratory distress and pneumonia that is non-responsive to anti-Rhodococcal agents.

CAUSES AND RISK FACTORS

• Primary fungal pneumonia is caused by inhalation of the infectious form of pathogen fungi such as *Blastomyces dermatiditis, Coccidioides immitis, Cryptococcus neoformans,* and *Histoplasma capsulatum,* and can affect clinically healthy animals. These species are seen in discreet geographical ranges; care should be taken to obtain a travel history on any animal that shows signs of one of these diseases.
• Secondary fungal pneumonia is caused by environmental (ubiquitous) fungi, and occurs only in horses profoundly immunocompromised by conditions such as neoplasia, neutropenia, severe systemic disease, or primary immunodeficiency. Agents identified in horses with secondary pneumonia include *Aspergillus, Phycomytes, Rhizopus, Mucor*, *Acremonium, Paecilomyces,* and *P. jiroveci* in foals. Aspergillosis is frequently secondary to an episode of severe enterocolitis, and is typically seen after broad-spectrum antibiotic use.

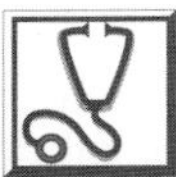

DIAGNOSIS

DIFFERENTIAL DIAGNOSIS

• Bacterial pneumonia/pleuritis • Interstitial pneumonia • Heaves • Intrathoracic neoplasia

CBC/BIOCHEMISTRY/URINALYSIS

Nonspecific inflammatory leukogram

OTHER LABORATORY TESTS

• Serology for *C. neoformans, C. immitis,* and *H. capsulatum* can be supportive of the diagnosis, but previous exposure can cause titers in unaffected animals. • In patients infected with a nonpathogenic fungus, tests of immune function should be ordered.

IMAGING

• Thoracic radiographs typically show significant abnormalities, although no individual pattern is diagnostic. Interstitial, miliary, nodular, and patchy bronchoalveolar patterns have all been described.
• Pleural fluid and areas of consolidation may be seen ultrasonographically.

OTHER DIAGNOSTIC PROCEDURES

• Special care should be taken not to overdiagnose this disease in the field; up to 70% of transtracheal washes have evidence of fungal elements which are considered normal, and should not be overinterpreted, nor treated with antifungal medication unless additional evidence of fungal pneumonia is obtained. • Lung biopsy is frequently diagnostic, although associated with significant complications including fatal hemorrhage.
• Large numbers of fungal material in BAL fluid with consistent clinical signs and radiographs are also acceptable to make the diagnosis.

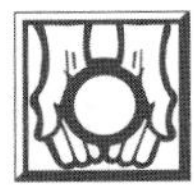

TREATMENT

Supportive care for pneumonia is indicated, such as intranasal oxygen, therapeutic pleurocentesis when necessary, and symptomatic and definitive treatment of other body systems with fungal disease, or comorbidities such as neoplasia or enteric disease.

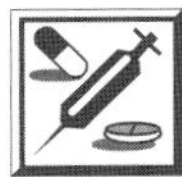

MEDICATIONS

DRUG(S)

• A recent report describes successful treatment of two cases of coccidioidomycosis with compounded fluconazole at a loading dose of 14 mg/kg PO and 5 mg/kg daily thereafter.
• Amphotericin B at a dose of 0.1–0.5 mg/kg IV 3 times a week has also been used successfully.
• Iodides, 5-fluorocytosine, and other drugs in the azole family have also been used. • For *Pneumocystis* infection in foals, trimethoprim-sulfamethoxazole is used at 25 mg/kg PO BID, although oral dapsone can be a useful alternative treatment. • NSAIDs may be added at the clinician's discretion.

CONTRAINDICATIONS/POSSIBLE INTERACTIONS

• Fluconazole (and other azole drugs) have been associated with hepatoxicity. • Amphotericin B is potentially nephrotoxic; kidney function should be monitored closely.
• Trimethoprim-sulfamethoxazole has been associated with colitis in horses and foals.

FOLLOW-UP

PATIENT MONITORING

• Repeated radiographs are useful for monitoring course of disease. • Resolution of clinical signs, BAL, and decreasing serum titers (where applicable) may also be helpful.

PREVENTION/AVOIDANCE

Horses should be housed in areas with low dust levels, as the majority of dust particles are of fungal origin.

POSSIBLE COMPLICATIONS

Most complications are associated with the chronic, severe pneumonia, or the primary cause of immunodeficiency.

EXPECTED COURSE AND PROGNOSIS

• The prognosis for fungal pneumonia is generally poor, although mild infection with some of the primary pathogens may be self-limiting. • Treatment is often unrewarding, and involves long-term (2–4 months) administration of antifungal agents and supportive care. There are several reports of curative therapy for the primary fungal pneumonias, but secondary fungal pneumonia cases are often euthanized shortly after diagnosis, preventing accurate data regarding prognosis with treatment.

MISCELLANEOUS

ASSOCIATED CONDITIONS

• Many of the primary fungal pathogens also cause disease of other organs such as the skin, liver, meninges, or bone. • Infection with typically nonpathogenic fungi is almost always secondary to immunosuppression or severe enterocolitis.

AGE-RELATED FACTORS

P. jiroveci has been diagnosed in foals only.

ZOONOTIC POTENTIAL

Although many of the primary fungal pathogens are zoonoses, the infective stages are generally environmental, and infected animals carry organisms that are of low virulence to humans. Nonetheless, immune compromised humans should be advised to avoid contact with these patients.

PREGNANCY

H. capsulatum and *C. neoformans* are associated with abortion in mares. Many anti-fungals are teratogens, and should be avoided during pregnancy if possible.

ABBREVIATION

• BAL = bronchoalveolar lavage

The author and editors with to acknowledge the contribution of Corinne R. Sweeney, author of this chapter in the previous edition.

Suggested Reading

Ainsworth DM, Hackett RP. Disorders of the respiratory system: fungal pneumonia. In: Reed SM, Bayly WM, Sellon DC, ed. Equine Internal Medicine, 2nd Ed. Elsevier: Saunders, 2004.

Author Rose Nolen-Walston
Consulting Editor Daniel Jean

FUSARIA

BASICS

OVERVIEW

• The *Fusarium* spp. produce a number of mycotoxins, including the trichothecenes, zearalenone, and fumonisins. Fumonisins are produced by *F. verticilloides* (formerly *F. moniliforme*) and are discussed elsewhere.
• The trichothecene class is produced predominantly by *F. sporotrichioides*, and consists of approximately 150 mycotoxins including deoxynivalenol (DON, vomitoxin), T-2 toxin, diacetoxyscirpenol (DAS), and nivalenol. Of these, DON is the most likely to be encountered at clinically relevant concentrations. • The trichothecenes are potent inhibitors of protein synthesis. • The trichothecenes are most commonly found in Canada and the north central United States and primarily in corn and wheat. Humid environmental conditions with alternating warm and cool temperatures favor trichothecene production • Zearalenone, which functions as a weak estrogen, is produced by a number of *Fusarium* spp., primarily *F. roseum (F. graminearum)* in corn, but has also been reported in wheat, barley, rice, and sorghum. Zearalenone toxicosis has not been widely documented in horses. • Zearalenone concentrations in cereal grains are low in the field, but tend to increase under storage conditions with moisture concentrations greater than 30%–40%. • Feeds may be co-contaminated with multiple mycotoxins. Fungal infection of grain, with or without toxin production, reduces nutrient quality leading to poor production and nutritional impairment of animals.

SIGNS

• Horses appear to be resistant to the effects of DON; feed refusal is reported in sensitive species. • Experimentally, T-2 and DAS can cause dermal irritation and necrosis, lymphoid depletion, gastroenteritis, diarrhea, shock, cardiovascular failure and death at concentrations which are unlikely to occur in the field. • In one case, zearalenone was associated with edematous vulvas, prolapsed vaginas, oversized uteruses, and internal hemorrhage in mares and severe flaccidity of the genitals in two male horses fed corn screenings for 30 days. Affected horses rapidly collapsed and died following respiratory paralysis and sudden blindness. Fumonisin was not recognized as a cause of equine illness at the time of the report and thus fumonisin concentrations in the feed were not ruled out. In general, zearalenone is not considered a likely cause of toxicosis in horses.

CAUSES AND RISK FACTORS

• Ingestion of contaminated grain or processed feed. Trichothecene mycotoxins and zearalenone are resistant to the heat and pressure of food processing, and are stable in the environment.
• Unusually cool weather conditions in late summer and early fall coupled with heavy rainfall can result in trichothecene production.
• Initial field production of zearalenone is associated with alternating low temperature and wet weather in late summer. High concentrations of zearalenone usually result from improper storage at high moisture concentrations.

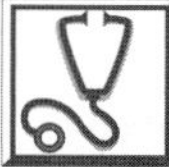

DIAGNOSIS

DIFFERENTIAL DIAGNOSIS

• For the gastrointestinal effects of the trichothecenes
  ○ Cantharidin toxicosis—detection of cantharidin in gastric contents or urine, evidence of insects in hay or GI contents, characteristic lesions
  ○ *Ranunculus* spp.—blistering of skin and mouth, erythema and swelling of muzzle and lips, evidence of ingestion
  ○ NSAIDs—history of use, detection of drug in tissues, gross and histopathology
  ○ Arsenic—arsenic concentration in liver, kidney, urine, hair, feed, hemorrhagic gastroenteritis
  ○ Castor bean (*Ricinus communis*) and other toxic lectins—clinical signs, detection of ricin in tissues, evidence of beans in GI contents, histopathology
  ○ Salmonellosis—clinical signs, isolation of salmonellae from feces, blood, or tissues
  ○ *Clostridium* associated enterocolitis—history of recent antibiotic use, presence of *C. difficile* toxin A and/or B in a freshly passed or frozen fecal sample
• For the reproductive effects of zearalenone
  ○ Fescue toxicosis—history of exposure to *Neotyphodium coenophialum*-infected fescue during late gestation, detection of *N. coenophialum* in plant tissues, determination of ergovaline concentrations in forage or hay, clinical signs
  ○ Endometritis and pyometra— endometrial cytology or biopsy samples, ultrasonographic demonstration of intraluminal free fluid, isolation of potentially pathogenic bacteria from endometrium

CBC/BIOCHEMISTRY/URINALYSIS

No clinically significant changes are expected in horses exposed to either DON or zearalenone.

OTHER LABORATORY TESTS

Feed can be tested for mycotoxins at a veterinary diagnostic laboratory.

OTHER DIAGNOSTIC PROCEDURES

N/A

PATHOLOGICAL FINDINGS (OPTIONAL)

• No pathognomonic lesions are expected from DON. • T-2 and DAS—dermal and mucosal irritation, necrosis, intestinal inflammation
• Zearalenone—swelling of vulva and uterus, ovarian atrophy

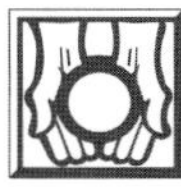

TREATMENT

• Removal of contaminated feed and replacement with high-quality, clean feed. Animals should return to normal performance in weeks to months following removal from toxin.
• There is no specific treatment for the trichothecenes or zearalenone. Symptomatic and supportive treatment is recommended.

MEDICATIONS

DRUG(S) OF CHOICE N/A

CONTRAINDICATIONS/POSSIBLE INTERACTIONS N/A

FOLLOW-UP

PATIENT MONITORING N/A

PREVENTION/AVOIDANCE

• Feed should be visually inspected and tested for the presence of mycotoxins from time to time.
• Avoiding late harvests, removing overwintered stubble from fields, and avoiding a corn/wheat rotation that favors *Fusarium* growth in crop residue can reduce contamination of grains.
• Store grains at less than 13%–14% moisture to prevent mycotoxin production. • Once produced, the trichothecenes and zearalenone are environmentally stable compounds.

POSSIBLE COMPLICATIONS

Poor performance in exposed animals

EXPECTED COURSE AND PROGNOSIS

The clinical effects are expected to resolve following removal of the toxin.

MISCELLANEOUS

ASSOCIATED CONDITIONS N/A

AGE-RELATED FACTORS

Neonatal animals are more susceptible to effects of the trichothecenes.

ZOONOTIC POTENTIAL N/A

PREGNANCY

Although not specifically documented in the horse, failure of implantation and early embryonic death were reported in swine administered zearalenone. Swine are considered the most sensitive species.

SEE ALSO

Fumonisins

Suggested Reading

Mostrom MS. Zearalenone. In: KH Plumlee, ed. Veterinary Toxicology, Basic and Clinical Principles. New York: Elsevier, 2007:977.
Mostrom MS, Raisbeck MF. Trichothecenes. In: RC Gupta, ed. Veterinary Toxicology, Basic and Clinical Principles. New York: Elsevier, 2007: 951.
Osweiler GD. Mycotoxins. Vet Clin North Am Equine Pract Toxicol 2001;17:547–566.
Villar D, Carson TL. Trichothecene mycotoxins. In: KH Plumlee, ed. Clinical Veterinary Toxicology. St. Louis: Mosby, 2004:270.

Author Petra A. Volmer
Consulting Editor Robert H. Poppenga

GAMMA-GLUTAMYLTRANSFERASE (GGT)

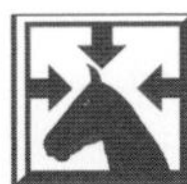

BASICS

DEFINITION

• Serum GGT is a marker for both cholestasis and hepatocellular injury and is one of the most sensitive measures of hepatobiliary disease. But normal values do *not* rule out significant disease.
• Some studies indicate serum increases may be associated with training, particularly overtraining or poor racing performance.
• Urine GGT can be used as a marker for renal tubular degeneration or necrosis.

PATHOPHYSIOLOGY

• GGT is a membrane-bound carboxypeptidase that catalyzes amino acid transfers between peptides and plays a major role in glutathione metabolism.
• High tissue concentrations are found in kidney, liver, and pancreas. Lower concentrations in many other tissues do not appear to affect serum activity appreciably.
• With renal injury, GGT is released into urine, not blood.
• Equine pancreatitis is uncommon, and its contribution to increased serum GGT apart from associated hepatobiliary alterations is unclear. Thus, increases in serum GGT are considered relatively specific for hepatobiliary disease.
• Liver GGT activity is greatest along the brush border of biliary epithelial cells.
• Increased membrane release or increased synthesis (i.e., induction) contributes to increased serum activity.
• The mechanism of release into the blood is proposed to involve membrane solubilization by bile salts, release of membrane fragments/vesicles, or biliary regurgitation.
• The serum half-life is ≅3 days.
• The greatest serum GGT elevations are associated with cholestasis or chronic liver disease, but hepatocellular injury also increases serum activity. Experimentally, bile duct ligation causes 8–10-fold increases by 10 days; cellular injury induced by carbon tetrachloride is associated with peak increases (4–5-fold) within 2 days. In acute cholestasis, bile salts and possibly conjugated bilirubin may precede serum GGT elevations, which depend in part on enzyme induction. Serum GGT also increases with biliary epithelial proliferation which, in chronic diseases, can be marked.
• The mechanism for increased serum GGT associated with training (i.e., overtraining) is unclear, but GGT values >100 U/L tend to be associated with compromised performance. Standard muscle injury markers (e.g., CK, AST, LDH-5) also may be elevated. Affected horses are often recovering from viral infections, upper respiratory disease, or mild lameness; however, they typically do not have elevations in other hepatobiliary parameters.
• Given their large muscle mass, small amounts of GGT in equine muscle might contribute to increased serum activity. Increased GGT activity typically is not reported with more severe muscle injury, however, its source in association with lesser injury remains equivocal.

SYSTEMS AFFECTED

• Hepatobiliary—increases are associated with cholestasis (with or without biliary hyperplasia) and cell injury.
• Renal—tubular epithelial injury increases urinary, but not serum, GGT.
• Musculoskeletal—increases reportedly are associated with overtraining; GGT source is equivocal.
• Pancreas—pancreatitis (uncommon) is a potential source of increased serum GGT.

SIGNALMENT

Neonates—healthy neonatal values during the first 2–3 weeks of life may exceed adult values by 2–3-fold. The change may reflect biliary proliferation. Foals do not absorb GGT from colostrum, as seen in ruminants.

SIGNS

General Comments

Signs do not directly result from increased serum GGT activity but from the underlying disease process.

Historical Findings

• Owners may report icterus, dark-yellow/orange urine, anorexia, weight loss, listlessness, and behavioral changes associated with hepatic failure in conditions associated with cholestasis or hepatocellular injury.
• Abdominal pain (e.g., sweating, rolling) may occur with acute hepatopathies (i.e., capsular swelling) or biliary obstructions.

Physical Examination Findings

• Icterus is frequently observed.
• Increased pulse and respiratory rates, fever, photosensitization, weight loss, and obesity vary and depend on the underlying disease process.

CAUSES

Hepatobiliary System

• Metabolic—secondary to severe anemia (see Hematopoietic System), hyperlipemia, fasting (<50% increase by 2–3 days, nonpathological), or diabetes mellitus
• Immune-mediated, infectious—chronic active hepatitis, Theiler's disease (i.e., serum hepatitis), amyloidosis, endotoxemia, viral (e.g., EIA, EVA, EHV in perinatal foals), bacterial (e.g., Tyzzer's disease, salmonellosis), fungal, protozoal (*Theileria equi, Babesia cabelli*), and parasitic (e.g., liver flukes, with or without strongyle larval migrans)
• Nutritional—hepatic lipidosis; ferrous fumarate toxicity in neonates
• Degenerative—cirrhosis; cholelithiasis
• Toxic—pyrrolizidine alkaloid–containing plants (e.g., senecio, crotalaria), alsike clover, kleingrass, aflatoxin, rubratoxin, *Fusarium* mycotoxins; chemical toxins (e.g., arsenic, chlorinated hydrocarbons, monesin, phenol, paraquat); mild increases are inconsistently reported with halothane anesthesia.
• Anomaly—biliary atresia; portovascular shunts
• Neoplastic—primary liver tumors (rare); metastatic neoplasia (uncommon)

Musculoskeletal System

Possibly associated with overtraining, but no convincing evidence

GI System

• Potentially associated with pancreatitis
• Proximal enteritis: elevated GGT 12-fold more likely versus small intestine strangulation obstruction
• Right displacement of descending large colon: compresses bile duct causing increased GGT in ~50% of cases, versus 2% for left displacement

Hematopoietic System

• Severe anemia (e.g., acute EIA, red maple leaf toxicity, onion toxicity, postparturient hemorrhage) leads to hypoxic injury and hepatocellular swelling, with subsequent cholestasis.
• Hepatic lymphosarcoma, leukemias, etc.

RISK FACTORS

• Pregnancy—some liver diseases causing increased GGT are more common in pregnant mares (e.g., hyperlipemia, Theiler's disease associated with receiving tetanus toxoid, etc.).
• Ponies and donkeys—particularly susceptible to hyperlipemia and hepatic lipidosis
• Antiserum donors—horses used long term as hyperimmunized serum donors (e.g., for *Escherichia coli, P. multocida*) tend to develop amyloidosis.
• Fasting—See Causes.
• Other factors—those associated with any disease leading to cholestasis or hepatocellular injury

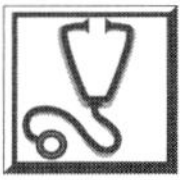

DIAGNOSIS

DIFFERENTIAL DIAGNOSIS

• Consider pancreatitis and overtraining. Otherwise, increased serum GGT is considered specific for hepatobiliary disease. However, it is not specific for the type of hepatobiliary condition.
• Highest elevations are associated with long-standing conditions with severe cholestasis or biliary hyperplasia—chronic active hepatitis, cirrhosis, cholelithiasis, and lipidosis.
• Concurrent obesity and high enzyme activities suggest hyperlipemia/lipidosis; anorexia and weight loss are typical of most other differentials.

CBC/BIOCHEMISTRY/URINALYSIS

• Serum is the preferred sample type, but heparin or EDTA plasma can be used. Other anticoagulants (e.g., citrate, oxalate, fluoride) depress human GGT activity by 10%–15%.
• Serum samples are stable for 3 days at 4° C or for at least 1 month at −20° C.
• Extreme icterus, severe lipemia, and marked hemolysis may affect values.
• No routine lab tests provide an etiologic diagnosis for increased GGT.

Erythrocytes

• Nonregenerative anemia may be seen with liver disease.
• Microcytosis is associated with portosystemic shunts.
• Acanthocytes, schistocytes (from liver microvascular disease), etc. are associated with decreased RBC survival and may contribute to mild hemolytic anemia.
• Any severe hemolytic anemia can cause hypoxic injury, leading to hepatocellular swelling and secondary cholestasis.

GAMMA-GLUTAMYLTRANSFERASE (GGT)

• A severe hemolytic crisis can occur terminally with liver failure.

Leukocytes

• Neutrophilia or neutropenia and monocytosis may occur with inflammatory hepatobiliary disease.
• Evidence of antigenic stimulation may be seen—lymphocytosis or reactive lymphoid cells.

Glucose

• Postprandial hyperglycemia or fasting hypoglycemia may occur with hepatic insufficiency/shunts.
• Hypoglycemia with liver disease carries a guarded prognosis.

Albumin

• Decreased production with hepatic insufficiency may decrease serum concentrations; this usually occurs late.
• Albumin is a negative acute-phase reactant; mild decreases may occur with inflammation.

BUN

Decreases (especially relative to creatinine) with hepatic insufficiency/shunts because of decreased conversion of ammonia to urea

SDH

Increases specifically with hepatocellular injury

AST

Increases with hepatocellular or muscle injury

ALP

Increases primarily with cholestasis

Bilirubin

• Conjugated—increases with cholestasis
• Unconjugated—increases with increased RBC destruction (i.e., hemolysis) and defective hepatocellular uptake (e.g., injured hepatocytes, hepatic insufficiency, vascular shunting); increases with fasting because of a nonpathological decrease in uptake

Cholesterol

• May be decreased with hepatic insufficiency/shunts
• Commonly increased with cholestasis and lipid metabolism disorders—hyperlipemia

Triglycerides

Increased with hyperlipemia

Urinalysis

• Bilirubinuria indicates cholestasis.
• Ammonia urates may be observed with hepatic insufficiency/shunt.

OTHER LABORATORY TESTS

Bile Acids

• Sensitive indicator of decreased hepatobiliary function, but not specific for this process
• Concentrations depend on adequate enterohepatic circulation, hepatobiliary function, and hepatocellular perfusion.
• More sensitive than GGT for acute cholestasis

Ammonia

Serum concentrations are affected by hepatic uptake and correlate inversely with hepatic functional mass.

Clearance Tests (BSP, ICG)

• Prolonged clearance intervals with decreased functional mass or cholestasis
• Accelerated clearance (possibly masking insufficiency) with hypoalbuminemia

Serology

Depends on degree of suspicion for specific diseases—viral, fungal, and so on

Coagulation Tests

May be prolonged with hepatic insufficiency/shunting—prothrombin time; activated partial thromboplastin time

IMAGING

Ultrasonography—useful for assessing liver size, shape, position, and parenchymal texture; may help to detect focal parenchymal lesions (e.g., abscesses, neoplasms) and abnormalities in the biliary tree (e.g., dilatations, obstructions) or large vessels (e.g., shunts, thrombosis)

OTHER DIAGNOSTIC PROCEDURES

Aspiration cytology or use of biopsied tissue for microbiologic testing, cytologic imprints, and histopathological evaluation may provide specific diagnostic information.

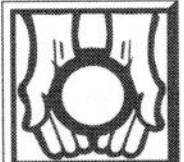

TREATMENT

• Decision regarding outpatient versus inpatient treatment depends on severity of disease, intensity of supportive care required, and need for isolation of infectious conditions.
• Fluid and nutritional support may be needed.
• Anorexic and hypoglycemic cases may benefit from IV dextrose (5%, 2 mL/kg per hour). Otherwise, fluid support depends on specific electrolyte and acid–base abnormalities.
• Avoid negative energy balance, especially in ponies and donkeys, to avoid/treat hyperlipemia and hepatic lipidosis.
• Toxicities or hepatic insufficiency may warrant efforts to reduce production/absorption of toxins.
• Mineral oil given by nasogastric tube helps to reduce toxin absorption.
• Lactulose (0.3 mL/kg q6 h by nasogastric tube) is suggested to combat GI ammonia production/absorption but causes diarrhea.
• A high-carbohydrate, low-protein diet reduces ammonia production.
• Specific therapy, including surgery, depends on the specific underlying cause.

MEDICATIONS

DRUG(S) OF CHOICE

Depend on the suspected cause and observed complications

CONTRAINDICATIONS

Depend on the suspected cause and observed complications

PRECAUTIONS

• Depend on the suspected caused
• With suspected hepatic insufficiency, assess coagulation profiles before invasive procedures.

POSSIBLE INTERACTIONS

Depend on the underlying cause

ALTERNATIVE DRUGS

Depend on the underlying cause

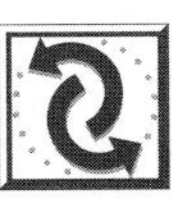

FOLLOW-UP

PATIENT MONITORING

• Serial chemistries can help to establish a prognosis by characterizing disease progression and identifying evidence of improvement.
• Initial evaluation at 1–2-day intervals helps to establish disease course.
• Subsequent testing can be at increasing intervals, depending on signs and severity.
• Cholangiohepatitis/cholelithiasis: Consider use of antibiotics until GGT is normal. Clinical improvement may precede this by days to weeks.

PREVENTION/AVOIDANCE

Depends on cause

EXPECTED COURSE AND PROGNOSIS

• Depend on cause
• Risk of nonsurvival appears to increase with GGT >399 IU/L (hazard's ratio = 4.54).

POSSIBLE COMPLICATIONS

Depend on the underlying cause

MISCELLANEOUS

ASSOCIATED CONDITIONS

Depend on the underlying cause

AGE-RELATED FACTORS

See Signalment.

ZOONOTIC POTENTIAL

Depends on the underlying cause

PREGNANCY

See Risk Factors.

SYNONYMS

γ-Glutamyltranspeptidase

SEE ALSO

• See Causes.

ABBREVIATIONS

• BSP = sulfobromophthalein
• CK = creatine kinase
• EHV = equine herpesvirus
• EIA = equine infectious anemia
• EVA = equine viral arteritis
• ICG = indocyanine green
• SDH = sorbitol dehydrogenase

Suggested Reading

Barton MH, Morris DD. Disorders of the liver. In: Reed S, Bayly W, Sellon D, eds. Equine Internal Medicine, ed 2. St. Louis: WB Saunders, 2004.

Durham AE, Newton JR, Smith KC, Hillyer MH, Hillyer LL, Smith MRW, Marr CM. Retrospective analysis of historical, clinical, ultrasonographic, serum biochemical and haematological data in prognostic evaluation of equine liver disease. Equine Vet J 2003;35:542–547.

The author and editor wish to acknowledge the contribution to this chapter by Armando Irizarry-Rovira, author in the previous edition.

Authors John A. Christian
Consulting Editor Kenneth W. Hinchcliff

GASTRIC DILATION/DISTENTION

BASICS

DEFINITION

Accumulation of excessive amounts of gas, fluid, or solid material in the stomach, resulting in dilatation.

PATHOPHYSIOLOGY

- Horses are not able to regurgitate; therefore, horses are predisposed to excessive distention of the stomach followed by possible rupture. Causes of gastric dilation can be primary, secondary, or idiopathic.
- Primary causes of gastric dilation include diseases of the stomach, feed engorgement, and rapid intake of water. The dilation results in decreased motility and a failure to discharge the stomach contents into the proximal duodenum.
- Overeating of easily fermentable food such as grain, fresh grass, beets, or beet pulp can lead to production of lactic acid and volatile fatty acids by the gastric flora. Gastric emptying is inhibited by increased concentrations of volatile fatty acids, resulting in further fermentation and production of gas.
- Primary gastric dilation may also result from local infestation of *Gasterophilus* larvae or habronemiasis, especially in the area of the pylorus.
- Primary gastric distention can also be caused iatrogenically following passage of a nasogastric tube and overloading the stomach with liquids.
- Gastric dilation can be secondary to an obstructive lesion of the small intestine, resulting in retrograde movement of intestinal fluid and bile, or nonobstructive small intestinal ileus (e.g., proximal duodeno-jejunitis).

SYSTEMS AFFECTED

- Gastrointestinal—Gastric dilation may results in dehydration or rupture. Gastric rupture results in endotoxemia, shock, and death.
- Respiratory—Abdominal distention and pressure on the diaphragm may affect breathing.

INCIDENCE/PREVALENCE

No data available

SIGNALMENT

No sex or breed disposition, but the age might assist in the identification of a primary cause. For example, foals are more predisposed to gastric ulceration.

SIGNS

General Comments

A gastric dilation/distention can lead to gastric rupture.

Historical

Depend on the severity of the dilation/distention. Signs of abdominal pain may occur abruptly following excessive or rapid consumption of large amount of liquid or food. There may be a history of ingestion of highly fermentable food. If secondary to a distal obstruction, the clinical signs are initially related to the primary problem. Mild to severe signs of abdominal pain (see Acute Abdominal Pain) may be observed. The animal may assume a dog-sitting position and present with retching or gurgling sounds.

Physical Examination

The following findings may accompany the clinical signs of abdominal pain—increase in heart and respiratory rates, sour smell to the breath, and possibly some ingesta at the nares. Cyanosis and pale mucous membranes may be present, likely due to the local increase in gastric space occupation, thus reducing venous return. There may be signs of dehydration or toxic shock as the disease progresses. Rectal examination may reveal the spleen to be displaced caudally. If the condition is secondary to an obstruction aborally, other abnormalities such as distention of the small intestines may be palpated. On passage of the nasogastric tube, large amounts of gas, fluid, or ingesta may escape. Gastric reflux of more than 2 L is considered significant. Spontaneous reflux may also be present. Passage of the nasogastric tube may be difficult due to distortion of the gastroesophageal junction. If gastric rupture occurs, the signs of colic will initially subside. Sudden massive sweating occurs, depression and severe signs of shock will develop, and once endotoxemic shock occurs, the signs of colic may return.

CAUSES

See Pathophysiology.

RISK FACTORS

- Overeating
- Intestinal obstructions

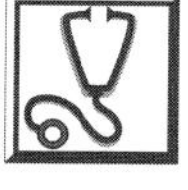

DIAGNOSIS

N/A

DIFFERENTIAL DIAGNOSIS

Any other cause of colic

CBC/BIOCHEMISTRY/URINALYSIS

Elevated PCV and TP and azotemia if dehydration or endotoxemic shock. Also occasionally seen—hypoproteinemia secondary to protein loss in the abdominal cavity; mild to moderate hypochloremia if gastric reflux is present, resulting in metabolic alkalosis; metabolic acidosis secondary to severe endotoxemic shock; moderate to severe leukopenia secondary to the acute peritonitis with gastric rupture.

OTHER LABORATORY TESTS

pH

pH of reflux might help determine the origin of the problem. Normal gastric pH varies between 3 and 6. pH of fluid originating from the small intestine is between 5 and 7 and has a bilious color.

Abdominocentesis

- Abdominocentesis is usually normal if there is a primary gastric dilation without rupture.
- There may be an increase in protein, and WBC may be present if there is some devitalized bowel (stomach or small intestine).
- Sanguineous fluid may be indicative of a strangulated obstructive lesion of the small intestine or devitalization of the stomach.
- Plant material in the sample in the absence of an enterocentesis suggests intestinal rupture.
- No leukocytes or cells should be present if an enterocentesis is performed.

IMAGING

Radiology

Radiography may identify an impacted stomach pushing on the diaphragm. In foals, a contrast study can help in outlining the gastric wall for detection of gastric ulcers and possibly strictures and determining the gastric emptying time.

Gastroscopy

Gastroscopy is useful for identification of impacted stomach, parasites, gastric ulcer, and neoplasm. In small horses, the duodenum also may be inspected for presence of ulceration and strictures.

Laparoscopy

Laparoscopy is useful for visual inspection of the visceral part of stomach and small intestine for lesions.

Ultrasonography

- May be useful to identify a primary lesion in the small intestine by evaluation of its wall thickness and diameter
- Abnormal findings such as intussusception, abscess, and adhesions may sometimes be identified
- Evaluation of the amount, quality, and characteristics of abdominal fluid is also possible.

DIAGNOSTIC PROCEDURES

Exploratory laparotomy is useful to treat small intestinal lesions and possibly some gastric problems.

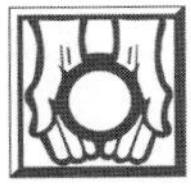

TREATMENT

Supportive therapy for treatment of shock

Primary Gastric Dilation/Impaction

Primary gastric dilatation consists of deflating the stomach regularly by passage of the nasogastric tube. If impaction is present, lavage of the stomach followed by administration of DSS (10–30 mg/kg of a 10% solution) acts as a surfactant and allows water to penetrate the impaction. It may be necessary to repeat this procedure. Care should be taken not to give too much DSS. Following resolution of an impaction the horse should be kept off feed for 48–72 hr.

Secondary Gastric Dilation

Secondary gastric dilatation consists of leaving the nasogastric tube in place and performing periodic decompression until resolution of the primary problem by medical or surgical treatment (see Small Intestinal Obstruction).

IV Fluid Therapy

Intravenous fluid may be administered to treat the dehydration.

MEDICATIONS

DRUG(S) OF CHOICE

Analgesics may be necessary to control the abdominal pain. They include:

- NSAIDs—flunixin meglumine (0.5–1.1 mg/kg IV, IM q8h or q12h) and α_2-agonists, such as xylazine 0.25–0.5 mg/kg IV, IM, detomidine 5–10 μg/kg IV, IM, or romifidine 0.02–0.05 mg/kg IV, IM.
- Narcotic or narcotic-derivative analgesics such as butorphanol 0.02–0.04 mg/kg IV, which can be given alone or in combination with xylazine. There is potentiation of these two drugs. Analgesics should be used judiciously as they may mask clinical signs and may lead to postponement of a needed surgery. Parenteral fluid treatments (100–200 mL/kg/day)
- When cardiovascular shock is present, administer hypertonic saline IV (in the adult horse, 2 L of 7% NaCl; 4 mL/kg) prior to balanced electrolyte solutions (e.g., lactated Ringer's).

PRECAUTIONS

The nasogastric tube should be manipulated gently; avoid overloading the stomach.

FOLLOW-UP

PATIENT MONITORING

The patient should be monitored for any increase in heart rate or discomfort indicating that the stomach may need to be further decompressed.

POSSIBLE COMPLICATIONS

- Gastric rupture
- Endotoxemic shock
- The use of NSAIDs may aggravate preexisting gastric ulcers.

ASSOCIATED CONDITIONS

Primary Conditions

- Gastric ulceration
- Parasitism
- Neoplasia

Secondary Conditions

- Small intestinal obstruction (strangulated or nonstrangulated)
- Anterior duodeno-jejunitis

AGE-RELATED FACTORS

Gastric ulceration is often the primary cause of gastric dilatation/distention in young foals.

ABBREVIATION

- DDS = dioctyl sodium succinate

Suggested Reading

Carter GK. Gastric diseases. In: Robinson NE. Current Therapy in Equine Medicine, ed 2. Philadelphia: WB Saunders, 1987:41–44.

Kiper ML, Traub-Dargatz J, Curtis CR. Gastric rupture in horses: 50 cases (1979–1987). JAVMA 1990;196:333–336.

Murray MJ. Diseases of the stomach. In: Mair T, Divers T, Ducharme N. Manual of Equine Gastroenterology. Philadelphia: WB Saunders, 2001:241–248.

Todhunter RJ, Erb HN, Roth L. Gastric rupture in horses: a review of 54 cases. Equine Vet J 1986:18;288–293.

Author Nathalie Coté

Consulting Editors Henry Stämpfli and Olimpo Oliver-Espinosa

GASTRIC NEOPLASIA

BASICS

DEFINITION

• Neoplasia of the gastrointestinal tract of horses is rare; however, different types of tumors affect the horse stomach and include SCC, adenocarcinoma, lymphosarcoma, leiomyosarcoma, and leiomyoma.
• SCC usually originates in the nonglandular (squamous) portion of the stomach, infiltrates the wall, and projects into the lumen.
• Adenocarcinoma of the glandular part of the stomach may affect the pylorus and the fundic region.
• Leiomyosarcoma has been reported to affect the cranial aspects of the stomach. Although SCC is the most common gastric neoplasm, only 3% of carcinomas in horses are of gastric origin, which is in marked contrast to the incidence in humans.
• The tumors may cause physical obstruction within the stomach and may occasionally be associated with severe intraluminal hemorrhage.
• Other signs may be related to the effects of metastases (e.g., pleural effusion).
• SCC lesions of the stomach may reach a considerable size due to local invasiveness and have a proliferative appearance. They are often ulcerated and secondarily infected. In these circumstances, the surface may have a grayish-white and hemorrhagic appearance. There may be adhesions of stomach to adjacent liver, spleen, or diaphragm, and there are frequently metastatic nodules in the abdominal and thoracic cavities; however, this metastatic form is slow to progress.
• Although adenocarcinomas may project into the gut lumen, the predominant feature is growth from the mucosa into the submucosa and the muscularis to the serosa.

SIGNALMENT

• Horses of middle age and older (range, 8.6–14.6 years with an increased risk between 11 and 12 years) are susceptible to SCC, and a 4:1 male:female ratio has been reported.
• Breeds with an increased risk to develop SCC are draft horse breeds, Appaloosas, American Paints, Pintos, and mixed breeds.
• Adenocarcinoma and lymphosarcoma have a similar age distribution.

SIGNS

• Affected horses have a history of gradual weight loss, anorexia, halitosis, dysphagia ptyalism, and lethargy extending over a period of 2–6 weeks.
• Abdominal pain and difficulty in eating or swallowing are not usually features of gastric neoplasia.
• Pallor of mucous membranes and an increase in heart rate may be seen due to anemia resulting from hemorrhage to the stomach or depressed erythrogenesis.
• Recurrent episodic pyrexia up to 40° C may occur as the result of necrosis in the neoplasm, and the respiratory rate may be raised in response to metastatic masses or pleural effusion in the thorax.
• Ascites and ventral edema may be primary signs in a few horses, so that despite the weight loss the abdomen appears distended.

CAUSES/RISK FACTORS

None known

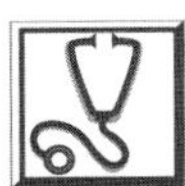

DIAGNOSIS

A definitive diagnosis is made on histologic examination of tissue obtained at autopsy or by biopsy.

DIFFERENTIAL DIAGNOSIS

See Chronic Weight Loss.

CBC/BIOCHEMISTRY/URINALYSIS

The PCV may be as low as 12%–28% in horses with anemia, secondary to gastric carcinoma.

OTHER LABORATORY TESTS

- Feces may test positive for occult blood.
- Neoplastic cells may be found in fluid recovered by gastric lavage, in peritoneal fluid, or in pleural fluid.

IMAGING

- Endoscopy using a video or fiber endoscope of 2 m in length or more enables direct visualization and biopsy of the tumor.
- Exploratory laparotomy or standing laparoscopy allows an examination of the serosal surface of the stomach, determines the extent of the spread of the tumor if any, and allows biopsy of primary mass or metastatic nodules.
- Radiographs of the thorax may reveal pleural effusion. A pneumogastrogram may be of value in delineating the intraluminal portion of the tumor.
- Ultrasonography from the left cranial abdomen may show thickening and abnormal echogenicity of the stomach wall.

DIAGNOSTIC PROCEDURES

Rectal examination may indicate metastatic masses or increased abdominal fluid.

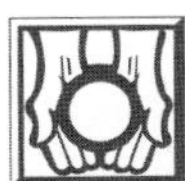

TREATMENT

By the time a diagnosis is made the tumors have usually progressed beyond the point where any treatment is feasible, and euthanasia is the only option.

MEDICATIONS

N/A

CONTRAINDICATIONS/POSSIBLE INTERACTIONS

N/A

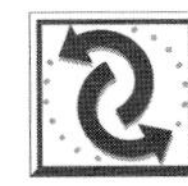

FOLLOW-UP

N/A

MISCELLANEOUS

ABBREVIATION

- SCC = squamous cell carcinoma

Suggested Reading

East LM, Savage CJ. Abdominal neoplasia (excluding urogenital tract). Vet Clin North Am Equine Pract 1998;14;475–493.

Head KW, et al. Tumors of the alimentary tract. In: Meuten DJ, ed. Tumors in Domestic Animals, ed 4. Ames, IA: Iowa State University Press, 2002:401–481.

Meagher DM, Wheat JD, Tennant B, Osburn BI. Squamous cell carcinoma of the equine stomach. JAVMA 1974;164:81–84.

Authors Olimpo Oliver-Espinosa and Garry B. Edwards

Consulting Editors Henry Stämpfli and Olimpo Oliver-Espinosa

GASTRIC ULCERS AND EROSIONS (EQUINE GASTRIC ULCER SYNDROME)

BASICS

DEFINITION

• Gastric ulcers are defects in the gastric mucosa that extend into the muscularis mucosa. Erosions are less severe and do not extend into the muscularis mucosa. Endoscopically, it can be difficult to distinguish erosions from ulcers in some cases.
• The equine stomach consists of a proximal portion lined with stratified squamous epithelium (nonglandular region) and a ventral portion lined with a glandular epithelial mucosa (glandular region).

PATHOPHYSIOLOGY

• Gastric ulcers are thought to occur when there is an imbalance of aggressive and protective factors. The aggressive factors are primarily hydrochloric acid and pepsin. Protective factors include the gastric mucosal barrier (mucus, bicarbonate), prostaglandins, mucosal blood flow, and mucosal restitution.
• The proximal third of the equine stomach or nonglandular region is covered by stratified squamous epithelium and has no mucus or bicarbonate layer to protect it against acid induced injury. Gastric ulcers are common in this region in horses in training, which is primarily a mechanical phenomenon, due to an increased exposure of that region of the stomach to acidic gastric contents during exercise. In addition, in horses fed high concentrate diets that are high in fermentable carbohydrates, the production of short-chain fatty acids by resident bacteria in the presence of a low stomach pH may also play an important role in the pathogenesis of stratified squamous epithelium destruction.
• Restitution is the process in which existing mucosal cells migrate rapidly to replace damaged mucosal cells and occurs in minutes to hours. Mucosal protective factors are important primarily in the glandular mucosa. The stratified squamous mucosa has less-advanced protective properties.

SYSTEMS AFFECTED

Gastrointestinal

"Equine gastric ulcer syndrome" has been adopted in reference to a number of specifically unique problems that can manifest as mucosal erosion and ulceration within the esophagus, stomach or upper duodenum, or some combination thereof. However, primarily the gastric stratified squamous mucosa and less often the glandular mucosa are affected in adult working horses. Esophageal mucosal inflammation and erosions/ulcers would primarily be seen in foals when gastroesophageal reflux is present.

Cardiovascular

Although hemorrhage is often visible on gastroscopic examination, blood loss sufficient to affect the cardiovascular system is rare.

Respiratory

Foals with gastroesophageal reflux may develop aspiration pneumonia.

Hepatobiliary

Ascending cholangitis is possible with duodenal ulceration.

INCIDENCE/PREVALENCE

Equine gastric ulcers have been reported from most parts of the world. The reported prevalence is 25–50% of foals, 80–90% of racehorses in training, and >90% of weanlings after housing in stalls and halter breaking. Ulcers identified endoscopically are primarily in the stratified squamous mucosa. However, it is often difficult to visualize large portions of the glandular mucosa in the standing horse, and therefore the true frequency of glandular ulcers may be underestimated. Necropsy results in racehorses indicate a 10% prevalence of glandular mucosal ulcers, and as many as 40% of foals 2–90 days old may have glandular mucosal lesions. Ninety-two percent of horses showing clinical signs had visible gastric ulceration. Approximately 5% of foals necropsied had duodenal ulceration.

SIGNALMENT

Breed Predilections

Although Thoroughbred racehorses in training appear to be overrepresented, all breeds appear to be affected.

Mean Age and Range

Horses of all ages are affected; however, severity is higher in horses ≥3 years of age than in 2-year-old horses. Relative risk for ulceration increases with age in castrated males.

Predominant Sex

N/A

SIGNS

General Comments

Asymptomatic in many animals. Signs may vary with the age group involved and are not specific for the condition.

Historical

• Poor appetite
• Decrease in performance
• Weight loss
• Low-grade colic or abdominal discomfort (rare—depends on the severity of the ulceration)

Physical Examination

• Foals—Many are asymptomatic, with poor appetite, intermittent nursing (may nurse for short period and then act mildly uncomfortable), episodes of mild colic, diarrhea, pot-bellied appearance, bruxism, salivation, and dorsal recumbency. Salivation and bruxism are usually indicative of severe glandular or duodenal ulcers with concurrent gastroesophageal reflux and delayed gastric emptying.
• Adults—Many are asymptomatic, with poor appetite, lethargy, poor body condition, rough hair coat, low-grade colic, and weight loss.

CAUSES

Probably multifactorial—any illness, surgery, intense training, halter breaking, confining and handling of young horses, NSAIDs, fasting, lack of roughage in diet in racehorses

RISK FACTORS

• Significant illness
• Intense training
• Administration of NSAIDs
• Halter breaking and confinement
• Fasting

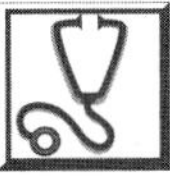

DIAGNOSIS

Although a definitive diagnosis can be reached with gastroscopic examination, a tentative diagnosis can be made based on clinical signs and response to therapy.

DIFFERENTIAL DIAGNOSIS

The clinical signs and physical examination findings with gastric ulcers are not pathognomonic and can be associated with many other conditions. In addition, gastric ulcers are often secondary to other diseases.

CBC/BIOCHEMISTRY/URINALYSIS

There are no changes in CBC/biochemistry/urinalysis associated with equine gastric ulcers. Anemia and hypoproteinemia are not associated with gastric ulcers and when present, other causes should be pursued.

OTHER LABORATORY TESTS

Fecal occult blood tests are often negative because colonic microflora digest hemoglobin.

IMAGING

Abdominal Radiography

Abdominal radiographs usually do not demonstrate gastric ulcerations. In foals, positive contrast studies might outline gastric ulcers but more effective methods should be used.

DIAGNOSTIC PROCEDURES

Gastroscopic Examination

Gastroscopic examination is the most effective diagnostic procedure. For foals, a 10-mm diameter, 1-m gastroscope is adequate. However, for optimum gastroscopic examination in the adult horse, a 2- to 3-m gastroscope is necessary. Fasting is necessary to ensure gastric emptying for adequate visualization. Young foals may require minimum fasting. However, older foals and adults eating roughage require a fasting period of 4–18 hr. Lesions in the stratified squamous mucosa are easily identified. Glandular mucosal lesions are frequently not visible because they are covered by ingesta and gastric secretions remaining in the stomach.

GASTRIC ULCERS AND EROSIONS (EQUINE GASTRIC ULCER SYNDROME)

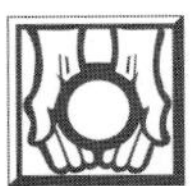

TREATMENT

APPROPRIATE HEALTH CARE

Treat as outpatient if stable and any underlying conditions have been corrected.

NURSING CARE

Treat any underlying medical conditions. Use NSAIDs with caution.

ACTIVITY

Decrease level of intense training if possible.

DIET

Turn out on pasture if practical.

CLIENT EDUCATION

- Decrease intensity of training
- Allow as much pasture time as possible
- Minimize NSAID administration
- Minimize periods of fasting
- Ulcers will likely recur when intense training is resumed.

SURGICAL CONSIDERATION

Surgical intervention is not indicated in uncomplicated cases. Foals with chronic gastric outflow disease caused by stricture of the pylorus or duodenum post-ulcer healing may require gastrojejunostomy.

MEDICATIONS

N/A

DRUG(S) OF CHOICE

- Proton pump inhibitors (omeprazole and lansoprazole)—significantly inhibit gastric acid secretion by the inhibition of hydrogen-potassium adenosine triphosphatase (H^+,K^+-ATPase). This enzyme in gastric parietal cells is believed to be the terminal step in the acid secretory pathway. These compounds have a long-term antisecretory effect that lasts for at least 24 hr. Omeprazole is administered 1–4 mg/kg PO once daily. Omeprazole has a time- and dose-related effect on healing of gastric ulcers. Therefore, higher doses result in more rapid and complete healing. However, lower doses are frequently effective in relieving clinical signs and promoting healing. Omeprazole requires 3–5 days of treatment for maximum antisecretory effect to occur. There are currently no data available on the use of lansoprazole in horses.
- Histamine H_2 receptor antagonists (cimetidine, ranitidine, and famotidine)—inhibit gastric acid secretion by blocking the effect of histamine on the parietal cell. These compounds rapidly inhibit secretion after oral or intravenous administration. However, the effect is short-lived and they must be administered q6–8h. Cimetidine is administered at 20–25 mg/kg PO or at 4–6 mg/kg IV body weight q6–8h. Ranitidine is administered at 6–8 mg/kg PO or 1.5–2.0 mg/kg IV every q6–8h.

CONTRAINDICATIONS

Use NSAIDs with caution. These compounds may increase the severity of squamous mucosal lesions and cause lesions in the glandular mucosa.

PRECAUTIONS

Clinical signs of gastric ulcers usually diminish quickly with appropriate therapy. If signs or condition worsen while on appropriate treatment, pursue an alternate diagnosis or concurrent disease.

POSSIBLE INTERACTIONS

Cimetidine and, to a lesser extent, omeprazole are hepatic cytochrome P450 inhibitors and might slow the metabolism of concurrently administered compounds that require this enzyme for metabolism and elimination. Drugs whose metabolism might be inhibited include phenylbutazone, diazepam, phenytoin, theophylline, and others.

ALTERNATIVE DRUGS

Antacid Compounds

Antacid compounds buffer gastric acid and are impractical to use in most instances. They must be administered 4–6 times daily and at approximately 250 mL/450-kg horse.

Sucralfate

Likely to be ineffective for treatment of stratified squamous lesions, but possibly effective in glandular lesions. Administer as crushed tablets in syrup at 1g/100 lb body weight PO q6–8h.

FOLLOW-UP

PATIENT MONITORING

Clinical Signs

- Diminished appetite
- Interrupted nursing
- Mild colic
- Teeth grinding

Signs of colic should be monitored frequently. If colic is more than low-grade or persists for >24–48 hr, an alternate diagnosis should be pursued. Endoscopic examination should be repeated after 14 days of treatment and, if not healed, again at 28 days.

PREVENTION/AVOIDANCE

Horses may require prophylactic treatment with omeprazole or histamine H_2 receptor antagonists during periods of intense training/racing. Horses with access to pasture have fewer gastric ulcers than horses in confinement. Avoid chronic administration of NSAIDs and minimize periods of fasting.

POSSIBLE COMPLICATIONS

Pyloric or duodenal stricture in foals; gastric or duodenal perforation (rare). Severe hemorrhage is rare but has been reported in one foal. Recurrence is frequent when intense training resumes.

EXPECTED COURSE AND PROGNOSIS

Most uncomplicated gastric ulcers heal after 14–28 days of treatment. The prognosis is generally good for uncomplicated cases. However, recurrence is frequent when intense training is resumed. Foals that develop pyloric or duodenal strictures and require surgical intervention have a guarded prognosis.

MISCELLANEOUS

ASSOCIATED CONDITIONS

Any disease process has the potential to have secondary gastric ulceration.

AGE-RELATED FACTORS

Foals have a higher incidence of glandular mucosal and duodenal ulcers.

ZOONOTIC POTENTIAL

N/A

PREGNANCY

There is inadequate data on the use of histamine H_2 receptor antagonists or omeprazole in pregnant mares. However, clinical cases of gastric ulcers in pregnant mares have been treated successfully with these compounds with no apparent adverse effects on the mare or the fetus.

SYNONYMS

N/A

ABBREVIATIONS

N/A

Suggested Reading

Jones WE. Understanding gastric ulcers in horses. J Equine Vet Sci 2002;22:330.

Lester GD, Smith RL, Robertson ID. Effects of treatment with omeprazole or ranitidine on gastric squamous ulceration in racing Thoroughbreds. JAVMA 2005;227:1636–1639.

Merrit AM. The equine stomach: a personal perspective (1963–2003). Proc 49th annu AAEP Meeting 2003;49:75–102.

Dionne RM, Vrins A, Doucet MY, Paré J. Gastric ulcers in standardbred racehorses: prevalence, lesion description, and risk factors. J Vet Intern Med 2003;17:218–222.

MacAllister CG. Medical therapy for equine gastric ulcers. Vet Med 1995:168–176.

Murray MJ. Gastroduodenal ulceration. In: Reed SM, Bayly WM, eds. Equine Internal Medicine. Philadelphia: WB Saunders, 1998.

Author Modest Vengust

Consulting Editors Henry Stämpfli and Olimpo Oliver-Espinosa

GASTRIC ULCERS, NEONATE

BASICS

DEFINITION

Areas of erosions that can occur in the nonglandular stratified squamous mucosa, margo plicatus, glandular mucosa, and pylorus of the stomach

PATHOPHYSIOLOGY

• Gastric ulcers are caused by an imbalance between mucosal aggressive factors (hydrochloric acid, pepsin, bile acids) and mucosal protective factors (mucosal blood flow, mucus-bicarbonate layer, mucosal prostaglandin E_1, epidermal growth factor production and gastroduodenal motility). • Ulcers in the squamous mucosa are primarily due to prolonged exposure to hydrochloric acid, pepsin, and bile acids. Foals secrete hydrochloric acid as early as the second day of life. The equine gastric squamous mucosa has no surface barrier against hydrochloric acid. The squamous mucosa near the margo plicatus is constantly exposed to these acids and gastric ulcers are commonly located in this region.
• Gastric ulcers may also be related to desquamation of the squamous epithelium that occurs in 80% of normal foals of up to 40 days of age. • Milk has a buffering effect on gastric acid and recumbency may increase exposure of the squamous mucosa to gastric acid. Therefore, infrequent nursing and recumbency may contribute to squamous ulceration in foals.
• Delayed gastric emptying or decreased gastric motility could increase exposure of the squamous mucosa to gastric acids leading to ulceration, especially during periods of cell desquamation.
• Blocking prostaglandin synthesis (by endogenous corticosteroids or NSAID treatment) causes decreased mucosal blood flow, inhibits bicarbonate secretion, and stimulates gastric acid secretion leading to glandular ulceration. • Glandular ulceration typically is considered the most clinically significant in neonatal foals. The mucus-bicarbonate layer covers the surface of the glandular mucosa. Ulcers in this region are primarily due to disruption of blood flow and decreased secretion of mucus and bicarbonate. • Although critically ill foals are able to secrete HCl by the first day of life, the 24-hr gastric pH profile of critically ill recumbent foals is primarily alkaline. Therefore, alterations in gastric perfusion may play a more significant role in the development of gastric ulcers than hydrochloric acid secretion in this patient population. • Mucosal blood flow is probably the most important element of gastric mucosal protection. Septic shock and hypovolemia leading to hypoperfusion and reduced oxygen delivery may be involved in the pathogenesis of glandular mucosal injury. Hypoperfusion results in reduced secretion of sodium bicarbonate or mucus. • Nitric oxide may also be involved in the pathogenesis of gastric ulceration as it is the primary regulator of gastric mucosal blood flow and other mediators such as prostaglandins. • Foals may also have ulcers in the pylorus or proximal duodenum that can lead to gastric and esophageal ulcers secondary to delayed gastric emptying.

SYSTEM AFFECTED

Gastrointestinal

INCIDENCE/PREVALENCE

• The reported prevalence of gastric ulcers in foals varies from 25% to 57%. • Endoscopic surveys of normal foals 2–85 days of age revealed that 50% had ulcers in the squamous mucosa and 4%–9% had ulcers in the glandular mucosa.

SIGNALMENT

No breed or sex predilection

SIGNS

General Comments

• Neonatal foals with gastric ulceration are often asymptomatic until ulceration is severe or gastric rupture has occurred. • In foals, there are 4 separate clinical syndromes:

1. Silent (subclinical) ulcers are the most common syndrome.
   - Silent squamous ulcers are most commonly found in foals younger than 4 mo.
   - Silent glandular ulcers are usually seen in foals with concurrent illness.
   - Ulcers may heal spontaneously and may be found incidentally at necropsy.
2. Active (clinical) ulcers
   - Primarily in the squamous mucosa
   - Clinical signs include depression, anorexia, bruxism, ptyalism, dorsal recumbency, and colic.
3. Perforating ulcers with diffuse peritonitis
   - Uncommon
   - Occur most frequently in the squamous mucosa
   - Clinical signs are almost always absent until just before rupture.
   - Severity cannot be predicted by endoscopic appearance.
   - Once ruptured, foals show progressive evidence of endotoxemia and may have abdominal distention and colic.
4. Pyloric strictures associated with gastric outflow obstruction
   - Uncommon
   - Can result in stricture formation, gastric outflow obstruction, and reflux esophagitis
   - Bruxism, ptyalism, drooling of milk, postprandial colic, aspiration pneumonia, dehydration, and systemic hypochloremic alkalosis
   - This syndrome can affect foals of all ages, but foals 3–5 mo of age tend to be more susceptible.

Historical

Poor growth, rough hair coat, potbellied appearance, and history of prior illness, including diarrhea, colic, lethargy, or anorexia

Physical Examination

• Depression and intermittent nursing are the most commonly observed clinical signs. • Colic • Diarrhea • Bruxism and ptyalism

CAUSES

• Increased exposure to gastric acid • Mucosal blood flow disruption

RISK FACTORS

• Fasting, decreased gastric motility, and delayed gastric emptying may lead to ulcers in the squamous mucosa. • Disruption of mucosal blood flow due to hypovolemia, endotoxic shock, stress, and NSAID use may cause glandular ulceration.

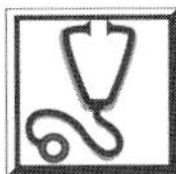

DIAGNOSIS

• Recognition of the clinical signs may lead to a presumptive diagnosis. • A definitive diagnosis is confirmed via gastroendoscopy.

DIFERENTIAL DIAGNOSIS

Any disorder resulting in signs of colic—small intestinal intussusceptions, small intestinal volvulus, peritonitis, pyloric hypertrophy, large colon impaction, diaphragmatic hernia, abdominal abscess, and enterocolitis

CBC/BIOCHEMISTRY/URINALYSIS

• Gastric ulcers can be associated with other diseases; therefore, obtain a CBC, chemistry panel, blood electrolytes, acid-base status and urinalysis. • Hematology values are usually normal but may show on a stress leukogram.
• Anemia may be present if blood loss is substantial. • In cases of gastric rupture and peritonitis, the CBC may show leukocytosis or leukopenia and hyperfibrinogenemia, dehydration, and hypochloremic metabolic acidosis.

OTHER LABORATORY TESTS

Fecal or gastric occult blood may be also suggestive of bleeding ulcers; these tests are neither sensitive nor specific.

IMAGING

• Abdominal radiographs may help rule out other causes of colic. • Contrast radiographs should be taken in foals with suspected gastric outflow obstruction. • Abdominal ultrasonography should be performed to evaluate the thickness of the intestinal wall and to evaluate for ileus and peritoneal effusion.

OTHER DIAGNOSTIC PROCEDURES

• Gastroscopy or gastroduodenoscopy will definitively confirm the diagnosis. Use a 1-m-long endoscope with a maximal outer diameter of 9mm. The squamous mucosa of neonatal foals is thin at birth, it has a light pink color and it becomes hyperplastic and parakeratotic within days. The glandular portions appear red. • In cases where pyloric stenosis is suspected, measurement of gastric emptying can be helpful in diagnosing the condition. This may be achieved with nuclear scintigraphy, acetaminophen absorption, and postconsumption [^{13}C]octanoic acid blood or breath testing.

PATHOLOGICAL FINDINGS

Phenylbutazone toxicity produces ulcers in the glandular and nonglandular stomach. The size of the ulcers is highly variable, ranging from 2 mm to 2 cm in diameter. The larger ulcers may be 1–2mm in depth and surrounded by hyperemia.

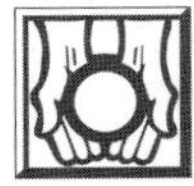

TREATMENT

AIMS OF TREATMENT

• Suppression or neutralization of gastric acid
• Supportive therapy for the critically ill foal
• Foals with mild to moderately severe gastric ulcers should respond to treatment within 24–48 hr.

APPROPRIATE HEALTH CARE

• Patients with gastric ulcers can be treated in the field. • With dehydration or electrolyte imbalance, peritonitis, toxic clinical signs, esophageal reflux, and uncontrolled pain, the animal should be hospitalized.

NURSING CARE

• In severely compromised, critically ill neonatal foals, supportive care may provide protection against ulcer formation more so than treatment to suppress HCl. • In a referral hospital, indirect blood pressure, arterial and venous blood gas analysis, and blood lactate should be monitored. Fluid therapy and ionotropic support may be needed to optimize organ perfusion.

ACTIVITY

Normal

DIET

• Normal diet in cases without esophageal reflux
• In case of gastroesophageal reflux, parenteral nutrition is sometimes necessary.

CLIENT EDUCATION

• Avoid use of NSAIDs without veterinary supervision. • Ensure animal has a regular feeding program.

SURGICAL CONSIDERATIONS

• Foals with severe gastroduodenal ulcer disease can develop duodenal strictures. If medical therapy is unsuccessful, then surgical correction is necessary. • Surgical techniques include pyloroplasty or bypass techniques.

MEDICATIONS

DRUG(S) OF CHOICE

Histamine H_2 Receptor Antagonists (ranitidine)

• Suppress HCl secretion by binding and competitively inhibiting the histamine H_2 receptor in the parietal cell.
  ◦ Cimetidine—6–20 mg/kg PO q8h or q6h or 6.6 mg/kg IV q6h
  ◦ Ranitidne—6.6 mg/kg PO q8h and 1.5–2 mg/kg IV q8h or q6h
  ◦ Famotidine—10 –15 mg/kg/day
• Continue therapy for 14–21 days.

Proton Pump Inhibitors

• Block secretion of H^+ at the parietal cell membrane H^+/K^+-ATPase pump (proton pump) • Acid secretion is completely suppressed for up to 27 hr. • Omeprazole—4.0 mg/kg PO q24h for treatment of gastric ulcers; the preventative dose is 2.0 mg/kg PO q24h.

Antacids

• Aluminum hydroxide, magnesium hydroxide, and calcium carbonate • They can be used to ameliorate the clinical signs or to prevent recurrence; efficacy not determined • Dose is 200–250 ml PO q6h. • Use is not recommended.

Sucralfate

• It adheres to ulcerated glandular mucosa, forms a proteinaceous bandage, and stimulates prostaglandin E_1 synthesis and mucus secretion.
• Efficacy in treatment of squamous mucosa lesions has not been determined. • Best used in addition to H_2 antagonists • Dose is 10–20 mg/kg PO TID or QID.

Prostaglandin Analogs

• Misoprostol (Cytotec)—1–4 mg/kg PO q24h
• Synthetic replacement for PGE_1 • PGE_1 inhibits hydrochloric acid and gastrin secretion; increases gastric mucus formation and blood flow to the mucosa • May aid in the treatment and prevention of gastric ulcers induced by NSAIDs

Prokinetics

• May be administered to foals with duodenal ulcers, with gastroesophageal reflux, and when delayed gastric emptying without a physical obstruction is suspected.
• Bethanecol—0.25–0.30 mg/kg SQ q3–4h; cholinergic that increases the rate of gastric emptying in horses

CONTRAINDICATIONS

• Prokinetics should not be used if there is a suspicion of mechanical obstruction of the bowel.

PRECAUTIONS

• Side effects of prostaglandin analog use (in humans) include abdominal pain, diarrhea, bloating, and cramping. • Bethanecol—adverse effects include diarrhea, inappetence, salivation, and colic.

POSSIBLE INTERACTIONS

• Cimetidine may inhibit the hepatic microsomal enzyme system and thereby reduce metabolism, prolong half-lives, and increase serum levels of some drugs, e.g., metronidazole.
• Do not use bethanecol concomitantly with other cholinergic or anticholinesterase agents.

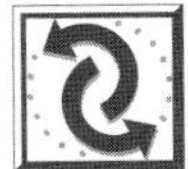

FOLLOW-UP

PATIENT MONITORING

• Recheck gastroendoscopy 14–21 days after initiating treatment. • If gastroendoscopy is unavailable, the efficacy of treatment can be based on clinical signs. • Signs of colic or diarrhea that result from gastric ulcers usually resolve within 48 hr. Appetite, bodily condition, and attitude improve within 1–3 weeks.

PREVENTION/AVOIDANCE

• Because critically ill foals are at risk of gastric perforation, prophylactic antiulcer therapy is routinely administered in this population. Some critically ill foals have a predominantly alkaline gastric pH profile and because gastric acidity may be protective against bacterial translocation in neonates, the need for prophylactic ulcer therapy is controversial. • Avoid NSAID use in foals.

POSSIBLE COMPLICATIONS

• Pyloric stricture • Acute hemorrhage • Gastric rupture and peritonitis

EXPECTED COURSE AND PROGNOSIS

• Outcome is variable. • Foals with gastric ulcers that respond favorably to therapy for a primary problem have a good prognosis. Ulcers may heal in 2–3 weeks. • Foals with duodenal ulcers have a guarded prognosis, because of the potential for duodenal strictures, fibrosis, and gastric outflow obstruction. • Foals with perforating ulcers have a grave prognosis. • Mortality from gastric ulceration ranges from 7.1% to 16.2%.

MISCELLANEOUS

ASSOCIATED CONDITIONS

• Septicemia • Septic arthritis • Hypoxic ischemic encephalopathy

AGE-RELATED FACTORS

Frequently seen in neonatal foals with concomitant disease

SYNONYMS

• Gastroduodenal ulcer syndrome • Peptic ulcers

SEE ALSO

• Gastric ulcers, adults • NSAID toxicity

ABBREVIATIONS

• HCl = hydrochloric acid
• PGE_1 = prostaglandin E_1

Suggested Reading

Andrews F, Nadeau J. Clinical syndromes of gastric ulceration in foals and mature horses. Equine Vet J Suppl 1999;29:30–33.

Magdesian G. Gastrointestinal problems in the neonatal foal. In: Paradis M, ed. Equine Neonatal Medicine: A Case-Based Approach. Philadelphia: Elsevier Saunders, 2006:208.

Murray MJ. Pathophysiology of peptic disorders in foals and horses: a review. Equine Vet J Suppl 1999;29:14–18.

Ryan C, Sanchez C. Nondiarrheal disorders of the gastrointestinal tract in neonatal foals. Vet Clin North Am 2005;21:313–332.

Author Sandra C. Valdez-Almada
Consulting Editor Margaret C. Mudge

GETAH VIRUS INFECTION

BASICS

OVERVIEW

Getah virus is an RNA alphavirus of the family *Togaviridae*. It is widely distributed throughout Southeast Asia and surrounding areas. In tropical areas, it is believed to be maintained in a mosquito-pig-mosquito cycle. Pigs are considered important amplifying hosts of the virus in endemic regions. Clinical signs associated with infection with the virus have been described only in horses and occasionally pigs. Although serologic evidence indicates equine exposure to the virus in Hong Kong, Korea, Japan, and India, and in other mammals over a much wider area, clinical signs associated with infection in horses have only been reported from Japan and India. There have been two significant outbreaks in Japan (1978 and 1983) and one localized outbreak in India (1990).

SIGNALMENT

Horses of any breed can be infected experimentally, but reported outbreaks have been mostly in Thoroughbreds. Few cases have been reported in foals.

SIGNS

- Anorexia
- Fever
- Limb and preputial edema
- Urticarial rash
- Serous nasal discharge
- Submandibular lymphadenopathy
- Stiff gait

Not all horses display all clinical signs, and in the Indian outbreak, rash and lymphadenopathy were absent. Fever usually develops 2–6 days after exposure and lasts 3–4 days. Clinical signs resolve within 7–10 days after onset. In pigs, the virus can cause a fatal peracute illness in neonatal piglets associated with depression, tremors and diarrhea. Infection in other animals is usually asymptomatic.

CAUSES AND RISK FACTORS

Getah virus is transmitted by mosquitoes, and hence is prevalent in areas with an appropriate mosquito population and reservoir host population. However, some cases of infection in Japan have been reported when the mosquito population is very low, suggesting other means of transmission, such as direct contact or indirectly, through contaminated fomites.

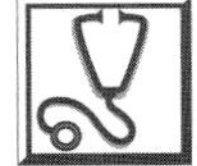

DIAGNOSIS

DIFFERENTIAL DIAGNOSIS

Equine viral arteritis can clinically mimic Getah virus infection in horses. However, abortions have not been a reported feature of Getah virus infection. The two diseases can be distinguished based on virus detection and serologic testing of acute and convalescent (paired) sera. Mild cases of African horse sickness (African horse sickness fever) can present with similar signs, although the geographic distribution of the two etiologic agents is very different.

CBS/BIOCHEMISTRY/URINALYSIS

The only consistent laboratory finding is a lymphopenia in the early phase of the disease. Serum biochemistry is usually normal.

OTHER LABORATORY TESTS

In the acute phase of infection, Getah virus can be detected in the blood and, in some horses, in nasal secretions by virus isolation and/or RT-PCR. A diagnosis can also be confirmed by testing acute and convalescent (paired) sera for antibodies to the virus by various serologic procedures.

IMAGING

N/A

DIAGNOSTIC PROCEDURES

N/A

PATHOLOGIC FINDINGS

Moderate enlargement of lymph nodes and scattered maculae in the dermis and subcutaneous edema. Histologically, there is lymphoid hyperplasia in the lymph nodes and spleen. In the dermal maculae, there is perivascular infiltration of lymphocytes, histiocytes, and eosinophils, with edema of blood vessel walls and hemorrhagic foci.

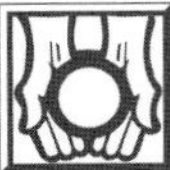

TREATMENT

N/A

MEDICATIONS

DRUG(S) OF CHOICE

Not usually necessary since this is not a life-threatening illness. Nonsteroidal anti-inflammatory agents may be helpful in anorexic horses during the febrile period.

CONTRAINDICATIONS/POSSIBLE INTERACTIONS

N/A

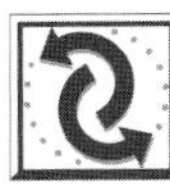

FOLLOW-UP

PREVENTION/AVOIDANCE

A killed vaccine is available in Japan and should be used prior to the onset of the mosquito season.

EXPECTED COURSE AND PROGNOSIS

Clinical signs last about 6–10 days and resolve without any reported sequelae.

MISCELLANEOUS

Suggested Reading

Timoney PJ. Getah virus infection. In: Infectious diseases of livestock – Volume Two. Coetzer JAW and Tustin RC (eds.). Oxford University Press, 2004:1023–1026.

Authors Christopher M. Brown and Peter J. Timoney

Consulting Editors Ashley G. Boyle and Corinne R. Sweeney

GLANDERS

BASICS

OVERVIEW

Glanders, a zoonosis, is a contagious disease of equids caused by *Burkholderia mallei* and is characterized by pneumonia and ulcerative nodules of the skin and upper respiratory tract. The mortality rate is high, although some animals remain asymptomatic and serve as a source of infection. The disease has been eradicated from North America, Western Europe, and Australia but still occurs in parts of Asia, the Middle East, Eastern Europe, and North Africa.

SIGNALMENT

Horses, donkeys, and mules of all ages are susceptible to glanders.

SIGNS

- Acute cases develop fever, depression, weight loss, cough, a mucopurulent or sanguinous nasal discharge, enlarged submandibular lymph nodes, ulceration of the nasal septum, and death within a few days. This form is most common in donkeys and mules.
- Chronic glanders is typically seen in horses and is marked by intermittent fever, cough, weight loss, purulent nasal discharge, and epistaxis. Submucosal nodules of the nasal septum and turbinates open and form ulcers that heal with a characteristic stellate scar.
- Some cases are asymptomatic.
- The cutaneous form, known as *farcy*, is characterized by nodules and thickened lymphatic vessels. The nodules frequently ulcerate and drain a honey-like fluid. The medial hock and thigh are the most common sites of cutaneous infection, and edema of the lower limb is a common sequela. Cases may have both respiratory and cutaneous involvement.

CAUSES AND RISK FACTORS

- The source of infection is nasal and cutaneous discharges from infected equids. Ingestion of feed or water contaminated by *B. mallei* is believed to be the primary route of infection, although inhalation and cutaneous exposure may occur.
- *Burkholderia mallei* does not survive in the environment more than a few weeks.
- Stresses including hard work, extreme weather, and gathering of animals increase the severity of the disease.
- *Burkholderia mallei* causes nodules in the lymph nodes and lungs. The upper airway, skin, liver, and other organs may also be involved.

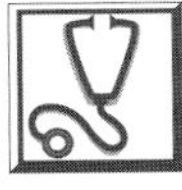

DIAGNOSIS

DIFFERENTIAL DIAGNOSIS

- Melioidosis, caused by *Burkholderia pseudomallei,* has similar signs. Identification of the organism is necessary to confirm the diagnosis because melioidosis patients may be positive on mallein test or serology for glanders.
- Lymphangitis caused by *Histoplasma farcimosum, Corynebacterium pseudotuberculosis,* or *Sporothrix schenkii* may have similar cutaneous lesions. Pneumonia and nasal lesions do not occur, however, and the causative agent is usually readily identified by culture or microscopic examination of exudate or tissue.
- Strangles (*Streptococcus equi*) is usually marked by abscessation and drainage of submandibular or retropharyngeal lymph nodes in contrast to glanders in which the submandibular lymph nodes rarely open. Culture of the nasopharynx or abscess should yield *S. equi.*

CBC/BIOCHEMISTRY/URINALYSIS

- Leukocytosis with neutrophilia
- Hyperfibrinogenemia
- Anemia in chronic cases

OTHER LABORATORY TESTS

- Bacterial culture of material from exudates, nodules, ulcers, or blood may yield *B. mallei,* especially in acute cases. *Burkholderia mallei* is a gram-negative, nonencapsulated, nonmotile rod. Precautions should be taken to prevent exposure of laboratory personnel to infective material.
- Complement fixation (CF) is considered the most reliable serologic test, although animals may not seroconvert until 4–12 weeks postinfection. False-positive CF may result from mallein testing or *B. pseudomallei* infection.

IMAGING

N/A

OTHER DIAGNOSTIC PROCEDURES

The mallein test is commonly used to diagnose glanders. An injection of 0.1 mL of mallein (*B. mallei* purified protein derivative) is made intradermally, often in the lower eyelid. A positive test is characterized by fever, pain, or swelling, 48–72 hr post-injection.

PATHOLOGIC FINDINGS

- The acute form is characterized by severe bronchopneumonia, enlarged bronchial lymph nodes, and widespread petechial hemorrhage.
- The chronic form is marked by miliary nodules in the lungs as well as lymphadenopathy and ulcerative nodules in the skin and upper respiratory tract.

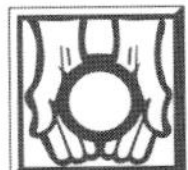

TREATMENT

Regulatory officials should be notified if glanders is suspected. Affected animals should be destroyed and all exposed animals quarantined for further testing. Treatment of animals should not be attempted.

MEDICATIONS

DRUG(S) OF CHOICE

A combination of enrofloxacin and trimethoprim-sulfadiazine is reportedly effective; however, treatment is not usually permitted.

CONTRAINDICATIONS/POSSIBLE INTERACTIONS

N/A

FOLLOW-UP

- Management of an outbreak includes destruction of clinical cases, mallein testing of all exposed horses with destruction of reactors, and destruction or disinfection of bedding and equipment associated with infected horses.
- No vaccine for glanders is available.
- All equids should be tested prior to entering a glanders-free area.

MISCELLANEOUS

ZOONOTIC POTENTIAL

People who handle infected horses and laboratory personnel working with *B. mallei* may be infected via breaks in skin or inhalation. Gloves and masks should be worn when handling clinical cases, and special biosecurity procedures should be followed in the laboratory.

SYNONYMS

- Farcy is often used to indicate the cutaneous form of glanders.
- *Burkholderia mallei* was formerly classified as *Pseudomonas, Actinobacillus* and *Malleomyces mallei.*

Suggested Reading

Muhammad G, Khan MZ, Athar M. Clinico-microbiological and therapeutic aspects of glanders in equines. J Equine Sci 1998; 9:93–96.

Pritchard DG. Glanders. Equine Vet Educ 1995; 7: 29–32.

Radostitis OM, Blood DC, Gay CC, et al Veterinary medicine. Philadelphia: Balliere Tindall. 1994:854–856.

Schlater LK. Glanders. In: Robinson NE, ed. Current therapy in equine medicine. Philadelphia: Saunders. 1992:761–762.

Author Laura K. Reilly

Consulting Editors Ashley G. Boyle and Corinne R. Sweeney

GLAUCOMA

BASICS

OVERVIEW

• The glaucomas are a group of diseases resulting from alterations of aqueous humor dynamics that cause an IOP increase above that which is compatible with normal function of the retinal ganglion cells and optic nerve.
• Glaucoma in horses is being recognized with increased frequency, although the prevalence of glaucoma in the horse is surprisingly low given the horse's propensity for ocular injury and marked intraocular inflammatory responses.
• All glaucomas consist of five stages: (1) an initial event or series of events that influences the aqueous humor outflow system; (2) morphological alterations of the aqueous outflow system that eventually lead to aqueous outflow obstruction and IOP elevation; (3) elevated IOP or ocular hypertension that severely reduces retinal ganglion cell sensitivity and function; (4) subsequent retinal ganglion cell and optic nerve axon degeneration; and (5) progressive visual deterioration that eventually leads to blindness.
• The glaucomas are frequently categorized into primary, secondary, and congenital types. While all types of glaucoma have a causative mechanism, primary glaucomas possess no overt ocular abnormality to account for the increase in IOP, whereas secondary glaucomas have an identifiable cause, such as intraocular inflammation, neoplasia, or lens luxation.
• Primary bilateral glaucoma has been rarely reported in the horse.
• Secondary glaucomas due to anterior uveitis and intraocular neoplasia are most commonly recognized in the horse.
• Congenital glaucoma is reported in foals and associated with developmental anomalies of the iridocorneal angle.

SIGNALMENT

• Glaucoma is reported in the Appaloosa, Paso Fino, Thoroughbred, and Warmblood, although all ages and breeds of horses are at risk.
• There appears to be an increased incidence of glaucoma in horses with previous or concurrent ERU, horses >15 years old, and Appaloosas.

SIGNS

• Equine glaucoma may not be easily recognized in the early stages of the disease due to the subtle nature of the clinical signs.
• There is generally a low index of suspicion for glaucoma in horses, the pupils are often only slightly dilated, and overt discomfort is uncommon.
• Afferent pupillary light reflex deficits, corneal striae, blockage of the drainage angle, decreased vision, lens luxations, mild iridocyclitis, and optic nerve atrophy/cupping may also be found in eyes of horses with glaucoma.
• The presence of corneal striae, or corneal endothelial "band opacities," in nonbuphthalmic horse eyes warrants a high degree of suspicion for the finding of elevated IOP, which may also be found in eyes that are normotensive at the time of examination. Corneal striae are linear, often interconnecting, white opacities found deep in the cornea, caused by stretching or rupture of Descemet's membrane, and may be associated with increased IOP.

CAUSES AND RISK FACTORS

• Aqueous humor is produced in the ciliary body by energy dependent and independent mechanisms. The ciliary enzyme carbonic anhydrase plays an important role in aqueous production. Aqueous humor passes into the posterior chamber, through the pupil into the anterior chamber, and then exits through the iridocorneal angle (conventional) outflow pathway or through the uveovortex and uveoscleral (unconventional) outflow pathways.
• Perfusion and morphologic studies indicate potentially extensive unconventional aqueous humor outflow pathway involvement in the horse. The extensive low-resistance equine conventional aqueous humor outflow pathway and the prominent unconventional outflow pathways in the horse may minimize development of glaucoma in many cases of anterior uveitis.
• However, anterior uveitis can lead to formation of preiridal fibrovascular membranes that limit aqueous absorption by the iris and to physical and functional obstruction of the iridocorneal angles with inflammatory cells and debris.
• Iridal and ciliary body neoplasms and endophthalmitis can cause secondary glaucoma by infiltration of the outflow pathways.

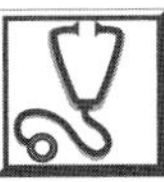

DIAGNOSIS

DIFFERENTIAL DIAGNOSIS

ERU and corneal ulceration may be associated with corneal edema, ocular pain, and blindness in horses.

CBC/BIOCHEMISTRY/URINALYSIS

N/A

OTHER LABORATORY TESTS

Serologic tests for infectious diseases causing the anterior uveitis in horses with glaucoma may identify the causative organism.

IMAGING

B-scan ultrasound can demonstrate intraocular tumors associated with glaucoma in horses.

DIAGNOSTIC PROCEDURES

• The diagnosis of equine glaucoma is made with the tonometric documentation of elevated IOP, and the presence of clinical signs specific to glaucoma, such as a mydriatic pupil and buphthalmia. ERU, in contrast, generally has a low IOP and a miotic pupil.
• The accurate measurement of IOP in the horse requires applanation tonometry. The mean IOP in the horse ranges from 17 to 28 mm Hg. The IOP can vary at different times of day in glaucoma horses and horses with ERU.

PATHOLOGIC FINDINGS

Preiridal fibrovascular membrane formation with secondary iridocorneal angle closure, and trabecular meshwork sclerosis and collapse are noted.

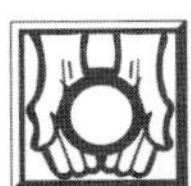

TREATMENT

Various combinations of drugs and surgery may be necessary to reduce the IOP to levels that are compatible with preservation of vision in horses with glaucoma. Glaucoma is particularly aggressive and difficult to control in the Appaloosa.

MEDICATIONS

DRUG(S) OF CHOICE

- Aqueous production should be reduced with the systemically administered carbonic anhydrase inhibitor acetazolamide (1–3 mg/kg QD PO), a β-adrenergic blocker such as 0.5% timolol maleate, and a topical carbonic anhydrase inhibitor such as 2% dorzolamide. Topical cholinergics and prostaglandin drugs may exacerbate iridocyclitis and should only be used with caution.
- Anti-inflammatory therapy, consisting of topically and systemically administered corticosteroids and/or topically and systemically administered nonsteroidal anti-inflammatories (phenylbutazone 1mg/kg BID PO; flunixin meglumine 250 mg BID PO) also appears to be beneficial in the control of IOP.
- When medical therapy is inadequate, neodymium:yttrium-aluminum-garnet (Nd:YAG) or diode laser cyclophotoablation may be a viable alternative for long-term IOP control. Nd:YAG laser cyclophotoablation is very effective at controlling IOP and maintaining vision in the horse. The author recommends 55 laser sites per eye for contact Nd:YAG laser cyclophotoablation in the horse, 5–6 mm posterior to the limbus, at a power setting of 12 W for 0.3-second duration per site. Diode lasers may be used at 55–70 sites for 1500 mW at 1500 msec per site.

CONTRAINDICATIONS/POSSIBLE INTERACTIONS

Conventional glaucoma treatment with miotics may provide varying amounts of IOP reduction in horses. A number of horses have *increased* IOP when administered topical miotics. As miotics can potentiate the clinical signs of uveitis, miotic therapy is generally considered to be contraindicated in glaucoma secondary to uveitis, and should be used cautiously, with careful IOP monitoring, in horses with mild or quiescent anterior uveitis.

FOLLOW-UP

PATIENT MONITORING

- Serial tonometry is required to document IOP spikes in horses with anterior uveitis and secondary glaucoma.
- Continued pupillary dilation is a sign of continued IOP elevation and optic nerve damage.
- Horses with glaucoma should be stall-rested until the condition is under control. Intraocular hemorrhage and increased severity of uveitis are sequelae to overexertion.
- Diet should be consistent with the training level of the horse.
- Self-trauma should be avoided by use of hard- or soft-cup hoods.

PREVENTION/AVOIDANCE

Breeding of horses with glaucoma is not recommended.

POSSIBLE COMPLICATIONS

Chronic pain and blindness are complications.

EXPECTED COURSE AND PROGNOSIS

The horse eye seems to tolerate elevations in IOP for many months to years that would blind a dog; however, blindness is the end result. Buphthalmia can be associated with exposure keratitis.

MISCELLANEOUS

ASSOCIATED CONDITIONS

- ERU
- Exposure keratitis and persistent corneal ulcerations

AGE-RELATED FACTORS

Older horses are at risk of developing glaucoma.

ZOONOTIC POTENTIAL

N/A

PREGNANCY

N/A

SYNONYMS

N/A

SEE ALSO

Recurrent uveitis

ABBREVIATIONS

- ERU = equine recurrent uveitis
- IOP = intraocular pressure

Suggested Reading

Brooks DE. Ophthalmology for the Equine Practitioner. Jackson, WY; Teton NewMedia, 2002.

Brooks DE, Matthews AG. Equine ophthalmology. In: Gelatt KN, ed. Veterinary Ophthalmology, ed 4. Philadelphia; Lippincott Williams and Wilkins, 2007.

Gilger BC, ed. Equine Ophthalmology. Philadelphia; WB Saunders, 2005.

Author Dennis E. Brooks
Consulting Editor Dennis E. Brooks

GLUCOSE TOLERANCE TEST

BASICS

DEFINITION

- Performed to evaluate a horse's ability to metabolize glucose appropriately.
- In normal horses, insulin secretion is closely tied to blood glucose concentrations. Fasted insulin concentrations are quite low but increase rapidly when the horse receives glucose. In turn, this rapidly causes blood glucose to return to the normal range.
- Administer dextrose (0.5 g/kg as a 50% solution IV). Either blood glucose alone or glucose and insulin are determined before and every 30 min after administration for 4 hr. Glucose is not given orally to remove the confounding effects of poor intestinal absorption or delayed gastric emptying. Serum glucose should be normal within 3 hr of administration.
- A common disease process causing abnormal results is insulin resistance in horses with pars intermedia tumors or hyperplasia (i.e., equine Cushing's disease, PPID) and idiopathic insulin resistance (equine metabolic syndrome), leading to prolonged elevation in blood glucose levels. Blood glucose also will be elevated longer than 3 hr in horses with diabetes mellitus caused by insulin deficiency.
- Also advocated as a means to assess maturity in neonatal foals. An insulin response of 250% over baseline at 5 min is associated with a good prognosis for life; a response of 100% or less at 15 min is associated with prematurity and a poor prognosis for life.

PATHOPHYSIOLOGY

- Pancreatitis leading to destruction of beta cells and development of type 1 diabetes mellitus leads to low insulin and increased glucose tolerance test times. This is very rare in equids.
- Increased serum insulin levels in euglycemic or hyperglycemic horses may result from peripheral insulin resistance, which may be idiopathic or caused by type 2 diabetes mellitus or an insulin antagonist (e.g., cortisol) in horses with PPID, stressed horses, or those receiving glucocorticoid therapy.
- Poor response to insulin in premature foals reflects immaturity of the pancreatic beta cells and poor homeostatic mechanisms.

SYSTEM AFFECTED

The endocrine system is primarily affected by abnormal blood glucose response tests—slow return of blood glucose to the normal range indicates either insulin deficiency or resistance.

SIGNALMENT

- Ponies tend to have a physiologic degree of insulin resistance; thus, blood glucose returns to normal levels more slowly than in adults.
- No sex differences
- Obese animals, particularly ponies, are more insulin resistant than are thinner animals.
- PPID disease tends to occur in old horses (>18 years).
- Premature foals are those born before 320 days of gestation.
- Dysmature foals are those born after 320 days of gestation but with signs of prematurity.

SIGNS

- In horses with an abnormal test caused by PPID—hirsutism and failure to shed winter coat
- Also common—abnormal fat distribution, pendulous abdomen, weight loss, polyuria and polydipsia, laminitis, and tendency to chronic infections
- The eyelids can look swollen, and the supraorbital fat pad may look bulging.
- The owner may report the horse is dull or depressed.
- Similar clinical signs, but without hirsutism or abnormal hair coat, are seen in horses with type II diabetes mellitus and equine metabolic syndrome
- In horses with type 1 diabetes mellitus—weight loss, polyuria and polydipsia, and lethargy or depression
- Prematurity—low body weight, weakness, short or silky hair coat, increased joint range of motion, bulging forehead, incomplete cartilage formation of the ears, and incomplete ossification of the tarsal and carpal bones.

CAUSES

- The primary cause for abnormal results is insulin antagonist. Exogenous or endogenous corticosteroids are the most common, although other hormones (e.g., growth hormone) may also have this effect.
- When insulin resistance occurs without a predisposing cause, equine metabolic syndrome is diagnosed.
- The most common reason for type 1 diabetes mellitus is pancreatic damage, secondary to parasite migration.
- The most common reason for prematurity is an adverse uterine environment, often placentitis or placental insufficiency.
- Some sedatives, particularly xylazine and detomidine, can cause a transient hyperglycemia that confounds results; hence, avoid these sedatives when performing these tests.
- High-carbohydrate diets may increase serum glucose while complete fasting may cause stress with cortisol release. Thus, the test should be performed on horses consuming grass hay or other low-carbohydrate feeds.

RISK FACTORS

- A pituitary tumor is the most common risk factor for abnormal test results.
- Glucocorticoid administration or increased cortisol from a stress response also leads to insulin resistance and hyperglycemia.
- Obesity, particularly in ponies, is associated with insulin resistance.

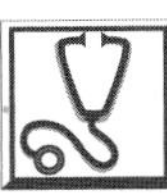

DIAGNOSIS

DIFFERENTIAL DIAGNOSIS

- Polyuria, polydipsia, and glucosuria in horses with suspected endocrine disorders indicate a disorder in glucose homeostasis.
- Weak foal—sepsis and neonatal maladjustment syndrome
- History of gestational length allows a diagnosis of prematurity to be established. Additionally, premature foals are often septic and have other medical conditions, so this diagnosis of prematurity does not preclude others.

LABORATORY FINDINGS

Drugs That May Alter Laboratory Results

N/A

Disorders That May Alter Laboratory Results

Delayed separation of serum from cells falsely lowers blood glucose values.

Valid If Run in a Human Lab?

Yes

CBC/BIOCHEMISTRY/URINALYSIS

- Horses with abnormal glucose response caused by PPID exhibit a stress response with mature neutrophilia, lymphopenia, and eosinopenia. They also may have glucosuria.
- Horses with type 1 or 2 diabetes mellitus have hyperglycemia. Horses with metabolic syndrome have normal blood glucose levels in the face of increased insulin concentrations.
- Premature foals have variable leukogram results. Good prognosis for life is associated with WBC counts >cells/mL and fibrinogen levels <400 mg/dL.

OTHER LABORATORY TESTS

- Pituitary function—endogenous ACTH determination and dexamethasone suppression tests. If these results are consistent with PPID, that diagnosis is supported; if these results do not indicate PPID, suspect either a stress response or equine metabolic syndrome.
- Check IgG levels in all neonatal foals; give plasma if <600 mg/dL.
- Arterial blood gas determination to assess the foal's ability to ventilate and oxygenate its tissues.

IMAGING

- Increased pituitary gland size may be visualized with specialized modalities—computed tomography or venous contrast.
- Lung maturity may be partially assessed in premature foals by thoracic radiography.

DIAGNOSTIC PROCEDURES

Exploratory laparotomy or abdominocentesis may reveal a damaged pancreas. However, these tests should be considered extremely low yield, because the pancreas normally is difficult to visualize and pancreatic tumors are too small to distort the pancreas so that they can be localized.

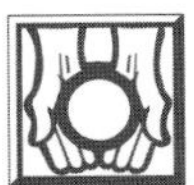

TREATMENT

APPROPRIATE HEALTH CARE

- Premature foals require inpatient treatment if severely affected—IV fluids, and nutritional support to maintain blood glucose at adequate levels. Also, they often require insufflation with oxygen or ventilatory support.
- Horses with hyperlipemia require inpatient treatment with IV dextrose, balanced electrolyte solutions, caloric replacement, heparin, and exogenous insulin.
- All other horses with abnormal test results can be treated as outpatients.

NURSING CARE

- Premature foals need extensive nursing care. They are prone to complications such as corneal ulcers, gastric ulcers, and pressure sores; they need aggressive, proactive care to minimize such occurrences.
- Horses with laminitis need corrective hoof trimming and shoeing and dietary management.

ACTIVITY

- Limit the activity of horses with laminitis.
- Increase the activity of sound, obese horses in an effort to lose weight.

DIET

- Horses with laminitis generally benefit from a low-carbohydrate, high-fiber diet.
- Keep horses with insulin resistance on a low-carbohydrate diet.
- Restrict or increase caloric intake in all horses until a condition score of 4–6 out of 10 is achieved.

CLIENT EDUCATION

- Long-term prognosis for life and work is good in premature foals if they can survive and develop to the point of no longer needing nursing care.
- Horses with PPID may be managed with medication and nursing care, but their prognosis is quite variable. Some do well for several years; others are refractory to treatment. Inform owners that treatment of such horses is palliative and required for life.
- Encourage clients to maintain horses at condition scores of 4–6 out of 10 and to prevent obesity.

SURGICAL CONSIDERATIONS

N/A

MEDICATIONS

DRUG(S) OF CHOICE

- The agent most commonly used to alter symptoms of PPID is pergolide (0.50–2 mg/day).
- Horses with insulin deficiency (i.e., type 1 diabetes mellitus) require insulin supplementation. Protamine zinc insulin (0.5 IU IM BID) was reported to normalize blood glucose in a case report of a pony.
- Hyperlipemia—protamine zinc insulin (0.075–0.4 IU/kg SQ or IM BID or daily). Regular insulin (0.4 IU/kg) has also been recommended.
- Regard these doses as starting points that should be changed in response to blood glucose levels.

CONTRAINDICATIONS

N/A

PRECAUTIONS

- Dextrose for injection should always be available when administering insulin to any horse. If signs of hypoglycemia occur, treat immediately with IV dextrose.
- Horses that receive overdoses of pergolide may exhibit anorexia, lethargy, and ataxia.

POSSIBLE INTERACTIONS

N/A

ALTERNATIVE DRUGS

N/A

FOLLOW-UP

PATIENT MONITORING

- Test horses with PPID every 12–20 weeks by endogenous ACTH determination or dexamethasone response testing. Abnormal results indicate the need for an increased dose of the compound the horse is receiving or change in medication.
- Check the blood glucose level of horses with diabetes mellitus on insulin therapy twice a day. Increase or decrease insulin doses in response to blood glucose values outside the normal range.

POSSIBLE COMPLICATIONS

N/A

MISCELLANEOUS

ASSOCIATED CONDITIONS

- Hirsutism, chronic infections, and laminitis are commonly associated with PPID.
- Obesity, laminitis, and hyperlipemia are commonly associated with insulin resistance.
- Sepsis is common in premature foals.

AGE-RELATED FACTORS

N/A

ZOONOTIC POTENTIAL

N/A

PREGNANCY

N/A

SYNONYMS

N/A

SEE ALSO

- Insulin levels/tolerance test
- Pituitary tumors
- Premature foals
- Equine metabolic syndrome

ABBREVIATIONS

- ACTH = adrenocorticotrophic hormone
- PPID = pituitary pars itermedia dysfunction

Suggested Reading

Beech J. Endocrine system. In: Colahan PT, Mayhew IG, Merritt AM, Moore JN, eds. Equine Medicine and Surgery, ed 5. St. Louis: Mosby, 1999:1947–1968.

Fowden AL, Silver M, Ellis L, *et al*. Studies on equine prematurity: III. Insulin secretion in the foal during the perinatal period. Equine Vet J 1984;16:286–291.

Freestone JF, *et al*. Insulin and glucose response following oral glucose administration in well conditioned ponies. Equine Vet J 1992;11;13–17.

Author Janice Sojka

Consulting Editor Michel Lévy

GLUCOSE

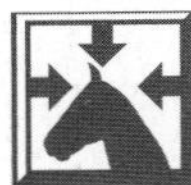

BASICS

DEFINITION

The glucose concentration is greater than the laboratory reference interval.

PATHOPHYSIOLOGY

• Serum glucose concentration depends on a variety of factors, with a net result from rate of entry and removal as influenced by intestinal absorption, hepatic production, hormonal regulation, and tissue utilization.
• Hyperglycemia may result from an absolute (rare) or relative insulin deficiency, reduced utilization of glucose in peripheral tissue, increased gluconeogenesis, or increased glycogenolysis. Glucocorticoids, catecholamines, glucagon, growth hormone, and thyroid hormone can increase gluconeogenesis and glycogenolysis.
• During cortisol release, cellular insulin receptors are down-regulated (i.e., insulin resistance); this can result from a marked endogenous cortisol release "stress response" or hypercortisolemia from pituitary adenomas.
• Epinephrine can mediate hyperglycemia during the "fight-or-flight" response.
• Physiologic, transient, postprandial hyperglycemia may be seen.
• Hyperglycemia may be associated with some stages of endotoxemia/septicemia due to decreased cellular glucose utilization. Glucose and energy metabolism varies depending on the stage, severity, and other conditions impacting energy metabolism and cortisol release (stress).
• Early in shock, increased catecholamines, glucagon, and glucocorticoids can increase hepatic gluconeogenesis leading to hyperglycemia.

SYSTEMS AFFECTED

• Endocrine/metabolic—hormonal regulation of gluconeogenesis and glycogenolysis
• Renal/urologic—PU/PD caused by glucosuria, resulting in osmotic diuresis
• Nervous—Severe hyperglycemia may result in CNS dysfunction because of increased osmolality.

GENETICS

Not usually a genetic basis

INCIDENCE/PREVALENCE

• May be variably associated with described syndromes, such as stress, sepsis/endotoxemia
• High incidence of hyperglycemia in diabetes and functional pituitary adenomas

GEOGRAPHIC DISTRIBUTION

N/A

SIGNALMENT

Any horse, but older horses are candidates for pituitary adenomas, with or without clinical signs.

SIGNS

Historical

• Variable
• PU/PD, depression, weight loss, obesity, polyphagia, hirsutism (i.e., pituitary adenoma), and underlying disease resulting in severe stress
• Asymptomatic if transient physiologic or stress response

Physical Examination

Dependent on the underlying cause—Obesity, hirsutism, weight loss, muscle wasting, pendulous abdomen, hyperhidrosis, or laminitis may be associated with functional pituitary adenomas.

CAUSES

• Hypercortisolemia can result in increased gluconeogenesis, decreased peripheral glucose utilization, sparing of glucose because of increased mobilization of free fatty acids, and insulin resistance.
• Insulin resistance because of cortisol release and down-regulation of insulin receptors; usually, significant glucose concentrations result from functional pituitary adenomas, with release of pituitary ACTH and POMC and subsequent cortisol release. Pituitary adenomas are significant when adverse clinical signs with metabolic abnormalities occur. Note, not all pituitary adenomas lead to adverse clinical metabolic disorders; the lesion may be asymptomatic and only found at necropsy.
• Absolute insulin deficiency (i.e., hypoinsulinemia) from diabetes mellitus is uncommon in horses and thought to be secondary to chronic pancreatitis that destroys pancreatic islets.
• Physiologic—postprandial, exertion or excitement that is epinephrine mediated, or stress response that is cortisol-mediated; can be from a severe disease process (e.g., painful colic)
• When giving parenteral nutrition, concurrent sepsis, shock, and major trauma can lead to insulin resistance and reduced glucose utilization.
• Iatrogenic because of dextrose-fluid administration or parenteral nutrition
• Acquired non–insulin-dependent diabetes mellitus (type 2) in obese ponies
• Administration of corticosteroids, xylazine, or detomidine

RISK FACTORS

• Obesity
• Pancreatitis
• Old age
• Severe disease
• Colic

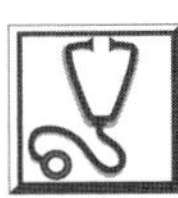

DIAGNOSIS

DIFFERENTIAL DIAGNOSIS

• Physiologic—Mild, transient hyperglycemia can be associated with cortisol or epinephrine release or postprandial fluctuations.
• Colic—Hyperglycemia has been reported in colic, with concentrations >300 mg/ L indicating a poorer prognosis.

CBC/BIOCHEMISTRY/URINALYSIS

Hyperglycemia may be the only laboratory finding.

CBC

• Inflammatory leukogram if underlying inflammatory disease
• Stress leukogram with neutrophilia and lymphopenia if cortisol mediated
• Mature neutrophilia if epinephrine induced

Biochemistry/Urinalysis

• Dependent on the underlying disease
• Functional pituitary adenoma—possible hyperglycemia, azotemia, elevated CK and AST because of muscle catabolism, and electrolyte abnormalities because of PU/PD or anorexia; decreased urine specific gravity; glucosuria if renal threshold (180–200 mg/L) is exceeded
• Diabetes mellitus—hyperglycemia; glucosuria

OTHER LABORATORY TESTS

• ACTH stimulation test—often an exaggerated response in pituitary-dependent hypercortisolemia, but not completely reliable; plasma ACTH measurement may be more useful.
• Dexamethasone suppression test—the cortisol concentration will be suppressed (80% after 1 hr) in normal horses, but will not suppress or have only modest suppression in horses with functional pituitary adenomas; not completely reliable because of the complexity of pituitary adenoma secretion
• Glucose tolerance test—used after pituitary adenoma is ruled out. Recommended method is to give IV glucose versus the oral route to prevent confounding effects of GI motility. Published recommendation is a 50% glucose solution (0.5 g/kg IV), and serum concentrations of glucose and insulin are then

measured. In cases of primary insulin-dependent diabetes mellitus, sustained, elevated glucose concentrations are found, with no rise in insulin. In cases of insulin resistance, the insulin concentration rises, but return of the glucose concentration to normal is delayed more than 3 hr.

- Measurement of plasma insulin—low in diabetes; high-normal or high in hypercortisolemia (i.e., insulin resistance)
- Insulin tolerance test—published recommendation is soluble regular insulin (1–8 IU/kg IV), with assay of the glucose concentration every 15 min for 3 hr; failure of insulin to lower the glucose concentration to normal suggests insulin-resistant diabetes.

IMAGING

Ultrasonography or radiology can be used to detect underlying diseases.

OTHER DIAGNOSTIC PROCEDURES

N/A

PATHOLOGICAL FINDINGS

Pituitary adenomas

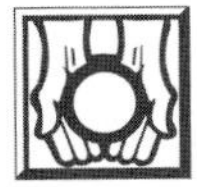

TREATMENT

AIMS OF TREATMENT

- Manage stress or the situation inducing epinephrine release—sample when calm.
- Resolve the underlying disease condition.
- Medical management of pituitary adenomas—correct any biochemical abnormalities with appropriate fluid therapy and diet supplementation.
- Medical management of diabetes mellitus

APPROPRIATE HEALTH CARE

Management of underlying cause

NURSING CARE

As applicable

ACTIVITY

None

DIET

May be applicable for management of diabetes mellitus or pituitary adenomas, especially to correct any metabolic imbalance

CLIENT EDUCATION

Education regarding the underlying cause. Diabetes mellitus or pituitary adenomas may require long-term medical and dietary treatment

SURGICAL CONSIDERATIONS

Can be applicable if correcting underlying cause. Surgery for pituitary adenomas has a minimal success rate in horses.

MEDICATIONS

DRUGS OF CHOICE

- Diabetes mellitus—insulin, but long-term therapeutic success has been limited.
- Functional pituitary adenomas—dopamine agonists or serotonin antagonists

CONTRAINDICATIONS

- Corticosteroids
- Dextrose-containing fluids

PRECAUTIONS

- Hyperglycemia may lead to laminitis and other complications depending on the underlying disease.
- Avoid abruptly decreasing serum glucose concentrations.
- High glucose concentrations above the renal threshold from severe disease can lead to cell deprivation of glucose for energy and may indicate a poorer prognosis for recovery.
- Ketosis may develop during diabetes mellitus.

POSSIBLE INTERACTIONS

N/A

ALTERNATIVE DRUGS

N/A

FOLLOW-UP

PATIENT MONITORING

- Monitor blood glucose concentrations after treatment.
- Monitor for signs associated with the underlying disease.
- Monitor urine specific gravity, glucosuria, ketonuria or other abnormalities, and electrolytes if PU/PD.

PREVENTION/AVOIDANCE

Appropriate use of dextrose fluids or parenteral nutrition

POSSIBLE COMPLICATIONS

- Hypercortisolemia and diabetes mellitus can predispose to secondary infections.
- Severe hyperglycemia can result in hyperosmolality and possible CNS depression.

EXPECTED COURSE AND PROGNOSIS

Guarded if prolonged hyperglycemia, since cells are deprived of glucose for energy. Several diseases have a guarded prognosis: those that are associated with hyperglycemia, such as diabetes mellitus, pituitary adenomas that have clinical signs, and diseases that result in severe and prolonged cortisol release.

MISCELLANEOUS

ASSOCIATED CONDITIONS

- Electrolyte concentration abnormalities
- Complications of diabetes mellitus—cataracts, glomerulopathies, ketosis, and acidosis

AGE-RELATED FACTORS

- Young foals can be prone to transient, increased glucose concentrations because of excitability and epinephrine release.
- Middle-aged to older horses have an increased incidence of pituitary adenomas.

ZOONOTIC POTENTIAL

N/A

PREGNANCY

N/A

SYNONYMS

N/A

SEE ALSO

- Diabetes mellitus
- Hypercortisolemia
- Pituitary adenoma

ABBREVIATIONS

- AST = aspartate aminotransferase
- CK = creatine kinase
- CNS = central nervous system
- GI = gastrointestinal
- POMC = pro-opiolipomelanocortin
- PU/PD = polyuria/polydipsia

Suggested Reading

Kaneko JJ. Carbohydrate metabolism and its diseases. In: Kaneko JJ, Harvey JW, Bruss ML, eds. Clinical Biochemistry of Domestic Animals, ed 5. San Diego: Academic Press, 1997:61–75.

Hollis AR, Boston RC, Corley KT. Blood glucose in horses with acute abdominal disease. J. Vet. Int. Med 2007;21:1099–1103.

Parry BW. Prognostic evaluation of equine colic cases. Compend Cont Educ Pract Vet 1986;8:S98–S104.

Toribio RE. Pars intermedia dysfunction (equine Cushing's disease). In: Reed SM, Bayly WM, Sellon DC, eds. Equine Internal Medicine, Ed 2. St. Louis: Saunders Elsevier, 2004:1327–1339.

Toribio RE. Endocrine pancreas. In: Reed SM, Bayly WM, Sellon DC, eds. Equine Internal Medicine, ed 2. St. Louis: Saunders Elsevier, 2004:1362–1365.

Author Claire B. Andreasen

Consulting Editor Kenneth.W. Hinchcliff

GLYCOGEN BRANCHING ENZYME DEFICIENCY

BASICS

OVERVIEW

- This is a genetically inherited autosomal recessive disease of Quarter Horses and Paints that results in a nonsense mutation in the gene coding for glycogen branching enzyme (GBE), rendering the enzyme ineffective.
- Also known as glycogen storage disease-IV (GSD-IV), which is also reported in humans and Norwegian Forest Cats.
- GBE is needed for the formation of a 1,6 branch points in glycogen. This defect in glycogen can lead to abnormal glucose homeostasis in cardiac and skeletal muscle and liver.
- Foals typically exhibit weakness and hypotonia and die shortly after birth.

SIGNALMENT

- Quarter Horse and Paint neonatal foals
- Clinical signs are generally seen from the time of birth.

SIGNS

- Many affected foals present for other illness such as septicemia. Concurrent disease such as pneumonia is common in this age group of foals.
- Late-term abortion
- Stillbirths or persistent recumbency
- Transient flexural limb deformities
- Seizures—due to inadequate glucose metabolism in neurons
- Cardiorespiratory failure—due to muscular weakness and cardiomyopathy

CAUSES AND RISK FACTORS

- It is a heritable trait among certain Quarter Horse and Paint lines.
- Defective gene is on chromosome 26 that encodes the GBE.
- In 2004, the genetic basis of the defective GBE gene was identified by cDNA sequences: A single C-to-A substitution at base 102 of codon 34 of exon 1.
- When evaluated in 11 affected foals, all were homozygous for the defective *X34* allele. When the gene is expressed, the mRNA product encodes for a 699 amino acid protein with a nonsense mutation, rendering the GB enzyme ineffective. The affected foal pedigrees had a common ancestry and contained prolific stallions who are likely to be heterozygous for the recessive *X34* allele.
- Up to 10% of all Quarter Horses may have at least one defective gene.

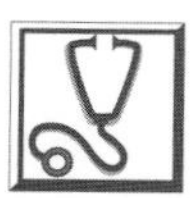

DIAGNOSIS

- Genetic testing using DNA from tail/mane hair (PCR technique)
- Muscle biopsy—PAS stain is decreased; polysaccharide accumulates in skeletal muscle with amorphous PAS-positive inclusions.
- Pedigree analysis—likely inherited as a simple autosomal recessive condition

DIFFERENTIAL DIAGNOSIS

- Neonatal septicemia—may also exhibit weakness and hypoglycemia, but should have characteristic changes in leukogram (neutropenia or neutrophilia), fever, and signs of infection
- Congenital myotonia—Progressive myotonia may have similar weakness, but progresses to muscle stiffness and atrophy with prolonged contraction of the affected muscles after stimulation. Apparent as early as 1 month of age, but usually not apparent from birth. Specific histologic changes in muscle
- Hyperkalemic periodic paralysis—muscular weakness is episodic rather than progressive; clinical signs rarely seen in neonatal foals. Serum potassium may be increased during episodes of muscle fasciculation. Autosomal dominant condition of Quarter Horses—genetic testing (DNA) is indicated if HYPP is suspected.

CBC/BIOCHEMISTRY/URINALYSIS

- CBC is usually normal, or reflects concurrent disease.
- Biochemistry is useful. Affected foals tend to have intermittent or persistent hypoglycemia, elevated serum liver enzyme activities, and increases in CK, AST, and GGT.

OTHER LABORATORY TESTS

N/A

IMAGING

N/A

OTHER DIAGNOSTIC PROCEDURES

N/A

PATHOLOGICAL FINDINGS

- Skeletal and cardiac muscle specimens show an absence of normal glycogen staining with PAS stain and myonecrosis.
- Accumulation of unbranched glycogen inclusion bodies in many tissues, including skeletal muscle, liver, myocardium, and Purkinje fibers
- Paucity of any normal glycogen content in skeletal muscle. Often normal glycogen content in liver

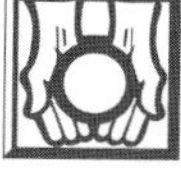

TREATMENT

This is a fatal condition of neonatal foals, with no known treatment.

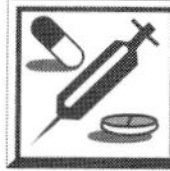

MEDICATIONS

DRUG(S) OF CHOICE

N/A

CONTRAINDICATIONS/POSSIBLE INTERACTIONS

N/A

FOLLOW-UP

PATIENT MONITORING, PREVENTION/AVOIDANCE, POSSIBLE COMPLICATIONS

N/A

EXPECTED COURSE AND PROGNOSIS

- Grave prognosis
- Most foals die during hospitalization or shortly after discharge. This is a fatal disease of neonates.

MISCELLANEOUS

ASSOCIATED CONDITIONS

N/A

AGE-RELATED FACTORS

- Clinical signs are seen from the time of birth.

ZOONOTIC POTENTIAL

N/A

PREGNANCY

N/A

SEE ALSO

- Seizures
- HYPP

ABBREVIATIONS

- GB = glycogen branching
- GBE = glycogen branching enzyme
- GBED = glycogen branching enzyme deficiency
- HYPP = hyperkalemic periodic paralysis
- PAS = periodic acid–Schiff
- PCR = polymerase chain reaction

Suggested Reading

Valberg SJ, Ward TL, Rush B, Kinde H, Hiraragi H, Nahey D, Fyfe J, Mickelson JR. Glycogen branching enzyme deficiency in Quarterhorse foals.J Vet Intern Med 2001;15:572–580.

Wagner ML, Valberg SJ, Ames EG, Bauer MM, Wiseman JA, Penedo CMT, Kinde H, Abbitt B, Mickelson JR. Allele frequency and likely impact of the glycogen branching enzyme deficiency gene in quarter horse and paint horse populations.J Vet Intern Med 2006;20:1207–1211.

Author Samuel D.A. Hurcombe

Consulting Editor Margaret C. Mudge

BASICS

OVERVIEW

• Goiter is enlargement of the thyroid gland to 2 times its normal size.
• Goiter is further classified as either diffuse or nodular. If it is nodular, it may be either uninodular or multinodular and either functional or nonfunctional. Nodular goiter is the result of thyroid tumors within the parenchyma of the gland. Diffuse goiter is caused by either excess or deficient iodine in the diet or by ingestion of goitrogens, which make ingested iodine unavailable.
• Goiter is most frequently congenital, seen in foals born to mares ingesting excess amounts of iodine throughout pregnancy. The endocrine system is the primary system affected.
• Horses with diffuse goiter are generally hypothyroid. Nodular goiter is usually caused by thyroid adenomas that are nonfunctioning and are not associated with clinical signs.

SIGNALMENT

• There are no breed or sex predilections. Most horses with goiter are foals born with congenital goiter. This is due to ingestion of goitrogens or unbalanced amounts of iodine by the dam.
• Goiter is not a genetic condition.

SIGNS

The defining characteristic of a goiter is a thyroid gland enlarged to 2 times its normal size.

CAUSES AND RISK FACTORS

• The cause of diffuse goiter is ingestion of either too much or too little iodine. If pregnant mares receive high-iodine diets, they will be clinically normal while their offspring will have enlarged thyroid glands.
• Thyroid adenoma or adenocarcinoma most often causes nodular goiter.
• Goiter is uncommon in horses.
• Endemic goiter may occur in broodmare farms if dietary iodine is unbalanced. Idiopathic hypothyroidism and goiter occur in foals born to mares pastured in the northwestern portion of the North American continent. The cause of this syndrome is not known, although an ingested goitrogen is suspected.

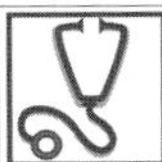

DIAGNOSIS

• Diagnosis can be made on physical examination by observing and palpating a grossly enlarged thyroid gland.
• Differential diagnosis includes other structures that might cause swelling in the proximal neck, including abscess, enlarged lymph node, guttural pouch, or generalized edema, or cellulitis.

CBC/BIOCHEMISTRY PANEL/URINALYSIS

These tests are generally normal.

OTHER LABORATORY TESTS

Serum T_3 and T_4 levels may be low if the animal is hypothyroid.

IMAGING

An enlarged thyroid gland may be seen as a soft tissue mass on radiographs of the proximal neck. The enlarged thyroid can also be imaged via ultrasound examination.

DIAGNOSTIC PROCEDURES

Fine needle biopsy or aspirate of the goiter may be performed to confirm that the structure in question is indeed the thyroid gland.

PATHOLOGICAL FINDINGS

• Nodular goiter—A tumor in the thyroid gland is often found on pathological examination.
• Diffuse goiter—Enlarged follicles filled with colloid and few or no resportion vesicles are seen on histopathological examination.

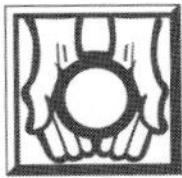

TREATMENT

• As dietary factors are most commonly implicated in goiter, the dietary iodine concentration of affected horses and their dams if they are foals should be determined.
• From 35 to 40 mg/day iodine in a pregnant mare's diet may cause congenital goiter in her foal. NRC recommendations for daily iodine intake are 1–2 mg/day.
• Once the diet is corrected to a proper iodine level, the goiter general resolves.
• It is important to recommend to broodmare owners that they do not feed supplements to pregnant mares containing excessive amounts of iodine. If a pregnant mare is pastured in the geographic area associated with idiopathic goiter (northwestern United States, particularly the states of Washington and Oregon, and northwestern Canada), removal from pasture or supplementation with hay may be preventative.
• Removal of a thyroid tumor in instances of nodular goiter is curative.

MEDICATIONS

If the horse is hypothyroid, supplementation with thyroxine is curative. Synthetic thyroxine at a dose of 20 μg/kg will maintain normal thyroid hormone levels for 24 hr.

CONTRAINDICATIONS/POSSIBLE INTERACTIONS

N/A

FOLLOW-UP

• If goiter is due to a benign tumor, removal of the tumor will be curative.
• If goiter is due to excess or deficient iodine, correcting the diet to an acceptable level should result in resolution of the symptoms.
• Foals with goiter should be carefully monitored to make sure that any skeletal abnormalities associated with hypothyroidism do not cause angular limb deformities.
• The expected course is for the goiter to resolve and for the thyroid gland to regain its normal size once the cause has been removed.

MISCELLANEOUS

SEE ALSO

• Hypothyroidism
• T_3 T_4 determination
• Thyroid tumors

ABBREVIATIONS

• T_4 = thyroxine
• T_3 = triiodothyronine

Suggested Reading

Driscoll J, Hintz HF, Schryer HF. Goiter in foals caused by excessive iodine. JAVMA 1968;153:1618–1630

Author Janice Sojka
Consulting Editor Michel Lévy

GRANULOMATOUS ENTERITIS

BASICS

DEFINITION

GE represents one of several types of chronic inflammatory bowel diseases affecting the mature horse. The disease is characterized by a diffuse and circumscribed infiltration of the lamina propria and submucosa of the gastrointestinal tract with lymphocytes, macrophages, and epithelioid cells with occasional plasma cells and multinucleated giant cells. The ileum is the most consistently and most severely affected site. The presence of marked villous atrophy and clubbing contributes to malabsorption of carbohydrates due to the loss of absorptive surface area and the loss of absorptive epithelial cells at the tips of the villi. Other features of the small bowel mucosa include ulceration, lymphoid hyperplasia, crypt abscesses, and lymphangiectasia. In GE, gross lesions involving small intestine are common (40/42), but also may involve large intestine (21/42). Granulomatous changes are also found in the mesenteric lymph nodes of most affected horses. Clinically, this condition is associated with carbohydrate malabsorption and excessive protein loss into the gastrointestinal tract.

SIGNALMENT

Granulomatous enteritis can occur at any age or in any breed, or either sex. GE appears to be most common in young adult horses (mean, 2.2 years; range, 1–5 years), and the Standardbred is the most commonly reported breed. A familial tendency for the development of GE has been suggested in Standardbreds.

SIGNS

- Chronic, insidious weight loss over several months' duration is the most common presenting sign. Horses present in thin or emaciated body condition.
- Appetite variable; may be increased, normal, or decreased. Initially, appetite is usually increased.
- Edema of the ventral thorax, ventral abdomen, and distal extremities may develop as animal becomes hypoproteinemic.
- Multiple, firm nodules or masses (5- to 10-cm diameter) within the mesentery or small intestine may be palpated consistently on per-rectal examination.
- Roughened hair coat; alopecia; skin dry and flaky. Skin lesions usually involve head and limbs, especially coronet.
- Diarrhea is not usually present unless there is involvement of large intestine and rectum. Intermittent diarrhea with semi-formed feces recorded in 24% (4/17) of cases.
- Bright and alert initially, but become depressed with debilitation.
- Decreased exercise tolerance may be the first clinical sign observed.

CAUSES AND RISK FACTORS

The etiologic agent or the initiating pathophysiologic mechanism is unknown. It has been hypothesized that the granulomatous lesions may result from an aberrant host immune-mediated response to dietary, parasitic, or bacterial antigens.

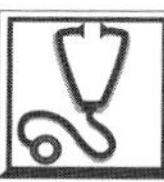

DIAGNOSIS

DIFFERENTIAL DIAGNOSIS

Rule out other diseases that cause significant protein loss into the pleural or peritoneal cavities or urinary system, and other causes of chronic weight loss.

- Chronic eosinophilic gastroenteritis
- Intestinal lymphosarcoma
- Abdominal abscessation
- Lymphocytic–plasmacytic enterocolitis

CBC/BIOCHEMISTRY/URINALYSIS

- Hypoalbuminemia (moderate to severe) (8–22g/L; normal 26–35g/L) is the most consistent laboratory finding being reported in 90% of GE cases. In the initial stages of GE, intestinal protein loss involves relatively larger quantities of albumin than globulins.
- Hypoproteinemia reported in approximately 65% of GE cases.
- Mild to moderate hypoglobulinemia. Varying serum gamma-globulin levels.
- Anemia reported in 87% (41/47) of GE cases or normal complete blood counts.
- Moderate neutrophilia with mild left shift
- Urinalysis normal

DIAGNOSTIC PROCEDURES

- Decreased D-xylose and glucose absorption tests if there is significant small intestine involvement. Malabsorption of carbohydrates occurs if there is diffuse and severe villous atrophy occurring throughout the small intestine. If small intestinal lesions are focal there may be a normal carbohydrate absorption test.
- Abdominocentesis is usually normal, except occasionally peritoneal macrophages may exhibit evidence of decreased phagocytic activity.
- Rectal mucosal biopsy may provide a diagnosis in approximately 50% of GE cases and depends on whether rectum is involved. Granulomatous changes in rectal mucosa.
- Intravenous administration of [^{51}Cr]albumin documents increased fecal radioactivity due to gastrointestinal protein loss.
- Ileal biopsy through a standing left-flank laparotomy is necessary for a definitive diagnosis; however, surgery on a debilitated, hypoproteinemic animal is not without risk.

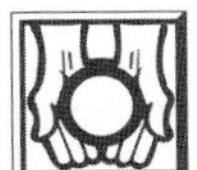

TREATMENT

Poor prognosis.

MEDICATIONS

DRUG(S) OF CHOICE

- Medical therapies have been generally unsuccessful in resolving the chronic inflammatory lesions. Long-term survival with any medical treatment has not been reported.
- Prednisolone 0.5–2.0mg/kg PO q24h has been ineffective. As malabsorption is a feature of this disease, parenteral administration should be considered.
- Long-term parenteral dexamethasone sodium phosphate administration—40mg IM q96h for 4 weeks; 35mg IM q96h for 4 weeks; 30mg IM q96h for 4 weeks; 20mg IM q96h for 2 weeks; 10mg IM q96h for 2 weeks has been used successfully in one case reported in the literature.
- Total parenteral nutrition may be indicated in very valuable patients.

CONTRAINDICATIONS/POSSIBLE INTERACTIONS

There is alleged risk of laminitis following parenteral dexamethasone administration.

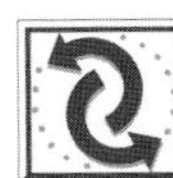

FOLLOW-UP

- Monitor body weight, total serum protein, and serum albumin levels following dexamethasone therapy.
- Repeat per-rectal examinations and D-xylose absorption test.
- Feed free-choice, high-quality ration.
- Prognosis—poor in the long-term

MISCELLANEOUS

ABBREVIATION

- GE = granulomatous enteritis

Suggested Reading

Cimprich RE. Equine granulomatous enteritis. Vet Pathol 1974;11:535–547.

Duryea JH, Ainsworth DM, Mauldin EA, Cooper BJ, Edwards RB. Clinical remission of granulomatous enteritis in a Standardbred gelding following long term dexamethasone administration. Equine Vet J 1997;29:164–167.

Lindberg R. Pathology of equine granulomatous enteritis. J Comp Pathol 1984;94:233–247.

Lindberg R, Persson SGB, Jones B, Thoren-Tolling K, Ederoth M. Clinical and pathophysiological features of granulomatous enteritis and eosinophilic granulomatosis in the horse. Zbl Vet Med A 1985;32:526–539.

Meuten DJ, Butler DG, Thomson GW, Lumsden JH. Chronic enteritis associated with the malabsorption and protein-losing enteropathy in the horse. JAVMA 1978;172:362–333.

Schumacher J, Edwards JF, Chen ND. Chronic idiopathic inflammatory bowel disease of the horse. J Vet Intern Med 2000;14:258–265.

Sweeney RW, Sweeney CR, Saik J, Lichtensteiger CA. Chronic granulomatous bowel disease in three sibling horses. JAVMA 1986;188;1192–1194.

Author John D. Baird

Consulting Editors Henry Stämpfli and Olimpo Oliver-Espinosa

GRASS SICKNESS

BASICS

DEFINITION

GS is a frequently fatal equine dysautonomia of unknown etiology that causes severe alterations of the gastrintestinal tract. It is associated with severe changes in neurons of the autonomic nervous system, the enteric nervous system, and in certain selected somatic ganglia and nuclei of the central nervous system.

PATHOPHYSIOLOGY

- There are widespread changes in autonomic neurons, the enteric plexuses, and some central neurons. The major signs are related to alimentary dysfunction due to to the damage of the autonomic nervous system. Dysphagia and muscular tremors may reflect a central involvement. Dysphagia is generated by either cranial nerve or brain stem involvement. The most severe lesions are encountered in the submucosal and myenteric plexus of the ileum, resulting in ileus and subsequent colonic impaction due to either decrease or cessation of intestinal peristalsis. The rapid functional alterations precede structural lesions.
- It has been suggested that a neurotoxin is responsible for damaging the enteric plexus. Recently, *Clostridium botulinum* type C has been implicated in GS. *C. botulinum* type C was shown to be present in 48% of ileum samples and 40% of fecal sample of horses with grass sickness, compared with 7% of ileum samples and 8% of fecal samples from control animals. On a farm where GS has occurred twice within 8mos, grass and soil samples and necropsy specimens of one horse were tested for the presence of bacterial forms and toxin of *C. botulinum*. Different types and type mixtures (A–E) of *C. botulinum* and botulinum neurotoxin were found.
- Mycotoxins and depletion of plasma sulfur amino acids have also been suggested to play a role in the pathogenesis of GS.

SYSTEM AFFECTED

- Gastrointestinal
- Autonomic, enteric, and central nervous systems

INCIDENCE/PREVALENCE

- GS is currently recognized in many European countries, including Great Britain, Norway, Sweden, Denmark, France, Switzerland, and Germany. In the Southern Hemisphere of the Americas, mal seco has been reported in the Patagonian region of Argentina, the Falkland Islands, and Chile. Mal seco is a syndrome indistinguishable from grass sickness. A similar clinical disease has been reported in Colombia and is called "tambora," but there has not been adequate histopathological documentation to establish a final diagnosis.
- Studies from Scotland have indicated that GS affects from 0.5% to 4% of the local horse population. It accounts for 18.3% of all fatal colics and it has been estimated that up to 1% of horses die of GS annually in some areas of Scotland. A case-control study in Wales determined that 1.3% of all colic cases were due to GS.

SIGNALMENT

GS is a disease of young adult horses with a peak range of 2–7 years. However, horses may be affected as early as 4 mo of age. There is no breed or gender predisposition.

SIGNS

Grass sickness may be classified into 3 groups based on disease duration. Horses survive < 2 days in the acute form, between 2 and 7 days when subacute, and they usually survive >7 days with chronic presentation.

Acute

- The clinical signs in the acute form are dullness, anorexia and different degrees of colic. At presentation, the horses are usually in good physical condition. Depression is more common in this clinical form. Abdominal distension becomes evident and is accompanied by reduced or absent abdominal sounds. Muscle tremors occur in approximately 74% of the cases, may vary from mild to severe, and occur more commonly over the shoulders, triceps, and flank areas. Sweating is also present. Heart rate is elevated, up to100 bpm; the heart rate seems to be more elevated than would be expected for the abdominal discomfort. Rectal temperature may be normal or elevated (up to 39.5° C/103.5° F).
- Affected horses may show various degrees of dehydration, and the mucous membranes are usually injected. Ptyalism is frequently observed. Spontaneous gastric reflux may occur and is manifested by green or brown malodorous regurgitation on the nares. Nasogastric intubation yields moderate to abundant amounts of gastric reflux. If not relieved, rupture of the stomach may follow.
- Dysphagia is frequent, but is not very obvious at the beginning of the disease due to lack of appetite.
- On rectal examination, there usually are small dry fecal balls present covered with abundant mucus. The rectal wall feels dry. In most cases, an impaction of the large left ventral and dorsal colon may be palpated. In some cases, distended loops of small intestine are present.

Subacute

Findings are very similar to those observed in the acute form but signs are less severe. Heart rate is usually elevated, but the animal does not appear to be distressed. Dry feces are commonly found. Slow mastication can be seen, and gastric reflux is usually absent in this form.

Chronic

The onset of clinical signs is more protracted and may be a progression from the subacute form. The animals lose physical condition to emaciation; have a sleepy appearance, a "tucked up" abdomen, a weak gait, and a tendency to stand with all four feet together. In males, the penis may be flaccid and pendulous. As in the acute form, there are different degrees of muscular tremors, colic signs, sweating, dysphagia, and decrease in intestinal sounds. Heart rate can be normal to increased. Horses are hungry, but dysphagic. Mastication is slow, and swallowing may be followed by esophageal spasm. There may be intermittent diarrhea, chronic rhinitis, and bilateral nasal discharge. Rectal examination reveals empty intestines and possibly splenomegaly.

CAUSES

A definitive etiology has not been identified. There is epidemiologic evidence that a possible agent is related to pasture. A neurotoxin of 30 kD has been detected in serum of affected horses that may reach the ganglions through retrograde ascension from the intestines. Mycotoxins have also been suggested as etiologic agents. However, there are recent reports supporting that *C. botulinum* type C toxins may be the cause.

RISK FACTORS

- GS occurs mainly in grazing horses, but there have been reports in horses without access to pasture. It occurs all year round. In Europe it peaks in May, with a high incidence between April and July. However, in Argentina, mal seco tends to occur mainly from October to February.
- GS usually affects animals in good body condition. Mares seem to be at a slightly reduced risk. Animals with a history of contact with a horse with grass sickness and high frequency of anthelmintic therapy appear to increase the risk of the disease. Moving animals to new pastures favors the occurrence of the disease. There are premises with greater incidence of GS, but it has not been possible to associate it to a specific type of pasture.
- In east Scotland, dry and cool weather with mean average temperatures of 7–11° C that lasts for at least 10 days and irregular ground frosts are conditions favoring the outbreak of grass sickness. An association between GS and increased soil nitrogen content, pasture disturbance, and previous occurrence of GS on the premises has been identified. There is also strong evidence for space time clustering of GS cases, and this may be attributed to contagious or other spatially and temporally localized processes such as local climate and/or pasture management practices.

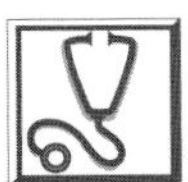

DIAGNOSIS

DIFFERENTIAL DIAGNOSIS

GS should be differentiated from other gastrointestinal conditions associated with surgical colic (see Acute Colic and Chronic Colic). A horse presenting with changing degrees of colic pain and dysphagia is very suggestive of acute GS. In chronic cases, the rapid weight loss accompanied with dysphagia, rhinitis, colic, and abnormal sweating indicates the possible diagnosis. GS and motor neuron disease may occur simultaneously.

CBC/BIOCHEMISTRY/URINALYSIS

- The CBC and biochemical profile alterations are similar to the observed with other colic causes.
- Haptoglobin and orosomucoid are elevated in horses with GS but not in other causes of colic. However, these changes are not specific as they may be elevated in various inflammatory processes. Ceruloplasmin and a $_2$-macroglobulin are increased in acute cases of grass sickness, but may also be elevated in colic cases.
- Peritoneal fluid of horses shows significantly higher specific gravity, protein creatinine and glucose concentrations and a significantly lower pH than that of horses with colic from other causes.

OTHER LABORATORY TESTS

Diagnosis of GS is provided by the demonstration of the pathologic changes in the autonomic or enteric nervous system. This has prompted the use of full-thickness ileal biopsies for making an antemorten diagnosis. As an alternative, rectal biopsy has been proposed, but the neuronal lesion is not very evident in the rectum, and at this time is not a reliable diagnostic tool.

Pathological Changes

- The gross pathological and histopathological changes described for grass sickness, mal seco, and the Colombian grass sickness–like disease are indistinguishable, and are most obvious in the alimentary tract. The esophageal wall may be edematous and the mucosa may show longitudinal bands of congestion. If the stomach has not ruptured, it may be severely distended with fluids. There is excess fluid in the small intestine, which may have hemorrhage and edema. The large intestine is often impacted with very dry contents.
- The intestinal wall may have a blackened surface. The small colon and rectum have small dry fecal balls. Histologic lesions occur mainly in the neurons of the enteric nervous system; the autonomic ganglia, especially the celiacomesenteric; and brain stem nuclei. The neuronal changes include chromatolysis resulting in cytoplasmic eosinophilia, cytoplasmic vacuolization, pyknosis, karyorrhexis, or apparent loss of nuclei. In the enteric nervous system, the typical neuronal lesion is observed in the stomach and intestine. However, it is the ileum where the most severe changes occur. The ileum is affected in both acute and chronic grass sicknesses. This is the only area that is usually affected in chronic cases. Brain lesions occur in several nuclei, but these lesions do not seem to be specific for grass sickness.

DIAGNOSTIC PROCEDURES

Phenylephrine (phenylephrine 10% w/v diluted to 0.5% with normal saline) applied (0.5mL) to the conjuntiva has been used for the antemortem diagnosis of grass sickness. In 23 affected horses, phenylephrine increased the size of the palpebral fissure, measured as the change in the angle of eyelashes, to a greater extent than seen in 12 control horses.

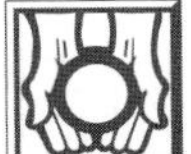

TREATMENT

A mortality of 100% have been reported in acute and subacute cases, and is only slightly lower in chronic cases. However, reports from Scotland and Colombia suggest that therapy may be warranted in selected chronic cases. The probability of success improves when horses are alert, able to swallow, and have not become cachectic.

DIET

Scottish researchers have suggested the following management regimen:

- Housing is advisable, and there should be short hand-walks daily.
- High-energy, high-protein diets should be provided. Sweet feed, crushed oats, and high-energy cubes fed wet or dry are preferable.
- Providing up to 500 mL of cotton oil to increase dietary fat content
- Feeding by nasogastric tube has not been successful.

MEDICATION

- Cisapride at a dose of 0.5–0.8 mg/kg PO TID a day for 7 days has been found to increase intestinal motility in chronic cases. It may cause mild colic, which occurs during feeding however.
- Treatment is usually prolonged. Signs of recovery are detected when the patient starts gaining weight 2–5 weeks from the onset of the disease. In a recent study on long-term prospects for horses with chronic GS, the owners thought that treated animals were capable of strenuous work, regained weight, and returned to normal life, apart from few residual problems such as difficulty in ingesting dry, fibrous food.
- There are no reports of recovery in animals with mal seco. However, in the Colombian disease there are reports of cases that recovered.

PREVENTION

In areas with high prevalence, the only method known to reduce the incidence of GS is to keep the horses stabled during dry cool days as well as during the time of high incidence of the disease, and to avoid pastures where the disease is known to occur.

ABBREVIATION

- GS = grass sickness

Suggested Reading

Böhnel H, Wernery U, Gessler F. Two cases of equine grass sickness with evidence for soil-borne origin involving botulinum neurotoxin. J Vet Med B 2003;50:178–182.

Doxey DL, Milne EM, Gilmour JS, Pogson DM. Clinical and biochemical features of grass sickness (equine dysautonomia). Equine Vet J 1991;23:360–364.

Doxey DL, Milne EM, Ellison J, Curry PJ. Long-term prospects for horses with grass sickness. Vet Rec 1998;142:207–209.

Fintl C, Milne EM, McGorum BC. Evaluation of urinalysis as an aid in the diagnosis of equine grass sickness. Vet Rec 2002;14:721–724.

Gerber H, Gerber V. Epidemiological findings in cases with simultaneous lesions of grass sickness and of motor neuron disease. Proceedings of the First International Workshop on Grass Sickness, Equine Motor Neuron Disease and Related Disorders. Bern, Switzerland. October 26–27, 1995:47–49.

Hahn CN, Mayhew IG. Phenylephrine eyedrops as a diagnostic test in equine grass sickness. Vet Rec 2000;147:603–606.

Hunter LC, Miller JK, Poxton IR. The association of Clostridium botulinum type C with euine grass sickness: toxic infection? Equine Vet J 1999;31:492–499.

McCarthy HE, French NP, Edwards GB, Miller K, Proudman CJ. Why are certain premises at increased risk of equine grass sickness? A matched case-control study. Equine Vet J 2004;36:130–134.

Ochoa R, Velandia S. Equine grass sickness: serologic evidence of association with *Clostridium perfringens* type A enterotoxin. Am J Vet Res 1978;39:1049–1051.

Uzal FA, Robles CA. Mal seco, a grass sickness-like syndrome of horses in Argentina. Vet Res Comm 1993;17:449–457.

Author Olimpo Oliver-Espinosa

Consulting Editors Henry Stämpfli and Olimpo Oliver-Espinosa

GUTTURAL POUCH EMPYEMA

BASICS

OVERVIEW

Definition

• Guttural pouches are diverticula of the auditory tubes that communicate with the pharynx through the pharyngeal orifice of the auditory tube.
• Accumulation of mucopurulent material within the guttural pouch usually results from a secondary bacterial infection of the upper respiratory tract.

Pathophysiology

• Upper respiratory tract infection associated with b -hemolytic streptococci invading the guttural pouch often follows abscessation of the retropharyngeal lymph nodes.
• Under normal head standing position, the guttural pouch opening to the pharynx is situated slightly more dorsally compared to the ventral portion of the medial and lateral compartment reducing proper drainage.
• Infections of the guttural pouches occur uni- or bilaterally.
• Any condition of the upper airways causing stenosis or occlusion of the guttural pouch pharyngeal opening will predispose to poor drainage and potential infections.

SIGNALMENT

• Guttural pouch infection occurs in horses of any breed or age.
• Retropharyngeal lymph node abscessation caused by *Streptococcus equi* var *equi* draining into the guttural pouches is reportedly more frequent in foals and yearlings than in adults.

SIGNS

Historical Findings

• Commonly associated as a complication of strangles infection.
• Chronic, unilateral, mucopurulent nasal discharge of unknown cause

Physical Examination Findings

• Intermittent nasal discharge
• Swelling of adjacent lymph nodes; painful lymph nodes on palpation
• Occasional difficulty in swallowing (i.e., dysphagia) or breathing (i.e., stertorous noise)

CAUSES AND RISK FACTORS

• Most frequently *S. equi* var *equi* and var *zooepidemicus*
• Outbreaks of strangles
• Congenital stenosis of the pharyngeal orifice of the auditory tube

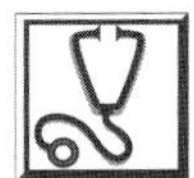

DIAGNOSIS

DIFFERENTIAL DIAGNOSIS

• Guttural pouch mycosis
• Trauma to the guttural pouch

CBC/BIOCHEMISTRY/URINALYSIS

• If associated with an upper respiratory bacterial infection (e.g., *S. equi* var *equi*), the leukogram shows a leukocytosis, and the fibrinogen level is elevated.
• If the guttural pouch infection is without systemic effect, the leukogram is in the normal range.

OTHER LABORATORY TESTS

Bacterial culture and sensitivity as well as cytology of purulent material are obtained through a catheter from the guttural pouches.

IMAGING

• Radiography—a standing, lateral projection is useful to identify a distinct fluid line representing the exudate within the pouch.
• Ultrasonography—potential diagnostic value if fluid can be identified in the dependent area of the guttural pouch; however, the scientific literature supporting the comparison is very limited.

OTHER DIAGNOSTIC PROCEDURES

• Pharyngeal endoscopy identifies a purulent discharge from the orifice of the affected guttural pouch; however, direct visualization of the guttural pouch itself confirms the presence of mucopurulent debris and the formation of chondroids.
• During endoscopy of the guttural pouch, a polyethylene catheter can be passed through the biopsy channel of the endoscope and mucopurulent debris collected for cytology and bacterial culture.

PATHOLOGIC FINDINGS

If related to strangles there is possible abscessation of the retropharyngeal lymph nodes draining directly into the guttural pouches; these lesions are frequently observed in foals and yearlings infected with *S. equi* var *equi*.

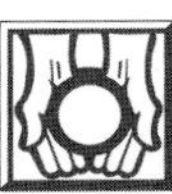

TREATMENT

• Placement of an indwelling catheter to facilitate irrigation of the guttural pouch is paramount to successful treatment.
• During the first 2 days, irrigate the affected pouch with a weak solution (1–3%) of povidone iodine (500 mL) twice daily, then

continue irrigation with sterile saline twice a day until mucopurulent debris no longer is visible during the irrigation procedure.
• Unless the affected horse is dysphagic or dyspneic, no particular care is needed.
• Rest is advised until the condition resolves.
• Activity is not recommended during therapeutic flushing of the guttural pouches.
• If the cause was strangles, provide specific advice relating to the condition (see the section on *S. equi* var *equi*).
• When treatment involves combination systemic antibiotic, local irrigation of the guttural pouch has been unsuccessful, and if chondroids have formed, surgical drainage of the guttural pouch is the intervention of choice.
• The hyovertebrotomy approach, which is a lateral approach to the guttural pouch combined with a ventral approach through the Viborg's triangle, assures maximal drainage of the guttural pouch.

MEDICATIONS

DRUG(S) OF CHOICE

• Antibiotics, depending on bacterial culture and sensitivity results.
• Affected horses usually respond to most b-lactam antibiotics (e.g., penicillin, cephalosporins, etc.) administered for a period of 10 days.

CONTRAINDICATIONS/POSSIBLE INTERACTIONS

Avoid irrigation with irritating solutions (e.g., strong iodine solution) and placement of traumatic catheter. This may damage several cranial nerves that course through the pouch wall, leading to a variety of signs—dysphagia, dorsal displacement of the soft palate, and occasionally, head tilt.

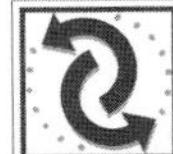

FOLLOW-UP

PATIENT MONITORING

• Repeat endoscopy 1–2 weeks after the last irrigation therapy.
• Ground feeding to encourage natural drainage

PREVENTION/AVOIDANCE

Encourage annual strangles vaccination in foals, yearlings, and mature horses on farms where the infection is endemic.

POSSIBLE COMPLICATIONS

• Chondroid formation necessitating surgical removal
• Neurologic injury to the glossopharyngeal, vagus, accessory, and hypoglossal nerves, leading to pharyngeal paralysis, dysphagia, and dyspnea

EXPECTED COURSE AND PROGNOSIS

• Duration of the condition depends on the causal agent if empyema results from abscessation of retropharyngeal lymph nodes or simple infection of the guttural pouch mucosa.
• Prognosis is favorable with early diagnosis and treatment.
• Chondroid formation with neurologic injury carries a poor prognosis.

MISCELLANEOUS

ASSOCIATED CONDITIONS

• Strangles
• *S. equi* var *equí* infection (strangle) of the upper respiratory tract

AGE-RELATED FACTORS

Retropharyngeal lymph node abscessation caused by strangles draining in the guttural pouches is reportedly more frequent in foals and yearlings than in adults.

SEE ALSO

• Guttural pouch mycosis
• Purulent nasal discharge
• Strangles

Suggested Reading

Lepage OM. Disorders of the guttural pouches. In: Lekeux P, ed. International Veterinary Information Service, Ithaca, NY (www.ivis.org), June 2007.

Author Laurent Viel
Consulting Editor Daniel Jean

GUTTURAL POUCH MYCOSIS

BASICS

OVERVIEW

• A fungal disease of the auditory tube diverticulum • Usually affects one guttural pouch, but bilateral lesions are possible.
• Clinical signs relate to damage to the arteries and nerves. • Spontaneous epistaxis in a resting horse usually is the first sign of this life-threatening condition. • Organ systems—respiratory, nervous, hemic/lymphatic/immune, and cardiovascular

SIGNALMENT

• Although described in horses as young as 6 months, this condition is more common in mature horses. • No breed or sex predilection • Believed to be more common in stabled horses

SIGNS

• May be asymptomatic • Epistaxis—the most frequent clinical sign; not related to exercise; severity varies from a mild, blood-tinged nasal secretion to fatal hemorrhage. Bleeding usually is unilateral but may be bilateral with severe hemorrhage; bleeding can stop spontaneously but, in most untreated cases, recurs in the following days or weeks. Premonitory bleeding often, but not always, precedes fatal hemorrhage.
• Ingesta in nasal discharge. Dysphagia results from lesions involving the vagus and glossopharyngeal nerves and may lead to aspiration pneumonia. • Other neurologic deficits—laryngeal hemiplegia, facial paralysis, and Horner's syndrome • Less commonly seen—nasal discharge, head shaking, abnormal head posture, visual disturbances, and parotid pain

CAUSES AND RISK FACTORS

• An initiating factor that predisposes to growth of opportunistic fungi in the affected guttural pouch has not been determined. • Different fungal species have been incriminated, with *Aspergillus nidulans* the most frequently isolated.
• Major blood vessels in the guttural pouch wall include internal and external carotids, maxillary, caudal auricular, and superficial temporal arteries. Mycotic diphtheritic membranes usually are in the caudodorsal part of the medial compartment of the guttural pouch, involving the internal carotid artery more frequently.
• Cranial nerves (IX, X, XI, XII), cranial cervical ganglion, and sympathetic trunk are in a mucous membrane fold in the caudal aspect of the medial compartment, and a small portion of the facial nerve (VII) crosses the dorsal aspect of the guttural pouch. The fungal plaque may invade one or more of these structures.

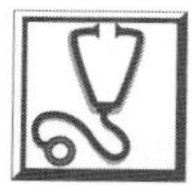

DIAGNOSIS

DIFFERENTIAL DIAGNOSIS

• Epistaxis—exercise-induced pulmonary hemorrhage, ethmoid hematoma, head trauma, foreign bodies, upper airway neoplasia, abscess rupture, longus capitis muscle rupture, and coagulopathy. Longus capitis muscle rupture usually is associated with a recent history of trauma. Epistaxis caused by coagulopathy is rare in horses and usually associated with other clinical signs and hemorrhages at other sites.
• Dysphagia—esophageal obstruction, megaesophagus, fracture of the hyoid apparatus, inflammatory reaction, cyst or neoplasia in the pharyngeal area, and cleft palate. Empyema or tympanism of the guttural pouch may lead to dysphagia in severe cases. Bacterial, viral, or mycotic infection of the central nervous system: neuritis of cranial nerves IX, X, and XI; botulism; lead or plant poisoning; hepatic encephalopathy; and leukoencephalopathy may also cause dysphagia in horses • Guttural pouch hemorrhage—longus capitis muscle rupture, iatrogenic trauma, and neoplasia

CBC/BIOCHEMISTRY/URINALYSIS

• Anemia is observed 12–24 hours after severe blood loss, but PCV may remain within normal ranges initially. • Biochemistry profile and urinalysis— unremarkable unless the affected horse is dehydrated because of an inability to drink.

OTHER LABORATORY TESTS

Fungal cultures, but these are not routinely done.

IMAGING

• Endoscopy—mycotic lesions of affected guttural pouches appear as a white, black, and yellow paste on the surface of the mucosa. Perform a thorough examination of both guttural pouches to determine which vessels are affected, and take care to avoid dislodging a thrombus on the affected artery. Preparing surgical facilities before endoscopic examination is a good precautionary measure as the tip of the endoscope may dislodge the thrombus and cause hemorrhage. No relationship exists between lesion size and severity of the clinical signs. Large quantities of blood in the guttural pouch may be present, precluding visualization of affected nerves and arteries. Blood may flow back into the trachea and must not be misinterpreted as coming from the lung. • Radiography of head is little value.

PATHOLOGIC FINDING

Involvement of deeper structures (e. g., hyoid apparatus, petrous temporal bones, and atlanto-occipital joint) have been described in severe cases.

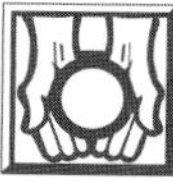

TREATMENT

• The first goal is to prevent spontaneous fatal hemorrhage. Perform arterial occlusion as soon as possible. In life-threatening emergency, ligature of the common carotid artery may in some cases prevent fatal bleeding. However, proximal ligature of the artery does not negate the risk of fatal hemorrhages owing to possible retrograde flux of blood from the circle of Willis. The aim of surgical treatment is to stop blood flow distally and proximally to the lesion. Because distal access to arteries is very difficult, different techniques of internal occlusion have been developed. At this time the best technique seems to be trans-arterial coil embolization. Dacron fiber coated stainless coils are placed under fluoroscopic guidance from the common carotid artery to cause embolization on both sides of the damaged arteries. Angiography allows the identification and occlusion of aberrant actively bleeding branches of arteries.
• Mycotic lesions usually resolve without specific treatment after arterial occlusion. • Intravenous administration of polyionic fluids and blood transfusion from an appropriate donor may be required before surgery in horses with profuse bleeding.

MEDICATIONS

DRUGS

• Medical treatment has been used with variable results. • In most cases, the risk of fatal hemorrhage is still present during long-term medical treatment.

CONTRAINDICATIONS/POSSIBLE INTERACTIONS

Development of dysphagia during apparently successful medical treatment suggests that topical drugs may have an irritating or neurotoxic effect.

FOLLOW-UP

• Although spontaneous regression of mycotic lesion has been reported in few horses, 50% of horses with guttural pouch mycosis left untreated die from fatal hemorrhage. • Surgical treatment provides a good prognosis for the treatment of hemorrhage. • Prognosis for recovery of neurologic dysfunction is more guarded depending on the reversibility of the damages to nerves.

MISCELLANEOUS

SEE ALSO

Hemorrhagic nasal discharge

ABBREVIATION

• PCV = packed cell volume

Suggested Reading

Lepage OM, Picot-Crézollet C. Trans-arterial coil embolization in 31 horses (1999–2002) with guttural pouch mycosis: A 2-year follow-up. Equine Vet J 2005;37:430–434.

Author Vincent J. Ammann
Consulting Editor Daniel Jean

GUTTURAL POUCH TYMPANY

BASICS

OVERVIEW

Nonpainful and tympanic swelling in the parotid and laryngeal region due to distention of one or both guttural pouches with air. The enlarged guttural pouch may displace the pharynx, larynx, and trachea ventrally and to the contralateral side.

SIGNALMENT

- Observed only in foals and weanlings; Most common between 2 and 4 months of age
- Fillies are predominantly affected with a female-to-male ratio of 2:1 to 4:1.
- Most frequently reported in Standardbreds, Thoroughbreds, Arabians, Quarter Horses, Appaloosas, Paints, American Saddle Horses, and Warmbloods.
- A genetic predisposition has been reported in Arabian horses.

SIGNS

- Nonpainful and tympanic swelling over the parotid region
- In severe cases, stertorous breathing and dysphagia may develop.
- Secondary guttural pouch empyema and aspiration pneumonia are common findings.
- Unilateral involvement of the guttural pouches is most frequently observed, although the parotid region is usually bilaterally distended.

CAUSES AND RISK FACTORS

- Exact etiology of the condition is unknown.
- It is considered to be a congenital dysfunction of the pharyngeal orifice of the affected guttural pouch.
- During respiration, the ingress of air within the guttural pouch is allowed but not its egress.
- Excessive accumulation of air within the affected guttural pouch results.

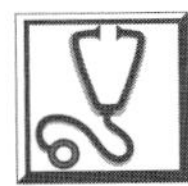

DIAGNOSIS

DIFFERENTIAL DIAGNOSIS

- *Streptococcus equi* infection (strangles) causing extreme swelling of the submandibular or retropharyngeal lymph nodes, retropharyngeal abscesses, and cellulitis is easily distinguished from guttural pouch tympany because these former conditions are associated with pain, fever, leukocytosis, and hyperfibrinogenemia.
- Primary guttural pouch empyema most often due to *Streptococcus zooepidemicus* is differentiated by the presence of nasal discharge, recognition of fluid within the guttural pouch on standing lateral radiographs and on endoscopic examination. Primary guttural pouch empyemas uncommonly cause tympanic swelling in the parotid region.

CBC/BIOCHEMISTRY/URINALYSIS

- Stress leukocytosis may be present with significant respiratory distress.
- Leukocytosis and hyperfibrinogenemia are found in the presence of aspiration pneumonia.

OTHER LABORATORY TESTS

- N/A

IMAGING

Endoscopic Examination

- Decreased airway size is observed when the nasopharynx and oropharynx are examined.
- Protrusion of either the roof alone or the roof and the wall of the pharynx on the affected side into the pharyngeal lumen are present.
- Introduction of the endoscope in the affected guttural pouch will deflate it and help to distinguish between unilateral and bilateral tympany.
- Secondary guttural pouch empyema may be observed.

Radiography

- Enlargement of air-filled guttural pouches is noticed on lateral radiographic examination of the head and neck (rostral portion). With guttural pouch tympany, the affected pouch extends caudally beyond the ventral tubercule of the atlas on lateral radiographs.
- Collapse of the pharynx can also be noted. Evidence of a fluid line is also observed when secondary guttural pouch empyema is present.
- Ventrodorsal radiographic examination of the head and neck (rostral portion) can help distinguishing between unilateral and bilateral tympany.

Thoracic Radiography

Standing lateral thoracic radiography to rule out aspiration pneumonia

OTHER DIAGNOSTIC PROCEDURES

Bacterial culture ad antimicrobial sensitivity of fluid accumulated in the guttural pouch may be performed in cases of secondary empyema.

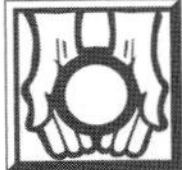

TREATMENT

- External deflation of the guttural pouch by needle aspiration is not recommended because of the possibility of causing hemorrhage or damaging the nerves that traverse the walls of the guttural pouch.
- Temporary alleviation can be achieved by applying a gentle pressure bilaterally on the parotid area or through an indwelling catheter placed in pharyngeal orifice of the affected pouch. Definitive treatment is surgical.
- Two surgical treatments performed under general anesthesia are described. One consists of the fenestration of the median septum that separates the two guttural pouches. The other consists of the resection of a small segment of the medial lamina of the eustachian tube and its associated mucosal fold to create a larger opening of the affected guttural pouch into the pharynx. Fenestration of the median septum is used in unilateral guttural pouch tympany; both procedures are performed when bilateral involvement is present.
- Fenestration of the median septum and creation of a fistula between the pharynx and the Eustachian tube with the use of laser equipment or electrosurgery can also be performed under endoscopic guidance with the affected animal sedated and standing.

MEDICATIONS

DRUG(S)

- Preoperative and postoperative medication consist of the administration of systemic antibiotics (procaine penicillin G 20,000 U/kg IV BID or trimethoprim sulfamethoxazole 30 mg/kg IV BID) and NSAIDs (flunixin meglumine 1 mg/kg IV BID).
- In cases complicated by aspiration pneumonia or guttural pouch empyema, administration of broad-spectrum antibiotics based on sensitivity tests is required.
- Control aspiration pneumonia when present if surgical correction of the tympany is performed under general anesthesia.

CONTRAINDICATIONS/POSSIBLE INTERACTIONS

a_2-Agonists agents, such as xylazine, detomidine, and romifidine, should be used with caution in horses with guttural pouch tympany as they may worsen upper airway obstruction by relaxing nasal alar, pharyngeal, and laryngeal muscles.

FOLLOW-UP

- In the absence of aspiration pneumonia or guttural pouch empyema, the prognosis for a unilateral guttural pouch tympany is favorable.
- Recurrence rate following a surgical correction of guttural pouch tympany is 30%. The prognosis for a bilateral guttural pouch tympany is guarded.
- Aspiration pneumonia or guttural pouch empyemas warrant a poor prognosis.

Suggested Reading

Blazyczek I, Hamann H, Deegen E, et al. Retrospective analysis of 50 cases of guttural pouch tympany in foals. Vet Rec 2004;154:261–264.

Blazyczek I, Hamann H, Ohnesorge B, et al. Inheritance of guttural pouch tympany in the Arabian horse. J Hered 2004;95:195–199.

Ragle CA. Guttural pouch disease. In: Robinson NE, ed. Current Therapy in Equine Medicine V. East Lansing: WB Saunders, 2003.

Author Ludovic Bouré
Consulting Editor Daniel Jean

HEAD TRAUMA

BASICS

DEFINITION

Trauma to the skull and/or associated soft tissues results in primary damage to the brain. Secondary brain injury results from the primary injury and causes physiologic changes in brain tissue. Secondary brain injury can be prevented or lessened, whereas primary injury cannot.

PATHOPHYSIOLOGY

- Following a traumatic insult to the brain, a cycle of cellular events occurs, including membrane disruption, ischemia, hypoxia, edema, and hemorrhage. The severity of these abnormalities is dependent on the type and extent of the initial primary injury. The traumatic insult is also responsible for increased permeability of brain capillary endothelial cells resulting in vasogenic edema. This is the most common type of edema found following head trauma, and white matter is especially prone to vasogenic edema. Vasogenic edema results in displacement of cerebral tissue and increased ICP. Ultimately, these changes may produce brain herniation.
- Cytotoxic edema results from swelling of the cellular elements of the brain. This type of edema occurs in gray and white matter and often results in decreased cerebral function, with stupor and coma as signs. A cycle occurs when increased ICP leads to decreased cerebral blood flow, resulting in further ischemia and brain swelling.
- The types of cranial trauma from least to most severe are concussion, contusion, laceration, and hemorrhage. Concussion is short-term loss of consciousness and is often reversible and occurs without anatomical lesions. Contusion is associated with vascular and neural tissue damage without major structural disruption. Laceration and hemorrhage result from penetrating wounds, fractures, or direct blunt trauma. Cerebral hemorrhage in horses may be subdural (rare), intracerebral, or subarachnoid (common).
- Fracture of the basisphenoid/basioccipital bones is not uncommon after trauma to poll (falling over backward).
- Hematoma formation is potentially devastating as hemorrhage results in expansion within the rigid skull with herniation, pressure necrosis, and brainstem compression possible.

SYSTEMS AFFECTED

- Behavioral—altered mentation
- Cardiovascular—arrhythmias/bradycardia due to dysfunction of central cardiovascular centers
- Musculoskeletal—skull fracture(s); postural/gait abnormalities due to disruption of central motor pathways; other lacerations/ fractures from traumatic episode
- Nervous—disruption of neural pathways resulting in changes in behavior, heart rate and rhythm, respiratory rate and rhythm, and neurologic testing
- Ophthalmic—abnormal eye position, movements and reflexes, and changes in vision
- Respiratory—apneustic and/or erratic breathing due to dysfunction of respiratory regulatory center in the caudal medulla oblongata.

SIGNALMENT

- Breed predilections—N/A
- Mean age range—N/A
- Predominant sex—N/A

SIGNS

Historical

- Ascertain if any known episode of trauma or physical evidence of trauma to the horse or its environment.
- Potentially abnormal behavior, gait changes, sudden blindness, or recumbency

Physical Examination

- The initial evaluation should be directed toward identification and stabilization of life-threatening problems such as open skull fractures, airway obstruction, hemorrhage, cardiovascular collapse, pneumothorax, and other fractures.
- Look for evidence of head trauma. Palpation of the skull may reveal fractures.
- Blood from the ears, mouth, or nostrils suggests potential basisphenoid or basioccipital fractures.
- Occasionally, CSF may be seen draining from the ears with basilar fractures.
- Bradycardia and/or arrhythmias may be present with apneustic or erratic breathing with injury to the central cardiac and respiratory centers.

Neurologic

- Neurologic deficits may range from inapparent to recumbency with profound depression, dementia, and tetraparesis. Injury to the cerebrum may manifest as behavior changes, obtundation, coma, circling or wandering, seizures, and blindness with normal pupillary reflexes. Injury to the cerebellum may manifest as altered behavior, ataxia, hypermetria, intention tremor, hypertonicity, and lack of menace without blindness. Injury to the diencephalons (thalamus) may manifest as depression to stupor, normal to mild tetraparesis, deviation of the head and eyes with circling toward the side of a unilateral lesion, and bilateral nonreactive pupils with blindness. Midbrain trauma may demonstrate stupor to coma with hemiparesis, tetraparesis or tetraplegia, and changes in pupils such as myosis, mydriasis (if mydriatic and unresponsive, sign of poor prognosis) or anisocoria. Trauma to the pons and rostral medulla oblongata (including the inner ear) often shows obtundation, ataxia with tetraparesis or tetraplegia, and head tilt, nystagmus, facial paralysis and medial strabismus. Trauma to the caudal medulla oblongata may manifest as obtundation, ataxia with hemiparesis to tetraparesis, abnormal respiratory patterns, and dysphagia with a flaccid tongue.

CAUSES

Head trauma

RISK FACTORS

- Young age
- Fractious behavior
- Unsafe environment

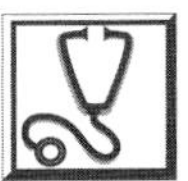

DIAGNOSIS

DIFFERENTIAL DIAGNOSIS

- Consider other primary brain disorders such as seizures, infection, inflammation, neoplasia, degenerative disease, and congenital problems.
- Syncope from cardiovascular disease, metabolic diseases, toxin exposure, adverse drug reactions, and nutritional deficiencies may also affect brain function.

CBC/BIOCHEMISTRY/URINALYSIS

Changes in any of these tests may reflect changes in other organ systems secondary to the effects of trauma or due to other underlying disease processes. There are no specific changes in any of these tests for head trauma.

IMAGING

- Skull radiographs may reveal fractures, luxations, and subluxations. Radiography of other areas of the body (long bones, chest) that have evidence of trauma is warranted.
- Computed tomography or magnetic resonance imaging of the head may reveal fractures, hemorrhage, or foreign bodies lodged in the skull or brain.
- Scintigraphy is useful for diagnosis of nondisplaced and occult fractures and soft tissue lesions.

DIAGNOSTIC PROCEDURES

- CSF analysis in cases of trauma may show xanthochromia with mild to moderate increases in protein. In acute or chronic cases, CSF may be normal. A cisternal CSF tap is contraindicated if increased ICP is suspected due to the possibility of brain herniation.
- Lumbosacral tap safer but may not reflect changes in intracranial CSF.
- Brainstem auditory evoked potentials are evaluated to determine brainstem function.
- ECG evaluation aids in determining cardiac rhythm dysfunction.

PATHOLOGIC FINDINGS

- Gross and histopathologic findings may include skull fractures, brain laceration/ foreign body, hemorrhage, edema, and evidence of hypoxia.
- Contusion and concussion may be seen.

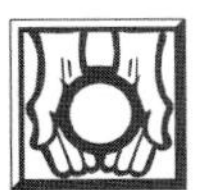

TREATMENT

APPROPRIATE HEALTH CARE

Usually requires intensive inpatient care—often on an emergency basis

NURSING CARE

- Treat shock first as neurologic status may improve once the shock is corrected.
- Adhere to the ABCs of trauma management.
- Monitor oxygenation with pulse oximetry and supplement oxygen as necessary.
- Consider controlled ventilation of horse if stuporous, comatose, or if rapid neurologic deterioration occurs.
- Maintain normal PCO_2 and PO_2.
- Elevate the head up to an angle of 20 degrees to help prevent increased ICP. Do not put the head at an angle greater than this to avoid pressure on the jugular vein as this increases ICP.
- Institute fluid therapy to avoid hypotension. Overzealous administration of crystalloids (shock doses of 40–90 mL/kg/hr) may exacerbate increased ICP. Possibly the use of colloids (hetastarch, dextran 70, or hypertonic saline) is preferable to restore normal blood volume while preventing increases in ICP. The use of colloids is contraindicated if intracranial hemorrhage is ongoing. Hypertonic saline (4–6 mL/kg IV over 15 minutes) is the preferred fluid choice for head trauma horses in shock. Isotonic fluids may then be used for maintenance requirements (60 mL/kg/day). In recumbent horses, physical therapy is critical to prevent myositis, decubital sores, and hypostatic pulmonary congestion.
- Lubricate the eyes and turn the horse every 2–4 hours.
- Use deep bedding.
- Hydro/massage therapy and therapeutic ultrasound are useful to maintain circulation to the large muscle groups.
- Ensure normothermia and especially avoid hyperthermia.

ACTIVITY

- Restricted with strict stall confinement.
- Once stable, controlled exercise is useful for physical therapy/rehabilitation.

DIET

- Allow access to food and water if the mental status allows.
- Provide supplemental tube feedings or parenteral nutrition if the horse is unable/unwilling to eat and drink.
- Adequate nutrition must be maintained to provide for the increased metabolic demands of the recovery period.

CLIENT EDUCATION

- True neurologic status may not be evident for several days, and intensive and potentially costly care may be required.
- Full recovery may take months and residual deficits may persist.
- An ataxic and demented horse is a potential hazard to humans.

SURGICAL CONSIDERATIONS

- Consider intervention of open or depressed skull fractures, and for retrieval of foreign bodies.
- Possible usefulness of craniectomy for decompression if suspect increased ICP despite medical treatment, and for midbrain signs with a history of cerebral trauma or bleeding. Practicality of this in the horse is suspect.

MEDICATION

DRUG(S) OF CHOICE

- DMSO not documented to be useful
- Sedation with α_2-agonist if patient delirious and thrashing
- Diuretics if horse remains in a coma or semicoma and recumbent for more than a few minutes—mannitol 0.25–2 mg/kg IV over 20 minutes
- If fracture of cranium obvious, tetanus prophylaxis and systemic antibiotics such as penicillin should be considered.

CONTRAINDICATIONS

- Glucocorticoids in human head trauma are considered contraindicated and their use should be judicious in horses with head trauma until further studied.
- Avoid drugs that may increase ICP such as ketamine or cause hypertension.

PRECAUTIONS

Avoid overzealous fluid administration, which may cause hypertension.

FOLLOW-UP

PATIENT MONITORING

- Evaluate progress with serial neurologic examinations.
- Perform examinations several times a day initially and taper the frequency based on the stability of the horse.

PREVENTION/AVOIDANCE

- Keep area that horses are housed free of clutter.
- Tranquilize fractious horses as necessary to perform procedures.

POSSIBLE COMPLICATIONS

- Increases in ICP may lead to further hemorrhage and ultimately herniation.
- Problems associated with recumbent horses (myositis, decubital sores, corneal lacerations, hypostatic pulmonary congestion leading to pneumonia, fecal and urine scalding)
- Malnutrition, seizures, cardiac and respiratory abnormalities, and death

EXPECTED COURSE AND PROGNOSIS

The best prognosis is with minimal injury that is identified early post injury in which prompt treatment is sought. Horses that show rapid improvement with stabilization of signs have a better prognosis.

SYNONYMS

Brain trauma, brain injury, traumatic brain injury

SEE ALSO

Basisphenoid-basioccipital fracture, coma and stupor, recumbency, weakness

ABBREVIATIONS

- CSF = cerebrospinal fluid
- ECG = electrocardiogram
- ICP = intracranial pressure

Suggested Reading

Alderson P, Roberts I. Corticosteroids for acute traumatic brain injury. Cochrane Database Syst Rev 2005;(1):CD000196.

Feary DJ, Magdesian KG, Aleman MA, et al. Traumatic brain injury in horses: 34 Cases (1994–2004). J Am Vet Med Assoc 2007;231:259–266.

Hahn CN, Mayhew IG, MacKay RJ, The nervous system. In: Collahan PT, Mayhew IG, Merritt AM, Moore JN, eds. Equine Medicine and Surgery, ed 5. St. Louis: Mosby, 1999.

The author and editors wish to acknowledge the contribution of Hilary K. Matthews, author of this chapter in the previous edition.

Author Caroline N. Hahn

Consulting Editor Caroline N. Hahn

HEAVES (RECURRENT AIRWAY OBSTRUCTION)

BASICS

DEFINITION

An inflammatory condition of the lower airways characterized by bronchospasm, excess mucus production, and airway remodeling, leading to partially or totally reversible airway obstruction.

PATHOPHYSIOLOGY

- Feeding dusty hay leads to inflammation and obstruction of the lower airways in susceptible horses.
- Hypoxemia, presumably resulting from ventilation and perfusion inequalities, is common.
- A hypersensitivity reaction to thermophilic molds and actinomyces antigens in dusty hay has been suggested.
- The role of viral infections and nonspecific environmental dust particles (e.g., endotoxins) on the induction and maintenance of heaves is currently ill-defined.

SYSTEM AFFECTED

Respiratory

GENETICS

Unknown, but a genetic susceptibility has been demonstrated in selected breeds.

INCIDENCE/PREVALENCE/ GEOGRAPHIC DISTRIBUTION

- Unknown
- Common in countries with temperate and cold climates, where horses are stabled for prolonged periods

SIGNALMENT

- No clear sex or breed predilections demonstrated to date.
- Incidence increases with age; uncommonly diagnosed in horses <7 years.

SIGNS

- Affected horses are alert and afebrile.
- Anorexia and weight loss may occur with respiratory distress.
- Signs may be limited to exercise intolerance, with an occasional cough at the onset of exercise or when eating when horses are in clinical remission. The frequency and severity of coughing episodes increase as the disease progresses, finally becoming paroxysmal bouts of deep, nonproductive coughs.
- During clinical exacerbation, increased respiratory rate, flared nostrils, and double expiratory effort may be present, and emaciation and a "heave line," caused by hypertrophy of the external abdominal oblique muscles, may develop.
- Appearance and severity of the clinical signs wax and wane. The duration of attacks varies from days to weeks, and some horses are asymptomatic between attacks. Reduced exercise capacity often persists even if horses are in clinical remission.
- Thoracic auscultation may be normal during remission periods.
- Increased breath sounds, wheezes throughout the lung fields, and expiratory crackles are common findings when labored breathing or during forced breathing using a rebreathing bag or after exercise in less severely affected horses.
- Bronchovesicular lung sounds may be decreased during severe episodes.
- Thoracic percussion may reveal hyperresonance of the ventral and caudal borders of the lung fields because of air trapping.

CAUSES

- Unknown
- Inhalation of organic dust particles from moldy hay and straw causes clinical exacerbation.
- Close contact between horses and chickens has been associated with clinical signs closely resembling those of heaves.

RISK FACTORS

- Moldy hay and straw
- Prolonged stabling

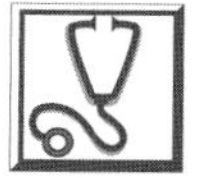

DIAGNOSIS

DIFFERENTIAL DIAGNOSIS

- Pharyngitis and mild dysphagia may cause chronic cough. Pharyngitis usually affects young horses and is associated with normal lung sounds; dysphagia is diagnosed on the basis of food particles in the airways and nasal secretions.
- Horses with IAD may be presented with clinical signs suggestive of heaves. However, there is no history of episodes of labored breathing in IAD.
- Viral and bacterial airway infections may lead to cough and increased respiratory effort. These conditions can be differentiated from heaves on the basis of febrile episodes, other signs of infection, and duration of clinical signs.
- Summer pasture associated chronic pulmonary disease occurs when horses are pastured and is controlled by stabling.
- Lungworm infection—larvae infeces or trachael secretions.

CBC/BIOCHEMISTRY/URINALYSIS

Usually within normal ranges

OTHER LABORATORY TESTS

- Increased percentage of neutrophils (generally > 25%) in BAL cell cytology. Cytology maybe normal when horses are clinically asymptomatic. Presence of bacteria and fungal elements in BAL cytology are common but indicate impaired mucociliary clearance rather than an ongoing intrapulmonary septic process.
- Cytology of transtracheal washes or tracheal aspirates also reveals neutrophilia, but this is less specific than similar findings in BAL cell cytology. Bacterial culture of tracheal secretions commonly yields bacterial growth, but without other signs of infection, this may represent colonization of the lower airways because of impaired mucociliary clearance.
- Arterial blood gases provide an easy assessment of the degree of respiratory dysfunction in affected horses—PaO_2 values are <80 and may be as low as 40 mm Hg in horses with labored breathing; $PaCO_2$ values may be slightly elevated.
- Routine lung biopsy for diagnosis of heaves is not recommended because of the uncommon but severe bleeding that may occur with this test.

IMAGING

- Endoscopy reveals copious mucopurulent exudate in lower airways.
- Thoracic radiography often is unremarkable but may reveal an increased bronchointerstitial pattern. Horses with heaves may also develop bronchiectasis.
- Thoracic ultrasonography usually unremarkable

OTHER DIAGNOSTIC PROCEDURES

- The diagnosis is established on the basis of signalment, history, and clinical findings combined with exclusion of other common diseases affecting the respiratory tract and response to therapy.
- The diagnosis is confirmed by >25% neutrophils in BAL fluid in horses presenting the clinical signs suggestive of heaves.

PATHOLOGIC FINDINGS

- Histologic lesions are of a chronic active bronchiolitis, with intraluminal accumulation of mucus and neutrophils, epithelial hyperplasia with goblet cell metaplasia, lymphocyte and plasma cell infiltration and increased airway smooth muscle mass.
- Interstitial emphysema, mostly in the cranial regions, and patchy areas of alveolar hyperinflation may be seen.

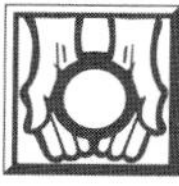

TREATMENT

AIMS OF TREATMENT

Control airway inflammation and decrease airway obstruction

APPROPRIATE HEALTH CARE

In- or outpatient medical management

NURSING CARE

- The disease is reversible with proper control of environmental dust, which is best achieved by keeping horses outdoors, preferably on pasture or replacing hay with cubed or pelleted food, haylage, or hydroponic hay, and use of shredded paper or good-quality wood shavings instead of straw.
- Respiratory signs usually recur within days to weeks of re-exposure to dusty hay and bedding.
- Without drug therapy, a few weeks to months of environmental dust control may be required before affected horses become free of respiratory signs.

• In horses with profound hypoxemia (PaO_2 <60 mm Hg), inhaled oxygen supplementation via a nasopharyngeal tube may be required until ventilation is improved by environmental dust control and medication.

ACTIVITY

• Adjust exercise level according to the degree of respiratory dysfunction.
• Rest is indicated in horses with severely compromised respiratory function.

DIET

• Cubed or pelleted food or haylage is preferred if pasture not available.
• Hay soaked in water for 2–3 hours may be an adequate alternative for some horses, but is usually less effective at control signs.

CLIENT EDUCATION

• Maintaining affected horses in a dust free environment is paramount for the long-term management.
• Place susceptible horses stabled in barns in paddocks when other horses are fed, the boxstalls are cleaned, or the aisles are brushed.
• Never feed moldy hay to horses.

SURGICAL CONSIDERATIONS

N/A

MEDICATIONS

DRUG(S) OF CHOICE

Corticosteroids

• Systemic corticosteroids allow effective control.
• Expect a delay of a few days between initiation of therapy and maximal clinical response.
• For severe attacks, dexamethasone (initial dose of 0.05 mg/kg IV or IM, or 0.05–0.15 mg/kg PO, until control of clinical signs and then decrease and administer on alternate days for 10–20 days) may be used.
• A single dose of triamcinolone acetonide (20–40 mg IM) also reverses clinical signs of airway obstruction for 3–5 weeks, but is less desirable because of increased risk of side effects.
• For mild cases, oral prednisolone (1–4 mg/kg) often is recommended, but its efficacy in affected horses has not been documented. Prednisone is poorly absorbed orally in horses.
• Inhaled corticosteroids allow maximal concentration of drug at the effector sites and minimize side effects. Masks (Equine Aeromask and EquineHaler) have been designed for use of MDIs. May be initially poorly tolerated in horses with labored breathing.
• Inhaled beclomethasone diproprionate (initial dose of 3500 mμg per 500 kg q12h) and fluticasone propionate (2000 μg per 500 kg q12h) have been shown to be both efficacious and well tolerated but have few residual effects. A delay in response of 7 days or longer should be expected before maximal response with inhaled corticosteroids.

Bronchodilators

• Bronchodilators are used to relieve small airway obstruction caused by the airway smooth muscle contraction. They also improve delivery of inhaled corticosteroids to the distal airways.
• Long-term administration of bronchodilators should be combined with strict environmental dust control or corticosteroid, because inflammation of the lower airways may progress despite the improvement of clinical signs observed with these drugs.
• Clenbuterol (0.8–3.2 μg/kg BID), a β_2-adrenergic agonist, has bronchodilator effects and increases mucociliary transport. Clinical efficacy is inconsistent if exposure to dusty hay and bedding is maintained.
• Ipratropium bromide (0.4–1 μg/kg q6h), albuterol (1–2 μg/kg), salmeterol (0.5–1 μg/kg, q6h), and pirbuterol (1.3 μg/kg q6h) are bronchodilators that can be used by inhalation with MDIs.
• Aminophylline (5–10 mg/kg), a xanthine derivative, has limited efficacy in heaves.
• Pentoxifylline (16 g/500-kg horses, BID) has proven effective to improve airway function in heaves, but cost limits its usage.

Expectorant, Mucolytic, and Mucokinetic Agents

Evidence of efficacy for these agents in improving clinical signs is sparse.

CONTRAINDICATIONS

Corticosteroid administration in the face of sepsis or laminitis

PRECAUTIONS

Administer potassium iodide with caution in affected horses, because it irritates the respiratory tract and can induce or worsen bronchospasm.

POSSIBLE INTERACTIONS

N/A

ALTERNATIVE DRUGS

• Inhaled sodium cromoglycate (80–200 mg q12–24h) in some horses in clinical remission prevents the appearance of clinical signs for as long as 3 weeks after introduction to a dusty environment.
• Nedocromil sodium (24 mg q12h), another cromone, may be used by inhalation.

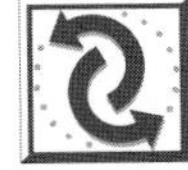

FOLLOW-UP

PATIENT MONITORING

Sequential Pao_2 determination to monitor response to therapy in horses with severely compromised respiratory function.

PREVENTION/AVOIDANCE

Dust-free environment

POSSIBLE COMPLICATIONS

• Heaves is a wasting disease that may rarely lead to death in severe cases if proper environmental control and effective medication are not provided.
• Bronchiectasis and right heart failure is a rare complication in severe cases.

EXPECTED COURSE AND PROGNOSIS

• The clinical signs at rest are reversible with prolonged environmental control and therapy. Some degrees of exercise intolerance may persist.
• Pulmonary neutrophilia often persists even if the horse is clinically asymptomatic in absence of strict environmental dust control.

MISCELLANEOUS

ASSOCIATED CONDITIONS

N/A

AGE-RELATED FACTORS

• Rarely seen in horses <7 years
• Incidence increases with age.

ZOONOTIC POTENTIAL

None

PREGNANCY

• Anecdotal reports suggest clinical signs may improve in some mares during pregnancy.
• Fetal growth retardation may occur in mares with severely compromised respiratory function.

SYNONYMS

• RAO
• Improper terminologies: COPD, chronic bronchitis, chronic bronchiolitis, broken wind

SEE ALSO

• Expiratory dyspnea
• Summer pasture–associated obstructive pulmonary disease
• Inflammatory airway disease

ABBREVIATIONS

• BAL = bronchoalveolar lavage
• COPD = chronic obstructive pulmonary disease
• IAD = inflammatory airway disease
• MDI = metered dose inhaler
• RAO = recurrent airway obstruction

Suggested Reading

Lavoie JP. Recurrent airway obstruction (heaves) and summer-pasture-associated obstructive pulmonary disease. In: McGorum BC, Dixon PM, Robinson NE, Schumacher J, eds. Equine Respiratory Medicine and Surgery. Edinburgh: Saunders Elsevier, 2007:565–589.

Robinson NE. International Workshop on Equine Chronic Airway Disease. Michigan State University 16-18 June 2000. Equine Vet J 2001;33:5–19.

Author Jean-Pierre Lavoie

Consulting Editor Daniel Jean

HEMANGIOSARCOMA

BASIC

OVERVIEW

• A malignant neoplasm originating from the vascular endothelium of horses
• Sometimes termed angiosarcoma or malignant hemangioendothelioma
• Can be focal, locally invasive, cutaneous, or disseminated
• Common primary sites in horses include lung, pleura, right heart, and spleen.
• Metastases can be found in respiratory tract, musculoskeletal system, gastrointestinal tract, skin, and central nervous system.

SIGNALMENT

• Disseminated hemangiosarcoma reported to be more common in middle-aged horses (age range 3–26 years; mean 12 years).
• No apparent breed or gender predilection

SIGNS

• Vary depending on location and often attributable to hemorrhage.
• Predominantly referable to respiratory and musculoskeletal systems including dyspnea (hemothorax), epistaxis, cough, subcutaneous edema/swelling, lameness, tachycardia, tachypnea, and pale/icteric mucous membranes.
• Cutaneous form includes generally solitary dermal or subcutaneous lesions that are poorly circumscribed with necrosis, ulceration, or bleeding.
• Rectal examination may reveal pelvic mass and/or splenomegaly, enlarged kidney, or ovarian mass.

CAUSES AND RISK FACTORS

No specific or perceived causes or risk factors

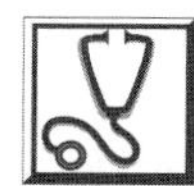

DIAGNOSIS

DIFFERENTIAL DIAGNOSIS

• Hemangiomas, which are the most benign endothelial cell tumor, generally occur in horses <1 year old with predilection for distal limbs.
• If dyspnea observed, consider infectious or obstructive respiratory disease including nasal or thoracic tumors. Endoscopy, ultrasonography, or radiography may be useful procedures to differentiate these conditions.
• If epistaxis observed, consider trauma, infection including guttural pouch mycosis, neoplasia, and exercise-induced pulmonary hemorrhage. Endoscopy or radiography may help differentiate.
• If lameness and/or intramuscular swelling observed, consider multiple causes including trauma and degenerative conditions, abscessation, or other forms of neoplasia.

CBC/BIOCHEMISTRY/URINALYSIS

• The most common laboratory abnormality is anemia (PCV <25%).
• Neutrophilic leukocytosis and thrombocytopenia also common
• Variable total protein, although hypoproteinemia accompanied by hypoalbuminaemia is common.
• Elevated globulin fractions (>4.0 g/dL or 40 g/L) with normal to slightly elevated fibrinogen
• Biochemical abnormalities may include mild to moderate azotemia and hyperbilirubinemia, increases in muscle enzyme activities (creatinine kinase and aspartate aminotransferase) along with mild electrolyte abnormalities.
• Urinalysis generally within normal limits or microscopic hematuria

OTHER LABORATORY TESTS

• Immunohistochemistry may be useful in differentiating hemangiosarcoma from other carcinomas. Specifically, factor VIII–related antigen (vWF), an endothelial cell marker, has been successfully used to identify endothelial-cell origin cutaneous tumors.
• aPTT may be mildly prolonged but generally within reference intervals.

IMAGING

A variety of imaging techniques may be useful, including endoscopy, radiography, ultrasonography, pleuroscopy, and cystoscopy, but they typically lack specificity.

OTHER DIAGNOSTIC PROCEDURES

- Antemortem diagnosis of hemangiosarcoma is difficult without direct visualization and biopsy.
- Cytological evaluation of various biological fluids (e.g., peritoneal fluid, pleural fluid, tracheal aspiration or bronchoalveolar lavage fluid, cerebrospinal fluid, tissue aspirate) is frequently consistent with hemorrhage or inflammation and not specifically diagnostic.
- Bone marrow aspirates may show erythroid hyperplasia.
- Localization of signs to a specific system (e.g., respiratory, urogenital) may allow for endoscopic/pleuroscopic/cystoscopic/laparoscopic-guided biopsy.
- Biopsy or fine needle aspiration may be diagnostic. Both histopathological (endothelial cells with numerous mitotic figures) and immunohistochemistry (factor VIII–related antigen) are helpful in differentiating hemangiosarcoma from hemorrhage and inflammation.
- Diagnosis is frequently established during postmortem examination.

PATHOLOGIC FINDINGS

- Common primary sites for disseminated hemangiosarcoma in horses include lung, pleura, skeletal muscle, right heart, and spleen. The kidney and brain also are reported to be invaded, but the primary tumor site is often not identified.
- Postmortem findings commonly include large volumes of blood in the thoracic and abdominal cavities and hemorrhage within affected muscle groups. Tumors are friable, dark red to black masses within the affected organ or tissue.
- Histologically, tumors consist of multiple, poorly organized vascular channels lined by plump, spindle-shaped cells. Neoplastic endothelial cells have large, ovoid, vesicular hyperchromic nuclei and prominent nucleoli with multiple and often bizarre mitotic figures.
- Neutrophils, lymphocytes, hemosiderin-filled macrophages, or free hemosiderin pigment may be present in some tumors.

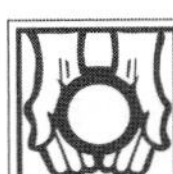

TREATMENT

- For cutaneous or well-localized lesions, surgical excision may be beneficial.
- A variety of supportive treatments have been used, including steroidal and nonsteroidal anti-inflammatory drugs, fluid therapy, blood transfusions, plasma, and antibiotics. Often, despite initial favorable responses, horses are eventually euthanized due to progression of clinical signs.

MEDICATIONS

DRUG(S)

No established protocols or approved medical therapy for treatment of hemangiosarcoma in horses

FOLLOW-UP

PATIENT MONITORING

Following surgical excision of cutaneous or localized lesions, horses should be carefully monitored for recurrence.

EXPECTED COURSE AND PROGNOSIS

Clinical deterioration is generally rapid with the disseminated form and the long term prognosis is poor. Median time from onset of clinical signs to euthanasia/death is 17 days (range, 0 days to 4 years).

MISCELLANEOUS

ABBREVIATIONS

- aPTT = activated partial thromboplastin time
- PCV = packed cell volume
- vFW = von Willebrand factor

Suggested Reading

Southwood LL, Schott HC, Henry CJ, Kennedy FA, Hines MT, Geor RJ, Hassel DM. Disseminated hemangiosarcoma in the horse: 35 cases. J Vet Intern Med 2000;14:105–109.

Author Mark V. Crisman

Consulting Editors Jennifer Hodgson and David Hodgson

HEMORRHAGE, ACUTE

BASICS

DEFINITION

Rapid loss of blood internally (e.g., into thoracic/abdominal cavities) or externally (including loss from the GIT) over usually <24 hr

PATHOPHYSIOLOGY

• Acute loss of >30% of circulating blood volume (≈12 L of blood in a 500-kg horse) results in hypovolemic shock with immediate triggering of compensatory mechanisms. Rapid loss of >40%–50% of circulating blood volume represents a severe, irreversible physiologic insult usually resulting in death. • Compensatory mechanisms include generalized vasoconstriction, increased cardiac contractility and rate, expansion of blood volume via increased water and sodium resorption from the kidney and GIT, and fluid movements from the intracellular and interstitial spaces into the vascular pool. • Additionally, RBCs are released into the circulation via catecholamine-induced splenic contraction ($^1/_3$ total RBC mass stored in the spleen). • There is little change in PCV and other erythrocyte indices for 12–24 hr after hemorrhage as RBCs and plasma are lost but there is release of stored splenic RBCs. True severity of blood loss can be determined only after 36–48 hr. • There is a decrease in TP within 6 hr as fluids move into the intravascular compartment. • With internal hemorrhage, ≈$^2/_3$ of RBCs are autotransfused back to the circulation within 24–72 hr. • Depending on severity, a regenerative bone marrow response is demonstrable from 3–42 days. Complete restoration of RBC mass requires 1–3 months.
• Replacement of plasma proteins occurs more rapidly, with albumin taking ≈5–10 days and globulins ≈3–4 weeks to return to normal.

SYSTEMS AFFECTED

• Cardiovascular and respiratory • Hemic/lymphatic/immune • Hepatobiliary, renal, GI, musculoskeletal, and central nervous systems may be involved due to hypoxia and ischemia.

SIGNS

General Comments

Signs vary with the duration and severity of blood loss, site of hemorrhage, and underlying disease.

Historical

• Evidence of trauma or recent difficult birth in neonatal foals with hemothorax • History of low-grade colic in adult horses (intra-abdominal hemorrhage) • Sudden collapse or distress in stallions; aortic root rupture • Recent intense exercise in racehorses (EIPH)

Physical Examination

• Signs of shock (loss of >30% of circulating blood volume) may include tachycardia, polypnea, mucous membrane pallor, systolic heart murmur, slowed jugular filling, reduced pulse pressure, and oliguria. Agitation, generalized weakness, and sweating may occur. Ataxia and collapse occur when there is >40% blood volume loss. • Epistaxis, respiratory distress, decreased or absent ventral lung sounds, and pluerodynia may occur if lung/thorax are involved. • Signs of low-grade colic and decreased GIT motility may occur if there is sufficient decreased organ perfusion or intra-abdominal hemorrhage. • Sudden death may be the only sign in cases of aortic root rupture.

CAUSES

Internal Abdominal Hemorrhage and Hemoperitoneum

• Splenic and hepatic rupture following trauma
• Rupture of the middle uterine artery following dystocia or uterine eversion/prolapse • Rupture of caudal vena cava (after incarceration of the small intestine in the epiploic foramen)
• Mesenteric arterial hemorrhage secondary to verminous arteritis, strangulating lipoma, coagulopathy, or previous GI surgery • Uterine bleeding secondary to birth trauma
• Hemorrhage from ovarian arteries • Iliac arterial rupture secondary to a displaced pelvic fracture • Neoplasia, e.g., hemangiosarcoma
• After surgery or biopsy

Internal Thoracic Hemorrhage

• Thoracic trauma, e.g., rib fractures, lacerated heart or vessels during lung biopsy
• Aortic root or other large vessel rupture
• Diaphragmatic hernia with vascular tearing
• Pulmonary hemorrhage
• Neoplasia
• Coagulopathy

External Hemorrhage

• Epistaxis due to guttural pouch mycosis with erosion of the carotid artery, EIPH, severe trauma
• Trauma, e.g., wounds
• Surgical complications, e.g., post-castration
• Cellulitis with erosion through a major vessel
• Umbilical hemorrhage
• Coagulopathy
• Ethmoid hematoma—usually chronic rather than acute hemorrhage

RISK FACTORS

• Horses undertaking high intensity exercise are at risk of EIPH.
• Previous periparturient hemorrhage in mares is a risk factor for bleeding during future pregnancies.
• Older breeding stallions may have a higher risk for acute aortic root rupture.
• Neonatal foals are at greater risk of rib fractures and umbilical cord hemorrhage.

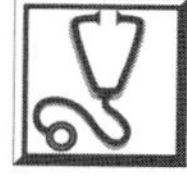

DIAGNOSIS

DIFFERENTIAL DIAGNOSIS

• Endotoxemia
• Low-grade colic may be differentiated by rectal examination, abdominal ultrasonography, and abdominocentesis.
• Acute severe hemolytic anemia may be differentiated on basis of history, serology (Coggins), examination of blood smears, or Coombs test.
• Sudden death may be differentiated by history, physical, and post-mortem examinations.

CBC/BIOCHEMISTRY/URINALYSIS

• Few changes to PCV or plasma TP concentration are noted for 12–24 hr post-hemorrhage with PCV reaching lowest values (<20%) around 36–48 hr.
• Few changes to MCV, MCH, and MCHC occur, but moderate increases in RDW may take place.
• Transient thrombocytopenia and leukocytosis with neutrophilia
• Increased serum creatinine and urea nitrogen concentrations reflecting prerenal or renal azotemia
• Increased AST and CK activities if significant musculoskeletal trauma has occurred.
• Oliguria and increased urine specific gravity (>1.040) may occur with hypovolemic shock.

OTHER LABORATORY TESTS

• Coagulation tests (e.g., platelet count, PT, aPTT) should be performed if a coagulopathy is suspected.
• With hemothorax, arterial blood gas analysis may demonstrate impaired ventilatory function.

IMAGING

Radiography

Thoracic radiography if hemothorax, rib fractures, or pneumothorax are suspected.

Ultrasonography

• Thoracic and abdominal ultrasonography to demonstrate fluid accumulation
• Splenic ultrasonography to identify masses (e.g., hematomas, abscesses, tumors)
• Transrectal ultrasonography to examine abnormalities of the caudal abdomen (e.g., swelling of the broad ligament)
• Echocardiography in stallions with suspected aortic root rupture

OTHER DIAGNOSTIC PROCEDURES

• Abdominocentesis and thoracocentesis. Evidence of erythrophagocytosis rules out inadvertent splenic or subcutaneous vessel puncture during sampling.
• Rectal palpation if intra-abdominal hemorrhage suspected
• Airway endoscopy to localize the source of hemorrhage in horses with epistaxis
• Laparoscopy to differentiate causes of intra-abdominal hemorrhage
• Measurement of blood pressure; systolic pressure <80 mm Hg indicates hypotension.

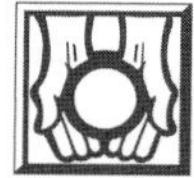

TREATMENT

AIMS OF TREATMENT

• Severe acute hemorrhage often constitutes an emergency. Controlling hemorrhage and replacing blood volume should be priorities.
• External hemorrhage may be controlled by application of pressure bandages or ligating ruptured vessels. Control of internal hemorrhage is more difficult and a "wait and see" approach may be necessary.

APPROPRIATE HEALTH CARE

Fluid Therapy

• Balanced isotonic IV fluid therapy (initially 20 mL/kg/hr or 10L/hr for a 500-kg horse) is indicated if the horse exhibits tachycardia, poor pulse quality, and cool extremities and has low blood pressure. If blood loss can be estimated, total volume administered should be ≥2–3 times the estimated loss.

• If high-volume isotonic fluid replacement is not practical, small volumes of hypertonic saline (7% NaCl at 2–5 mL/kg) can be administered IV over 15min *if hemorrhage has been controlled*. Additionally, isotonic fluids in sufficient volume to replace estimated deficits should follow within a few hours.

• A 6% hydroxyethyl starch solution (8–10 mL/kg) IV may be used *when hemorrhage has been controlled* to improve intravascular oncotic pressure.

Blood Transfusion

• Indications for blood transfusion include poor clinical response to crystalloid therapy, persistent severe tachycardia, profound hypotension, ongoing hemorrhage, PCV decreasing to <20% within 12 hr or if PCV falls to <12% over 24–48 hr.

• Donors should be selected based on compatibility testing, but if an immediate transfusion is needed blood may be collected from an available gelding of similar breed with no history of blood/plasma therapy. Initial transfusions rarely are associated with adverse reactions, but subsequent transfusions (after ≈3 days) may be associated with severe reactions.

• A healthy adult horse can donate 8–10L of blood (or 20%–25% of their total blood volume) every 4–5 weeks without adverse clinical or physiological consequences. Blood should be collected into bags containing ACD anticoagulant (15 mL of ACD for every 100 mL of blood).

• The transfusion volume should be based on degree of hypovolemia and estimates of blood loss. For adult horses weighing ≈500 kg, 6–8 L (or 15 mL/kg) usually is required, but volume should not exceed 20% of blood volume (i.e., 20% × 0.08 × body weight [kg] ≈ 8L) to ensure circulatory overload does not occur.

• Transfusion should be slow initially (0.1 mL/kg/min) and if no adverse clinical reactions occur can be increased to 20 mL/kg/h.

• Transfused red cells are cleared within 2–6 days.

NURSING CARE AND ACTIVITY

• Horses with severe, acute hemorrhage require inpatient care for treatment and further diagnostic evaluation.

• In horses with hemothorax and respiratory distress blood can be removed by thoracocentesis, but rapid refilling may occur.

• Nasal administration of oxygen is indicated in hypoxemic patients.

• Vital signs, TP, and PCV should be monitored and fluid rates adjusted to prevent dilution of blood and exacerbation of anemia and hypoproteinemia. Reduction of TP <45 g/L (4.5 g/dL) necessitates discontinuation of isotonic fluids.

DIET

A balanced diet should provide the necessary minerals and vitamins for an optimal bone marrow regenerative response.

SURGICAL CONSIDERATIONS

Horses with acute severe hemorrhage are poor anesthetic risks and should be stabilized prior to emergency surgery.

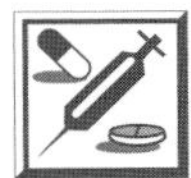

MEDICATIONS

DRUG(S)

• Several drugs have been used to control hemorrhage, but their efficacy in horses has not been established.

• Aminocaproic acid (20–80 mg/kg IV diluted in 0.9% saline and administered over 30–60 min) and tranexamic acid (1g IV) have been used in mares with postpartum uterine artery hemorrhage.

• Oxytocin (20 IU IM q30 min) also has been used for hemorrhage in mares postpartum to decrease bleeding from the myometrium. However, oxytocin has no effect on hemorrhage from the uterine arteries.

• Naloxone (0.01–0.02 mg/kg IV) may be used to antagonize the effects of endogenous opioids on cardiovascular function.

• Flunixin meglumine (0.5–1.0 mg/kg q8–12 h) may be used for its anti-inflammatory and analgesic activity.

CONTRAINDICATIONS

• Oxytocin use is contraindicated in horses with hematoma of the broad ligament.

• Parenteral iron dextran preparations can cause death.

PRECAUTIONS

• Synthetic colloidal products (e.g., dextrans, hetastarch) may inhibit platelet aggregation and decrease coagulation protein concentration and function.

• Intravenous formaldehyde (0.37%) should be used with caution as higher doses can result in adverse effects (e.g., muscle fasciculations, agitation, restlessness). No evidence exists supporting its efficacy.

• Acepromazine should be used with extreme caution in hypotensive animals.

• Hypertonic saline in horses with uncontrolled hemorrhage may increase blood loss and risk of mortality.

ALTERNATIVE DRUGS

Stromal free bovine hemoglobin (30 mL/kg; Biopure Corp., Boston, MA) has been used as an alternative to whole-blood transfusion.

FOLLOW-UP

PATIENT MONITORING

• Heart rate, pulse quality, and blood pressure should be monitored frequently during the initial 12–24 hr of treatment.

• Ongoing hemorrhage and the bone marrow response can be assessed by determining PCV regularly for 1–3 days after acute hemorrhage. A regenerative response is indicated by increases in PCV whereas PCV remaining low suggests continuing bleeding.

POSSIBLE COMPLICATIONS

• Blood transfusion should be stopped if signs of an immediate transfusion reaction are observed and appropriate therapy administered (see Blood Transfusion Reactions).

• Bacterial sepsis

• Laminitis

EXPECTED COURSE AND PROGNOSIS

• The prognosis for horses suffering acute hemorrhage depends on the severity, rate, and cause of blood loss.

• Anemia can resolve within 4–12 weeks in cases where hemorrhage is controlled and hypovolemic shock is successfully managed.

• Rupture of major vessels (e.g., aorta, middle uterine artery) has a higher case-fatality rate.

MISCELLANEOUS

PREGNANCY

Severe hypovolemic shock may compromise the fetus, particularly during the last trimester. Follow-up monitoring should include evaluation of fetal viability.

SEE ALSO

• Anemia

• Blood transfusion reactions

• Hemorrhage, chronic

ABBREVIATIONS

• aPTT = activated partial thromboplastin time
• AST = aspartate aminotransferase
• CK = creatine kinase
• EIPH = exercise-induced pulmonary hemorrhage
• GIT = gastrointestinal tract
• MCH = mean cell hemoglobin
• MCHC = mean cell hemoglobin concentration
• MCV = mean cell volume
• PCV = packed cell volume
• PT = prothrombin time
• RDW = red cell distribution width
• TP = total protein

Suggested Reading

Collatos C. Blood loss anemia. In: Robinson NE, ed. Current Therapy in Equine Medicine, ed 5. Philadelphia: WB Saunders, 2003:340–344.

Hurcombe SD, Mudge MC, Hinchcliff KW. Clinical and clinicopathologic variables in adult horses receiving blood transfusions: 31 cases (1999–2005). J Am Vet Med Assoc 2007;231;267–274.

Malikides N, Kessell A, Hodgson JL, Rose RJ, Hodgson DR. Bone marrow response to large volume blood collection in the horse. Res Vet Sci 1999;67:285–293.

Schmall LM, Muir WW, Robertson JT. Haemodynamic effects of small volume hypertonic saline in experimentally induced haemorrhagic shock. Equine Vet J 1990;22:273–277.

Author Nicholas Malikides
Consulting Editors Jennifer Hodgson and David Hodgson

HEMORRHAGE, CHRONIC

BASICS

OVERVIEW

• Chronic hemorrhage occurs most frequently as a result of low grade bleeding into the GIT.
• The resulting physiologic adaptations often obscure clinical signs until the PCV is <0.12 L/L (12%). • Bone marrow regenerative responses usually compensate for losses unless the rate of erythropoiesis is exceeded by the rate of blood loss, or if chronic blood loss occurs externally, where eventual iron deficiency causes maturation arrest of marrow erythroid precursors. • Chronic internal hemorrhage (e.g., into pleural or peritoneal cavities) allows reutilization of some RBCs, which are reabsorbed into lymphatic vessels, as well as iron and plasma protein. In contrast, horses with chronic external hemorrhage, including GIT and urinary tract bleeding, often develop deficiencies of these blood constituents.

SIGNALMENT

• There is no breed, sex, or age predilection for chronic hemorrhage. However, some underlying primary diseases may be more common in some types of horses (e.g., nonsteroidal anti-inflammatory toxicosis and GIT bleeding in ponies).

SIGNS

• Overt signs of anemia (e.g., tachycardia, tachypnea, or weakness) may not be seen until PCV <0.12 L/L (<12%). • Pale mucous membranes, exercise intolerance, and marked increases in heart and respiratory rates may be observed if the horse is subjected to stress.
• Other signs of an underlying disease process (e.g., weight loss in horses with neoplasia, parasite-induced diarrhea) may be observed.

CAUSES AND RISK FACTORS

• Risk factors for chronic hemorrhage depend on those for the primary disease process (e.g., inadequate anthelmintic use, phenylbutazone administration, exposure to relevant toxins).

Gastrointestinal Causes

• Severe parasitism (e.g., large and small strongyles) • GIT ulceration • NSAID toxicity resulting in GIT ulceration • Gastric and/or duodenal ulcers in foals • Neoplasia (e.g., gastric squamous cell carcinoma, lymphosarcoma)
• Bleeding abdominal abscess • Granulomatous intestinal disease (e.g., granulomatous enteritis)

Renal/Urologic Causes

• Hemorrhagic, erosive cystitis or urolithiasis
• Renal or bladder neoplasia • Vascular anomaly—idiopathic urethral hemorrhage in geldings • Pyelonephritis

Respiratory Causes

• Exercise-induced pulmonary hemorrhage
• Ethmoid hematoma • Guttural pouch mycosis
• Pulmonary or paranasal sinus abscess • Fungal rhinitis • Upper respiratory tract neoplasia
• Pulmonary neoplasia

Miscellaneous Causes

• Immune-mediated thrombocytopenia
• Coagulopathies

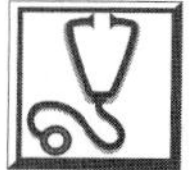

DIAGNOSIS

DIFFERENTIAL DIAGNOSIS

• Causes of anemia of chronic disease, e.g., inflammation, infection, or neoplasia. These are differentiated by evidence of nonregenerative anemia and clinical identification of the primary, chronic disease process. • Causes of low-grade chronic hemolytic anemia (due to oxidant, infectious, or immune-mediated causes). These are differentiated by Coombs test, Coggins test, blood smear examination, and evaluation of history and clinical signs.

CBC/BIOCHEMISTRY/URINALYSIS

• Hemogram findings are inconsistent.
• Microcytic, hypochromic anemia with low serum iron, low marrow iron stores, and increased TIBC may be present, especially if chronic GIT hemorrhage has occurred.
• Hypoproteinemia may indicate external blood loss (e.g., from GIT, urogenital or respiratory tract) although plasma total protein concentration may be normal due to liver compensation. • Increased total and indirect bilirubinemia suggests internal blood loss.
• Chronic tissue hypoxia (PCV < 12%) may cause increased serum hepatic enzyme activities and increased serum creatinine concentrations indicative of hypoxic hepatopathy and nephropathy. • Microscopic or gross hematuria may indicate a primary renal/urologic problem.

OTHER LABORATORY TESTS

Low serum iron, low bone marrow iron stores, and increased TIBC may be noted following chronic external hemorrhage.

IMAGING

• Ultrasonography may be useful in identifying NSAID-induced right dorsal colitis or may identify intra-abdominal or intrathoracic masses.
• Upper respiratory tract radiography may reveal sinus or ethmoidal masses.

OTHER DIAGNOSTIC PROCEDURES

• Bone marrow aspirate. If the myeloid:erythroid ratio is <0.5, the anemia is regenerative. Other causes of chronic regenerative anemia (e.g., chronic hemolytic anemia or anemia of chronic disease) should be ruled out. • Positive fecal occult blood indicates significant GIT hemorrhage or blood swallowed from the respiratory tract. However, this test has low sensitivity and specificity. • Positive fecal examination for parasitic ova supports a diagnosis of parasitism when accompanied by weight loss, diarrhea, or poor deworming history, and possibly a positive fecal occult blood test. • Gastroscopy may reveal gastroduodenal ulceration or gastric squamous cell carcinoma.
• Cystoscopy may identify urethral, bladder, or ureteral hemorrhage. • Upper airway endoscopy may demonstrate rhinitis, neoplasia, guttural pouch mycosis, ethmoid hematoma, or blood in the trachea. • Erythrocytophagia and hemosiderophages may be identified in abdominal fluid, tracheal aspirate, or bronchoalveolar lavage fluid. • Ultrasound-guided biopsies of masses may characterize the primary disease process as infectious or neoplastic.

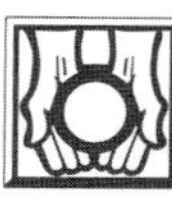

TREATMENT

• Appropriate management is based on identification and elimination of the source of the underlying disease, which may necessitate inpatient care. • Blood transfusion usually is unnecessary unless PCV is <8% (<0.08 L/L) or clinical and laboratory signs of tissue hypoxia are present. • If there is evidence of true iron deficiency, ferrous sulfate can be administered at 2 mg/kg PO daily.

MEDICATIONS

DRUG(S) OF CHOICE

Medications to treat the underlying disease

CONTRAINDICATIONS/POSSIBLE INTERACTIONS

Parenteral iron dextran solutions should be avoided due to the possibility of fatal reactions.

FOLLOW-UP

PATIENT MONITORING

• The response to treatment of the underlying disease should be assessed. • Additionally, the anemia should be monitored by weekly evaluation of PCV. A gradual increase of PCV to values within the reference range should be expected over 6–12 weeks. • Serial bone marrow aspiration is rarely necessary. • Client education should include recommendations regarding the underlying disease (e.g., parasite control).
• Prognosis depends on accurately identifying the underlying disease.

MISCELLANEOUS

SEE ALSO

• Anemia
• Hemorrhage, acute

ABBREVIATIONS

• GIT = gastrointestinal tract
• NSAID = nonsteroidal anti-inflammatory drug
• PCV = packed cell volume
• TIBC = total iron-binding capacity

Suggested Reading

Collatos C. Blood loss anemia. In: Robinson NE, ed. Current Therapy in Equine Medicine, ed 5. Philadelphia: WB Saunders, 2003:340–344.

The author and editors wish to acknowledge the contributions of Chrysann Collatos, author of this topic in the previous edition.

Author Nicholas Malikides
Consulting Editors Jennifer Hodgson and David Hodgson

HEMORRHAGIC NASAL DISCHARGE

BASICS

OVERVIEW

• May be composed of frank blood or blood mixed with secretions—mucus, pus, froth, and necrotic debris • May be caused by lesions within the respiratory tract or adjacent structures and by hemostatic dysfunctions; the latter, particularly thrombocytopenia and DIC, often are associated with mucosal petechia and ecchymotic hemorrhages and prolonged bleeding from venipuncture sites. • Unilateral discharge—usually results from lesions rostral to the nasopharynx (e. g., nasal passage, paranasal sinuses). • Bilateral discharge—usually due to lesions caudal to the nasopharynx or from hemostatic dysfunctions.

SYSTEMS AFFECTED

Hemic and respiratory

SIGNS

• Bleeding—acute or chronic • Discharge may be composed of blood only (i.e. epistaxis) or blood mixed with seromucoid, mucopurulent, or frothy nasal discharge. • Mucopurulent or foul smelling discharges suggest an infectious or necrotic origin. • Bilateral frothy discharge is consistent with pulmonary edema.
• Hemorrhage from the nasal passage, turbinates, or paranasal sinuses manifests as an ipsilateral discharge; hemorrhage originating caudal to the nasal septum, including the nasopharynx, guttural pouch, and lower respiratory tract, usually causes bilateral discharge. • Hemostatic disorders may also result in bleeding diatheses from other organs.
• Thrombocytopenia and DIC often are associated with mucosal petechiation, ecchymotic hemorrhages, and occult blood from the GI or urinary tracts. • DIC frequently leads to thrombophlebitis; spontaneous epistaxis is less common. • Coagulation factor deficiencies tend to result in hemorrhages into body cavities (e.g., joints, abdomen, thorax), epistaxis, melena, excessive bleeding and hematoma formation after trauma, venipuncture or surgery.

CAUSES AND RISK FACTORS

• Hemostatic dysfunction— thrombocytopenia (e.g., immune-mediated, DIC, myelophthisic disease, bone marrow aplasia), DIC (e.g., sepsis, GI and renal disease, hemolytic anemia, neoplasia), coagulation factor deficiency (e.g., inherited coagulopathies, warfarin and sweet-clover toxicosis), or envenomation (e.g., rattlesnake). • Respiratory tract disease—upper respiratory disease may result from bacterial or fungal infections (e.g., guttural pouch mycosis, sinusitis), neoplasia or idiopathic diseases (e.g. nasal polyp, nasal amyloidosis, ethmoid hematoma); relevant lower respiratory diseases include exercise-induced pulmonary hemorrhage, pleuropneumonia, pulmonary edema, primary lung tumors (e.g., myoblastoma, pulmonary carcinoma, bronchial myxoma), and metastatic neoplasms (e.g., hemangiosarcoma, adenocarcinoma). • Trauma—nasal intubation, facial bone and skull base fractures, longus capitis muscle rupture secondary to falling backward, transtracheal puncture, and lung biopsy • Other—vasculitis (e.g., purpura hemorrhagica), fibrous dysplasia, periocular bleeding, and dacryohemorrhea

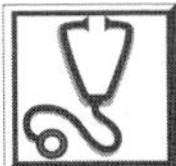

DIAGNOSIS

CBC/BIOCHEMISTRY/URINALYSIS

• Anemia may result from blood loss.
• Neutrophilia or neutropenia may accompany inflammatory diseases. • Leukemia may be evident with myeloid neoplasia. • Occult blood in the feces and urine may result from a bleeding diathesis.

OTHER LABORATORY TESTS

Assessment of hemostasis requires platelet count (reference range: 100,000–600,000 cells/μL), plasma fibrinogen (reference range, 200–400 mg/dL), prothrombin and activated partial thromboplastin time (reference range, 75%–125% of control values), and D-dimer concentration.

IMAGING

• Skull radiography may reveal bone fracture, mass, or fluid accumulation in the sinuses or guttural pouches. • Thoracic radiography may help to identify pleuropneumonia, exercise-induced pulmonary hemorrhage, pulmonary edema, and lung tumors. • Thoracic ultrasonography is a sensitive means to pleural fluid—blood or purulent effusion.

OTHER DIAGNOSTIC PROCEDURES

• Endoscopy of the respiratory tract may help to identify the cause; trephination provides access to paranasal sinuses using a flexible or rigid endoscope. • Fluid cytology from tracheobronchial aspirates, bronchoalveolar lavage, thoracocentesis or percutaneous centesis of the paranasal sinuses may reveal the source or cause of bleeding. • Biopsy should help to identify the nature of a mass; full-thickness punch biopsies of the skin in the affected areas may confirm a diagnosis of vasculitis.

PATHOLOGIC FINDINGS

• Depend on the primary disease process.
• Nasal and paranasal neoplasms are malignant in 68% of cases.

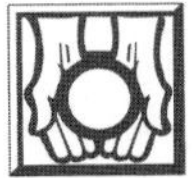

TREATMENT

• Treat the primary disease. • Stall rest is recommended and sedation if horse is agitated.
• Treat severe blood loss with IV administration of sodium-containing crystalloid solutions to maintain the circulating blood volume. However, if the hemorrhage is not controlled, volume expansion may worsen blood loss. Perform blood transfusion when the RBC mass is insufficient to maintain tissue oxygenation (e.g., >30% blood volume lost acutely). • Patients with hemostatic disorders may benefit from fresh plasma transfusion. • Consider surgical resection of a nasal or paranasal mass. • Radiation therapy may be useful with paranasal neoplasm. • Guttural pouch mycosis may be treated surgically by occlusion of the affected artery.

MEDICATIONS

DRUG(S) OF CHOICE

• Immunosuppressive therapy with corticoids (e.g., dexamethasone 0.05–0.2 mg/kg IM or IV q24 h) is useful in cases of immune-mediated coagulopathy or vasculitis. • Heparin (20–80 IU/kg SQ or IV q6–12 h) and low-dose aspirin (15 mg/kg PO q24–48 h) may reduce complications of DIC. • Warfarin and sweet-clover toxicosis—treat with vitamin K_1 (0.5–1 mg/kg SC q6 h) until the clinical signs resolve and the prothrombin time is normal for at least 2 days. • Antifibrinolytics may help decrease blood loss (Aminocaproic acid 10–20 mg/kg IV; tranexamic acid 1 g IV).
• Institute appropriate antimicrobial or antifungal therapy for underlying infectious diseases. • Pulmonary edema—treat with furosemide (1 mg/kg IV) and respiratory support.

FOLLOW-UP

PATIENT MONITORING

• Monitor hematocrit and hydration status.
• Monitor the condition both qualitatively and quantitatively.

POSSIBLE COMPLICATIONS

Severe, fatal bleeding may occur if a major artery is involved.

EXPECTED COURSE AND PROGNOSIS

Depend on the underlying cause

MISCELLANEOUS

SEE ALSO

• Exercise-induced pulmonary hemorrhage
• Guttural pouch mycosis • Pleuropneumonia
• Sinusitis

ABBREVIATIONS

• DIC = disseminated intravascular coagulation
• GI = gastrointestinal

Suggested Reading

Collatos C. Blood loss anemia. In: Robinson NE, ed. Current Therapy in Equine Medicine. Philadelphia: WB Saunders, 2003:340–342.

Author Laurent Couëtil
Consulting Editor Daniel Jean

HEMOSPERMIA

BASICS

DEFINITION/OVERVIEW
Contamination of an ejaculate with blood

ETIOLOGY/PATHOPHYSIOLOGY
- Injury to the urethral process (from lacerations by tail hair, abrasion with a phantom during semen collection procedure, cutaneous habronemiasis, squamous cell carcinoma)
- Lacerations to the glans or body of the penis
- Tears in the urethral mucosa
- Infection/inflammation of the accessory sex glands

SYSTEM AFFECTED
Urogenital

GENETICS
Quarter Horse breed—tears in the urethral mucosa

SIGNS
- General physical examination of the stallion at rest is usually unremarkable. • Discoloration of semen ranging from pink-tinged to frank hemorrhage is the most common sign. • In natural breeding situations, blood may be seen dripping from the penis on dismount, at the vulvar lips of the mare following breeding, or mares may not become pregnant following breeding. • Some stallions will concurrently have hematuria.

CAUSES
- Top two causes
  - *Trauma*: laceration of the urethral process, glans penis or body of penis (usually from tail hair); stricture of the urethra from chronic placement without monitoring/cleaning of a stallion ring
  - *Urethral defects*
- Urethritis • Infection/inflammation of the accessory sex glands • Neoplasia
  - Squamous cell carcinoma
  - Papilloma
- Cutaneous habronemiasis

RISK FACTORS
- Breeding activity (infection, lacerations to external penis) • Hot, humid environmental conditions (cutaneous habronemiasis)

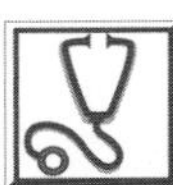

DIAGNOSIS

Differentiating Causes
- Semen collected with an AV permits visualization of hemorrhage within the ejaculate.
- Fractionation of the ejaculate, using an open-ended AV, allows direct visualization of the source of hemorrhage in some cases, e. g., with a penile laceration. • Fractionation may also aid in determining from which portion of the ejaculate hemorrhage originates:
  - Blood in the gel fraction likely originates from the vesicular glands.
  - WBCs predominate over RBCs with infections of the accessory sex glands.

CBC/BIOCHEMISTRY/URINALYSIS
- CBC and chemistry panel are generally unaffected. • Urinalysis might reveal RBCs.

IMAGING

U/S
- Transrectal U/S may be useful in diagnosing abnormalities of the vesicular glands:
  - Normal glands can vary significantly in appearance. Range from flat in the nonaroused state to enlarged and filled with hypoechoic fluid after sexual stimulation.
  - Inflamed vesicular glands may be thickened and filled with echogenic fluid.
  - Note: Echogenic luminal content does not always indicate pathology of the glands, as some stallions produce normal gel that is echogenic on U/S examination.
- Ancillary tests such as culture, cytology, and endoscopy should be considered for definitive diagnosis of accessory sex gland infection/inflammation.

OTHER DIAGNOSTIC PROCEDURES
- Endoscopy: useful tool to diagnose urethral abnormalities (urethritis, rents) and vesicular gland inflammation • Bacterial culture and cytology of semen are beneficial for determination of accessory sex gland infection.
- Biopsy and histopathology can be used to diagnose neoplasia or cutaneous habronemiasis.

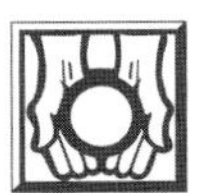

TREATMENT

All conditions warrant sexual rest.

- *Trauma:* usually outpatient care, palliative therapy aimed at hygiene and parasite control
- *Urethral defects*:
  - Conservative approach: sexual rest (limited success)
  - Surgical approach: ischial urethrotomy and a minimum of 2 mo of sexual rest.
- *Urethritis*: antibiotic therapy
- *Infection/inflammation of the accessory sex glands*:
  - Antibiotic therapy (local, systemic)
  - Lavage of the glands (endoscopically)
  - Intrauterine infusion of semen extender containing appropriate antibiotics
- *Neoplasia*
  - Cryotherapy
  - Hyperthermia
  - Local excision
  - Reefing operation
  - Phallectomy
- *Cutaneous habronemiasis*
  - Parasite control
  - Cryotherapy
  - Surgical removal of affected sites

CLIENT EDUCATION
Sexual rest until problem is completely resolved—essential.

SURGICAL CONSIDERATIONS
Refer to individual etiologies, Treatment.

MEDICATIONS

DRUG(S) OF CHOICE

Drugs and Fluids
- Anti-inflammatory therapy (phenylbutazone, flunixin meglumine) is indicated in most cases.
- Antibiotic therapy is directed at the organism identified to cause bacterial urethritis, culture and sensitivity. • Systemic antibiotic therapy for vesicular gland infection is often ineffective due to poor diffusion of the drug into the affected area. • Antibiotic of choice for systemic treatment is trimethoprim-sulfamethoxazole (15–30 mg/kg PO BID) if the identified organism is susceptible to it. • Lavage of the glands and infusion of an antibiotic directly into the vesicular glands may be a more effective treatment. • Antiparasitic therapy for cutaneous habronemiasis (ivermectin 0.2 mg/kg PO q30 days until resolution of lesions)

PRECAUTIONS
- Trimethoprim-sulfamethoxazole at higher doses may cause colitis. • Decrease the dosage or discontinue the drug if the horse shows signs of colitis (diarrhea).

FOLLOW-UP

PATIENT MONITORING
Semen collection for identification of RBC or WBC in the ejaculate

POSSIBLE COMPLICATIONS
- Infertility • Urethral stricture or adhesions
- Adhesions of the vesicular glands • Ruptured urinary bladder

EXPECTED COURSE AND PROGNOSIS
Dependent on etiology

MISCELLANEOUS

ASSOCIATED CONDITIONS
Hematuria

PREGNANCY
Blood in the ejaculate can be harmful to spermatozoa and thus conception rates may decrease.

ABBREVIATIONS
- AV = artificial vagina • CBC = complete blood count • RBC = red blood cell • U/S = ultrasound • WBC = white blood cell

Suggested Reading

Varner DD, Schumacher J, Blanchard T, Johnson L. Diseases and Management of Breeding Stallions. Goleta: American Veterinary Publications, 1991:257–340.

Voss JL, McKinnon AO. Diagnosis of pregnancy. In: McKinnon AO, Voss JL, eds. Equine Reproduction. Philadelphia: Lea & Febiger, 1993:864–870.

Author Margo L. Macpherson

Consulting Editor Carla L. Carleton

HENDRA VIRUS

BASICS

OVERVIEW

• Hendra virus (HeV; formerly known as equine morbillivirus) is an acute and frequently fatal viral pneumonia in horses. An outbreak of HeV pneumonia was first reported in 1994 in Hendra, Queensland, Australia. Two horses in a separate occurrence, remote from the outbreak, were diagnosed retrospectively. Both outbreaks were associated with human fatalities and illness. Since these initial reports there have been three separate outbreaks of the HeV pneumonia resulting in fatalities of all horses affected and a nonfatal illness of an attending veterinarian.
• The outbreaks have been isolated and the virus does not appear to be highly contagious.
• HeV is a member of the genus *Henipavirus* in the Paramyxoviridae family.
• Flying foxes (fruit bats or Pteropodidae) are the likely wildlife reservoirs of HeV.

SIGNALMENT

Nonspecific

SIGNS

• The incubation period in experimentally infected horses is 5–10 days. The clinical course is very acute, with death occurring 1–3 days after onset of clinical signs.
• Initial signs include anorexia, depression, fever (up to 41° C), edema around the lips and head, cyanosis, and slightly jaundiced mucous membranes. Clinical signs indicative of respiratory distress include shallow, rapid respiration and nasal discharge that varies from clear to serosanginous.
• Terminal signs include headpressing, dependent edema, ataxia, and copious frothy nasal discharge.
• Two of the recovered horses showed mild transient neurologic signs.

CAUSES AND RISK FACTORS

• No outbreaks of HeV have been identified in countries other than Australia. HeV is not endemic in the Queensland horse population.
• HeV has been isolated from flying fox uterine fluid and fetal tissue. It is postulated that the source of infection for the horse is food or water contaminated by infective fetal fluids.
• Very close contact appears necessary for disease transmission via infected aerosols, nasal secretions, contaminated tack or handlers.

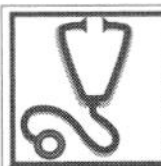

DIAGNOSIS

DIFFERENTIAL DIAGNOSIS

• African horse sickness is differentiated by serology, virus isolation, histopathology, and immunofluorescence.
• Equine influenza has a lower mortality; coughing is a more common clinical sign and is differentiated by virus culture from acute-phase collection of nasal secretions, ELISA antigen detection, or immunofluorescence.
• Equine viral arteritis is differentiated by virus isolation from nasal or conjunctival swabs, heparinized blood, and virus neutralization on serum.
• The encephalitides' clinical signs relate to the nervous system, as do postmortem findings and serology.
• Anthrax is differentiated by postmortem findings, black tarry exudates, and organisms in blood smears.
• Hantavirus infection is differentiated by serology.
• Toxins—paraquat, monensin, heavy metals, mycotoxins—are differentiated by a history of exposure; presence of the toxin in the stomach, urine, or feed; lack of supportive serology; and postmortem findings.

CBC/BIOCHEMISTRY/URINALYSIS

No characteristic abnormalities have been detected.

OTHER LABORATORY TESTS

• Serum neutralization test or indirect ELISA should be performed for antibody determination. Death may occur prior to seroconversion.
• Virus isolation from fresh specimens of the lung, liver, spleen, and kidney. Duplicate tissues in 10% formalin for histopathology.

IMAGING

N/A

DIAGNOSTIC PROCEDURES

N/A

PATHOLOGIC FINDINGS

Significant gross lesions are dilated pulmonary lymphatics, severe pulmonary edema and congestion and airways filled with blood-stained stable froth. Histologically, the main lesion is an acute interstitial pneumonia. Syncytial giant cells, which are typical of HeV infection, are found in the endothelium of pulmonary capillaries and arterioles.

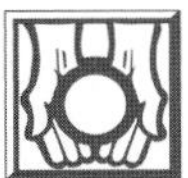

TREATMENT

No known treatment

MEDICATIONS

There is no medication for HeV.

CONTRAINDICATIONS/POSSIBLE INTERACTIONS

N/A

FOLLOW-UP

Control of outbreak by quarantine, containment, early identification of the causal agent, and disinfection of the area

MISCELLANEOUS

ZOONOTIC POTENTIAL

• Infections and deaths have occurred from close contact with HeV-infected body fluids in live and dead horses at post mortem.
• Clinical signs in humans are flu-like signs, which may progress to respiratory and renal failure and cardiac arrest, or acute progressive encephalitis.
• Persons in close contact with affected animals should wear protective facemasks, goggles, and gloves and avoid contact with body fluids.

ABBREVIATIONS

• ELISA = enzyme-linked immunosorbent assay
• HeV = Hendra virus

Suggested Reading

Hooper PT, Williamson MM. Hendra and Nipah virus infections. Vet Clin North Am Equine Pract 2000;16:597-603.
Queensland Department of Primary Industries. Available at: www.dpi.qld.gov.au/health/3892.html.

Author Jane E. Axon
Consulting Editors Ashley G. Boyle and Corinne R. Sweeney

HEPATIC ABSCESS AND SEPTIC CHOLANGIOHEPATITIS

BASICS

OVERVIEW

Discrete hepatic abscesses are not common in horses but ascending septic cholangiohepatitis is common in the horse. Discrete abscesses may occur, although rarely, from intestinal-hepatic adhesions with necrosis, parasite migration, *Rhodococcus* or *Streptococcus*-disseminated infections in younger horses, neoplastic abscessation, septic portal vein thrombosis, or extension of an umbilical vein abscess into the liver.

SIGNALMENT

• Cholangiohepatitis is most commonly diagnosed in adult horses without any age predilection.
• There is no sex predilection. Focal abscesses are sporadic and may affect the rare foal, e.g., *Rhodococcus*, umbilical vein infection, or an adult horse, e.g., tumor necrosis.

SIGNS

The signs of cholangiohepatitis may include weight loss, icterus, abdominal pain, fever, and dermatitis. Focal hepatic abscesses may cause ill thrift.

CAUSES

• Cholangiohepatitis is thought to be the result of ascending infection from enteric gram-negative bacteria.
• There is generally no historical intestinal crisis to explain the ascending infection.
• The inflammation of the bile epithelium and enzymes released from the bacteria may cause calcium bilirubinate calculi to form.

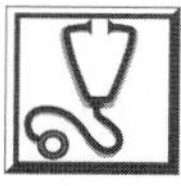

DIAGNOSIS

DIAGNOSTIC PROCEDURES

• The most important invasive diagnostic procedure is needle aspirate and/or biopsy for aerobic/anaerobic culture and sensitivity and microscopic examination of the liver.
• This can be safely performed using a biopsy needle after outlining the location of the liver via ultrasound examination.

DIFFERENTIAL DIAGNOSIS

• The differential diagnosis for chronic colic would be extensive. However, colic with marked jaundice and moderately to markedly elevated liver enzymes would have a short differential diagnosis list and would include cholangiohepatitis, chronic displacement of the large colon and neoplasia.
• Fever, leukocytosis, and elevated serum globulins, in addition to the above, would be nearly pathognomonic for cholangiohepatitis.

LABORATORY TESTS

• Serum laboratory abnormalities in horses with cholangiohepatitis include marked elevation in GGT (generally >300 U/L), less dramatic elevation in hepatocellular enzymes, elevations in conjugated bilirubin (which may, on a few occasions, approach ≥50% of the total bilirubin), and elevated serum globulins.
• CBC generally reveals a mature neutrophilia with mild elevation in plasma fibrinogen.
• Foals and horses with discrete hepatic abscess(es) may have mild elevations only in GGT without increases in hepatocellular enzymes or bilirubin.
• Neutrophil counts are generally increased and may be dramatic with *Rhodococcus equi* abscess(es).
• Fibrinogen and globulins are generally increased with any abscess, although they may not be abnormal with neoplasia-related abscess and *R. equi*.

IMAGING

• Ultrasound examination of the liver (both right and left side) is the imaging procedure of choice.
• Cholangitis may cause distended bile ducts (in ≈60% of cases), calculi with acoustic shadowing, sludge with acoustic enhancement and a subjective hepatomegaly.
• In more long-standing cases, increased echogenicity (fibrosis) may be apparent.
• In horses or foals with focal abscesses, the echogenicity of the abscess is variable.
• Only a small percentage of the liver can be visualized on abdominal ultrasonography in the adult; a greater percentage can be visualized in the foal. Computed tomography scanning can be used in imaging the foal's liver if discrete lesions are suspected.

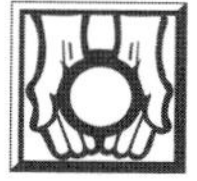

TREATMENT

• Hospitalization may not be required unless intravenous fluids are required.
• Icteric horses should not be exposed to sunlight.

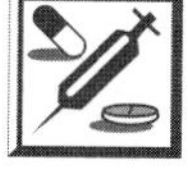

MEDICATIONS

DRUGS AND FLUIDS

• The primary treatment for septic cholangiohepatitis is long-term, appropriate treatment with antibiotics (based upon culture and sensitivity). Several drugs have been used successfully in treating the condition. These include trimethoprim-sulfa (30 mg/kg q12h) (>50% of the organisms may be resistant), enrofloxacin (7.5 mg/kg q24h) and metronidazole (15 mg/kg PO q8–12h), ceftiofur (3 mg/kg q12h), and gentamicin (6 mg/kg q24h) combination. Antimicrobials that can be given per os are preferred since long-term treatment (3 weeks to 6 mo) is generally required.
• Parenterally administered antibiotics, fluids, and DMSO may be required for some cases with biliary sludge and persistent fevers.
• NSAID treatment (e.g., flunixin meglumine) should be used at routine dosages for abdominal pain and during the first 3–5 days of antimicrobial therapy.
• Since hepatoencephalopathy rarely occurs, a normal diet can be fed. However, exposure to sunlight should not occur until the bilirubin has returned to a normal range.
• If obstructing calculi are observed and/or there is no response to medical therapy, surgery might be necessary to remove an obstructing stone. This has been successfully accomplished with full recovery on a few cases.
• Horses with marked hepatic fibrosis are not surgical candidates.
• Discrete or focal abscess(es) should be treated with appropriate antibiotics based upon culture and sensitivity of aspirated fluid or knowledge of suspected pathogen.
• Large abscess(es) or infected umbilical veins should be drained or removed.

FOLLOW-UP

• Antimicrobial therapy is ideally continued until the GGT has returned to normal range or at least <100 U/L.
• After discontinuing antimicrobials, a follow-up measurement of GGT should be performed.

PROGNOSIS

• The prognosis of septic suppurative cholangitis is good with medical therapy if no obstructing calculi are found and echogenicity of the liver is normal. Horses with GGT >2500 U/L have recovered.

ABBREVIATIONS

• DMSO = dimethylsulfoxide
• GGT = γ-glutamyltransferase

Suggested Reading

Johnston JK, Divers TJ, Reef VB, Acland H. Cholelithiasis in horses: ten cases (1982-1986). JAVMA 1989;194:405-409.

Author Thomas J. Divers
Consulting Editor Michel Lévy

HEPATIC ENCEPHALOPATHY

BASICS

OVERVIEW

• Clinical syndrome in which animals have altered mentation caused by hepatic insufficiency • Animals may have inappropriate behavior and impaired conscious proprioception (forebrain disease with cerebral dysfunction).
• Can be acute, subacute, or chronic • >80% of liver function must be impaired to develop clinical signs. • Possible mechanisms:
  ○ Toxic metabolites may act as false neurotransmitters (i.e., ammonia, mercaptans, phenols, fatty acids).
  ○ There may be an imbalance between excitatory (i.e., glutamate) and inhibitory (i.e., GABA) neurotransmission.
  ○ Increase in AAA increases false neurotransmitters, some of which (i.e. serotonin) can cause sedation with corresponding decrease in BCAA, which decreases neurotransmitters (norepinephrine, dopamine).
  ○ There may also be increased permeability of blood-brain barrier.
  ○ Ammonia—inhibits Na/K^+-ATPase activity in nerve membrane, which decreases ATP; causes changes in TCA cycle, resulting in a decrease in alpha-ketoglutarate and increased glutamine, which causes cell swelling and cerebral edema; downregulates glutamate receptor, which decreases excitatory transmission; increases nitric oxide and peroxides, causing oxidative stress and neuronal cell damage

SIGNALMENT

• No breed or sex predilection

SIGNS

• Behavior changes (depression, somnolence, progressing to aggressive or violent behavior mixed with stupor as disease progresses)
• Head pressing • Circling • Ataxia
• Wandering/aimless movements • Anorexia
• Recumbency • Icterus • Photosensitization
• Pyrexia • Weight loss • Colic—chronic
• Coagulopathy • Blindness • Yawning
• Inspiratory stridor (laryngeal paralysis)

CAUSES AND RISK FACTORS

• Toxic hepatopathy, including pyrrolizidine alkaloids, mycotoxins, iron • Acute necrotizing hepatitis—Theiler's disease • Cholelithiasis
• Chronic active hepatitis • Tyzzer's disease
• Hyperlipemia—ponies; miniature horses more at risk • Neoplasia • Hyperammonia (adult horses, portosystemic shunts, Morgans)

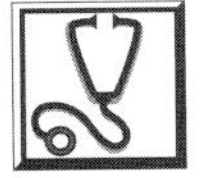

DIAGNOSIS

DIFFERENTIAL DIAGNOSIS

• Viral encephalitis (e.g., EEE, WEE, West Nile virus) —rule out by viral isolation, serology, virus neutralization, IgM (West Nile virus) titers and/or CSF tap cytology (EEE,WEE: increased neutrophils, protein in CSF) and titer
• Rabies—rule out by IFA on tactile hairs or brain; possible xanthochromia on CSF • Trauma—rule out based on history, palpation, radiographs, and CSF tap • Aberrant parasite migration (verminous encephalitis)—xanthochromia +/− increased white blood cells in CSF; can affect kidneys • Electrolyte abnormalities—hyponatremia, hypernatremia, hypocalcemia, hypomagnesemia
• Abscess—vision loss contralateral eye, cortical signs, depression, seizures, leukocytosis, neutrophilia, hyperfibrinogenemia, hyperglobulinemia • Meningitis—increased or decreased white blood cell count +/− left shift, CSF increased neutrophils and protein, xanthochromia • Hypoxic-ischemic encephalopathy—foals, history • Metabolic (foals: hypoglycemia, acidosis)
The following diseases are differentials, but the progression of these diseases can lead to HE:
• Theiler's disease—history of antitoxin 4–10 weeks prior • Cholangiohepatitis—adults, most >9 years old

CBC/BIOCHEMISTRY/URINALYSIS

• Azotemia—may be secondary to changes in mentation/appetite/drinking • BUN—may be decreased in liver failure • Glucose—may be decreased in advanced liver failure
• Liver-specific changes—elevated bilirubin, increased GGT, SDH, GLDH, hypoalbuminemia, hypoproteinemia, elevated resting ammonia levels, and elevated bile acids, bromsulfthalein clearance delayed • Animals with encephalopathy from hyperlipemia—have increased cholesterol and triglycerides
• Secondary hypocalcemia, hypokalemia, and metabolic acidosis

OTHER LABORATORY TESTS

Coagulation profiles—may or may not be prolonged

IMAGING

• Ultrasonography may help to assess size, changes in the parenchyma (i.e., fibrosis, bile duct dilatation), portosystemic shunts; scan for abscesses and masses, and assist with biopsy.
• Radiographs—rule out fractures
• CT/MRI—assess for trauma, abscesses, tumors, hydrocephalus

OTHER DIAGNOSTIC PROCEDURES

• CSF tap might be considered to rule out other infectious causes of abnormal neurological behavior, including cytology, culture, and viral titers • Feed analysis to assess for toxins

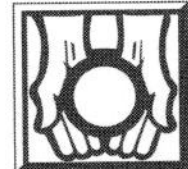

TREATMENT

• It should be remembered that the prognosis for recovery of a horse that has liver failure to the point of showing hepatoencephalopathy is poor.
• For dysphoric or demented animals, sedation may be necessary. *Caution:* Xylazine and detomidine can occasionally exacerbate signs. Valium and/or phenobarbital for seizures but can potentiate GABA effect and exacerbate HE signs.
• Correction of fluid and electrolyte deficits caused by dehydration followed by correction of acid-base deficits • For anorectic or hypoglycemic animals, give 5% dextrose (2 mL/kg/hr) to start, then 2.5% in half-strength saline. • High-carbohydrate, low-protein (i.e., 10%) diet with branched chain amino acids; need some fiber (i.e., oat, grass hay, beet pulp) to decrease gastrointestinal dysfunction. • Feed small amounts frequently (q2–4h). • Vitamin B and C supplementation
• Protect from sunlight to prevent photosensitization.

MEDICATIONS

DRUG(S) OF CHOICE

• Lactulose (0.3 mL/kg q6h) • Hyperlipemic horses can be given insulin, glucose/galactose, and heparin. • Mannitol if suspect cerebral edema • Pentoxifylline if inflammatory disease present • Mineral oil or magnesium sulfate if suspect toxins ingested • Septic cholangiohepatitis—Antibiotics are warranted.
• SAMe (*S*-adenosylmethionine) if expect oxidative injury

CONTRAINDICATIONS/POSSIBLE INTERACTIONS

Avoid drugs that require hepatic metabolism.

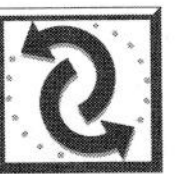

FOLLOW-UP

• Prognosis depends on the primary cause.
• Animals with hyperlipidemia/hyperlipemia may respond well to aggressive treatment.
• Animals with HE from toxins probably experienced the initial insult several weeks/months prior; determine if signs are still progressing. These animals may be stabilized, but if signs continue to progress or recur, a poor prognosis is indicated. • Poor prognosis for recumbent animals

MISCELLANEOUS

PREGNANCY

Small percentage of pregnant animals will be hyperlipemic.

ABBREVIATIONS

• AAA = aromatic amino acids • BCAA = branched chain amino acids • CSF = cerebrospinal fluid • EEE = Eastern equine encephalopathy • EPM = equine protozoal myelitis • GABA = γ-aminobutyric acid
• GGT = γ-glutamyltransferase • GLDH = glutamate dehydrogenase • HE = hepatic encephalopathy • IFA = indirect fluorescent antibody • SDH = sorbitol dehydrogenase
• TCA = tricarboxylic acid cycle • WEE = Western equine encephalopathy
• WNV = West Nile virus

Suggested Reading

Reed SM, Bayly WM, Sellon DC. Equine Internal Medicine, ed 2. St. Louis: Elsevier, 2004.

Author S. G. Witonsky
Consulting Editor Caroline N. Hahn

HEREDITARY EQUINE REGIONAL DERMAL ASTHENIA

BASICS

OVERVIEW
HERDA ("hyperelastosis cutis") is a disease that occurs early in life in horses.

SIGNALMENT
Most affected horses are American Quarter Horses, but registered Paints and Appaloosas with Quarter Horse lineage have been reported with this disease. Many of the Quarter Horses are from high-quality cutting lines. The disease (or something very similar) has also been reported in a cross-bred Arabian mare, a Thoroughbred gelding, a Hanoverian foal, and a Hafflinger horse. The condition is almost certainly present at birth but may not be noticed until around 2 years of age, when horses start being trained with tack, saddle, etc, and the friction/trauma of this may induce the typical lesions. However, not all cases have an immediate history of trauma.

SIGNS
Typically, the areas over the back (especially the saddle area) and the sides of the neck are affected. Less commonly, lesions may be observed on the pastern areas (these are almost always seen in association with dorsal body lesions). The skin in these areas seems to be easily torn, stretched, or often develops seromas and hematomas (described by owners as "blisters" filled with either serum or blood). Healing per se is usually adequate, but often leaves rather unsightly scars, or hair which grows in white.

CAUSES AND RISK FACTORS
The working hypothesis is that these horses have a defect in their collagen fibers, in the way those fibers are structurally organized, or in the ability of these fibers to repair, in the mid to deep dermis. In the American Quarter Horse, this disease follows an autosomal recessive mode of inheritance, so in order for the foal to be affected, both the sire and the dam carry the gene, and if they were bred to each other again, there would be an approximately 25% chance that the next foal would also be affected.

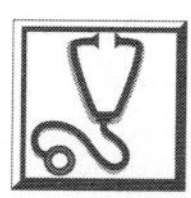

DIAGNOSIS

DIFFERENTIAL DIAGNOSIS
Trauma

CBC/BIOCHEMISTRY/URINALYSIS
Normal

OTHER LABORATORY TESTS
N/A

IMAGING
N/A

OTHER DIAGNOSTIC PROCEDURES
- A genetic marker was determined for this disease. The Veterinary Genetics Laboratory at UC Davis offers a diagnostic test to determine carrier or affected status (www.vgl.ucdavis.edu/service/horse/index.html). Hair with roots attached from the mane or tail should be submitted.
- Skin biopsy—This is much less accurate than finding evidence of the genetic marker (see below).

PATHOLOGICAL FINDINGS
Histologic findings are sometimes subtle, but "clumped" or poorly organized collagen fibers below the level of the hair follicles may be seen. A zone of mid to deep dermal separation has been reported in two horses, and has been present in some of the biopsy samples the author has seen. However, comparing age-matched tissues from normal appearing skin in affected versus normal horses has not been diagnostic.

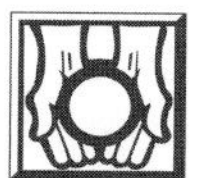

TREATMENT

As with many genetic diseases, there is no effective treatment of cure. Affected and carrier animals should be removed from the breeding pool. Some affected horses have been maintained as "pasture pets." In those cases, fly control is important, because if the horse rolls on its back to relieve pruritus, great damage to the skin is possible.

MEDICATIONS

DRUG(S) OF CHOICE
N/A

CONTRAINDICATIONS/POSSIBLE INTERACTIONS
N/A

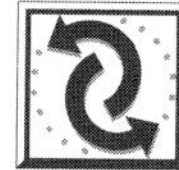

FOLLOW-UP

PATIENT MONITORING
N/A

PREVENTION/AVOIDANCE
N/A

POSSIBLE COMPLICATIONS
Secondary infections from ulcerations

EXPECTED COURSE AND PROGNOSIS
- For affected: Poor—Some horses may be maintained as "pasture pets."
- For carriers: Excellent—These horses have no known health problems related to carrier status.

MISCELLANEOUS

ASSOCIATED CONDITIONS
N/A

AGE-RELATED FACTORS
N/A

ZOONOTIC POTENTIAL
N/A

PREGNANCY
Mares with HERDA have had successfully completed pregnancies, without damage to the mare's reproductive tract or the foal.

ABBREVIATION
- HERDA = hereditary equine regional dermal asthenia

Suggested Reading

Tryon RC, White SD, Bannasch DL. Homozygosity mapping approach identifies a missense mutation in equine cyclophilin B (PPIB) associated with HERDA in the American Quarter Horse. Genomics 2007;90:93–102.

Tryon RC, White SD, Famula TR, et al. Inheritance of hereditary equine regional dermal asthenia (HERDA) in the American Quarter Horse. Am J Vet Res 2005;66:437–442.

White SD, Affolter V, Bannasch DL et al. Hereditary equine regional dermal asthenia (HERDA; 'Hyperelastosis cutis') in 50 horses: clinical, histologic and immunohistologic findings. Vet Dermatol 2004;15:207–217.

White SD, Affolter VK, Schultheiss PC, et al. Clinical and pathological findings in a HERDA-affected foal for 1.5 years of life. Vet Dermatol 2007;18:36–40.

Author Stephen D. White
Consulting Editor Gwendolen Lorch

HERNIAS (UMBILICAL AND INGUINAL)

BASICS

OVERVIEW

Umbilical Hernia

• Umbilical hernias are the most common type of abdominal hernia in the horse. • At birth, linea alba is noncontinuous and the umbilical ring normally closes within the first days of life. • Incidence of umbilical hernias is 0.5%–2%. Although defects in the abdominal lining are seen fairly commonly, incarceration of intestine is seen only in about 4% of cases. • Small hernias (usually <5 cm) close within first weeks of life.
• Large defects (>10 cm) and hernias persisting at the age of 4 mo warrant surgical repair.
• Classified as reducible or nonreducible, simple or complicated • Complicated hernias—bowel becomes incarcerated and cannot be reduced.
• The affected segment of bowel is usually small intestine, but herniation of large colon and cecum has been reported. • Intestinal incarceration warrants emergency surgery.

Inguinal Hernia

• Inguinal hernia is caused by abdominal contents passing through the vaginal ring.
• Most commonly, herniation is caused by small intestine, but herniation of urinary bladder, omentum, small colon, and large colon is possible. • If the contents pass through the external inguinal ring, the term *scrotal hernia* may be used. • Indirect hernia—Abdominal contents penetrate the inguinal opening within the vaginal tunic.
• Direct hernia—Abdominal contents penetrate ruptured peritoneum or ruptured vaginal tunic gaining access to the subcutaneous tissues. More common in neonatal foals and often seen at the time of birth or within the first few days of life.
• Usually unilateral

SIGNALMENT

Umbilical Hernia

• Palpable umbilical ring is usually noticed in the neonatal foal during initial physical exam. Weakening of the fibrous plate may lead to umbilical hernia formation as the foal matures.
• Umbilical hernias can be seen in any breed horse of either gender.

Inguinal Hernia

• Many breeds can be affected but Standardbreds, American Saddlebreds, and Tennessee Walking Horses have been reported to have higher prevalence of inguinal hernias.
• Neonatal foals are more likely to suffer from direct inguinal or scrotal hernias. Inguinal hernias are most commonly seen as a congenital condition in colts.

SIGNS

Umbilical Hernia

• Simple hernias do not necessarily cause any clinical signs and the hernia is usually soft, nonpainful, and reducible on palpation.
• Complicated hernias involve incarceration of bowel resulting in abdominal discomfort.
• Swollen, firm, warm, and painful hernia sacs are typical signs when incarceration is present and indicating need for urgent intervention.

Inguinal Hernia

• Foals with indirect inguinal hernia may be asymptomatic but a soft, easily reducible swelling can be palpated at the scrotal area.
• Foals with direct inguinal hernia may show abdominal discomfort and swelling extending from the inguinal region to the prepuce. Usually the intestines can be palpated in the subcutaneous space.

CAUSES AND RISK FACTORS

Umbilical Hernia

• May have a genetic predisposition • Increased abdominal pressure at birth, umbilical infection, umbilical trauma at birth, and excessive straining due to abdominal discomfort may be predisposing factors.

Inguinal Hernia

Increased pressure during delivery may cause rupture of the peritoneum or vaginal tunic and therefore predispose to direct inguinal herniation.

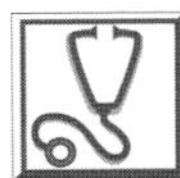

DIAGNOSIS

DIFFERENTIAL DIAGNOSIS

Umbilical Hernia

• Omphalophlebitis—Foal may have signs of systemic illness (fever, lethargy, leukocytosis); palpation reveals thickened and warm umbilicus; ultrasonographic examination reveals enlargement of the umbilical remnants.
• Urachal disruption and subsequent urine leakage subcutaneously—Swelling is not reducible; skin quickly becomes irritated and macerated.

Inguinal Hernia

Swelling due to trauma or testicular problems

IMAGING

Umbilical Hernia

• Ultrasonography allows evaluation of the hernia size and contents; secondary distention of intestine.
• Ultrasound of the umbilical stalk, arteries, and veins may help to rule out omphalophlebitis.

Inguinal Hernia

• Ultrasonography may be beneficial in confirming the abdominal structures involved in the herniation, especially if significant edema is present.

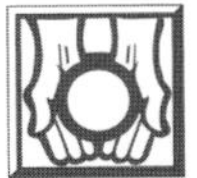

TREATMENT

UMBILICAL HERNIA

• Reducible umbilical hernias <5 cm in diameter usually close spontaneously within days to weeks after birth. • Digital reduction of the hernia on a daily basis may be beneficial and allows changes in size or consistency to be noted. • Hernia clamps are successfully used by some practitioners in case of small, simple hernias. However, intestine may be entrapped while placing the elastic band around the neck of the hernial sac, risking intestinal obstruction/strangulation, peritonitis, and enterocutaneous fistula. • Hernias that persist at the age of 4 months or hernias >10 cm in diameter should be surgically corrected.
• Incarcerated hernias require immediate emergency surgery.

INGUINAL HERNIA

• Initial management of a reducible, indirect inguinal hernia consists of frequent manual reductions or application of a figure-eight bandage.
• Surgery should be considered if the hernia is >10 cm in size or reduction is not achieved with conservative management by the age of 4 months. • Nonreducible direct hernias require immediate surgical treatment. If the herniated abdominal contents become nonviable, a ventral midline approach is necessary to allow resection of the necrotic bowel. The vaginal tunic and external inguinal ring are closed during the surgery, and removal of the testicle on the affected side is recommended.

MEDICATIONS

DRUG(S) OF CHOICE

• No drug therapy needed for nonsurgical hernias
• Perioperative antibiotics can be used as a prophylactic measure.

FOLLOW-UP

PATIENT MONITORING

Umbilical Hernia

• Simple, small umbilical hernias should be evaluated on a daily basis until the ring is closed in order to allow early recognition of changes in size or consistency of the umbilical sac.
• If colic occurs, consider the hernia as a possible cause.

Inguinal Hernia

• Indirect inguinal hernias should be evaluated and manually reduced on a daily basis. • If colic occurs, consider the hernia as a possible cause.

EXPECTED COURSE AND PROGNOSIS

Umbilical Hernia

• Most foals with small hernias have a good prognosis for resolution, generally within the first weeks or months of life. • Larger hernias have a greater chance of not fully resolving and of requiring surgical correction.

Inguinal Hernia

• Most foals with small, indirect hernias have a good prognosis for resolution, generally within the first weeks or months of life. • Larger hernias have a greater chance of not fully resolving and of requiring surgical correction.

MISCELLANEOUS

SEE ALSO

Omphalophlebitis

Suggested Reading

Stick JA. Abdominal hernias. In: Auer JA, Stick JA, eds. Equine Surgery, ed 3. St. Louis: Saunders Elsevier, 2006.

Author Laura Hirvinen
Consulting Editor Margaret C. Mudge

HERPESVIRUS MYELOENCEPHALOPATHY

BASICS

DEFINITION

A central nervous system disease associated with EHV-1 infection

PATHOPHYSIOLOGY

- EHV-1 infection of pregnant mares can produce syndromes of late gestational abortion, stillbirth, and weak neonatal foals. Only rarely does it result in overt neurologic disease.
- The primary inflammatory target is the vascular endothelium, with secondary ischemic and hemorrhagic infarction of neutropil. Thus, this disease is referred to as a myeloencephalopathy rather than myeloencephalitis.
- Cell-mediated immunity is reported to be more important than humoral immunity because of the high degree of cell association in infection and the ability to have cell-to-cell infection without release of virons.
- The propensity of certain viral strains to induce neurologic signs does not seem to be the result of those viruses having specific neurotropism.
- Variation in one specific nucleotide within different EHV-1 strains has shown a highly significant association with paralytic and nonparalytic disease.

SYSTEMS AFFECTED

- Nervous system
- Respiratory tract infections may also be observed
- Reproductive—abortions possible
- Hemic/lymphatic/immune—Limb edema is common.
- Gastrointestinal—Diarrhea occasionally observed
- Ophthalmic—Chorioretinitis is possible.

INCIDENCE/PREVALENCE

Can occur sporadically or in outbreaks

GEOGRAPHIC DISTRIBUTION

Worldwide

SIGNALMENT

There is no breed or sex predilection; however, adult horses seem to be more likely affected than very young horses.

SIGNS

Historical

- Horses may or may not have a current vaccination record.
- Respiratory disease or abortion may, or may not, be evident in exposed horses and herd mates.

Physical Examination

- The latent period is approximately 7 days in experimental studies of EHV–1 infection. Clinical examination may reveal evidence of concurrent respiratory disease, distal limb edema, fever or hypothermia, and enteritis.
- Pregnant mares may abort immediately before, during, or sometime after development of neurologic signs.
- Pelvic limb ataxia and paresis are usually symmetrical, but thoracic limbs can less frequently be involved.
- Frequently, urinary bladder paralysis with dribbling of urine, and sometimes repeated erections in males, occurs. In many cases, there is urinary incontinence.
- Decreased tail tone and perineal hypalgesia are variably seen.
- Evidence of brain lesions, such as stupor, diffuse face, jaw, tongue, and pharyngeal weakness, and signs of vestibular involvement occur less frequently.
- Enteritis and chorioretinitis associated with EHV-1 have been described.

CAUSES AND RISK FACTORS

Contact with affected herd mates. There is now good evidence that neurologically affected horses can be the source of new transmission of EHV-1 myeloencephalopathy up to a week or more from onset of clinical neurologic signs. Thus it is recommended that strict isolation protocols remain in place for 21 days after evidence of active (ie new cases) of EHV-1 disease.

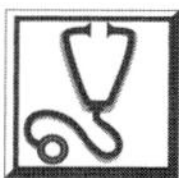

DIAGNOSIS

A presumptive diagnosis of EHV-1 myeloencephalitis can be made in horses with peracute spinal cord deficits, incontinence, and bladder distention.

DIFFERENTIAL DIAGNOSIS

Trauma, equine protozoal myeloencephalitis, polyneuritis equi, other viral encephalitis (i.e., Eastern, Western, and Venezuelan equine encephalopathy)

CBC/BIOCHEMISTRY/URINALYSIS

No consistent abnormalities

OTHER LABORATORY TESTS

- EHV virus can be isolated from pharyngeal or nasal secretions; this strongly suggests that this particular virus strain is the cause of the neurologic disease.
- PCR testing can be used to look for viral DNA shedding in pharyngeal or nasal secretions, and its presence in peripheral blood buffy coat indicating current or recent

viremia. A significant rise in anti–EHV-1 viral neutralization, complement fixation, or ELISA antibody titers between acute and convalescent samples indicates recent virus infection.

OTHER DIAGNOSTIC PROCEDURES

Cerebrospinal fluid, especially from the lumbosacral space, may have xanthochromia and elevated protein content (0.01–0.04 g/L), reflecting the leakage of blood pigments from vasculitis.

PATHOLOGIC FINDINGS

- A brown discoloration may be seen grossly in the spinal cord. Histopathologic examination indicates that these are areas of ischemic and hemorrhagic infarction, with perivascular edema, necrosis, and hemorrhage.
- There is a vasculitis with endothelial and perivascular lymphocytes, plasma cells, and macrophages in the meninges and parenchyma.
- Intranuclear inclusions may occur in other areas, such as the respiratory tract and the fetus.
- Immunologic staining with EHV polyclonal antiserum may also be useful.

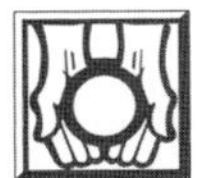

TREATMENT

AIMS OF TREATMENT

Many horses with EHV-1 myeloencephalitis can recover if given time and any necessary supportive treatment such as rolling animals and use of supportive slings for the recumbent horses.

NURSING CARE

Ensure animal is able to urinate. Care for dysphagia if cranial nerves are affected.

CLIENT EDUCATION

Isolate new animals coming into premise, and isolate animals with respiratory signs.

MEDICATIONS

DRUG(S)

- Glucocorticosteroids such as 0.05–0.1 mg/kg dexamethasone IM BID for 1–3 days in the acute phase of the disease appear to be useful.
- Treatment with acyclovir appears useful, but its efficacy is not proven.

ALTERNATIVE DRUGS

- None proven

FOLLOW-UP

PREVENTION/AVOIDANCE

- Segregation and isolation of affected horses are important in containing an outbreak.
- Some data support vaccination as also possibly reducing the risk of an individual horse developing EHV-1 myeloencephalopathy.

POSSIBLE COMPLICATIONS

- Complications include trauma associated with weakness and attempts at rising, decubital sores, and paralytic bladder with secondary urinary tract infection.
- Recovered horses may remain latently infected, and viral recrudescence and shedding may occur.

EXPECTED COURSE AND PROGNOSIS

- Many horses with EHV-1 myeloencephalitis recover completely. The time to recovery depends on the severity of the lesion signs and ranges from several days to more than 1 year.
- Urinary tract function returns before gait abnormalities resolve.
- The prognosis is poor if horses become recumbent.

MISCELLANEOUS

ASSOCIATED CONDITIONS

Secondary urinary tract infection

PREGNANCY

Mares may coincidentally abort.

ABBREVIATIONS

- EHV-1 = equine herpesvirus 1

Suggested Reading

Divers TJ, Mayhew IG. Neurology. Clin Tech Equine Pract 2006;5(1).

Goodman LB, et al. A point mutation in herpesvirus polymerase determines neuropathogenicity. PLoS Pathog, 2007, 3: e60.

Wilkins PA, Henninger R, Reed SM, Piero Fd. Acyclovir as treatment for EHV-1 myeloencephalopathy. AAEP Proc 2003.

The author and editor wish to acknowledge the contribution of Joseph J. Bertone, author of this chapter in the previous edition.

Author Caroline N. Hahn

Consulting Editor Caroline N. Hahn

HERPESVIRUS TYPES 1 AND 4

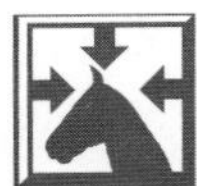

BASICS

DEFINITION

A ubiquitous, contagious viral equine pathogen that most frequently causes respiratory tract disease but may also cause abortion, fatal neonatal illness, or neurologic disease.

PATHOPHYSIOLOGY

Equine herpesvirus 1 (EHV-1) and 4 (EHV-4) infect the respiratory tract; however, EHV-1 may also infect white blood cells, subsequently causing a viremia and dissemination of the virus to the reproductive tract or central nervous system (CNS). EHV-4 infections are usually limited to the upper respiratory tract and are a common cause of respiratory disease in young horses. Following resolution of clinical signs, either virus may become dormant (latent infection), only to recrudesce during periods of stress, such as shipping, weaning, training, or competition. The ability of the virus to evade the immune system and establish latent infection is important in the propagation of the disease and has made control by immunization difficult. It is unknown why EHV-1 periodically induces reproductive tract or CNS disease; infectious dose, immune status of the horse, and viral strain are likely factors. Recently, clearer identification of neurotropic strains has become possible. These strains seem to share a common mutation in their genetic code and also appear to result in more prolonged viremia, perhaps contributing to the development of neurologic disease.

SYSTEMS AFFECTED

Respiratory

Reproductive

Following infection of the upper respiratory tract and subsequent viremia, EHV-1 may infect endometrium and fetal tissues, resulting in fetal death and abortion.

Nervous

Both isolated cases and outbreaks of CNS disease occur. Viremic spread of EHV-1 to the CNS endothelium leads to thrombosis, ischemic neural damage, and characteristic clinical signs.

GENETICS

No known genetic predisposition.

INCIDENCE/PREVALENCE

Worldwide wherever large groups of horses are present.

SIGNALMENT

The median age of horses hospitalized for the neurologic form of EHV-1 infection is 3 years. However, horses of any age or breed are susceptible to EHV-related diseases. Respiratory tract disease due to EHV-4 is extremely common in young horses.

SIGNS

In horses with partial immunity to EHV, silent infections occur in which the only signs are fever and depression. Distal limb edema may accompany EHV-1 infection due to associated vasculitis and decreased ambulation.

Respiratory Disease

Respiratory tract disease, manifested by cough, mucopurulent nasal discharge, fever (102–106°F, 38.9–41°C), depression, and abnormal lung sounds, is the most common form of EHV-1 and 4 infection. Rarely, infection of the respiratory vascular endothelium occurs, resulting in severe disease that is potentially fatal. This form is known as the "pulmonary vasculotropic form" of herpesvirus infection.

Reproductive Tract Disease

Abortions usually occur late in gestation (7–11 months) with or without other signs of EHV-related disease. Abortions may be either sporadic or multiple mares may be affected. The lesions in the infected aborted fetus may include pulmonary edema, pleural and peritoneal effusions, multifocal hepatic necrosis, icterus, and petechiation. Alternatively, the fetus may have no lesions and be uninfected.

Neurologic Disease

Neurologic deficits may be symmetric or asymmetric. Fever usually precedes an acute onset of hindlimb ataxia, proprioceptive deficits, and weakness. In the most severe form, hindlimb paralysis leads to a dog-sitting posture or recumbency. Although the hindlimbs are most commonly affected, cranial nerve abnormalities (head tilt, tongue weakness, nystagmus, blindness) also occur. Bladder atony, fecal retention, perineal sensory deficits, and decreased tail tone are common. Ophthalmologic examination may reveal retinal hemorrhages due to optic neuritis.

CAUSES

Equine herpesvirus types 1 and 4

RISK FACTORS

Outbreaks and isolated cases of EHV-related disease are frequently associated with stress, such as transportation, weaning, overcrowding, surgery, other illnesses, or competition. The risk of infection may be increased by poor ventilation, which increases the concentration of viral particles and causes the accumulation of noxious gases, thus impairing respiratory immune function.

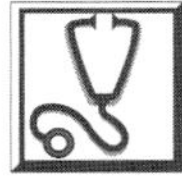

DIAGNOSIS

DIFFERENTIAL DIAGNOSIS

Respiratory Disease

• Influenza • Equine viral arteritis • Adenovirus • Bacterial pneumonia • Heaves

Reproductive Tract Disease

Abortion—Equine viral arteritis, bacterial or fungal placentitis

Neurologic Disease

Equine protozoal myeloencephalitis, aberrant parasite migration, trauma, West Nile virus infection or cauda equina syndrome. Fever is an aspect of herpesvirus myeloencephalopathy that is uncommon in the equine neurologic diseases above, excepting West Nile virus.

CBC/BIOCHEMISTRY

CBC and serum biochemistry are frequently normal at the onset of clinical signs.

OTHER LABORATORY TESTS

PCR testing for herpesvirus using nasopharyngeal swabs and whole blood at the time of first examination may be rapidly diagnostic, frequently within 48 hours of submission to an appropriate laboratory.A rapid PCR test specifically designed to detect the neurologic strains of EHV-1 has recently been reported in use. A four-fold increase in convalescent serum neutralizing antibody titer to EHV-1/4 collected over a 2-week period is diagnostic. Because most horses have been exposed to, or vaccinated against, EHV-1/4, positive titers are common, making interpretation of a single sample difficult. Natural infection usually causes a rapid and dramatic increase in titer such that serum must be collected early in the course of the disease to demonstrate an increasing titer.

IMAGING

Thoracic ultrasonography or radiology when secondary bacterial pneumonia is suspected.

DIAGNOSTIC PROCEDURES

Virus Isolation

Virus can be isolated from nasopharyngeal swabs. Veterinarians should contact their diagnostic laboratory for transport media and specific collection and transportation procedures. One method is to use a sterile gauze swab attached to a flexible metal wire placed in the nasal passages and pharynx to obtain material for virus isolation. Swabs should be placed immediately in media and refrigerated or frozen until transported to the laboratory. Virus may also be isolated from the buffy coat of whole blood preserved with EDTA. Viremia frequently occurs during clinical signs of respiratory tract, CNS, or reproductive tract disease. Nasopharyngeal secretions may be evaluated by immunoperoxidase staining for EHV-1/4 antigen.

Cerebrospinal Fluid Aspirate

Typically reveals an increase in protein concentration and normal or only mildly increased nucleated cell concentration with herpesvirus myeloencephalopathy. Xanthochromia, a yellow discoloration of CSF due to breakdown of red blood cells, is common. Virus is rarely isolated from CSF.

PATHOLOGIC FINDINGS

EHV-1/4 infection of the respiratory epithelium can be inapparent or cause epithelial necrosis, thrombi formation, and petechiation. If viremia occurs and the reproductive tract is affected, lesions may be present in the endometrium. The virus may also infect the fetus, resulting in abortion, and an aborted fetus typically shows evidence of vasculitis. In the neurologic syndrome, characteristic lesions secondary to EHV-1 infection of CNS endothelium include vasculitis of the small arteries and veins of the white matter of the spinal cord resulting in hemorrhage, thrombosis, and secondary ischemic degeneration.

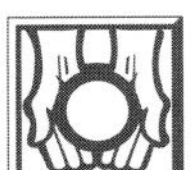

TREATMENT

APPROPRIATE HEALTH CARE

Rhinopneumonitis

Fever lasting more than 3 days, persistent cough, abnormal lung sounds, depression, or anorexia may indicate secondary bacterial bronchopneumonia. Horses recovering from respiratory tract disease caused by EHV-1/4 should not be trained and should be maintained in well-ventilated areas. Caution should also be used when transporting horses for long distances following viral respiratory tract infection due to the possibility of severe pleuropneumonia associated with impaired respiratory tract immune function.

Abortion

Mares that abort due to herpesvirus infection should have a reproductive tract examination to rule out retained fetal membranes or trauma.

Neurologic Disease

Recumbent horses should be placed in a well-bedded stall, kept sternal, and repositioned frequently. Many horses remain standing or can stand with the assistance of a sling. Horses should be monitored for urinary incontinence, and if bladder atony is suspected, abdominal palpation per rectum may reveal a distended bladder. Urinary catheterization should then be performed at least twice daily by aseptic technique or an indwelling urinary catheter may be placed. If fecal incontinence is present, feces should be evacuated manually. If dysphagia is present, hydration should be monitored and fluids given intravenously or by nasogastric tube as needed.

ACTIVITY

With severe infections it may take the respiratory epithelium as long as 1 month to regain normal function. Mucociliary clearance is impaired during this time, leading to accumulation of respiratory secretions and inhaled antigens in the lower airways. Persistent airway inflammation may occur when training is resumed prematurely. Lung sounds should be normal, and spontaneous cough should have resolved prior to training. Many horses require 2–4 weeks of rest to recover from uncomplicated rhinopneumonitis.

CLIENT EDUCATION

Owners should be advised about sources of EHV-1/4 (other horses) and risk factors for infection. Vaccination of horses at risk is effective in reducing severity and frequency of EHV-1/4–associated respiratory and reproductive tract disease.

MEDICATIONS

DRUG(S) OF CHOICE

Respiratory Disease

No specific antiviral therapy has been proven effective in the treatment of rhinopneumonitis. Nonsteroidal anti-inflammatory drugs (flunixin meglumine 1 mg/kg, IV or PO, q24h) can be given to combat inflammation and fever. Antimicrobials (trimethoprim-sulfamethoxazole 30 mg/kg, PO, q12h) should be administered if secondary bacterial infections are suspected.

Abortion

No specific drug therapy.

Neurologic Diseases

Corticosteroids (dexamethasone, 0.05–0.25 mg/kg, IV or IM, q12h in decreasing doses for 7–14 days) may be necessary for severely affected horses due to the immune-mediated nature of this disease. Dimethyl sulfoxide (1 g/kg IV diluted in saline to a concentration of 10%, daily for 3 days), nonsteroidal anti-inflammatory drugs (flunixin meglumine 1 mg/kg PO or IV q12h) and broad-spectrum antimicrobials (ceftiofur 5 mg/kg IV or IM q12h) are indicated in recumbent horses due to potential for pneumonia, cystitis, and decubital ulceration. The antiviral drug acyclovir has been show to be effective against some equine herpesvirus isolates. Acyclovir may be administered intravenously at 10 mg/kg twice daily given in 1 liter of crystalloid fluid (Not 5% dextrose) over 1 hour.

PRECAUTIONS

Laminitis is a rare complication of corticosteroid administration in horses. Acyclovir may result in anaphylactic-like reaction if administered intravenously in large concentrations rapidly.

ALTERNATIVE DRUGS

Administration of acyclovir at 20 mg/kg, PO, 3 times daily appears to be safe although of unknown efficacy due to poor oral bioavailability.

FOLLOW-UP

PATIENT MONITORING

Most horses recover from rhinopneumonitis uneventfully. Aborting mares should be isolated for at least 2 weeks but may be bred 1 month following abortion. Recumbent horses with the neurologic form should be monitored for dehydration, decubital ulcers, pneumonia, bladder atony, cystitis, fecal incontinence, and self-trauma.

PREVENTION/AVOIDANCE

Providing adequate ventilation, decreasing stress, and ensuring quarantine of new horses may prevent herpesvirus disease in horses. Vaccination of animals at risk every 3 months is effective at reducing the severity and frequency of respiratory disease and decreases the likelihood of abortion. Broodmares should be vaccinated during their fifth, seventh, and ninth months of pregnancy with a vaccine specifically designed for pregnant mares. Vaccination of unexposed horses in the face of the outbreak may decrease the spread of disease. Currently available vaccines do not claim protection against neurologic disease. Vaccination of animals with the neurologic syndrome is contraindicated; however, horses that are not yet exposed may benefit from vaccination. Horses recovering from herpesvirus infections may shed the virus from nasal secretions for 2 weeks after infection and therefore should remain quarantined. The aborted fetus and fetal membranes are major sources of virus and therefore should be placed in a sealed container and removed to decrease contamination of the environment.

EXPECTED COURSE AND PROGNOSIS

Respiratory Disease

Most horses recover from an uncomplicated infection in 2–4 weeks.

Reproductive Tract Disease

Mares recover readily and subsequent fertility is not impaired.

Neurologic Disease

Following acute onset of previously described signs, many horses stabilize in 24–48 hr, and if they remain standing, slow improvement usually occurs over a period of weeks to months. Some horses may have long-term residual neurologic deficits. Horses that become recumbent and cannot rise with assistance have a poor prognosis. There is no apparent correlation between outcome and CSF characteristics.

MISCELLANEOUS

PREGNANCY

Caution should be used when administering corticosteroids to pregnant mares with herpesvirus myeloencephalopathy.

SYNONYM

Rhinopneumonitis

Suggested Reading

Donaldson MT, Sweeney CR. Equine herpes myeloencephalopathy. Compendium on continuing education for the practicing veterinarian. 1997;19:864–871.

Wilkins PA, Papich M, Sweeney RW. Acyclovir pharmacokinetics in adult horses. Journal of Veterinary Emergency and Critical Care 2005;15:174–178.

Author Pamela A. Wilkins
Consulting Editors Ashley G. Boyle and Corinne R. Sweeney

HERPESVIRUS 3

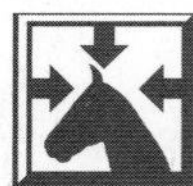

BASICS

OVERVIEW

EHV-3 causes equine coital exanthema, a highly contagious venereal disease resulting in vesicular lesions on the penis and prepuce of stallions and on the vulva of mares. The disease is generally limited to the reproductive tract, and infection does not appear to affect fertility. Lesions have been reported in the nostril of a foal by the side of a dam with coital exanthema, an example of horse-to-horse transmission of coital exanthema virus without coitus. Although coital exanthema is uncommon and resolves spontaneously, some stallions may not be willing to breed mares when affected, leading to economic losses. Like other herpesviruses, a short-lived immunity develops after infection. The disease occurs sporadically worldwide.

SIGNALMENT

The primary route of infection is by genital contact; thus, horses most frequently affected are of breeding age.

SIGNS

Occasionally, stallions are more severely affected than mares and become dull, anorectic, and febrile. Vesicles appear within 2–5 days on the penis and later on the prepuce. Vesicles become pustules, which then slough, leaving ulcerated areas up to 1.5 cm in diameter. Ulcers heal within a few weeks, leaving depigmented areas. Mares develop multifocal areas of sharply demarcated vulval erosions that subsequently develop scabs that heal in a similar manner. Aged broodmares may develop recurrent coital exanthema during late gestation or in the early postparturient period, but a relationship with viral recrudescence has not been established. Lesions rarely occur on the oral and nasal mucosa.

CAUSES AND RISK FACTORS

Coital exanthema is caused by EHV-3. Horses of breeding age are at risk due to viral transmission by genital contact. Iatrogenic transmission by contaminated instruments is also possible.

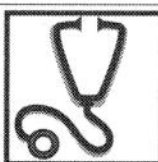

DIAGNOSIS

DIFFERENTIAL DIAGNOSIS

Coital exanthema lesions are characteristic; however, inflammation of the penis or vulva may also occur due to trauma, bacterial infection, or contact hypersensitivities. Vesicular stomatitis may also uncommonly affect genitalia.

CBC/BIOCHEMISTRY/URINALYSIS

N/A

OTHER LABORATORY TESTS

Diagnosis can be made based on clinical signs. Serum neutralizing antibodies peak 2–3 weeks after infection and may remain detectable for up to 1 year later; however, complement fixing antibodies are not present beyond 60 days after infection.

IMAGING

N/A

DIAGNOSTIC PROCEDURES

Virus can be isolated from erosions and characteristic herpesvirus inclusions can be seen during histologic evaluation of biopsy samples.

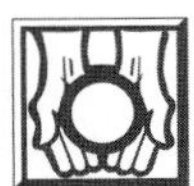

TREATMENT

Specific treatment is not necessary, as lesions are self-limiting. Application of topical antimicrobial ointments to affected areas may reduce chances of secondary bacterial infections.

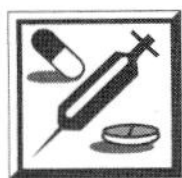

MEDICATIONS

No specific antiviral therapy has been evaluated for the treatment of EHV-3 infections. The use of topical antimicrobial ointments may decrease secondary bacterial infections.

FOLLOW-UP

Sexual rest of infected stallions for at least 3 weeks after infection decreases spread of the EHV-3. If the breed registry permits, semen may be collected directly from the urethra through an open-ended artificial vagina and artificially inseminated, so as to reduce the chance of viral transmission to the mare. Silent recrudescence of the virus in stallions is likely, and may contribute to propagation of the disease. Iatrogenic transmission is possible; therefore, instruments that are disposable or easily cleaned should be used when working with affected horses.

MISCELLANEOUS

ABBREVIATION

- EHV = equine herpesvirus

Suggested Reading

Blanchard TL, Kenney RM, Timoney PJ. Venereal disease. Vet Clin North Am Equine Pract 1992;8:191–203.

Author Pamela A Wilkins

Consulting Editors Ashley G. Boyle and Corinne R. Sweeney

HIGH-RISK PREGNANCY, NEONATE

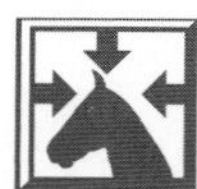

BASICS

OVERVIEW

• High-risk pregnancies are most often recognized when the mare has a history of periparturient problems or develops a new problem during pregnancy. Illness in the mare, problems with the placenta, prolonged pregnancy, premature delivery, and dystocia can lead to significant problems in the neonatal foal.
• The specific conditions of high-risk pregnancy often involve decreased perfusion and/or oxygen delivery to the placenta, ascending infection to the fetal-placental unit, and lack of readiness of the fetus for parturition.
• Conditions most commonly associated with high-risk pregnancy are prematurity, septicemia, and perinatal asphyxia syndrome.

SIGNALMENT

• Pregnant mare and neonatal foal
• Any breed
• Older mares may have a higher incidence of high-risk pregnancy.

SIGNS

Mare

• Vaginal discharge
• Premature udder development/secretions
• Endotoxemia
• Large abdominal size (disproportionate for stage of gestation)—hydrops; pendulous abdomen—prepubic tendon rupture
• There may be no premonitory signs.

Foal

The neonate born from a high-risk pregnancy can show signs of prematurity, sepsis, or perinatal asphyxia syndrome.

CAUSES AND RISK FACTORS

• Mares that have historical problems with pregnancies are considered high risk. Examples include previous dystocia, premature delivery, premature placental separation, placentitis, early embryonic loss, and prolonged pregnancy (including fescue toxicosis).
• Illness in the mare during gestation can predispose to placental and fetal problems. Examples include colic, endotoxemia, and malnutrition.
• Late-term abortion: MRLS, EHV1, twins, umbilical cord torsion, hydoallantois, placentitis (*Streptococcus zooepidemicus, Escherichia coli, Pseudomonas aeruginosa, Klebsiella pneumoniae, Aspergillus* spp.)
• Uterine conditions that interfere with normal gestation and foaling are associated with high-risk pregnancy. Examples include twins, abdominal hernias, uterine torsion, pelvic abnormalities, hydrops amnion, and hydrops allantois.
• Subsequent pregnancies should be monitored closely, and any contributing risk factors identified and managed.

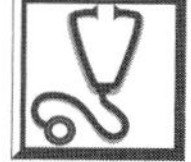

DIAGNOSIS

DIFFERENTIAL DIAGNOSIS

Prolonged or shortened gestation can be normal for some mares. Check breeding dates.

CBC/BIOCHEMISTRY/URINALYSIS

• Mare—Illness during pregnancy with neutropenia or evidence of organ dysfunction (azotemia or elevated liver enzymes) should be considered high risk for the fetus/foal. Anemia and low arterial oxygen content may place the foal at risk of hypoxic damage.
• Foal—Significantly elevated creatinine concentration may indicate placental insufficiency. Neutropenia or neutrophilia and elevated fibrinogen are suggestive of in utero infection.

OTHER LABORATORY TESTS

• Evaluation of fetal fluids—Amniocentesis carries a high risk of abortion.
• Evaluation of mammary secretions—The use of electrolyte concentrations in mammary secretions is not reliable for determining impending parturition in the high-risk mare.

IMAGING

• Transabdominal ultrasound of uterus and fetus—can detect fetal heart rate, presence of excessive fetal fluids
• Ultrasound of uterus, placenta, and fetus per rectum—early in pregnancy, can detect presence of twins; placental detachment and fetal positioning can be determined in later pregnancy.

OTHER DIAGNOSTIC PROCEDURES

• Fetal ECG—Electrodes are placed on the mare's sacrum and flank regions in order to obtain maximum amplitude of the fetal ECG. Normal fetal heart rate near the end of gestation can range between 65 and 115 beats per minute.
• Per rectum palpation of fetus—Determine positioning and viability of the fetus.
• Vaginal examination of mare—indicated if uterine culture is needed or parturition is imminent. It is not recommended routinely due to possible introduction of contamination to the uterus and disruption of the cervix.

PATHOLOGICAL FINDINGS

• Placenta—should be examined for signs of placentitis and placental insufficiency

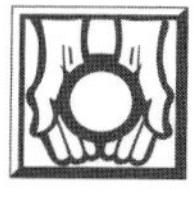

TREATMENT

MARE

• Supportive care for the mare to ensure adequate hydration and nutrition
• Improve oxygen delivery to the fetus—intranasal supplementation to the mare; blood transfusions if significant anemia is present in mare
• Prevent oxidant injury to the foal (PAS) by administering antioxidants to the mare—There is no evidence that this strategy is protective, but higher antioxidant concentrations in the fetus may mitigate some of the hypoxic injury to the foal.

• Induction of labor may be indicated if the mare is no longer able to safely support the pregnancy (debilitating disease, prepubic tendon rupture, etc); however, induction of labor without complete fetal readiness for birth is generally riskier for the foal.

FOAL

• Ex utero intrapartum (EXIT) procedures—includes intubation and oxygen supplementation/ventilation if the foal is accessible but unable to be delivered due to dystocia
• Foal resuscitation—secure an airway, intubate and ventilate, if needed. Chest compressions and epinephrine if a nonperfusing cardiac rhythm is present.
• Resuscitation fluids—balanced electrolyte solution given IV—glucose free for initial resuscitation
• Postresuscitation fluids and nutritional supplementation may be required.

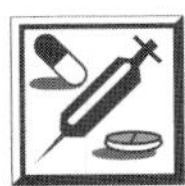

MEDICATIONS

DRUG(S)

Mare

• Trimethoprim sulfa for antimicrobial coverage of high-risk mare—25 mg/kg PO q12h
• Flunixin meglumine for anti-inflammatory treatment in mare—0.5–1.1 mg/kg PO or IV q12h
• Altrenogest for tocolytic effects—0.44 mg/kg PO daily—not useful in late gestation
• Vitamin E as an antioxidant—6000–10,000 IU PO daily

Foal

• Epinephrine 0.01–0.02 mg/kg IV (low dose) or 0.1–0.2 mg/kg IV (high dose) for resuscitation
• Broad-spectrum antimicrobials if in utero sepsis is suspected (see Septicemia, neonatal)

CONTRAINDICATIONS/POSSIBLE INTERACTIONS

Trimethoprim sulfa should be discontinued if the mare develops diarrhea.

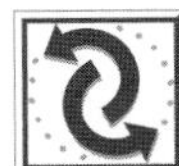

FOLLOW-UP

PATIENT MONITORING

• The mare should be monitored closely (with walkby or video monitor, at least every 30–60 min) for signs of parturition and should be assisted if needed.
• Neonatal foals from high-risk pregnancies should be monitored for signs of weakness, septicemia, altered mentation, and abnormal behavior. Associated abnormalities in the foal are usually recognized by 24–48 hr after parturition.

PREVENTION/AVOIDANCE

• Recognition of the high-risk mare
• Coordinated delivery plan for high-risk mares

POSSIBLE COMPLICATIONS

Neonatal Foal

• Perinatal asphyxia syndrome
• Septicemia

EXPECTED COURSE AND PROGNOSIS

In a recent publication (Lynch Norton), survival to discharge of high-risk pregnancy foals was 79%, compared to 10%–13% of foals delivered from emergency dystocia mares.

MISCELLANEOUS

ASSOCIATED CONDITIONS

N/A

AGE-RELATED FACTORS

• At-risk foals will generally be identified in late gestation, in the periparturient period, or in the early neonatal period.
• Older mares are at increased risk of high-risk pregnancy due to poor perineal conformation, risk of uterine artery bleed, and other placental and systemic factors.

ZOONOTIC POTENTIAL

Leptospirosis

PREGNANCY

N/A

SEE ALSO

• High-risk pregnancy, mare
• Perinatal asphyxia syndrome
• Fluid therapy, neonate

ABBREVIATIONS

• ECG = electrocardiogram
• EHV1 = equine herpesvirus 1
• MRLS = mare reproductive loss syndrome

Suggested Reading

Lynch Norton J, Dallap BL, Johnston JK, Palmer JE, Sertich PL, Boston R, Wilkins PA. Retrospective study of dystocia in mares at a referral hospital. Equine Vet J 2007;39:37–41.

Wilkins PA. Disorders of foals. In: Reed SM, Bayly WM, Sellon DC, eds. Equine Internal Medicine, ed 2. St. Louis: Saunders, 2004: 1381–1431.

Author Margaret C. Mudge
Consulting Editor Margaret C. Mudge

HIGH-RISK PREGNANCY

BASICS

DEFINITION/OVERVIEW

Pregnancy prone to early termination, delivery of a compromised foal, and/or prolongation by virtue of maternal, fetal, and/or placental abnormalities (structure or function)

ETIOLOGY/PATHOPHYSIOLOGY

Maternal systemic disease, fetal abnormalities, and/or placental infection, insufficiency, separation, or other abnormalities result in maternal and/or fetal death, premature initiation of the labor, prolonged gestation.

SYSTEMS AFFECTED

• Reproductive • Other organs systems, depending on the nature of maternal/systemic disease; complications, e.g., dystocia, retained fetal membranes

INCIDENCE/PREVALENCE

Sporadic

SIGNALMENT

• Nonspecific • Thoroughbred, Standardbreds, draft and related breeds (for twinning) • Mares >15 years • American Miniature Horses

SIGNS

Historical

• Maternal gestational disease—colic, hyperlipidemia, prepubic tendon rupture, uterine torsion • Previous problem pregnancy—placentitis or fetal compromise • Mucoid, hemorrhagic, serosanguinous, or purulent vulvar discharge • Premature udder development and dripping of milk • History of abortion, high-risk pregnancy, or dystocia • Delivery of small, dysmature, septicemic, or congenitally malformed foal • Preexisting maternal disease at conception—laminitis, equine Cushing's-like disease, endometrial inflammation, or fibrosis • Exposure to abortigenic infections or xenobiotics, e.g., EHV, Eastern tent caterpillars, fescue toxicosis

Physical Examination

• Anorexia, fever, other signs of concurrent, systemic disease • Abdominal discomfort • Mucoid, hemorrhagic, serosanguinous, or purulent vulvar discharge • Premature udder development and dripping of milk • Fetal distress, delayed development, other abnormalities by transrectal or transabdominal U/S • Placentitis, placental separation, or fetal hydrops (U/S) • Excess swelling ventral midline, ventral body wall weakening (TRP, transabdominal U/S); excess abdominal distention

CAUSES AND RISK FACTORS

• Pre-existing maternal disease—Cushing's-like disease; chronic, moderate to severe endometrial inflammation or fibrosis; laminitis • Gestational maternal disease—malnutrition, colic, endotoxemia, hyperlipidemia, prepubic tendon rupture, uterine torsion, granulosa cell tumor, laminitis, musculoskeletal disease, equine fescue toxicosis, exposure to xenobiotics • Fetal conditions—twins, fetal abnormalities (hydrocephalus), delayed fetal development (small for gestational age, IUGR), fetal trauma
• Placental conditions:
  ○ Placentitis
  ○ Insufficiency
  ○ Separation
  ○ Fetal hydrops

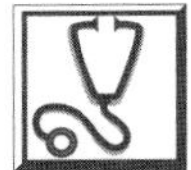

DIAGNOSIS

DIFFERENTIAL DIAGNOSIS

• Other organ system involvement depends on presence of placentitis, stage of gestation, presence of maternal disease, infection, and/or toxemia. • Hyperlipidemia—special concern: American Miniature Horse, ponies, and donkeys

CBC/BIOCHEMISTRY/URINALYSIS

• CBC and profile indicated based on physical examination findings • Assessment for presence of inflammatory, stress, or left shift leukocyte response, other organ system involvement.

OTHER LABORATORY TESTS

Maternal P4

• If history of abortion or high-risk pregnancy; old mare with endometrial inflammation and fibrosis in biopsy specimen taken prebreeding; cases of suspected maternal, fetal, placental disease • P4 (ELISA or RIA) <80 days of gestation
  ○ Acceptable level—varies >1 to >4 ng/L; depends on reference lab.
  ○ >100 days' gestation, RIA for P4 detects both P4 (may be very low >150 days) and cross-reacting 5α-pregnanes of uterofetoplacental origin (maternal levels decreased with equine fescue toxicosis)
• Acceptable levels of 5α-pregnanes vary by stage of gestation and laboratory.

Maternal Estrogens

• Reflection of fetal estrogen production and viability, especially conjugated estrogens (estrone sulfate) • Normal values vary by laboratory.

Maternal Relaxin

• Decreases with placental abnormalities • No commercial assay available

Maternal T_3/T_4

• Anecdotal reports—decreased levels in mares with history of conception failure, EED, abortion; significance of low T_4 is unclear.

Maternal Peritoneal Fluid Analysis

• Useful in late gestation, mare with abdominal discomfort (torsion of GI tract or uterus), obstetrics cases

Maternal Xenobiotics

• In cases of specific intoxications, submit whole blood, plasma, or urine.

Allantoic/Amniotic Fluid

• To assess fetal karyotype, pulmonary maturity, measure fetal proteins, detect bacteria, meconium, or inflammatory cells • Equine sampling technique of higher risk than in humans • Utility not established

Feed

• Analysis indicated:
  ○ Specific xenobiotics—ergopeptine alkaloids, phytoestrogens, heavy metals
  ○ Endophyte—*Neotyphodium coenophialum*

IMAGING

General Comments

Transrectal and transabdominal U/S to confirm pregnancy, diagnose twins, evaluate fetal viability and development, assess placental health, diagnose other gestational abnormalities (fetal hydrops)

Confirm Pregnancy and Diagnose Twins

• With serious disease or considering surgical intervention in mare bred within the last 11 mo.
• Twin pregnancy—presence of 2 fetuses (<90 days' gestation by transrectal U/S) or by presence of nonpregnant uterine horn (transabdominal U/S) in late gestation

Fetal Viability and Development

• Best by transabdominal U/S in late gestation
• View fetus—active and resting states, record fetal presentation and position

Fetal Activity and Normal Muscle Tone

• *<330 days of gestation*—normal FHR is ≤100 bpm after activity; ≥60 bpm resting rate • *>330 days of gestation*—normal FHR is ≥50 bpm resting and ≤40 bpm between resting and active rates

Normal Fetal Heart Rhythm

Assessed by ECG

Appropriately Sized Fetus for Gestational Stage

• Fetal aortic diameter—≅2.1 cm at 300 and 2.7 cm at 330 days of gestation • Record length and width of fetal orbit.

Normal Quantities of Fetal Fluids

• Maximum normal range:
  ○ Allantoic fluid depth—4.7–22.1 cm
  ○ Amniotic fluid depth—0.8–14.9 cm

Placental Health

• Normal uteroplacental thickness, by transabdominal US—7–20 mm • Normal uteroplacental thickness by transrectal U/S:
  ○ 271–300 days of gestation—≤8 mm
  ○ 300–330 days—≤10 mm
  ○ >330 days—≤12 mm
• Look for evidence of absence or very small areas of uteroplacental discontinuity.

OTHER DIAGNOSTIC PROCEDURES

• Prebreeding reproductive evaluation—indicated in mares predisposed to problem pregnancies, e.g., barren, old mares; mares with history of abortion • Fetal ECG—detect twins; assess fetal viability and distress; now largely replaced by transabdominal U/S

PATHOLOGICAL FINDINGS

Endometrial biopsy—moderate to severe, chronic endometritis and/or fibrosis

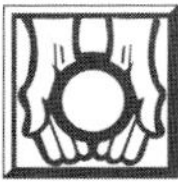

TREATMENT

GENERAL COMMENTS

• If history of abortion, evidence of moderate to severe endometritis and/or fibrosis, evaluate and treat the mare prebreeding. • Consider progestin supplementation, especially *if*:

- ○ Clinical diagnosis—luteal insufficiency (anecdotal)
- ○ Premature CL regression (possibly involved in early pregnancy loss)
- ○ History of abortion
- ○ Supplementation indicated with diagnosis of placentitis, maternal endotoxemia

• ET—means to continue breeding high-risk mare • Fescue toxicosis and prolonged gestation—treat with D2-dopamine receptor antagonists • Induction of parturition or cesarean section, indicated in specific instances of:

- ○ Maternal disease
- ○ Fetal stress/distress/viability
- ○ Placental separation

• Close supervision of parturition; the neonatal foal may need treatment as well.

APPROPRIATE HEALTH CARE

• Detected early, high-risk pregnancies may be treated on an ambulatory basis. • Close supervision of foaling in all cases • Consider facilities equipped for foaling high-risk pregnancies.

NURSING CARE

Nursing care—required for mare and neonatal foal, depends on maternal disease, fetal distress, need for surgical intervention

ACTIVITY

• Limited/supervised exercise • Prepubic tendon rupture, laminitis, hydrops of fetal membranes—may need complete exercise restriction

DIET

Mare—adequate, late-gestation diet; appropriate energy, protein, vitamins, minerals, unless contraindicated by concurrent maternal disease

CLIENT EDUCATION

Pregnant mare is at added risk, poorer prognosis for reaching term; neonate may need extended intensive care and a nurse mare.

SURGICAL CONSIDERATIONS

Cesarean section indicated if vaginal delivery is not possible.

MEDICATIONS

DRUG(S) OF CHOICE

• See specific conditions.
• Endotoxic/gram-negative septicemic mares <80 days of gestation—altrenogest (initially—0.088 mg/kg PO daily, then 0.044 mg/kg daily; to ≥100 days' gestation); decrease dose over 14 days at end of treatment period • Endometritis/previously aborted mare (without active infectious component) and/or mare with fibrosis—altrenogest (0.044–0.088 mg/kg PO daily); commence 2– 3 days after ovulation or upon diagnosis of pregnancy, continue to ≥100 days gestation, decrease dose over 14 days at end of treatment period.
• Altrenogest—may start later, continue longer, or use only short periods depending on serum P4 levels during first 80 days of gestation (>1 to >4 ng/mL), clinical circumstances, risk factors, clinician preference • Near term, discontinue altrenogest 7–14 days before expected foaling date, case dependent, unless otherwise indicated by assessment of fetal maturity/viability or questions regarding accuracy of gestational age.
• Domperidone (1.1 mg/kg PO daily)—begin when fescue toxicosis is diagnosed or with prolonged gestation diagnosis.

- ○ Continue domperidone to parturition, with anticipated normal mammary development and lactation.

CONTRAINDICATIONS

Altrenogest

• Only to prevent abortion with demonstration of fetus in utero • Not recommended to prevent spontaneous, infectious abortion other than those caused by placentitis and endotoxemia

PRECAUTIONS

• Initially, weekly monitor fetal viability.
• Retention of dead fetuses has been reported to result from continued treatment with supplemental progestins. • Altrenogest—absorbed across skin; wear nitrile gloves and wash hands. • Supplemental progestins for pregnancy maintenance—success is anecdotal.
• Depending on etiology of at-risk pregnancy, progestin supplementation may be unsuccessful.

ALTERNATIVE DRUGS

• Injectable P4 (150– 500 mg IM daily, oil base), alternative to oral product • Flunixin meglumine (0.25 mg/kg IM or IV daily to QID), prophylaxis if endotoxin release is anticipated

- ○ Increase dose—for analgesia and anti-inflammatory effect.
- ○ May help decrease premature uterine contractions

• Thyroxine supplementation—anecdotal treatment success in subfertile mares.

- ○ Use is controversial; considered deleterious by some

FOLLOW-UP

PATIENT MONITORING

• Monitor frequently to completion of pregnancy. • Vaginal speculum examination, uterine cytology and culture—may be useful 7–10 days postpartum. • Postpartum uterine biopsy—may identify etiology of mare's problem, define reproductive prognosis and appropriate treatment decisions

PREVENTION/AVOIDANCE

• Early recognition of high-risk pregnancy
• Correction of poor VC, especially mare with history of placentitis • Records—complete, prior double ovulations • Early diagnosis of twins
• Selective embryonic or fetal reduction
• Prebreeding resolution of endometritis
• Remove mares from fescue pasture or ergotized grasses or grains, minimum 30 days prepartum.
• Cull problem mares from population.
• Embryo transfer • Prudent use of medications in pregnant mares • Avoid exposure to known toxicants and infectious diseases.

POSSIBLE COMPLICATIONS

• Abortion, dystocia, retained fetal membranes, metritis, laminitis, septicemia, endometritis, reproductive tract trauma, impaired fertility
• Neonatal foal from high-risk pregnancy—more likely dysmature, septicemic, subject to angular limb deformities than with normal foal/pregnancy

EXPECTED COURSE AND PROGNOSIS

• Resolution/progression of maternal systemic, fetal, or placental disease determines outcome of the pregnancy. • Generally—guarded prognosis for high-risk pregnancy • Guarded to poor prognosis—pregnancy maintenance in mare with a history of abortion or preexisting, moderate to severe chronic endometritis and/or fibrosis

MISCELLANEOUS

ASSOCIATED CONDITIONS

• Abortion, spontaneous, infectious and noninfectious • Dystocia • Endometritis • Fetal distress/stress/viability • Hydrops, allantois and amnion • Metritis, postpartum • Prepubic tendon rupture • Placental insufficiency
• Placentitis • Premature placental separation
• Uterine torsion

AGE-RELATED FACTORS

• Chronic endometritis and endometrial fibrosis in old mares • Old mares generally have more chronic health problems.

SEE ALSO

• Abortion, spontaneous, infectious • Abortion, spontaneous, noninfectious • Dystocia
• Endometrial biopsy • Endometritis • Embryo transfer • Fetal stress/distress/viability • High risk pregnancy, neonate • Hydrops allantois/amnion • Metritis • Placental insufficiency • Placentitis • Premature placental separation • Prepubic tendon rupture
• Retained fetal membranes • Twin pregnancy
• Uterine torsion

ABBREVIATIONS

• CL = corpus luteum • ECG = electrocardiogram • EED = early embryonic death • EHV = equine herpesvirus • ELISA = enzyme-linked immunosorbent assay • ET = embryo transfer • FHR = fetal heart rate
• GI = gastrointestinal • IUGR = intrauterine growth retardation • P4 = progesterone
• RIA = radioimmunoassay • SFGA = small for gestational age • T_3 = triiodothyronine
• T_4 = thyroxine • TRP = transrectal palpation
• U/S = ultrasound, ultrasonography
• VC = vulvar conformation

Suggested Reading

Sertich PL. Fetal ultrasonography. In: Reef VB, ed. Equine Diagnostic Ultrasound. Philadelphia: WB Saunders, 1999:425–445.

Author Tim J. Evans
Consulting Editor Carla L. Carleton

HYDROCEPHALUS

BASICS

DEFINITION

• In horses, hydrocephalus generally refers to increased volume of CSF within the ventricular system (internal hydrocephalus).
• Increased volume of the subarachnoid space (external hydrocephalus) is rare in this species and often a post-mortem artifact.
• The spinal equivalent of hydrocephalus is hydromyelia.

PATHOPHYSIOLOGY

• Internal hydrocephalus is due to enlargement of the ventricular system within the brain with any resulting cavity being lined by ependyma.
• It is unusual in horses compared with in dogs, but it can be a rare inherited trait in Standardbred horses or an isolated occurrence in all breeds.
• CSF production is independent of pressure, and hydrocephalus can accompany numerous diseases that result in prenatal or postnatal loss of brain tissue or obstruct the aqueductal drainage of CSF.
• In adults, it can be associated with traumatic or infectious inflammation or space-occupying lesions (e. g., abscess, neoplasia).

SYSTEMS AFFECTED

Central nervous system

SIGNALMENT

Acquired disease is evident at any stage, but congenital disease often manifests slowly.

SIGNS

Historical

• A history of central nervous system disease and/or trauma can be seen with acquired disease. However, there may be no historical association.
• In foals, severe hydrocephalus can on occasion be noted as an incidental finding after sudden death, due to vascular instability in the hydrocephalic brain.

Physical Examination

• Clinical signs can be very subtle even with minimal cerebral mantle remaining but usually include failure to thrive, somnolence and aimless activity, poor suck reflex, poor swallowing, and central blindness.
• Additional signs can accompany additional lesions present in individual disease types.
• Just like in dogs, a ventrolateral deviation of the eyeballs can also occur. Presumably, this is the result of a change in shape and position of the bony orbits.
• Normal eyeball movements may be seen.

CAUSES
See Pathophysiology.

RISK FACTORS
- Similar for the primary central nervous system disease processes that may be associated with acquired disease.
- There may be a genetic relationship in congenital disease.

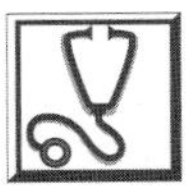

DIAGNOSIS

Classically, plain lateral radiographs have a homogeneous ground-glass appearance of the calvaria.

DIFFERENTIAL DIAGNOSIS
Any inflammatory or metabolic disease that can induce stupor or seizures

CBC/BIOCHEMISTRY/URINALYSIS
No pathognomonic abnormalities

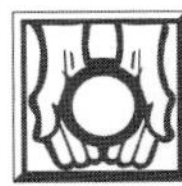

TREATMENT

Euthanasia should be considered.

ASSOCIATED CONDITIONS
Any inflammatory, traumatic, or space-occupying central nervous system disorder

AGE-RELATED FACTORS
- Acquired hydrocephalus can occur at any age.
- Congenital disease often manifests at birth.

ABBREVIATION
- CSF = cerebrospinal fluid

Suggested Reading

Bester RC, et al. Hydrocephalus in an 18-month-old colt. JAVMA 1976;168:1041–1042.
Foreman JH, et al. Congenital internal hydrocephalus in a Quarter Horse foal. J Equine Vet Sci 1983;3:154–164.
Ojala M, Huikku I. Inheritance of hydrocephalus in horses. Equine Vet J 1992;24:140–143.

The author and editors wish to acknowledge the contribution of Joseph J. Bertone, author of this chapter in the previous edition.

Author Caroline N. Hahn
Consulting Editor Caroline N. Hahn

HYDROPS ALLANTOIS/AMNION

BASICS

DEFINITION/OVERVIEW

• Excessive fluid accumulation in either the allantoic or amniotic cavity of the pregnant uterus
• Hydrops allantois is related primarily to placental dysfunction/insufficiency.
• Hydrops amnion is attributable to abnormalities of the fetus, contributing directly to fluid accumulation by virtue of congenital anomalies. Segmental aplasias (primarily GI in origin) preclude swallowing and processing and/or recycling of amniotic fluid. The fetus may be delivered alive but is nonviable.

ETIOLOGY/PATHOPHYSIOLOGY

• Dysfunction of either the placenta or the fetus results in accumulation of excessive amounts of allantoic or amniotic fluid, undermining the dam's health by excessive weight of modest to rapid accumulation, contributing to her dehydration, compromised GI function, and labored respiration.
• Clinical management for both conditions is the same—induction of parturition, to save the dam's life, to prevent rupture of the ventral abdominal wall and/or the uterus.

SYSTEMS AFFECTED

Reproductive, dam and fetus

GENETICS

There may be a hereditary role in development of hydropic conditions.

INCIDENCE/PREVALENCE

Rare

SIGNALMENT

• No breed or age predisposition, although more cases have been reported in draft mares.
• Abnormal accumulation of fluid (up to 100 L) in the allantoic cavity; abdominal size is abnormally large for stage of gestation.
• Commonly occurs from 6 to 10 mo of gestation
• Frequently has a rapid onset occurring over a few days to a few weeks
• Most mares develop a tremendous amount of ventral abdominal edema.
• Abdominal and/or uterine rupture can result due to the excessive weight of allantoic or amniotic fluid.

SIGNS

• Modest to rapid accumulation of fluid within the uterus (allantoic or amniotic)
• Rapid increase in abdominal size/shape
• Abdominal pain (moderate to severe), severe ventral edema, elevated pulse, labored respiration due to pressure on the diaphragm, difficulty walking, recumbency as the condition progresses
• TRP reveals an abnormal accumulation of fluid.
• The fetus is difficult or impossible to detect.

CAUSES

N/A

RISK FACTORS

Draft mares

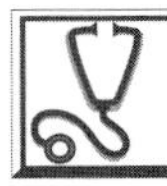

DIAGNOSIS

DIFFERENTIAL DIAGNOSIS

• Twin pregnancy: mid-to-late gestation
• Prepubic tendon rupture
• Herniation or rupture of ventral abdominal wall
• Possibly, uterine torsion

CBC/BIOCHEMISTRY/URINALYSIS

• Possible increased or decreased PCV (secondary to hypovolemia or dehydration, respectively)
• Possible increase in BUN and creatinine secondary to dehydration

OTHER LABORATORY TESTS

N/A

IMAGING

U/S

• Fluid compartments are grossly enlarged, either allantoic or amniotic.
• Torso/abdomen of the hydramnios fetus may have a grossly widened diameter as a result of ascites.

OTHER DIAGNOSTIC PROCEDURES

• u/s and TRP
• Abdominocentesis, U/S-guided, may be of use to detect abnormal free fluid in abdomen and in cases of uterine rupture.

PATHOLOGIC FINDINGS

• Placental insufficiency secondary to placentitis
• Hydrops amnion—fetal swallowing defects (segmental aplasia(s) preventing swallowing and processing of amniotic fluid, which leads to its accumulation in excessive amounts
• Fetal defects such as growth retardation and hydrocephalus have been reported, as well as brachygnathia.
• Torsion of the umbilical cord and amnion has been reported.

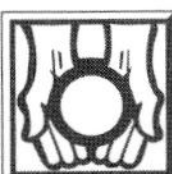

TREATMENT

APPROPRIATE HEALTH CARE

• Manual dilation of the cervix, completed gradually over a 10- to 20-min period.
• Measured, controlled drainage of allantoic/amniotic fluid via aseptic insertion of a sterile drain tube through the cervix and fetal membranes.
• Slow removal of fluid is important to prevent hypovolemic shock in the mare.
  ○ A sudden loss of pressure on the abdominal vessels may result as the uterus is drained, and lead to vascular pooling. Monitor PCV and plasma proteins throughout.
  ○ If removal can be well managed, achieving a gradual decrease in volume over a 12- to 24-hr period is best.
  ○ One method—manually dilate cervix, serial cloprostenol administration (250 μg at 12-hr interval; 2–4 doses). Place nasogastric tube tube through membranes and tie off around tubing to facilitate controlled fluid removal, 5–10 L at a time, clamping off in between increments to keep mare stabilized.
  ○ Continue with IV fluid delivery and care, as follows.
• For the dam:
  ○ IV fluids—balanced electrolyte solutions, LRS, or hypertonic saline solution
  ○ Corticosteroids—Solu-Delta-Cortef (prednisolone sodium succinate). Initial dose is 50–100 mg IV or IM. Initial IV should be given slowly (30 second to 1 min).
  ○ Dexamethasone—0.1–0.5 mg/kg; use at the higher end of the dose range to decrease the likelihood of hypovolemic shock.
  ○ Oxytocin is often ineffective due to chronic stretching (uterine atony/inertia).
• Once sufficient fluid has been removed by a slow, controlled rate removal, the CA membrane should be ruptured and the fetus removed by forced extraction.
  ○ Note—In some cases the CA membrane may be thickened and difficult to rupture, in which case, the membrane should be pulled caudally, into the anterior vagina, to facilitate easier opening of the membrane and extraction of the fetus.
  ○ Continue monitoring the mare, fluids and antibiotic administration, as indicated.

NURSING CARE

Close monitoring of the mare for signs of shock and/or infection after removal of fluids and fetus.

ACTIVITY

Limited by inability of dam to move

DIET

N/A

CLIENT EDUCATION

Mares that appear excessively large for stage of gestation should be evaluated, particularly if signs of systemic disease or disability develop.

SURGICAL CONSIDERATIONS

- Induction of parturition
- Caesarean section, but keep in mind that fetal survival is unlikely

MEDICATIONS

DRUG(S) OF CHOICE

- Since most hydrops mares spontaneously abort, treatment should be directed at terminating the pregnancy.
- The use of oxytocin is usually not effective since most of these mares will have uterine inertia (atony) due to the stretching of the uterine musculature.

CONTRAINDICATIONS

N/A

PRECAUTIONS

N/A

POSSIBLE INTERACTIONS

N/A

ALTERNATIVE DRUGS

N/A

FOLLOW-UP

PATIENT MONITORING

- Once a diagnosis is made, termination of pregnancy is the appropriate follow-up.
- Monitor for respiratory distress, stability of dam's vital signs.

PREVENTION/AVOIDANCE

- Hydrops amnion: breed to different sire once mare recovers from either controlled vaginal deliver or caesarean section.
- Hydrops allantois: as the abnormal placentation may reflect ineffective placental attachment because of an abnormal endometrium, placentitis, or primary placental failure, rebreeding may result in a similar outcome.
- Adventitious placentation has been reported in cattle and is an effort by the placenta to generate additional, however ineffective, sites for placental transfer (oxygen in, removal of fetal waste).

POSSIBLE COMPLICATIONS

- Loss of pregnancy
- Prepubic tendon rupture
- Rupture of ventral belly wall
- Maternal death

EXPECTED COURSE AND PROGNOSIS

- Prognosis for fetal survival is poor.
- Prognosis for survival of the dam is guarded, if parturition is induced before more serious damage occurs.
- Prognosis for future reproduction:
  - Guarded for hydrops allantois
  - Guarded for hydrops amnion mare, with the recommendation that she be bred to a different stallion

MISCELLANEOUS

ASSOCIATED CONDITIONS

- Placentitis
- Adventitious placentation has been reported in cattle.

AGE-RELATED FACTORS

Older, multiparous mares, but has been reported in all ages

ZOONOTIC POTENTIAL

N/A

PREGNANCY

A pregnancy-related condition

SYNONYMS

N/A

SEE ALSO

- Dystocia
- Placentitis
- Placental basics
- Placental insufficiency
- Premature placental separation

ABBREVIATIONS

- BUN = blood urea nitrogen
- CA = chorioallantoic
- LRS = lactated Ringer's solution
- PCV = packed cell volume
- TRP = transrectal palpation
- U/S = ultrasound examination

Suggested Reading

Honnas CH, et al. Hydramnios causing uterine rupture in a mare. J Am Vet Med Assoc 1988;193:332–336.

Immegart HM, Threlfall WR. In: Reed SM, Bayly WM, eds. Equine Internal Medicine. Philadelphia: WB Saunders, 1998:763–766.

Löfstedt RM. Miscellaneous diseases of pregnancy and parturition. In: McKinnon AO, Voss JL, eds. Equine Reproduction. Philadelphia: Lea & Febiger, 1993:596–597.

Vandeplassche M, et al Dropsy of the fetal sacs in the mare: induced and spontaneous abortion. Vet Rec 1976;99:67–69.

Reimer JM. Use of transcutaneous ultrasonography in complicated latter-middle to late gestation pregnancies in the mare: 122 cases. Proc Am Assoc Eq Pract 1997;259–261.

Palmer JE. The high risk mare. Presented to Belgian Eq Practitioners Society, 2005. IVIS, Ithaca, NW; P2001.1105

Author Carla L. Carleton

Consulting Editor Carla L. Carleton

HYPERKALEMIC PERIODIC PARALYSIS

BASICS

OVERVIEW

• HYPP is an autosomal dominant trait affecting Quarter Horses, Quarter Horse crosses, American Paint Horses, and Appaloosas worldwide. • HYPP is caused by a point mutation in the skeletal muscle sodium channel resulting in persistent depolarization of skeletal muscle cells, temporary weakness, and increased serum potassium concentrations. • The trait is linked to a Quarter Horse stallion named "Impressive," and approximately 4% of the Quarter Horse breed may be affected.

SYSTEMS AFFECTED

• Endocrine/metabolic • Neuromuscular
• Cardiovascular • Ophthalmic

SIGNALMENT

• Quarter Horses or Quarter Horse–related breeds that are descendants of a sire or dam with the genetic mutation • Horses with hypertrophied muscles • Clinical signs usually commence by 2–3 years of age.

SIGNS

• Clinical sings range from asymptomatic to daily muscle fasciculations and weakness. • In mild disease, muscle fasciculations on the flanks, neck, and shoulders and/or facial muscle spasm and generalized muscle tension • Third eyelid prolapse • In severe disease, severe muscle cramping, weakness with swaying, staggering, dogsitting, or recumbency • +/− Tachycardia
• Tachypnea, respiratory stridor or distress
• Death

CAUSES AND RISK FACTORS

• Caused by a point mutation resulting in a phenylalanine/leucine substitution in the skeletal muscle sodium channel alpha subunit. This results in excessive inward flux of sodium and outward flux of potassium, resulting in persistent depolarization and weakness of muscle.
• Descent from the stallion "Impressive" on the sire's or dam's side in a horse with episodic muscle tremors is strongly suggestive of HYPP.
• Risk factors include sudden dietary changes or ingestion of diets high in potassium (>1.1%), (e.g., alfalfa hay, molasses, electrolyte supplements, and kelp-based supplements), fasting, anesthesia or heavy sedation, trailer rides, and stress. • Exercise does not appear to stimulate clinical signs and may even relieve them.

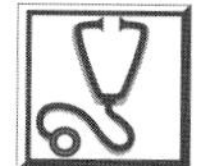

DIAGNOSIS

DIFFERENTIAL DIAGNOSIS

• Most clinical signs of HYPP are not specific for the disease. Confirmation is achieved by elimination of other differentials and DNA analysis. • Differential diagnoses for clinical signs include colic, exertional rhabdomyolysis, tetanus, botulism, laminitis, seizures, and upper airway obstruction. • Differential diagnoses for hyperkalemia include delay before serum centrifugation, hemolysis, ruptured bladder, chronic renal failure, and severe rhabdomyolysis.

CBC/BIOCHEMISTRY/URINALYSIS

• Hyperkalemia (6–9 mEq/L) during an episode
• Hemoconcentration • Hyponatremia • Serum CK is usually normal or mildly increased.

OTHER LABORATORY TESTS

Definitive diagnosis requires DNA testing of mane or tail hair samples (including the hair bulb) or whole blood (EDTA) for the genetic defect.

OTHER DIAGNOSTIC PROCEDURES

Electromyographic examination of affected horses between episodes reveals abnormal fibrillation potentials, complex repetitive discharges with occasional myotonic potentials, and trains of doublets.

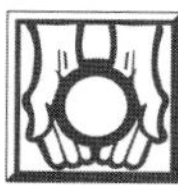

TREATMENT

• Often spontaneous recovery in 20 minutes • Early mild episodes may be halted using low-grade exercise or feeding grain or corn syrup to stimulate insulin-mediated movement of potassium across cell membranes. • Dietary management—decreasing dietary potassium to between 0.6% and 1.1% of the total ration and increasing renal loss of potassium. Pasture such as later cuts of timothy or Bermuda grass hay and grains such as oats, corn, wheat, and barley, and beet pulp will provide lower levels of potassium in the diet and should be fed in small meals several times a day. • Complete feeds for HYPP horses are commercially available.
• Regular exercise and/or frequent access to a large paddock may be beneficial. • With severe clinical signs, aggressive medical therapy may be needed. • With severe respiratory obstruction, a tracheostomy may be necessary.

HYPERKALEMIC PERIODIC PARALYSIS

MEDICATIONS

DRUG(S)

• During an episode, epinephrine (3 mL/500 kg 1:1000 formulation IM) • In severe cases, administration of calcium gluconate (0.2–0.4 mL/kg 23% solution diluted in 1 L of 5% dextrose) or IV dextrose (6 mL/kg of a 5% solution) alone or combined with sodium bicarbonate (1–2 mEq/kg) will often provide immediate improvement. • If clinical signs cannot be controlled with dietary changes, acetazolamide (2–4 mg/kg PO q8–12 h) or hydrochlorthiazide (0.5–1 mg/kg PO q12 h) may be helpful.

CONTRAINDICATIONS/POSSIBLE INTERACTIONS

• Care should be taken during anesthesia or heavy sedation as this may precipitate signs.
• Glucocorticoids may be contraindicated in susceptible horses as they induce episodes in humans with similar disorders.

FOLLOW-UP

PATIENT MONITORING

• Serum potassium concentrations are usually normal between episodes. • Success of therapy is evaluated based on the absence of clinical signs.
• Affected horses require frequent monitoring for clinical signs.

PREVENTION/AVOIDANCE

• See Treatment/Medications. • Avoid high-potassium feeds such as alfalfa hay, brome hay, canola oil, soybean meal or oil, and sugar molasses and beet molasses. • Due to the autosomal transmission of this disorder, owners of affected animals should be discouraged from breeding these animals. • Horses under or recovering from general anesthesia appear to be particularly at risk.

POSSIBLE COMPLICATIONS

• Death during acute severe episodes
• Respiratory distress due to paralysis of upper respiratory muscles • Aspiration pneumonia may occur due to laryngeal dysfunction, particularly in foals. • Cardiac arrhythmias (ventricular fibrillation) may occur due to hyperkalemia.

EXPECTED COURSE AND PROGNOSIS

• Prognosis for life for most affected horses is good, although there may be recurrence of clinical signs and severe episodes may be fatal.
• Severely affected animals can be managed in the long term with low-potassium diets and maintenance diuretic therapy.

MISCELLANEOUS

PREGNANCY

• Due to the autosomal transmission of this disorder, owners of affected animals should be discouraged from breeding these animals.

SEE ALSO

• PSSM

ABBREVIATION

• CK = creatinine kinase
• HYPP = hyperkalemic periodic paralysis

Suggested Reading

MacLeay JM. Diseases of the musculoskeletal system. In: Reed SM, Bayly WM, Sellon DC, eds. Equine Internal Medicine, ed2. St. Louis; Saunders, 2004;461–531.

Author Anna M. Firshman
Consulting Editor Elizabeth J. Davidson

HYPERLIPIDEMIA/HYPERLIPEMIA

BASICS

DEFINITION

• *Hyperlipidemia* refers to the detection of elevated blood concentrations of lipids including TG or cholesterol. • *Hypertriglyceridemia* is abnormally high serum or plasma TG concentration. • *Hyperlipemia* is a clinical condition characterized by elevated serum TG concentrations (>500 mg/dL), depression, anorexia, and organ dysfunction.
• Hyperlipidemia is an incidental finding in healthy nursing foals and results from normal chylomicron production after feeding.
• Congenital hyperlipidemia occurs in newborn foals born to mares affected by hyperlipemia prior to parturition.

PATHOPHYSIOLOGY

• Negative energy balance or stress stimulates lipolysis within adipose tissues, causing mobilization of FFAs (also called NEFAs) and glycerol. • Lipolysis is mediated by HSL under the influence of several hormones—glucagon, insulin, and glucocorticoids. • Mobilization of FFAs from adipose tissues is a normal physiologic response to fasting. • Hyperlipemia is driven by excessive mobilization of FFAs from adipose tissue TG stores and is caused by two major problems—an overabundance of substrate (i.e., TG) in the obese animal and IR. • Insulin normally dampens the activity of HSL after feeding, but affected horses or ponies can be insulin resistant. • Most circulating FFAs are removed from the blood by the liver and serve as substrates for energy production or are esterified to TG. In turn, TG is stored within hepatocytes or packaged into VLDLs and exported to other tissues via the blood. The transported TG is utilized by peripheral tissues under the action of LPL, an enzyme found on endothelial surfaces.
• FFAs are generated from TG hydrolysis by LPL and used as a source of energy. • If a high rate of lipolysis within adipose tissue persists, blood FFA concentrations rise and uptake of FFAs into the liver accelerates. Rates of TG-rich VLDL synthesis and export substantially increase and accumulation of TG-rich VLDL within the blood (i.e., hyperlipidemia) develops as hepatic production exceeds the maximal clearance rate of lipid by LPL. • In severe cases, accumulation of TG within the liver results in hepatic lipidosis and TG deposits in other tissues, causing fatty infiltration followed by organ dysfunction. A vicious cycle then develops as elevated serum TG concentrations further suppress appetite.

SYSTEMS AFFECTED

• Endocrine/metabolic • Blood • Hepatobiliary
• Renal • Gastrointestinal

GENETICS

• Ponies, miniature horses, and donkeys are at greatest risk. • Shetland ponies are particularly predisposed.

INCIDENCE/PREVALENCE

Incidence generally is considered to be low, but depends upon the breed of horse and feeding practices.

GEOGRAPHIC DISTRIBUTION

No geographic variations in incidence are reported.

SIGNALMENT

• Ponies, donkeys, and miniature horses are more susceptible. • Occurs at all ages, including foals that may be born with congenital hyperlipidemia • Mares are more susceptible during pregnancy and lactation.

SIGNS

• Early signs are nonspecific—lethargy, inappetence, and depression. • As the disease progresses, patients cease eating and drinking and develop clinical signs associated with organ dysfunction. Fetid, fat-covered feces (steatorrhea) are produced (eventually in the form of diarrhea) and neurologic signs consistent with hepatic encephalopathy develop—severe depression, head pressing, ataxia, and sham drinking. Renal dysfunction develops. • Some animals exhibit mild colic caused by stretching of the liver capsule. • Pregnant mares may abort.
• Severely affected patients show progressive deterioration in neurologic status and require euthanasia. • Newborn foals with congenital hyperlipemia are normal in appearance.

CAUSES

• Most often develops in animals that are in negative energy balance and have recently been stressed • Often occurs as a secondary complication in patients suffering from a disease that suppresses feed intake—enterocolitis, parasitism, dental problems, dysphagia, and esophageal obstruction • Endotoxemia directly stimulates adipose mobilization. • The additional strain of pregnancy and lactation on energy metabolism predispose to hyperlipidemia. • Insulin-resistant patients are more likely to develop hyperlipemia.

RISK FACTORS

• Ponies, donkeys, and Miniature Horses are most commonly affected. • EMS • PPID
• Pregnancy • Stress • Concurrent disease
• Endotoxemia • Parasitism • Lactation

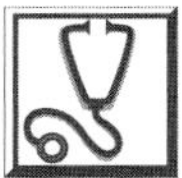

DIAGNOSIS

DIFFERENTIAL DIAGNOSIS

• Acute infectious diseases with nonspecific signs of depression and inappetence • Liver disease
• Neurologic disease • Gastrointestinal disease

CBC/BIOCHEMISTRY/URINALYSIS

Note: Markedly elevated blood lipid concentrations may interfere with analyzer functions, particularly biochemical analysis.
• A simple diagnostic test can be performed by standing a blood sample (collected in EDTA) upright and examining the plasma once the RBC mass has settled. Opaque (milky) plasma develops when the TG concentration exceeds 500 mg/dL and it is not possible to read newsprint through the tube. • Triglyceride concentrations may be reported in mmol/L and the conversion factor is approximately 89 (500 mg/dL is equivalent to 5.6 mmol/L). • The reference range for adult horses is 11–65 mg/dL, but higher concentrations are detected in healthy donkeys and pregnant ponies. • Hypoglycemia
• Abnormalities associated with hepatic dysfunction/damage—elevated concentrations of total bilirubin, GGT, ALP, AST, and SDH
• Abnormalities associated with renal dysfunction—elevated BUN and azotemia with normal urinalysis. Assessment of BUN should account for the adequacy of hepatic function at the time. • Metabolic acidosis is sometimes detected.

OTHER LABORATORY TESTS

• Elevated serum insulin concentration consistent with IR
• Insulin resistance detected using the combined glucose-insulin test (CGIT)
• Elevated blood ammonia concentration
• Elevated serum bile acid concentration
• Prolonged coagulation profile—advanced liver failure
• Diagnostic evaluation for PPID

IMAGING

Ultrasonography—liver enlargement and alterations in echogenicity are associated with hepatic lipidosis.

OTHER DIAGNOSTIC PROCEDURES

Liver biopsy to confirm hepatic lipidosis in advanced cases.

PATHOLOGIC FINDINGS

• Findings are consistent with fatty infiltration of tissues.
• Liver and kidneys may be pale and swollen, with a greasy, cut surface.
• Capsular rupture and hemorrhage in severe cases.
• Additional sites of fatty infiltration—skeletal muscle, myocardium, and adrenal glands.
• Histopathologic findings indicate the degree of fatty infiltration of tissues.
• Pituitary adenoma(s) may be present in older horses.

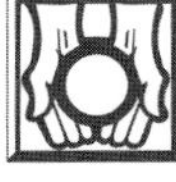

TREATMENT

AIMS OF TREATMENT

• To reverse the negative energy balance by providing more calories
• To inhibit lipolysis within adipose tissues and reduce the mobilization of FFAs
• To minimize damage to the liver and kidneys
• To control side effects of hepatic failure including hepatic encephalopathy

APPROPRIATE HEALTH CARE

• In mild cases detected early, appropriate care can be provided on the farm.
• Patient assessment is based on serum TG concentrations, duration of inappetence, and seriousness of concurrent disease conditions.
• Regardless of the initial presentation, monitor patients closely and provide treatment early in the course of disease.
• Hospitalize severely affected patients immediately.

NURSING CARE

The primary goal of these recommendations is to reverse the patient's negative energy balance.

Increase Feed Intake

- Mildly affected patients improve as their feed intake increases.
- Provide a large variety of feedstuffs or treats until a preferred diet is identified.
- If a preferred feed is identified, provide fresh samples frequently to maintain interest.
- Provide access to pasture.
- In more depressed patients, hand feeding may be necessary.

Enteral and Parenteral Feeding

- A commercial enteral diet such as Osmolite can be used for smaller patients.
- If a larger-diameter nasogastric tube can be passed, liquid preparations of alfalfa meal or soaked, pelleted feedstuffs with added dextrose can be carefully pumped into the stomach. Administer small quantities frequently (as often as q4h).
- *Caution:* Colic, enterocolitis, or laminitis may be induced, so intravenous nutritional support is the preferred treatment option.

IV Fluid/Nutritional Support

- Administer 5%–10% dextrose within polyionic fluids as a continuous infusion. An initial rate of 60 mL/kg body weight per day is recommended.
- Ideally, blood glucose measurements and urine dipstick testing should be used to establish a rate that minimizes renal overflow of glucose.
- Regular insulin can be administered as a CRI if blood glucose concentrations exceed 200 mg/dL or glucose is detected in the urine. Add 1.0 mL (100 units) regular insulin (100 units/mL) to 1 L saline (final concentration 0.1 unit/mL) and begin the CRI at rate of 2 mL/min (0.2 unit/min). Monitor blood glucose concentrations. Clinical signs of hypoglycemia include sweating, muscle fasciculations, and weakness.
- PPN can be provided using a solution composed of 50% dextrose and amino acids.

ACTIVITY

No specific restrictions but minimize stress

DIET

See Nursing Care.

CLIENT EDUCATION

- Inform clients who keep high-risk animals about hyperlipidemia and instruct them to seek veterinary advice if inappetence develops.
- Clients should recognize obesity as a serious predisposing factor, particularly in pregnant animals.

SURGICAL CONSIDERATIONS

Not applicable

MEDICATIONS

DRUG(S)

Insulin

- Increases cellular uptake of glucose, and inhibits HSL
- Reduction of lipolysis and promotion of TG synthesis within adipose tissue reduce the rate of FFA production. However, the extent to which exogenous insulin can overcome IR at times of high glucagon (i.e., fasting) or glucocorticoid (i.e., stress) activity is questionable.
- Regular insulin can be administered as described above (see Nursing Care).

Heparin Sulfate

- Potentiates LPL activity, resulting in increased VLDL clearance from the blood. However, if LPL activity is already maximized, as several reports suggest, administration of heparin would be ineffective.
- Can be administered at a dose of 10–20 IU/kg body weight IV or SQ TID
- Note that heparin lowers hematocrit levels and can inhibit hemostasis.

Other Drugs

- Consider medications such as lactulose that are administered in cases of liver failure and hepatic encephalopathy.
- After recovery, anthelmintics should be administered to remove intestinal parasites.

CONTRAINDICATIONS

- Insulin administration in hypoglycemic patients
- Use of heparin sulfate in patients that may require surgery (e.g., cesarean section)
- Corticosteroids are contraindicated as they can exacerbate insulin resistance

PRECAUTIONS

Monitor blood glucose concentrations.

POSSIBLE INTERACTIONS

N/A

ALTERNATIVE DRUGS

N/A

FOLLOW-UP

PATIENT MONITORING

Repeated measurement of serum TG concentration

PREVENTION/AVOIDANCE

- Maintain appropriate body condition and avoid obesity.
- Minimize stressful conditions for high-risk breeds, particularly when metabolic demands are high—pregnancy or lactation.
- Awareness of the disease, and early intervention when feed intake is reduced

POSSIBLE COMPLICATIONS

- Liver and renal failure
- Neurologic deficits
- Death
- Colic and laminitis may result from dietary changes.

EXPECTED COURSE AND PROGNOSIS

- The course of this disease is rapid.
- Mildly affected patients can recover quickly if the disease is detected early and the negative energy balance is reversed.
- Severely affected patients with signs of organ failure or neurologic deficits have a poorer prognosis
- Mortality rates of 57–85% have been reported, but these figures do not reflect recent advances in the treatment of this disorder. Many patients can be successfully managed with aggressive intravenous fluid therapy and PPN. If hepatic encephalopathy has not developed, the prognosis for a patient with hyperlipemia is fair, provided that finances are sufficient.

MISCELLANEOUS

ASSOCIATED CONDITIONS

- Hepatic lipidosis and subsequent liver failure
- Hepatic encephalopathy
- Renal failure

AGE-RELATED FACTORS

N/A

ZOONOTIC POTENTIAL

N/A

PREGNANCY

In pregnant animals, organ failure, metabolic acidosis, and stress may compromise the fetus, resulting in abortion.

SYNONYMS

- Hyperlipoproteinemia
- Hypertriglyceridemia

SEE ALSO

- Pituitary pars intermedia dysfunction/equine Cushing's disease
- Equine metabolic syndrome/insulin resistance
- Hepatic encephalopathy
- Liver disease

ABBREVIATIONS

- ALP = alkaline phosphatase
- AST = aspartate aminotransferase
- CRI = continuous rate infusion
- EMS = equine metabolic syndrome
- FFA = free fatty acid
- GGT = γ-glutamyltransferase
- HSL = hormone-sensitive lipase
- IR = insulin resistance
- LPL = lipoprotein lipase
- NEFAs = nonesterified fatty acids
- PPID = pituitary pars intermedia dysfunction
- PPN = partial parenteral nutrition
- SDH = sorbitol dehydrogenase
- TG = triglyceride
- VLDL = very low-density lipoprotein

Suggested Reading

Oikawa S, McGuirk S, Nishibe K, *et al*. Changes of blood biochemical values in ponies recovering from hyperlipemia in Japan. J Vet Med Sci 2006;68:353-359.

Hughes KJ, Hodgson DR, Dart AJ. Equine hyperlipaemia: a review. Aust Vet J 2004;82:136-142.

Mogg TD, Palmer JE. Hyperlipidemia, hyperlipemia, and hepatic lipidosis in American miniature horses: 23 cases (1990–1994). J Am Vet Med Assoc 1995;5:604-607.

Moore BR, Abood SK, Hinchcliff KW. Hyperlipemia in miniature horses and miniature donkeys: 1990-1993. J Vet Intern Med 1994:8;376-381.

Author Nicholas Frank
Consulting Editor Michel Lévy

HYPERTHERMIA

BASICS

DEFINITION

- An abnormally high body temperature in which the hypothalamic temperature set-point is not altered but the heat-dissipating mechanisms are overwhelmed or fail.
- Different from a fever, in which the body temperature is elevated because of upward resetting of the set-point with the heat-dissipating mechanisms remaining intact.
- Heat stroke occurs when hyperthermia is combined with dehydration and electrolyte derangement.
- Multi-organ compromise and failure will occur without medical intervention.
- Critical temperature above which the CNS becomes impaired—106° F (41° C)

PATHOPHYSIOLOGY

- The normal physiologic body temperature is set by the hypothalamic thermoregulatory center at 99.5°–101.5° F (37.5°–38.5° C).
- With fever, the set-point is altered upward by the pyrogenic effects of mediators (e.g., IL-1) released during disease states.
- With hyperthermia, the mechanisms of heat dissipation are overwhelmed or inadequate.
- Body heat is generated by working muscles and solar radiation.
- Horse muscle generates massive heat loads during work. From 70% to 80% of energy expended is in the form of heat.
- Horses have a low surface area–to–body mass ratio, so heat dissipation mechanisms can be overwhelmed.
- Evaporative loss is through sweating and breathing.
- Heat is dissipated by conduction, convection, radiation, and evaporation.
- Dilation of surface vasculature allows heat to be lost by convection.
- Heat from the body core is dissipated to the cooler surface tissues by the circulation of blood (i.e., conduction).
- Heat is lost from the body surface to cooler ambient air by radiation.
- Electrolytes, as well as water, are lost with profuse sweating and result in dehydration and metabolic derangements.
- A body temperature >103° F (39.5° C) can be considered hyperthermia.
- Heat denaturation of cellular proteins results in organ dysfunction, failure, and death. The central nervous system is most sensitive to hyperthermic damage. As the temperature continues to increase and/or persist, other systems also become affected.

SYSTEMS AFFECTED

All systems are susceptible to damage by hyperthermia.

GENETICS

Genetic predisposition to hyperthermia during anesthesia (i.e., MH) and rhabdomyolysis.

INCIDENCE/PREVALENCE

Greater in hot, humid weather

SIGNALMENT

Breeds with a massive body size–to–skin ratio have increased heat production with a relatively smaller surface area for heat dissipation.

SIGNS

Historical

- Excessive sweating or lack of sweating
- Prolonged muscular exertion (endurance rides)
- Weakness
- Stilted gait
- Fatigue
- Depression
- Impaired performance
- Respiratory distress
- Seizures
- Anesthesia
- Transport
- Foal on erythromycin

PHYSICAL EXAMINATION

- Elevated temperature associated with panting, tachypnea, tachyarrhythmia, and tachycardia
- Parameters remain elevated in spite of cessation of exercise
- Excessive, patchy, or lack of sweating associated with dehydration
- Weakness with ataxia, collapse, muscle rigidity
- SDF
- Decreased anal tone
- Prolapsed penis
- Colic
- Ileus
- Diarrhea
- Seizures
- Decreased urine production
- Dark urine
- Atrial fibrillation
- Dilated cutaneous vasculature
- Loss of appetite for food or water

CAUSES

- Excessive muscular activity—prolonged work
- Generalized seizures
- Hypocalcemic tetany associated with transit or lactation
- Drugs—erythromycin, halothane anesthesia (i.e., MH), phenothiazine tranquilizers
- Toxins–endophyte-infested tall fescue
- Anhidrosis
- Confinement in closed trailers or buildings during hot weather

RISK FACTORS

- Poor physical fitness, insufficient conditioning, and lack of acclimatization
- High ambient temperature and relative humidity
- No air movement and high solar radiation
- Foal on erythromycin, especially in hot ambient temperatures and exposed to direct solar heat
- Large body mass relative to body surface area and prolonged work
- Long hair coat (i.e., equine Cushing's syndrome), anhidrosis, and obesity
- Dehydration—no access to drinking water during work
- Airway disease (cannot dissipate heat)
- Possible risk of hyperthermia during anesthesia of horses with HPP
- MH genetic predilection
- Halothane anesthesia

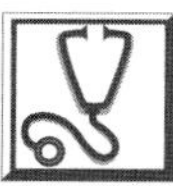

DIAGNOSIS

DIFFERENTIAL DIAGNOSES

- Fever from diseases such as infectious, inflammatory and neoplastic (usually does not exceed 106° F).
- Rule out RAO (heaves), anhidrosis, exertional rhabdomyolysis, and equine Cushing's syndrome.

CBC/BIOCHEMISTRY/URINALYSIS

- CBC—stress, hemoconcentration
- Biochemistry—elevated muscle enzymes (i.e., CK and AST) with exertional rhabdomyolysis
- Electrolyte depletion (i.e., Ca^{2+}, K^{+}, Mg^{2+})
- Sodium can be increased or decreased
- Elevated K^{+} with HPP
- Metabolic alkalosis
- Azotemia with dehydration, elevated renal and hepatic enzymes with organ damage
- Urinalysis (may be oliguric)—concentrated urine; possibly myoglobinuria

OTHER LABORATORY TESTS

- Intradermal epinephrine/terbutaline test for decreased sweating—anhidrosis
- Genetic-marker blood test for HPP
- Blood gas disorders—possible alkalosis or acidosis
- Clotting profile—development of DIC, liver failure, thrombocytopenia, prolonged clotting time, and elevated FDPs.
- Halothane—caffeine contracture test to identify individuals with MH

IMAGING

N/A

DIAGNOSTIC PROCEDURES

N/A

PATHOLOGICAL FINDINGS

N/A

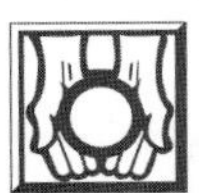

TREATMENT

- Stop exercising/activity.
- Provide shade or remove from direct sunlight.
- Enhance cooling mechanism by providing air movement—fans.
- Provide misting fans.
- Repeatedly applying cold water can be used to provide rapid cooling. This does not lessen heat loss.
- Correct dehydration by providing drinking water if patient is not critical and IV fluids if heat stroke has occurred.
- Oral and IV sources of K^+, Na^+, Cl^-, Ca^{2+}, Mg^{2+} as indicated
- IV saline, lactated Ringer's solution to restore blood volume and renal function
- Identify and correct electrolyte and acid-base derangements.
- Clip long hair coat.
- Identify and treat accordingly other conditions—rhabdomyolysis, renal failure
- Monitor rectal temperature and continue cooling until <104° F (40° C) for 15–30 min.
- SDF—Administer 300 mL of 20% calcium borogluconate in a 1:4 ratio with saline or 5% dextrose.

MEDICATIONS

DRUG(S) OF CHOICE

- Appropriate adjunctive therapy with rhabdomyolysis—muscle relaxants, anti-inflammatories
- Antipyretic drugs usually are not indicated for nonpyrogenic hyperthermia but may be useful for their anti-inflammatory properties.
- MH—dantrolene sodium 10 mg/kg loading dose PO, then 2.5 mg/kg PO q2h

CONTRAINDICATIONS

Supplemental K^+ in cases of HPP

PRECAUTIONS

- Use NSAIDs cautiously in cases of renal compromise or dehydration.
- Do not administer bicarbonate without knowing blood gas status. Note that these horses are most often alkalotic.

POSSIBLE INTERACTIONS

N/A

ALTERNATIVE DRUGS

N/A

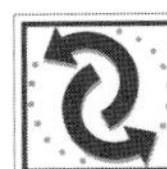

FOLLOW-UP

PATIENT MONITORING

- Monitor body temperature frequently.
- Assess for renal compromise and urination.
- Assess hydration, PCV, and total solids.
- Assess response of electrolyte and blood gas adjustments.

PREVENTION/AVOIDANCE

- A period of acclimation (15 days has been shown to be beneficial) to hot and humid conditions will help reduce the risk of heat related disorders.
- Condition animals appropriately for the level of work they are expected to do.
- Avoid riding in very hot and humid weather.
- Identify MH and HPP individuals prior to anesthesia.
- Keep foals on erythromycin in a shaded, cool environment.

POSSIBLE COMPLICATIONS

- CNS failure—seizures, coma, death
- Renal and hepatic failure
- DIC
- Laminitis
- Pulmonary edema
- May be more prone to subsequent hyperthermia

EXPECTED COURSE AND PROGNOSIS

Favorable to grave—depending on early detection and reversal of hyperthermia, correction of dehydration and electrolyte derangements, and prevention of organ failure

MISCELLANEOUS

ASSOCIATED CONDITIONS

N/A

AGE-RELATED FACTORS

N/A

ZOONOTIC POTENTIAL

N/A

PREGNANCY

Abortions may occur with prolonged hyperthermia.

SYNONYMS

- Exhausted horse syndrome
- Heat exhaustion
- Heat stress

SEE ALSO

- Anhidrosis
- Rhabdomyolysis
- Fever
- Seizures
- SDF
- MH

ABBREVIATIONS

- AST = aspartate aminotransferase
- CK = creatinine phosphokinase
- CNS = central nervous system
- DIC = disseminated intravascular coagulation
- FDPs = fibrinogen degradation products
- HPP = hyperkalemic periodic paralysis
- IL-1 = interleukin 1
- MH = malignant hyperthermia
- PCV = packed cell volume
- SDF = synchronous diaphragmatic flutter

Suggested Reading

Cohn CW, Hinchcliff KW, McKeever KH. Evaluation of washing with cold water to facilitate heat dissipation in horses exercised in hot, humid conditions. Am J Vet Res 1999;60:299–305.

Foreman JH. The exhausted horse syndrome. Vet Clin North Am Equine Pract 1998;14:205-219.

Hines MT. Changes in body temperature. In: Reed SM, Bayly WM, Sellon DC, eds. Equine Internal Medicine, ed 2. St. Louis: Saunders, 2004:148-155.

White SL. Alterations in body temperature. In: Smith BP, ed. Large Animal Internal Medicine, ed 3. St. Louis: Mosby, 2002:36-45.

Author Wendy Duckett
Consulting Editor Michel Lévy

HYPOXEMIA

BASICS

DEFINITION

- A decreased amount of oxygen carried in the arterial blood (oxygen content)
- Can be measured indirectly as a Pa_{O_2} of <80 mm Hg or as arterial hemoglobin saturation levels <95%
- Cellular function is adversely affected at a Pa_{O_2} of <60 mm Hg.
- Venous oxygen tension of <40 mm Hg is highly suggestive of arterial hypoxemia.

PATHOPHYSIOLOGY

- Can develop by several mechanisms—hypoventilation; diffusion impairment from interstitial exudate, edema, or fibrosis; right-to-left cardiac or intrapulmonary shunt; and $\dot{V}/\dot{Q}$ mismatch
- Low levels of inspired oxygen as seen at high altitudes result in hypoxemia.
- Abnormalities of hemoglobin structure or function (e.g., methemoglobinemia) decrease the oxygen-carrying capacity of hemoglobin (Sa_{O_2}); however, Pa_{O_2} may be normal.
- More than one mechanism often is present in many patients.
- $\dot{V}/\dot{Q}$ mismatch is the most frequent and significant cause in anesthetized or recumbent patients, because many factors contribute to this phenomenon—any alteration of pulmonary blood flow or ventilation as well as the matching of these two components can limit the amount of oxygen transferred.

SYSTEMS AFFECTED

- Cardiovascular
- Nervous
- Respiratory

SIGNALMENT

- Any horse
- Most anesthetized horses maintained on room air develop hypoxemia from $\dot{V}/\dot{Q}$ mismatch, which develops from atelectasis and variations in pulmonary blood flow, which develop with recumbency.

SIGNS

Historical Findings

Owners may report signs of exercise intolerance, respiratory difficulty, coughing, lethargy, and other signs referable to the primary problem.

Physical Examination Findings

- Tachypnea and tachycardia usually are present.
- Cyanosis does not develop until P_{O_2} is <40 mm Hg.
- Mucous membranes may be pale, hyperemic, or muddy with endotoxemia or cardiovascular disease/compromise.
- Other clinical signs relative to primary disease states may be present—nasal discharge, coughing, and abnormal lung sounds with respiratory disease; jugular vein distention, murmurs, arrhythmias, and ventral edema with cardiac failure or congenital defects.

CAUSES

- Hypoventilation has many causes (see Acidosis, Respiratory) but rarely is the sole factor responsible for hypoxemia, because a Pa_{O_2} of <60 mm Hg stimulates respiration and increases minute ventilation. This may correct hypercapnia but often does not improve oxygen levels. Oxygen does not diffuse as quickly as CO_2 and is more dependent on the matching of blood flow to ventilation to obtain normal levels.
- High altitude reduces the inspired oxygen tension, but it is uncommon, although not unknown, for horses at high altitude.
- Diffusion impairment results from respiratory diseases such as viral, bacterial, or interstitial pneumonia; allergic small airway disease; heaves; and inhalation of toxic substances (e.g., smoke). Pulmonary edema is uncommon in horses but may occur with anaphylaxis, airway obstruction, chordae tendinea rupture, or cardiac failure.
- $\dot{V}/\dot{Q}$ inequality develops with changes in pulmonary blood flow locally, as with pulmonary hypertension, or systemically, as with hypotension. Atelectasis and other causes of hypoventilation also contribute to $\dot{V}/\dot{Q}$ mismatch.
- General anesthesia is a major cause of both atelectasis and alterations of pulmonary blood flow; mismatch generally is always present in anesthetized horses and can be severe enough to result in hypoxemia even when the F_{IO_2} is 100%.
- Right-to-left cardiac shunts (e.g., tetralogy of Fallot, truncus arteriosus, tricuspid atresia) produce hypoxemia, because pulmonary blood flow is greatly diminished. Persistent fetal circulation produces hypoxemia via right-to-left shunting through the foramen ovale and ductus arteriosus and pulmonary hypertension.
- Cardiac failure is uncommon in horses but results in hypoxemia via pulmonary edema and pulmonary hypertension and, sometimes, hypoventilation if pleural or peritoneal effusion is significant.
- Endotoxic shock produces hypoxemia via several mechanisms—pulmonary hypertension, endothelial cell damage, decreased cardiac contractility, systemic hypotension, and so on.

RISK FACTORS

- All horses are susceptible to hypoxemia during general anesthesia, especially if oxygen supplementation is not utilized.
- Premature foals or term neonates born to mares with systemic illness during pregnancy or that experience dystocia or asphyxia during parturition are predisposed.
- Horses with allergic airway diseases may develop hypoxemia with acute attacks or with progression of the disease.
- Acidotic patients and those with cardiovascular compromise are more likely to develop hypoxemia.

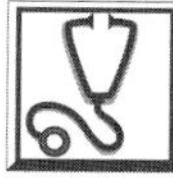

DIAGNOSIS

DIFFERENTIAL DIAGNOSIS

Diseases that present with tachypnea, dyspnea, or cyanosis

LABORATORY FINDINGS

Drugs That May Alter Lab Results

N/A

Disorders That May Alter Lab Results

- With poor peripheral perfusion or cardiovascular shunt, results of blood gas analysis on samples taken from peripheral arteries may differ from those taken elsewhere or may not reflect the patient's overall systemic condition.
- Exposure to room air via air bubbles in arterial blood samples increases the P_{O_2} tension, because the sample equilibrates with the air.
- Ideally, arterial samples should be collected into glass syringes and stored on ice for <2 hr.

Valid If Run in Human Lab?

Yes, if properly submitted

CBC/BIOCHEMISTRY/URINALYSIS

N/A

OTHER LABORATORY TESTS

- Arterial blood gas analysis is the definitive method for documenting hypoxemia.
- Take a heparinized blood sample anaerobically, cap with a rubber stopper, and analyze within 15–20 min.
- If the sample is stored on ice, results are valid for up to 3–4 hr if analysis must be delayed.
- Handheld analyzers are available for use with equine patients, or the sample may be sent to a commercial laboratory or hospital.

IMAGING

Radiography or ultrasound (with or without contrast enhancement) is very helpful in evaluating cardiac and pulmonary disease.

DIAGNOSTIC PROCEDURES

- Pulse oximetry can be used to measure and monitor hemoglobin saturation.
- The oximeter calculates the amount of oxygenated versus deoxygenated hemoglobin in blood based on light absorption.
- Inaccurate readings can be seen with decreased blood flow in the area where the probe is attached because of hypotension, vasoconstriction, or local or systemic hypothermia.
- Probes designed for the tongue or earlobe of other species can be used on the tongue of anesthetized horses.
- Conscious patients require use of a nasal probe.

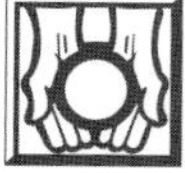

TREATMENT

Resolution of the primary cause of hypoxemia is the most effective therapy.

OXYGEN THERAPY

- Oxygen therapy via nasal insufflation can be quite effective in elevating the Pa_{O_2}. Inspired concentrations are limited to 30%–45% with nasal insufflation. Higher levels may be obtained via insufflation directly into the trachea.
- Inspired gases must be humidified to avoid damage to mucous membranes from desiccation. This is readily accomplished by use of a humidifier or passing the oxygen through a bottle of sterile water before exposure to the airway. The bottle must be secured in an upright position to prevent inspiration of fluid.
- To avoid oxygen toxicity, maintain the F_{IO_2} at the lowest level that produces a P_{O_2} of >80 mm Hg. If insufflation eliminates hypoxemia, P_{CO_2}

levels may increase if the low Po_2 was the primary stimulus of respiratory drive.
• Begin insufflation at 3–5 L/min in foals and 5–10 L/min in adults.

POSTURAL THERAPY AND THORACIC PERCUSSION

• Helpful to improve ventilation and drainage of secretions, especially in foals.
• Maintenance in sternal recumbency is best; turning every few hours is necessary for those in lateral recumbency.

MECHANICAL VENTILATION

• Necessary in patients with severe hypoventilation (Pco_2 persistently >65 mm Hg) and hypoxemia, and feasible in foals and anesthetized adults.
• Conscious foals can be intubated nasotracheally and connected to the rebreathing circuit of a small-animal anesthesia machine.
• Two flowmeters (or one that allows mixing of O_2 and room air) are necessary, as is a monitor that can measure Fio_2 level.
• Assisted rather than controlled ventilation usually is better, because most foals are more comfortable and respiratory drive is not eliminated, making weaning somewhat easier.
• Sedation may be necessary in some patients, but many relax once ventilation improves.
• Periodic suctioning of the nasotracheal tube is necessary to prevent obstruction from accumulated secretions.
• After weaning from mechanical ventilation, temporary nasal insufflation of oxygen is recommended in foals, because their functional residual capacity will decrease and hypoxemia may recur.

SUPPLEMENTAL OXYGEN

• Should improve Pao_2 levels with all causes of hypoxemia, except right-to-left cardiac shunts, persistent fetal circulation, and severe $\dot{V}/\dot{Q}$ mismatch, which is essentially an intrapulmonary physiologic shunt.

MEDICATIONS

DRUG(S) OF CHOICE

• Supportive therapy aimed at improvement in any factors contributing to hypoxemia is useful.
• Hypovolemic or hypotensive patients benefit from fluid therapy and inotropes—dobutamine or dopamine.
• Endotoxemic patients may improve with anti-inflammatory therapy.
• Bronchodilation may help in some respiratory conditions, especially small airway diseases.
• Methylxanthines or β_2-agonists (e.g., clenbuterol, albuterol) PO or via aerosol therapy may improve gas exchange in some cases if bronchospasm exists.
• Infusions of doxapram or methylxanthines (e.g., aminophylline, caffeine) may improve respiratory function in neonates.

CONTRAINDICATIONS

• *Do not* use doxapram to improve respiratory function in healthy anesthetized patients, especially during weaning. Its effects are temporary, and if the patient's CO_2 levels are still low or the patient remains depressed once it wears off, apnea may occur.
• Mechanical ventilation for meconium aspiration because of the risk of air-trapping behind obstructed bronchioles and subsequent alveolar damage.

PRECAUTIONS

• Do not allow combustible materials or smoking in the vicinity of the patient or the oxygen tanks.
• Securely attach tanks to a wall or other immovable structure, because they can rupture or explode violently if knocked over.
• Wear safety glasses, and the operator should keep his or her face out of range of the valves during setup and disconnection.
• Use aseptic techniques in handling endotracheal tubes to prevent secondary pneumonia.
• Side effects of methylxanthines and β_2-agonists are not uncommon; therapeutic doses are close to toxic doses. Monitor patients for restlessness, sweating, tachycardia, and arrhythmia.
• Use fluid therapy carefully in neonates and cardiac patients to avoid volume overload.
• Arrhythmias are not uncommon with inotrope therapy; monitor cardiac rhythm closely.
• Oxygen toxicity can occur with administration of >50% O_2 or maintenance of a Pao_2 >100 mm Hg for long periods.

POSSIBLE INTERACTIONS

• Cimetidine, erythromycin, and other inhibitors of hepatic microsomal activity may decrease clearance and increase serum levels of methylxanthines.
• Rifampin, chloramphenicol, and other inducers of hepatic metabolism decrease serum levels of xanthine derivatives by increasing clearance.

ALTERNATIVE DRUGS

N/A

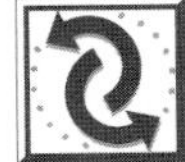

FOLLOW-UP

PATIENT MONITORING

• Serial evaluation of arterial Po_2
• Pulse oximetry can be used to monitor hemoglobin saturation. However, measure blood gases intermittently, because the hemoglobin O_2 cannot be >100% even when the Fio_2 may be much higher.
• As the Pao_2 improves, provide decreasing levels of Fio_2. Eventually, periodic trials on room air can be attempted.
• Evaluate patient demeanor and degree or quality of respiratory effort as blood gas levels. When the patient can maintain a Po_2 of >70 mm Hg (>60 mm Hg in premature neonates) on room air, oxygen therapy can be discontinued.

POSSIBLE COMPLICATIONS

• Damage to nervous tissue from prolonged periods of hypoxemia may result in brain damage as exhibited by altered consciousness, blindness, seizures, and so on.
• Cardiac arrhythmias may be caused by hypoxemic damage to the myocardium.

MISCELLANEOUS

ASSOCIATED CONDITIONS

Metabolic acidosis caused by accumulation of lactic acid from anaerobic glycolysis may develop with prolonged hypoxemia, especially if hypotension exists.

AGE-RELATED FACTORS

Premature neonates are highly predisposed to hypoxemia.

PREGNANCY

• Heavily pregnant mares are at greater risk of hypoxemia under general anesthesia.
• Prolonged hypoxemia during gestation may result in fetal growth retardation and hypoxic-ischemic syndrome at parturition.

ABBREVIATIONS

• $\dot{V}/\dot{Q}$ = ventilation-perfusion ratio
• Fio_2 = fractional percent inspired oxygen concentration
• Pao_2 = partial pressure of arterial oxygen tension, mmHg
• $Paco_2$ = partial pressure of arterial carbon dioxide tension, mmHg
• Sao_2 = arterial oxygen saturation—the % of hemoglobin sites that are bound to oxygen
• HbO_2 = hemoglobin saturation

Suggested Reading

Palmer J. Ventilatory support of the neonatal foal. Vet Clin North Am Equine Pract 1994:10:167–186.

Picandet V, Jeanneret S, Lavoie J-P. Effects of syringe type and storage temperature on results of blood gas analysis in arterial blood of horses. J Vet Intern Med 2007:21;476–481.

Tranquilli WJ, et al., eds. Lumb & Jones' Veterinary Anesthesia and Analgesia, ed 4. Ames, IA: Blackwell Publishing Ltd, 2007:495–532.

Tranquilli WJ, et al., eds. Lumb & Jones' Veterinary Anesthesia and Analgesia, ed 4. Ames, IA: Blackwell Publishing Ltd, 2007:533–560.

Tranquilli WJ, et al., eds. Lumb & Jones' Veterinary Anesthesia and Analgesia, ed 4. Ames, IA: Blackwell Publishing Ltd, 2007:117–152.

Author Jennifer G. Adams
Consulting Editor Kenneth W. Hinchcliff

ICTERUS (PREHEPATIC, HEPATIC, AND POSTHEPATIC)

BASICS

DEFINITION

Icterus is caused by hyperbilirubinemia with concomitant bilirubin deposition in tissues. It is characterized by yellow discoloration of the sclerae, nonpigmented skin, and mucous membranes.

PATHOPHYSIOLOGY

• Bilirubin, derived from breakdown of heme, is first converted to biliverdin and then to unconjugated bilirubin, which is bound to albumin in plasma for transfer to the liver. Uncongugated bilirubin is not filtered by the kidneys but is taken up by hepatocytes, where it is conjugated. •Conjugated bilirubin is secreted into the bile and enters the intestine where most of it is converted by anaerobic bacteria to urobilinogen. Some conjugated bilirubin, which is water soluble, enters the general circulation. If the concentration is high enough, it is filtered by the kidneys and appears in the urine.
• Hyperbilirubinemia can result from increased bilirubin production, impaired hepatic uptake or conjugation of bilirubin, or impaired bilirubin excretion.

SYSTEMS AFFECTED

• Skin/exocrine—Bilirubin has an affinity for elastic tissues; thus icterus is most evident in the sclerae and vulva.
• Hepatobiliary—Accumulated bilirubin may contribute to hepatocellular injury and cholestasis. • Renal/urologic—Bile casts may cause tubular injury. • Nervous—Bilirubin accumulation may cause degenerative lesions (e.g., kernicterus, a rare condition reported in neonates).

INCIDENCE/PREVALENCE

Depends on primary disease condition

GEOGRAPHIC DISTRIBUTION

Depends on primary disease condition

SIGNALMENT

Depends on primary disease condition

SIGNS

Clinical Findings

• Depression • Anorexia • Icterus • Severely altered mentation—HE is attributed to hypoglycemia, hyperammonemia, decreased BCAA:AAA ratio, increased concentrations of mercaptans, sulfur-containing amino acids, and short-chain fatty acids in plasma. • Weight loss —due to anorexia or failure of hepatic metabolic functions in chronic hepatic insufficiency
• Acute or recurrent subacute abdominal pain—caused by hepatic swelling or biliary obstruction (e.g., cholelithiasis)

Less Frequent

• Photodermatitis—from accumulation of phylloerythrin in skin • Diarrhea—with chronic hepatic insufficiency and caused by altered intestinal microflora or portal hypertension
• Bleeding diathesis—caused by inadequate hepatic synthesis of clotting factors • Dependent edema—associated with hypoalbuminemia or portal hypertension • May include ascites, tenesmus, pruritus, fever, pale mucous membranes, pigmenturia, and polydypsia

CAUSES

Prehepatic (Hemolytic) Icterus

Associated with intravascular hemolysis and/or extravascular hemolysis or with massive intracorporeal hemorrhage where the rate of bilirubin production exceeds the liver's ability to conjugate and excrete it.
• Oxidative injury—red maple leaf (*Acer rubrum*), wild onion (*Allium* sp.), phenothiazine toxicosis, and nitrate poisoning • Immune mediated—neonatal isoerythrolysis, IMHA (secondary to *Clostridium perfringens* septicemia, purpura hemorrhagica, lymphosarcoma, penicillin administration, etc.), AIHA, DIC (i.e., microangiopathic hemolytic anemia)
• Infectious—EIA, equine piroplasmosis, equine granulocytic ehrlichiosis, leptospirosis
• Iatrogenic—concentrated DMSO (>10%) IV, hypotonic or hypertonic fluids
• Miscellaneous—snake venoms (rattlesnake, copperhead, water moccasin) and terminal hepatic failure

Hepatic (Retention) Icterus

Impaired uptake and/or conjugation of bilirubin by the liver

Hepatic Causes of Hepatic Icterus

Acute Hepatic Diseases (Adult Horses)
• Idiopathic—serum hepatitis (Theiler's disease)
• Bacterial—primary or secondary bacterial cholangiohepatitis, bacterial endotoxemia, and infectious necrotic hepatitis caused by *Clostridium novyi* type B • Viral—EIA and EVA
• Parasitic—migration of *Strongylus equinus* and *S. edentatus* or thromboembolic disease from *S. equinus* • Toxic—arsenic, carbon tetrachloride, chlorinated hydrocarbons, monensin, pentachlorophenols, phenol, phosphorus, paraquat, aflatoxin, and rubratoxin
• Drugs—anabolic steroids and erythromycin
Acute Hepatic Diseases (Foals)
• Bacterial—Tyzzer's disease (*Bacillus piliformis*), bacterial septicemia, and bacterial endotoxemia
• Viral—EHV-1 • Parasitic—*Parascaris equorum* and strongyles • Toxic—ferrous fumarate and toxins listed for adults
Chronic Hepatic Diseases (Adults)
• Idiopathic—chronic active hepatitis
• Bacterial—hepatic abscessation (*Streptococcus equi*) • Metabolic—hyperlipemia and hepatic lipidosis • Neoplastic—primary (e.g., cholangiocarcinoma, hepatocellular carcinoma) and secondary (e.g., lymphosarcoma)
• Immunologic—amyloidosis • Toxic—chronic megalocytic hepatopathy caused by *Senecio* sp., *Crotolaria* sp., or *Heliotropium* sp.
Chronic Hepatic Diseases (Foals)
• Bacterial—hepatic abscessation (secondary to septicemia or omphalophlebitis)
• Neoplastic—mixed hamartoma

Extrahepatic Causes of Hepatic Icterus

• Anorexia • Heparin administration
• Prematurity

Posthepatic (Obstructive) Icterus

Partial or complete obstruction of the biliary tree that decreases biliary excretion of conjugated bilirubin. Usually accompanied by bilirubinuria.
• Adults—cholelithiasis, large colon displacement, cholangitis, neoplastic infiltration, fibrosis or hyperplasia of the biliary tract, and hepatitis • Foals—acquired biliary obstruction (e.g., healing duodenal ulcer adjacent to hepatopancreatic ampulla) or congenital biliary atresia

RISK FACTORS

• Previous administration of equine-origin biologic (i.e., tetanus antitoxin)—serum hepatitis • Septicemia or omphalophlebitis in foals • Duodenal ulceration • Poor parasite control • Inadequate vaccination • Exposure to toxic plants and environmental toxins • Use of certain drugs • Anorexic, obese pony or Miniature Horse

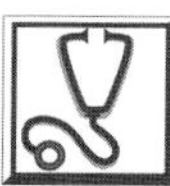

DIAGNOSIS

DIFFERENTIAL DIAGNOSIS

Prehepatic Icterus

• Prehepatic icterus generally is characterized by an abrupt onset of exercise intolerance, weakness, fever, tachypnea and dyspnea, tachycardia, mucous membrane pallor, mild jaundice, and, in some cases, pigmenturia. • The hemolytic crisis that occurs in some horses with terminal liver failure could lead to a misdiagnosis of prehepatic icterus.

Hepatic and Posthepatic Icterus

• History and clinical signs for hepatic and posthepatic icterus are quite similar and may include chronic weight loss, diarrhea, abdominal pain, altered mentation, photodermatitis, and pruritus. These signs are usually not observed in prehepatic icterus. • Icterus is more pronounced in posthepatic than hepatic icterus because conjugated bilirubin causes more pronounced icterus than unconjugated bilirubin. • Recurrent abdominal pain is a frequent feature of posthepatic icterus as is pyrexia caused by secondary bacterial cholangitis.

CBC/BIOCEHEMISTRY/URINALYSIS

Prehepatic Icterus

• Severe anemia (usually regenerative), Heinz bodies, or spherocytes • Marked increase in unconjugated bilirubin with some increase in conjugated bilirubin • Mildly increased ALP and SDH • Normal to low glucose • Normal to high BUN • Normal albumin • Bilirubinuria

Hepatic Icterus

• Mild, nonregenerative anemia. • Moderate increase in unconjugated bilirubin (rarely >25 mg/dL) and mild to moderate increase in conjugated bilirubin (up to 25% of total bilirubin) • Mild to moderate increases in GGT, AST, and SDH; mild increase in ALP • Normal to low glucose • Normal to low BUN • Normal to low albumin • Normal to slight increase in urinary bilirubin • Normal to low urinary urobilinogen

Posthepatic Icterus

• Mild, nonregenerative anemia • Normal to mild increase in unconjugated bilirubin and marked increase in conjugated bilirubin (>25%–50% of total bilirubin) • Normal to

ICTERUS (PREHEPATIC, HEPATIC, AND POSTHEPATIC)

mild increase in AST and SDH, moderate to marked increase in GGT and marked increase in ALP • Albumin, glucose, and BUN often are normal • Marked bilirubinuria • Urinary urobilinogen (absent) with complete bile duct obstruction

OTHER LABORATORY TESTS

Prehepatic Icterus

• Giemsa or NMB stain for intraerythrocytic parasites • Saline agglutination test • Direct antiglobulin (Coombs) test • Osmotic fragility test

Hepatic and Posthepatic Icterus

• Serum bile acids—highest in obstructive liver disease but not discriminating • Blood ammonia concentration not correlated with severity of hepatic encephalopathy and not discriminating • Serum prothrombin time may be prolonged but not discriminating • Serology for infectious diseases in patients with hepatic icterus • Serum triglycerides—marked increased in hyperlipemia

IMAGING

Utrasonography

• To determine liver size, presence of abscesses, cysts, choleliths, dilated bile ducts, or neoplasms • To demonstrate (sometimes) abnormal intrahepatic or extrahepatic blood flow • To guide liver biopsy

OTHER DIAGNOSTIC PROCEDURES

Liver Biopsy

• Yields diagnostic, prognostic, and therapeutic information • Samples—obtained using ultrasound-guided percutaneous or blind techniques and placed in formalin for histopathology and transport media for microbiology • Complications—hemorrhage, pneumothorax, spread of infectious hepatitis, and peritonitis (e.g., through contamination with bile or colonic ingesta). • Complications minimized by performing hemostasis profile and using ultrasound guidance

PATHOLOGIC FINDINGS

• Yellow discoloration of mucous membranes and body fat stores • Other findings depend on the primary disease condition.

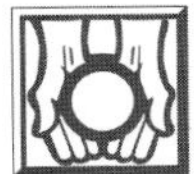

TREATMENT

APPROPRIATE HEALTH CARE

Varies, depending on the underlying cause

NURSING CARE

• In the first 24 hr, use IV fluid therapy (5% dextrose at 2 mL/kg per hour) for hypoglycemic patients with signs of HE. • After 24 hr, substitute 2.5%–5% dextrose in lactated Ringer's solution (60 mL/kg per day). • In anorexic patients, add potassium chloride (20–40 mEq/L) to fluids. • Treatment can best be accomplished in a hospital environment.

ACTIVITY

Restrict activity, and avoid sunlight.

DIET

For patients with hepatic and posthepatic icterus, a diet that provides 40–50 kcal/kg in the form of low-protein, high-energy feeds rich in BCAAs (e.g., milo, sorghum, beet pulp) is recommended.

CLIENT EDUCATION

Depends on primary disease condition

SURGICAL CONSIDERATIONS

• Foals with acquired bile duct obstruction
• Horses with colonic displacement causing acute bile duct obstruction

MEDICATIONS

DRUG(S) OF CHOICE

Prehepatic Icterus

• Treatment of IMHA (corticosteroids)
• Whole-blood transfusion if indicated • Fluid therapy (lactated Ringer's solution 60 mL/kg per day) to promote diuresis

Hepatic and Posthepatic Icterus

• Manage clinical signs of HE with sedation (e.g., xylazine,or diazepam) if the patient is convulsing, and decrease production and absorption of toxic metabolites (mineral oil via nasogastric tube: lactulose 0.3 mL/kg PO q6 h or neomycin 10–100 mg/kg PO q6 h). Oral BCAA concentrates can be formulated, and IV preparations are available. • Weekly supplementation with vitamin K_1 (40–50 mg/450 kg daily) as well as vitamin B_1 and folic acid when cholestasis is present
• Antimicrobial therapy based on results of culture and sensitivity. Empiric therapy for suppurative cholangitis includes trimethoprim-sulfamethoxazole or a β-lactam and an aminoglycoside. Use metronidazole if an anaerobic infection is suspected. • Chronic active hepatitis is treated with corticosteroids—dexamethasone (0.05–0.1 mg/kg per day for 4–7 days, then gradually tapering the dose over 2–3 weeks), followed by prednisolone (1 mg/kg per day for several weeks).

CONTRAINDICATIONS

• Hepatotoxic drugs—anticonvulsants, anabolic steroids, phenothiazines, and macrolides (e.g., erythromycin) • Tetracyclines, which suppress hepatic protein synthesis • Drugs eliminated primarily by the liver—analgesics, anesthetics, barbiturates, and chloramphenicol

PRECAUTIONS

• Avoid use of drugs listed above. • Use sedatives that are metabolized by the liver at reduced dosages. • Use corticosteroids cautiously as they may exacerbate intercurrent infections.

POSSIBLE INTERACTIONS

For many drugs, duration and intensity of action may be increased in patients with hepatobiliary disease.

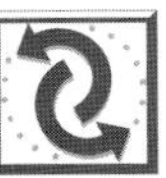

FOLLOW-UP

PATIENT MONITORING

Prehepatic Icterus

• Recheck PCV as needed. • Repeat transfusions if required.

Hepatic and Posthepatic Icterus

• Monitor liver enzyme activities and bilirubin concentration to assess progression. • Repeat biopsies to monitor progression.

PREVENTION/AVOIDANCE

Depends on primary disease condition

POSSIBLE COMPLICATIONS

Horses that are icteric because of anorexia or cholestatic drugs (e.g., heparin) do not suffer long-term complications.

EXPECTED COURSE AND PROGNOSIS

Depends on primary disease condition

MISCELLANEOUS

ASSOCIATED CONDITIONS

Prehepatic Icterus

• Hemoglobinemic nephrosis • Hemic murmur

Hepatic and Posthepatic Icterus

• See Clinical Findings.

AGE RELATED FACTORS

• See Differential Diagnosis.

ZOONOTIC POTENTIAL

Leptospirosis may be transmitted to people.

PREGNANCY

Pregnant or lactating, obese ponies and Miniature Horses are predisposed to hyperlipemia.

SYNONYMS

• Hyperbilirubinemia • Jaundice

SEE ALSO

• Hemolytic anemia • Liver disease topics

ABBREVIATIONS

• AAA = aromatic amino acids • AIHA = autoimmune-mediated hemolytic anemia • ALP = alkaline phosphatase • AST = aspartate aminotransferase • BCAA = branched-chain amino acid • DIC = disseminated intravascular coagulation • EIA = equine infectious anemia • EHV-1 = equine herpesvirus 1 • EVA = equine viral arteritis • GGT = γ-glutamyltransferase • HE = hepatoencephalopathy • IMHA = immune-mediated hemolytic anemia • NMB = new methylene blue • PCV = packed cell volume • SDH = sorbitol dehydrogenase

Suggested Reading

Barton MH. Disorders of the liver. In: Reed SM, Bayly WM, Sellon DC, eds. Equine Internal Medicine. Philadelphia: WB Saunders, 2004.

Author Jeanne Lofstedt
Consulting Editor Michel Lévy

IDIOPATHIC COLITIS

BASICS

DEFINITION

A severe undifferentiated active inflammatory condition within the large colon associated with local and systemic pathophysiologic events resulting in a variety of clinical signs, the most prominent of which is diarrhea. The cause is not known, and it was formerly referred to as *colitis X*.

PATHOPHYSIOLOGY

In the adult horse, colitis is commonly observed after a disturbance of the normal colonic flora upsetting homeostasis of absorption, secretion, permeability, and motility. This will result in net colonic fluid accumulation, systemic electrolyte imbalances, protein loss, overactivity, or loss of coagulation factors with a net intestinal wall inflammation. These alterations result in diarrhea. Underlying infectious agents causing disease are suspected but are often not identified.

SYSTEMS AFFECTED

Gastrointestinal

The main clinical sign in idiopathic colitis is diarrhea. Signs of colic varying from mild to severe may be present. Abdominal distention can also occur. Intestinal hyperactivity or ileus may be present.

Cardiovascular

Varying degrees of dehydration and cardiovascular shock may be observed. Systemic and local thromboembolic events, including venous thrombosis of injection or catheter sites, have been described.

Musculoskeletal

Laminitis may develop in affected animals. Peripheral edema if severe hypoproteinemia.

Respiratory

Septic emboli leading to pulmonary abscess formation may be observed in the lungs.

GENETICS

There is no known genetic basis for idiopathic colitis.

INCIDENCE/PREVALENCE

Idiopathic colitis is a sporadic condition

SIGNALMENT

There is no reported breed, age, or sex predilection. Foals as young as 24 hr of age may be affected.

SIGNS

Historical

Occasionally, animals may be presented before the development of diarrhea with colic, abdominal distension, depression, anorexia, and pyrexia. When present, diarrhea can range from cow-pie consistency to profuse and watery to hemorrhagic. There may or may not be a history of recent antibiotic use. Feeding, recent deworming, transport, surgery, and other management changes (stressors) may have occurred.

Physical Examination

Diarrhea is present in most cases. Dehydration, fever, and tachycardia are common. Gastrointestinal sounds auscultate fluid, and may be hypermotile or hypomotile. Characteristic sounds may be detected on auscultation of the ventral abdomen in colitis secondary to chronic sand impaction. Signs of endotoxemia such as hyperemic mucous membranes may be present. Marked intestinal distention may be seen, especially in peracute, severe cases, and may cause colic. Gastric reflux can occur as consequence of ileus. Peripheral edema may be present secondary to hypoproteinemia or vasculitis. This disease often has a very fulminant character and horses may succumb to it within 8–24 hr.

CAUSES

A variety of enteric pathogens are likely to be involved but are not identified with common diagnostic procedures.

RISK FACTORS

Antibiotic use is a well-documented risk factor. Additional postulated causes include transportation, dietary changes, surgery, and other gastrointestinal disorders (e.g., impactions).

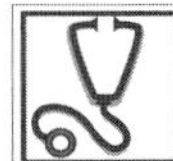

DIAGNOSIS

DIFFERENTIAL DIAGNOSES

• Salmonellosis • *Clostridium difficile* enterocolitis • *Clostridium perfringens* enterocolitis • Potomac horse fever
• Cyathostomiasis • NSAID-induced colitis
• Cantharidin toxicosis • Chronic sand impaction

CBC/BIOCHEMISTRY/URINALYSIS

CBC

Elevated PCV from dehydration and splenic contraction is common. Serum protein levels may be increased due to hemoconcentration, although hypoproteinemia due to protein loss into the gastrointestinal wall and lumen is more frequent. Leukopenia with neutropenia and a left shift is often present early. Toxic changes may be present in neutrophils. At later stages of disease or in milder cases, a leukocytosis and neutrophilia may be present.

Biochemistry

Serum sodium and chloride levels are typically decreased. Potassium levels may be increased in animals with a metabolic acidosis, or decreased concurrently with sodium and chloride, especially in anorexic animals. Hypocalcemia and hypoalbuminemia are also common. These changes are likely due to electrolyte and protein loss into the intestinal lumen. A prerenal azotemia is common in dehydrated animals.

Urinalysis

An increase in urine specific gravity is frequently present as a response to dehydration.

OTHER LABORATORY TESTS

• Acid-base assessment—In severe cases a marked metabolic acidosis develops, and the extent of negative base excess has been used as a prognostic indicator for survival.
• As idiopathic colitis is a diagnosis of exclusion, appropriate samples should be submitted to rule out the common infectious causes of colitis. In endemic areas, hay should be inspected for the presence of *Epicauta* beetles.

IMAGING

Abdominal Ultrasonography

The large colon may appear fluid filled and excess motility may be observed. Edematous large colon may be identified.

DIAGNOSTIC PROCEDURES

Rectal palpation should be performed to ensure that other problems, such as a surgical lesion, are not present. This should be performed with caution, as the rectal mucosa may be friable.

PATHOLOGICAL FINDINGS

Marked exfoliation of colonic and cecal mucosal epithelial cells and hemorrhagic colitis-typhlitis, with thrombosis of the intestinal mucosal capillaries, are common. Pulmonary and renal tissues lesions when present are suggestive of endotoxemia.

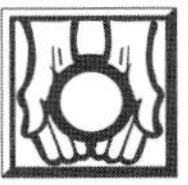

TREATMENT

APPROPRIATE HEALTH CARE

This condition is best managed with intensive inpatient care. Cases with mild diarrhea and adequate hydration may be treated at the farm but require close monitoring as a rapid deterioration of the horse 's condition may occur.

NURSING CARE

• Intravenous fluid therapy using a balanced electrolyte solution (e.g., lactated Ringer's solution) is mandatory in most cases. The rate of fluid administration depends on the degree of dehydration and the fluid loss through diarrhea. The use of two large-bore catheters in separate veins may help deliver a large volume of fluid for the rapid correction of fluid deficits in severely dehydrated horses. After correction of dehydration, intravenous administration of maintenance fluids (50–100 mL/kg/day) plus the estimated fluid loss through diarrhea should be continued. Once the diarrhea begins to resolve, the rate of fluid administration can be decreased. Hydration status should be assessed frequently because affected animals may become dehydrated even in the presence of fluid therapy. Mild to moderate cases of metabolic acidosis typically resolve with fluid therapy. Sodium bicarbonate administration may be required with severe metabolic acidosis. In severely hypokalemic horses, 20–40 mEq/L of KCl can be added to lactated Ringer's solution or saline. Intravenous administration of KCl should not exceed 0.5 mEq/kg/hr. An oral electrolyte solution containing 35 g KCl and 70 g NaCl in 10 L of water should be provided, along with clean, fresh drinking water and a salt block. Intravenous administration of hypertonic saline (4–6 mL/kg of 5%–7.5% NaCl) may be indicated in severely dehydrated animals. It is essential that isotonic fluid therapy follow the use of hypertonic saline.
• Due to the high incidence of venous thrombosis in colitis, the catheter site should be monitored frequently.

• If distal limb edema develops due to hypoproteinemia, leg wraps should be applied and changed daily.
• Deep bedding should be provided if there are any signs of laminitis.

ACTIVITY

Due to the need for continuous intravenous fluid therapy in most cases, stall confinement is required. Diarrheic horses should be considered infectious and managed appropriately.

DIET

• Affected horses should be provided with free-choice hay. It is recommended to feed hay in a hay-net because hypoproteinemic horses eating off the ground may develop severe facial and head edema.
• Higher-energy feeds can also be provided, but should be introduced slowly. Large amounts of grain should be avoided.
• Anorexic animals may benefit from forced enteral feeding. Partial or total parenteral nutrition may be indicated, but is expensive.

CLIENT EDUCATION

Clients should be made aware that colitis is a potentially life-threatening condition, often associated with the development of secondary problems, such as laminitis and jugular vein thrombosis. In multi-horse environments, it is important to explain the risk of infection to other animals and to be made aware that salmonellosis and *C. difficile* colitis are possibly zoonotic.

SURGICAL CONSIDERATION N/A

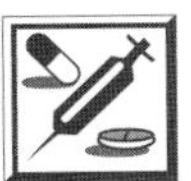

MEDICATIONS

DRUG(S) OF CHOICE

Antimicrobial Agents

The use of these drugs in idiopathic colitis is controversial. In a noncontrolled clinical trial, metronidazole 15–25 mg/kg q6–8 h has been reported to be useful in the treatment of idiopathic colitis. Zinc bacitracin (11 mg/kg of the active principal BID the first day and then daily for 3–4 days or until diarrhea has resolved) has been used by some clinicians successfully in the treatment of idiopathic colitis, although controlled clinical trials supporting this treatment are lacking. Administration of broad-spectrum antibiotics to severely neutropenic patients has been suggested to prevent systemic bacterial seeding to various organs, although this appears to be a rare event. Ceftiofur sodium 2–5 mg/kg IV or IM q12 h may be used; however, this drug has been implicated anecdotally as a cause of clostridial colitis. Trimethoprim-sulfamethoxazole 24 mg/kg IV q12 h also provides broad-spectrum antibiotic coverage; gentamicin 6.6 mg/kg daily administered IV for a short (3–5 days) course can also be used provided renal function is normal and fluid deficits are addressed.

Flunixin Meglumine

• A dose of 0.25–0.5 mg/kg q8 h can be used for its purported antiendotoxic effects. A higher dosage (1.1 mg/kg) may be necessary for analgesia in horses displaying signs of colic.
• Fresh-frozen plasma is beneficial in severely hypoproteinemic animals (<40 g/L); 3–10 L of plasma can be given intravenously, with close attention paid to the recipient for signs of transfusion reaction.

Hyperimmune Serum

Administration of serum from horses hyperimmunized to *E. coli* J5 strain has been proposed to moderate the effects of endotoxemia.

Colloidal therapy

• Colloidal solutions (e.g., whole blood, plasma, hetastarch, dextrans) can be used to maintain the fluid in the vascular space. Colloids should be initiated when plasma proteins are less than 4 g/dL (40 g/L). Colloids should be from a commercial source or from appropriate donors (Aa and Qa isoantibody–negative). Plasma provides protein, anticoagulants, and procoagulant substances.

Laminitis Treatment

See Laminitis.

CONTRAINDICATIONS

Metronidazole may be teratogenic and therefore is contraindicated in pregnant mares.

PRECAUTIONS

At a dose of 1.1 mg/kg, flunixin meglumine may be nephrotoxic in dehydrated animals. Bacitracin and metronidazole should not be used concurrently; combined effects of these two antibiotics on the intestinal microflora are unknown.

POSSIBLE INTERACTIONS

Cimetidine should not be used concurrently with metronidazole because there is interaction through hepatic inhibition.

ALTERNATIVE DRUGS N/A

FOLLOW-UP

PATIENT MONITORING

Patients should be monitored frequently. Initially, PCV and total plasma protein levels should be evaluated at least daily. If azotemia was present on presentation, this should be reevaluated after rehydration to ensure it was prerenal and not due to renal failure. Serum or plasma electrolytes should be monitored to determine whether supplementation, especially with potassium and calcium, is required. The intravenous catheter site should be monitored frequently. The feet should be checked frequently for evidence of discomfort and increased digital pulses or hoof wall temperature, indicative of laminitis.

PREVENTION/AVOIDANCE

Antibiotics should be used judiciously to decrease the risk of disruption of the gastrointestinal microflora.

POSSIBLE COMPLICATIONS

• Endotoxemia
• Laminitis
• Jugular vein thrombosis
• Renal failure
• Pulmonary abscessation

EXPECTED COURSE AND PROGNOSIS

There is a wide variety in the severity of idiopathic colitis. Overall mortality rates for colitis in animals presented to referral centers has been reported to range from 10% to 40%.

MISCELLANEOUS

ASSOCIATED CONDITIONS

• Laminitis
• Venous thrombosis

AGE-RELATED FACTORS

None

ZOONOTIC POTENTIAL

All affected horses should be treated as zoonotic until shown to be negative for *Salmonella* spp. and *C. difficile.*

PREGNANCY

Metronidazole should not be administered to pregnant mares. An increased risk of abortion may be present due to endotoxemia and hypovolemic shock.

SYNONYMS

Colitis X

SEE ALSO

• Laminitis
• Salmonellosis
• *Clostridium difficile* enterocolitis
• Potomac horse fever
• Sand impaction
• Cantharidin toxicosis
• Endotoxemia

Suggested Reading

Cohen ND, Divers TJ. Acute colitis in horses. Part 1. Assessment. Compend Cont Educ Pract Vet 1998;20:92–98.

Cohen ND, Divers TJ. Acute colitis in horses. Part II. Initial management. Compend Cont Educ Pract Vet 1998;20:228–233.

Cohen ND, Woods A. Characteristics and risk factors for failure of horse with acute diarrhea to survive: 122 cases (1990–1996). JAVMA 1999;214:382–390.

McGorum BC, Dixon PM, Smith DG. Use of metronidazole in equine acute idiopathic toxaemic colitis. Vet Rec 1998;142:635–638.

Oliver-Espinosa O, Stämpfli HR. Acute diarrhea in the adult horse: case example and review. Vet Clin North Am Equine Pract 2006;22;73–84.

Staempfli HR, Prescott JF, Carman RJ, McCutcheon LJ. Use of bacitracin in the prevention and treatment of experimentally-induced idiopathic colitis in horses. Can J Vet Res 1992;56:233–236.

Staempfli HR, Townsend HGG, Prescott JF. Prognostic features and clinical presentation of acute idiopathic enterocolitis in horses. Can Vet J 1991;32:232–237.

Authors Olimpo Oliver-Espinosa and Henry Stämpfli

Consulting Editors Henry Stämpfli and Olimpo Oliver-Espinosa

IDIOPATHIC SYSTEMIC GRANULOMATOUS DISEASE (SARCOIDOSIS)

BASICS

OVERVIEW

- ISGD is an uncommon disease in horses often called sarcoidosis. However, idiopathic systemic granulomatous disease is more accurate and avoids confusion with equine sarcoids.
- ISGD is characterized by exfoliative dermatitis, severe wasting, and granulomatous inflammation of multiple organ systems. The following organs (listed in order of decreasing frequency) are affected: skin, lungs, lymph nodes, liver, gastrointestinal tract, spleen, kidneys, bones, and central nervous system.

SIGNALMENT

Rare disorder with no apparent age, breed, or sex predilections

SIGNS

- Clinical signs vary, depending on the organ involved.
- Onset of the disease is typically slowly progressive but may be explosive.
- Nonpruritic exfoliative dermatitis is the primary clinical sign followed by severe wasting in most horses.
- Skin lesions take two forms with scaling, crusting, and alopecia representing the most common form. Lesions usually start on the face or legs before progressing to generalized disease. The mane and tail are usually unaffected. Skin lesions may rarely include nodules or large tumor-like masses.
- Most affected horses develop exercise intolerance, weight loss, and low-grade fever. Many have granulomatous inflammation of the internal organs confirmed at necropsy, which would explain the wasting syndrome.

CAUSES AND RISK FACTORS

- The etiologic agent or the initiating pathophysiologic mechanism is currently unknown. Too few cases have been reported to allow valid genetic, infectious, or environmental associations to be made. Disease likely occurs because of an abnormal host-immune response to either an ingested or inhaled environmental antigen or an underlying infectious or neoplastic process resulting in chronic antigenic stimulation.
- Possible triggers include infectious diseases such as mycobacterium or *Borrelia* spp. and hairy vetch (*Vicia* sp.) toxicoses. However, neither culturing nor electron microscopy has revealed viral, bacterial, or fungal agents.

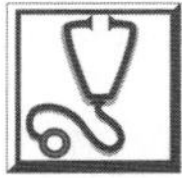

DIAGNOSIS

DIFFERENTIAL DIAGNOSIS

Rule out other common causes of nonpruritic scaling and crusting dermatoses.

- Dermatophilosis
- Dermatophytosis
- Contact dermatitis
- Idiopathic seborrhea

Less common causes that may also have systemic signs of illness.

- Drug reaction
- Pemphigus foliaceus
- Cutaneous and systemic lupus erythematosus
- Epitheliotropic lymphoma
- Multisystemic eosinophilic epitheliotropic disease
- Toxicoses caused by arsenic, mercury, selenium, or iodide

CBC/BIOCHEMISTRY/URINALYSIS

May be normal; some affected horses have leukocytosis, mild nonregenerative anemia, hyperfibrinogenemia, hyperglobulinemia, and hypoalbuminemia depending on organs involved and chronicity.

OTHER LABORATORY TESTS

- Multiple, full-thickness punch biopsies of the affected skin and peripheral lymph nodes
- A pathologist experienced with the histopathological findings of equine dermatoses should examine biopsy specimens.
- Confirmation of a diagnosis is obtained when typical granulomatous changes exist and other granulomatous diseases secondary to bacterial or fungal organisms have been ruled out by appropriate cultures and/or special stains.

IMAGING

Thoracic radiography, abdominal ultrasonography, and percutaneous needle biopsies of the lungs and/or liver may be helpful in determining the presence and extent of systemic involvement. In horses with lung involvement, findings on thoracic radiographs may include interstitial infiltration.

OTHER DIAGNOSTIC PROCEDURES

May depend on organs involved and clinical signs

PATHOLOGICAL FINDINGS

- The major histologic changes in affected organs are aggregates of epithelioid cells and multinucleated giant cells (i.e., sarcoidal granulomas). Granulomas in the skin tend to involve the superficial and perifollicular dermis.

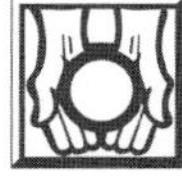

TREATMENT

Topical therapies include antibacterial and antiseborrheic shampoos.

MEDICATIONS

DRUG(S)

Corticosteroids at immunosuppressive doses are the preferred treatment in most cases and administration should be continued for several weeks to months with a slow taper when remission is achieved. The relative benefits and risks of long-term corticosteroid therapy should be considered in cases with only cutaneous involvement as resolution with conservative management has been reported.

- Prednisolone at 2.2–4.4 mg/kg PO q24h
- Dexamethasone 0.2–0.4 mg/kg PO q24h

CONTRAINDICATIONS/POSSIBLE INTERACTIONS

The use of corticosteroids may cause increased susceptibility to infections, polydipsia, polyuria, poor wound healing, decreased muscle mass, weight loss, behavioral changes, and diabetes mellitus. There are anecdotal reports of an increased risk of laminitis.

FOLLOW-UP

PATIENT MONITORING

Evaluate response to therapy to allow for tapering of corticosteroids to lowest effective dose.

PREVENTION/AVOIDANCE

None

POSSIBLE COMPLICATIONS

Secondary to corticosteroid treatment

EXPECTED COURSE AND PROGNOSIS

- Response to therapy is not well documented. The prognosis varies with chronicity and severity of the disease but is generally considered to be poor.
- Horses with only cutaneous involvement may have a better long-term prognosis.

MISCELLANEOUS

ASSOCIATED CONDITIONS

None

AGE-RELATED FACTORS

None

ZOONOTIC POTENTIAL

None documented

PREGNANCY

Corticosteroid treatment is contraindicated.

SEE ALSO

- Pemphigus foliaceus
- Multisystemic eosinophilic epitheliotropic disease
- Dermatophilosis

ABBREVIATION

- ISGD = idiopathic systemic granulomatous disease

Suggested Reading

Sargent SJ, Buchanan BR, Frank LA, Sommardahl CS, Kania SA, Rotstein DS. Idiopathic systemic granulomatous disease. Compend Cont Educ Vet Equine Ed 2007;2(1):23–30.

Scott DW, Miller WH: Equine Dermatology. St. Louis: Saunders, 2003, 675.

Spiegel IB, White SD, Foley JE, et al. A retrospective study of cutaneous equine sarcoidosis and its potential infectious etiological agents. Vet Dermatol 2007;17(1):51–62.

Author Sandra J. Sargent
Consulting Editor Gwendolen Lorch

ILEAL HYPERTROPHY

BASICS

OVERVIEW

Ileal hypertrophy is hypertrophy of the muscular layers of the ileum and results in a decrease in the luminal diameter. It is either a primary idiopathic condition or occurs secondary to an aboral stenosis. Suggested etiologies for the primary idiopathic hypertrophy include inflammation of the ileal mucosa, including mucosal edema, an imbalance in the autonomic nervous system, and dysfunction of the ileocecal valve. Ileocecal intussusception is a cause of distal stenosis that can in turn cause a compensatory muscular hypertrophy of the ileum. Parasitic damage may be associated with mucosal irritation. There is an increased risk of ileal impaction in horses with tapeworm burdens, and the same may be true of ileal hypertrophy. Hemomelasma ilei is a common finding in horses with ileal hypertrophy. Failure of normal cecal motility has also been proposed as an etiologic factor.

SIGNALMENT

Occurs in adult horses of all ages, but tends to be more frequent in horses 5 years and older. There is no sex or breed predilection.

SIGNS

- Clinical signs are dependent on the degree of luminal obstruction.
- Most commonly, horses have a history of recurrent, low-grade colic with decreased appetite, and weight loss.
- If complete obstruction occurs, horses develop a more severe, continuous colic with ileus and nasogastric reflux.

CAUSES AND RISK FACTORS

Risk factors for idiopathic hypertrophy are unknown, although poor parasite control and poor-quality roughage may be contributory factors. With compensatory ileal hypertrophy, risk factors also include parasitism and poor-quality roughage, as well as intestinal neoplasia, lipoma formation, and previous abdominal surgeries (adhesions).

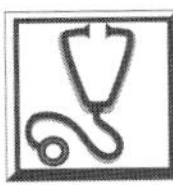

DIAGNOSIS

DIFFERENTIAL DIAGNOSIS

- Ileal impactions and ileocecal intussusception often present with a similar history and similar clinical signs on presentation. Ileocecal intussusceptions are more commonly observed in horses 3 years and younger. There is little evidence that these conditions can be differentiated by examination per rectum; however, ileocecal intussusception has a characteristic ultrasonographic "target" image.
- Adhesions may be detected per rectum, and may be suspected following previous abdominal surgery.
- Small intestinal displacement (epiploic foramen) and strangulating lipomas can be difficult to diagnose, but the acute onset and severe colic signs differentiate them from ileal hypertrophy, and further diagnosis is often made via exploratory celiotomy.
- The diagnosis of small intestinal inguinal herniation is made via scrotal palpation.

CBC/BIOCHEMISTRY/URINALYSIS

There are no specific laboratory tests for ileal hypertrophy.

OTHER LABORATORY TESTS

Abdominocentesis is useful, but there are no abnormalities specific to ileal hypertrophy. Biopsy of the ileum at the time of exploratory celiotomy may be used to confirm the diagnosis.

IMAGING

Ultrasound images of the ileum may detect ileal hypertrophy and are likely to reveal the presence of small intestinal distension orally and small intestinal hypermotility. The hypertrophied wall of the ileum is usually between 15 and 25 mm thick, becoming less thick orally. Narrowing of the ileal lumen may also be discernible. Ultrasonography of the ileum is usually performed from the right dorsal paralumbar fossa, but transrectal ultrasound may be beneficial, particularly when the thickened ileum is palpable.

DIAGNOSTIC PROCEDURES

Rectal examination findings may include a thickened ileum palpable in the right dorsal quadrant and loops of distended small intestine. Not all cases have these findings, and the diagnosis may only be revealed after evaluation of a biopsy of the ileum taken at the time of exploratory celiotomy. Passage of a nasogastric tube is mandatory to test for the presence of reflux.

PATHOLOGICAL FINDINGS

There is muscular hypertrophy of both circular and longitudinal smooth muscle layers for variable lengths along the ileum, and possibly also the jejunum. Individual muscle cells are enlarged, with elongated vesicular nuclei. Mucosal diverticula through the muscularis layer were found in approximately half of the specimens from one study. Fibrosis of the mucosa is often present, and may indicate parasitic damage or damage from a resolved intussusception.

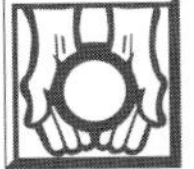

TREATMENT

- Conservative therapy is attempted, but progression of clinical signs, and in particular increasing small intestinal distension, are indicators for surgical intervention. One study found a relationship between duration of colic signs prior to surgery and rate of survival for ileal impaction; however, successful medical treatment has also been reported.
- Surgical treatments include ileal myotomy, ileocecal bypass, and jejunocecostomy. Ileal myotomy consists of longitudinal incisions made through the serosa and muscularis to allow expansion of the submucosa and relief of the ileal obstruction. This technique is not considered the treatment of choice, particularly if there are abnormalities in ileal motility, or if there is a dysfunction of the ileocecal valve. Ileocecal bypass has been used, but ingesta may still pass through the ileum, causing pain. In addition, complications associated with the anastomosis are more likely if the ileum is markedly thickened at the anastomosis. A jejunocecostomy with blind stumping of the ileum distally and removal of the proximal ileum may be the treatment of choice.
- A laxative diet may be palliative in horses in which surgery is not an option.

MEDICATIONS

DRUG(S) OF CHOICE

Medical therapy for colic and ileus is mentioned elsewhere. There is no specific medication for ileal hypertrophy.

CONTRAINDICATIONS/POSSIBLE INTERACTIONS

Prokinetics may exacerbate colic pain severity if there is a partial or complete intestinal obstruction. Similarly, gastrointestinal osmotic cathartics, such as Epsom salts, may increase proximal small intestinal distension.

FOLLOW-UP

Routine postsurgical monitoring for colic cases is required. Prognosis after surgical correction is considered good, provided that the hypertrophy is focal (i.e., the proximal small intestine is normal).

MISCELLANEOUS

ASSOCIATED CONDITIONS

See Differential Diagnosis.

AGE-RELATED FACTORS

There are little data on age-related factors, but whereas compensatory ileal hypertrophy may occur in horses of any age, idiopathic muscular hypertrophy appears to be more common in mature horses. In one study of 11 cases of idiopathic ileal muscular hypertrophy, the age range was 5–18 years with a median age of 10 years.

Suggested Reading

Chaffin MK, Carmen Fuenteabla I, Schumacher J, *et al*. Idiopathic muscular hypertrophy of the equine small intestine: 11 cases (1980–1991). Equine Vet J 1992;24:372–378.

Authors Judith B. Koenig and Simon G. Pearce
Consulting Editors Henry Stämpfli and Olimpo Oliver-Espinosa

ILEUS

BASICS

DEFINITION

Gastrointestinal ileus has been defined as the functional inhibition of propulsive intestine activity, irrespective of its pathophysiology, which results in impaired aboral transit of ingesta. Using the duration of clinical signs for classification, ileus can be characterized as either adynamic, resulting from short-term alterations of gastrointestinal motility, or paralytic, when motility is lost for longer than 72 hr. Obstructive intestinal diseases are sometimes referred to as *obstructive ileus.*

PATHOPHYSIOLOGY

- In general, regulation of motility occurs as a complex interaction of central innervation, autonomic innervation, and the enteric nervous system. The enteric nervous system is a collection of neurons in the gastrointestinal tract that control motility, exocrine and endocrine secretions, and microcirculation. It exerts its influences on the gastrointestinal tract either directly through neurotransmitters or indirectly through intermediate cells, such as the interstitial cells of Cajal, cells of the immune system, or endocrine cells.
- Acetylcholine is the main excitatory neurotransmitter in the gut. Sympathetic stimulation (norepinephrine) inhibits acetylcholine release from the cholinergic fibers, resulting in inhibition of motility. Nonadrenergic–noncholinergic neurotransmitters like adenosine triphosphate, vasoactive intestinal peptide, substance P, nitric oxide, and others also play a role in regulating gastrointestinal activity.
- Many reflexes are present that are essential to proper functioning of intestinal motility, some of which occur locally within the enteric nervous system and are responsible for peristalsis and mixing contractions. Other reflexes travel to sympathetic ganglia, the spinal cord, or the brainstem to coordinate more complex activities, such as the gastrocolic reflex, where distention of the stomach causes contraction of the colon to promote emptying of the contents.
- Knowledge of normal control mechanisms of intestinal motility allows for insight into some of the causes of ileus. For example, pain can cause a systemic release of norepinephrine from the adrenal glands, which inhibits acetylcholine release in the intestine and decreases intestinal motility. Ileus can develop from diseases directly involving the digestive system, or it can be a consequence of conditions in other body systems, such as trauma to retroperitoneal structures or irritation of the peritoneum. Shock, electrolyte imbalances, hypoalbuminemia, peritonitis, endotoxemia, and distention, ischemia, or inflammation of the intestinal tract have all been implicated as contributing to the pathophysiology of ileus in the horse.
- POI occurs in up to 21% of horses after laparotomy, with those in which a small–intestinal resection and anastomosis were performed had an even greater risk of POI (42% of horses), with the small intestine being more commonly affected than the large intestine.

SYSTEMS AFFECTED

- Gastrointestinal
- Cardiovascular—Hypovolemia due to fluid sequestration in the intestinal tract and endotoxemia can result in depressed cardiovascular function. Endotoxemia can further contribute to depressed cardiac function.

SIGNALMENT

POI is more common in the Arabian breed and horses over 10 years of age.

SIGNS

Historical

Depression, mild to moderate signs of abdominal pain, anorexia, and decreased fecal output. Ileus can occur secondary to many diseases (see Causes). Historical findings that are consistent with a primary disease may also be present.

Physical Examination

Heart rate and respiratory rate are often elevated due to abdominal discomfort, and the horse usually exhibits mild to severe signs of colic. Clinical signs associated with dehydration are often present due to intestinal sequestration of fluids. Abdominal auscultation usually reveals an absence or reduction of borborygmi. On palpation per rectum, distention of either the small or large intestine depending on the affected bowel segment may be present. Passage of a nasogastric tube is an important diagnostic and therapeutic tool. Buildup of fluid in the stomach occurs because of a lack of progressive motility. Decompression with a nasogastric tube not only prevents gastric rupture and provides pain relief, but it also allows for the volume of fluid to be quantified for intravenous replacement fluid therapy, thereby providing a rough estimate of the severity of disease.

CAUSES

Ileus can be induced by virtually any intestinal insult. Causes of ileus include intestinal distention or impaction, enteritis/colitis, and serosal irritation from abdominal surgery or peritonitis. Ileus can also be caused by vascular or obstructive intestinal injuries, endotoxemia, pain, shock, hypoproteinemia, or electrolyte imbalances.

RISK FACTORS

Any factor that predisposes the development of a previously mentioned cause of ileus can be considered a risk factor. Electrolyte imbalances (hypokalemia or hypocalcemia) can alter intestinal smooth muscle function and have a deleterious effect on motility. Certain drugs (α_2-agonists or opioid analgesics) also inhibit intestinal motility.

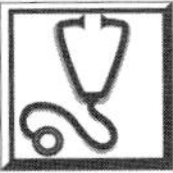

DIAGNOSIS

DIFFERENTIAL DIAGNOSIS

Adynamic/paralytic ileus should be differentiated from obstructive diseases that require immediate surgical intervention.

CBC/BIOCHEMISTRY/URINALYSIS

- Increase in PCV due to dehydration and/or splenic contraction. Azotemia may also be present.
- Hypoproteinemia or hyperproteinemia, depending on the underlying cause of ileus and degree of dehydration. Colitis or enteritis can cause a loss of protein-rich fluid into the intestines, which results in hypoproteinemia. If an inflammatory response is present, hyperproteinemia can result.
- Leukopenia may be present if ileus is associated with an acute inflammatory response. A long-standing inflammatory response can cause leukocytosis.
- Hypokalemia, hypocalcemia, hypomagnesemia, hypochloremia, and hyponatremia may be present due to sequestration of fluid in the intestines and inflammation of the intestinal wall.

OTHER LABORATORY TESTS

Abdominocentesis

Ileus usually results in no detectable abnormalities except in cases of duodenitis/proximal jejunitis. In these cases, an elevation of abdominal protein is usually present. In cases of ileus secondary to peritonitis, a marked increase in white blood cells and protein is usually present. If an obstructive ileus is present, the peritoneal fluid can be serosanguinous due to intestinal compromise and the cellular and protein levels are often high.

IMAGING

Ultrasonography

The intestine can be assessed for presence of movement, mural thickness, and dilation. Normal small intestinal wall thickness is $\leq$3 mm.

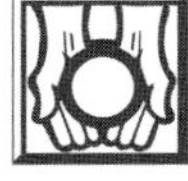

TREATMENT

AIMS OF TREATMENT

The main goals for treatment of ileus are to decompress the gastrointestinal tract, reduce inflammation and pain, stimulate motility, maintain hydration, and keep electrolytes balanced to both promote motility and maintain the gastrointestinal barrier, as well as to prevent cardiovascular impairment.

APPROPRIATE HEALTH CARE

Inpatient intensive care management with 24-hr monitoring

NURSING CARE

- Parenteral fluid therapy is vital due to the inability to administer oral fluids. Fluid rates should be calculated based on fluid deficit + maintenance + ongoing loss. The fluid deficit can be calculated as percent dehydration × body weight (kg) = fluid deficit (liters).
- Maintenance fluid requirements for adult horses are 50–60 mL/kg/day, and for foals, 70–80 mL/kg/day. Ongoing losses can be determined by quantifying the amount of fluid lost as gastric reflux.
- Horses suffering from hypovolemic or endotoxemic shock may benefit from hypertonic saline administration to rapidly expand the vascular fluid volume. Hypertonic saline (5%–7%) can be administered at a dose of 4 mL/kg as a rapid bolus, followed by isotonic fluids because the volume expansion by hypertonic fluids is short-lived (<30 min).
- Horses with severe hyponatremia (<120 mmol/L) should not be given hypertonic saline due to the potential for cerebral edema to develop.
- Electrolyte imbalances should be addressed due to the negative effect of hypokalemia, hypomagnesemia and hypocalcemia on motility. KCl may be added to parenteral fluids. The rate of potassium administration should not exceed 0.5 mEq/kg/hr due to the potential for cardiac effects.
- When treating an adult horse, a potassium concentration of 20 mEq/L in parenteral fluids results in a rate of administration <0.5 mEq/kg/hr, even at fast fluid rates.
- To correct hypocalcemia, 200–500 mL of 23% calcium borogluconate can be administered slowly (diluted in lactated Ringer's solution).
- To correct hypomagnesemia, 150mg/kg per day of $MgSO_4$ (0.3 mL/kg of a 50% solution) is administered diluted in lactated Ringer's solution.
- Gastric decompression via a nasogastric tube should be performed to relieve discomfort and to prevent gastric rupture.

ACTIVITY

Frequent hand-walking (4–6 times daily) may help stimulate the gastrointestinal tract.

DIET

Feed and water should be withheld.

SURGICAL CONSIDERATIONS/CLIENT EDUCATION

If ileus persists, an exploratory laparotomy for surgical decompression can be performed to relieve discomfort. If the horse appears to deteriorate clinically with medical management, then surgery is indicated due to the potential for an obstructive/ischemic lesion.

MEDICATIONS

DRUG(S) OF CHOICE

Analgesics

Pain relief is important when correcting ileus. NSAIDs are a good choice for analgesia because they do not inhibit motility. If additional analgesia is needed, then α_2-agonists can be given alone or in conjunction with butorphanol (opioid). α_2-Agonists appear to function synergistically with butorphanol; however, these drugs can inhibit motility for <2 hr and should be used judiciously.

- NSAIDs—flunixin meglumine 0.5–1.1 mg/kg IV q8–12h, phenylbutazone 2.2–4.4 mg/kg IV q12–24h
- α_2-Agonists—xylazine 0.25–0.5 mg/kg IV or IM, detomidine 5–10 μg/kg IV or IM, romifidine 0.02–0.05 mg/kg IV or IM
- Opioids—butorphanol 0.02–0.04 mg/kg IV or continuous-rate infusion of butorphanol 13 μg/kg/hr IV

Prokinetic Agents

- Bethanechol chloride—improves gastric and cecal emptying by stimulation of muscarinic receptors on the smooth muscle and myeneteric plexus. Recommended dose—0.025 mg/kg IV or SQ q6h. Side effects—salivation, abdominal cramps, diarrhea
- Cisapride—improves motility of the entire gastrointestinal tract by increasing acetylcholine release from enteric nerves through 5-HT_4 receptor agonism and 5-HT_3 receptor antagonism. Recommended dose—0.1 mg/kg IM q8h. Side effects in people are cardiotoxicity. Related drugs like tegaserod or mosapride appear to be effective in horses as well.
- Erythromycin lactobionate—improves small and large intestinal motility by stimulating intestinal motilin receptors, but its efficacy is questionable in the presence of inflammation of the intestine. Recommended dose—0.5 mg/kg IV q6h. Side effect—diarrhea
- Metoclopramide—improves gastric and proximal small intestinal motility by increasing acetylcholine release from intestinal neurons through dopamine receptor antagonism, 5-HT_4 receptor antagonism, and 5-HT_3 receptor antagonism. Recommended dose—0.04 mg/kg/hr IV in saline as a continuous-rate infusion. Side effects—excitement, restlessness, sweating, abdominal cramps
- Lidocaine—decreases the amount and duration of gastric reflux in horses with ileus, possibly through suppression of sympathetic neurotransmission. Recommended dose—1.3 mg/kg IV as a slow bolus, followed by 0.05 mg/kg/min IV in saline or lactated Ringer's solution as a continuous-rate infusion over 24 h. Side effects—muscle fasciculations, trembling ataxia

CONTRAINDICATIONS

Oral drug administration is contraindicated in horses with ileus of the small intestine (nasogastric reflux or with distended small intestine on rectal palpation).

PRECAUTIONS

N/A

POSSIBLE INTERACTIONS

N/A

ALTERNATIVE DRUGS

Acupuncture may be successful in promoting motility in horses.

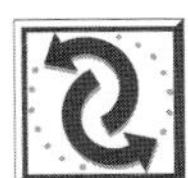

FOLLOW-UP

PATIENT MONITORING

The patient should be monitored closely to ensure that intravenous fluid therapy is appropriate and that decompression of gastric and small intestinal distention is adequate.

PREVENTION/AVOIDANCE

N/A

POSSIBLE COMPLICATIONS

- Circulatory shock
- Gastrointestinal rupture

EXPECTED COURSE AND PROGNOSIS

In one study, 13% of horses that developed POI died during short-term hospitalization.

MISCELLANEOUS

AGE-RELATED FACTORS

N/A

ZOONOTIC POTENTIAL

N/A

ABBREVIATION

- POI, postoperative ileus

Suggested Reading

Guyton A, Hall J. General principles of gastrointestinal function—motility, nervous control, and blood circulation. In: Guyton A, ed. Textbook of Medical Physiology, ed 10. Philadelphia: WB Saunders; 2000:718–727.

Hardy J, Rakestraw PC. Postoperative care and complications associated with abdominal surgery. In: Auer J, Stick, JA, ed. Equine Surgery, ed 3. Philadelphia: WB Saunders Company; 2006:499–506.

Lester G. Gastrointestinal ileus. In: Smith B, ed. Large Animal Internal Medicine. St. Louis: Mosby; 2002:674–679.

Author Judith B. Koenig

Consulting Editors Henry Stämpfli and Olimpo Oliver-Espinosa

IMMUNE-MEDIATED KERATITIS

BASICS

OVERVIEW

IMMK is characterized by chronic (>3 months) corneal opacities with mild to moderate cellular infiltrate and vascularization. In general, no secondary uveitis, severe ocular discomfort, and associated infectious agents are present.

SYSTEM AFFECTED

Ophthalmic

SIGNALMENT

All ages and breeds of horses can be affected.

SIGNS

- Corneal opacities with mild to moderate cellular infiltrate and vascularization. The infiltrate can appear yellow to white.
- Depending on the corneal plane affected, IMMK is classified as (a) superficial stromal keratitis, (b) mild or deep stromal keratitis, or (c) endotheliitis.
- Epithelial keratopathy has also been reported.
- Corneal endotheliitis is characterized by diffuse corneal edema.
- Equine IMMK is usually a unilateral disease, but both eyes can be affected.

CAUSES AND RISK FACTORS

Immune mediated

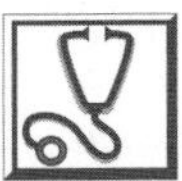

DIAGNOSIS

DIFFERENTIAL DIAGNOSIS

- Other nonulcerative keratopathies such as onchocerciasis, bacterial or fungal stromal infections (stromal abscesses), viral keratitis, infiltrative neoplasia, corneal degeneration or dystrophy, calcific band keratopathy, eosinophilic keratoconjunctivitis, and bullous keratopathy
- Infectious keratitis is usually more acute in onset and associated with secondary anterior uveitis and more severe ocular discomfort.

CBC/BIOCHEMISTRY/URINALYSIS

N/A

OTHER LABORATORY TESTS

- Rule out infectious causes (bacterial or fungal) by corneal scrapings of superficial lesions for cytology, culture, and possibly histopathology.
- Deeper lesions cannot be sampled unless penetrating keratoplasty is performed.

IMAGING

N/A

DIAGNOSTIC PROCEDURES

N/A

PATHOLOGIC FINDINGS

Histopathology reveals stromal fibrosis, vascularization, and cellular infiltrates consisting mainly of lymphocytes and plasma cells but also neutrophils.

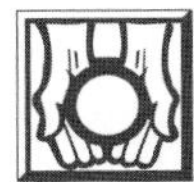

TREATMENT

Even though most cases of IMMK respond well to topical medication, a complete cure may only be achieved by surgical removal of the cellular infiltrates followed by a grafting procedure (e.g., conjunctival graft). Of all the IMMK forms, endotheliitis is the least amenable to medical treatment.

MEDICATIONS

DRUG(S) OF CHOICE

Topical corticosteroids (1% prednisolone acetate or 0.1% dexamethasone QID to effect) or cyclosporine A BID. Complete or incomplete clinical improvement with topical anti-inflammatory medication helps to confirm the diagnosis.

CONTRAINDICATIONS/POSSIBLE INTERACTIONS

N/A

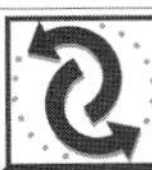

FOLLOW-UP

EXPECTED COURSE AND PROGNOSIS

Unless surgical options are considered, long-term topical treatment SID or BID may be required to control the disease and prevent recurrences.

MISCELLANEOUS

ASSOCIATED CONDITIONS

Superficial corneal ulcers can develop secondary to chronic corneal edema due to endotheliitis.

SEE ALSO

- Corneal stromal abscesses
- Eosinophilic keratitis
- Calcific band keratopathy
- Nonulcerative keratouveitis
- Ocular/adnexal squamous cell carcinoma

ABBREVIATION

- IMMK = immune-mediated keratitis

Suggested Reading

Brooks DE. Ophthalmology for the Equine Practitioner. Jackson, WY; Teton NewMedia, 2002.

Brooks DE, Matthews AG. Equine ophthalmology. In: Gelatt KN, ed. Veterinary Ophthalmology, ed 4. Philadelphia; Lippincott Williams and Wilkins, 2007.

Gilger BC, ed. Equine Ophthalmology. Philadelphia; WB Saunders, 2005.

Gilger BC, Miller Michau T, Salmon JH. Immune-mediated keratitis in horses: 19 Cases (1998–2004). Vet Ophthalmol 2005;8:233–239.

Matthews AG. Nonulcerative keratopathies in the horse. Equine Vet Educ 2000;12:271–278.

Author Andras M. Komaromy

Consulting Editor Dennis E. Brooks

IMMUNOGLOBULIN DEFICIENCIES

BASICS

OVERVIEW

• Rare disorders of the immune system that are commonly primary, rarely secondary. • SIgMD is associated with decreased or absent serum IgM with no abnormalities of other immunoglobulins. • AG is associated with a lack of mature B lymphocytes and plasma cells with failure to synthesize immunoglobulins or specific antibodies after immunization or infections.
• FPIS is associated with low concentrations of immunoglobulins in serum, low numbers of B lymphocytes in blood, and severe anemia.

SIGNALMENT

• SIgMD occurs mainly in Arabians but also is observed in other breeds (e.g., Thoroughbred, Standardbred, Quarter Horse, Paso Fino).
• Primary SIgMD occurs usually in horses <2 years of age, but a secondary form can occur in older horses. • SIgMD has no apparent sex predilection. • AG has been described in Thoroughbreds Quarter Horses, and Standardbreds and only occurs in male foals.
• FPIS has only been described in Fell Ponies that are usually <4 mo old.

SIGNS

• Recurrent bacterial infections are common in all 3 syndromes. These may respond to aggressive antimicrobial therapy, but frequently relapse a few weeks after cessation of treatment.
• The infections often involve organisms that are low-grade pathogens. • Common manifestations include pneumonia, arthritis, and enteritis.
• Foals or weanlings often present with ill thrift, nasal discharge, cough, and/or diarrhea • Two main presentations of SIgMD occur—the most common occurs in foals <10 mo old (usually 2–8 mo). • Most of these foals die by 8 mo of age—those surviving >1 year have poor growth rates/stunting. • The second form of SIgMD occurs in horses older than 2 years and is usually secondary to lymphoreticular neoplasia, which may not be apparent at the time of presentation.
• Horses with this form present with ill thrift, weight loss, or chronic recurrent infections.
• Foals with AG may survive for months with appropriate therapy, due to the existence of intact T-lymphocyte function, but they invariably die. • Foals with FPIS are normal at birth but by 2–4 weeks develop weight loss, become severely anemic, and die or are euthanized by 3 mo of age.

CAUSES AND RISK FACTORS

• A genetic basis is suspected in primary cases of all 3 disorders, but the specific molecular defects are not known. • The mechanism for SIgMD may involve a mutation of the immunoglobulin μ chain. • In humans, AG is due to a mutation in the gene encoding tyrosine kinase and is inherited as an X-linked trait; the occurrence of this disorder only in male horses indicates a similar X-linked mechanism in this species. • A single, autosomal recessive gene defect is thought to be the basis of FPIS, which results in impaired development of B cells in bone marrow and secondary lymphoid organs (e.g., lymph nodes and spleen).
• The association with neoplasia in some cases of SIgMD in adults and the reporting of spontaneous recovery in others may be interpreted to suggest that this is a secondary, not primary, immunodeficiency disorder.

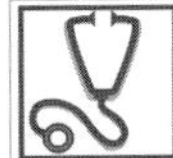

DIAGNOSIS

DIFFERENTIAL DIAGNOSIS

• Differential diagnoses that may resemble these disorders include SCID and FPT.
• SCID is typically found in young Arabian foals with low immunoglobulins and a total lymphopenia (both B and T lymphocytes).
• FPT is observed in neonates as compared to the older age of presentation for foals with Ig deficiencies that are genetically based.

CBC/BIOCHEMISTRY/URINALYSIS

• In both AG and FPIS blood lymphocyte counts may be normal (due to presence of T lymphocytes) or decreased.
• The hemogram may be normal in horses with SIgMD and AG or reflect an infectious or inflammatory process (i.e., leukocytosis, neutrophilia, hyperfibrinogenemia).
• Marked anemia occurs in foals with FPIS together with mild to moderate lymphopenia and thrombocytopenia in some cases.

OTHER LABORATORY TESTS

• For all 3 syndromes, serum IgM should be measured once the foal is >4 weeks of age and will be <2 standard deviations below mean of age-matched normal animals (4–8 mo, <15 mg/dL; >8 mo, <25 mg/dL).
• With SIgMD only IgM is decreased; other globulins are normal to increased.
• With AG, diagnosis is supported by absence or a significant decrease in serum IgA, IgG, Ig(T), and IgM and a decrease in B (but not T) lymphocytes.
• Similarly, FPIS is associated with decreased IgM, IgGa, IgGb, and IgG(T) together with decreased B (but not T) lymphocytes.
• Blood lymphocyte counts are normal for SIgMD and lymphocytes respond adequately to mitogens.
• Total B-cell counts in blood are severely depleted in foals with AG and FPIS, but remaining T lymphocytes are responsive to mitogens at normal concentrations.

OTHER DIAGNOSTIC PROCEDURES

As indicated for lymphosarcoma if the secondary form of SIgMD is suspected in older horses

PATHOLOGICAL FINDINGS

• Lymphoid tissues are grossly and histologically normal in cases of SIgMD.
• Foals with AG have a depletion of lymphoid tissues and regions containing these cells are severely disarranged.
• Glossal hyperkeratosis, erythroid hypoplasia, peripheral ganglionopathy, and depletion of B lymphocytes in lymphoid tissues are seen in foals with FPIS.

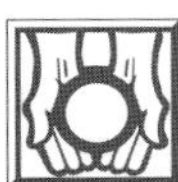

TREATMENT

• No specific treatment is available for immunoglobulin deficiencies. • Appropriate antimicrobial therapy for treatment of concurrent bacterial infections may ameliorate presenting signs, but these can recur with cessation of antibiotics. • Plasma transfusions may provide an exogenous source of antibodies and provide short-term benefit, prolonging the life of affected foals. • Foals and horses with these disorders invariably die or are euthanized.

MEDICATIONS

DRUG(S) OF CHOICE

Treat infections with appropriate antibiotics after culture and sensitivity testing.

FOLLOW-UP

PATIENT MONITORING

Confirmation of the diagnosis may be made by repeating IgM assay.

POSSIBLE COMPLICATIONS

Infections

EXPECTED COURSE AND PROGNOSIS

• Prognosis is poor to grave, although rare cases of SIgMD have spontaneously recovered. • In these cases, the secondary form of SIgMD is likely and these horses have been reported to resolve infections and develop normal serum IgM concentrations after several months. • The mechanism for this improvement is unknown, and therefore the ability to predict which cases will respond is difficult. • No cases of AG or FPIS have been reported to recover.

MISCELLANEOUS

ASSOCIATED CONDITIONS

Bacterial infections

AGE-RELATED FACTORS

Predominantly observed in foals and weanlings

SEE ALSO

- Lymphosarcoma
- SCID
- Lymphopenia

ABBREVIATIONS

- AG = agammaglobulinemia
- FPIS = Fell Pony immunodeficiency syndrome
- FPT = failure of passive transfer
- SCID = severe combined immunodeficiency
- SIgMD = selective IgM deficiency

Suggested Reading

Perryman L. Primary immunodeficiencies of horses. Vet Clin North Am 2000;16:105.

Author Jennifer Hodgson
Consulting Editors David Hodgson and Jennifer Hodgson

IMPACTION

BASICS

DEFINITION

An impaction is obstruction of the alimentary tract, and depending on the portion affected, may result in a variety of clinical signs. The obstruction may consist of feed material, fecal material, or foreign matter that slows or stops the movement of ingesta. This may result in distention of a viscus, causing abdominal pain. Impactions may be primary or secondary, and may cause partial to complete obstructions.

PATHOPHYSIOLOGY

- Any disease that causes decreased gastric or intestinal motility may cause an impaction (see Ileus).
- There are feed-associated factors (coarse, high-fiber, low digestible feedstuffs), insufficient water intake, poor dentition, or a change in diet that may affect the breakdown of feed material resulting in delayed passage.
- Factors such as dehydration, change in exercise, and transport are thought to be important in initiating an obstruction.
- In addition, general anesthesia and surgical manipulations may affect the gastrointestinal motility; therefore, postanesthetic impactions are not uncommon.
- Portions of the bowel where the intestinal lumen size narrows are common areas for impactions. These include the stomach, distal small intestine, cecum, pelvic flexure, right dorsal colon, transverse colon, and small colon.
- Impactions may also occur in areas where pacemakers controlling motility are located (cecum, pelvic flexure).
- In some cases, the cause of impactions may not be delineated.

SYSTEMS AFFECTED

Gastrointestinal

- Decreased appetite
- Decreased fecal output
- Increased or decreased borborygmi
- Abdominal distention
- Colic
- Other signs caused by primary disease

Behavioral

Behavioral changes range from vague changes in demeanor to severe signs of colic and toxemia.

Cardiovascular

- Normal to increased heart rate and capillary refill time
- Tacky mucous membranes
- Greater signs of cardiovascular compromise as severity increases

Renal/Urologic

Changes associated with hypovolemia

Reproductive

Cecal impaction following parturition

Respiratory

- Mild tachypnea
- Shallow respiration due to pain and abdominal distention

Skin/Exocrine

Sweating

SIGNALMENT

Any age, breed, or sex
- Ascarid impactions—occur in foals, weanlings, and yearlings
- Small colon impactions—may be more common in ponies and American Miniature Horses
- Cecal impaction—more common in post-parturient mares and in horses following general anesthesia

SIGNS

- Abdominal distention
- Anorexia (partial to complete)
- Decreased fecal output
- Diarrhea—sand impaction, although may occur in course of treatment of other impactions
- Feces—firm/hard, dry, mucus covered
- Flank watching
- Frequent attempts to defecate
- Increased or decreased borborygmi
- Lethargy
- Nasogastric reflux
- Pawing
- Rectal prolapse
- Recumbency
- Rolling
- Straining to defecate
- Tail swishing

CAUSES

Gastric Impaction

Abrupt increase in amount of concentrates fed, especially those that swell; outflow obstructions due to pyloric dysfunction or small intestinal ileus or other disease that decreases small intestinal motility.

Small Intestine Impaction

Associated with coarse feed, such as coastal Bermuda grass, or with mesenteric vascular disease; ascarid impactions in young horses with heavy worm burdens are usually associated with anthelmintic treatments that cause sudden die-off or sudden paralysis of a large number of parasites (organophosphates, piperazine, pyrantel pamoate), or cause hyperexcitability of the parasite prior to death (ivermectin).

Cecal Impaction

Multifactorial problem that occurs in the adult horse and is rare in foals. May occur as a primary problem due to an abrupt change in feed or may be secondary to altered motility due to general anesthesia, surgery, parturition, or sand ingestion. Parasitic or vascular damage affecting the cecal pacemaker may alter cecal motility.

Large Colon Impaction

- Decreased water intake
- Diet alteration
- Poor dentition
- Decreased exercise
- Sand ingestion
- Enteric parasitism

Small Colon Impaction

Similar to causes of large colon impaction.

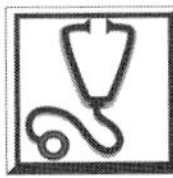

DIAGNOSIS

DIFFERENTIAL DIAGNOSIS

Determination of the cause of colic should include a thorough collection of historical information (including management, exercise, and prior treatments), physical examination, abdominal palpation per rectum, and passage of a nasogastric tube.

Gastric Impaction

Rule out many other causes of colic, including causes of small intestinal/gastric reflux.

Small Intestine Impaction

Ileal hypertrophy, ileum-associated mass, small intestinal or ileal–cecal intussusception. Other causes of small intestinal distention include proximal duodenitis/jejunitis, small intestinal volvulus, and strangulating lipoma.

Cecal Impaction

Differentials for cecal distention include cecocecal intussusception and cecocolic intussusception. For a "simple" cecal impaction, a cecum that is distended with ingesta should be palpable in the upper right abdominal quadrant. A medial and ventral band may be palpated. The cecum should be palpated to course cranioventral as palpate from the base toward the apex. An apical impaction, early in the disease process, may not be palpable.

Large Colon Impaction

Displacements, early large colon/cecal torsions. Impaction of the left large colons should be palpable per rectum. The impacted pelvic flexure is usually located within the pelvic inlet and is positioned with the dorsal and ventral colon in a horizontal plane. An NSE may closely resemble a simple impaction of the left colons. With an NSE, the position of the left colons is often reversed (ventral colon located in a dorsal position), and the colon and associated bands may be palpated from the pelvic brim to the nephrosplenic space. Ultrasound examination is very helpful in making the diagnosis. Palpation of impactions of the right dorsal or transverse colon is not possible, and diagnosis would require a celiotomy or necropsy.

Small Colon Impaction

Major differential is impaction of the small intestine. Differentiation requires the detection of the large antimesenteric band on the small colon. Multiple loops of impacted small colon are usually palpable.

CBC/BIOCHEMISTRY/URINALYSIS

Usually normal; abnormalities may occur with progressive disease due to hypovolemia and debilitation of the bowel.

IMPACTION

Abdominal Fluid Analysis

Abdominal fluid should be collected judiciously if an impaction is suspected because enterocentesis may cause rupture of a distended viscus. Consider identifying fluid pocket with ultrasound prior to centesis and using a blunt tipped cannula such as a 4-in. teat cannula. The fluid should be normal in appearance and have normal cytologic parameters. Abnormal cell count, cell differential, protein level, presence of bacteria or foreign material consistent with compromised bowel or another problem.

IMAGING

Radiographs

Radiographs are helpful in assessing foal abdomens or searching for foreign bodies, enteroliths, or sand in adult horses.

Ultrasound

Ultrasound is a useful tool in evaluating foal and adult abdomens. Can be used transcutaneously or per rectum to assess intestinal distention (may include loss of sacculations with large colon impaction), intestinal wall thickness, and intestinal motility. Possible to detect intussusceptions and masses. Select areas can be evaluated in adult horses, but there are limitations due to size of adult abdomen and inability to penetrate through cecum or colon. Hyperechoic fluid may have high cell count, protein level, or feed/fecal material and can also assess presence of fibrin deposition and peripheral abscess formation.

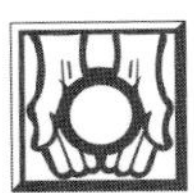

TREATMENT

Gastrointestinal Impactions

Resolve primary problem (feed, dentition, hydration, exercise). Medical therapy should include withholding feed; however, small amounts of feed may help maintain gastrointestinal motility and may be considered in impactions of the large or small colon. Grass or grass hay should be considered. Further medical therapy may include intravenous crystalloid fluids given at a high rate to increase the fluid content in the bowel to break down impaction. If tolerated, fluids may be given via an indwelling nasogastric tube at rates up to 6 L/hr in a 450-kg horse. Medications may be given orally to soften the feces and analgesics may be administered as needed. Exploratory surgery may be required depending on the type of disease and its severity, duration, and progression. Factors that should be considered include deteriorating signs of pain, increasing heart rate, retrieving gastric reflux, increased abdominal distention, increased distention of viscera on rectal examination, lack of fecal production, and indications of loss of visceral integrity, such as increased nucleated cells, protein level, presence of bacteria, or presence of feed material in peritoneal fluid.

Gastric

Medical therapy should include withholding feed and maintenance of the hydration status. The stomach may be lavaged through a nasogastric tube; however, caution must be used to prevent further gastric distention and rupture.

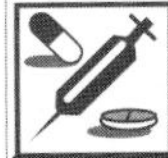

MEDICATIONS

Laxatives

- Mineral oil—2–4L/450-kg horse, q12h via nasogastric tube
- DSS—120–240 mL/450-kg horse of 4% DSS with water
- Psyllium hydrophilic mucilloid—0.25–0.5 kg/450-kg horse

Cathartics

- Magnesium sulfate (Epsom salts)—0.5–1.0 kg q24h
- Sodium sulfate (Glauber's salts)—0.25–0.5 kg q24h

DRUGS OF CHOICE

NSAIDs

- Flunixin meglumine—0.5–1.1 mg/kg IV q24h/12h/8h.
- Ketoprofen—2.2 mg/kg IV q24h/12h/8h
- Phenylbutazone—2.2–4.4 mg/kg IV q24h/12h

Analgesia and Sedation

- Xylazine—Use α_2-adrenergic agonist sparingly due to decreased motility.
- Romifidine—40–80 μg/kg IM, IV
- Detomidine—10–30 μg/kg IM, IV
- Butorphanol—0.01–0.05 mg/kg (some horses may need prior or concurrent α-adrenergic agonist treatment to prevent tremors)
- *N*-Butylscopolammonium (spasmolytic)—0.3 mg/kg IV

CONTRAINDICATIONS

NSAIDs

NSAIDs may cause renal papillary necrosis or gastrointestinal ulceration; side effects may be worse in a dehydrated animal. Decreasing order of toxicity: ketoprofen, flunixin, phenylbutazone.

α-Adrenergic Agonists

Side effects include transient hypertension followed by longer-lasting hypotension, bradycardia, second-degree atrioventricular blockade, decreased gastrointestinal motility, sweating, and diuresis.

Salt Cathartics

Animal must be well hydrated; may cause distention and more severe colic. Toxic to enterocytes with repeated administration

POSSIBLE DRUG INTERACTIONS

N/A

ALTERNATIVE DRUGS

N/A

SURGERY

Consider abdominal surgery for unmanageable pain, displacement of intestine, abnormal peritoneal fluid, or deterioration in condition.

PROGNOSIS

- Good for cecal impaction if primary and detected and treated early in disease
- Guarded for cecal impaction if it persists for >24–48 hr
- Very good for pelvic flexure impaction
- Guarded for ileal and small colon impactions

FOLLOW-UP

PATIENT MONITORING

N/A

POSSIBLE COMPLICATIONS

Magnesium sulfate therapy can lead to hypermagnesemia, especially if there is deficiency in renal function, hypocalcemia, or compromised vascular integrity.

MISCELLANEOUS

ASSOCIATED CONDITIONS, AGE-RELATED FACTORS, ZOONOTIC POTENTIAL, PREGNANCY

N/A

SEE ALSO

Colic

ABBREVIATION

- DSS = dioctyl sodium succinate
- NSE = nephrosplenic entrapment

Suggested Reading

White NA, Dabareiner RM. Treatment of impaction colics. Vet Clin North Am [Equine Prac] 1997;13:243–259.

Hanson RR, et al. Medical treatment of horses with ileal impactions: 10 cases (1990–1994). J Am Vet Med Assoc 1996;208:898–900.

Dart AJ, et al. Abnormal conditions of the equine descending (small) colon: 102 cases (1979–1989). J Am Vet Med Assoc 1992;200:971–978.

Snyder JR, Spier SJ. Disorders of the small intestine associated with acute abdominal pain. In: Smith BP, ed: Large Animal Internal Medicine, 2nd ed. St. Louis, Mosby 1996;755–783.

Blikslager AT. Surgical disorders of the small intestine. In: Smith BP, ed: Large Animal Internal Medicine, 3rd ed. St. Louis, Mosby 2002;649.

Author Daniel G. Kenney

Consulting Editors Henry Stämpfli and Olimpo Oliver-Espinosa

INFECTIOUS ANEMIA (EIA)

BASICS

DEFINITION

- An infectious disease caused by equine infectious anemia virus (EIAV), a lentivirus of the family Retroviridae.
- EIAV is closely related to HIV-1, the cause of AIDS in humans.

PATHOPHYSIOLOGY

- EIAV is transmitted primarily by blood-feeding insects, especially tabanids (i.e., horseflies and deerflies); iatrogenic transmission can occur via contaminated needles, syringes, and surgical instruments as well as through contaminated semen and transfusion of contaminated blood or plasma.
- Once infected, a horse remains so for life.
- EIAV infects cells of the monocyte/macrophage lineage and can be detected in the cytoplasm of this cell type in the liver, spleen, lymph nodes, lung, bone marrow, and circulation.
- EIAV can be characterized by three clinical syndromes—acute, chronic, and inapparent carrier; not all horses progress through all three syndromes.
- Acute disease—usually occurs 1–4 weeks after infection; is associated with high levels of viremia; can be characterized by fever, anorexia, lethargy, ventral edema, thrombocytopenia, anemia, and occasionally, epistaxis and death; and is usually <1 week in duration and sometimes mild enough to go completely unnoticed.
- Chronic disease—associated with recurrent episodes of viral replication, causing repeated bouts of clinical signs; classic signs of anemia, ventral edema, and weight loss occur during this phase.
- With time, episodes of clinical disease decrease in duration and severity, and most horses control the infection within 1 year, becoming inapparent carriers.
- Inapparent carriers show no clinical signs, are seropositive, and are reservoirs of infection, capable of transmitting the virus to uninfected horses.

SYSTEMS AFFECTED

- Hemic/lymphatic/immune—anemia caused by immune-mediated intravascular and extravascular hemolysis as well as bone marrow suppression. Likewise, thrombocytopenia is caused by both bone marrow suppression and enhanced platelet destruction; severe thrombocytopenia can lead to mucous membrane petechiae and epistaxis.
- Cardiovascular—immune-mediated vasculitis leads to hemorrhage, thrombosis, and edema.
- Hepatobiliary—accumulations of lymphocytes and macrophages in the liver can result in hepatomegaly, fatty degeneration, and hepatic cell necrosis.
- Renal/urologic—immune complex deposition can result in glomerulonephritis.
- Neurologic—vasculitis and lymphocyte accumulation in meninges occasionally result in ataxia.

GENETICS

N/A

WORLDWIDE DISTRIBUTION

- In the United States, the true prevalence is unknown, because less than 25% of the total U.S. horse population is tested. Prevalence varies by state, and ranges from 0 – 0.14% of horses tested. The prevalence is usually higher in the Gulf Coast states, because the climate is favorable for virus transmission.

SIGNALMENT

- Horses, ponies, mules, and donkeys are susceptible; however, donkeys and mules appear to be less severely affected.
- No breed, age, or sex predilections

SIGNS

General Comments

- Clinical signs—vary, depending on the stage of disease.
- Inapparent carriers—clinically normal.
- Chronic stage—affected animals may show no signs between clinical episodes.

Historical Findings

- Signs can go unnoticed.
- May be a history of inappetence, lethargy, and fever.
- Severely affected horses may have a history of high fever (40.5–41.5°C; 105–106°F), depression, ventral edema, weight loss, ataxia, and epistaxis.

Physical Examination Findings

Normal, or could include poor body condition, lethargy, fever, mucosal petechiation, ventral edema, pale mucous membranes, epistaxis, and ataxia

CAUSES

Infection with EIAV

RISK FACTORS

Contact with other equids during warm weather, when tabanids are abundant. Transfusion of contaminated blood or plasma.

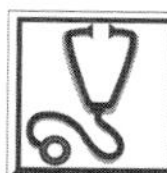

DIAGNOSIS

DIFFERENTIAL DIAGNOSIS

- List of differential diagnoses depends on the predominant clinical signs.
- Horses affected with these other diseases are seronegative for EIAV and easily differentiated from those infected with EIAV.
- Anemia/thrombocytopenia—blood loss, anemia of chronic disease, red-maple intoxication, immune-mediated thrombocytopenia/hemolytic anemia, and neoplasia
- Fever—other viral/bacterial/inflammatory diseases and neoplasia
- Weight loss—inadequate feed intake, dental abnormalities, parasitism, other chronic diseases, and neoplasia
- Ventral edema—hypoalbuminemia, pleuropneumonia, vasculitis, neoplasia, protein-losing enteropathy, and peritonitis
- Ataxia—cervical stenotic myelopathy, EHV-1 myeloencephalitis, and equine protozoal myeloencephalitis

CBC/BIOCHEMISTRY/URINALYSIS

- Thrombocytopenia—the first laboratory abnormality detected in acutely infected horses, occurs coincidentally with fever, resolves along with resolution of the clinical disease, but recurs with subsequent disease cycles.
- Decreases in PCV and RBCs can occur shortly after infection but generally are more severe during the chronic stage; leukopenia, lymphocytosis, and monocytosis are observed in many infected horses.
- Hypergammaglobulinemia may be present.
- Increases in liver enzyme activities may occur.

OTHER LABORATORY TESTS

- Diagnosis confirmed by serologic testing—AGID (Coggins test) and several ELISA tests are approved by the USDA and detect serum antibody to the EIAV core protein, Gag p26.
- Acute infection produces detectable antibody within 45 days.
- Coggins test—the most widely used and 95% accurate in diagnosing EIAV infection; occasional false-negative results may occur.
- ELISA is more sensitive than AGID, leading to possible false-positive results.
- All horses testing positive with either test should be retested for confirmation.

IMAGING

N/A

DIAGNOSTIC PROCEDURES

N/A

PATHOLOGIC FINDINGS

- In horses that die or are euthanized during a febrile episode, lesions include splenomegaly, hepatomegaly, accentuated hepatic lobular structure, lymphadenopathy, mucosal and visceral hemorrhages, ventral subcutaneous edema, and vessel thrombosis.
- Accumulations of lymphocytes and macrophages in the periportal regions of the liver and in the spleen, lymph nodes, adrenal gland, lung, and meninges
- Lymphoproliferative lesions are thought to result from the spread of virus-reactive T lymphocytes to control infection.
- Fatty degeneration of the liver and hepatic cell necrosis
- Glomerulitis can be present.
- Necropsy of inapparent carriers—unremarkable

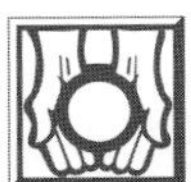

TREATMENT

APPROPRIATE HEALTH CARE

- No effective treatment
- Immediately isolate seropositive horses from other equids.

NURSING CARE

- Provide general supportive care during clinical episodes; the nature of this care varies, depending on the types and severity of signs.
- Whole-blood transfusions may benefit horses with severe anemia or thrombocytopenia.
- Standing leg wraps may benefit horses with ventral pitting edema.
- Cold-water hosing may decrease the temperature in horses with high fever that is nonresponsive to NSAIDs.

ACTIVITY

N/A

DIET

N/A

CLIENT EDUCATION

- A reportable disease in many countries, including the United States
- Federal law prohibits interstate travel of infected animals, except for slaughter, return to place of origin, or transport to a recognized research facility or diagnostic laboratory.
- Individual states regulate intrastate travel, and most control measures include the following options for seropositive horses—euthanasia, permanent identification and life-long quarantine, or transport to a recognized research facility.

SURGICAL CONSIDERATIONS

N/A

MEDICATIONS

DRUGS OF CHOICE

- Because no treatment for EIAV is effective and infected horses remain so for life, only rarely is treatment attempted.
- NSAIDs may be administered for control of fever and inflammation during viremic, febrile episodes—flunixin meglumine (1.1 mg/kg IV q12h).

CONTRAINDICATIONS

- Corticosteroids will exacerbate viremia and clinical disease, and are therefore contraindicated.

PRECAUTIONS

N/A

POSSIBLE INTERACTIONS

N/A

ALTERNATIVE DRUGS

N/A

FOLLOW-UP

PATIENT MONITORING

N/A

PREVENTION/AVOIDANCE

- Federal and state control measures have lowered the prevalence of EIAV in the U.S., but outbreaks still occur.
- Veterinarians, horse owners, and others in the equine industry can reduce the chance of exposure by requiring an EIAV test as part of every prepurchase examination; a recent, negative EIAV test before admitting any new horse to a farm; recent, negative EIAV tests for horses entering shows, sales, race tracks, and other events; annual testing of all horses for EIAV exposure; never injecting different horses with a common needle or syringe; ensuring that blood and blood products used for transfusions are from EIAV-negative donors; thoroughly disinfecting instruments that come into contact with blood; and practicing rigorous fly control.

POSSIBLE COMPLICATIONS

N/A

EXPECTED COURSE AND PROGNOSIS

- Occasionally, horses may die of EIAV, but most eventually control the infection and become life-long, inapparent carriers.
- Inapparent carriers are clinically normal but remain reservoirs of infection.

MISCELLANEOUS

ASSOCIATED CONDITIONS

N/A

AGE-RELATED FACTORS

N/A

ZOONOTIC POTENTIAL

N/A

PREGNANCY

- EIAV can be transmitted transplacentally in pregnant mares and may cause abortion.
- EIAV also may be transmitted via colostrum or milk.

SYNONYMS

Swamp fever

ABBREVIATIONS

- AGID = agar gel immunodiffusion
- AIDS = acquired immunodeficiency syndrome
- ELISA = enzyme-linked immunosorbent assay
- EHV = equine herpesvirus
- EIAV = equine infectious anemia virus
- HIV = human immunodeficiency virus
- NSAID = nonsteroidal anti-inflammatory drug
- PCV = packed cell volume
- USDA = United States Department of Agriculture

Suggested Reading

Mealey RH. Equine Infectious Anemia Virus. In Sellon DC and Long MT, eds. Equine Infectious Diseases.St. Louis: Saunders-Elsevier, 2006:213–219.

Montelaro RC, Ball JM, Rushlow KE. Equine retroviruses. In: Levy JA, ed. The retroviridae. New York: Plenum Press, 1993:257–360.

Sellon DC, Fuller FJ, McGuire TC. The immunopathogenesis of equine infectious anemia virus. Virus Res 1994;32:111–138.

Author Robert H. Mealey

Consulting Editors Ashley G. Boyle and Corinne R. Sweeney

INFECTIOUS ARTHRITIS (NONHEMATOGENOUS)

BASICS

DEFINITION

Inflammatory process within a joint caused by direct invasion of microorganisms such as bacteria or in rare occasions viruses or fungi

PATHOPHYSIOLOGY

Organisms such as bacteria invade the joint by direct inoculation, such as during intra-articular injections, traumatic wounds and surgery, or by dissemination from neighboring infected tissue such as with peri-articular septic cellulitis.

SYSTEM AFFECTED

Musculoskeletal—joint

GENETICS

N/A

INCIDENCE/PREVALENCE

Although any breed can be affected, Standardbreds show a higher incidence due to the greater number of joint injections this breed receives compared to others.

GEOGRAPHIC DISTRIBUTION N/A

SIGNALMENT

Breed Predilections

Standardbreds are overrepresented due to the higher incidence of intra-articular injections.

Mean Age None

Predominant Sex None

SIGNS

Historical Findings

• Lameness +/− joint effusion • Traumatic wound involving a joint • Draining wound over or near a joint • Recent intra-articular injection

Physical Examination Findings

• Lameness, often severe • Joint effusion
• Periarticular edema and/or cellulitis • Heat
• Extreme pain on palpation and manipulation of the affected joint • With open joint lacerations, lameness and effusion are minimal.

CAUSES

• Traumatic articular wounds* • Inoculation during intra-articular injection* • Postsurgical infection • Idiopathic • Isolates from penetrating wounds are often polymicrobial.
• Common gram-negative organisms—Enterobacteriaceae including *Escherichia coli, Pseudomonas, Acinetobacter, Proteus, Klebsiella, Citrobacter, Salmonella, Enterococcus*
• Common gram-positive organisms—coagulase-positive *Staphylococcus**, coagulase-negative *Staphylococcus*, β-hemolytic *Streptococcus*, non–β-hemolytic *Streptococcus, Rhodococcus equi, Corynebacterium* • *Staphylococcus aureus* is the most common after surgery or injection.
• Anaerobic contaminations such as *Clostridium**, *Bacteroides, Fusobacterium*, and *Peptostreptococcus* are common in wounds near the foot.

RISK FACTORS

• Performance horse • Intra-articular injection

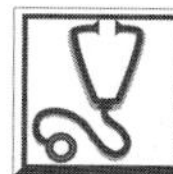

DIAGNOSIS

DIFFERENTIAL DIAGNOSIS

• Aseptic synovitis ("flare")—Rule out with synovial fluid analysis. • Traumatic osteochondral fragmentation—Rule out with radiography and synovial fluid analysis.

CBC/BIOCHEMESTRY/URINALYSIS

+/− Hyperfibrinogenemia

OTHER LABORATORY TESTS

Synovial Fluid Analysis

• Gross abnormalities—watery, turbid, and cloudy fluid, +/− flocculent material
• Nucleated cell count—>30,000 cells/μL
• Nucleated cell distribution—>80% neutrophils, +/− toxic and degenerative changes • Total protein level—≥4.0g/dL; in acute cases, >3.5g/dL

Synovial Fluid Culture

• Only 60%–75% of synovial fluid cultures from infected joints will yield a positive culture. For this reason, it is imperative that fluid be submitted for cytology.
• To increase the likelihood of obtaining a positive culture, synovial sample must be obtained prior to the administration of antibiotics and submitted in broth culture medium with the largest volume of synovial fluid sample possible such as 5–10mL.

IMAGING

Radiography

• Often normal in early infection • +/− Concomitant fracture • +/− Osteolysis or other signs of bone infection (osteomyelitis)
• Serial radiography is used to identify preexisting or developing osteoarthritis and to monitor progression, particularly in chronic infection.

Ultrasound

• Abnormalities include synovial effusion, intra-articular fibrinous material, and synovial proliferation, +/− cartilaginous defects.
• It can be very helpful with the diagnosis when extensive edema and swelling of the periarticular tissues or joint location (hip or shoulder) make visual assessment of joint difficult.

Nuclear scintigraphy

• Abnormalities include increased radiopharmaceutical uptake in the subchondral and/or periphyseal bone. • Areas of reduced radioactivity (photopenia) with sequestra

CT/MRI

Abnormalities include synovial proliferation and cartilage defects.

OTHER DIAGNOSITC PROCEDURES

Digital Exploration of the Wound

• This should be performed with sterile gloves and after the wound and surrounding skin have been thoroughly and aseptically prepared. • It confirms the wound communicates with the joint when articular cartilage is palpated. • Caution should be taken to avoid creating a previously nonexistent communication between the wound and the joint.

Distention of the Joint with Sterile Saline

• Easiest and most effective means of determining wound communication
• Procedure—Asepticly prepare the joint, place a sterile needle into the joint at a point distant from the wound, distend the joint with sterile saline. • Leakage of fluid from the wound confirms communication with the joint.

Contrast Radiography

• Similar to distending the joint with saline, except that an iodinated contrast agent is injected into the joint and radiographs are obtained. • The presence of contrast agent outside the synovial compartment indicates involvement with the wound.

PATHOLOGICAL FINDINGS

• Synovial thickening • Hyperemia of the synovium • Cartilage degradation • Bone necrosis • Fibrin within the joint

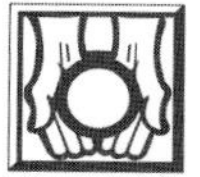

TREATMENT

AIMS OF TREATMENT

• Eliminate infection within the joint.
• Avoid or minimize articular damage.
• Reduce joint pain and inflammation.
• Return horse to previous level of soundness.

APPROPRIATE HEALTH CARE

• Should be regarded as a medical emergency
• Inpatient medical management is desirable.
• Typical case management consists of antimicrobial therapy, joint lavage +/− debridement, and pain management. Periodic synovial fluid analysis, lameness evaluation, and radiographic assessment are also performed.
• Antimicrobial therapies:
  ○ Systemic antimicrobial therapy—broad-spectrum antimicrobial until infection has completely resolved. Initial choices can be adjusted following bacterial culture and sensitivity results. Treatment should continue for a minimum of 2–4 weeks beyond clinical resolution.
  ○ Local antimicrobial therapy—intra-articular antimicrobials via single injection, constant rate infusion, and/or antimicrobial impregnated polymethylmethacrylate beads; daily treatment initially and then as needed

○ Regional perfusion of joint—delivery of high antimicrobial concentration via intravenous or interosseous delivery;

• Procedure—Placing a tourniquet proximal to the affected joint, antimicrobials diluted into 60mL of saline are administered slowly via venous or interosseous injection; after 30–35min, tourniquet is removed; performed on a daily or every other day basis until resolution of the infection

• Pain management—daily systemic NSAIDs, intra-articular NSAIDs, epidural narcotics

NURSING CARE

• Bandaging—Important to reduce soft tissue swelling, edema, and joint effusion. This can result in an increased level of comfort for the animal and better visual assessment of the infected structure(s). • Physical therapy—passive joint flexion once acute inflammation has resolved

ACTIVITY

Rest and controlled exercise—A minimum of 4 weeks of stall rest with only hand-walking exercise should be recommended in cases of acute synovial infections that respond readily to intervention. Chronic cases, particularly those with associated degenerative changes and other sequelae, might require a more-extended convalescence.

DIET

• Reduce high-energy feeds during convalescent period. • Monitor hay intake in order to prevent large colon or cecal impactions.

CLIENT EDUCATION

• Infectious arthritis is a medical emergency and should be treated as such. • Any wound near a joint should be fully investigated.
• Any unexpected lameness and/or effusion soon after joint injections should be fully investigated. • Multiple therapies are common and treatment is frequently prolonged.
• Without proper treatment, joint sepsis may result in chronic lameness, refractory infection, and contralateral limb laminitis.

SURGICAL CONSIDERATIONS

• Joint lavage—Copious lavage is the most important intervention along with antimicrobials; performed immediately and then daily or as needed depending on the severity of the infection; procedure—copious balanced electrolyte solution infused under pressure, +/− antimicrobials or anti-inflammatories, multiple large (14–18)-gauge needles placed on opposite sides of joint; performed in the sedated standing horse with local anesthesia or in the anesthetized horse • Arthroscopic lavage and debridement—allows visualization of the joint and removal of foreign debris, fibrin, infected synovium; also an effective method of lavage
• Joint drainage—considered in chronic cases and those in which lavage alone has not provided the desired results; drainage via arthroscopic stab incisions, preexisting wound tract, open arthrotomy, or closed suction drainage systems

MEDICATIONS

DRUG(S) OF CHOICE

• Systemic antimicrobial therapy—broad-spectrum combination (penicillin or cephalosporin and aminoglycoside)
  ○ Penicillin—potassium penicillin (22,000–44,000 IU/kg IV QID)
  ○ Cephalosporin—ceftiofur sodium (2.2–4.4 mg/kg IV daily to BID)
  ○ Aminoglycoside—gentamicin sulfate (6.6–8.0 mg/kg IV SID)
  ○ Fluroquinolone—enrofloxacin (5 mg/kg PO SID)
• Intra-articular antimicrobial therapy
  ○ Amikacin sulfate (250–500mg)
  ○ Gentamicin sulfate (500mg)
  ○ Sodium penicillin (1×10^6 units)
  ○ Cefazolin (500mg)
  ○ Ceftiofur sodium (500mg)
• Antimicrobials for regional limb perfusion
  ○ Amikacin sulfate, ceftiofur sodium, cefazolin, ceftazidime
  ○ All at 1-g concentrations diluted into 60 mL of saline
• Dimethyl sulfoxide can be added to the lavage as a 10% solution as a free radical scavenger and anti-inflammatory agent.
• Systemic NSAID—phenylbutazone (2.2–4.4 mg/kg IV or PO daily to BID)
• Topical NSAID—1% diclofenac sodium cream (5-inch ribbon of cream over the affected joint BID for up to 10 days)
• Epidural narcotics—morphine (0.1 mg/kg SID) or detomidine (0.05 mg/kg daily to QID)

CONTRAINDICATIONS

• Fluoroquinilones should not be used systemically in neonates due to the potential for significant osteochondrosis.
• Fluoroquinilones should not be used intra-articularly due to its toxic effects on chondrocytes.

PRECAUTIONS

• Systemic NSAIDs can be ulcerogenic. Monitor for abnormal clinical signs such as inappetence, diarrhea, and colic. • NSAIDs and aminoglycosides can be nephrotoxic; therefore, renal function (via serum creatinine levels) should be evaluated and rechecked periodically.

POSSIBLE INTERACTIONS

None

ALTERNATIVE DRUGS

None

FOLLOW-UP

PATIENT MONITORING

• The joint is evaluated on a daily basis during bandage change. Joint effusion, drainage, heat, and swelling are assessed. • General comfort and lameness are initially monitored daily and then as needed. • To assess disease progression and response to therapy, periodic synovial fluid analysis and synovial fluid culture and sensitivity are performed.
• Periodic radiographic and ultrasonographic evaluations are also performed.

PREVENTION/AVOIDANCE

• Avoid unnecessary joint injections. • Good husbandry to reduce the likelihood of accidents and lacerations

POSSIBLE COMPLICATIONS

• Osteoarthritis • Osteomyelitis • Lameness, inability to return to previous level of performance • Contralateral limb laminitis
• If severe, complications could necessitate euthanasia.

EXPECTED COURSE AND PROGNOSIS

• Prognosis is good for survival and return to athletic soundness as long as the infection is recognized early. • Preexisting osteoarthritis or cartilage damage secondary to the infection will negatively affect return to performance.
• Prompt recognition and aggressive treatment often result in good prognosis.
• Delayed recognition, minimal therapy, and drug-resistant organisms will negatively affect the prognosis.

MISCELLANEOUS

ASSOCIATED CONDITIONS

• Osteoarthritis • Lameness • Traumatic articular fracture

AGE-RELATED FACTORS

None

ZOONOTIC POTENTIAL

N/A

PREGNANCY

None

SYNONYMS

Septic arthritis, joint infection

SEE ALSO

• Osteochondrosis • Laminitis
• Osteoarthritis

Suggested Reading

Bertone AL. Infectious arthritis. In: Ross MW, Dyson SJ, eds. Diagnosis and Management of Lameness in the Horse. Philadelphia: WB Saunders, 2003:598–606.

Schneider RK. Synovial and osseous infections. In: Auer JA, Stick JA, eds. Equine Surgery, ed 3. Philadelphia: WB Saunders, 2006:1121–1130.

Author José M. García-López
Consulting Editor Elizabeth J. Davidson

INFLAMMATORY AIRWAY DISEASE

BASICS

DEFINITION

• A recurrent and reversible airway obstruction caused by accumulation of inflammatory cells leading to excess mucus production and airway hyperresponsiveness.
• Shares similar features with heaves. The signs are less severe, however, and it may also affect young horses.
• If no action is taken, may progress to clinical signs of heaves over several years.

PATHOPHYSIOLOGY

Horses develop an increased sensitivity to dust, molds, pollens, and other irritants, causing mast cells, neutrophils, eosinophils, lymphocytes, and alveolar macrophages to release potent mediators. Relationship between the presence of increased population of inflammatory cells and airway hyperreactivity has been documented. Further, lung biopsies obtained from actively racing horses with IAD demonstrated changes in the small airways in a pattern similar to heaves, i.e., peribronchiolar inflammatory cell infiltration, goblet cells hyperplasia and accumulation of mucus and neutrophils in the airway lumen.

SYSTEM AFFECTED

• Strictly limited to the respiratory system.
• Pathologic changes occur in the small airways (i.e., bronchioles). The alveoli are not affected.

GENETICS

Thus far there has not been any study linking genetic traits to a specific breed.

INCIDENCE/PREVALENCE

Widespread worldwide, where horses are stabled or trained in enclosed environments.

GEOGRAPHIC DISTRIBUTION

Inflammatory airway disease in performing horses has been identified in North America (USA and Canada), United Kingdom, Iceland, Europe and Australia.

SIGNALMENT

• Any breed
• May be recognized in horses <1 year of age.
• Seems to progress to a chronic form such as heaves with age.

SIGNS

Historical

• In athletic horses, reduced exercise tolerance or poor performance, with a prolonged recovery period after exercise is the most commonly reported clinical sign.
• Other observations—intermittent to frequent coughing while the horse is eating or early in exercise, nasal discharge, and occasionally increased respiratory rate (>15 breaths/min).

Physical Examination

• The vital signs are within the normal range, except on occasion, when the resting respiratory rate may exceed 18 breaths/min or when a prolonged return to normal respiratory rate after exercise is observed.
• Nasal discharge—uncommon but occasionally a serous to mucopurulent discharge may be observed.
• Significant increase in bronchial sounds over both lung fields.
• With a rebreathing bag, wheezes are frequently detected over the dorsal area of the lung field and coughing may be elicited.
• Lung-field percussion may identify dorsal and caudal areas of hyperresonance, detectable beyond the 16th rib.
• A keen observer may notice a slight abdominal lift on expiration.
• No clinical signs of other systemic illness and CBC/biochemistry profile are normal.

CAUSES

• Airborne environmental allergens and irritants are believed to be the primary causative agents—mold and dust from hay and bedding, airborne endotoxins and noxious gases such as ammonia from stagnant bedding.
• Persistent airway inflammation post respiratory viral infections.
• Development and progressive airway inflammation following onset of exercise-induced pulmonary hemorrhage.
• Persistent airway inflammation following a bacterial bronchitis in weanlings and occasionally yearlings.

RISK FACTORS

• Predisposing and exacerbating factors include respiratory viral infections (e. g., equine influenza virus, rhinovirus and herpesvirus) and bacterial bronchitis in weanlings.
• Higher incidence during hot summer days with high humidity.
• High intensity training and racing.

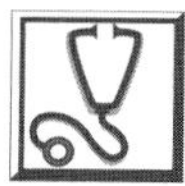

DIAGNOSIS

DIFFERENTIAL DIAGNOSIS

• Respiratory viral infections (e. g., equine influenza virus, rhinovirus and herpesvirus) generally affect several horses in the same stable within a defined period of time, whereas inflammatory airway disease affects and persists in one to two horses and worsens over time or resolves spontaneously.
• Bacterial tracheitis and bronchitis, usually secondary to respiratory viral infection, normally are responsive to a 5–7-day course of broad-spectrum antibiotic.
• Any persistence of respiratory clinical signs without elevated body temperature suggests inflammatory airway disease.
• Localized pulmonary abscess may present a similar history, but clinical signs indicate fever, inappetence, and pain on chest percussion over the anteroventral area of the lung fields.
• Relapsing bacterial bronchitis in weanlings due to *Streptococcus equi* var *zooepidemicus* following a 2–3-week treatment with antibiotics.

CBC/BIOCHEMISTRY/BLOOD GAS ANALYSIS/URINALYSIS

Normal

OTHER LABORATORY TESTS

• Bronchoscopy and bronchoalveolar lavage to retrieve cells of the lower airways and alveoli.
• Total count and differential of cells counts harvested from bronchoalveolar lavage fluid. These cells are analyzed quantitatively and qualitatively to determine major changes in the inflammatory cell.
population—neutrophils, mast cells, eosinophils, lymphocytes, and exfoliated epithelial cells.
• Lung biopsies permit histologic examination of the small airways and provide information on severity and prognosis but are not routinely done.
• Histamine provocation is a specific test that determines the degree of airway hyperresponsiveness, which manifests as increased sensitivity to a wide variety of allergic and nonallergic agents resulting from the underlying airway inflammation. Histamine provocation test is highly correlated to increased number of mast cells and neutrophils from BAL (from referral center).

IMAGING

Thoracic radiography has little value except to demonstrate small, 2–4-mm-diameter, donut-shaped lesions representing accumulation of inflammatory cells in the periphery of bronchioles.

OTHER DIAGNOSTIC PROCEDURES

• Lung biopsy to assess alveoli and small airway pathology
• Histamine provocation test to assess airway hyperresponsiveness
• Breath and breath condensate analysis is an indicator of airway inflammation but presently restricted to few academic institutions.
• Pulmonary scintigraphy may have some potential as an adjunct diagnostic tool but not presently accessible at most academic institutions or specialized equine clinics.

PATHOLOGIC FINDINGS

• Lesions are restricted to the small airways (<5 mm).
• Accumulation of inflammatory cells in the airways and mucus plugging of the airways caused by goblet cell hyperplasia are early changes.
• Smooth muscle hyperplasia from frequent constriction or spasm of the airways.

- Persistent small airway inflammation has led the histopathologist to use the term "airway remodeling" referring to dynamic pathological changes during the course of persistent ongoing inflammation. Such changes have been recognized in heaves affected horses but not defined in IAD.

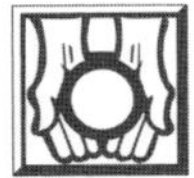

TREATMENT

AIMS OF TREATMENT

To control the airway inflammation leading to improvement in pulmonary function and reduction in airway hyperreactivity and in mucus production.

APPROPRIATE HEALTH CARE

- Make all possible attempts to avoid environmental dust from low quality hay and bedding.
- Encourage outdoor living with opened shelter access.

NURSING CARE

N/A

ACTIVITY

No limitations with proper therapeutic plans and environmental management control.

DIET

Generally there is no need to alter the diet of high performing horses as their diet is largely composed of high concentrate grain ration and lower quantity of hay for the source of roughage. Haylage has not been widely utilized in North America due to the fear of botulism.

CLIENT EDUCATION

- The disease may not be curable and may remain active for the horse's life in some cases; however, the condition can be kept under control allowing the horse to maintain an active and maximal performance athletic career.
- Well ventilated stall environment, rubber flooring with highly efficient urine absorbent materials, complete pelleted ration with small amount of soaked or wetted hay.
- Outdoor living if at all possible.
- Long term therapy with metered dose inhaler (MDI) is preferable as the medication is directly deliver to the lung with minimal systemic effect, i.e., reduction of adrenal suppressive effects and reduced risk of laminitis.
- Maintain an up to date vaccination schedule for respiratory viral infections particularly influenza and herpesviruses.

SURGICAL CONSIDERATIONS

N/A

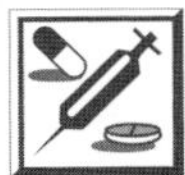

MEDICATIONS

DRUGS OF CHOICE

Corticosteroids (Mature Horses)

- Oral—prednisolone (400 mg BID for 15 days, then 300 mg once a day for 15 days, and a maintenance dose of 300 mg once a day on alternate days for as long as needed)
- Metered dose inhalers with special delivery devices—fluticasone proprionate (250 μg/puff; eight puffs BID for 2 weeks, then on alternate days for as long as needed) or beclomethasone dipropionate (250 μg/puff; 12 puffs BID for 2 weeks, then on alternate days for as long as needed).

Mast Cell Stabilizer

Nedocromil sodium (2 mg/puff; 12 puffs BID for 2 weeks, then on alternate days for as long as needed) (Not available in Canada)

Bronchodilators

- Clenbuterol (see the label recommendation; dosage varies from country to country)
- Ipatropium bromide (20 μg/puff; 5–6 puffs given 10–15 min before exercise)
- Salbutamol/albuterol (100 μg/puff; 5–10 puffs given 10–15 min before exercise)

CONTRAINDICATIONS

Do not use high doses of corticosteroids in cases with suspected concomitant viral or bacterial infection, or with active laminitis.

PRECAUTIONS

- Oral corticosteroids are not recommended in mares while in late gestation; however, inhaled corticosteroids appear safe because of their very low systemic effect.
- Verify medication regulations for withdrawal times before racing and or competition.

POSSIBLE INTERACTIONS

N/A

ALTERNATIVE DRUGS

Herbal therapy and allergen desensitization have not been shown to control the airway inflammatory process and be effective.

FOLLOW-UP

PATIENT MONITORING

N/A

PREVENTION/AVOIDANCE

- Avoid moldy hay and straw.
- Maximize fresh-air periods and reduce stabling time. Outdoor living with shelter is an ideal environment.
- Change diet—haylage, complete feed, or hay cubes with low-dust content and soaking/watering hay prior to feeding to better control dust contents.

POSSIBLE COMPLICATIONS

Acute exacerbation similar to heaves if the horse is exposed to an environment rich in mold and dust.

EXPECTED COURSE AND PROGNOSIS

The disease is a lifelong condition, and prognosis largely depends on early diagnosis and owner compliance with maintaining a low-allergen environment and a therapeutic corticosteroid regimen.

MISCELLANEOUS

ASSOCIATED CONDITIONS

N/A

AGE-RELATED FACTORS

The condition tends to progress with age.

ZOONOTIC POTENTIAL

N/A

PREGNANCY

See Medications and Precautions.

SYNONYMS

- Nonseptic inflammatory airway disease
- Allergic lower airway disease
- Allergic small airway disease

SEE ALSO

Heaves

ABBREVIATIONS

- BAL = bronchoalveolar lavage
- IAD = inflammatory airway disease

Suggested Reading

Conclusions of the Havemeyer Workshop. Inflammatory airway disease: Defining the syndrome. Equine Vet Educ 2003;15: 61–63.

Couetil LL, Hoffman AM, Hodgson J, et al. Inflammatory airway disease of horses. J Vet Intern Med 2007;21, 356–361.

Author Laurent Viel

Consulting Editor Daniel Jean

INFLUENZA

BASICS

DEFINITION

• Infection of the respiratory tract by the equine influenza virus. • Highly contagious • Most economically important contagious respiratory disease of the horse

PATHOPHYSIOLOGY

• Inhalation of aerosolized virus allows deposition of viral particles throughout respiratory tract. • Virus enters epithelial cells lining respiratory tract, replicates, and is released into the airways. • Infected cells undergo apoptosis. • Rapid spread of virus causes desquamation and denudation of respiratory epithelial cells and clumping of cilia. • Impaired mucociliary clearance results and may persist for 4 weeks postinfection.
• Secondary bacterial infections may occur.

SYSTEMS AFFECTED

• Respiratory • Musculoskeletal (rare)
• Cardiac (rare)

INCIDENCE AND PREVALENCE

• Endemic in North America and Europe
• First outbreak in Australia in 2007 • Not present in New Zealand or Iceland
• Outbreaks occur among large groups of susceptible horses, often young racehorses.
• Prevalence depends on age of animals in the group and previous exposure to the virus (either via natural exposure or vaccination).
• Morbidity can approach 100% in a population of young naïve horses.

SIGNALMENT

• Equidae of all ages are susceptible. • Young horses (1–3 years) are more commonly affected.

CLINICAL SIGNS

• One- to 2-day incubation period • Fever
• Frequent dry cough • Mucoid nasal discharge. May become mucopurulent to purulent if secondary bacterial infection occurs • Anorexia • Depression • Limb edema
• Conjunctivitis, epiphora • Submandibular lymphadenopathy • Muscle stiffness, soreness
• Clinical signs typically less severe in vaccinated horses.

CAUSES

• The disease is caused by an influenza A virus, which is a member of the family Orthomyxoviridae, genus *Influenza virus A and B*.
• Subtypes are identified by surface antigens HA and NA, which are primary determinants of antigenicity.
• Two subtypes of the virus exist.
  ○ A/equine/1 (H7N7)—has not been identified since 1979
  ○ A/equine/2 (H3N8)—currently identified virus
• Virus undergoes antigenic drift (minor changes of the HA and NA surface proteins) and antigenic shift (major change).
• Two antigenically distinct but related influenza A viruses co-circulate in horse populations in America and Europe.

RISK FACTORS

• All horses living in areas where influenza virus has been reported are at risk.
• Risk of developing the disease depends on age and immunity.
• Epidemics often occur when young, susceptible horses congregate, for example, at racecourses, sales, and shows.
• The spread of equine influenza throughout the world is believed to have been facilitated by international transport of horses for competition. Subclinically infected horses may introduce the virus into previously naïve populations, causing large epidemics.
• Donkeys are more severely affected than horses.

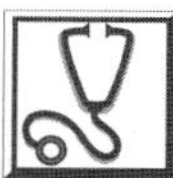

DIAGNOSTICS

DIFFERENTIAL DIAGNOSES

• Infections with EHV-1, EHV-4, EVA, and *Streptococcus equi* subsp *equi* can cause respiratory disease similar to equine influenza.
• The rapidity with which influenza spreads can help differentiate infection with this virus from other contagious respiratory pathogens.
• In addition, cough is less commonly observed in animals infected with EHV, EVA, or *S. equi.*
• The lymphadenopathy seen in cases of *S. equi* infection is typically more marked than that reported for influenza infections.

CBC/BIOCHEMISTRY/URINALYSIS

• An early lymphopenia and eosinopenia followed by a monocytosis may be seen, although these changes are transient and may be missed.
• Leukocytosis and hyperfibrinogenemia may occur if a secondary bacterial pneumonia develops.
• Increased creatine phosphokinase and aspartate aminotransferase have been rarely reported in horses which develop severe myopathies.

OTHER LABORATORY TESTS

• Diagnosis is typically based on classic clinical signs but can be confirmed by a number of different methods.
• Virus isolation from nasopharyngeal swabs/washings—Infected horses may shed virus for up to 7–10 days, but swabs should be taken within 24 hours of the development of a fever to maximize chances of isolating the virus. Samples should be placed in cool transport media.
• Directigen Flu-A Test—A commercial immunoassay (ELISA) developed for rapid in vitro recognition of influenza A nucleoprotein in human specimens has been used for the detection of equine influenza. The disease can be confirmed within 20–30 minutes of a nasopharyngeal swab being obtained from a horse.
• Reverse transcription–polymerase chain reaction from nasopharyngeal swabs/washings—allows rapid detection of viral antigen. It is highly sensitive but false positivity possible.
• Seroconversion—A 4-fold increase in antibody titer between acute and convalescent samples obtained 10–14 days apart is considered diagnostic. HI, VN, and SRH are tests used to detect antibodies against equine influenza.
• Diagnosis of secondary bacterial pneumonia can be made via culture of transtracheal wash specimens.

IMAGING

Ultrasonographic or radiographic evaluation of the thorax can be used to diagnose pneumonia as a sequela to influenza infection.

PATHOLOGIC FINDINGS

• Pharyngitis, laryngitis, tracheitis
• Bronchitis, bronchiolitis
• Interstitial pneumonia, congestion, edema, and neutrophilic inflammation

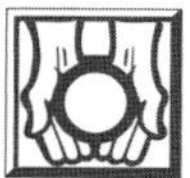

TREATMENT

APPROPRIATE HEALTH CARE

• Affected animals should be isolated to prevent spread.
• Most horses will recover from equine influenza infection within 1–3 weeks.

NURSING CARE

Horses should be housed in well-ventilated stalls.

ACTIVITY

• Stall rest or limited exercise is important until the respiratory epithelium has healed.
• One week of rest is suggested for each day the horse is febrile.
• Early return to exercise can delay recovery, and may lead to serious long-term and possibly life-threatening complications, such as myocarditis.

DIET

Horses should be fed palatable feeds with low dust content.

CLIENT EDUCATION

• Animals new to a population or potentially exposed horses returning to a group (such as horses attending a show or other event) should be isolated for at least several days (ideally, 2 weeks) and monitored closely for development of a fever or nasal discharge.
• If an outbreak of influenza or other respiratory disease is suspected, a quarantine should be established, and arrivals and departures from the premise should be prevented.
• Owners should be aware that vaccination of horses does not prevent infection.

SURGICAL CONSIDERATIONS

N/A

MEDICATIONS

DRUGS(S) OF CHOICE

- No antiviral drugs are marketed for the treatment of equine influenza.
- Antiviral drugs such as amanatadine and rimantadine may be useful but have not been evaluated extensively.
- Treatment is supportive—NSAIDs such as flunixin meglumine (1.1 mg/kg PO, IV q12h) or phenylbutazone (2.2–4.4 mg/kg IV, PO q12h) can be used to alleviate fever, depression, and muscle soreness.
- Secondary bacterial pneumonia should be treated with antimicrobials based on sensitivity pattern of organisms identified from a transtracheal wash. Pending culture results, broad-spectrum antimicrobial combinations targeted at commonly isolated organisms (*Streptococcus* spp. and *Actinobacillus* spp.) can be used (such as ceftiofur, penicillin, and gentamicin; trimethoprim-sulfamethoxazole).

CONTRAINDICATIONS

Corticosteroids are immunosuppressive, and because recovery from influenza depends largely on an effective immune response, these drugs should not be used.

PRECAUTIONS

NSAIDs should be used judiciously in horses that are inappetent and dehydrated, due to the potential development of gastrointestinal (gastric ulcers, right dorsal colitis) and renal toxicity (medullary crest necrosis).

POSSIBLE INTERACTIONS

N/A

ALTERNATE DRUGS

N/A

FOLLOW-UP

PATIENT MONITORING

Monitoring of vital signs, appetite, and attitude will allow horses that develop secondary sequelae such as bacterial pneumonia to be identified.

PREVENTION/AVOIDANCE

- Implementation of a quarantine program for newly introduced horses will decrease the likelihood of an influenza outbreak.
- Long-lived (12-month) immunity exists after natural infection with influenza virus. This immunity is independent of circulating antibody levels.
- The protection provided by traditional vaccines is dependent on generation of short-lived antibodies to the surface glycoproteins HA and NA.
- Vaccination can be used to decrease the risk of contracting the disease and reduce the severity of infection in at-risk horses but cannot be reliably used to prevent infection in individual animals.
- A number of different vaccines are available, containing varying strains of the virus as well as different viral preparations (killed, modified live).
- In order to be effective, it is important that vaccines contain viruses similar to strains circulating in the field.
- Novel live vaccines, delivered via the intranasal route, are available and are expected to generate a cellular immune response, more closely mimicking the protection afforded by natural infection. There is no method by which the cellular immunity generated by these vaccines can be easily measured.
- Traditional inactivated virus vaccines are administered intramuscularly, with a booster 3–4 weeks later. The vaccine manufacturers recommend a yearly booster, although it is generally accepted that levels of antibody generated by this schedule will be insufficient in most animals to prevent disease. More frequent administration, as often as every 2–3 months, may be needed to maintain antibody levels at a level considered protective. For horses considered at high risk of being exposed to influenza (such as young racehorses) this program may be recommended.
- The intranasal vaccines are licensed for use in animals over 9 months of age for one product, and 11 months for the other.
- Vaccination programs for foals depend on the vaccination status of the mare.
    - For foals from unvaccinated mares, using the intramuscularly inactivated products, an initial dose at 6 months, followed by two further doses at monthly intervalsis
    - For foals from vaccinated mares, the program should begin at 9 months, so that there is no interference from maternally derived antibodies.
- Regardless of vaccine used or program implemented, horses can still shed virus if exposed.
- Vaccinated, subclinically affected animals are known to have introduced the virus into susceptible populations, resulting in influenza epidemics.
- Isolation of affected horses and biosecurity measures aimed at preventing fomite transmission of the virus are important factors during an outbreak.

POSSIBLE COMPLICATIONS

- Secondary bacterial infections, causing pneumonia and pleuropneumonia, are potential sequelae. The destruction of the mucociliary apparatus by the virus removes one of the major defenses of the respiratory tract.
- In addition, the development of a mucopurulent to purulent nasal discharge is suggestive of bacterial infection.
- Auscultation of the thorax may reveal abnormal lung sounds such as wheezes and crackles in the case of pneumonia, or dull ventral sounds if pleural effusion develops.
- Myocarditis and immune-mediated myositis have been rarely reported as a sequela to influenza infection.
- Persistent coughing and an increased incidence of heaves in affected animals have been anecdotally reported.

EXPECTED COURSE AND PROGNOSIS

- Most horses will recover from influenza infection within 1–3 weeks.
- However, recovery of the respiratory tract can take longer than this, and horses are often lost to competition for >3 months.
- The prognosis for recovery is excellent, as long as sufficient rest is provided.
- Horses that develop secondary bacterial pneumonia or pleuropneumonia have a worse prognosis, although most of these horses will recover, provided that aggressive treatment and prolonged rest are implemented.

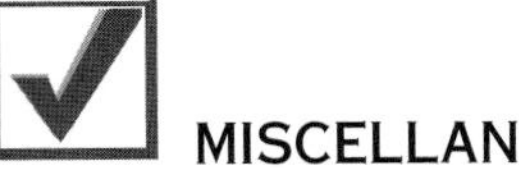

MISCELLANEOUS

AGE-RELATED FACTORS

- Foals without maternal antibodies against influenza can develop severe viral pneumonia.
- Prognosis is generally guarded in these foals, even with intensive care.

ZOONOTIC POTENTIAL

Equine influenza virus has not been shown to infect humans.

PREGNANCY

- Pregnant mares that become infected may abort.
- NSAIDs may help prevent abortion in exposed mares.

ABBREVIATIONS

- EHV = equine herpesvirus
- ELISA = enzyme-linked immunosorbent assay
- EVA = equine viral arteritis
- HA = hemagglutinin
- HI = hemagluttinin inhibition
- NA = neuraminidase
- SRH = single radial hemolysis
- VN = virus neutralization

Suggested Reading

Daly JM, Newton JR, Mumford JA. Current perspectives on control of equine influenza. Vet Res 2004;35:411–423.

Robinson NE. Current Therapy in Equine Medicine, ed 5. Philadelphia: WB Saunders, 2003:42–44.

Author Imogen Johns
Consulting Editors Ashley G. Boyle and Corinne R. Sweeney

INSECT HYPERSENSITIVITY

BASICS

DEFINITION

IH is a severely pruritic seasonal dermatitis that results in secondary self-inflicted trauma and sometimes urticaria. Hypersensitivity results from salivary proteins, venoms, excrement, or other proteinaceous body parts of biting arthropods such as midges (*Culicoides* spp.), and black flies (*Simulium* spp.). Other implicated insects include but are not limited to the horse fly (*Tabanus* spp.), common stable fly (*Stomoxys calcitrans*), mosquitoes (*Aedes*), wasps, bees, hornets *(Hymenoptera)*, and the filarial nematode *(Onchocerca cervicalis)*.

PATHOPHYSIOLOGY

Susceptible animals become sensitized to arthropod antigens by producing allergen-specific IgE, which binds to receptor sites on mast cells; further allergen exposure (inhalation, bites, percutaneous absorption) leads to mast cell degranulation, inducing an IgE-mediated immediate reaction, and results in the release of histamine and many other inflammatory mediators. Late phase (4–12 hr) and cell-mediated delayed reactions (24–72 hr) are also involved.

SYSTEM AFFECTED

Skin

GENETICS

A genetic basis for insect hypersensitivity has been demonstrated in Icelandic horses imported from Iceland and German Shire horses.

INCIDENCE/PREVALENCE

• Insect hypersensitivity is the most common cause of equine recurrent seasonal allergic pruritic skin disease worldwide. • Incidence rates range from 2.8% in the United Kingdom to 32% in Australia. • In cooler climates, IH presents as recurrent and seasonal and is most prevalent during the peak of the fly breeding season. • In warmer climates the incidence may present strictly as a nonseasonal disease. • Arthropod breeding sites add a localized prevalence, as weak fliers do not travel long distances to feed.

GEOGRAPHIC DISTRIBUTION

• Widespread but limited to areas conducive to respective arthropod breeding sites • *Culicoides* spp. require still water or marshy areas that also support mosquito development. • *Simulium* spp. require moving water for larval development.
• *S. calcitrans* breeds in decaying materials, indicating a hygiene issue for that stable.

SIGNALMENT

Breed Predilections

Breeds possibly at risk include Arabians, Connemaras, and Quarter Horses.

Mean Age and Range

Typically seen in horses between 2 and 4 years of age as previous sensitization is required. May find clinical signs as early as 6 mo of age but this is rare

Predominant Sex

No known sex predilection

SIGNS

General Comments

Owners may not witness the feeding of the insects if nocturnal but find wheals and skin lesions secondary to the insect bites. Clinical signs of IH reflect intense pruritus in specific distribution patterns. Primary acute lesions are papules or crusted papules and rarely papular urticaria. Chronic pruritus results in typical lesions of self-trauma such as excoriation, represented as erosions and ulcers, serous effusions, scale, crusts, exfoliation, lichenification, pigmentary disturbances, and various degrees of patchy alopecia represented by mild hypotrichosis to severe hair loss. The mane and tail are composed of sparse, broken, and distorted hairs that give the appearance of a "roached mane" and "rat tail."

Historical

• Note the age of onset of disease, seasonality, duration, locations of the initial disease, and how it has progressed. • Inquire if a response to strict insect control and/or administration of anti-inflammatory therapy has had an effect.

Physical Examination

• IH can have various clinical presentations based on the offending insect(s). Often there is no clinical feature to permit a definitive clinical diagnosis. • In general, the appearance of three dermatitis lesional distribution patterns can be recognized:

1. Dorsal—involves the face, pinnae, poll, mane, withers and tail head; insects implicated are various *Culicoides* spp. among others.
2. Ventral—involves the intermandibular space, ventral thorax and abdomen, axillae, ventral midline, and groin; insects implicated are *Haematobia irritans, Simulium* spp., and some *Culicoides* spp.
3. A combination of 2 and 3

Distribution may reflect the feeding patterns of various insects; for example, the caudal lateral aspects of both the front and hindlimbs are preferred feeding areas of *Aedes* and *S. calcitrans.*
• Secondary moderate to severe bacterial dermatitis is common.

CAUSES

• Exposure and sensitization to insect salivary protein, venom, excrement, or other proteinaceous body parts • Other flies not previously mentioned—horn, deer, and sand flies

RISK FACTORS

• Proximity to insect habitat • Flies require decaying bedding and manure, and standing water to breed; thus poor hygiene is a risk factor for any stable. • Concurrent pruritic dermatoses, such as atopic dermatitis or ectoparasitic disease (summation effect)

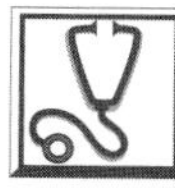

DIAGNOSIS

DIFFERENTIAL DIAGNOSIS

• Atopic dermatitis • Cutaneous adverse reaction to food or supplements • *Onchocerciasis* (uncommon with ivermectin use) • Cutaneous drug reaction • Contact hypersensitivity • Oxyuriasis • Ectoparasitic disease (acariosis, pediculosis, trombiculosis, strongyloidosis)
• Dematophytosis • Dermatophilosis

CBC/BIOCHEMISTRY/URINALYSIS

NA

IMAGING

NA

OTHER DIAGNOSTIC PROCEDURES

• Cytology from erosions or ulcers shows a neutrophilic exudate with cocci representative of a secondary folliculitis. • Perform skin scrapings to rule out ectoparasites. • Perform bacterial and DTM cultures to determine bacterial species and susceptibility and/or dermatophyte infections.
• Following the initial diagnosis of IH, confirmation of allergen-specific hypersensitivity to the offending insect(s) by intradermal testing can be used to institute avoidance practices and environmental management changes.

PATHOLOGIC FINDINGS

• The histologic pattern of IH has variable degrees of orthokeratotic to parakeratotic hyperkeratosis, epidermal hyperplasia, eosinophilic and lymphocytic epidermal exocytosis, erosion, ulceration, and a predominantly eosinophilic superficial and deep perivascular to interstitial dermatitis and folliculitis.
• Dermal fibrosis may be present in chronic lesions.
• Findings can support a diagnosis of IH but will not conclusively rule out differentials such as atopic disease, food allergy, or some ectoparasites.

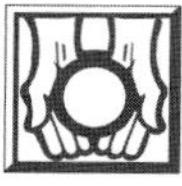

TREATMENT

AIMS OF TREATMENT

• Resolve secondary infections
• Control pruritus
• Institute integrated pest management including the use of topical pesticides, protective fly wear, avoidance measures, and stable modifications

APPROPRIATE HEALTH CARE

Outpatient medical management

NURSING CARE

• Judicious use of long-acting fly repellent such as those containing DEET or a citrus extract is imperative. Many of the topical spot-on formulations contain up to 50% permethrin and claim 7- to 14-day protection.
• Frequent cool water bathing with antimicrobial, keratolytic and keratoplastics shampoos can remove surface irritants, bacteria, allergens, and pruritogenic substances and provide temporary soothing.
• Application of topical antipruritics such as colloidal oatmeal help to raise the pruritic threshold by cooling and moisturizing dry skin.
• Products that contain local anesthetics such as pramoxine HCl, lidocaine, benzoyl peroxide, and tars have short duration of action but can provide relief.
• Avoidance of bites through physical interventions, such as habitat alterations or fans,

and some chemical interventions, such as repellents on the horse or insecticide fogs during feeding times. In lieu of fans, timed misters can emit pulses of insecticide fogs targeting the flying midges.

ACTIVITY

• Stable horse at the time the predominant insect is feeding. For example, *Simulium* spp. are daytime feeders and weak fliers, thus stable in daytime; *Culicoides* spp. are night feeders, thus stable at night and with fans to create light breezes as these are weak fliers.
• Relocation may be the best option.

DIET

Essential fatty acid supplementation may be beneficial.

CLIENT EDUCATION

• Essential that the client understand the feeding habits of the offending arthropod in order to time the appropriate interventions
• Successful control of the disease may be represented by an 80% control of pruritus.
• Discuss that therapeutic modifications over the life of the horse are to be expected and finding the most successful treatment protocol will take time.
• Due to the potential hereditary factor, owners should be advised to remove affected individual from breeding stock.
• Advise disease is not curable, but rather manageable and life long therapy may be needed.

MEDICATIONS

DRUG(S)

Corticosteroids

• Best selection—prednisolone, greater bioavailability than prednisone, tablets or syrup (compounded) at 0.5–1.5 mg/kg q24h until control achieved; then reduce to lowest-dose alternate-day regimen, for example, 0.2–0.5 mg/kg q48h
• For horses that do not respond to prednisolone, try dexamethasone powder or injectable. Initial loading oral or IV dose of 0.02–0.1 mg/kg q24h for 3–5 days; then taper to 0.01–0.02 mg/kg q48–72h for maintenance.
• Repository injectable corticosteroids should be avoided as withdrawal upon an adverse reaction is not possible.

Antihistamines—A Nonsteroidal Alternative for Long-Term Control

• Not useful when moderate to severe pruritus is present; rather use as a preventative either before the onset of severe pruritus or in a maintenance regimen to suppress pruritus once controlled.
• Pharmacokinetic data for the use of antihistamines in horses is limited. Anecdotal reports suggest that H_1-receptor antagonist hydroxyzine hydrochloride/pamonate (0.5–1 mg/kg q8h), chlorpheniramine (0.25 mg/kg q12h), diphenhydramine (0.75–1.0 mg/kg q12h), or pyrilamine malate (1 mg/kg q12h) may decrease pruritus and provide a steroid sparing effect.
• Antihistamines should be given at least 10–14 days before efficacy is determined. If no response, select another class of antihistamine.

CONTRAINDICATIONS

Due to the anticholinergic properties of antihistamines and tricyclic antidepressants, do not use in horses with a history of cardiac arrhythmias, colic, glaucoma, or urinary retention disorders. Antihistamines may thicken mucous in the respiratory tract. Extra caution should be used in horses with respiratory problems due to excess mucus.

PRECAUTIONS

• Pyrethroid insecticides have toxicities to cats, birds, bats, reptiles, amphibians, and fish—thus need to be used with caution.
• Corticosteroids—Use judiciously to avoid laminitis, iatrogenic hyperglucocorticism, diabetes mellitus, polydipsia and polyuria, aggravation of bacterial folliculitis, decreased muscle mass, weight loss, poor wound healing, and behavior changes.
• Antihistamines—can produce sedation and/or behavior changes, whole body or fine tremors or seizures. High doses of antihistamines cause birth defects in laboratory animals. Do not administer antihistamines intravenously in the horse due to potential CNS stimulation.
• Note drug withdrawal times and regulations pertaining to horse show or racing associations.

POSSIBLE INTERACTIONS

• Prednisolone interacts with phenytoin, phenobarbital, rifampin, erythromycin, and the anticholinesterase drugs, neostigmine and pyridostigmine.
• Antihistamines have an additive effect when combined with other CNS-depressant drugs, such as tranquilizers.

ALTERNATIVE DRUGS

• Citronella aromatics as repellents. Avon's Skin So Soft Bug Guard Plus line of sprays are effective repellents.
• Polyunsaturated omega 3 and 6 fatty acids—variable response in decreasing pruritus, provide support for epidermal barrier function and anti-inflammatory properties. Use as adjunctive therapy. Response noted within 2–8 weeks after starting therapy. Exact dosing for horse is lacking; the consulting editor uses 180 mg of EPA/10 lb q24h.
• ASIT—no long-term (≥1 year) double-blinded placebo-controlled studies with statistically significant numbers of horses have been conducted using ASIT formulated from insect extracts; therefore the benefit of ASIT in horses with IH is unclear.

FOLLOW-UP

PATIENT MONITORING

Observe animals for bites and reactions indicating the onset of midge season.

PREVENTION/AVOIDANCE

• Alter insect breeding habitat if possible; use fans to create light drafts over animals and fine mesh screen/netting doubled over in front of and over stalls. Spray screens daily with repellents. Use repellents on horses and/or misters with timers to emit fog of short-acting pyrethrins during feeding times. Use full coverage protective fly apparel, i.e., sheets with belly bands, neck and face masks.
• Use of a propane-powered CO_2 and octenol trap, such as the Mosquito Magnet, provides coverage up to 1 acre and attracts biting insects but not beneficial insects.

POSSIBLE COMPLICATIONS

Development of severe secondary infections and permanent scarring

EXPECTED COURSE AND PROGNOSIS

• Not life-threatening unless intractable pruritus persists
• No reports of spontaneous remission exist.

MISCELLANEOUS

ASSOCIATED CONDITIONS

Often concurrent association with atopic dermatitis

AGE-RELATED FACTORS

• Severity of clinical signs may progress as the horse ages.
• Disease may commence in middle aged horses if the horse has been moved to an area with a heavier insect burden.

ZOONOTIC POTENTIAL

N/A

PREGNANCY

Avoid corticosteroid and antihistamine use during pregnancy and lactation unless the benefits outweigh the risks.

SYNONYMS

• Sweet itch
• Summer itch
• Queensland itch
• No-see-um hypersensitivity

SEE ALSO

• Ectoparasites
• Atopic dermatitis

ABBREVIATIONS

• ASIT = allergen-specific immunotherapy
• CNS = central nervous system
• IH = insect hypersensitivity

Suggested Reading

Gray P. Parasites and Skin Diseases. London: JA Allen, 1995.

Lloyd DH, Littlewood JD, Craig JM, Thomsett LR. Practical Equine Dermatology. Oxford: Blackwell Science, 2003:17.

Scott DW, Miller WH Jr. Equine Dermatology. St. Louis: Saunders, 2003:458.

Author Cliff Monahan
Consulting Editor Gwendolen Lorch

INSPIRATORY DYSPNEA

BASICS

DEFINITION

• Dyspnea is a term that describes the sensation of difficult breathing. • In animals, dyspnea is used to describe clinical signs associated with respiratory distress, which can be present throughout the respiratory cycle or be primarily associated with either inhalation (i.e., inspiratory dyspnea) or exhalation (i.e., expiratory dyspnea).

PATHOPHYSIOLOGY

• Generally a sign of impaired gas exchange, with the increased effort to inhale being associated with an increased need to ventilate the lung. • Primary causes – failure of delivery of air into the lung (i.e. alveolar hypoventilation) and of exchange between the lung and blood (i.e., an exchange problem). The former can result from airway obstruction, pleural disease, chest wall or diaphragmatic injury, pneumothorax, encroachment of the abdomen on the thorax (e. g., advanced pregnancy), or CNS disease. Relevant exchange problems primarily are those causing alveolar disease (e. g., pneumonia, pulmonary edema). • Can also be a sign of decreased oxygen delivery to the tissues (e. g., cardiovascular disease, anemia) and of the need to eliminate more carbon dioxide to correct a metabolic acidosis. • The most severe cases usually result from obstruction of the extrathoracic airway, because the negative pressure generated in the airways during inhalation tends to collapse these structures. Thus, cases originating in the extrathoracic airway often become worse during exercise.

SYSTEMS AFFECTED

• Respiratory • Cardiovascular
• Hemic/lymphatic/immune
• Endocrine/metabolic—response to metabolic acidosis • Nervous

INCIDENCE/PREVALENCE

Unknown

GEOGRAPHIC DISTRIBUTION

Worldwide

SIGNALMENT

Depends on the underlying cause—foals with guttural pouch tympany, young mature horses with pleuritis, and old animals with neoplasia encroaching on the airway.

SIGNS

Inspiratory dyspnea is a sign, but associated signs can indicate the source of the dyspnea.

HISTORICAL

• Sudden onset of inspiratory dyspnea can indicate acute inflammatory disease of the lung or pleural space; trauma to the chest wall, diaphragm, or extrathoracic airway; or acute blood loss. • Dyspnea of slower onset may result from a space-occupying mass encroaching on the respiratory system. • Inappetence indicates inflammatory disease or inability to eat as a consequence of severe dyspnea. • Cough indicates inflammation of the tracheobronchial tree and can be a sign of pneumonia. • Bilateral mucopurulent nasal discharge usually indicates inflammation of the lower airway. • Unilateral nasal discharge, either purulent or hemorrhagic, suggests nasopharyngeal (including the sinuses and guttural pouches) disease. • Noisy breathing (stridor) indicates obstruction of the extrathoracic airway.

PHYSICAL EXAMINATION

• Flared nostrils, increased excursions of the thorax during breathing, and retractions (i.e., "sinking in") of the intercostals spaces, particularly if the horse is laboring against a severe upper airway obstruction. • Exaggerated excursions of the diaphragm are indicated by increased movement of the anal sphincter.
• Nasal obstruction—unilateral nasal discharge, foul breath, or noisy breathing
• Strangles—fever, mucopurulent nasal discharge, swollen, or draining lymph nodes
• Guttural pouch tympany—fluctuant, air-filled swelling of the parotid region (usually bilateral)
• Pharyngeal or laryngeal paralysis—if severe or bilateral, severe inspiratory dyspnea and inspiratory noise. • Laryngeal hemiplegia does not produce signs in resting animals, but reduced exercise tolerance is associated with inspiratory noise (i.e., "roaring") during strenuous exercise.
• Pneumonia —fever, tracheal sensitivity or increased breath sounds audible by stethoscope over the affected region (can be silent if consolidation is extensive or there is overlying pleural fluid) • Pulmonary edema—fine, inspiratory crakles • Pneumothorax—lack of breath sounds, possible resonance on percussion, and little air movement despite large effort.
• Pleural effusion/pleuritis—lack of lung sounds ventrally, harsh sounds dorsally, can be friction rubs, abducted elbows indicating pain, fever, or depression. • Fractured ribs—signs of trauma, sounds of air entering and leaving wounds, or signs of pain. • Diaphragmatic hernia—reduction in lung sounds, signs of colic, or borborygmi audible in chest.
• Anemia—pallor • Cardiac disease—murmurs, thrills, or arrhythmias

CAUSES

Respiratory Causes

- Extrathoracic airway
  - Paresis of the external nares
  - Severe atheroma
  - Congestion of the nasal mucosa—Horner's syndrome; inflammatory disease.
  - Deviation of the nasal septum
  - Space-occupying lesion affecting the nasal cavity—foreign body, intraluminal mass, ethmoid hematoma, or extraluminal mass or swelling.
  - Congenital pharyngeal cysts
  - Pharyngeal or laryngeal paresis
  - Space-occupying masses encroaching on the pharynx—enlarged lymph nodes; guttural pouch enlargement (usually by tympanites).
  - Trauma to the hyoid bone or larynx—edema; chondritis
  - Laryngeal or pharyngeal paresis—degenerative nerve disease, lead poisoning, or trauma to recurrent laryngeal nerves by jugular perivascular injection
  - Tracheal foreign body or collapse—Shetland ponies; miniatures horses
- Intrathoracic respiratory tract
  - Heaves— accompanied by expiratory dyspnea, which is more pronounced
  - Pulmonary edema—cardiogenic or noncardiogenic
  - Pneumonia—bacterial, viral or fungal
  - Pleuritis/pleuropneumonia
  - Accumulation of pleural fluid
  - Pneumothorax
  - Diaphragmatic hernia
  - Fractured ribs
  - Flail chest
  - Mediastinal masses

Nonrespiratory Causes

• Cardiovascular—congenital cardiac defect with right-to-left shunt, right sided failure, or pulmonary embolus • Hemic—anemia, methemoglobinemia, or carbon monoxide or cyanide poisoning
• Endocrine/metabolic—metabolic acidosis; hyperthermia • Nervous—trauma to recurrent laryngeal nerves or pharyngeal plexus, lead poisoning, phrenic nerve injury, or diaphragmatic paralysis
• Reproductive—advanced pregnancy; hydrops amnion

RISK FACTORS

See the individual conditions causing inspiratory dyspnea.

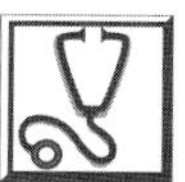

DIAGNOSIS

DIFFERENTIAL DIAGNOSIS

Differentiating Similar Signs

• Expiratory dyspnea is characterized by an enhanced abdominal component to exhalation, with a tucking up of the abdomen toward the end of exhalation. • Tachypnea, a rapid breathing in response to severe heat stress, is not accompanied by prolonged inhalation. • Deep breathing with a marked inspiratory effort also follows strenuous exercise.

Differentiating Causes

• Upper airway obstructions can produce severe respiratory distress and often are accompanied by inspiratory noise. • Lung and pleural disease often is inflammatory and, therefore, accompanied by fever, malaise, and inappetence.
• Damage to the respiratory pump (i.e., chest and diaphragm) may result in strenuous efforts to breathe, with little movement of air. • Cardiac disease usually is accompanied by other signs—murmurs, thrills, and irregularities of rate and rhythm. • Metabolic acidosis is accompanied by signs of disease of the kidneys, gastrointestinal, or endocrine systems.

CBC/BIOCHEMISTRY/URINALYSIS

A hemogram identifies anemia and inflammatory disease.

OTHER LABORATORY TESTS

• Arterial blood gas analysis identifies hypoventilation (i.e., increased $Paco_2$) and hypoxemia (i.e., low PaO_2). • Elevated $PaCO_2$ (>45 mm Hg) accompanied by hypoxemia (PaO_2 <85 mm Hg) indicates severe upper airway obstruction, damage to the respiratory pump, or severe lung disease. • Low $PaCO_2$ (<40 mm Hg) accompanied by decreased pH and elevated PaO_2 (>100 mm Hg) indicates metabolic acidosis; low $PaCO_2$ accompanied by hypoxemia indicates pulmonary disease.

IMAGING

Radiography

• Skull—nasal obstructions; sinus disease • Throat—guttural pouch tympany and empyema, hyoid bone injury, or laryngeal injury. • Neck—tracheal damage, foreign bodies, or tracheal collapse • Thorax—pleuritis, pleural fluid, pneumonia, pulmonary edema, pneumothorax, cardiac enlargement, fractured ribs, or diaphragmatic hernia.

Ultrasonography

• Very useful for identifying pleural fluid or focal loculated regions of pleural effusion • Also may identify masses in the lung—abscesses; neoplasia • Echocardiography can identify chamber enlargement, congenital defects, and valvular disease. • Doppler flow can determine the severity of regurgitant blood flow.

Endoscopy

• Essential for diagnosing space-occupying lesions of the extrathoracic airway • Videoendoscopy during exercise may be necessary to determine the significance of pharyngeal or laryngeal collapse. • Endoscpopy also can assess for mucopurulent exudates in the trachea, which is a sign of inflammation of the lower airways and lung.

OTHER DIAGNOSTIC PROCEDURES

• Cytology of lower airways, preferably with bronchoalveolar lavage, can determine the presence of lower airway inflammation. • Bronchoalveolar lavage may overlook a focal lesion if the lavage tube is not lodged specifically in the affected region. • Bacterial culture of tracheal mucus of tracheal lavage revealing a relatively pure culture of a known pathogen is significant. • Pleurocentesis determines the presence and nature of air or fluid in the pleural space.

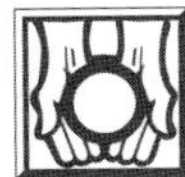

AIMS OF TREATMENT

Relieving Upper Airway Obstruction

• Relieve upper airway obstruction sufficient to cause panic or life-threatening hypoxemia (indicated by cyanosis) by tracheotomy • Nasotracheal intubation can be used to bypass the obstruction, especially if that obstruction will be corrected surgically within a short time. • NOTE: Tracheotomy is not useful for relief of dyspnea originating in the lower airway, lungs, or thorax.

Support Ventilation

• Animals with hypoventilation resulting from thoracic damage may need positive-pressure ventilation, which can be accomplished via nasotracheal tube until the horse is anesthetized for correction of the injury. • Ventilation to maintain gas exchange in an animal with pulmonary disease is difficult.

APPROPRIATE HEALTH CARE

In- or outpatient medical management

NURSING CARE

Oxygen Therapy

• Supplemental oxygenation via a nasotracheal or nasopharyngeal catheter relieves hypoxemia and accompanying distress when dyspnea results from lung disease. • In cases of upper airway obstruction or thoracic trauma, oxygen can be life-saving until the problem is surgically corrected. • Anemia (PCV < 10) sufficient to cause dyspnea requires administration of blood to restore the PCV; without hemoglobin, blood cannot carry oxygen.

Chest Tap

• Can be both diagnostic and therapeutic. • Drainage of pleural fluid allows lung expansion. • Removal of air in cases of pneumothorax restores the negative pressure necessary for breathing.

ACTIVITY

See the individual conditions causing inspiratory dyspnea.

SURGICAL CONSIDERATIONS

See the individual conditions causing inspiratory dyspnea.

MEDICATIONS

DRUG(S) OF CHOICE

Depend on cause of the dyspnea

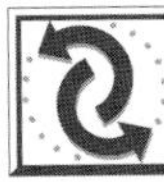

FOLLOW-UP

PATIENT MONITORING

• After surgery for upper airway obstruction, monitor patients carefully for signs of further obstruction caused by postoperative swelling. • Tracheotomy tubes need to be removed and cleaned regularly to prevent occlusion by mucus and exudates. • Once tracheotomy tubes are removed, strictures at the site of tracheotomy may lead to further inspiratory dyspnea. • Carefully monitor for redevelopment of pleural effusion and recurrence of pneumothorax.

EXPECTED COURSE AND PROGNOSIS

Depend on cause of the dyspnea

MISCELLANEOUS

PREGNANCY

Fetal growth retardation and fetal death may be observed in mares with severely compromised respiratory function.

SEE ALSO

• Acute epiglottiditis • Arytenoid chondopathy • Aspiration pneumonia • Atheroma of the false nostril • Diaphragmatic hernia • Expiratory dyspnea • Guttural pouch tympany • Pleuropneumonia • Pneumothorax • Acute respiratory distress syndrome • Thoracic trauma

Suggested Reading

Barakzai S. Treadmill endoscopy. In: McGorum BC, Dixon PM, Robinson NE, Schumacher J, eds. Equine Respiratory Medicine and Surgery. Oxford: Saunders, 2007:235–247.

Hannas CM, Derksen FJ. Principles of emergency respiratory therapy. In: Colahan PT, Mayhew IG, Merritt AM, Moore JM, eds. Equine Medicine and Surgery, ed 4. Goleta: American Veterinary Publications, 1991:1:372–374.

Laverty S. Thoracic trauma. In: Robinson NE, ed. Current Therapy in Equine Medicine, ed 4. Philadelphia: WB Saunders, 1997:463–465.

McGorum BC, Dixon PM. Clinical examination of the respiratory tract. In: McGorum BC, Dixon PM, Robinson NE, Schumacher J, eds. Equine Respiratory Medicine and Surgery. Oxford: Saunders, 2007:103–117.

Parente EJ. Diagnostic techniques for upper airway obstruction. In: Robinson NE, ed. Current Therapy in Equine Medicine, ed 4. Philadelphia: WB Saunders, 1997:401–403.

Author N. Edward Robinson
Consulting Editor Daniel Jean

INSULIN LEVELS/INSULIN TOLERANCE TEST

BASICS

DEFINITION

- Serum insulin concentrations may be measured to appropriately evaluate a horse's ability to regulate its blood glucose.
- In normal horses, insulin secretion is closely tied to blood glucose concentrations. Insulin concentrations are quite low when the horse is fasting but increase rapidly when the horse receives glucose or eats a meal high in soluble carbohydrates.
- Blood insulin concentrations may be consistently elevated in horses with pars intermedia tumors or equine metabolic syndrome.
- Because insulin concentrations are so labile, insulin response or tolerance tests may give a better picture of the horse's endocrine status than a one-time measurement.
- Insulin tolerance test—give crystalline insulin (0.05 U/kg IV) or regular insulin (0.4–8 IU/kg IV) and determine blood glucose at baseline and then every 15 min for 3 hr. In normal horses, expect to see a decrease =50% in blood glucose at 30 min.
- Serum insulin response can also be measured after administering dextrose (0.5 g/kg IV). Insulin should be low when starting, increase within 5 min of the dextrose load, and then decrease rapidly once blood glucose levels begin to drop. Serum glucose should normalize within 3 hr after dextrose administration.
- The most common pathologic process leading to abnormal results is insulin resistance in horses with idiopathic insulin resistance (equine metabolic syndrome) and pars intermedia tumors—equine Cushing's syndrome, PPID.

PATHOPHYSIOLOGY

- Inappropriately low insulin levels–pancreatitis, leading to destruction of beta cells and development of type 1 diabetes mellitus
- Increased insulin levels in hypoglycemic horse—insulin-secreting tumor (i.e., insulinoma) or iatrogenic insulin administration
- Increased serum insulin levels in hyperglycemic horses—peripheral insulin resistance caused by type 2 diabetes mellitus or an insulin antagonist (e.g., cortisol)
- Increased serum insulin levels in euglycemic horses without PPID—equine metabolic syndrome
- Increased blood cortisol—PPID, stress, or glucocorticoid therapy
- Horses with hyperlipemia also exhibit insulin resistance.

SYSTEM AFFECTED

The endocrine system is primarily affected by abnormal blood insulin and insulin response tests—decreased insulin is diagnostic of diabetes mellitus; increased insulin is most commonly associated with insulin antagonists.

SIGNALMENT

- Ponies tend to have higher blood insulin levels than horses and are more prone to hyperlipemia.
- No sex difference
- Obese animals, particularly ponies, are more insulin resistant than are thinner animals.
- PPID tends to occur in old horses (>18 years).

SIGNS

- The most common signs in horses with an abnormal insulin response test are those of equine metabolic syndrome—obesity with abnormal fat distribution, infertility, and laminitis.
- The eyelids can look swollen, and the supraorbital fat pad may look bulged.
- Owners may report the horse is dull or depressed.
- Similar clinical signs, with the addition of hirsutism or an abnormal hair coat, weight loss, polyuria and polydipsia, and tendency to suffer chronic infections particularly sinusitis and hoof abcess, are seen in horses with PPID.
- Clinical signs in horses with type 1 diabetes mellitus—weight loss, polyuria and polydipsia, lethargy, or depression
- Signs of excess insulin caused by exogenous overdose or insulinoma are those of hypoglycemia—muscle trembling, ataxia, nystagmus, depression, and facial twitching, leading to convulsions, coma, and death
- Signs of hyperlipemia include depression, anorexia, and icterus.

CAUSES

- The primary known cause of increased serum insulin, abnormal response to an insulin response test, or increased insulin after IV glucose is the presence of insulin antagonists. Exogenous or endogenous corticosteroids are the most common insulin antagonists but other hormones (e.g., growth hormone, epinephrine) also have this effect.
- When insulin resistance occurs without a predisposing cause, equine metabolic syndrome is diagnosed.
- The most common reason for increased blood insulin without insulin resistance is an insulin-secreting tumor.
- The most common reason for type 1 diabetes mellitus is pancreatic damage, secondary to parasite migration.

RISK FACTORS

- Pituitary tumor is the most common risk factor for the development of abnormal insulin secretion.
- Glucocorticoid administration or increased cortisol from a stress response may also lead to insulin resistance and hyperglycemia.
- Obesity, particularly in ponies, is associated with insulin resistance, as is hyperlipidemia.

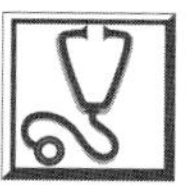

DIAGNOSIS

DIFFERENTIAL DIAGNOSIS

- Polyuria, polydipsia, and glucosuria in horses with suspected endocrine disorders should alert the practitioner to a disorder in glucose homeostasis and, thus, in insulin levels.
- Hypoglycemia from excess insulin—myositis, neurologic disease, and colic
- Determination of abnormally low blood glucose should cause the practitioner to suspect inappropriate insulin levels.

LABORATORY FINDINGS

Drugs That May Alter Lab Results

N/A

Disorders That May Alter Lab Results

Delayed separation of serum from cells falsely lowers blood glucose values, making interpretation of insulin levels more difficult.

Valid If Run in Human Lab?

Yes

CBC/BIOCHEMISTRY/URINALYSIS

- Horses with abnormal insulin levels caused by PPID may have a stress response with mature neutrophilia, lymphopenia, and eosinopenia. They may also have increased blood glucose and glucosuria.
- Horses with type 1 or 2 diabetes mellitus have hyperglycemia.
- Horses with insulinoma or exogenous insulin overdose have hypoglycemia.
- Horses with hyperlipemia have high serum bilirubin and lipid levels.

OTHER LABORATORY TESTS

- Pituitary function—endogenous ACTH determination and dexamethasone suppression test
- If these results are consistent with PPID, this supports that diagnosis; if they do not indicate PPID, suspect stress response or equine metabolic syndrome.

IMAGING

Increased pituitary gland size may be depicted with specialized modalities—computed tomography or venous contrast

DIAGNOSTIC PROCEDURES

Exploratory laparotomy or abdominocentesis may reveal a damaged pancreas but should be considered extremely low yield procedures, because the pancreas is normally difficult to visualize and pancreatic tumors often are microscopic.

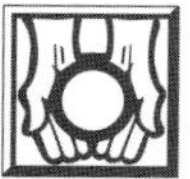

TREATMENT

APPROPRIATE HEALTH CARE

- Horses with hypoglycemia require inpatient medical management if the disease is severe and IV dextrose to maintain blood glucose at adequate levels.
- Horses with hyperlipemia also require inpatient medical management that includes IV dextrose, balanced electrolyte solutions, caloric replacement, heparin, and exogenous insulin.
- All other horses with abnormal insulin levels may be treated as outpatients.

NURSING CARE

- Carefully monitor hypoglycemic animals to prevent them from collapsing and injuring themselves.
- Horses with laminitis need corrective hoof trimming and shoeing and an appropriate diet.

ACTIVITY

- Limit the activity of horses with laminitis.
- Increase the activity of sound, obese horses in an effort to lose weight.

DIET

- Horses with laminitis generally benefit from a low-carbohydrate, high-fiber diet.
- Keep any horse with insulin resistance on a low-carbohydrate diet.
- Restrict or increase caloric intake until a condition score of 4–6 out of 10 is achieved.

CLIENT EDUCATION

- Horses with PPID may be managed with medication and nursing care, but their prognosis is quite variable. Some do well for several years; others are refractory to treatment. Owners need to understand that treatment of PPID is palliative and is required for life.
- Encourage clients to maintain their horses at condition scores of 4–6 out of 10 and to prevent obesity from developing.

SURGICAL CONSIDERATIONS

N/A

MEDICATIONS

DRUG(S) OF CHOICE

- The agent most commonly used to alter the symptoms of PPID is pergolide (0.5–2 mg/day).
- Insulin-deficient horses (i.e., type 1 diabetes mellitus) require insulin supplementation, with the dose being changed in response to the blood glucose level. Protamine zinc insulin (0.5 IU IM BID) normalized blood glucose in a case report of a pony with insulin deficiency.
- Exogenous insulin for the treatment of hyperlipemia—protamine zinc insulin (0.075–0.4 IU/kg SQ or IM BID or SID). Regular insulin (0.4 IU/kg) has also been recommended.

CONTRAINDICATIONS

N/A

PRECAUTIONS

- Dextrose for injection should always be available when administering insulin to any horse. If signs of hypoglycemia occur, treat immediately with IV dextrose.
- Horses that receive an overdose of pergolide may exhibit anorexia, lethargy and ataxia.

POSSIBLE INTERACTIONS

N/A

ALTERNATIVE DRUGS

N/A

FOLLOW-UP

PATIENT MONITORING

- Retest horses with PPID every 12–20 weeks with endogenous ACTH determination or dexamethasone response testing. Abnormal results indicate the need for an increased dose or a change in medication.
- Check the glucose level of horses with diabetes mellitus receiving insulin therapy twice a day. Insulin doses should be increased or decreased in response to blood glucose values outside the normal range.

POSSIBLE COMPLICATIONS

N/A

MISCELLANEOUS

ASSOCIATED CONDITIONS

- Hirsutism, chronic infections, and laminitis are commonly associated with PPID.
- Obesity, laminitis, and hyperlipemia are commonly associated with insulin resistance.

AGE-RELATED FACTORS

N/A

ZOONOTIC POTENTIAL

N/A

PREGNANCY

Pregnant mares tend to have higher blood insulin levels than nonpregnant horses. This tendency is most profound early during gestation, but blood glucose levels remain normal.

SYNONYMS

N/A

SEE ALSO

- ACTH
- Pituitary tumors
- Equine metabolic syndrome
- Glucose

ABBREVIATION

- PPID = pituitary pars intermedia dysfunction

Suggested Reading

Beech J. Endocrine system. In: Colahan PT, Mayhew IG, Merritt AM, Moore JN, eds. Equine Medicine and Surgery, ed 5. St. Louis: Mosby, 1999:1947–1968.

Beech J, Garcia M. Hormonal response to thyrotropin-releasing hormone in healthy horses and in horses with pituitary adenoma. Am J Vet Res 1985;46:1941–1943.

Coffman JR, Colles CM. Insulin tolerance in laminitic ponies. Can J Comp Med 1983;47:347–351.

Ruoff WW, Baker DC, Morgan SJ, et al. Type II diabetes mellitus in a horse. Equine Vet J 1986;18:143–144.

Author Janice Sojka
Consulting Editor Michel Lévy

INTERNAL ABDOMINAL ABSCESSES

BASICS

DEFINITION

Internal abdominal abscesses can be defined as an insidious clinical disease characterized by internal sepsis in different localizations presenting in two typical distinct clinical presentations, characterized by weight loss or prolonged colic; both may be accompanied by fever.

PATHOPHYSIOLOGY

- The pathogenesis of mesenteric abscesses has not been elucidated; however, it has been proposed that the development of the internal infection is associated with the inability of the animal to develop adequate immune response to the microorganism involved, thereby allowing systemic spread of the infection.
- It is thought by some authors that given the high frequency of these abscesses being caused by *Streptococcus equi,* treatment with penicillin prior to abscess maturation and drainage in strangles results in more frequent occurrence of metastatic abscesses. Other authors have pointed out that withholding therapy to allow maturation of the abscess does not help in preventing hematogenous spread of the organisms. However, internal abdominal abscesses can occur in horses with no history of a respiratory disease or contamination of the abdominal cavity in areas close to penetration of the intestine or nearby anastomosis sites.
- Once the internal abdominal abscess has developed, it can remain dormant as an abscess or peritonitis may develop. This seems to be responsible for the different clinical presentations. Colic events seem to be due to prolonged tension on the mesentery or from adhesions or scarring of the small intestine with acute or chronic obstruction.

SYSTEMS AFFECTED

The internal abdominal abscesses usually involve the mesentery but can also occur in parenchymatous abdominal organs such as liver, spleen, kidneys, and uterus.

INCIDENCE AND PREVALENCE

There is no information regarding incidence or prevalence.

SIGNALMENT

Internal abscessation may affect any domestic species. In the equine, all individuals at any age or either sex are at risk. In a study of 25 cases, it was observed that horses <5 years of age were more commonly affected.

SIGNS

- Usually, horses with internal abdominal abscesses present with one of two chief complaints. The first is a history of intermittent or prolonged colic. However, there are cases with history of colic of sudden onset. These animals show depression, congested mucous membranes, increased rectal temperature (>38.6° C), increased and shallow respiratory rate, groaning on expiration, partial or complete anorexia, constipation, decreased peristaltic sounds, and dehydration. Dysuria can be noticed in some cases.
- In the second form of presentation of internal abdominal abscesses, the chief complaint is chronic ongoing weight loss. The body condition in these animals ranges from the cachectic horse to the thin horse that is unable to gain weight. Some animals are depressed, inconsistently anorexic, and have poor shaggy hair coats. The rectal temperature and heart and respiratory rates may be elevated. Abdominal peristaltic sounds are usually normal. Combinations of the two forms can occur.
- In some cases there is evidence of diarrhea, and this seems to be more commonly associated with abscesses caused by *Rhodococcus equi* infection in foals and in growing horses.

CAUSES

The agents more commonly involved are *Streptococcus equi* subsp. *equi, Streptococcus equi* subsp. *zooepidemicus, Corynebacterium pseudotuberculosis, Salmonella* spp., *E. coli,* very rarely *Serratia marcescens* and *R. equi* in foals, and obligate anaerobes (*Bacteroides* spp.,*Clostridium novyi* type A and *Fusobacterium necrophorum*); there has been a report of internal abdominal abscess in association with *Parascaris equorum* in a foal.

RISK FACTORS

There have no been epidemiologic studies that have determined specific risk factors yet. However, it has been indicated that heavily parasitized animals are more prone to internal abdominal abscessation. In a review of clinical cases it was noted that many affected animals had a previous history of respiratory disease or lymphadenitis. The problem is more likely to occur on farms where infections with *Streptococcus equi* subsp. *equi* and *R. equi* are common. Abdominocentesis should be considred a risk factor when enterocentesis has occurred.

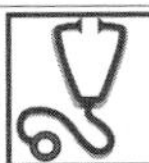

DIAGNOSIS

DIFFERENTIAL DIAGNOSIS

Internal abdominal abscessation must be differentiated from the different cases of chronic weight loss, such as pleuropneumonia, neoplasia, chronic hepatic disease, chronic intestinal malabsorption disease, chronic renal failure, severe parasitism, and dental problems. In the colic presentation, it must be differentiated from peritonitis of different origin or surgical or medical colics.

CBC/BIOCHEMISTRY/URINALYSIS

The CBC may indicate a slight to moderate anemia of chronic inflammation. The PCV can be <0.3 L/L (30%). The WBC count shows a leukocytosis with neutrophilia and a left shift evident in most horses. Plasma fibrinogen concentration is frequently increased, with values close to 1000 mg/dL (10 g/L). Plasma proteins are increased, usually due to increased globulin fractions; albumin may be below normal levels. The albumin:globulin (A:G) ratio is below normal, ranging from 0.17 to 0.63 (normal 0.65–1.46).

OTHER LABORATORY TESTS

Peritoneal fluid is usually determined to be an exudate based on a specific gravity (>1.017), protein level (>2.5 g/dL [25 g/L]), and WBC count (>10,000 cells/μL [>10^9 cells/L]). The protein levels, WBC, and fibrinogen can be as high as 8.5 g/dL (85 g/L), 400,000 cells/μL (365 × 10^9 cells/L), and 500 mg/dL (5 g/L), respectively. Intracellular bacteria (both cocci and bacilli) can be observed, but only on rare occasions are free bacteria observed.

IMAGING

Ultrasonography, conducted transrectally or percutaneously, can be useful in diagnosing these abscesses when they can be located during rectal examination. Nuclear scintigraphy using technetium-99 m or ^{111}indium labeled WBCs can be potentially used to locate abscesses that are difficult to localize.

DIAGNOSTIC PROCEDURES

- Rectal palpation may be limited by the fact that some animals often show severe abdominal straining and rectal expulsive efforts during the colic episodes. In both clinical presentations, detailed rectal examination may allow the detection of an abdominal mass.

• Abdominal laparoscopy could well be indicated in these instances and may allow visualization of the mass. Fine-needle aspirate of the abscess could be done percutaneously with ultrasound guidance or by laparoscopy.
• A Gram stain and culture of the peritoneal fluid should be carried out. The clinician should request anaerobic and aerobic methods for bacterial isolation from the cultures submitted. In some instances, exploratory laparotomy might be indicated.

PATHOLOGICAL FINDINGS

Abdominal abscessation can involve the mesentery or several internal organs, such as intestines, spleen, liver, or kidneys. When localized in the mesentery, adhesions to various organs might be present.

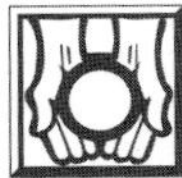

TREATMENT

APPROPRIATE HEALTH CARE

Most cases can be managed in a farm setting.

ACTIVITY

Animals with internal abdominal abscesses should have stall or pasture rest until the problem has resolved.

DIET

Normal diet

CLIENT EDUCATION

Cases that are managed with long-term antibiotic therapy can be treated by the owner. If owners are unfamiliar with the administration of medication to horses, they must be trained to do this. Compliance can be a problem, particularly with parenteral therapy, as many horses rapidly become intolerant of twice-daily intramuscular injections.

SURGICAL CONSIDERATIONS

• In cases in which colic presentation is the chief complaint, the severity of the colic may warrant intensive care management and even surgical management in some cases.
• Surgical treatment could be attempted in cases with a grave prognosis, but it is complicated by the need to drain the abscess without contaminating the abdominal cavity. It is usually very difficult to excise the abscess. In cases of abdominal obstruction, it may be necessary to bypass the abscess. Abdominal lavage is indicated in cases when rupture of the abscess occurs. This procedure is not without constraints and difficulties. There have been reports of marsupialization of the abscesses when close to the abdominal wall.

MEDICATIONS

DRUG(S) OF CHOICE

• Medical treatment of abdominal internal abscesses is usually preferred. For the most part it is empirical, as the causative organism(s) is not usually positively identified. Farm history and clinical findings are the basis for antibiotic selection. Antibiotic therapy should last for a minimum of 30 days and may extend up to 90 days in some cases, depending on the response to therapy.
• Procaine penicillin 40,000–100,000 UI/kg divided in 2 doses daily has been recommended. It may be combined with trimethoprim-sulfadiazine 16–30 mg/kg body weight.
• In the author's experience, the combination of rifampin 10 mg/kg BID PO and trimethoprim-sulfadiazine 30 mg/kg BID PO for minimum of 30 days has been very successful.
• Rifampin may alternatively be combined with erythromycin estolate 15 mg/kg BID to TID.
• Metronidazole 20–25 mg/kg TID could be added in the case of a suspected or isolated anaerobic pathogen.

FOLLOW-UP

PATIENT MONITORING

In order to follow up the patient evolution, repeated rectal examinations, abdominocentesis, and ultrasound examinations are necessary.

PREVENTION/AVOIDANCE

On problem farms, careful monitoring of all horses may lead to early detection of the problem. If *Streptococcus equi* subsp. *equi* is the etiologic agent, then consideration should be give to a vaccination program.

POSSIBLE COMPLICATIONS

• Peritonitis
• Purpura hemorrhagica

EXPECTED COURSE AND PROGNOSIS

The prognosis is usually guarded to good when there has been good response within 2 weeks of treatment. The prognosis becomes grave if there is either intestinal obstruction or internal rupture of the abscess, lack of response to the treatment, and evidence of intestinal adhesions.

Suggested Reading

Byars DT. Miscellaneous acute abdominal diseases. In: White NA, ed. The Equine Acute Abdomen. Philadelphia: Lea & Febiger, 1990:403–404.
Golland LC, Hodgson DR, Hodgson JL, Brownlow MA, Hutchins DR, Rawlinson RJ, Collins MB, McClintock SA, Riasis AL. Peritonitis associated with *Actinobacillus equuli* in horses: 15 cases. JAVMA 1994;205:340–343.
Hawkins JF, Bowman KF, Roberts MC, Cowe P. Peritonitis in horses: 67 cases. JAVMA 1993;203:284–288.
Koblik PD, Lofsted J, Jakowski RM, Johnson KL. Use of ^{111}In- labeled autologous leukocytes to image an abdominal abscess in the horse. JAVMA 1985:186;1319–1322.
Mogg TD, Rutherford DJ. Intra-abdominal abscess and peritonitis in an Appaloosa gelding. Vet Clin North Am Equine Pract 2006;22:e17-e25.
Rigg DL, Gatlin SL, Reinertson EL. Marsupialization of an abdominal abscess caused by *Serratia marcescens* in a mare. JAVMA 1987;191:222–224.
Rumbaugh GE, Smith BF, Carlson GP. Internal abdominal abscesses in the horse: a study of 25 cases. JAVMA 1978;172:304–308.
Tevillian CJ, Anderson BH, Collett MG. An unusual paracaecal abscess associated with *Fusobacterium necrophorum* in a horse. Aust Vet J 1998;76:659–662.

Author Olimpo Oliver-Espinosa
Consulting Editors Henry Stämpfli and Olimpo Oliver-Espinosa

INTESTINAL ABSORPTION TESTS

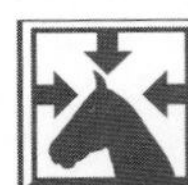

BASICS

These tests assess the absorptive integrity of the small intestine, by measuring the efficiency of sugar absorption from the intestinal lumen. They are indicated in weight loss cases where an overt cause is not established and there is apparent adequate food intake.

PATHOPHYSIOLOGY

Weight loss can result from many different clinical conditions (see Chronic Weight Loss section).

SYSTEM AFFECTED

Small intestine

DIAGNOSTIC PROCEDURES

OGAT

Glucose is absorbed from the small intestine by specific transport processes and thus it assesses small intestinal function. It provides empiric evidence of the absorptive capacity of the small intestine. The test is easily performed, inexpensive and necessitates readily available reagents.

Test Procedure

The horse is weighed as accurately as possible (e. g., scale or girth weight tape). It is fasted overnight (14–16 hr) and kept on inedible bedding. Access to water is restricted starting 2 hr prior to the test. Anhydrous or monohydrate D-glucose (1 g/kg of body weight), mixed in warm water to form a 20% (20 g/dL) solution w/v, is administered via stomach tube. Since the test depends on the rapid entry of the given glucose solution into the small intestine, and because gastric emptying is delayed by excessive glucose concentration, the quantity of glucose and the concentration of the solution are paramount. Blood samples are collected by direct venipuncture into fluoride oxalate glass vacutainers immediately prior to glucose administration and 30, 60, 90, 120, 150, 180, 240, 300, and 360 min later. Samples are submitted to the laboratory for glucose measurement or analyzed by a handheld glucometers. Access to food is denied until the end of the sampling; if the patient is not adequately fasted the presence of food in the stomach will mix with the solution and then interfere with the availability of the glucose in the small intestine, thus causing spurious results.

Curve Plotting

The glucose values at each time period are plotted arithmetically.

Test Interpretation

- The absorption curve in normal conditions has two phases. Glucose absorption from the small intestine occurs continuously during the first 2 hr and the fasting plasma glucose concentration almost doubles (>85% increase in normal horses) during this period. This phase is dependent on mucosal integrity, the rate of gastric emptying, intestinal transit time, previous dietary history, and age. It has been reported that altering the diet, from pasture to hay and concentrate and vice versa, in the week previous to testing, results in different oral glucose tolerance curves. The second phase (>2 hr) is insulin-dependent and is characterized by a progressive decline to resting levels by 6 hr. A late but normal-sized glucose peak may occur in cases of delayed gastric emptying.
- The interpretation of abnormal curve is dependent on the characteristics of the curve. A flat line is indicative of a total malabsorption state and is associated with progressive inflammatory or neoplastic cellular infiltration of the small intestinal wall; this constitutes generally a grave prognosis. The diseases include lymphosarcoma, granulomatous enteritis, eosinophilic gastroenteritis, and intestinal mycobacteriosis. The definitive diagnosis of these conditions is made by histopathological examination of a small intestinal biopsy.
- A curve positioned between causes associated with normal absorption and total malabsorption suggests partial malabsorption. It may be caused by several reversible or nonspecific entities, such as villous atrophy, circulatory disturbances, and inflammatory reversible changes due to intestinal parasitism. Partial malabsorption, when associated with normal small intestinal histology, may result from delayed gastric emptying, rapid intestinal transit, intestinal bacterial overgrowth, or abnormalities in cellular uptake and metabolism as is believed to occur in equine motor neuron disease.

D-Xylose Absorption Test

- D-Xylose is a pentose sugar that is absorbed in the small intestine by passive diffusion and active transport by a sodium-absorption carrier.
- The oral D-xylose absorption test has been used widely as an index of the small intestine absorptive function. Since it is not a normal constituent of the plasma, its absorption curve is not affected by the endogenous metabolic events influencing blood glucose concentration. Based on these characteristics, the D-xylose absorption test is considered to provide a more accurate assessment of absorption than the glucose absorption test.

Test Procedure

The horse is weighed and fasted as for the OGAT. A commercial-grade xylose solution at 10% (10 g/dL) is prepared and administered at a dose of 0.5 g/kg via a nasogastric tube. The sampling protocol is started with a pretest sample (time 0) followed ideally by sampling at 30, 60, 90, 120,180, 240, 300, and 360 min after dosing. However, a 2-hr sampling period is considered adequate in a clinical practice. The samples are taken into potassium oxalate–sodium fluoride anticoagulant vacutainers. Ideally, the laboratory conducting the analysis of samples has established a laboratory-specific normal reference ranges for horses.

Test Interpretation

- Blood xylose concentration rises from zero to a peak concentration of 1.37–1.67 mmol/L (Bolton et al., 1976) or 0.68–0.85 mmol/L (Roberts and Norman, 1979) 60–90 min after dosing. As with OGAT, it is easy to determine a total malabsorption and a normal absorption curves, but an intermediate curve is difficult to interpret.
- The shape of the xylose plasma concentration curve can also be affected by a number of factors others than absorption per se. Factors identified include rate of gastric emptying, intestinal transit time, mucosal blood flow, renal clearance, bacterial overgrowth, cellular or intraluminal metabolism of sugar, and composition of previous diets.
- Most commercial labs do not process these samples routinely. Thus, the OGAT is more commonly performed.

OLTT

- The OLTT is an indirect assay use to determine if persistent maldigestion and diarrhea in a foal are secondary to milk intolerance associated with lactase deficiency. This may follow intestinal epithelial damage caused by enteric disease such as rotavirus infection and *Clostridium difficile* enterocolitis.
- Lactase (neutral β-galactosidase), a disaccharidase produced by small-intestine mucosal cells, hydrolyzes lactose to monosaccharide glucose and galactose. This hydrolytic process is essential for milk digestion.

Test Procedure

The foal is weighed as accurately as possible. It is fasted for 4 hr before lactose administration and for the duration of the test. The foal should not be allowed to have access to water especially in the first hour of the test, as it may dilute the lactose and alter its digestion. Then, 1 g/kg of body weight of a 20% (20 g/dL) solution of lactose monohydrate (in warm water) is administered via stomach tube. The sampling protocol is started with a pretest sample (time 0) and followed by samplings at 30, 60, 90, 120,180, 240, and 300 min after dosing. The samples are taken into potassium oxalate–sodium fluoride anticoagulant vacutainers.

Test Interpretation

- The general shape of this curve is similar to those reported for sugar tolerance tests. The mean peak in glucose level occurs approximately 1 hr after dosing, with a return to fasting values by 3 hr. The initial increase in plasma glucose indicates that it is absorbed from the intestine at a faster rate than it is removed from blood. As blood glucose increases, it enters the cells (particularly hepatic cells that convert glucose to glycogen), facilitated by the insulin activity. An increase of >1.4 mmol/L within 30 minutes of lactose administration is indicative of normal digestion and absorption. There are some variations with age, with the absorption being higher in older foals.
- When an appropriate increase in blood glucose is not observed, an oral glucose or xylose test should be performed and will help to differentiate maldigestion from malabsorption.

ABBREVIATIONS

- OGAT = oral glucose absorption test
- OLTT = oral lactose tolerance test

Suggested Reading

Jacobs KA, Norman P, Hodgson DRG, Cymbaluk N. Effect of diet on the oral D-xyose absorption test in the horse. Am J Vet Res 1982;43:1856–1858.

Mair TS, Hillyer MH, Taylor FGR, Pearson GR. Small intestinal malabsorption in the horse: an assessment of the specificity of the oral glucose tolerance test. Equine Vet J 1991; 23:344–346.

Mair TS, Perason GR, Divers TJ. Malabsorption syndromes in the horse. Equine Vet Educ 2006;8:383–394.

Martens RJ, Malone PS, Brust DM. Oral lactose tolerance test in foals: technique and normal values. Am J Vet Res 1985;46:2163–2165.

Murphy D, Reid SWJ, Love S. The effect of age and diet on the oral glucose tolerance test in ponies. Equine Vet J 1997;29:467–470.

Rice L, Ott EA, Beede DK, Wilcox CJ, Johnson EL, Lieb S, Borum P. Use of oral tolerance tests to investigate disaccharide digestion in neonatal foals. J Anim Sci 1992;70:1175–1181.

Roberts MC. Small intestinal malabsorption in horses. Equine Vet Educ 2000;2:269–274.

Roberts MC, Hill FWG. The oral glucose tolerance test in the horse. Equine Vet J 1973;5:171–173.

Roberts MC, Norman P. A re-evaluation of the D(+)xylose absorption test in the horse. Equine Vet J 1979;11:239–243.

Weese JS, Parsons DA, Staempfli HR. Association of Clostridium difficile with enterocolitis and lactose intolerance in a foal. JAVMA 1999;214:229–231.

Authors Olimpo Oliver-Espinosa and Henry Stämpfli

Consulting Editors Henry Stämpfli and Olimpo Oliver-Espinosa

INTRA-ABDOMINAL HEMORRHAGE IN HORSES

BASICS

DEFINITION

Accumulation of blood in the abdominal cavity

PATHOPHYSIOLOGY

Acute Abdominal Hemorrhage

Acute massive blood loss of 30% or more of total blood volume results in hypovolemic shock. Loss of blood results initially in a decrease in venous pressure and in venous blood return to the heart. Consequently, the cardiac output and arterial pressure decrease. Physiologic compensation for hypovolemic shock includes redistribution of interstitial fluid from tissue spaces into capillaries to expand circulating fluid volume and increased sympathetic activity. Tachycardia and peripheral vasoconstriction to increase cardiac output result from this physiologic compensation. Splenic contraction subsequent to the increased sympathetic activity occurs. This results in initial maintenance of PCV concentrations. As the hemorrhage progreses, more vital organs, such as the kidneys and the pancreas, followed by the intestines and liver, undergo vasoconstriction and the oncotic pressure and the oxygen-carrying capacity of the blood decrease. Due to lack of oxygen, the cells go into to anaerobic metabolism, which results in the production of organic acids such as lactic acid. Blood flow to the most vital organs such as the brain and the heart is maintained for the longest period.

Chronic Abdominal Hemorrhage

More than 30% of total blood volume must be lost with chronic or slow hemorrhage before clinical signs become evident. This compensation can be attributed to an immediate release of erythrocytes via splenic contracture, redistribution of interstitial fluid intravascularly over a 12- to 24-hr time span, and enhanced erythropoiesis within 1 week.

SYSTEMS AFFECTED

Cardiovascular

Since abdominal hemorrhage may result in hypovolemic shock, the main affected system is the cardiovascular system. The systolic pressure is decreased. The diastolic pressure is increased. The difference between these two pressures determines if strength of the pulse is decreased.

Urinary

Urine output is decreased because of vasoconstriction.

GENETICS

N/A

INCIDENCE/PREVALENCE

Hemoperitoneum is an infrequent condition in horses.

GEOGRAPHIC DISTRIBUTION

N/A

SIGNALEMENT

Breed Predilections

Arabians seem to be more affected with hemoperitoneum associated with neoplasia than any other breeds. In one study, Thoroughbreds were most commonly affected.

Mean Age and Range

Older horses (>13 years) are more frequently affected. Multiparous broodmares >11 years of age are the prime candidates for hemoperitoneum due to reproductive tract bleeding.

Predominant Sex

Blood loss from the reproductive tract occurs in broodmares.

SIGNS

General Comments

Clinical manifestations are frequently nonspecific and can be easily misinterpreted. Abdominal discomfort is the primary complaint in horses with hemoperitoneum.

Historical

Initial clinical signs include colic, shock, pale membranes, depression, lethargy, and partial or complete anorexia.

Physical Examination

As the anemia and the hypovolemia intensify, tachycardia, tachypnea, weak peripheral pulses, pale mucous membranes, and a holosystolic murmur develop. Ileus and abdominal distention may be observed if a large volume of blood accumulates.

CAUSES

- Idiopathic
- Trauma
- Disseminated intravascular coagulopathy
- Mesenteric injury
- Hemorrhage from the reproductive tract
  - The most common location from which intra-abdominal bleedings occurs in females
  - The ovaries, uterus, or utero-ovarian blood vessels may be involved.
  - Ovarian hemorrhage can originated from rupture of the capsule of granulosa cell tumors and from ovarian follicular hematomas.
  - Uterine bleeding can be associated with birth-related trauma to the uterine vessels or with uterine neoplasia such as leiomyomas or leiomyosarcoma.
- Hemorrhage from the GI tract
  - Rupture of the mesenteric arteries secondary to *Strongylus vulgaris* larval migration. This condition is less frequent since the use of ivermectin.
  - Splenic rupture secondary to blunt trauma to the left caudal abdomen or to splenic neoplasia
  - Entrapment of the small intestine within the epiploic foramen
  - GI vascular leakage secondary to neoplasia or abscessation, coagulopathies, surgery, renal trauma, and hepatic disease.

RISK FACTORS

Age

- Peri-parturient hemorrhage associated with the rupture of the uterine or ovarian arteries is most frequently observed in older broodmares. There is an age-related degeneration within the arterial walls, which leads to aneurysm formation. Arterial rupture, at the aneurysm site, occurs subsequent to uterine contractions and fetal movement during late gestation and parturition.
- Particularly in older horses in epiploic foramen entrapment, rupture of the caudal vena cava occurs.

Pregnancy

Peri-partum hemorrhage can occur before, during, or after foaling.

Blunt External Trauma

Splenic rupture

Parasitism

Infestation by *S. vulgaris*

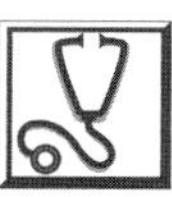

DIAGNOSIS

DIFFERENTIAL DIAGNOSIS

- All disorders resulting in colic in the horse should be included in the differential diagnoses.
- In broodmares, peri-partum conditions such as uterine torsion, uterine rupture, and dystocia should be considered. Rectal palpation and ultrasonography will help to differentiate these disorders.

CBC/BIOCHEMISTRY/URINALYSIS

- Hematologic abnormalities in acute blood loss will be seen after the initial 24 hr and include anemia (decrease in PCV, erythrocyte count, and hemoglobin concentration) and decreased total plasma protein. These changes are observed when intercompartmental fluid shifts or IV fluid replacement occurs. Hypoproteinemia usually is noted prior to the decline in hematocrit. In the anemic horses, there is no evidence of a regenerative response in the peripheral blood (no reticulocytosis). Sequential measurement of PCV will be helpful in determining whether the blood loss and resulting anemia are progressive or controlled.
- Evaluation of the coagulation profile reveals thrombocytopenia in conjunction with a normal activated partial thromboplastin time and prothrombin time. Thrombocytopenia is secondary to blood loss.

OTHER LABORATORY TESTS

Abdominal Paracentesis

Hemoperitoneum is definitively diagnosed by abdominal paracentesis. The fluid collected has an elevated erythrocyte count, which in the early stages will generally be less than or equal to the erythrocyte count in the peripheral blood. On cytologic examination, platelets are not typically present unless the hemorrhage is peracute. However, blood may be introduced into the peritoneal fluid during sampling by aspiration of splenic blood or by laceration of a subcutaneous vessel. Cytologic evidence of erythrophagocytosis suggests that the hemorrhage occurred before paracentesis unless fluid is not analyzed promptly. Normally, splenic blood readily clots because of increased concentration of fibrinogen. In chronic intra-abdominal hemorrhage, the erythrocyte count is usually equal to or greater than the erythrocyte count in peripheral blood and the protein content is less due to resorption. On cytologic examination, hypersegmented pyknotic neutrophils and hemosiderophages are observed.

Blood Gas Analysis

Measurement of arterial or venous P_{CO_2}, P_{O_2}, pH, and HCO_3^- provide useful information in hypovolemic shock states. Lactic acidosis, resulting from anaerobic metabolism, causes a nonrespiratory acidosis (decreased pH and HCO_3^- concentration) with respiratory compensation (decreased Pco_2). The diagnosis of respiratory compensation is made from arterial blood. Decrease in arterial (normal, 80–100 mm Hg) or venous (normal, 40 mm Hg) Po_2 indicates that normal cellular oxygenation is not maintained.

IMAGING

Abdominal Ultrasonography

Ultrasonographic evaluation of the abdomen, performed transabdominally or transrectally, reveals hyperechoic fluid within the abdominal cavity and permits assessment of the distribution of fluid. Occasionally, particularly when a neoplasia is present, the origin of the hemorrhage can be identified.

OTHER DIAGNOSTIC PROCEDURES

Rectal Palpation

Fluid accumulation within the abdomen, abnormal (neoplastic) masses, abnormalities within the reproductive tract or other lesions associated with the site of hemorrhage, and gas-distended intestine may be noted on rectal palpation.

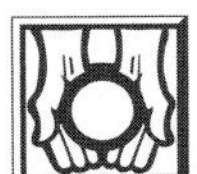

TREATMENT

AIMS OF TREATMENT

Primary aims of treatment of hemoperitoneum consist of restoring perfusion and oxygen delivery to tissues, correcting hypovolemia and controlling the hemorrhage. Normal intravascular volume is restored by the administration of crystalloid fluids and/or plasma. Blood transfusion is required when anemia becomes life threatening.

APPROPRIATE HEALTH CARE

Emergency inpatient intensive care is required in horses with hemoperitoneum. Most cases will respond favorably to this type of medical treatment. However, exploratory laparotomy may be needed in patients with hemorrhage from tumors, rupture of viscus, or leaking gastrointestinal vessel. Surgery should be performed only when the patients are stabilized.

NURSING CARE

Fluid Therapy

- When hypovolemic shock is present, the condition is addressed by prompt IV therapy with isotonic crystalloid solutions (lactated Ringer's solution, 20–40 mL/kg/hr) to increase vascular volume. Replacement fluid volume necessary to maintain perfusion in hemorrhagic shock is usually 2–7 times greater than the actual blood loss, because redistribution within the entire extracellular space occurs. Monitoring the clinical response to fluid replacement is mandatory. Improvement in jugular distensibility and capillary refill time, increased pulse strength, and decreased heart rate are indications of improved cardiovascular status.
- Replacement of intravascular volume may also be accomplished with hypertonic saline (5%–7.5%). Hypertonic saline (7.5% NaCl, 4 mL/kg) expands vascular volume, enhances vascular tone and restore intravascular pressure. However, when blood loss is not controlled, hypertonic saline increases bleeding from the mesenteric vasculature and decreases mean arterial pressure.

Blood Transfusion

In most instances, only crystalloid solution is used to successfully treat acute abdominal hemorrhage but when the packed cell volume is decreased to 15% (0.15 L/L) or the hemoglobin concentration falls below 5 g/dL (50 g/L), whole blood transfusion is required to increase oncotic pressure and oxygen-carrying capacity. The volume of blood transfusion will depend on the rate and quantity of blood loss. Whole blood should be administered at 15– 25 mL/kg of body weight and repeated if necessary. Balanced crystalloid solutions should be administered concurrently to maintain perfusion. Transfused red cells survive only 4–6 days in the horse, so the increase in PCV is only transient. It will also blunt the bone marrow response to anemia.

ACTIVITY

Horses with acute hemoperitoneum should be strictly rested. Horses surviving a large blood loss should not be exercised for 90 days.

SURGICAL CONSIDERATION

Patients not responding to conservative medical treatment and requiring surgical exploration of the abdominal cavity have a low percentage survival rate.

MEDICATION

DRUG(S) OF CHOICE

Use of procoagulant and antifibrinolytic agents in horses with bleeding disorders is empirical and their efficacy is not proven. The following drugs may be use in attempt to control the hemorrhage:

- Opioid antagonist (naloxone, one treatment of 8 mg IV)
- Ten to 30 mL of 10% buffered neutral formalin added to 500 mL of 0.09% NaCl. This solution is administered through an intravenous catheter placed in the jugular vein.

CONTRAINDICATIONS

Phenothiazine tranquilizers (acepromazine) are contraindicated in horses with hemorrhagic shock because these drugs decrease systemic arterial blood pressure.

PRECAUTIONS

α_2-Agonists (xylazine and detomidine) should be use with extreme caution in horses with intra-abdominal hemorrhage because these drugs decrease the cardiac output.

ALTERNATIVE DRUGS

Adjunctive treatments included NSAIDs, broad-spectrum antimicrobials, conjugated estrogens, aminocaproic acid, vitamin K, and propanolol. The use of these drugs in horses with hemoperitoneum is empirical and their impact on clinical outcome is not proved.

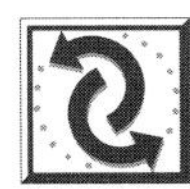

FOLLOW-UP

PATIENT MONITORING

Cardiovascular status should be assessed by monitoring heart rate, pulse strength, capillary refill time, and jugular vein distensibility. Frequency of assessment may vary from every 5 min to a few times a day depending whether the hemorrhage is controlled or not.

POSSIBLE COMPLICATIONS

Cardiovascular collapse and death

EXPECTED COURSE AND PROGNOSIS

The overall survival rate for horses with hemoperitoneum is between 50% and 70%. Horses with high respiratory rate (>30 breaths/min), neoplasia, mesenteric injury, or disseminated intravascular coagulopathy are less likely to survive. In post-parturient broodmares with rupture of the utero-ovarian artery, two clinical outcomes are possible depending on whether the hemorrhage is confined in the uterine broad ligament. In the former, a large hematoma develops in the broad ligament and the mare survives. In the latter, death can occur within minutes to days after parturition.

MISCELLANEOUS

ASSOCIATED CONDITIONS

N/A

ZOONOTIC POTENTIAL

N/A

ABBREVIATIONS

- GI = gastrointestinal
- PCV = packed cell volume

Suggested Reading

Dechant JE, Nieto JE, Le Jeune SS. Hemoperitoeum in horses: 67 cases (1989–2004). JAVMA 2006;229:253–258.

Pusterla N, Fecteau M-E, Madigan J, Wilson WD, Magdesian KG. Acute hemoperitoneum in horses: a review of 19 cases. J Vet Intern Med 2005;19:344–347.

Hurcombe SD, Mudge MC, Hinchcliff KW. Clinical and clinicopathologic variables in adult horses receiving blood transfusions: 31 cases (1999–2005). JAVMA 2007;231:267–274.

Author Ludovic Bouré

Consulting Editors Henry Stämpfli and Olimpo Oliver-Espinosa

INTRACAROTID INJECTION

BASICS

DEFINITION

Accidental injection of drugs into the carotid artery associated with acute neurologic signs

PATHOPHYSIOLOGY

- Drugs are accidentally injected into the carotid artery. The proximity of the common carotid artery to the jugular vein and patient movement make this a real hazard. The injected material often travels via the carotid artery and distributes to the ipsilateral forebrain supplied by the middle cerebral artery and is associated with acute, and possibly severe, cerebral disturbances.
- Marked cardiovascular changes, such as bradycardia, arrhythmias, and blood pressure fluctuations, may accompany CNS signs.
- Local cerebral pathology and clinical signs are dependent on the potential of the drug to induce tissue abnormalities and the rate of and quantity injected (see Expected Course and Prognosis).

SYSTEMS AFFECTED

CNS—Cardiovascular signs may include bradycardia, ectopia, and hypotension. Ophthalmic, ipsilateral ocular lesions may be present.

GENETICS

N/A

INCIDENCE/PREVALENCE

N/A

GEOGRAPHIC DISTRIBUTION

N/A

SIGNALMENT

No breed, sex, or age predisposition

SIGNS

Historical

A very recent history of parenteral drug administration

Physical Examination

- A violent reaction typically occurs within 5–30 seconds from the time of initiating the injection.
- Signs range from apprehension, facial twitching, head shaking, kicking, propulsive circling, to recumbency, loss of consciousness, seizures.
- The episodes can be variable in length, and death occurs on occasion.

CAUSES

See Pathophysiology.

RISK FACTORS

Fractious animals and attempts at an intravenous injection

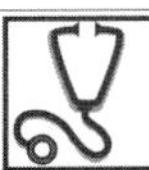

DIAGNOSIS

History and onset of clinical signs

DIFFERENTIAL DIAGNOSIS

The preacute onset after attempted intrajugular injection should rule out other causes of encephalopathies. Initial clinical signs may suggest anaphylaxis.

CBC/BIOCHEMISTRY/URINALYSIS

No specific abnormalities

OTHER LABORATORY TESTS

No specific abnormalities

IMAGING

- N/A

OTHER DIAGNOSTIC PROCEDURES

- N/A

PATHOLOGIC FINDINGS

It is unusual for these horses to not recover. However, in horses that do not survive, diffuse perivascular necrosis with marked edema, vascular endothelial damage, hemorrhage, and neuronal degeneration are evident.

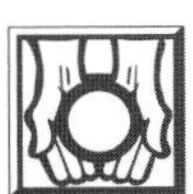

TREATMENT

- Treatment is largely supportive and symptomatic. Padding and sedation are indicated for thrashing, delirious horses.
- Dexamethasone 0.1–0.25 mg/kg IV, DMSO 1 g/kg diluted in physiologic saline 1–6 L IV, and anticonvulsant therapy may be useful.
- Hypertonic (7%) saline solution may be useful.
- Use of mannitol may be considered in horses that do not rapidly improve despite the risk of cerebral hemorrhage.
- Status epilepticus may be treated with diazepam 0.01–0.4 mg/kg IV.

MEDICATIONS

DRUG(S)

None proven

CONTRAINDICATIONS/POSSIBLE INTERACTIONS

N/A

PRECAUTIONS

It is surprisingly easy to inject the carotid artery by mistake and it behooves clinicians, particularly those who are not highly experienced, to use a large-gauge needle (i.e., 18 gauge) and to take the needle off the hub after insertion, ensuring that the blood that flows out is slow dripping and dark colored.

POSSIBLE COMPLICATIONS

Complications often arise from self-induced trauma if the horse falls or has seizures.

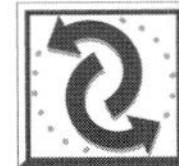

FOLLOW-UP

PATIENT MONITORING

Regular detailed neurologic examinations

PREVENTION/AVOIDANCE

Always use a large-bore needle and insert needle into vein before attaching syringe.

EXPECTED COURSE AND PROGNOSIS

- Injection of water-soluble drugs (e. g., xylazine, butorphanol, acetylpromazine) is usually associated with complete recovery within hours. Some horses may require up to 7 days to recover and, on rare occasion, some die.
- Common signs during recovery are facial hypalgesia, blindness, and poor menace response contralateral to the side of injection.
- Intracarotid injection of procaine penicillin, phenylbutazone, and oil-based or poorly water-soluble drugs is associated with a poorer prognosis. Intracarotid injection of such drugs is often associated with prolonged intractable seizures, coma, or stupor.

MISCELLANEOUS

ASSOCIATED CONDITIONS

N/A

AGE-RELATED FACTORS

N/A

ZOONOTIC POTENTIAL

NONE

PREGNANCY

N/A

SYNONYMS

None

Suggested Reading

Hahn CN, Mayhew IG, MacKay RJ, The nervous system. In: Collahan PT, Mayhew IG, Merritt AM, Moore, JN, eds. Equine Medicine and Surgery, ed 5. St. Louis: Mosby, 1999.

The author and editors wish to acknowledge the contribution of Joseph J. Bertone, author of this chapter in the previous edition.

Author Caroline N. Hahn
Consulting Editor Caroline N. Hahn

IONOPHORE TOXICOSIS

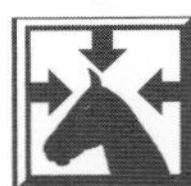

BASICS

DEFINITION

• Horses are sensitive to the toxic effects of the ionophore antimicrobials such as monensin, salinomycin, laidlomycin propionate, and lasalocid. • Several polyether ionophorous drugs (ionophores) are approved for use as coccidiostats, growth promotants. or both. Those currently in use are laidlomycin propionate (Cattlyst), lasalocid (Avatec, Bovatec), maduramycin (Cygro), monensin (Coban, Rumensin), narasin (Maxiban, Monteban), and salinomycin (Biocox, Coxistat, Saccox). • Ingestion of toxic amounts of ionophore drugs can result in a physicochemical and/or pathologic disruption of cardiac muscle, skeletal muscle, nerves, liver, and kidney.
• Although some of the ionophores have not been evaluated in the horse, all should be considered toxic and clinical effects should be similar. The LD_{50} doses for monensin, lasalocid and salinomycin are 2–3 mg/kg, 21.5 mg/kg, and 0.6 mg/kg body weight, respectively.

PATHOPHYSIOLOGY

• Ionophores are used are growth promoters in cattle and as coccidiostats for poultry. • The LD_{50} of these drugs in horses is much lower than that in cattle. • Ionophores embed in the biological membranes of cells and subcellular organelles. There they transport ions across the membrane, down concentration gradients. This results in the loss of ionic gradients across the membranes of excitable cells (muscle and nervous) as well as across the mitochondrial membrane. • Monensin has a higher affinity for sodium ions than potassium ions, whereas salinomycin has higher affinity for potassium than sodium. Lasalocid binds to calcium and magnesium ions. • For each ion transported into a cell, another ion has to be transported out in order to maintain the solubility in the membrane. Loss of the ion gradients across the mitochondrial membrane prevents oxidative metabolism. • Loss of intracellular potassium suppresses ATP production and decreases cell energy production; increases in intracellular sodium lead to cellular water influx and mitochondrial swelling; ionophores potentiate intracellular calcium influx, and all of these effects contribute to cell death. • Clinical effects and case-fatality rates are influenced by the quantity of ionophore ingested.

- With large amounts, the progression can be extremely rapid with death ensuing within 1–15 hr. Cardiac and skeletal lesions are not necessarily found in horses that die acutely.
- With lesser amounts, signs and pathological abnormalities related to skeletal and cardiac myopathy are observed.
- More mildly affected horses can develop a delayed form of cardiomyopathy that, depending on its severity, can lead to variable degrees of cardiac compromise evident weeks or months after initial exposure.

SYSTEMS AFFECTED

• Cardiovascular—Mitochondrial damage results in loss of aerobic ATP production and myocardial necrosis. Loss of ion gradients alters the polarity of the excitable tissues. Cardiac function, including conductance through the heart muscle, is altered. In animals that survive acute intoxication, connective tissue replaces necrotic myocardial cells, which can result in permanent myocardial dysfunction.
• Musculoskeletal—Effects on skeletal muscle are similar to the myocardial muscles. However, skeletal muscle damage is frequently less severe. Muscle fibrosis can occur in animals that survive acute intoxication. • Nervous system—The ionophores can alter nerve conduction and conduction through the muscle fibers. This results in altered reflexes and muscle coordination. • Renal/urologic—Renal tubular damage can occur. This is generally associated with myoglobin casts. In addition, distention of the urinary bladder can be seen.
• Hepatobiliary—Hepatocellular necrosis and decreased function can occur. • Gastrointestinal system

INCIDENCE/PREVALENCE

Ionophore poisoning in horses is not as common now as when ionophores were first introduced.

SIGNALMENT

There are no breed, age, or sex predilections.

SIGNS

General Comments

The severity and speed of onset of signs reflect the amount of ionophore ingested.

Historical

• Several horses in a group can be affected.
• Feed refusal, colic, ataxia, weakness, and recumbency are early signs.

Physical Examination

• Sudden death • Tachycardia • Cardiac arrhythmias • Tachypnea • Muscle weakness and ataxia • Profuse sweating • Epistaxis • Signs of congestive heart failure (peripheral and ventral edema, venous distention, jugular pulsation)
• Exercise intolerance

CAUSES

Horses are exposed to ionophores due to accidental contamination of feed at feed mills or when horses inadvertently gain access to feed formulated for cattle or poultry.

RISK FACTORS

Vitamin E and/or selenium deficiency can predispose to more severe tissue damage, but adequate concentrations do not prevent toxicosis.

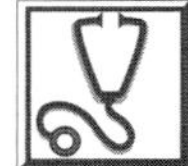

DIAGNOSIS

DIFFERENTIAL DIAGNOSIS

• Acute gastrointestinal diseases • Acute neurologic diseases • Rhabdomyolysis • Vitamin E/selenium deficiency • Viral, bacterial, or other toxic forms of myocardial failure

CBC/BIOCHEMISTRY/URINALYSIS

• Increased serum activity of CK, AST, and LDH • Increased serum concentrations of BUN and indirect bilirubin • Hyperglycemia
• Hypocalcemia, hypokalemia, hypomagnesemia, and hypochloremia
• Myoglobinurina

OTHER LABORATORY TESTS

• Elevated serum cardiac isoenzymes (CK-MB, HBDH or LDH 1 and 2) or cardiac troponin I can be present but absence of increases in these biomarkers does not rule out ionophore toxicosis. • Blood lactate can be increased, reflecting poor tissue perfusion.

Electrocardiography

Paroxysmal or sustained supraventricular and/or ventricular arrhythmias can be present.

Echocardiography

Echocardiographic abnormalities can range in severity and include: • Dilation of the left and/or right ventricle using two-dimensional and M-mode echocardiography. The ventricles can be rounded at their apices and adopt a globoid shape. • Regional or generalized hypokinesis or dyskinesis • Decreases in fractional shortening
• Marked spontaneous contrast (this is sometimes also noted in horses with no cardiac dysfunction) • Increases in the mitral E point—septal separation • Increased preejection period and decreased left ventricular ejection period • Flattening of the aortic root, reduced aortic root diameter • Mild, usually anechoic, pericardial effusion

Thoracic Ultrasonography

With pulmonary edema, irregularity of the periphery of the lungs (comet tails) is visible.

Thoracic Radiography

Pulmonary edema

OTHER DIAGNOSTIC PROCEDURES

• Radiotelemetric ECG monitoring—This is indicated for real-time monitoring of horses with unstable cardiac rhythms. • Continuous 24-hour Holter monitoring— This is particularly helpful in identifying intermittent or paroxysmal cardiac arrhythmias, in quantifying numbers of isolated premature depolarizations and in assessing response to therapy. • Exercising electrocardiography— Characterization of the effect of exercise on cardiac arrhythmias is important in assessing their clinical significance. This should be undertaken 2–3 mo after exposure in horses that show minimal signs at the time of exposure. • Toxicology—Stomach contents and feedstuffs should be analyzed for the presence of ionophores. Accumulation of ionophores in tissues is low. Thus, tissue testing is often unproductive.

PATHOLOGIC FINDINGS

• No lesions can be associated with sudden death. • Heart and skeletal muscle—vacuolation, swollen mitochondria, lipid vesicles, hypereosinohpilia, pyknosis, mineralization, and loss of fiber striation progressing to myocardial fibrosis and chamber dilation in more chronically affected cases
• Nervous system—polyneuropathy of peripheral nerves with axonal degeneration and neuronal vaculation. Wallerian degeneration in the dorsal funiculi of the spinal cord has been documented in other species. • Additional findings—Widespread petechial hemorrhages are found in the lungs, heart, gastrointestinal tract, and spleen. With congestive heart failure,

IONOPHORE TOXICOSIS

there can be pleural and peritoneal effusion, pulmonary edema, and peripheral edema. Distention of the urinary bladder can be seen.

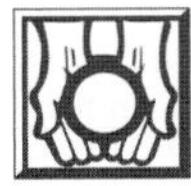

TREATMENT

AIMS OF TREATMENT

• There is no specific antidote. • Prevent further absorption of the toxin. • Supportive therapy is aimed at restoration of cardiac output and improved tissue perfusion, stabilization of cell membranes, and antiarrhythmic therapy if unstable, life-threatening arrhythmias are present.

APPROPRIATE HEALTH CARE

• Severely affected cases should be managed as inpatients. • Mildly affected cases may not require specific emergency treatment but should be rested until the degree of cardiac damage can be determined.

NURSING CARE

• Continuous electrocardiographic monitoring should be performed if horse is showing signs of active myocardial disease, particularly if the cardiac rhythm is unstable. • Horses should be kept quiet and not moved if showing signs consistent with low cardiac output. • Severely ataxic horses may benefit from protective measures such as head protectors, bandaging, and housing in a padded area.

ACTIVITY

• Horses should be rested, initially in a stable and subsequently, depending on the severity of clinical signs, for 2–3 mo after exposure to ionophores. An echocardiogram and exercising ECG should be performed in order to identify signs of chronic cardiomyopathy. • Caution is advised, since permanent myocardial damage can occur.

DIET

Supplementation of vitamin E and selenium has been shown to be effective as a pretreatment in cattle and pigs. However, its efficacy after exposure to ionophores has not been established.

CLIENT EDUCATION

• Ionophore toxicosis can have significant medicolegal implications. The client should be advised to make detailed records of events leading up to the onset of signs and to have these corroborated by third parties where possible.
• Where a group of horses has been exposed to ionophores, it can be impossible to determine which horses ingested the ionophore and how much they consumed. Horses that do not show clinical signs in the acute stages may be at risk for developing cardiac compromise later. Clients should be advised not to use the horses for riding activities for 2 mo, and after this time, an echocardiogram and exercising ECG should be performed in order to identify signs of chronic cardiomyopathy.

MEDICATIONS

DRUG(S)

• Gastric lavage and activated charcoal and a saline cathartic, administered by nasogastric tube, can reduce further absorption of the toxin.
• Intravenous fluid therapy should be used with care as it can exacerbate pulmonary edema if acute myocardial failure is present. • Thiamine (0.5–5.5 mg/kg IM), vitamin E (up to 20 IU/kg daily PO), and selenium (0.01 mg/kg IM) might promote stabilization of cell membranes.
• Antiarrhythmic drugs are described in Supraventricular Arrhythmias and Ventricular Arrhythmias elsewhere in this text.

CONTRAINDICATIONS

• Digoxin acts synergistically with ionophores through inhibition of Na^+,K^+-ATPase and increases in cellular calcium influx, promoting cell death and myocardial necrosis.
• Chloramphenicol, sulfonamides, and macrolides can also potentiate ionophore toxicity.

PRECAUTIONS

All antiarrhythmic drugs have the potential to be proarrhythmic, particularly in the unstable myocardium. The ECG should be monitored, in real-time, continuously during antiarrhythmic therapy.

POSSIBLE INTERACTIONS

See Contraindications.

FOLLOW-UP

PATIENT MONITORING

In the acute stages, frequent assessment of heart and respiratory rate, pulse quality, blood pressure (using noninvasive methods), blood lactate concentrations, and continuous ECG monitoring are indicated.

PREVENTION/AVOIDANCE

Most outbreaks occur due to accidents at feed mills. It is incumbent on feed manufacturers to take every possible precaution to ensure that ionophores are not accidentally included in feeds destined for the equine market.

POSSIBLE COMPLICATIONS

Congestive heart failure can occur in horses that survive the initial stages.

EXPECTED COURSE AND PROGNOSIS

• Reported mortality ranges from 60% to 100%. However, it is extremely difficult to determine whether horses that have had access to ionophores have actually ingested it. The bitter taste may deter many individuals, particularly if they have access to alternative feed sources.
• Some horses that show no signs in the acute stages develop congestive heart failure, whereas others may have milder degrees of decreased cardiac function that may be performance-limiting without leading to death.

MISCELLANEOUS

PREGNANCY

There is a high risk of fetal compromise if mares develop low cardiac output during pregnancy.

SYNONYMS

Monensin toxicosis, salinomycin toxicosis, et cetera

SEE ALSO

• Myocardial disease • Supraventricular arrhythmias • Ventricular arrhythmias

ABBREVIATIONS

• AST = aspartate transaminase
• ATP = adenosine 5ψ-triphosphate
• CK-MB = MB isoenzyme of creatine kinase
• ECG = electrocardiography
• HBDH = α-hydroxybutyrate dehydrogenase
• K^+ = potassium • LDH = lactate dehydrogenase • LD_{50} = median lethal dose
• Na^+ = sodium

Suggested Reading

Hall JO. Feed-associated toxicants: ionophores. In: Plumless KH, ed. Clinical Veterinary Toxicology. St. Louis: Mosby, 2004.

Hall JO. Toxic feed constituents in the horse. Vet Clin North Am Equine Pract 2001;17:479–489.

Peek SF, Marques FD, Morgan J, Steinberg H, Zoromski DW, McGuirk S. Atypical acute monensin toxicosis and delayed cardiomyopathy in Belgian Draft horses. J Vet Intern Med 2004;18:761–764.

Authors Celia M. Marr and Jeff Hall
Consulting Editor Celia M. Marr

IRIS PROLAPSE

BASICS

OVERVIEW

• Iris prolapse in the horse most frequently follows acute ocular trauma (TIP), particularly sharp perforating corneal injuries, or blunt injuries causing rupture of the cornea, limbus, and/or sclera. • Corneal perforation can also occur secondary to rapid enzymatic degradation of stromal collagen and ground substance due to infectious and noninfectious ulcerative iris proiapse (UIP).

SIGNALMENT

All ages and breeds of horses in all types of environments are at risk.

SIGNS

• The eye may be cloudy, red, and painful. Blepharospasm and tearing are present. Slight droopiness of the eyelashes of the upper eyelid may be a subtle sign of corneal ulceration.
• Corneal edema may be focal or generalized.
• A brown to red structure protruding through a corneal or scleral laceration is diagnostic. • The anterior chamber will be shallow or collapsed due to loss of aqueous humor.

CAUSES AND RISK FACTORS

Corneal perforation with iris prolapse may be a sequel to traumatic insult to the globe or orbit, as well as ulcerative infectious and noninfectious corneal ulcerations.

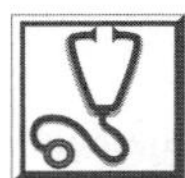

DIAGNOSIS

DIFFERENTIAL DIAGNOSIS

Ocular pain may be found with corneal ulcers, uveitis, conjunctivitis, glaucoma, blepharitis, and dacryocystitis.

DIAGNOSTIC PROCEDURES

• Fluorescein dye will indicate the site of a corneal perforation, and the dye may leak into the anterior chamber. • A Seidel's test where the orange color of fluorescein is changed to green by leaking aqueous humor can be seen.

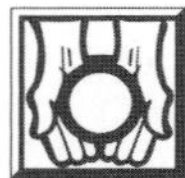

TREATMENT

SURGICAL THERAPY

• Clinical and surgical guidelines for the treatment of iris prolapse in horses, based upon the possibility of useful vision and ocular survival, will assist in choosing a therapeutic plan of action. Replacement of missing cornea with a corneal transplant is recommended. The transplant site should be covered with a conjunctival flap graft.
• Key techniques in repairing an iris prolapse:
1. Remove as much necrotic cornea as possible before placing the corneal graft. Replace missing cornea with a larger- diameter frozen corneal donor graft. Suture the cornea in place.
2. Make the CF thin. CF fibrosis and failure may be associated with iris prolapse under the flap. Aqueous humor leakage induces fibroplasia of the corneal side of the flap such that this surface becomes thickened and fibrotic and does not completely adhere to the wound. The flap may still partially adhere but vascularization of the cornea may fail.
3. Flap bruising manifesting as purple areas of the CF may indicate flap ischemia.
4. A white CF has become avascular.
5. CF bulging may indicate iris prolapse. Check for low intraocular pressure and positive Seidel's test.
6. Continue antiproteinases after flap placement or absorbable sutures may be dissolved prematurely.
7. Anchor CF with sutures at the limbus to reduce tension.
8. *Streptococcus* and *Aspergillus* can melt a flap and leave the sutures intact.

MEDICATIONS

DRUG(S) OF CHOICE

• Topically applied antibiotics (chloramphenicol, bacitracin-neomycin-polymyxin B, gentamicin; QID), atropine (1%; QID), and serum (QID) are recommended. Systemic NSAIDs (phenylbutazone, 2 mg/kg BID PO; flunixin meglumine 1 mg/kg BID, PO, IM, IV), and broad-spectrum parenteral antibiotics are also indicated. • Intensive postoperative medical therapy, especially use of systemic NSAID, is critical for successful management of the profound iridocyclitis and endophthalmitis in these cases. By inhibiting the cyclooxygenase inflammatory pathway, flunixin meglumine reduces uveal prostaglandin synthesis and, subsequently, vasodilation and permeability of the uveal vasculature.

CONTRAINDICATIONS/POSSIBLE INTERACTIONS

Horses receiving topically administered atropine should be monitored for signs of colic.

FOLLOW-UP

PATIENT MONITORING

• Horses with iris prolapse and secondary uveitis should be stall-rested until the condition is healed. Intraocular hemorrhage and increased severity of uveitis are sequelae to overexertion.
• The horse should be protected from self-trauma with hard- or soft-cup hoods.
• Horses should be monitored for signs of eye pain and colic. The ocular pain should gradually diminish following surgical repair. • Diet should be consistent with the training level of the horse.

POSSIBLE COMPLICATIONS

Infectious endophthalmitis and blindness are complications that will require enucleation.

EXPECTED COURSE AND PROGNOSIS

• Prognosis of perforating corneal lacerations is generally considered guarded depending on the size, location, and mechanism of injury. Perforating lacerations caused by sharp injuries are generally associated with a better prognosis than those caused by blunt or missile injuries. High-energy blunt ocular trauma may result in hyphema and/or globe rupture, most often occurring at the limbus or equator where the sclera is the thinnest. • Uncontrolled, iridocyclitis may predispose to fibropupillary membrane formation, with subsequent posterior synechiae and cataract development. • Prognosis for horses with corneal lacerations and mild hyphema is slightly more favorable, albeit guarded, compared with horses with corneal lacerations and total hyphema. Eyes with TIP and hyphema comprising greater than an estimated 10% of the anterior chamber often result in blindness, phthisis bulbi, or enucleation. • In horses with TIP, corneal wound lengths 15 mm or less may have a positive visual outcome. Wound lengths greater than 15 mm result in either blindness, phthisis bulbi, or enucleation. • There is a direct relationship between a prolonged duration of ulcerative keratitis prior to UIP, and poor visual outcome. Eyes with perforating corneal ulcers due to ulcerative keratitis greater than 2 weeks' duration, and melting ulcers and/or ulcers with concomitant fungal and bacterial infections, tend to have a poor visual outcome or result in enucleation due to endophthalmitis in a majority of such cases.

MISCELLANEOUS

ASSOCIATED CONDITIONS

Ulcerative keratitis in the horse frequently incites severe anterior uveitis mediated by reflex axonal pathways and/or infection.

ABBREVIATIONS

• CF = conjunctival flap • TIP = traumatic iris prolapse • UIP = ulcerative iris prolapse

Suggested Reading

Brooks DE. Ophthalmology for the Equine Practitioner. Jackson, WY; Teton NewMedia, 2002.
Brooks DE, Matthews AG. Equine ophthalmology. In: Gelatt KN, ed. Veterinary Ophthalmology, ed 4. Philadelphia; Lippincott Williams and Wilkins, 2007.
Gilger BC, ed. Equine Ophthalmology. Philadelphia; WB Saunders, 2005.

Author Dennis E. Brooks
Consulting Editor Dennis E. Brooks

IRON TOXICOSIS

BASICS

OVERVIEW

• Iron is an essential mineral required for a variety of physiologic functions involving oxidation–reduction reactions. • Horses often are supplemented with various iron salts, either in their feed or via parenteral administration. • Intoxication is often associated with oral exposure to iron-containing supplements, with most documented cases occurring in neonates <3 days of age from oral administration of a digestive inoculant containing ferrous fumarate. • Toxicity of iron salts depends on the amount of elemental iron present—ferrous sulfate is 20% elemental iron; ferrous gluconate is 12% elemental iron. • Ingestion of iron salts causes corrosive damage to the GI mucosa, resulting in edema, ulceration, and hemorrhage. • After absorption, ferrous iron (Fe^{2+}) is converted to ferric iron (Fe^{3+}), releasing an unbuffered hydrogen ion and causing metabolic acidosis. • Intracellularly, iron disrupts oxidative phosphorylation and causes free-radical formation and lipid peroxidation, resulting in cell death. • Periportal hepatocytes are especially vulnerable to damage and necrosis. • Iron also can result in a coagulopathy from inhibition of thrombin. • Iron is cardiotoxic, resulting in decreased cardiac output. • Hypovolemia from GI fluid loss and decreased cardiac output contribute to circulatory shock.

SIGNALMENT

• Most reported cases involve neonates. • The sensitivity of neonates is believed to result from their lower capacity to bind iron to transferrin and their increased absorption of orally administered iron. • The toxicity of elemental iron to horses is uncertain, but toxic doses for neonates are estimated to be 25-fold less than those for adults.

SIGNS

• Early signs associated with oral ingestion include colic, diarrhea, and melena.
• Intoxicated horses often present with anorexia, lethargy, and icterus. • Signs of hepatoencephalopathy (e.g., ataxia, head pressing, coma) may be seen.

CAUSES AND RISK FACTORS

Iron is more toxic in selenium- or vitamin E–deficient individuals.

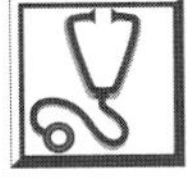

DIAGNOSIS

DIFFERENTIAL DIAGNOSIS

Adult Horses

• Other hepatotoxicants—aflatoxins (detection in feed, histopathologic lesions), blue-green algae toxins (presence of algal bloom, detection of toxins, histopathologic lesions), PAs (evidence of PA-containing plant consumption, histopathologic lesions) • Theiler's disease—history of equine immune serum administration • Causes of hemolytic anemia—red maple ingestion (evidence of plant consumption, Heinz bodies, methemoglobinemia); equine infectious anemia (positive Coggin's test) • Immune-mediated thrombocytopenia—positive Coomb's test
• DIC—detection of underlying disease, thrombocytopenia, moderately prolonged PT and aPTT, and increased serum FDPs
• Bacterial cholangiohepatitis—liver biopsy
• Lymphosarcoma—evaluation of blood smears, cytologic evaluation of bone marrow, and enlarged lymph nodes or tumor masses

Foals

• Septicemia—fever; neutrophilia • Neonatal isoerythrolysis—low PCV; positive Coomb's test
• Tyzzer's disease—histopathologic examination
• Equine herpesvirus—histopathologic lesions, serology, virus identification or isolation

CBC/BIOCHEMISTRY/URINALYSIS

• Thrombocytopenia, lymphopenia, and prolonged PT and aPTT • Increased serum GGT, ALP, total and conjugated bilirubin, bile acids, fibrinogen, FDP, and ammonia • Anion gap metabolic acidosis

OTHER LABORATORY TESTS

• High serum iron concentration, high saturation of iron binding, and high free iron in tissues • Post-mortem interpretation of high liver iron concentrations is difficult in the absence of compatible histopathologic lesions.

IMAGING N/A

DIAGNOSTIC PROCEDURES N/A

PATHOLOGICAL FINDINGS

Gross

Lesions include icterus, small livers with dark red areas or tan discoloration and uneven surfaces, GI hemorrhages, and thymic atrophy in foals.

Histopathologic Findings

• Lesions include hepatocellular necrosis that is primarily periportal or panlobular, varying degrees of bile duct proliferation, fibrous connective tissue proliferation, mixed inflammatory cell infiltration, and cholestasis.
• There may be multifocal to locally extensive areas of necrosis and hemorrhage in the gastric glandular mucosa and areas of necrosis in the lamina propria of the small intestine. • Mild to severe lymphoid lesions, including thymic lymphoid necrosis and necrosis in splenic lymphoid follicles

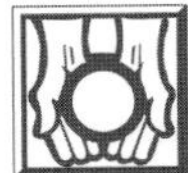

TREATMENT

• Stabilize the patient, paying particular attention to cardiovascular support and acid-base status. • GI decontamination is unlikely to be beneficial because of the inability of AC to bind iron.

MEDICATIONS

DRUG(S) OF CHOICE

• Use of the specific iron-chelator deferoxamine mesylate is possible. Appropriate dosage regimens have not been determined and efficacy and safety studies in horses are lacking. • For mild intoxications, chelation therapy probably offers little advantage compared with supportive care. • A suggested deferoxamine dosage based on experience in humans and dogs is 15 mg/kg/hr IV; if used, therapy probably should be limited to 24 hr.

CONTRAINDICATIONS/POSSIBLE INTERACTIONS

• Do not give deferoxamine to patients with renal impairment. • Rapid administration of deferoxamine can cause cardiac dysrhythmias and exacerbate existing hypotension. • Do not give deferoxamine to pregnant animals because of possible fetal skeletal abnormalities. • Do not give corticosteroids to iron-intoxicated patients because of possible increased serum free-iron concentrations.

FOLLOW-UP

PATIENT MONITORING

Monitor serum iron concentrations, liver function, and cardiovascular status.

PREVENTION/AVOIDANCE

• Do not oversupplement iron in individuals without confirmed iron deficiency. • A normal dietary requirement of iron in adult horses is 40 ppm.

POSSIBLE COMPLICATIONS

N/A

EXPECTED COURSE AND PROGNOSIS

• Individuals with mild liver pathology have a good prognosis with good supportive care.
• Individuals with severe liver pathology or hepatoencephalopathy have a guarded prognosis.

ABBREVIATIONS

• AC = activated charcoal
• ALP = alkaline phosphatase
• aPTT = activated partial thromboplastin time
• DIC = disseminated intravascular coagulation
• FDP = fibrin degradation product
• GGT = γ-glutamyltransferase
• PA = pyrrolizidine alkaloid
• PCV = packed cell volume
• ppm = parts per million
• PT = prothrombin time

Suggested Reading

Edens LM, Robertson JL, Feldman BF. Cholestatic hepatopathy, thrombocytopenia and lymphopenia associated with iron toxicity in a Thoroughbred gelding. Equine Vet J 1993;25:81–84.

Mullaney TP, Brown CM. Iron toxicity in neonatal foals. Equine Vet J 1988;20:119–124.

Author Robert H. Poppenga
Consulting Editor Robert H. Poppenga

ISCHEMIC OPTIC NEUROPATHY

BASICS

OVERVIEW

Atrophy of the optic nerve as a sequel to infarction or injury to the vascular supply to the optic nerve

ORGAN SYSTEM

Ophthalmic

SIGNALMENT

N/A

SIGNS

- Rapidly developing blindness
- Dilated pupil
- Absent PLR
- No signs of pain
- Following sudden loss of blood supply, the optic disc at first appears slightly pale. Within 3–5 days, there is a papilloedema due to ischemia and infarction of the optic nerve. This may progress to white, raised lesions overlying the optic nerve and its margins. After several weeks, there is ophthalmoscopic signs of optic nerve atrophy with pallor and vascular attenuation of the optic disc.
- Peripapillary retinal ischemia results in microinfarcts of the nerve fiber layer, which appear clinically as whitish indistinct spots. These are areas of a thickened nerve fiber layer consisting of aggregates of ruptured and swollen axons. With time, there are increasing signs of retinal atrophy.

CAUSES AND RISK FACTORS

- Head trauma
- Severe systemic hemorrhage
- Septic embolism
- Optic neuritis
- Surgical ligation of the internal carotid, external carotid, and greater palatine arteries for treatment of epistaxis caused by guttural pouch mycosis

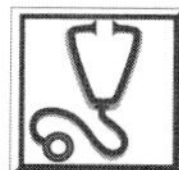

DIAGNOSIS

DIFFERENTIAL DIAGNOSIS

- Traumatic neuropathy
- Exudative optic neuritis
- Retinal detachment
- ERU

CBC/BIOCHEMISTRY/URINALYSIS

N/A

OTHER LABORATORY TESTS

N/A

IMAGING

N/A

DIAGNOSTIC PROCEDURES

ERG will be normal initially but reduced to absent as the ischemia becomes prolonged.

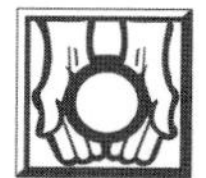

TREATMENT

Treatment is symptomatic depending on the cause and whether any specific etiological agent has been determined.

MEDICATIONS

CONTRAINDICATIONS/POSSIBLE INTERACTIONS

N/A

FOLLOW-UP

EXPECTED COURSE AND PROGNOSIS

Poor prognosis for return of vision

MISCELLANEOUS

SEE ALSO

- Exudative optic neuritis
- Recurrent uveitis

ABBREVIATIONS

- ERG = electroretinogram
- ERU = equine recurrent uveitis
- PLR = pupillary light reflex

Suggested Reading

Brooks DE. Ophthalmology for the Equine Practitioner. Jackson, WY; Teton NewMedia, 2002.

Brooks DE, Matthews AG. Equine ophthalmology. In: Gelatt KN, ed. Veterinary Ophthalmology, ed 4. Philadelphia; Lippincott Williams and Wilkins, 2007.

Gilger BC, ed. Equine Ophthalmology. Philadelphia; WB Saunders, 2005.

Authors Maria Källberg and Dennis E. Brooks

Consulting Editor Dennis E. Brooks

ISOCOMA WRIGHTII (RAYLESS GOLDENROD) TOXICOSIS

BASICS

OVERVIEW

- In the past, *Isocoma wrightii* (rayless goldenrod) has been known as *Haplopappus heterophyllus*.
- The plant is an erect, bushy, unbranching perennial shrub that grows 2–4 feet in height.
- The leaves are alternate and linear and generally have a smooth margin but can be toothed; the leaves also may have a sticky feel to them.
- The flowers are yellow, tubular, and terminal and number 7–15 per head.
- The plant prefers the arid Southwest and is found in dry rangelands of southern Colorado, through New Mexico and Arizona, western Texas, and into northern Mexico.
- The plant grows well in river valleys, along drainage areas, and is abundant along the Pecos River.
- Tremetone, a ketone, is reportedly the toxic agent.

SIGNALMENT

N/A

SIGNS

- No cases of *I. wrightii* intoxication have been documented in horses although intoxication is suspected to recur.
- The toxin is the same as that found in *Eupatorium rugosum* (white snakeroot), and presumptive evidence exists that the same clinical signs could be expected—heart muscle degeneration, muscle tremors, ataxia, reluctance to walk, heavy sweating, myoglobinuria, and depression.
- Horses that eat *E. rugosum* have an onset of clinical signs within 2–3 weeks after ingestion; generally, 2–3 days of ingestion is required.
- Affected horses stand with their legs wide apart and develop swelling near the thoracic inlet and along the ventral neck.
- There may be a jugular pulse and associated tachycardia.
- ECG changes—increased heat rate, ST elevation, and variable QRS complexes
- Cardiac arrhythmias often are present and detectable on auscultation.

CAUSES AND RISK FACTORS

- Environmental conditions such as drought result in less desirable forages or weeds being consumed.
- Hungry or thirsty horses that are unfamiliar with a given area are more likely to consume *I. wrightii*.

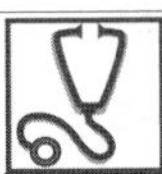

DIAGNOSIS

DIFFERENTIAL DIAGNOSIS

- Evidence of consumption and occurrence of compatible clinical signs remain the best way of diagnosing intoxication.
- Examination of the pasture may reveal that the plant has been browsed.
- Selenium/vitamin E deficiency (white muscle disease)—measurement of selenium and vitamin E in whole blood, serum, or liver
- Ionophore intoxication—detection of ionophore in feed or GI contents

CBC/BIOCHEMISTRY/URINALYSIS

- Horses intoxicated with *E. rugosum* have elevated serum CK, AST, and AP activities.
- Presumably, horses consuming *I. wrightii* have similar abnormalities.

OTHER LABORATORY TESTS

- ECG changes may be noted as described above.
- Detection of toxin may be possible.

IMAGING

N/A

DIAGNOSTIC PROCEDURES

N/A

PATHOLOGICAL FINDINGS

- Horses ingesting *E. rugosum* have nonspecific histopathologic lesions.
- Lesions associated with suspected *I. wrightii* intoxication—myocardial degeneration, necrosis, and fibrosis
- The pericardial sac may contain straw-colored fluid, and the subendocardium may have extensive pale areas.

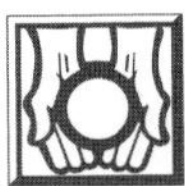

TREATMENT

- Decontamination with AC and a saline cathartic may be helpful.
- Monitor ECG and treat arrhythmias accordingly.
- Animals that survive may be left with a severely scarred heart and circulatory dysfunction; therefore, symptomatic and supportive care is always appropriate.

MEDICATIONS

DRUG(S) OF CHOICE

- AC (1–4 g/kg PO in a water slurry [1g of AC per 5 mL of water)]
- Sodium or magnesium sulfate (250 mg/kg PO as a 20% solution)

CONTRAINDICATIONS/POSSIBLE INTERACTIONS

N/A

FOLLOW-UP

PATIENT MONITORING

N/A

PREVENTION/AVOIDANCE

- Preventing access to the plant is the best solution for avoiding intoxication.
- Herbicides can be used to control plant growth.

POSSIBLE COMPLICATIONS

N/A

EXPECTED COURSE AND PROGNOSIS

N/A

MISCELLANEOUS

ASSOCIATED CONDITIONS, AGE-RELATED FACTORS, ZOONOTIC POTENTIAL, PREGNANCY

N/A

SEE ALSO

E. rugosum (white snakeroot)

ABBREVIATIONS

- AC = activated charcoal
- AST = aspartate aminotransferase
- AP = alkaline phosphatase
- CK = creatine kinase

Suggested Reading

Olson CT, Keller WC, Gerken Reed SM. Suspected tremetol poisoning in horses. J Am Vet Med Assoc 1984;185:1001–1003.

Sanders M. White snakeroot poisoning in a foal: a case report. Equine Vet Sci 1983;3:128–131.

Author Tam Garland

Consulting Editor Robert H. Poppenga

JUGLANS NIGRA (BLACK WALNUT) TOXICOSIS

BASICS

OVERVIEW

Juglans nigra (black walnut) is a large tree native to the eastern United States whose wood is prized for furniture and gun stocks. When fresh black walnut shavings are used as bedding, horses can develop laminitis and pyrexia within 12–24 hr. It usually presents as a stable-wide outbreak, but not all horses in contact with black walnut–contaminated bedding will develop problems.

SIGNALMENT

No breed, age, or sex predilection

SIGNS

- Laminitis (can be severe)
- Pyrexia
- Depression
- Limb edema
- Colic

CAUSES AND RISK FACTORS

- An unknown compound in fresh black walnut shavings
- Toxicity decreases with exposure of shavings to light and air.
- Problems can occur when as little as 5%–20% of bedding is black walnut.

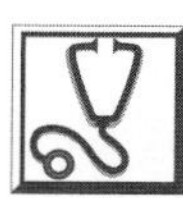

DIAGNOSIS

DIFFERENTIAL DIAGNOSIS

- Other causes of laminitis—history, no evidence of exposure to black walnut
- *Berteroa incana* (hoary alyssum) ingestion—evidence of exposure
- History will indicate multiple horses bedded with black walnut shavings develop laminitis over a relatively short period of time.

CBC/BIOCHEMISTRY/URINALYSIS

N/A

OTHER LABORATORY TESTS

- Black walnut shavings can be identified by their dark brown color (with a hint of purple).
- Samples can be submitted to diagnostic laboratories or forestry departments for positive identification by microscopy.

IMAGING

N/A

DIAGNOSTIC PROCEDURES

N/A

PATHOLOGICAL FINDINGS

Laminitis

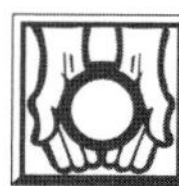

TREATMENT

- Remove all animals from suspect bedding.
- Wash legs with mild soap and water.
- Treat for laminitis.

MEDICATIONS

DRUG(S) OF CHOICE

- If ingested, administer oral AC at 1–4 g/kg body weight in a water slurry.
- Treat for laminitis.

CONTRAINDICATIONS/ POSSIBLE INTERACTIONS

N/A

FOLLOW-UP

PATIENT MONITORING

N/A

PREVENTION/AVOIDANCE

Inspect bedding deliveries for black walnut contamination.

POSSIBLE COMPLICATIONS

Ventral rotation of the third phalanx

EXPECTED COURSE AND PROGNOSIS

Good with no complications

MISCELLANEOUS

ASSOCIATED CONDITIONS, AGE-RELATED FACTORS, ZOONOTIC POTENTIAL, PREGNANCY

N/A

SEE ALSO

Laminitis

ABBREVIATION

- AC = activated charcoal

Suggested Reading

Uhlinger, C. Black walnut toxicosis in ten horses. J Am Vet Med Assoc 1989;195: 343–344.

Author Larry J. Thompson

Consulting Editor Robert H. Poppenga

JUNCTIONAL EPIDERMOLYSIS BULLOSA

BASICS

OVERVIEW

• JEB is an inherited fatal disease of newborn Belgian and other draft horse breed foals that is similar to the lethal Herlitz subtype of JEB (H-JEB) in humans. In horses, the condition has also been called EI, EIN, and JMBD. • The heritable forms of EB are characterized by fragility of the skin as well as other epithelial surfaces, including the mucous membranes of the gastrointestinal, respiratory, and urinary tracts. • JEB refers to the group of inherited blistering diseases in which blister formation takes place within the lamina lucida of the dermal-epidermal basement membrane.

SYSTEMS AFFECTED

• Skin, respiratory, gastrointestinal, and urologic

SIGNALMENT

• Breeds affected—Belgian draft horse, American Cream draft horse, Trait Breton, Trait Comtois, Vlaams Paard, Belgische Koudbloed Flander. American Saddlebreds, and Appaloosas have also been documented with H-JEB. Other breeds may be affected. • There is no sex predilection. • Disease may be apparent at birth or within the first 10–14 days of life. • Inherited as an autosomal recessive trait

SIGNS

• Erosions and ulceration of the skin and mucous membranes seen in the first few days of life • Primary skin lesions are vesicles and bullae, but these are transient, easily ruptured, and usually absent when the foals are examined.
• The predominant clinical lesions are well-demarcated ulcers with variable degrees of peripheral epidermal and mucosal collarettes.
• Exudation and crusting are pronounced.
• Lesions typically present on the coronets; the mucocutaneous junctions of the lips, anus, vulva, eyelids, nostrils, and oral cavity. • Skin lesions occur over bony prominences of the hock, stifle, hip, elbow, carpus, and fetlock.
• Erosions over pressure points may rapidly develop into deep ulcerative lesions. • Some foals are born with a complete loss of the epidermis on distal extremities and rump.
• Teeth erupt prematurely, so incisor teeth are visible at birth. • Abnormally shaped teeth—teeth have irregular serrated edges.
• Enamel hypoplasia with pitting of teeth
• Coronary band separation in one or more limbs • Exungulation (loss of the hoof capsule) in one or more limbs • Foals are depressed, cachectic, and pyrexic. • Death due to secondary sepsis

CAUSES AND RISK FACTORS

• In the draft horse breeds, JEB results from a mutation that causes a defect in the formation of laminin-5. Laminin-5 is an anchoring filament attachment protein that is widely distributed within the basement membrane zone of epithelial tissues and is critical in anchoring the epidermis to the dermis. In addition, it is essential for adhesion of ameloblasts to the enamel matrix of the teeth as well as attachment of the gingiva to the tooth surface. Laminin-5 consists of three polypeptide subunits—the α3, ε3, and γ2 chains, encoded by the *LAMA3*, *LAMB3*, and *LAMC2* genes, respectively. • In the Belgian, and other draft horse breeds, JEB is caused by a homozygous single base (cytosine) insertion at position 1368 of the *LAMC2* gene. This frame shift mutation results in the transcription of a premature termination codon that gives rise to a truncated N-terminal γ2 polypeptide that is lacking the α-helical C-terminal domain. The C-terminal domain of the protein is essential for assembly of laminin-5. The *LAMC2* gene is located on equine chromosome 5. • The genetic defect responsible for EI (H-JEB) in American Saddlebred horses has yet to be elucidated; however, it is not the same as in the draft horse breeds. Genetic analysis by linkage disequilibrium has shown that the EI disease locus was located on equine chromosome 8q, at the location of the *LAMA3* gene.

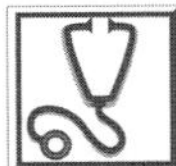

DIAGNOSIS

DIFFERENTIAL DIAGNOSIS

• Clinical presentation is highly suggestive.
• Trauma • Septicemia • Pemphigus vulgaris, bullous pemphigoid, systemic lupus erythematosus—
immune-mediated diseases are unlikely to occur as congenital or neonatal disorders. • Drug reaction

OTHER DIAGNOSTIC PROCEDURES

Perform skin biopsy for histopathology at the margin of affected areas. Other suggested biopsy sites include intact vesicles or bullae. Obtain the entire vesicle or bullae by punch biopsy or by wedge resection if necessary. Do NOT surgically prepare the site before the biopsy.

PATHOLOGICAL FINDINGS

Histopathology reveals subepidermal cleft and vesicle formation with minimal inflammation except in locations of ulceration and infection. Periodic acid–Schiff staining may be positive representing basement membrane zone attachment to the floor of clefts associated with vesicles or bullae.

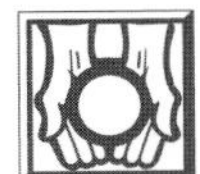

TREATMENT

• Fatal inherited disease • Euthanasia recommended • Intensive care may prolong life of foal.

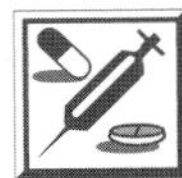

FOLLOW-UP

PATIENT MONITORING

Erosions and ulcerations become more extensive with age.

PREVENTION/AVOIDANCE

• Determine if breeding stock are carriers of the *LAMC2* mutation. • Commercial test is available through breed registry/associations, Veterinary Genetics Laboratory, University of California, Davis, California (www.vgl.ucdavis.edu). • Do not breed carrier sire and carrier dam. • Approximately 12%–13% of North American Belgian draft horse breed, 13% of Breton breed and 8% of Comtois breed are carriers of the *LAMC2* mutation (as of May 2007).

POSSIBLE COMPLICATIONS

• Sepsis • Exungulation

EXPECTED COURSE AND PROGNOSIS

Foals invariably die within first 2 weeks of life.

MISCELLANEOUS

ABBREVIATIONS

• EB = epidermolysis bullosa
• EI = epitheliogenesis imperfecta
• EIN = epitheliogenesis imperfecta neonatorum • H-JEB = Herlitz subtype of junctional epidermolysis bullosa
• JEB = junctional epidermolysis bullosa
• JMBD = junctional mechanobullous disease
• *LAMC2* = gene encoding for the formation of γ2 chain of laminin-5

Suggested Reading

Baird JD, Millon LV, Dileanis S, et al. Junctional epidermolysis bullosa in Belgian draft horses. Proc Am Assoc Equine Pract 2003;49:122–126.

Lieto LD, Cothran EG. The epitheliogenesis imperfecta locus maps to equine chromosome 8 in American Saddlebred horses. Cytogenet Genome Res 2003;102:207–210.

Milenkovic D, Chaffaux S, Taourit S, et al. A mutation in the *LAMC2* gene causes the Herlitz junctional epidermolysis bullosa (H-JEB) in two French draft horse breeds. Genet Sel Evol 2003;35:249–256.

Schott HC, Petersen AD. Cutaneous markers of disorders affecting young horses. Clin Tech Equine Pract 2005;4:314–323.

Spirito F, Çharlesworth A, Linder K, et al. Animal models for skin blistering conditions: absence of laminin 5 causes hereditary junctional mechanobullous disease in the Belgian horse. J Invest Dermatol 2002;119:684–691.

Author John D. Baird

Consulting Editor Gwendolen Lorch

LAMINITIS

BASICS

DEFINITION

Laminitis is failure of the hoof-distal phalanx attachment apparatus.

PATHOPHYSIOLOGY

- The lamellae suspend P3 within the hoof capsule. Epidermal lamellae extend like sheets from the stratum medium of the hoof wall, interdigitating with dermal lamellae, which are connected to P3. Each primary lamella has multiple secondary lamellae, increasing the surface area and strength of attachment. The intricate architecture is required to withstand the forces of weight bearing and athletic performance. The basement membrane separates the epidermal and dermal lamellae and is a key structural component of the apparatus. Hoof growth occurs almost exclusively at the coronary band; therefore, the lamellae must also allow the hoof wall to slide downward past P3.
- MMPs reside in normal lamellar tissue and are responsible for controlled detachment and remodelling, facilitating constant hoof growth. There is an extensive sublamellar blood supply, rich in arteriovenous anastamoses; however, the epidermal lamellae lack a direct blood supply and rely on diffusion of nutrients, metabolites, and oxygen from the dermis. The lamellae have a high demand for glucose as an energy substrate; however, lamellar glucose uptake appears to be independent of insulin.
- Laminitis generally occurs secondary to disease processes remote from the foot. Although endotoxin alone has not produced laminitis experimentally, diseases that are complicated by the development of acute laminitis share endotoxemia as a common feature.
- It may also develop as a consequence of excessive weight bearing on one limb.
- The exact pathophysiology of laminitis is unclear, and there may be several different mechanisms that cause lamellar failure. Upregulation and activation of MMPs within lamellar tissue occur during the acute phase of laminitis. Uncontrolled degradation of the basement membrane by MMPs is likely the end cause of lamellar separation; however, the triggering events leading to this remain a mystery.
- Digital hypoperfusion and ischemia due to vasospasm, microthrombosis, or edema has been the traditional basis for pathophysiological theories; however, no molecular or biochemical evidence of lamellar ischemia has been found in the developmental phase of experimentally induced laminitis.
- Gut-derived bacterial exotoxins or endogenous molecules released into circulation after tissue damage have been suggested as possible trigger factors for MMP activation. Upregulation of inflammatory cytokines and other inflammatory mediators, as well as an influx of leukocytes into the lamellar tissue early in experimental laminitis, has led to the suggestion that laminitis occurs as part of a systemic inflammatory response syndrome. The lamellae have a high requirement for glucose, and reducing the availability of glucose causes lamellar separation in vitro.
- Once the lamellar attachments are weakened, the pathological processes that ensue are the result of mechanical damage associated with the forces of weight bearing. By the onset of lameness, significant architectural damage has already occurred. The nature and severity of the resultant pathology are determined by the extent of lamellar damage. Wholesale acute lamellar detachment can result in downward "sinking" of P3 within the hoof capsule. When the rate of onset is modest, the pull of the deep flexor tendon and the proliferating epidermal lamellar tissue result in palmar rotation of P3 away from the hoof wall. The growth of the hoof wall is disrupted and vascular structures are crushed. With further progression the sole prolapses and P3 may eventually penetrate the sole. Necrosis of the solar margin of P3 from ischemia and pressure often occurs. In many cases, horses with clinical signs of acute laminitis do not develop any detectable displacement of P3 and can revert to soundness. The lamellar interface is often weakened, however, and some of these horses are unable to engage in athletic pursuits without recurrence of foot pain.

SYSTEMS AFFECTED

Musculoskeletal—foot

GENETICS

N/A

INCIDENCE/PREVALENCE

N/A

GEOGRAPHICAL DISTRUBUTION

N/A

SIGNALMENT

- Rare (absent?) in foals or weanlings
- Pony breeds may be more susceptible to chronic laminitis.
- Chronic laminitis is also common in broodmares.

SIGNS

General Comments

- Clinical signs are usually diagnostic, except in very mild cases.
- Frequently develops secondarily to a primary disease process
- Laminitis is divided into three phases: developmental, acute, and chronic.

Historical

- Acute onset of lameness of variable severity in one or more feet
- Extremely reluctant to move
- +/− Recumbency
- Lameness worse when circling or on hard ground
- Recent systemic disease or access to excess grain or lush pasture
- +/− Severe, often prolonged contralateral limb lameness

Physical Findings

- Developmental phase
    - No clinical signs; however, the primary disease and the pathological processes that lead to lamellar damage are under way.
- Acute laminitis
    - Increase in digital pulse amplitude and temperature of the hoof wall and coronary band
    - +/− Distal limb edema
    - Shifting weight incessantly in the fore and hind limbs
    - In mild cases, subtle lameness
    - With increasing severity, obvious lameness at the walk exacerbated by turning on a hard surface
    - Most often, one or both front feet are affected; less severe in the hind
    - Characteristic stance— forelimbs extended forward and hindlimbs underneath the body
    - In severe cases, unwillingness to move and recumbency
    - +/− Difficulty lifting the limbs off the ground due to the horse's reluctance to bear weight on the opposite limb
    - Tachycardia, tachypnea, and sweating may be profound.
    - Response to hoof testing is highly variable. There may be generalized pain across the hoof or more focally over the toe region. The horse may react to tapping of the hoof wall.
- Chronic laminitis
    - Is defined by ≥48 hr of clinical laminitis and/or radiographic displacement of P3 within the hoof capsule
    - Increased digital pulse amplitude
    - Varying degrees of lameness
    - +/− Prolonged periods in recumbency
    - Palpable cleft at the coronary band
    - Prolapse of the sole in the toe region; +/− P3 penetration through the sole
    - In longstanding cases, growth rings in the hoof wall are noted. The rings are wider apart in the quarter/heel regions and closer at the dorsal wall.
    - Characteristic "dished" appearance to the dorsal hoof wall
    - +/− Separation at the white line with seedy toe and abscess formation
    - Depending on the severity, +/− persistent tachycardia and hypertension
    - Weight loss is common in moderate to severe cases.

CAUSES

- Acute colitis—salmonellosis, Potomac horse fever, etc.
- Anterior enteritis
- Colonic volvulus
- Septic peritonitis
- Pneumonia, pleuropneumonia
- Acute metritis/retained fetal membranes

• Excessive grain intake, access to pasture high in nonstructural carbohydrates (fructans)
• Equine Cushing's disease
• Hyperinsulinemia associated with obesity ("equine metabolic syndrome")
• Excessive weight bearing on a limb due to pain or dysfunction of the opposite limb
• Exertional rhabdomyolysis
• Exposure to black walnut (*Juglans nigra*) heartwood shavings
• Ingestion of the toxic plant hoary alyssum (*Berteroa incana*) in hay or pasture
• Excessive work on hard surfaces
• Corticosteroid administration (empirical reports only)
• Excessive intake of cold water (empirical reports only)

RISK FACTORS

See Causes.

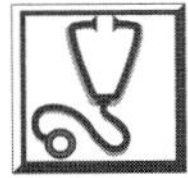

DIAGNOSIS

DIFFERENTIAL DIAGNOSIS

• Laminitis affecting both front feet or the front and hind feet must be differentiated from other painful conditions such as rhabdomyolysis, tetanus, or pleurodynia secondary to pleuropneumonia. Rule out by absence of increased digital pulse amplitude and digital hyperthermia.
• Laminitis affecting a single digit, or laminitis that is more severe in one digit, must be differentiated from a hoof abscess or fracture of the third phalanx. Rule out by hoof testing and radiographs.

CBC/BIOCHEMISTRY/URINALYSIS

• Abnormalities due to the inciting cause
• +/− Stress leukogram

OTHER LABORATORY TESTS

• Testing of the pituitary adrenal axis in cases of suspected Cushing's disease. Baseline ACTH concentration, TRH response test, or domperidone stimulation should be used in preference to a dexamethasone suppression test initially.
• Baseline insulin concentration, glucose tolerance testing, or other modified techniques may be used to determine insulin sensitivity in cases of suspected "metabolic syndrome."
• Determination of the plasma creatinine and albumin concentrations in cases where NSAIDs are to be administered is prudent in order to monitor for toxicity.

IMAGING

• Standard lateral to medial radiographic view should be obtained to examine the position of P3 relative to the hoof capsule. A radiopaque marker should be placed on the dorsal hoof wall and at the coronary band to aid in measurements. A steel rod of known length can be used to correct for magnification.
• Radiographs should be obtained as soon as possible after the onset of clinical signs in order to document progression.
• The angle of P3 within the capsule, the dorsal hoof wall to P3 distance, and the distance from the coronary band to the extensor process of P3 can be used as a guide to progression and prognosis.
• Retrograde digital venography can be useful in chronic cases to determine areas of venous compression or thrombosis. This may help to determine the need for hoof wall resection. Close adherence to published descriptions of this technique will help to avoid common artifacts.

DIAGNOSTIC PROCEDURES

Perineural anesthesia should be avoided unless there is difficulty isolating the source of lameness to the foot.

PATHOLOGICAL FINDINGS

• Sagittal sectioning of the feet will reveal the characteristic gross changes of chronic laminitis: formation of the lamellar wedge and palmar rotation of P3 within the hoof capsule.
• Even in the most severe acute cases there may be little gross evidence of pathology. In acute cases where confirmation of the diagnosis is required, lamellar histopathology should be performed.

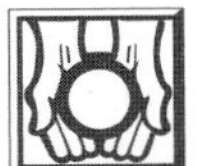

TREATMENT

AIMS OF TREATMENT

• Limit mechanical damage and control inflammation during the acute phase.
• Provide mechanical support and encourage normal hoof growth during the chronic phase.
• Provide adequate analgesia and supportive care.

APPROPRIATE HEALTH CARE

Developmental Phase

• Laminitis is irreversible; therefore, focus should be placed on prevention during the developmental phase and minimizing progression in the early acute phase.
• Aggressive treatment of the primary disease is most important to minimize the lamellar insult. Anti-endotoxic and anti-inflammatory therapy should be administered in cases where endotoxemia is apparent.
• Cooling of the feet during the developmental phase has successfully ameliorated laminitis in experimental models and there are empirical reports of efficacy in preventing laminitis in clinical cases. Ideally, an ice and water mixture is applied from the proximal metacarpal/metatarsal region to (and including) the hooves, in order to consistently cool the feet to the required temperature. The distal limbs can be cooled constantly in this way for at least 3 days without detrimental effect.
• Preemptive removal of shoes and application of frog/sole support in cases that are at high risk of developing acute laminitis

Acute Phase

• Once clinical signs are apparent, efforts must be directed at limiting mechanical damage.
• Strict stall confinement
• Light sedation may encourage recumbency.
• If regular shoes are present, they should be removed (in less painful horses only) and excessive toe conservatively trimmed.
• Attempts should be made to unload the hoof wall by loading the frog and sole: bed on sand or apply silicone impression material or Styrofoam padding to the sole of the foot.
• Styrofoam pads should be cut to fit the foot and taped on overnight. Once crushed down, the pad can be removed and the anterior (toe) portion cut off. The pad can then be refitted with a second pad underneath. This preferentially loads the caudal aspect of the sole and the frog.
• +/− Heel elevation (10–20 degrees) to reduce tension in the deep flexor tendon and redistribute some of the distracting forces from the dorsal wall to the quarters and heels
• NSAIDs should be used judiciously; excessive analgesia may encourage locomotion and increase mechanical damage.
• +/− Distal limb cold therapy in the early acute phase
• +/− Sling support during standing periods especially where rapid P3 sinking is occurring

Chronic Phase

• Ongoing farriery and a close client/veterinarian/farrier relationship are required for successful management.
• Radical trimming or shoeing practices should be avoided. Any changes should be made gradually over more than one shoeing interval to avoid destabilizing the foot and worsening of clinical signs.
• There are several available shoes and techniques for treatment of chronic laminitis. The basic principles are the same: redistribute weight from the hoof wall to the frog and caudal sole, minimize the forces of breakover, and reduce tension on the deep flexor tendon.
• Radiographs should be used as a guide for trimming and shoeing.

NURSING CARE

• Deep bedding, particularly if recumbent for prolonged periods
• Sling support can be useful to facilitate procedures such as trimming and shoeing.

ACTIVITY

• In the acute phase, absolute strict stall confinement
• Stall rest should continue for at least 1 mo, and up to ≥6 mo, after an acute episode of laminitis, depending on the severity.

LAMINITIS

• Care should be exercised when contemplating returning a horse to athletic activity after apparent recovery from laminitis. Very gradual reintroduction to exercise is advisable.

DIET

• Excessive carbohydrate in grain, hay, and pasture should be avoided.
• Horses suffering from obesity and hyperinsulinemia will benefit from controlled, gradual weight loss.

CLIENT EDUCATION

• Clients should be made aware of the potentially life-threatening nature of the disease.
• Frequently the client will have preconceptions about laminitis based on a previous experience with the disease. A client that has previously had a pony with mild chronic laminitis may have difficulty understanding the severity of the problem when faced with acute severe laminitis in a horse suffering from colitis. It is therefore important to explain each case based on the possible and probable outcomes.

SURGICAL CONSIDERATIONS

• In chronic cases where there is significant palmar rotation of P3 (>15 degrees) or where the cranial aspect of P3 is penetrating the sole or causing solar prolapse, a deep flexor tenotomy may be of benefit.
• In chronic cases, coronary grooving or dorsal hoof wall resection can relieve tension on the coronary band, reduce sublamellar venous compression and allow for better quality regrowth of the hoof wall.

MEDICATIONS

DRUG(S) OF CHOICE

• NSAIDs—Phenylbutazone (2.2–4.4 mg/kg BID) tends to provide superior analgesia to flunixin meglumine (1 mg/kg BID).
• Acepromazine (0.02–0.04 mg/kg IV or IM QID) during the acute phase to reduce ambulation

CONTRAINDICATIONS

Administration of corticosteroid should be avoided.

PRECAUTIONS

Patients requiring long-term NSAID therapy for chronic laminitis should be monitored carefully for signs of toxicity.

POSSIBLE INTERACTIONS

N/A

ALTERNATIVE DRUGS

• Constant rate infusion of drugs such as lidocaine, ketamine, and morphine, alone or in combination, can provide more potent short-term analgesia in acute and chronic cases.
• Alternate analgesic drugs such as gabapentin and phenytoin should be used with extreme caution, as they are not labeled for use in horses and are associated with potentially severe side effects.

FOLLOW-UP

PATIENT MONITORING

• Daily monitoring of acute cases
• Chronic cases require consistent monitoring, the frequency of which may depend upon the experience of the owner or trainer and disease severity.
• Initially, repeat radiographs should be obtained at each trimming/shoeing interval (2 weeks) and subsequently at 4-week intervals.

PREVENTION/AVOIDANCE

• Aggressive and early treatment of primary disease
• Identify horses prone to obesity and hyperinsulinemia and subsequently avoid hay/grain and pasture high in soluble carbohydrate.
• For those horses at high risk, avoid turnout on pasture when fructan levels are likely to be highest: mid morning to late afternoon, spring and fall, during flowering and early seeding or after frosts.
• Consider the use of a grazing muzzle during high-risk periods.

POSSIBLE COMPLICATIONS

• Severe acute/subacute cases may completely detach and slough the hoof wall.
• Progressive rotation and sinking in chronic cases can lead to penetration of the sole by P3 and subsequent necrosis and osteomyelitis.
• Longstanding chronic cases may develop persistent hypertension with cardiac hypertrophy.
• Renal failure and right dorsal colitis can result from long-term NSAID use.

EXPECTED COURSE AND PROGNOSIS

• Depends entirely on the extent of the lamellar damage
• "Sinking" of P3 within the hoof capsule results in a poor prognosis for survival.
• Penetration of the sole by P3 significantly worsens the prognosis.
• Chronic cases that have >15 degrees of palmar rotation of P3 carry a guarded prognosis for survival and a grave prognosis for future soundness.
• Return to athletic activity is highly variable. Generally, cases with >5 degrees of palmar rotation, or cases where sinking of P3 has occurred, are unlikely to return to athletic activity at previous levels.

MISCELLANEOUS

ASSOCIATED CONDITION, AGE-RELATED FACTORS, ZOONOTIC POTENTIAL, PREGNANCY

N/A

SYNONYMS

Founder

ABBREVIATIONS

• ACTH = adrenocorticotropic hormone
• MMP = matrix metalloproteinase
• P3 = third phalanx
• TRH = thryrotropin-releasing hormone

Suggested Reading

Linford RL. Laminitis. In: Smith BP, ed. Large Animal Internal Medicine, ed 3. St. Louis: Mosby, 2002:1116–1124.
Pollitt CC. Equine laminitis. Clin Techn Equine Pract 2004;3:34–44.

Author Andrew W. van Eps
Consulting Editor Elizabeth J. Davidson

LANTANA CAMARA (LANTANA) TOXICOSIS

BASICS

OVERVIEW

- *Lantana camara* (lantana or red sage) is an herbaceous, perennial, ornamental shrub.
- It is erect or sprawling, clumped, stout, and hairy and grows to 210 cm tall, with several stems arising out of the base.
- It has square twigs or stems that have small, scattered spines.
- The leaves are simple, opposite or whorled, and are oval shaped, with a petiole up to 1.5 cm long.
- The net-veined leaf blade is aromatic when crushed; the blades are broadly lanceolate and between 5 and 11 cm long and 2.5 and 6 cm wide, with a wedge-shaped base and regularly spaced, toothed margins.
- The flowers most often consist of two colors, ranging from white, yellow, or orange to red, blue, or even dark violet; the flowers are small and tubular in flat-topped clusters.
- A green, immature, berry-like fruit also is found, with hard seeds that turn blue to black at maturity.
- The plant is regarded as ornamental, but some varieties have escaped cultivation. These most often are found in fence lines and around old houses or fields over most of the United States.
- This plant is known to grow in southern Florida and into the northern United States and Canada and as far west as California.
- The green berry apparently is the most toxic, although the entire plant is toxic.
- The toxins are polycyclic triterpenoids—lantadene A and lantadene B.
- Lantana toxins cause intrahepatic cholestasis, characterized by inhibition of bile secretion without extensive hepatocyte necrosis.
- The plant has been extensively studied in ruminants and produces secondary or hepatogenous photosensitization secondary to hepatobiliary damage.
- Horses are suspected of developing liver disease, but not photosensitization, after ingestion.

SIGNALMENT

N/A

SIGNS

- Anecdotally, horses develop nonspecific liver and renal dysfunction after ingestion that is evident on clinicopathologic tests and at necropsy.
- Horses are not believed to develop photosensitization with lantana intoxication, but one report of ingestion by horses described associated crusty, contact-type lesions around the muzzles and light-skinned areas.
- Some owners report icterus of the sclera and mucous membranes after ingestion.

CAUSES AND RISK FACTORS

- Plants accessible to animals are subject to being consumed and animals that are hungry or unfamiliar with the plants are more likely to consume *L. camara*.
- Hepatic metabolism differences between species may account for differences in susceptibility to lantana toxins.
- Injury to the liver cells could result from the action of metabolite rather than the parent compound.

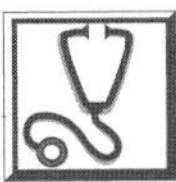

DIAGNOSIS

DIFFERENTIAL DIAGNOSIS

- Consider other hepatotoxins—aflatoxin (detection in feed and histopathology), PAs (ingestion of alkaloid-containing plants and histopathology), and iron toxicosis (tissue iron concentrations and histopathology).
- In addition to PA-containing plants, consider exposure to other hepatotoxic plants—*Nolina texana, Agave lecheguilla, Panicum* spp., and *Trifolium hybridum*.
- A nontoxic differential includes Theiler's disease (history and histopathology).

CBC/BIOCHEMISTRY/URINALYSIS

Hyperbilirubinemia (conjugated) is the most consistent finding.

OTHER LABORATORY TESTS

- Lantadenes may be detected in stomach contents if death occurs close to the time of consumption.
- Portions of the plant may be identified in the stomach contents by a competent microscopist.
- The most valuable tool is a good history.

IMAGING

N/A

DIAGNOSTIC PROCEDURES

N/A

PATHOLOGICAL FINDINGS

- Liver lesions—cholestasis, pigmentation and degeneration of hepatocytes, and fibrosis
- Kidney lesions—vacuolation and degeneration of convoluted tubule epithelium and presence of various casts. Occasionally, multifocal, interstitial, mononuclear cell infiltration and fibrosis may be evident.

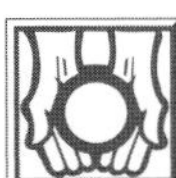

TREATMENT

- No specific treatment
- Consider GI decontamination.
- Symptomatic and supportive care

MEDICATIONS

DRUGS

AC (2–4 g/kg in a water slurry [1 g of AC per 5 mL of water])

CONTRAINDICATIONS/POSSIBLE INTERACTIONS

N/A

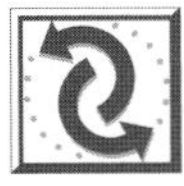

FOLLOW-UP

PATIENT MONITORING

- Monitor hepatic function.

PREVENTION/AVOIDANCE

- Preventing access to the plant is the best solution for avoiding toxicosis.
- Herbicides can be used to control the plant.

POSSIBLE COMPLICATIONS

N/A

EXPECTED COURSE AND PROGNOSIS

N/A

MISCELLANEOUS

ASSOCIATED CONDITIONS, AGE-RELATED FACTORS, ZOONOTIC POTENTIAL, PREGNANCY

N/A

ABBREVIATIONS

- AC = activated charcoal
- GI = gastrointestinal
- PA = pyrrolizidine alkaloid

Suggested Reading

Pass MA. Poisoning of livestock by lantana plants. In: Keeler RF, Tu AT, eds. Toxicology of Plant and Fungal Compounds: Handbook of Natural Toxins. New York: Marcel Dekker, 1991:297–311.

Author Tam Garland
Consulting Editor Robert H. Poppenga

LARGE COLON TORSION

BASICS

DEFINITION

- Rotation of the large colon about the mesocolic axis in a dorsomedial or dorsolateral direction
- Most commonly located at the level of the cecocolic fold
- Less commonly involves the sternal and diaphragmatic flexures
- The transverse colon or cecum may also be involved.
- Most torsions are in a dorsomedial direction.
- A rotation of 90–270 degrees will cause partial obstruction of lumen and passage of ingesta.
- A rotation of 270–360 degrees results in complete obstruction, and torsions >360 degrees result in strangulating obstruction of the colon.

PATHOPHYSIOLOGY

- The large colon consists of 4 parallel limbs separated by 3 flexures. The order is: right ventral colon, ventral diaphragmatic flexure, left ventral colon, pelvic flexure, left dorsal colon, dorsal diaphragmatic flexure, and right dorsal colon.
- The dorsal and ventral portions of the large colon are joined by the ascending mesocolon.
- The only attachment of the large colon to the body wall is through continuity with the cecum and transverse colon, and the retroperitoneal anchoring of these parts.
- Because of its lack of anchoring attachments, the large colon is mobile, predisposing it to displacement.
- Torsion causes varying degrees of mechanical bowel obstruction, decreasing normal colonic absorption and resulting in electrolyte imbalances and hypomotility, which in turn may contribute to further twisting of the colon.
- Blood supply to the colon is via the colic arteries, which branch from the cranial mesenteric artery. Strangulation of the large colon is typically hemorrhagic rather than ischemic, i.e., venous drainage of the colon is compromised but arterial inflow is relatively intact.
- With venous obstruction, blood accumulates in the veins and, eventually, extravasates into the submucosa and colonic lumen. This extravasation disrupts the colonic epithelium that sloughs into the lumen, and these phenomena produce increased gas and fluid accumulation within the colonic lumen. The accumulation of gas results in painful distention of the colon.
- Vascular damage results in degeneration of blood vessels and intraluminal hemorrhage.
- With damage to the bowel wall, bacteria and endotoxins, as well as fluid and protein, leak into the peritoneal cavity, which results in endotoxemia, hypovolemia, and hypoproteinemia. Within 4–5 hours, the colonic mucosa undergoes complete necrosis.
- Severe systemic shock leads to cardiovascular collapse and death.
- With complete arterial and venous obstruction, tissue perfusion decreases, with resultant hypoxia and ischemia that cause reduced absorption and hypomotility. Prolonged ischemia causes bowel necrosis, with leakage of bacteria and endotoxins into the peritoneal cavity.
- Endotoxemia and hypovolemia result in severe systemic shock, cardiovascular collapse, and death.

SYSTEMS AFFECTED

- GI
- Cardiovascular

GENETICS

No known genetic basis

INCIDENCE/PREVALENCE

The reported incidence ranges between 11% and 26% of horses undergoing surgical treatment of colic.

SIGNALMENT

Old horses and broodmares, especially during the post-parturient period, appear to be more commonly affected.

SIGNS

Historical

Owners typically report a sudden onset of severe abdominal pain.

Physical Examination

- With strangulating large colon torsion, horses usually present with acute, severe abdominal pain that is nonresponsive to analgesia.
- With progression of clinical signs, horses may become depressed.
- Horses typically have tachycardia and tachypnea, although some have normal heart and respiratory rates.
- As the condition progresses, abdominal distention is evident.
- Borborygmi are reduced to absent in all GI quadrants.
- Mucous membranes may be normal initially, with progression to pallor or congestion.
- Signs of shock become rapidly evident in strangulating torsions.

CAUSES

- The exact cause is unknown, but hypomotility and increased intraluminal gas accumulation are theorized to initiate a dorsomedial or dorsolateral rotation of the left or right ventral colon. Nonstrangulating obstructions may progress to strangulating obstructions by this mechanism as well.
- Horses undergoing a sudden dietary change may be predisposed to increased gas production and altered GI motility. Similarly, horses fed lush pasture or large volumes of grain have significant fermentation processes within the ventral colon, producing excessive amounts of gas that may initiate torsion.
- Post-parturient broodmares are thought to be predisposed because of increased space within the abdomen.

RISK FACTORS

A diet high in grain, rich grass, or a sudden change in feed may predispose because of increased fermentation, subsequent gas production, and hypomotility.

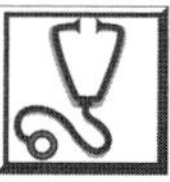

DIAGNOSIS

DIFFERENTIAL DIAGNOSIS

- Nonstrangulating obstruction—torsion <360 degrees
- Right dorsal colon displacement
- Left dorsal colon displacement
- Large colon impaction
- Enterolithiasis
- Adhesions
- Colonic or cecal tympany
- Strangulating obstruction—torsion ≥360 degrees
- Large intestinal intussusception
- Incarceration of the large intestine through the epiploic foramen, gastrosplenic space, or mesenteric rents
- Colonic or cecal tympany
- A definitive preoperative diagnosis may be difficult to establish, because significant gas distention within the large colon may preclude thorough rectal examination. However, the severe, unrelenting abdominal pain, tachycardia, and abnormal rectal findings allow recognition of need for surgical intervention, and a definitive diagnosis may be established at the time of exploratory surgery.

CBC/BIOCHEMISTRY/URINALYSIS

- CBC and biochemistry may be normal or show evidence of hemoconcentration (i.e., elevated PCV and serum proteins) and prerenal or renal azotemia.
- With endotoxemia, a leukopenia characterized by neutropenia, with or without a left shift, may be evident.
- A mild metabolic acidosis may be exacerbated by a respiratory acidosis secondary to severe abdominal distention.
- In chronic, nonstrangulating obstruction or strangulating obstruction, hypovolemia and shock, if they ensue, may cause prerenal or renal azotemia, which can result in isosthenuria, glucosuria, proteinuria, and casts or RBCs at urinalysis.

OTHER LABORATORY TESTS

- Attempt abdominocentesis with caution, because distended large intestines increase the risk of enterocentesis.
- Peritoneal fluid may be normal or reveal elevated protein concentration and RBC count.

IMAGING

Nonspecific, but may be used for differentiation from other causes of nonstrangulating obstructions—

enterolithiasis (i.e., abdominal radiography) and left dorsal colon displacement (i.e., abdominal ultrasonography).

DIAGNOSTIC PROCEDURES

- Nasogastric intubation and rectal examination
- Nasogastric reflux has been reported in as much as 35% of cases because of tension on the duodenocolic fold.
- Findings at rectal examination may be normal early during the course of the disease. With progression, increasing gaseous distention of the large colon is found, and tight colonic bands may be palpable.
- With careful palpation, sacculations of the ventral colon may be palpable dorsally, indicating colon torsion.
- Colonic edema may be palpable as thickening of the colonic wall.
- In some cases, gas distention is so severe that it fills the abdomen, preventing a complete rectal examination.

PATHOLOGICAL FINDINGS

- The torsion, its origin, and its direction are determined during surgery or at postmortem examination.
- Varying degrees of large colon and cecal necrosis or rupture may be present, depending on the level, degree, and duration of the torsion.

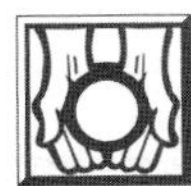

TREATMENT

APPROPRIATE HEALTH CARE

- Successful treatment of colonic torsion is reported only after surgery.
- Initial evaluation—physical examination, nasogastric intubation, and rectal examination
- Nonstrangulating torsion often results in progression to strangulation and worsening clinical signs with time, requiring emergency surgical intervention.
- Strangulating torsion is a rapidly progressive condition and represents a surgical emergency; early recognition and prompt surgery are paramount for patient survival.

NURSING CARE

Refer affected horses to a surgical facility immediately after initial diagnosis.

ACTIVITY

- Limit activity to stall rest with hand-walking.
- Stall rest with hand-walking is recommended for the first 4 weeks after surgery.
- Full return to exercise or breeding is not recommended for at least 6 mo.

DIET

- Discontinue oral intake until the postoperative period.
- Gradually reintroduce feed postoperatively.

CLIENT EDUCATION

- Inform clients that prompt diagnosis and surgical intervention maximize the outcome for survival.
- Varying degrees of endotoxemia, hypovolemia, and abdominal distention pose added risks for general anesthesia.
- Many potential postoperative complications may worsen the prognosis—laminitis and colitis.
- Inform clients of the 5%–8% recurrence rate.
- Advise owners of pregnant mares regarding the risk of fetal compromise.

SURGICAL CONSIDERATIONS

Surgical correction is performed via exploratory laparotomy.

MEDICATIONS

DRUGS OF CHOICE

- Administer a single dose of flunixin meglumine or similar NSAID.
- Further analgesics may be administered based on severity of the clinical signs.

CONTRAINDICATIONS

As described for other causes of colic

PRECAUTIONS

- Worsening of symptoms may be masked by repeated administration of analgesics.
- Avoid repeated dosing of drugs because of the potential for toxicity.

POSSIBLE INTERACTIONS N/A

ALTERNATIVE DRUGS N/A

FOLLOW-UP

PATIENT MONITORING

- Perform routine postoperative monitoring for alterations in attitude or appetite, recurrence of colic, and laminitis.
- Initially (1–2 weeks after surgery) monitor rectal temperature daily; fever may be an early indication of impending colitis, pleuropneumonia, thrombophlebitis, incisional infection, or peritonitis.

PREVENTION/AVOIDANCE

- Employ careful feeding practices that avoid large quantities of lush pasture and large amounts of grain wherever possible.
- Make all dietary changes gradually over a period of several days.

POSSIBLE COMPLICATIONS

- Because of the rapid progression of colonic torsion, bowel necrosis and rupture may occur before surgical intervention, resulting in death. Similarly, severe endotoxic and hypovolemic shock may ensue before treatment, resulting in cardiovascular collapse and death.
- Postoperative complications—recurrence of colic, laminitis, thrombophlebitis, pleuropneumonia, incisional infections or herniation, colitis, and peritonitis

EXPECTED COURSE AND PROGNOSIS

- Prognosis for survival after conservative, medical management is poor.
- Historically, the prognosis has been poor despite surgical intervention, with a short-term survival rate of 21%–42%. A 1996 study, however, reported that early diagnosis, rapid referral, and prompt surgery improve short-term survival rate to 83%.
- No data have been reported regarding long-term survival rates for horses undergoing surgical treatment.

MISCELLANEOUS

ASSOCIATED CONDITIONS

Endotoxemia

AGE-RELATED FACTORS N/A

ZOONOTIC POTENTIAL N/A

PREGNANCY

- Broodmares appear to be predisposed, especially during the post-parturient period.
- In affected pregnant mares, severe systemic deterioration and the added stress of general anesthesia and surgery pose a significant risk to the fetus.

SYNONYMS

Large colon volvulus

SEE ALSO

- Acute abdomen
- Dorsal colon displacements
- Endotoxemia

ABBREVIATIONS

- CBC = complete blood cell count
- GI = gastrointestinal
- PCV = packed cell volume
- RBC = red blood cell

Suggested Reading

Embertson RM, Cook G, Hance SR, *et al.* Large colon volvulus: surgical treatment of 204 cases (1986–1995). Proc AAEP 1996;42:254–255.

Fischer AT, Meagher DM. Strangulating torsions of the equine large colon. Compend Contin Educ 1986;8:S25–S30.

Harrison IW. Equine large intestinal volvulus: a review of 124 cases. Vet Surg 1988;17:77–81.

Hughes FE, Slone DE. Large colon resection. Vet Clin North Am Equine Pract 1997;13:341–349.

Johnston JK, Freeman DE. Diseases and surgery of the large colon. Vet Clin North Am Equine Pract 1997;13:317–339.

Author Nicola C. Cribb

Consulting Editors Henry R. Stämpfli and Olimpo Oliver-Espinosa

LARGE OVARY SYNDROME

BASICS

DEFINITION/OVERVIEW

• Includes a number of conditions, both normal and abnormal, that result in one or both ovaries achieving a size that is significantly larger than considered normal, as detected by TRP and/or U/S • Definition of the cause is reached by a systematic process that considers:
- ○ History
- ○ Season/time of year
- ○ Behavior
- ○ Physical examination findings (TRP and U/S)
- ○ Hormone analysis
- ○ Response to some routine treatments to elicit alterations in either size of the enlarged gonad or a change in behavior

Most common causes of LOS:
• Persistent follicles • Hematoma • Pregnancy
Less common/rare causes:
• GCT/GTCT • Teratoma • Dysgerminoma
• Cystadenoma • Abscess • Multiple single reports of additional tumor types

ETIOLOGY/PATHOPHYSIOLOGY

Physiology

• Equids are long-day breeders, i.e., estrous cycles and the ovulatory period normally occur during spring and summer.
• Light is the predominant influence on ovarian activity and estrous cycles.
• Outside the optimal season for breeding activity, the gonads are waxing or waning relative to follicular activity and the occurrence of ovulation.
- ○ Light is perceived by the pineal gland, a neuroendocrine transducer, and relays its perception of available light by increasing or decreasing the production of GnRH from the hypothalamus.
- ○ Increasing GnRH (springtime) increases circulating FSH and LH, and thus ovarian activity.
- ○ There is a lag time of 60–90 days following the winter equinox (late December, shortest day of year in the Northern Hemisphere) for the increasing light to be reflected in consistent/regular estrous cycles and ovulation.
- ○ After the summer solstice (late June, longest day of the year), day length begins to decrease, GnRH production tapers, followed by decrease in LH and FSH to a point that their available levels are insufficient to complete maturation and/or induce ovulation of follicles.

• *Persistent follicles in vernal (spring) transition*
- ○ Variable sizes throughout transition. Those late in vernal transition may regress after persisting for a month or more, or,
- ○ Eventually ovulation will occur (of its own accord, if time is not an issue) with sufficient light, FSH, and LH.
- ○ Ovulation, late in spring transition, may be stimulated by the administration of hCG.

• *Persistent follicles in autumnal (fall) transition*
- ○ Early in fall transition it is possible to stimulate additional ovulations, especially those identified in the first half of autumnal transition and ≥35 mm.
- ○ All will eventually regress (decrease in size) as daylight wanes and endogenous GnRH, LH and FSH decrease, and the mare slips into winter anestrus (bilateral small, inactive ovaries).

Normal Ovary, Persistent Follicles

• The most common cause cited for LOS
• May be single or multiple, present on one or both ovaries
• Presence/characteristics are primarily due to season (late spring/early fall) and increasing or decreasing duration of light.
• Their presence does not indicate ovarian disease, i.e., normal structures that will resolve if left alone.

Normal Ovary, Hematoma

• Second most common cause of LOS
• Enlargement resolves without assistance over time unless treated with prostaglandin to stimulate earlier initiation of estrous cyclic activity.
• Only considered pathological if the hematoma causes sufficient destruction of ovarian tissue that future normal activity is precluded

Abnormal Ovary, Tumors and Other Causes

• Hormone treatments fail to elicit a desirable response (PGF, hCG, deslorelin).
• TRP, U/S, radiography—reveal appearance inconsistent with normal ovarian structures
• Systemic illness of the mare
• Type of cell identified on histopathological examination of ovarian tissue following OVX

SYSTEM AFFECTED

Reproductive

GENETICS

N/A

INCIDENCE/PREVALENCE

Persistent Follicles

• Potentially 80% of reproductively normal mares
• Approximately 20% of Northern Hemisphere mares continue to experience estrous cycle activity year-round, albeit with some variation in length from the "normal" of 21 days.

Hematoma

Uncommon, but a few cases a year will be recognized within a normal population of mares during the breeding season.

Tumors

• GCT/GTCT is the most common ovarian tumor, but its occurrence is rare.
• All other tumors occur even less frequently (all rare).

SIGNALMENT

• Females of breeding age (post-pubertal and pre-ovarian senescence)
• All breeds

SIGNS

Persistent Follicles

• Seasonal component—typically during one of the two transition periods
• Usually *tease in*, demonstrate a positive response to a stallion, for extended periods of time (1+ mo)
• Estrus behavior persists longer than during a normal estrous cycle (>12–14 days in the spring).
• TRP and U/S reveal the presence of follicles, may be multiple of varying size; their appearance is still as follicles, i.e., they do not take on the irregular appearance of the multilocular/ fenestrated spaces typical of a granulosa cell tumor.
• May increase in size/diameter with time, but the increase is slower than observed with dominant follicles (5–6 mm/day) during the ovulatory period

CAUSES

Persistent Follicles

• Vernal transition—increasing day length between winter anestrus and the ovulatory period
• Autumnal transition—decreasing day length between the ovulatory period and winter anestrus

RISK FACTORS

N/A

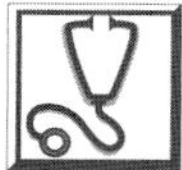

DIAGNOSIS

DIFFERENTIAL DIAGNOSIS

Ovaries During Pregnancy (>37–40 Days' Gestation)

• With formation of endometrial cups and subsequent production of eCG, secondary follicles luteinize to become secondary CL. The ovaries of the pregnant mare become bilaterally enlarged.
• Mare's behavior may mimic the aggression of some mares with a GCT/GTCT.
- ○ Most likely related to increased circulating testosterone stemming from fetal gonads.
- ○ May be >100 pg/mL by 60–90 days' gestation.
- ○ Peaks at approximately 200 days' gestation; declines to basal levels by time of foaling.

Ovarian Hematoma

• This event occurs following estrus and ovulation.
• The CH increases to a size substantially larger than the follicle that preceded it.
• Usually by the time of diagnosis, the acute pain associated with the rapid stretch of the ovarian tunic has subsided, and the mare's behavior is that of a diestrus mare, i.e., normal (teases out; rejects the stallion's advances).
• Although the initial rise of progesterone may be delayed slightly compared with a normal CH, blood progesterone will rise (>1 ng/mL) by 5–6 days post-ovulation, confirmation that ovulation occurred.
• Contralateral ovary is normal.
• U/S of hematoma is eventually similar to a CH, albeit a large one.
• The rapid size increase of the hematoma causes stretching of the tunic surrounding the ovary and the mare may exhibit pain/colic in the short term.
• Resolution—time or prostaglandin. Complete luteinization may be delayed and thus delay

responsiveness to PGF (>6 days post-ovulation; often as long as 2 weeks).

GCT/GTCT

- TRP—characterized by a unilateral gonad enlargement (rate of tumor growth varies significantly by case)
  - Surface of tumor remains smooth, but may have gentle lobulations.
  - Ovulation fossa disappears [fills in] early in development of tumor.
  - Over time, contralateral ovary shows evidence of suppression. Early on the number/size of follicles decreases, then the total volume/size of parenchyma decreases.
  - Chronic GCT/GTCTs will be coupled with a contralateral ovary that may become so small it is difficult for the novice to detect.
  - Rare contralateral ovary will continue to experience follicular activity and ovulations.
- Circulating levels of inhibin (produced by the granulosa cells) are elevated in 90% of GCT/GTCT.
- Behavior
  - Mares typically exhibit one of 3 primary behaviors—chronic anestrus (80%), stallion-like (increased aggression, 15%), persistent estrus (*nymphomanic*, 5%).
  - Because of the slower increase of size stretching the ovarian tunic, mares rarely exhibit pain (contrast with the rapid formation of a hematoma).
  - Mare may exhibit discomfort at the trot or refuse to go over jumps. Weight of the enlarging ovary coupled with impact bounces ovary; felt as a sharp, painful stretching of the mesovarium and may elicit behavioral changes (pain, anger, reticence to perform).

Teratoma/Dysgerminoma

- Rare, not hormonally active
- TRP—contralateral ovary is normal. Surface of teratoma may exhibit some sharper protuberances reflecting its contents.
- No effect on behavior or estrous cycle activity
- Teratoma is benign.

Dysgerminoma

- Rare
- Initial presentation for intermittent chronic colic, weight loss, stiff extremities
- Presence of tumor may only be discovered once mare's health deteriorates due to metastases.
- Potentially/can be highly malignant.

Cystadenoma

- Unilateral, no effect on contralateral ovary.
- No effect on behavior.
- Appearance—large, cystic structures, may confuse early on with persistent follicles, remains nonresponsive to hCG.
- Rare hormonal impact. If it does occur, it is usually as elevated testosterone.

Ovarian Abscess

- Rare
- Early reports may have been associated with attempts to reduce the size and number of persistent follicles via a flank approach aspiration.
- Contralateral ovary is normal.
- No effect on behavior or estrous cycle activity

CBC/BIOCHEMISTRY/URINALYSIS

N/A

OTHER LABORATORY TESTS

GCT/GTCT

- Elevation of circulating inhibin levels (>0.7 ng/mL) in 90% of GCT/GTCT
- Elevation of testosterone (>50–100 pg/mL) in 50%–60% of affected mares
- Progesterone levels are usually <1 ng/mL.

Ovarian Hematoma

Blood progesterone will increase by 5–7 days of hematoma formation.

Dysgerminoma

- Reports of hypertrophic pulmonary osteoarthropathy developing secondary to metastatic dysgerminoma
- Initial presentation for intermittent chronic colic, weight loss, stiff extremities
- Radiography, biopsies for metastasis

IMAGING

U/S

One of the most important adjunct tools to evaluate/differentiate cases of LOS.

- *Persistent follicle*—except for larger size, appearance is similar to normal follicles.
- *Hematoma*
  - Recent—fluid-filled space (black)
  - 2–10 days hyperechoic areas began to appear; ongoing clotting of blood and contraction of clot and invasion of luteal cells
  - Eventually takes on the uniform hyperechoic appearance of a CH, a large one
- *GCT/GTCT*
  - Multicystic, the spaces of which can appear quite irregular; sizes of fluid pockets range from a few mm to multiple centimeters.
  - Size/location of tumor during U/S scan can range from readily accessible off tip of uterine horn, to very pendulous (dependent on weight and stretch of mesovarium/broad ligament).
  - Recorded weights have ranged from <1 to 45+ kg (MSU clinic, over a 20-year period).
  - At the time of detection, the majority will be <30 cm diameter.
- *Teratoma*
  - Variable echogenicity, reflecting the nature of its contents, i.e., soft tissue, fluid, hair, bone, teeth

OTHER DIAGNOSTIC PROCEDURES

In addition to serial TRP and U/S, blood hormone evaluations are valuable:

Hormone	Normal range	GCT/GTCT
Progesterone, estrus	<1 ng/mL	
Progesterone, diestrus	>1 ng/m	
Progesterone,		<1 ng/mL
Testosterone		>50–100 pg/mL
Inhibin	0.1–0.7 ng/mL	>0.7 ng/mL

PATHOLOGICAL FINDINGS

- Persistent follicles—N/A
- Hematoma—N/A
- Neoplasms can potentially arise from any of the tissue types present in the ovary.
- Classification is based on their origin in surface epithelium—sex cord-stromal tissue, germ cell, or mesenchymal tissue.
- *GCT/GTCT*—sex cord-stromal tumor, endocrine effects, specific in mare—inhibin production by thecal cells (GTCT)
- *Teratoma*—many tissue types, including germ cells, within the mass; can include hair, skin, respiratory epithelium, tooth, and bone. High metastatic potential in mice and humans, not a routine concern in the mare. Immature teratomas—tissue resembles embryonic origins; mature teratomas are also known as dermoid cysts.
- *Cystadenoma*—from epithelium; forms cystic neoplastic masses
- *Dysgerminoma*—from germ cells, analogous to seminoma of the testis; cells are arranged in sheets and cords with a dense population of large pleomorphic cells; all malignant.

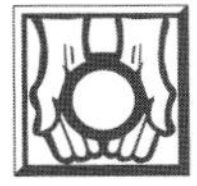

TREATMENT

APPROPRIATE HEALTH CARE

Only as specified for particular conditions within text above

NURSING CARE

- None specific to conditions
- General postoperative medical care recommended following an OVX

ACTIVITY N/A

DIET N/A

CLIENT EDUCATION

- Importance of conducting serial examinations to reach an accurate diagnosis of LOS and thus avoid an unnecessary ovariectomy.
- Vast majority of LOS cases are due to persistent follicle/s and hematoma.
- GCT/GTCTs are the most common tumor causing ovarian enlargement, but they are still an uncommon/rare occurrence.
- *History*
  - Season—during transitional periods, persistent follicle/s is first rule out.
  - Estrous activity—e.g., a mare recently showing estrus, is now out of estrus, may be painful, and an enlarged ovary is detected. Hematoma is the first rule out.
  - Response to treatment—progesterone supplementation, prostaglandin, hCG
  - Behavior changes—prolonged anestrus, increased aggression, nymphomania
- *Serial TRP*
  - At an interval of 7–10 days, may require 3–5 examinations.
  - Avoids too frequent examinations (at intervals too short to expect significant increase or decrease in size of affected ovary); avoids unnecessary cost and/or surgery. Allows examination 2× within the span of a potential estrus period—(1) for comparison of affected and contralateral ovary, (2) rate of size increase, and (3) activity of opposite gonad.
- U/S is a most effective tool to evaluate the internal characteristics of the enlarging gonad. See Imaging.

LARGE OVARY SYNDROME

- *Circulating hormone levels*
  - Inhibin, testosterone, progesterone
  - Inhibin assay developed at UC Davis Endocrinology Lab, Davis, CA, offers an ovarian tumor *panel* to evaluate for most likely rule-outs.

SURGICAL CONSIDERATIONS

• OVX • See rule-outs as listed in Expected Course and Prognosis.

MEDICATIONS

DRUG(S) OF CHOICE

Hematoma

- No treatment, wait for ovary to regress in size and other follicular activity to develop, or,
- $PGF_2\alpha$, 5–10 mg IM, when >7–10 days post-ovulation and formation of the hematoma
- May be unresponsive to treatment within first 2+ weeks • Successful treatment is noted by the mare returning to estrus within 2–5 days.

Persistent Follicles

- Can elect "no treatment, but for time"—wait for estrous activity to begin (vernal transition) or cease (autumnal transition) on its own.
- To shorten duration of vernal transition—
  - Regu-Mate, do not institute treatment before significant follicular activity is present. In transition, mare is experiencing behavioral, not physiologic estrus. See Estrus, abnormal intervals. Wear protective gloves. Dosed PO at 0.044 mg/kg (1 mL per 110 lb body weight) daily for 15 days. Can be delivered by dose syringe PO or placed on grain at feeding time.
  - hCG 2500–3000 IU, IV; may induce ovulation late in vernal transition. See Estrus, abnormal intervals. Wait until a follicle of ≥35 mm is present. Anticipate ovulation within 36–44 hr.
  - Deslorelin, GnRH analogue, is available as an injectable product. Results in ovulation within 38–60 hr. Little difference (other than cost, deslorelin is more expensive) in percent of mares responding (≈80%), time to ovulation, and conception rate, compared to hCG. As a decapeptide, it does not stimulate antibody production as can hCG. A subset of mares will experience persistent anestrus if PGF is administered 1 week after deslorelin administration.
  - Progesterone + estradiol-17β—10 days—Results in more effective ovulation and follicular suppression than progesterone alone. Administered IM daily 150 mg/day progesterone and 10 mg/day estradiol-17β; PGF on the last day of treatment. hCG may be used once a ≥35-mm follicle has been detect for ovulation induction.
  - Other progesterone products are available—P4 in oil (100 mL vial for IM injection); Bio Release P+ LA (long-acting) also in a 100 mL vial (150 mL progesterone + estradiol-17β IM); and P+ in oil (50 mg/mL progesterone + 3.3 mg/mL estradiol-17β IM).
  - Future products to come on the market with a 2-week interval of administration—P+ microspheres and SABER progesterone for injection.

CONTRAINDICATIONS

N/A

PRECAUTIONS

- Some behavior changes can be dramatic. Use caution around mares that are showing aggressive behavior; may need individual paddock, distance from other mares in estrus, separation from foals, stallions.
- Large ovarian tumors can develop extensive blood supplies. Intraoperative time can be significantly lengthened due to time required to properly ligate vessels supplying the tumor; increases surgical risks.

POSSIBLE INTERACTIONS

N/A

ALTERNATIVE DRUGS

N/A

FOLLOW-UP

PATIENT MONITORING

Routine postoperative care for OVX

PREVENTION/AVOIDANCE

N/A

POSSIBLE COMPLICATIONS

- Any operative procedure/anesthesia holds potential risk for death.
- GCT/GTCT—Time from OVX to resumption of estrous cycle activity is influenced by the mo/years of suppression.
  - Usually <1–3 years
  - Rare cases of suppression being permanent
  - Rare case of remaining ovary also developing into a GCT/GTCT
  - Few mares with this tumor will continue to develop follicles and ovulate on the contralateral ovary.

EXPECTED COURSE AND PROGNOSIS

Prognosis, Poor

- *Dysgerminoma*—potential for metastasis
  - Usually advanced state of disease by the time of diagnosis

Prognosis for Future Reproduction, Good

- *Hematoma*—Large size returns nearly to normal over 1–6 mo.
  - Rare hematoma will destroy remaining ovarian tissue.
  - Some mares will develop hematoma on subsequent cycles within a season.
- *Persistent follicles*—100% resolution with time and season

Prognosis for Life, Good

- GCT/GTCT
- Abscess
- Cystadenoma
- Teratoma

Recommendation for OVX

- GCT/GTCT—removal of affected gonad for reproductive function to return, prognosis fair to good depending on size of tumor, surgical route, duration of suppression of contralateral ovary
- Cystadenoma—rare, reported testosterone production
- Abscess, teratoma—dysfunctional ovary

MISCELLANEOUS

ASSOCIATED CONDITIONS

- Dysgerminoma—hypertrophic osteoarthropathy developing secondary to metastatic dysgerminoma; initial presentation was for intermittent chronic colic, weight loss, stiff extremities.
- Behavior modification with GCT/GTCT

AGE-RELATED FACTORS

Of breeding age (capable of estrous activity):
- Hematoma
- Persistent follicles

Tumors:
- No age limitation

ZOONOTIC POTENTIAL

N/A

PREGNANCY

N/A

SYNONYMS

N/A

SEE ALSO

- Abnormal estrus intervals
- Anestrus
- Ovulation failure
- Pregnancy
- Prolonged diestrus

ABBREVIATIONS

- CH = corpus hemorrhagicum
- CL = corpus luteum
- eCG = equine chorionic gonadotropin
- FSH = follicle-stimulating hormone
- GCT = granulosa cell tumor
- GTCT = granulosa theca cell tumor
- GnRH = gonadotropin releasing hormone
- hCG = human chorionic gonadotropin
- LH = luteinizing hormone
- LOS = large ovary syndrome
- OVX = ovariectomy
- PGF = prostaglandin F (natural prostaglandin)
- TRP = transrectal palpation
- U/S = ultrasound, ultrasonography

Suggested Reading

Carleton CL. Atypical, asymmetrical, but abnormal? Large ovary syndrome. Proceedings of Mare Reproduction Symposium, American College of Theriogenologists/Society for Theriogenology, 1996:27–39.

Foley GL. Proceedings of Reproductive Pathology Symposium, American College of Theriogenologists/Society for Theriogenology,1997:60–65.

McCue PM. Review of ovarian abnormalities in the mare. Proc Am Assoc Equine Pract 1998;125–133.

Schlafer DH. Non-neoplastic lesions of the ovaries of the mare. Proceedings of Reproductive Pathology Symposium, American College of Theriogenologists/Society for Theriogenology, 1997:69–72.

Stangroom JE, Weevers R. Anticoagulant activity of equine follicular fluid. J Reprod Fert 1962;3:269–282.

Author Carla L. Carleton
Consulting Editor Carla L. Carleton

LARGE STRONGYLE INFESTATION

BASICS

OVERVIEW

- In the past, infections with the large strongyles (i.e., *Strongylus vulgaris, S. edentatus,* and *S. equinus*) were considered to be the most common and important equine intestinal parasites.
- Their perceived importance has decreased, and that of the small strongyles (i.e., cyathostomes) has increased.
- The worms can cause significant damage and, in combination with cyathostomes, probably are responsible for many cases of equine colic.
- Eggs are passed in the feces of infected horses.
- The rate of strongyle development depends on climatic conditions and is favored by warm, moist conditions.
- Development of the infective L3 larvae occurs after larval growth and a molt. The L3 are ensheathed and, under moist conditions, migrate up to the tips of grass blades, increasing the likelihood of ingestion by a grazing horse.
- Dry, hot conditions lead to rapid desiccation of larvae.
- The larvae exsheath in the intestine and penetrate the walls of the small intestine, cecum, and colons.
- In ≅8–11 days, L4 larvae are produced, inducing a marked inflammatory response in the bowel wall. The larvae then begin to migrate, the pattern of which varies with each species.
- *S. vulgaris* larvae penetrate the intima of the arterioles and migrate within the vessel wall to the cranial mesenteric artery, arriving there ≅14 days after infection. Severe arteritis, with fibrosis and thrombus formation, is noted. Rarely, an aneurysm occurs. At ≅45 days postinfection, larvae migrate back to the subserosa of the large intestine, where they encyst for ≅45 more days and develop into L5 larvae. These larvae enter the lumen of the gut and mature, with egg production starting ≅6–7 mo postinfection.
- *S. edentatus* larvae penetrate the cecal mucosa, enter the hepatic portal system, and then enter the liver. Here, they molt to L4 larvae, which by the 10th week postinfection may have migrated to various sites, such as the body wall, where they cause nodules, and L5 larvae develop. They then migrate back to the cecum and colon and mature. Egg production starts ≅11 mo postinfection, although it can be as short as 6 mo.
- *S. equinus* larvae follow a similar path to that of *S. edentatus,* but the migration of L4 larvae is more likely to involve the pancreas and peritoneal cavity. The prepatent period of this latter parasite is ≅9 mo.
- Clinical signs caused by larval migration are thought to result from direct damage to the tissues through which the larvae migrate, release of various inflammatory mediators, and potential impacts on blood flow to the bowel. This latter aspect is thought to be particularly important with *S. vulgaris* infection, in which reduced blood flow is speculated to arise due to vasoconstriction and thromboembolism, which then lead to ischemia, altered motility and colic. This hypothesis has not been totally supported by experimental findings.
- Adult worms attach to the mucosa and feed on mucosal cells, blood, and tissue fluids.

SIGNALMENT

- All ages, breeds, and sexes
- Young animals, particularly those with little previous exposure to enteric parasites, are more susceptible than old horses.

SIGNS

- Infections often are mixed, with both large and small strongyles, so clinical signs cannot be attributed to a specific infestation.
- In experimental infections with infective larvae of one species, specific clinical signs have been observed.
- With *S. vulgaris,* an acute syndrome has been described, characterized by colic, fever, and diarrhea, that may coincide with the initial invasion of the intestinal mucosa by the infective larvae.
- With *S. equinus,* experimental heavy infections caused colic, anorexia, and depression, and a similar infection with *S. edentatus* larvae caused peritonitis, jaundice, and fever. These latter three syndromes often are not recognized in the clinical setting. More typically there are signs of colic, which can be severe and acute or, more commonly, recurrent and moderate. In addition, signs of ill thrift and, occasional diarrhea may be noted. These nonspecific signs may be the result of the mixed infection.
- Rarely, aberrant larval migration and clinical signs may ensue—into the central nervous system, renal artery, or iliac artery.

CAUSES AND RISK FACTORS

- Grazing pasture with infective larvae is the primary risk factor.
- Lack of a coordinated parasite monitoring and control program on a particular farm is likely to sustain pastures as high risk.

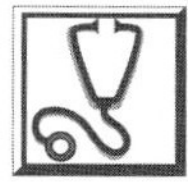

DIAGNOSIS

DIFFERENTIAL DIAGNOSIS

- Many conditions can cause signs of colic—impactions, ileus, bowel displacements and strangulations, incarcerated hernias, enteroliths, severe enteritis, and peritonitis
- Strongyle infestations may play a significant role in development of some of these conditions, but not others.
- Detailed evaluation of the GI system helps to determine the most likely cause of the problem.
- Vague signs of ill thrift and weight loss also can have a wide range of causes and be differentiated based on physical and laboratory findings.

CBC/BIOCHEMISTRY/URINALYSIS

Possible neutrophilia during the early stages and an eosinophilia later

OTHER LABORATORY TESTS

- Serum β- and α-globulins may be elevated later during the disease, but not consistently.
- Fecal analysis may reveal eggs in patent infections. This may have little diagnostic value, however, because most damage occurs during the prepatent period.

IMAGING

N/A

DIAGNOSTIC PROCEDURES

N/A

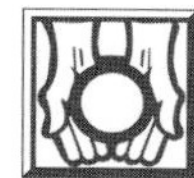

TREATMENT

- Pasture management may help to reduce exposure to infective larvae.
- Regular manure removal (e. g., every 2 days) significantly reduces the numbers of infective larvae on the pasture.
- Mixed grazing, using cattle or sheep, also may help to reduce the pasture load.

MEDICATIONS

DRUG(S) OF CHOICE

- A cornerstone of treating strongyle infections is an appropriate anthelmintic regimen both with respect to drug selection and frequency of use.
- The efficacy of drugs against larvae dictates their frequency of use—pyrantel 6.6 mg/kg every 4 weeks, ivermectin 0.2 mg/kg every 8 weeks, or moxidectin 0.4 mg/kg every 12 weeks.

FOLLOW-UP

- Develop a parasite monitoring and management plan for all horses on a farm; this should include regular fecal analysis for eggs as well as a coordinated use of appropriate anthelmintics.
- Prognosis for individual horses with large strongyles infections varies, depending on the extent and severity of the damage caused by migrating larvae. Those with massive bowel infarcts and ischemia may die, but most do not and, with appropriate immediate care and follow-up, they recover.

MISCELLANEOUS

ASSOCIATED CONDITIONS

Usually a mixed infection with cyathostomes

AGE-RELATED FACTORS, ZOONOTIC POTENTIAL, PREGNANCY

N/A

ABBREVIATIONS

- GI = gastrointestinal

Suggested Reading

Uhlinger CA. Equine strongyle disease. In: Smith BP, ed. Large Animal Internal Medicine, ed 2. Philadelphia: Mosby, 1996:1689–1693.

Author Christopher M. Brown
Consulting Editors Henry Stämpfli and Olimpo Oliver-Espinosa

LARYNGEAL HEMIPARESIS/HEMIPLEGIA

BASICS

DEFINITION

• This disease is a result of neuropathy of the recurrent laryngeal nerve.
• Failure of an anatomically normal left (rarely right) arytenoid cartilage to abduct fully during forced inspiration results in inspiratory respiratory obstruction.
• The cause generally is unknown; therefore, the disease is referred to as idiopathic laryngeal hemiparesis/hemiplegia.
• The condition is graded from I to IV, with IV being the most severe.

PATHOPHYSIOLOGY

• Trauma to the left recurrent laryngeal nerve can produce the condition, but in most cases, the underlying pathologic basis is peripheral neuropathy characterized by distal loss of large myelinated fibers (i.e., distal axonopathy). This neuropathy affects long nerves of large-statured horses.
• Because the left recurrent laryngeal nerve is the longest equine nerve, it is the most severely affected, resulting in clinical signs of left-sided laryngeal hemiparesis/hemiplegia. Interestingly, the right recurrent laryngeal nerve and long nerves in the limbs also are affected histologically. Lesions in these latter nerves are far less severe, however, and clinical signs rarely, if ever, are associated with these abnormalities. • The peripheral neuropathy is progressive and accompanied by attempts at axonal regeneration such that both axonal degeneration and regeneration are observed histologically. • Patterns of denervation and reinnervation are seen histologically in the laryngeal muscles innervated by the recurrent laryngeal nerve. • Distal axonopathy of the left recurrent laryngeal nerve leads to neurogenic atrophy of the intrinsic laryngeal muscles supplied by this nerve. • The loss of abductory function associated with neurogenic atrophy of the CAD muscle causes the clinical signs. Impaired CAD function leads to inability of the left arytenoid cartilage to abduct and to resist pressure swings in the upper airway during exercise. As a result, negative pressure during inspiration leads to adduction of the left arytenoid cartilage, and positive pressure during expiration leads to abduction of the left arytenoid cartilage. The paradoxic adduction during inspiration obstructs the airway, leading to inspiratory stridor and diminished airflow during inspiration, which in turn results in decreased ventilation and, therefore, hypoxemia, hypercarbia, and consequent impaired athletic performance. • Horses respond to inspiratory obstruction by modifying their breathing strategies during exercise to restore minute volume. Strategies include more negative inspiratory (i.e., driving) pressure, increased inspiratory time, and increased tidal volume.

SYSTEM AFFECTED

Respiratory—upper respiratory tract

GENETICS

Evidence beyond the tendency to have tall offspring suggests this is an inheritable defect.

INCIDENCE/PREVALENCE

• Worldwide in horses • Rarely affects ponies

GEOGRAPHIC DISTRIBUTION

Worldwide

SIGNALMENT

• Males are more commonly affected.
• Horses of large height, particularly Thoroughbreds, Warmbloods, and Draft horses, are predisposed. • Approximately 5% (range, 1.8%–9.5%) of Thoroughbreds and up to 42% of draft breeds are affected; the condition is far less common in Standardbreds and almost nonexistent in ponies. • In Thoroughbreds, the incidence is reported to increase from 6.5% in 2-year-old horses to 9.5% in 6-year-olds.

SIGNS

• Horses are presented for upper respiratory noise, exercise intolerance, or both.
• Laryngeal hemiplegia significantly interferes with ventilation in horses that perform at high speed. The higher the speed of exercise, the more severe the hypoventilation; therefore, the horse does not finish well. • In show horses, loss of points during competition because of upper respiratory noise is the main owner concern. Upper airway noise at low airflow or speeds is best described as a soft whistle that increases in intensity as airway pressures become more negative during high-intensity exercise.

CAUSES

• Most commonly idiopathic on the left arytenoid cartilage
• Genetic predisposition • Any abnormality affecting the left or right recurrent laryngeal nerve can result in laryngeal hemiparesis/hemiplegia—perivenous jugular vein injection, jugular thrombophlebitis, common carotid artery puncture, cervical trauma, guttural pouch mycosis, esophageal rupture and subsequent cellulitis, and any surgical procedure in the vicinity of the recurrent laryngeal nerve. • Viral neuritis • Neurologic diseases (e. g., equine lower motor neuron disease) that may affect neurons of the nucleus ambiguous • Intoxications (e.g., organophosphate, lead) may cause bilateral paresis of the laryngeal nerves.

RISK FACTORS

• Perivenous injection—look for damage to vagosympathetic trunk (e.g., Horner's syndrome). • Cervical trauma • Surgical procedures near the left recurrent nerve

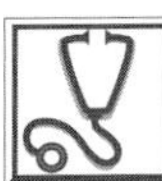

DIAGNOSIS

DIFFERENTIAL DIAGNOSIS

• Unlike horses with arytenoid chondritis, horses with laryngeal hemiparesis/hemiplegia have a normally shaped arytenoid cartilage.
• Right-sided hemiplegia is rare. If it is detected careful examination of the arytenoid cartilage shape is necessary to identify horses with arytenoid chondritis. In addition, be suspicious for congenital malformation of the muscular process of the arytenoid cartilage or of the thyroid lamina in right-sided paresis/paralysis. • Other causes of upper respiratory obstruction • Other causes of diminished athletic performance

CBC/BIOCHEMISTRY/URINALYSIS

Of no value

OTHER LABORATORY TESTS

Arterial blood gases during exercise, with which hypoventilation can be evaluated—in affected horses at maximal exercise, $Paco_2$ can be >55 mm Hg and Pao_2 can be <65 mm Hg.

IMAGING

• Lateral radiographs of the larynx in older (>8 years) horses may reveal ossification of the laryngeal cartilage, which may interfere with placement of laryngeal prosthesis sutures or degree of abduction obtained with surgery.
• Laryngeal ultrasound allows identification of reduction in movement of vocal fold and arytenoid cartilage. There may also be characteristic changes in the echogenicity and pattern in the ipsilateral cricoarytenoid lateralis muscle.

OTHER DIAGNOSTIC PROCEDURES

Videoendoscopy at Rest

• Diagnosis of complete laryngeal hemiplegia (i.e., grade IV) is confirmed by videoendoscopy at rest. Marked laryngeal asymmetry is observed with the left arytenoid cartilage in the midline or paramidline position. No substantial movement of the left arytenoid cartilage is observed during any phase of respiration.• Diagnosis of laryngeal hemiparesis (i.e., grade III) also is obtained by videoendoscopy at rest. These horses have asynchronous movement (e.g., hesitation, flutter, adductor weakness, etc.) of the left arytenoid cartilage during inspiration or expiration, and they cannot achieve and maintain full abduction of the left arytenoid cartilage by swallowing or nasal occlusion.
• Horses with laryngeal grade I and II are generally normal at exercise:
 ○ Grade I—synchronous, full abduction and adduction of the left and right arytenoid cartilages
 ○ Grade II—asynchronous movement (e.g., hesitation, flutter, adductor weakness, etc.) of the left arytenoid cartilage during inspiration or expiration; full abduction of

the left arytenoid cartilage (compared with the right) inducible by swallowing or nasal occlusion
- On external palpation, the left CAD muscle may be atrophied compared to the right.
- "Slap" test—Normally, reflex adduction of the contralateral arytenoid cartilage occurs when the withers are slapped with the hand; loss of this reflex suggests recurrent laryngeal nerve dysfunction.

Examination at Exercise

- Videoendoscopy at exercise determine the degree of laryngeal collapse as well as additional structural collapse such as right aryepiglottic fold and right focal fold.
- Arterial blood gases during exercise, with which hypoventilation can be evaluated—in affected horses at maximal exercise, $Paco_2$ can be >55 mm Hg and Pao_2 can be <65 mm Hg. • Respiratory mechanics—during exercise, affected horses have more negative inspiratory tracheal pressures than normal horses as well as loss of the linear relationship between tracheal and pharyngeal pressures during inspiration and increased translaryngeal pressures during inspiration.

PATHOLOGICAL FINDINGS

Gross

- Atrophy of all intrinsic laryngeal muscles innervated by the left recurrent laryngeal nerve—lateral cricoarytenoideus, dorsal cricoarytenoideus, vocalis, and ventricularis muscles • Atrophy of the left lateral cricoarytenoideus lateralis usually is most severe and is best detected by laryngeal ultrasound. • Atrophy of the dorsal cricoarytenoideus dorsalis muscle is most obvious clinically and can be estimated by manual palpation of the dorsal aspect of the cricoid and muscular process of the arytenoid cartilage.

Histopathologic

- Distal loss of large, myelinated fibers in the left recurrent laryngeal nerve • Left intrinsic laryngeal muscles exhibit angular fiber atrophy and fiber-type grouping.

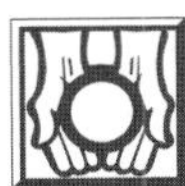

TREATMENT

AIMS OF TREATMENT

- Reduce or eliminate abnormal upper respiratory sound associated with the dilated ventricle. • Improve airway patency by preventing collapse (adduction) of arytenoid cartilage during inhalation and by increasing the cross sectional diameter of the larynx by abduction of the arytenoid cartilage.

APPROPRIATE HEALTH CARE N/A

NURSING CARE N/A

ACTIVITY N/A

DIET N/A

CLIENT EDUCATION

Unless a traumatic or iatrogenic cause is identified, clients should be informed of the possible genetic basis for this disease and that breeding to affected horses may not be indicated.

SURGICAL CONSIDERATIONS

- Treatment is not necessary if exercise intolerance is not present and owners are willing to tolerate the upper respiratory noise.
- Placement of laryngeal prosthesis that fixes the left arytenoid cartilage in near-maximal abduction coupled with cordectomy or ventriculocordectomy is the treatment of choice in horses used for strenuous athletic activities. Chronic coughing during eating is seen in as many as 20% of horses after this surgery. • Unilateral or bilateral ventriculocordectomy is superior to laryngoplasty in reducing or eliminating the abnormal upper respiratory noise associated with this condition. • Unilateral or bilateral ventriculocordectomy can improve exercise tolerance in selected horses with laryngeal grade III, in which arytenoid abduction is adequate yet vocal cord collapse is present and in sport horses where the exercise is less intense. • Laryngeal reinnervation of the CAD muscle in yearlings

MEDICATIONS

DRUGS OF CHOICE

None, other than routine, perioperative antimicrobial and anti-inflammatory agents

CONTRAINDICATIONS N/A

PRECAUTIONS N/A

POSSIBLE INTERACTIONS N/A

ALTERNATIVE DRUGS N/A

FOLLOW-UP

PATIENT MONITORING

- Upper airway endoscopy is required 6 weeks after surgery to monitor response to surgery.
- Determining final response to treatment or monitoring of affected horses is made on the basis of evaluating exercise tolerance and upper respiratory noise.

PREVENTION/AVOIDANCE

N/A

POSSIBLE COMPLICATIONS

Horses undergoing laryngeal prosthesis may experience chronic coughing and, rarely, aspiration pneumonia.

EXPECTED COURSE AND PROGNOSIS

- Laryngeal hemiplegia—horses with grade IV will not exhibit any further deterioration of athletic activity or upper respiratory noise.
- Laryngeal hemiparesis—horses with grade III may exhibit further deterioration of athletic activity or upper respiratory noise.

MISCELLANEOUS

ASSOCIATED CONDITIONS

Untreated horses may be predisposed to EIPH if submitted to strenuous exercise. In addition, it is likely that untreated horses are distressed by the marked hypoxia associated with this condition during intense exercise.

AGE-RELATED FACTORS N/A

ZOONOTIC POTENTIAL N/A

PREGNANCY N/A

SEE ALSO

- Dynamic collapse of the upper airway
- EIPH

ABBREVIATIONS

- CAD = dorsal cricoarytenoid muscle
- EIPH = exercise-induced pulmonary hemorrhage

Suggested Reading

Brown DL, Derksen FJ, Stick JA, et al. Ventriculocordectomy reduces respiratory noise in horses with laryngeal hemiplegia. Equine Vet J 2003;35:570–574.

Chalmers HJ, Cheetham J, Yeager AE, et al. Ultrasonography of the equine larynx. Vet Radiol Ultrasound 2006;47:476–481.

Duncan ID, Griffith IR. A light and electron microscopic study of the neuropathy of equine idiopathic laryngeal hemiplegia. Acta Neuropathol 1978;4:483–501.

Greet TR, Jeffcott LB, Whitwell KE, Cook WR. The slap test for laryngeal adductory function in horses with suspected cervical spinal cord damage. Equine Vet J 1980;12:127–131.

Parente EJ, Martin BB, Tulleners EP, Ross MW. Upper respiratory dysfunctions in horses during high-speed exercise. Proc Am Assoc Equine Pract 1994;40:81–82.

Rakestraw PC, Hackett RP, Ducharme NG, et al. Arytenoid cartilage movement in resting and exercising horses. Vet Surg 1991;20:122–127.

Shappel KK, Derksen FJ, Stick JA, Robinson NE. Effects of ventriculectomy, prosthetic laryngoplasty, and exercise on upper airway function in horses with induced left laryngeal hemiplegia. Am J Vet Res 1988;49:1760–1766.

Taylor SE, Barakzai SZ, Dixon P. Ventriculocordectomy as the sole treatment for recurrent laryngeal neuropathy: Long-term results from ninety-two horses. Vet Surg 2006;35:653–657.

Authors Norm G. Ducharme and Richard P. Hackett

Consulting Editor Daniel Jean

LAVENDER FOAL SYNDROME

BASICS

OVERVIEW

LFS, or CCDL, is an as yet poorly characterized tetanic neurologic syndrome of neonatal foals of Egyptian Arabian breeding. The disease is rare, and the outcome is uniformly fatal in affected individuals. A familial tendency has been reported, and an autosomal recessive mode of inheritance is suspected based on a limited number of cases.

SIGNALMENT

• LFS affects neonatal Arabian foals of pure Egyptian lineage, with clinical signs of disease noted immediately after birth. • Cases involving other breeds have not been reported, and there is no apparent sex predilection.

SIGNS

• Persistent seizure-like activity (often provoked with auditory or tactile stimulation, indicating an intact sensorium) with pronounced extensor rigidity, opisthotonus, and frequent paddling • Apparent blindness • Failure to stand or assume sternal recumbency • Preserved, often strong, suckle reflex • Dilute coat color (classically silver-gray ["lavender"] but may also be dilute chestnut or pale slate gray) • Affected foals are not always of "lavender" coloration.

CAUSES AND RISK FACTORS

• A genetic basis is highly suspected based on the breed exclusivity, and an autosomal recessive mode of inheritance is suspected based on analysis of a limited number of cases. However, the gene(s) involved is not known, and inheritance may be complex. • The disease is clinically similar to tetanic syndromes identified in polled Hereford cattle and Paso Fino horses that result from inherited glycine receptor deficiency in spinal cord motor neurons (glycine is the predominant inhibitory neurotransmitter active in the spinal cord, and lack of glycine signaling disinhibits, or "releases," lower motor neurons; extensor tone predominates, and extensor rigidity is noted clinically).

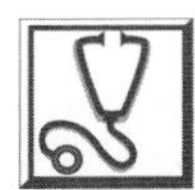

DIAGNOSIS

DIFFERENTIAL DIAGNOSIS

• Hypoxic ischemic encephalopathy— Affected foals are often apparently normal at birth and within 24–48 hr display signs of varying degrees of cerebral dysfunction (loss of affinity for the mare, loss of suckle reflex, seizures, etc.). These foals typically improve with treatment, and most survive. • Neonatal septicemia—Most affected foals are clinically normal at birth, and, if not, infection in utero is often evident (gross and/or histological evidence of placentitis, such as placental thickening, associated exudate, and hemorrhage); additionally, affected foals often display marked clinicopathological abnormalities and may have a positive blood culture (confirmatory). Lavender foals may also develop signs and lesions of sepsis if kept alive for several days, however. • Idiopathic epilepsy of Arabian foals—also noted in Arabian foals of Egyptian breeding, but affected foals are normal at birth and between episodes. Epileptic foals often "outgrow" the seizure disorder by 12–18 mo of age and are thereafter clinically normal. Affected foals rarely die, and coat color is unaffected.
• Occipitoatlantoaxial malformation—also noted more commonly in Arabian foals. Tetanic episodes are not characteristic, and palpation and diagnostic imaging (radiography) confirm this diagnosis. Again, coat color is unaffected.
• Hydrocephalus—Seizures are characteristic, and affected foals often (but not always) display prominent doming of the skull.

CBC/BIOCHEMISTRY/URINALYSIS

The CBC is typically unremarkable, unless septicemia develops in foals that have been maintained for several days. Serum biochemistry analysis is usually normal, but it may display evidence that the foal has not nursed its dam or been administered colostrum (hypoproteinemia, hypoglobulinemia, and hypoglycemia).

OTHER LABORATORY TESTS

IgG will be low if there has been inadequate ingestion of colostrum.

IMAGING

Skull and cervical spinal radiography may be performed to rule out congenital bony malformations in these regions, but no imaging modality is diagnostic for LFS.

OTHER DIAGNOSTIC PROCEDURES

Histopathological analysis of skin biopsy specimens may reveal melanin clumping and follicular dysplasia in affected individuals.

PATHOLOGICAL FINDINGS

No gross or histological lesions of the central nervous system have been noted during post-mortem examination of affected foals. Evidence of self-trauma inflicted during paddling and changes associated with recumbency (dependent pulmonary atelectasis, decubital ulceration) are often the only gross post-mortem findings. Melanin clumping in the dermal follicular bulbs and hair shafts may be noted histologically.

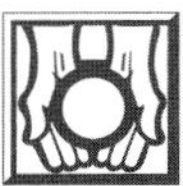

TREATMENT

Affected foals are often referred to a tertiary care facility for evaluation and treatment for hypoxic-ischemic encephalopathy or sepsis. Failure to respond to conventional treatment for these diseases, as well as the characteristic signalment and appearance of these foals, is often diagnostic. There is no treatment for LFS, and the prognosis is hopeless for affected individuals.

MEDICATIONS

DRUG(S) OF CHOICE

N/A

CONTRAINDICATIONS/POSSIBLE INTERACTIONS

N/A

FOLLOW-UP

PATIENT MONITORING

A lack of response to treatment and recognition of the likely diagnosis based on breed and color should prompt euthanasia in most cases.

PREVENTION/AVOIDANCE

Although the precise genetic defect and the mode of inheritance of LFS are not definitively known, a familial tendency has been documented, and certain mares and stallions have been reported to produce multiple affected foals. Therefore, it is recommended that individuals who have produced an affected offspring be removed from breeding programs in an attempt to prevent the disease.

EXPECTED COURSE AND PROGNOSIS

Affected foals do not recover and are invariably euthanized in the hours or days following birth.

MISCELLANEOUS

ASSOCIATED CONDITIONS

Mares and stallions that have produced affected foals have also produced foals with juvenile epilepsy. The relationship, if any, between these two syndromes is not clear, but they do not occur concurrently.

SEE ALSO

Septicemia, neonatal
Hypoxic ischemic encephalopathy
Juvenile epilepsy of Arabians
Occipitoatlantoaxial malformation
Hydrocephalus, congenital

ABBREVIATIONS

• LFS = lavender foal syndrome
• CCDL = coat color dilution lethal

Suggested Reading

Fanelli HH. Coat colour dilution lethal ('lavender foal syndrome'): a tetany syndrome of Arabian foals. Equine Vet Educ 2005;17:260–263.

Page P, Parker R, Harper C, Guthrie A, Nesser J. Clinical, clinicopathologic, postmortem examination findings and familial history of 3 Arabians with lavender foal syndrome. J Vet Intern Med 2006; 20:1491–1494.

Author Teresa A. Burns
Consulting Editor Margaret C. Mudge

LAWSONIA INTRACELLULARIS INFECTION IN FOALS

BASICS

OVERVIEW

PE is a transmissible enteric disease caused by *Lawsonia intracellularis*, an obligate intracellular bacterium. It affects a number of animal species and has a worldwide distribution. Equine cases of PE have been reported so far in North America, Europe, and Australia. A fecal-oral transmission and spread via drinking water and food are likely to be the main sources of infection. The incubation period of the disease is believed to be 2–3 weeks in foals. Isolated cases are most common but outbreaks also occur. The infection is limited to the gastrointestinal system, although the presence of concurrent medical problems affecting other body systems is not uncommon.

SIGNALMENT

- Foals 3–13 mo may be affected, but weanling foals, 4–7 mo of age, are most susceptible to the infection.
- There appear to be no sex or breed predisposition to the disease.

SIGNS

Depression, fever, anorexia, weight loss, diarrhea, edema, and colic are commonly observed. Concomitant conditions such as upper or lower respiratory tract infection, intestinal parasitism, gastric ulcers, and dermatitis are common in severely affected foals.

CAUSES AND RISK FACTORS

- Weaning is currently the only known identified predisposing factor.
- As in pigs, overcrowding, lack of specific immunity, commingling of animals, and introduction of new animals on the premises may also predispose foals to PE.

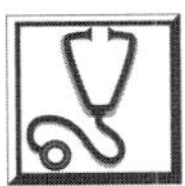

DIAGNOSIS

DIFFERENTIAL DIAGNOSIS

- Parasitism, gastroduodenal ulcers, sand impaction, acute intestinal obstruction, infiltrative bowel disease including neoplasia (lymphoma), eosinophilic gastroenteritis, and intoxication with plants and chemicals, including pharmacological agents such as NSAIDs
- Infectious diarrhea caused by *Salmonella* spp., *Rhodococcus equi*, *Clostridium* spp., *Ehrlichia risticii*, *Campylobacter jejuni*, rotavirus, and adenovirus

CBC/BIOCHEMISTRY/URINALYSIS

Hypoproteinemia (<50 g/L) and, occasionally, leucocytosis, neutrophilia, hyperfibrinogenemia, increased creatinine kinase, hypocalcemia, hyponatremia, azotemia, and anemia. Urinalysis and glucose absorption tests are within the normal range.

OTHER LABORATORY TESTS

- Serology using immunofluorescence may help confirming exposure to the bacteria. Serology may be positive when the clinical signs are first detected, and foals may remain seropositive for more than 6 mo.
- Positive PCR on feces will confirm the presence of *L. intracellularis* in the intestine. Fecal excretion of *L. intracellularis* detected by PCR ended soon (<4 days) after the beginning of an effective antimicrobial administration however.
- *L. intracellularis* do not grow on conventional bacteriological media. Thus, bacterial cultures are not used for the diagnosis of the disease.

IMAGING

Abdominal ultrasonography often reveals thickening of segments of the small intestinal wall.

OTHER DIAGNOSTIC PROCEDURES

N/A

PATHOLOGICAL FINDINGS

- Marked thickening of the small intestine mucosa, giving its surface an irregular and corrugated appearance.
- Thickened mucosa and severe hyperplasia of crypt epithelium.
- Silver-stained sections reveal numerous short and slightly curved bacterial rods in the apical cytoplasm of the immature epithelial cells. Diagnosis is confirmed by immunohistochemistry.

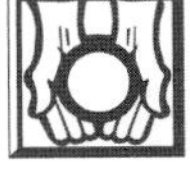

TREATMENT

- Less severely affected foals may be treated as outpatients.
- Transfusion of fresh or fresh-frozen plasma may be required in foals with severe hypoproteinemia.
- Additional symptomatic treatment such as antiulcer therapy, intravenous crystalloid or colloid fluid therapy, and parenteral feeding may be indicated in some cases.

MEDICATIONS

DRUG(S) OF CHOICE

- Erythromycin estolate (25 mg/kg PO q8h, alone or combined with rifampin 10 mg/kg PO q12–24h), administered for 2–3 weeks. Azithromycin 10 mg/kg PO q24h, chloramphenicol 50 mg/kg PO q6h, and tetracyclines (doxycycline 10 mg/kg PO q12h) may also be viable alternatives to erythromycin.
- Drugs should also target concurrent infections, if present.

CONTRAINDICATIONS/POSSIBLE INTERACTIONS

N/A

FOLLOW-UP

PATIENT MONITORING

- A rapid improvement in attitude, appetite, weight gain, and colic signs or diarrhea is observed in most foals, following administration of appropriate antimicrobials.
- Hypoproteinemia will slowly resolve with therapy.

PREVENTION/AVOIDANCE

Environmental contamination by fecal shedding from infected foals is likely to be minimal once antimicrobial treatment is initiated.

POSSIBLE COMPLICATIONS

N/A

EXPECTED COURSE AND PROGNOSIS

Prognosis for *Lawsonia intracellularis* infection in foals is favorable with therapy unless severe concurrent medical complications are present.

MISCELLANEOUS

ASSOCIATED CONDITIONS

Marked hypoproteinemia may lead to thromboembolic diseases.

AGE-RELATED FACTORS

Weaning time is a predisposing factor suggesting that ration changes, mixing, and transportation may contribute to equine PE.

ZOONOTIC POTENTIAL

PE is not currently considered to be a zoonosis, although it affects nonhuman primates.

PREGNANCY

N/A

ABBREVIATIONS

- PCR = polymerase chain reaction
- PE = proliferative enteropathy

Suggested Reading

Lavoie JP, Drolet R, Parsons D, Leguillette R, Sauvageau R, Shapiro J, Houle L, Hallé G, Gebhart CJ. Equine proliferative enteropathy: a cause of weight loss, colic, diarrhea and hypoproteinemia in foals on three breeding farms. Equine Vet J 2000;32:418–425.

Sampieri F, Hinchcliff KW, Toribio RE. Tetracycline therapy of *Lawsonia intracellularis* enteropathy in foals. Equine Vet J 2006;38:89–92.

Author Jean-Pierre Lavoie

Consulting Editors Henry Stämpfli and Olimpo Oliver-Espinoza

LEAD (PB) TOXICOSIS

BASICS

OVERVIEW

- Lead (Pb) toxicosis, also referred to as "plumbism," involves adverse effects on the nervous, musculoskeletal, gastrointestinal, hematopoietic, and renal systems.
- Horses are less susceptible to plumbism than either cattle or dogs. Lead intoxication in horses is relatively uncommon in the United States.
- Acute (rare) and chronic forms result from exposures to Pb-contaminated forages in habitats adjacent to mines and smelters or environments with buildings or fences built prior to 1977 and/or coated with Pb-based paints.
- The ingestion of Pb from Pb-acid batteries, leaded gasoline, soil contaminated with Pb-containing products, or the ashes of combusted older buildings also poses a risk of Pb intoxication to horses.
- Lead binds to sulfhydryl groups and mimics calcium, thereby disrupting heme synthesis, neurotransmission, and vitamin D metabolism.

SIGNALMENT

- No breed predilections
- Young, growing foals absorb 10%–20% of ingested Pb.
- Pregnant and lactating mares have enhanced GI absorption of Pb and transfer Pb to the fetus or neonate when the diet is marginally adequate in mineral content.

SIGNS

- Peripheral neuropathies including abnormal lip and tongue movements, laryngeal hemiplegia ("roaring") or paralysis, dysphagia, esophageal obstruction ("choke"), aspiration pneumonia
- Anorexia
- Depression
- Weight loss
- Weakness
- Ataxia
- Muscle fasciculations
- Hyperesthesia
- Lameness and swollen joints (young, growing horses or Pb-containing foreign bodies near joint surfaces)
- Colic, diarrhea
- Anemia
- Seizures
- Death

CAUSES AND RISK FACTORS

- Acute exposures to >500–750 mg/kg
- Chronic exposures to 1.7–7 mg/kg/day
- Whole-blood Pb concentrations >0.20 ppm
- Habitats near smelting or mining operations
- Housing in or around barns or fences built prior to 1977 that contain Pb-lined pipes and/or surfaces coated with Pb-based paints
- Premises contaminated with Pb-containing batteries, shot, solder, gasoline, oil, or ashes of combusted older buildings
- Diets deficient in calcium, zinc, iron, or vitamin D
- Trauma from Pb-containing objects

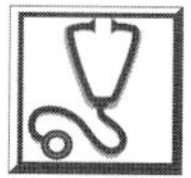

DIAGNOSIS

DIFFERENTIAL DIAGNOSIS

- Laryngeal hemiplegia or paralysis ("roaring"), esophageal obstruction ("choke"), and EIPH not associated with plumbism—physical examination, endoscopy, radiography, no identified sources of Pb exposure, history of trauma, only one animal on the premises affected
- Rabies and other viral encephalitides
- EMND and EDM
- Fumonisin B_1 intoxication ("moldy corn poisoning" or ELEM)
- Botulism
- Intoxications by *Centaurea* sp.
- Arsenic toxicosis

CBC/BIOCHEMISTRY/ URINALYSIS

- Anemia
- Nucleated red blood cells
- Basophilic stippling and Howell-Jolly bodies
- Proteinuria (uncommon)

OTHER LABORATORY TESTS

- Ante-mortem—Whole-blood concentrations of Pb >0.35 ppm in the presence of appropriate clinical signs, alterations in erythrocyte ALAD activity (decreased), zinc protoporphyrin concentrations (increased), and increased urinary excretion of coproporphyrin and uroporphyrins (ALAD and porphyrin analyses not performed in many veterinary diagnostic laboratories)
- Post-mortem—concentrations of Pb in liver or kidney >10 ppm on a wet-weight basis (>5 ppm in chronic cases), bone concentrations of Pb > 40 ppm on a dry-matter basis in chronic cases

IMAGING

- Radiography to detect Pb-containing objects in the GI tract of small foals or around joints
- Radiographic visualization of "Pb lines" at epiphyseal plates of long bones in young, growing horses

DIAGNOSTIC PROCEDURES

- Endoscopy to diagnose laryngeal hemiplegia or to visualize Pb-containing foreign bodies in the stomach
- Measurement of 24-hr urinary excretion of Pb following chelation therapy (logistically challenging)

PATHOLOGICAL FINDINGS

- Gross—inconsistent gross pathologic changes in horses, aspiration pneumonia, and emaciation in chronic cases
- Histologic—peripheral neuropathy with segmental degeneration of axons and myelin in distal motor fibers, pulmonary changes consistent with aspiration pneumonia, reports of renal tubular disease in chronic cases

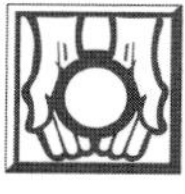

TREATMENT

- Prevent further Pb exposure
- Administer sulfate-containing cathartics to bind Pb in GI tract (decrease absorption) and to increase elimination of Pb

- Enhance urinary Pb excretion with chelation
- Control pain and hyperexcitability
- Treat aspiration pneumonia with appropriate antibiotics and NSAIDs
- Provide supportive care for dehydration, circulatory shock, and dysphagia

MEDICATIONS

DRUG(S) OF CHOICE

- Sodium or magnesium sulfate administered by nasogastric tube (250–500 mg/kg)
- Dimercaprol (British anti-lewisite [BAL]) to chelate intracellular and extracellular Pb at a BAL loading dose of 4–5 mg/kg given by deep IM injection, followed by 2–3 mg/kg q4h for 24 hr and then 1 mg/kg q4h for 2 days; adverse reactions include tremors, convulsions, and coma.
- Ca-EDTA to chelate Pb at a dosage of 75 mg/kg/day divided into two or three equal treatments and administered for 5 days by slow intravenous infusion as a 6.6% solution in normal saline or 5% dextrose (1.1 mL of 6.6% EDTA solution/kg); if deemed necessary, retreatment with Ca-EDTA after a 2-day "rest"; adverse effects include depletion of zinc and essential electrolytes.
- Thiamine hydrochloride at dosages of 2 to 10 mg/kg twice daily IM for 2 weeks in cattle; efficacy not clearly demonstrated in horses
- Flunixin meglumine at 0.55–1.1 mg/kg IV q12–24h and/or butorphanol tartrate at 0.02–0.1 mg/kg IV q3–4h up to 48 hr for abdominal discomfort
- Xylazine hydrochloride at 0.3–1.1 mg/kg IV alone (higher dosage) or with butorphanol at 0.01–0.02 mg/kg IV (lower dosage of xylazine) for sedation or control of severe pain
- Diazepam administered to adults (25–50 mg IV) or foals (0.05–0.4 mg/kg IV) for hyperesthesia, muscle tremors, and seizures (can repeat in 30 min)
- Appropriate fluid therapy as necessary

CONTRAINDICATIONS/POSSIBLE INTERACTIONS

- Depletion of essential cations and electrolytes by excessive chelation
- Sedatives in ataxic horses
- NSAIDs in GI and renal disease British anti-lewisite

FOLLOW-UP

- Identification of source of Pb
- Proper disposal of or limited access to Pb sources
- Recheck Pb concentration in whole blood 2 weeks after final chelation; chelate again if >0.35 ppm.
- Monitor serum electrolytes and supplement as needed.

PATIENT MONITORING

- Monitor hemogram and whole blood Pb concentrations.
- Periodic neurologic assessments

PREVENTION/ AVOIDANCE

- Prevent exposure to habitats near smelters or mines.
- Avoid use of Pb-containing paints.
- Clean up Pb-contaminated pastures or paddocks.

POSSIBLE COMPLICATIONS

- Aspiration pneumonia
- Concurrent exposure to other toxic metals

EXPECTED COURSE AND PROGNOSIS

Long-term neurologic deficits possible following removal from Pb source and partial recovery of neurologic function

MISCELLANEOUS

ASSOCIATED CONDITIONS

- · Other metal intoxications
- · Laryngeal hemiplegia
- · EIPH
- · Esophageal obstruction

AGE-RELATED FACTORS

Young, growing horses

ZOONOTIC POTENTIAL

N/A

PUBLIC HEALTH IMPORTANCE

Appropriate regulatory agencies should be notified of Pb-contaminated water sources used by humans and food-producing animals.

PREGNANCY

Lead can cross the placenta and, potentially, have adverse effects on the fetus.

ABBREVIATIONS

- ALAD = d-aminolevulinic acid dehydratase
- Ca-EDTA = calcium disodium ethylenediaminetetraacetic acid
- EDM = equine degenerative myeloencephalopathy
- EIPH = exercise-induced pulmonary hemorrhage
- ELEM = equine leukoencephalomalacia
- EMND = equine motor neuron disease
- GI = gastrointestinal
- Pb = lead
- ppm = parts per million

Suggested Reading

Casteel SW. Metal toxicosis in horses. Vet Clin North Am Equine Pract 2001;17:517–527.

Gwaltney-Brant S. Lead. In: Plumlee KH, ed. Clinical Veterinary Toxicology. St. Louis: Mosby, 2004:204–210.

Author Tim J. Evans

Consulting Editor Robert H. Poppenga

LENS OPACITIES/CATARACTS

BASICS

OVERVIEW

- The transparency of the lens is made possible by layers of perfectly aligned linear cells or lens fibers.
- Disruption of the precise anatomical arrangement of these lens fibers results in opacification or cataract formation of the lens.
- The basic mechanism of cataract formation is a decrease in soluble lens proteins, failure of the lens epithelial cell sodium pump, a decrease in lens glutathione, and lens fiber swelling and fiber membrane rupture.
- These lens opacities or cataracts can vary in size depending on the number of lens fibers damaged. Very small incipient lens opacities are common and not associated with blindness.
- As cataracts develop or mature, they become more opaque, and blindness develops.

SIGNALMENT

All ages and breeds of horses are at risk for cataract development. Cataracts are a frequent congenital ocular defect in foals.

SIGNS

- Horses manifest varying degrees of blindness as cataracts mature. The tapetal reflection is seen with incipient, immature, and hypermature cataracts but is not seen in mature cataracts. The rate of cataract progression and development of blindness cannot be predicted in most instances.
- Blepharospasm and lacrimation may accompany cataracts in horses due to associated uveitis.
- Assessment of visual function can be made by distant observation of the horse walking, feeding, and interacting with other horses. Visually impaired horses may demonstrate a reluctance to run or even walk, although some horses with bilateral cataracts appear to do quite well in a familiar environment. Differences in head posture may be associated with cataracts, as a unilaterally blind horse may attempt to keep its sighted eye toward activity in its environment.

CAUSES AND RISK FACTORS

- Heritable, traumatic, nutritional, and postinflammatory etiologies have been proposed.
- Cataracts may be associated with microphthalmos.
- Cataracts secondary to ERU or trauma are frequently seen, while juvenile onset cataracts are uncommon in horses. True senile cataracts that interfere with vision are found in horses older than 20 years.
- Dominant inheritance has been reported for cataracts in Belgian and Thoroughbred horses. Morgan horses have nonprogressive, nuclear, bilaterally symmetrical cataracts that do not generally interfere with vision.

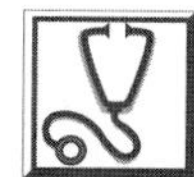

DIAGNOSIS

DIFFERENTIAL DIAGNOSIS

- Increased cloudiness of the lens occurs with age and is called nuclear or lenticular sclerosis. It is common in older horses, but vision is clinically normal as nuclear sclerosis does not cause vision loss.
- Blindness in horses is also due to ERU, glaucoma, and retinal disease.

CBC/BIOCHEMISTRY/URINALYSIS

N/A

OTHER LABORATORY TESTS

N/A

IMAGING

B-scan ultrasound is beneficial in assessing the anatomic status of the retina if a cataract is present.

DIAGNOSTIC PROCEDURES

Electroretinography is beneficial in assessing the functional status of the retina if a cataract is present.

PATHOLOGIC FINDINGS

Epithelial cell metaplasia, liquefaction of lens material, and lens fiber swelling are noticed.

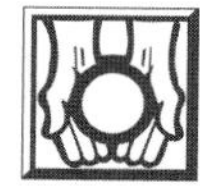

TREATMENT

- Most veterinary ophthalmologists recommend surgical removal of cataracts in foals less than 6 months of age if the foal is healthy, no uveitis or other ocular problems are present, and the foal's personality will tolerate aggressive topical therapy, but adults with visual impairment due to cataracts are also candidates for cataract surgery.
- Therapy for cataracts is necessarily surgical, although some degree of spontaneous cataract resorption may occur with hypermature cataracts. Horses considered for lens extraction should be in good physical condition. Complete ophthalmic and general physical examinations should be performed. Preoperative complete blood counts and serum chemistries are important for evaluating systemic organ function. A complete ophthalmic examination is necessary.
- Slow or absent pupillary light reflexes may indicate active iridocyclitis with or without posterior synechiation, retinal disease, optic nerve disease, or iris sphincter muscle atrophy.
- Afferent pupillary defects in a cataractous eye cannot be attributed to the cataract alone, as well as the fact that normal PLRs do not exclude some degree of retinal or optic nerve disease.
- Any signs of anterior uveitis should delay cataract surgery until the cause of the inflammation is diagnosed and has been successfully treated. Cataract surgery should also be delayed in the presence of active eyelid, conjunctival, or corneal disease.
- Examination of the fundus may be difficult due to the cataract. Preoperative electroretinography and B-scan ultrasonography are beneficial to evaluate outer retinal function and the integrity of intraocular structures, respectively.
- Phacoemulsification cataract surgery is most useful for equine cataract surgery as it involves a small corneal incision of 3.2 mm. Immature, mature and hypermature cataracts have been successfully removed in horses with this technique.
- Intraocular lenses of 25 diopters (D) have been used in horses following cataract surgery but are often associated with postoperative iridocyclitis.

MEDICATIONS

DRUG(S) OF CHOICE

- Topically applied antibiotics, such as chloramphenicol, gentamicin, ciprofloxacin, or tobramycin ophthalmic solutions, may be used preoperatively and postoperatively. Frequency of medication varies from q2h to q8h.
- Topically applied 1%–2% atropine is effective in stabilizing the blood-aqueous barrier, minimizing pain from ciliary muscle spasm, and causes pupillary dilatation. Atropine may be used as often as q4h, with the frequency of administration reduced as soon as the pupil dilates.
- Topically applied corticosteroids, such as prednisolone acetate (1%), are beneficial to suppress preoperative and postoperative inflammation.
- Systemically administered NSAIDs, such as phenylbutazone (2 mg/kg BID PO) or flunixin meglumine (1 mg/kg BID IV, IM or PO), can be used orally or parenterally, and are effective in reducing anterior uveitis in horses with cataracts.
- Topically administered NSAIDs, such as flurbiprofen and suprofen, can be used TID to QID to suppress signs of anterior uveitis.

PRECAUTIONS

Horses receiving topically administered atropine should be monitored for signs of colic.

CONTRAINDICATIONS/POSSIBLE INTERACTIONS

- Infectious endophthalmitis is a devastating complication.
- General anesthesia with its attendant risks is required for cataract surgery.

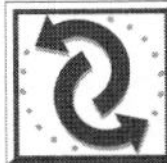

FOLLOW-UP

PATIENT MONITORING

- Horses with cataracts should be monitored for blepharospasm and lacrimation as cataracts can cause uveitis.
- Blind horses should be monitored in their environment.
- Horses that have had cataract surgery should be monitored for signs of eye pain, self-trauma, a reoccurrence of blindness, and colic.

PREVENTION/AVOIDANCE

Breeding of horses with cataracts is to be avoided.

POSSIBLE COMPLICATIONS

Postoperative complications include persistent iridocyclitis and plasmoid aqueous, fibropupillary membranes, synechiae, iris bombé, corneal ulceration, corneal edema, corneal fibrovascular infiltrates, posterior capsular opacification, retained lens cortex, wound leakage, vitreous presentation into anterior chamber, retinal degeneration, retinal detachment, and infectious endophthalmitis.

EXPECTED COURSE AND PROGNOSIS

- Foals are easiest to perform surgery on because the globe size is small enough that the standard cataract surgical equipment is of a satisfactory size, general anesthesia is less of a risk in foals, and foals heal very quickly following cataract surgery. Early return of vision is paramount in foals for development of the higher visual centers.
- Slight corneal edema is usually present from 24 to 72 hours postoperatively. One week following surgery the pupil should be functional, any fibrin in the anterior chamber resorbing, and the fundus visible. Three weeks following surgery the eye should be nonpainful, the patient visual, pupillary movement normal, and the ocular media clear.
- Most reliable reports of vision in successful cataract surgery in horses indicate vision is functionally normal postoperatively. From an optical standpoint, the aphakic eye should be quite far-sighted or hyperopic postoperatively, and was +9.94 D in one study. Images close to the eye would be blurry and appear magnified.

MISCELLANEOUS

ASSOCIATED CONDITIONS

Retinal detachment
ERU

AGE-RELATED FACTORS

N/A

ZOONOTIC POTENTIAL

N/A

PREGNANCY

N/A

ABBREVIATIONS

- ERU = equine recurrent uveitis
- PLR = pupillary light reflex

Suggested Reading

Brooks DE. Ophthalmology for the Equine Practitioner. Jackson, WY; Teton NewMedia, 2002.

Brooks DE, Matthews AG. Equine ophthalmology. In: Gelatt KN, ed. Veterinary Ophthalmology, ed 4. Philadelphia; Lippincott Williams and Wilkins, 2007.

Gilger BC, ed. Equine Ophthalmology. Philadelphia; WB Saunders, 2005.

Author Dennis E. Brooks
Consulting Editor Dennis E. Brooks

LEPTOSPIROSIS

BASICS

DEFINITION

Leptospirosis is a worldwide disease caused by pathogenic serovars of the spirochete *Leptospira interrogans.* It affects wildlife and domestic animals and has a zoonotic potential. Serologic surveys show that equine exposure to leptospires is common but clinical disease is uncommon. Clinical leptospirosis in horses is primarily associated with recurrent uveitis, abortions, stillbirths, and neonatal disease. Hepatic and renal disease in adults is uncommon.

PATHOPHYSIOLOGY

Leptospires are spirochetes that are both host and non–host adapted. Infection by host-adapted serovars results in an increase in endemic disease or clinical disease in immunologically naïve animals. Infection by non–host-adapted serovars results in sporadic infections or disease outbreaks. If the serovar is host adapted, then infection is often for life; if the serovar is non–host adapted, then infection and shedding are usually brief. *L. interrogans* serovar *bratislava* is the presumed host-adapted serovar of horses. Leptospires penetrate mucosal and skin surfaces and result in a bacteremia and an invasion of internal organs 4–10 days later. Outcome of infection depends on the horse's humoral response and the pathogenicity of the serovar. Organisms multiply in organs and release metabolites that, combined with immune-mediated damage, cause the clinical signs associated with the disease. Leptospires evade the immune system in the proximal renal tubules, genital tract, central nervous system, and eyes. Leptospires are shed into the environment in high concentrations in the urine, although all body secretions may contain leptospires during the bacteremic phase.

SYSTEMS AFFECTED

- Ophthalmic—recurrent uveitis
- Reproductive—abortion, stillbirth
- Renal/urologic—renal disease and pyuria
- Neonatal disease—hepatic and renal disease, weakness, pulmonary hemorrhage
- Hepatobiliary–liver disease and jaundice

GENETICS

N/A

INCIDENCE/PREVALENCE

Serologic surveys have identified worldwide exposure to leptospires. Predominant serovars vary with geographic area and leptospire antigens used in the surveys.

SIGNALMENT

Nonspecific

SIGNS

Signs associated with the bacteremia include pyrexia, depression, lethargy, and anorexia. Signs associated with organ invasion are indicative of the specific organ involved. Usually no premonitory signs are observed prior to abortion. Chronic disease is associated with recurrent uveitis. Subclinical infections and carrier states are asymptomatic.

Physical Examination

- Ophthalmic: initially, blepharospasm, excessive tearing, photophobia, chemosis, miosis, aqueous flare, hypopyon, and corneal edema. Chronic sequelae include synechia formation, retinal detachment, chorioretinitis, cataracts, atrophy of corpora nigra, and phthisis bulbi.
- Reproductive: abortion (usually late gestation), stillbirth, or premature birth or neonatal disease depending on stage of gestation and infection
- Renal/urologic: azotemia, polyuria/polydipsia, pyuria, hematuria, pyrexia
- Neonatal disease: weakness, icterus, renal failure, hematuria. One outbreak also reported respiratory distress, pyrexia, and depression.
- Hepatobiliary: jaundice, pyrexia, lethargy

CAUSES

- Pathogenic serovars of *L. interrogans*
- In North America, most abortions have resulted from infections by leptospires in the serovar *kennewicki* and less frequently serovars *grippotyphosa* and *hardjo.* Leptospiral abortions previously reported as *L. pomona* have been reclassified as *L. interrogans* serovar *kennewicki.* In northern Ireland, the serovar *bratislava* is identified most frequently.

RISK FACTORS

- Direct transmission with host-to-host contact via infected urine, exposure to postabortion discharge, and aborted fetuses
- Indirect transmission via contaminated environment from exposure to shedding maintenance hosts. Skunk and raccoons are maintenance hosts for serovars *kennewicki* and *grippotyphosa,* and cattle for serovar *hardjo.*
- Warm, moist environment; neutral to slightly alkaline soil pH; and a high density of carrier and susceptible animals

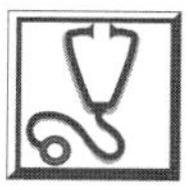

DIAGNOSIS

DIFFERENTIAL DIAGNOSIS

Recurrent Uveitis

- *Toxoplasma* spp., *Onchocerca cervicalis, Streptococcus* spp., viral agents, ocular trauma
- *Onchocerca* microfilariae and viral inclusion bodies are found in conjunctival scraping and biopsy.
- Rising serum titers are associated with *Toxoplasma* spp.

Abortion

- Infectious causes—EHV-1 is differentiated by characteristic histologic lesion of intranuclear eosinophilic inclusion bodies and indirect immunofluorescent tests. Placentitis (bacterial and fungal) is differentiated by gross evidence of placentitis, isolation of organisms from the placenta and fetal organs, especially the stomach. EVA is differentiated by viral isolation from placental and fetal tissues. *Ehrlichia risticci* is differentiated by histopathology of the fetus and isolation of the organism from the fetus.
- Noninfectious causes—placental abnormalities, twinning, twisted umbilical cord, and maternal systemic disease

Renal/Urologic

- Bacterial pyelonephritis is identified by pyuria and the presence of bacteria in the urine.
- Hemodynamic renal dysfunction is differentiated by other physical examination findings.
- Nephrotoxicity is identified by exposure to a source.

Neonatal Disease

- Neonatal isoerythrolysis is associated with hemolytic anemia.
- Tyzzer's disease is seen in older foals; organisms are seen in the liver with Warthin-Starry stain.
- EHV-1 is differentiated from severe leukopenia and pneumonia.
- Septicemia is differentiated by other physical examination findings, blood culture and post-mortem specimens.

Hepatobiliary

- Hemolytic anemia, fasting, cholelithiasis, neoplasia, hepatic abscess, acute and chronic hepatitis
- Differentiated on ultrasonographic findings, hematology, and serum biochemistry

CBC/BIOCHEMISTRY/URINALYSIS

- Serum biochemistry profile reflects specific organ involvement; leukocytosis, hyperfibrinogenemia.
- Urinalysis (if renal involvement) shows red and white blood cells and casts.

OTHER LABORATORY TESTS

- Culture of *Leptospira* is difficult due to fastidious growth requirements and length of time required for culture. Dark-phase microscopy and FAT are also used.
- Antemortem body fluids (urine, blood, aqueous humor) or postmortem tissues (kidney, liver, fetus, placenta) must be placed in transport media recommended by the diagnostic laboratory. The collection of midstream urine samples from second urination after furosemide administration enhances isolation, and repeat sampling increases the chances of isolation.

• MAT results need to be interpreted with caution as normal adults can have titers >1:100. Paired samples take 2–4 weeks apart showing a 4-fold increase also need cautious interpretation as the duration and strength of the response are variable. Comparison with other farm individuals may assist with interpretation. Mares with MAT titers > 1:6400 that are in contact with a mare that has aborted should be isolated and treated accordingly.
• MAT and culture can be performed on vitreous humor samples.
• No PCR is available, at this stage, for routine use.

IMAGING

Ultrasonography may assist in the evaluation of hepatic and renal disease.

PATHOLOGY FINDINGS

Fetus and neonates—Most common findings are icterus, generalized petechial and ecchymotic hemorrhages, and microabscesses of kidneys. Placenta is edematous with a necrotic chorion covered with mucous exudates. Allantoic membrane may contain cystic nodular masses.

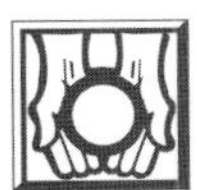

TREATMENT

APPROPRIATE HEALTH AND NURSING CARE

Reproductive

Aborting mares should be isolated and the area they inhabited disinfected. Contaminated bedding and fetal and placental tissues should be rapidly removed and appropriately disposed. Mares can shed leptospires in urine for up to 4 months post abortion.

Renal/Urologic

Appropriate antimicrobials and supportive care to ensure adequate renal function should be administered.

Neonatal Disease

Appropriate antimicrobials and supportive care should be administered. Foals should be isolated as high numbers of leptospires are shed in urine.

Hepatobiliary

Appropriate antimicrobials and supportive care should be administered.

ACTIVITY

Activity should be restricted to decrease environmental contamination.

CLIENT EDUCATION

The client should be informed as to the zoonotic potential. Infection can occur through contact of mucous membranes or skin lesions with urine or tissue from an infected animal.

MEDICATIONS

DRUG(S) OF CHOICE

• Effectiveness of treatment for leptospirosis in horses in unknown.
• Combination of penicillin (200,000 IU/mL) and dihydrostreptomycin (250 mg/mL) 20 mL IM BID for 7 days resulted in no urine shedding. Potassium penicillin (20,000 IU/kg IV q6h) has been recommended in infected pregnant mares to prevent infection of the fetus.

Ophthalmic

Therapy is aimed at reducing immune-mediated inflammation and providing mydriasis and analgesia.

Reproductive

Antimicrobial therapy is indicated to prevent and decrease shedding of spirochetes in urine or for prophylactic treatment of pregnant in-contact mares with high titers.

CONTRAINDICATIONS

N/A

PRECAUTIONS

Avoid use of potentially nephrotoxic drugs if renal disease is suspected.

POSSIBLE DRUG INTERACTIONS

N/A

ALTERNATIVE DRUGS

Oxytetracycline (5–10 mg/kg) for 7 days has been used.

FOLLOW-UP

PATIENT MONITORING

Ophthalmic

Recurrent episodes of uveitis.

Reproductive

Therapy should be instituted if fetal membranes are retained or if signs of systemic illness become evident. Monitor in-contact mares' serum titer levels and consider antibiotic therapy of in-contact pregnant mares.

Renal/Urologic/Neonatal Disease/Hepatobiliary

Monitor hepatic and renal function.

PREVENTION/AVOIDANCE

• Approved vaccinations are not available for use in horses in North America.
• Extra label uses of vaccines are being investigated as prevention for recurrent uveitis.
• Isolate affected animals, and consider antibiotic therapy for in-contact pregnant mares.
• Limit access to wet environments, and avoid contamination with other domestic animals and wildlife.

POSSIBLE COMPLICATIONS

• Ophthalmic—blindness associated with recurrent uveitis
• Reproductive—abortion outbreak
• Neonatal disease—Foals from infected dams may be born with clinical disease.

EXPECTED COURSE AND PROGNOSIS

• Ophthalmic—alternating periods of acute and quiescent disease
• Reproductive—uneventful recovery of mare
• Neonatal disease, renal/urologic, and hepatobiliary—Prognosis is guarded in severe acute disease and depends on the extent of organ invasion and the severity of tissue injury.

MISCELLANEOUS

ASSOCIATED CONDITIONS

N/A

ZOONOTIC POTENTIAL

Clinical signs are variable from asymptomatic infection to sepsis and death. Most common complaints are flu-like symptoms and vomiting; however, neurologic, respiratory, cardiac, ocular, and gastrointestinal manifestations can occur.

PREGNANCY

Abortion, stillbirths, and neonatal disease can be sequelae, depending on the stages of infection and gestation.

ABBREVIATIONS

• EHV = equine herpesvirus
• ELISA = enzyme-linked immunosorbent assay
• EVA = equine viral arteritis
• FAT = fluorescent antibody test
• MAT = mixed agglutination test

Suggested Reading

Bernard WV. Leptospirosis. Vet Clin North Am Equine Pract 1993;9:435–444.
Donahue JM, Williams NM. Emergent causes of placentitis and abortion. Vet Clin North Am Equine Pract 2000;16:443–456.

Author Jane E. Axon
Consulting Editors Ashley G. Boyle and Corinne R. Sweeney

LETHAL WHITE FOAL SYNDROME

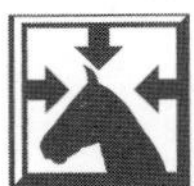

BASICS

OVERVIEW

Lethal white foal syndrome, or ileocecocolonic aganglionosis, is a fatal heritable syndrome of horses with white patterning (usually APH) occurring most frequently in foals of Overo-Overo Paint crosses. Failure of proper development of neural crest–derived cell populations results in lack of both melanocytes in the skin and myenteric ganglia cells in the caudal gastrointestinal tract. Clinically, affected foals are completely white and show signs of progressive colic within 24 hr of birth. The syndrome is inherited as an autosomal recessive trait, and the outcome is invariably fatal. A genetic test is available to test breeding stock for the heterozygous carrier state.

SIGNALMENT

• Neonatal foals of Overo-cross-Overo APH breeding • Signs of colic usually noted by 12–24 hr of age • White coloration • No sex predisposition • Genetic disease, inherited as an autosomal recessive trait

SIGNS

• White color (some foals have a small amount of pigmented hair, usually on the mane and/or tail) • Blue eyes, usually • Typically normal, vigorous foals, which stand and nurse normally after birth • Failure to pass meconium after birth • Progressive signs of colic beginning within 12–24 hr of birth (exacerbated with ingestion of colostrum and/or milk) • Progressive abdominal distention • Death within 48–72 hr of birth • May also have congenital deafness

CAUSES AND RISK FACTORS

• LWFS is caused by a mutation in the EDNRB gene. The mutation is likely a complete loss-of-function mutation. • Function of the EDNRB and its ligand, endothelin-3, is vitally important for the proper migration of certain neural crest–derived cell populations, particularly melanocytes and the cells of many autonomic ganglia. Failure of the neural crest cells to migrate and mature properly in foals affected with LWFS results in the characteristic disease phenotype (a nonpigmented foal with functional ileus due to an abnormal enteric nervous system). • Affected foals are homozygous for the mutation, while their parents are heterozygotes at that locus. The gene is likely involved, or linked closely to other genes involved, with white patterning in horses; as such, the carrier state has been identified only in horse breeds which commonly register individuals with white patterning. The heterozygous carrier state appears to be highest among Overo Paint horses, especially frame Overos.

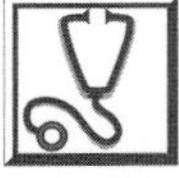

DIAGNOSIS

DIFFERENTIAL DIAGNOSIS

• Not all white foals of APH breeding have LWFS. White foals should not be euthanized if they fail to develop signs of colic and are otherwise clinically normal. However, a white foal with colic in the immediate neonatal period, especially of Overo breeding, is highly likely to be affected. • Other causes of colic in neonatal foals include:
 ○ Meconium retention/impaction (most common)—may be diagnosed via digital rectal examination and/or abdominal radiographs; should respond to enema administration
 ○ Congenital atresia of the gastrointestinal tract
  • Atresia coli—barium contrast radiography may be helpful for diagnosis.
  • Atresia ani—visual examination of perineum is diagnostic.
 ○ Intussusception—may be visible via abdominal ultrasonography; abdominal radiographs show an obstructive pattern.
 ○ Mesenteric volvulus
 ○ Enterocolitis—signs of systemic disease with changes noted in CBC, serum biochemistry; usually older foals (>24 hr of age)
 ○ Birth hypoxia with subsequent ileus—often other systems concurrently affected (CNS, renal)
 ○ Rupture of the urinary bladder with subsequent uroperitoneum—ultrasonography of umbilicus, urinary bladder and evaluation of peritoneal fluid are diagnostic.

CBC/BIOCHEMISTRY/URINALYSIS

Often within normal limits. It is not helpful diagnostically.

OTHER LABORATORY TESTS

PCR test to detect DNA mutation (affected horses and carriers)—whole blood or hair (with roots) can be submitted.

IMAGING

Abdominal radiographs may reveal gas distention of the cranial gastrointestinal tract, and barium contrast studies may be useful to rule out congenital atresias. However, imaging studies are rarely required to make the diagnosis.

OTHER DIAGNOSTIC PROCEDURES

Exploratory laparotomy confirms the diagnosis but is rarely indicated. The diagnosis is usually made on the basis of clinical findings (white foal of Overo breeding with severe, progressive colic).

PATHOLOGIC FINDINGS

• Post-mortem examination reveals hypoplasia of the ileum, cecum, and the ascending and descending colon to varying degrees. While the extent of grossly affected intestine is variable, the transverse and descending colon sections are typically most severely affected. Affected segments are very small (reported luminal diameters from $\frac{1}{4}$ inch to $\frac{1}{2}$ inch) and contain no ingesta. The more orad regions of the gastrointestinal tract are grossly normal but may be distended with gas and/or ingesta.
• Histologically, an absence of myenteric and submucosal ganglia characterizes the abnormal intestine; the enteric nervous system is normal in the stomach and proximal small intestine. Sections of skin show an absence of melanocytes and melanin; while the iris is typically nonpigmented, the retinas of affected foals usually contain melanin.

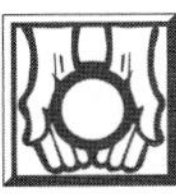

TREATMENT

LWFS is inevitably fatal with no known viable treatment options. Humane euthanasia is recommended if the syndrome is strongly suspected.

MEDICATIONS

None

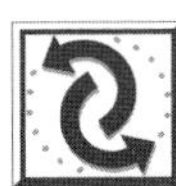

FOLLOW-UP

PREVENTION/AVOIDANCE

A PCR-based genetic test for the heterozygous carrier state is available for use in breeding stock. Although most carriers are Overo Paints, the trait has also been identified in Tobiano Paints, Thoroughbreds, American Miniature Horses, and Quarter Horses. Any horse that is a product of white-patterned horses, or itself is a white-patterned horse, is a potential carrier (including solid-colored "breeding stock" Paint horses). As LWFS is inherited as an autosomal recessive trait, the offspring of two carriers has a 1:4 chance of being affected. Carriers should either not be bred or bred only to noncarriers to avoid the production of a lethal white foal.

EXPECTED COURSE AND PROGNOSIS

Affected foals inevitably die within 48–96 hr of birth (most within 48 hr). Although surgical intervention has been attempted, no reports of successfully treated foals exist. Humane euthanasia is recommended in any case in which LWFS is strongly suspected based on clinical findings.

MISCELLANEOUS

AGE-RELATED FACTORS

Congenital syndrome—signs are seen soon after birth.

SEE ALSO

• Meconium retention • Colic in foals

ABBREVIATIONS

• APH = American Paint Horse • EDNRB = endothelin-B receptor • LWFS = lethal white foal syndrome • PCR = polymerase chain reaction

Suggested Reading

Parry NMA. Overo lethal white foal syndrome. Comp Contin Ed Pract Vet 2005;27:945–950.

Author Teresa A. Burns
Consulting Editor Margaret C. Mudge

LEUKOCYTOCLASTIC PASTERN VASCULITIS

BASICS

OVERVIEW

- Specific dermatitis that affects the lateral and medial aspects of nonpigmented lower limbs of horses at pasture
- The condition is most likely an immune-mediated disorder, although the exact etiology has not been clarified.

SIGNALMENT

- No sex or breed predilections, but observed in adults and the majority of cases occur in horses with nonpigmented lower limbs; occurrence in pigmented limbs is rare.
- There may be a genetic predisposition; in some farms with many related horses the incidence of this normally sporadic disease can be much higher.

SIGNS

- Often multiple and reasonably well-demarcated skin lesions with oozing and erythema. Crusting erosions and superficial ulcerations develop almost exclusively on the lateral and medial aspects of the pastern, the fetlock, and the canon.
- Lesions are (very) painful but not pruritic.
- Sometimes the lesions coalesce and affect larger, less well-defined areas.
- The affected limb(s) is often significantly edematous.

CAUSES AND RISK FACTORS

- Horses at summer pasture; most likely, grass plays a significant etiologic role either by ingestion or direct contact.
- Photoexacerbation may be a factor.
- Restriction of the lesions to nonpigmented lower limbs suggests a role of direct sunlight (ultraviolet radiation) in the pathogenesis. However, horses with a known history of leucocytoclastic pastern vasculitis do not show lesions when kept in a paddock instead of at pasture.

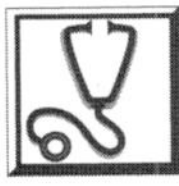

DIAGNOSIS

DIFFERENTIAL DIAGNOSIS

- Any inflammatory dermatosis of the nonpigmented lower limb including “scratches” or “greasy heel,” although all of these disorders are almost always located on the palmar/plantar aspect of the lower limb
- Photosensitization mostly affects all white parts of the horse (limbs, nose, etc.); a careful history will eliminate plant etiology and a check on liver function is indicated.

CBC/BIOCHEMISTRY/URINALYSIS

No significant abnormalities in blood or urine

OTHER LABORATORY TESTS

None

IMAGING

None

OTHER DIAGNOSTIC PROCEDURES

Skin biopsy under local anesthesia; the lesions are often extremely painful and heavy sedation is necessary before a local anesthesia can be administered (regional blocks can be effective, but sometimes disappointing)

PATHOLOGICAL FINDINGS

Perivascular edema and (peri)vascular lymphohistiocytic inflammation in the superficial dermis with very localized vascular necrosis and thrombosis

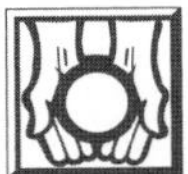

TREATMENT

- Remove from pasture and limit exposure to strong sunshine.
- Topical treatment is of limited value and may be dangerous as these patients are very painful.
- Clipping the affected areas may reveal the full extent of the disorder but is not advisable as secondary infections may occur as result of clipping; healing is probably no faster than without clipping.

MEDICATIONS

DRUG(S)

- Prednisolone (1 mg/kg PO q24h), to be given between 7:00 and 9:00 A.M.
- In severely affected limbs with significant edema, antimicrobials (e.g., trimethoprim sulfa 30 mg/kg q12h) may be helpful.

CONTRAINDICATIONS/POSSIBLE INTERACTIONS

In cases with a history of laminitis, corticosteroids should be used with care.

FOLLOW-UP

PATIENT MONITORING

- If horses with lesions are not removed from pasture, lesions will deteriorate and the horse eventually will become lame.
- Significant improvement occurs within 2 weeks following stabling and treatment with corticosteroids.

PREVENTION/AVOIDANCE

- Horses known to have this problem should preferably not be at pasture (at least during day time) in subsequent years.
- Bandaging the horse may prevent or limit the severity of the condition.

POSSIBLE COMPLICATIONS

Lameness may occur in severe cases.

EXPECTED COURSE AND PROGNOSIS

If vulnerable horses are not at pasture but stabled or in a paddock, they do not show the symptoms; this makes direct sunlight as a primary cause less likely.

MISCELLANEOUS

ASSOCIATED CONDITIONS

Not known

AGE-RELATED FACTORS

Only recognized in adult horses; very rarely in youngsters and never in foals

ZOONOTIC POTENTIAL

Nil

PREGNANCY

Not known

SEE ALSO

- Photosensitization
- Greasy heel

Suggested Reading

Stannard A. Pastern leucocytoclastic vasculitis. Vet Dermatol 2000;11:217–220.

Authors Marianne M. Sloet van Oldruitenborgh-Oosterbaan
Consulting Editor Gwendolen Lorch

LEUKOENCEPHALOMALACIA

BASICS

DEFINITION

A generally fatal, rapidly progressing neurologic disease caused by ingestion of fumonisin mycotoxin and characterized by liquefactive necrosis of subcortical white matter of the cerebral hemispheres. Fumonisin B_1 is the most abundant fumonisin in corn naturally infected with *Fusarium verticillioides.*

PATHOPHYSIOLOGY

Fumonisin mycotoxins interfere with sphingolipid metabolism, resulting in damage to the vascular endothelium of the brain and, with some animals, in hepatocellular necrosis and vacuolization.

SYSTEMS AFFECTED

- CNS—damage to vascular endothelium
- Hepatobiliary—pathogenesis not definitively known
- An association has been detected among experimentally induced fumonisin neurologic disease and decreased cardiovascular function in horses.

GENETICS

N/A

INCIDENCE/PREVALENCE

• Sporadic but one of the most common equine toxicoses • Worldwide, most often in humid climates after a dry summer and wet harvest season • Outbreaks are seasonal, most occurring from fall through early spring • Although variable, 15%–25% or more of horses in a group can be affected.

SIGNALMENT

• Affects horses and other equids • Mature horses appear most susceptible.

SIGNS

Neurologic Syndrome

• Anorexia • Depression, with little response to stimuli
• Frantic behavior such as head pressing, agitation, and hyperexcitability • Progressive ataxia and proprioceptive defects • Delirium • Blindness
• Aimless wandering; tendency to lean to one side
• Eventual recumbency • Coma • Body temperature generally normal • Death from 12 hours to as long as 1 week after onset of signs

Hepatotoxic Syndrome

• Occurs occasionally and may occur concurrently with neurologic syndrome • Icterus • Swelling of the lips and nose • Petechiae in mucous membranes • Lowered head • Reluctance to move • Abdominal breathing
• Cyanosis • Hemoglobinuria • Death within hours to a few days

CAUSES

Ingestion of corn products contaminated (>5 ppm) with fumonisin mycotoxins, especially fumonisin B_1 (FB1), which are produced by *F. verticillioides* (synonym *F. moniliforme*) and *F. proliferatum* molds growing on corn.

RISK FACTORS

• Fumonisins are produced in corn during hot, dry weather at pollination, and increase when temperature and moisture remain high into harvest resulting in contaminated corn products used for horse feed.
• Corn screenings contain small, shrunken, and broken kernels— often heavily contaminated with fumonisin. • Development of disease depends on fumonisin concentration in feed and duration of exposure. • Death may result from the ingestion of 10 ppm for 30 days. • Onset of clinical disease generally occurs 2–9 weeks after start of continuous consumption of fumonisin-containing feeds.

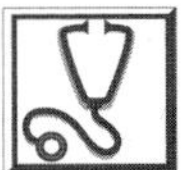

DIAGNOSIS

DIFFERENTIAL DIAGNOSIS

• Rabies • Equine encephalomyelitis
• Hepatoencephalopathy • Head trauma • Bacterial meningoencephalitis • Pyrrolizidine alkaloid hepatotoxicosis • Aflatoxicosis

CBC/BIOCHEMISTRY/URINALYSIS

• Inconsistent parameters between affected horses
• Anemia may occur • Variable WBC counts • Total bilirubin often is elevated with hepatotoxicosis, especially with icterus • Elevations of GGT and AST vary with amount of liver damage
• CSF may be normal but often shows elevated total protein and neutrophils. Horses with experimentally induced neurologic disease had high CSF protein, albumin, IgG concentrations, and albumin quotients.

OTHER LABORATORY TESTS

• Feed analysis for fumonisin (FB_1); >5 ppm of FB_1, is significant; may contain 40–100 ppm. • Alteration of the sphinganine:sphingosine ratio in serum or tissues—consistent with fumonisin ingestion.

PATHOLOGIC FINDINGS

• The primary lesions consist of softening and liquefactive necrosis, chiefly of the white matter of the cerebrum. • Massive softening of the interior of the hemispheres may create large cavitations of liquefactive necrosis. • Microscopically, liquefaction and proliferation of macrophages in response to the necrosis are seen.

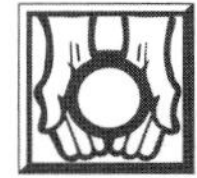

TREATMENT

APPROPRIATE HEALTH CARE

• Horses with neurologic signs usually die or are euthanized. • When clinical signs appear, significant and irreversible cerebral necrosis may be present, therapy may be an option in selected clinical cases.

NURSING CARE

• Supportive therapy—tube feeding and PO and IV fluids for rehydration • Sedate excited horses to prevent injury to themselves and caregivers. • Oral activated charcoal with saline cathartic may help to eliminate toxin already in GI tract.

DIET

Immediately ELIMINATE feeds suspected of contamination with fumonisin.

MEDICATIONS

DRUGS OF CHOICE

No specific antidote.

FOLLOW-UP

PATIENT MONITORING

• Continue supportive care. • Monitor for progression or remission of neurologic signs.

CLIENT EDUCATION/PREVENTION/ AVOIDANCE

• Inform clients of risk of using corn-based feeds, specifically containing corn screenings or moldy feeds.
• Inform clients of risk in years with drought stress during growing season and periods of high moisture at harvest. • Feed containing corn needs to be kept dry and protected from moisture when stored to prevent levels of fumonisins from increasing. • Corn and corn by-products used in horse feed should contain <5 ppm fumonisins and comprise no more than 20% of the dry weight of the total ration. • Do not use corn screenings in horse feed.

POSSIBLE COMPLICATIONS

Neurologic deficits may remain if horses recover.

EXPECTED COURSE AND PROGNOSIS

• Treatment of horses with significant neurologic signs rarely is successful; death generally occurs from 12 hours to 1 week after onset of signs, regardless of treatment. • Euthanasia of advanced cases often is advised.

MISCELLANEOUS

ASSOCIATED CONDITIONS

Corn infected with *Fusarium* spp. molds may contain DON, but feeds with ≤14 ppm have no effect on horses.

SYNONYMS

• Corn stalk poisoning • Fumonisin toxicosis • Moldy corn poisoning • Equine leukoencephalomalacia
• *Fusarium verticillioides* (synonym *F. moniliforme*)

ABBREVIATIONS

• AST = aspartate transaminase • CSF = cerebrospinal fluid • DON = deoxynivalenol, vomitoxin • GGT = γ-glutamyltransferase • GI = gastrointestinal

Suggested Reading

Foreman JH, Constable PD, Waggoner AL, et al. Neurologic abnormalities and cerebrospinal fluid changes in horses administered fumonisin B1 intravenously.
J Vet Intern Med 2004;18:223–230.

McCue PM. Equine leukoencephalomalacia. Compend Contin Educ Pract Vet 1989;11:646.

Smith GW, Constable PD, Foreman JH, et al. Cardiovascular changes associated with intravenous administration of fumonisin B1 in horses. Am J Vet Res 2002;63:538–545.

Uhlinger C. Leukoencephalomalacia. Vet Clin North Am Equine Pract 1997;13:13.

Author Steven T. Grubbs
Consulting Editor Caroline N. Hahn

LINEAR KERATOSIS AND LINEAR ALOPECIA

BASICS

OVERVIEW

Relatively uncommon and poorly understood diseases. These diseases have classic clinical and histologic presentations. Both are characterized by linear, vertically oriented areas of hyperkeratosis and/or alopecia. They can coexist in some horses, suggesting the possibility of variable presentations of the disease or a progression of keratosis to alopecia.

SIGNALMENT

- Affects all ages and breeds of horses; however, most horses develop lesions between 6 mo and 5 years of age.
- Quarter Horses and Thoroughbreds are thought to be predisposed.
- Rarely encountered in pony breeds
- Equal distribution exists between males and females.

SIGNS

- Linear keratosis are small areas of asymptomatic, one or multiple, unilateral, linear, vertically orientated bands of hyperkeratotic papules that progress to marked hyperkeratosis and alopecia. The lesions vary from 0.25 to 3.5 cm in width and from 5 to 70 cm in length. Lesions are most common on the neck, shoulder, lateral thorax, and hip. The lesions from this initial stage may resemble dermatophytosis. Gradual replacement of the prominent hyperkeratosis with permanent partial to complete alopecia may ensue. This disease is NOT associated with pain, pruritus, or evidence of an inflammatory reaction.
- Linear alopecia is a gradual development of one or more annular areas of alopecia usually in a linear, vertically orientated configuration. One to multiple areas may be present. Varying degrees of scaling or crusting are present. The lesions are typically 2–10 mm in width and vary in length from a few centimeters to over 1 m. Common locations are the neck, shoulder, lateral thorax, and hip.
- The appearance of typical vertical lesions suggests some external factor that "dripped" down the skin surface, causing the lesion.
- Atypical lesions of linear alopecia can appear as multifocal and confined to a localized region with no evidence of a linearization.
- In both clinical presentations, affected horses are otherwise healthy.

CAUSES AND RISK FACTORS

The etiopathogenesis of linear alopecia is thought to be an immunological attack by T lymphocytes on the follicular wall, with the inciting cause unknown. The gross linear configurations of the lesions do not follow blood or lymphatic vessels, nerves, or dermatomes.

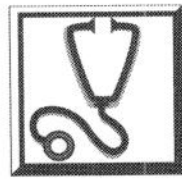

DIAGNOSIS

DIFFERENTIAL DIAGNOSIS

- Diagnosis is often made from clinical appearance and rule-out of differentials. Confirmation of clinical diagnosis is obtained from histopathology.
- Linear epidermal nevus is very hyperkeratotic and has a "rough appearance."
- Contact reaction from topical application of medication or chemical solution
- Occult sarcoid
- Dermatophilosis
- Early dermatophytosis
- Alopecia from skin scald secondary to wound discharge
- Linear alopecia must be differentiated from linear trauma (scratches, whip marks, etc.).

CBC/BIOCHEMISTRY/URINALYSIS

Not necessary

OTHER LABORATORY TESTS

N/A

IMAGING

N/A

OTHER DIAGNOSTIC PROCEDURES

- Skin biopsy for histopathology will confirm the diagnosis. Do NOT surgically prepare the site before using a 4- to 6-mm punch biopsy. Preservation of the lesion surface is imperative. Changes may be subtle, and unless the pathologist is familiar with this type of process, important changes may overlooked.
- Skin cytology obtained from skin scrapes and crusts may help rule out dermatophilosis. Skin scrapes will be negative for microorganisms and parasites with both linear keratosis and alopecia.
- A DTM culture of the hair and scale or crust is the gold standard to rule out dermatophytosis.

PATHOLOGICAL FINDINGS

- Linear keratosis histopathological findings are of a regular or irregular epidermal hyperplasia in association with marked compact hyperkeratosis. Mild lymphohistocytic superficial perivascular dermatitis is possible.
- Linear alopecia histopathological findings are an infiltrative lymphocytic mural folliculitis with subsequent damage to the wall and possibly sebaceous glands. Mild to severe edema of the follicular walls can be present. In well-developed or older lesions, epithelioid cells and giant cells can infiltrate the outer root sheath of affected follicles. Varying degrees of perivascular eosinophilic infiltration may also be present. In end-stage disease, complete follicular destruction is present resulting in permanent nonreversible alopecia.

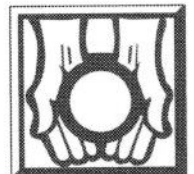

TREATMENT

- Owners should be aware of no cure.
- Linear keartosis responds poorly to treatment.
- Topical keratoplastic and keratolytic shampoos (sulfur–salicylic acid containing shampoos) or 50% propylene glycol can be used q3–4days to reduce hyperkeratosis but must be continued for life.
- As neither condition is life-threatening or symptomatic, observation without treatment is acceptable.

MEDICATIONS

DRUG(S) OF CHOICE

Anecdotal reports of topical or systemic corticosteroid therapy slowing the progression of linear alopecia in the acute lesions have been reported; however, recurrence is probable.

CONTRAINDICATIONS/POSSIBLE INTERACTIONS

N/A

FOLLOW-UP

PATIENT MONITORING

Not necessary

PREVENTION/AVOIDANCE

Advise owner of potential hereditary nature of disease; therefore, removal from breeding stock should be considered.

POSSIBLE COMPLICATIONS

N/A

EXPECTED COURSE AND PROGNOSIS

- Condition may be progressive and self-limiting.
- Prognosis for resolution is poor as lesions persist with no tendency for spontaneous regression.

MISCELLANEOUS

ASSOCIATED CONDITIONS, AGE-RELATED FACTORS, ZOONOTIC POTENTIAL, PREGNANCY

N/A

SEE ALSO

- Sarcoid
- Dermatophilosis

ABBREVIATION

- DTM = dermatophyte test medium

Suggested Reading

Scott DW, Miller WH Jr. Equine Dermatology. St. Louis: Saunders, 2003:582

von Tscharner C, Kunkle GA, Yager JA; Stannard's illustrated equine dermatology notes. Alopecia in the horse—an overview. Vet Dermatol 2000;11:193–195.

Author Gwendolen Lorch

Consulting Editor Gwendolen Lorch

LOCOMOTOR STEREOTYPIC BEHAVIORS

BASICS

DEFINITION

• A stereotypy is as an invariant, repetitive pattern of movement with no apparent purpose.
• It arises from a normal maintenance behavior (e.g., walking), but it is performed excessively and out of context, to the exclusion of normal behaviors.
• Performance of the stereotypy usually interferes with the animal's well-being.
• Equine locomotor stereotypies include head shaking, swinging, or bobbing; stall walking; weaving; fence running; and stall kicking.

PATHOPHYSIOLOGY

• Unclear
• Proposed mechanisms implicate serotonergic and dopaminergic dysfunction; the exact contribution of each system is undetermined.
• Endogenous endorphin concentrations are suspected to be aberrant among horses engaging in stereotypic behaviors with a self-injurious component, such as self-mutilation or wall kicking.

SYSTEMS AFFECTED

• Behavioral—may interfere with expression of normal maintenance behaviors or with performance of learned responses
• CNS—Proposed causes involve serotonergic, dopaminergic, or endogenous opioid system abnormalities at the gross anatomic or molecular level.
• Musculoskeletal—uneven hoof wear or muscle development, or decreased performance if the behavior is performed to the point of fatigue or self-injury

GENETICS

A genetic component is suspected, but the precise contribution of inheritance has not been determined.

INCIDENCE/PREVALENCE

Reported as low as 2% and as high 7.32% depending on breed and stereotypy

GEOGRAPHIC DISTRIBUTION

Worldwide

SIGNALMENT

• No age or sex predilection
• Warmbloods and Thoroughbreds may be at increased risk of developing stereotypic behaviors.
• Onset may be more common at the time of social maturity (≅4–5 years) but can occur at any age.

SIGNS

General Comments

• Time spent performing the behavior varies. The behaviors are often elicited by increased emotional arousal or social stimulation—being led to and from barns or pastures, toward or away from herdmates; or in anticipation of pleasurable experiences (e.g., feeding time). The intensity of a stereotypy may be exaggerated during situations of increased emotional arousal.
• Head shaking, swinging, or bobbing—side to side, circular, or up-and-down motions of the head, neck, or both when the horse is at rest, moving at liberty, or under saddle
• Stall walking—circular pacing when confined to a stall. The horse may circle in one or both directions, when severe.
• Weaving—rhythmic stepping in place with the front limbs, alternating from foot to foot, usually accompanied by a side-to-side swaying of the head and neck. The hindlimbs also may march, in which case the foot placing corresponds to a trot, without any moment of suspension.
• Fence running—the horse walks, trots, or canters in a repetitive pattern along a fence line or before a gate, with the distance traveled and the location and features of the turns being invariant.
• Stall kicking—the horse repetitively strikes the stall walls, with one or both hind legs, with a hoof, the plantar aspect of the metatarsus, or the tarsometatarsal joint.

Historical

• Owners may report a gradual onset or an inciting event after which the behavior was seen or became more noticeable.
• Information on related horses (e.g., dam, or full- or half-siblings) sometimes reveals other affected individuals.

Physical Examination Findings

Unremarkable, except for lesions from self-injurious behavior or uneven shoe or hoof wear or muscle development secondary to increased ambulation

CAUSES

• Environments or management practices that inhibit expression of normal behaviors
• An association between stereotypies and dysregulation of neurotransmitter systems and functions is suspected.

RISK FACTORS

Offspring of affected horses and dominant mares may be at a higher risk.

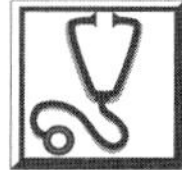

DIAGNOSIS

DIFFERENTIAL DIAGNOSIS

• Stall kicking—any painful medical condition (e.g., colic, nephroliths) may cause a horse to strike with or toward the affected area.
• Do not confuse anxiety specific to separation from herdmates with a locomotor stereotypy, unless the signs fit the diagnostic criteria.
• Head shaking—rule out trigeminal neuritis, photophobia, orodental disease, auricular disease, guttural pouch and tracheopharyngeal disease, poor horsemanship or myopathies (if the behavior occurs while under saddle or in harness), and response to airborne allergens.
• A learned response reinforced by a reward (e.g., a horse bangs the stall door at feeding time and is fed first by the caretaker; thus, door banging occurs only at feeding time).

CBC/BIOCHEMISTRY/URINALYSIS

Ancillary tests to rule out medical problems; results should be unremarkable if no underlying disease is present.

OTHER LABORATORY TESTS

Aggression associated with equine hypothyroidism has been reported; if other clinical signs suggest the possibility of hypothyroidism in a horse exhibiting self-injurious stereotypies, the clinician may consider assessing thyroid function of the horse.

IMAGING

Ultrasonic examination of the urogenital tract, if signs are suggestive of reproductive abnormalities

OTHER DIAGNOSTIC PROCEDURES

Endoscopy of the oropharynx, larynx, and related structures may be indicated to rule out medical problems in headshaking horses.

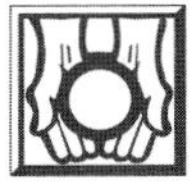

TREATMENT

AIMS OF TREATMENT

• Ethologically based approaches address behavioral needs.
• Devices and management measures that focus on preventing performance of the behavior without addressing the psychologic well-being of the horse do not constitute treatment. Anti-weaving stall doors prevent neck swaying, but the horse will continue to march with its feet. Chains on the horse's pasterns may temporarily decrease kicking, but the anxiety level may increase from an inability to kick and may express itself in a different way. Horses have rearranged obstacles placed on the stall floor, such as tires, in order to continue stall walking.

APPROPRIATE HEALTH CARE

• Treatment plan focuses on management practices that allow the horse to express a wider range of normal behaviors while decreasing confinement, isolation, and emotional arousal.
• Manage as an outpatient.
• Recommended modifications in management practices—increased turnout time, preferably with a compatible companion; increased grazing time; increased opportunities for social contact within the confines of the stall.
• Rubber mats or padding on stall floors and walls decrease wear and tear on the stall and the horse's feet and extremities.
• Stall toys can be useful with young horses. Toys that release food when moved about by the horse can help to direct locomotive patterns into an activity that resembles the walk-and-nibble sequence of a grazing

horse. Food dispensed this way gets mixed with the bedding. This problem can be solved by using the device in a small, dirt-floored paddock if available.

- Placing hay in nested hay bags can approximate grazing. Before pulling the drawstring tight, a second and a third bag are placed inside the first, always with some hay between the added hay bags. Two or three nested bags of hay can be hung at a safe height in different corners of the stall.

NURSING CARE N/A

ACTIVITY

Increase grazing, turnout, and aerobic activity.

DIET

Increased roughage:concentrate ratio in feed and replacement of sweet feed (or other highly palatable grain) with a complete pelleted or extruded feed.

CLIENT EDUCATION

- Caution owners against reinforcing undesirable, repetitive behaviors.
- Rewards may promote stereotypic behaviors.
- Scientific evidence does not support that stereotypies cause unthriftiness.

SURGICAL CONSIDERATIONS N/A

MEDICATIONS

DRUGS OF CHOICE

- Use of medications is limited by drug's cost and/or its frequency and route of administration and that none are approved for use in horses for these problems.
- Opioid antagonists, such as naltrexone and naloxone, may have a role in treatment of self-injurious stereotypies (e.g., self-mutilation) and may help in cases of stall kicking, but their short half-life, cost, and route of administration (IV) make currently available forms impractical for the long-term treatment.
- Tricyclic antidepressants and selective serotonin-reuptake inhibitors have been used to treat obsessive-compulsive disorders in humans and small animals and may have a place in treatment of locomotor stereotypies in horses. Such drugs include amitriptyline, clomipramine, doxepin, fluoxetine, and imipramine. Few (if any) uses of these drugs in horses are reported. There is a single case report of a mare that exhibited a reduction of weaving behavior (57% improvement over baseline in stressful situations) when treated with paroxetine at 0.5 mg/kg PO q24h.
- Other anxiolytics may help, but their use in treatment of stereotypies is underexplored.
- Doxepin, a tricyclic antidepressant, and selegiline, a monoamine oxidase inhibitor, are specifically banned in competition horses (as may be the use of all psychotropic drugs). Imipramine can induce sedation, erection, and masturbation.
- Individual response to drugs varies greatly.

CONTRAINDICATIONS

- Tricyclics have anticholinergic and antihistaminic properties; in humans, their use is contraindicated in patients receiving thyroxine supplementation or in cases of cardiac conduction abnormalities, glaucoma, seizures, and urinary and fecal retention. Horses with a history of recurrent ileus may be at higher risk of an adverse reaction.
- Concurrent hepatic or renal disease warrants adjustment of starting dosages and careful monitoring of serum chemistry values and clinical signs.

PRECAUTIONS

- Owners should be aware that use of psychotropic medication constitutes experimental and off-label use.
- Owners should sign an informed consent form and receive an explanation (preferably in writing) of the medication, selection rationale, expected benefits, and possible side effects.
- CBC and serum chemistry panel are recommended before initiating drug therapy and repeated approximately 6 weeks later.
- Cardiac conduction abnormalities are a contraindication for use of tricyclic antidepressants, which are arrhythmogenic in humans and companion animals and may be so in horses.
- Laboratory diagnostics can be repeated 6 weeks after start of medication or whenever clinical signs warrant.

POSSIBLE INTERACTIONS

- Phenothiazines may potentiate the effect of buspirone through inhibition of dopaminergic function.
- Combinations of tricyclics and serotonin-reuptake inhibitors may be synergistic, so initial dosages should be lowered if the two drug classes are used together.

ALTERNATIVE DRUGS

N/A

FOLLOW-UP

PATIENT MONITORING

- Drug dosages may need adjustment, so weekly follow-up is recommended. If long-term use of medication is intended, semiannual or annual monitoring of CBC and serum chemistry is recommended.
- Monitor owner compliance regarding management recommendations. Intervals for follow-up vary depending on the severity of the problem.

PREVENTION/AVOIDANCE

See Aims of Treatment and Appropriate Health Care.

POSSIBLE COMPLICATIONS

Any situations that may increase stress and anxiety may exacerbate locomotor stereotypies.

EXPECTED COURSE AND PROGNOSIS

Very little is known about the actual neurochemical and genetic basis of stereotypic disorders in horses. Treatment is aimed at improving welfare and minimizing the display of the behaviors, but owners must be cautioned that complete elimination cannot be guaranteed.

MISCELLANEOUS

ASSOCIATED CONDITIONS

- Lameness
- Impaired performance
- If stereotypies lead to self-injury, it can become a welfare issue.

AGE RELATED FACTORS

N/A

ZOONOTIC POTENTIAL

N/A

PREGNANCY

- Avoid the above mentioned drugs during pregnancy.
- Use of tricyclics is contraindicated in pregnant individuals.

SYNONYMS

- Compulsive disorders
- Obsessive-compulsive disorders
- Stable vices
- Stereotypies

SEE ALSO

- Oral stereotypic behaviors
- Self-mutilation

Suggested Reading

Crowell-Davis SL, Murray T. Veterinary Psychopharmacology. Ames, IA: Blackwell Publishing, 2006.

Dallmeyer BS, et al. Theriogenology question of the month. J Am Vet Med Assoc 2006;229:511–513

Dodman NH, Normile JA, Shuster L, Rand W. Equine self-mutilation syndrome (57 cases). J Am Vet Med Assoc 1994;204:1219–1223.

Dodman NH, Shuster L, Court MH, Patel J. Use of a narcotic antagonist (nalmefene) to suppress self-mutilative behavior in a stallion. J Am Vet Med Assoc 1988;192:1585–1587.

McDonnell SM. Is it psychological, physical, or both? AAEP Proc 2005;51:231–238.

McGreevy P. Equine Behavior: A Guide for Veterinarians and Equine Scientists. Sydney: Saunders, 2004.

Mills DS, et al. Weaving, headshaking, cribbing, and other stereotypies. AAEP Proc 2005;51:220–230.

Valentine BA. Diagnosis and treatment of equine polysaccharide storage myopathy. J Equine Vet Sci 2005;25:52–61.

Author Soraya V. Juarbe-Díaz

Consulting Editors Victoria L. Voith and Daniel Q. Estep

LUNGWORM—PARASITIC BRONCHITIS AND PNEUMONIA

BASICS

OVERVIEW

The development of an inflammatory response in the airways and lung parenchyma due to an infection with the lungworm *Dictyocaulus arnfieldi.*

SIGNALMENT

- Donkeys and mules are most likely to harbor patent lungworm infections.
- There is no breed or sex predilection.
- All ages can be affected, but the prepatent period for *D. arnfieldi* is 6 weeks; therefore, disease is less likely in very young foals.

SIGNS

- Chronic, nonprogressive cough that is unresponsive to antibiotic or anti-inflammatory therapy.
- An elevated respiratory rate and bilateral nasal discharge may also be associated with lungworm infection.
- Donkeys and mules do not typically exhibit clinical signs of infection.

CAUSES AND RISK FACTORS

- Ingestion of infective larvae of *D. arnfeldi* from contaminated pasture.
- Horses kept on green or irrigated pastures that concurrently or previously contained donkeys or mules.
- Infections usually occur during warm, wet weather in temperate climates.

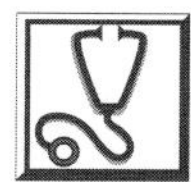

DIAGNOSIS

DIFFERENTIAL DIAGNOSIS

- Heaves, inflammatory airway disease, tumor or polyp in the airway, tracheobronchial foreign body, chronic bacterial pneumonia, pulmonary abscess, postviral airway hyperreactivity. Signs are often indistinguishable from those associated with heaves.
- Audible wheezes and crackles may be evident during thoracic auscultation providing evidence of lower airway involvement.

CBC/BIOCHEMISTRY/URINALYSIS

- Complete blood count— peripheral eosinophilia is variable but if present is strongly suggestive of a parasitic infection.
- Routine biochemistry and urinalysis are unremarkable.

OTHER LABORATORY TESTS

The definitive diagnosis is established with the identification of larvae in a TTA or identification of larvae recovered from feces using the modified Baermann technique. The TTA fluid can be concentrated in a cytospin to improve the likelihood of finding larvae. Cytologic examination of the TTA will reveal a mixed inflammatory response with eosinophilia. Horses will likely be negative for larvae using the modified Baermann technique but co-pastured donkeys should be tested and will likely be positive.

IMAGING

Thoracic radiography can be useful to rule out chronic bacterial pneumonia or pulmonary abscesses.

OTHER DIAGNOSTIC PROCEDURES

Endoscopy may reveal an increase in mucus production in the airways. Rarely, an adult worm may be seen.

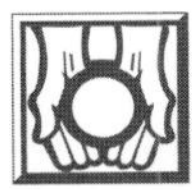

TREATMENT

Lungworm infection in the horse can be successfully treated with anthelmintic therapy and removal of horses from the contaminated pasture.

MEDICATIONS

DRUG(S) OF CHOICE

- Ivermectin (200 μg/kg PO) and moxidectin (200 μg/kg PO) have been confirmed to be highly effective against the mature and larval forms of *D. arnfeldi.* Moxidectin is highly lipophilic and persists in the tissues far longer than ivermectin. Moxidectin (400 μg/kg) was found to be 99.9% effective in treating lungworm infections in donkeys.
- Larvicidal doses of fenbendazole (10 mg/kg) daily for 5 consecutive days would be a reasonable alternate drug choice.

CONTRAINDICATIONS/POSSIBLE INTERACTIONS

N/A

FOLLOW-UP

PATIENT MONITORING

- If donkeys are treated, then repeating the modified Baermann technique on feces will allow the practitioner to monitor the efficacy of therapy.
- Horses can be monitored for the resolution of clinical signs.

PREVENTION/AVOIDANCE

Do not pasture horses with donkeys that are not on a helminth control program.

EXPECTED COURSE AND PROGNOSIS

Lungworm infection in the horse has an excellent prognosis for full recovery post-treatment. Resolution of clinical signs should be seen in 7–10 days after treatment.

MISCELLANEOUS

ABBREVIATION

- TTA = transtracheal aspirate

Suggested Reading

Ainsworth DM, Hackett RP. Equine lungworms. Disorders of the respiratory system. In: Reed, SM, Bayly, WM, Sellon, DC, Ed. Equine Internal Medicine. Second edition. St-Louis: Saunders, 2004, 337–338.

Dolente, B. Equine Lungworms. In: Smith, BP, Ed. Large Animal Internal Medicine. St. Louis: Mosby, 2002:500–504.

Author Joie L. Watson

Consulting Editor Daniel Jean

LYME DISEASE

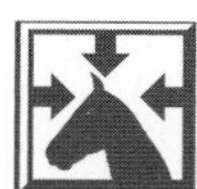

BASICS

DEFINITION

• Lyme disease is caused by the spirochete *Borrelia burgdorferi.* It is the most frequent tick-borne disease of humans in the United States and has been reported in cats, dogs, cattle, and horses. Serologic surveys indicate the disease is endemic in various regions of the United States and United Kingdom; however, only isolated clinical cases of Lyme disease in horses have been documented.
• Definitive diagnosis in horses is difficult and clinical diagnosis is usually presumptive, based on clinical signs, a history of tick exposure in an endemic region, supportive serology, PCR testing, elimination of other possible causes, and response to treatment.
• Shifting lameness and behavioral changes are the most common presenting complaints. Associated clinical signs include polyarthritis, limb edema, stiffness, hyperesthesia, lethargy, unwillingness to work, and low-grade fever. Uveitis and neurologic disease have been described in a pony and horse, and there is a possibility that multiorgan involvement and transplacental transmission may occur.

PATHOPHYSIOLOGY

• The pathogenesis is not completely understood. • The ticks become infected with *B. burgdorferi* with their first blood meal from an infected host. The spirochete penetrates the gut epithelium and invades the salivary gland where it resides until transmission. *B. burgdorferi* cause a localized skin infection after the tick has been feeding for 24 hours. A transient bacteremia may follow, disseminating the spirochete. • Post-mortem findings from experimentally infected ponies suggest a possible migration of the organism through connective, perineural, and perivascular tissues in the skin, fascia, muscle, and synovial membrane. It is currently unknown how *B. burgdorferi* induces the pathological changes and subsequent clinical signs, but it is likely to be secondary to an inflammatory reaction against the borrelial antigen. The differences in host reaction to the presence of the organism may explain the relatively few infected horses that develop clinical signs. • Experimental infection of ponies resulted in detectable antibody levels at 5–6 weeks and 3–4 months after tick infection; the KELA units were 200–300. Infected ponies became positive on WB at 10–12 weeks.

SYSTEMS AFFECTED

• Musculoskeletal—polyarthritis, stiffness, lameness • Hemic/lymphatic/immune—distal limb edema • Ophthalmic—uveitis
• Nervous—encephalitis, meningitis

INCIDENCE/PREVALENCE

B. burgdorferi has a worldwide distribution in humans, with reports of disease in horses limited to the United States and the United Kingdom. Seroprevalence from horses in the United States has ranged from <1% in nonendemic areas to 75% in endemic areas.

SIGNALMENT

Nonspecific

SIGNS

• Suspected clinical cases of Lyme disease have been reported only from endemic areas. The common reported clinical findings are shifting lameness, behavioral changes, arthritis, polyarthritis, stiffness, hyperesthesia, distal limb edema, low-grade fever, and lethargy. It has been proposed that the low-grade fever and distal limb edema may be a result of *Anaplasma phagocytophilia* infection rather than *B. burgdorferi* as many ticks are infected with both organisms. • The lameness can be associated with joint or periarticular pain without swelling, lasting hours to a few days in each location; or it can be overt arthritis, with swelling of one or more joints, lasting days to a few weeks and often reoccurring. Reoccurring episodes can lead to chronic inflammatory arthritis. • Behavior changes may be seen with reluctance to work and lethargy. • Panuveitis with the clinical signs of blepharospasm, photophobia, aqueous flare, hypopyon, and miosis has been reported in one pony. This may reoccur, resulting in chronic sequelae associated with recurrent uveitis. • Neurologic diseases with clinical signs relating to meningitis and encephalitis and multiorgan system involvement with clinical signs relating to the organ systems involved have been reported but are extremely rare. • *B. burgdorferi* have been isolated from the kidney, liver, and brain of two foals and a yearling in which transplacental transmission was suspected to have occurred; the clinical significance of the findings is questionable.

CAUSES

• *B. burgdorferi* is maintained in a 2-year enzootic lifecycle with three stages. The usual life cycle for *B. burgdorferi* involves an *Ixodes* tick as the vector and a small mammal as the intermediate host for the larval and nymph stages, with a deer as the final host for the adult. The deer and white footed mouse (*Peromyscus leucopus*) are the most common mammals involved in maintaining the life cycle. *Ixodes pacificus* (Western black-legged tick) is the principal vector for *B. burgdorferi* in the western United States and *I. scapularis* (black-legged tick or deer tick) is the principal vector in the upper midwestern and eastern United States. • The tick can become infected at any stage of the lifecycle by feeding on an infected small mammalian host. In most cases, transmission of *B. burgdorferi* usually occurs only after at least 24 hours of feeding. It is not known whether the larva or nymph stages can transmit *B. burgdorferi* to the horse.

RISK FACTORS

Contact with *Ixodes* ticks in Lyme endemic areas. Contact transmission has not been reported between horses.

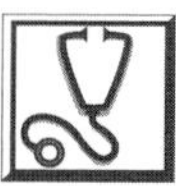

DIAGNOSIS

DIFFERENTIAL DIAGNOSIS

• Lyme arthritis should be differentiated from infectious causes of arthritis by synovial fluid cytology and culture. Traumatic causes of arthritis can be differentiated by history, radiographic findings, scintigraphy, and lack of response to antibiotic therapy. Immune-mediated causes of arthritis can be differentiated on the presence of other systemic clinical signs, synovial fluid cytology, synovial biopsy, and laboratory data, including antinuclear antibodies, lupus erythematosus preparations, and rheumatoid arthritis factor. • Distal limb edema due to Lyme disease should be differentiated from cellulitis, vasculitis (purpura hemorrhagica, EVA, EIA, *Anaplasma phagocytophilia*), stocking up from inactivity, and systemic diseases that are immune-mediated or associated with hypoproteinemia. The presence of other physical examination findings, laboratory data, and serologic tests assist in differentiation. • Cervical vertebral malformation, the encephalitides, rabies, equine protozoal myeloencephalitis, cauda equina syndrome, spinal nematodiasis, space-occupying lesion, and equine herpes virus 1 are differentiated from the neurologic manifestation of Lyme disease by radiographs, serology, and cerebrospinal fluid analysis.
• Muscle stiffness is differentiated from polysaccharide storage myopathy, chronic intermittent rhabdomyolysis, thoracic spinous process osteoarthritis by serum biochemistry (pre and post exercise), muscle biopsies and radiographs. • Causes of uveitis, including ocular trauma and infectious agents such as *Toxoplasma, Onchocerca cervicalis, Leptospira* spp., *Streptococcus,* and viral agents, should be investigated. *Onchocerca* microfilariae and viral inclusion bodies can be found in conjunctival scraping and biopsy. Rising serum titers may be associated with *Leptospira* spp. and *Toxoplasma.*

CBC/BIOCHEMISTRY/URINALYSIS

Hematologic and biochemical analysis of blood is usually unremarkable. Serum biochemistry profile may reflect specific organ involvement.

OTHER LABORATORY TESTS

• Culture and isolation of *B. burgdorferi* are difficult and require special media. It may be possible from blood, urine, and CSF. IFA, ELISA, and WB have been used to detect *B. burgdorferi* antibodies in serum, CSF, synovial fluid, and aqueous humor.

• Horses with ELISA titers >440 KELA units have a high probability (>95%) of being infected. Horses with lower KELA units or that may have received the canine vaccine should have the disease confirmed by WB. • Positive serologic results indicate exposure to *B. burgdorferi* but do not indicate clinical disease. • False-negative results can occur in first few weeks of infection prior to seroconversion and with concurrent use of antibiotics. False-positive results may occur due to cross-reactivity with other *Borrelia* spp. • PCR has been used to detect *B. burgdorferi* DNA. PCR detection of the organism in the synovial membrane of a painful joint is indicative of active infection.

IMAGING

Radiographs are useful in assisting with the differential diagnosis of lameness and neurologic dysfunction, as well as in evaluating chronic Lyme arthritis.

DIAGNOSTIC PROCEDURES

• Synovial fluid analyses may have a neutrophilic inflammation: 10,000–25,000 neutrophils. • Synovial biopsy and histopathology with IFA or PCR • CSF analysis and WB.

PATHOLOGIC FINDINGS

Gross findings in cases with suspected Lyme disease in horses relate to the organ system involved. Joints from Lyme arthritis and polyarthritis may have a congested hyperplastic synovial membrane. Histopathology of affected tissues may show a lymphoplasmacytic infiltrate. Immunohistochemical staining and PCR may detect *B. burgdorferi* in affected tissues.

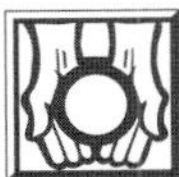

TREATMENT

APPROPRIATE HEALTH CARE

Horses with Lyme disease can be treated as outpatients.

NURSING CARE

• Polyarthritis and distal limb edema—cold hosing, supportive standing wraps
• Acupuncture may be useful in horses with hyperesthesia that do not respond to NSAIDs.

ACTIVITY

Reduced activity until clinical signs have resolved

DIET

No diet change necessary

CLIENT EDUCATION

• Examine horse after riding through bush and remove ticks with tweezers or gloves.
• Spirochetes are not transferred from the ticks until at least 24 hours of feeding has occurred.

SURGICAL CONSIDERATIONS

Synovial biopsy via arthroscopic guidance for assistance with diagnosis

MEDICATIONS

DRUG(S) OF CHOICE

• The recommended antibiotics for treatment are intravenous tetracycline (6.6 mg/kg IV q12h) or oral doxycycline (10 mg/kg PO q12h). Tetracycline for 1 week prior to starting doxycycline may provide a more rapid response. Infections are usually treated for 4 weeks. Tetracycline in experimentally infected animals resulted in elimination of the infection. Doxycycline therapy (10 mg/kg PO q24h) had inconsistent results and may inhibit the proliferation of the organism but not eliminate it. The efficacy of tetracycline may be different in chronic infections.
• Doxycycline has anti-inflammatory properties that may temporarily relieve clinical symptoms without eliminating the etiologic agent. • NSAID therapy may be used with antibiotic therapy, but can make monitoring response to treatment difficult by masking clinical signs. • Chondroprotective agents may be useful with chronic disease. • Therapy for uveitis is aimed at reducing inflammation and providing mydriasis and analgesia.

PRECAUTIONS

Colitis may occur secondary to antimicrobial therapy.

POSSIBLE INTERACTIONS

Jarisch-Herxheimer reactions have been reported in humans during the treatment of spirochetal disease. This reaction involves the exacerbation of clinical signs with antibiotic therapy and is believed to be an immune-associated reaction caused by the release of products of lysed spirochetes. Pyrexia associated with the initiation of tetracycline therapy has been documented in one equine case.

ALTERNATIVE DRUGS

Corticosteroid therapy remains controversial and is not recommended.

FOLLOW-UP

PATIENT MONITORING

A marked improvement in clinical signs should be seen after the commencement of antibiotic therapy.

PREVENTION/AVOIDANCE

• No commercially available vaccine is available for horses. A vaccine using recombinant Osp-A antigen is currently being investigated. • Avoid tick-infested areas endemic for Lyme disease. The horse should be carefully groomed daily to remove ticks.
• Use appropriate insecticide sprays (not Amitraz) for horses. No adverse effects have been reported with the use of commercially available canine tick sprays (e.g., Fipronil) in the horse. • Isolation of horses suspected of having Lyme disease is not necessary.

POSSIBLE COMPLICATIONS

• Chronic inflammatory arthritis
• Recurrent episodes of uveitis

EXPECTED COURSE AND PROGNOSIS

• Recovery should be expected within 1 week of commencement of antibiotic therapy.
• Horses with arthritis may be unable to return to previous athletic performance.

MISCELLANEOUS

AGE-RELATED FACTORS

No reported age predisposition

ZOONOTIC POTENTIAL

No zoonotic potential. Humans in contact with infected horses may have increased risk of infection due to increased exposure from animals bringing ticks into their environment.

PREGNANCY

Intrauterine infection of foals has been reported with *B. burgdorferi* isolated from the kidney and brain of one foal with positive serum titers and from the kidney from another foal without serum titers. The significance of the isolated organisms is questionable.

SYNONYMS

• Borreliosis
• Lyme arthritis
• Lyme borreliosis

ABBREVIATIONS

• EIA = enzyme immunoassay
• ELISA = enzyme-linked immunosorbent assay
• EVA = equine viral arteritis
• IFA = immunofluorescence assay
• NSAID = nonsteroidal anti-inflammatory drug
• PCR = polymerase chain reaction
• KELA = kinetics-based, enzyme-linked immunosorbent assay
• WB = Western immunoblot

Suggested Reading

Chang Y-F, Ku KW, Chang CF, et al. Antibiotic treatment of experimentally Borrelia burgdorferi–infected ponies. Vet Microbiol 2005;107:285–294.
Chang Y-F, Novosol V, McDonough SP, et al. Experimental infection of ponies with *Borrelia burgdorferi* by exposure to Ixodid ticks. Vet Pathol 2000;37:68–76.
Divers TJ, Chang Y-F, McDonough PL. Equine Lyme disease: A review of experimental disease production, treatment efficacy and vaccine protection. AAEP Proc 2003;49:391–393.
Fritz CL, Kjemtrup AM. Lyme borreliosis. JAVMA 2003;223:1261–1270.

Author Jane E. Axon
Consulting Editors Ashley G. Boyle and Corinne R. Sweeney

LYMPHADENOPATHY

BASICS

OVERVIEW

- Lymphadenopathy is a disease of LNS, which may be local, regional, or generalized and usually results in LN enlargement. It may be primary or secondary in nature.
- LNs can be enlarged due to benign (lymphoid hyperplasia, lymphadenitis) or malignant (primary or metastatic neoplasia) causes.
- LN enlargement may cause obstruction to lymphatic drainage, leading to peripheral edema, pleural effusion, or ascites.

SIGNS

- History and clinical signs depend on underlying cause and location of enlarged LNs.
- Owners should be questioned about previous infections, wounds, and vaccination for strangles.
- The peripheral LNs most accessible for examination in horses are the submandibular and prescapular. Enlarged LNs may be warm, soft, and painful on palpation and be draining purulent material. Enlargement may cause obstruction to lymphatic drainage with subsequent local edema.
- Additional signs associated with enlargement of peripheral LNs are variable; submandibular and retropharyngeal lymphadenopathy (e.g., *Streptococcus equi* ss *equi* infection) may cause anorexia and dysphagia. Anthrax (due to *Bacillus anthracis)* may initially present as a cervical lymphadenopathy with considerable inflammation and swelling in the pharynx and neck.
- When there is generalized lymphadenopathy, enlarged internal LNs may cause obstruction of the pharynx, esophagus, trachea, or bronchi in the neck and thorax and intestinal obstruction in the abdomen. Clinical signs in these cases may include dyspnea, anorexia, reflux, diarrhea, or other signs of organ dysfunction. Dyschezia, abdominal pain, and urinary dysfunction may be observed in young horses if anorectal LNs are involved.
- Nonspecific signs reported with lymphadenopathies include pale mucous membranes, signs of depression, anorexia, weight loss, tachypnea, tachycardia, respiratory distress, elevated rectal temperature, ventral edema, edema of the peripheral limbs, ascites, and pleural effusion.

CAUSES AND RISK FACTORS

- There are 3 common causes of LN enlargement—lymphoid hyperplasia due to immune stimulation associated with regional drainage of a nearby pathological process; lymphadenitis due to inflammation/infection within the LN itself (primary) or drainage of purulent site (secondary); and neoplasia, which may be due to primary lymphoid neoplasia (lymphoma) or metastatic spread (e.g., melanoma, leukemia).
- LN enlargement associated with lymphoid hyperplasia is characterized by a variable population of lymphocytes including increased proportions of plasma cells. Idiopathic lymphoid hyperplasia may be observed in lymphoid follicles or LNs in young horses in the pharyngeal and anorectal regions. Occasionally, LN enlargement due to lymphoid hyperplasia may be generalized due to systemic and/or widespread infection and antigenic stimulation.
- LN enlargement due to lymphadenitis is characterized by increased proportions of neutrophils, macrophages, or eosinophils depending on the cause and chronicity of the process.
- Lymphoid neoplasia (lymphosarcoma) will have a monomorphic population of abnormal lymphocytes that may obliterate the normal LN architecture, while the cells in metastatic neoplasia will reflect the primary neoplasm.
- Generalized enlargement of LNs usually reflects a neoplastic process or systemic infection.
- Infectious agents that may be associated with either localized or generalized LN enlargement include *S. equi* ss *equi* (strangles), *S. equi* ss *zooepidemicus* (lymphadenitis), *Corynebacterium pseudotuberculosis* (ulcerative lymphangitis), *Burkholderia mallei* (glanders), *B. anthracis* (anthrax), *Mycobacterium avium-intracellulare*, *Histoplasma capsulatum* var. *farciminosum* (epizootic lymphangitis*)*, *Echinococcus granulosus* var *equinus* (echinococcosis), and *Trypansoma evansi* and *T. equiperdum* (trypanosomiasis).
- Risk factors may include recent introduction of new horses, exposing horses to infected animals (e.g., during competition), or transporting naïve horses to areas with endemic disease.

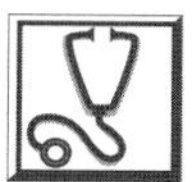

DIAGNOSIS

DIFFERENTIAL DIAGNOSIS

- If LN enlargement is the primary presenting sign, lymphoid hyperplasia, lymphadenitis (primary or secondary), or neoplasia must be differentiated.
- If nonspecific signs (due to involvement of other body systems) are primary presenting signs, appropriate and thorough investigation of these signs is warranted (e.g., full workup of abdominal pain, dyspnea, etc.).

CBC/BIOCHEMISTRY/URINALYSIS

- Highly variable depending on cause of LN enlargement and LNs involved.
- An inflammatory leukogram (i.e., leukocytosis, neutrophilia, hyperproteinemia, hyperfibrinogenemia) may be present in cases of lymphoid hyperplasia and lymphadenitis.
- Neoplastic lymphocytes may be present in peripheral blood if lymphoma is cause of LN enlargement (=lymphosarcoma cell leukemia; leukemic phase of lymphoma).

OTHER LABORATORY TESTS

- Evaluation of LN aspirate or biopsy to determine if LN is reactive (lymphoid hyperplasia), inflamed (lymphadenitis), or neoplastic (primary or metatstatic).
- Culture if lymphadenitis is observed.
- Evaluation of bone marrow aspirate or biopsy for neoplastic cells
- Abdominocentesis and/or thoracocentesis to determine if inflammatory or neoplastic cells are present
- Serology for infectious agents

IMAGING

- Ultrasonography of local and regional drainage areas (thorax or abdomen) to assess size, detect extent if multiple LN involvement, detect infiltrative disease, and allow for guided biopsy
- Thoracic radiography for suspected pulmonary lymphadenopathy

OTHER DIAGNOSTIC PROCEDURES

Rectal palpation to palpate accessible internal LNs

PATHOLOGICAL FINDINGS (OPTIONAL)

Histologic evaluation of the enlarged LN can confirm underlying cause (i.e., lymphoid hyperplasia, lymphadenitis, or neoplasia) if cytology is equivocal.

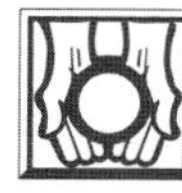

TREATMENT

- Aimed at underlying disease process
- Should include surgical drainage or removal of LN if abscessed and accessible

MEDICATIONS

DRUG(S)

- Vary with the underlying cause and may include appropriate antibiotics or antiparasitics
- Anti-inflammatory medication (e.g., fluxinin meglumine 0.5–1mg/kg) as required

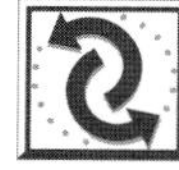

FOLLOW-UP

EXPECTED COURSE AND PROGNOSIS

Depends on underlying cause

MISCELLANEOUS

ASSOCIATED CONDITIONS

Lymphadenopathy is frequently associated with other underlying disease processes; a complete diagnostic work-up is warranted to evaluate the extent of these diseases.

SEE ALSO

- *Streptococcus equi* ss *equi* (strangles)
- *Corynebacterium pseudotuberculosis* (ulcerative lymphangitis)
- Lymphosarcoma

ABBREVIATION

- LN = lymph node

Suggested Reading

Cowell R, Tyler D, Dorsey K, Guglick M. Lymph nodes. In: Cowell R, ed. Diagnostic Cytology and Hematology of the Horse, ed 2. St. Louis: Mosby, 2007:99–106.

Author Jennifer Hodgson
Consulting Editors David Hodgson and Jennifer Hodgson

LYMPHOCYTIC–PLASMACYTIC ENTEROCOLITIS

BASICS

OVERVIEW

• LPE is a pathological description of a type of infiltrative intestinal disease within the complex of idiopathic IBD in the horse. Malabsorption and protein-losing enteropathy result due to the diffuse infiltration of well-differentiated lymphocytes and plasma cells into the lamina propria, between crypts, and sometimes in the submucosa of the small intestine and to a lesser extent the large intestine. Lesions involving the small intestine (13/16) are more common than lesions involving the large intestine (7/16). Normal fecal consistency indicates that the majority of the large intestine is functional.
• LPE is an uncommon equine intestinal disease that is difficult to diagnose antemortem.

SIGNALMENT

• No breed, age, or sex predisposition
• Median age 12 years ($n = 14$)

SIGNS

• Chronic weight loss (95%)
• Thin to emaciated
• Generalized weakness
• Lethargy (20%)
• Inappetence (50%)
• Normal feces consistency or diarrhea (35%). Diarrhea indicates that LPE involves the large intestine.
• Normal vital signs
• Recurrent colic (20%)
• Per-rectal examination: Firm mass in craniodorsal abdomen suggestive of mesenteric lymphadenopathy in the region of the cranial mesenteric artery (3/12)

CAUSES AND RISK FACTORS

Exact cause is unknown, although there is a strong probability that LPE is an immune-mediated disorder.

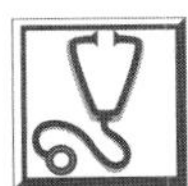

DIAGNOSIS

DIFFERENTIAL DIAGNOSIS

• Malnutrition
• Internal parasitism
• Granulomatous enteritis
• Alimentary lymphosarcoma
• Eosinophilic enteritis
• Multisystemic eosinophilic epitheliotropic complex
• Tuberculosis
• Histoplasmosis
• Basophilic enterocolitis

CBC/BIOCHEMISTRY/URINALYSIS

• Hypoalbuminemia (<30 g/L) (11/20)
• Hypoproteinemia (<60 g/L) (7/20)
• Hyperbilirubinemia if horse is inappetent
• Increased plasma fibrinogen (5/8)
• Normal urinalysis

OTHER LABORATORY TESTS

• D-Xylose absorption test/oral glucose tolerance test abnormal (14/17)
• Serum protein electrophoresis abnormal

IMAGING

N/A

DIAGNOSTIC PROCEDURES

• Rectal mucosal biopsy—abnormal (3/7). Moderate to large numbers of lymphocytes and plasma cells seen in the lamina propria. Unlikely to be diagnostic as lymphoid and plasma cells may also be found in rectal tissue of horses with granulomatous disease, cyathostomiasis, and malignant lymphoma
• Definitive diagnosis by small intestine biopsy—Standing flank or laparoscopy; infiltration with lymphocytes and plasma cells

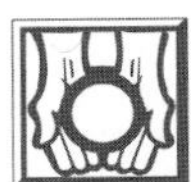

TREATMENT

Poor prognosis

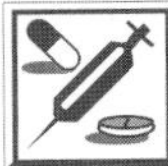

MEDICATIONS

DRUG(S) OF CHOICE

Corticosteroids (e. g., prednisolone 1 mg/kg PO q12 h or dexamethasone 0.1 mg/kg IM q24 h for 3 day, then 0.02 mg/kg IM). Anecdotal reports of brief resolution of diarrhea in some cases when given for several weeks.

CONTRAINDICATIONS/POSSIBLE INTERACTIONS

Corticosteroids at this dosage are immunosuppressive and also may have significant metabolic side effects. Therapy should be withdrawn gradually.

FOLLOW-UP

N/A

MISCELLEANEOUS

ABBREVIATIONS

• IBD = inflammatory bowel disease
• LPE = lymphocytic–plasmacytic enterocolitis

SYNONYM

Lymphocytic–plasmacytic enteritis

Suggested Reading

Chandler K, McNeill PM, Murphy D. Small intestinal malabsorption in an aged mare. Equine Vet Educ 2000;12:166–171.

Clark ES, Morris DD, Allen D, Tyler DE. Lymphocytic enteritis in a filly. JAVMA 1988;193:1281–1283.

Kemper DL, Perkins GA, Schumacher, Edwards JF, Valentine BA, Divers TJ, Cohen ND. Equine lymphocytic-plasmacytic enterocolitis: a retrospective study of 14 cases. Equine Vet J Suppl 2000;32:108–112.

MacAllister CG, Mosier D, Qualls CWJr, Cowell RL. Lymphocytic-plasmacytic enteritis in two horses. JAVMA 1990;196:995–1998.

Schumacher J, Edwards JF, Cohen ND. Chronic idiopathic inflammatory bowel diseases of the horse. J Vet Intern Med 2000;14:258–265.

Author John D. Baird

Consulting Editors Henry Stämpfli and Olimpo Oliver-Espinosa

LYMPHOCYTOSIS

BASICS

DEFINITION

- Lymphocyte count in peripheral blood greater than the upper limit of the laboratory reference interval; usually >5500 cells/mL (5.5×10^9 cells/L)
- Lymphocytes constitute the second most common WBC in peripheral blood and lymphocyte counts are usually stable in healthy horses.
- Lymphocytes are a heterogenous group of cells that have an essential role in adaptive immune responses and also contribute to innate immunity.
- Broadly, lymphocytes are divided into T cells (responsible for cell-mediated immunity), B cells (responsible for humoral immunity), and null cells (killer and NK cells); however, function of the different cells types is strongly interrelated.
- Lymphocyte count can change rapidly due to physiologic influences, disease, or administration of drugs.
- Young animals have higher lymphocyte counts than adults.

PATHOPHYSIOLOGY

- Lymphopoiesis occurs in central (bone marrow and thymus) and peripheral (lymph nodes, spleen, and MALT) lymphoid tissues.
- Bone marrow pluripotential stem cells provide lymphoid stem cells that populate central lymphoid organs to form two functionally different populations; these cells then migrate to the peripheral lymphoid organs to give rise to T and B lymphocytes and possibly null cells.
- B cells are involved in antigen presentation and production of antigen-specific immunoglobulins.
- Immunoglobulins are secreted by terminally differentiated B cells called plasma cells.
- T cells regulate immune responses and are responsible for cell-mediated immunity.
- Most lymphocytes in blood originate from the peripheral lymphoid tissues. Both B and T cells circulate, although T cells are predominant.
- Less than 5% of the total body lymphocyte pool is in blood.
- B and T cells cannot be differentiated on examination of a blood smear.
- Among leukocytes, a unique feature of lymphocytes (principally T cells) is the ability to recirculate between the blood and tissues. Recirculation facilitates exposure of T cells to antigens in tissues and distribution of sensitized cells throughout the body for appropriate adaptive immune responses.
- Antigenic exposure triggers memory T and B cells and subsequent clonal proliferation of effector T and B cells of the adaptive immune response.
- The lymphocyte count in blood is influenced by rates of production, recirculation, utilization, and destruction.
- Lymphocytosis may be associated with physiologic states, chronic antigenic stimulation, or neoplasia.

SYSTEMS AFFECTED

- Hemic/lymphatic/immune
- Involvement of other body systems is dependent on the underlying cause of the lymphocytosis.
- Lymphosarcoma may occur in generalized, multicentric, alimentary, cutaneous, or mediastinal (thymic) forms.

SIGNS

General Comments

Depend on the cause of lymphocytosis

Historical

- Physiologic causes may be associated with a history of an excited or apprehensive demeanor or (intense) exercise.
- Chronic antigenic stimulation and lymphoproliferative disorders may be associated with a history of weight loss, lethargy, inappetence.

Physical Examination

- Physiologic causes—increased heart rate, alert mentation
- Chronic antigenic stimulation and lymphoproliferative disorders—signs of specific organ involvement, pyrexia.
- Enlargement of peripheral lymph nodes may or may not be associated with lymphocytosis. When present, lymph node enlargement may be localized or generalized. Localized enlargement is due to lymphoid hyperplasia or lymphadenitis, while generalized lymphadenopathy is rarer and due to systemic infections or lymphoproliferative disorders.

CAUSES

Physiologic Causes

- Fear, excitement, or (intense) exercise.
- Lymphocytosis is transient (<30min) and occurs more frequently in horses <2 years of age.
- Blood lymphocyte count may reach 15,000 cells/mL (15×10^9 cells/L), and concurrent neutrophilia is common.
- Results from release of epinephrine and mobilization of rapidly accessible pool of lymphocytes due to increased blood flow in the microvasculature
- In addition, uptake of lymphocytes by lymphoid tissues may be reduced.

Chronic Antigenic Stimulation (Reactive Lymphocytosis)

- Bacterial infection—e.g., pneumonia, peritonitis, abscess
- Viral infection—e.g., EIA, EVA
- Fungal infection—rarer than bacterial or viral infections
- Vaccination
- Reactive lymphocytes (immunocytes or plasma cells) may be observed in peripheral blood smears.

Neoplasia

- Lymphoid neoplasia—lymphosarcoma or lymphocytic leukemia
- Primary lymphocytic leukemia may occur as an acute or a chronic form; both are very rare.
- Secondary lymphoid leukemia is an occasional finding in horses with lymphosarcoma. This leukemic phase of lymphoma is also called lymphosarcoma cell leukemia.
- Occasionally, marked lymphocytosis may be observed in these horse (up to 250,000 cells/mL [250×10^9 cells/L]).
- The morphology of circulating lymphocytes is variable and ranges from atypical, immature, or blast cells to well-differentiated lymphocytes.

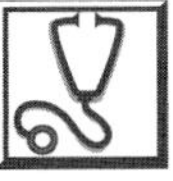

DIAGNOSIS

DIFFERENTIAL DIAGNOSIS

- Underlying cause of lymphocytosis (physiologic versus inflammatory versus lymphoproliferative) should be determined.
- If inflammatory, site and cause of inflammatory process should be determined.

CBC/BIOCHEMISTRY/URINALYSIS

- Lymphocyte count >5500 cells/mL (>5.5×10^9 cells/L)
- If a mature neutrophilia is concurrently observed, consider physiologic response or chronic antigenic stimulation.
- If a left shift +/− morphologic (toxic) changes in neutrophils are observed, consider inflammatory condition, especially bacterial infections.
- The presence of antigenically stimulated lymphocytes (immunocytes) suggests reactive lymphocytosis.
- If atypical, blast, or poorly differentiated lymphocytes are observed, consider acute lymphocytic leukemia; however, reactive lymphocytosis needs to be excluded. Examination of peripheral blood smears by a veterinary hematologist or oncologist may facilitate diagnosis and assist in case management.
- If anemia, thrombocytopenia, and granulocytopenia are noted, consider myelophthisis due to lymphocytic leukemia or lymphosarcoma with bone marrow involvement.
- If hemolytic anemia is present, consider lymphosarcoma.
- If hypercalcemia is reported, consider lymphosarcoma (paraneoplastic syndrome due to release of PTHrP by neoplastic lymphocytes).
- If hyperglobulinemia is present, consider chronic antigenic stimulation or neoplasia.

OTHER LABORATORY TESTS

- Serum protein electrophoresis to determine if a polyclonal or monoclonal gammopathy is present. If polyclonal, consider chronic antigenic stimulation or neoplasia; if

monoclonal, consider lymphosarcoma or multiple myeloma.
- Coombs test for EIA
- Serology for EVA or other viral infections
- Quantification of individual immunoglobulin classes. Horses with lymphosarcoma may have IgM deficiency. However, recent evidence suggests this test is unreliable.

IMAGING

- Ultrasonography of the thorax and abdomen for detection of organomegaly, abscess, neoplasia, and effusions. Mediastinal or splenic masses may be reflective of lymphosarcoma.
- Radiography of the thorax for detection of pneumonia, abscess, or lymphosarcoma
- Radiography of the skeleton for detection of inflammatory or neoplastic lesions
- Scintigraphy using radiolabeled autologous neutrophils for detection of occult abscesses

OTHER DIAGNOSTIC PROCEDURES

- Abdominocentesis or thoracocentesis to determine if inflammatory or neoplastic processes are present
- CSF collection to determine if inflammatory or neoplastic processes are present
- Bone marrow biopsy to detect lymphoproliferative disorders
- Fine needle aspirate/biopsy and cytology/histopathology of internal or external tumor
- Rectal biopsy for detection of lymphosarcoma
- Endoscopy (airways, esophagus/stomach, bladder) to determine if inflammatory or neoplastic processes are present
- Laparoscopy/thoracoscopy if abscess/tumor is suspected
- Aspirate of lymph nodes and cytology/histology if lymphadomegaly is present

PATHOLOGICAL FINDINGS

- Dependent on the underlying cause.
- Sarcomatous masses involving the mediastium, spleen, liver, alimentary tract, and/or lymph nodes are consistent with lymphosarcoma.

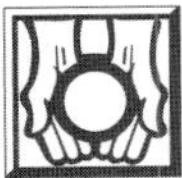

TREATMENT

AIMS OF TREATMENT

- Elimination of the underlying cause
- Varies with the nature of the underlying cause and may include elimination of infection, resolution of inflammation, or treatment of neoplasia. Medical and/or surgical treatment may be required.

APPROPRIATE HEALTH CARE

- Physiologic causes of lymphocytosis require no treatment.
- Reactive lymphocytosis associated with vaccination requires no treatment.
- Inpatient medical and/or surgical management of horses with reactive lymphocytosisis (due to infection) or neoplasia may be required.
- Megavoltage radiation can be attempted for treatment of lymphosarcoma. This is most suitable for treatment of solitary tumors.

NURSING CARE

- Depends on the underlying cause
- If pleural effusion is present, therapeutic paracentesis/drainage may be required if respiration is affected.

CLIENT EDUCATION

- Persistent lymphocytosis denotes the presence of an underlying disease that will require appropriate diagnostic assessment and treatment.
- Neoplasia has poor to grave prognosis.

SURGICAL CONSIDERATIONS

Depend on the underlying cause

MEDICATIONS

DRUG(S) OF CHOICE

- Bacterial or fungal infections require antimicrobial therapy based on culture and sensitivity testing.
- Corticosteroids may be used for treatment of lymphosarcoma.
- Antineoplastic chemotherapeutic regimens for lymphosarcoma using cytotoxic drugs have been described (see Lymphosarcoma).

CONTRAINDICATIONS

Avoid corticosteroids in cases with infectious disease or laminitis.

PRECAUTIONS

Use of cytotoxic drugs requires appropriate use of personal protection equipment during preparation, administration, and disposal to minimize exposure of personnel to the drugs.

FOLLOW-UP

PATIENT MONITORING

Serial monitoring of CBC and lymphocyte morphology

EXPECTED COURSE AND PROGNOSIS

- Depends on the underlying cause
- Reactive lymphocytosis resolves with removal of chronic antigenic stimulation. Therefore, prognosis depends on the response of the underlying disease to treatment.
- Prognosis for lymphoproliferative disorders is hopeless.

MISCELLANEOUS

AGE-RELATED FACTORS

- Lymphocyte counts increase gradually after birth over the first 3 mo.
- Physiologic lymphocytosis is more common in horses <2 years of age.

SEE ALSO

- Leukemia, lymphoid
- Lymphosarcoma
- Lymphadenopathy
- Pancytopenia

ABBREVIATIONS

- CSF = cerebrospinal fluid
- EIA = equine infectious anemia
- EVA = equine viral arteritis
- MALT = mucosa-associated lymphoid tissue
- NK = natural killer
- PTHrP = parathyroid hormone–related peptide

Suggested Reading

Jain NC. The lymphocytes and plasma cells. In. Essentials of Veterinary Hematology. Philadelphia: Lea & Febiger, 1993.

Latimer KS. Diseases Affecting Leukocytes. In: Colahan PT, et al, eds. Equine Medicine and Surgery, 5th Ed. St Louis: Mosby, 1999; 2025–2034.

Mair TS, Couto CG. The use of cytotoxic drugs in practice. Equine Veterinary Education 2006;18:149–156.

McClure JT, Young KM, Fiste M, Sharkey LC and Lund DP. Immunophenotypic classification of leukemia in 3 horses. Journal of Veterinary Internal Medicine 2001;15:144–152.

Perkins GA, Nydam DV, Flaminio MJBF, Ainsworth DM. Serum IgM concentrations in normal, fit horses and horses with lymphoma and other medical conditions. Journal of Veterinary Internal Medicine 2003;17:337–342.

Author Kristopher Hughes

Consulting Editors Jennifer Hodgson and David Hodgson

LYMPHOID HYPERPLASIA (PHARYNGITIS)

BASICS

OVERVIEW

• Acute and chronic forms of pharyngitis are recognized. Acute inflammation of the lymphoid (and surrounding) tissues in the pharynx is termed pharyngitis and chronic inflammation of the pharynx is defined as a pharyngeal lymphoid hyperplasia; • Pharyngeal lymphoid hyperplasia is commonly recognized in young athletic horses; • It is not generally considered to be a specific disease entity but rather a response to other diseases and to a lesser extent to local physical, chemical, or allergic causes; • The pharyngeal tonsil consists of discrete lymphoid follicles diffusely distributed in the dorsal and lateral walls of the pharynx. In response to local or lymphogenous spread of infection, the tonsillar tissue becomes inflamed, and the tonsillar crypts become filled with desquamated epithelium, leukocyte, and bacteria.

SIGNALMENT

Pharyngeal lymphoid hyperplasia is commonly observed in weaning to performance horses 2–3 years of age.

SIGNS

• Some authors have implicated pharyngeal lymphoid hyperplasia as a performance- limiting entity, although now the consensus states that this condition has little consequence on the athletic ability of the horse or on the function of the upper respiratory tract, unless severe. • In acute pharyngitis, signs may included pharyngeal pain (dysphagia), nasal discharge (serous, seromucous, mucopurulent, purulent, feed- contaminated), regional lymphadenopathy (submandibular, retropharyngeal nodes), respiratory noise (often inspiratory), pharyngeal swelling, and cough. • There may also be odor (breath and/or nasal discharge) if pharyngitis results from local pharyngeal trauma (with foreign bodies or not).

CAUSES AND RISK FACTORS

• The cause of chronic pharyngitis is not known but is probably multifactorial. • Many clinicians attribute pharyngeal lymphoid hyperplasia to a local immune response to inhaled or ingested antigens. • In the horse, *Streptococcus* spp., myxovirus (influenza A/equi 1, A/equi 2), herpesvirus (EHV-1 and EHV-4), picornavirus (rhinovirus 1 and 2), and paramyxovirus (parainfluenza 3) have been incriminated as specific causes of pharyngitis. But the role and the specificity of microbial pathogens as causative agents remain unknown. • Physical and chemical causes of pharyngitis have been identified. • Fungal infections caused by *Conidiobolus coronatus* are also reported as etiologic agents in equine pharyngitis.

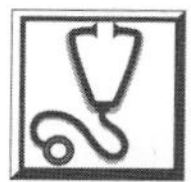

DIAGNOSIS

DIFFERENTIAL DIAGNOSIS

• Rhinitis and laryngitis • Dysphagia—Tongue foreign bodies, fractures of the hyoid apparatus or jaws, and disease of guttural pouches should be considered. • If exercise intolerance is the primary complaint, pharyngitis should only be considered after all other possible causes of impaired performance have been eliminated.

CBC/BIOCHEMISTRY/URINALYSIS

Changes in the hemogram and the biochemical profile are likely to result from a concurrent respiratory disease (leukopenia or leukocytosis, hyperfibrinogenemia, anemia) or reflect abscess formation (neutrophilia, hyperfibrinogenemia) or dehydration and fasting associated with dysphagia.

OTHER LABORATORY TESTS

Microbial culture of nasopharynx swab samples is helpful for the identification of the causative organism in acute upper respiratory tract infections. The interpretation of results may be difficult because (1) the pharynx normally has a resident microflora, and (2) many of the microorganisms isolated are capable of opportunistic infections.

IMAGING

• Endoscopy—Evidence of more pronounced hyperplasia of the lymphonodular follicles within the pharyngeal mucosa and single or multiple lymphonodular masses may be within, or protrude from, the pharyngeal mucosa.
• Radiography of the pharynx can provide information on the presence of radiodense foreign bodies, soft tissue masses, fractures, and in the guttural pouch diseases.
• Ultrasonography of the pharynx area may identify abnormal images (masses, inflammation, abscesses).

OTHER DIAGNOSTIC PROCEDURES

N/A

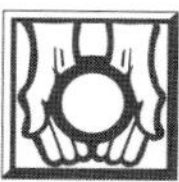

TREATMENT

• Treatment is empiric and generally palliative for pharyngeal lymphoid hyperplasia. • When pharyngeal angina is causing inappetence or dysphagia, administration of nonsteroidal anti-inflammatory drugs should be considered.
• Dehydration and dysphagia should be managed by either parenteral or enteral fluid administration. • Soft feeds, especially green grass, should be offered when available to encourage animals with pharyngeal discomfort to eat. • Infections secondary to foreign body injuries should be treated with antibiotics having a broad aerobic and anaerobic spectrum. • Daily lavage of any cavitary wounds, debridement, and removal of feed material may be necessary.
• Topical antifungal and systemic fungal treatment is indicated in cases with documented fungal infection. • Rest from training for 4–8 weeks.

MEDICATIONS

DRUG(S) OF CHOICE

Custom topical preparations, usually containing an antibiotic, an anti-inflammatory drug, and a hygroscopic agent (glycerine) or dimethyl sulfoxide, are often used for palliation of clinical signs. There are several combinations used by equine clinicians. These preparations are administered 2 or 3 times daily through a transnasal catheter and sprayed onto the pharyngeal surface. Despite their frequent use, it is not known if this form of therapy is effective or if the response reflects natural resolution of the predisposing cause.

FOLLOW-UP

PATIENT MONITORING

• Repeat upper respiratory endoscopy at 3–4 weeks post-treatment. • Reevaluation of CBC if there were inflammatory modifications initially.

PREVENTION/AVOIDANCE

Methods used to control and prevent most of the common viral (influenza and herpesvirus 1 and 4) and bacterial respiratory diseases should limit herd problems with acute pharyngitis. However, there are no substantive data to support this contention. Nevertheless, racetrack veterinarians maintain that frequent immunization against influenza and rhinopneumonitis markedly reduces the severity of pharyngeal lymphoid hyperplasia and improves exercise tolerance.

EXPECTED COURSE AND PROGNOSIS

Depend of the cause of pharyngitis

MISCELLANEOUS

ASSOCIATED CONDITIONS

N/A

AGE-RELATED FACTORS

N/A

ZOONOTIC POTENTIAL

N/A

PREGNANCY

Equine herpesvirus may cause abortion.

SEE ALSO

• Herpesvirus types 1 and 4
• Influenza

Suggested Reading

Ainsworth DM, Hackett RP. Pharyngeal and laryngeal disorders. In: Reed SM, Bayly WM, Sellon DC, ed. Equine Internal Medicine, ed 2. Philadelphia: WB Saunders, 2004:302–303.

Pascoe JR. Pharyngitis. In: Smith BP, ed. Large Animal Internal Medicine, ed 3. St. Louis: Mosby, 2002:530–532.

Sullivan EK, Parente, EJ. Disorders of the pharynx. Vet Clin Equine 2003;19:159–167.

Author Daniel Jean
Consulting Editor Daniel Jean

LYMPHOPENIA

BASICS

OVERVIEW

• Lymphocyte count in peripheral blood less than the lower limit of the laboratory reference interval—usually <1500 cells/μL ($<1.5 \times 10^9$ cells/L) • Lymphocytes constitute the second most common WBC in peripheral blood.
• Lymphocytes are a heterogeneous group of cells that have an essential role in adaptive immune responses and also contribute to innate immunity. • Broadly, lymphocytes are divided into T cells (responsible for cell-mediated immunity), B cells (responsible for humoral immunity), and null cells (killer and NK cells); however, function of the different cells types is strongly interrelated. • Lymphocyte count can rapidly change due to physiologic influences, disease, or administration of drugs.
• Lymphopenia can be caused by corticosteroids, acute infectious disease, increased loss, or decreased production.

SIGNALMENT

• Lymphopenia can occur in horses of any breed or age and in either sex. • SCID occurs in Arabian and Arabian cross foals and is an autosomal recessive disorder. • FPIS occurs in Fell Pony foals; an autosomal recessive mode of inheritance is suspected. • AG has been described in Thoroughbred, Quarter Horse, and Standardbred horses and is only seen in male foals.

SIGNS

• Depends on the cause • Foals with SCID, FPIS, or AG often present with signs of ill thrift, pyrexia, lethargy, rough coat, and respiratory and/or GIT infections with associated coughing, nasal discharge, and/or diarrhea.

CAUSES AND RISK FACTORS

Corticosteroid-Induced

• Endogenous (stress) or exogenous corticosteroids predictably induce lymphopenia.
• Mechanism involves redistribution of circulating lymphocytes (predominantly T cells) to body compartments (including the bone marrow) and lympholysis. • Lymphopenia occurs within a few hours of corticosteroid exposure and may resolve within 12–24 hr.

Acute Infection

• Viral infection—e.g., EI, EHV • Bacterial infection—e.g., bacteremia, septicemia, peritonitis, pleuropneumonia • Mechanism is complex and may involve endogenous corticosteroid release (stress) and sequestration of lymphocytes in lymphoid and other tissues. Increased blood flow to lymphoid tissues and temporary obstruction of efferent lymphatic vessels also facilitates trapping of lymphocytes.

Increased Loss

Loss of lymphocyte-rich lymph into the thorax (chylothorax) is rarely reported in horses.

Decreased Production

• SCID is a genetic disorder that results in an inability of lymphocyte progenitor cells to mature and results in a profound lymphopenia involving both T and B cells. • FPIS is a congenital impairment of development of B cells in bone marrow and secondary lymphoid organs (e.g., lymph nodes and spleen). • AG is associated with a lack of mature B lymphocytes and plasma cells with failure to synthesize immunoglobulins or specific antibodies after immunization or infections. • Use of cytotoxic chemotherapeutic agents • Radiation toxicity

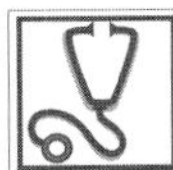

DIAGNOSIS

CBC/BIOCHEMISTRY/URINALYSIS

• Lymphocyte count <1500 cells/μL ($<1.5 \times 10^9$ cells/L)
• If concurrent neutrophilia and eosinopenia are reported, consider stress or administration of exogenous corticosteroids.
• Presence of neutropenia/neutrophilia, increased band neutrophil count, and toxic changes in neutrophils are consistent with acute infection.
• Persistent marked lymphopenia (<1000 cells/μL [$<1.0 \times 10^9$ cells/L]) in an Arabian or Arabian cross foal is consistent with SCID.
• Anemia, thrombocytopenia, and lymphopenia in a Fell Pony foal are consistent with FPIS.
• Lymphopenia may or may not be present in foals with AG due to complete lack of B cells but normal numbers of T cells.

OTHER LABORATORY TESTS

• Genetic testing (PCR) for SCID
• Quantification of individual immunoglobulin subtypes where lack of IgM in presuckle blood or after 30 days of age is consistent with SCID and FPIS while hypogammaglobulinemia is consistent with AG.
• Serology for viral or bacterial pathogens

IMAGING

Ultrasonography and/or radiography of the thorax or abdomen if infection is suspected

OTHER DIAGNOSTIC PROCEDURES

• Abdominocentesis, thoracocentesis, CSF collection, or blood culture if infectious disease is suspected
• Fecal examination for identification of opportunistic *Cryptosporidium parvum* infection in foals with SCID, FPIS, or AG
• Bone marrow aspirate/biopsy, where increased myeloid:erythroid ratio in Fell Pony foals is consistent with erythroid hypoplasia.
• Lymphocyte proliferation assays will detect impaired lymphocyte responses in foals with SCID.

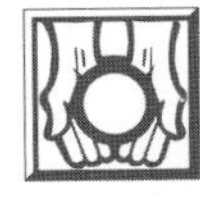

TREATMENT

• Corticosteroid-induced lymphopenia does not require treatment.
• Lymphopenia associated with acute infection, increased loss, or decreased production often requires inpatient medical treatment until the underlying condition is stabilized.

MEDICATIONS

DRUG(S)

Bacterial infections require antimicrobial therapy based on culture and sensitivity testing.

FOLLOW-UP

PATIENT MONITORING

• Serial monitoring of the CBC and lymphocyte count
• Corticosteroid-induced lymphopenia usually resolves within 24 hr.
• Persistent marked lymphopenia in Arabian or Arabian cross foals is consistent with SCID.

EXPECTED COURSE AND PROGNOSIS

• Depends on underlying cause
• Corticosteroid-induced lymphopenia is transient.
• SCID is invariably fatal, despite supportive therapy, due to recurrent infections unless provision of histocompatible lymphoid stem cells by bone marrow transplantation is performed (seldom practical in horses).
• The genetic basis of SCID and implications of further breeding of the mare and stallion should be discussed with owners.
• FPIS and AG are invariably fatal due to the effects of immunodeficiency and nonregenerative anemia in case of FPIS.
• Foals with SCID, FPIS, and AG succumb to secondary infections usually by 3 mo of age.

MISCELLANEOUS

ASSOCIATED CONDITIONS

• SCID
• AG
• FPIS
• Acute viral/bacterial infections

AGE-RELATED FACTORS

Lymphocyte counts are low in foals in the first week of the postnatal period and then increase gradually over the next 3 mo in normal foals.

SEE ALSO

• SCID
• Immunoglobulin deficiencies

ABBREVIATIONS

• AG = agammaglobulinemia
• CSF = cerebrospinal fluid
• EHV = equine herpesvirus
• EI = equine influenza
• FPIS = Fell Pony immunodeficiency syndrome
• SCID = severe combined immunodeficiency

Suggested Reading

Latimer KS. Diseases Affecting Leukocytes. In: Colahan PT, et al, eds. Equine Medicine and Surgery, ed 5. St Louis: Mosby, 1999;1992–2001, 2025–2034.

Author Kristopher Hughes
Consulting Editor Jennifer Hodgson and David Hodgson

LYMPHOSARCOMA

BASICS

DEFINITION

A malignant, neoplastic disorder of lymphoid tissue

PATHOPHYSIOLOGY

- The neoplastic cells in equine lymphoid tumors have been evaluated by histopathology and immunohistochemistry and consist primarily of B or T cells. Equine lymphoid tumors have been described as B cell lymphoma (most common), T cell lymphoma, B cell–rich T-cell lymphoma, T cell–rich B-cell lymphoma, or non–B-cell, non–T-cell lymphoma.
- Clinical signs of lymphoma may be caused by organ and tissue dysfunction resulting from the infiltration of lymphocytes, physical obstruction from tumor masses or cytokines released by tumor cells.
- Some horses with lymphoma have compromised humoral or cellular immunity, which may predispose them to secondary infection.

SYSTEMS AFFECTED

- Four forms of equine lymphoma have been described based on the location of tumors. These forms include multicentric (generalized), intestinal (alimentary), mediastinal (thymic), and cutaneous.
- Lymphocytic leukemia (also called lymphosarcoma cell leukemia), characterized by lymphocytosis with circulating atypical lymphocytes, is rare and usually reflects bone marrow infiltration.
- Most common sites for tumors include lymph nodes, skin/subcutis, spleen, mediastinum, liver, intestine, heart, lungs, and kidneys. Other body systems affected occasionally include nervous, vision, and reproductive.

INCIDENCE/PREVALENCE

Lymphoma is the most common tumor of the equine hemolymphatic system. However, in abattoir and necropsy studies the prevalence of affected horses is less than 5%.

SIGNALMENT

Mean Age and Range

Usually affects horses between 5 and 10 years of age with a range from birth to 25 years. The alimentary form appears to be more common in younger horses.

Breed and Predominant Sex

There are no breed or sex predilections reported.

SIGNS

General Comments

- The clinical signs are variable and depend on the organ or system affected by neoplastic infiltrate.
- The clinical signs may have a gradual or sudden onset but often progress slowly over weeks to months.

Historical

The chief complaints often include signs of dullness, weight loss, inappetence, and decreased performance.

Physical Examination

- The most common clinical findings include fever, poor body condition, pallor of mucous membranes, ventral edema and lymphadenomegaly, which may be internal, external, regional, or generalized.
- Intestinal (alimentary) form may have a history of colic or diarrhea and physical examination may demonstrate ventral edema, abdominal lymphadenomegaly, and/or splenomegaly.
- Mediastinal (thymic) form may have tachypnea, dyspnea, and pleural effusion.
- Cutaneous form often has multiple dermal or subcutaneous nodules (1- to 20-cm diameter), which may appear suddenly, grow slowly, remain static, or regress and recur. Local lymph nodes often are enlarged, but internal organs are infiltrated rarely.

CAUSES

Virus-like particles were detected in a lymph node from a foal with lymphoma, but a viral cause of lymphoma in the horse has not been established.

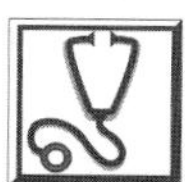

DIAGNOSIS

DIFFERENTIAL DIAGNOSIS

- Chronic inflammatory diseases, including internal abscessation or pleuropneumonia, often present with signs of dullness, inappetence, and weight loss. In addition, there is often fever, pallor, and ventral edema. Localization of site of inflammation and demonstration of inflammatory process and its cause are required for differentiation.
- Infectious diseases including EIA and babesiosis (piroplasmosis) often cause fever, pallor, and weight loss. Serology (e.g., Coggins test for EIA) and/or demonstration of organisms in blood smears (e.g., babesiosis).
- Immune-mediated disorders including immune-mediated hemolytic anemia and immune-mediated thrombocytopenia may be associated with lymphoma. Coombs test to verify the presence of immune-mediated hemolytic anemia. Platelet factor-3 (PF-3) test may be used as an indirect test for immune-mediated thrombocytopenia.

CBC/BIOCHEMISTRY/URINALYSIS

- Laboratory findings are highly variable and often nonspecific and usually indicate a chronic inflammatory condition.
- CBC usually reveals neutrophilic leukocytosis and hyperfibrinogenemia.
- Anemia is common and may be caused by suppression of erythropoiesis, bone marrow infiltration, or immune-mediated hemolytic anemia/immune-mediated thrombocytopenia.
- Lympohocyte counts are usually normal or mildly decreased. The presence of atypical or obviously neoplastic lymphocytes on a peripheral blood smear occurs in 30%–50% of cases, but lymphocytic leukemia (increased lymphocyte counts) is rarer.
- Biochemistry usually reveals hypoalbuminemia and hyperglobulinemia, which may be caused by a polyclonal gammopathy (common) or a monoclonal gammopathy (rare).
- Hypercalcemia associated with pseudohyperparathyroidism of malignancy has been reported occasionally.
- A reduction in IgM has been reported in less than 50% of horses with lymphoma.
- Increased activities of liver-derived enzymes (AST, GGT) may be caused by neoplastic infiltration of the liver.

OTHER LABORATORY TESTS

- Aspiration of bone marrow may reveal myelophthisis characterized by decreased red and white blood cell precursors and infiltration by neoplastic lymphocytes.
- Oral glucose or xylose absorption tests may have abnormal results due to neoplastic infiltration of the small intestine.
- Coombs test and PF-3 test may be positive with immune-mediated hemolytic anemia and immune-mediated thrombocytopenia, respectively, associated with lymphoma.

IMAGING

- Thoracic ultrasound examination may detect pleural effusion.
- Abdominal ultrasound examination may detect ascites, enlargement/infiltration of the spleen, liver, and kidneys. This technique may aid when taking biopsy samples from these organs.

OTHER DIAGNOSTIC PROCEDURES

- A definitive diagnosis of lymphoma is based on the observation of neoplastic lymphocytes in peripheral blood, an aspirate of a lymph node, bone marrow or fluid from the thoracic or abdominal cavity, or a biopsy sample of a lymph node or internal organ.
- Histopathological examination of a biopsy is preferred as it may be difficult to distinguish neoplastic versus reactive lymphocytes in a fine needle aspirate.
- Laparoscopy, exploratory laparotomy, or postmortem examination may be required to make a definitive diagnosis.

PATHOLOGICAL FINDINGS

- Gross lesions may include lymphadenomegaly and neoplastic masses in the spleen, liver, kidney, intestine, heart, lung, thymus, and/or skin.
- Affected lymph nodes are red-gray and glisten on cut surface.
- Impression smears of the cut surface of an infiltrated lymph node or organ often reveal variable sized lymphocytes that are larger and darker-staining (cytoplasmic basophilia) than normal and contain a variable ratio of nucleus:cytoplasm, prominent or multiple

nucleoli, clumping of nuclear chromatin, indented or binucleate nuclei, and mitotic figures.
• Histologically, the neoplastic cellular morphology also varies, but destruction of normal tissue architecture by a population of lymphoid cells aids the diagnosis.

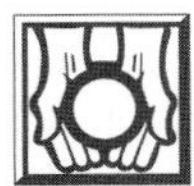

TREATMENT

AIMS OF TREATMENT

The aim of treatment using combination chemotherapy is to reduce the size of neoplastic tissue.

CLIENT EDUCATION

• The prognosis for a horse with the multicentric, intestinal, or mediastinal form of lymphoma generally is poor as most untreated horses do not survive beyond 6 mo following diagnosis.
• The treatment of horses with these forms of lymphoma using combination chemotherapy has been reported and may have prolonged the life of the affected horse by a few months.
• Horses with the cutaneous form of lymphoma usually have a better prognosis and a longer clinical course.

SURGICAL CONSIDERATIONS

Surgical removal of a solitary mass attached to the wall of the intestine and intestinal resection has prolonged the life of a few horses with the intestinal form of lymphoma that did not have evidence of metastasis.

MEDICATIONS

DRUG(S) OF CHOICE

• Chemotherapeutic agents including cytosine arabinoside, cyclophosphamide, and vincristine have been administered intravenously every 1–2 weeks in an alternating regimen in conjunction with prednisolone administered orally daily. However, the long-term response to therapy is poor for horses with the multicentric, intestinal, or mediastinal forms.
• The cutaneous form of lymphoma has proved responsive to the oral administration of a progestin (altrenogest) or progestogen (megestrol) and systemic or intralesional administration of a glucocorticoid. However, cutaneous or subcutaneous masses tend to recur (and may be more aggressive and rapidly progressive) in horses that are treated with systemic glucocorticoids for inadequate periods.
• Glucocorticoids have been used to treat horses with lymphoma that have immune-mediated hemolytic anemia or immune-mediated thrombocytopenia.

PRECAUTIONS

Horses with lymphoma that are being treated with combination chemotherapy should have a CBC and biochemical profile performed periodically to assess side effects such as bone marrow and organ dysfunction.

FOLLOW-UP

PATIENT MONITORING

A reduction in the size of a lymph node(s) or mass(es) and improved attitude, appetite, and weight gain can be interpreted to suggest a positive response to treatment.

EXPECTED COURSE AND PROGNOSIS

• The prognosis for life beyond 6 mo following diagnosis is grave for a horse with the multicentric, intestinal, or mediastinal form of lymphoma.
• The prognosis for a horse with the cutaneous form of lymphoma that is treated appropriately is better as the lesions may regress and the affected horse can often survive beyond 6 mo post-diagnosis.

MISCELLANEOUS

ASSOCIATED CONDITIONS

• Immune-mediated hemolytic anemia
• Immune-mediated thrombocytopenia
• Immunosuppression

PREGNANCY

Combination chemotherapy may pose a risk to the fetus, especially when administered during the first trimester. However, combination chemotherapy administered to one mare from months 6–11 of pregnancy and discontinued 1 week prior to foaling had no adverse effects on the foal.

SYNONYMS

Malignant lymphoma

SEE ALSO

• Immunoglobulin deficiencies
• Lymphadenopathy

ABBREVIATIONS

• AST = aspartate aminotransferase
• GGT = γ-glutamyl transferase
• IgM = immunoglobulin M

Suggested Reading

Byrne BA, Yvorchuk-St. Jean K, Couto CG, Kohn CW. Successful management of lymphoproliferative disease in two pregnant mares. Proc Vet Cancer Soc 1991;8–9.

Carlson GP. Lymphoma (lymphosarcoma) in horses. In: Smith BP, ed. Large Animal Internal Medicine, ed 3. St. Louis: Mosby. 2002:1071–1072.

Diseases of the hemolymphatic and immune systems. In: Radostits O, Gay C, Hinchcliff K, Constable P, eds. Veterinary Medicine, ed 10. Philadelphia: WB Saunders, 2007;439–469.

Madewell BR, Theilen GH. Equine lymphosarcoma. In: Theilen GH, Madewell BR, eds. Veterinary Cancer Medicine, ed 2. Philadelphia: Lea & Febiger, 1987:431–437.

Rebhun WC, Bertone A. Equine lymphosarcoma. J Am Vet Med Assoc 1984;184:720–721.

Sellon DC. Disorders of the hematopoietic system. In: Reed SM, Bayly WM, Sellon DC, eds. Equine Internal Medicine, ed 2. Philadelphia: Saunders, 2004:740–742.

Author W. Kent Scarratt

Consulting Editors Jennifer Hodgson and David Hodgson

MAGNESIUM DISORDERS

BASICS

DEFINITION

• Serum magnesium concentration above or below reference range • Anorexia results in hypomagnesemia, but whole-body magnesium deficiency is unusual. • Hypermagnesemia is secondary to overdose of magnesium-containing laxatives.

PATHOPHYSIOLOGY

• Magnesium is the second most abundant intracellular cation and fourth most abundant electrolyte in the body. • Adult horses are ≅0.05% magnesium by weight, 60% of which is in the bones. • Magnesium in serum is present in ionized, protein-bound, and complexed forms.
• Serum concentration is not a good indicator of total-body magnesium. • There is no storage pool of readily available magnesium. • There is no specific homeostatic regulation system for magnesium. Hormones that regulate calcium have a lesser effect on magnesium metabolism.
• Magnesium is excreted by the kidneys, which regulate magnesium balance by controlling tubular reabsorption. This is the primary means of maintaining magnesium homeostasis.
• Magnesium is secreted in the milk of lactating mares. • Magnesium has numerous physiologic functions. It is part of the ATP complex and is essential for all energy metabolism. Magnesium is important for muscle contraction and problems with impulse transmission at the neuromuscular junction account for most of the clinical signs of inappropriate concentration.
• Magnesium is antagonistic to the actions of calcium. • Low magnesium levels increase the release of acetylcholine at nerve endings, which can induce tetany. • Low magnesium levels have been associated with insulin resistance. • High magnesium alters the resting membrane potential of muscles and neurons, resulting in muscle relaxation. • Decreased glomerular filtration, as with prerenal azotemia, often results in hypermagnesemia.

SYSTEMS AFFECTED

• Neuromuscular • Nervous
• Endocrine/metabolic • Cardiovascular

SIGNALMENT

• Hypermagnesemia
• Horses or foals administered magnesium sulfate or other magnesium-containing laxatives
• Hypomagnesemia
• Lactating mares • Hard-working draft horses
• Horses suffering from blister beetle toxicosis
• Anorexic horses

SIGNS

• In most instances, altered serum magnesium is an incidental finding with no apparent ill effects.
• In horses with colic, low magnesium is not predictive of days of hospitalization or survival.
• There is an association between postoperative ileus and hypomagnesemia.
In rare instances, signs of hypermagnesemia are:
• Ataxia • Muscle weakness • Poor response to stimuli • Diarrhea
In rare instances, signs of hypomagnesemia include:
• Muscle fibrillation • Weakness • Hyperreflexia
• Arrhythmias • Hyperpnea • Tetany

CAUSES

• Insufficient intake due to poor diet, severe anorexia, or small intestinal disease prevents adequate absorption of magnesium to replace the continual endogenous losses in the intestinal secretions. • The most common causes of low serum magnesium are lack of food intake, diets low in available magnesium, gastrointestinal disturbances, lactation, and exhaustion.

RISK FACTORS

• Anorexia • Transport • Surgery • Lactation
• Diuretics • Ingestion of blister beetle–contaminated hay • Risk factors for hypermagnesemia—administration of magnesium laxatives

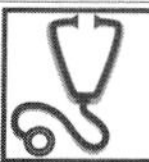

DIAGNOSIS

DIFFERENTIAL DIAGNOSIS

• Differential diagnoses for hypermagnesemia include other causes of diarrhea and other neuromuscular conditions. • Signs of hypomagnesemia vary, so conditions associated with neuromuscular abnormalities must be considered. • Other conditions that must be investigated and may be more common are eclampsia, botulism, equine lower motor neuron disease, blister beetle toxicity, and other less common neuromuscular conditions.

LABORATORY FINDINGS

Disorders That May Alter Lab Results

Hemolysis may increase serum magnesium concentrations.

Valid If Run in Human Lab?

Yes

CBC/BIOCHEMISTRY/URINALYSIS

• Calcium—if low, may accentuate signs
• Decreased fractional excretion of magnesium indicates inadequate intake. • High fractional excretion of magnesium indicates renal disease.
• Other electrolytes (sodium, potassium) often abnormal

OTHER LABORATORY TESTS

• Fractional excretion of magnesium, as determined by comparing urinary magnesium and creatinine to serum magnesium and creatinine, helps differentiate renal from dietary causes. • Ionized magnesium concentrations, although rarely available, may provide a better indication of the amount of metabolically available magnesium.

DIAGNOSTIC PROCEDURES

- An accurate history of food intake and recent activity is more useful than other invasive tests.
- An electromyogram may reveal the effect of hypomagnesemia on the muscles; however, it will not reveal the cause.

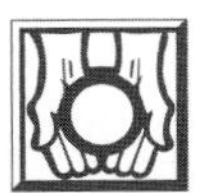

TREATMENT

HYPERMAGNESEMIA

- IV fluids and diuretics until magnesium is within normal ranges

HYPOMAGNESEMIA

- Initiate treatment of the underlying cause or the condition will persist. • Increase dietary intake of magnesium; total-body stores may be depleted and the condition will reoccur.
- Intravenous magnesium supplementation using commercial cattle products is possible. Dosage is empirical and should be given to effect.

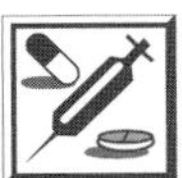

MEDICATIONS

DRUG(S) OF CHOICE

If the serum magnesium level is low enough to cause clinical signs, administer 20% $MgSO_4$ in water or glucose at 1 mEq/kg IV or to effect; a 10% solution of $MgCl_2$ also can be used.

CONTRAINDICATIONS

Magnesium can potentiate the toxic effect of aminoglycosides.

PRECAUTIONS

Administer solutions slowly if given IV.

POSSIBLE INTERACTIONS

- Magnesium sulfate is incompatible with sodium bicarbonate and hydrocortisone solutions. • Calcium-containing compounds lower serum magnesium concentrations.

FOLLOW-UP

PATIENT MONITORING

- Determine serum magnesium and calcium concentrations once or twice a day to detect overdosage or recurrence. • ECG is helpful if arrhythmias are detected. • Monitor TPR and presenting physical signs both during and after treatment.

POSSIBLE COMPLICATIONS

- Severe hypomagnesemia or hypermagnesemia can lead to coma and death. • Cardiac arrhythmias

MISCELLANEOUS

ASSOCIATED CONDITIONS

- Hypocalcemia • Hyponatremia
- Hypokalemia

AGE-RELATED FACTORS

Adult horses, especially lactating mares, and nursing foals are more susceptible to hypermagnesemia.

PREGNANCY

Effect on the fetus is the same as that on the dam.

SYNONYMS

Transport tetany

ABBREVIATION

- ECG = electrocardiogram
- TPR = temperature, pulse, and respiration

Suggested Reading

Garcia-Lopez JM, Provost PJ, *et al*. Prevalence and prognostic importance of hypomagnesemia and hypocalcemia in horses that have colic surgery. Am J Vet Res 2001;62:7–12

Henninger RW, Horst J. Magnesium toxicosis in two horses. JAVMA 1997;211:82–85.

Author Erwin G. Pearson and Janice Sojka
Consulting Editor Michel Lévy

MALABSORPTION

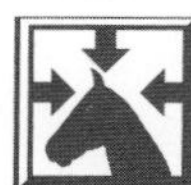

BASICS

DEFINITION

Malabsorption or malassimilation from the intestine occurs when there is diffuse or localized intestinal disease that inhibits the transference of nutrients from the intestinal lumen to the vasculature. Transient malabsorption occurs with enteritis caused by viral and bacterial agents. Chronic malabsorption is caused by parasitism, infiltrative bowel diseases, amyloidosis, and neoplasia. Besides parasitism, the causes of chronic inflammatory bowel disease are uncommon. The small intestine is usually affected in the chronic diseases; however, the large intestine may also be involved.

PATHOPHYSIOLOGY

- Malabsorption is caused by loss of the intestinal absorptive area (villous atrophy), loss of absorptive villous epithelial cells, and enlargement of junctional areas between epithelial cells. Thickening of the intestinal wall with edema, inflammatory cells, or fibrous tissue inhibits the absorptive capacity. Blockage of normal lymphatic drainage (lymphangiectasia) and decreased intestinal blood flow due to verminous arteritis may be involved. Horses that have had extensive small intestinal resection may also suffer from malabsorption.
- Viral and bacterial infections of the bowel wall can result in the temporary loss of the absorptive capacity of the small intestine. Chronic malabsorption is caused by uncontrolled immune reactions (infiltrative bowel diseases, such as lymphocytic/plasmacytic enteritis, granulomatous enteritis, or eosinophilic granulomatous enteritis). The initiating factors in this group of diseases are unknown; however, allergens or infectious agents may be stimuli. Chronic diseases include infections with *Mycobacterium avium* ssp. *avium, Mycobacterium avium* ssp. *paratuberculosis,* and fungi (*Aspergillus* spp., *Histoplasma* spp.). Alimentary neoplasia may also cause similar signs.
- Transient malabsorption may result in short-term weight loss, delayed growth, and diarrhea. These problems should resolve once the infection and immune reaction subside and the intestines achieve normal structure and function. The signs of chronic malabsorption persist; however, the progression and severity may vary. A hallmark of chronic disease is hypoproteinemia resulting from decreased protein intake (due to inappetence), malabsorption of nutrients, and protein loss into the bowel. Decreased albumin production may occur due to negative feedback mechanisms in response to elevated globulin levels, thus maintaining plasma oncotic pressure. Other disease entities cause protein-losing enteropathy rather than malabsorptive diseases.

SYSTEMS AFFECTED

Gastrointestinal

Normal feces or diarrhea if diffuse colonic involvement with weight loss

Endocrine/Metabolic

Altered protein levels and ratios

Hemic/Lymphatic/Immune

Lymphadenopathy with neoplasia or granulomatous disease

Hepatobiliary

Decreased feed intake may cause mild increase in bilirubin; eosinophilic epitheliotropic disease may affect many organs, including the liver.

Musculoskeletal

- Weight loss
- Muscle atrophy

Skin/Exocrine

Due to malnutrition, vasculitis, or inflammatory cell infiltration

Behavioral

Mildly-depressed demeanor

SIGNALMENT

Any breed or sex; younger horses usually involved (1–6 yr)

SIGNS

- Colic
- Cutaneous lesions—alopecia; rough, dry hair coat
- Dermatitis
- Coronitis
- Depressed demeanor
- Diarrhea or normal feces
- Edema
- Lethargy
- Lymphadenopathy
- Pyrexia
- Weakness
- Weight loss

CAUSES

Parasitic damage due to *Strongylus* spp. or cyathostomes. *Parascaris equorum* may cause disease in young horses. Infiltrative diseases may be due to an allergic response or uncontrolled response to infectious agent. Infection with *Lawsonia intracellularis* has been increasingly identified in the young horse. Familial occurrence has been reported. The causes of alimentary neoplasia, such as lymphosarcoma, are unknown.

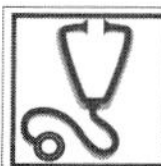

DIAGNOSIS

DIFFERENTIAL DIAGNOSIS

- A detailed history and physical examination are required. Initially, common causes of weight loss should be considered, such as inadequate nutritional intake for metabolic demands (poor feed quality, bad dentition, competition for food). Many other diseases should be considered using a systematic approach.
- Differential diagnosis for hypoproteinemia include decreased protein absorption (inadequate intake, gastroenteric disease), decreased production (liver failure), sequestration into third spaces (pleural cavity, peritoneal cavity, abscesses), or loss (alimentary or renal). Protein-losing enteropathy may be caused by acute/subacute colitis, parasitism, NSAID toxicity, gastrointestinal neoplasia (lymphosarcoma, adenocarcinoma), infiltrative bowel disease, tuberculosis, or congestive heart failure, chronic inflammatory bowel disease with lymphocytic/plasmacytic enteritis, eosinophilic granulomatous enteritis, and granulomatous enteritis.

CBC/BIOCHEMISTRY/URINALYSIS

CBC

Common findings include neutrophilia, anemia (due to chronic inflammatory disease or blood loss from ulcerations), and hypoproteinemia. The neutrophil level can be high, normal or low.

Biochemistry

- Hypoalbuminemia
- Globulin level—low, normal, or elevated
- Fibrinogen—mild elevation
- Hypocalcemia (due to loss of protein-bound calcium)
- Elevations of hepatobiliary parameters—γ-glutamyl transferase, aspartate aminotransferase, alkaline phosphatase, bilirubin (conjugated), lactate dehydrogenase, glutamate dehydrogenase, inositol dehydrogenase (sorbitol dehydrogenase), bile acids

Urinalysis

Normal

Abdominal Fluid Analysis

Normal

Fecal Examination

Fecal egg counts. Identification of large or small strongyles do not necessarily pinpoint parasites as the cause of malabsorption.

Ultrasound Imaging

Determine thickness of wall of small intestine and the presence of masses.

Carbohydrate Absorption Tests

Horse should be fasted for at least 12 hr but not >24 hr. A blood sample should be collected before the administration of the sugar, then at 30-min intervals for up to 4 hr. Water intake should be restricted for the initial 2 hr of the test period. Low or no absorption levels are consistent with delayed gastric emptying, enteric disease, or delayed intestinal transit. In addition to absorption, distribution, metabolism, and excretion are important factors to consider.

D-Xylose Absorption Test

Give 0.5 g/kg as a 10% solution via nasogastric tube. Samples may be collected into heparinized tubes. A peak is expected at approximately 60 min.

Glucose Absorption Test

Give 1 g/kg as a 20% solution via nasogastric tube. Collect blood samples into tubes containing sodium fluoride to prevent cellular metabolism of glucose. Heparinized samples can be used if the glucose level is determined immediately after collection. Normal absorption is a 2-fold increase in the baseline glucose level within 90–120 min. Low levels may occur if there is metabolism of the glucose in the lumen. Levels also reflect the metabolic/endocrinologic status of the animal.

Rectal Mucosal Biopsy

Use uterine biopsy forceps or other instrument (bottlecap, syringe-case cap); collect mucosal sample from dorsal or lateral rectal wall in region of retroperitoneal space (30-cm orad to anus). Samples with infiltration of lymphocytes, plasmacytes, eosinophils, and/or histocytes represent diffuse disease. Negative sample is nondiagnostic, necessitating intestinal biopsy.

Small Intestinal Biopsy

Requires general anesthesia, celiotomy, and wedge biopsies. Risks of anesthesia, surgery, and poor wound healing due to catabolic state with hypoalbuminemia

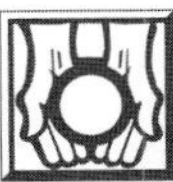

TREATMENT

Symptomatic care or specific treatment for transient diseases

DIET

Consider feeding highly digestible feed; high-quality fiber should be fed for colonic digestion. Multiple small feedings should be given. Intestinal resection for localized small intestinal disease.

MEDICATION

Anthelmintics

Treatment should be aimed for appropriate worm; repeat treatment may be required for encysted stages of nematode.

- Ivermectin—0.2 mg/kg PO
- Moxidectin—0.4 mg/kg PO
- Fenbendazole—10 mg/kg PO once daily for 5 days. Consider prior treatment with dexamethasone if treating for encysted cyathostomes.
- Pyrantel tartrate—2.2 mg/kg/day. Used as a preventative; other anthelmintics should be used to kill adult worms.

Corticosteroids

- Infiltrative bowel disease
- Prednisolone—1–2 mg/kg, PO, IM BID
- Dexamethasone—0.1–0.2 mg/kg PO SID or by parenteral administration

Antibiotics

Trimethoprim–sulfonamide 30 mg/kg PO or IV, sulfasalazine

CONTRAINDICATIONS

Corticosteroids have been associated with laminitis.

POSSIBLE DRUG INTERACTIONS

N/A

ALTERNATIVE DRUGS

N/A

PROGNOSIS

- Parasitism—poor to good
- Infiltrative bowel disease—poor
- Neoplasia—poor

FOLLOW-UP

PATIENT MONITORING

- Appetite
- Demeanor
- Feces
- Body condition

POSSIBLE COMPLICATIONS

Drug associated (immunosuppression; laminitis; Cushing's or Addison's disease)

MISCELLANEOUS

ASSOCIATED CONDITIONS

N/A

AGE-RELATED FACTORS

N/A

ZOONOTIC POTENTIAL

May be possible if shedding mycobacterial organisms or *Salmonella* spp.

PREGNANCY

Debilitation may lead to infertility, early embryonic death, or abortion.

SYNONYMS

- Chronic inflammatory bowel disease
- Granulomatous bowel disease
- Infiltrative bowel disease

SEE ALSO

- Colic

ABBREVIATIONS

N/A

Suggested Reading

Brown CM. The diagnostic value of the D-xylose absorption test in horses with unexplained chronic weight loss. Br Vet J 1992;148:41–44.

Lindberg R, Nygren A, Persson SG. Rectal biopsy diagnosis in horses with clinical signs of intestinal disorders: a retrospective study of 116 cases. Equine Vet J 1996;28:275–284.

MacAllister CG, *et al.* Lymphocytic-plasmacytic enteritis in two horses. JAVMA 1990;196:1995–1998.

Schumacher J, *et al.* Effect of intestinal resection on two juvenile horses with granulomatous enteritis. J Vet Int Med 1990;4:153–156.

Sweeney RW. Laboratory evaluation of malassimilation in horses. Vet Clin North Am [Equine Pract] 1987;3:507–515.

Author Daniel G. Kenney

Consulting Editors Henry Stämpfli and Olimpo Oliver-Espinosa

MALICIOUS INTOXICATION

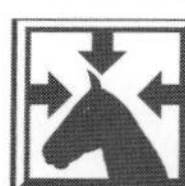

BASICS

OVERVIEW

• Determination of underlying etiologies for sudden and/or unexplained equine deaths has significant medicolegal importance. • Equine insurance mortality policies often contain exclusions, especially for death due to intoxication. • It is critical to determine the cause and manner of death in order to substantiate claims and the ultimate liability of insurers. • A systematic and thorough post-mortem examination is essential to confirm death due to toxicant exposure, whether accidental or due to malicious intent.
• Documentation of proper sample collection, storage, and laboratory submission is crucial.

SIGNALMENT

N/A

SIGNS

• Signs vary considerably depending on the specific toxicant used. However, most malicious intoxications are associated with the administration of highly toxic drugs or chemicals intended to kill quickly. • A ideal toxicant used maliciously would cause rapid death, not result in specific post-mortem lesions and be difficult to detect in post-mortem tissue or fluid samples.
• Most toxicants that result in sudden death impair the central or peripheral nervous systems, cardiovascular system, or respiratory system. Thus, if any signs are noted prior to death, they will generally be related to failure of one or more of these systems. • Depending on the toxicant used, there may be evidence of struggle before death. Alternatively, some toxicant-induced deaths are associated with no struggle prior to death. • While most malicious deaths follow the administration of a single dose of a highly toxic compound, it is possible that repeated administration of a less toxic or cumulative drug or chemical has occurred.

CAUSES AND RISK FACTORS

• The list of potential toxicants is long. Potential toxicants include strychnine, phosphides, cholinesterase-inhibiting insecticides (OPs and carbamates), nicotine, metaldehyde, cyanide, fluoroacetate, illicit drugs such as amphetamines, cocaine, heroin, and morphine, metals such as mercury, arsenic, lead, selenium, and iron, drugs such as insulin, barbiturates, reserpine, and succinylcholine, electrolytes such as potassium or calcium, and vitamins A, D, and E. • Although less common, exposure to extremely toxic plants such as *Nerium oleander* (oleander), *Taxus* spp. (yew), *Conium maculatum* (poison hemlock), or *Cicuta* spp. (water hemlock), among others, should be considered as should zootoxins such as cantharidin. • Potentially all horses are at risk, but there is likely to be more incentive to kill horses that are insured or are involved in some form of competition.

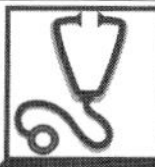

DIAGNOSIS

DIFFERENTIAL DIAGNOSIS

• There are many causes of sudden and/or unexplained death other than those due to a toxicant. • Physical causes include trauma, electrocution, lightning strike, suffocation, heat stroke, and gunshot. • Natural or genetic causes include hyperkalemic periodic paralysis, cardiac conductive disturbances, acute myocardial necrosis, cerebral thromboembolism, aortic aneurysm or other vessel rupture, and neoplasia.
• Infectious or parasitic causes include acute clostridial diseases, salmonellosis, Tyzzer's disease, anthrax, equine monocytic ehrlichiosis, foal actinobacillosis, babesiosis, and verminous arteritis. • Metabolic and nutritional causes include hypoglycemia, hypocalcemia, hypomagnesemia, and selenium and vitamin E deficiencies.

CBC/BIOCHEMISTRY/URINALYSIS

• When possible, whole blood, serum, plasma, and urine should be collected prior to death in order to perform routine clinical pathological tests. This will help delineate pathophysiologic processes that aid in refining an initial differential list. • If there is the opportunity to obtain these samples, additional quantities beyond those needed for clinical pathology should be collected for possible toxicologic analysis.

OTHER LABORATORY TESTS

• In addition to any samples collected for clinical pathological testing, other samples for toxicologic analysis include stomach contents, urine, liver, kidney, brain, eye, and heart blood. • If there is any suspicion of an injection site or sites, tissue from around the site should be saved. • Representative feed and water samples should also be collected. • Because of medicolegal considerations, all samples should be handled under chain-of-custody procedures. Chain-of-custody records specifically identify all specimens, document their condition and container in which packaged, the time and date of transfer and receipt of samples, and all individuals involved in the handling, transferring, or receiving of samples.

IMAGING N/A

DIAGNOSTIC PROCEDURES N/A

PATHOLOGICAL FINDINGS

• Consideration should be given to transporting animals to a veterinary diagnostic facility for a complete and thorough post-mortem examination. If this is not an option, a thorough field post-mortem should be conducted and any abnormalities or suspected abnormalities recorded. • GI contents should be examined carefully for evidence of toxic plant fragments or unexpected grain or forage ingestion. • Formalin-fixed samples should be collected from all major organ systems and any gross lesions and submitted to a veterinary pathologist for histopathological examination. • Lesions may suggest specific target organs and help narrow the list of differentials.

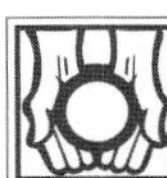

TREATMENT

• In many situations, treatment is not possible. However, if an animal is alive, treatment is directed toward stabilization of vital organ systems. Once stabilized, oral and dermal decontamination procedures should be initiated if appropriate. This includes the administration of AC and a cathartic or washing skin. • Antidotes are not available for many toxicants but fortunately, many animals survive with timely decontamination and appropriate symptomatic and supportive care.

MEDICATIONS

DRUG(S)

Activated charcoal at 1–4 g/kg body weight in water slurry (1 g AC in 5 mL water) PO. One dose of cathartic PO with AC if no diarrhea or ileus (70% sorbitol at 3 mL/kg or sodium or magnesium sulfate at 250–500 mg/kg). Administration of other drugs is dependent on each situation.

CONTRAINDICATIONS POSSIBLE INTERACTIONS N/A

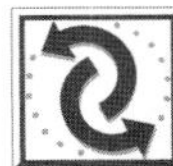

FOLLOW-UP

An appropriate follow-up is dependent on the specific toxicant under suspicion or analytically confirmed. It is possible that residual neurologic or cardiac damage may result.

PATIENT MONITORING

Dependent on the situation. Monitoring of vital functions is critical.

PREVENTION/AVOIDANCE N/A

POSSIBLE COMPLICATIONS

Potential complications are dependent on the toxicant involved

EXPECTED COURSE AND PROGNOSIS

Dependent on the toxicant involved

MISCELLANEOUS

ASSOCIATED CONDITIONS, AGE-RELATED FACTORS, ZOONOTIC POTENTIAL, PREGNANCY N/A

ABBREVIATION

• AC = activated charcoal • GI = gastrointestinal • OP = organophosphate

Suggested Reading

Haliburton JC, Edwards WC. Medicolegal investigation of the sudden or unexpected equine death: toxicologic implications. In: Robinson, NE, ed. Current Therapy in Equine Medicine, ed 4. Philadelphia: WB Saunders, 1997:657.

Author Robert H. Poppenga
Consulting Editor Robert H. Poppenga

MASTITIS

BASICS

DEFINITION

Inflammation of the mammary gland is most commonly caused by bacterial colonization within the gland; other causes are nematode migration, mycotic infection, and neoplasia.

PATHOPHYSIOLOGY

Pathophysiology of mastitis depends on the pathogen and route of infection. Initial infection occurs via three possible routes: hematogenous, adjacent dermatologic inflammation, or, most commonly, ascending via the teat canal. Bacterial colonization of the teat cistern does not automatically lead to mastitis. This suggests that failure of the immune system either locally at the teat canal or systemically as seen with endotoxemia is necessary for mastitis to occur. The equine mammary gland consists of two glands separated by a fascial septum. Each gland is divided into two or three lobes by fibroelastic capsules, with one teat cistern emptying each lobe. Inflammation may involve one or several lobes of one or both glands. In the case of ascending infection via the canal a cycle is created, with cellular debris clogging the teat canal and leading to an increase in pressure and no effective drainage of the infected material, thus encouraging it to spread into surrounding tissues.

SYSTEM AFFECTED

Mammary—However, other systems may be affected if primary mammary gland infection leads to systemic endotoxemia or if the mastitis is secondary to infection in other systems.

GENETICS

No genetic predisposition has been documented.

INCIDENCE/PREVALENCE

The incidence of infectious mastitis in the mare is quite low, and several factors may play a role in this, such as frequent nursing by the foal, which keeps the mammary gland empty. Also, the mare's lactation period is often less than 6 months, and mares have small teats, which are concealed and less likely to be traumatized. In addition, mares experience less human manipulation of teats than other species, such as cattle, in which mastitis is more common.

SIGNALMENT

Most clinical cases are in lactating mares, but it has been documented in nonlactating mares and has also been observed in foals.

SIGNS

Historical

Owners report reluctance to allow the foal to nurse the lactating mare; they may also report depression, anorexia, and severe adverse behavior when udder is palpated.

Physical Examination

- Abnormal size or swelling of the mammary gland
- Heat or pain associated with palpation
- Abnormal mammary secretions, serous, purulent, or bloody in nature
- Fever
- Ventral edema
- Hindlimb lameness or circumduction of the ipsilateral limb if one gland is affected or bilateral if both glands are affected
- Signs associated with concurrent disease

Note: Not all signs are seen in every animal; any combination may occur.

CAUSES

Infectious

Agents that cause infectious mastitis are most often bacterial. The most common isolate is *Streptococcus zooepidemicus.* Other isolates are *Staphylococcus, Actinobacillus, Pseudomonas, Klebsiella,* and *Escherichia coli.* Fungi documented to cause mastitis are *Aspergillus* spp. and *Coccidioides immitis.* Aberrant parasitic migration is also a cause.

Noninfectious

Neoplasia, the most common being primary mammary adenocarcinoma

RISK FACTORS

- Primary infection of the mammary gland occurs most commonly via the teat canal. Lactation, trauma to the teats, or insects feeding on the teats allow for colonization through this route.
- Hematogenous spread due to other disease process within the body
- Dermatologic route via cellulitis, wounds on the abdomen, culicoides hypersensitivity
- Recent surgical incision
- Lactation does not appear to be a significant predisposing factor; mastitis can occur in any female horse of any age or breed.

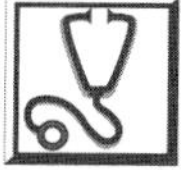

DIAGNOSIS

DIFFERENTIAL DIAGNOSIS

Other Causes of Mammary Heat, Pain, or Abnormal Secretions

Mammary abscess is differentiated from diffuse mastitis by palpation of the udder, which indicates a focal site of inflammation. Mares may show signs of pain on palpation of the udder if their foal has suddenly stopped nursing and the udder is transiently distended. These signs of discomfort should resolve completely with stripping of the udder.

Other Causes of Abnormal Udder Development

Placentitis in the pregnant mare is differentiated by history and reproductive examination findings. Impending parturition or abortion is differentiated by history and response to treatment. Hyperplasia of the mammary gland.

CBC/BIOCHEMISTRY

All laboratory data may be normal or there may be a leukocytosis with neutrophilia and hyperfibrinogenemia. Other abnormalities such as azotemia, leukopenia, increased nonsegmented white cell count, or toxic changes in neutrophils may be seen if systemic endotoxemia, bacteremia, or concurrent disease is present. Anemia of chronic disease may also be present.

IMAGING

Sonographic imaging of the mammary gland may be useful to identify and document a mammary abscess and its subsequent response to treatment.

OTHER DIAGNOSTIC PROCEDURES

Culture and cytology of mammary secretions and/or milk are necessary for a definitive diagnosis. Samples from each teat cistern should be collected, with attention paid to aseptic technique. Each sample should be submitted for cytologic examination and culture. Cytology is important because culture results may be negative with clinical mastitis. Cytologic examination of milk from normal mares is often acellular or with rare neutrophils present. During the drying-off period, normal mammary secretions contain macrophages with vacuoles present, often called *foam cells,* and lymphocytes. Smears of milk or mammary secretions from mares with signs of mastitis show numerous intact and degenerated neutrophils and cellular debris, and may show large numbers of bacteria or fungal hyphae if a mycotic infection is present. Gram-stain preparations of mammary secretions or milk may guide initial treatment until culture results are available. Aerobic culture and sensitivity are recommended. Anaerobes are not considered significant bacterial pathogens in equine mastitis, so anaerobic culture is not necessary.

Mammary gland biopsy may be indicated if clinical signs are not responsive to initial treatment for bacterial infection, or if cytologic examination of mammary secretions is not suggestive of infectious mastitis. Biopsy may show other causes of mastitis, such as parasitic migration, mycotic infections, or neoplasia.

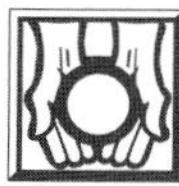

TREATMENT

- Most important therapy is local treatment, consisting of frequent stripping out of the affected lobes to remove pathogens and inflammatory cells.
- Hot packing
- Hydrotherapy
- Mild exercise, consisting of hand walking, to decrease edema formation

• Surgery may be indicated if sonographic examination reveals a mammary abscess requiring drainage, or if neoplasia is the causative agent and removal of the neoplasm is attempted.

MEDICATIONS

DRUG(S) OF CHOICE

• Local antimicrobial therapy with lactating cow intramammary treatments
• Choice of antimicrobial agent is dictated by culture and sensitivity results.
• Prior to local infusions, the teat orifice must be cleaned and disinfected with povidone-iodine solution or chlorhexidine solution. Intramammary infusions of 0.1% gentamicin solutions made from 100 mg gentamicin added to 100 mL of sterile saline have been used. Caution is needed when administering intramammary treatments because the equine teat canal is smaller and shorter than the bovine, for which the teat cannulas are designed.
• Systemic antimicrobial therapy may not be necessary in every case—Trimethoprim sulfadiazine (15 mg/kg q12 h) pending culture and sensitivity results. Penicillin alone is often not effective, but if used in combination with an aminoglycoside, it is effective in most cases. Procaine penicillin 30,000 units/kg IM q12 h. Gentamicin 8 mg/kg IM q24 h.

ALTERNATIVE MEDICATIONS

Anti-inflammatory treatment with flunixin meglumine 1.1 mg/kg IV or PO q24 h or phenylbutazone 2–4 mg/kg IV or PO q24 h

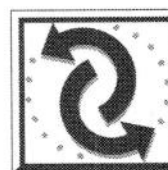

FOLLOW-UP

PATIENT MONITORING

The udder should be palpated manually daily. Initial treatment should be aimed at bacterial infection unless another etiology is suggested. Only if the patient does not respond to treatment should other causes of mastitis be considered and further diagnostic tests, as outlined above, be performed. Response to treatment should be seen within 3 days. Resolution of signs should be seen within 5–7 days. Treatment should be continued until 24 hours after signs have resolved or for 5–7 days. If abnormalities in the peripheral blood were noted, follow-up CBC or fibrinogen should be checked within 1 week of discontinuing treatment. Monitor renal function with sequential serum creatinine measurements when long-term systemic aminoglycoside or nonsteroidal anti-inflammatory administration is administered. Rectal temperature should be evaluated at least once a day for 14 days if the mare was febrile prior to treatment.

POSSIBLE COMPLICATIONS

Possible complications include sepsis, bacteremia, endotoxemia, laminitis, colitis, lymphadenopathy, lymphangitis, and fibrosis of the affected mammary glands with subsequent decreased milk production.

MISCELLANEOUS

ASSOCIATED CONDITIONS

There is one reported case of acute mastitis that was followed by abortion; however, no association was found.

AGE-RELATED FACTORS

No age predilection has been documented.

ZOONOTIC POTENTIAL

N/A

PREGNANCY

N/A

ABBREVIATIONS

N/A

Suggested Reading

McCue PM, Wilson WD. Equine mastitis—A review of 28 cases. Equine Vet J 1989;2:351–353.

Perkins N, Threlfall WR. Mastitis. In: Reed S, ed. Equine Internal Medicine. Philadelphia: WB Saunders, 1998:804–806.

Author Kerry Beckman
Consulting Editors Ashley Boyle and Corinne R. Sweeney

MATERNAL FOAL REJECTION

BASICS

OVERVIEW
• Two major forms—rejection of the foal's attempts to suckle and overt aggression toward the foal
• Because a mare's identification of her foal largely depends on smell, iatrogenic foal rejection can occur if the foal's odor changes because of extensive clinical treatments.
• Can occur without any physical pathology; however, any painful condition (e.g., mastitis) may cause this behavior.

SYSTEM AFFECTED
Central nervous system—mechanism unknown

SIGNALMENT
• More common in primiparous and Arabian mares but can occur in any breed at any age.
• Most common immediately postpartum but can occur hours or days after initial acceptance.

SIGNS
• Rejection of attempts to suckle—squealing by mare and signs of fear and avoidance, including repeatedly moving the hindquarters away from the foal or walking away from the foal, especially when the foal moves its head toward the teats
• Aggressive rejection—squealing by mare, head-threat (i.e., ears laid back against the neck), threatening to bite, biting, threatening to kick, kicking, threatening to strike, and striking

CAUSES AND RISK FACTORS
• Genetics may be a contributing factor; the problem has been identified as being more common in Arabians and in certain pedigrees.
• Turgid udders and lack of experience in primiparous mares probably are the most relevant factors in failure to allow suckling with a first birth; the mare has not yet learned that allowing the foal to suckle relieves her discomfort.
• First birth
• Arabians, especially if relatives have exhibited this behavior
• Previous foal rejection
• A highly disrupted environment or unusual circumstances at the time of birth

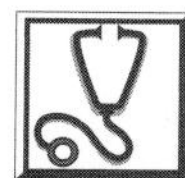

DIAGNOSIS

DIFFERENTIAL DIAGNOSIS
Any pathological condition that might cause pain or discomfort (e.g., mastitis or musculoskeletal disease)

CBC/BIOCHEMISTRY/URINALYSIS
• Should be normal if the problem is purely behavioral
• Abnormalities supporting the diagnosis of a physical pathology suggest that rejecting behavior is secondary to pain.

OTHER LABORATORY TESTS
N/A

IMAGING
N/A

DIAGNOSTIC PROCEDURES
N/A

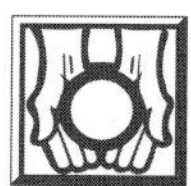

TREATMENT

PRIMIPAROUS MARES
• Restrain the mare until the foal can suckle allows the mare to learn that suckling relieves the discomfort in her udder and familiarizes her with the process of standing for nursing.
• Punishment of the mare is contraindicated. She already is fearful and may associate the presence of the foal with the physical punishment.

AGGRESSIVE MARES
• Restrain the mare to prevent injury of the foal. Cross-tying the mare still allows the mare to kick. Separating the foal and mare with a pole or partition allows the foal to reach under to suckle while the mare is held in place and reduces the likelihood she can kick the foal.
• Provide close supervision for at least the first 24 hr.
• Restrain the mare during all interactions with the foal for at least 3 days; if the mare's behavior does not improve in 7 days, acceptance of the foal is unlikely.

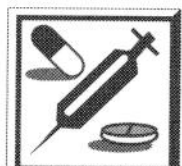

MEDICATIONS

DRUGS OF CHOICE
• Acepromazine (0.02–0.06 mg/kg IV, IM, or SC q2–4h to effect)
• Butorphanol (0.05 mg/kg IV) to relieve pain from turgid udder; if no complicating painful conditions are present, do not repeat

CONTRAINDICATIONS/POSSIBLE INTERACTIONS
• Benzodiazepines (e.g., diazepam) are contraindicated in aggressive animals, because these drugs may disinhibit aggression.
• Administration of anxiolytics and progestins for foal rejection constitutes extra-label use, and owners should be so informed.
• Review all side effects, and prepare an informed consent form for the owner to sign.

ALTERNATIVE DRUGS
• Anxiolytics (e.g., diazepam) may help with fearful mares.
• Progestins may help with aggressive mares.

FOLLOW-UP

PATIENT MONITORING
Intensive monitoring until the mare consistently allows the foal to suckle and fails to show aggression for several hours

POSSIBLE COMPLICATIONS
Inadequate supervision and restraint of an aggressive mare may result in injury to or death of the foal.

MISCELLANEOUS

ASSOCIATED CONDITIONS
Mastitis

AGE-RELATED FACTORS
Most common in primiparous mares

ZOONOTIC POTENTIAL
N/A

PREGNANCY
N/A

SYNONYMS
N/A

SEE ALSO
• Aggression

Suggested Reading

Crowell-Davis SL, Houpt KA. Maternal behavior. Vet Clin North Am Equine Pract 1986;2:557–571.

Houpt KA. Foal rejection—a review of 23 cases. Equine Pract 1984;6:38–40.

Houpt KA. Foal rejection and other behavioral problems in the postpartum period. Compend Cont Educ Pract Vet 1984;6:S144–S148.

Houpt KA, Lieb S. A survey of foal rejecting mares. Appl Anim Behav Sci 1994;39:188.

Juarbe-Diaz SV, Houpt KA, Kusunose R. Prevalence and characteristics of foal rejection in Arabian mares. Equine Vet J 1998;30:424–428.

Author Sharon L. Crowell-Davis
Consulting Editors Victoria L. Voith and Daniel Q. Estep

MAST CELL TUMOR

BASICS

OVERVIEW
Mast cell tumor is a rare neoplastic disorder arising from mast cells that affects the skin and/or subcutaneous tissue. The disease is usually localized. Metastasis to local lymph nodes and abdominal and thoracic cavity can occur but has been rarely reported.

SIGNALMENT
- No age predilection (range 1–18 years).
- No breed predilection, although Arabian horses may be predisposed and Thoroughbred horses may have a lower predisposition.
- Males have a higher predisposition.

SIGNS
- Usually mast cell tumors are single, solitary, raised, well-demarcated, and movable cutaneous nodules that range from 0.5 to 20 cm in diameter commonly affecting the head, neck, trunk, and limbs. The nodules may be ulcerated.
- Mast cell tumors also may be present as a diffuse, firm, and poorly demarcated swelling involving the distal extremities with focal aggregation of eosinophils, fibrinoid necrosis, collagen accumulation, and mineralization.
- Few cases of extracutaneous location and malignant behavior of mast cell tumors have been reported, including trachea, nasopharynx, ocular, interosseous, synovial joint, and metastasis to local lymph nodes or abdominal and thoracic cavity.

CAUSES AND RISK FACTORS
Unknown

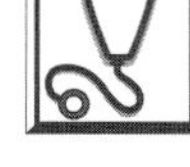

DIAGNOSIS

DIFFERENTIAL DIAGNOSIS
- Sarcoids
- Eosinophilic granuloma
- Equine collangenolytic granuloma
- Allergic or insect bite/sting reaction

CBC/BIOCHEMISTRY/URINALYSIS
Laboratory findings usually within the normal limits and nonspecific

OTHER LABORATORY TESTS
- Fine needle aspirate for cytology to reveal predominantly a population of mast cells, which are round cells with variable numbers of distinctive small, purple-staining granules in the cytoplasm. The presence of eosinophils, scattered mesenchymal cells, and degenerated collagen may be seen. Histopathology always is recommended for obtaining a definitive diagnosis.

IMAGING
Radiographs from the distal lesions of the extremities reveal usually soft tissue swelling in proximity to the joint with areas of mineralization.

OTHER DIAGNOSTIC PROCEDURES
- Evaluation of local lymph nodes should be performed; if enlarged, cytology or biopsy for histopathology should be submitted.
- If local metastasis is detected, involvement of distant lymph nodes and abdominal organs (such as spleen and liver) and presence of abdominal or pleural effusion should be determined.

PATHOLOGICAL FINDINGS
Mast cell tumors are characterized by the presence of well-differentiated mast cells affecting the dermis and subcutaneous tissue and usually accompanied by numerous eosinophils with presence of collagenolysis, necrosis, fibrosis, and mineralization. The mitotic index usually is low.

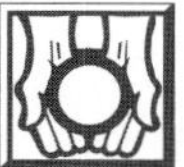

TREATMENT

- Complete surgical excision for solitary, well-demarcated nodules more often is curative, although incomplete surgical excision followed by spontaneous remission may occur in some cases.
- In tumors where surgical resection is not an option, treatment with radiation therapy or intralesional administration of triamcinolone acetonide (5–10 mg) can be tried.
- Treatment for disseminated or metastatic mast cell tumors has not been reported.

MEDICATIONS

DRUG(S) OF CHOICE
Intralesional administration of triamcinolone acetonide can be used for localized, solitary masses where surgery or radiation therapy is not an option.

CONTRAINDICATIONS/POSSIBLE INTERACTIONS
N/A

FOLLOW-UP

PATIENT MONITORING
N/A

PREVENTION/AVOIDANCE
N/A

POSSIBLE COMPLICATIONS
N/A

EXPECTED COURSE AND PROGNOSIS
- The prognosis is good for localized, solitary, well-demarcated nodules where a complete surgical excision can be achieved.
- The prognosis is guarded to poor for tumors where surgical excision is not an option without any response to radiation therapy or intralesional administration of glucocorticoids; cases with distant metastasis have a poor prognosis.

MISCELLANEOUS

ASSOCIATED CONDITIONS, AGE-RELATED FACTORS, ZOONOTIC POTENTIAL, PREGNANCY
N/A

Suggested Reading

Brown HM, Cuttino E, LeRoy BE. A subcutaneous mass in the neck of a horse. Vet Clin Pathol 2007;36:109–113.

Cole R, Chesen AB, Pool R, et al. Imaging diagnosis: equine mast cell tumor. Vet Radiol Ultrasound 2007;48:32–34.

Scott DW, Miller WH Jr. Equine Dermatology. St. Louis: Saunders, 2003.

Seeliger F, Heb O, Probsting M, et al. Confocal lasser scanning of an equine oral mast cell tumor with atypical expression of tyrosinase kinase receptor c-kit. Vet Pathol 2007;44:225–228.

Taylor S, Martinelli MJ, Trostle SS, et al. Articular mastocytosis in the tarsocrural joint of a horse. Equine Vet Educ 2005;17:207–211.

Author Francisco J. Alvarez-Berger

Consulting Editor Gwendolen Lorch

MECONIUM RETENTION

BASICS

OVERVIEW

• Meconium refers to the fetal feces made up of cellular debris, amniotic fluid, intestinal secretions, and bile. • Meconium is normally passed within 3 hr of birth, and is considered retained if the foal has not passed all meconium by 12 hr after birth. • Most meconium impactions are in the small colon at the pelvic inlet, but they also occur in the right dorsal colon or transverse colon.

SIGNALMENT

• All breeds • Possible higher incidence in colts
• This is a condition of neonatal foals, usually 6–36 hr of age.

SIGNS

• Abdominal pain (colic)—tail flagging, kicking at abdomen, rolling • Straining to defecate; tenesmus—resulting in mild rectal prolapse and/or reopening of the urachus • Failure to pass meconium. The foal may pass some meconium but retain enough meconium to cause an impaction. • Depression and decreased nursing
• More severe or advanced impactions can cause abdominal distention and severe signs of colic.
• Initial signs are usually within 6–24 hr of birth.

CAUSES AND RISK FACTORS

• Narrow pelvic canal (more common in colts)
• Delayed colostrum ingestion • Systemic disease, such as hypoxia or sepsis, can result in decreased intestinal motility. • Dehydration, prolonged recumbency, and drugs that slow GI motility may also contribute. • Meconium impaction is the most common cause of colic in neonatal foals.

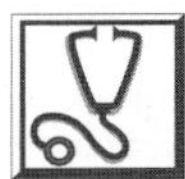

DIAGNOSIS

DIFFERENTIAL DIAGNOSIS

• Atresia coli—similar signs initially, but no meconium staining is seen after repeated enemas. • Intestinal aganglionosis (lethal white foal syndrome)—in white foals, offspring of Overo Paint breeding; usually no meconium production • Other gastrointestinal causes of neonatal colic—enterocolitis, small intestinal volvulus, intussusception • Uroperitoneum—foal may posture and strain in a similar manner; free fluid in abdomen and electrolyte abnormalities help to confirm uroabdomen. Excessive straining from meconium impaction causes bladder tears in some foals.

CBC/BIOCHEMISTRY/URINALYSIS

• No consistent abnormalities • Conditions that predispose to meconium retention (dehydration, sepsis) may lead to hemoconcentration or low IgG.

IMAGING

• Abdominal radiography—gas-filled large and small colon with radiodense fecal material in distal small colon; barium enema can help to confirm the site of obstruction and barium also acts as an osmotic agent inis the enema.
• Abdominal ultrasound—dense fecal material in small colon; can rule out enteritis, uroabdomen, or other causes of colic/abdominal distention

OTHER DIAGNOSTIC PROCEDURES

• Abdominal palpation—identify abdominal distention; firm fecal material/meconium may be recognized on deep abdominal palpation when there is not significant gas distention. • Digital rectal examination—use a well-lubritated, gloved finger—hard feces may be identified in the rectum; rule out atresia ani.

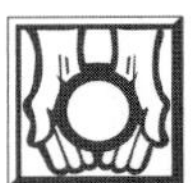

TREATMENT

• Foals with mild meconium impaction may be treated with enemas at the farm. Foals with more severe impactions or with concurrent medical problems should be admitted for inpatient medical care. • Enemas—Administration of soapy water or sodium phosphate enemas is usually effective. Acetylcysteine retention enemas are used for impactions that are refractory to soapy water or sodium phosphate enemas. Acetylcysteine (4%) will cleave disulfide bonds in the mucoprotein of the meconium, causing the surface to become slippery. Acetylcysteine retention enemas are administered via Foley catheter with inflated bulb. Gravity flow is used to administer 100–200 mL of solution, and it is retained for approximately 30–40 min. Enemas will cause some rectal irritation, and continued straining due to irritation should not be confused with persistent meconium impaction. Use of phosphate enemas should be limited in order to avoid hyperphosphatemia. • Oral laxatives—Mineral oil can be administered via nasogastric tube in order to encourage passage of feces. Colostrum also appears to have a laxative effect. In more refractory cases of impaction, osmostic agents such as sodium sulfate can be given via nasogastric tube; however, these can be irritating to the intestinal tract, and may place the foal at risk of sepsis secondary to bacterial translocation. Mineral oil and other laxatives should not be used in foals less than 24 hr of age.
• IV fluids to correct dehydration
• Nutrition—If the foal is colicky and has a continued obstruction, supplementation with intravenous fluids and dextrose or with parenteral nutrition should be initiated. • Foals that have not nursed well or that have meconium retention secondary to lack of colostrum intake should be treated with hyperimmune plasma if indicated by low IgG. • Surgical treatment—very rarely necessary; ventral midline celiotomy with guided enema and bowel massage is usually sufficient to resolve the impaction. Severe cases may require eneterotomy to remove hard meconium or other obstructive material.

MEDICATIONS

DRUG(S) OF CHOICE

• NSAIDs such as flunixin meglumine (0.5–1.1 mg/kg IV or PO q12–24h) or ketoprofen (1.1–2.2 mg/kg IV q12–24h) can be given for analgesia. • Sedation and analgesia are often needed for administration of the enema—xylazine (0.5–1.1 mg/kg IV), butorphanol (0.02–0.1 mg/kg IV) or valium (0.1 mg/kg IV).

CONTRAINDICATIONS/POSSIBLE INTERACTIONS

• NSAIDs should be used with caution in neonates, especially if there are signs of dehydration or renal compromise. • The foal should be monitored closely for changes in condition—Analgesics and sedation may mask a more serious underlying condition.

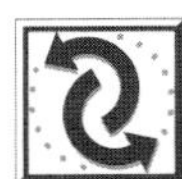

FOLLOW-UP

PATIENT MONITORING

• Progression of colic signs and abdominal distention—take serial measurements of the abdomen. • Passage of fecal material—pasty yellow "milk" feces are passed after all meconium has been passed.

PREVENTION/AVOIDANCE

• Ensure adequate colostrum intake. • Routine administration of a warm soapy water enema is recommended if the foal has not passed its meconium within 3 hr of birth.

POSSIBLE COMPLICATIONS

• Rectal tear • Secondary ileus • Bacterial translocation and sepsis from irritated GI mucosa • Foals that require surgical correction of the impaction are at risk of abdominal adhesions.

EXPECTED COURSE AND PROGNOSIS

Meconium impactions have a very good prognosis, and rarely require surgery. Generally, 1 or 2 enemas will resolve mild meconium impactions.

MISCELLANEOUS

ASSOCIATED CONDITIONS

Neonatal hypoxia and sepsis can contribute to meconium retention.

AGE-RELATED FACTORS

This is a condition of neonatal foals.

SEE ALSO

• Lethal white foal syndrome • Colic in foals

ABBREVIATIONS

• GI = gastrointestinal

Suggested Reading

Ryan CA, Sanchez LC. Nondiarrheal disorders of the gastrointestinal tract in neonatal foals. Vet Clin Equine 2005;21:313–332.

Author Margaret C. Mudge
Consulting Editor Margaret C. Mudge

MELANOMA

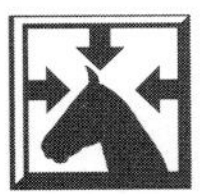

BASICS

DEFINITION

Neoplasm arising from melanocytes or melanoblasts (melanin-producing cells)

PATHOPHYSIOLOGY

• Locally invasive • Often multifocal • Metastasis occurs late in disease course in up to 70%. • More aggressive in non-gray horses

SYSTEMS AFFECTED

• Skin/exocrine • Hemic/lymphatic/immune • Gastrointestinal (salivary gland)

GENETICS

A heritable component is suggested in Lipizzaners—mode unknown.

INCIDENCE/PREVALENCE

• Up to 15% of all equine tumors • Very common in gray horses—up to 80% may eventually be affected. • Rare, and typically more aggressive in non-gray horses

SIGNALMENT

Breed Predilection

• Common in gray horses • Arabians, Lipizzaners, and Percherons may be overrepresented.

Mean Age and Range

Usually >5 years old— incidence increases with age

Predominant Sex

None

SIGNS

Historical

• Slowly progressive mass(es), often in perineum or ventral tail or parotid area • Often initially solitary, progressing to multifocal • Usually clinically silent unless very large/metastatic

Physical Examination Findings

• Multifocal, darkly pigmented cutaneous masses, most commonly in perineum or on ventral tail • May be concurrent involvement of parotid salivary gland(s) • Rectal examination may reveal intrapelvic extension/lymphadenopathy in late stages.

CAUSES

Unknown

RISK FACTORS

Unknown, other than gray coat color

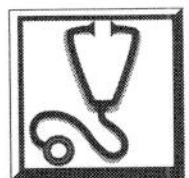

DIAGNOSIS

DIFFERENTIAL DIAGNOSIS

• Abscess • Other neoplasia • Histopathology or cytology necessary to confirm

CBC/BIOCHEMISTRY/URINALYSIS

Usually normal

IMAGING

Abdominal ultrasound considered in select cases, especially prior to major perineal surgery

PATHOLOGICAL FINDINGS

• Often contained within a fibrous pseudocapsule • Usually black on cut surface • Heavily pigmented intradermal and subcutaneous areas in proximity to sweat glands and other adnexal structures • Mixture of epithelioid, spindloid, and balloon-shaped pigmented cells with coarse granularity • Mitotic figures are rare. • "Amelanotic," sparsely pigmented, or nonpigmented forms can be seen in non-gray horses.

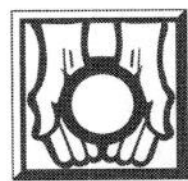

TREATMENT

AIMS OF TREATMENT

• Reduce tumor burden to prevent anatomic abnormality. • Delay tumor progression if possible.

APPROPRIATE HEALTH CARE

Inpatient or outpatient surgery may be appropriate based on extent of disease.

ACTIVITY

No restrictions

DIET

No restrictions

CLIENT EDUCATION

Disease will almost uniformly progress, but few animals will die as a result of melanoma.

SURGICAL CONSIDERATIONS

Thorough familiarity with anatomy of perineum and parotid area important to ensure that operative morbidity is minimized

MEDICATIONS

DRUG(S)

• Cimetidine 2.5–5 mg/kg PO BID–TID: believed to act as a biologic response modifier • Cisplatin in sesame oil and sorbitol monooleate 3.3 mg/mL by intratumoral injection q2weeks for 4 treatments • Therapy with NSAIDs may be theoretically useful. • An autologous tumor cell vaccine has been used in some patients—efficacy is questionable.

PRECAUTIONS

Veterinarians administering chemotherapy should be familiar with potential hazards to personnel associated with its administration. Appropriate personal protection should be used.

FOLLOW-UP

PATIENT MONITORING

• Quarterly to biannual rechecks for progression is reasonable if benign neglect or oral medical therapy is elected. • If intratumoral cisplatin is performed, recheck every 2 weeks prior to injection and then 1 mo following completion of injections—quarterly to biannual rechecks thereafter are reasonable.

POSSIBLE COMPLICATIONS

• Difficulties associated with bridle fit, parturition, urination, or defecation are possible with disease progression. • Effects of eventual metastasis depend on body system involved. Sites of metastasis include abdominal lymph nodes, visceral organs, lungs, and central nervous system, among others.

EXPECTED COURSE AND PROGNOSIS

• Short- to intermediate-term prognosis is generally excellent. • Over years, some animals may develop metastatic disease or local disease progression that can lead to diminished quality of life/utility or, occasionally, acute decompensation.

MISCELLANEOUS

AGE-RELATED FACTORS

Incidence increases with age.

PREGNANCY

Avoid cisplatin during first trimester of pregnancy.

SYNONYMS

• Melanocytoma • Melanocytic nevus • Melanomatosis • Malignant melanoma

SEE ALSO

• Sarcoid • Mast cell tumor

Suggested Reading

Hare JE, Staempfli HR. Cimetidine for the treatment of melanomas in horses: efficacy determined by client questionnaire. Equine Pract 1994;16:18–21.

MacGillivray KC, Sweeney RW, Del Piero F. Metastatic melanoma in horses. J Vet Intern Med 2002;16:452–456.

Rowe EL, Sullins KE. Excision as treatment of dermal melanomatosis in horses: 11 cases (1994–2000). J Am Vet Med Assoc 2004;225:94–96.

Smith SH, Goldschmidt MH, McManus PM. A comparative review of melanocytic neoplasms. Vet Pathol 2002;39:651–678.

Theon AP, Wilson WD, Magdesian KG, Pusterla N, Snyder JR, Galuppo LD. Long-term outcome associated with intratumoral chemotherapy with cisplatin for cutaneous tumors in equidae: 573 cases (1995–2004). J Am Vet Med Assoc 2007;230:1506–1513.

Valentine BA. Equine melanocytic tumors: a retrospective study of 53 horses (1998 to 1991). J Vet Intern Med 1995;9:291–297.

Author Douglas H. Thamm
Consulting Editor Gwendolen Lorch

MELENA AND HEMATOCHEZIA

BASICS

OVERVIEW

• Melena results from bleeding from the mouth to the colons into the GIT. This includes also blood coughed up from the respiratory tract and swallowed. The dark, black, or tarry appearance of feces is caused by oxidation (microbial digestion) of the iron in hemoglobin passing through the gut. Large quantities of blood must be present for melena to be evident, and fecal occult blood tests are frequently negative despite the loss of blood into the GIT. • Hematochezia is defined as presence of undigested blood in the feces. The probable bleeding sites include the distal parts of large colon, small colon and rectum.

PATHOPHYSIOLOGY

• Gastrointestinal bleeding may be occult, slow, and/or rapid bleeding. Occult bleeding is usually not visible. The total volume loss depends on the duration of bleeding, which may be substantial despite the lack of clinical symptoms. A major concern is the loss of iron.
• Slow bleeding may arise de novo or be superimposed on chronic occult blood loss. It may eventually lead to hemodynamic instability or shock. • Rapid bleeding may lead to hypovolemic shock and death. Therefore, hemodynamic stability must be promptly restored with appropriate treatments.

SIGNALMENT

There is no age, breed, or sex predisposition for this condition.

SIGNS

Historical

Clients frequently have observed dark or bloody feces. In cases of chronic or severe bleeding, exercise intolerance and/or pale mucous membranes may be present. Low-grade colic or abdominal discomfort has been observed.

Physical Examination

Dark or tarry feces or frank blood in feces. If substantial blood loss has occurred, mucous membranes may become pale and capillary refill time extended. In patients with occult bleeding sometimes anemia is observed. Additional signs present depend on underlying cause.

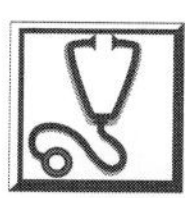

DIAGNOSIS

CAUSES, RISK FACTORS, AND DIFFERENTIAL DIAGNOSIS

History of exposure to risk factors is helpful in establishing the diagnosis:
• Rectal examination—rectal tears • Nasogastric intubation—upper gastrointestinal tract trauma or trauma to nasal passages • NSAIDs treatment—gastritis, duodenitis, gastroduodenal erosions, and colitis • Exposure to toxins (acorn, aflatoxin, arsenic, cantharidin, *Crotolaria* spp., mycotoxin, oak, organophosphate, warfarin)
Other causes/differential diagnoses include:
• Parasitism • Enteritis/colitis syndrome
• Gastric neoplasia • Small or large bowel neoplasia • Lymphoma • Colonic hematomas
• Swallowed blood from the respiratory tract
• Gastroduodenal ulcers • Purpura hemorrhagica • Thrombocytopenia
• Coagulopathies • Vasculitis • Mesenteric arterial aneurysm
Although gastric ulcers are widely present in the working horse population, melena is rarely observed.

CBC/BIOCHEMISTRY/URINALYSIS

• Hemogram may show anemia from blood loss. Leukopenia is present in many bacterial enterocolitis cases. Hypoproteinemia possible from loss of protein into the GIT lumen. Thrombocytopenia if present may result in significant GIT hemorrhage. Electrolyte and acid–base abnormalities with many diarrheas. Mild azotemia may be associated with dehydration. Urine typically concentrated from fluid retention, with the exception of cantharidin toxicosis. With cantharidin toxicosis there is frequently hyposthenuria (SG 1.003–1.006) despite clinical dehydration. • Anemia may be associated with decreased bone marrow iron, which can be appreciated with a Prussian blue staining of the bone marrow specimen. Serum iron may be decreased, whereas iron-binding capacity may increase. Eventually microcytic, hypochromic erythrocytes are seen on the CBC.

OTHER LABORATORY TESTS

• Fecal examination for parasites and bacterial cultures • Coagulation profile may reveal primary or secondary clotting abnormality
• Commercial (fecal occult) tests for detection of presence of fresh or digested blood in feces (fecal occult blood tests are often negative because colonic microflora digest hemoglobin)

DIAGNOSTIC PROCEDURES

Gastroscopic Examination

Check for the presence of origin for bleeding in the upper respiratory tract, esophagus, stomach, and duodenum. *Caution!* It is not uncommon for mild iatrogenic hemorrhage to occur with gastric ulcers in the stratified squamous mucosa when the stomach is insufflated for gastroscopy. In addition, it is rare to have melena from bleeding gastric ulcers in the horse.

Proctoscopy

Useful in hematochezia

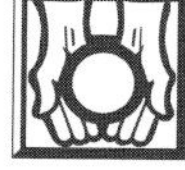

TREATMENT

Most patients with melena or hematochezia should be hospitalized to determine a cause of the condition and provide supportive care. Fluid electrolyte and acid–base abnormalities should be corrected.

MEDICATIONS

Blood transfusion should be considered if the PCV is <12%, 0.12 L/L, or is low and rapidly falling. A 1000-lb (454-kg) horse with a PCV <12% should receive 5–8 L of whole blood.

DRUG(S) OF CHOICE N/A

CONTRAINDICATIONS

NSAIDs should not be administered to patients with suspected or proven NSAID toxicosis.

PRECAUTIONS

NSAIDs should not or should be used with caution in patients diagnosed with GIT mucosal lesions.

POSSIBLE INTERACTIONS N/A

ALTERNATIVE DRUGS N/A

FOLLOW-UP

PATIENT MONITORING

PCV should be monitored twice daily until stabilized

POSSIBLE COMPLICATIONS

Right dorsal colitis and chronic, low-grade colic with NSAID toxicosis

MISCELLANEOUS

Administration of bismuth compounds such as bismuth subsalicylate turns the feces black and can be misinterpreted as melena.

ASSOCIATED CONDITIONS

N/A

AGE-RELATED FACTORS

N/A

ZOONOTIC POTENTIAL

The zoonotic potential of *Salmonella* spp. and *Cryptosporidium* (foals) should be considered when treating patients with diarrhea of unknown etiology.

PREGNANCY

Mares receiving blood transfusions develop alloantibody to the transfused RBCs. The alloantibody may be transferred to subsequent foals via the colostrum. If sufficient quantities of the alloantibody are present in the colostrum and the foal's RBCs contain the same antigens as the transfused RBCs, the foal could develop neonatal isoerythrolysis.

ABBREVIATIONS

• GIT = gastrointestinal tract
• PCV = packed cell volume

Suggested Reading

Pearson EG, Smith BB, McKim JM. Fecal blood determinations and interpretations. Proc Am Assoc Equine Pract 1987:77–81.
Smith BP. Alterations in alimentary and hepatic function. In: Smith B, ed. Large Animal Internal Medicine. St. Louis: Mosby, 1996:118–141.

Author Modest Vengust
Consulting Editors Henry Stämpfli and Olimpo Oliver-Espinosa

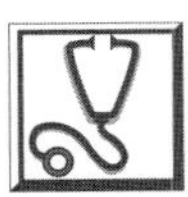

BASICS

OVERVIEW

- A toxic syndrome involving the GI and renal systems, resulting primarily from the ingestion or dermal absorption of blistering agents containing inorganic mercury salts (e.g., mercuric iodide or mercuric chloride)
- Toxicosis from ingesting seeds treated with mercury-containing fungicides is unlikely, because such fungicides are no longer used.
- Mercury binds to a variety of sulfhydryl-containing enzymes resulting in nonspecific cell injury and death.

SIGNALMENT

No breed, age, or sex predilections

SIGNS

- Depression
- Colic
- Diarrhea
- Weakness
- Skin erosions, ulcerations, and crusting
- Dehydration
- Oliguria
- Laminitis

CAUSES AND RISK FACTORS

- Excessive application of mercury-containing blistering agent
- Application of mercury-containing blistering agent to damaged skin
- Failure to prevent the animal from ingesting a dermally applied mercury-containing agent
- Application of mercury-containing blistering agent in combination with DMSO

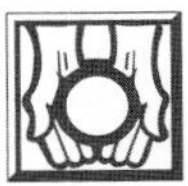

DIAGNOSIS

DIFFERENTIAL DIAGNOSIS

- Lead toxicosis—likely evidence of neurologic dysfunction; measurement of whole-blood or tissue lead concentrations
- Arsenic toxicosis—measurement of whole-blood, urine, or tissue arsenic concentrations
- NSAID toxicosis—history of previous use; measurement in plasma or serum
- Cantharidin toxicosis—evidence of cystitis; detection of cantharidin in stomach contents or urine
- *Quercus* spp. (oak) toxicosis—detection of plant material in the GI tract; evidence of oak consumption
- Salmonellosis—fecal cultures
- Ehrlichial colitis—serology
- Acute cyathastomiasis—fecal egg counts
- Clostridial colitis—isolation of pathogenic clostridia; identification of toxins
- Antimicrobial-induced colitis (e.g., lincomycin, tetracycline)—history of drug use

CBC/BIOCHEMISTRY/URINALYSIS

- Increased PCV
- Hyperfibrinogenemia
- Serum electrolyte changes—hyponatremia, hypochloremia, hyperphosphatemia, and hyperkalemia
- Hyperglycemia
- Azotemia
- Urinalysis—glycosuria, proteinuria, isosthenuria, hematuria, waxy or granular casts
- Occult blood in feces

OTHER LABORATORY TESTS

- Ante-mortem—measurement of mercury in urine or blood
- Post-mortem—measurement of mercury in liver or kidney tissue

IMAGING

N/A

DIAGNOSTIC PROCEDURES

N/A

PATHOLOGICAL FINDINGS

Gross

- Watery feces
- Intraluminal hemorrhage
- GI mucosal edema
- Mucosal ulcerations in the oral cavity, stomach, and colon
- Subcutaneous edema
- Pale, soft, and swollen kidneys

Histopathologic

- Acute, severe renal tubulonephrosis
- Severe, extensive ulcerative colitis and enteritis

TREATMENT

- Remove source of mercury.
- Treat for dehydration, circulatory shock, and renal failure.
- Provide a bland diet containing reduced amounts of high-quality protein.

MEDICATIONS

DRUGS

- Enhance mercury elimination with a chelator.
  - Dimercaprol (British anti-lewisite) is classic mercury chelator—loading dose of 4–5 mg/kg by deep muscular injection followed by 2–3 mg/kg q4h for 24 hr and then 1mg/kg q4h for 2 days; adverse reactions include tremors, convulsions, and coma.
  - Succimer is a less toxic chelator—dose is not established for horses, but 10 mg/kg PO q8h is suggested.
- Control abdominal pain.
  - Flunixin meglumine (1.1 mg/kg IV q12–24h) or butorphanol tartrate (0.1 mg/kg IV q3–4h up to 48 hr)
  - Xylazine hydrochloride (1.1 mg/kg IV) may be used in conjunction with butorphanol (0.01–0.02 mg/kg IV).
- Demulcents—mineral oil; kaolin-pectin

CONTRAINDICATIONS/POSSIBLE INTERACTIONS

Use NSAIDs cautiously because of possible adverse GI and renal effects.

FOLLOW-UP

PATIENT MONITORING

Monitor renal function.

PREVENTION/AVOIDANCE

- Identify and properly dispose of the source of exposure.
- Avoid use of mercury-containing blisters.

POSSIBLE COMPLICATIONS

N/A

EXPECTED COURSE AND PROGNOSIS

- Dependent on the severity of clinical signs
- Renal impairment suggests a poor prognosis.
- One equine case report described brain neuronal degeneration.
- Long-term neurologic deficits are possible after recovery.

MISCELLANEOUS

ASSOCIATED CONDITIONS

N/A

AGE-RELATED FACTORS

N/A

ZOONOTIC POTENTIAL

N/A

PREGNANCY

- Most forms of mercury can cross the placenta.
- The significance of fetal exposure after use of mercury salts on pregnant mares is unknown.

ABBREVIATIONS

- DMSO = dimethylsulfoxide
- GI = gastrointestinal
- PCV = packed cell volume

Suggested Reading

Guglick MA, MacAllister CG, Sundeep Chandra AM, Edwards WC, Qualls CW, Stephens DH. Mercury toxicosis caused by the ingestion of a blistering compound in a horse. J Am Vet Med Assoc 1995;206:210–213.

Author Robert H. Poppenga

Consulting Editor Robert H. Poppenga

METACARPO- (METATARSO-) PHALANGEAL JOINT DISEASE

BASICS

OVERVIEW

• Any disease localized to the MCPJ/MTPJ
• The MCPJ/MTPJ is intensely loaded and has the greatest range of motion of any equine joint. The high degree of mobility makes this joint particularly susceptible to exercise-induced wear and tear. Hyperextension, high compressive, and torsional forces result in injury. • The term "osselets" is used to describe the thickening associated with synovitis and capsulitis of the MCPJ and, less commonly, the MTPJ.
• Musculoskeletal— fetlock

SIGNALMENT

• All breeds and types of horses • Most common in horses used for racing or other high-impact sports

SIGNS

• Lameness is variable in onset, often bilateral with one limb affected more than the other.
• Pain, heat, synovial distention of the MCPJ/MTPJ • Stiff gait and shortened stride
• Resentment and decreased range of motion during MCPJ/MTPJ flexion

CAUSES AND RISK FACTORS

• Sports that require maximal speed, i.e., racing
• Poor conformation • Specific diseases that may cause MCPJ/MTPJ synovitis or arthritis:
  ○ Dorsal osteochondral fragmentation of the first phalanx ("chip fracture")
  ○ Articular fractures of the proximal first phalanx, proximal sesamoid bones, or distal third metacarpal/metatarsal bone
  ○ Osteochondrosis of the MCPJ/MTPJ
  ○ Subchondral bone disease of the distal palmar/plantar aspects of MCPJ/MTPJ
  ○ Traumatic rupture of the suspensory apparatus
  ○ Luxation of the MCPJ/MTPJ

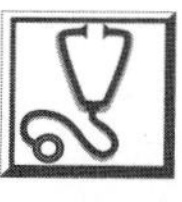

DIAGNOSIS

DIFFERENTIAL DIAGNOSIS

• Positive lower limb flexion is not specific to MCPJ/MTPJ disease. Lower limb abnormalities should be ruled out with imaging and/or diagnostic analgesia procedures. • Joint distention may be a false localizing sign. Diagnostic analgesia procedure will confirm or rule out MCPJ/MTPJ disease.

IMAGING

• Radiography—In early or acute disease, radiographic evaluation may be normal. Periarticular osteophyte formation, loss of joint space, and subchondral bone sclerosis are signs of chronic disease. • Nuclear scintigraphy—Generalized increased radiopharmaceutical uptake of the MCPJ/MTPJ with disease. Focal increased radiopharmaceutical uptake of specific location(s) for corresponding fracture(s) Focal increased radiopharmaceutical uptake of the distal palmar/plantar aspect of MCIII/MTIII in subchondral bone injury • MRI—Excellent imaging modality for assessment of subchondral bone and articular cartilage

OTHER DIAGNOSTIC PROCEDURES

• Diagnostic analgesia—intra-articular analgesia of the MCPJ/MCTJ and low palmar/plantar analgesia • Arthroscopy—Global visualization of the articular cartilage and articular lesions of the MCPJ/MTPJ. Removal of offending osteochondral fragmentation is common.
• Synovial fluid analysis to rule out infectious arthritis

PATHOLOGICAL FINDINGS

Periarticular osteophyte formation, thin cartilage, cartilaginous fibrillation, osteochondral fragmentation, thickened or enlarged dorsal synovial pad, subchondral sclerosis and/or lysis

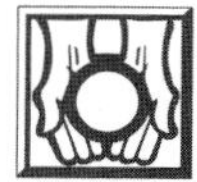

TREATMENT

• Intra-articular anti-inflammatory medication(s) of the MCPJ/MTPJ • Rest periods from weeks to several months
• Reduction in workload and expectations for the horse • Arthroscopic removal of osteochondral fragmentation(s) when appropriate • Surgical fixation of articular fracture(s) of the proximal first phalanx, distal MCIII/MTIII, or proximal sesamoid bones. Screws placed in lag fashion, bone plates, or both depending on fracture configuration • Surgical arthrodesis of the MCPJ/MTPJ using a dorsal bone plate and tension band wiring on the palmar aspect joint is indicated in advanced disease or as a salvage procedure in horses with traumatic rupture of the suspensory apparatus.

MEDICATIONS

DRUG(S) OF CHOICE

• NSAIDs—phenylbutazone (2.2 mg/kg daily to BID for 7–10 days) • Intra-articular corticosteroids— methylprednisolone acetate (20–40 mg) or triamcinolone (3–6 mg)
• Intra-articular sodium hyaluronate (10–20 mg) • Combination of intra-articular corticosteroids and sodium hyaluronate
• Systemic chondroprotective drugs—polysulfated glycosaminoglycan (500 mg IM q4days for 7 treatments) or sodium hyaluronate (40 mg IV q7days for 3 treatments)
• Oral chondroprotective medications—glucosamine/chondrotin sulfate powder (1 scoop [3.3 g] BID)

CONTRAINDICATIONS/POSSIBLE INTERACTIONS

Intra-articular corticosteroids use is not recommended in horses with a previous history of laminitis.

FOLLOW-UP

PATIENT MONITORING

• Resolution or decreased amount of synovial distension of MCPJ/MTPJ is expected after rest or intra-articular anti-inflammatories. • Periodic lameness evaluation as clinical signs dictates

PREVENTION/AVOIDANCE

• Appropriate training and conditioning for desired sport • Recognition of acute disease and appropriate treatment in a timely manner
• Avoid the use of horseshoes with toe grabs.
• Reduction in workload or alterative sport may prolong athletic career albeit at a lower level.

POSSIBLE COMPLICATIONS

Inability to perform expected sport due to chronic lameness

EXPECTED COURSE AND PROGNOSIS

• For MCPJ/MTPJ disease, early recognition and response to treatment may prolong the intended use of the horse. • Osteoarthritis of the MCPJ/MTPJ is progressive and a reduction in athletic soundness is expected. • In advanced MCPJ/MTPJ disease or traumatic rupture of suspensory apparatus, surgical arthrodesis is indicated. After arthrodesis, horses may be salvaged for breeding purposes or retired to pasture.

MISCELLANEOUS

AGE-RELATED FACTORS

Uncommon in weanlings, yearlings, and 2-year-olds unless associated with osteochondrosis

SEE ALSO

• Osteoarthritis • Osteochondrosis

ABBREVIATIONS

• MCPJ = metacarpophalangeal joint
• MTPJ = metatarsophalangeal joint
• MCIII = third metacarpal bone
• MTIII = third metatarsal bone

Suggested Reading

Richardson DW. The metacarpophalangeal joint. In: Ross MW, Dyson SJ, eds. Diagnosis and Management of Lameness in the Horse. St. Louis: Saunders, 2003:348–362.

Author Elizabeth J. Davidson
Consulting Editor Elizabeth J. Davidson

METALDEHYDE TOXICOSIS

BASICS

OVERVIEW

• Metaldehyde toxicosis is referred to as the "shake and bake" syndrome in domestic animals and involves adverse effects on the nervous and musculoskeletal systems ("classically" caudal-to-cranial progression of signs), GI tract, liver and kidneys, as well as disrupted thermoregulation and coagulation. • Metaldehyde is a polycyclic tetramer of acetaldehyde and is primarily available in molluscacides containing less than 5% metaldehyde. • Although intoxication is relatively uncommon in horses, this species seems to be particularly sensitive (rapid onset within as little as 15 min and usually within 2 hr). • Intoxication usually results from mishandling of pelleted baits. • Intoxication is associated with decreased brain concentrations of inhibitory neurotransmitters (e.g., GABA, norepinephrine, 5-hydroxytryptamine, and 5-hydroxyindoleacetic acid), as well as possibly increased concentrations of excitatory neurotransmitters.

SIGNALMENT

No age, sex, or breed predilections

SIGNS

• Salivation • Agitation • Profuse sweating • Colic • Tachycardia and weak pulse • Tachypnea • Dyspnea • Hyperesthesia and muscle fasciculations • Tremors • Ataxia • Exaggerated leg movements • Violent continuous convulsions • Hyperthermia • DIC • Organ failure • Death

CAUSES AND RISK FACTORS

• Acute exposures of horses to greater than 60–100 mg/kg of metaldehyde • Mishandling of pelleted baits • Coastal or low-lying areas enzootic to snails and slugs

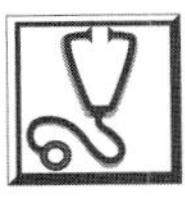

DIAGNOSIS

DIFFERENTIAL DIAGNOSIS

• Strychnine toxicosis:
  ○ Organochlorine insecticide toxicosis
  ○ AChE-inhibiting insecticides
• Plant intoxications—physical examination, history of *Cicuta* (water hemlocks), verticillate-leaved *Asclepias* (whorled milkweeds), *Conium* (poison hemlocks), or *Nicotiana* (tobacco) species, plant identification in habitat or GI contents, pathological lesions, analysis for toxins (when possible) in GI contents and tissues
• Cranial or cervical trauma • Rabies
• Fumonisin B_1 intoxication • Hepatic encephalopathy • Tetanus

CBC/BIOCHEMISTRY/ URINALYSIS

• Increased PCV and total protein • Elevations in serum concentrations of liver and muscle enzymes, BUN, and creatinine (especially with hyperthermia) • Metabolic acidosis

OTHER LABORATORY TESTS

• Ante-mortem—analysis of metaldehyde in serum, plasma, urine, retrieved GI contents, feces (may not be completed until after death or resolution) • Post-mortem—analysis of metaldehyde in GI contents and feces

IMAGING

N/A

DIAGNOSTIC PROCEDURES

N/A

PATHOLOGICAL FINDINGS

• Gross—generalized renal, hepatic, GI and pulmonary congestion, petechial and ecchymotic hemorrhages throughout the body, subepicardial and subendothelial hemorrhages, hyperemia of the GI mucosa, and mild enteritis • Histologic—swollen medullary axons and mild hepatic degeneration

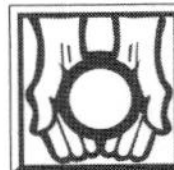

TREATMENT

• Prevent further metaldehyde exposure.
• Gastric lavage immediately after exposure
• Administer AC soon after ingestion.
• Administer mineral oil to enhance elimination of metaldehyde and acetaldehyde.
• Provide supportive care for dehydration, hypovolemic shock, acidosis, and hyperthermia.

MEDICATIONS

DRUG(S) OF CHOICE

• Xylazine hydrochloride at 0.3–1.1 mg/kg IV alone (higher dosage) or in conjunction with acepromazine maleate at 0.02–0.05 mg/kg IV (lower dosage of xylazine) can be used as needed for sedation in the absence of convulsions. • AC (1–4 g/kg), possibly followed by 2–4 L of mineral oil via nasogastric tube • Diazepam can be administered to adults (25–50 mg IV) or foals (0.05–0.4 mg/kg IV) for muscle tremors and convulsions (can repeat in 30 min).
• Phenobarbital (1–10 mg/kg IV) can be administered along with diazepam to control convulsions. • General anesthesia may be indicated for the control of convulsions in some instances. • Slow IV infusion of methocarbamol (15–25 mg/kg; up to 55 mg/kg recommended by manufacturer) for muscle relaxation • Fluid therapy (lactated Ringer's solution, 0.9% saline, or saline with dextrose), with or without sodium bicarbonate, to control dehydration, acidosis, and hyperthermia

CONTRAINDICATIONS/POSSIBLE INTERACTIONS

• Sedatives and anesthetics should be used prudently in ataxic horses. • Acepromazine has been associated with lowered seizure thresholds and hypotension and should be avoided in the presence of convulsions or circulatory collapse.

FOLLOW-UP

• Identification of source of metaldehyde
• Proper disposal of or limited access to metaldehyde-containing products

PATIENT MONITORING

• Monitor pulse rate, quality, and rhythm, as well as capillary refill time and mucous membrane color, continuously to assess the cardiovascular system. • Monitor body temperature, PCV, total protein, and acid-base status. • With severe hyperthermia, monitor liver and kidney function and blood clotting for several days.

PREVENTION/AVOIDANCE

• Use molluscacides according to label instructions. • Properly store metaldehyde-containing products. • Use alternative products for control of populations of snails and slugs.

POSSIBLE COMPLICATIONS

• DIC • Multiorgan failure

EXPECTED COURSE AND PROGNOSIS

In the absence of hyperthermia-associated complications, the prognosis for long-term survival is good with immediate and aggressive therapy.

MISCELLANEOUS

ASSOCIATED CONDITIONS

• Acidosis • Hyperthermia • DIC
• Multiorgan failure

AGE-RELATED FACTORS N/A

ZOONOTIC POTENTIAL

N/A

PREGNANCY

N/A

ABBREVIATIONS

• AC = activated charcoal
• AChE = acetylcholinesterase
• DIC = disseminated intravascular coagulation
• GI = gastrointestinal
• PCV = packed cell volume

Suggested Reading

Talcott PA. Metaldehyde. In: Plumlee KH, ed. Clinical Veterinary Toxicology.St. Louis: Mosby, 2004:182–183.

Author Tim J. Evans
Consulting Editor Robert H. Poppenga

METHEMOGLOBINEMIA

BASICS

DEFINITION

- Methemoglobinemia occurs when the normal regulatory mechanisms maintaining RBC hemoglobin in a reduced state (as hemoglobin-Fe^{2+}) are overwhelmed resulting in excessive production of methemoglobin (hemoglobin-Fe^{3+}), exceeding a concentration of 3% of hemoglobin.
- Horses have a relatively poor erythrocyte reductive capacity and are highly susceptible to the effects of oxidizing agents that cause methemoglobinemia.

PATHOPHYSIOLOGY

- Methemoglobin is a form of hemoglobin spontaneously formed in small quantities during the normal process of oxygen binding to the RBC iron-hemoglobin molecule with conversion of the ferrous iron (Fe^{2+}) to ferric iron (Fe^{3+}).
- Methemoglobin is unable to bind oxygen.
- Under normal circumstances methemoglobin is continuously reduced back to hemoglobin by several protective enzyme systems, namely NADH-dependent methemoglobin reductase (or cytochrome b_5 reductase), which is the principal conversion mechanism, and NADPH-methemoglobin reductase (or NADPH diaphorase). Although of minor importance, the latter enzymatic system utilizes glutathione reductase, glucose-6-phosphate dehydrogenase, and glutathione peroxidase to reduce methemoglobin to hemoglobin.
- Ascorbic acid and reduced glutathione also play a role in methemoglobin reduction.
- Most cases of methemoglobinemia are due to excessive production of methemoglobin when these normal physiological regulatory mechanisms are overwhelmed. In horses, this can occur following exposure to oxidant drugs, chemicals or toxins, or because of a deficiency in key RBC enzymes including glutathione reductase (resulting in familial methemoglobinemia and hemolytic anemia) and RBC flavin adenine dinucleotide, which is a required cofactor for both enzymatic conversion systems.
- Methemoglobinemia results in a reduced oxygen-carrying capacity of blood, which may be fatal in horses with concentrations of 22% methemoglobin, as occurs with red maple (*Acer rubrum*) leaf toxicity.
- The reduced oxygen-carrying capacity of RBCs in horses with methemoglobinemia results in functional anemia, while hemolysis caused by methemoglobin producing oxidant toxins results in "true" anemia.

SYSTEMS AFFECTED

- Hemic/lymphatic/immune system: although PCV is usually within reference range, non–oxygen-carrying RBCs produce a functional anemia and cyanotic muddy-brown mucous membranes.
- Cardiovascular and respiratory systems may be involved reflected by increased heart and respiratory rates.
- Hepatobiliary system may be involved due to centrilobular degeneration associated with hypoxia.
- Renal insufficiency may be identified due to hypoxic injury and pigmenturia.
- Gastrointestinal tract may be involved due to hypoxic damage to intestines resulting in motility disorders, impaction, and colic.
- Nervous system may be involved with hypoxia causing signs of depression and weakness.
- Musculoskeletal system involvement includes laminar hypoxia resulting in laminitis.

GENETICS

Inheritance is suggested by a report of familial methemoglobinemia in a mare and its dam.

INCIDENCE/PREVALENCE

- No incidence or prevalence data currently is available for methemoglobinemia in horses.
- In a study of red maple leaf toxicosis, 19 of 32 horses died (case-fatality rate ≈60%), but there was no relationship between death and initial blood methemoglobin concentrations.

SIGNALMENT

- Can occur in any age, breed, or sex
- Rarely, familial methemoglobinemia and hemolytic anemia have been reported in association with decreased erythrocyte glutathione concentrations and glutathione reductase activities.

SIGNS

Historical

- Access to wilted or dried leaves or bark of red maple (*A. rubrum*) or nitrate-containing plants
- Sudden onset of lethargy, inappetence, and signs of depression are common presenting signs.

Physical Examination

- Vary with the severity and organ systems involved
- Muddy-brown cyanotic mucous membranes may be noted in addition to brownish discoloration of the blood (methemoglobin content of blood >10%) and urine.
- Clinical signs usually become evident when methemoglobin concentrations are ≈30%. Signs include weakness, lethargy, ataxia, tachycardia, polypnea, exercise intolerance, and icterus. Signs of colic or laminitis also may be observed.
- Coma and death may result when the methemoglobin content of blood reaches or exceeds 80%. However, death can occur in active animals with only 50%–60% methemoglobin concentrations.
- Salivation, diarrhea, colic, or increased urination also may be noted in horses with nitrate/nitrite toxicity.

CAUSES

- Red maple (*Acer rubrum*) toxicity, which also causes Heinz body hemolytic anemia
- Other oxidant toxins (phenothiazine and onions) may induce a degree of methemoglobinemia, although they predominantly cause Heinz body hemolytic anemia.
- Nitrite/nitrate poisoning (rare in horses: being hindgut fermenters, they convert less nitrate to nitrite compared to ruminants)
- Rarely, deficiencies in RBC enzymes involved in normal regulatory reduction of methemoglobin into hemoglobin. Glutathione reductase and flavin adenine dinucleotide deficiencies have been confirmed in horses.

RISK FACTORS

- Access to dry or wilted red maple leaves or bark, often during autumn
- Exposure to nitrate/nitrite sources (e.g., plants, forages, silages, fertilizer spills)
- Familial history of methemoglobinemia

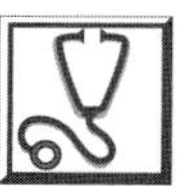

DIAGNOSIS

DIFFERENTIAL DIAGNOSIS

- Other diseases causing anemia must be differentiated from methemoglobinemia.
- Immune-mediated hemolytic anemia can be differentiated by autoagglutination of RBC, bilirubinemia, and bilirubinuria.
- Infectious causes of anemia include EIA (positive Coggins test or C-ELISA test), piroplasmosis (organisms observed in Giemsa-stained smears or positive serology), and anaplasmosis (*Anaplasma phagocytophila*, formerly *Erhlichia equi*) (granular inclusions observed in neutrophils in Giemsa-stained smears).
- Administration of hypertonic or hypotonic solutions; history of use
- History of exposure is also helpful to differentiate other toxicities, including intravenous DMSO, heavy metal toxicosis, and snake envenomation.
- Other causes of mild colic and lameness may be ruled out through a thorough systematic investigation of presenting signs.
- End-stage hepatic disease may mimic severe methemoglobinemia (signs of depression and coma) but can be differentiated by increases in bile acid concentrations and chronic weight loss.

CBC/BIOCHEMISTRY/URINALYSIS

- It is important to note that post-collection hemolysis of the blood sample may falsely elevate the methemoglobin value.
- In horses with methemoglobinemia caused by wilted red maple leaf toxicity, CBC may reveal Heinz body hemolytic anemia, hemoglobinemia, and inflammatory neutrophilic leukocytosis.
- Depending on severity, results of clinical chemistry analysis can demonstrate evidence of hypoxic injury to various organ systems with elevations in BUN, creatinine, and bilirubin concentrations and/or liver enzymes.
- Urinalysis may reveal hemoglobinuria, bilirubinuria, and proteinuria.

OTHER LABORATORY TESTS

- Determination of methemoglobin content requires rapid submission to an appropriate laboratory as concentrations decrease quickly in vitro, even in cold storage. Addition of a phosphate buffer helps preserve methemoglobin concentrations. Many co-oximeters report methemoglobin concentrations.
- The methemoglobin spot test consists of comparing a drop of patient blood, which is placed on absorbent paper, to that of a normal control horse. Methemoglobin content >10% results in a brown discoloration of patient blood

compared with the frank red color of control blood.
• The brown discoloration of blood, combined with the normal to high Po_2 content of arterial blood, aids in establishing the diagnosis by distinguishing methemoglobinemia from hypoxemia (where the arterial Po_2 is low).

OTHER DIAGNOSTIC PROCEDURES

• A blood smear stained with New Methylene Blue should be examined for Heinz bodies, which indicate concurrent Heinz body hemolytic anemia. Wright-Giemsa–stained smears should also be examined for eccentrocytes and pyknocytosis, which may be indicative of RBC enzyme deficiency.
• Specially handled blood samples may be submitted to appropriate specialist laboratories for RBC enzyme assays.

PATHOLOGICAL FINDINGS

Histopathological lesions may include centrilobular hepatic degeneration, hemoglobinemic renal tubular nephrosis, icteric tissues, and erythrophagocytosis by splenic, adrenal, and hepatic phagocytes.

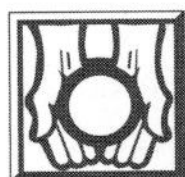

TREATMENT

AIMS OF TREATMENT

• Treatment of methemoglobinemia involves identification and removal of the oxidant source (if underlying cause) and provision of supportive care.
• Access to toxin sources, such as red maple leaves or other oxidants, should be eliminated and mineral oil or activated charcoal should be administered to reduce further absorption of toxin.

APPROPRIATE HEALTH CARE

• In-hospital medical management may be necessary depending on severity and rapidity of onset of the anemia.
• Balanced IV fluid therapy with isotonic crystalloid solutions should be administered for vascular volume expansion, increased tissue perfusion, prevention of hemoglobin-induced nephropathy and to promote diuresis. Correction of electrolyte or acid–base disturbance may be required in horses with evidence of renal insufficiency. Other appropriate therapy for renal failure may be warranted including dopamine and/or furosemide.
• Cross-matched blood transfusion may be considered if PCV decreases to <8% or if there is persistent tachycardia, tachypnea, prolonged CRT, mucous membrane pallor, and weak pulse pressure and if poor response to isotonic fluid therapy occurs.
• NSAIDs may be indicated to control inflammation and provide analgesia in horses with adequate renal function.

NURSING CARE

• Close monitoring of vital signs, fluid rates (to avoid hemodilution), and blood hematology and clinical chemistry is essential.
• Concomitant monitoring for renal failure induced by hemoglobinuria or hypoxia and for laminitis also is necessary.

ACTIVITY

Minimize or eliminate activity and stress, but allow the animal access to fresh air and sunshine if possible.

DIET

• Make efforts to keep the horse eating a balanced diet, with good-quality hay and grain.
• Fresh water should be available ad libitum.

CLIENT EDUCATION

The hazards of exposure to wilted red maple leaves (including red maple hybrids) and nitrate/nitrite-containing plants or fertilizer spills should be explained.

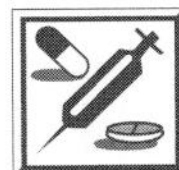

MEDICATIONS

DRUG(S) OF CHOICE

If nitrate/nitrite poisoning is suspected, Methylene Blue (4.4 mg/kg) may be administered slowly IV as a 1%–2% solution in isotonic saline, and repeated if necessary after 30 minutes.

PRECAUTIONS

• Although Methylene Blue and other reductive therapy can be used, these agents are relatively ineffective in enhancing methemoglobin reduction and may exacerbate concurrent Heinz body hemolytic anemia.
• There is little evidence that ascorbic acid is of clinical benefit. Corticosteroids should be used with caution as there is some evidence that their use may be associated with decreased survival.

FOLLOW-UP

PATIENT MONITORING

• If Methylene Blue is administered, carefully monitor PCV over 3 days to ensure severe anemia does not develop because of Heinz body formation.
• Serial determination of PCV may allow assessment of bone marrow regeneration and response to treatment. The PCV should remain stable or slowly increase over time.
• Renal function should also be reassessed and signs of laminitis monitored.

PREVENTION/AVOIDANCE

Limiting access to excess oxidant-containing plants and nitrate/nitrite sources

POSSIBLE COMPLICATIONS

Coma and death if methemoglobin content of blood exceed 80%

EXPECTED COURSE AND PROGNOSIS

• As little as 22% methemoglobin content of blood may be fatal in horses with red maple leaf poisoning, which may result from the concurrent Heinz body hemolytic anemia.
• Cyanosis should resolve if methemoglobin content of blood falls below critical levels, and blood should again become red (using the spot test) if the content falls below 10%. However, in general, the prognosis for horses with methemoglobinemia, particularly from red maple leaf toxicosis, is guarded.

MISCELLANEOUS

ASSOCIATED CONDITIONS

Heinz body hemolytic anemia

SEE ALSO

• Anemia
• Anemia, Heinz body

ABBREVIATIONS

• BUN = blood urea nitrogen
• CBC = complete blood count
• CRT = capillary refill time
• DMSO = dimethylsulfoxide
• EIA = equine infectious anemia
• IV =intravenous
• NSAID = nonsteroidal anti-inflammatory drug
• PCV = packed cell volume
• RBC = red blood cell

Suggested Reading

Alward A, Corriher CA, Barton MH, Sellon DC, Blikslager AT, Jones SL. Red maple (*Acer rubrum*) leaf toxicosis in horses: A retrospective study of 32 cases. J Vet Intern Med 2006; 20:1197–1201.
Corriher CA, Parvianen AKJ, Gibbons DS, Sellon DC. Equine red maple leaf toxicosis. Compend Contin Educ Pract Vet 1999; 21:74–80.
George LW, Divers TJ, Mahaffey EA, Suarez JH. Heinz body anemia and methemoglobinemia in ponies given red maple (*Acer rubrum*) leaves. Vet Pathol 1982;19:521–533.
Harvey JW, Stockham SL, Scott MA, Johnson PJ, Donald JJ, Chandler CJ. Methemoglobinemia and eccentrocytosis in equine erythrocyte flavin adenine dinucleotide deficiency. Vet Pathol 2003; 40:632–642
Jain NC. Hemolytic anemias of noninfectious origin. In: Essentials of Veterinary Hematology. Philadelphia: Lea & Febiger, 1993: 196–197.
Schmitz DG. Toxicologic problems. In: Reed SM, Bayly WM, eds. Equine Internal Medicine. Philadelphia: WB Saunders, 1998: 1019–1020.

Author Nicholas Malikides
Consulting Editors Jennifer Hodgson and David Hodgson

METHYLXANTHINE TOXICOSIS

BASICS

OVERVIEW

- Methylxanthines include theobromine, caffeine, and theophylline.
- Generally, they cause release of catecholamines (i.e., epinephrine, norepinephrine), increased muscular contractility, and stimulation of the CNS.
- Only theobromine (from cocoa bean hulls) has been associated with clinical intoxication and death in horses; the diagnosis is established based on a history of ingestion and determination of theobromine in serum, plasma, urine, or stomach contents.
- Use and detection in race horses are of concern.

SIGNALMENT

All Equidae are susceptible to theobromine intoxication, but the few reported cases of theobromine poisoning in horses do not allow for determination of breed or sex predilections.

SIGNS

- One case of theobromine ingestion by horses has been reported with "violent excitement" as the outstanding clinical sign.
- The sole other case in the literature reported only sudden death.
- Clinical signs of toxicosis reported in other species (primarily dogs)—hyperactivity, diarrhea, diuresis, muscle tremors, ataxia, cardiac arrhythmias, and death

CAUSES AND RISK FACTORS

- Theobromine is found in cocoa bean hulls, chocolate, chocolate-containing bakery waste, and, formerly, in some diuretics.
- Toxicoses and deaths have been reported through ingestion of cocoa bean hulls used as bedding or in feed.
- Roughly, a dose of 100 mg/kg of theobromine given over 4 days as cocoa bean hulls in feed has been reported to cause death; the possibility of toxicosis at lower doses has not been investigated.
- Cocoa bean hulls are reported to contain as much as 0.5% theobromine by weight.
- Theobromine and caffeine have been detected in the urine of race horses fed small amounts of chocolate candy or incorporated into feed.

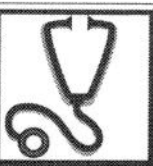

DIAGNOSIS

DIFFERENTIAL DIAGNOSIS

Other causes of rapid/sudden death in horses from cardiac arrhythmias include accidental ingestion of ionophore feed supplements (test for ionophores in the feed), ingestion of *Eupatorium rugosum* or white snakeroot (history; evidence of ingestion and myocardial necrosis), or ingestion of bark and leaves of *Robinia pseudoacacia* or black locust (history; evidence of ingestion).

CBC/BIOCHEMISTRY/URINALYSIS

No abnormalities have been reported with theobromine toxicoses.

OTHER LABORATORY TESTS

N/A

IMAGING

N/A

DIAGNOSTIC PROCEDURES

- The diagnosis of theobromine toxicosis is established based on clinical history, evidence of ingestion, and presence of theobromine in serum, plasma, urine, or stomach contents.
- ECG can monitor for possible cardiac arrhythmias.

METHYLXANTHINE TOXICOSIS

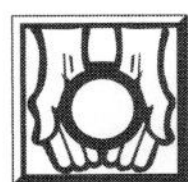

TREATMENT

- Eliminate exposure.
- Restrict activity because of possible cardiac arrhythmias.

MEDICATIONS

DRUGS

- Administer AC unless contraindicated (1–4 g/kg in a water slurry).
- Because of the limited number of reported cases, pharmacologic intervention in equine theobromine toxicosis has not been evaluated.

CONTRAINDICATIONS/POSSIBLE INTERACTIONS

N/A

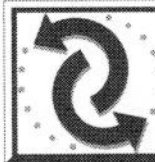

FOLLOW-UP

PATIENT MONITORING

Monitor ECG to evaluate cardiac status.

PREVENTION/AVOIDANCE

Do not allow horses to eat cocoa bean hulls or chocolate products.

POSSIBLE COMPLICATIONS

N/A

EXPECTED COURSE AND PROGNOSIS

The rarity of theobromine toxicosis precludes generalization to all prospective equine cases; however, when less than toxic amounts are ingested and ECG abnormalities are not present, the prognosis is excellent.

MISCELLANEOUS

ASSOCIATED CONDITIONS, AGE-RELATED FACTORS, ZOONOTIC POTENTIAL, PREGNANCY

N/A

SEE ALSO

N/A

ABBREVIATION

- AC = activated charcoal
- ECG = electrocardiogram (graph)

Suggested Reading

Blakemore F, Shearer GD. The poisoning of livestock by cacao products. Vet Rec 1943;55:165.

Harkins JD, Rees WA, Mundy GD, Stanley SD, Tobin T. An overview of the methylxanthines and their regulation in the horse. Equine Pract 1998;20:10–16.

Author Stephen B. Hooser

Consulting Editor Robert H. Poppenga

MITRAL REGURGITATION

BASICS

DEFINITION

• Occurs when the mitral (left AV) valve allows blood to leak into the left atrium during systole and creates a systolic murmur with its PMI in the mitral to aortic valve area
• The murmur radiates toward the left base or dorsally and caudally.

PATHOPHYSIOLOGY

• The mitral leaflets do not form a complete seal between the left atrium and ventricle.
• During systole, blood regurgitates into the left atrium, causing increased left atrial pressure and a left atrial and ventricular volume overload.
• As the regurgitation becomes more severe, further increases in left atrial pressure produce increased pulmonary venous pressure, increased pulmonary capillary pressure, pulmonary edema, pulmonary hypertension, and clinical signs of left-sided congestive heart failure.
• As the pulmonary hypertension becomes more severe, clinical signs of right-sided congestive heart failure appear.

SYSTEMS AFFECTED

Cardiovascular

GENETICS

N/A

SIGNS

General Comments

Often an incidental finding during routine auscultation. Mitral regurgitation can develop as a physiologic adaptation to athletic training, and in these horses there is no effect on performance. The severity of signs is dependent on the nature and severity of any valvular pathology.

Historical

• Often poor performance
• Sometimes congestive heart failure

Physical Examination

• Grade 2–6/6, band-shaped, crescendo or musical holosystolic or pansystolic murmur with PMI in the mitral to aortic valve area (left fifth to fourth intercostal space) and radiating dorsally to the left heart base
• Other, less common findings—atrial premature depolarizations, atrial fibrillation, accentuated third heart sounds, tachypnea, cough, and congestive heart failure
• Degenerative changes of the mitral leaflets
• Nonvegetative valvulitis
• Ruptured chordae tendineae
• Infective endocarditis
• Congenital malformation
• Physiologic adaptations to athletic training

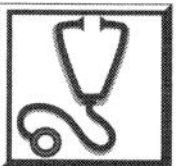

DIAGNOSIS

DIFFERENTIAL DIAGNOSIS

• Physiologic ejection murmur—common; murmur is typically grade 1–3/6 and localized to the aortic valve; differentiate echocardiographically.
• Aortic stenosis—rare; murmur radiates up the carotid arteries and to the right side; weak arterial pulses; differentiate echocardiographically.

CBC/BIOCHEMISTRY/URINALYSIS

May have neutrophilic leukocytosis and hyperfibrinogenemia with infective endocarditis.

OTHER LABORATORY TESTS

• Elevated cardiac isoenzymes may be present (e. g., cardiac troponin I, CK-MB, HBDH, LDH-1, and LDH-2) with concurrent myocardial disease.
• Positive blood culture may be obtained from horses with infective endocarditis.

IMAGING

Electrocardiography

• Atrial premature depolarizations may be present in horses with acute onset of severe regurgitation and left atrial enlargement.
• Atrial fibrillation often is present in affected horses with significant left atrial enlargement.
• Ventricular premature depolarizations may be present in affected horses with diffuse myocardial disease.

Echocardiography

• Affected horses may have thickened mitral valve leaflets. Diffuse thickening of the leaflet free edge is more common than nodular thickening.
• Prolapse of a mitral leaflet (usually an accessory leaflet) into the left atrium is detected frequently.
• A ruptured chorda tendinea, flail mitral leaflet, or bacterial endocarditis are detected infrequently.
• Left atrium—enlarged and dilated, with a rounded appearance
• Left ventricle—enlarged and dilated, with a rounded apex
• Thinning of the left ventricular free wall and interventricular septum
• Subjective ventricular hyperkinesis, dilation and increased fractional shortening are suggestive of left ventricular volume overload.
• Normal or decreased fractional shortening in a horse with left ventricular enlargement is consistent with myocardial dysfunction.
• Dilatation of the pulmonary veins and, later, the pulmonary artery in severely affected horses
• Pulsed-wave and color-flow Doppler reveals a jet or jets of regurgitation in the left atrium. Size and extent of the regurgitation jet are a good method of semiquantitating severity, as is the strength of the regurgitation signal.

Thoracic Radiography

• Left-sided cardiac enlargement may be detected.
• Pulmonary edema may be detected in horses with left-sided congestive heart failure.

DIAGNOSTIC PROCEDURES

Cardiac Catheterization

• Right-sided catheterization can be performed to directly measure pulmonary arterial and pulmonary capillary wedge pressures.
• Severely affected horses have elevated pulmonary capillary wedge pressures and pulmonary arterial pressures, with normal oxygen saturation.
• Right atrial and ventricular pressures also may be elevated with right-sided heart failure.

Continuous 24-Hour Holter Monitoring

Useful in the diagnosis of horses with suspected atrial or ventricular premature depolarizations

PATHOLOGIC FINDINGS

• Where the regurgitation relates to physiological adaptation to athletic training, no pathological findings are expected.
• Focal or diffuse thickening or distortion of one or more mitral leaflets may be present.
• Ruptured chordae tendineae, flail mitral leaflets, infective endocarditis, or congenital malformations of the mitral valve infrequently are detected.
• Jet lesions usually are detected in the left atrium.
• With significant regurgitation, left atrial enlargement and atrial myocardial thinning, as well as left ventricular enlargement and thinning of the left ventricular free wall and interventricular septum
• Dilatation of the pulmonary veins in severely affected horses
• Dilatation of the pulmonary artery in horses with pulmonary hypertension
• Pale areas may be seen in the atrial and/or ventricular myocardium, with areas of atrial fibrosis detected histopathologically.
• Inflammatory cell infiltrate has been documented in affected horses with myocarditis.
• Myocardial necrosis occasionally is detected in affected horses with primary myocardial disease.

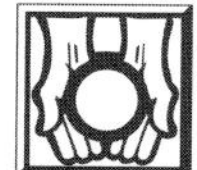

TREATMENT

AIMS OF TREATMENT

• Management by intermittent monitoring in horses with mitral regurgitation that is mild or moderate in severity

• Palliative care in horses with severe mitral regurgitation.

APPROPRIATE HEALTH CARE

• Most affected horses require no treatment and can be monitored on an outpatient basis.
• Horses with moderate to severe regurgitation may benefit from long-term vasodilator therapy, particularly with ACE inhibitors.
• Treat horses with severe regurgitation and congestive heart failure for the congestive heart failure with positive inotropic drugs, vasodilators, and diuretics on an inpatient basis, if possible, and monitor response to therapy.

NURSING CARE

N/A

ACTIVITY

• Affected horses are safe to continue in full athletic work until the regurgitation becomes severe or ventricular arrhythmias develop.
• Monitor horses with moderate to severe regurgitation by ECG during high-intensity exercise to ensure they are safe to continue in ridden work. These horses can be used for lower-level athletic activities until they begin to develop congestive heart failure.
• Horses with significant ventricular arrhythmias or pulmonary artery dilatation are no longer safe to ride.

CLIENT EDUCATION

• Regularly monitor the cardiac rhythm; any irregularities other than second-degree AV block should prompt ECG.
• Carefully monitor for exercise intolerance, respiratory distress, prolonged recovery after exercise, increased resting respiratory or heart rate, or cough; if detected, seek a cardiac reexamination.

SURGICAL CONSIDERATIONS

N/A

MEDICATIONS

DRUG(S) OF CHOICE

• Severe regurgitation—enalapril (0.25–0.5 mg/kg PO daily or BID) or another ACE inhibitor
• ACE inhibitors prolong the time to valve replacement in humans with moderate to severe regurgitation.
• The bioavailability of enalapril is poor but horses with mitral regurgitation have experienced a decrease in severity of regurgitation and increase in stroke volume with ACE inhibitors.
• Affected horses in heart failure—Treat with digoxin, furosemide, and vasodilators.

CONTRAINDICATIONS

ACE inhibitors and other vasodilators must be withdrawn before competition to comply with the medication rules of the various governing bodies of equine sports.

PRECAUTIONS

ACE inhibitors can cause hypotension; thus, do not give a large dose without time to accommodate to this treatment.

POSSIBLE INTERACTIONS

N/A

ALTERNATIVE DRUGS

Most other vasodilatory drugs should have some beneficial effect in horses with moderate to severe regurgitation but may be less effective than ACE inhibitors.

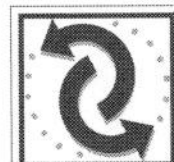

FOLLOW-UP

PATIENT MONITORING

• Frequently monitor cardiac rhythm and respiratory system.
• Horses with mild to moderate regurgitation should be reexamined echocardiographically every year.
• Horses with severe regurgitation should be reexamined echocardiographically every 3–6 months, depending on severity of the regurgitation and its probable speed of progression, to ensure the horse continues to be safe to ride.

PREVENTION/AVOIDANCE

N/A

POSSIBLE COMPLICATIONS

Chronic and/or severe regurgitation—atrial fibrillation; congestive heart failure

EXPECTED COURSE AND PROGNOSIS

• Many affected horses have a normal performance life and life expectancy.
• Prognosis for horses with mitral valve prolapse and mild regurgitation is excellent; in many, the amount of regurgitation remains unchanged for years.
• Progression of regurgitation associated with degenerative valve disease usually is slow; if the regurgitation is mild, these horses also have a good prognosis.
• Horses with ruptured chordae tendineae, flail mitral valve leaflets, or infective endocarditis have a more guarded prognosis, because regurgitation usually becomes more severe and results in shortened performance life and life expectancy.
• Affected horses with congestive heart failure usually have severe underlying valvular heart and myocardial disease and a guarded to grave prognosis for life.
• Most affected horses being treated for congestive heart failure respond to supportive therapy and improve. This improvement usually is short lived, however, and most are euthanized within 2–6 mo of initiating treatment.

MISCELLANEOUS

ASSOCIATED CONDITIONS

N/A

AGE-RELATED FACTORS

Old horses are more likely to be affected.

ZOONOTIC POTENTIAL

N/A

PREGNANCY

• Affected mares should not experience any problems with pregnancy unless the regurgitation is moderate to severe.
• The volume expansion of late pregnancy places an additional load on the already volume-loaded heart and may precipitate the onset of congestive heart failure in mares with severe regurgitation.
• Pregnant mares affected with congestive heart failure should be treated for the underlying cardiac disease with positive inotropic drugs and diuretics; ACE inhibitors are contraindicated because of potential adverse effects on the fetus.

SYNONYMS

Mitral insufficiency

SEE ALSO

• Atrial fibrillation
• Infective endocarditis

ABBREVIATIONS

• ACE = angiotensin-converting enzyme
• AV = atrioventricular
• CK-MB = MB isoenzyme of creatine kinase
• HBDH = α-hydroxybutyrate dehydrogenase
• LDH = lactate dehydrogenase
• PMI = point of maximal intensity

Suggested Reading

Gehlen H, Vieht JC, Stadler P. Effects of the ACE inhibitor quinapril on echocardiographic variables in horses with mitral valve insufficiency. J Vet Med A Physiol Pathol Clin Med. 2003;50:460–465.

Reef VB. Cardiovascular ultrasonography. In: Reef VB, ed. Equine Diagnostic Ultrasound. Philadelphia: WB Saunders, 1998:215–272.

Reef VB. Heart murmurs in horses: determining their significance with echocardiography. Equine Vet J 1995;19(suppl):71–80.

Reef VB, Bain FT, Spencer PA. Severe mitral regurgitation in horses: clinical, echocardiographic, and pathologic findings. Equine Vet J 1998;30:18–27.

Young LE, Wood JL. Effect of age and training on murmurs of atrioventricular valvular regurgitation in young thoroughbreds. Equine Vet J. 2000;32:195–199.

Author Virginia B. Reef
Consulting Editor Celia M. Marr

MONOCYTOSIS

BASICS

DEFINITION

Monocyte count greater than the upper limit of the laboratory reference interval; usually >600 cells/μL (>0.6 × 10^9 cells/L)

PATHOPHYSIOLOGY

- Monocyte production and kinetics have not been studied in horses. They are assumed to be similar to other mammalian species.
- Monopoiesis occurs in the bone marrow and commences with a bipotential stem cell (CFU-GM).
- Differentiation of CFU-GM into CFU-M and sequentially to monoblasts, promonocytes and monocytes is under the influence of IL-3, GM-CSF, and M-CSF.
- GM-CSF and M-CSF are produced by endothelial cells, fibroblasts, lymphocytes, and also cells of monocyte origin. Hence monocytes have a role in regulation of monopoiesis and production of other bone marrow cells lineages.
- Monopoiesis is rapid—monocytes are released into blood within 6 days of initiation of stem cell division.
- Monocytes have a short marrow transit time (<2.5 days). A bone marrow storage pool is absent for monocytes and these cells are released shortly after their last division.
- In blood, monocytes are thought to be unevenly distributed between a circulating pool and a marginated pool (1:3.5 in humans). However, the presence of a marginated pool has been questioned.
- Monocytes have a circulating half-life of ≈3 days and they account for ≈5% of peripheral blood leukocytes.
- During periods of inflammatory demand, increased monopoiesis and release of monocytes into the circulation occur and the circulating half-life of monocytes is shortened.
- Monocytes migrate from blood to tissues and body cavities either in a random manner or at specific sites of inflammation due to the presence of chemotactic agents. They do not reenter the circulation.
- Chemotaxis of monocytes and free macrophages to areas of acute or chronic inflammation occurs in response to microbial products and varied endogenous chemokines, many of which also recruit neutrophils.
- Within the tissues and body cavities, monocytes undergo transformation into macrophages, accompanied by numerous morphologic, metabolic and functional changes.
- Although tissue macrophages are capable of mitosis, de novo production usually accounts for <5% of the resident macrophage population.
- Considerable heterogeneity exists in the morphologic, metabolic, and functional characteristics of tissue macrophages at various locations throughout the body.
- Tissue macrophages are classified as free or fixed. Free macrophages are located primarily in mesothelial cavities and synovial cavities, alveoli (alveolar macrophages), and inflammatory sites. Fixed macrophages are found in most tissues, in particular the spleen, liver (Kupffer cells), bone (osteoclasts), skin (Langerhans cells), connective tissue (histiocytes), lymph nodes, lung, brain (microglia), and GIT.
- Monocytes and their precursors in bone marrow and macrophages comprise the mononuclear phagocytic system, which is an integral component of the reticuloendothelial system (RES).
- Resident macrophages are long-lived, whereas tissue macrophages have a life span of days to months. In contrast, monocytes/macrophages involved in inflammatory processes are short-lived.
- Monocytes/macrophages have numerous functions—phagocytosis and microbiocidal activity, phagocytosis of cellular debris and particulate matter, orchestration and regulation of immune and inflammatory responses, cytotoxicity against tumor and foreign cells, coagulation, fibrinolysis, and tissue repair and remodeling.
- Monocytes/macrophages have an important role in the body's defense against a diverse array of microorganisms, in particular intracellular bacteria, fungi, protozoa, and viruses.
- Macrophages may fuse to form multinucleated giant cells in response to infection with mycobacteria, fungi, or certain viruses and localization of foreign material in tissues.
- Monocytosis usually arises from an increased rate of monopoiesis and release of monocytes from the bone marrow. Monocytosis may be appropriate (in response to increased tissue demand) or inappropriate (unassociated with tissue demand).

SYSTEMS AFFECTED

- Hemic/lymphatic/immune
- Other body systems can be involved by an underlying infectious disease causing monocytosis.
- In monocytic myeloproliferative diseases, bone marrow, lymph nodes, spleen, and liver may be infiltrated with neoplastic cells.

SIGNS

General Comments

- Signs are referable to the underlying disease resulting in monocytosis.
- Clinical abnormalities observed may assist in determining which body system(s) is/are affected.

Historical

Inflammatory or myeloproliferative disorders may cause weight loss, inappetence, lethargy, and pyrexia.

Physical Examination

- Pyrexia is common with inflammatory and myeloproliferative disorders.
- Signs of specific organ involvement may be present.
- Enlargement of peripheral lymph nodes may occur occasionally with myeloproliferative disorders and can be detected upon palpation.

CAUSES

Inflammation

- Any acute, subacute, or chronic inflammatory process that stimulates neutrophilia will also cause monocytosis as monocytes and neutrophils share the bipotential stem cell, CFU-GM.
- Causes include suppurative inflammation, pyogranulomatous inflammation, necrosis, hemorrhage, hemolysis, and neoplasia.
- In contrast to dogs, corticosteroids do not consistently induce monocytosis in horses.

Myeloproliferative Disease (Neoplasia)

Monocytic and myelomonocytic forms of leukemia are rare causes of monocytosis in horses. Most cases are acute and progress rapidly and affected animals have leukocytosis caused by immature monocytoid cells (often blast forms) with bizarre morphology.

Miscellaneous

Administration of recombinant CSF-GM or CSF-M in other species can result in monocytosis.

RISK FACTORS

Immunodeficiency syndromes in foals, e.g., FPT or SCID

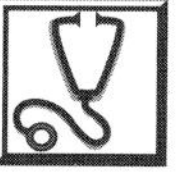

DIAGNOSIS

DIFFERENTIAL DIAGNOSIS

- Underlying cause of monocytosis (inflammatory versus myeloproliferative) should be determined.
- If inflammatory, site and cause of inflammatory process should be determined.

CBC/BIOCHEMISTRY/URINALYSIS

- Monocyte count in peripheral blood >600 cells/μL (>0.6 × 10^9 cells/L)
- If concurrent neutrophilia +/−left shift is present, consider acute or chronic inflammatory process.
- If immature or bizarre monocytes/blast forms are observed, consider myeloproliferative disease.
- Marked monocytosis (>10,000 cells/μL [>10.0 × 10^9 cells/L]) with anemia, thrombocytopenia, and neutropenia is associated with monocytic myeloproliferative disorder and myelophthisis.
- If concurrent anemia is noted, consider hemorrhage, hemolysis, or myelophthisis.
- Biochemical analysis may reveal evidence of specific organ involvement.

OTHER LABORATORY TESTS

- Coombs test for immune-mediated hemolytic anemia
- Genetic testing (PCR) for SCID
- Quantification of individual immunoglobulin subtypes—lack of IgM in

presuckle blood or after 30 days of age is consistent with SCID, while in neonatal foals a concentration of IgG <400 mg/dL is consistent with FPT.
- Serology for viral (e.g., EIA virus) or bacterial pathogens

IMAGING

- Thoracic and abdominal ultrasonography to detect morphologic lesions of inflammatory processes
- Thoracic radiography to detect pneumonia, lung abscess, neoplasia

OTHER DIAGNOSTIC PROCEDURES

- Abdominocentesis for detection of intraperitoneal inflammatory or neoplastic disease
- Thoracocentesis for detection of intrathoracic inflammatory or neoplastic disease
- Endoscopy (e.g., respiratory tract, stomach, bladder) to determine if inflammatory or neoplastic processes are present
- Bone marrow aspirate/biopsy to detect myeloproliferative disease
- Aspirate of lymph nodes if lymphadomegaly is present to determine if inflammatory or neoplastic processes are present
- Laparoscopy/thoracoscopy if abscess/tumor is suspected

PATHOLOGICAL FINDINGS

Dependent on the underlying cause of monocytosis

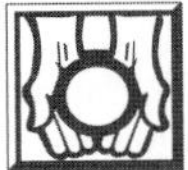

TREATMENT

AIMS OF TREATMENT

- Elimination of the underlying cause of monocytosis (± neutrophilia)
- Often directed toward resolution of infectious disease and accompanying inflammation
- Correction of any body fluid and electrolyte deficits consequent to the underlying disease. May require enteral or IV fluid therapy

APPROPRIATE HEALTH CARE

- Depends on the severity of the underlying disease
- Often inpatient medical management is required.
- Surgical management may be appropriate to address specific infectious conditions (e.g., removal/drainage of an abscess) once the condition of the patient is stable.

NURSING CARE

- Depends on the underlying cause of monocytosis
- If pleural effusion is present, therapeutic paracentesis/drainage may be required if respiration is affected.
- Enteral/IV fluid therapy if required

CLIENT EDUCATION

- Persistent monocytosis denotes the presence of an underlying disease that will require appropriate diagnostic assessment and treatment.
- Myeloproliferative disorders have a grave prognosis.

SURGICAL CONSIDERATIONS

Depend on the underlying cause of the monocytosis

MEDICATIONS

DRUG(S) OF CHOICE

- Bacterial infections require antimicrobial therapy based on culture and sensitivity testing.
- Immune-mediated hemolytic anemia may require the use of immunosuppressive doses of corticosteroids.

CONTRAINDICATIONS

Corticosteroids should be avoided in horses with laminitis or infectious disease.

FOLLOW-UP

PATIENT MONITORING

Periodic monitoring of CBC to determine monocyte and neutrophil counts

EXPECTED COURSE AND PROGNOSIS

- Depends on the underlying cause of monocytosis
- Prognosis for infectious/inflammatory disease is variable and ranges from good to guarded/poor dependent on the etiology, severity, and response to treatment.
- Myeloproliferative disorders have a hopeless prognosis.

MISCELLANEOUS

AGE-RELATED FACTORS

Monocyte counts are not affected by age.

ZOONOTIC POTENTIAL

Certain microorganisms that may stimulate tissue +/−blood monocytosis (e.g., *Mycobacterium* spp., *Rhodococcus equi*) have zoonotic potential.

SEE ALSO

Neutrophilia

ABBREVIATIONS

- CFU-GM = colony-forming unit–granulocyte-macrophage
- CFU-M = colony-forming unit–macrophage
- EIA = equine infectious anemia
- FPT = failure of passive transfer
- GIT = gastrointestinal tract
- GM-CSF = granulocyte-macrophage colony-stimulating factor
- IgG = immunoglobulin type G
- IgM = immunoglobulin type M
- M-CSF = macrophage colony-stimulating factor
- SCID = severe combined immunodeficiency

Suggested Reading

Bienzle D. Monocytes and macrophages. In: Feldman BF, et al., eds. Schalm's Veterinary Hematology, ed 5. Baltimore: Williams & Wilkins, 2000;318–325.

Jain NC. The monocytes and macrophages. In: Essentials of Veterinary Hematology. Philadelphia: Lea & Febiger, 1993.

Latimer KS. Diseases affecting leukocytes. In: Colahan PT, et al., eds. Equine Medicine and Surgery, ed 5. St Louis: Mosby, 1999:1992–2001, 2025–2034.

McClure JT. Leukoproliferative disorders in horses. Vet Clin North Am Equine Pract 2000;16:165–182.

Newlands CM, Cole D. Monocytic leukemia in a horse. Can Vet J 1995;36:765–766.

Author Kristopher Hughes

Consulting Editors Jennifer Hodgson and David Hodgson

MOTOR NEURON DISEASE

BASICS

DEFINITION

An acquired neurodegenerative disease primarily affecting somatic motor neurons.

PATHOPHYSIOLOGY

The cause of equine motor neuron disease (EMND) is unproven, although there is a strong association between the disease and vitamin E deficiency. Lower motor neuron cell bodies in the spinal cord and brainstem degenerate, presumably from oxidative damage. The oxidative damage is likely a result of an imbalance in pro-oxidants and anti-oxidants and the disease is associated with a low vitamin E status. Early dysfunctional changes in the motor neuron cells may be associated with mitochondrial damage, followed by disintegration of the nucleus and neurofibrillary accumulation. Dead motor neurons may eventually be removed by glial cells. Clinical signs only become apparent when approximately 30% of the motor neurons become dysfunctional. Ventral horn motor neurons that supply postural muscles (those muscles with predominantly type 1 fibers) are preferentially affected: this is believed to occur because of the higher oxidative activity of predominant type I muscle and its corresponding parent motor neuron. The oxidative disease causes lipopigment (ceroid) accumulation in the endothelium of spinal cord capillaries, neurons and retinal pigment epithelium (RPE). The RPE ceroid can generally be seen on fundoscopic exam as brown streaks. Excessive lipopigment may also, on occasion, be found in the liver of affected horses.

SYSTEM AFFECTED

- Neuromuscular–motor neuron cell dysfunction causing neurogenic muscular atrophy and weakness
- Ocular–lipopigment accumulation in the RPE causes electroretinographic abnormalities and undoubtedly affects vision, although this is rarely reported by the owners.
- Gastrointestinal – a functional abnormality in carbohydrate absorption occurs in severely affected horses and may be related to a mitochondrial dysfunction in the enterocyte. There are rarely abnormal light microscopic changes. Hepatic lipofuscinosis occurs in a few cases.

GENETICS

There is no known genetic basis to the disease. Although superoxide dismutase activity is abnormally low in red cells and nervous tissue, this is believed to be a result of excessive oxidative stress. Abnormal polymorphism in the SOD gene in affected horses versus controls have not been found.

INCIDENCE/PREVALENCE

Affects approximately one horse per 10,000 per year in the Northeastern U. S. (between 1990 and 1996).

GEOGRAPHIC DISTRIBUTION

EMND is seen worldwide but is most common in those geographic areas less likely to have alfalfa hay, e. g., Northeastern U.S. and Canada, and lack of pasture (urban areas). Clusters may occur on certain premises.

SIGNALMENT

- Environment: Most horses have a history of being kept without pasture and leafy green hay for at least one year, however increasingly horses in Europe are presented with EMND even though they have had access to grass (those tested however are still low in vitamin E).
- Breed Predilection: All breeds of horses and ponies may be affected.
- Age: Mean age is 12 years. Range 2 to 25 years.
- No gender predisposition.

SIGNS

Clinical signs vary depending upon the stage/duration of the disorder and are due to neuromuscular weakness. EMND cases do not have proprioceptive deficits ie they are not ataxic. Signs are best summarized by dividing into subacute and chronic forms.

- Subacute Form

Horses develop an acute onset of trembling, fasciculations, lying down more than normal, frequent shifting of weight in the pelvic limbs and abnormal sweating. Head carriage may be abnormally low. Horses may appear less comfortable when standing than walking. Appetite and gait are usually not noticeably affected. The owners may mention that the horses had been losing weight (loss of muscle mass) for one month prior to the trembling, etc.

- Chronic Form

The trembling and fasciculations subside and the horse stabilizes but with varying degrees of muscle atrophy. In some cases, the atrophy is so severe that the horse looks emaciated. In other cases, there is noticeable improvement in muscle mass and/or fat deposition. The tail head is frequently in an abnormally high resting position.

HISTORICAL FINDINGS

In many cases lack of access to grass. Low serum alpha-tocopherol.

CAUSES

Unproven. Probably oxidative stress.

RISK FACTORS

Low access to vitamin E or increased exposure to putative oxidant

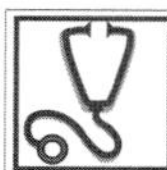

DIAGNOSIS

Finding evidence of neurogenic atrophy in a muscle biopsy of the sacrocaudalis dorsalis medialis muscle (tail head muscle) is a reliable diagnostic tests for EMND. A more invasive test is biopsy of the spinal accessory nerve looking for wallerian degeneration.

DIFFERENTIAL DIAGNOSIS

- Colic is often considered because of the propensity of the horses to stand for only brief periods during the subacute form. The normal appetite and fecal production should serve to rule out an abdominal disorder.
- Laminitis is another consideration because of the almost constant shifting of weight in the subacute form. The ease of motion and even desire to walk as seen in EMND is contradictory to the diagnosis of laminitis.
- Other neuromuscular disorders such as botulism, myositis/myopathy may have similarities to EMND. The normal appetite, elevated tail head and lack of cranial nerve dysfunction and dysphagia should separate EMND from botulism. Chronic myopathies, e. g., polysaccharide storage myopathy (PSSM), may appear very similar to EMND and a muscle biopsy may be required to delineate between the two. EMND causes symmetric muscle weakness and atrophy without ataxia and as opposed to EPM.

The severe muscle wasting with a normal appetite in the chronic form may look similar to intestinal malabsorption syndrome. Plasma albumin is low in most infiltrative bowel syndromes but is normal in EMND.

CBC/BIOCHEMISTRY/URINALYSIS

The CBC is generally within normal range. The most common abnormal biochemical finding is a moderate elevation in muscle enzymes in the subacute case. A few horses may have elevated liver enzymes. The urinalysis is normal in most cases, although some may have myoglobinuria. CBC, biochemistry and urinalysis are all normal in the chronic cases.

OTHER LABORATORY TESTS

- In the subacute cases, plasma or serum Vitamin E (alpha-tocopherol) is abnormally low (mean 0.56 ug/ml). Serum ferritin is often abnormally high.
- In chronic cases, alpha-tocopherol values may have returned to normal.
- Fundoscopic examination frequently reveals brown streaking of the retina. This is specific for vitamin E deficiency and only supportive for EMND.
- Glucose malabsorption is generally present in subacute cases, but is only supportive for EMND.

IMAGING

N/A

OTHER DIAGNOSTIC FINDINGS

As above

PATHOLOGIC FINDINGS

- There are few or no gross lesions in EMND. An abnormal paleness of some muscles (e. g., vastus intermedius) containing most type I fibers may be observed. Body fat stores are variable.
- Microscopically, central nervous system lesions are confined to the spinal cord ventral horn cells, and cranial nerves nuclei V, VII, VIII, IX, X, XI and XII. Degeneration of corresponding motor nerves and neurogenic muscle atrophy are found.
- There is lipofuscinosis of the retinal pigment epithelial layer and spinal cord endothelium in all cases and of the liver in a few cases.
- There are no light microscopic lesions in the intestine in 90% of the cases, but ultrastructural changes may be seen.

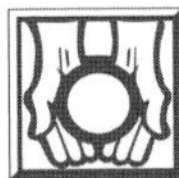

TREATMENT

AIMS OF TREATMENT/ APPROPRIATE HEALTH CARE

Horses with EMND can be treated either on the farm or in the hospital. Transporting can worsen the clinical signs.

- Activity – The affected horse should not have free movement restricted but should not be exercised and/or ridden.
- Diet – Leafy green hay or grass with additional Vitamin E (2,000 to 7,000 units/day) should be provided.

CLIENT EDUCATION

Regular access to grass for all horses that are deficient

SURGICAL CONSIDERATIONS

N/A

MEDICATIONS

DRUG(S)

Oral vitamin E supplements 2000–7000 units/day

CONTRAINDICATIONS

- N/A

PRECAUTIONS

- N/A

POSSIBLE INTERACTIONS

- N/A

ALTERNATIVE DRUGS

Other oral antioxidants may be helpful

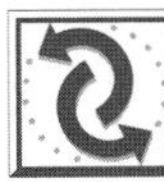

FOLLOW-UP

PATIENT MONITORING

- With the subacute form, improvement in clinical signs often corresponds to return of serum muscle enzymes to normal values. Vitamin E concentrations should be monitored to determine that levels return to normal. It should be kept in mind however that neurons that have been lost will never be replaced, and an increase in weight is likely to be due to fat deposition rather than muscle hypertrophy.

PREVENTION/AVOIDANCE

- All other horses kept under similar conditions should be supplemented with vitamin E.

POSSIBLE COMPLICATIONS/ EXPECTED COURSE AND PROGNOSIS

- Of horses subacutely affected with EMND approximately 40% will stabilize within 3 to 8 weeks and regain some loss of muscle mass. Other horses will have progressive deterioration in clinical signs or no improvement, in spite of vitamin E treatment.
- Horses with the chronic and more stabilized form may have several years of quality life but not performance. Their life expectancy would be shorter than normal and another acute onset of clinical signs may occur years later (similar to the human post-polio paresis). Horses diagnosed with EMND should not be ridden as they can be unsafe and moderate to severe exercise will likely shorten their life expectancy.

MISCELLANEOUS

ASSOCIATED CONDITIONS

- N/A

AGE-RELATED FACTORS

- N/A

ZOONOTIC POTENTIAL

- None

PREGNANCY

- N/A

SYNONYMS

- None

SEE ALSO

Degenerative myelencephalopathy

ABBREVIATIONS

- RPE: Retinal pigment epithelium
- SOD: Superoxide dismutase
- PSSM: Polysaccharide storage myopathy

Suggested Reading

Divers, TJ, Cummings, J. E. *et al.* Evaluation of the risk of motor neuron disease in horses fed a diet low in vitamin E and high in copper and iron. Am J Vet Res 2006;67:120–6.

Ledwith A and McGowan CM. Muscle biopsy: a routine diagnostic procedure. Equine Veterinary Education. 2003 2004; 16:62–67.

McGorum, BC, Mayhew IG, Amory, H *et al.* Horses on pasture may be affected by equine motor neuron disease. Equine Vet J 2006;38:47–51.

The author and editors wish to acknowledge the contribution of Thomas J. Divers, author of this chapter in the previous edition.

Author: Caroline N Hahn

Consulting Editor: Caroline N Hahn

MULTIPLE ENDOCRINE NEOPLASIA

BASIC

OVERVIEW

MEN syndrome is the development of hyperplasia, neoplasia, or both of 2 or more endocrine glands. This rare syndrome is well described in humans and has been reported in dogs, cats, and cattle. The disease is rare in horses. The functional significance of these tumors in the horse is unclear at present.

SYSTEMS AFFECTED

Endocrine/Metabolic

- Thyroid
- Pituitary gland
- Parathyroid
- Adrenals

Other systems may be affected if the tumors compress or displace other organs (e.g., ocular globe).

SIGNALMENT

- No sex or breed predisposition reported
- Diagnosed in aged horses

SIGNS

- Signs are related to the different endocrine effects of neoplasms, if active, or to a mass effect.
- Thyroid gland—usually no clinical signs other than enlargement of the gland. Weight loss may be present.
- Pituitary gland—hirsutism, polyuria and polydipsia, weight loss, potbelly appearance, chronic laminitis
- Parathyroids—intermittent weakness, weight loss possible
- Adrenals—sweating, tachycardia, tachypnea, abdominal pain, mydriasis, muscle tremors if the tumor is functional
- Exophthalmos in case of orbital neoplasm

CAUSES AND RISK FACTORS

Unknown.

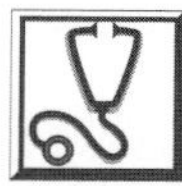

DIAGNOSIS

DIFFERENTIAL DIAGNOSIS

MEN should be suspected in horses presented with signs of PPID, thyroid enlargement, or when a mass of neuroendocrine origin is diagnosed.

CBC/BIOCHEMISTRY/URINALYSIS

Laboratory findings are variable and depend on the types of neoplasms present:

- With a pituitary adenoma—stress leukogram and/or hyperglycemia
- With a functional parathyroid neoplasm—hypercalcemia, hypophosphatemia, and hyperphosphaturia
- With a functional pheochromocytoma—hyponatremia, hyperkalemia, metabolic acidosis, hypocalcemia, hyperphosphatemia, azotemia, hyperglycemia, glucosuria, and occult hematuria

OTHER LABORATORY TESTS

Endocrine tests may help in the diagnosis of the different types of tumors.

- Serum T_3 or T_4 may be increased or decreased with a thyroid tumor.
- Endogenous plasma ACTH levels or dexamethasone suppression test if suspicion of a pituitary adenoma.
- Plasma or urinary catecholamines levels when suspecting a pheochromocytoma.
- Serum parathyroid hormone may be elevated in case of a neoplastic parathyroid gland.

IMAGING

- Thyroid tumors may be imaged via ultrasound.
- Parathyroid neoplasia may be detected using nuclear scintigraphy.

OTHER DIAGNOSTIC PROCEDURES

Fine needle aspirate can identify a thyroid tumor; a biopsy can provide a definitive diagnosis.

PATHOLOGICAL FINDINGS

MEN syndrome is mainly diagnosed at necropsy. Most cases identified at necropsy had a combination of C-cell thyroid adenoma and pheochromocytoma. Pituitary pars intermedia adenoma, orbital paraganglioma have also been associated with these tumors.

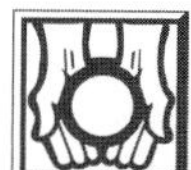

TREATMENT

Surgical excision when warranted. Medical treatment and management of clinical signs associated with primary tumors.

MEDICATIONS

DRUG(S) OF CHOICE

Indicated for the type of endocrine tumors diagnosed—pergolide if pituitary adenoma, diuretics to promote urinary calcium excretion if hypercalcemia associated with a parathyroid gland adenoma or adenocarcinoma

CONTRAINDICATIONS/POSSIBLE INTERACTIONS

Depend on the tumor

FOLLOW-UP

Standard postoperative follow-up if a tumor is removed surgically

MISCELLANEOUS

In humans, MEN syndrome is classified into 2 principal categories:

- MEN type 1 (MEN 1)—usually the association of parathyroid, enterohepatic endocrine, and pituitary neoplasia
- MEN type 2 (MEN 2)—usually involves C-cell thyroid adenoma/carcinoma, pheochromocytoma, and parathyroid hyperplasia/adenomas. Two subtypes of MEN 2 are identified.

ABBREVIATIONS

- ACTH = adrenocorticotrophic hormone
- MEN = multiple endocrine neoplasia
- PPID = pituitary pars intermedia dysfunction

Suggested Reading

De Cock HEV, MacLachlan NJ. Simultaneous occurrence of multiple neoplasms and hyperplasias in the adrenal and thyroid gland of the horse resembling multiple endocrine neoplasia syndrome: case report and retrospective identification of additional cases. Vet Pathol 1999;36:633–636.

Author Michel Lévy
Consulting Editor Michel Lévy

Multiple Myeloma

BASICS

OVERVIEW

• A rare neoplasm • A malignant proliferation of plasma cells or plasmacytoid lymphocytes (plasma cell myeloma) characterized by diffuse or multifocal bone marrow involvement and bone destruction.

SIGNALMENT

• Quarter Horses are overrepresented.
• Reported age range is 3 mo to 25 years (median, 16 years). • No sex predilection • No genetic predisposition

SIGNS

• Nonspecific signs—weight loss most commonly reported • Other nonspecific signs may include anorexia, fever, limb edema, pneumonia, rear leg paresis/ataxia, epistaxis, lymph node enlargement, bone pain, muscle atrophy, soft feces, swollen head, cough, and delayed shedding of hair coat.

CAUSES AND RISK FACTORS

The cause is unknown. No risk factors identified in horses

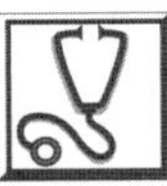

DIAGNOSIS

DIFFERENTIAL DIAGNOSIS

• Lymphosarcoma and lymphoid leukemia are differentiated by identification of neoplastic lymphocytic proliferation on tissue cytology, bone marrow aspirate or biopsy, and immunofluorescent or immunohistochemical staining. • Chronic inflammation, infection, liver disease, and neoplasia are differentiated by a polyclonal gammopathy and absence of atypical plasma cell populations. • Benign, transient monoclonal gammopathy is differentiated by the absence of homogenous plasma cell populations on cellular morphology or immunohistochemistry.

CBC/BIOCHEMISTRY/URINALYSIS

• Hyperproteinemia characterized by hyperglobulinemia and hypoalbuminemia
• Anemia, occasionally macrocytic
• Thrombocytopenia • Leukopenia • Plasma cell leukemia • Hypercalcemia • Hyponatremia
• Proteinuria • Azotemia (rare)

OTHER LABORATORY TESTS

• Serum or urine electrophoresis, immunoelectrophoresis, or immunodiffusion indicative of a monoclonal gammopathy. Paraproteins are predominantly IgG and less commonly IgA. There is an associated, variable decrease in other paraproteins. • Bence Jones proteinuria may be present. • Hyperviscosity of serum may be present. • Normal PTH activity and elevated PTHrP concentration are associated with malignancy. PTHrP is synthesized in normal cells activated by the presence of neoplastic cells and can be directly correlated with serum calcium concentrrations. Concurrent demonstration of high serum PTHrP concentration, hyperglobulinemia, and hypercalcemia is suspicious of multiple myeloma.

IMAGING

• Radiography—may see focal, punctuate bone lysis, adjacent periosteal reaction and sclerosis, diffuse osteoporosis, and pathological bone fractures • Ultrasound—may visualize masses in the abdominal and thoracic cavities and may assist in collection of tissues for cytologic analysis of plasmacytoid accumulations. Increased wall thickness of the esophagus, stomach, small intestine, and rectum also has been reported. This is thought to be associated with concurrent, idiopathic, multifocal hypertrophy of the alimentary tract or amyloidosis.

OTHER DIAGNOSTIC PROCEDURES

• Bone marrow aspirate—identification of plasmacytosis (>10% of cells) and atypical plasma cells with nuclear-cytoplasmic asynchrony are the most common features. Repeated bone marrow aspirates at several sites may be needed to identify abnormalities if focal bone involvement exists. • Aspirates or biopsy of extraosseous tissues—plasmacytosis or neoplastic plasmacytoid cells may be identified in some cases. The spleen, liver, lymph nodes and kidney are most commonly involved.
• Immunofluorescence or immunohistochemical labeling of cytoplasmic or surface immunoglobulins can be used to identify homogeneous plasma cell populations suggestive of malignant plasmacytosis.

PATHOLOGICAL FINDINGS

• Multifocal or diffuse bone lesions including osteoporosis, cortical erosion, pathological fractures, and grossly visible tumor with normal to increased number of plasma cells or atypical plasma cells histologically • Extraosseus plasmacytoid infiltration of tissues, particularly the spleen, liver, lymph nodes, and kidney
• Immunofluorescence or immunohistochemical staining may be required to identify neoplastic plasma cell populations.

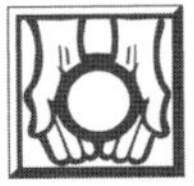

TREATMENT

• No successful treatment has been reported. In humans and dogs, chemotherapy is rarely curative but may result in clinical improvement and remission (median survival 24–30 mo in humans). • Initial therapy requires inpatient care to provide supportive therapy to relieve associated clinical problems and side effects of chemotherapeutic agents.

MEDICATIONS

DRUG(S) OF CHOICE

• The protocol of choice in humans and dogs is melphalan and prednisone. Suggested dose rates of melphalan in horses are 3.5–7.0 mg/m^2 PO q24 h for 5–10 days, then every 3 weeks. Short-term stabilization of disease (7–12 mo) has been reported in 2 horses. Cyclophosphamide and prednisolone (prednisone is not effective in the horse) were administered to 1 of these horses. The dose rates were not reported.
• Vincristine, carmustine, cyclophosphamide, and doxorubicin also have been used in dogs. Recent use of bortezomib, thalidomide, and lenalidomide in conjunction with melphalan and steroids has improved response rates in affected humans. • Plasmapharesis • Treatment of acquired secondary infections

CONTRAINDICATIONS/POSSIBLE INTERACTIONS

• Bone marrow suppression, gastrointestinal upset, and laminitis are potential side effects of therapy.

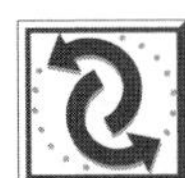

FOLLOW-UP

PATIENT MONITORING

• Pancytopenia becomes more common with disease progression due to progressive myelopthisis. • Serial monitoring of PTHrP concentrations in horses with suspected multiple myeloma may be useful. Elevations in PTHrP concentrations despite normal PTH concentrations with concurrent hyperglobulinemia and hypercalcemia increase suspicion of multiple myeloma.

POSSIBLE COMPLICATIONS

Acquired secondary infections, particularly pneumonia, may occur due to leukopenia and impaired immunologic function associated with disease progression or side effects of chemotherapy.

EXPECTED COURSE AND PROGNOSIS

• Median life expectancy after diagnosis is 3 mo in reported cases (range, 1.5 mo to 2 years). • Advances in chemotherapeutics in human patients have resulted in higher rates of remission, but the condition remains rarely curable.

MISCELLANEOUS

ASSOCIATED CONDITIONS

• Systemic light-chain (AL) amyloidosis has been reported in one case of multiple myeloma in a horse. In contrast, AL amyloidosis is frequently associated with multiple myeloma in humans. • Idiopathic multifocal smooth muscle hypertrophy has been reported in one case.

PREGNANCY

Melphalan, cyclophosphamide, and the majority of other chemotherapeutic agents have embryolethal and teratogenic effects.

SEE ALSO

Lymphosarcoma

ABBREVIATIONS

• PTH = parathyroid hormone • PTHrP = parathyroid hormone–related protein

Suggested Reading

Edwards DF, Parker JW, Wilkinson JE, Helman RG. Plasma cell myeloma in the horse. A case report and literature review. J Vet Intern Med 1993;7:169–176.

Author Rachel H. Tan
Consulting Editors Jennifer Hodgson and David Hodgson

MULTISYSTEMIC EOSINOPHILIC EPITHELIOTROPIC DISEASE

BASICS

DEFINITION

A chronic debilitating generalized, progressive condition of unclear etiology usually associated with weight loss, dermatitis, eosinophilia, and the presence of eosinophilic infiltrates in multiple organs including the skin, alimentary tract, lungs, liver, and spleen

PATHOPHYSIOLOGY

The precise pathophysiology is unknown. In humans, a similar condition exists, and parasitic, allergic, autoimmune, viral, and toxic causes have all been implicated. The coexistence of T-cell lymphosarcoma and the syndrome in horses has led some authors to suggest the production by clonal neoplastic cells of cytokines (such as interleukin-5) that stimulate production and proliferation of eosinophils.

SYSTEMS AFFECTED

Multiple organ and tissue involvement, often including skin, lungs, liver, and alimentary tract

GENETICS

No genetic link has been identified.

INCIDENCE/PREVALENCE

• Rare • Precise incidence and prevalence unknown

GEOGRAPHIC DISTRIBUTION

Worldwide

SIGNALMENT

• Breed predilections—none known • Younger horses ranging from 3–13 years old • Both sexes are affected.

SIGNS

• Most horses present with weight loss of several weeks' or months' duration. • Examination often, although not always, shows concomitant crusting and exfoliating dermatitis and alopecia over whole body and coronary bands.

CAUSES

• Multiple etiologies have been proposed. • May be secondary to T-cell lymphosarcoma producing cytokines that stimulate bone marrow proliferation and tissue infiltration of eosinophils

RISK FACTORS

None known

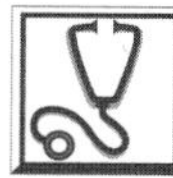

DIAGNOSIS

DIFFERENTIAL DIAGNOSIS

Note: Tissue biopsy and hematologic and biochemical testing help differentiate this disease from other diseases that present with similar signs such as:

• Other causes of chronic weight loss, including dental problems, poor nutrition, and parasitism
• Other causes of dermatitis including dermatophilosus (rain scald) and dermatophytosis (ringworm). • Infiltrative bowel diseases including alimentary lymphosarcoma • Other organ-specific causes of weight loss • Sarcoidosis (not to be confused with the common equine skin tumor) • Autoimmune skin diseases

CBC/BIOCHEMISTRY/URINALYSIS

Signs usually, but not always include some or all of the following:

• Hypereosinophilia • Hypoproteinemia
• Hypoalbuminemia • Hyperfibrinogenemia
• Evidence of other organ involvement including increased GGT, ALP, or creatinine

OTHER LABORATORY TESTS

• Abdominocentesis may reveal a modified transudate containing some eospinophils.
• Liver biopsy or bone marrow biopsy may reveal large clusters of proliferating eosinophils or eosinophilic granulomas, often with a lymphocytic infiltrate.

IMAGING

• Radiography of the thorax may reveal patterns consistent with either miliary or granulomatous infiltrates. • Ultrasound of liver, spleen, or kidneys may suggest similar granulomatous changes.

OTHER DIAGNOSTIC PROCEDURES

• Skin biopsy—ulceration and acanthosis with infiltrating neutrophilic and lymphocytic exudate and eosinophilic granulomas • Glucose or xylose gastrointestinal absorption test—may be abnormal • Exploratory laparotomy may reveal focal or disseminated lymphosarcoma.

PATHOLOGICAL FINDINGS

Multiorgan involvement—see above

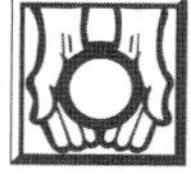

TREATMENT

AIMS OF TREATMENT

Attempt to reduce eosinophilic infiltrates.

APPROPRIATE HEALTH CARE

• Most cases are refractory to treatment • In one reported case, the condition resolved following treatment with dexamethasone, trimethoprim-sulfamethoxazole, and antihistamine. • Hydroxyurea administered to one horse without success

MULTISYSTEMIC EOSINOPHILIC EPITHELIOTROPIC DISEASE

NURSING CARE

• Encourage appetite. • Treat/manage skin problems and any ulceration.

ACTIVITY

Affected horses should be rested.

DIET

Any

CLIENT EDUCATION

Owners should be warned that the condition generally has a grave prognosis and leads to euthanasia in most cases.

SURGICAL CONSIDERATIONS

Consider exploratory laparotomy to rule out other intestinal involvement or theoretically to resect a primary alimentary lymphosarcoma.

MEDICATIONS

DRUG(S) OF CHOICE

Attempt treatment with dexamethasone (0.05–0.1 mg/kg IV or PO daily, reducing over several weeks) or other anti-inflammatory medications.

CONTRAINDICATIONS

None

PRECAUTIONS

None

POSSIBLE INTERACTIONS

None

ALTERNATIVE DRUGS

See above.

FOLLOW-UP

PATIENT MONITORING

• Monitor the horse's weight. • Monitor response to medication through hematology and biochemistry and/or through imaging.

EXPECTED COURSE AND PROGNOSIS

Most horses require euthanasia after several months of poor response to treatments.

MISCELLANEOUS

ASSOCIATED CONDITIONS

Lymphosarcoma

SYNONYMS

• Chronic eosinophilic gastroenteritis • Chronic eosinophilic dermatitis

Suggested Reading

Hillyer MH, Mair TS. Multisystemic eosinophilic epitheliotropic disease in a horse: attempted treatment with hydroxyurea and dexamethasone. Vet Rec 1992;130:392–395.

La Perle KM, Piercy RJ, Long JF, Blomme EA. Multisystemic, eosinophilic, epitheliotropic disease with intestinal lymphosarcoma in a horse. Vet Pathol 1998;35:144–146.

McCue ME, Davis EG, Rush BR, Cox JH, Wilkerson MJ. Dexamethasone for treatment of multisystemic eosinophilic epitheliotropic disease in a horse. J Am Vet Med Assoc 2003;223:1320–1323.

Nimmo Wilkie JS, Yager JA, Nation PN, Clark EG, Townsend HG, Baird JD. Chronic eosinophilic dermatitis: a manifestation of a multisystemic, eosinophilic, epitheliotropic disease in five horses. Vet Pathol 1985;22:297–305.

Singh K, Holbrook TC, Gilliam LL, Cruz RJ, Duffy J, Confer AW. Severe pulmonary disease due to multisystemic eosinophilic epitheliotropic disease in a horse. Vet Pathol 2006;43:189–193.

Author Richard J. Piercy

Consulting Editor Gwendolen Lorch

MYELOPROLIFERATIVE DISEASES

BASICS

OVERVIEW

• Rare (<1% of all reported neoplasms) tumors of horses involving an increase in neoplastic myeloid hematopoietic cells (nonlymphoid) either within the bone marrow or in extramedullary tissues. They result in the pathological destruction of normal tissue architecture and ultimately the loss of normal marrow elements and myelosphthisis.
• Malignant histiocytosis and myeloid leukemia are the 2 forms of myeloproliferative disease reported in horses. Myeloid leukemia can be further classified into 4 forms—monocytic and myelomonocytic leukemia, granulocytic leukemia, megakaryocytic leukemia, and primary erythrocytosis.
• Malignant histiocytosis involves proliferation of mononuclear phagocytes, which are intermediate in differentiation between monoblasts and tissue histiocytes.
• Single-cell leukemias reported in horses include monocytic leukemia, myelomonocytic leukemia, granulocytic leukemia, and eosinophilic myeloproliferative disorder.
• Familial megakaryocytic hypoplasia has been described in Standardbred horses, but other forms of leukemia of the megakaryocyte have not been described.
• Primary erythrocytosis is very rare.
• A genetic predisposition has been described in humans but not demonstrated in the horse.

SIGNALMENT

• Seen in a younger population than other neoplastic lesions
• Age range reported for monocytic leukemia is between 2 and 11 years
• Other myeloproliferative disorders reported between 10 mo and 16 years.
• No breed or sex predisposition

SIGNS

• Most clinical signs are related to destruction of tissue by invasive neoplastic cells and are often nonspecific.
• Signs may include fever, weight loss, signs of depression, and exercise intolerance.
• Ventral and peripheral edema, lymphadenopathy, pallor of mucous membranes, and/or petechial hemorrhages and oral ulceration may be observed.
• Less common signs include epistaxis, dyspnea, and colic.
• Icterus may be seen is cases with secondary immune-mediated hemolytic anemia.

CAUSES AND RISK FACTORS

Remain undefined. Possibly similar to causes found in humans include ionizing radiation and exposure to certain chemicals.

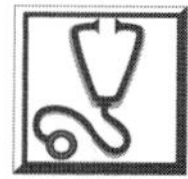

DIAGNOSIS

DIFFERENTIAL DIAGNOSIS

• Lymphoid neoplasia may present with similar signs. Lymph node and/or bone marrow aspirates or biopsies can help differentiate. Abnormal circulating lymphocytes (although uncommon) may be observed and would indicate lymphoid neoplasia.
• Other causes of nonspecific clinical signs can include pleuritis, peritonitis, colitis, pneumonia, and abdominal abscessation and must be ruled out by a thorough physical examination. Immune suppression and secondary infections (commonly respiratory) may occur in horses with myeloproliferative disorders and may complicate diagnosis.
• Ventral and limb edema also may be observed in vasculitis, impaired lymph drainage, hypoproteinemia, or purpura hemorrhagica. CBC and biochemistry may help differentiate together with detection of underlying cause.

CBC/BIOCHEMISTRY/URINALYSIS

• Nonregenerative anemia is often an early finding.
• Leukopenia, leukocytosis, or a normal white cell count may be seen depending on whether the patient is leukemic, subleukemic, or aleukemic. Abnormal leukocytes invariably occur in peripheral blood.
• Thrombocytopenia or pancytopenia may be observed.
• Immune-mediated hemolytic anemia and thrombocytopenia may coexist.
• Gammopathy or mild hypoproteinemia may be present.

OTHER LABORATORY TESTS

• Blood gas analysis and erythropoietin concentration for diagnosis of primary erythrocytosis
• Decreased concentrations of erythropoietin with a normal Pao_2 and elevated hematocrit are observed.
• May be accompanied by thrombocytosis or leukocytosis.

IMAGING

• Abdominal ultrasound detects lymphadenopathy, hepatomegaly, or splenomegaly.
• Thoracic ultrasound and radiographs may demonstrate secondary respiratory infections in some horses.

OTHER DIAGNOSTIC PROCEDURES

• Bone marrow aspirates or biopsies may demonstrate an elevated myeloid:erythroid ratio (normal 0.5–3.75) and neoplastic cells occurring as a monomorphic population.
• Serum lysozyme (muramidase) concentrations can be measured and should be <5 μg/mL in normal horses. Myeloid cells contain almost no lysozyme, while monocytes and neutrophils have large amounts, which may be reflected in increased serum concentrations in myeloproliferative disorders.
• Cytochemistry—Nonspecific myeloid markers include Sudan black B, PAS stain, alkaline phosphatase, peroxidase, and chloroacetate esterase, and uptake by neoplastic cells helps confirm myeloid lineage. Monocytic markers such as the esterase stains, α-naphthyl-butyrate esterase, and α-naphthyl acetate esterase can then be used to differentiate granulocytic cells from monocytic and megakaryocytic cells. Megakaryocyte stain (Megacolor) is used to differentiate monocytic and megakaryocytic cells.

PATHOLOGICAL FINDINGS

• Gross findings include generalized lymphadenopathy, hepatomegaly, and splenomegaly. In severe cases, hemorrhages can be found throughout the body. Discoloration of myeloid tissue is also described.
• Histopathology may demonstrate immature myeloblastic cells in a number of tissues including bone marrow, lymph nodes, spleen, liver, kidneys, lungs, and heart. Leukostasis has been described whereby white cell accumulation causes blood vessel occlusion.

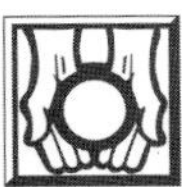

TREATMENT

• A limited response to treatment is reported, and euthanasia is usually warranted in these cases and should be timely.
• Inpatient care is required if treatment is to be attempted.
• The client should be made aware of the poor prognosis and limited treatment options available.

MEDICATIONS

DRUG(S)

• Most antineoplastic agents are not effective in these cases and treatment options are limited. In addition, the available drugs are expensive with little guarantee of success.
• Cytosine arabinoside (10 mg/m^2 q12 h for 3 weeks) has shown most promise.
• Broad-spectrum antibiotics as needed to treat secondary infections in patients undergoing chemotherapy.

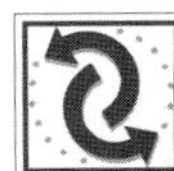

FOLLOW-UP

PATIENT MONITORING

Horses with myeloproliferative disorders treated with chemotherapy should have a CBC and biochemical profile performed periodically to assess side effects such as bone marrow and organ dysfunction.

POSSIBLE COMPLICATIONS

Immunosuppression occurs commonly in affected horses resulting in secondary infections that can affect any body system.

EXPECTED COURSE AND PROGNOSIS

• Prognosis is poor.
• Rapid progression of clinical signs can be expected, and most horses will die within weeks of initial presentation.

MISCELLANEOUS

SEE ALSO

• Anemia
• Anemia, aplastic
• Lymphosarcoma
• Multiple myeloma
• Pancytopenia
• Thrombocytopenia

Suggested Reading

Diseases of the hemolymphatic and immune systems. In: Radostits O, Gay C, Hinchcliff K, Constable P, eds. Veterinary Medicine, ed 10. Philadelphia: WB Saunders, 2007;439–469.

Savage CJ. Lymphoproliferative and myeloproliferative disorders. Vet Clin North Am Equine Pract 1998;14:563–578.

Author Laura C. Lee

Consulting Editors Jennifer Hodgson and David Hodgson

MYOCARDIAL DISEASE

BASICS

DEFINITION

• Myocardial disease can consist of myocardial degeneration, ischemia, necrosis, inflammation, fibrosis, or a combination of these pathological processes. • It may be focal or generalized, and clinical signs are generally more severe when widespread pathology is present.

PATHOPHYSIOLOGY

• Focal myocardial disease usually leads to arrhythmias, which, if rapid, reduce the diastolic filling time and thereby compromise cardiac output. • Generalized myocardial disease leads to compromise of the heart's pumping ability, and pump failure, reduced cardiac output, and poor perfusion ensue.
• Reduction of cardiac output has widespread effects as there is failure of perfusion of vital organs and tissues, including the myocardium.
• Lack of forward flow can lead to congestion of pulmonary circulation, pulmonary edema, and signs of acute left-sided heart failure.

SYSTEMS AFFECTED

• Cardiovascular—primary • Renal—secondary • Gastrointestinal tract and liver—secondary • Musculoskeletal system—secondary • Neurologic system—secondary

GENETICS N/A

INCIDENCE/PREVALENCE

Uncommon

GEOGRAPHIC DISTRIBUTION N/A

SIGNALMENT

There are no specific breed, age, or sex predilections.

SIGNS

General Comments

The severity of clinical signs generally reflects the nature and extent of myocardial pathology. With focal pathology, signs may be relatively mild.

Historical

• Poor performance • Collapse and distress
• Fever may be present.

Physical Examination

• Tachycardia • Arrhythmias • Weakness
• Weak peripheral pulses, pale mucous membranes • Pulse deficits • Respiratory distress, tachypnea, cough, and frothy nasal discharge • Moist crackles on auscultation of the lung fields suggesting pulmonary edema

CAUSES

• Focal fibrosis is commonly found either as an incidental finding at post-mortem examination or occasionally in horses known to have persistent arrhythmias. The cause is unknown. • Bacterial infection (localized to the myocardium or by extension of infection from endocardial or pericardial lesions)
• Viral infection • Fungal infection
• Aberrant parasite migration • Immune-mediated disease • Toxins such as ionophores and snake venom • Neoplastic infiltration, e. g., lymphosarcoma, hemangiosarcoma
• Myocardial failure occurs with MODS and SIRS. This is principally due to dysregulation of systemic vascular function and is accompanied by microthrombosis. However, a direct myocardial depressant effect mechanism may also come into play. • Streptococcal toxic shock • Brain-heart syndrome (a syndrome in which massive release of catecholamines at nerve endings within the myocardium follows brain trauma) • White muscle disease (linked to selenium deficiency and seen mainly in young animals) • Coronary artery disease, the most common cause of myocardial ischemia in human beings, has not been well documented in horses but may occur.

RISK FACTORS

• No specific risk factors have been identified.

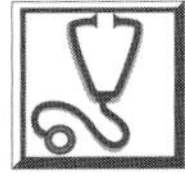

DIAGNOSIS

DIFFERENTIAL DIAGNOSIS

• Secondary causes of arrhythmias such as hypoxia, toxemia, septicemia, or metabolic disturbances • Vavular heart disease including infective endocarditis—Cardiac murmurs are usually present, differentiate echocardiographically. • Pericarditis—Differentiate echocardiographically. • Severe skeletal myopathies such as atypical myoglobinuria and increases in serum activities of total CK and myoglobinuria are present. • Pneumonia—Differentiate with thoracic ultrasonography and radiography.
• Hemoperitoneum or hemothorax—Differentiate ultrasonographically.

CBC/BIOCHEMISTRY/URINALYSIS

• Increased serum creatinine concentration and BUN suggest prerenal dysfunction or, if marked, concurrent renal dysfunction.
• Neutrophilic leukocytosis and hyperfibrinogenemia may be present.

OTHER LABORATORY TESTS

• Elevated cardiac isoenzymes (CK-MB, HBDH, or LDH-1 and LDH-2) or cardiac troponin I may be present. These biomarkers are often normal in horses with other evidence of focal myocardial disease such as arrhythmias. They are released into the peripheral circulation only with myocardial cell necrosis and may be present only in the early stages of myocardial disease, quickly returning to normal. Marked increases are likely to be indicative of myocardial disease, but mild increases are nonspecific. Equally, myocardial disease cannot be ruled out on the basis that there are no increases in these biomarkers. • Blood lactate may be increased, reflecting poor tissue perfusion. • Blood culture and viral serology may be indicated in some cases. • Submission of additional samples such as transtracheal aspirates for bacterial or fungal culture may also be useful in selected cases. • Measurement of serum selenium and glutathione peroxidase concentrations can be useful if white muscle disease is suspected.

IMAGING

Electrocardiography

Supraventricular and/or ventricular arrhythmias may be present. These may be paroxysmal or sustained.

Echocardiography

• With focal myocardial disease, the echocardiogram may be unremarkable. Occasionally, focal areas of increased echogenicity are observed which may indicate myocardial fibrosis. These are also sometimes observed in horses with related clinical signs.
• With generalized myocardial disease, echocardiographic abnormalities are more obvious:
  ○ Dilation of the left and/or right ventricle is noted on two- dimensional and M-mode echocardiography. The ventricles can be rounded at their apices and adopt a globoid shape.
  ○ Regional or generalized hypokinesis or dyskinesis.
  ○ Decreases in fractional shortening.
  ○ Marked spontaneous contrast (this is sometimes also noted in horses with no cardiac dysfunction).
  ○ Increases in the mitral E point-septal separation.
  ○ Increased pre-ejection period and decreased left ventricular ejection period.
  ○ Flattening of the aortic root, reduced aortic root diameter.
  ○ Mild, usually anechoic, pericardial effusion.
• With myocardial neoplasia, extensive nodular masses with mixed echogenicity may be visible, often partially obliterating the walls of the chambers and in the case of lymphoma, can also involve valve cusps.

THORACIC ULTRASONOGRAPHY

With pulmonary edema, irregularity of the periphery of the lungs (comet tails) is visible.

THORACIC RADIOGRAPHY

Pulmonary edema may be evident.

OTHER DIAGNOSTIC PROCEDURES

Radiotelemetric ECG Monitoring

This is indicated for real-time monitoring of horses with unstable cardiac rhythms.

Continuous 24-Hour Holter Monitoring

This is particularly helpful in identifying intermittent or paroxysmal cardiac arrhythmias, in quantifying numbers of isolated premature depolarizations and in assessing response to therapy.

Exercise Electrocardiography

Characterization of the effect of exercise on cardiac arrhythmia is important in assessing clinical significance.

Noninvasive Blood Pressure Measurement

This can serve as a useful means of monitoring horses with generalized myocardial disease.

Toxicology

Stomach contents and feedstuffs should be analyzed for the presence of ionophores, particularly in group outbreaks of myocardial disease.

PATHOLOGICAL FINDINGS

• Grossly, there may be focal or diffuse areas of discolored, pale myocardium.
• Histologically, there may be focal or diffuse myocardial degeneration, ischemia, necrosis, inflammation, and/or fibrosis. • Neoplastic infiltration is generally visible grossly, but its nature must be confirmed histologically.
• Evidence of poor perfusion may be evident on histologic examination of other body systems such as the kidneys, liver, and intestine. • With left-sided heart failure, there may be accumulation of frothy pink-tinged fluid in the alveoli and small and large airways.

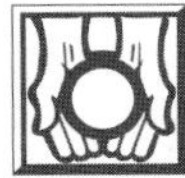

TREATMENT

AIMS OF TREATMENT

• Restoration of cardiac output and improved tissue perfusion • Specific therapy aimed at cause if relevant. • Antiarrhythmic therapy if unstable, life-threatening arrhythmias are present.

APPROPRIATE HEALTH CARE

• Anti-inflammatories, antiarrhythmics, and, if necessary, pressor support may be useful in generalized myocardial disease, in addition to specific measures aimed at the cause in individual cases. • With focal myocardial disease, rest with or without corticosteroid therapy is helpful in around 40% of cases. In the remainder the problem may persist, but provided the cardiac rhythm is not unstable during exercise, the horse may still be able to be used for some level of ridden exercise.

NURSING CARE

• Continuous ECG monitoring should be performed while showing signs of active myocardial disease, particularly if the cardiac rhythm is unstable. • Horses should be kept quiet and not moved if showing signs consistent with low cardiac output.

ACTIVITY

Horses with active focal or generalized myocardial disease should be rested until there is significant improvement in their clinical status, echocardiogram and ECG.

DIET

• In white muscle disease, selenium, vitamin E, and other antioxidants should be added to the diet. • If feed-derived toxins are suspected, the source of feed should be changed.

CLIENT EDUCATION

Clients must be warned of the grave prognosis and potential complications associated with generalized myocardial disease.

SURGICAL CONSIDERATIONS N/A

MEDICATIONS

DRUG(S) OF CHOICE

• Antiarrhythmic drugs are described in the sections Supraventricular Arrhythmias and Ventricular Arrhythmias elsewhere in this text. • Broad-spectrum antimicrobials, such as penicillin and gentamicin, are indicated if bacterial myocarditis is diagnosed.
• Furosemide (1 mg/kg IV TID) may relieve pulmonary congestion. • Dobutamine (1–5 μg/kg/min continuous rate infusion) may improve cardiac output, and digoxin (0.011 mg/kg PO BID) has potentially beneficial postive inotropic and negative chronotropic effects. • Corticosteroids may be useful in horses with immune-mediated or other forms of inflammatory myocarditis; either prednisolone 1 mg/kg PO every other day or dexamethasone 0.05–0.1 mg/kg IV or 0.1 mg/kg PO once a day for 3 or 4 days and then continued every 3–4 days in decreasing dosages is recommended. • Vitamin E supplementation at up to 10 IU/kg PO SID may be beneficial.

CONTRAINDICATIONS

• Digoxin is contraindicated if ionophore toxicity is suspected. • Corticosteroids are contraindicated in horses with concurrent pituitary pars intermedia dysfunction.

PRECAUTIONS

• Potentially nephrotoxic drugs such as aminoglycosides should be use cautiously in horses with poor tissue perfusion.
• Therapeutic drug monitoring is recommended.

POSSIBLE INTERACTIONS

Digoxin can interact with other drugs, notably quinidine, and care should be taken to monitor plasma concentrations when both are used concurrently.

ALTERNATIVE DRUGS N/A

FOLLOW-UP

PATIENT MONITORING

• Monitoring systemic blood pressure and blood lactate is helpful in assessing the early response to therapy. • If biomarkers are increased, these can be a useful tool for monitoring resolution of the myocardial disease in the early stages of recovery.
• Frequent echocardiographic and 24-hour Holter ECG recordings should be obtained in the convalescent period.

POSSIBLE COMPLICATIONS

Renal failure and congestive cardiac failure

EXPECTED COURSE AND PROGNOSIS

• Focal myocardial disease can have limited clinical significance, although cardiac arrhythmias may persist. • Generalized myocardial disease is life-threatening and therefore a grave prognosis is warranted. Horses can return to athletic activity if they survive the acute stages of myocardial failure. Persistent echocardiographic evidence of reduced ventricular function such as low fractional shortening and regional or global hypokinesis and persistent arrhythmias during exercise indicate that the horse should be retired from ridden activities.

MISCELLANEOUS

ASSOCIATED CONDITIONS

Myocardial disease can be associated with respiratory infection, SIRS, or MODS.

AGE-RELATED FACTORS N/A

ZOONOTIC POTENTIAL N/A

PREGNANCY

• There is a high risk of fetal compromise if mares develop low cardiac output during pregnancy.

SEE ALSO

• Ventricular arrhythmias • Supraventricular arrhythmias • Infective endocarditis
• Ionophore toxicosis

ABBREVIATIONS

• CK-MB = MB isoenzyme of creatine kinase
• HBDH = α-hydroxybutyrate dehydrogenase • LDH = lactate dehydrogenase • MODS = multiple organ dysfunction syndrome • SIRS = systemic inflammatory response syndrome

Suggested Reading

Bowen IM, Marr CM, Elliott JE. Cardiovascular pharmacology. In: Bertone J, Horspool L, eds. Clinical Pharmacology of the Horse. Philadelphia; WB Saunders, 2004:193–216.

Dolente BA, Seco OM, Lewis ML. Streptococcal toxic shock in a horse. J Am Vet Med Assoc 2000;217:64–67, 30.

Marr CM. Heart failure. In: Marr CM, ed, Cardiology of the Horse. Philadelphia: WB Saunders, 1999:289.

Reef VB. Myocardial disease. In: Robinson NE, ed. Current Therapy in Equine Medicine, ed 3. Philadelphia: WB Saunders, 1992:393.

Reef VB. Pericardial and myocardial diseases. In: Kobluk CN, Ames TR, Geor RJ, eds. The Horse: Diseases and Clinical Management. Philadelphia: WB Saunders, 1995:185.

Author Celia M. Marr
Consulting Editor Celia M. Marr

NARCOLEPSY AND CATAPLEXY

BASICS

DEFINITION

Rapid eye movement (REM) sleep disorders resulting in excessive daytime sleepiness and paroxysmal sleep attacks with rapid eye movements (narcolepsy) or complete loss of muscle tone and reflexes (cataplexy)

PATHOPHYSIOLOGY

In laboratory species and dogs, it has been shown that the neuropeptide hypocretin (orexin) is central to the control of sleep and arousal. Hypocretin neurons project to areas involved in these processes, including the ascending reticular activating system, and hypocretin levels fluctuate across the sleep-wake cycle and increase with sleep deprivation. Hypocretin neurons activate brainstem "REM-off" neurons and reduce the activity of "REM-on" neurons, acting as a gate to entry into REM sleep. In humans, narcolepsy has been associated with reduced hypocretin levels, and in dogs, narcoleptic lines that lack hypocretin receptors have been bred. This has not been demonstrated in horses, and animals with "sleep attacks" may simply be REM sleep deficient (i.e., not lying down enough).

SYSTEM AFFECTED

Central nervous system

SIGNALMENT

Narcolepsy-like episodes can be seen transiently in foals, particularly in miniature horses, Fell Ponies, Shetland and Welsh Ponies, and Appaloosas. Usually, the episodes resolve with time. More commonly, it is seen in aged horses.

SIGNS

Foals

- An attack may progress from buckling at the knees without falling, to sudden and total collapse and areflexia, usually with maintenance of some eye and facial responses and normal cardiorespiratory function.
- Each recumbent episode may last hours if the foal is totally undisturbed, but the patient usually can be aroused from this state with varying degrees of difficulty.

Adults

- Most commonly, this includes horses resting in the back of a field that can seem to "buckle" at the knees but rarely collapse.
- Excessive somnolence is easily noted by owners with the patient often resting the head or hind quarters on objects.
- Most times the animal awakes with the [impending] fall within 1 minute to resume the somnolent state or revert to wakefulness.
- Some horses have had relentless persistence of the syndrome to the point of severe knee and face trauma.
- In some patients, episodes may be triggered by specific stimuli such as saddling, hosing down or feeding, with no permanent consequences. Only occasionally do episodes occur with the excitement of being ridden.

CAUSES

- No specific cause has been identified, but rigorous assessment of hypocretin levels has not been undertaken.
- In some older horses, the cause may well be due to sleep deprivation, perhaps because the horse is unwilling to lie down as a result of joint pain or fear of enclosed spaces.

RISK FACTORS

Not identified

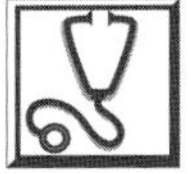

DIAGNOSIS

Diagnosis by exclusion only. It is worthwhile getting the owner to set up a 24-hour video recording to assess how often these episodes occur, and whether the animal appears to go into normal REM sleep (≈20 minutes per day total, in lateral recumbency).

DIFFERENTIAL DIAGNOSIS

Cardiac arrhythmias, seizures

CBC/BIOCHEMISTRY/URINALYSIS

No specific abnormalities

PATHOLOGIC FINDINGS

No associated findings

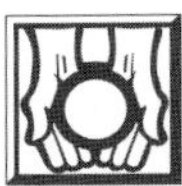

TREATMENT

Long-term therapy is inappropriate, although short-term responsiveness to the tricyclic antidepressant imipramine (1–2 mg/kg IM or IV q6–12 h) and other drugs can alter the severity of the clinical syndrome.

DRUGS

See Treatment.

PROGNOSIS

Poor for the persistent form, and excellent for the neonatal form

ABBREVIATIONS

REM = rapid eye movement

Suggested Reading

Baumann CR, Bassetti CL. Hypocretins (orexins) and sleep-wake disorders. Lancet Neurol 2005;4:673–682.

Lunn DP, et al.: Familial occurrence of narcolepsy in miniature horses. Equine Vet J 1993;25:483–487.

Parkes JD, Chen SY, Clift SJ, Dahlitz MJ, Dunn G. The clinical diagnosis of the narcoleptic syndrome. J Sleep Res 1998;7:41–52.

Sutcliffe JG, de Lecea L. The hypocretins: setting the arousal threshold. Nat Rev Neurosci 2002;3:339–349.

The author and editors wish to acknowledge the contribution of Joseph J. Bertone, author of this chapter in the previous edition.

Author Caroline N. Hahn

Consulting Editor Caroline N. Hahn

NAVICULAR SYNDROME

BASICS

OVERVIEW

• Lameness originating from the caudal third of the foot caused by pain from injury to the navicular bone and/or the navicular suspensory apparatus (impar ligament, collateral suspensory ligament, DDFT near the navicular bone) and/or the navicular bursa.
• Biomechanical theory suggests that degenerative changes within the navicular bone result from abnormal forces exerted on the navicular bone, its surrounding ligaments and the DDFT within the hoof.
• Faulty distal limb conformation, improper hoof balance, and poor shoeing lead to these abnormal forces in the navicular area. • Vascular occlusion of the navicular arteries may lead to ischemic necrosis of the navicular bone.

SYSTEM AFFECTED

Musculoskeletal—foot

SIGNALMENT

• Middle-aged horses • Quarter Horses but also Thoroughbreds, Warmbloods, mixed breeds
• Rare in ponies, donkeys, mules, Arabians, draft breeds

SIGNS

Historical

• Initially intermittent, slowly progressive lameness
• Lameness is more apparent on hard ground
• Bilateral forelimb lameness • +/− Unilateral forelimb lameness, rare in hindlimbs • Short, choppy stride • Stumbling • Increased lameness immediately after shoeing • +/− Point affected limb • With recent soft tissue injury, unilateral acute lameness

Physical Examination

• Long toe-low heel hoof conformation
• Increased heat in hoof capsule • Increased digital pulses in affected foot • Hoof tester application elicits pain in central frog region and across caudal third of hoof capsule at the medial and lateral aspect of navicular bone. • Atrophied frog • Lameness, frequently bilateral, although predominates in one limb

CAUSES AND RISK FACTORS

• Hoof imbalance* • Poor or inadequate shoeing*
• Poor hoof conformation (long toe–low heel, excessive toe length, underrun heel)* • Lack of heel support
• Quarter Horse breed • Big horse with small feet
• Faulty distal limb conformation • Mismatched front feet— one foot may be smaller and narrower.
• Excessive work on hard ground

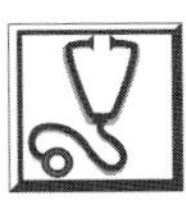

DIAGNOSIS

DIFFERENTIAL DIAGNOSIS

• Laminitis— acute, severe bilateral forelimb lameness. Hoof tester pain at the point of the frog in toe region
• Sheared heels—one heel higher than opposite heel on same foot • Bruised feet especially in the heel region of the foot termed a "corn"

IMAGING

Radiography—Navicular Bone

• Variation in synovial foramina size and shape
• Osteolysis or osseous cyst formation
• Enthesiophyte formation at collateral suspensory ligament attachment • Flexor cortex erosion
• Loss of corticomedullary distinction
• DDFT calcification • Osseous fragments associated with avulsion of the impar ligament

Ultrasound—Transcuneal Approach

• Tendonitis of the distal aspect of DDFT
• Desmitis of the impar ligament near the flexor surface of the navicular bone • Navicular bursitis

Nuclear Scintigraphy

• Increased radiopharmaceutical uptake in the caudal aspect of the foot • Lateral pool (soft tissue) phase and solar bone phase images of the front feet improve accuracy of diagnosis.

MRI

• Best diagnostic tool for imaging soft tissue injury within the navicular area such as DDFT, collateral suspensory ligament, impar ligament, distal annular ligament, and navicular bursa
• Navicular bone edema

OTHER DIAGNOSTIC PROCEDURES

• Diagnostic analgesia—palmar digital analgesia, intra-articular analgesia of DIP, and analgesia of the navicular bursa may all alleviate pain due to navicular syndrome.
• Endoscopic evaluation of the navicular bursa
• Contrast radiography of the navicular bursa

PATHOLOGICAL FINDINGS

• Erosive cartilaginous lesions on navicular bone
• Linear or core lesions in the DDFT fibers
• Adhesion(s) between DDFT and navicular bone

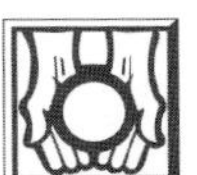

TREATMENTS

• Rest
• Improve/restore hoof balance, shorten toe, and ease breakover of the foot.
• Increase heel support, 2-degree wedge shoe or pad, eggbar shoe
• Intrasynovial anti-inflammatory medication(s) of DIP or navicular bursa
• Reduction in workload and expectations
• Palmar digital neurectomy as a last resort

MEDICATIONS

DRUG(S)

• NSAIDs—phenylbutazone (2.2 mg/kg daily for 7–10 days) • Isoxsuprine hydrochloride (1 mg/kg PO BID for 3 weeks then 1 mg/kg daily PO for 3 weeks, then 1 mg/kg PO every other day for 3 weeks)
• Intrasynovial corticosteroids— methylprednisolone acetate (20–40 mg) or triamcinolone (3–6 mg)
• Intrasynovial sodium hyaluronate (10–20 mg)
• Combination of intra-synovial corticosteroids and sodium hyaluronate • Systemic chondroprotective drugs—polysulfated glycosaminoglycan (500 mg IM q4days for 7 treatments) or sodium hyaluronate (40 mg IV q7days for 3 treatments) • Oral chondroprotective medications—glucosamine/chondrotin sulfate powder (1 scoop [3.3 g] BID)

CONTRAINDICATIONS/POSSIBLE INTERACTIONS

Intrasynovial corticosteroid use is *not* recommended in horses with previous history of laminitis.

FOLLOW-UP

PATIENT MONITORING

• Reevaluate lameness after several weeks of medical treatment. • NSAIDs may be necessary prior to excessive use. • Intra-articular medication(s) of DIP or navicular bursa may need to be repeated 2 to 3 times per year.
• Therapeutic trimming and shoeing every 6 weeks

PREVENTION/AVOIDANCE

• Reduction in workload or alterative sport
• Frequent and proper trimming and shoeing

POSSIBLE COMPLICATIONS

• Laminitis can occur secondary to intra-articular corticosteroids. • Gastric ulceration, right dorsal colon inflammation, or kidney damage can occur secondary to chronic NSAID use. • Neuroma formation, nerve regrowth, and DDFT rupture may occur following palmar digital neurectomy.

EXPECTED COURSE AND PROGNOSIS

• In early mild disease, horses can return to previous athletic use with continued medical therapy including trimming and shoeing, systemic medications, and/or medication of DIP or navicular bursa. • The syndrome is usually progressive, and increased severity in lameness and navicular bone degeneration is expected.
• After palmar digital neurectomy, horses may remain sound for approximately 2 years. Surgery is reserved as a last resort due the serious postoperative complications. • DDFT injuries carry a poor prognosis for returning to athletic use.

MISCELLANEOUS

ASSOCIATED CONDITIONS

• Sheared heels or chronic heel bruising in poorly conformed foot • Concurrent DIP disease or arthritis

AGE-RELATED CONDITIONS

• Uncommon in horses <5 years • Palmar digital neurectomy is not recommended in younger horses.

SYNONYMS

• Caudal heel pain • Navicular disease • Palmar foot pain

ABBREVIATIONS

• DDFT = deep digital flexor tendon • DIP = distal interphalangeal joint

Suggested Reading

Dabareiner RM, Carter GK. Diagnosis, treatment, and farriery for horses with chronic heel pain. In: O'Grady SE, ed. Vet Clin N Am Equine Pract 2003;19:417–441.

Author Robin M. Dabareiner
Consulting Editor Elizabeth J. Davidson

NEONATAL ISOERYTHROLYSIS

BASICS

DEFINITION

Alloimmune-mediated destruction of a neonatal foal's erythrocytes, caused by ingesting maternally (colostral) derived anti–foal erythrocyte antibodies.

PATHOPHYSIOLOGY

• First, a naïve mare is sensitized to a new RBC antigenic sequence. This can occur during blood transfusion or exposure to fetal RBCs that express the new antigenic sequence. Exposure may occur at parturition, or possibly secondary to in utero disease such as placentitis. Following exposure, the mare develops unique antibody targeted against the fetal RBC surface antigen.
• Second, the mare conceives a subsequent foal, sired by a stallion with that particular RBC surface antigen, and the foal inherits the stallion's RBC surface antigen. • At birth, the foal ingests antibody rich colostrum and absorbs anti-foal RBC antibodies that cause destruction of RBCs. • Antibodies attach to the foal erythrocytes, which results in hemolysis and/or premature removal of damaged RBC by the reticuloendothelial system. • Results in anemia

SYSTEMS AFFECTED

• Hemic/lymphatic/immune—intravascular and extravascular hemolysis leading to anemia, jaundice and hemoglobinemia
• Renal/urologic—hemoglobinuria leading to pigment nephropathy, acute tubular necrosis and acute renal failure • Cardiovascular—tachycardia from hypoxic anemia • Nervous—hypoxic anemic shock causing weakness, hyperbilirubinemia causing basal ganglia dysfunction and seizures (kernicterus)

GENETICS

• Genetic diversity between the dam and sire/foal is the underlying cause for disease. The dam lacks the specific genetic sequence that codes for foal/stallion erythrocyte surface antigen, resulting in incompatibility. • There are many RBC surface antigen factors, and in theory any of these can be involved in NI development. However two factors are of notable importance—Aa in the A system and Qa in the Q system—and represent the majority of cases.
• In mules, the "donkey factor," which is unique to all donkeys and not horses, is commonly involved.

INCIDENCE/PREVALENCE

• Among Thoroughbreds and Standardbreds, the prevalence of disease is ≈1%–2%. • In mule foals, the prevalence is as high as 10%–25%.
• Breed variability reflects the frequency of specific genes involved in erythrocyte antigenicity or blood groups found in each breed. • Most horse mares bred to donkey jacks are at high risk (see Risk Factors).

GEOGRAPHIC DISTRIBUTION

Worldwide

SIGNALMENT

Breed Predilections

• The antigenic factors are not specific for, or limited to, any particular breed of horse.
• Most mule pregnancies are incompatible regarding the blood group factor, "donkey factor," in which donkeys express and horses do not.

Age and Range

• Usually foals born to multiparous mares
• Most foals present during the first 4 days of life (mean range 0–8 days)

Predominant Sex

Both sexes are equally affected.

SIGNS

General Comments

The severity and magnitude of clinical signs vary depending on the magnitude and rate of hemolysis.

Historical

• Affected foals are generally healthy at birth and nurse appropriately from the mare.
• Nonspecific signs such as lethargy begin within hours to days of colostral ingestion and immunoglobulin absorption. These signs may mimic other common neonatal disorders such as septicemia. • Icterus and generalized pallor soon develop. • Mare may have a history of producing jaundiced or NI-confirmed foals from previous pregnancies, especially if the same stallion had sired these foals. • Previous administration of transfused blood or other blood products can help identify "at risk" mares.

Physical Examination

• Lethargy, disinterest in suckling • Tachypnea; tachycardia • Pallor (acute stages) often progressing to jaundice • Pigmenturia (hemoglobinuria) • Recumbency • Mild fever is often present. • Systemic signs of hypoxic insult and/or hyperbilirubinemia including colic, melena, and seizure activity (hypoxia; kernicterus)

CAUSES

• Maternal production of anti-foal erythrocyte immunoglobulin from exposure of incompatible fetal blood because of placentitis, trauma/exposure at parturition, sensitization from the stallion at conception, or incompatible blood transfusion

RISK FACTORS

• Mares lacking erythrocyte factors Aa and/or Qa are at greater risk (>90%) of producing antibodies to these blood types if exposed than are mares with incompatibilities against other blood types. • Mares bred to donkeys are at a very high risk for the production of immunoglobulin to donkey factor. • Qa antigen is rare in Standardbreds—Ca antigen is more common (present in ≈20% Standardbred and 10% Thoroughbreds) but does not appear to be associated with clinical disease. • *Donkey RBC antigen "donkey factor"*—The risk of an incompatible mating between a horse and a donkey (or the chance of a mare becoming sensitized to this antigen) is 100%. Because clinical NI in mule foals only occurs ≈8%–10% of the time, it is suggested that many mule foals may have subclinical NI.

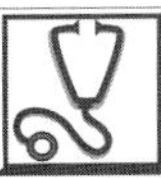

DIAGNOSIS

DIFFERENTIAL DIAGNOSIS

• Anemia due to blood loss • Hepatopathy—icterus may be present with Tyzzer's disease (*Clostridium piliforme* infection), cholangiohepatitis, obstructive cholestatic disease; severe anemia is usually not present with hepatic disease. • Neonatal maladjustment syndrome—weakness, lethargy present; icterus and anemia should differentiate. • Neonatal septicemia—icterus, leukocytosis, and weakness may be present, but significant anemia is uncommon with septicemia. • In endemic areas, consider neonatal babesiosis (piroplasmosis).

CBC/BIOCHEMISTRY/URINALYSIS

• Anemia—decreased PCV (usually <20%), decreased hemoglobin concentration, and decreased erythrocyte number
• Hemoglobinemia • Hemoglobinuria
• Hyperbilirubinemia (primarily indirect, unconjugated fraction); kernicterus is associated with total bilirubin >20 mg/dL. • Mild leukocytosis • Mild thrombocytosis
• Hypoglycemia is often present.

OTHER LABORATORY TESTS

• Coomb's testing (direct antiglobulin test)
  ○ Detects immunoglobulin coated erythrocytes, and may remain positive for several weeks, until maternal antibody is utilized and metabolized.
  ○ Detects antierythrocyte factor in mare's serum and colostrum. A sample from the mare may be preferred as all maternally derived immunoglobulin in the foal may be bound to erythrocytes and not free in the serum.
• JFA test—This is a field screen test to detect NI. The foal's RBCs are exposed to the mare's colostrum or serum. If the cells agglutinate, then NI may develop. • Saline agglutination or complement-mediated hemolytic test can be performed by some laboratories. • Fluorescence antibody cell sorting on erythrocytes (FACS) has also been reported.

OTHER DIAGNOSTIC PROCEDURES

• Foal IgG determination will provide useful information to determine if the foal has ingested colostrum from the mare. • Clinical evidence of jaundice with complete failure of transfer of passive immunity makes NI less likely.

PATHOLOGICAL FINDINGS

• If the foal dies acutely, pallor and icterus may be observed throughout the body. If the foal dies later, the conversion of free hemoglobin to bilirubin leads to widespread jaundice of the body. • Splenomegaly • Pigment nephropathy related to hemoglobinuric nephrosis • Bone marrow hypoplasia

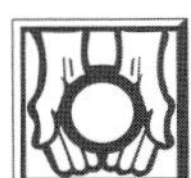

TREATMENT

AIMS OF TREATMENT

• Restore oxygen-carrying capacity with transfusion of whole blood, packed RBCs, or hemoglobin-based oxygen carrier. • Prevent further intake of maternal colostrum.

APPROPRIATE HEALTH CARE

• If the foal is showing signs of icterus and lethargy/weakness, emergency inpatient intensive care management may be required, and inpatient medical management including blood transfusion is recommended. • If there is early recognition of the problem, withholding further maternal colostrum and providing supportive care in the field may be adequate.

NURSING CARE

Blood Transfusion

• Blood transfusion with packed RBCs should be considered in foals where the PCV is <12%–15% and/or the foal is showing clinical signs of decompensatory anemic hypoxia. Transfusion is not essential to all cases of NI, only those where it is considered a life-saving measure. • Washed and irradiated erythrocytes from the mare are immunologically anergic and are the ideal donor cells. The stallion is the most unsuitable blood donor. • Previously blood-typed animals negative for Aa or Qa antibodies are also suitable blood donors.
• Where compatible donor capabilities are limited, cautious transfusion with blood from a horse breed other than Thoroughbred or Standardbred is recommended. Ideally, these should be geldings and have not had a blood transfusion themselves. • For a 50-kg foal, give whole blood 2–4 L slowly over 1–2 hr or packed erythrocytes 1–2 L slowly over 1–2 hr.

Intranasal Oxygen

Nasal insufflation with humidified oxygen (5–10 L/min) may be used to increase inspired oxygen concentration, although this is not a substitute for transfusion in severely anemic foals.

Additional Treatment

• To treat the pigment nephropathy (hemoglobin nephropathy), balanced polyionic crystalloid fluids should be administered to promote renal perfusion and diuresis (with or without diuretic medication). • Supplement IV/PO dextrose/glucose where appropriate.

ACTIVITY

Foals should not be stressed and exercise should be at a minimum to conserve oxygen.

DIET

• If recognized before the 24 hr of age, the foal should be muzzled to prevent from ingesting further colostral antibodies. The mare should be milked out and the milk discarded. • Affected foals should be supplemented with mare's milk replacer for the first 24–36 hr from birth; then resume nursing from the mare. • Enteral feeding with mare's milk free of colostrum is preferred whether unassisted or via nasogastric tube. If a foal develops ileus secondary to anemic hypoxia, parenteral nutrition should be considered.

CLIENT EDUCATION

Mares of NI foals are likely to produce NI foals in subsequent pregnancies, especially if the same stallion is used. Preventative strategies should be exercised to minimize the chance of having an NI foal.

MEDICATIONS

DRUG(S) OF CHOICE

Seizure control where appropriate using benzodiazepines (diazepam bolus 0.1–0.4 mg/kg IV or midazolam infusion 0.02–0.2 mg/kg/hr and/or phenobarbital 2–10 mg/kg IV).

PRECAUTIONS

• Cautiously administer plasma transfusions where serum IgG concentrations are low. Frequent assessment for disease exacerbation (i.e., hemolytic crisis) is necessary.
• Nephrotoxic drugs such as aminoglycoside antimicrobials and NSAIDs should be avoided.

ALTERNATIVE DRUGS

Oxyglobin administration has clinical utility in providing oxygen transportation with little immunologic reactivity. Suitable as bridging treatment until blood is available. Availability and expense of this drug may limit its use for the treatment of NI in foals.

FOLLOW-UP

PATIENT MONITORING

• CBC, PCV, and lactate to monitor anemia. In acute cases, monitoring may be required every 4–8 hr. • Heart rate, arterial oxygen levels, and attitude are also useful for determining response to therapy. • BUN and creatinine concentrations to monitor pigment nephropathy. Perform daily until stable. • Serum glucose should be evaluated every 6 hr. Supplement if necessary.

PREVENTION/AVOIDANCE

• Identify broodmares that are negative for the Qa and/or Aa erythrocyte antigens by blood typing. These mares are at highest risk for developing alloantibodies to antigens on the sire's or foal's RBCs. • Identify sires that are positive for the Qa and Aa antigens by blood typing. This will help prevent broodmares from becoming sensitized to these two main offending antigens. • Determine the probability of NI in unintended or potentially incompatible matings. The mare's serum is collected 2 weeks prior to parturition and tested against known blood cell groups or against the sire's RBCs. The presence of hemolysis or agglutination suggests that NI will develop. • In high-risk cases, withhold colostrum from the foal derived from its dam. Transfer of passive immunity can be accomplished by foster feeding the foal provided that the maternal colostrum (from another mare or plasma) is devoid of antibodies that could result in NI. The foal should be foster fed for 2–3 days until gut closure occurs. • Perform a JFA test. Positive reactions at 1:16 or greater suggest incompatibility and the risk of NI.

POSSIBLE COMPLICATIONS

• Renal failure due to pigment nephropathy
• Cerebral hypoxia with neurologic sequelae
• Secondary septicemia

EXPECTED COURSE AND PROGNOSIS

• Peracute cases—Prognosis is poor due to the rapidity of onset and severity of disease. • Acute cases—Prognosis is good providing early recognition and diagnosis are established and appropriate therapy is instituted. • Subacute cases–Prognosis is excellent. Even without treatment, most foals are expected to survive.

MISCELLANEOUS

ASSOCIATED CONDITIONS

• Neonatal immune-mediated thrombocytopenia • Evan's syndrome

AGE-RELATED FACTORS

Affected foals are typically 2–3 days of age at the onset of clinical signs.

SYNONYMS

• Hemolysis of newborns • Jaundiced foal disease

ABBREVIATIONS

• JFA = jaundice foal agglutination test
• NI = neonatal isoerythrolysis
• PCV = packed cell volume • RBC = red blood cell

Suggested Reading

Boyle AG, Magdesian KG, Ruby RE. Neonatal isoerythrolysis in horse foals and a mule foal: 18 cases (1988–2003). J Am Vet Med Assoc 2005;227:1276–1283.

McClure JJ. Strategies for prevention of neonatal isoerythrolysis in horses and mules. Equine Vet Educ 1997;9:118–122.

Traub-Dargatz JL, McClure JJ, Koch C, Schlipf JW Jr Neonatal isoerythrolysis in mule foals. J Am Vet Med Assoc 1995;206:67–70.

Author Samuel D. A. Hurcombe
Consulting Editor Margaret C. Mudge

NERIUM OLEANDER (OLEANDER) TOXICOSIS

BASICS

OVERVIEW

• *Nerium oleander* (oleander) is an evergreen shrub (family Apocynaceae) with leathery, dark, gray-green, sharply pointed leaves 4–12 inches long with a prominent midrib and parallel secondary veins.
• Oleander is native to Asia but now is a common ornamental in the southern United States and other parts of the world. Oleander contains several cardiac glycosides and ingestion can cause severe cardiac abnormalities and sudden death. The plant remains toxic when dry.

SIGNALMENT

All animals are susceptible.

SIGNS

• Onset usually several hours after ingestion
• Anorexia
• Colic
• Diarrhea
• Cardiac arrhythmias
• Tremors
• Seizure-like activity
• Coma
• Death

CAUSES AND RISK FACTORS

• Cardiac glycosides including oleandrin, oleandroside, nerioside, digitoxigenin, and others.
• Cardiac glycosides inhibit Na^+/K^+-ATPase.
• Ingestion of 0.005% of plant by body weight may be lethal.

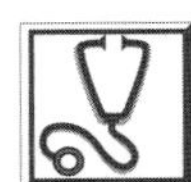

DIAGNOSIS

DIFFERENTIAL DIAGNOSIS

• *Taxus* (yew) toxicosis (evidence of consumption)
• Other cardiac glycoside-containing plants (evidence of consumption)
• Other causes of sudden death

CBC/BIOCHEMISTRY/URINALYSIS

N/A

OTHER LABORATORY TESTS

• Identification of oleander leaves in ingesta
• Chemical analysis of ingesta or serum for oleandrin

IMAGING

N/A

DIAGNOSTIC PROCEDURES

ECG disturbances are supportive—widening of the QRS wave, ST-segment depression, enlarged P waves, and a variety of ventricular arrhythmias.

PATHOLOGICAL FINDINGS

• Identification of oleander leaves in ingesta
• Often no lesions in peracute cases
• Endocardial hemorrhages
• Increased pericardial fluid
• Necrosis of subendocardium, most often involving the left ventricle
• Pulmonary edema or hepatic congestion may be present.

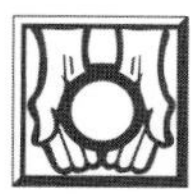

TREATMENT

- Keep animal quiet.
- Supportive care

MEDICATIONS

DRUGS

- Evaluate cardiac function (ECG) and treat appropriately.
- AC at 1–4 g/kg body weight PO as a water slurry

CONTRAINDICATIONS/POSSIBLE INTERACTIONS

N/A

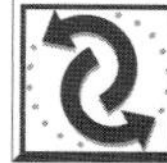

FOLLOW-UP

PATIENT MONITORING

ECG evaluation

PREVENTION/AVOIDANCE

Remove oleander from animal access.

POSSIBLE COMPLICATIONS

N/A

EXPECTED COURSE AND PROGNOSIS

N/A

MISCELLANEOUS

ASSOCIATED CONDITIONS, AGE-RELATED FACTORS, ZOONOTIC POTENTIAL, PREGNANCY

N/A

ABBREVIATIONS

- AC = activated charcoal
- ECG = electrocardiogram (graph)

Suggested Reading

Galey FD, Holstege DM, Plumlee KH, Tor E, Johnson B, Anderson ML, Blanchard PC, Brown F. Diagnosis of oleander poisoning in livestock. J Vet Diagn Invest 1996;8:358–364.

Author Larry J. Thompson
Consulting Editor Robert H. Poppenga

NEUTROPENIA

BASICS

DEFINITION

• Neutrophil count in peripheral blood less than the lower limit of the laboratory reference interval—usually <3000 cells/μL (<3 × 10^9 cells/L)
• Neutrophils are the predominant WBC in peripheral blood of horses—neutropenia is usually synonymous with leukopenia.
• Neutropenia is clinically important as it predisposes to infection.
• Acute or chronic
• May be accompanied by a left shift (≥10% of total blood neutrophil pool composed of immature cells) and toxic cytoplasmic changes—basophilia, vacuolation, toxic granulation, and Döhle bodies.

PATHOPHYSIOLOGY

• Granulopoiesis occurs continuously in the bone marrow to maintain appropriate numbers of neutrophils in blood and tissues.
• The transit time for granulopoiesis is ≈5.5 hr—however, times are shorter with increased demand.
• Granulopoiesis is stimulated by cytokines (IL-3, IL-6) and hemopoietic factors (GM-CSF and G-CSF) produced by monocytes, T cells, endothelial cells, and fibroblasts.
• Neutrophils in peripheral blood are distributed evenly between the CNP and cells adhered to the endothelium of small vessels (MNP)—it is the CNP that is sampled during blood collection.
• Circulating neutrophils have a half-life of ≈10.5 hr, after which they migrate to tissues and body cavities to undertake physiological functions.
• Once recruited to tissues, neutrophils survive for up to 4 days after which they undergo apoptosis and are phagocytosed by mononuclear cells or are lost from the body via mucosal surfaces.
• Neutropenia may result from defective or ineffective granulopoiesis, neutrophil shift from the CNP to the MNP, increased migration to tissues, or reduced survival of neutrophils.
• Increased margination and migration (usage) of neutrophils at a rate that exceeds the rate of production and release from the bone marrow are the most common cause of neutropenia in horses. It is often due to endotoxemia associated with GIT disease (e.g., strangulating lesion, acute colitis).
• Severe disease can rapidly exhaust the bone marrow pool of mature neutrophils and result in increased immature cells (bands +/− metamyelocytes +/− myelocytes) in the circulation—*left shift*.
• *Regenerative* left shift (immature cells < mature cells) is an appropriate response to tissue demand for neutrophils.
• When immature cells > mature cells, the left shift is *degenerative* indicating tissue use exceeds the capacity of the bone marrow production. This is a poor prognostic indicator.

SYSTEMS AFFECTED

• Hemic/lymphatic/immune
• Other system involvement is dependent on any underlying cause and development of secondary infections.

SIGNALMENT

Mean Age and Range

• Animals of any age can be affected.
• Neutropenia is common in foals with sepsis or dysmaturity.

SIGNS

General Comments

• Depend on the underlying disease
• Signs of localized or systemic infection may be present.

Historical

• A history of colic, diarrhea or metritis may be associated with endotoxemia.
• Lethargy, inappetence, pyrexia, weight loss, exercise intolerance may be associated with pancytopenia.
• Foals may be born prematurely or have FPT. Mares may have a history of metritis.

Physical Examination

• Signs of endotoxemia include congested or cyanotic mucous membranes, tachycardia, tachypea, pyrexia or hypothermia, bleeding diathesis or vessel thrombosis.
• Signs of infection
• Pyrexia
• Signs of pancytopenia may include mucous membrane pallor, petechial hemorrhages, epistaxis, mucosal bleeding, blood in feces, hematomas or prolonged bleeding from wounds.

CAUSES

Defective/Ineffective Granulopoiesis

• Rare
• Myelophthisis may involve leukoproliferative disorders, infiltrative neoplasia, myelofibrosis, myelodysplasia, bone marrow necrosis, granulomatous disease.
• Aplastic anemia may be due to toxins, drugs (e.g., estrogens, chloramphenicol, trimethoprim-sulfa drugs), chemicals, infections (e.g., EIA), radiation.
• Myeloid and megakaryocytic hypoplasia has been reported in related Standardbreds.
• Left shift is absent.

Redistribution from the CNP to the MNP

• Most common cause of neutropenia
• Usually associated with endotoxemia/SIRS caused by GIT disease (strangulating lesion, enteritis, colitis), peritonitis, metritis, or pleuropneumonia.
• Results from upregulation of adhesion molecules on neutrophils and endothelial cells +/− increased migration into tissues.
• Leukoembolization and sequestration of neutrophils in the microvasculature may occur in endotoxemia/SIRS.
• Total blood neutrophil pool may be unchanged.
• Left shift usually present

Increased Migration to Tissues

• Common
• Rate of tissue migration exceeds bone marrow production of neutrophils.
• Observed in bacterial diseases such as neonatal septicemia, devitalized GIT, colitis (salmonellosis, *Clostridium* spp., *Neorickettsia risticii*), acute pleuropneumonia, peritonitis, etc.
• May be observed in viral diseases including EIA, EHV-1, equine influenza
• Total blood neutrophil pool is reduced and left shift is usually present.

Reduced Survival of Neutrophils

• Increased migration of neutrophils to tissues with subsequent rapid destruction observed in bacterial infections (see above)
• Immune-mediated neutropenia due to presence of alloantibodies to neutrophils in neonates
• Viral infection in foals including EHV-1, EVA virus
• Total blood neutrophil pool is reduced and left shift is usually present.

RISK FACTORS

• Placentitis, umbilical infection, and FPT are risk factors for bacterial sepsis in foals.
• Induction of parturition is a risk factor for dysmaturity.
• Protracted administration of sulphadiazine-pyrimethamine drugs is a risk factor for folate deficiency and bone marrow suppression.

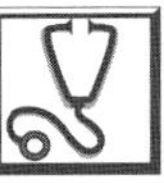

DIAGNOSIS

DIFFERENTIAL DIAGNOSIS

• Laboratory error may result from failure to mix blood sample properly before analysis.
• Sampling error may result from collection through an IV catheter used for fluid administration with dilution of blood sample.
• Leukocyte aggregration or entrapment in a partially clotted sample

CBC/BIOCHEMISTRY/URINALYSIS

• Neutropenia +/− left shift
• Toxic changes in the cytoplasm may be present.
• Additional hematological and blood biochemical changes are dependent on underlying condition.
• Anemia and thrombocytopenia may occur with EIA virus infection, aplastic anemia, myelophthisis, and EGE.
• Neutrophil cytoplasmic inclusions (morulae) may be observed in EGE.
• Lymphopenia may occur in EHV-1.

OTHER LABORATORY TESTS

• Serology for EIA, EHV-1, EVA, equine influenza, and *Anaplasma phagocytophilum* (EGE)
• PCR for EHV-1
• Tests of hemostasis and fibrinolysis if endotoxemia suspected
• Analysis of body fluids (peritoneal, pleural, pericardial, synovial, or CSF).
• Microbiological culture of body fluids or tissue samples
• Blood culture
• Quantification of blood immunoglobulin G for detection of FPT.
• Flow cytometry for detection of neutrophil surface-associated antibodies

IMAGING

- Abdominal, thoracic, and soft tissue ultrasonography for detection of effusion or space-occupying lesion
- Thoracic and skeletal radiography for detection of a space-occupying lesion

OTHER DIAGNOSTIC PROCEDURES

- Abdominocentesis, thoracocentesis, pericardiocentesis or CSF collection if indicated, followed by fluid analysis, cytology, and bacterial culture
- Bone marrow aspirate/biopsy to investigate unexplained neutropenia, pancytopenia, or abnormal circulating cells
- Fecal culture for *Salmonella* spp. and *Clostridium* spp.
- Fecal ELISA or PCR for *Clostridium difficile* toxins A and B and *Clostridium perfringens* enterotoxin
- Laparoscopy/thoracoscopy if space-occupying lesion suspected

PATHOLOGICAL FINDINGS

Depend on underlying cause and presence of any secondary infection

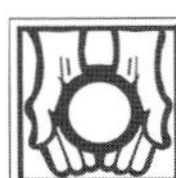

TREATMENT

AIMS OF TREATMENT

- Resolution of underlying condition and correction of neutropenia
- Resolution of any secondary infection
- Medical and/or surgical treatment may be required.

APPROPRIATE HEALTH CARE

- Inpatient medical management is usually ideal until the condition and neutropenia are stabilized.
- Some cases require surgical management either as an emergency (e.g., strangulating GIT lesion) or once the patient is stabilized (e.g., peritonitis).

NURSING CARE

- IV fluid therapy is required if fluid, electrolyte and acid-base deficits are present.
- Enteric or parenteral nutrition may be required for nutritional support.
- Peritonitis and pleuritis may require therapeutic paracentesis/drainage.
- Foals with sepsis and/or dysmaturity require aggressive supportive treatment, e.g., fluid, oxygen and nutritional therapy, postural support, and climate control.

ACTIVITY

Foals with sepsis/dysmaturity and horses with systemic disease require confinement.

CLIENT EDUCATION

Neutropenia is often associated with diseases with a guarded to poor prognosis, especially if a degenerative shift and toxic changes are present.

SURGICAL CONSIDERATIONS

Neutropenia increases the risk of postoperative infections, including surgical incisions and sites of IV catheterization.

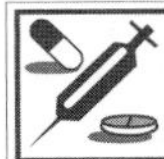

MEDICATIONS

DRUG(S) OF CHOICE

- Bacterial disease requires administration of appropriate antimicrobials based on culture and sensitivity testing.
- Several drugs can be used in the treatment of endotoxemia/SIRS including NSAIDs, hyperimmune plasma or serum, polymyxin B, pentoxifylline, heparin, free radical scavengers, and positive ionotropes.
- Corticosteroids are indicated if immune-mediated disease is diagnosed.
- Treatment for EGE includes oxytetracycline (7 mg/kg IV once daily for 5–7 days).

CONTRAINDICATIONS

Avoid use of corticosteroids if infection is suspected.

PRECAUTIONS

The use of NSAIDs, aminoglycosides, trimethoprim-sulfonamide drugs, and polymyxin B should be avoided until fluid deficits are corrected.

ALTERNATIVE DRUGS

- Poor response of confirmed bacterial infection to treatment may precipitate alteration of the antimicrobial regimen.
- Canine recombinant G-CSF has been used successfully to increase blood neutrophil count of foals. Expense may be limiting.

FOLLOW-UP

PATIENT MONITORING

- Clinical monitoring is important to document clinical improvement and response of the underlying condition to treatment.
- CBC once/twice daily until neutropenia stabilized and improving and then as required
- Leukocyte and neutrophil counts increasing to reference intervals and resolution of left shift and toxic changes are indicative of improvement.
- Rebound neutrophilia is common after recovery from neutropenia.

POSSIBLE COMPLICATIONS

Secondary infections (usually bacterial)

EXPECTED COURSE AND PROGNOSIS

- Depend on underlying condition and presence of secondary infections
- Endotoxemia/SIRS with evidence of failure of ≥1 organ is associated with a poor prognosis.
- Marked leukopenia and neutropenia in foals with sepsis increase the risk of mortality.
- In premature/dysmature foals, neutrophil: lymphocyte ratio has prognostic value—a ratio that remains <1.3:1 is associated with a high risk of mortality, while foals with a ratio that increases to >3:1 within 18 hr often survive.
- The prognosis of myeloproliferative disorders is hopeless.
- Presence of degenerative left shift and/or severe toxic changes denotes a poor prognosis.
- Improvement in the leukogram is often associated with a guarded to good prognosis.

MISCELLANEOUS

ASSOCIATED CONDITIONS

Secondary infections (usually bacterial)

AGE-RELATED FACTORS

- Foals with incomplete adrenal maturation (premature/dysmature) have leukopenia and neutropenia and neutrophil:lymphocyte is usually <1:1.
- After birth of normal foals, neutrophil count tends to decrease by 4 mo of age and may remain below adult values until 12 mo of age.

SEE ALSO

- Anemia, aplastic
- Colitis
- Equine granulocytic ehrlichiosis
- Myeloproliferative disorders
- Pancytopenia
- Salmonellosis
- Septicemia

ABBREVIATIONS

- CNP = circulating neutrophil pool
- EGE = equine granulocytic ehrlichiosis
- EHV1 = equine herpesvirus type 1
- EIA = equine infectious anemia
- EVA = equine viral arteritis
- FPT = failure of passive transfer
- G-CSF = granulocyte colony–stimulating factor
- GM-CSF = granulocyte-macrophage colony-stimulating factor
- IL-3 = interleukin 3
- IL-6 = interleukin 6
- MNP = marginated neutrophil pool
- SIRS = systemic inflammatory response syndrome

Suggested Reading

Davis EG, Rush B, Bain F, Clark-Price S, Wilkerson MJ. Neonatal neutropenia in an Arabian foal. Equine Vet J 2003;35:517–520.

Latimer KS. Diseases affecting leukocytes. In: Colahan PT, et al., eds. Equine Medicine and Surgery, ed 5. St Louis: Mosby, 1999:2025–2034.

Peek SF, et al. Prognostic value of clinicopathologic variables obtained at admission and effect of antiendotoxin plasma on survival in septic and critically ill foals. Vet Intern Med 2006;20:569–574.

Smith GS. Neutrophils. In: Feldman BF, et al., eds. Schalm's Veterinary Hematology, ed 5. Baltimore: Williams & Wilkins, 2000;281–296.

Welles EG. Clinical interpretation of equine leukograms. In: Feldman BF, et al., eds. Schalm's Veterinary Hematology, ed 5. Baltimore: Williams & Wilkins, 2000;405–410.

Author Kristopher Hughes

Consulting Editors Jennifer Hodgson and David Hodgson

NEUTROPHILIA

BASICS

DEFINITION

• Neutrophil count in peripheral blood greater than the upper limit of the laboratory reference interval—usually >6000 cells/μL (>6.0 × 10^9 cells/L) • May be caused by physiologic, pathological, or xenobiotic mechanisms
• Neutrophils are the predominant WBC in peripheral blood of horses—neutrophilia is usually synonymous with leukocytosis.
• Neutrophilic response to inflammation in horses is usually less marked compared to responses in dogs and cats. • Blood neutrophil count is dependent on the rate of supply from the bone marrow (rate of granulopoiesis and release from the marrow), distribution between the CNP and MNP pools and rate of efflux of neutrophils into tissues. • Neutrophils comprise a critical component of the innate immune system, forming the first line of cellular defense against pathogens. • Neutrophils can contribute to host tissue damage and morbidity if the underlying insult cannot be resolved.
• Neutrophil count does not provide evidence of functional capacity of the cells in blood or tissues. • A neutrophil count within the reference interval does not preclude the presence of inflammation. • The WBC count can be used to categorize neutrophilic leukocytosis as moderate (14,000–20,000 cells/μL [14.0–20.0 × 10^9 cells/L]), marked (20,000–30,000 cells/μL [20.0–30.0 × 10^9 cells/L]), or extreme (>30,000 cells/μL [>30.0 × 10^9 cells/L]).

PATHOPHYSIOLOGY

• Granulopoiesis occurs continuously in the bone marrow to maintain concentrations of neutrophils in blood and tissues.
• Granulopoiesis is stimulated by cytokines (IL-3, IL-6) and hemopoietic factors (GM-CSF and G-CSF) produced by monocytes, T cells, endothelial cells, and fibroblasts. • The transit time for granulopoiesis is ≈5.5 hr—however, times are shorter with increased demand.
• Neutrophils in peripheral blood are distributed evenly between the CNP and cells adhered to the endothelium of small vessels (MNP)—it is the CNP that is sampled during blood collection.
• Circulating neutrophils have a half-life of ≈10.5 hr, after which they migrate to tissues to undertake physiologic functions. • Once recruited to tissues, neutrophils survive for up to 4 days after which they undergo apoptosis and are phagocytosed by mononuclear cells or are lost from the body via mucosal surfaces.
• Neutrophilia results from ≥1 of the following—increased granulopoiesis and neutrophil release from the bone marrow, neutrophil movement from the MNP to the CNP, increased neutrophil intravascular survival, decreased neutrophil migration into tissues or leukemia. • Movement from the MNP to the CNP is due to corticosteroids or catecholamines.
• Increased release from the bone marrow is due to inflammatory demand, corticosteroids or leukemia. • During inflammation, mature (segmented) neutrophils are released from the bone marrow storage pool in response to inflammatory cytokines. • Inflammatory mediators promote neutrophil margination, adhesion to vascular endothelium and migration into tissues. • If demand is > bone marrow storage pool, a *left shift* occurs as immature neutrophils (predominantly bands) are released into the circulation. • Marked neutrophilia with a left shift that includes metamyelocytes and myelocytes indicates intense inflammation and is termed a *leukemoid response*. • Immature neutrophils, and those with toxic changes, have decreased functional capacity compared to mature neutrophils.

SYSTEMS AFFECTED

• Hemic/lymphatic/immune • Other involvement is dependent on any underlying cause.

SIGNS

General Comments

• Vary with the cause of the neutrophilia
• Clinical abnormalities may assist in determining which body system(s) is/are affected.

Historical

Inflammatory or myeloproliferative disorders may cause weight loss, inappetence, lethargy, and pyrexia.

Physical Examination

• Excitable mentation may be associated with physiologic neutrophilia. • Pyrexia is common with inflammatory and myeloproliferative disorders. • Signs of specific organ involvement may be present.

CAUSES

The causes of neutrophilia are physiologic changes including stress or corticosteroid-induced changes, tissue inflammation, myeloproliferative disorders, and administration of specific xenobiotics.

Physiologic Neutrophilia

• Fear, excitement and brief, strenuous exercise can result in a transient (usually 20–30 min) mature neutrophilia. • Neutrophils move from the MNP to the CNP due to decreased adhesion to the endothelium and increased flow through the microvasculature. • Because the MNP approximates the CNP, the measured neutrophil count can double. • Total blood neutrophil pool size, neutrophil release from the bone marrow and circulating half-life all remained unchanged.
• May be accompanied by lymphocytosis

Corticosteroid-Induced Neutrophilia

• Endogenous release of corticosteroids (stress response) or exogenous corticosteroids cause mild to moderate leukocytosis and neutrophilia.
• Characterized by neutrophilia without a left shift, lymphopenia, eosinopenia, and variable monocyte count. • Neutrophilia is caused mainly by increased release of mature neutrophils from the bone marrow resulting in an expanded total blood neutrophil pool. To a lesser extent, decreased tissue migration and increased movement from the MNP to the CNP contribute. • Stress response may contribute to the neutrophilia of inflammation. • Rarely, hypercortisolemia of PPID is associated with mature neutrophilia and hypersegmented neutrophils due to prolonged half-life in circulation.

Inflammation-Associated Neutrophilia

• Inflammation may occur in response to infectious agents, exogenous noninfectious antigens, tissue damage/necrosis, or immune-mediated responses.
• Inflammation can affect any body tissue or space—common conditions include abscess, pleuropneumonia, peritonitis, cyathastominosis, colitis, hepatopathy, traumatic wounds, and immune-mediated disease.
• Infectious agents include bacteria, viruses, fungi, and parasites.
• Tissue damage/necrosis can be a result of external forces or underlying disease.
• Immune-mediated causes include vasculitis, pemphigus, lupus erythematosis, and IMHA.
• Release of cytokines and granulopoietic factors result in neutrophilia of varying severity and maturity.
• The hallmark of inflammation is neutrophilia and left shift.
• Sustained neutrophilia occurs when the rate of neutrophil release from the bone marrow storage pool is > rate of emigration into the tissues—both total blood pool and CNP are increased.
• Left shift occurs when demand is > bone marrow storage pool of mature neutrophils.
• The size of a left shift depends on mature neutrophil numbers in the bone marrow, rate of neutrophil release from the bone marrow and rate of granulopoiesis.
• Generally the degree of the left shift indicates the severity of disease and has prognostic relevance.
• If immature count > mature count, the left shift is *degenerative* and prognosis is often guarded to poor.
• If immature count < mature count, the left shift is *regenerative* and prognosis is often better.
• Chronic or mild inflammation may be devoid of a left shift if increased granulopoiesis replenishes the bone marrow store and only mature neutrophils are released.

Myeloproliferative Diseases

• Granulocytic or myelomonocytic leukemia
• Acute leukemia has poorly differentiated cells/blasts in circulation.

Xenobiotic-Associated Neutrophilia

Administration of recombinant G-CSF causes marked leukocytosis and neutrophilia.

Other

• Hemolytic anemia—neutrophilia due to the release of free iron, endogenous corticosteroids, increased bone marrow neutrophil release, or immune-mediated disease
• Hemorrhage is associated with increased release of neutrophils from the bone marrow.
• Secretion of G-CSF and GM-CSF by malignant neoplastic cells is very rare.

RISK FACTORS

Depend on the underlying cause

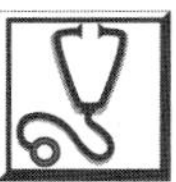

DIAGNOSIS

DIFFERENTIAL DIAGNOSIS

• Underlying cause of neutrophilia must be determined.

• If inflammatory, site and cause of inflammatory process must be determined.

CBC/BIOCHEMISTRY/URINALYSIS

• Neutrophil count > upper limit of laboratory reference interval (usually >6000 cells/μL [>6.0 × 10^9 cells/L]).
• A left shift denotes the presence of inflammation.
• A substantial left shift occurs when the band count is >300 cells/μL [>0.3 × 10^9 cells/L] and the neutrophil count is ≥ the reference interval.
• If neutropenia is present, a considerable left shift is present if the band count is ≥10% of total neutrophil count.
• Toxic changes in neutrophils indicate severe local/systemic infection, endotoxemia, or severe noninfectious inflammatory disorders.
• Toxic changes most commonly affect the cytoplasm—cytoplasmic basophilia, foamy vacuolation, toxic granulation, and Döele bodies.
• Döele bodies usually indicate serious infection.
• Resolution of toxic changes is a favorable prognostic finding.
• Nuclear toxic changes (karyolysis) are uncommon and are most commonly associated with endotoxemia.
• Sequential leukograms are important as neutrophil count and morphology can change substantially within hours.
• Trends for increasing, persistent or decreasing neutrophil counts and change in neutrophil morphology assist in establishing diagnosis and prognosis.
• Physiologic neutrophilia is mature in nature.
• Corticosteroids cause a mature neutrophilia, lymphopenia, and eosinopenia.
• Myeloproliferative disorders may result in circulating neutrophil blast cells. Blood counts of other WBC types, RBCs, and platelets may be reduced due to myelophthisis.
• Biochemical analysis for evidence of underlying organ involvement and/or dysfunction.

OTHER LABORATORY TESTS

• Coombs test for suspected IMHA
• Serology for viral, bacterial, or rickettsial agents
• Immunophenotypic techniques for classification of leukemia

IMAGING

• Ultrasonography of the thorax, abdomen, soft tissues for detection of space-occupying lesions, organomegaly, and effusions
• Radiography of the thorax or skeleton for detection of inflammatory or neoplastic lesions
• Scintigraphy using radiolabelled autologous neutrophils for detection of an occult abscess

OTHER DIAGNOSTIC PROCEDURES

• Abdominocentesis, thoracocentesis, and/or CSF collection with analysis of peritoneal fluid, pleural fluid, or CSF
• Microbiological culture of body fluids or tissue samples
• Bone marrow biopsy to detect myeloproliferative disorders
• Fine needle aspirate/biopsy of internal/external space-occupying lesion
• Endoscopy (airways, esophagus/stomach, bladder)
• Laparoscopy/thoracoscopy if abscess/tumor is suspected

PATHOLOGICAL FINDINGS

Depend on the underlying cause

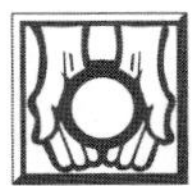

TREATMENT

AIMS OF TREATMENT

• Elimination of the underlying cause
• Varies with the nature of the underlying cause and may include elimination of infection, resolution of inflammation and correction of fluid, electrolyte, and acid-base derangements
• Medical and/or surgical treatment may be required.

APPROPRIATE HEALTH CARE

• Physiologic neutrophilia and stress neutrophilia do not require treatment.
• Mild forms of inflammation-associated neutrophilia can often be addressed by outpatient medical care.
• Inflammation-associated neutrophilia may require inpatient medical and/or surgical treatment and some forms (e.g., acute sepsis, IMHA) require emergency intensive care.

NURSING CARE

Depend on the underlying cause

ACTIVITY

Depend on the underlying cause

CLIENT EDUCATION

Neutrophilia often denotes the presence of an underlying disease that is the focus of diagnostic assessment and treatment.

SURGICAL CONSIDERATIONS

Depend on the underlying cause

MEDICATIONS

DRUG(S) OF CHOICE

• Bacterial or fungal infections require antimicrobial therapy based on culture and sensitivity testing.
• Parasitism requires the use of anthelmintics.
• NSAIDs to reduce inflammation
• Corticosteroids for treatment of immune-mediated disease

CONTRAINDICATIONS

Avoid corticosteroids in cases with infectious disease or laminitis.

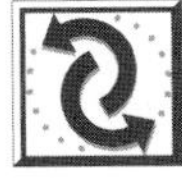

FOLLOW-UP

PATIENT MONITORING

Horses with inflammation-associated neutrophilia may require daily leukograms until stable.

POSSIBLE COMPLICATIONS

Neutropenia develops if rate of tissue migration is > rate of bone marrow production.

EXPECTED COURSE AND PROGNOSIS

• Depend on the underlying cause
• Prognosis for marked inflammation or severe tissue trauma is guarded.
• Prognosis for myeloproliferative disorders is hopeless.

MISCELLANEOUS

AGE-RELATED FACTORS

• In healthy foals up to 30 days of age, neutrophil counts may be >6000 cells/μL (>6.0 × 10^9 cells/L).
• Neutrophil:lymphocyte ratios of healthy foals decrease from >2.5:1 at birth to ≈1:1 at 30 days.

SEE ALSO

• Anemia, immune-mediated
• Myeloproliferative disorders
• Neutropenia

ABBREVIATIONS

• CNP = circulating neutrophil pool
• G-CSF = granulocyte colony-stimulating factor
• GM-CSF = granulocyte-macrophage colony-stimulating factor
• IL-3 = interleukin 3
• IL-6 = interleukin 6
• IMHA = immune-mediated hemolytic anemia
• MNP = marginated neutrophil pool
• PPID = pituitary pars intermedia dysfunction

Suggested Reading

Latimer KS. Diseases affecting leukocytes. In: Colahan PT, el al., eds. Equine Medicine and Surgery, 5th Ed. St Louis: Mosby, 1999;2025–2034.
Latimer KS, Rakich PM. Peripheral blood smears. In: Cowell RL, Tyler RD eds. Diagnostic Cytology and Hematology of the Horse, ed 2. St Louis: Mosby, 2002; 200–216.
Smith GS. Neutrophils. In: Feldman BF, et al., eds. Schalm's Veterinary Hematology, ed 5. Baltimore: Williams & Wilkins, 2000;281–296.
Welles EG. Clinical interpretation of equine leukograms. In: Feldman BF, et al., eds. Schalm's Veterinary Hematology, ed 5. Baltimore: Williams & Wilkins, 2000;405–410.
Zinkl JG, et al. Haematological, bone marrow and clinical chemical changes in neonatal foals given canine recombinant granulocyte-colony stimulating factor. Equine Vet J 1994;26:313–318.

Author Kristopher Hughes
Consulting Editors Jennifer Hodgson and David Hodgson

NITRATE/NITRITE TOXICOSIS

BASICS

OVERVIEW

- Nitrate intoxication is primarily a problem in ruminants because of their efficient reduction of nitrate to nitrite within the rumen.
- Monogastrics generally tolerate rather high concentrations of nitrate because it is not rapidly reduced to nitrite in the GI tract.
- Nitrite is approximately 3- and 10-fold more toxic than nitrate for ruminants and monogastrics, respectively.
- Nitrate is found in plants, water, fertilizers, and animal wastes.
- Horses are most likely to be intoxicated after exposure to high concentrations of nitrate or nitrite in fertilizers, but no cases of equine nitrate/nitrite intoxication have been published.
- Nitrite converts Fe^{2+} in hemoglobin to Fe^{3+}, forming methemoglobin, which cannot bind and transport oxygen. In turn, this leads to generalized tissue hypoxia.

SIGNALMENT

- No breed or sex predispositions
- Neonates may be more sensitive because of their more efficient reduction of nitrate to nitrite, but data are lacking.

SIGNS

- Polypnea
- Dyspnea
- Cyanotic or muddy mucous membranes
- Weakness
- Muscle tremors
- Reluctance to move
- Terminal convulsions
- Death

CAUSES AND RISK FACTORS

The most likely cause is acute exposure to a concentrated source of nitrate or nitrite (e.g., fertilizers or contaminated water source); a horse is unlikely to be exposed to sufficient nitrate from other sources to cause intoxication.

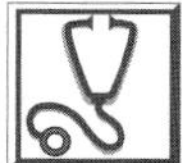

DIAGNOSIS

DIFFERENTIAL DIAGNOSIS

Other causes of methemoglobin formation such as *Acer rubrum* (red maple) toxicosis (clinical signs of icterus and anemia) or chlorate toxicosis (identified source of exposure to a chlorate salt, e. g., potassium or sodium chlorate).

CBC/BIOCHEMISTRY/URINALYSIS

- Methemoglobin imparts a brown discoloration to blood.
- All routinely measured parameters are normal.

OTHER LABORATORY TESTS

- Significant methemoglobinemia (>30%)
- High plasma, serum, or ocular fluid nitrate or nitrite concentrations—diagnostic concentrations have not been determined for horses.
- Measurement of high nitrate/nitrite in an environmental source has been associated with a suspected fertilizer spill.

IMAGING

N/A

DIAGNOSTIC PROCEDURES

N/A

PATHOLOGICAL FINDINGS

No specific post-mortem findings except for a dark red to brown discoloration of the blood and muscle as a result of methemoglobin pigmentation.

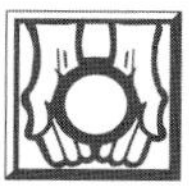

TREATMENT

Treat acidosis and ischemia-induced ECG changes.

MEDICATIONS

DRUGS

Reduce methemoglobin to hemoglobin.

- The standard treatment for methemoglobinemia is methylene blue, which is not believed to be efficacious in horses (although this conclusion is based on limited data).
- Ascorbic acid (30 mg/kg BID given in IV fluids) may be beneficial in reducing methemoglobin, but as with methylene blue, studies of clinical efficacy are lacking.

CONTRAINDICATIONS/POSSIBLE INTERACTIONS

N/A

FOLLOW-UP

PATIENT MONITORING

Monitor methemoglobin concentrations, acid–base status, and ECG.

PREVENTION/AVOIDANCE

N/A

POSSIBLE COMPLICATIONS

N/A

EXPECTED COURSE AND PROGNOSIS

Because methylene blue may not be efficacious; prognosis is guarded.

MISCELLANEOUS

ASSOCIATED CONDITIONS

N/A

AGE-RELATED FACTORS

More efficient reduction of nitrate to nitrite might occur in neonates.

ZOONOTIC POTENTIAL

N/A

PREGNANCY

Fetal hypoxia is a concern in pregnant animals.

SEE ALSO

Acer rubrum (Red Maple) Toxicosis

Suggested Reading

Osweiler GD, Carson TL, Buck WB, Van Gelder GA. Clinical and Diagnostic Veterinary Toxicology. 3rd ed. Dubuque: Kendall Hunt Publishing, 1985:460–467.

Author Robert H. Poppenga
Consulting Editor Robert H. Poppenga

NONULCERATIVE KERATOUVEITIS

BASICS

OVERVIEW

NKU is characterized by a paralimbal corneal stromal infiltrate combined with a pronounced anterior uveitis.

SYSTEM AFFECTED

Ophthalmic

SIGNALMENT

All ages and breeds of horses can be affected.

SIGNS

- Nonulcerated, fleshy, stromal infiltrate involving the limbus
- Uveitis presents with signs such as miosis, aqueous flare, corneal edema, and blepharospasm.

CAUSES AND RISK FACTORS

Immune mediated

DIAGNOSIS

DIFFERENTIAL DIAGNOSIS

- Stromal abscesses, onchocerciasis, keratomycosis, infiltrating limbal neoplasms, ERU
- While NKU generally improves with topical steroids, stromal abscesses tend to deteriorate.

CBC/BIOCHEMISTRY/URINALYSIS

N/A

OTHER LABORATORY TESTS

Rule out infectious causes (bacterial or fungal) with corneal scrapings for cytology, culture, and possibly biopsy.

IMAGING

N/A

DIAGNOSTIC PROCEDURES

N/A

PATHOLOGIC FINDINGS

Corneal epithelial thickening, dermal fibrosis, and mild to moderate suppurative cellular infiltrate are noted histologically. No evidence of stromal necrosis or infection.

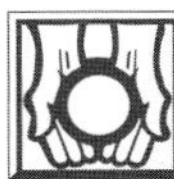

TREATMENT

- Beta-irradiation
- Enucleation due to the inability to control pain is often the result.

MEDICATIONS

DRUG(S) OF CHOICE

- Topical corticosteroids (1% prednisolone acetate or 0.1% dexamethasone 4–6 times daily), cyclosporin A BID, and mydriatics/cycloplegics (1% atropine daily to QID). Systemic nonsteroidal anti-inflammatory drugs (e.g., flunixin meglumine 0.25–1 mg/kg BID PO or phenylbutazone 1 mg BID PO or IV).
- Topical cyclosporine A (2%) has been beneficial in some eyes with NKU.

PRECAUTIONS

Horses receiving topically administered atropine should be monitored for signs of colic.

CONTRAINDICATIONS/POSSIBLE INTERACTIONS

N/A

FOLLOW-UP

EXPECTED COURSE AND PROGNOSIS

Persistent, painful uveitis results in enucleation.

MISCELLANEOUS

ASSOCIATED CONDITIONS

Severe iridocyclitis

SEE ALSO

- Corneal ulceration
- Corneal/scleral lacerations
- Corneal stromal abscesses
- Eosinophilic keratitis
- Burdock pappus bristle keratopathy
- Calcific band keratopathy
- Corneal stromal abscesses
- Glaucoma
- Recurrent uveitis

ABBREVIATIONS

- ERU = equine recurrent uveitis
- NKU = nonulcerative keratouveitis

Suggested Reading

Brooks DE. Ophthalmology for the Equine Practitioner. Jackson, WY; Teton NewMedia, 2002.

Brooks DE, Matthews AG. Equine ophthalmology. In: Gelatt KN, ed. Veterinary Ophthalmology, ed 4. Philadelphia; Lippincott Williams and Wilkins, 2007.

Gilger BC, ed. Equine Ophthalmology. Philadelphia; WB Saunders, 2005.

Authors Andras M. Komaromy and Dennis E. Brooks

Consulting Editor Dennis E. Brooks

NUTRITION IN FOALS

BASICS

DEFINITION

• Enteral nutrition is milk or feed consumed orally or administered through an NG feeding tube. • PN is an intravenous solution of dextrose, protein (amino acids), lipid emulsion, electrolytes, and multivitamins. Partial PN can consist of only dextrose and amino acids in a balanced electrolyte solution.

PATHOPHYSIOLOGY

• Neonatal foals have very little energy reserves and can become rapidly dehydrated and hypoglycemic if they are unable to nurse regularly. Sepsis, musculoskeletal abnormalities or injuries, and neurologic disease may prevent the foal from nursing regularly. Foals that are unable to nurse on their own, but that have functional GI tracts, may be fed orally or via an NG tube. • Foals with enterocolitis may not be able to tolerate a milk diet that is high in lactose. Foals with colic or ileus may also be unable to tolerate enteral feeding until the underlying cause of GI dysfunction has been treated. Severely debilitated foals may require PN until GI function can be better assessed.

SYSTEM AFFECTED

GI

GENETICS

N/A

INCIDENCE/PREVALENCE

N/A

GEOGRAPHIC DISTRIBUTION

N/A

SIGNALMENT

There are no significant breed or sex differences for nutritional requirements in foals. Most of the information about nutritional requirements in healthy foals has been collected from Thoroughbred populations.

SIGNS

General Comments

The following are findings associated with the need for supplemental nutrition:

Historical

• Decreased nursing • Weight loss or failure to gain weight • Agalactia in mare—Foal may make frequent, short attempts to nurse, and mare may become agitated by foal's attempts.
• Debilitation or feed restriction in the mare

Physical Examination

• Dehydration, weakeness/depression
• Angular limb or flexural limb deformity—difficulty rising or remaining in standing position for prolonged periods
• Dried milk on head—may indicate milk streaming from dam's udder when foal does not adequately nurse • Diarrhea, colic, or abdominal distention

CAUSES

Indications for Enteral Nutrition Supplementation

• Musculoskeletal abnormalities that limit activity—severe angular or flexural limb deformity • Neurologic dysfunction or dysphagia—PAS/HIE, botulism • Orphan foals

Indications for PN Supplementation

• Enterocolitis • Lactose intolerance, including rotavirus infection • Colic—GI obstruction, ileus, or intolerance of enteral feeding • GI dysfunction—secondary to sepsis, ischemic damage (PAS)

RISK FACTORS

• Perinatal hypoxic episodes may place the foal at risk of hypoxic GI injury or to neurologic dysfunction that prevents normal nursing behavior. • Septicemia—Foals should be monitored closely for signs of enterocolitis or poor GI perfusion.

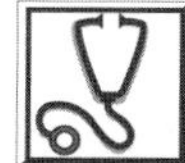

DIAGNOSIS

DIFFERENTIAL DIAGNOSIS

N/A

CBC/BIOCHEMISTRY/URINALYSIS

• Hypoglycemia (blood glucose <80 mg/dL) will occur quickly in neonates that have no access to the mare or are unable to nurse.
• Hemoconcentration (elevated packed cell volume) due to dehydration

OTHER LABORATORY TESTS

Low IgG (<800 mg/dL)—failure of transfer of passive immunity

IMAGING

N/A

OTHER DIAGNOSTIC PROCEDURES

Lactose tolerance test—Oral milk feedings with serial blood glucose measurements can help to identify foals with lactose intolerance.

PATHOLOGICAL FINDINGS

N/A

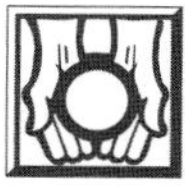

TREATMENT

AIMS OF TREATMENT

• Provide adequate nutrition for growth. Normal foals (<30 days of age) generally consume 20%–30% of their body weight in milk each day (≈135 kcal/kg/day). • GI rest for foals with malabsorption diarrhea, hypoxic GI injury, or GI obstruction or other dysfunction

APPROPRIATE HEALTH CARE

• Enteral nutrition via feeding tube, bottle, or bucket can be administered in a farm or hospital setting. Bottle feeding and NG tube feedings must be given frequently (every 1–2 hr) in the neonate; therefore, inpatient medical management may be more appropriate. The underlying disease (e.g., sepsis, PAS, musculoskeletal abnormality) may require more intensive management in a hospital setting. • PN should be administered as part of inpatient medical management.

NURSING CARE

Orphan Foal Options

• Nurse mare—may be expensive and limited in availability but can provide ideal nutrition and companionship for an orphan foal.
• Bottle feeding—Neonatal foals may accept a bottle readily, but this method of feeding is very labor intensive and can place the foal at risk of aspiration pneumonia (especially in debilitated foals). Syringe feeding should never be performed due to the risk of aspiration and inability to deliver adequate volumes. • Bucket feeding—Foal may be slower to accept this feeding method, but it is much less labor intensive than bottle feeding and reduces the risk of behavioral problems that can be associated with bottle feeding (excessive human contact). • Initial frequency of feeding is every 2 hr, although this can be increased to every 4 hr as the foal reliably consumes the milk or milk replacer. Acidified mare's milk replacer (see below) may be fed in larger quantities less frequently.

Enteral Feeding via NG Tube

• Pliable enteral feeding tubes (14 Fr) can remain in place and are well tolerated by foals.
• Placement should be confirmed by palpation, endoscopy, or radiography prior to feeding. • The tube should also be aspirated prior to feeding to check for gastric reflux.
• The foal should be fed in the standing or sternal position to reduce the risk of aspiration. • Feeding requirements for normal foals are 20%–30% of body weight in milk per day, but in sick foals, enteral feeding may begin at 5%–10% of body weight per day (supplemented with PN). • Frequency of feeding is every 1–2 hr, although a CRI may be used if bolus feedings are not well tolerated.

PN

• A jugular intravenous catheter should be placed in sterile fashion for administration of PN. Over-the-wire polyurethane catheters are preferred. • Although energy requirements in normal foals are approximately 120–140 kcal/kg/day, sick foals appear to require far less (30 kcal/kg/day of nonprotein energy).
• Parenteral feeding should begin at 25% of the target rate, increasing to the target rate within 24 hr. • When PN is discontinued (change to enteral nutrition), the foal should be "weaned off" over 12–24 hr in order to avoid hypoglycemia. • Supplemental intravenous fluids are needed to supply the balance of the maintenance requirements of the foal. • The mare should be milked every 2–4 hr while the foal is receiving PN so that lactation continues and the foal can be reintroduced to the mare.

Trophic Feeding

• Small enteral feedings (20 ml q2–6h) are recommended in foals on PN unless all enteral feeding is contraindicated (i.e., intestinal obstruction). • Trophic feedings are meant to assist with intestinal development and barrier function (reduce the risk of bacterial translocation).

ACTIVITY

• There are no specific restrictions for foals receiving nutritional supplementation. Foals receiving PN should be disconnected from the intravenous solution as infrequently as possible to avoid contamination and changes in blood glucose levels. • Orphan foals should get adequate exercise and socialization.

DIET

Enteral Nutrition Formulations

- Mare's milk—ideal nutrition if enteral feeding is tolerated. The mare can be milked, and this can be fed via NG tube or bottle if the foal is unable to nurse on its own.
- Milk substitutes
  - Mare's milk replacer—should mimic mare's milk as closely as possible. Mare's milk has approximately 25% crude protein, 17% crude fat, 11% total solids, and 0.5 kcal/mL digestible energy. Mare's Milk Plus (Buckeye Nutrition) is an acidified milk replacer that can be fed every 12 hr. Other milk replacers should be made fresh before each feeding (every 2–4 hr). Proper dilution of the milk replacer (according to manufacturer's instructions) is very important to help avoid diarrhea or constipation.
  - Cow's milk and goat's milk—higher in fat, protein, and total solids, but have been used effectively in foals
  - Lactose-free cow's milk—can be valuable in foals with lactose intolerance
- Solid feeds—Milk pellets can be introduced to the foal immediately as free choice feeding, although the majority of nutrition requirements will be provided by milk feedings initially. Small amounts of good-quality hay and 16% protein grain may also be introduced to the foal. By 8 weeks of age, the foal may be weaned off of milk replacer and onto solid feed.

PN Formulations

• Total energy and nutrition requirements are usually not met, but total PN consists of dextrose, amino acids, lipid emulsion, vitamins, and electrolytes. Partial PN may be provided as dextrose and amino acids.
• Dextrose—up to a 5% solution may initially be given alone, but this is not appropriate for long-term nutritional needs. Dextrose solutions should always be diluted to at least 10% as higher concentrations are irritating and hypertonic. • Amino acids—approximately 4–6 g per 100 kcal nonprotein should be added to the PN formulation. • Lipid emulsion—a 10% emulsion supplies 1 kcal/mL.

CLIENT EDUCATION

Owners should be instructed on proper introduction of bucket or bottle feeding and warned of the risks of behavioral problems in orphan foals that do not have proper socialization.

SURGICAL CONSIDERATIONS

N/A

MEDICATIONS

DRUG(S) OF CHOICE

• Insulin may be needed to treat hyperglycemia secondary to PN. Administer 0.1–0.5 IU/kg SC or IV, or alternatively a CRI of 0.01–0.02 IU/kg/hr. Preferable to decrease rate of glucose administration • Lactase tablets may be used in foals with lactose intolerance (e.g., rotavirus diarrhea)—for a 50-kg foal, 3000–6000 U PO with each feeding. Relatively ineffective treatment
• Domperidone (1.1 mg/kg PO q24h) can be administered to mares with suspected fescue toxicity or poor milk production in order to help stimulate lactation.

CONTRAINDICATIONS

N/A

PRECAUTIONS

Hypoglycemia can occur with the use of insulin. Use caution especially if administering a separate CRI of insulin (PN solution may stop while insulin continues to flow).

POSSIBLE INTERACTIONS

N/A

ALTERNATIVE DRUGS

N/A

FOLLOW-UP

PATIENT MONITORING

• Daily weight measurements—Foals should gain approximately 1.5 kg per day (<30 days of age). • Glucose measurements should be performed frequently (q2–4h) when PN is started in order to prevent hyperglycemia. Electrolytes should be monitored q24–48h unless there have been significant abnormalities (check more frequently). • NG tube placement should be confirmed prior to enteral feedings. • Sick or debilitated foals should be monitored for abdominal distention, colic, and NG reflux. Enteral feeding should be reduced or discontinued if these complications occur. • IV catheter should be monitored for signs of thrombophlebitis and other catheter site problems. The catheter should be removed if there are any concerns about thrombophlebitis.

PREVENTION/AVOIDANCE

N/A

POSSIBLE COMPLICATIONS

• Enteral nutrition—Aspiration can occur with bottle feeding but is also a risk with NG tube feeding in debilitated/recumbent foals. Transient diarrhea can occur when the foal is introduced to milk replacer. • PN—hyperglycemia, phlebitis, and hyperlipidemia. Complications occur more frequently in severely ill foals.

EXPECTED COURSE AND PROGNOSIS

• The goal of parenteral and supplemental enteral feeding is to act as a "bridge" until the foal can be reintroduced to nursing the mare.
• Foals with uncomplicated diarrhea often show improvement with 24 hr of parenteral feeding, although PN may need to be continued for 3–5 days as the underlying cause of the diarrhea is addressed and the foal regains the ability to digest lactose. Less commonly, foals may continue to require lactose-free milk even after the primary disease is resolved. • The foal should continue to have contact with the mare in order to facilitate reintroduction after a period of NG or parenteral feeding.

MISCELLANEOUS

ASSOCIATED CONDITIONS

• Diarrhea • Prematurity

AGE-RELATED FACTORS

Although solid feeds (grain and hay) can be introduced early, these should not make up the majority of the diet until the foal is at least 8 weeks of age.

ZOONOTIC POTENTIAL

N/A

PREGNANCY

N/A

SYNONYMS

Feeding

SEE ALSO

Diarrhea, neonatal

ABBREVIATIONS

- CRI = constant rate infusion
- GI = gastrointestinal
- HIE = hypoxic-ischemic encephalopathy
- NG = nasogastric
- PAS = perinatal asphyxia syndrome
- PN = parenteral nutrition

Suggested Reading

Buechner-Maxwell VA. Nutritional support for neonatal foals. Vet Clin North Am Equine Pract 2005;21:487–510.

Krause JB, McKenzie HC. Parenteral nutrition in foals: a retrospective study of 45 cases (2000–2004). Equine Vet J 2007;39:74–78.

Author Margaret C. Mudge
Consulting Editor Margaret C. Mudge

NUTRITIONAL SECONDARY HYPERPARATHYROIDISM (NHP)

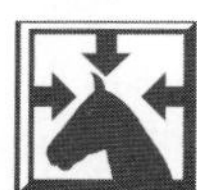

BASICS

OVERVIEW

• A skeletal disease that occurs in horses fed a ration with an excess of phosphorus or a deficiency in digestible calcium. Also called big head, bran disease, or miller's disease. • Three basic mechanisms may result in NHP. First, sustained consumption of diets containing excess phosphorus (e.g., wheat bran) that binds calcium in the gut, resulting in decreased calcium absorption. Second, diets high in cereal grain contain excess phosphorus but, more important, are calcium deficient. Third, oxalate crystals in certain plants combine with calcium in the gut and cannot be absorbed. • In all cases, decreased plasma ionic calcium stimulates PTH secretion and inhibits calcitonin secretion, leading to increased calcium and phosphorus mobilization from bone. • Over time, minerals mobilized from bone are replaced by a larger volume of fibrous connective tissue, leading to fibrous osteodystrophy and weakened bones.

SIGNALMENT

• Any breed and sex • Clinical signs are seen in foals to old, mature animals.

SIGNS

Historical

Intermittent or shifting lameness, enlarged jaws, loose teeth, difficult and painful mastication, weight loss, and weakness

Physical Examination

• Intermittent lameness usually is an early sign and may result from periosteal avulsion, tendon or ligament tear, articular pain, and fractures. • Swelling of the distal limbs • Constant shifting of weight at rest from one side to the other • Bilateral facial swelling resulting from maxillary and mandibular enlargement in advanced NHP • A stertorous sound can be heard on sinus percussion. Extreme deformation of nasal turbinates may impair nasal airflow and result in dyspnea. • Obstruction of the lacrimal duct results in epiphora. • Resorption of bone from the laminae durae may cause loose teeth and difficulty in chewing and weight loss.

CAUSES AND RISK FACTORS

• High phosphorus intake with a diet rich in grain byproducts—wheat bran • Rations with a calcium:phosphorus ratio <1:3 (e.g., high–cereal grain diet with grass hay) can cause the disease even with adequate calcium intake. However, the lower the calcium intake, the more severe is the disease. • Calcium combined with oxalate crystals contained in grass or leaves cannot be absorbed in the gut. Plants more commonly cited are setaria grass, buffel grass, and purple pigeon grass.

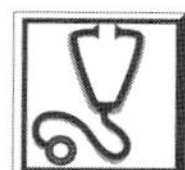

DIAGNOSIS

DIFFERENTIAL DIAGNOSIS

• The major differential diagnosis for fibrous osteodystrophy is primary hyperparathyroidism. In both cases, PTH secretion is increased. However, hypercalcemia is characteristic of primary hyperparathyroidism, whereas serum calcium may be normal or decreased in NHP.

• Chronic renal failure may result in renal secondary hyperparathyroidism in dogs and human beings. However, it has not been reported in horses.

CBC/BIOCHEMISTRY/URINALYSIS

• Serum calcium may be below or in the lower limits of the reference range. • Serum phosphorus may be within or above the reference range. • Increased urinary fractional excretion of phosphorus is characteristic of NHP (reference range, 0–0.5%). • Excretion of calcium is decreased, but accurate measurement is difficult because of the formation of calcium carbonate crystals in horse urine.

OTHER LABORATORY TESTS

• Analysis of dietary calcium and phosphorus is important to determine the cause and correct any imbalance. • Increased serum PTH is a sensitive indicator of NHP.

IMAGING

• Decreased bone density may be visualized radiographically. However, a minimum decrease of 30% is necessary for detection. • Loss of laminae durae usually is detected first and is particularly evident on a ventrodorsal view of the rostral end of the mandible. • Long bone cortical thinning and demineralization are only seen in long-lasting cases.

PATHOLOGICAL FINDINGS

• Bone minerals are replaced by fibrous tissue (osteodystrophia fibrosa), resulting in increased bone volume but decreased bone density. • Bone resorption is more pronounced in cancellous bone of the skull, ribs, and metaphyses of long bones. • Parathyroid gland hypertrophy and hyperplasia are evident in prolonged cases.

NUTRITIONAL SECONDARY HYPERPARATHYROIDISM (NHP)

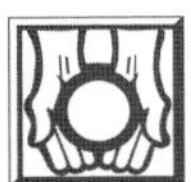

TREATMENT

ACTIVITY

Confine affected horses for several months, until radiographic evidence indicates bone density normalization.

DIET

• Total dietary calcium and phosphorus intake should be twice the horse's requirement with a calcium:phosphorus ratio between 1:1 and 3:1 for an initial 2- to 3-mo period. Afterward, feed the horse a normal ration that meets its calcium and phosphorus requirements. • Legume hay (e.g., alfalfa) is a good source of calcium.
• Mineral supplements (e.g., ground limestone) supply large amounts of digestible calcium (0.38 g calcium/g limestone). • Treat cases secondary to excess oxalate intake by removing oxalate-containing plants from the diet or by supplementing calcium and phosphorus. A weekly supplementation with 1 kg of a mixture containing 1 part ground limestone for every 2 parts dicalcium phosphate effectively prevents or treats clinical signs in horses grazing oxalate-rich pastures.

MEDICATIONS

Use NSAIDs with caution—Decreasing pain may result in increased physical activity and skeletal trauma.

FOLLOW-UP

PATIENT MONITORING

Radiography helps assess a return to normal bone density. If care is taken to match for age, gender, and activity, radiographs may be compared to those of nonaffected horses.

PREVENTION/AVOIDANCE

• Avoid large amounts of bran in the diet. • For horses fed large amounts of grain, supplement the diet with the amount of calcium required to ensure a calcium:phosphorus ratio >1:1.
• Either deny access to pastures containing oxalate-accumulating plants or supplement the diet with calcium and phosphorus.

POSSIBLE COMPLICATIONS

In advanced cases, horses may lose teeth or suffer skeletal trauma—fractures of long bones, compression fractures of vertebrae, and periosteal avulsions

EXPECTED COURSE AND PROGNOSIS

• In most cases, lameness disappears after 4–6 weeks on the corrected diet. However, some severely affected horses or long-lasting cases may never completely recover. • Lameness resolves before bone density actually returns to normal. Full recovery of bone strength may take as long as 9 mo to a year. • In most cases, enlarged skull bones remain deformed or show little regression after the diet is corrected.

MISCELLANEOUS

PREGNANCY

• Mares in the last 3 mo of pregnancy and early lactation are particularly susceptible because of their higher calcium requirements at these times.
• Mares may raise a healthy foal once their diet is corrected.

ABBREVIATION

• PTH = parathyroid hormone

Suggested Reading

Joyce JR, Pierce KR, Romane WM, Baker JM. Clinical study of nutritional secondary hyperparathyroidism in horses. JAVMA 1971;158:2033–2042.

Author Laurent Couëtil
Consulting Editor Michel Lévy

OCULAR/ADNEXAL SQUAMOUS CELL CARCINOMA

BASICS

DEFINITION

A malignant epithelial tumor of the equine eyelids, nictitans, conjunctiva, cornea, or corneal limbus that is locally invasive but typically slow to metastasize

PATHOPHYSIOLOGY

The etiopathogenesis is unknown. Suggested predisposing factors include solar radiation, reduced or absent periocular pigmentation, viral agents, and hormonal, genetic, and immunologic factors. The most plausible carcinogenic agent is the UV component of solar radiation, as it targets the tumor suppressor gene *p53,* which is altered in equine SCC. Malignant lesions are usually preceded by actinic keratosis, solar elastosis, and epithelial dysplasia.

SYSTEMS AFFECTED

• Ophthalmic—eyelids, nictitans, conjunctiva, cornea, limbus • Other systems or tissues may be affected by local extension and invasion or by metastasis. Any squamous epithelial cell in the body may undergo malignant transformation; however, those exposed to higher levels of UV radiation or those with minimal pigment are most susceptible.

GENETICS

• No proven genetic basis, but apparent breed predispositions suggest possible heritability, and affected horses have mutant forms of the tumor suppressor gene. • Reduced or absent periocular pigmentation inherited in certain breeds may predispose to ocular SCC.

INCIDENCE/PREVALENCE

• Most common is equine ocular/adnexal tumor
• The nictitating membrane and medial canthus are the most commonly affected sites, followed by the limbus and the eyelid. • One study has indicated that of all the horses presented for evaluation of ocular disease, 10% were afflicted with SCC.

GEOGRAPHIC DISTRIBUTION

A national survey of equine ocular/adnexal SCC revealed an increased prevalence with increase in longitude, altitude, or mean annual solar radiation.

SIGNALMENT

Species

Ocular/adnexal SCC is reported in horses, cats, cattle, dogs, and sheep. Any species, however, has the potential to develop this tumor under the right circumstances.

Breed Predilections

• An increased prevalence for SCC has been reported in Belgians, Clydesdales, and other draft horses, followed by Haflingers, Appaloosas, and Paints, with the lowest prevalence found in Arabians, Thoroughbreds, and Quarter Horses.
• White, gray-white, and palomino hair colors predispose to ocular/adnexal SCC, with less prevalence in bay, brown, and black hair coats.

Mean Age and Range

• Prevalence increases with age. • Mean age around 10 years

Predominant Sex

No proven sex predilection, although a recent study found geldings to be at higher risk.

SIGNS

Historical

• Horse may manifest excessive tearing or ocular discharge, squinting, redness or cloudiness of the cornea, or redness or ulceration of the eyelid margins or nictitans. • In advanced cases, raised, ulcerated, or proliferative masses, sometimes resembling granulation tissue, of the eyelids, nictitans, or the globe may be found.

Physical Examination

• Nonspecific findings may include serous to mucopurulent ocular discharge, blepharospasm, nictitans prolapse, and conjunctival hyperemia.
• Closer inspection may reveal red to white plaque-like, proliferative, or pedunculate lesions of the eyelids, nictitans, conjunctiva, or corneal limbus. These lesions may be ulcerated or nonulcerated, and there may be associated infection or hemorrhage. On the eyelids, alopecia and pyoderma may accompany SCC. On the cornea, SCC may be associated with corneal vascularization, cellular infiltration, edema, fibrosis, and occasionally ulceration. Corneal SCC is typically limited to the superficial cornea, though chronic SCC may invade intraocular structures. Chronic SCC of any periocular location may invade the deep tissues of the eyelids and orbit, including the bony orbit. Thorough palpation is essential to evaluate the extent of the lesion and typically requires topical anesthesia as well as an auriculopalpebral nerve block. Diagnostic imaging such as radiography, ultrasound, or computed tomography may be necessary to determine which and to what extent the periocular tissues are involved.

CAUSES

Unknown

RISK FACTORS

• UV radiation • Lack of periocular pigmentation • Possible genetic risk factors

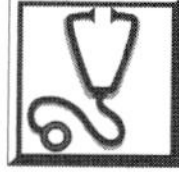

DIAGNOSIS

DIFFERENTIAL DIAGNOSIS

• Diagnosis is made on the basis of biopsy results; however, a characteristic clinical appearance is helpful in differentiating SCC from other periocular diseases. • Differentials include other tumors such as papilloma, sarcoid, schwannoma, adenoma, adenocarcinoma, angiosarcoma, mastocytoma, melanocytoma, plasmacytoma, fibroma, fibrosarcoma, lymphoma, and liposarcoma; parasites such as habronema, onchocerca, and thelazia; and inflammatory lesions such as abscesses, granulation tissue, and foreign body reactions.

CBC/BIOCHEMISTRY/URINALYSIS

Results usually normal

OTHER LABORATORY TESTS

Azostix placed over conjunctival, corneal, or nictitans lesions may reveal higher-than- normal tear protein levels and hemorrhage, possibly differentiating active lesions with leaky vessels from inactive scars.

IMAGING

• Skull radiographs may be required if orbital or bony involvement is suspected. • Thoracic radiographs are indicated if metastasis is suspected based on supporting clinical signs of systemic involvement and unthriftiness.
• Orbital ultrasound may also be helpful in determining extent of orbital invasion.

OTHER DIAGNOSTIC PROCEDURES

• Cytologic evaluation of cells obtained by aspiration or scraping followed by Giemsa or Wright's staining may reveal abnormal epithelial cells suggestive of SCC. • Aspiration of or histopathologic examination of biopsy specimens from the regional lymph nodes is often useful in determining presence of metastatic disease.

GROSS AND HISTOPATHOLOGIC FINDINGS

• The gross appearance varies from erosive to proliferative. Proliferative lesions range from small nodules to firm, sessile masses. The outer surface may demonstrate inflammation secondary to trauma or bacterial infection, and the mass may be covered by a purulent exudate. There may be secondary invasion by parasitic or fungal organisms. • Histologically, the tumor consists of nests or cords of epithelial cells with varying degrees of dermal infiltration. Mitotic figures are common, and intercellular bridges may be present. Well-differentiated tumors form epithelial "pearls" consisting of rings of cells with central areas of keratinization. Poorly differentiated tumors usually lack epithelial pearls but may exhibit individual cell dyskeratosis. Inflammatory cells and fibrosis may be present.

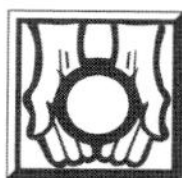

TREATMENT

INPATIENT VERSUS OUTPATIENT

• Very small, superficial lesions of the eyelids and nictitans may be removed standing with sedation and local anesthesia. Larger, more invasive lesions of the eyelids or nictitans, or lesions involving the conjunctiva or cornea, require hospitalization for surgery. • Alternatively, eyelid lesions may be treated under sedation and local anesthesia using intralesional chemotherapy.

ACTIVITY

Restrict during immediate postoperative period. The eye should be protected from self-trauma and secondary infection. A soft- or hard-cup hood can be applied.

CLIENT EDUCATION

• If postoperative medication is required, the client should wait at least 5 minutes between topical eye medications. • If intralesional chemotherapy is used, the client should be instructed to wear gloves when handling the periocular region for several days postinjection.
• The client should be made aware of clinical signs suggesting recurrence of SCC, tumor metastasis, or the development of new lesions on the fellow eye. • The client should also be made

aware of the possible role of UV radiation in the formation of ocular SCC, and appropriate steps should be taken to minimize exposure to solar radiation.

SURGICAL CONSIDERATIONS

• Tumors may be removed by surgical excision alone if adequate margins can be obtained. However, adjunctive therapy is often recommended to improve the chance for a complete cure, especially with large or invasive tumors. Adjunctive therapies include cryotherapy, irradiation, radiofrequency hyperthermia, CO_2 laser ablation, and intralesional chemotherapy. Additionally, reconstructive eyelid surgery may be required when eyelid margins are lost following tumor excision, and conjunctival or amniotic membrane grafts may be required following keratectomy to protect the surgical wound. • Cryosurgery with liquid nitrogen or nitrous oxide induces cryonecrosis of malignant cells when temperatures of −20° to −40° C are achieved using a double freeze-thaw technique. Radiotherapy with beta-irradiation (strontium 90) is most beneficial in superficial SCC of the cornea and limbus following superficial keratectomy, with reported success rates approaching 80%. Brachytherapy using cesium 137, radon 222, cobalt 60, or iridium 192 may be used following surgical debulking of invasive eyelid tumors. Interstitial radiation therapy has the advantage of providing continuous exposure of the tumor to high levels of radiation over a period of time. Small, superficial tumors may be treated with radiofrequency hyperthermia, killing malignant cells with local temperatures of 41° to 50° C following surgical excision. Excision of corneal limbal SCC followed by CO_2 laser ablation has also been advocated.

MEDICATIONS

DRUGS AND FLUIDS

Topical and Intralesional Immunotherapy/Chemotherapy

• Immunotherapy with bacillus Calmette-Guerin (BCG) cell wall extract has been used successfully for large periocular SCCs in horses. • Chemotherapy of invasive eyelid SCC with intralesional, slow-release cisplatin has also been used with very effective results, with and without surgical debulking. One-year relapse-free rates approach 90%. At least four sessions (and sometimes several more until tumor-free biopsy results are obtained) at 1- to 2-week intervals using 1 mg/cm^3 of tumor is necessary. Tumors up to 20 cm^3 may be treated using 3.3 mg/mL cisplatin (10 mg Platinol in 1 mL water and 2 mL purified medical-grade sesame oil). If this therapeutic modality is chosen, the owner must be committed to the entire course of therapy because if the injections are prematurely discontinued, the tumor that recurs often will be resistant to treatment thereafter. • Piroxicam (150 mg PO daily) can be beneficial in some ocular SCCs. The drug is begun once a day and then reduced to every other day. Therapy with piroxicam should be continued for at least several months. • Topical 5-FU (1% TID) or topical mitomycin C (0.02% QID) may be effective for corneal SCC in situ and may be beneficial for extensive periocular SCC.

Antibiotics

Topical and systemic antibiotics may be required to prevent infection following surgical and adjunctive therapy of ocular/adnexal SCC. A broad-spectrum ophthalmic antibiotic such as neomycin, polymyxin B, and bacitracin (Trioptic P) is an excellent choice for topical prophylactic therapy. Broad spectrum systemic antibiotics such as trimethoprim-sulfamethazone are used for more-invasive procedures of the eyelids or orbit.

Atropine

Atropine 1% ophthalmic ointment or solution (q8h to q24h) may be used to treat "reflex anterior uveitis" following keratectomy for corneal limbal SCC. It is used with sufficient frequency to affect mydriasis.

Analgesic/Anti-inflammatory Agents

NSAIDs may be indicated following surgical excision or intralesional chemotherapy. Flunixin meglumine (0.5–1 mg/kg q12h to q24h PO) can be used, depending on the degree of intraoperative trauma.

FOLLOW-UP

PATIENT MONITORING

Patients should be observed closely for recurrence of lesions, new lesions, and signs of metastasis. Long-term follow-up may be necessary as tumor recurrence has been reported months to years post-treatment.

PREVENTION/AVOIDANCE

Reduction of solar radiation exposure, through either avoidance of light (stalling during daytime, nighttime turnout) or use of protective headgear (fly masks), may reduce the incidence of recurrence or new tumor growth.

POSSIBLE COMPLICATIONS

• Tumor progression may lead to orbital involvement with subsequent exophthalmos, necessitating orbital exenteration. • Local invasion usually occurs in the orbit, guttural pouch, or nasal cavity, causing bony destruction. • Limbal SCC may invade intraocular structures with secondary glaucoma, retinal detachment, uveitis, and globe rupture, necessitating enucleation. • Chronic ulceration or tissue necrosis may lead to secondary bacterial or fungal infection and possible septicemia. • Metastasis occurs in 10%–15% of horses with SCC, with regional lymph nodes, parotid salivary glands, and thorax being the most frequently affected sites.

EXPECTED COURSE AND PROGNOSIS

• Prognosis is generally good provided treatment is early in the course of disease and owners are committed to long-term follow-up therapy and monitoring. • Factors affecting prognosis include tumor location, degree of invasiveness, presence or absence of metastasis, and the number of tumors present at the time of diagnosis. • The initial treatment modality does not appear to affect survival time. • Recurrence rates following therapy range from 25% to 42%. • Third eyelid tumors and eyelid tumors tend to spread and metastasize more frequently than does limbal SCC.

MISCELLANEOUS

ASSOCIATED CONDITIONS

Precancerous changes include actinic keratosis, solar elastosis, and epithelial dysplasia.

SEE ALSO

Periocular sarcoid

ABBREVIATIONS

• 5-FU = 5 fluorouracil • SCC = squamous cell carcinoma

Suggested Reading

Brooks DE. Ophthalmology for the Equine Practitioner. Jackson, WY; Teton NewMedia, 2002.

Brooks DE, Matthews AG. Equine ophthalmology. In: Gelatt KN, ed. Veterinary Ophthalmology, ed 4. Philadelphia; Lippincott Williams and Wilkins, 2007.

Gilger BC, ed. Equine Ophthalmology. Philadelphia; WB Saunders, 2005.

Author Caryn E. Plummer
Consulting Editor Dennis E. Brooks

OCULAR EXAMINATION

BASICS

OVERVIEW

• Obtaining a thorough history is important before performing the ophthalmic examination. If some form of visual disability is suspected, it is of value to know how the horse performs under different lighting conditions. An ophthalmic examination for pre-purchase is designed to detect any ophthalmic disease which may recur, or that is associated with decreased vision. The purpose for which the horse is to be used determines the emphasis placed on any ocular lesion seen. • The head is examined for symmetry, ocular discharge, and blepharospasm. The general appearance of the eyes and adnexa is noted. The size, movement and position of the globe in relation to the orbit should be assessed. • It can be useful to examine the angle of the eyelashes on the upper lid to the cornea of the two eyes, as droopiness of the lashes of the upper lid may well indicate blepharospasm, ptosis, enophthalmos, or exophthalmos. Normally, the eyelashes are almost perpendicular to the corneal surface. The first sign of a painful eye often is the eyelashes pointing downward. • The palpebral reflex is tested by touching the eyelids and observing for a blink response. • The menace response is tested by making a quick, threatening motion toward the eye to cause a blink response and/or a movement of the head. Care is taken not to create air currents toward the eye when performing this test. The menace reflex is a very crude indicator of vision potential. • The dazzle reflex consists of shining a bright light at the eye and watching for a quick blink reflex. This reflex is a very good indicator of retinal function and is very useful in evaluating vision potential in scarred or edematous corneas. • Vision could be further assessed with maze testing, with blinkers alternatively covering each eye. Maze tests should be done under both dim and light conditions. • The pupillary light reflex (direct and indirect) should also be tested. The normal equine pupil responds somewhat sluggishly and incompletely unless the stimulating light is particularly bright. • Intravenous sedation, a nose or ear twitch, and supraorbital sensory and auriculopalpebral motor nerve blocks may be necessary to facilitate the rest of the examination. • The margins, outer and inner surfaces of the upper and lower eyelids, should be examined with the light source, as well as the position and the outer surface of the third eyelid. • The cornea should be clear, smooth and shiny. Schirmer tear tests can be used if the cornea is dry in appearance. The normal Schirmer tear test values in horses is 22 +/− 6 mm wetting per minute. • Cultures and cytology of the cornea also aid the diagnosis of eye problems in horses. • In most horses, there is an obvious gray line at the medial and lateral limbus, which represents the insertion of the pectinate ligaments into the posterior cornea. This pectinate ligament area should have open spaces between the linear ligaments indicating the potential for aqueous outflow. This area will be more solid in eyes with glaucoma. • Placing fluorescein dye in the eye to identify corneal ulcers should be routine in every eye examination of the horse. Small corneal ulcers will stain that might otherwise be undetected. • Rose Bengal dye should be used immediately following fluorescein dye instillation to evaluate the integrity of the tear film. • To determine the patency of the nasolacrimal system it is best to use irrigation, which is most easily accomplished from the nasal orifice, although fluorescein dye penetration through the nasolacrimal system may also indicate patency. • The anterior chamber is filled with aqueous humor and should be optically clear, and is best examined with a slitlamp. Any discoloration of the cornea or sign of aqueous flare should be cause for concern. • The IOP is measured with applanation tonometry and is 17 to 28 mm Hg with a Tonopen applanation tonometer. • Persistent pupillary membrane remnants are common and are of no significance unless they span the pupil or attach to lens and cornea. The pupillary margin should be examined for any posterior synechiae (adhesions) as a consequence of uveitis. • Pupillary dilatation is necessary in order to examine the whole lens in detail. • A mydriatic should be applied to the eye once the pupillary light response has been evaluated. The agent of choice is topical 1% tropicamide, which takes some 15–20 minutes to produce mydriasis in normal horses and has an action that persists for approximately 4–6 hours. The lens should be checked for position and any opacities or cataract. • To be able to perform a proper ophthalmic examination, it is necessary to have a good focal light source, such as a transilluminator and a direct ophthalmoscope. Magnification with the direct ophthalmoscope is ×79 lateral and ×84 axial, in horses, and with the indirect ophthalmoscope and a 20-D lens, it is ×0.79 lateral and ×0.84 axial. • There are a number of lens opacities that may be regarded as normal variations: prominent lens sutures, the point of attachment of the hyaloid vessel (Mittendorf's dot), refractive concentric rings, fine "dustlike" opacities, and sparse "vacuoles" within the lens substance. Normal aging of the horse lens will result in cloudiness of the lens nucleus beginning at 7–8 years of age, but this is not a true cataract. The suture lines and the lens capsule may also become slightly opaque as a normal feature of aging. • Cataracts are always important. They can be secondary to previous uveitis, congenital, progressive or nonprogressive. In some horses, they may rarely be hereditary. • The adult vitreous should be free of obvious opacities. Vitreal floaters can develop with age or be a sequela to ERU. They are generally benign in nature. • The fundus should be examined for any signs of ERU, such as peripapillary depigmentation. The nontapetal region ventral to the optic disc should be carefully examined with a direct ophthalmoscope as this is the area where focal retinal scars are seen. Retinal detachments may be congenital, traumatic, or secondary to ERU and are serious faults due to their association with complete or partial vision loss. • Optic nerve atrophy can be related to ERU, glaucoma, or trauma and is associated with blindness. • Proliferative lesions of the optic nerve may be noted in older horses but are generally not sight or life threatening.

ORGAN SYSTEM

Ophthalmic

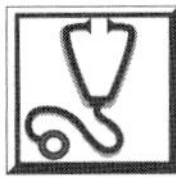

DIAGNOSIS

IMAGING

ERG, ultrasound (B-scan)

DIAGNOSTIC PROCEDURES

• Culture • Schirmer tear test • Cytology • Tonometry

MEDICATIONS

DRUG(S) OF CHOICE

• Tropicamide 1% for mydriasis • Topical local anesthetic for cytology

MISCELLANEOUS

SEE ALSO

All other ocular topics

ABBREVIATIONS

• ERG = electroretinogram • ERU = recurrent uveitis • IOP = intraocular pressure

Suggested Reading

Brooks DE. Ophthalmology for the Equine Practitioner. Jackson, WY; Teton NewMedia, 2002.

Brooks DE, Matthews AG. Equine ophthalmology. In: Gelatt KN, ed. Veterinary Ophthalmology, ed 4. Philadelphia; Lippincott Williams and Wilkins, 2007.

Gilger BC, ed. Equine Ophthalmology. Philadelphia; WB Saunders, 2005.

Authors Maria Källberg and Dennis E. Brooks
Consulting Editor Dennis E. Brooks

OCULAR PROBLEMS IN THE NEONATE

BASICS

OVERVIEW

• The equine neonatal eye has many features of immaturity that over time resolve to yield a healthy adult eye. Despite normal embryogenesis and a fully developed adnexa and globe, a newborn foal may exhibit lagophthalmos, low tear secretion, a round pupil, reduced corneal sensitivity, lack of a menace reflex for up to 2 weeks, hyaloid artery remnants possibly containing blood for hours after birth, prominent lens Y sutures, and a round optic disc with smooth margins. • Tapetal color is related to coat color and is usually blue-green but may be partially red, orange, or blue. Color dilute foals have a red fundic reflection from lack of a tapetum and consequential exposure of choroidal vessels.

DEFINITION

Knowing the accepted presentation of the neonatal ophthalmic system as previously mentioned, any further evidence of ocular pathology either from abnormal embryogenesis or progression of ocular and periocular inflammation from any cause may define a true neonatal ophthalmic disorder.

PATHOPHYSIOLOGY

• Congenital, inherited, and acquired diseases have been identified. • These problems may be inactive or dynamic and may or may not have a significant impact on vision.

SYSTEMS AFFECTED

• Ophthalmic • Central nervous system • Skin

GENETICS

• Belgian and Thoroughbred horses can get cataracts with a dominant mode of inheritance.
• CSNB of Appaloosas and Quarter Horses is inherited through a recessive or sex-linked recessive mode of transmission with the defect on the X chromosome.

INCIDENCE/PREVALENCE

Esotropia (crossed eyes) in mules has an incidence of 0.5%.

SIGNALMENT

Equine species

BREED PREDILECTIONS

• Congenital and dorsomedial strabismus and CSNB are reported in Appaloosas. • Limbal dermoids have been noted with iridal hypoplasia and cataracts in Quarter Horses.
• Heterochromia iridis, or dual coloration of the iris (usually blue and brown), is common to the Appaloosa, palomino, chestnut, gray, spotted, and white horses and is not considered a true pathologic condition. • Aniridia, or the complete absence of the iris, is reported in Quarter Horses and Belgians and is also seen with congenital cataracts in Thoroughbreds. • Morgan horses have nonprogressive, nuclear, bilaterally symmetrical cataracts that do not seriously interfere with vision. • Superficial, irregular corneal epithelial opacities may be found in one or both eyes in Thoroughbred foals. These do not appear painful and resolve with age.
• Goniodysgenesis and neonatal glaucoma have no breed predilection in the horse.

SIGNS

• Because there are numerous disease processes—each with a specific set of signs—emphasis is placed on the serious (vision-threatening) and treatable problems of the neonate eye, namely, ulcerative keratopathies and iridocyclitis. • A variety of congenital/inherited and acquired disorders are briefly mentioned.

Historical

• In many instances, the newborn may be suffering from more serious, life-threatening problems and in addition develops traumatic or progressive inflammatory ocular or periocular disease. • In other circumstances, the neonate may not be adjusting well to the new environment, gazing off into space with little physical activity, or may be easily startled and running into things with reluctance to move. Neonatal maladjustment syndrome should be a consideration. • On occasion, the owner or trainer may notice an abnormal appearance to one or both eyes without any visual or behavioral problems.

Physical Examination

• Note it is sometimes helpful to sedate a fractious foal for examination with diazepam (Valium 5–10mg IV in a 50-kg foal) and to have a few people present to handle the mare and assist with restraining the foal. • Both eyes should be compared for symmetry. Any nystagmus or strabismus should be noted. The menace reflex is unreliable in neonates, but pupillary light responses should be recorded.
• Any painful eye needs a thorough examination of the eyelids, the nictitans, the conjunctiva, the cornea, and the anterior chamber. Upper cilia (eyelashes) tend to point downward in a painful eye. Epiphora, blepharospasm, and photophobia may indicate trauma, a foreign body, and possible ocular inflammation and infection.
• On rare occasions, serious keratitis and blepharitis are noted without any signs of ocular pain. • Iris prolapse with or without panophthalmitis has a poor prognosis and is seen in acute severe trauma or aggressive infection.
• Congenital and developmental abnormalities have a myriad of clinical features that may or may not affect vision. Each disorder will be listed with its possible etiologies.

CAUSES

- Corneal ulcers*
  - Fungal or bacterial keratitis, *Pseudomonas, Streptococcus*, *Aspergillus*
  - Entropion
  - Lagophthalmos
  - Deficient palpebral reflex
  - Sicca
  - Distichia or ectopic cilia (rare)
- Iridocyclitis*
  - Ulcerative keratitis
  - Sepsis, from immune-mediated causes or from *Rhodococcus equi, Escherichia coli, Streptococcus equi*, *Actinobacillus equuli*, adenovirus, and EVA
- Conjunctivitis and subconjunctival hemorrhage*
  - Environmental irritants
  - Secondary to pneumonia caused by adenovirus, EHV-1, EVA, influenza virus, *Streptococcus equi* subspecies *equi*, *Rhodococcus equi*, and *Actinobacillus* spp.
  - Trauma
  - Neonatal maladjustment syndrome
- Glaucoma*
  - Goniodysgenesis
  - Trauma
- Microphthalmos
  - Congenital
- Strabismus
  - Congenital
  - Post trauma
- Blepharitis*
  - Fly strike
  - Dermatophytosis
  - Dermatophilus
  - Staphylococcal folliculitis
  - Trauma
- Entropion*
  - Microphthalmia
  - Dehydration
  - Malnutrition
  - Prematurity/dysmaturity
  - Eyelid trauma
  - Cicatrices
- Dermoids
  - Congenital
- Nasolacrimal system atresia
  - Congenital
- Dacryocystitis*
  - Systemic illness
  - Nasolacrimal system atresia
- Heterochromia iridis
  - Congenital
- Aniridia, iridal hypoplasia, enlarged corpora nigra, iridal colobomata
  - Congenital
- Persistent pupillary membranes
  - Congenital
- Lens luxation
  - Congenital
  - Post trauma
- Cataracts
  - Congenital
  - Uveitis
  - Penetrating trauma/lens rupture or perforation
- Retinal dysplasia
  - In utero inflammation
- Retinal detachments
  - Congenital
  - Inflammatory
  - Traumatic
- Chorioretinitis
  - Possibly maternal systemic disease late in gestation
- Optic nerve head colobomas
  - Congenital
- Optic nerve hypoplasia and optic nerve atrophy
  - Developmental
  - Inflammation in utero

RISK FACTORS

• "Downer" foals are more prone to develop entropion, blepharitis, conjunctivitis, and infected or persistent corneal ulcers. • Risk factors in these neonates include malnourishment, sepsis, contact with soiled shavings, and invariable pressure and friction placed on the eyes and eyelids from chronic recumbency. • Protection of the eyes in these neonates (padding, eye lubricant) is critical if secondary ophthalmic disorders are to be avoided.

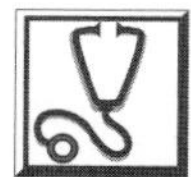

DIAGNOSIS

DIFFERENTIAL DIAGNOSES

• It is important to distinguish active disease requiring treatment (*most of the causes previously marked with an asterisk) from inactive problems that do not need intervention. • Consulting with a veterinary ophthalmologist is helpful to identify treatable eye diseases in a neonate. • Careful ophthalmic examination is the most important way to localize disease in an eye and decide on the appropriate diagnostic tests and treatment.

CBC/BIOCHEMISTRY/URINALYSIS

Usually normal in pure primary eye disorders

OTHER LABORATORY TESTS

Cytology and microbial (bacterial and fungal) culture of infected tissue, especially melting corneas, cellular aqueous humor, or purulent ocular or nasolacrimal discharge

IMAGING

Radiographs or dacryocystorhinography is helpful to identify nasolacrimal system atresia.

DIAGNOSTIC PROCEDURES

• Sterile corneal scrapings from the edge and base of the ulcer for culture and cytology, Schirmer's tear test, and fluorescein stain are indicated in painful eyes with suspect ulceration. Topical anesthesia should be applied before deep scrapings are attempted. • Aqueocentesis may identify pathogens in cases of severe idiopathic anterior uveitis. • A complete ophthalmic examination includes measuring intraocular pressure with applantation tonometry, slit lamp biomicroscopy, pupil dilation, and a funduscopic examination. Many suspected congenital abnormalities are confirmed by these special tests. • Diagnostic tests for all cataract surgery candidates include ocular ultrasound and electroretinography.

PATHOLOGIC FINDINGS

• Findings will be consistent with the disease process. Infections will yield a suppurative inflammation with or without large numbers of organisms. Enucleated eyes that were blind and painful with hypopyon may show panophthalmitis with or without bacterial sepsis.

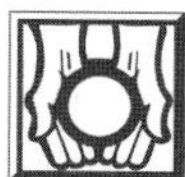

TREATMENT

APPROPRIATE HEALTH CARE

• Severe ulcerative keratitis and uveitis need aggressive therapy to preserve vision and eliminate pain. Initially hourly or bihourly instillation of medication is required to halt a melting ulcer and prevent corneal perforation. These eyes need to be examined several times daily until the clinical signs improve. Hospitalization of the foal and the mare is sometimes indicated to administer the frequent medication and enable examination by the veterinarian several times each day. • Usually the patient can be managed at home when medications are given 4 times daily or less often. Some farms or stables have round-the-clock staff that can give the medications in a less stressful environment. • Deep ulcers need to be watched very closely; they may progress to descemetoceles and perforate in a matter or hours. • Glaucoma must be managed on a day-to-day basis until the disease is under control. • Most other types of neonatal problems, if they need medical therapy, can be managed on an outpatient basis.

NURSING CARE

• A "downer" foal with eye disease not only needs correct medical management but also may benefit from a protective eye hood or plenty of padding and supplemental lubrication in the form of artificial tear ophthalmic ointment applied on the eye 2–6 times daily depending on other topical medication. • All foals in intensive care should be monitored daily for corneal ulceration.

ACTIVITY

In general, activity is restricted until the eye lesions are healed.

DIET

Good nutrition is essential for the neonate to have enough energy not only for growth but also for wound healing and recuperation.

CLIENT EDUCATION

• Some diseases threaten vision more than others. Severe inflammatory disease without therapy often results in a phthisical or septic eye that may have to be removed. Hospitalization for a period of time may be necessary to initiate aggressive therapy. Treatment can be over days to weeks for the most severe inflammatory conditions, and surgery may be necessary to preserve vision in the cases of deep ulcerations and uncontrolled glaucoma. • Neonatal anesthesia is a high-risk event and must be weighed heavily against the benefits of surgery, especially if the newborn is debilitated in any way. • Often a full workup including CBC determination of serum IgG concentration and chest radiographs is standard even for elective procedures such as cataract removal. • Genetic information listed earlier should be shared with clients as necessary.

SURGICAL CONSIDERATIONS

• Surgery under general anesthesia in the neonate is risky and should be done only if the owner concedes to the dangers involved and understands the potential consequences of the whole procedure. • Conjunctival grafting is a common surgery to aid in the healing of deep corneal ulcers and descemetoceles.
• Magnification and proper ophthalmic instrumentation are essential to a successful surgical outcome. • Corneal scarring is a sequela to surgery but may diminish as the foal matures.
• Entropion in the neonate is corrected by placing a temporary suture perpendicular to the eyelid margin in the affected areas (2–3 mm from the edge of the eyelid) in a vertical mattress pattern. These sutures remain in until the cause of the entropion is gone. Hotz-Celsus procedures should NOT be done on neonatal eyelids: the foal usually outgrows neonatal entropion but may need temporary tacking in the meantime.
• Cataract surgery is performed in foals as young as 1 week of age if no other ocular pathology (e.g., retinal detachment or degeneration) is discovered during the diagnostic workup. A veterinary ophthalmologist does this procedure with phacofragmentation. • Glaucoma can be surgically treated with valve implants or laser surgery when medical therapy does not control the progression of the disease. This procedure is reserved for the veterinary ophthalmologist.
• Eyelid trauma needs to be corrected with maximal preservation of eyelid tissue. Adequate flushing with a 1:50 povidone-iodine solution followed by a two-layer closure of skin-orbicularis muscle and tarsal-conjunctival layers is recommended. Systemic antibiotics are administered. • Keratectomy or blepharoplasty is indicated in the diagnosis of dermoids.

• Restoration of atretic nasal or palpebral puncta is done by flushing and cannulating the duct through one opening, and after creating a new opening at the other end, leaving the polyethylene tubing or silicone in the entire duct for several weeks to allow epithelialization of the new puncta and resolution of any dacryocystitis. • Anterior lens luxation requires lens removal by a veterinary ophthalmologist to prevent secondary glaucoma. Posterior lens luxation does not necessitate surgical intervention. • Persistent corneal ulcers in foals may need repeated debridement with topical anesthesia and a dry cotton swab every 3–4 days in addition to medical therapy. If that is unsuccessful, a grid keratotomy can be carefully made over the ulcer bed with topical anesthesia and a sterile 20-gauge needle at a very shallow angle dragged across the ulcer in a grid of linear patterns.

MEDICATIONS

DRUG(S) OF CHOICE

• Drugs for ulcerative keratitis and iridocyclitis have been thoroughly outlined in the other sections of this book under the topics of uveitis and corneal ulceration. Please refer to these pages for preferred drugs used in these diseases. • Medical management of glaucoma is discussed in the section on equine glaucoma. • Anti–gastric ulcer medications should be given to all hospitalized foals, especially if they are on systemic NSAIDs for iridocyclytis. • In foals, subconjunctival injections of medications and subpalpebral and nasolacrimal lavage systems effectively deliver drugs to the eye without frequent manual manipulation of the eye.

CONTRAINDICATIONS

Topical steroids must *not* be used on eyes with ulcerative keratitis.

PRECAUTIONS

• Foals on topical atropine should be carefully watched for signs of colic. Persistent dilation of the contralateral pupil indicates systemic absorption of the atropine. When this is observed, the atropine should be discontinued or given less frequently until the contralateral pupil function returns to normal. • Topical ophthalmic gentamicin (Gentocin) may retard corneal epithelialization. • Topical ophthalmic medications are not intended for subconjunctival injection and will cause a severe inflammatory response if they are injected under the conjunctiva. • Using topical steroids to reduce scarring on a cornea with prior fungal or bacterial ulcerative keratitis is dangerous and may cause a relapse of the infection.

POSSIBLE INTERACTIONS

N/A

ALTERNATE DRUGS

N/A

FOLLOW-UP

PATIENT MONITORING

• Not necessary for inactive ophthalmic disorders • Rechecks are advised for most inflammatory disorders until the eye shows no sign of active disease. If recurrence of infection or inflammation is apparent, a thorough workup is recommended to document relapse of microbial infection or other inflammation.A new or nosocomial infection may also be possible. • Other reasons for recurrence of the problem may also be failure to correct the underlying cause (e.g., entropion-induced ulcers).

PREVENTION/AVOIDANCE

• A clean, well-ventilated stall where the neonate can nurse and move about readily will help prevent any infectious or traumatic ocular problems. • Some congenital lesions such as retinal dysplasia may be less likely if the mare maintains good health during pregnancy.

POSSIBLE COMPLICATIONS

• Any ocular anomaly or disease can impair vision, even if it has been successfully treated. • Modifications to activity and the environment of the neonate may be necessary when eye disorders are diagnosed.

EXPECTED COURSE AND PROGNOSIS

• With accurate diagnosis and timely treatment, most vision-threatening problems in the neonate can be successfully managed. • Aphakic (meaning "without a lens") foals who had cataracts removed will adjust to their environment but will remain permanently hyperopic (farsighted). • Even with complete recovery from an inflammatory disease in the eye, the owner needs to be observant for and report any recurrence of ocular pain. The veterinarian should do a brief ophthalmic examination during routine check-ups to assess the eye's health. • When the vision cannot be saved in a neonatal eye, ocular comfort becomes the long-term goal of therapy.

MISCELLANEOUS

ASSOCIATED CONDITIONS

• Sepsis • Pneumonia

AGE-RELATED FACTORS

N/A

SYNONYMS

• Anterior uveitis = iridocyclitis

SEE ALSO

• Orbital disease • Eyelid diseases • Glaucoma • Ulcerative keratomycosis • Recurrent uveitis • Chorioretinitis

ABBREVIATIONS

• CSNB = congenital stationary night blindness • EHV = equine herpesvirus • EVA = equine viral arteritis • NMS = neonatal maladjustment syndrome

Suggested Reading

Brooks DE. Ophthalmology for the Equine Practitioner. Jackson, WY; Teton NewMedia, 2002.

Brooks DE, Matthews AG. Equine ophthalmology. In: Gelatt KN, ed. Veterinary Ophthalmology, ed 4. Philadelphia; Lippincott Williams and Wilkins, 2007.

Gilger BC, ed. Equine Ophthalmology. Philadelphia; WB Saunders, 2005.

Author Dennis E. Brooks
Consulting Editor Dennis E. Brooks

OMPHALOPHLEBITIS

BASICS

OVERVIEW

• Omphalophlebitis, or "navel ill," is an infection of one or more of the umbilical structures. The structures that comprise the umbilicus—the umbilical vein, umbilical arteries, and urachus—can become infected alone or in combination, with the urachus most commonly affected. Infection of the umbilicus more often occurs secondary to ascending bacterial invasion from open umbilical structures, although it can also occur from hematogenous seeding in a septicemic foal.
• The normal umbilicus should not be patent beyond 24 hr and should become dry and involute by 3–7 days. The umbilicus should be essentially nonexistent by 3–4 weeks of age. The bacteria most commonly associated with septic omphalophlebitis are β-hemolytic streptococci, *Escherichia coli*, and *Actinobacillus* sp.

SIGNALMENT

• Most commonly seen in neonatal foals, usually several days of age, although umbilical abscesses have been reported in older foals and horses (reported up to 16 mo of age).
• No breed or sex predisposition.

SIGNS

• External abnormalities are seen in approximately 50% of cases.
• Swollen, warm, and painful umbilicus
• Ventral edema may be present in more chronic cases.
• Purulent discharge may be seen, and urine may leak due to presence of a patent urachus.
• Deeper palpation may reveal thickened umbilical arteries and/or vein.
• Fever, lethargy, and poor nursing are often recognized first. Secondary complications such as septicemia, septic arthritis, septic physitis, and pneumonia may be the most obvious clinical signs—the umbilicus should be carefully examined in these cases.

CAUSES AND RISK FACTORS

• Failure of transfer of passive immunity
• Poor hygiene in the foaling environment
• Septicemia
• Contamination of the umbilical remnant or improper care of the umbilicus

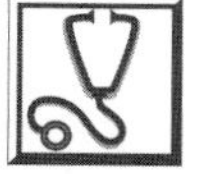

DIAGNOSIS

DIFFERENTIAL DIAGNOSIS

• Patent urachus—This may occur secondary to omphalophlebitis especially if it is an acquired patent urachus; can occur as a primary congenital condition in the absence of omphalophlebitis—history and ultrasonographic examination can help to differentiate.
• Umbilical hernia—An uncomplicated hernia should not have palpable heat, drainage, or enlargement of external or internal umbilical remnant structures. Foals with uncomplicated hernias generally do not have signs of systemic illness such as fever or lethargy.

CBC/BIOCHEMISTRY/URINALYSIS

• An increase in WBC count and fibrinogen is commonly seen.
• If the urachus is involved, urinalysis may reveal WBCs and bacteria.

OTHER LABORATORY TESTS

IgG should be checked, as failure of transfer of passive immunity is a common risk factor for omphalophlebitis.

IMAGING

Ultrasonography

• Ultrasound of umbilical remnants using a 7.5-MHz probe—The urachus, umbilical arteries, umbilical vein, and bladder should be evaluated.
• Normal umbilical vein should measure <1 cm in diameter, and normal umbilical arteries should measure <1.3 cm. The combined umbilical arteries and urachus should measure <2.5 cm at the apex of the bladder.
• Affected structures will generally be enlarged with a fluid-filled core, and often with gas shadowing.

Abdominal Radiography

Positive-contrast radiographs of the urinary tract (retrograde via the urethra) can help to identify any urachal tears that may be present secondary to umbilical sepsis.

OTHER DIAGNOSTIC PROCEDURES

• Blood cultures in neonatal foals to confirm septicemia and guide antimicrobial therapy
• Culture of umbilical stump to guide antimicrobial therapy

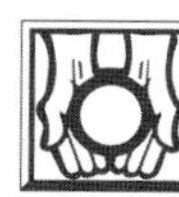

TREATMENT

• Surgical resection of umbilical remnants—Surgery is indicated if there is not adequate response to medical treatment, the umbilicus is severely enlarged and unlikely to respond quickly to medical therapy, or there is leakage of urine from the urachus. Surgical marsupialization of the umbilical vein remnant has been reported in cases where complete resection of the infected remnant was not possible.
• Nursing care—The foal should be supported systemically if there is concurrent septicemia, inappetence, or dehydration. Septicemic foals should be hospitalized and may require emergency medical care.

MEDICATIONS

DRUG(S)

• Systemic antimicrobials—Broad-spectrum antibiotics should be continued as required for resolution of the infection, often for at least 2 weeks. The choice of antimicrobials will be guided by culture results, but a common initial choice is a penicillin (22,000 IU/kg IV QID) and an aminoglycoside

(amikacin 25 mg/kg IV daily). If long-term antimicrobials are needed, the choice of an oral antimicrobial may be guided by culture results, and the foal should be monitored closely to ensure that there is not a recurrence of infection.
• NSAIDs—as needed for treatment of umbilical inflammation, fever, and discomfort or postoperatively to reduce the risk of adhesion formation and to reduce incisional discomfort. Flunixin meglumine (0.25–1.1 mg/kg IV BID) or ketoprofen (0.5–1.1 mg/kg IV BID)

CONTRAINDICATIONS/POSSIBLE INTERACTIONS

• Aminoglycosides should be used with caution in dehydrated foals or foals with renal compromise. Alternatively, a cephalosporin such as ceftiofur (10 mg/kg IV QID) may be used.
• Gastroduodenal ulcer prophylaxis may be needed when NSAIDs are used.

FOLLOW-UP

PATIENT MONITORING

• Foals should be monitored closely with palpation and serial ultrasound examinations for response to therapy.
• Twice-daily physical examinations should be performed to monitor for septic arthritis, septic physitis, and other possible complications.
• Follow-up blood work should reveal a decrease in fibrinogen and normalization of the leukogram.

PREVENTION/AVOIDANCE

• Provide good hygiene in the foaling environment.
• Ensure adequate transfer of passive immunity—Check IgG and administer plasma if needed.
• Dipping of the umbilical stump with dilute chlorhexidine or dilute povidine-iodine (Betadine) may help to prevent ascending infection.

POSSIBLE COMPLICATIONS

• Primary or secondary septicemia can occur in association with omphalophlebitis, with septic arthritis being the most common complication.
• Septic physitis, osteomyeltis, and pneumonia may also occur in combination with omphalophlebitis.
• Acquired patent urachus is a possible sequela.
• Infection of the urachus can lead to necrosis and possible uroabdomen.
• Extension of venous abscess to the liver

EXPECTED COURSE AND PROGNOSIS

• Foals with small, focal umbilical remnant infections usually respond to medical therapy. In foals with more extensive infection of the umbilical structures, surgical resection of the umbilical remnants appears to improve survival due to the reduced incidence of secondary infections.
• The presence of infected joints worsens the prognosis.

MISCELLANEOUS

ASSOCIATED CONDITIONS

• Patent urachus
• Septicemia
• Septic arthritis

AGE-RELATED FACTORS

Umbilical remnant infection is most commonly a condition of neonatal foals, and this population should also be evaluated critically for signs of generalized septicemia or other foci of infection.

ZOONOTIC POTENTIAL

N/A

PREGNANCY

N/A

SEE ALSO

• Sepsis, neonatal
• Septic arthritis, neonatal

ABBREVIATION

• WBC = white blood cell

Suggested Reading

Adams SB, Fessler JF. Umbilical cord remnant infections in foals: 16 cases (1975–1985). J Am Vet Med Assoc 1987;190:316–318.
Edwards RB, Fubini SL. A one-stage marsupialization procedure for management of infected umbilical vein remnants in calves and foals. Vet Surg 1995;24:32–35.
Reef VB, Collatos CA. Ultrasonography of umbilical structures in clinically normal foals. Am J Vet Res 1988;49:2143–2146.
Reef VB, Collatos CA, Spencer PA, et al. Clinical, ultrasonographic and surgical findings in foals with umbilical remnant infections. J Am Vet Med Assoc 1989;195:69–72.

Author Margaret C. Mudge
Consulting Editor Margaret C. Mudge

OPTIC NERVE ATROPHY

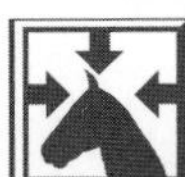

BASICS

OVERVIEW

Atrophy of the optic nerve due to inflammatory or noninflammatory causes. In the early stages, the ophthalmoscopic appearance of the optic nerve head may be normal although the eye is blind. With time, the optic disc becomes pale with profound vascular attenuation and an obvious granularity of the optic disc due to exposure of the scleral lamina cribrosa.

SYSTEM AFFECTED

Ophthalmic

SIGNALMENT

N/A

SIGNS

Blindness and pupil dilatation

CAUSES AND RISK FACTORS

Inflammatory—optic neuritis, equine recurrent uveitis, chorioretinitis
Noninflammatory—trauma to head and orbit, glaucoma, toxins, neoplasia, blood loss

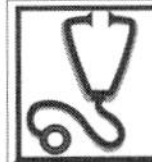

DIAGNOSIS

DIFFERENTIAL DIAGNOSIS

- Optic nerve hypoplasia
- Orbital trauma
- Retinal detachment
- Glaucoma
- Cataract

CBC/BIOCHEMISTRY/URINALYSIS

N/A

OTHER LABORATORY TESTS
N/A

IMAGING
Ultrasound

DIAGNOSTIC PROCEDURES
Electroretinogram

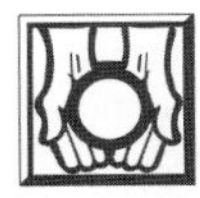

TREATMENT

There is no therapy for this condition.

MEDICATIONS

N/A

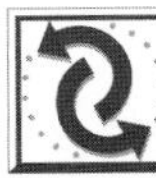

FOLLOW-UP

EXPECTED COURSE AND PROGNOSIS
Poor prognosis

MISCELLANEOUS

ASSOCIATED CONDITIONS
See Causes and Risk Factors.

SEE ALSO
Optic nerve hypoplasia

Suggested Reading

Brooks DE. Ophthalmology for the Equine Practitioner. Jackson, WY; Teton NewMedia, 2002.

Brooks DE, Matthews AG. Equine ophthalmology. In: Gelatt KN, ed. Veterinary Ophthalmology, ed 4. Philadelphia; Lippincott Williams and Wilkins, 2007.

Gilger BC, ed. Equine Ophthalmology. Philadelphia; WB Saunders, 2005.

Authors Maria Källberg and Dennis E. Brooks
Consulting Editor Dennis E. Brooks

ORAL NEOPLASIA

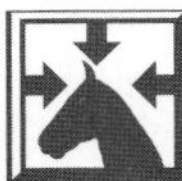

BASICS

DEFINITION

Neoplasia is uncommon in horses, however with the increase in the geriatric horse population, practioners may see an increase in incidence. A significant proportion of equine neoplasia will occur in the head and neck. Neoplasms of the oral cavity may originate from dental tissue (odontogenic), bone (osteogenic) and soft tissue (gums, tongue, lips, and oropharynx) and may extend into surrounding tissues.

Odontogenic

The classification systems have emphasized the tissue differentiation suggesting the origin of the neoplasm. Odontogenesis begins with the ingrowth of oral ectoderm into the mesenchyme of the jaw.

- Tumors of odontogenic epithelium without odontogenic mesenchyme
  - Ameloblastoma (adamantinoma)—benign but locally invasive. Often interosseal distorting the mandible
  - Keratinizing ameloblastoma—It is the same tumor but with an increased tendency toward keratin expression.
- Tumors of odontogenic epithelium with odontogenic mesenchyme
  - Ameloblastic odontoma (odontoameloblastoma)—benign, slowly expanding, and locally invasive
  - Complex odontoma—contains all the elements of a normal tooth but structure is disorganized
  - Compound odontoma—contains all the elements of a normal tooth. Forms a tooth-like structure—denticles. Often regarded as a malformation
- Tumors composed primarily of odontogenic ectomesenchyme
  - Cementoma—dense, mineralized structure
  - Cementifying fibroma—is analogous to ossifying fibroma but the components have lines of cementum

Osteogenic

Osteogenic tumors are usually benign and have a predilection for the mandibular symphysis.

- Osteomas
- Osteosarcomas
- Fibro-osteoma
- Ossifying fibromas
- Hemangiosarcoma

Soft tissue

- Squamous cell carcinoma—tongue, gingiva, pharynx, and hard palate
- Lymphosarcoma—horse palate
- Fibrosarcoma—tongue
- Myosarcoma
- Melanomas
- Adenomas

PATHOPHYSIOLOGY

N/A

SYSTEMS AFFECTED

The neoplasms affect most commonly the digestive system but may also invade the respiratory tract.

GENETICS

N/A

INCIDENCE

Malignant bone tumors are extremely rare in the horse, but more than 80% of osteosarcomas occur in the head region. Neoplasia of the oral cavity or pharynx is extremely uncommon. In one study of 141 cases with squamous cell carcinomas, only 5% involved the oral or pharyngeal mucosa.

SIGNALMENT

- The age of the horse may suggest the type of neoplasm. There is a high incidence of ameloblastic odontomas in young animals (6 weeks to 1 year of age). Ameloblastomas occur in older horses (5–20 yr of age), whereas osteogenic neoplasms have no age predilection.
- Horses with osteogenic tumors of the intramembranous bone of the head are young, 2–14 mo of age. Squamous cell carcinoma, which is by far the most common type of soft-tissue tumor, occurs in older horses.
- No breed or sex susceptibility has been suggested for any of the neoplasms.

SIGNS

Historical

- The clinical signs of oral cavity and oropharyngeal neoplasia are dependent on the location and size of the neoplasm and may include dysphagia, difficulty in prehension or mastication, halitosis, oral discharge, and lymphadenopathy. Nasal discharge may be evident if the tumor has expanded to involve the nasal chamber or paranasal sinuses.
- The anatomy of the oral cavity allows for considerable progression and expansion of the lesion before it causes major clinical signs. Therefore, the majority of neoplasms in this region are usually well advanced with extensive local infiltration before clinical signs become apparent.

Physical Examination

- Odontogenic neoplasms usually present as slowly developing, firm, immobile swellings of the mandible or maxilla.
- The most common presentation of osteogenic tumors is proliferation of bony tissue on the rostral mandible in the young horse. The syndrome has been classified as equine juvenile mandibular ossifying fibroma, and usually presents as a rapidly growing subgingival mass of the rostral mandible or, much less commonly, the premaxilla. The mucosa covering the mass is usually ulcerated. The proliferation can be symmetric or may only involve the rostral aspect of one hemimandible. On palpation, the teeth may be loose but the mass is usually nonpainful. Prehension and mastication are initially unaltered, but become apparent when the tumor reaches a large size.
- The typical appearance of squamous cell carcinoma of the oral cavity is a partially ulcerated multilobular mass projecting from the mucosa. The tumor is usually locally invasive and metastasis can occur. Displacement and loosening of the teeth are present. Horses with squamous cell carcinoma and lymphosarcoma of the hard palate commonly have a foul, fetid odor to their breath.
- Although lesions of the rostral mandible are readily identified, those affecting the more caudal part of the oral cavity and pharynx require a more detailed examination. Sedation and the use of a Houssmann gag and headlamp or pen flashlight allow the presence of a tumor to be determined visually or by palpation and a biopsy taken in many cases, but in others general anesthesia is necessary. The regional lymph nodes should be examined.

CAUSES

N/A

RISK FACTORS

N/A

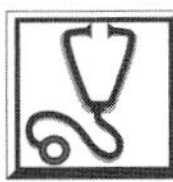

DIAGNOSIS

The definitive diagnosis depends on histologic examination of tissue removed by biopsy or at necropsy.

DIFFERENTIAL DIAGNOSIS

- Swellings of the mandible or maxilla due to underlying dental disease, especially periapical abscessation
- Foreign bodies in the oropharynx causing dysphagia and halitosis

CBC/BIOCHEMISTRY

N/A

OTHER LABORATORY TESTS

N/A

IMAGING

- Radiography is of considerable value in evaluating the nature and extent of the neoplasm and in differentiating it from a dental problem.
- Ameloblastomas appear as a radiolucent multiloculated mass often well marginated by thick, sclerotic bone with cortical expansion on the lingual and buccal surfaces. The tooth roots may appear shortened and lytic with loss of lamina diva and periodontal membrane.
- Ameloblastic odontomas are radiopaque masses that may appear to fill the maxillary sinus, obstructing the nasal passage on the affected side. The maxilla and teeth are usually displaced laterally.
- Radiographically osteogenic tumors are characterized by a smooth, bony proliferation of the rostral mandible with or without

osteolytic change involving the roots of the teeth.

• Horses with squamous cell carcinoma of the hard palate show dental displacement and loss of alveolar bone. Extension into the paranasal sinuses results in loss of the normal radiolucent appearance. Radiography of the pharynx may show its dorsal wall to be deformed and thickened, particularly when affected by lymphosarcoma.

• Endoscopy is of value in determining the extent of palatine and nasal involvement. In cases of lymphosarcoma, the pharyngeal wall may be edematous with moderately severe lymphoid hyperplasia and ulceration of the soft palate. Guttural pouch empyema may be noted, particularly if the pharyngeal walls are affected. In some cases an oronasal fistula may be present. Oral endoscopy carried out under general anesthesia allows a thorough examination that may not be possible by other means.

DIAGNOSTIC PROCEDURES

Biopsy

• Biopsies of masses involving the mandible or maxilla enable differentiation between odontogenic and osteogenic tumors.

• Biopsy of squamous cell carcinoma of the mouth can be obtained without difficulty by breaking off a piece of the proliferative tissue, whereas biopsies of pharyngeal or palatine tissues may be accomplished with a biopsy instrument through an endoscope or using uterine biopsy forceps under general anesthesia. If lymph node enlargement is present, a fine-needle aspirate or biopsy is necessary to determine if metastasis has occurred.

PATHOLOGICAL FINDINGS

Histology

• Ameloblastomas contain odontogenic islands set in well-vascularized connective tissue. The periphery of the follicle is composed of a layer of columnar cells with distinct polarization of nuclei away from the basement membrane, resembling ameloblasts. Toward the center of the follicles the cells form a loose network similar to the stellate reticulum of the developing tooth. Differentiation of this tumor from other odontogenic epithelial tumors is based on the degree of stellate reticulum formation without intracellular bridges.

• Ameloblastic odontomas differ from ameloblastomas in that the islands of epithelium are smaller, so that the formation of cysts is less frequent and the stellate reticulum is less extensive.

• The term *odontoma* implies that there has been induction of both dentine and enamel within the lesion and their presence is evident histologically.

• It should be noted, however, that these tumor classifications are subjective, and because of their rarity and difficulties in their histologic recognition, a degree of inconsistency exists with respect to their nomenclature.

• Two reports of rostral mandibular enlargement in young horses were described as osteosarcomas, but there were no mitotic cells observed histologically and it is possible that these lesions were related to the equine juvenile ossifying fibroma syndrome.

• Histologic diagnosis of oral and pharyngeal neoplasms is much less complicated.

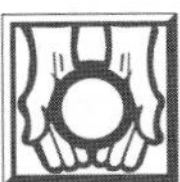

TREATMENT

• Whereas neoplasms of the mouth and pharynx, such as squamous cell carcinoma and lymphosarcoma, are usually too advanced when diagnosed to consider anything but euthanasia, there have been several reports of attempted surgical removal of odontogenic and osteogenic tumors of the mandible and maxilla. The ease of surgical debridement is dependent on the size and location of the tumor. Surgical excision and curettage are often followed by recurrence, although this may be delayed for several years. Because the growth of ameloblastic odontomas is by expansion rather than infiltration, theoretically they may represent a better prognosis than ameloblastomas. Radical tumor resection in conjunction with partial mandibulectomy and possible stabilization of the resulting defect with internal or external orthopedic devices has met with greater success. Recurrence is more common when the neoplasm is located in the maxilla. Cryosurgery has been used as an adjunct to surgical excision. This has the potential advantage of destroying neoplastic cells at the surgical margins without removing additional bone. The amount of dead space is decreased, and scaffolding is provided for new bone development by creeping substitution.

• As previously mentioned, many neoplasms of the oral cavity and oropharynx are advanced before detection; consequently, surgical removal often leads to poor success rates because of difficult access and incomplete removal of the lesion. Confirmation of malignancy by histologic examination in an extensive lesion is an indication for euthanasia.

• The use of laser surgery had been advocated for the ablation of certain soft-tissue neoplasms of the oropharynx or nasopharynx, but the success of this therapy is largely dependent on early tumor recognition.

NURSING CARE/ACTIVITY/DIET

Horses that have undergone radical surgical excision, including mandibulectomy, may have difficulty prehending short grass; however, prehending longer grass and mastication have not been complications. Cosmetically, the postoperative appearance of the horses is acceptable, even though all horses have some flaccidity of the lower lip. Horses with a mandibulectomy have been able to return to their intended uses, including racing.

MEDICATIONS

CONTRAINDICATIONS, PRECAUTIONS, POSSIBLE INTERACTIONS, ALTERNATIVE DRUGS

N/A

FOLLOW-UP

PATIENT MONITORING, PREVENTION/AVOIDANCE, POSSIBLE COMPLICATIONS

N/A

EXPECTED COURSE AND PROGNOSIS

Successful treatment depends on complete removal/destruction of the neoplasm.

MISCELLANEOUS

ASSOCIATED CONDITIONS, AGE-RELATED FACTORS, ZOONOTIC POTENTIAL, PREGNANCY

N/A

Suggested Reading

Head KW, Else RW, Dubielzig. Tumors of the alimentary tract In: Meuten DJ (ed). Tumors in domestic animals 4th edition Iowa State Press 2002 pg 401–481

Pirie RC, Tremaine WH. Neoplasia of the mouth and surrounding structure. In: Robinson NE (Ed.): Current therapy in equine medicine, 4th ed. WB Saunders & Co. 199X:153–155.

Richardson DW, Evans LH, Tulleners EP. Rostral mandibulectomy in five horses. JAVMA 1991;174;734.

Authors Olimpo Oliver-Espinosa and Garry B. Edwards

Consulting Editors Henry Stämpfli and Olimpo Oliver-Espinosa

ORAL STEREOTYPIC BEHAVIORS

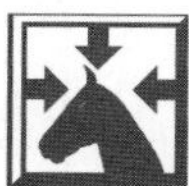

BASICS

DEFINITION

- Repetitive, apparently functionless behavior that may be considered to be compulsive
- Oral stereotypies that are common include: cribbing (grasping a horizontal surface with the incisors, flexing the neck and making a grunting sound), tongue flapping, and sucking; those less common include: lip licking, lip flapping, noise making with the head, and teeth grinding.

PATHOPHYSIOLOGY

- Cribbing is the only stereotypy in which the pathophysiologic mechanism has been elucidated with endoscopy and fluoroscopy. Air is usually not completely swallowed, but stays in the upper esophagus causing transient dilation. The grunting noise is produced when air rushes through the cricopharynx. Contraction of the ventral neck muscles produces negative pressure in the esophagus that allows air to move in; the air then is expelled from the pharynx rostrally, with only a small amount passing into the lower esophagus.
- Endogenous opiates may be involved, because administration of an opiate blocker inhibits cribbing for several hours. Cribbing does not cause release of endogenous opiates and measurement of opiates in cribbers in comparison to non-cribbers has yielded contradictory results, but opiates are necessary for cribbing to occur.
- Young horses that crib have more severe gastric ulcers compared to those who do not crib; therefore cribbing may either cause ulcers due to vagally stimulated gastric acid secretion resulting from the chewing movements, or stimulation of the lips and mouth during cribbing. The alternate hypothesis is that cribbing is a homeostatic response to ulcers and may lead to more saliva production.
- Little is known concerning the pathophysiology of repetitive tongue movements.

SYSTEMS AFFECTED

Gastro Intestinal, Neurologic and Musculoskeletal

- Behavioral cribbing is repetitive, apparently functionless behavior involving the head. Tongue and lip movements are repetitive, apparently functionless behavior involving the tongue or lips usually preceding feeding.
- Wear of the upper incisors is one definite outcome of cribbing as is neck thickening. Some horses exhibit colic ("gas colic") and a few suffer from epiploic foramen entrapment. Tooth grinding can lead to wear of the molars. Oral problems may cause tongue protrusion.
- A greater percentage of horses with neurological problems such as equine motor neuron disease seem to be affected.
- Musculoskeletal thickening of the neck muscles can be a cosmetic problem.

GENETICS

There is a definite breed predilection and, within Thoroughbreds, familial tendencies have been observed. The mode of inheritance may be recessive.

INCIDENCE/PREVALENCE

The prevalence of cribbing is approximately 2%. The mortality rate is unknown. The prevalence of tongue movements and tooth grinding is unknown.

GEOGRAPHIC DISTRIBUTION

Cribbing has been observed worldwide.

SIGNALMENT

Usually an adult horse confined in a stall, fed a high concentrate diet, and used for different activities such as flat racing, jumping, three day eventing or dressage.

Breed Predilections

Thoroughbreds have a higher risk of cribbing. Standardbreds have a very low incidence. There is no known breed predilection for tongue movements and teeth grinding.

Mean Age and Range

The age of onset is at weaning and the frequency of diagnosis increases with age. There is no known age predilection for tongue movements and teeth grinding.

Predominant Sex

Males are more likely to crib, especially young horses. Older mares are more likely to crib than old geldings or stallions. There is no sex predilection for tongue movements and tooth grinding.

SIGNS

General Comments

- Cribbing: the horse grasps a horizontal surface with its incisors, flexes its neck, and allows air to pass into the upper esophagus. A few horses do not grasp a horizontal surface, but flex their neck and make a grunting sound. These are called wind suckers.
- Tongue movements are not as frequent in horses as in cattle, probably because horses do not use their tongues to prehend food as cattle do. Some horses simply protrude their tongue, which probably relates to food-anticipating movements that occur when horses are expecting palatable food, and free-lunged. Other horses move the tongue in and out or flap the tongue.
- Teeth grinding—The horse presses its teeth together and moves the jaw laterally producing an audible sound. This usually occurs when the horse is being groomed or saddled. Purposeless stereotypic behavior must be differentiated from purposeful behavior. Tongue movements may have been rewarded by the present or a previous owner or be a result of dental problems or by misfitted tack. If the oral behavior occurs mostly before feeding, consider it anticipatory and not stereotypic behavior.

Historical Findings

Stereotypic behavior usually begins with an abrupt change in the environment; e.g taking a horse from pasture and immediately limiting its access to hay can be the initiating factor to cribbing.

Physical Examination Findings

- Cribbing: well developed neck muscles and wear of the upper incisors. Rarely, the horse is very thin, because it spends so much time cribbing that it does not have time to ingest the calories it needs.
- Tongue movements: usually none, but dental problems should be eliminated as a cause.
- Tooth grinding: grinding can be a sign of pain, so the cause of the pain should be identified and eliminated.

CAUSES

- The cause of stereotypic behavior is unknown.
- Boredom probably is not a cause, because providing stall toys usually does not help and an increase in exercise load increases time spent cribbing.
- The horse is thwarted in some goal, usually grazing, and the frustration leads to repetition of a behavior that is part of the appetitive portion of that behavior (e.g., cribbing as part of biting a mouthful of grass as the first step of ingestion).
- Feeding sweet feed or other highly palatable food stimulates cribbing.
- The causes of other oral stereotypies are unknown but they are thought to be anticipatory.

RISK FACTORS

- Genetic predisposition for Thoroughbreds. Certain families of Thoroughbreds have a much higher frequency of cribbing.
- Stall confinement with limited (<7 kg) forage, <40 L/day of water, bedding other than straw, and minimal visual or tactile contact with other horses.
- Race, dressage, jumping and eventing horses are at greater risk than endurance horses.
- In only 10% of cases has another horse begun to crib after a cribber arrived in the barn or pasture. There is little evidence that horses learn to crib by observing other horses; if the environment is conducive to cribbing and the horse has the genetic predisposition, it may learn to crib by observation.

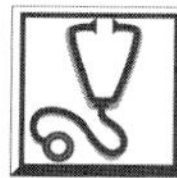

DIAGNOSIS

DIFFERENTIAL DIAGNOSIS

- Differentiate cribbing from wood chewing. The cribbing horse grasps wooden edges but does not ingest them; the wood-chewing horse does. The cribbing horse makes a loud noise when the air passes through the pharynx; the only sound made by the wood-chewing horse is that of wood being splintered.
- Differentiate tongue movements and tooth grinding from oral pathologies. Tooth grinding of sudden onset also can be a sign of pain elsewhere in the body.

Oral Stereotypic Behaviors

CBC/BIOCHEMISTRY/URINALYSIS

Perform a chemistry screen and CBC to determine presence of an underlying disease and to judge whether medication can be administered safely.

OTHER LABORATORY TESTS

N/A

IMAGING

May be necessary to rule out GI tract problems as a cause of cribbing.

DIAGNOSTIC PROCEDURES

Endoscopy of the nasal cavity and pharynx to rule out medical causes of tongue movements and to determine if ulcers are present.

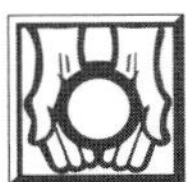

TREATMENT

AIMS OF TREATMENT

The objectives of treatment are to decrease the horse's motivation to crib or engage in other stereotypies. The secondary aim is to prevent gastrointestinal problems that are associated with oral stereotypies.

- Diet change has the most impact especially in horses that have just begun to crib. Feeding a hay diet with another source of forage and no sweet feed results in the lowest rate of cribbing. Substitution of fat (e.g., corn oil) for carbohydrates (e.g., molasses and grain) can be done for horses, that expend more calories than hay provides.
- Other treatments are aimed at creating a normal equine environment, which means the horse has physical contact with other horses and available forage at all times. The best environment for the horse is to remove it from the stall and put it in a compatible social group with access to pasture or hay free choice. When the use of the horse precludes keeping it in a group with a run-out housing situation, eliminating risk factors (e.g., limited forage, wood shavings as bedding) helps. Stall toys generally are ineffective as are taste repellents. Punishment is not the preferred method of treatment, but clinicians should be aware of this option. Several types of collars (wide leather straps, a nutcracker or metal collar or one on a headstall to prevent slipping) can pinch the horse when it cribs or mechanically prevent neck flexion. A metal muzzle prevents the horse from making contact with a horizontal surface. A remotely triggered shock collar is available, but the operator must be present to punish cribbing each time it occurs. An automatically triggered electronic shock collar was available, which shocked the horse when it flexed its neck, but some horses would flex their necks in response to the shock and become highly agitated.
- Providing a padded horizontal bar on which the horse can bite without damaging his teeth or the stall fixtures is the best approach and will eliminate damage to fences and stall equipment.
- Provide oral stimulation in the form of several types of forage, pasture, or a barrel the horse can turn to receive pelleted feed or grain. If the behavior occurs before feeding, the horse probably is frustrated by hunger (i.e., undernourishment); if it occurs after feeding, the horse probably is frustrated from the lack of a specific dietary component (i.e., malnourishment).
- Counterconditioning—training the horse to do something incompatible with the oral behavior (e.g., teaching horse to hold something in its mouth for a food reward so it does not scrape the teeth on metal or bite and toss the feed bucket)
- Tongue protrusion under saddle is usually treated with a dropped nose band.

APPROPRIATE HEALTH CARE

Outpatient care should be sufficient.

NURSING CARE

NA

ACTIVITY

Forced exercise may increase cribbing behavior.

DIET

The diet should be high in roughage and low in carbohydrates and grains other than oats.

CLIENT EDUCATION

The owners should be told that cribbing and other oral stereotypies are not "vices", but rather responses to the unnatural environment in which we keep them. Managers of broodmares should know that weaning on pasture greatly reduces the risk of the foal beginning to crib.

SURGICAL CONSIDERATIONS

- Accessory neurectomy, strap muscle myectomy, or a combination of the two have been used. Reserve these surgical approaches for horses that experience colic when they crib or are emaciated because they crib rather than eat. Wire staples in the gums that extend beyond the incisors can be inserted in the upper gums to prevent the horse from making contact with its incisors.

MEDICATIONS

DRUGS OF CHOICE

Opiate blockers such as naloxone (0.02–0.04 mg/kg IV), naltrexone (0.04 mg/kg or SC), or nalmefene (0.08 mg/kg IM) inhibit cribbing, but these drugs are too expensive and too short acting to be practical. Recently intravenous dextromorphan of 1 mg/kg has been used to reduce cribbing.

CONTRAINDICATIONS

Mares during late pregnancy

PRECAUTIONS

GI side effects, including diarrhea, inappetence, and behaviors indicative of colic, are seen after naloxone administration.

POSSIBLE INTERACTIONS

N/A

ALTERNATIVE DRUGS

- Acupuncture

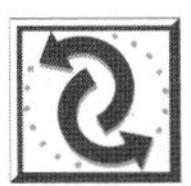

FOLLOW-UP

PATIENT MONITORING

Regular follow-up after 2 weeks of treatment to evaluate the owner's compliance and the success of the treatments given.

POSSIBLE COMPLICATIONS

N/A

MISCELLANEOUS

ASSOCIATED CONDITIONS

N/A

AGE-RELATED FACTORS

Usually a disease of mature horses

ZOONOTIC POTENTIAL

N/A

PREGNANCY

N/A

SYNONYMS

- Crib biting
- Wind sucking

SEE ALSO

- Locomotor stereotypic behaviors
- Pica

Suggested Reading

Dodman NH, Shuster L, Court MH, Dixon R. An investigation into the use of narcotic antagonists in the treatment of a stereotypic behaviour pattern (crib-biting) in the horse. Am J Vet Res 1989;48:311–319.

Gillham SB, Dodman NH, Shuster L, Kream R, Rand W. The effect of diet on cribbing behavior and plasma endorphin in horses. Appl Anim Behav Sci 1994;41:147–153.

Luescher UA, McKeown DB, Halip J. Reviewing the causes of obsessive compulsive disorders in horses. Vet Med 1991:527–530.

McGreevy PD, Richardson JD, Nicol CJ, Lane JG. Radiographic and endoscopic study of horses performing an oral based stereotypy. Equine Vet J 1995;27:92–95.

Rendon RA, Shuster L, Dodman NH. The effect of the NMDA receptor blocker, dextromethorphan, on cribbing in horses. Pharm Biochem Behav 2001:68:49–51.

Author Katherine Albro Houpt

Consulting Editors Olimpo Oliver-Espinosa and Henry Stämpfli

ORAL ULCERS

BASICS

DEFINITION

Oral ulcers are disruptions in the integrity of the oral mucosa that may be preceded by lesions such as vesicles, bullae, crusts, or traumatic injury.

PATHOPHYSIOLOGY

- The pathophysiologic events that lead to oral ulceration are variable and depend on the inciting cause. In the case of vesicular stomatitis, a viral disease caused by a vesiculovirus, a short incubation period of 24 hr, and invasion of oral epithelial cells by the virus occurs. The lesions progress rapidly from blanched maculae to vesicles and soon rupture, leaving sloughed epithelium and ulcers.
- Phenylbutazone is known to inhibit prostaglandin synthesis by inhibition of cyclooxygenase. This inhibition of prostaglandin synthesis in the gastrointestinal tract results in a depletion of PGE_1 and PGE_2, which is thought to cause vasoconstriction of the microvasculature of the mucosa, leading to ischemia and ulcer formation.
- The mechanism of action of cantharidin to induce ulcers is not well understood yet, but acantholysis and vesicle formation occur as a result of damage to cell membrane due to interference with oxidative enzymes bound to mitochondria.
- The oral ulcers caused by facial paralysis and dental problems are due to impaction of food material between the teeth and the cheek, as well as direct traumatic damage by the teeth.
- In uremia, oral ulcers develop as a consequence of increased excretion of urea into the oral cavity, degradation of urea into ammonia by bacterial urease and subsequent disruption of oral mucosa integrity.

SYSTEMS AFFECTED

- The different systems affected vary depending on the initial cause. When oral ulcers are the result of vesicular stomatitis, the locomotor system is usually affected. The vesicular lesions are also present on the coronary band, and lameness is observed.
- In cases of phenylbutazone toxicity, several sections of the gastrointestinal tract are affected, causing gastric and intestinal ulceration and colitis of the right dorsal colon. The kidney is also affected, causing renal medullary crest necrosis. Ventral and peripheral edema may also be observed.
- Blister beetle toxicosis (cantharidin toxicosis), besides affecting the mucosal surface, also affects the gastrointestinal tract, causing colic. There is hypocalcemia and hypoproteinemia, and the kidney is slightly affected. Myocardial necrosis is a common finding in affected horses. Some horses show stilted gait, as seen in myositis.
- In the uremic syndrome, weight loss is the most common affliction; there is PU/PD due to kidney damage. Gastric ulceration, coagulation disorders, and halitosis (urine odor) have been reported. There is excessive dental tartar, and there is ventral edema because of a decrease in oncotic pressure, increased vascular permeability, and increased hydrostatic pressure. Bone marrow, the endocrine system, and the CNS might be affected.
- The other causes of oral ulceration are local phenomena limited to the buccal mucosa.

SIGNALMENT

Oral ulcers can occur at any age, and there is no sex or breed predisposition.

SIGNS

Historical

The history of oral ulceration cases is quite variable and is dependent on the initial cause. In the cases of vesicular stomatitis, it starts as an outbreak. The owner usually reports that the affected animals have excessive salivation, inappetence, and lameness. In the cases where toxicity is involved, there is history of ingestion of toxic material. With phenylbutazone toxicity, the history indicates that an excessive dosage for several days or accidental administration of large amounts has occurred. Facial nerve paralysis is usually preceded by some history of trauma or CNS disease. The main complaint with uremia is usually PU/PD.

Physical Examination

- In the majority of the cases of oral ulcers regardless of the cause, there is ptyalism, different degrees of anorexia, and dysphagia due to pain. Halitosis is common.
- Vesicular stomatitis starts with oral vesicles that with time coalesce and turn into ulcers. Lameness of different degrees is observed due to involvement of the coronary band, which has vesicles and is swollen (see Vesicular Stomatitis).
- In phenylbutazone toxicity there are signs typical of oral ulcers, but also there may be ventral and peripheral edema, bruxism, diarrhea (see Colitis), melena, ulceration of the digestive tract, and weight loss (see NSAID Toxicity).
- In addition to oral ulcers, cantharidin toxicosis is also manifested by depression; colic, fever, profuse diarrhea, stranguria, synchronous diaphragmatic flutter, and a stiff gait (see Cantharidin Toxicosis). Oral ulcers in uremia are accompanied by all the signs that distinguish the uremic syndrome (see Chronic Renal Failure).

CAUSES

- Vesicular stomatitis
- Phenylbutazone toxicity
- Uremia
- Cantharidin toxicosis
- Chemical stomatitis
- Periodontal disease
- Foxtail and plant thorn stomatitis
- Oral foreign body
- Oral ulcers secondary to yellow star thistle grass
- Food impaction between molar teeth and cheek (facial nerve paralysis, dental problems)
- Equine herpesvirus type II
- *Actinobacillus lignieresii*

RISK FACTORS

The risk factors involved in oral ulcers are related to the primary cause (see each clinical entity).

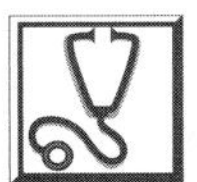

DIAGNOSIS

DIFFERENTIAL DIAGNOSIS

See Ptyalism.

CBC/BIOCHEMISTRY/URINALYSIS

No findings are specific to oral ulceration, but changes may reflect the underlying causes.

IMAGING

- Radiographic studies are indicated when there is suspicion of dental problems or trauma has caused facial paralysis.
- Ultrasonographic examination of the kidneys may help in determining the cause of chronic renal failure.

DIAGNOSTIC PROCEDURES

- A thorough physical and oral examination is indicated to rule out the different causes of oral ulceration.
- To diagnose vesicular stomatitis, virus isolation from biopsy of the vesicles is done. A complement fixation test, fluorescent antibody test, and virus neutralization test in tissue culture are used for virus identification. An ELISA is also available.
- Cantharidin toxicosis diagnosis is based on detecting cantharidin in stomach contents or in urine or finding blister beetles in the forage.
- The diagnosis of phenylbutazone toxicity is suggested by history of inappropriate drug administration and clinical picture compatible with it.
- The diagnosis of chronic renal failure is based on serum urea and creatinine measurement, ultrasonographic examination of the kidneys, urinalysis, sodium fractional excretion, and kidney biopsy. Biopsy and histologic examination of lesions may assist in narrowing differential diagnosis and rule out associated neoplastic events.
- In the case of infection by *Actinobacillus lignieresii*, aspirate material should be cultured in specific media.

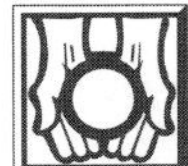

TREATMENT

- Specific therapy for particular conditions may be indicated. The treatment strategies for oral ulcers involve local therapy to relieve pain and irritation, such as mild antiseptic mouthwashes with potassium permanganate (2%), hydrogen peroxide (0.5%), saturated solution of boric acid, or povidone-iodine solution (1% v/v). If present, thorns or any foreign body should be extracted. There is also need to remove any chemical irritant that may be causing oral ulceration. This also applies for all toxicoses. When dental problems are the cause, appropriate dental prophylactic measures are indicated.
- The treatment of *A. lignieresii* is done with 150 mL of 20% sodium iodide IV; one treatment seems sufficient if accompanied by other antibiotics.

ZOONOTIC POTENTIAL

Among the causes of oral ulcers, only vesicular stomatitis has zoonotic potential.

SYNONYMS

- Vesicles
- Crusts
- Growths

ABBREVIATIONS

- PD/PU = polydipsia/polyuria
- PGE = prostaglandin E

Suggested Reading

Baun KH, Shin SJ, Rebhun WC, Patten VH. Isolation of *Actinobacillus lignieresii* from enlarged tongue of a horse. JAVMA 1984;185:792–793.

Green S. Vesicular stomatitis in the horse. Vet Clin North Am Equine Pract 1993;9:349–353.

Letchworth GJ, Rodriguez LL, Barrera J Del C. Vesicular stomatitis. Vet J 1999;157:239–260.

Meschter CL, Giñbert M, Krook L, Maylin G, Corradino R. The effects of phenylbutazone on the intestinal mucosa of the horse: a morphological, ultrastructural and biochemical study. Equine Vet J 1990;22:255–263.

Scmitz DG. Cantharidin toxicosis in horses. J Vet Intern Med 1989;3:208–215.

Scrutchfield WL, Schumacher J. Examination of the oral cavity and routine dental care. Vet Clin North Am Equine Pract 1993;9:123–131.

White SD. Diseases of the lips and oral cavity of domestic animals. Clin Dermatol 1987;5:190–201.

Author Olimpo Oliver-Espinosa

Consulting Editors Henry Stämpfli and Olimpo Oliver-Espinosa

ORBITAL DISEASE

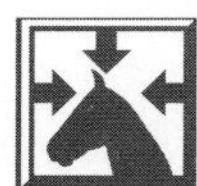

BASICS

OVERVIEW

• An assortment of diseases and conditions that lead to dysfunction of the anatomical orbit. The orbit is composed of several bones forming a series of canals, fissures, and foramina that communicate with the extraorbital compartments. It is a closed conical cavity with a broad opening anteriorly. Within the orbit are the globe and numerous types of extraocular supportive tissue: fascia, nerves, blood vessels, muscle, fat, and glands. Pathology of any of these extraocular tissues—including the bony orbit—broadly defines orbital disease. • Orbital disease progresses as tissue within or adjacent to the orbit loses its ability to function. Vision is consequently endangered. Compression by a space-occupying lesion, anatomical rearrangement by trauma or disease, or invasion of a systemic illness into the orbit highlights the major mechanisms of orbital disease.

SYSTEMS AFFECTED

Opthalmic, musculoskeletal, vascular, nervous, and upper respiratory systems including sinuses can be involved.

SIGNALMENT

Older horses tend to develop neoplasia, whereas foals and yearlings may be prone to acute trauma.

SIGNS (variable according to disease process)

- Exophthalmos, or anterior displacement of the globe, is associated with nictitans protrusion, lagophthalmos, and corneal ulceration.
- Enophthalmos, or posterior displacement of the globe due to atrophy of tissue behind the globe, may also be found following orbital fractures.
- Phthisis bulbi (globe atrophy)
- Nasal discharge or epistaxis
- Blepharedema, chemosis, corneal edema
- Epiphora or other ocular discharge
- Strabismus with associated visual difficulties and abnormal head posture
- Vision loss (usually unilateral)
- Orbital asymmetry from fractures, cellulitis, and orbital emphysema
- Fever, pain

CAUSES AND RISK FACTORS

- Trauma causing orbital fractures and proptosis
- Foreign bodies leading to orbital abscesses
- (Pyo)granulomatous diseases
- Guttural pouch disease
- Sinusitis involving frontal, maxillary, sphenopalatine sinuses
- Tooth root abscesses
- Orbital neoplasia—meningioma, neuroendocrine tumor, lipoma, adenocarcinoma, lymphoma, melanoma, sarcoid, squamous cell carcinoma, hemangiosarcoma, multilobular osteoma, medulloepithelioma, schwannoma, and neurofibroma have all been found in the equine orbit.
- Varices or abnormal distention of venules causing a displacement of normal tissue
- Retro-orbital cysts
- Parasitism as in hydatid cysts

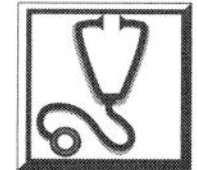

DIAGNOSIS

DIFFERENTIAL DIAGNOSES

- Any cause of ocular pain
- Exophthalmos, a sign of orbital disease, can be confused with buphthalmos, which is a marked increase in globe diameter associated with advanced glaucoma.
- Primary extraorbital disease close to but not affecting the orbit—sinusitis, guttural pouch disorders, tooth problems

CBC/BIOCHEMISTRY/URINALYSIS

- CBC may show elevated fibrinogen or other nonspecific inflammatory indicators if the disease is extensive.
- Systemic illness should be taken into consideration.

OTHER LABORATORY TESTS

N/A

IMAGING

Skull radiographs, retro-orbital ultrasound, computed tomography or magnetic resonance imaging where available (foals and small ponies primarily)

OTHER DIAGNOSTIC PROCEDURES

- Digital retropulsion of affected and unaffected eyes is helpful in confirming retro-orbital masses.
- Aspiration of fluid or biopsy of tissue should be performed.
- Cytology, microbial culture, and sensitivity and histopathology are recommended as part of an orbital disease workup.
- Orbitotomy can be diagnostic and therapeutic; however, it is difficult surgery that may require orthopedic instruments.
- Trephination into paranasal sinuses may be indicated for microbial culture, irrigation, and drainage.
- In cases of proptosis, careful ophthalmic examination will dictate viability of the eye. Miosis with severe hypotony and hyphema indicates severe trauma and poor visual prognosis.

GROSS AND HISTOPATHOLOGIC FINDINGS

Varies greatly depending on the particular disease

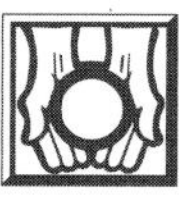

TREATMENT

- Orbital diseases, once identified, may be treated medically as in minor trauma or may need surgical attention (e.g., orbital neoplasia) and short hospital stays until the owner or trainer can monitor and treat the patient at home.
- Activity is based on degree of vision impairment and comfort of horse. Some of these diseases are very painful especially after invasive surgery. Stall rest may be indicated for the short term.
- No change in diet is necessary unless malnutrition is a cause of the atrophy of orbital contents.
- Long-term damage may be sustained in orbital trauma, including eyelid paralysis, chronic keratitis, or intermittent nasal or ocular discharge.
- Recurrence of retrobulbar tumors or infections is possible after primary treatment depending on the definitive diagnosis.
- For primary orbital disease, prognosis for vision is guarded initially. In severe, painful orbital disease with irreversible blindness and orbital neoplasia, the best management may be orbital exenteration.
- In a sighted eye, orbitotomy is best for discrete, solitary retrobulbar masses that do not invade the optic nerve.

• Enucleation may be recommended to remove a painful, blind, pathologic eye and its associated conjunctiva and nictitans. An intraorbital prosthesis may be placed in the orbit to replace the globe if risk of infection or tumor recurrence is low. Intrascleral prostheses are an acceptable alternative to enucleation and can be placed in an eviscerated scleral shell as long as the cornea is not severely diseased and there is no residual lagophthalmos or exophthalmos. Orbital bleeding should be minimized by careful hemostasis.
• Periorbital fractures should be repaired quickly as fibrous union can occur as soon as one week post trauma. Tarsorrhaphies are beneficial to proptosed eyes and should not be removed until most of the periorbital swelling has subsided, usually 5–7 days.

MEDICATIONS

DRUG(S) OF CHOICE

• Systemic antibiotics should be administered in cases of trauma or suspected orbital infection.
• The globe itself may benefit from topical ophthalmic lubricants or antibiotics.
• Periorbital swelling can be alleviated by judicious use of anti-inflammatories.
• Occasionally uveitis is seen with orbital trauma and should be treated with topical or systemic anti-inflammatories.
• Flunixin meglumine at a dose of 1 mg/kg IV, IM, or PO BID or phenylbutazone at a dose of 4.4–8.8 mg/kg PO once daily can be given for pain associated with the orbital disease.

CONTRAINDICATIONS

Topical steroids are contraindicated in ulcerative keratitis.

PRECAUTIONS

Long-term flunixin meglumine or phenylbutazone use may cause an ulcerative gastroenteritis.

POSSIBLE INTERACTIONS

N/A

ALTERNATE DRUGS

Intralesional iridium implants or cisplatin chemotherapy into the orbital tumor may be beneficial in some types of neoplasia.

FOLLOW-UP

• Recheck visits are indicated for more extensive diseases, especially if orbital surgery is performed as for an aggressive tumor.
• Providing a safe environment with good training may decrease the opportunity for trauma.
• Recurrence of tumor, reinfection of orbit, and persistent pain and swelling can all occur during and after the treatment period.
• Blindness and loss of eye are possible sequelae of severe orbital disease.
• Highly variable outcomes are based on correct diagnosis and appropriate treatment. Some orbital diseases such as trauma are one-time events with possible long-term side effects. Other diseases such as tumors can never be cured, only treated palliatively.

MISCELLANEOUS

SEE ALSO

• Skull fractures
• Central nervous system diseases
• Sinus and guttural pouch disorders
• Ocular neoplasia

Suggested Reading

Brooks DE. Ophthalmology for the Equine Practitioner. Jackson, WY; Teton NewMedia, 2002.
Brooks DE, Matthews AG. Equine ophthalmology. In: Gelatt KN, ed. Veterinary Ophthalmology, ed 4. Philadelphia; Lippincott Williams and Wilkins, 2007.
Gilger BC, ed. Equine Ophthalmology. Philadelphia; WB Saunders, 2005.

Author Dennis E. Brooks
Consulting Editor Dennis E. Brooks

ORGANOPHOSPHATE AND CARBAMATE TOXICOSIS

BASICS

DEFINITION

• Toxicosis caused by exposure to AChE-inhibiting OP or carbamate compounds • These compounds are active ingredients in many animal oral and topical parasiticides, as well as in numerous household and agricultural pesticide products. There are dozens of different, but structurally similar, OP and carbamate compounds with hundreds of different formulations, containing varying concentrations of active ingredient. • The toxicity among individual compounds varies tremendously. • Oral ingestion is the most common form of exposure in horses, either from ingesting pasture grass or hay where pesticide spills or drift have occurred or from overdosing with oral parasiticide products. Inhalation or dermal exposure leading to poisoning is not common but can occur. • BE CAREFUL—Not all pesticides labeled as "carbamates" inhibit AChE.

PATHOPHYSIOLOGY

• Most OP and carbamate pesticides are rapidly absorbed by the respiratory or GI systems and dermally. • Some are direct acting compounds; others require metabolic activation by the liver to a toxic metabolite. The underlying biochemical change responsible for the clinical syndrome is an inhibition of AChE activity in the nervous system resulting in accumulation of acetylcholine at synapses and myoneural junctions. Inhibition of the enzyme by OPs is considered irreversible, particularly once covalent bonding or aging has occurred. • Inhibition of the enzyme by carbamates is reversible. In order to restore AChE activity following pesticide exposure, the enzyme must either be reactivated or synthesized.

SYSTEMS AFFECTED

• Nervous and musculoskeletal—Excess acetylcholine at synapses and myoneural junctions initially excites, then paralyzes, transmission in cholinergic synapses found in the CNS and at parasympathetic and a few sympathetic nerve endings (muscarinic effects) and somatic nerves and ganglionic synapses of autonomic ganglia (nicotinic effects). • Respiratory—Buildup of secretions from the muscarinic effects can lead to respiratory difficulties, perfusion problems, and secondary bacterial invaders.

INCIDENCE/PREVALENCE

Poisonings with these compounds in horses seem to be not as common as observed in other species. However, most cases occur in the spring and summer when agricultural and household pesticide use is highest. Poisonings can occur from eating hay that was baled several months previously; any pesticide spilled or drifted onto the hay and then baled will have a slower rate of degradation, and some pesticides have been known to persist in baled hay for up to 6 mo.

SIGNALMENT

There are no breed, age, or sex predilections.

SIGNS

General Comments

There is considerable variation in clinical signs between different species of animals despite the fact that the mechanism of action is the same. In the horse, GI signs predominate and nervous signs may be absent altogether. The severity of the clinical syndrome and time to onset depend on exposure dose, route of exposure, and formulation of the pesticide product. Clinical signs can be immediate, following inhalation or oral exposure, or may be delayed by several hours (oral or dermal route).

Physical Examination

• Abdominal pain, accompanied by restlessness, anxiety, and sweating • Markedly increased intestinal sounds • Watery diarrhea • Weakness and depression • Mild to severe muscle tremors (seizures uncommon) • Tachycardia or bradycardia • Myosis or mydriasis • Dyspnea • Excessive salivation can occur.

CAUSES

Most cases of poisoning occur via ingestion of pesticide-contaminated grass or hay or from overdosing of oral parasiticide products. Horses also can be poisoned by accidental access to spilled or improperly used, stored, or discarded pesticides. Dermal and inhalation exposure can also occur.

RISK FACTORS

Some of these compounds are lipophilic and are slowly released, so animals with a lean body mass may exhibit more severe signs.

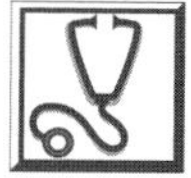

DIAGNOSIS

DIFFERENTIAL DIAGNOSIS

• Bacterial or viral gastroenteritis (physical exam, bacteriology, serology), intestinal compromise such as a twist, torsion, or intussusception (physical examination) • Peritonitis (physical examination, abdominocentesis) • Inorganic arsenic poisoning (urine, whole blood, or tissue arsenic determination)

OTHER LABORATORY TESTS

• Inhibition of blood, brain, or retinal AChE activity is suggestive of exposure, particularly if the activity is reduced to <50% of what is considered normal. Assessment of AChE activity can be done up to several days after the suspect exposure. • Carbamate binding can be reversed during sample transit to a laboratory facility so lack of enzyme inhibition does not necessarily rule out carbamate exposure. In peracute to acute, high-dose exposures, an animal may die of respiratory compromise before sufficient brain enzyme activity can be inhibited. In addition, some OPs and carbamates poorly penetrate the CNS, so that lack of brain AChE inhibition cannot totally rule out exposure to these compounds. • Tissue residue testing (liver, kidney, stomach contents, skin, fat, urine) is readily available at most diagnostic facilities and can confirm exposures.

PATHOLOGICAL FINDINGS

Visible evidence of insecticide granules in the stomach contents. Most OP and carbamate pesticides have a strong sulfur or "chemical" odor. There are no specific gross or histopathologic changes—pulmonary edema and effusions are sometimes reported.

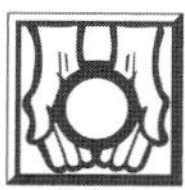

TREATMENT

APPROPRIATE HEALTH CARE

Prompt and aggressive treatment is essential to a favorable outcome. Samples of blood, urine or stomach reflux should be saved for toxicologic analysis before any specific treatments are initiated.

NURSING CARE

• Administration of IV fluids is important to correct intestinal fluid and electrolyte losses and to assist in renal excretion of the parent compound or its metabolites. Fluids should be continued until the fluid losses are under control and the horse can eat and drink on its own. • Decontamination procedures following oral exposures include administration of AC and a laxative/cathartic via stomach tube (laxatives should only be given if diarrhea is NOT present). AC is administered at 2–5 g/kg body weight (1 g AC in 5 mL water) PO. Leave in the stomach for 20–30 min and then give a laxative (e.g., mineral oil) to hasten removal of the toxicant. Alternatively, an osmotic cathartic can be given (70% sorbitol at 3 mL/kg or sodium or magnesium sulfate at 250–500 mg/kg, the latter two given in a water slurry). • Care should be used in administering laxatives or cathartics to patients who are severely dehydrated due to diarrhea, and possibly these should be avoided. For cases of dermal exposure, bathe the patient with warm soapy water and follow up with a thorough rinse.

MEDICATIONS

DRUGS OF CHOICE

• Diazepam (adults: 25–50 mg IV; foals: 0.05–0.4 mg/kg IV) can be used in those patients that are overly anxious or restless or have muscle tremors or seizures. • Atropine sulfate (0.22 mg/kg *slow* IV, remainder SQ or IM, as needed) can be used to control the muscarinic signs. Some have suggested not exceeding 65 mg atropine total in horses because of the risk of developing ileus. • Xylazine (0.3–1.1 mg/kg IV, repeat as necessary) can be used as a sedative/analgesic to control signs associated with colic but should not be used in conjunction with tranquilizers. • Butorphanol (0.1 mg/kg IV q3–4hr) is an alternative analgesic to relieve the pain associated with colic. • Pralidoxime chloride (20–35 mg/kg *slow* IV, repeat q4–6h as necessary) reactivates AChE that has been inactivated by phosphorylation secondary to most OP exposures and is most effective in controlling muscle fasciculations within the first 24 hr of exposure. Cost can be an issue in treating adult horses, but most patients require no more than 1–3 treatments.

• Bronchoconstriction, pulmonary edema, and respiratory muscle weakness may occur. In these cases, the use of a diuretic (e.g., furosemide at 0.25–1.0 mg/kg IV), a bronchodilator (e.g., aminophylline at 2–7 mg/kg POq8h) and mechanical respiratory support may be necessary.

CONTRAINDICATIONS

Phenothiazine tranquilizers may potentiate the signs associated with some OP poisonings.

PRECAUTIONS

Avoid overzealous use of atropine and aminophylline.

POSSIBLE INTERACTIONS

The use of OP anthelmintics in the horse may potentiate the action of succinylcholine chloride for up to 1 mo after administration of the OP.

FOLLOW-UP

PATIENT MONITORING

Continuously monitor heart rate and rhythm, respiratory system, urination, defecation, and hydration and electrolyte status.

PREVENTION/AVOIDANCE

Care should be taken to read the label carefully on all products containing OPs and carbamates. Make sure they are used, stored and disposed of in the appropriate manner.

POSSIBLE COMPLICATIONS

An intermediate syndrome has been described in animals where muscle weakness occurs several days after the pesticide exposure. Delayed neuropathy may occur following some OP exposures but this is not common. Bilateral laryngeal paralysis has been reported to occur in foals after dosing with an OP anthelmintic.

EXPECTED COURSE AND PROGNOSIS

Good in horses that have received prompt and aggressive therapy. Most animals recover uneventfully over a period of 24–48 hr.

MISCELLANEOUS

ASSOCIATED CONDITIONS, AGE-RELATED FACTORS, ZOONOTIC POTENTIAL, PREGNANCY

N/A

ABBREVIATIONS

• AC = activated charcoal • AChE = acetylcholinesterase • CNS = central nervous system • GI = gastrointestinal • OP = organophosphate

Suggested Reading

Anticholinesterase insecticides. In: KH Plumlee, ed. Clinical Veterinary Toxicology. St. Louis: Mosby, 2003:178–180.

Organophosphorus compounds and carbamates. In: Radostits OM, Blood DC, Gay CC, eds. Veterinary Medicine: A Textbook of the Diseases of Cattle, Sheep, Pigs, Goats and Horses. Philadelphia: Bailliere Tindall, 1994:1514–1517.

Author Patricia A. Talcott

Consulting Editor Robert H. Poppenga

OSMOLALITY, HYPEROSMOLALITY

BASICS

DEFINITION

- Osmolality (mOsm/kg) represents the number of solute particles per kilogram of solvent (e.g., the concentration of a solution expressed as mOsm/kg).
- Osmolality is a thermodynamically more precise term than osmolarity, because it is based on weight, which is temperature independent, versus volume (i.e., osmolarity), which is temperature dependent.
- Osmolarity (mOsm/L) represents the number of solute particles per liter of solvent (e.g., the concentration of a solution expressed as mOsm/L).
- Osmotic pressure governs the movement of water across membranes because of differences in solute content.
- Hyperosmolarity and hyperosmolality are defined in horses as serum concentrations >270–300 mOsm/L or >270–300 mOsm/kg.
- One osmole is the gram molecular weight of a nondissociable substance and contains Avogadro's number of particles.
- A solvent is a liquid holding another substance in solution; for osmolality, this would be water.
- A solute is the dissolved substance in the solution.
- A solution, in this discussion, contains solutes within a solvent.

PATHOPHYSIOLOGY

- In serum/plasma, Na^+ is primarily responsible for osmotically active particles, as well as associated Cl^- and HCO_3^-, with lesser contributions by glucose and urea.
- Anything causing water loss increases the concentrations of solutes in plasma/serum, thereby increasing serum osmolality.
- Dissolved particles that cannot move between adjacent compartments exert osmotic pressure and cause water to move to dilute differences in solute concentrations between compartments.
- Serum osmolality is a measure of ECF osmolality but is not a measure of total body water. The ECF compartment comprises one-third of total body weight, with the remaining two-thirds in the ICF compartment.
- The osmolalities of ICF and ECF are equal, but the ionic compositions differ. ECF is primarily Na^+ and Cl^-, with small concentrations of HCO_3^-, K^+, phosphate, Ca^{2+}, and Mg^{2+}, whereas ICF is high in K^+ and phosphate, with lower concentrations of Na^+, Cl^-, and Ca^{2+}.
- Blood volume, hydration status, and ADH are involved in controlling the ECF volume. Low circulating blood volume stimulates carotid and aortic baroreceptors to respond to changes in blood pressure, causing ADH secretion.
- Hyperosmolality affects osmoreceptors in the hypothalamus and stimulates ADH secretion from the neurohypophysis. The kidney's ability to produce urine of various concentrations maintains body regulation of osmolality. The hypothalamic thirst center also is stimulated and causes an increase in water consumption to counteract serum hyperosmolality. Therefore, regulation is by modifying water loss in urine or water intake.
- Rapid increases in serum osmolality cause water movement along its concentration gradient, from ICF to ECF spaces, resulting in neuronal dehydration, cell shrinkage, and cell death.
- Hypo-osmolality is associated with hyponatremia.

SYSTEMS AFFECTED

- Nervous—because of fluid shifts (changes in neuronal volume–brain swelling)
- Cardiovascular—hypotension and depressed ventricular contractility
- Renal/urologic—low urine output

GENETICS

N/A

INCIDENCE/PREVALENCE

N/A

GEOGRAPHIC DISTRIBUTION

N/A

SIGNALMENT

Any age

SIGNS

General Comments

- Excessive thirst may be the first sign of hyperosmolality.
- Signs are primarily neurologic and behavioral.
- Severity of signs relates more to how quickly hyperosmolality occurs rather than to the absolute magnitude of change.
- Signs are most likely to develop with serum osmolality >350 mOsm/kg, and they usually are severe if >375 mOsm/kg.

Historical

- Anorexia
- Lethargy
- Vomiting
- Weakness
- Disorientation
- Ataxia
- Seizures
- Coma
- Polydipsia, followed by hypodipsia

Physical Examination

- Abnormalities reflect the underlying disease.
- Dehydration, tachycardia, hypotension, weak pulse, and fever may be present.

CAUSES

- Increased solutes—hypernatremia; hyperglycemia; severe azotemia; ethylene glycol toxicosis (potential); propylene glycol toxicosis; salt poisoning; shock; administration of ethanol, mannitol, radiographic contrast solution, and parenteral nutrition solutions; lactate in patients with lactic acidosis; and acetoacetate and β-hydroxybutyrate ketones (rare in horses)
- Decreased ECF volume—dehydration (e.g., GI loss, cutaneous loss, third-space loss, low water consumption) and polyuria without adequate compensatory polydipsia

RISK FACTORS

- Predisposing medical conditions—renal failure, diabetes insipidus, diabetes mellitus, hyperadrenocorticism, hyperaldosteronism, and heat stroke
- Therapeutic hyperosmolar solutions—hypertonic saline, sodium bicarbonate, and mannitol
- High environmental temperatures
- Fever
- Limited access to water

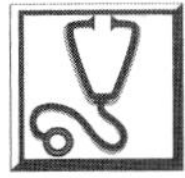

DIAGNOSIS

DIFFERENTIAL DIAGNOSIS

- Primary CNS disease from a variety of causes—neoplasia, inflammation, or trauma; serum osmolality usually is normal.
- Assess hydration status, and obtain information regarding previous treatment that may have included sodium-containing fluids or hyperosmolar solutions.

CBC/BIOCHEMISTRY/URINALYSIS

- High PCV, hemoglobin, and plasma proteins in dehydrated patients; serum electrolytes also may be high.
- Hyperosmolality is an indication to evaluate serum sodium, BUN, and glucose concentrations. Estimated serum osmolality can be calculated from serum biochemistries as $2(\text{Na}) + \text{BUN}/2.8 + \text{glucose}/18$. Sodium concentration provides an estimate of the total electrolyte concentrations and, thus, is multiplied by two. The remaining calculation is to convert concentrations into mmol/L; therefore, BUN is divided by 2.8 and glucose by 18.
- Normally, measured osmolality should not exceed the calculated osmolality by more than 10 mOsm/kg. If it does, calculate the osmolar gap (i.e., measured osmolality-calculated osmolality).

• High measured osmolality with a high osmolar gap indicates the presence of unmeasured solutes—not Na^+, K^+, glucose, or BUN.
• High measured osmolality and high calculated osmolality with a normal osmolar gap usually indicate that hyperosmolality results from measured solutes—Na^+, K^+, glucose, or BUN
• Serum sodium may be low in patients with severe hyperglycemia and hyperosmolality.
• Fasting hyperglycemia and glucosuria support a diagnosis of diabetes mellitus.
• Numerous calcium oxalate monohydrate crystals in urine suggest ethylene glycol toxicosis, but this is not well documented in horses.
• High urine specific gravity rules out diabetes insipidus; low urine specific gravity, especially hyposthenuria, suggests diabetes insipidus.

OTHER LABORATORY TESTS

Urine osmolality less than serum osmolality suggests diabetes insipidus, whereas concentrated urine rules out diabetes insipidus.

IMAGING

Renal ultrasonography may differentiate renal disease.

OTHER DIAGNOSTIC PROCEDURES

N/A

PATHOLOGICAL FINDINGS

Dependent on cause

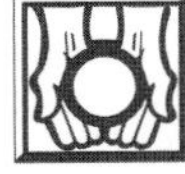

TREATMENT

AIMS OF TREATMENT

Correction of hyperosmolality

APPROPRIATE HEALTH CARE

• Mild hyperosmolality without clinical signs may not warrant specific treatment; however, any underlying diseases should be diagnosed and treated.
• Patients with moderate to high osmolality (>350 mOsm/kg) or exhibiting clinical signs should be hospitalized and their serum osmolality gradually lowered with IV fluid administration while a definitive diagnosis is pursued.

NURSING CARE

• D_5 W or 0.45% saline should be administered slowly IV.
• Initially, 0.9% saline may be used to restore normal hemodynamics and to replace dehydration deficits.

ACTIVITY

N/A

DIET

N/A

CLIENT EDUCATION

Dependent on cause and prognosis

SURGICAL CONSIDERATIONS

N/A

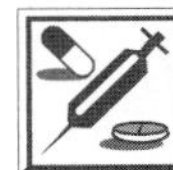

MEDICATIONS

DRUG(S) OF CHOICE

Seizures can be controlled with appropriate anticonvulsants.

CONTRAINDICATIONS

Hypertonic saline and hyperosmolar solutions

PRECAUTIONS

• Normal saline may be used initially, but rapid administration may worsen neurologic signs.
• Rapid administration of hypotonic fluids (e.g., D_5 W, 0.45% saline) also may cause cerebral edema and worsen neurologic signs.

POSSIBLE INTERACTIONS

N/A

ALTERNATIVE DRUGS

N/A

FOLLOW-UP

PATIENT MONITORING

• Monitor hydration status; avoid overhydration.
• Monitor urine output and breathing patterns during IV fluid administration.
• Anuria and irregular breathing patterns may be signs of deterioration.
• Monitor mentation and behavior.

PREVENTION/AVOIDANCE

N/A

POSSIBLE COMPLICATIONS

Altered consciousness and abnormal behavior

EXPECTED COURSE AND PROGNOSIS

Dependent on cause

MISCELLANEOUS

ASSOCIATED CONDITIONS

• Azotemia
• Hyperglycemia
• Hypernatremia

AGE-RELATED FACTORS

N/A

ZOONOTIC POTENTIAL

N/A

PREGNANCY

N/A

SYNONYM

Hyperosmolarity

SEE ALSO

• Diabetes mellitus
• Glucose, hyperglycemia
• Sodium, hypernatremia

ABBREVIATIONS

• ADH = antidiurectic hormone
• ECF = extracellular fluid
• GI = gastrointestinal
• ICF = intracellular fluid
• PCV = packed cell volume

Suggested Reading

Carlson GP. Fluid, electrolyte, and acid-balance. In: Kaneko JJ, Harvey JW, Bruss ML, eds. Clinical Biochemistry of Domestic Animals. San Diego: Academic Press, 1997:512–513.

DiBartola SP, Green RA, Autran de Morais HS. Osmolarity and osmolar gap. In: Willard MD, Tvedten H, Turnwald GH, eds. Small Animal Clinical Diagnosis by Laboratory Methods, ed 2. Philadelphia: WB Saunders, 1994:106–107.

Johnson PJ. Physiology of body fluids in the horse. Vet Clin North Am Equine Pract 1998;14:1–22.

Author Claire B. Andreasen
Consulting Editor Kenneth W. Hinchcliff

OSTEOARTHRITIS

BASICS

DEFINITION

Progressive deterioration and nonseptic inflammation of the articular cartilage accompanied by changes in the soft tissues and bone of the joint

PATHOPHYSIOLOGY

• Abnormal forces, such as repetitive trauma, overwhelm the normal metabolic repair functions of the joint. This leads to a net cartilage matrix loss and chondromalacia. Unchecked, this cycle creates further damage and loss of the viscoelastic properties of the remaining cartilage. • Synovitis results from biomechanical damage and is often part of the disease process of OA. The inflamed synovium contributes a variety of inflammatory mediators and degradative enzymes (prostaglandins such as prostaglandin E_2, cytokines such as interleukin-1, and matrix-degrading enzymes such as matrix metalloproteinases). The viscous shock-absorbing and lubricating synovial fluid, rich in hyaluronan, loses viscosity in this inflammatory milieu, reducing its protective abilities. • The subchondral bone plate provides shock absorption. It remodels and becomes less compliant if repetitive trauma overwhelms its ability to heal microdamage normally. The stiffer subchondral bone offers less shock absorption to the articular cartilage, further traumatizing it. • In addition to cartilage thinning and joint capsule thickening, remodeling occurs within the joint. Osteophytes are formed at the articular cartilage margins. These fibrocartilage-covered bony outgrowths can fracture to become osteochondral fragments (chip fractures). Presence of the fragments free in the joint can increase the inflammatory process within the joint.

SYSTEM AFFECTED

Musculoskeletal—diarthrodial joints

GENETICS

None elucidated

INCIDENCE/PREVALENCE

Undefined, lameness to joint disease is the most significant factor responsible for loss of racehorses' performance.

GEOGRAPHIC DISTRIBUTION

N/A

SIGNALMENT

• No breed predilection other than some breeds are more likely to be trained in a way that overwhelms repair mechanisms, e. g., Thoroughbreds in race training. • Young horses undergoing training can develop OA. The chronic, progressive nature of the disease means that it can affect horses of all ages.
• No sex predilection

SIGNS

General

The hallmark of OA is the degeneration of articular cartilage, a process occurring in a tissue devoid of innervation. Lameness is generally attributed to the involvement of periarticular soft tissue structures. Pain originating from subchondral bone changes is controversial at present.

Historical

• Intra-articular fractures, previous septic arthritis, osteochondrosis, dislocation, or ligamentous damage can predispose a joint to OA. • Low-motion joints such as the distal intertarsal and tarsometatarsal joints may have insidious onset OA-related lameness. High-motion joints, like the fetlock, are more likely to have acute onset lameness. • Horses often have a history of becoming less lame after a period of rest.

Physical Examination

• Lameness at high speeds, but also evident at a walk in severe cases • Lameness is rarely acute and severe in onset. • Pain on flexion
• Synovial effusion will be present depending on the location. For example, joint effusion is a common finding in fetlock OA but in the small joints of the distal tarsus this would not be a clinical feature. • Acute synovitis will cause the joint to be warm to the touch, but periarticular swelling and edema are not a feature of noninfectious arthritis. • Chronic OA joints will have thickened joint capsules and a reduced range of motion. Crepitation can be appreciated upon palpation. The joint will be grossly thickened and may have palpable bony abnormalities.

CAUSES

The exact cause of OA is unknown. It is a combination of traumatic events that involve the soft tissue, bone, and cartilage of diarthrodial joints.

RISK FACTORS

• Poor limb conformations that increase joint stress, collateral ligament strain, or even weight bearing are considered risk factors. For example carpal varus or flexural tendon laxity ("back-at-the-knees"). • Intense high-speed training is a risk factor.

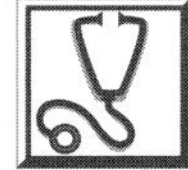

DIAGNOSIS

DIFFERENTIAL DIAGNOSIS

• Septic arthritis should always be ruled out in cases of joint swelling and acute lameness. Joint fluid analysis is helpful to rule out sepsis.
• In young horses with joint effusion, osteochondrosis should be ruled out with radiography.

CBC/BIOCHEMISTRY/URINALYSIS

For research purposes only, urine excretion of various "joint markers" have been studied. Their clinical application remains uncertain.

OTHER LABORATORY TESTS

• Analysis of synovial fluid protein content or nucleated cell counts is unremarkable compared to normal joints. • +/− Reduced joint viscosity

IMAGING

• Good-quality radiographs remain the mainstay of OA diagnosis. Standard four views should always be use. Flexed lateral views should be included for carpi and fetlocks. For changes on the dorsal articular margins of the carpal bones dorsal, proximal to dorsal-distal (skyline) views should be included.
• Radiographic changes include:
  ○ Narrowing or loss of joint space
  ○ Marginal osteophyte formation or fragmentation
  ○ Periosteal bone proliferation
  ○ Subchondral bone sclerosis
  ○ +/− Ankylosis
  ○ Osteolysis is a feature of OA of the distal intertarsal or tarsometatarsal joints.
• It is important to remember that radiological findings of OA alone do not mean that the lameness is arising from the abnormal joint. Further diagnostic procedures are necessary.
• Nuclear scintigraphy can be helpful if lesions are metabolically active. In the case of subchondral bone disease, it is the diagnostic tool of choice. Abnormalities include generalized increased radiopharmaceutical uptake associated with affected joint and/or focal increased radiopharmaceutical uptake associated with the affected subchondral bone.
• Diagnostic arthroscopy can be used to directly view the articular cartilage. This is important since cartilage damage cannot be seen on radiographs, and evaluation of articular damage has prognostic relevance.
• MRI is a useful modality to clearly see pathological changes in articular cartilage, subchondral bone, and periarticular soft tissue structures. Currently, good-quality images are best acquired with stationary magnets, thereby requiring general anesthesia and specialist equipment. This modality is not yet commonplace but nevertheless available for horses.

OTHER DIAGNOSTIC PROCEDURES

Perineural and /or intra-articular anesthesia are the gold standard to localize pain causing lameness.

PATHOLOGICAL FINDINGS

• Articular cartilage thinning, erosion, fibrillation, and scoring • Osteophyte and enthesiophyte formation • Reduced synovial fluid viscosity • Subchondral bone sclerosis

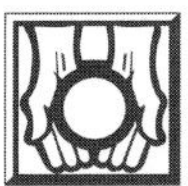

TREATMENT

AIMS OF TREATMENT

Reduce inflammation in the joint and facilitate restoration of joint homeostasis.

APPROPRIATE HEALTH CARE

• The mainstay of treatment is early recognition and medical management. • Numerous medications and combinations of medications are used. Decisions regarding treatment are multifactorial and may include the specific joint, stage of OA, performance type, treatment costs, response to therapy, and regulations regarding medication use in competition. • Cartilage resurfacing techniques are in advanced experimental stages and are available at certain university teaching hospitals for clinical cases. They may play a role in OA management in the future.

NURSING CARE

• +/– Local cryotherapy (ice, cold water) during acute phases of inflammation and joint swelling • +/– Passive motion (flexion) in the immediate postoperative period

ACTIVITY

• Reduce activity to reduce repetitive injury to the joint. • In well-trained horses, maintaining cardiovascular fitness while sparing the joints can be achieved with swimming. This is not a substitute and should be carefully considered and integrated into a horse's program by experienced professionals.

DIET

Diet is only relevant in the prevention of osteochondrosis, which is a predisposing factor for OA.

CLIENT EDUCATION

Valuable in terms of monitoring lameness, watching for signs of OA exacerbation and the judicious use of intra-articular corticosteroids

SURGICAL CONSIDERATIONS

• Arthroscopic surgery is essential for the treatment of loose osteochondral fragments and can be helpful in severe joints where removal of damaged cartilage and forage of subchondral bone can encourage fibrocartilage healing of defects. • In end-stage OA joints, surgical arthrodesis techniques can prolong the horse's activity and comfort level.

MEDICATIONS

DRUG(S) OF CHOICE

• There is no one drug of choice. • Systemic NSAIDs, such as phenylbutazone (2.2 mg/kg daily to BID) and flunixin meglumine (0.5 mg/kg daily to BID). Daily oral phenylbutazone can be used long term. Side effects may include gastric ulceration, right dorsal colitis, and renal papillary necrosis. • Intra-articular HA—10–20 mg of high molecular weight (>1 × 10^6 Daltons) • Intravenous HA—40 mg daily q14–28days, as needed • Intramuscular polysulfated glycosaminoglycan—500 mg every 5 days for 5 treatments • Intra-articular corticosteroids make up the mainstay of intra-articular anti-inflammatory drug use. They are powerful anti-inflammatory agents but have deleterious effects on articular cartilage and should be used with care. This effect is dose dependent. Magnitude and clinical effects vary between drugs and between cases. Commonly used drugs and doses include betamethasone sulfate (3–18 mg/joint), triamcinolone acetate (6–18 mg/joint), and methylprednisolone acetate (20–40 mg/joint). • In high-motion joints, it is generally accepted to try to use a short-acting drug such as betamethasone or triamcinolone. • In low-motion joints where facilitated ankylosis is desirable, such as the distal intertarsal and tarsometatarsal joints, longer-acting drugs are desirable such as methylprednisolone acetate. • Corticosteroids and HA are often injected intra-articularly simultaneously. • IRAP is now available for clinical use. A kit is obtained and IRAP is purified from a sample of the horse's blood. It can be aliquoted and used fresh or stored frozen. The exact efficacy of this technique is yet to be defined.

CONTRAINDICATIONS

• Do not use NSAIDs in dehydrated horses. • In horses with laminitis, intra-articular corticosteroids may exacerbate their laminitis.

PRECAUTIONS

• Strict aseptic technique should be used for all joint injections. • Some practitioners use 125 mg of amikacin sulfate in each intra-articular injection to reduce the risk of iatrogenic sepsis. • Patient sedation and adequate restraint are critical to successful injection. • Horses are generally given a few days of NSAID therapy and rest after a joint injection. • Where possible, joints are bandaged after intra-articular medication to prevent surface contamination. • Frequent repetition of intra-articular corticosteroid medication can cause cartilage thinning and damage.

ALTERNATIVE DRUGS

Oral nutraceuticals that contain chondroitin sulfate and glucosamine are marketed. There is limited evidence to suggest that they may help OA in horses. Further studies are required.

FOLLOW-UP

PATIENT MONITORING

• Following an intra-articular injection the horse should be monitored for any signs of increased lameness or inflammation in that joint due to iatrogenic introduction of bacteria. In joints that have been treated with corticosteroids, their potent anti-inflammatory effect can delay this process by up to 21 days. • Periodic lameness and radiographic evaluations are performed to assess progression of OA.

POSSIBLE COMPLICATIONS

• "Joint flare" can be seen after intra-articular injections. It should be distinguished from iatrogenic joint sepsis and treated with ice and NSAID therapy. The use of high quality HA can reduce this chance. • Corticosteroids can cause laminitis in horses. The exact dose or mechanism is not understood.

EXPECTED COURSE AND PROGNOSIS

• OA may progress as part of the aging process, especially horses in work or horses that have joints medicated with corticosteroids repeatedly. • Prognosis is extremely variable and depends on the location and severity of OA, use of the horse, and duration of clinical signs. Horses with mild OA in a low-motion joint such as a tarsometatarsal joint may respond favorably to treatment and maintain performance for years. Horses with severe OA in a high-motion joint such as a metacarpophalangeal joint often respond poorly to therapy and may be candidates for arthrodesis.

MISCELLANEOUS

ASSOCIATED CONDITIONS

N/A

ZOONOTIC POTENTIAL

None

PREGNANCY

N/A

SYNONYMS

• Osteoarthrosis • Degenerative joint disease • Arthritis

SEE ALSO

Infectious arthritis

ABBREVIATIONS

• HA = hyaluronic acid
• IRAP = interleukin receptor antagonist protein
• OA = osteoarthritis

Suggested Reading

Caron JP. Osteoarthritis. In: Ross MW, Dyson SJ, eds. Diagnosis and Management of Lameness in the Horse. St. Louis: Saunders, 2003:572–591.

Caron JP, Genovese RL. Principles and practices of joint disease treatment. In: Ross MW, Dyson SJ, eds. Diagnosis and Management of Lameness in the Horse. St. Louis: Saunders, 2003:746–764.

Frisbie DD. Synovial joint pathobiology and principles of treatment of joint disease. In: Auer JA, Stick JA, eds. Equine Surgery, ed 3. St. Louis: Saunders, 2006:1035–1073.

Goodrich LR, Nixon AJ. Medical treatment of osteoarthritis in the horse—a review. Vet J 2006;171:61–69.

McIlWraith CW, Trotter GW, eds. Joint Disease in the Horse. Philadelphia: Saunders, 1996.

Author Emma Adam
Consulting Editor Elizabeth J. Davidson

OSTEOCHONDROSIS

BASICS

DEFINITION

• Developmental disorder of bone and cartilage of unspecified etiology resulting in failure of endochondral ossification • The term OCD is generally reserved for a detachment or "flap" of abnormal cartilage, or cartilage and bone, from the surrounding tissue.

PATHOPHYSIOLOGY

• Failure of normal endochondral ossification results in thickening and retention of the hypertrophic zone of the growth cartilage. When this affects the articular-epiphyseal cartilage, the disorder can manifest either as a flap or fragment(s) of cartilage or cartilage and bone (OCD), or infolding of defective cartilage and formation of periarticular SBC. • These lesions may be precipitated by abnormal chondrocyte structure or function, abnormal extracellular matrix production, or a vascular disorder.
• What determines whether osteochondrosis results in the development of OCD or SBC is not fully understood. High-motion areas may subject the articular surface to shear forces predisposing to OCD, whereas SBCs tend to be located in areas of maximal compressive loads (i.e., maximal weight bearing). • Trauma leading to subchondral bone microfracture and necrosis, followed by cystic resorption and collapse of overlying articular cartilage, may also be part of the pathogenesis of SBC. • Full-thickness, linear defects in the articular cartilage at the points of maximal weight bearing can lead to SBC development.

SYSTEM AFFECTED

Musculoskeletal—epiphyseal cartilage and bone

GENETICS

• Although certain genetic lines have been shown to have a high heritability of osteochondrosis lesions, a specific genetic defect responsible for alteration of endochondral ossification has not yet been identified. • In Scandinavian Standardbred populations, heritability of tarsocrural osteochondrosis ranges from 0.24 to 0.52.

INCIDENCE/PREVALENCE

Unknown

GEOGRAPHIC DISTRIBUTION

Worldwide

SIGNALMENT

Breed Predilection

Although any breed can be affected, osteochondrosis is common in Standardbred, Thoroughbred, and Warmblood breeds.

Mean Age and Range

Commonly becomes clinically apparent in yearlings or weanlings with a range from neonates to 3 years of age, although it can occur at any time during bone development

Predominant Sex

None

SIGNS

General Comments

• Depends on its location, variable clinical signs, and physical examination findings
• Frequently bilateral with reported incidences between 45% and 60% • Type and location of osteochondrosis:
  - Tarsus (tarsocrural joint)—cranial distal intermediate ridge of the tibia, lateral trochlear ridge of the talus, medial malleolus of the tibia, lateral malleolus of the tibia, medial trochlear ridge of the talus
  - Stifle—lateral trochlear ridge of the femur, medial distal femoral condyle (SBC). Other locations are possible, albeit rare.
  - Fetlock—distal dorsal sagittal ridge of MCIII/MTIII, proximal palmar/plantar eminence of P1, proximal dorsal P1, distal MCIII/MTIII (SBC)
  - Shoulder—humeral head (OCD or SBC), distal scapula (SBC)
  - Other locations include proximal and distal P1, proximal and distal P2, proximal and distal radius, distal humerus, and distal tibia. These are infrequent and usually SBCs.
  - OCD also affects the cervical vertebral articular facets and is one of the recognized causes of cervical vertebral instability or stenosis in young horses ("Wobbler's syndrome").

Historical

• Variable findings depending on location; classically joint effusion without lameness
• Tarsus—mild to severe joint effusion without lameness • Stifle—mild to severe joint effusion (OCD lateral trochlear ridge), mild to no joint effusion (SBC of distal femur); mild to severe lameness • Fetlock—mild to moderate lameness and joint effusion • Shoulder—mild to severe lameness

Physical Examination

• Variable findings depending on location
• Tarsus—mild to severe joint effusion without lameness • Stifle—absent to severe joint effusion, mild to severe lameness, +/− muscle atrophy
• Fetlock—joint effusion, absent to moderate lameness • Shoulder—shortened cranial phase of the stride, scuffed toe, muscle atrophy

CAUSES

Developmental osteochondrosis has a complex, multifactorial etiology that is still incompletely understood. However, several factors have been identified as having a direct effect on its development.

Growth Rate

Rapid growth rate

Dietary Factors

• High carbohydrate load • Extremely low copper or excessive zinc levels • +/− Overfeeding phosphorus and calcium

Genetics

• A specific genetic defect responsible for alteration of endochondral ossification has not yet been identified, although it is highly suspected in certain breeding lines. • Heritability of a predisposition for fast growth and larger skeletal size might be the most important factor.

Trauma

• Trauma alone may not be the sole primary factor, but in susceptible cartilage may be the necessary contributing factor. • There seem to be time-dependent windows of vulnerability to trauma for growth cartilages in specific locations.

RISK FACTORS

See Causes

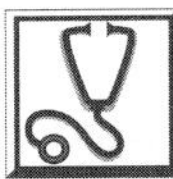

DIAGNOSIS

DIFFERENTIAL DIAGNOSIS

• Nonseptic synovitis—Rule out with radiography. • Septic synovitis—Rule out with radiography and synovial analysis.
• Osteomyelitis—Rule out with serial radiography and culture. • Traumatic fracture—Rule out with radiography and histology.

IMAGING

Radiography

• Subchondral radiolucency along an articular margin • Osseous fragment(s) separated from subchondral bone by a radiolucent area
• SBC—round subchondral radiolucency, often articular • In most instances, this modality will provide a definitive diagnosis. • Important to image contralateral joint

Nuclear Scintigraphy

Increased radiopharmaceutical uptake (SBC) but often normal with OCD

CT/MRI

In rare cases, occult SBCs can only be identified with these two modalities.

Ultrasound

Can be helpful for osteochondrosis of the cervical articular facets

OTHER DIAGNOSTIC PROCEDURE

Synovial fluid analysis and culture—to differentiate from septic arthritis

PATHOLOGICAL FINDINGS

Histology—persistence of chondrocytes in the mid-to-late hypertrophic zone, with failure of vascular invasion and subsequent osteogenesis resulting in retained cartilage cores

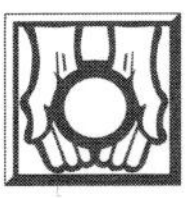

TREATMENT

AIMS OF TREATMENT

• Reduce or eliminate joint effusion • Avoid the development of or reduce or eliminate lameness
• Eliminate lesion as part of presale

APPROPRIATE HEALTH CARE

• No treatment when identified as an incidental finding or without active clinical signs • In young animals (foals, weanlings), conservative management via exercise restriction, anti-inflammatory medications, and diet modification for 6–10 mo can be useful.

NURSING CARE

Postoperative care—Surgical incisions are kept clean and bandaged until suture removal 10–14 days after surgery. Bandages are replaced and incisions inspected every 2–3 days or more often if wet, soiled, or dislodged. In areas where conventional bandaging is difficult or impossible, no bandage or an adhesive iodinated dressing is used.

ACTIVITY

• After surgery, stall confinement and controlled exercise program: The length of stall confinement and exercise restriction will vary depending on the severity and/or location of the lesion. In general, 2 weeks of strict stall rest followed by 4–8 weeks of stall rest with hand walking exercise. Then, limited turn-out in a small paddock for 4–6 weeks followed by another 4–6 weeks of regular paddock turnout. Horses with SBCs may require 6–12 mo of rest and controlled exercise before initiating or returning to regular training exercise. • Patients managed conservatively may also be managed with stall confinement and a controlled exercise program. Type and duration will depend on the location of the lesion.

DIET

• Foals and yearlings should not be fed in groups, since the more dominant individuals will consume more, leading to excessive energy (carbohydrate/protein) intake. • In young horses (weanlings to 2, year, olds) that are either at risk or identified as developing osteochondrosis, decrease or eliminate high-energy hay, such as alfalfa, and high-energy concentrate, such as 14% protein. • Mild to moderate caloric reduction of intake while stall confined or resting

CLIENT EDUCATION

• Avoid feeding high-energy feeds, which can lead to excessive rapid growth and secondary osteochondrosis development. • Breeders should monitor sires and mares suspect of yielding offspring with osteochondrosis. • Any young horse with persistent joint effusion should be fully evaluated, including with radiography. Horses with OCD and SBC that are identified and treated early may be athletic; however, if unrecognized, osteoarthritis and lameness may develop.

SURGICAL CONSIDERATIONS

• Arthroscopic removal of OCD lesions and debridement of SBC is the mainstay of treatment in clinically affected horses. • Specific surgical treatment based on location:
  ○ Tarsal lesions—arthroscopic removal
  ○ Stifle lesions—OCD: arthroscopic removal; SBC: arthroscopic debridement, mosaicoplasty, intralesional corticosteroids
  ○ Fetlock lesions—arthroscopic removal for articular lesions, routine removal for nonarticular lesions
  ○ Shoulder lesions—arthroscopic debridement and/or removal
  ○ Cervical facet lesions—ventral cervical vertebral stabilization using stainless steel basket filled with cancellous bone

• SBCs in locations not reachable arthroscopically may be debrided using osteostixis (forage) via an extra-articular approach +/− intralesional cancellous bone graft or corticosteroids.

MEDICATIONS

DRUG(S) OF CHOICE

• NSAIDs such as phenylbutazone (2.2–4.4 mg/kg PO or IV daily to BID) or flunixin meglumine (1.1 mg/kg PO or IV daily to BID) for affected horses treated both medically or surgically • For SBCs, intralesional corticosteroids—methylprednisolone acetate (20–40 mg) or triamcinolone (3–6 mg)

CONTRAINDICATIONS

In immature horses, oral and intravenous administration of fluoroquinilones may increase the incidence and severity of osteochondrosis.

PRECAUTIONS

NSAIDs can be ulcerogenic and nephrotoxic, especially in young patients and/or with chronic use.

FOLLOW-UP

PATIENT MONITORING

Radiographic Evaluation

• Provides an objective assessment of the progression of the condition • In horses managed surgically, radiographs are obtained immediately following surgery. Depending on the severity of the condition, additional radiographs may be obtained 2 and 6 mo following surgery. • In horses treated conservatively, radiographic evaluation in 6- to 8-week intervals is recommended.

Lameness Examination

• Should be performed on a regular basis in horses treated conservatively in order to assess response to treatment • In horses treated surgically, it should be performed once the patient is ready to begin controlled exercise, which can be anywhere from 3 to 12 mo.

PREVENTION/AVOIDANCE

• Diet modification in young horses at risk
• Caution when selecting for certain breeding lines

POSSIBLE COMPLICATIONS

• Lameness • Osteoarthritis • In horses intended to be sold, osteochondrosis may negatively affect the sale.

EXPECTED COURSE AND PROGNOSS

• Clinical signs become apparent in 1- to 3-year–olds. • In general, arthroscopic removal of OCD lesions is favorable. • SBCs have a less favorable prognosis and are more likely to develop arthritis with or without treatment.
• Joint effusion improves but may not resolve after surgery. • Prognosis depends on location and type of lesion:
  ○ Tarsus—Prognosis is favorable in most cases, particularly single lesions that are removed before lameness develops. Lesions involving the majority of the lateral trochlear ridge of the talus have the least favorable prognosis for racing soundness.
  ○ Stifle—Prognosis for OCD of the lateral trochlear ridge of the femur is fair to good depending on the size of the lesion. Prognosis is less favorable with extensive and/or bilateral disease. Young horses with SBC of the medial femoral condyle managed surgically have a fair to good prognosis. Horses with SBCs treated conservatively (i.e., rest for 6–12 mo with or without intra-articular corticosteroids) have a fair prognosis. Older horses (7- to 10-year-olds) with SBCs have a poor prognosis.
  ○ Fetlock—Depending on the degree of pathology and secondary degenerative changes, prognosis is fair to good for racehorses and very good to excellent in nonracehorses. Palmar/plantar eminence PI lesions have a good prognosis. Sagittal ridge lesions have a fair to good prognosis. Horses with SBCs have a similar prognosis as for SBC of the medial femoral condyle of the femur.
  ○ Shoulder—Prognosis is guarded at best for athletic use +/− surgical management.
  ○ The prognosis for osteochondrosis in other joints will vary depending on location, size, and concurrent degenerative changes.

MISCELLANEOUS

ASSOCIATED CONDITIONS

• Osteoarthritis • Cervical vertebral malformation with cervical osteochondrosis

AGE-RELATED FACTORS

Clinical signs apparent in young animal

PREGNANCY

None

SYNONYMS

• Osteochondritis • Osteochondritis dissecans

SEE ALSO

• Equine protozoal myeloencephalitis
• Infectious arthritis • Osteoarthritis • Cervical vertebral malformation

ABBREVIATIONS

• MCIII = third metacarpal bone • MTIII = third metatarsal bone • OCD = osteochondrosis dissecans • PI = first phalanx
• SBC = subchondral bone cyst

Suggested Reading

Douglas J. Pathogenesis of osteochondrosis. In: Ross MW, Dyson SJ, eds. Diagnosis and Management of Lameness in the Horse. Philadelphia: Saunders, 2003:534–543.

Van Weeren PR. Osteochondrosis. In: Auer JA, Stick JA, eds. Equine Surgery, ed 3. Philadelphia: Saunders, 2006:1166–1177.

Von Rechenberg B, Auer JA. Subchondral cystic lesions. In: Auer JA, Stick JA, eds. Equine Surgery, ed 3. Philadelphia: Saunders, 2006:1178–1183.

Author José M. García-López
Consulting Editor Elizabeth J. Davidson

OVULATION FAILURE

BASICS

DEFINITION/OVERVIEW

The ovulatory follicle in a mare is generally ≥35 mm in diameter. Follicles that obtain that size, but fail to ovulate, are addressed.

ETIOLOGY/PATHOPHYSIOLOGY

- During diestrus, waves or "clutches" of oocytes are recruited for development into antral follicles.
- Ultimately, one or two follicles become dominant and progress to ovulation, while the remaining follicles undergo atresia. The mechanism for this selection is not well understood.
- Estradiol (follicular origin) stimulates an increase in LH secretion (pituitary origin) that ultimately induces ovulation.
  - The LH rise in mares is prolonged compared to other species.
  - Deficiencies of either follicular estradiol or pituitary LH secretion can contribute to ovulation failure.

SYSTEM AFFECTED

Reproductive

GENETICS

N/A

INCIDENCE/PREVALENCE

N/A

SIGNALMENT

- Mares of any breed and age
- Multiple dominant follicle formation is more common in Thoroughbred, Standardbred, Warmblood, and draft mares.
- Multiple dominant follicles are most frequently observed from March through May in the Northern Hemisphere.

SIGNS

Historical

- Mares exhibit prolonged estrus behavior.
- Discomfort from ovarian enlargement can mimic pain associated with colic or a sore back under saddle, especially if the etiology causes a rapid stretching of the ovarian tunic.

Physical Examination

- TRP—at least one large (>35 mm) fluid-filled structure or simply an enlarged ovary
- Ovarian U/S—single or multiple follicle(s), polycystic structures typical of neoplasia, a fluid-filled cavity filled with echogenic particles or fibrin-like strands indicative of a hematoma, or, rarely, an ovarian abscess

CAUSES

Hemorrhagic Anovulatory Follicles

- Normal follicular development occurs, but ovulation does not. These follicles can become quite large (60–110 mm diameter), are filled with blood, and may or may not have luteinization of the follicular wall.
- Such follicles may be estrogen-deficient or result from insufficient hypothalamic GnRH release. Decreased pituitary LH secretion/synthesis may be involved in the pathogenesis.
- The occurrence of hemorrhagic anovulatory follicles is most common during the autumnal transition, but can occur during the equine breeding season (spring/summer).

Persistent Follicles

- These are not ovarian cysts, which rarely occur in the mare, but are follicles that fail to undergo final maturation and ovulation.
- Most common during late spring or early autumnal transition

Luteinized Follicles

- Described in humans, luteinized follicles may also occur in mares. An association with reproductive senility has been proposed.
- This form of ovulation failure may occur in the normal mare when secondary CLs form during pregnancy.

Diestrus Follicular Development

Large antral follicles can form during the luteal phase of the estrous cycle and frequently undergo atresia rather than proceeding to ovulation.

RISK FACTORS

N/A

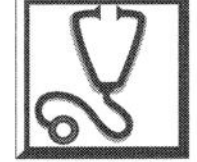

DIAGNOSIS

DIFFERENTIAL DIAGNOSIS

Differentiating Similar Signs

- If TRP is the sole means being used to determine follicular growth and ovulation, the presence of two or more adjacent follicles may be inaccurately interpreted to be one follicle that fails to ovulate.
- Ovarian neoplasia can mimic persistent follicular development due to similarities of behavior, cycling/teasing, and the presence of fluid-filled cavities on TRP and U/S (see Large Ovary Syndrome).
- Ovarian abscesses have been reported to occur secondary to invasive procedures or as a result of hematogenous infection. Abscesses may be confused with persistent follicles on palpation, but the contents are very echogenic (U/S). The mare is rarely systemically ill.
- Parovarian cysts can be confused with ovarian follicles if they are in close proximity to the ovary.
  - Distinguish from ovarian structures by careful TRP and U/S.

Differentiating Causes

- Historical review— Rule out problems related to season, sexual behavior, and teasing methods.
- TRP— Ovarian size, shape, and activity, uterine size and tone, and cervical relaxation may need to be evaluated three times per week over the course of 1–3 weeks to accurately characterize the mare's reproductive status.
- U/S— Essential tool to fully evaluate the abnormal ovary
  - Normal follicles exhibit increased echogenicity of follicular fluid and change their shape from spherical to pear/triangular shape as ovulation approaches.
  - Hematomas may have a distinctly echogenic fluid content with large, crisscrossing fibrin-like strands (see Large Ovary Syndrome).
  - Persistent follicles appear normal on U/S examination (see Large Ovary Syndrome).
  - Ovarian neoplasia varies depending upon the tumor type. The most common, the GCT/GTCT, frequently appears to be polycystic/multilocular (see Large Ovary Syndrome).

CBC/BIOCHEMISTRY/URINALYSIS

N/A

OTHER LABORATORY TESTS

- Serum progesterone concentration:
  - Basal levels of <1 ng/mL indicate no active/mature CL is present.
  - Active (mature) CL function is associated with levels of >4 ng/mL. Follicles can develop during diestrus when progesterone concentrations are >1 ng/mL.
- Serum testosterone and inhibin concentrations:
  - Mares typically have testosterone values <50–60 pg/mL and inhibin values <0.7 ng/mL.
  - Hormone levels suggestive of a GCT/GTCT (in a nonpregnant mare) are testosterone levels of >50 to 100 pg/mL, inhibin levels >0.7 ng/mL, with progesterone levels of <1 ng/mL.

IMAGING

Transrectal U/S is routinely used to evaluate the equine reproductive tract. The reader is referred to other texts for a comprehensive discussion on this technique.

OTHER DIAGNOSTIC PROCEDURES

N/A

PATHOLOGICAL FINDINGS

N/A

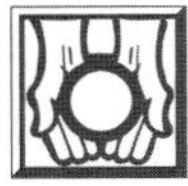

TREATMENT

- If ovulation failure is related to season (transition, anestrus), no treatment is necessary. Transitional follicles eventually regress (may require 30–45 days).
- Luteinized follicles and some hematomas may respond to prostaglandin treatment. Hematomas may be unresponsive to treatment for the first 2 weeks after development (due to insufficient luteal development).
- Ovulation of persistent follicles may be induced using either hCG or deslorelin, if persistent follicles are present late in vernal transition.
- Ovarian tumors or abscess—ovariectomy

MEDICATIONS

DRUG(S) OF CHOICE

- $PGF_{2\alpha}$ (Lutalyse [Pfizer] 10 mg IM) or its analogs to lyse persistent CL tissue
- Ovulation can be stimulated, if a follicle is $\geq$30 mm, by deslorelin (Ovuplant [Fort Dodge] 2.1 mg implant SC) or if $\geq$35 mm by hCG (2500 IU IV).
- Altrenogest (Regu-Mate [Intervet] 0.044 mg/kg PO daily, minimum 15 days) can be used to shorten the duration of vernal transition, providing follicles >20 mm diameter are present and the mare is demonstrating behavioral estrus.
  - $PGF_{2\alpha}$ (Lutalyse [Pfizer] 10 mg IM) on day 15 of the altrenogest treatment increases the reliability of this transition management regimen.

CONTRAINDICATIONS

$PGF_{2\alpha}$ and its analogs are contraindicated in mares with heaves or other bronchoconstrictive disease.

PRECAUTIONS

- Horses
  - $PGF_{2\alpha}$ causes sweating and colic-like symptoms due to its stimulatory effect on smooth muscle cells. If cramping has not subsided within 1 to 2 h, symptomatic treatment should be instituted.
  - Antibodies to hCG can develop after treatment. It is desirable to limit its use to no more than 2–3 times during one breeding season. The half-life of these antibodies ranges from 30 days to several months; they typically do not persist from one breeding season to the next.
  - Deslorelin implants have been associated with suppressed FSH secretion and decreased follicular development in the diestrus period immediately following use, leading to a prolonged interovulatory period in nonpregnant mares. Implant removal post-ovulation may decrease this possibility. The implant format is not currently sold in the United States, but the injectable product remains available.
  - Altrenogest, deslorelin, and $PGF_{2\alpha}$ should not be used in horses intended for food.
- Humans
  - $PGF_{2\alpha}$ or its analogs should not be handled by pregnant women, or persons with asthma or other bronchial diseases. Any accidental exposure to skin should be washed off immediately.
  - Altrenogest should not be handled by pregnant women, or persons with thrombophlebitis/thromboembolic disorders, cerebrovascular disease, coronary artery disease, breast cancer, estrogen-dependent neoplasia, undiagnosed vaginal bleeding or tumors that developed during the use of oral contraceptives or estrogen-containing products. Any accidental exposure to skin should be washed off immediately.

POSSIBLE INTERACTIONS

N/A

ALTERNATIVE DRUGS

- Cloprostenol sodium (Estrumate [Schering-Plough Animal Health] 250 µg/mL IM) is a prostaglandin analog.
  - This product is used in similar fashion to the natural prostaglandin, but has been associated with fewer side effects.
  - It is not currently approved for use in horses, but it is an analog in broad use in the absence of an alternative.

FOLLOW-UP

PATIENT MONITORING

Until normal cyclicity is established, regular TRP examinations are recommended.

POSSIBLE COMPLICATIONS

Individual mares may be prone to develop more than one hemorrhagic/anovulatory follicle in a season.

MISCELLANEOUS

ASSOCIATED CONDITIONS

N/A

AGE-RELATED FACTORS

N/A

ZOONOTIC POTENTIAL

N/A

PREGNANCY

- Prostaglandin administration to pregnant mares can cause CL lysis and abortion.
- Carefully rule out pregnancy before administering this drug or its analogs.

SYNONYMS

- Autumn follicles
- Hemorrhagic anovulatory follicles

SEE ALSO

- Abnormal estrus intervals
- Anestrus
- Large ovary syndrome

ABBREVIATIONS

- CL = corpus luteum
- FSH = follicle-stimulating hormone
- GCT = granulosa cell tumor
- GTCT = granulosa theca cell tumor
- GnRH = gonadotropin-releasing hormone
- hCG = human chorionic gonadotropin
- LH = luteinizing hormone
- $PGF_{2\alpha}$ = natural prostaglandin
- TRP = transrectal palpation
- U/S = ultrasound, ultrasonography

Suggested Reading

Carleton CL. Atypical, asymmetrical, but abnormal? Large ovary syndrome. Proc Mare Reprod Symp ACT/SFT 1996:27–39.

Ginther OJ. Ovaries. In: Ultrasonic Imaging and Animal Reproduction: Horses. Cross Plains: Equiservices, 1995:23–42.

Hinrichs K. Irregularities of the estrous cycle and ovulation in mares (including seasonal transition). In: Youngquist RS, Threlfall WR, eds. Current Therapy in Large Animal Theriogenology. St. Louis: Saunders Elsevier, 2007:144–152.

Pierson RA. Folliculogenesis and ovulation. In: McKinnon AO, Voss JL, eds. Equine Reproduction. Philadelphia: Lea & Febiger, 1993:161–171.

Sharp DC, Davis SD. Vernal transition. In: McKinnon AO, Voss JL, eds. Equine Reproduction. Philadelphia: Lea & Febiger, 1993:133–143.

Author Carole C. Miller

Consulting Editor Carla L. Carleton

PANCREATIC DISEASE

BASICS

OVERVIEW

- Clinical pancreatic disease is rarely recognized in the horse. Acute and chronic pancreatic disease has been reported.
- Equine pancreatic disorders include inflammatory disease, chronic eosinophilic pancreatitis, endocrine or exocrine insufficiency, and neoplasia.
- Fibrosis of the pancreas induced by parasitic migration of *Strongylus equinus* is probably the most common cause of pancreatic disease in the horse. Aberrant migration of *S. edentatus, S. vulgaris,* and *Parascaris equorum* may also occur.
- Pancreatitis has also been reported in horses with cholelithiasis.
- Diabetes mellitus is rare in the horse, and most cases are secondary to a demonstrable cause of insulin resistance, such as elevated concentrations of hormones, which antagonize the action of insulin. The most common etiology for the secondary diabetes mellitus in the horse is induced by dysfunction of the pars intermedia of the pituitary gland. Insulin-dependent diabetes mellitus, which is far less common in the horse, has been reported secondary to pancreatic fibrosis.
- There are a few rare reports of pancreatic neoplasia (adenocarcinoma, adenoma) in the horse. Typically, pancreatic adenocarcinoma occludes the common bile duct and causes cholestasis and severe liver dysfunction. Pancreatic fibrosis is seen in MEED.

SIGNALMENT

The few published reports of pancreatic neoplasia have been on aged horses and donkeys (>11 years).

SIGNS

The clinical signs of equine pancreatic disease are not specific. Signs of acute pancreatitis may include:

- Abdominal pain (moderate to severe) due to gastric distension, peritonitis, and hemoabdomen
- Gastric reflux
- Hypovolemic shock
- Signs of cardiovascular compromise (tachycardia, prolonged capillary refill, congested mucous membranes)

Signs of chronic pancreatitis may include:

- Weight loss
- Intermittent colic
- Icterus

Signs of diabetes mellitus may include:

- Polyuria, polydipsia
- Weight loss despite polyphagia
- Rough hair coat

Signs of pancreatic neoplasia may include:

- Pyrexia
- Depression
- Weight loss
- Icterus
- Ascites
- Per-rectal examination may be able to palpate neoplastic pancreas in the left kidney region.

CAUSES AND RISK FACTORS

Causes of pancreatitis that have been documented in the horse include parasitic migration (*Strongylus equinus, S. edentatus, S. vulgaris, Parascaris equorum*); ascending or hematogenous bacterial infections; viral (VEE, EIA) infections; immune-mediated disease; biliary or pancreatic duct inflammation; deficiencies of vitamin E or A; deficiencies of selenium and methionine; and vitamin D toxicity. The cause of acute pancreatitis is not known, but the autodigestion of pancreas by activated enzymes has been suggested. Pancreatic neoplasia (e.g., adenocarcinoma, adenoma) is very rare.

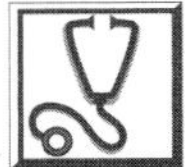

DIAGNOSIS

DIFFERENTIAL DIAGNOSIS

- Intra-abdominal abscessation
- Neoplasia

CBC/BIOCHEMISTRY/URINALYSIS

No specific abnormalities associated with pancreatic disease have been documented in the horse.

- Hyperglycemia (persistent)
- Glycosuria (persistent)
- Elevated serum GGT without elevation of other liver-specific enzymes may increase possibility of pancreatitis.
- Elevated serum amylase (normal, <35 U/L; pancreatitis, >700 U/L)
- Elevated serum lipase (normal, 400–1000 U/L) (variable)
- Hyperfibrinogenemia (acute pancreatitis)

OTHER LABORATORY TESTS

- Elevated peritoneal fluid amylase concentration (normal, 0–14 U/L) compared to serum amylase concentration (normal, <35 U/L) in acute pancreatitis
- Dexamethasone suppression test or beta-endorphin assay to rule out PIPD
- Serum insulin concentration—elevated in insulin resistance and reduced in insulin-dependent diabetes mellitus
- IV glucose tolerance test—0.5 g/kg glucose administered IV as 50% solution; serum glucose and insulin determined
- Insulin-dependent (type 1) diabetes mellitus—increased blood glucose without accompanying increase in insulin
- Insulin-resistance (type 2) diabetes mellitus—when blood glucose remains elevated for a prolonged period of time after infusion, despite high blood insulin levels. This is the most common type of diabetes mellitus in horses and ponies and is usually associated with PIPD.
- Abdominocentesis—abnormal cells in peritoneal fluid; elevated peritoneal fluid amylase activity (normal, 0–14 U/L)

IMAGING

- Abdominal ultrasound has been used to detect pancreatic neoplasia in the horse.
- Laparoscopy

OTHER DIAGNOSTIC PROCEDURES

Ultrasound-guided biopsy of pancreas

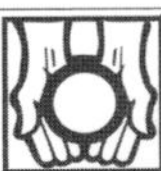

TREATMENT

- Symptomatic medical management
- Indwelling nasogastric tube to prevent gastric rupture; reflux every 2–4 hr

MEDICATIONS

DRUG(S) AND FLUIDS

Acute Pancreatitis

- Intravenous balanced polyionic electrolyte fluids
- Analgesics (NSAIDs such as flunixin meglumine 1.1 mg/kg q24h) and opiates (e.g., butorphanol 0.02 mg/kg q4h) for abdominal pain
- Broad-spectrum antibiotics to prevent secondary bacterial infection
- Plasma transfusion may be indicated.
- Calcium-containing fluids

CONTRAINDICATIONS/POSSIBLE INTERACTIONS

N/A

FOLLOW-UP

- Monitor hydration, serum calcium.
- Monitor abdominal pain.
- Prognosis poor to grave for acute pancreatitis

MISCELLANEOUS

ABBREVIATIONS

- EIA = equine infectious anemia
- GGT = γ-glutamyltransferase
- MEED = multisystemic eosinophilic epitheliotropic disease
- PIPD = pars intermedia pituitary dysfunction
- VEE = Venezuelan equine encephalitis

Suggested Reading

Baker RH. Acute necrotizing pancreatitis in a horse. JAVMA 1978;172:268–270.

Breider MA, Kiely RG, Edwards JF. Chronic eosinophilic pancreatitis and ulcerative colitis in a horse. JAVMA 1985; 186:809–811.

Furr MO, Robertson J. Two cases of equine pancreatic disease and a review of the literature. Equine Vet Educ 1992;4:55–58.

Johnson PJ, Scotty NC, Wiedmeyer C, Messer NT, Kreeger JM. Diabetes mellitus in a domesticated Spanish mustang. JAVMA 2005;226:584–588.

Waitt LH, Cebra CK, Tornquist SJ, Löhr CV. Panniculitis in a horse with peripancreatitis and pancreatic fibrosis. J Vet Diagn Invest 2006;18:405–408.

Author John D. Baird
Consulting Editors Henry Stämpfli and Olimpo Oliver-Espinosa

BASICS

OVERVIEW

• Term used to describe concurrent decrease in circulating erythrocytes (red blood cells), leukocytes (white blood cells) and thrombocytes (platelets). • Rarely reported in horses • Usually associated with disruption of hematopoiesis in the bone marrow due to either a failure of stem cells to undergo differentiation (aplastic anemia) or destruction of the bone marrow microenvironment by neoplastic, fibrous, or inflammatory diseases (myelophthisic anemia).
• Increased destruction, consumption, or sequestration of >1 cell line can occur occasionally, usually associated with infectious diseases.

SIGNS

• Clinical signs are referable to inadequate numbers of functional cells circulating in blood or in tissues. • Onset is often insidious with vague signs including weight loss, lethargy, poor performance, and intermittent pyrexia.
• Hemorrhagic diatheses due to thrombocytopenia may occur and include petechial hemorrhages, epistaxis, mucosal bleeding, blood in feces, hematomas, or prolonged bleeding from wounds. • Mucous membrane pallor, tachycardia, and a systolic heart murmur may be present dependant on the degree of anemia. • Secondary infections due to leukopenia may be present.

CAUSES AND RISK FACTORS

• Aplastic anemia may be congenital or acquired and can result from intrinsic stem cell failure or disruption of stem cell interactions with other cells in the bone marrow microenvironment. It is often idiopathic, but can also be (rarely) associated with administration of drugs (e.g., phenylbutazone, chloramphenicol, estrogens, trichloroethylene-extracted soybean meal, trimethoprim, pyrimethamine) or secondary to infectious/immune-mediated disease (e.g., infection with EIA virus or *Anaplasma phagocytophilum*). • Myelophthisic anemia has been associated with myelofibrosis, myelodysplasia, myeloproliferative disorders (monocytic, myelomonocytic, eosinophilic, myelogenous, or malignant histiocytosis), or lymphoproliferative disorders (multiple myeloma or lymphoid leukemia).

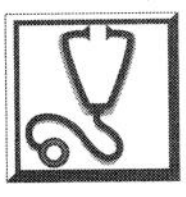

DIAGNOSIS

DIFFERENTIAL DIAGNOSIS

• See Causes and Risk Factors. • Hemorrhagic diatheses may also be observed with thrombocytopenia unassociated with bone marrow dysfunction or vasculitis. • Lethargy, pallor, petechiae, and edema may also be observed in horses with piroplasmosis (*Babesia caballi* or *Theileria equi* infection). • Familial megakaryocytic and myeloid hypoplasia is reported in Standardbred horses. • Concurrent immune-mediated anemia and thrombocytopenia

CBC/BIOCHEMISTRY/URINALYSIS

• Anemia, thrombocytopenia, and leukopenia
• Leukopenia is predominantly due to a neutropenia without a left shift.
• Lymphocyte count may be normal due to continued production of lymphocytes in lymphoid tissues.
• Anemia occurs after other hematologic derangements due to longer life span of circulating erythrocytes ($\approx$140 days) compared to thrombocytes ($\approx$5 days) and neutrophils ($\approx$12 hr).
• Examination of blood smears should be conducted for presence of *Anaplasma phagocytophilum* morulae in neutrophils, erythrocytic parasites (e.g., *B.caballi* or *T. equi*), absence of platelets, or abnormal leukocytes in subleukemic/leukemic neoplasia.

OTHER LABORATORY TESTS

• Serology for *B. caballi*, *T. equi*, or *Anaplasma phagocytophilum*
• Coggins test for EIA
• Coombs test
• Antiglobulin test

IMAGING

• Radiography of the skeleton and thorax for multiple myeloma
• Abdominal and thoracic ultrasonography for lymphoproliferative disorders

OTHER DIAGNOSTIC PROCEDURES

• Bone marrow aspiration/biopsy is indicated in the assessment of pancytopenia of undetermined cause.
• Best obtained from the sternum or proximal rib from adults and the sternum, rib, or tuber coxae in juveniles
• Biopsies are preferred for confirmation of bone marrow hypoplasia and myelofibrosis.
• Normal myeloid:erythroid ratio (M:E) is 0.5:1.5. A ratio <0.5 suggests a regenerative erythrocyte response or myeloid hypoplasia.
• Urine protein electrophoresis is indicated for the detection of Bence Jones proteins in cases where multiple myeloma is suspected.
• Monoclonal gammopathy on serum protein electrophoresis suggests lymphoproliferative neoplasia.
• Immunophenotypic techniques may be used for classification of leukemia.

PATHOLOGICAL FINDINGS

• Variable, dependant on the cause of pancytopenia.
• Neoplastic cells in bone marrow aspirates/biopsies are present in leukoproliferative disorders.
• Myelofibrosis is characterized by replacement of the bone marrow with fibrous tissue.
• Aplastic anemia is characterized by hypocellularity and fat infiltration of the bone marrow.

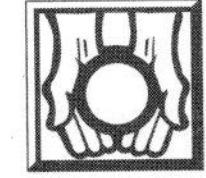

TREATMENT

• Remove suspected causative medications (e.g., phenylbutazone, chloramphenicol, estrogens).
• Supportive care; avoid trauma, rest

MEDICATIONS

DRUG(S)

• Immunosuppressive treatment (e.g., corticosteroids) if immune-mediated disease is suspected.
• Antimicrobial therapy if secondary infections develop.
• Blood or platelet-rich plasma transfusions provide only temporary improvement.
• Androgens may stimulate erythropoiesis in remaining hematopoietic tissue.
• No treatment for EIA exists.
• Treatment for *Anaplasma phagocytophilum* (oxytetracycline 7 mg/kg IV once daily for 5–7 days) or piroplasmosis (imidocarb diproprionate–*B. caballi* 2.2 mg/kg IM twice at 24-hr interval, *T. equi* 4 mg/kg IM q72h for 4–6 doses).

CONTRAINDICATIONS/POSSIBLE INTERACTIONS

Immune status may be compromised further by use of corticosteroid treatment.

FOLLOW-UP

PATIENT MONITORING

• Monitor for pyrexia, lethargy, worsening pallor, evidence of hemorrhagic diathesis.
• Regular hematologic monitoring

EXPECTED COURSE AND PROGNOSIS

• Anaplastic anemia; insufficient documented cases to provide a clear indication of prognosis.
• Myeloproliferative and lymphoproliferative disorders have a hopeless prognosis.

MISCELLANEOUS

ASSOCIATED CONDITIONS

Infectious disease (e.g., respiratory, skin) may occur due to neutropenia.

SEE ALSO

• Anemia
• Anemia, aplastic
• Equine granulocytic ehrlichiosis
• EIA
• Lymphosarcoma
• Multiple myeloma
• Myeloproliferative diseases
• Piroplasmosis

ABBREVIATION

• EIA = equine infectious anemia

Suggested Reading

Sellon DC. Disorders of the hematopoietic system. In: Reed SM, et al., eds. Equine Internal Medicine, ed 2. St Louis: Saunders, 2004:721–768.

Author Kristopher Hughes
Consulting Editors Jennifer Hodgson and David Hodgson

PANICUM COLORATUM (KLEINGRASS) TOXICOSIS

BASICS

OVERVIEW

- *Panicum coloratum* (kleingrass, kleingrass 75) is a tufted, perennial grass with stems usually 60–135 cm in height from a firm, knotty base.
- The blades are elongate, 2–8 mm in width, smooth or stiff, with bristly hairs on one or both surfaces.
- Loosely branched, pyramidal flower clusters are mostly 8–25 cm in length, with spikelets on spreading branches; the spikelets are 2.8–3.2 mm in length and smooth.
- The rootstock is hearty and easily develops rhizomes.
- *Panicum* spp. grow in Australia, New Zealand, South Africa, South America, Afghanistan, India, and Texas. In Texas, it reaches from the high plains to the Edward's Plateau and the Trans-Pecos area.
- *Panicum* spp. were introduced into the United States during the 1950s; *P. coloratum* was developed by Texas A & M University during the early 1970s and prefers improved pastures.
- Some native species found outside the United States generally are not toxic.
- The toxin is a saponin (saponins are composed of sapogenins and a sugar moiety) that is probably the same as that found in *Tribulus, Nolina*, and *Agave* spp.
- Horses have developed liver disease while grazing kleingrass or eating kleingrass hay, but they have not developed photosensitization.

SIGNALMENT

No known breed, sex, or age predispositions

SIGNS

- Horses develop liver disease and become icteric.
- Anorexia and weight loss
- Horses tend not to develop secondary or hepatogenous photosensitization.

CAUSES AND RISK FACTORS

N/A

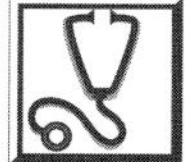

DIAGNOSIS

DIFFERENTIAL DIAGNOSIS

- History of grazing kleingrass; compatible clinical signs
- Other hepatotoxins—aflatoxin (detection in feed and histopathology), PAs (ingestion of alkaloid-containing plants and histopathology), and iron toxicosis (tissue iron concentrations and histopathology)
- In addition to PA-containing plants, exposure to other hepatotoxic plants—*Nolina texana, Agave lechuguilla, Panicum* spp., and *Trifolium hybridum* (identification in animal's environment, evidence of consumption)
- Nontoxic differential—Theiler's disease (history, histopathology)

CBC/BIOCHEMISTRY/URINALYSIS

- Horses on kleingrass have high serum GGT activity, total and direct bilirubin, blood ammonia, and sulfobromophthalein clearance times.
- Serum SDH, AST, and AP activities are variable.

OTHER LABORATORY TESTS

N/A

IMAGING

N/A

DIAGNOSTIC PROCEDURES

N/A

PATHOLOGICAL FINDINGS

- Histopathologically, chronic hepatitis with varying degrees of fibrosis, which is dependent on the length of exposure
- Characteristic lesions—bridging hepatic fibrosis, cholangitis, and hepatocellular regeneration

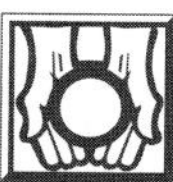

TREATMENT

- Remove animals from the kleingrass pastures or hay.
- Although horses have not shown photosensitization, shade may be helpful.
- Symptomatic and supportive care

MEDICATIONS

DRUG(S) OF CHOICE

No specific therapeutic interventions

CONTRAINDICATIONS/POSSIBLE INTERACTIONS

Impaired hepatic function may prolong clearance of drugs metabolized by the liver.

FOLLOW-UP

PATIENT MONITORING

Monitor hepatic function.

PREVENTION/AVOIDANCE

Do not allow horses to graze *Panicum* spp. or ingest hays containing the grass.

POSSIBLE COMPLICATIONS

Photosensitization

EXPECTED COURSE AND PROGNOSIS

Onset of clinical signs is associated with significant hepatic fibrosis, making the long-term prognosis guarded to poor.

MISCELLANEOUS

ASSOCIATED CONDITIONS, AGE-RELATED FACTORS, ZOONOTIC POTENTIAL, PREGNANCY

N/A

ABBREVIATIONS

- AP = alkaline phosphatase
- AST = aspartate aminotransferase
- GGT = γ-glutamyltransferase
- PA = pyrrolizidine alkaloids
- SDH = sorbitol dehydrogenase

Suggested Reading

Cornick JL, Carter GK, Bridges CH. Kleingrass-associated hepatotoxicosis in horses. J Am Vet Med Assoc 1988;193:932–935.

Author Tam Garland

Consulting Editor Robert H. Poppenga

PAPILLOMATOSIS

BASICS

OVERVIEW

• Papillomas are benign proliferative epithelial neoplasms associated with the presence of EPV. • Third most common cutaneous equine neoplasm and most common tumor in horses between 1 and 3 years of age • Two forms include papillomatosis (warts) affecting mucocutaneous or haired skin and ear papillomas (aural plaque, hyperplastic dermatitis of the ear).

SYSTEM AFFECTED

Skin

SIGNALMENT

• Papillomatosis can occur in horses of any age, but is more common in younger horses (<3 years of age). Multiple horses within a group may be affected. Congenital papillomas reported in a small number of neonatal foals • Ear papillomas are seen in horses of all ages and rarely occur in horses <1 year of age. • No apparent breed or sex predisposition

SIGNS

• The most commonly affected sites are the muzzle and lips; however, the eyelids, external genitalia, distal legs, and ears can also be involved. • Lesions may be solitary or multiple (up to 100) resembling papillomatosis of other species; can cause problems because of physical location and esthetics • Papillomas in any location, with the exception of the ear, are 0.2–2 cm in diameter, 0.5 cm in height, broad-based to pedunculated, gray, pink or white; surface is hyperkeratotic with numerous frond-like projections. Solitary lesions can be larger. • Ear papillomas usually occur on the inner surface of the pinna manifesting as well-demarcated, raised, white, smooth or hyperkeratotic plaques or papules, 1–3 cm in diameter. Asymptomatic, except during summer when the pinnal lesions may be aggravated by biting flies and secondary infections

CAUSES AND RISK FACTORS

• Two different types of EPVs believed to cause warts and ear papillomas, and a third EPV may be associated with penile papillomas • EPV (a DNA papovavirus)— infects stratified squamous epithelium. • Transmitted by direct and indirect contact (e. g., biting insects) • Damaged skin predisposes to natural infection by the virus. • Transmission of the virus from the dam to the foal may occur transplacentally (not proven) or inoculation of the skin may occur in the foal from infected sites on the dam during parturition.

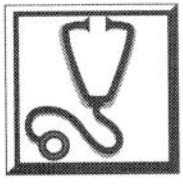

DIAGNOSIS

DIFFERENTIAL DIAGNOSIS

• The appearance and distribution of the lesions are strongly suggestive of a diagnosis of papillomatosis. • Verrucose sarcoid (extensive areas are usually affected with markedly thickened skin around and evidence of hypotrichosis at the periphery of the lesion) • Squamous cell carcinoma (especially facial and vulvar proliferative forms) • Papular dermatoses (e. g., hypersensitivity reaction, parasites, infectious disease) • Molluscum contagiosum

OTHER DIAGNOSTIC PROCEDURES

• Biopsy and histopathologic examination to establish definitive diagnosis • Immunohistochemistry to detect viral antigen within the lesion. Papillomavirus capsid antigens are well conserved among species; therefore antibodies directed against these antigens are used on formalin-fixed tissue to detect the presence of virus. • Electron microscopy—While not normally necessary to establish the diagnosis, hexagonal viral particles measuring 38–42 nm in diameter can be found in all forms of equine papillomatosis (except congenital form). • PCR for equine papillomavirus can be performed; however, this test is not usually necessary since clinical findings and biopsy are usually definitive; PCR was negative in aural plaques and congenital papillomas in one study.

PATHOLOGICAL FINDINGS

Histopathological

• Papillomatosis—early phase characterized by marked epidermal hyperplasia, mild to moderate acanthosis and hyperkeratosis, with the presence of very few viral inclusion bodies. Progression to the classical features—pronounced papillated epidermal hyperplasia and papillomatosis, koilocytosis (ballooning degeneration of keratinocytes), numerous mitoses, viral intranuclear inclusion bodies found in about 50% of lesions (most common in stratum corneum). With chronicity, the epidermis becomes more hyperplastic with the development of rete pegs. Regressing lesions contain increased proliferation of fibroblasts and infiltration of lymphocytes. • Ear papillomas—lesions similar to those described for papillomatosis except epidermal hyperplasia is only mildly papillated, papillomatosis is mild to absent, and hypomelanosis is striking

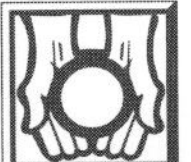

TREATMENT

• Papillomas (warts) typically regress spontaneously within 1–9 mo; therefore, treatment may not be necessary. • Ear papillomas do not regress spontaneously (see aural plaques). • Surgical excision is the treatment of choice, useful for health (e. g., lesion interferes with function) or esthetic reasons. • Cryosurgery is also effective. • Secondary infections may require treatment with topical antibacterial products (e. g., creams, gels, washes). • Efficacy of autogenous vaccines is not proved.

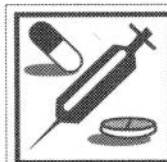

MEDICATIONS

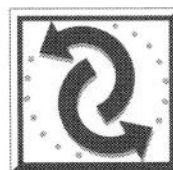

FOLLOW-UP

PREVENTION/AVOIDANCE

• Papillomaviruses are resistant to freezing or desiccation; however, formalin, detergents, or high temperatures may decrease infectivity. • Avoid transmission of the virus among horses that are stabled or pastured together by isolation of affected horses; prevent horses from rubbing on each other; dedicated grooming equipment and halters • Preventing insect bites (e. g., repellent sprays) may decrease irritation in the affected horse and limit spread of the virus among horses.

EXPECTED COURSE AND PROGNOSIS

• Spontaneous regression of warts is common within 1–9 mo. • Ear papillomas rarely, if ever, spontaneously regress. • Surgical excision—excellent prognosis and recurrence should not occur

MISCELLANEOUS

ASSOCIATED CONDITIONS

• Equine congenital papilloma is a hamartomatous lesion (epidermal nevus) and studies have been unable to find histopathological, immunohistochemical, or PCR evidence of papillomaviral infection. • Congenital papillomas are a cauliflower-like, flattened wart from 5 mm to 20 cm in diameter on the skin of a new foal. The lesions are usually single and located on the head, neck, or trunk.

ZOONOTIC POTENTIAL

None

PREGNANCY

EPV may be transmitted from an infected mare to the foal transplacentally (not proved) or from infected skin lesions on the mare to the foal during parturition.

SEE ALSO

• Sarcoid • Aural plaques

ABBREVIATIONS

• EPV = equine papillomavirus
• PCR = polymerase chain reaction

Suggested Reading

Scott DW, Miller Jr. WH. Neoplastic and Non-neoplastic Tumors. In: Equine Dermatology. St. Louis: Saunders, 2003;700.

Author Beverly Kidney
Consulting Editor Gwendolen Lorch

PARAPHIMOSIS

BASICS

DEFINITION

Prolapse of the penis and inner preputial fold with extensive penile and preputial edema and the inability to retract the penis into the prepuce

PATHOPHYSIOLOGY

- The anatomic location of the penis and prepuce affects how it reacts to injury. The effect of gravity magnifies the inflammatory reaction to an injury with the accumulation of edema, or with the formation of a hematoma or seroma.
- As the penis and prepuce prolapse, vascular and lymphatic drainage are impeded, leading to further edema accumulation.
- The inelasticity of the preputial ring further promotes fluid retention.
- Chronic prolapse may lead to penile/preputial trauma, balanoposthitis, or penile paralysis.

SYSTEMS AFFECTED

- Reproductive—Prolapse of the penis and prepuce exposes them to trauma. Chronic paraphimosis may result in penile paralysis, fibrosis of the CCP, and an inability to achieve an erection.
- Urologic—Urethral obstruction may be the inciting cause of paraphimosis, or it may occur secondary to edema.

SIGNALMENT

- Predominantly stallions, but geldings can also be affected
- No breed predilection
- Unlikely to occur in the first month of life, when normal adhesions exist between the free penis and inner lamina of the preputial fold

SIGNS

Historical

- Acute cases often present as traumatic injury to the penile or preputial area.
- Chronic cases—Delay in presentation for veterinary care may occur if owners believed an injury was minor and attempted care themselves or the injury may only recently have become obvious because of its slow increase in size, e. g., a slow developing enlargement of the penis or preputial area such as is seen with *Habronema* spp. infections or neoplastic growths.

Physical Examination

- Prolapse of the penis and prepuce with severe penile enlargement is readily apparent. Caudoventral displacement of the glans penis is common. A careful visual and digital exam is necessary to properly define the nature of the injury.
- Balanitis (inflammation of the penis), posthitis (inflammation of the prepuce), or balanoposthitis (inflammation of the prepuce and penis) may be present. Serous or hemorrhagic discharges on the surface of the penis and prepuce are common. Lacerations, excoriations, ulcerative lesions, or neoplastic masses may be evident.
- Hematomas, when present, are generally located on the dorsal surface of the penis and usually arise from blood vessels superficial to the tunica albuginea.
- Transrectal palpation may reveal an enlarged urinary bladder indicative of urethral blockage.
- Chronic prolapse may result in penile paralysis.

CAUSES

Noninfectious Causes

- Trauma—breeding injuries, fighting or kicks, improperly-fitting stallion rings, falls, movement through brush or heavy ground cover, whips, or abuse
- Priapism, penile paralysis, posthitis, or balanoposthitis
- Postsurgical complication—castration or cryptorchid surgery
- Neoplasia of the penis or prepuce—sarcoids, SCC, melanoma, mastocytoma, hemangioma, or papillomas
- Debilitation or starvation
- Spinal injury or myelitis
- Urolithiasis/urinary tract obstruction

Infectious Causes

- Bacterial—*Staphylococcus, Streptococcus*
- Viral—EHV-1, EHV-3, EIA, EVA
- Purpura hemorrhagica—vasculitis as a sequela to infection or vaccine administration
- Parasitic—*Habronema muscae, Habronema microstoma, Draschia megastoma, Onchocera* spp., *Cochliomyia hominivorax* (screw worm)
- Fungal—phycomycosis due to *Hyphomyces destruens*
- Protozoal— *Trypanosoma equiperdum* (Dourine)

RISK FACTORS

- Use of phenothiazine tranquilizers in stallions. Increased risk during transport.
- Open-range/pasture, not in-hand, stud management
- More aggressive stallions
- Poor management, unsanitary conditions, or malnutrition

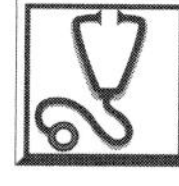

DIAGNOSIS

DIFFERENTIAL DIAGNOSIS

- Any injury or condition that leads to chronic protrusion of the penis or prepuce can lead to paraphimosis. The initial cause may be due to injury or disease, but because both cases result in accumulation of edema and leave the surfaces exposed to further injury, the underlying cause must be determined whenever possible.
- Diagnostic—the presence of visible lacerations or hematomas, or a history of trauma, or surgical intervention
- The presence of ulcerative or proliferative lesions warrants investigation to determine if the origin of the lesion is neoplastic, parasitic, or infectious.
- Systemic signs indicative of neurologic or systemic disease include ataxia, depression, lymph node enlargement, or increased rectal temperature.

CBC/BIOCHEMISTRY/URINALYSIS

- Generally, there are no abnormal findings unless the causative factor is an infectious agent, neoplastic disease, or severe debilitation/starvation.
- Urinalysis may indicate urolithiasis/cystitis.

OTHER LABORATORY TESTS

- Bacterial causes—culture (swab) of affected tissues
- EHV-1—rising antibody titers (paired sera, collected at a 14- to 21-day interval); virus isolation from nasopharyngeal swabs or blood (buffy coat) during the acute stage
- EHV-3—rising antibody titer (paired sera, collected at a 14- to 21-day interval); eosinophilic intranuclear inclusion bodies in cytologic smears; virus isolation from lesions during the acute stage
- EIA—AGID (Coggins) test
- EVA—rising antibody titer (paired sera collected at a 14- to 21-day interval); virus isolation from nasopharygneal swabs
- Protozoal—identification of the causative agent in urethral exudates; serology—CF

IMAGING

Ultrasound findings are generally unrewarding. In other species, fibrosis of the CCP has been visualized in chronic cases.

DIAGNOSTIC PROCEDURES

Cytology or biopsy of masses or lesions may provide a diagnosis in the case of parasitic, neoplastic, or fungal disease.

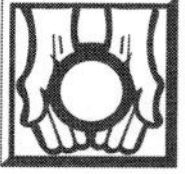

TREATMENT

- The primary goals—Reduce the inflammation and edema and return the penis to the prepuce to improve venous and lymphatic drainage. The initial management of the patient is intensive and may require hospitalization to allow adequate physical restraint and patient access.
- Ensure urethral patency. Catheterize or perform a perineal urethrostomy, if necessary.

• Methods of manual reduction of the prolapse:
  ○ Elastic or pneumatic bandaging may reduce edema prior to attempting reduction.
  ○ Preputiotomy if the preputial ring is preventing successful reduction.
  ○ Purse-string suture of umbilical tape around the preputial orifice, tightened to a one-finger opening, to hold the penis within the prepuce, has the additional benefit of maintaining pressure on the penis for sustained reduction of edema.
  ○ Additional support can be gained by putting on a net sling, which covers the cranial aspect of the prepuce but allows urine to drain.
• In cases resistant to manual reduction, support remains of primary importance. Wrap the exposed penis and prepuce to reduce edema. Support in the form of a sling is essential. Nylon slings raise and maintain the penis close to the ventral belly wall. Using netting with small perforations allows urine to drain.
• Hydrotherapy—Cold hydrotherapy for the first 4–7 days until edema and hemorrhage subside, then warm hydrotherapy. Generally applied for 15–30 min BID to QID.
• Massage the penis and prepuce BID to QID to reduce edema.
• Topical emollient ointment application—A & D ointment, lanolin, petroleum jelly, nitrofurazone
• Exercise—Confinement and limited activity until after active hemorrhage and edema subside, then slowly increase, aids in resolution of dependent edema.
• No sexual stimulation in the early stages of therapy. It may be necessary to prevent exposure to mares for up to 4–8 weeks.
• Local surgical resection, cryosurgery, or radiation therapy of neoplastic or granulomatous lesions, once the edema is resolved
• Chronic refractory paraphimosis may require surgical intervention, including circumcision (reefing or posthioplasty), penile retraction (Bolz technique), or penile amputation (phallectomy).

MEDICATIONS

DRUG(S) OF CHOICE

• NSAIDs including phenylbutazone (2–4 g/450 kg/day PO) or flunixin meglumine (1 mg/kg/day IV, IM, or PO) for symptomatic relief and to reduce inflammation
• Systemic or local antibiotics as indicated to treat local infection and prevent septicemia.
• Diuretics—furosemide (1 mg/kg IV daily or BID) if indicated in the acute phase for reduction of edema.
• Specific topical or systemic treatments for parasitic, fungal, or neoplastic conditions as indicated by results of diagnostic testing

CONTRAINDICATIONS

• Tranquilizers, particularly the phenothiazine tranquilizers, should be avoided in males to avoid drug-induced priapism.
• Nitrofurazone should not be used on horses intended for food.
• Avoid sexual stimulation in the early stages and usually for 4–8 weeks after treatment for paraphimosis has begun.

PRECAUTIONS

Diuretics are contraindicated if urinary obstruction is present. Their effectiveness in treating localized edema is in doubt.

POSSIBLE INTERACTIONS

N/A

ALTERNATIVE DRUGS

DMSO has been used topically (50/50 mixture by volume with nitrofurazone ointment) or systemically (1 g/kg IV as a 10% solution in saline BID to TID for 3–5 days) to reduce inflammation and edema. Note that the parenteral administration of DMSO is not approved and is considered extra-label use.

FOLLOW-UP

PATIENT MONITORING

• Initial management is intensive. Frequent evaluation is essential.
• Good prognostic indicators—reduction of edema, coupled with the horse's ability to retain penis in the prepuce

POSSIBLE COMPLICATIONS

• Excoriations/ulcerations or further trauma of exposed skin surfaces
• Fibrosis of tissues, leading to the inability to achieve erection or to a urethral obstruction
• Chronic paraphimosis
• Continued hematoma enlargement indicates that a rent may be present in the tunica albuginea. The hematoma should be surgically explored.
• Penile paralysis
• Frostbite due to exposure
• Myiasis
• Infertility

MISCELLANEOUS

ASSOCIATED CONDITIONS, AGE-RELATED FACTORS, ZOONOTIC POTENTIAL, PREGNANCY

N/A

SEE ALSO

• Viral diseases, infectious
• Penile lacerations
• Penile paralysis
• Penile vesicles/erosions
• Purpura hemorrhagica
• Priapism

ABBREVIATIONS

• AGID = agar gel immunodiffusion
• CCP = corpus cavernosum penis
• CF = complement fixation
• DMSO = dimethylsulfoxide
• EHV-1 = equine herpesvirus 1, equine rhinopneumonitis
• EHV-3 = equine herpesvirus 3, equine coital exanthema
• EIA = equine infectious anemia, swamp fever
• EVA = equine viral arteritis

Suggested Reading

Clem MF, DeBowes RM. Paraphimosis in horses. Part I. Compend Contin Educ 1989;11:72–75.

Clem MF, DeBowes RM. Paraphimosis in horses. Part II. Compend Contin Educ 1989;11:184–187.

De Vries PJ. Diseases of the testes, penis, and related structures. In: McKinnon AO, Voss JL, eds. Equine Reproduction. Philadelphia: Lea & Febiger, 1993:878–884.

Vaughan JT. Surgery of the penis and prepuce. In: Walker DF, Vaughan JT, eds. Bovine and Equine Urogenital Surgery. Philadelphia: Lea & Febiger, 1980:125–144.

Vaughan JT. Penis and prepuce. In: McKinnon AO, Voss JL, eds. Equine Reproduction. Philadelphia: Lea & Febiger, 1993:885–894.

Author Carole C. Miller
Consulting Editor Carla L. Carleton

PASTERN DERMATITIS

BASICS

DEFINITION

• Pastern dermatitis (commonly referred to as "grease heel") describes a variety of inflammatory skin conditions of the horse's distal extremity. Considered as a "syndrome or cutaneous reaction pattern" of the plantar/palmar aspects of the pastern and bulbs of the heels but may extend proximally to the mid-cannon.
• "Grease heel" is *not a specific disease entity*. Pastern dermatitis is often multifactorial.

PATHOPHYSIOLOGY

• Dermatitis is preceded by mechanical injury to the stratum corneum. Mechanical irritants include chronic moisture, frictional injury from bedding, tack, arenas and track soils, ectoparasites and microorganisms. Inflammation of the epidermis, dermis, and adnexa gives rise to crusts, scale, erosion, ulceration, alopecia, lichenification, fibrosis, exuberant, verrucous masses representing granulation tissue and scarring. Certain breeds are predisposed to develop alterations in proliferation and differentiation of keratinocytes in their pastern skin, resulting in progressive hyperplasia and production of excess keratin.

SYSTEMS AFFECTED

• Skin/Exocrine

GENETICS

• Genetics may play a role, as anatomical features correlate with disease severity in draft horses.

INCIDENCE/PREVALENCE

• The most prevalent form of the disease is mild.
• Syndrome described for many centuries
• True incidence is unknown but presumed to be within the top 10 equine dermatoses.

GEOGRAPHIC DISTRIBUTION

• Presumably worldwide

SIGNALMENT

• Occurs in all breeds. Chronic pastern dermatitis is most common in heavy draft horses.
• Breed predilections: Belgium and Rhenish German draft horses. • Mean age of onset is 9 years—range 2.5–26 years of age. • No reported sex predilection

SIGNS

• Clinical signs vary and are dependent to both the etiology and the stage of disease. Bilateral symmetrical involvement of the hind limb is the most common presentation. Unilateral disease is recognized. Signs begin on the palmar and plantar aspects of the fetlocks up to the carpal and tarsal joints and may progress to the metatarsal regions. All surfaces of the limbs can be involved. Earliest lesions are mild scale and crusts with erythema and alopecia. Other features are hyperkeratosis with hyperplastic plaque lesions and scaling. Verrucous masses, referred to as "grapes", have rugged surfaces with fissures, scale, crusts, excoriations, erosion, ulceration and varying degree of greasiness, malodor and exudate. Grapes represent chronic disease and are almost exclusively found in heavy draft horses. In advanced cases, removal of thick adherent scale and crusts can cause significant pain, erosion and ulceration. Serosanguinous or suppurative exudate is associated with erosion, ulceration, crusts or the presence of a vasculitis. Distal limb edema, cellulitis, lameness or reluctance to ambulate occurs in moderate to severe cases. Varying degrees of pruritus are present in all stages depending on the etiology. Distal extremities with white stockings may be more affected, although this does not appear to be the case in heavy draft breeds.

CAUSES

Pastern dermatitis has numerous potential causes. Categorizing factors that play a role in the development, initiation and maintenance of symptoms into respective groups will elucidate all causes and allow formulation of an appropriate therapeutic plan.

1. ***Factors and patient characteristics that provide the basis for the DEVELOPMENT of pastern dermatitis.***
   • In heavy draft horses
      ○ Circumference of cannon
      ○ Prominence of fetlock tufts of hair, chestnuts, ergots and if present, prominent bulges in the fetlock region
      ○ Poor hoof condition
   • Chronically moist conditions, abrasion from plants in the pasture or irritants in the soils of tracks or riding areas, sand or beddings • Alkaline soils • Poor stable hygiene • Use of irritant topical products, training devices or treated bedding • Keratinization disorder e. g. cannon keratosis and coronary band dystrophy
2. ***Factors that INITIATE dermatitis. These factors are considered primary disease etiologies.***
   • Parasitic
   - *Chorioptes* spp.—intense pruritus in the majority cases; however, some are non-pruritic. Exudation of serum among feathers of distal limb, dried crusts and scales, matted hair, thickening of the skin and self-inflicted trauma (excoriation, lichenification, and alopecia) are other clinical signs.
   - Trombiculidiasis—intense pruritus, clumped hair tufts, orange or brown sticky patches of serum which resembles resin
   - *Pelodera strongyloides*
   - *Strongyloides westerni* larvae
   - Habronemiasis
   • Infectious
   - Dermatophytosis
   - Mycetoma
   - Sporotrichosis
   - Spirochetosis
   - Vaccinia (horsepox)
   • Immune-mediated
   - Contact hypersensitivity
   - Photoactivated vasculitis (photosensitization due to phylloerythrin involves white pasterns and/or other white areas)
   - Leukocytoclastic pastern vasculitis
   - Cutaneous drug reaction
   - Pemphigus complex
   - Bullous pemphigoid
   • Iatrogenic
   - Application of blistering agents
   - Pin firing
   - Scald from urine or feces
   - Wire injury
   • Neoplastic
   - Fibroblastic or verrucose sarcoid
   - Squamous cell carcinoma
   - Cutaneous lymphoma
3. ***Features of the dermatitis that MAINTAIN, reinforce and strengthen the disease process.***
   • Bacterial
   - *Staphylococcus spp*, *Corynebacterium spp*, fusiform bacteria, botryomycosis infections
   - *Dermatophilus congolensis*
   • Environmental
   - Overvigorous washing and scrubbing after exercise
   - Application of occlusive ointments and dressings over necrotic skin and crusts resulting in opportunistic infection
   - UV light exposure
   - Insect bites
   • Chronic pathological changes to the epidermis, dermis and adnexa

RISK FACTORS

Risk factors are predisposing factors that increase susceptibility
• Environmental—climate (more common in the winter), moisture and stable and pasture hygiene • Iatrogenic—adverse reactions to topical medications, use of splint boots and other training devices • Genetic—nonpigmented or depigmented skin, excessive hair or feathering on pastern, keratinization defect

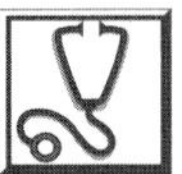

DIAGNOSIS

DIFFERENTIAL DIAGNOSIS

Diagnosis is based on history, physical examination, and findings from diagnostic tests. See Causes for specific differentials
In addition consider:
• Chronic progressive lymphedema
• Hepatocutaneous syndrome • Exfoliative eosinophilic dermatitis and stomatitis
• Idiopathic

CBC/BIOCHEMISTRY/URINALYSIS

• Perform if photosensitization, hepatopathy or vasculitis is suspected. • Use to screen for metabolic disorders.

OTHER LABORATORY TESTS

• Cytology with Diff-Quik stains collected from erosions or ulcers show a neutrophilic exudate with intra- and/or extracellular cocci and represents secondary folliculitis. • Perform skin scrapings to rule out ectoparasites. • Perform bacterial and DTM cultures to determine bacterial species and susceptibility and/or dermatophyte infections.

IMAGING

Radiographs may rule out other causes of lameness.

OTHER DIAGNOSTIC PROCEDURES

Obtain skin biopsies by wedge resection in horses with marked hyperkeratosis, nodular, or proliferative changes. Biopsies are essential for confirmation of pastern dermatitis due to immune-mediated or neoplastic disease, keratinization disorders, vasculopathies or contact hypersensitivities.

PATHOLOGIC FINDINGS

Histopathology from biopsies have mild to marked epidermal hyperplasia, orthokeratotic hyperkeratosis with foci of parakeratosis, and serocellular and neutrophilic crusts that may have cocci and/or *Chorioptic* mites. Mild disease may have neutrophilic intraepithelial pustules. In mild to marked disease, a focal to total absence of keratohyalin granules with focal to moderate spongiosis in addition to marked epidermal hyperplasia with prominent rete pegs and dermal papillae are present. Dermal changes range from superficial perivascular lymphocytic dermatitis to marked dermal fibrosis and dilation of the lymphatics.

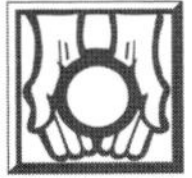

TREATMENT

AIMS OF TREATMENT

The primary goal is to establish and eliminate the predisposing, primary and perpetuating causes. No single therapy applies to all cases due to the variability of cause and clinical consequences. Many cases will have had previous therapy before presentation.

APPROPRIATE HEALTH CARE

- Outpatient medical management is appropriate for the majority of cases.

NURSING CARE

- Debridement—objective is to remove all necrotic and contaminated tissues. Keep the skin dry and free of irritation throughout the treatment. Debridement may require sedation or general anesthesia, as severe cases are usually painful. Remove excess hair. Simple hydrotherapy with the application of an antimicrobial, keratolytic and keratoplastic shampoo should be used in the initial debridement of the lesions. In mild cases, a conservative approach of cleansing lesions q 12 hr for 7–10 days may be all that is needed. Alternatively, in moderate to severe cases, debridement can be performed using creams with benzoic or salicylic acids and propylene glycol applied to the lesions, covered with thin plastic film and wrapped with a lightly padded clean stable bandage for 12 hr. Remove the dressing and gently wash with a mild antimicrobial shampoo. If significant crusting is still present, repeat the process. Make an assessment of the degree and depth of ulceration. Severely ulcerated skin will not heal if exposed to repeated wetting and trauma. • For exudative lesions, astringent solutions, such as Burrow's solution (aluminum acetate in water) can be applied to the area q 8–12 hr for 10 minutes; alternatively, soak the leg in an astringent solution for 15–30 minutes. Before application of astringent, wash extremities with an antimicrobial shampoo.
- If providing a dry environment for the patient is not possible, consider applying a light barrier cream, such as petroleum jelly or liquid bandages (Facilitator® Liquid Bandage, IDEXX Laboratories, Inc., or Nexcare™ Liquid Bandage Drops, 3M US). Liquid bandages may promote re-epithelization.

ACTIVITY

- Rest from work. Avoid areas that are wet, muddy, sandy, or have an abundance of sharp protruding roughage that initiates epidermal microtrauma.
- If predominantly white legs are affected suggestive of solar or photoactivated dermatitis, keep out of UV light until a definitive diagnosis is made.

DIET N/A

CLIENT EDUCATION

- Warn owners and plan for recurrence in periods of wet weather.
- Describe multifactorial nature of the disease.

SURGICAL CONSIDERATIONS

Surgical or cryosurgical intervention of exuberant granulation tissue may be required.

MEDICATIONS

DRUG(S)

- For localized bacterial dermatitis, consider topical antimicrobials such as silver sulfadiazine or 2% mupirocin ointment applied q 12 hr for 2 weeks past clinical cure.
- For mild to deep bacterial dermatitis involving all four legs, use systemic antimicrobials, such as sulfamethoxazole/trimethoprim 30 mg/kg PO q 24 hr × 21 days or 2 weeks past clinical cure. May need to administer 15 mg/kg PO q 12 hr to prevent diarrhea
- Dermatophytosis—topical rinses such as 2% lime sulfur, 2% miconazole/2–4% chlorhexidine and 2% enilconazole can be used.
- Ectoparasiticial therapies—topical pyrethorids, lime sulfur, 0.25% fipronil spray and avermectins. Fipronil spray has shown to be curative in one treatment. Apply spray from elbow and stifles down with 125 ml of the product applied to each leg. Apply a second treatment in 3 to 4 weeks. Treat all animals in contact with the infected animal simultaneously. Infestation with *Chorioptes* requires environmental decontamination.
- Judicious use of systemic steroids is indicated to reduce inflammation especially in idiopathic, contact, vasculitis, and immune-mediated conditions.

CONTRAINDICATIONS

Condition worsens by overzealous application of topical ointments on the surface of necrotic skin and crusts.

PRECAUTIONS

Use of fipronil spray constitutes extra-label use of an EPA-registered pesticide.

POSSIBLE INTERACTIONS N/A

ALTERNATIVE DRUGS

Holistic remedies of black tea bag or sauerkraut poultices

FOLLOW-UP

PATIENT MONITORING

Depends on severity and causes

PREVENTION/AVOIDANCE

- Prevention relies on avoidance to the exposure to recurrent wetting. Wet grass in the early summer morning can irritate and macerate the epidermis. Recurrent cases benefit from stalls with clean, dry bedding to prevent skin damage from ammonia and dampness. Simple avoidance of UV light may not be sufficient to prevent disease.
- Application of a light barrier creams such as petroleum jelly before exercise, combined with cleansing and drying after exercise may prevent recurrence.
- Asymptomatic carriers of dermatophytosis or *Chorioptes* may need to be treated.

POSSIBLE COMPLICATIONS

Lameness and/or excessive granulation tissue

EXPECTED COURSE AND PROGNOSIS

Prognosis depends on stage of the disease and if etiologies are identified. May take years for full recovery. Permanent thickening, hyperplasia, alopecia and recrudescence are common.

MISCELLANEOUS

ASSOCIATED CONDITIONS

N/A

AGE-RELATED FACTORS

Severity worsens with age.

ZOONOTIC POTENTIAL

Dermatophilosis, dermatophytosis and *Chorioptes* are zoonotic. Wear gloves when handling horse.

PREGNANCY

Corticosteroids—contraindicated during pregnancy

SYNONYMS

Terminology to describe this syndrome is numerous and changes with disease progression.

- Grease heel—early form
- Scratches- early form; colloquial term
- Mud Fever or Rash—early form; used in Europe and Australia
- Cracked Heels—exudative form
- Dew poisoning—exudative form
- Grapes—chronic proliferative form

SEE ALSO

- Pastern Leukocytoclastic Vasculitis
- Chronic Progressive Lymphedema
- Ectoparasite Dermatoses
- Dermatophilosis
- Bacterial dermatitis
- Pemphigus foliaceus
- Sarcoid

Suggested Reading

Geburek F, Ohnesorge B, Deegen E, et al. Alterations of epidermal proliferation and cytokeratin expression in skin biopsies from heavy draught horses with chronic pastern dermatitis. Veterinary Dermatology 2005;16:373–384.

Author Gwendolen Lorch
Consulting Editor Gwendolen Lorch

PATENT DUCTUS ARTERIOSUS

BASICS

DEFINITION

• A persistently patent vascular communication between the aorta and pulmonary artery.
• The ductus arteriosus is a vessel that allows blood to shunt from the pulmonary artery to the aorta in the fetus.
• The ductus arteriosus normally constricts after birth in response to increased local oxygen tension and prostaglandin inhibition, and closure should be complete within 4 days of birth.

PATHOPHYSIOLOGY

• When the ductus arteriosus remains patent, blood shunts from the higher-pressure aorta to the lower-pressure pulmonary artery, creating left atrial and left ventricular volume overload.
• Size of the patent ductus arteriosus determines severity of the volume overload—With a large PDA, stretching of the mitral annulus occurs over time, and mitral regurgitation develops; as mitral regurgitation becomes more severe, left atrial pressure increases, resulting in increased pulmonary venous pressure and clinical signs of left-sided congestive heart failure.
• PDA may also be a component of more complex congenital cardiac defects.

SYSTEM AFFECTED

Cardiovascular

GENETICS

• Not yet determined in horses
• The condition is heritable in other species but rare in horses.

INCIDENCE/PREVALENCE

PDA is a rare, isolated congenital defect, but it occurs more frequently in horses with complex congenital heart disease.

SIGNALMENT

• Arabian horses appear to be predisposed to complex congenital cardiac defects.
• Murmurs usually are detectable at birth.
• Diagnosed most frequently in neonates, foals, and young horses but can be found at any age

SIGNS

General Comments

May be an incidental finding but usually is part of a more complex congenital cardiac disorder

Historical

• Exercise intolerance—medium-size to large PDA and those associated with complex congenital cardiac defects
• Congestive heart failure—large PDA and those associated with complex congenital cardiac defects

Physical Examination

• A grade 3–6/6 continuous machinery murmur with point of maximal intensity over the main pulmonary artery between the pulmonic and aortic valve area
• Additional loud murmurs may be detected in complex congenital cardiac defects, with characteristics dependent on the exact nature of the defects.
• Bounding arterial pulses
• Premature beats or an irregularly irregular heart rhythm of atrial fibrillation may be present with larger PDA or those associated with complex congenital cardiac defects.

CAUSES

Lack of constriction of the ductus arteriosus

RISK FACTORS

• Premature foal
• Hypoxia
• Neonatal pulmonary hypertension
• Neonatal respiratory distress syndrome
• Mares treated with prostaglandin inhibitors during late gestation

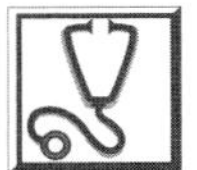

DIAGNOSIS

DIFFERENTIAL DIAGNOSIS

• Physiologic flow murmur—usually systolic rather than continuous murmur; differentiate echocardiographically.
• Ventricular septal defect with aortic regurgitation—pansystolic and holodiastolic murmur and point of maximal intensity of pansystolic murmur, usually in the tricuspid valve area; differentiate echocardiographically.
• Complex congenital cardiac disease—Differentiate echocardiographically.

CBC/BIOCHEMISTRY/URINALYSIS

N/A

OTHER LABORATORY TESTS

N/A

IMAGING

Electrocardiography

Atrial premature depolarizations or atrial fibrillation may be present in horses with left atrial enlargement.

Echocardiography

• Difficult to visualize
• The left atrium and ventricle are enlarged and dilated and have a rounded appearance.
• Pulmonary artery dilatation in horses with a large shunt.
• Color-flow Doppler may reveal the shunt from aorta to pulmonary artery through the PDA.
• Continuous, high-velocity, turbulent flow is detected with continuous-wave Doppler toward the main pulmonary artery.
• Retrograde, turbulent flow in the main pulmonary artery may be identified with color-flow and continuous-wave Doppler.
• Additional cardiac defects such as great vessel anomalies, right atrioventricular valve atresia, or hypoplastic left ventricle syndrome may be present. A segmental approach where each structure is identified and its connection to other structures documented echocardiographically is required to differentiate complex congenital cardiac defects. Color-flow and contrast echocardiography may allow documentation of the path of blood flow in affected horses.

Thoracic Radiography

• Increased pulmonary vascularity and cardiac enlargement may be detected.
• Pulmonary edema may be detected in foals or horses with congestive heart failure.

DIAGNOSTIC PROCEDURES

Cardiac Catheterization

• Right-sided cardiac catheterization to directly measure pulmonary arterial and capillary wedge pressures and to sample blood for oxygen content
• Elevated pulmonary arterial and capillary wedge pressures as well as increased oxygen saturation of pulmonary arterial blood are found in horses with patent ductus arteriosus.

24-Hour Holter Monitoring

Continuous monitoring is useful for establishing the diagnosis in horses with suspected atrial premature depolarizations.

PATHOLOGIC FINDINGS

• The PDA is present between the aorta and main pulmonary artery.
• Left atrial and ventricular enlargement and thinning of the left atrial and ventricular free wall in horses with a significant shunt
• Dilatation of the main pulmonary artery and right and left pulmonary arteries in those horses with a large shunt and in those with pulmonary hypertension.
• Thickened media of the pulmonary arterioles in horses with chronic pulmonary hypertension.
• Pulmonary edema in horses with congestive heart failure.
• PDA is often identified in conjunction with additional defects in a variety of complex congenital cardiac defects including hypoplastic left ventricle syndrome, transposition of the great arteries, critical pulmonic stenosis, and atresia of the right atrioventricular orifice.

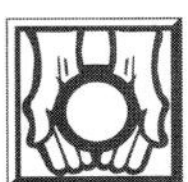

TREATMENT

AIMS OF TREATMENT

- Management by intermittent monitoring in horses with small isolated PDA
- Palliative care in horses with large PDA and those in which there are multiple cardiac defects

APPROPRIATE HEALTH CARE

- Most newborn foals with PDA should have the underlying pulmonary disease or pulmonary hypertension treated if present.
- Monitor affected horses on an annual basis.
- Horse with PDA and congestive heart failure could be treated for the congestive heart failure with positive inotropic drugs, vasodilators, and diuretics. Consider humane destruction, however, because only short-term, symptomatic improvement can be expected.

NURSING CARE

N/A

ACTIVITY

- Horses with small PDA may be able to perform successfully at lower levels of athletic activities, but they are unlikely to be able to perform satisfactorily at upper levels.
- Monitor affected horses echocardiographically on an annual basis to ensure they are safe to ride. Dilation of the pulmonary artery should prompt discontinuation of ridden activities as it can be a precursor to pulmonary artery rupture.
- Affected horses that develop atrial fibrillation need a complete cardiovascular examination to determine if lower levels of athletic performance are safe.

DIET

N/A

CLIENT EDUCATION

- Regularly monitor the horse's rhythm; any irregularities other than second-degree atrioventricular block should prompt an electrocardiographic examination.
- Carefully monitor the horse for exercise intolerance, respiratory distress, prolonged recovery after exercise, increased resting respiratory or heart rate, or cough; if detected, obtain a cardiac reexamination.

SURGICAL CONSIDERATIONS

- Closure of the PDA is possible with a transvenous umbrella catheter or coil having a diameter large enough to close the defect.
- Surgical closure is not financially feasible or practical for obtaining an equine athlete at this time.

MEDICATIONS

DRUGS OF CHOICE, CONTRAINDICATIONS, ALTERNATIVE DRUGS

N/A

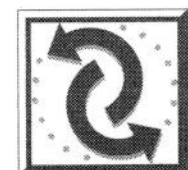

FOLLOW-UP

PATIENT MONITORING

Frequently monitor the horse's cardiac rate, rhythm, respiratory rate, and effort.

PREVENTION/AVOIDANCE

N/A

POSSIBLE COMPLICATIONS

Large PDA and those forming part of complex congential cardiac defects—atrial fibrillation, congestive heart failure, and pulmonary artery rupture

EXPECTED COURSE AND PROGNOSIS

- Horses with a small PDA may have a normal performance life for lower levels of athletic competition and a normal life expectancy.
- Horses with a moderate to large PDA may develop atrial fibrillation and have a guarded prognosis; these horses should have a shortened performance life at lower levels of athletic competition and a shortened life expectancy.
- Horses with pulmonary artery dilatation have a grave prognosis for life and are not safe to ride.
- Horses with associated congestive heart failure usually have a guarded to grave prognosis for life. Most horses with a PDA being treated for congestive heart failure should respond to the supportive therapy and transiently improve, but once congestive heart failure develops, euthanasia is recommended.

MISCELLANEOUS

ASSOCIATED CONDITIONS

- Complex congenital cardiac disease is the rule, rather than the exception, in affected horses.
- Mitral regurgitation can develop in horses with PDA associated with stretching of the mitral annulus secondary to significant left atrial and ventricular volume overload.
- Pulmonary artery rupture can occur secondary to the pulmonary artery dilatation and elevated pulmonary arterial pressures.

AGE-RELATED FACTORS

Young horses are more likely to be diagnosed with this defect.

ZOONOTIC POTENTIAL

N/A

PREGNANCY

Breeding affected horses should be discouraged even though the condition is rare and the heritable nature of this defect is not known.

SYNONYMS

N/A

SEE ALSO

Atrial fibrillation

ABBREVIATION

- PDA = patent ductus arteriosus

Suggested Reading

Buergelt CD, Carmichael JA, Tashjian RJ, Das KM. Spontaneous rupture of the left pulmonary artery in a horse with patent ductus arteriosus. J Am Vet Med Assoc 1970;157:313–320.

Carmichael JA, Buergelt CD, Lord PF, et al. Diagnosis of patent ductus arteriosus in a horse. J Am Vet Med Assoc 1971;158:767–775.

Marr CM. Cardiac murmurs: congenital heart disease. In Marr CM ed. Cardiology of the Horse. Philadelphia: WB Saunders, 1999:210–233.

Reef VB. Cardiovascular ultrasonography. In: Reef VB, ed. Equine Diagnostic Ultrasound. Philadelphia: WB Saunders, 1998:215–272.

Scott EA, Kneller SK, Witherspoon DM. Closure of ductus arteriosus determined by cardiac catheterization and angiography in newborn foals. Am J Vet Res 1975;36:1021–1023.

Author Virginia B. Reef
Consulting Editor Celia M. Marr

PATENT URACHUS

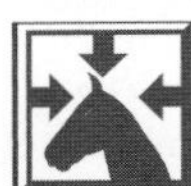

BASICS

OVERVIEW

The urachus is the umbilical structure that directs urine from the fetal bladder to the allantoic fluid. The urachus normally closes at the time of birth, but it can remain patent or can reopen secondary to inflammation or infection. The urachus that fails to close within hours of birth (congenital patent urachus) or that begins to leak urine after it has initially closed (acquired patent urachus) is considered a patent urachus.

SIGNALMENT

- Neonatal foals are affected by this condition.
- There does not appear to be a breed or sex predilection.

SIGNS

- Urine is seen streaming or dripping from the umbilicus when the foal urinates, or the umbilicus may be moist from urine leakage.
- Urine scalding may be noted on the inside of the hindlimbs. • When there is infection associated with a patent urachus, the umbilicus may also be enlarged, painful, or warm, and the foal may exhibit fever, lethargy, and poor appetite.

CAUSES AND RISK FACTORS

- Congenital factors such as excessive traction or twisting of the umbilical cord in utero may be related to congenital or persistent patent urachus. • After parturition, omphalophlebitis can lead to reopening or failure to close of the urachus. Debilitated and septicemic foals are at higher risk of developing omphalophlebitis.

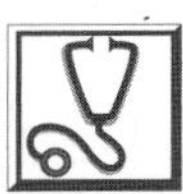

DIAGNOSIS

DIFFERENTIAL DIAGNOSIS

Omphalophlebitis—In the absence of patent urachus, there may be purulent drainage, but no urine leakage. The foal may show signs of systemic inflammation or infection (fever, lethargy, other sites of infection), and the umbilicus may be enlarged, warm, and painful. Ultrasound examination of the umbilicus can help to rule out omphalophlebitis.

CBC/BIOCHEMISTRY/URINALYSIS

- Uncomplicated patent urachus is not associated with any significant changes in blood work. • When patent urachus is complicated with omphalophlebitis, leukocytosis and hyperfibrinogenemia are often present.
- Occasionally, tears in the urachus can extend intra-abdominally and result in uroperitoneum. Azotemia, hyponatremia, and hyperkalemia may be seen in these cases.

OTHER LABORATORY TESTS

IgG levels—should be >800 mg/dL by 20 hr

IMAGING

- Ultrasonography—The umbilical remnants and bladder should be evaluated using a 7.5-MHz probe. Examination will confirm patency between the bladder and the urachus, and can determine whether omphalophlebitis or urachal abscess is present.
- Positive-contrast radiography—Contrast material delivered retrograde via the urethra can confirm patency between the bladder and the urachus and can also reveal any leakage from the urachus into the abdomen or subcutaneous tissues.

OTHER DIAGNOSTIC PROCEDURES

- Bacterial culture of the aseptically prepared umbilical stump if omphalophlebitis is suspected
- Blood cultures should be performed in neonates to rule out septicemia.

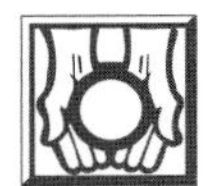

TREATMENT

- The umbilicus should be kept clean by dipping in dilute chlorhexidine (0.5%) or alternatively with dilute iodine (2%) twice daily until the umbilicus is no longer patent. Topical application of cauterizing compounds such as silver nitrate or strong iodine can be used for congenital uncomplicated patent urachus; however, these should never be used in cases of acquired patent urachus with omphalophlebitis.
- Foals with low IgG are at higher risk of septicemia, and should be treated with hyperimmune plasma IV. • Nursing care should also include protection of the skin from urine scalding. Petroleum jelly can be used on the foal's hindlimbs after the skin is thoroughly dried.
- Surgical resection of the umbilical remnants is recommended if infection is present with patent urachus or if the urachus has not closed after 5–7 days of medical treatment. Surgical treatment requires hospitalization for the perioperative period (usually for several days). Exercise should be restricted for 3–4 weeks if the umbilical structures are surgically removed.

MEDICATIONS

DRUG(S) OF CHOICE

- Systemic antimicrobials are recommended for congenital and acquired patent urachus.
- Uncomplicated (congenital) patent urachus may be managed with penicillin (22,000 IU/kg IV QID) or trimethoprim sulfa (30 mg/kg PO BID). • Patent urachus secondary to omphalophlebitis should be treated with broad-spectrum antimicrobials—usually a penicillin and an aminoglycoside (amikacin 25 mg/kg IV daily or gentamicin 6.6 mg/kg IV daily), and treatment should be guided by culture and sensitivity from umbilical or blood cultures.

CONTRAINDICATIONS/POSSIBLE INTERACTIONS

- Aminoglycosides should be used with caution in foals with renal compromise or dehydration.
- Other broad-spectrum parenteral antimicrobial choices include ceftiofur (10 mg/kg IV QID).

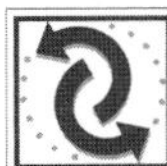

FOLLOW-UP

PATIENT MONITORING

- The foal should be monitored frequently for signs of systemic infection such as fever, lethargy, joint effusion, or lameness. • Umbilicus should be palpated to detect any changes in size or consistency. The foal should be monitored for signs of leakage or moisture at the umbilicus when urinating. • Serial ultrasound examinations of the umbilical remnants can detect development of omphalophlebitis.

PREVENTION/AVOIDANCE

- Adequate colostrum • Clean environment
- Avoid traction on the umbilicus during parturition. • Umbilical disinfection with 0.5% chlorhexidine solution

POSSIBLE COMPLICATIONS

- Foals with a patent urachus are at risk of ascending infection and bacteremia, and so should be monitored carefully for signs of septic omphalophlebitis, septicemia, and septic arthritis. • Treatment with cauterizing agents can lead to significant inflammation of the umbilicus, and can cause scalding of the ventral abdomen and prepuce if used incorrectly.

EXPECTED COURSE AND PROGNOSIS

- Most foals with congenital patent urachus will have resolution with medical management. If the urachus remains patent after 5–7 days of treatment or if there are signs of progressive infection, surgical removal of the umbilicus is recommended. • Prognosis for congenital patent urachus is excellent. Prognosis for acquired patent urachus is good provided there are no secondary complications with infection.
- Septicemia and septic arthritis will greatly reduce the prognosis.

MISCELLANEOUS

ASSOCIATED CONDITIONS

Omphalophlebitis

AGE-RELATED FACTORS

This is a condition of neonatal foals.

SEE ALSO

- Septicemia, neonatal • Omphalophlebitis

Suggested Reading

Nolen-Walston R. Umbilical and urinary disorders. In: Paradis MR, ed. Equine Neonatal Medicine: A Case-Based Approach. Philadelphia: Elsevier Saunders, 2006:231–245.

Robertson JT, Embertson RS: Congenital and perinatal abnormalities of the urogenital tract. Vet Clin North Am Equine Pract 1988;4:359.

Author Margaret C. Mudge
Consulting Editor Margaret C. Mudge

PENTACHLOROPHENOL (PCP) TOXICOSIS

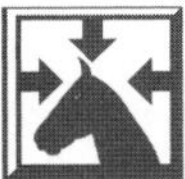

BASICS

OVERVIEW

- PCP causes uncoupling of oxidative phosphorylation and direct irritation to the skin and respiratory tract.
- Acute and chronic intoxication syndromes have been described in animals. The chronic syndrome may be due to PCDD and PCDF isomers found in PCP.
- Restrictions on the use of PCP due to environmental and toxicity concerns make exposure and toxicosis unlikely.

SIGNALMENT

N/A

SIGNS

- Acute—hyperthermia, restlessness, tachypnea, increased gastrointestinal motility, weakness, seizures, and collapse
- Chronic—anorexia, weight loss, dependent edema, alopecia, skin cracks and fissures, colic, joint stiffness, recurrent hoof problems, conjunctivitis, hematuria, and secondary opportunistic infections

CAUSES AND RISK FACTORS

- Most likely source of exposure is treated wood used for fences or feedbunks.
- Exposure to bedding from treated wood

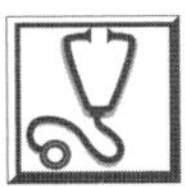

DIAGNOSIS

DIFFERENTIAL DIAGNOSIS

- Acute—infectious causes of pyrexia (CBC, bacterial culture, serology)
- Chronic—*Vicia villosa* toxicosis (skin biopsy)

CBC/BIOCHEMISTRY/URINALYSIS

- Acute—not reported for horses
- Chronic—changes consistent with hepatic dysfunction, anemia, and thrombocytopenia

OTHER LABORATORY TESTS

- Acute—ante-mortem detection of PCP in blood, serum/plasma or urine; PCP is rapidly cleared so measurement is useful only in acute intoxications; post-mortem detection of PCP in skin, liver, or kidney
- Chronic—measurement of PCDD or PCDF isomers in plasma/serum or tissues

IMAGING

N/A

DIAGNOSTIC PROCEDURES/ PATHOLOGICAL RESULTS

- Acute—not reported for horses
- Chronic—grossly, emaciation; alopecia; crusty, scaly dermatitis; cracks or fissures of the skin that exude clear serum-like fluid; splenomegaly; histologically, chronic nonsuppurative dermatitis; hepatic bile duct proliferation, inflammation and focal necrosis; splenic hemosiderosis; multifocal renal tubular necrosis; nonregenerative bone marrow

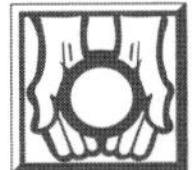

TREATMENT

- Acute—control hyperthermia; remove from source of exposure; if recent oral exposure, consider gastrointestinal decontamination; wash exposed skin.
- Chronic—remove from source of exposure; provide symptomatic and supportive care.

MEDICATIONS

DRUG(S) OF CHOICE

Acute—AC at 1–2 g/kg in water slurry (1 g AC in 5 mL water) PO and either magnesium sulfate at 250 mg/kg PO or sorbitol (70%) at 3 mL/kg PO, given once with AC

CONTRAINDICATIONS/POSSIBLE INTERACTIONS

N/A

FOLLOW-UP

PATIENT MONITORING

N/A

PREVENTION/AVOIDANCE

Avoid use of treated wood where animal contact is possible.

POSSIBLE COMPLICATIONS

N/A

EXPECTED COURSE AND PROGNOSIS

Poor prognosis and prolonged recovery in chronic intoxication due to dioxin

MISCELLANEOUS

Current environmental restrictions on the use of PCP make clinically significant exposure and toxicosis unlikely.

ASSOCIATED CONDITIONS

N/A

AGE-RELATED FACTORS

N/A

ZOONOTIC POTENTIAL

N/A

PREGNANCY

Chronic intoxication of pregnant horses with PCDD and PCDF can result in birth of weak foals susceptible to opportunistic infections.

ABBREVIATIONS

- AC = activated charcoal
- CBC = complete blood count
- PCDD = dibenzo-*p*-dioxin isomers
- PCDF = dibenzofuran isomers
- PCP = pentachlorophenol

Suggested Reading

Kerkvliet NI, Wagner SL, Schmotzer WB, Hackett M, Schrader WK, Hultgren B. Dioxin intoxication from chronic exposure of horses to penta-chlorophenol-contaminated wood shavings. J Am Vet Med Assoc 1992;201:296–302.

Author Robert H. Poppenga
Consulting Editor Robert H. Poppenga

PEMPHIGUS FOLIACEUS

BASICS

OVERVIEW

• PF is an autoimmune skin disease and the most common cause in the author's practice for noninfectious crusts in the horse. It is also the most commonly seen autoimmune skin disease in the horse, after purpura hemorrhagica.
• The exact pathomechanism has not been investigated in the horse, but it is presumed to be similar to that for humans and the dog—Autoantibodies are produced that attack the intercellular connections between the skin's epidermal cells. This leads to formation of transient pustules or bullae and subsequent crusts.

INCIDENCE/PREVALENCE

Geographic distribution of the disease is presumably worldwide. The incidence is unknown but the disease is relatively uncommon. In a study from California, 80% of the horses first exhibited signs between September and February; the reason for this is not known.

SYSTEMS AFFECTED

Skin and hemolymphatic system

SIGNALMENT

Breed Predilections

Appaloosa (in one study)

Mean Age and Range

8.6 years (2.5 mo to 25 years)

Age or Sex Predilection

None

GENETICS

It is unknown if there is a genetic basis for PF.

SIGNS

• Crusts, frequently starting on the face and legs and then become generalized. • Occasionally, crusts only on the coronary band • Alopecia
• Peripheral edema ("stocking up") • Fever
• Pustules • Lethargy • Anorexia

CAUSES AND RISK FACTORS

Unknown in most cases. One published case of possible causation by penicillin

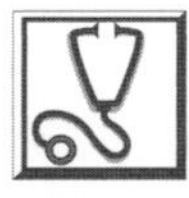

DIAGNOSIS

DIFFERENTIAL DIAGNOSIS

• Severe superficial staphylococcal dermatitis
• Dermatophytosis • Dermatophilosis
• Sarcoidosis (chronic granulomatous disease)

CBC/BIOCHEMISTRY/URINALYSIS

Low-grade anemia combined with a leukocytosis

OTHER LABORATORY TESTS

N/A

IMAGING N/A

OTHER DIAGNOSTIC PROCEDURES

• Skin biopsy for histopathology • Very important NOT to surgically prepare the area to be biopsied. It is acceptable to surgically prepare the site *after* taking the biopsy sample (i.e., before suturing the site) to limit chances of infection. • Choose multiple sites, and include the crust. • Provide the pathologist with the patient signalment, a brief history, descriptions and locations of the biopsied sites, as well as differential diagnosis. • Cytology of aspirates or impression smears from pustules and crusts may reveal acantholytic cells and neutrophils.
• Bacteriologic and fungal (DTM) cultures will identify secondary bacterial folliculitis or dermatophytosis, respectively.

PATHOLOGICAL FINDINGS

• Subcorneal or intracorneal pustules with acantholytic cells • Certain strains of the dermatophyte species *Trichophyton* may cause acantholysis; therefore, any histology suggestive of PF should have special stains for fungi performed.

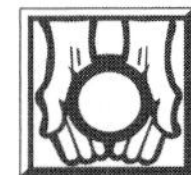

TREATMENT

• Control disease, reduce lesions, return horse to function • May not be able to eliminate all lesions

MEDICATIONS

DRUG(S) OF CHOICE

• Corticosteroids at immunosuppressive doses (prednisolone 1 mg/kg q12h, dexamethasone 0.05–0.1 mg/kg q24h) for 2 weeks, then taper to lowest effective dose • Azathioprine in combination with the above corticosteroids at 1 mg/kg q24h for 1 mo, then q48h. Usually takes 1 mo for effect. Anecdotal reports of using the gold salt sodium aurothiomalate in conjunction with the above corticosteroids—1 mg/kg IM q7 days until improvement, then taper to q14 days, q30 days, etc. May take 3 mo for a clinical response (generally a lag phase of 6–8 weeks)
• Both azathioprine and gold salts are used as steroid-sparing agents; both are moderately expensive. As they take effect, the corticosteroid dosage should be slowly reduced.

CONTRAINDICATIONS/POSSIBLE INTERACTIONS

• Horses with a predisposition to laminitis, or with a previous history of laminitis, should be monitored very closely for recurrence, or possibly just treated with azathioprine or gold salts, although this method of treatment has not be substantiated in equine PF. • Therapeutic precautions include the following—corticosteroids: laminitis; azathioprine: bone marrow suppression (rare); gold salts: bone marrow suppression, glomerulonephropathy (both very rare).

FOLLOW-UP

PATIENT MONITORING

• Physical examinations, especially looking for resolution of lesions as well as laminitis caused by corticosteroids • If initially anemic, monitor with CBC. • If using azathioprine, monitor CBC and platelets, once monthly. • If using gold salts, monitor CBC, platelets, and urine protein, once monthly. Gold toxicity, although rare, may be cumulative: a horse may receive the medication without problems for extended periods, and then develop adverse effects such as thrombocytopenia.

PREVENTION/AVOIDANCE

N/A

POSSIBLE COMPLICATIONS

• Corticosteroid-induced laminitis
• Immunosuppression can predispose animal to secondary cutaneous (pyoderma, dermatophytosis) and systemic infections, although rare.

EXPECTED COURSE AND PROGNOSIS

• Guarded to good, depending on response to treatment, and if corticosteroid-induced adverse effects occur • Some horses need life-long treatment, others may have treatment discontinued after complete resolution of lesions without the PF recurring. • Advise client of the controllable, rather than curable, nature of the disease. • In a minority of cases, it is possible to taper down and stop medication without relapse.
• Advise client of the adverse effects of medications (e.g., corticosteroids)—particularly potential for laminitis.

MISCELLANEOUS

PREGNANCY

• Anecdotal reports of affected mares giving birth to affected newborn foals • One report describes a female donkey in which PF occurred, then regressed, during 2 of its 5 pregnancies.

SEE ALSO N/A

ABBREVIATION

• PF = pemphigus foliaceus

Suggested Reading

Bourdeau P, Baudry J. [Pemphigus-type bullous dermatosis associated with pregnancy in a female donkey] [in French]. Informations Dermatologiques Vétérinaries 2005 October (11):19–24.

Scott DW. Marked acantholysis associated with dermatophytosis due to *Trichophyton equinum* in two horses. Vet Dermatol 1994;5:105–110.

Scott DW. Immune-mediated skin diseases in domestic animals: ten years after—Part I. Compend Cont Educ Pract Vet 1987;9:424–434.

Scott DW, Miller WH Jr. Equine Dermatology. St. Louis: Saunders, 2003:480.

Vandenabeele SIG, White SD, Kass P, et al. Pemphigus foliaceus in the horse: 20 cases. Vet Dermatol 2004;15:381–388.

Author Stephen D. White
Consulting Editor Gwendolen Lorch

PENETRATING INJURIES TO THE FOOT

BASICS

OVERVIEW

• A puncture of the solar surface or frog of the foot caused by nail, screw, or other sharp object. Also referred to as "street nail." • The penetrating object carries debris (manure, soil, rust) into deeper structures, initiating a bacterial infection. The infection can be within the soft tissues, bony structures, or synovial structures of the foot.

SYSTEMS AFFECTED

• Musculoskeletal—foot
  ○ Soft tissue structures—deep digital flexor tendon, hoof cushion
  ○ Bony structures—third phalanx, navicular bone
  ○ Synovial structures—DIP, navicular bursa, digital flexor tendon sheath

SIGNS

Historical

• Acute, non–weight bearing to toe-touching lameness • +/− Penetrating object in foot
• Initially, discharge comes from the wound, and the horse may quickly become more comfortable.
• Subsequently, the superficial aspect of the wound closes, causing a buildup of purulent discharge within the deeper structures leading to increased lameness.

Physical Examination

• Varying degrees of lameness—initially severely lame, then may improve • Chronic injuries (>1 week)—increasingly lame • Increased digital pulses and heat in affected limb • Hoof tester application elicits severe pain. • +/− Penetrating foreign body • Upon inspection of sole, wound tract may be seen, although it can be hard to identify if not examined acutely.
• +/− Discharge from the wound tract • +/− DIP or digital flexor tendon sheath effusion
• +/− Fever

CAUSES AND RISK FACTORS

Stepping on a sharp object

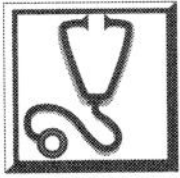

DIAGNOSIS

DIFFERENTIAL DIAGNOSIS

• Subsolar abscess—if no history of foreign body and no puncture wound • Third phalanx fracture—Rule out by radiography. • Deep digital flexor tendon injury—Severely affected horses may flip toe up at a walk; ultrasonography and radiography (DIP subluxation) will confirm the injury. • Navicular bone fracture—Rule out by radiography.

CBC/BIOCHEMISTRY/URINALYSIS

+/− Hyperfibrinogenemia if injury >24 hr

IMAGING

Radiography—Plain Films

• If foreign body is still present, obtain lateral and dorsopalmar views (minimally) of the foot with it in place to determine which deeper tissues are involved. • If the foreign body is not present, aseptically prepare the hoof and tract and insert a sterile malleable radiopaque probe into the tract and then obtain the above views to determine the course of the tract. • Additional views as needed to rule out third phalanx or navicular bone fracture or to further define the path of the foreign body.

Radiography—Contrast Radiography

• Contrast material can be injected into the wound tract using aseptic technique; a radiograph is obtained immediately to determine if synovial structures are involved. • Alternately, the DIP, digital flexor tendon sheath, and navicular bursa are injected with contrast material using aseptic technique; a radiograph is obtained to identify communication with the wound.

OTHER DIAGNOSTIC PROCEDURES

• Synovial fluid analysis (cytology, total nucleated cell count, total protein) • Microbial culture and sensitivity from the wound tract and/or synovial fluid. This should be done before antibiotic administration to direct future therapy.

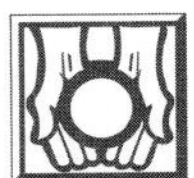

TREATMENTS

• Penetrating injuries to the foot can have life-threatening consequences; therefore, these injuries should be treated as an emergency. • If synovial involvement (i.e., DIP, navicular bursa, or digital flexor tendon sheath) is suspected, the horse should be referred for surgical treatment. Prior to referral, remove the foreign body, clean and bandage the foot, provide appropriate analgesia (with NSAIDs), +/− begin antibiotic therapy. Surgical treatment includes arthroscopic wound debridement and generous lavage of synovial structure(s). • If no synovial structures are involved, debride the wound tract, bandage the foot, and initiate medical treatment. This may be facilitated by using local anesthesia prior to debridement. • The foot bandage should keep the tract clean and dry. Duct tape covering the bottom of the foot will facilitate this. The foot bandage may require daily changing initially.
• +/− Regional limb perfusions with antibiotics
• Stall rest until the tract is healed
• If horse is severely lame, sole support for the contralateral foot

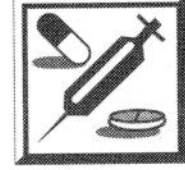

MEDICATIONS

DRUG(S) OF CHOICE

• Tetanus toxoid and antitoxin • NSAIDs (phenylbutazone 2.2–4.4 mg/kg daily to BID) as needed • Broad-spectrum antibiotics until tract has completely healed. Initial choices can be adjusted following bacterial culture and sensitivity results. • Anaerobic infections are common; therefore, include an antimicrobial with good anaerobic coverage (i.e., penicillin, metronidazole). • Daily regional limb perfusions with antibiotics—aminoglycosides (amikacin 2 g per adult horse diluted to 60 mL with sterile saline)

CONTRAINDICATIONS/POSSIBLE INTERACTIONS

These horses may require prolonged therapy with NSAIDs and aminoglycosides; therefore, renal function (via serum creatinine levels) should be evaluated before initiating treatment and rechecked periodically.

FOLLOW-UP

PATIENT MONITORING

• The degree of lameness should be monitored closely on a daily basis. In horses treated medically, if lameness does not improve quickly (within 3–5 days), or if the severity of lameness increases despite treatment, referral should be considered. • If the wound communicated with the third phalanx, follow-up radiographs should be obtained for possible sequestrum formation.

PREVENTION/AVOIDANCE

Routine pasture maintenance and inspection for foreign objects

POSSIBLE COMPLICATIONS

• Septic arthritis (DIP, navicular bursa), septic tenosynovitis (digital flexor tendon sheath), septic deep digital flexor tendonitis and subsequent rupture, third phalanx osteitis +/− sequestrum, navicular bone fracture • The above complications may cause severe lameness, inability to return to athletic soundness, and contralateral limb laminitis. • If severe, complications could necessitate euthanasia.

EXPECTED COURSE AND PROGNOSIS

• Without synovial involvement and with prompt medical treatment, prognosis is good to excellent for athletic soundness. • Synovial involvement with prompt (i.e., <48 hours) surgical treatment has a fair to good prognosis for athletic soundness.
• Prolonged synovial (i.e., >7 days) involvement without prompt surgical treatment has a poor prognosis for athletic soundness and poor to grave prognosis for life.

MISCELLANEOUS

ASSOCIATED CONDITIONS

Severely lame horses are at risk for contralateral limb laminitis.

PREGNANCY

In later gestation, increased weight may exacerbate lameness.

SEE ALSO

• Septic arthritis • Solar abscess

ABBREVIATION

• DIP = distal interphalangeal joint

Suggested Reading

Furst AE, Lischer CJ. Foot. In: Auer JA, Stick JA, eds. Equine Surgery, ed 3. St. Louis: Saunders, 2006:1193–1195.

Author Liberty Getman
Consulting Editor Elizabeth J. Davidson

PENILE LACERATIONS

BASICS

DEFINITION
Any wound to the penile epithelial surface

PATHOPHYSIOLOGY
N/A

SYSTEMS AFFECTED
- Reproductive
- Urinary

SIGNALMENT
No age or breed predilection

SIGNS
N/A

CAUSES
Trauma—breeding accidents, improperly fitted stallion rings, kicks, jumping injuries, masturbation, and improper surgical technique

RISK FACTORS
Aggressive stallions/colts housed or handled in unsafe conditions are more likely to injure themselves and others.

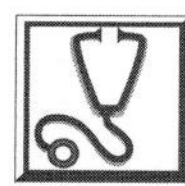

DIAGNOSIS

DIFFERENTIAL DIAGNOSIS

Differentiating Causes

- Visual inspection generally reveals the laceration.
- Paraphimosis may be present, but may be secondary to the laceration.
- Ulcerative lesions caused by neoplastic or parasitic diseases should not be considered lacerations for this discussion.

CBC/BIOCHEMISTRY/URINALYSIS
N/A

OTHER LABORATORY TESTS
N/A

IMAGING
N/A

DIAGNOSTIC PROCEDURES
N/A

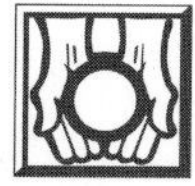

TREATMENT

- Ensure urethral patency. Placement of a urinary catheter may be indicated.
- Cleanse and debride the wound as dictated by location and severity.
- Acute post-trauma lacerations can be sutured for first intention healing.
- Old or grossly contaminated lacerations may have to heal by second intention, or delayed closure can be considered.
- Support the penis and prepuce with slings, hydrotherapy, and judicious exercise to prevent or eliminate extensive dependent edema.
- Sexual stimulation is absolutely contraindicated until healing is complete.

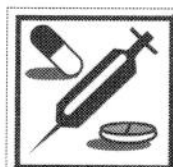

MEDICATIONS

DRUG(S) OF CHOICE
- NSAIDs including phenylbutazone (2–4 g/450 kg/day PO) or flunixin meglumine (1.1 mg/kg/day IV, IM, or PO) for patient comfort and to decrease inflammation. High initial dosages should be titrated to the lowest effective dose if more than 5 successive days of therapy is required.
- Systemic or local antibiotics for local infections and to prevent septicemia, if indicated
- Emollient application to the penile surface PRN to prevent or address urine scalding, if indicated

CONTRAINDICATIONS
Phenothiazine tranquilizers should never be used in the intact male.

PRECAUTIONS
N/A

POSSIBLE INTERACTIONS
N/A

ALTERNATIVE DRUGS
N/A

FOLLOW-UP

PATIENT MONITORING
- If the penis can be maintained within the prepuce without support, less frequent evaluation is necessary.
- If retraction of the penis is not possible, hospitalization may be required for frequent evaluation and care of the exposed penis.

POSSIBLE COMPLICATIONS
- Urine leakage with extensive tissue necrosis is possible if the penile urethra has been lacerated.
- Wounds that cannot be treated surgically are usually complicated by suppuration and cellulitis.
- Scar formation can result in phimosis, erectile dysfunction, impotence, or infertility.
- Hematomas generally arise from blood vessels superficial to the tunica albuginea. A hematoma that continues to enlarge is more likely attributable to a rent in the tunica albuginea, and closure of that defect is a priority.
- Paraphimosis is a common sequela to penile lacerations.
- Penile paralysis is possible as a result of the injury itself or secondary to paraphimosis.

MISCELLANEOUS

ASSOCIATED CONDITIONS
- Hemospermia
- Impotence
- Paraphimosis
- Penile paralysis
- Phimosis

AGE-RELATED FACTORS
N/A

ZOONOTIC POTENTIAL
N/A

PREGNANCY
N/A

SEE ALSO
- Paraphimosis
- Penile paralysis
- Phimosis

ABBREVIATION
- PRN = *pro re nata* (Latin); administer as needed

Suggested Reading

Ley WB, Slusher SH. Infertility and diseases of the reproductive tract of stallions. In: Youngquist RS, Threlfall WR, eds. Current Therapy in Large Animal Theriogenology. St. Louis: Saunders Elsevier, 2007:15–23.

Schumacher J, Varner DD. Surgical correction of abnormalities affecting the reproductive organs of stallions. In: Youngquist RS, Threlfall WR, eds. Current Therapy in Large Animal Theriogenology. St. Louis: Saunders Elsevier, 2007:23–36.

Schumacher J, Vaughan JT. Surgery of the penis and prepuce. Vet Clin North Am Equine Pract 1988;4:443–449.

Vaughan JT. Penis and prepuce. In: McKinnon AO, Voss JL, eds. Equine Reproduction. Philadelphia: Lea & Febiger, 1993:885–894.

Author Carole C. Miller

Consulting Editor Carla L. Carleton

PENILE PARALYSIS

BASICS

DEFINITION/OVERVIEW
Protracted extension of the penis in a flaccid state

ETIOLOGY/PATHOPHYSIOLOGY
Injury to the sacral nerves that innervate the penis and/or the retractor penis muscle results in the inability to retract the penis into the prepuce.

SYSTEMS AFFECTED
Reproductive

GENETICS N/A

INCIDENCE/PREVALENCE N/A

SIGNALMENT
Stallions (predominantly) or geldings of any age

SIGNS N/A

CAUSES
- Trauma—direct penile trauma, spinal cord injury or disease
- Infectious disease—EHV-1, rabies, EIA, purpura hemorrhagica, dourine (*Trypanosoma equiperdum*)
- Drug-induced—propiopromazine, acepromazine maleate, reserpine

RISK FACTORS
- Chronic paraphimosis or priapism
- Exhaustion or starvation
- Spinal cord lesion

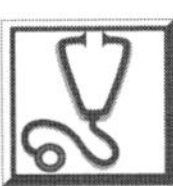

DIAGNOSIS

DIFFERENTIAL DIAGNOSIS

Differentiating Similar Signs
- Paraphimosis results in prolapse of the penis and prepuce, and dependent edema develops. The inability to retract the penis is generally due to the accumulated edema rather than true penile paralysis.
- Penile paralysis can be a sequela to chronic, severe paraphimosis. Long-standing penile paralysis can present as paraphimosis due to the formation of extensive dependent edema.
- Priapism, a persistent erection with engorgement of the corpus cavernosum penis, should not be confused with penile paralysis in which the penis is flaccid.

Differentiating Causes
- The presence of neurologic deficits other than the penile paralysis may link the penile problem with infectious causes and/or spinal cord injury as the primary problem.
- A recent history of respiratory disease (affected horse or on its farm) may implicate EHV-1 as a possible cause.

CBC/BIOCHEMISTRY/URINALYSIS
N/A

OTHER LABORATORY TESTS

EHV-1
- Rising antibody titers from paired sera, collected at a 14- to 21-day interval
- PCR testing or virus isolation from nasopharyngeal swabs or blood in the acute stage of the disease

EIA
AGID (Coggins) test

Dourine
- Identification of the causative agent in preputial or urethral exudates; serologic testing by complement fixation test
- Note—Dourine has been eradicated from North America and some areas of Europe.

IMAGING N/A

OTHER DIAGNOSTIC PROCEDURES
N/A

PATHOLOGICAL FINDINGS N/A

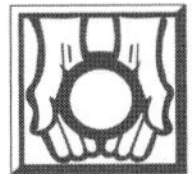

TREATMENT

- Replace the penis in the prepuce as soon as possible to prevent accumulation of dependent edema, drying of exposed surfaces, and traumatic injury. If replacement is impossible due to swelling, slings can be used to support the penis against the ventral abdominal wall.
- Lubricate the exposed mucosal surfaces with an emollient or antimicrobial ointment.
- In cases of chronic, nonresponsive penile paralysis, surgical intervention, including penile amputation or penile retraction (Bolz technique), should be considered. Castration generally precedes these surgical techniques.

APPROPRIATE HEALTH CARE, NURSING CARE, ACTIVITY, DIET, CLIENT EDUCATION, SURGICAL CONSIDERATIONS N/A

MEDICATIONS

DRUG(S) OF CHOICE
Anti-inflammatory medication (phenylbutazone 2–4 g/450kg/day PO) may be useful for patient comfort and to decrease inflammation.

CONTRAINDICATIONS
Phenothiazine tranquilizers should be avoided.

PRECAUTIONS N/A

POSSIBLE INTERACTIONS N/A

ALTERNATIVE DRUGS N/A

FOLLOW-UP

PATIENT MONITORING
- Initial management is intensive.
- Frequent evaluation is of paramount importance.
- Return of the ability to maintain the penis in the prepuce is a good prognostic indicator.

PREVENTION/AVOIDANCE N/A

POSSIBLE COMPLICATIONS
- Libido is often maintained, but if erection is impossible, live cover will not be possible without human intervention and assistance.
- Some affected stallions can still be trained to ejaculate into an artificial vagina or by an alternate system, e.g., application of hot compresses to the penis (glans and base), semen collection into a bag.
- Possible secondary complications of paralysis:
  - Paraphimosis due to the accumulation of dependent edema
  - Frostbite due to exposure
  - Surface excoriations (ulcers, secondary bacterial contamination, necrosis)

EXPECTED COURSE AND PROGNOSIS
N/A

MISCELLANEOUS

ASSOCIATED CONDITIONS
- Paraphimosis
- Balanoposthitis

AGE-RELATED FACTORS N/A

ZOONOTIC POTENTIAL N/A

PREGNANCY N/A

SYNONYMS N/A

SEE ALSO
- Herpesvirus (EHV) myeloencephalopathy
- Paraphimosis
- Priapism
- Psychogenic sexual behavior dysfunction

ABBREVIATIONS
- AGID = agar gel immunodiffusion
- EHV = equine herpevirus
- EIA = equine infectious anemia

Suggested Reading

Ley WB, Slusher SH. Infertility and diseases of the reproductive tract of stallions. In: Youngquist RS Threlfall WR, eds. Current Therapy in Large Animal Theriogenology. St. Louis: Saunders Elsevier 2007:15–23.

McDonnell SM, Turner RM, Love CC, LeBlanc MM. How to manage the stallion with a paralyzed penis for return to natural service or artificial insemination. In Proc AAEP 2003. Available at www.ivis.org, Document No. P0642.1103.

Memon MA, Usenik EA, Varner DD, Meyers PJ. Penile paralysis and paraphimosis associated with reserpine administration in a stallion. Therio 1988;30:411–419.

Vaughan JT. Surgery of the penis and prepuce. In: Walker DF, Vaughan JT, eds. Bovine and Equine Urogenital Surgery. Philadelphia: Lea & Febiger, 1980:125–144.

Wheat JD. Penile paralysis in stallions given propiopromazine. JAVMA 1966;148:405–406.

Author Carole C. Miller

Consulting Editor Carla L. Carleton

PENILE VESICLES, EROSIONS, AND TUMORS

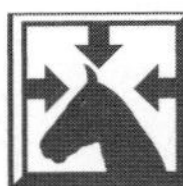

BASICS

DEFINITION/OVERVIEW

Any vesicular, ulcerative, or proliferative lesion associated with the penis or preputial folds

ETIOLOGY/PATHOPHYSIOLOGY

- Equine herpesvirus type 3 (EHV-3) is a relatively benign viral venereal disease of horses. Its common name is equine coital exanthema. The incubation period is typically 4–7 days.
    - No proof of a non–clinically apparent carrier state exists, although shedding has been reported to occur immediately prior to vesicle formation.
    - As with other herpes infections, virus recrudescence and formation of a new population of vesicles (infective stage) are associated with stress.
- Habronemiasis occurs when larvae of stomach nematodes are deposited on moist mucosal surfaces by stable flies. The larvae cause an influx of eosinophils to the affected tissues, resulting in granulomatous reactions and intense pruritis.
- Neoplasia—Appearance and progression vary with the type and size of neoplasia.

SYSTEMS AFFECTED

- Reproductive
- Urinary
- Lymphatic
- Dermatologic

GENETICS

N/A

INCIDENCE/PREVALENCE

N/A

SIGNALMENT

Any age and breed can be affected.

SIGNS

Historical

Most lesions are slow-growing. Size, location, and presentation of the lesions vary. Dysuria or hematuria may be observed. Stallions may be unwilling to complete intromission; libido may be normal or diminished.

Physical Examination

- May include visible lesions on the penis, prepuce, urethral process, fossa glandis, and on other mucocutaneous junctions
- Phimosis due to stricture formation, adhesions, or tumor proliferation
- Paraphimosis due to secondary edema formation or mechanical impedance
- Hematuria or hemospermia
- Enlargement of local lymphatics or draining sinuses

CAUSES

- Viral infections—EHV-3
- Parasites—*Habronema*
- Neoplasia—Squamous cell carcinoma, sarcoid, melanoma, papilloma, hemangioma
- Trauma—chronic wounds, local irritants, thermal injuries
- Bacteria—abscessation like that associated with bastard strangles

RISK FACTORS

- Because equine coital exanthema is a venereal disease, natural breeding programs are more likely to have an outbreak than programs using artificial insemination. Similarly, unsanitary breeding practices can put patients at greater risk.
- Unsanitary housing conditions or poor fly control can contribute to habronemiasis. It is more often seen in hot, humid locations in the spring or summer seasons.
- Gray-colored horses are the most likely to present with melanoma.
- Lightly pigmented horses are more likely to have squamous cell carcinoma, and geldings may be affected more than stallions.
- Quarter Horses are reportedly at higher risk for sarcoid development.

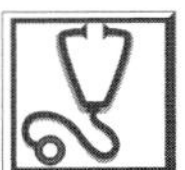

DIAGNOSIS

Biopsy should be used to confirm possible neoplasia.

DIFFERENTIAL DIAGNOSIS

Differentiating Causes

- EHV-3 infection, typical presentation—multiple, circular, 1- to 2-mm nodules that progress into vesicles and pustules and ultimately rupture to form ulcerations 5–10 mm in diameter on the penile/preputial mucosa. Systemic involvement is rare, although lesions have been found on other mucocutaneous junctions in some cases.
- Habronemiasis—Bollinger's granules, caseous masses in the exuberant granulation tissue, are diagnostic for habronemiasis. Lesions typically are extremely pruritic. *Summer sores,* the characteristic lesion, most often occur in the area of the urethral process or on the preputial ring.
- Neoplastic lesions can either be ulcerative or proliferative—squamous cell carcinomas usually are only locally invasive, although they can metastasize to regional lymph nodes and other body tissues.
- Chronic traumatic lesions can mimic any other disease process. Diagnosis is established by history, exclusion, or response to therapy.

CBC/BIOCHEMISTRY/URINALYSIS

N/A

OTHER LABORATORY TESTS

- Confirmation of EHV-3 by virus isolation from vesicular aspirates.
- Rising antibody titers for EHV-3 from paired sera, at a 14- to 21-day interval.

IMAGING

N/A

OTHER DIAGNOSTIC PROCEDURES

- Cytology—Intranuclear, eosinophilic inclusion bodies are indicative of EHV-3.
- Biopsy and histopathology can distinguish between the various tumor types and habronemiasis.

PATHOLOGICAL FINDINGS

N/A

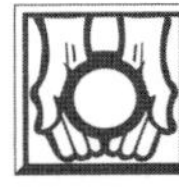

TREATMENT

- Coital exanthema is a self-limiting disease with a course of disease of 3–5 weeks. The lesions can be quite uncomfortable, and secondary bacterial infections can occur. Daily cleansing and the application of emollient or antimicrobial ointments may be indicated. Sexual rest while vesicles form, rupture, and heal prevents venereal transmission.
- Therapy for habronemiasis includes eradicating the infective larvae as well as controlling the local hypersensitivity reaction. Surgical resection of residual scar tissue may be necessary.
- Tumors may be surgically excised, or eliminated with cryosurgery, radiation therapy, hyperthermia, reefing, or phallectomy, dependent upon their size, location, invasiveness, and type.
- Papillomas often regress spontaneously in 3–4 mo.
- Topical or intralesional injections of chemotherapeutic agents have been used to address equine sarcoids and penile squamous cell carcinoma.
- Chronic wounds should be cleansed, debrided, and closed, when possible. Local irritants (i.e., povidone-iodine scrub) should be thoroughly rinsed off after application, if used.
- Streptococcal infections should be treated with systemic antibiotics.

APPROPRIATE HEALTH CARE, NURSING CARE, ACTIVITY, DIET, CLIENT EDUCATION, SURGICAL CONSIDERATIONS

N/A

MEDICATION

DRUG(S) OF CHOICE

- *Habronema* larvae can be eradicated using ivermectin (0.2 mg/kg PO). The use of prednisone to diminish localized pruritic reactions is in question because of questionable GI absorption.
- NSAIDs including phenylbutazone (2–4 g/450 kg/day PO) or flunixine meglumine (1 mg/kg/day IV, IM, or PO) are useful for symptomatic treatment of discomfort and to reduce local inflammation.
- Systemic (procaine penicillin G 20,000–22,000 IU/kg IM BID) or local (0.2% nitrofurazone ointment) antibiotics are used to treat primary or secondary bacterial infection.

PRECAUTIONS

- Chronic steroid use can result in iatrogenic Cushing's disease and may predispose the patient to developing laminitis due to systemic vasoconstrictive action.
- Phenothiazine tranquilizers should be used with caution, or not at all, due to the possibility of their causing priapism in intact stallions.

POSSIBLE INTERACTIONS

N/A

ALTERNATIVE DRUGS

- Trichlorfon (22 mg/kg diluted in 1–2 L of 0.9% NaCl slow IV) has been used to eliminate *Habronema* larvae. There is risk of clinical organophosphate toxicity.
- Topical application of trichlorfon in 0.2% nitrofurazone (4.5 g trichlorfon in 4 oz of 0.2% nitrofurazone) once daily to granulomatous lesions can be effective in the acute stage of habronemiasis.
- Autogenous vaccines have been suggested to deter the spread of papillomatosis within a herd.
- 5-Flurouracil in sesame oil has been reported to have some use as a topical sarcoid treatment.

FOLLOW-UP

PATIENT MONITORING

The frequency of reevaluation depends upon the inciting cause and severity of the lesion.

PREVENTION/AVOIDANCE

Avoid breeding activity in the presence of active EHV-3 lesions, but some shedding may occur prior to and immediately following the appearance of vesicles.

POSSIBLE COMPLICATIONS

- Chronic *Habronema* spp. infection involving the urethral process can result in periurethral fibrosis; if severe, it will necessitate amputation of the urethral process.
- Paraphimosis
- Phimosis
- Metastatic lesions in local lymph, lung, or other body tissues
- Progression of squamous papillomatous lesions to squamous cell carcinoma has been reported.
- Urethral blockage due to either the pathological condition or therapeutic intervention can occur; urethral patency should be closely monitored.

EXPECTED COURSE AND PROGNOSIS

N/A

MISCELLANEOUS

N/A

ASSOCIATED CONDITIONS

N/A

AGE-RELATED FACTORS

- Young horses are more likely to present with papillomatous lesions.
- Melanomas are more typically found in aged animals.

ZOONOTIC POTENTIAL

N/A

PREGNANCY

Coital exanthema does not cause abortion.

SYNONYMS

- EHV-3
- Equine coital exanthema
- Equine venereal balanitis
- Genital horse pox
- Habronemiasis
- Swamp cancer
- Genital bursatti
- Esponja
- Summer sores
- Warts

SEE ALSO

- Equine dermatology/neoplasia
- Equine venereal diseases
- Paraphimosis
- Penile lacerations
- Phimosis

ABBREVIATION

- EHV = equine herpesvirus

Suggested Reading

Couto MA, Hughes JP. Sexually transmitted (venereal) diseases of horses. In: McKinnon AO, Voss JL, eds. Equine Reproduction. Philadelphia: Lea & Febiger, 1993:845–854.

Fortier LA, Mc Harg MA. Topical use of 5-fluorouracil for treatment of squamous cell carcinoma of the external genitalia of horses: 11 cases (1988–1992). JAVMA 1994;205:1183–1185.

Gate DM, Cox JH, DeBowes RM. Diagnosis and treatment of acquired pathologic conditions of the equine penis and prepuce. Compend Cont Educ Pract Vet 1989;11:1498–1504.

May KA, Moll HD, Lucroy MD. Recognizing tumors of the equine external genitalia. Compend Cont Educ Pract Vet 2002;24:970–976.

Schumacher J, Varner DD. Surgical correction of abnormalities affecting the reproductive organs of stallions. In: Youngquist RS, ed. Current Therapy in Large Animal Theriogenology. Philadelphia: WB Saunders, 2007:23–36.

Vaughan JT. Penis and prepuce. In: McKinnon AO, Voss JL, eds. Equine Reproduction. Philadelphia: Lea & Febiger, 1993:885–894.

Vaughan JT. Surgery of the penis and prepuce. In: Walker DF, Vaughan JT, eds. Bovine and Equine Urogenital Surgery. Philadelphia: Lea & Febiger, 1980:125–144.

Author Carole C. Miller

Consulting Editor Carla L. Carleton

PERICARDITIS

BASICS

DEFINITION

Inflammation in the pericardial sac resulting in accumulation of fluid (transudate or exudate), fibrin, or both in the pericardial sac

PATHOPHYSIOLOGY

Accumulation of pericardial fluid compromises cardiac filling; beginning with compromised right atrial and ventricular filling, followed by impaired left ventricular filling and decreased cardiac output, resulting in generalized venous distention and ventral edema

SYSTEM AFFECTED

Cardiovascular

SIGNS

General Comments

Horse may be presented for colic.

Historical

• Colic • Fever • Exercise intolerance

Physical Examination Findings

• Depression • Lethargy • Tachycardia • Other, less common findings—anorexia; weight loss; fever; generalized venous distention; ventral, pectoral, or preputial edema; weak arterial pulse; pulsus paradoxus; arrhythmias; muffled heart sounds; pericardial friction rubs; and dull cranioventral lung field

CAUSES

• Septic—viral or bacterial • Bacterial infections—most frequently streptococcal or *Actinobacillus* sp. • Viral infections most frequently may result in immune-mediated pericarditis. • Idiopathic—Many of these also may be immune mediated.
• Idiopathic—potentially associated with outbreaks of mare reproductive loss syndrome involving ingestion of Eastern Tent caterpillars in the United States • Neoplastic—rare

RISK FACTORS

• Pleuritis or pneumonia has been reported in several horses with pericarditis. • Pericarditis may be secondary to the primary respiratory tract infection and be septic or immune mediated. • An epidemic of pericarditis was observed at the same time as outbreaks of mare reproductive loss syndrome in Kentucky.

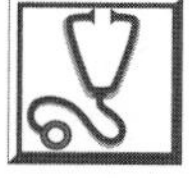

DIAGNOSIS

DIFFERENTIAL DIAGNOSIS

• Endocarditis—Many horses have a murmur, heart sounds are not muffled, and pericardial friction rubs are absent; differentiate echocardiographically. • Congestive heart failure—Murmurs are usually are detected; differentiate echocardiographically. • Cranial mediastinal abscess/mass—Heart sounds usually are not muffled; no venous distention caudally; differentiate echocardiographically and ultrasonographically.

CBC/BIOCHEMISTRY/URINALYSIS

• Neutrophilic leukocytosis and hyperfibrinogenemia are detected frequently.
• Anemia of chronic disease may be present.
• Prerenal azotemia may be present, with mildly elevated creatinine and BUN.

OTHER LABORATORY TESTS

• Virus isolation is indicated. • Paired serology may be performed, looking for a 4-fold increase in titer to equine viruses. • Elevated cardiac isoenzymes (i.e., cardiac troponin I, CK-MB, HBDH, or LDH-1 and LDH-2) indicate concurrent myocardial disease. • Perform cytologic evaluation of pericardial fluid along with culture and sensitivity testing. • Perform cytologic evaluation of transtracheal aspirate and pleural fluid sample along with culture and sensitivity testing of the fluid obtained with suspected concurrent pleuritis or pneumonia.

IMAGING

Electrocardiography

• Diminished amplitude of complexes occurs with significant pericardial effusion. • Electrical alternans may occur secondary to swinging of the heart in the fluid-filled sac. • Atrial or ventricular premature depolarizations occasionally occur with associated epicarditis or myocarditis.

Echocardiography

• The pericardial sac usually is distended with fluid and fibrin; the fluid is usually anechoic, with hypoechoic fibrin lining the epicardial surface and pericardial sac. • Fibrinous loculations may be present, and the pericardial sac may be thickened. • Occasionally, horses have a noneffusive pericarditis, with only a small amount of fibrin in the pericardial sac.
• Excessive swinging of the right ventricular free wall is present in horses with pericardial effusion.
• Right atrial and ventricular diastolic collapse (first visualized in the right ventricular outflow tract) occurs early with the development of pericardial effusion. • An inspiratory increase in right ventricle diameter and decrease in left ventricle diameter also occur in horses with cardiac tamponade. • Abrupt cessation of ventricular filling during early diastole with diastolic flattening of the left ventricular free wall indicates constrictive pericarditis—rare in horses.

Diagnostic Ultrasonography

• Evaluation of the pleural space reveals an anechoic pleural effusion in most horses with pericarditis. • In horses with pleuropneumonia, consolidation of the pulmonary parenchyma, a pulmonary abscess, or a composite pleural fluid may be present.

Thoracic Radiography

• A globoid cardiac silhouette is detected.
• Increased ventral lung field opacity and a pleural fluid line may be detected in horses with pleuropneumonia.

DIAGNOSTIC PROCEDURES

Cardiac Catheterization

• Elevated central venous pressure in horses with cardiac tamponade • Elevated right atrial pressure with a preserved systolic x descent and absence of or a diminutive diastolic y descent
• Right ventricular, pulmonary arterial systolic, and pulmonary capillary wedge pressures usually are elevated.

Pericardiocentesis

• Perform with ultrasound guidance to obtain a sample for cytology and culture and sensitivity testing. • If possible, insert a large-bore chest tube (26–32 F), and obtain the sample at that time. • After pericardial drainage and lavage, leave the large-bore chest tube in place.
• Obtain a sample of pleural fluid, if present, for cytology and culture and sensitivity testing.
• With suspected pneumonia, obtain a transtracheal aspirate for cytology and culture and sensitivity testing.

PATHOLOGIC FINDINGS

• Fibrin coating the parietal and visceral pericardial surfaces along with the pericardial effusion • A pleural effusion usually is present.
• Concurrent fibrinous pleuritis or pneumonia in some horses

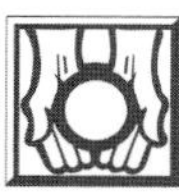

TREATMENT

AIMS OF TREATMENT

• Correct cardiac tamponade, if present, by establishing pericardial drainage. • Remove bacterial infection, if present, with appropriate broad-spectrum antimicrobials. • Control immune-mediated mechanisms, if present, using anti-inflammatory drugs.

APPROPRIATE HEALTH CARE

• Insert a large-bore, indwelling pericardial tube for drainage and lavage and direct instillation of antimicrobials if there is adequate space to do so safely, in particular if right atrial and ventricular collapse is present. • After drainage of the pericardial sac, instill 1–2 L of isotonic saline into the pericardial sac, leave in place for 30–60 min, drain, and then instill 1 L of isotonic saline with 10–20 million IU sodium penicillin and/or 1 g gentamicin. Leave this second liter of isotonic saline containing antimicrobials in place until the next drainage 12–24 hr later. Repeat the process until the initial drainage consistently recovers less fluid than is left in the pericardial sac at the time of the last instillation. At that time, the indwelling pericardial tube can be removed, and the horse should continue to improve with broad-spectrum antimicrobial coverage or systemic corticosteroids, if a septic cause has been ruled out. • Occasionally, little or no accumulation of fluid develops, and the pericarditis resolves without drainage.

ACTIVITY

Stall rest and hand walking during treatment for pericarditis and for several weeks after discontinuation of treatment

CLIENT EDUCATION

Closely monitor the horse after discontinuation of treatment for tachycardia, venous distention, or exercise intolerance; if detected, seek a cardiac reevaluation.

SURGICAL CONSIDERATIONS

Subtotal pericardiectomy has been tried in a horse with constrictive pericarditis but was not successful in the long term.

MEDICATIONS

DRUG(S) OF CHOICE

• Base the selection of antimicrobials for horses with septic pericarditis on culture and sensitivity results. Initially, until these results are available, IV bactericidal drugs (e. g., penicillin, gentamicin) are recommended for broad-spectrum coverage. • The most common causative bacterial organisms in horses are streptococci sp.; which are usually sensitive to penicillin, and gram-negative organisms (usually *Actinobacillus* sp.), which usually are sensitive to gentamicin. The drugs can also be directly instilled into the pericardial sac after lavage and drainage, which increases the drug concentration locally. • Once septic pericarditis has been successfully treated or ruled out, systemic corticosteroids may be administered to horses with idiopathic pericarditis. • If septic pericarditis is diagnosed, antimicrobial treatment for 4 weeks is indicated.

CONTRAINDICATIONS

Do *not* use corticosteroids in horses with an active bacterial or viral cause of pericarditis.

PRECAUTIONS

• Place an IV catheter before pericardiocentesis or placement of an indwelling pericardial tube so that rapid antiarrhythmic treatment can be performed, if necessary. • Monitor the horse electrocardiographically during pericardiocentesis and placement of a large-bore, indwelling chest tube to detect any cardiac arrhythmias induced during these procedures.
• Evaluate creatinine and BUN before starting aminoglycoside antimicrobials and use therapeutic drug monitoring to individualize dosage regimens.

ALTERNATIVE DRUGS

• Base use of alternative antimicrobial drugs on results of culture and sensitivity testing of the pericardial fluid. • With suspected septic pericarditis in a horse with pleuropneumonia and no growth obtained from culture and sensitivity testing of the pericardial fluid, the results obtained from a transtracheal aspirate or pleural fluid aspirate may be used, because the organisms likely are the same. • With pinpoint hyperechoic echoes visualized consistently with free gas, suspect an anaerobic infection, and treat with metronidazole. Anaerobic pericarditis, however, is rare in horses.

FOLLOW-UP

PATIENT MONITORING

• Monitor heart rate, which should decrease gradually and return to normal with the presence of little or no pericardial fluid. • Monitor peripheral veins, particularly the jugular, for venous distention and its severity. The generalized venous distention and ventral edema should gradually resolve with drainage of the pericardial sac. • Amplitude of ECG complexes should gradually increase with reduction in the pericardial fluid surrounding the heart.
• Monitor for any arrhythmias during pericardiocentesis and while the indwelling pericardial tube is in place. • Respiratory rate and temperature should return to normal as the pericarditis and any associated pleural effusion or pleuropneumonia resolve. • Monitor WBC count, fibrinogen, and creatinine until they return to normal.

PREVENTION/AVOIDANCE

Aggressive treatment of horses with pleuropneumonia may prevent pericarditis secondary to pleuritis.

POSSIBLE COMPLICATIONS

Horses with fibrinous pericarditis may develop constrictive pericarditis several months later due to scarring of the pericardial and epicardial surfaces and subsequent restriction to ventricular filling during late diastole.

EXPECTED COURSE AND PROGNOSIS

• Most horses with pericarditis treated aggressively with placement of an indwelling chest tube in the pericardial sac, pericardial lavage and drainage, direct instillation of appropriate antimicrobials, and broad-spectrum antibiotics or corticosteroids (if indicated) have an good prognosis for life and return to performance. • The indwelling pericardial tube is not removed until less fluid is recovered than was left in place for the previous 12–24 hr; in most horses, this varies from 3 to 5 days.
• Broad-spectrum antimicrobials are continued until cytology and culture reveal no evidence of bacterial infection, after which corticosteroid therapy is initiated. • With septic pericarditis, the horse should remain on IV bactericidal antimicrobials for at least 7–14 days, followed by a switch to appropriate oral antimicrobials for another 2–4 weeks. In most horses, the total length of antimicrobial treatment is at least 4–6 weeks. The horse then should receive another 4 weeks rest, followed by cardiac reevaluation before returning the horse to work.
• In most horses, any echocardiographic evidence of pericarditis is difficult to detect 1 mo after discontinuation of treatment.

MISCELLANEOUS

ASSOCIATED CONDITIONS

• Pleuritis and pleuropneumonia may result in direct extension of infection into the pericardial sac. • The pericardium also may be involved in horses with cranial mediastinal lymphosarcoma, mesothelioma, and hemangiosarcoma.

AGE-RELATED FACTORS

• Pericarditis can occur at any age. • In old horses, a neoplastic cause, although rare, must be considered.

PREGNANCY

• Pregnant mares are not particularly predisposed to pericarditis; however, if it occurs, it may result in fetal compromise if cardiac tamponade also is present. • Aim treatment at successful drainage of the pericardial sac and restoration of normal cardiac output and organ perfusion.

SEE ALSO

• Cranial mediastinal abscess/mass • Pleuritis
• Pleuropneumonia

ABBREVIATIONS

• BUN = blood urea nitrogen • CK-MB = MB isoenzyme of creatine kinase
• HBDH = α-hydroxybutyrate dehydrogenase
• LDH = lactate dehydrogenase

Suggested Reading

Bernard W, Reef VB, Clark ES, et al. Pericarditis in horses: six cases (1982–1986). J Am Vet Med Assoc 1990;196:468–471.

Hardy J, Robertson JT, Reed SM. Constrictive pericarditis in a mare: attempted treatment by partial pericardiectomy. Equine Vet J 1992;24:151–154.

Marr CM. Cardiovascular Infections. In Sellon DC, Long MT, eds. Equine Infectious Disease, Philadelphia: WB Saunders, 2007:21.

Reef VB, Gentile DG, Freeman DE. Successful treatment of pericarditis in a horse. J Am Vet Med Assoc 1984;185:94–98.

Worth LT, Reef VB. Pericarditis in horses: a review of 18 cases (1986—1995) J Am Vet Med Assoc 1998;212:248–253.

Author Virginia B. Reef
Consulting Editor Celia M. Marr

PERINATAL ASPHYXIA SYNDROME

BASICS

DEFINITION

• Neurologic, gastrointestinal, renal dysfunction with or without other organ dysfunction that occurs secondary to hypoxic events in the periparturient period • The predominant sign is usually neurologic or behavioral dysfunction, with underlying cause not infectious, traumatic, or genetic/congenital.

PATHOPHYSIOLOGY

• The exact pathophysiology of organ injury in neonates is unknown, but it is speculated that hypoxic events or limitations to placental blood flow such as dystocia and premature placental separation may initiate hypoxic-ischemic injury. Intrauterine infection may also contribute to a decrease in blood flow, oxygen delivery, and nutrient supply. • The syndrome of perinatal hypoxic-ischemic encephalopathy (HIE) is recognized in human infants, and is attributed at least in part to the accumulation of glutamate in synaptic clefts. Hypoxia leads to a breakdown of cerebral energy metabolism, leading to dysfunction of the Na+/K+ pump, and subsequent leakage of calcium into the cell. Hypoxic injury also stimulates release of glutamate due to cellular depolarization. Glutamate binds to NMDA receptors, opening calcium channels, and this inflow of calcium causes neuronal injury through activation of proteases, lipases, and endonucleases. Glutamate also activates receptors that regulate intracellular G-protein signal cascades, leading to a further increase in intracellular calcium. • Foals affected at birth have likely suffered hypoxia secondary to placental insufficiency or other in utero compromise. Foals that have peripartum asphyxia may not show neurologic signs until 3–24 hr after birth. The delay in clinical signs in these foals may be related to reperfusion injury.
• The renal and gastrointestinal systems can be affected when blood flow to the fetus is limited and redistributed to the brain and heart (away from kidneys and intestinal tract).

SYSTEMS AFFECTED

• Nervous—Encephalopathy is commonly recognized, with signs generally limited to the cerebrum. Behavioral abnormalities are common. • Gastrointestinal—Ischemic damage and reperfusion injury can lead to mucosal degeneration and subsequent ileus, bacterial translocation, and enterocolitis. • Renal—Acute renal failure (acute tubular necrosis) can occur after an ischemic episode. The risk of renal failure is increased with sepsis and NSAID use.
• The cardiovascular and respiratory systems are affected less commonly.

INCIDENCE/PREVALENCE

• Relatively common in the neonate; exact incidence unknown • PAS or HIE is the most common cause of acquired seizures in the neonatal foal.

SIGNALMENT

Breed Predilections

All breeds can be affected.

Mean Age and Range

Foals may be abnormal at birth, but others will appear normal at birth and develop signs at 24–48 hr of age.

Predominant Sex

No sex predisposition

SIGNS

General Comments

Signs vary from mild depression to severe seizures and generalized organ failure. Many foals do not show obvious signs until 12–24 hr of age.

Historical

• Dystocia, premature placental separation ("red bag"), placentitis, prepartum illness in the mare, induced labor, and prolonged gestation are maternal factors that can put the foal at risk of PAS.

Physical Examination

• Lack of interest in the mare or disorientation and "star-gazing" • Tongue protrution • Weak suckle or misdirected suckling
• Hyperresponsiveness • Focal or generalized seizures • Diarrhea or colic may be present if there is hypoxic injury to the gastrointestinal system.

CAUSES

Maternal Factors

• Placental insufficiency or dysfunction (including twins, placentitis, fescue toxicity, premature placental separation) • Compromised blood flow or oxygenation secondary to colic, endotoxemia, pulmonary disease, and anemia

Peripartum Factors

• Dystocia • Cesarean section and general anesthesia • Compression/torsion of the umbilical cord • Induction of labor with oxytocin • Uterine inertia

Foal Factors

• Congenital cardiac abnormalities • Pulmonary disease • Anemia • Sepsis

RISK FACTORS

• Fescue toxicity in mare—Alkaloids produced by *Acremonium coenephialum* can lead to prolonged gestation and placental abnormalities.
• High-risk pregnancies (see High-Risk Pregnancy, Neonate)

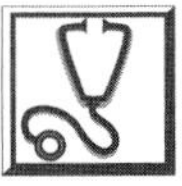

DIAGNOSIS

DIFFERENTIAL DIAGNOSIS

• Sepsis—Sepsis score, blood culture, and leukogram changes should differentiate. Foals can suffer concurrently from sepsis and PAS.
• Meningitis—fever, ataxia, depression; CSF analysis can confirm. • Trauma—Historical and physical exam information may help to differentiate. • Congenital neurologic abnormality (lavender foal syndrome, hydrocephalus, hydrancephaly)—lack of improvement in clinical signs; neurologic deficits may not be restricted to the cerebrum.
• Kernicterus—can occur with NI and very high serum bilirubin levels

CBC/BIOCHEMISTRY/URINALYSIS

• CBC and biochemistry are usually normal when the primary disorder is neurologic. • If there are significant abnormalities (neutropenia, azotemia), sepsis and multiple organ dysfunction should be suspected. • Hypoglycemia is common if the foal has not been able to nurse adequately.

OTHER LABORATORY TESTS

• Serum IgG—can be low if foal has not been able to consume adequate colostrum, if the foal's gastrointestinal tract cannot adequately absorb immunoglobulins, or if the mare has not produced good quality colostrum. • Blood gas analysis—Although hypoxic injury is usually limited to the cerebrum, hypoventilation can occur as a result of CNS damage. Hypercapnea with or without hypoxemia may be seen.

IMAGING

• Skull radiographs may be performed to rule out traumatic fracture as a cause of neurologic dysfunction. • MRI—Cerebral edema and necrosis may be seen with severe cases, although there may be no abnormalities seen in mild cases. There is limited information on the use of this imaging modality in foals with PAS.

OTHER DIAGNOSTIC PROCEDURES

• CSF aspirate—will usually be normal with PAS, although with significant necrosis and edema, increased RBCs and protein may be seen in the fluid. Necessary to rule out bacterial meningitis

PATHOLOGIC FINDINGS

• Consistent cerebral abnormalities have not been reported, although cerebral necrosis, edema, and hemorrhage may be seen. Uncomplicated cases have a good prognosis, so post-mortem information is limited.
• Hypoxic-ischemic injury to the kidneys may result in tubular necrosis. • Hypoxia and/or ischemia to the GI tract may cause necrosis and hemorrhage.

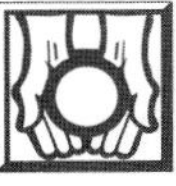

TREATMENT

AIMS OF TREATMENT

• Supportive care—mildly affected foals may only need to have adequate nutrition and immunoglobulin provided until they can nurse effectively on their own, usually within 2–3 days.
• Seizure control • Reduce or prevent further brain injury—anti-inflammatory and antiedema drugs. • Prevent sepsis in recumbent or debilitated foals. • Respiratory support may be needed if there is hypoventilation related to PAS.

APPROPRIATE HEALTH CARE

• Mildly affected foals may be managed with careful monitoring and tube feeding with colostrum and mare's milk, if needed. • The majority of affected foals require inpatient medical management.

NURSING CARE

• Oxygen therapy is clearly indicated when hypoxemia is present but may also be of benefit in at-risk foals. • Fluid therapy—Maintenance requirements may need to be provided in foals that are transiently unable to nurse.

Hypovolemia should be corrected in order to maintain cerebral perfusion pressure, renal blood flow, and intestinal perfusion; however, fluid overload has the potential to contribute to cerebral edema. • The foal should be protected from self-trauma during seizures or struggling activity and should be monitored carefully for the development of corneal ulcers or abrasions. • Transfusion with hyperimmune plasma may be required if the foal has not been able to ingest adequate colostrum within the first several hr of birth.

ACTIVITY

Activity will be limited by the treatments required and by the neurologic and metabolic status of the foal.

DIET

• Foals may need to be fed via nasogastric feeding tube until a strong suckle reflex and coordinated nursing is achieved. The mare can be milked or mare's milk replacer may be used, beginning with feedings of approximately 10%–15% of body weight per day, and increasing to 20%–25% of body weight per day. Feedings should be divided into every 1–2 hr. The foal should be weighed daily to help ensure that adequate nutrition is being provided. • Care should be taken if GI ischemia is suspected. Foals with GI injury or ileus may not be able to tolerate full enteral feedings and may require parenteral nutrition until intestinal function returns. Small ("trophic") enteral feedings can be used along with parenteral feeding until full enteral feeding is tolerated.

MEDICATIONS

DRUG(S) OF CHOICE

For Seizure Control (see Seizures in Foals for drug information and dosages)

• Diazepam • Midazolam • Phenobarbital • Phenytoin

For Treatment of Cerebral Asphyxia/Edema

• Magnesium sulfate (50 mg/kg/hr loading dose, then 25 mg/kg/hr CRI)—blocks NMDA production • Mannitol (0.25–1.0 g/kg as a 20% solution IV)—osmotic diuretic to reduce cerebral edema. This is useful for interstitial edema, but is not effective for intracellular edema. • DMSO (0.5–1.0 g/kg as a 10% solution IV)—given shortly after the initial insult to scavenge free radicals and mediate ischemia-reperfusion injury. There is no evidence of efficacy of DMSO, and many practitioners have eliminated DMSO from the routine treatment regimen. • Thiamine (5 mg/kg IV slowly or diluted in fluids q24h)—to support mitochondrial metabolism

For Treatment of Hypoventilation

Caffeine (10 mg/kg initial dose, then 2.5 mg/kg PRN, given PO or per rectum)—respiratory stimulant for centrally mediated hypoventilation.

Antioxidants

• Vitamin E (alpha-tocopherol)—500–1000 IU PO q24h • Vitamin C (ascorbic acid)—50–100 mg/kg PO q24h

For Renal Failure

Furosemide (1–2 mg/kg IV PRN)—if signs of fluid overload are present

For Prevention of Sepsis or Treatment of Enterocolitis

• Broad-spectrum parenteral antimicrobials. Penicillin (22,000 IU/kg IV q6h) and amikacin (25 mg/kg IV q24h) are commonly used. • Metronidazole (15 mg/kg PO q8h) may also be used if anaerobic infection is suspected or if necrotizing enterocolitis is present.

CONTRAINDICATIONS

• Corticosteroids are not indicated for the treatment of PAS. • Ketamine and xylazine increase intracranial pressure, and should be avoided, if possible. • Mannitol is contraindicated with cerebral hemorrhage.

PRECAUTIONS

Aminoglycoside antimicrobials and NSAIDs should be used with caution if renal damage is suspected. Therapeutic drug monitoring can be used to adjust the aminoglycoside dosages.

ALTERNATIVE DRUGS

If renal compromise is suspected, a third-generation cephalosporin can be used in place of the penicillin/amikacin combination (ceftiofur 10 mg/kg IV q6h; ceftazidime 50 mg/kg IV q6h; cefotaxime 40 mg/kg IV q6h). These drugs are also useful if septic meningitis has not been ruled out, as they are able to cross the blood-brain barrier.

FOLLOW-UP

PATIENT MONITORING

• The foal should be reevaluated at least daily for ability to stand and nurse. An adequate suckle reflex and ability to remain standing are required for reintroduction to nursing the mare. The foal may require assistance to stand as it is initially reintroduced to nursing. • The foal should be monitored closely for signs of sepsis, as many of the risk factors for PAS also place the foal at risk of sepsis. • Blood pressure should be monitored in more severe cases and hypotension treated in order to maintain perfusion to vital organs.

PREVENTION/AVOIDANCE

Any potential underlying causes such as placental insufficiency, ascending uterine infection, or prolonged gestation due to fescue toxicity should be investigated in order to help prevent PAS in future foals.

POSSIBLE COMPLICATIONS

• Septicemia • Enterocolitis • Ventilatory failure

EXPECTED COURSE AND PROGNOSIS

• Prognosis is good to excellent (approximately 75% survival) for uncomplicated PAS. Mildly affected foals generally respond to treatment within several days. Foals with additional organ dysfunction require more intensive and prolonged care. • Delayed treatment can result in failure of transfer of passive immunity and sepsis. Concurrent diseases such as sepsis will decrease the prognosis.

MISCELLANEOUS

ASSOCIATED CONDITIONS

• Sepsis • Enterocolitis/diarrhea

AGE-RELATED FACTORS

This is a condition of neonatal foals, with initial signs seen by 48hr of age.

SYNONYMS

• Neonatal maladjustment syndrome
• Hypoxic-ischemic encephalopathy
• Dummy foal • Barker foal • Neonatal encephalopathy

SEE ALSO

• Seizures in foals • High-risk pregnancy

ABBREVIATIONS

• CRI = constant rate infusion • CSF = cerebrospinal fluid • DMSO = dimethyl sulfoxide • MRI = magnetic resonance imaging • NMDA = *N*-methyl-D-aspartate • PAS = perinatal asphyxia syndrome

Suggested Reading

MacKay RJ. Neurologic disorders of neonatal foals. Vet Clin North Am Equine Pract 2005;21:387–406.

Paradis MR. Neurologic dysfunctions. In: Paradis MR, ed. Equine Neonatal Medicine: A Case-Based Approach. Philadelphia: Elsevier Saunders, 2006.

Wilkins PA. Perinatal asphyxia syndrome. In: Reed SM, Bayly WM, Sellon DC, eds. Equine Internal Medicine. St. Louis: Saunders, 2004.

Author Margaret C. Mudge
Consulting Editor Margaret C. Mudge

PERINEAL LACERATIONS/RECTO-VAGINAL-VESTIBULAR FISTULAS

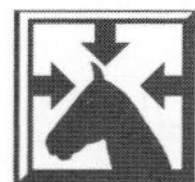

BASICS

DEFINITION/OVERVIEW

- A laceration of the perineal body
- First-degree laceration involves the mucous membrane of the vulva and skin.
- Second-degree laceration involves the next deeper layer of the vestibule and/or the vaginal wall, extending into the perineal body and deeper layers of the vulva.
- Third-degree laceration involves full-thickness tears through the perineal body, extending through the rectal wall and anal sphincter, and full-thickness through the vulva.
- RVVF are full-thickness tears through the rectal wall and, possibly, involving the perineal body, but not involving the anal sphincter or vulva.
- Recto-vestibular fistulas are much more common than RVFs.

ETIOLOGY/PATHOPHYSIOLOGY

- Perineal lacerations occur at parturition because of abnormal posture or position of the fetus, which predisposes the fetal extremities to be pushed more dorsal than normal, thus forcing the fetal feet into and/or through the wall of the vagina or vestibule.
- Lacerations of the rectum or vagina can occur at breeding, but perineal lacerations are rare at this time.

SYSTEM AFFECTED

Reproductive

GENETICS

Only if the mare has inherited a narrowing of the vagina

INCIDENCE/PREVALENCE

- No statistics available regarding incidence
- Not rare, but infrequent

SIGNALMENT

- All breeds
- All of breeding age

SIGNS

General Comments

- The condition is not an emergency.
- Because of the tearing, bruising, and edema occurring at and after injury, delay correction of these lacerations until the initial inflammation and bruising have subsided; generally at least 30 days

Historical

- The mare may have a history of assisted delivery, but this is not essential.
- Because of the excessive force developed by the abdominal musculature (*active labor*), it is possible for the mare to deliver a live foal unassisted while creating a perineal laceration.

Physical Examination

Careful physical examination of the perineum, perineal body, vagina, and rectum, including TRP and vaginal examination

CAUSES

- Abnormal posture or position of the fetus at parturition
- Fetal extremities are pushed more dorsal than normal within the birth canal, such that they penetrate and damage maternal soft tissue structures within the vagina, vestibule, and/or rectum.

RISK FACTORS

- Late or term gestation and parturition
- Abnormal fetal position or posture
- Because fetal posture and position can change within minutes before parturition, examinations conducted much before parturition are of little value.

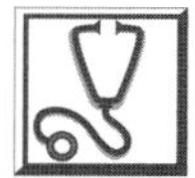

DIAGNOSIS

DIFFERENTIAL DIAGNOSIS N/A

CBC/BIOCHEMISTRY/URINALYSIS

N/A

OTHER LABORATORY TESTS

N/A

IMAGING N/A

OTHER DIAGNOSTIC PROCEDURES

N/A

PATHOLOGICAL FINDINGS

- Partial- to full-thickness lacerations of the vestibule, vagina, anal sphincter, and/or rectum
- Aspiration of air into the vagina and/or uterus secondary to damaged normal barrier tissues—vulvar lips; vestibular sphincter
- Fecal contamination of the vagina and vestibule, followed by inflammation of the vestibule, vagina, cervix, and possibly, the endometrium

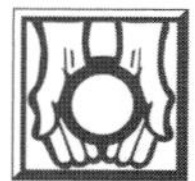

TREATMENT

APPROPRIATE HEALTH CARE

- Confirm whether the laceration extends into the peritoneal cavity— a rare occurrence with perineal laceration or RVF.
- Systemic antibiotics seldom are indicated or necessary to control infection in this area; client education is imperative.
- Local medication rarely is indicated.
- Repair lacerations before attempting to rebreed.
- Boost tetanus vaccination, if not recent.

NURSING CARE

N/A

ACTIVITY

No restrictions

DIET

No restrictions

CLIENT EDUCATION

- Advise regarding the importance of close/frequent observation of foaling mares.
- Many lacerations occur before a problem is detected, even in the presence of trained foaling attendants.

SURGICAL CONSIDERATIONS

General Comments

- Surgical repair once the inflammation and bruising have subsided is a minimum of 30 days.
- Imperative after surgery that feces remain soft until healing is complete.
- Early in the spring (preoperative), place the mare on pasture, and return it to pasture immediately after surgery. Green grass has a high-moisture content, which should soften stool.
- Other methods of stool softening include bran and mineral oil, but are less effective in the author's opinion.

Two-Stage Repair

Stage 1

- Epidural anesthesia and sedation of the mare
- The tail is wrapped and elevated over the mare and attached to a support directly above the animal.
- The rectum and vagina/vestibule are emptied of feces and thoroughly but gently cleaned. Use of irritating scrubs could stimulate postoperative straining and is contraindicated.
- Reconstruction of the perineal body:
  - An incision is made into the remaining shelf ≅2–3 cm anterior to the cranial limit of the laceration.
  - The incision is continued posteriorly along the sides of the existing laceration in a plane approximately equal to the original location of the perineal body.
  - The vestibular and vaginal mucosa is reflected ventrally ≅2 cm.
  - Simple interrupted sutures are placed through the area of the perineal body so that the perineal body is reapposed and the submucosal vaginal or vestibular tissue is brought together in the same suture pattern.
  - After placement of one or two of these sutures, a continuous suture pattern is begun in the reflected mucosal membrane to oppose the submucosal surfaces.
  - This suture pattern continues cranial to caudal, as additional simple interrupted sutures are placed.

Stage 2

- Completed after healing of stage 1
- Debride the anal sphincter and dorsal vulvar commissure, and place sutures in these tissues to reestablish the sphincters, if possible.
- Optimal success is achieved if sphincter tone is regained after repair.

One-Stage Repair

Similar to two-stage repair, except that repairs of the anal sphincter and dorsal vulvar commissure are completed at the time of the initial surgery

MEDICATIONS

DRUG(S) OF CHOICE

- Systemic antibiotics may be indicated immediately after laceration to prevent possible systemic involvement, but the laceration must be quite severe to warrant their use.
- Medications specific to accomplish the surgical repair

CONTRAINDICATIONS N/A

PRECAUTIONS N/A

POSSIBLE INTERACTIONS N/A

ALTERNATIVE DRUGS

Any agent designed for sedation and analgesia can be used during surgical correction.

FOLLOW-UP

PATIENT MONITORING

- An immediate examination is indicated with the possibility or concern that a laceration has occurred.
- If its presence is confirmed but it does not extend into the perineal cavity, reexamine the area in ≅2 weeks to assess degree of inflammation and formation of granulation tissue at the laceration site.

PREVENTION/AVOIDANCE

- Occurrence is difficult to predict.
- Cannot be prevented by other than not breeding a mare

POSSIBLE COMPLICATIONS

- Abscesses may develop in the laceration area, but this is uncommon, aided in part by the abundant surface area that facilitates drainage and formation of granulation tissue from the deeper layers outward.
- If the laceration is sutured immediately after the occurrence, the potential for abscessation may actually increase.

EXPECTED COURSE AND PROGNOSIS

- Without surgical correction, mares with third-degree lacerations and RVFs have a very low probability of conceiving and maintaining a pregnancy to term.
- Therefore, surgical correction is strongly recommended before attempting breeding.

MISCELLANEOUS

N/A

ASSOCIATED CONDITIONS

N/A

AGE-RELATED FACTORS

N/A

ZOONOTIC POTENTIAL

N/A

PREGNANCY

Occurs only after gestation and parturition

SYNONYMS

N/A

SEE ALSO

- Delayed uterine involution
- Dystocia
- Prolonged pregnancy
- Urine pooling/urovagina

ABBREVIATIONS

- RVF = recto-vaginal fistula
- RVVF = recto-vaginal-vestibular fistula
- TRP = transrectal palpation

Suggested Reading

Aanes WA. Surgical repair of third degree perineal lacerations and recto-vaginal fistulas in the mare. JAVMA 1964;144:485–491.

Belknap JK, Nickels FA. A one-stage repair of third-degree perineal lacerations and rectovestibular fistula in 17 mares. Vet Surg 1992;21:378–381.

Colbern GT, Aanes WA, Stashak TS. Surgical management of perineal lacerations and recto-vestibular fistulae in the mare: a retrospective study of 47 cases. J Am Vet Med Assoc 1985;186:265–269.

Heinze CD, Allen AR. Repair of third-degree perineal lacerations in the mare. Vet Scope 1966;11:12–15.

Stickle RL, Fessler JF, Adams SB, et al. A single stage technique for repair of recto-vestibular lacerations in the mare. J Vet Surg 1979;8:25–27.

Author Walter R. Threlfall

Consulting Editor Carla L. Carleton

PERIOCULAR SARCOID

BASICS

DEFINITION

A neoplasm of fibroblastic origin that generally has a low metastatic potential, yet is often locally aggressive. There are several clinical forms ranging simply from areas of alopecia and altered, flaky skin to more pronounced nodular lesions with or without overlying skin involvement or fleshy, proliferative masses with ulceration.

PATHOPHYSIOLOGY

- The etiopathogenesis is unknown, but BPV has been implicated as a potential inciting agent. Intradermal inoculation with cell-free extract from bovine skin tumors caused by BPV has caused lesions in horses resembling equine sarcoid, both clinically and histologically.
- Additionally, genetic susceptibility may exist with equine sarcoid. Animals that express certain MHC-encoded ELAs have increased incidence of occurrence and higher recurrence rates after surgery (MHC-I ELA W3 and B1 and MHC-II ELA W13 and A5). Flies have been implicated as vectors for transfer of sarcoid cells between animals.

SYSTEMS AFFECTED

- Eyelids and periocular skin
- Equine sarcoid can affect any cutaneous area, but approximately 32% of the tumors are located on the head and neck. As many as 14% of all the equine sarcoids are periocular.

GENETICS

- No proven genetic basis, but genes in or near MHC have been implicated as a predisposing factor.
- There has also been demonstrated a correlation between the development of sarcoids and heterozygosity for the equine severe combined immunodeficiency allele.

INCIDENCE/PREVALENCE

- Sarcoids are the most commonly reported equine tumor overall and the second most common periocular tumor of the horse.
- SCC is the most common tumor of the equine eye and periocular tissue.

GEOGRAPHIC DISTRIBUTION

No reported geographic distribution

SIGNALMENT

Species

Horses, donkeys, and mules

Breed Predilections

Nearly all breeds have been reported to have sarcoids. However, Quarter Horses, Appaloosas, Arabians, and Thoroughbreds are reported to have the highest risk for developing sarcoids, while Standardbreds and Lippizaners have the lowest.

Mean Age and Range

Mean age of affected animals is between 3 and 7 years, with a range of 1 to >15 years.

Predominant

No proven sex predilection

SIGNS

Historical

- Single or multiple, firm areas of dermal thickening or nodules in the eyelids or periocular region
- Lesions may be ulcerated, and those affecting the eyelid margins or canthi may cause secondary tearing, squinting, or ocular discharge.
- Ocular irritation often occurs because of either disruption of eyelid function or direct rubbing on the globe.
- Growth rate and biologic behavior are highly variable.

Physical Examination

- Nonspecific findings may include serous to mucopurulent ocular discharge, blepharospasm, and conjunctival hyperemia.
- Solitary or multiple areas of linear or focal dermal thickening in the eyelids or periocular skin can be found. Lesions may also appear as nodules or pedunculated masses. Cutaneous ulceration and infection may be present.

CAUSES

- Viral etiologies have been suggested.
- A predisposition associated with genes on or near the MHC has also been suggested.

RISK FACTORS

- Possible breed predilections, possible genetic risk factors.
- Epizootics in herds suggest an infectious risk, possibly associated with fly vectors.

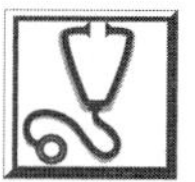

DIAGNOSIS

DIFFERENTIAL DIAGNOSIS

- Diagnosis depends on an index of clinical suspicion and the results of a surgical biopsy.
- Differentials include granulation tissue or scarring; granulomas including those caused by habronemiasis, onchocerciasis, or foreign body reactions; fungal dermatitis; dermatophilus; and other tumors such as SCC, papilloma, schwannoma, adenoma, adenocarcinoma, angiosarcoma, mastocytoma, melanocytoma, plasmacytoma, fibroma, and fibrosarcoma.

CBC/BIOCHEMISTRY/URINALYSIS

Results usually normal

OTHER LABORATORY TESTS

None

IMAGING

Skull radiographs may be required if orbital or bony involvement is suspected.

GROSS AND HISTOPATHOLOGIC FINDINGS

Gross

- Several morphologic types of sarcoid have been described.
- Occult lesions are those with alopecia, altered hair, and small miliary nodules or plaques.
- The verrucous ("warty") sarcoid is usually less than 6 cm in diameter, often with cauliflower edges and extensive flakiness of the skin with or without some ulceration.
- Nodular lesions may or may not have epidermal involvement (type A versus type B).
- Fibroblastic lesions may be sessile and pedunculated, or papillomatous. They often have a fleshy, ulcerated appearance and infection may be present.
- The mixed sarcoid is a combination of the previous types.
- Malignant sarcoids are unusual.

Histologic

- The tumor consists of a moderate to high density of fusiform or spindle-shaped, fibroblastic cells that form whorls, interlacing bundles, and haphazard arrays with one another (fibroblastic proliferation).
- Cells vary from slender, with elongated, pointed nuclei, to plump with large, irregular, pleomorphic nuclei.
- Cytoplasmic boundaries are ill defined, and the amount of collagen varies considerably.
- The mitotic rate is low.
- In many sarcoids, fibroblastic cells are oriented perpendicularly to the overlying epithelial basement membrane.
- Where the epidermis is present, it is often hyperplastic, with elongated rete pegs extending into the tumor.

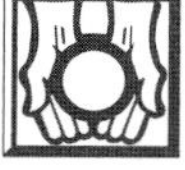

TREATMENT

INPATIENT VERSUS OUTPATIENT

- Very small, superficial lesions may be removed standing with sedation and local anesthesia.
- Larger, more invasive lesions, or lesions involving the eyelid margins or canthi, may require hospitalization for surgery.
- Alternatively, lesions may be treated under sedation and local anesthesia using intralesional chemotherapy or immunotherapy.

ACTIVITY

- Restrict during the immediate postoperative period.
- The eye should be protected from self-trauma and secondary infection. A soft- or hard-cup hood can be applied.

DIET

N/A

CLIENT EDUCATION

- If intralesional chemotherapy is used, the client should be instructed to wear gloves when handling the periocular region for several days post injection.
- The client should be made aware of clinical signs suggesting tumor recurrence.

SURGICAL CONSIDERATIONS

- Complete surgical excision of periocular sarcoid can be difficult or impossible, and recurrence rates of 50%–64% have been reported with surgical excision alone. When surgical excision is combined with adjunctive therapy, however, success rates range from 65% to 95%. Various adjunctive therapies include cryotherapy, hyperthermia, CO_2 laser photoablation, topical chemotherapy, radiotherapy, and intralesional chemotherapy and immunotherapy. Reconstructive eyelid have been surgery may also be necessary following excision of periocular sarcoids.
- Intralesional BCG injections require multiple injections spaced several weeks apart but have success rates ranging from 69% to 100%. Intralesional chemotherapy with either cisplatin or 5-FU can produce cures in up to 80% of cases. Cryotherapy uses temperatures of −20° to −40° C in a triple freeze-thaw cycle to induce cryonecrosis of sarcoid cells. Reported success rates are up to 75%. Radio-frequency hyperthermia has been reported to induce tumor regression when lesions are heated to 50° C for 30 seconds using a 2-MHz radiofrequency current. Multiple treatments may be necessary to prevent recurrence. One study reported an 81% success rate using CO_2 laser photoablation. Advantages included a clean, dry surgical site and a lack of postoperative pain and swelling. Radiation therapy has the highest success rates, in many cases approaching 100% depending upon the source of radiation used. Unfortunately, radiation therapy, while it is the gold standard, is a difficult modality to access due to hazards to involved personnel. Interstitial brachytherapy using iridium-192 has been reported with success rates ranging from 87% to 94%. Radium-226 and cobalt-60 have been used with remission rates greater than 60%, gold-198 had a remission rate of 83%, and radon-222 had a remission rate of 92%.

MEDICATIONS

DRUGS AND FLUIDS

Topical and Intralesional Immunotherapy/Chemotherapy

- Daily topical applications of podophyllum or topical 5-FU (1% TID) have been used with inconsistent results.
- Herbal pastes of blood root extracts can be used topically in some sarcoids and ocular SCC (XXTerra; Larson Labs, Fort Collins, CO).
- Intralesional chemotherapeutics including 5-FU and cisplatin have been used with success rates of approximately 80%. Intralesional cisplatin is administered in four sessions at 2-week intervals using 1 mg/cm^3 of tumor. Tumors up to 20 cm^3 may be treated using 3.3 mg/mL cisplatin (10 mg Platinol in 1 mL water and 2 mL purified medical-grade sesame oil). Success rates were lower for intralesional xanthate and recombinant human TNFα.
- Immunotherapy includes autogenous vaccines and immunomodulators using mycobacterial products. Intralesional injections of bovine papilloma virus vaccine have been successful in horses with sarcoids, but systemic side effects have been severe in a few horses. Immunomodulation using BCG-attenuated *Mycobacterium bovis* cell wall in oil, however, has produced remission rates approaching 100%. Using a 22- or 25-gauge hypodermic needle, 1 ml of BCG/cm^2 of tumor surface area is injected into the lesion. Therapy is repeated every 2–4 weeks for up to 9 injections. Anaphylaxis may occur and can be minimized with pretreatment using flunixin meglumine (1.1 mg/kg IV) and corticosteroids or diphenhydramine.

Antibiotics

- Topical and systemic antibiotics may be required to prevent infection following surgical and adjunctive therapy of periocular sarcoid.
- A broad-spectrum ophthalmic antibiotic such as neomycin, polymyxin B, and bacitracin (Trioptic P) may be used for prophylactic therapy if lesions involve the eyelid margins or canthi.
- Broad-spectrum systemic antibiotics such as trimethoprim/sulfamethazone (Tribrissen) may also be used.
- Culture of any obviously infected wound is recommended so that the most appropriate antibiotic choice can be made.

Analgesic/Anti-inflammatory Agents

NSAIDs may be indicated following surgical excision or adjunctive therapy. Flunixin meglumine (1.1 mg/kg) provides analgesic and anti-inflammatory effects, and it may reduce the severity of anaphylaxis associated with intralesional immunotherapy.

FOLLOW-UP

PATIENT MONITORING

- Patients should be observed for signs of anaphylaxis immediately post injection when immunomodulating agents are used.
- Long-term follow-up includes monitoring for tumor recurrence or failure of tumor regression.

PREVENTION/AVOIDANCE

Fly control may reduce the incidence of sarcoid in herds with affected animals.

POSSIBLE COMPLICATIONS

- Tumor progression may lead to eyelid deformation, possibly resulting in secondary keratitis and conjunctivitis.
- Ulceration of lesions may lead to secondary bacterial or fungal infections and possible septicemia. With ulcerated lesions, myiasis may also be a problem.

EXPECTED COURSE AND PROGNOSIS

- Prognosis for life is generally good for animals with single sarcoids, as these tumors do not metastasize.
- In animals with numerous sarcoids, seen rarely in the United States and more commonly seen in the United Kingdom, prognosis for life is poor.
- Factors affecting prognosis include tumor size, location, degree of local invasiveness, and the number of tumors present.
- Recurrence rates following therapy depend on the therapeutic modalities used, with remission rates approaching 100% for some modalities.

MISCELLANEOUS

ASSOCIATED CONDITIONS

N/A

ZOONOTIC POTENTIAL

No proven zoonotic potential, but multiple occurrences in some herds suggest that this is possible. If so, fly vectors may be involved, possibly necessitating fly control.

PREGNANCY

N/A

SEE ALSO

Ocular/adnexal SCC

ABBREVIATIONS

- BCG = bacillus Calmette-Guerin
- BPV = bovine papilloma virus
- ELA = equine leukocyte antigen
- 5-FU = 5-fluorouracil
- MHC = major histocompatibility complex
- SCC = squamous cell carcinoma
- TNFα = tumor necrosis factor alpha

Suggested Reading

Brooks DE. Ophthalmology for the Equine Practitioner. Jackson, WY; Teton NewMedia, 2002.

Brooks DE, Matthews AG. Equine ophthalmology. In: Gelatt KN, ed. Veterinary Ophthalmology, ed 4. Philadelphia; Lippincott Williams and Wilkins, 2007.

Gilger BC, ed. Equine Ophthalmology. Philadelphia; WB Saunders, 2005.

Author Caryn E. Plummer

Consulting Editor Dennis E. Brooks

PERIODONTAL DISEASE

BASICS

INTRODUCTION

The equine periodontium is a dynamic structure that constantly remodels, facilitating eruption of the horse's hypsodontic teeth. It comprises those structures that surround the tooth, namely the periodontal ligament, alveolar bone, gingiva and cementum. Periodontal disease encompasses those disorders occurring in the periodontium.

PATHOPHYSIOLOGY

- Unlike brachydont animals, primary periodontal disease does not appear to be a significant problem in the horse. A transient inflammation of the periodontal membrane and adjacent gingiva occurs in many horses and may be recognized by a marginal reddening of the gum around the erupting teeth; however, most authors now believe significant equine periodontal disease to be secondary to abnormalities in dental wear. These abnormalities include "angular malocclusions" (step-, shear-, or wave-mouth; missing or unopposed teeth, and hooks and ramps) and improperly shed deciduous premolars, which generate unevenly distributed forces that may in turn result in separation of the normally tightly aligned adjacent teeth. Food material that becomes impacted into this resultant diastema incites a focal gingivitis, leading to the development of a gingival sulcus. Impacted feed undergoes decay and bacterial fermentation within these sulci; this process and the resulting by-products cause progressive destruction of the periodontal ligament and the alveolar bone; support for the tooth is consequently decreased. Apical migration of the infection may result in periapical infection, abscessation and necrosis of the affected tooth.
- Horses with mandibular or maxillary fractures can develop periodontal disease as a direct result of exposure of the periodontium to food material and as an indirect result of alterations to normal mastication.

SYSTEMS AFFECTED

- Gastrointestinal
- Musculoskeletal
- Respiratory (maxillary sinusitis)

GENETICS

N/A

INCIDENCE/PREVELENCE

One study found evidence of periodontal disease in approximately one third of 500 equine skulls. An incidence of 60% has been reported in horses of greater than 15 years of age.

SIGNALMENT

Periodontal disease occurs more frequently in mature animals. However, disease as a result of retained deciduous teeth usually occurs between 2.5 and 4 years of age and disease of traumatic origin may occur at any age. Draft animals may be predisposed.

SIGNS

Horses with periodontal disease may exhibit no external clinical signs of disease. With increased severity of disease signs due to painful mastication may become evident. These include excessive salivation, slow eating, oral dysphagia (quidding), halitosis, abnormal positioning of the head during mastication, anorexia, and weight loss. If secondary maxillary sinusitis is present purulent nasal discharge, epiphora, epistaxis, and facial swelling may also be noted.

RISK FACTORS

- Domestic feeding practices and processed feeds often lead to abnormal mastication and decreased salivary fluid production with resultant abnormality of wear and lowered local mechanical defence function, respectively.
- Various conformational abnormalities become more common in geriatric horses; in addition, as horses age, there is progressive exposure of the reserve crown and consequently a less secure apposition between adjacent teeth.
- Cushing's syndrome and other systemic conditions that may alter immune function are common in older horses and may contribute to the occurrence of periodontal disease in affected animals.

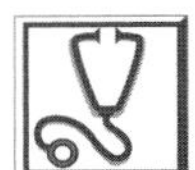

DIAGNOSIS

DIFFERENTIAL DIAGNOSIS

Differential diagnoses to consider include other causes of dental sepsis such as apical abscessation and infundibular necrosis, oral neoplasia and non-neoplastic masses such as abscesses, granulomas, phycomycosis, habronemiasis, and pharyngeal cysts. Disease of the salivary glands, including sialodentitis, sialothiasis, and salivary mucoceles, should also be considered.

CBC/BIOCHEMISTRY/URINALYSIS

Nonspecific

OTHER LABAROTORY TESTS

N/A

DIAGNOSTIC PROCEDURES

- A thorough oral examination is required for the diagnosis of periodontal disease. This should include palpation of the teeth through the cheeks, observation of the horse during mastication, assessment of lateral mandibular excursion, and a visual and digital examination of the oral cavity with the aid of a full mouth speculum. Rinsing the oral cavity is recommended *after* initial examination with a gag in place; this will allow assessment of areas of impacted or pocketed feed prior to their displacement.
- Palpation of the gingiva can identify areas of swelling, hyperaemia, recession, and pain; a gingival probe may be used to measure the extent of gingival sulci. While increased mobility of a tooth may be palpated, significant destruction of the periodontal tissues is required for detection of a loose tooth using this method. This is a consequence of the extensive support provided by adjacent teeth.
- A dental mirror is invaluable for the evaluation of the buccal, lingual, and interproximal spaces of the cheek teeth.

IMAGING

Radiographs of the teeth can detect destruction of the periodontal ligament as a loss of definition of the radiolucent ligament. Changes to the alveolus include bone lysis and production as well as clubbing of tooth roots in more advanced cases. Whereas septic processes in the maxilla tend to result in radiographically evident sclerosis, the mandible is more frequently characterized by radiolucency. Other radiographic abnormalities that may be detected in the periodontal tissues include soft tissue densities, the production of gas from bacterial fermentation, and fluid in the maxillary sinuses if the caudal three maxillary cheek teeth are involved. The radiographic lesions described above are seen with dental sepsis. Periodontal disease is the early stages in a continuum of dental sepsis. Computed tomography has been used to increase sensitivity of radiographic imaging, and nuclear scintigraphy has been suggested to be a sensitive method for diagnosis of apical abscessation in both the mandible and the maxilla.

PATHOLOGICAL FINDINGS

Focal gingival hyperplasia appears histologically as inflamed, well-vascularized, fibrous connective tissue covered by epitheliomatous hyperplasia. Ulcerated sections may also be present. In more advanced cases, destruction of the periodontal ligament and osteitis of the alveolus are present.

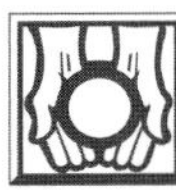

TREATMENT

- Treatment of secondary periodontal disease is aimed at addressing the underlying painful or mechanically restrictive lesion and as such promoting normal masticatory activity. Appropriate crown reduction with the use of a dental rasp and extraction of loose teeth may be performed on an outpatient basis. Extraction of the cheek teeth may, however, require general anesthesia and elective surgical management. The removal of severely diseased teeth eliminates periodontal pockets and potential sources of sepsis; pulling a tooth out of occlusion will also eliminate the abnormal forces acting upon it.
- Many mild cases of periodontal disease caused by feed impaction will resolve after the

diastema is cleaned and appropriate crown reduction is performed. Many practitioners advocate the use of a hand scaler, dental probe, and vigorous flushing with dilute chlorhexidine solution to achieve the removal of impacted feed material from the interproximal spaces.

NURSING CARE

N/A

ACTIVITY

N/A

DIET

Lateral excursion of the mandible, which is important for normal dental wear, is associated with fiber length. Adequate dietary roughage is therefore of importance for the prevention of periodontal disease. However, if periodontal disease is already present and extensive, a high-energy, pelleted diet may be required to provide adequate energy intake.

CLIENT EDUCATION

Periodontal disease is very common in older horses. Routine dental prophylaxis is the best method for preventing periodontal disease, whereas treatment of affected horses is limited. It is recommended that those horses at high risk for developing periodontal disease undergo biannual dental examination; this group includes horses under the age of 5 and those over the age of 15.

SURGICAL CONSIDERATIONS

High-quality preoperative radiographs are useful for identifying affected teeth, and intraoperative radiographs are useful for confirming correct placement of a dental punch. Following tooth repulsion, the resulting defect can be packed with dental wax or a similar preparation to prevent exposure of feed material to the alveolus. This packing should be removed in 6–8 weeks. When tooth repulsion requires entry into a sinus, a lavage system may be installed postoperatively. Postoperative radiographs are useful to confirm complete removal of the affected tooth.

MEDICATIONS

DRUG(S) OF CHOICE

- *Sedatives* may be required to complete a thorough and safe oral examination. α_2-Agonists (xylazine, romifidine, detomidine) provide adequate sedation; the addition of an opioid such as butorphanol can increase the reliability of the sedation achieved.
- NSAIDs (phenylbutazone, flunixin meglumine) administered prior to any dental work helps to minimize discomfort both during and after dental treatment, especially if soft-tissue damage is incurred.
- Little data exist on the effectiveness of *systemic antibiotics* in the treatment of equine periodontal disease. Antibiotics are unlikely to halt progression of the disease without removal of the underlying cause of the problem. Some practitioners advocate the use of doxycycline subgingivally in affected areas.

CONTRAINDICATIONS, PRECAUTIONS, POSSIBLE INTERACTIONS, ALTERNATIVE DRUGS

N/A

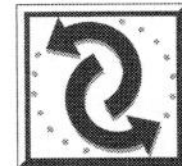

FOLLOW-UP

PATIENT MONITORING

Weight gain in horses with ill thrift should be monitored and is often impressive following successful treatment of periodontal disease. Otherwise, a good appetite, without evidence of quidding or undigested grain in the feces, should be noted following treatment.

PREVENTION/AVOIDANCE

Regular dental prophylaxis (see Client Education) can prevent the formation of dental conformational abnormalities as a result of abnormal wear. Feeding diets with adequate roughage may decrease abnormal dental wear.

POSSIBLE COMPLICATIONS

With conservative therapy, progression of the disease is common. Following tooth extraction, complications may include formation of a fistula between the oral cavity and a sinus, or externally through a trephination and formation of a sequestrum from a piece of alveolus or tooth not extracted at surgery. The dental wax may become dislodged postoperatively and require replacement. The opposing tooth requires additional floating to ensure that it does not become too long (step-mouth), causing malocclusion and further periodontal disease.

EXPECTED COURSE AND PROGNOSIS

Conservative treatment consisting of regular dental floating and a diet with sufficient high-quality roughage may successfully manage periodontal disease. However, the condition is generally considered progressive and is only completely resolved following tooth extraction. When the condition is extensive, removal of several teeth may not be practicable and management with a high-energy diet and regular dental care should be considered palliative. Periodontal disease is likely to be a life-limiting condition in wild horses. It is possible that mild periodontal disease in younger horses, with malocclusion due to abnormalities of permanent tooth eruption or mild abnormalities of dental wear, may be reversible following resolution of the underlying cause.

MISCELLANEOUS

ASSOCIATED CONDITIONS

Ill thrift and weight loss are commonly associated with periodontal disease.

AGE-RELATED FACTORS

As horses age, the reserve crown is exposed and the gap between adjacent teeth increases. This increases the potential for feed to become impacted between adjacent teeth.

ZOONOTIC POTENTIAL

N/A

PREGNANCY

N/A

SYNONYMS

- Periodontitis
- Alveolar periostitis
- Alveolar osteitis
- Gingivitis

SEE ALSO

- Abnormal dental wear
- Dental sepsis

ABBREVIATIONS

N/A

Suggested Reading

Crabill MR, Schumacher J. Pathophysiology of acquired dental disease of the horse. Vet Clin North Am 1998;14:291–307.

Kirkland KD, Maretta SM, Inoue OJ, Baker GL. Survey of equine dental disease and associated oral pathology. In Proceedings of the 40th Annual Convention of the American Association of Equine Practitioners, Vancouver, BC, 1994:119–120.

Lane JG. A review of dental disorders of the horse, their treatment and a possible fresh approach to management. Equine Vet Educ 1994;6:13–21.

Mueller POE, Lowder MQ. Dental sepsis. Vet Clin North Am 1998;14:349–363.

Author Hugo Hilton

Consulting Editors Henry Stämpfli and Olimpo Oliver-Espinosa

PERITONITIS

BASICS

OVERVIEW

Peritonitis is defined as inflammation of the peritoneal cavity. Peritonitis may be primary or secondary, and diffuse or localized. Peritonitis is caused by the presence of chemicals, infectious agents, or foreign matter within the peritoneal cavity. Inflammation involves the liberation of many mediators resulting in the decrease in vascular integrity and a flux of inflammatory cells, protein, red blood cells, and electrolytes into the peritoneal cavity. These components may help control the inciting cause (such as bacteria), but may also lead to adhesion or abscess formation if the disease becomes chronic. The disease may range from mild to severe, thereby causing hypovolemic and septic/toxic shock and, ultimately, death.

SYSTEMS AFFECTED

• Gastrointestinal • Musculoskeletal
• Behavioral • Cardiovascular • Respiratory
• Hemic/lymphatic/immune • Renal/urologic
• Reproductive • Skin/exocrine

SIGNALMENT

Any age, breed, or sex

SIGNS

Primary Disease

• Depressed demeanor • Inappetence • Fever
• Different degrees of dehydration • Altered gastrointestinal motility • Distended abdomen
• Splinting or guarding of abdomen • Mild colic
• Distended viscus; serosal fibrin deposition palpated per rectum

Secondary Disease

• Signs as listed previously • Moderate to severe colic
• Evidence of trauma • Laminitis

CAUSES AND RISK FACTORS

Primary

• Hematogenous spread • Immunocompromise (failure of passive transfer, combined immunodeficiency, transient immunodeficiency)

Secondary

• Loss of gastrointestinal integrity • Gastroduodenal ulceration, right dorsal colitis • Proximal enteritis, typhlitis, colitis • Gastric or intestinal rupture due to distension/devitalization • Vascular compromise thrombosis or intestinal torsion/volvulus • Trauma—iatrogenic (abdominal paracentesis/enterocentesis, rectal tear, surgery), foaling, foreign body • Loss of reproductive tract integrity • Breeding injury • Foaling injury • Wounds—penetrating • Surgery—castration, celiotomy with/without enterocentesis, enterotomy, resection and reanastamosis • Abscess rupture • Direct extension of other infection • Urine leakage
• Hemorrhage—rupture/tearing of spleen, liver, ovary
• Neoplasia • Parasite migration

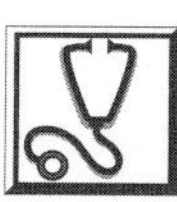

DIAGNOSIS

DIFFERENTIAL DIAGNOSIS

Includes any pain-causing, inflammatory, or infectious disease involving the gastrointestinal system. Ovulation, uterine torsion, urinary tract obstruction, cholelithiasis, and cholangitis should also be considered. Nonabdominal diseases such as pleuropneumonia may also present with similar signs.

CBC/BIOCHEMISTRY/URINALYSIS

CBC

• Neutrophilia • Neutropenia
• Hyperproteinemia • Hypoproteinemia

Biochemistry

• Hypoproteinemia (early loss of protein into abdominal cavity), hyperproteinemia (subacute to chronic inflammation). Albumin levels may be normal or decreased. Globulin levels may be normal, decreased, or increased.
• Urinalysis—reflects hemoconcentration

OTHER LABORATORY TESTS

Abdominal Paracentesis

• Appearance—turbid fluid may have elevated protein, nucleated cells, or foreign material; green or brown fluid likely contains feed or fecal material. • Cytology (collect into EDTA tube)—there may be an elevated protein level (>25 g/L; >2.5 g/dL) and nucleated cell count ($>10 \times 10^9$ nucleated cells/L;10^4 nucleated cells/μL), increased proportion of neutrophils, and the presence of toxic neutrophils. The presence of bacteria (intracellular or extracellular), feed material, and spermatozoa is also supportive of the presence of peritonitis. Puncture of the bowel while attempting to collect peritoneal fluid may result in a false-positive interpretation. • Culture and sensitivity (collect into clot tube)—Consider Gram stain and aerobic and anaerobic culture of fluid. False-negative results are frequent. • Other peritoneal fluid— Serum-to-peritoneal fluid glucose levels >50 mg/dL, decreased glucose level <30 mg/dL, pH < 7.3, elevated fibrinogen level >200 mg/dL support septic peritonitis even if bacterial culture does not yield any growth.

IMAGING

Radiographs

Radiographs are helpful in assessing foal abdomens or searching for foreign bodies in adult horses.

Ultrasound

Ultrasound is a useful tool in evaluating foal and adult abdomens. Hyperechoic fluid may have high cell count, protein level, or feed/fecal material. It can also assess presence of fibrin deposition and peripheral abscess formation.

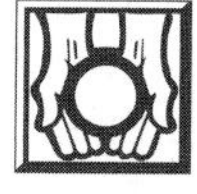

TREATMENT

• Resolve primary problem. • Abdominal drainage or lavage (standing horse; high risk of minor complications) • Abdominal exploration and lavage (anesthetized horse) • Fluid therapy (crystalloid fluid)
• Protein replacement (plasma, other oncotic agents)
• Laminitis prophylaxis

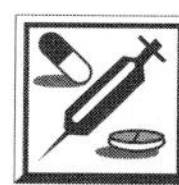

MEDICATIONS

DRUG(S) OF CHOICE

Antibiotic Therapy

• Broad spectrum initially (consider parenteral penicillin, cephalosporin, and aminoglycoside); a fluoroquinolone (enrofloxacin) may be indicated; macrolides with/without rifampin may be indicated in cases of abdominal abscessation; metronidazole should be used if anaerobic bacteria (especially *Bacteroides fragilis*) is suspected. • Antibiotic therapy—Adjust to sensitivity pattern of organisms isolated in culture. *Actinobacillus equuli* may be resistant to beta-lactam antibiotics. • NSAIDs (analgesia, decrease effects of toxins)

CONTRAINDICATIONS/POSSIBLE DRUG INTERACTIONS

• Corticosteroids are contraindicated in peritonitis because a bacterial infection is usually present.
• Aminoglycoside antibiotics such as gentamicin should be used with caution because nephrotoxicity may occur in the dehydrated animal. Periodic assessment of urine, serum creatinine, and serum blood urea nitrogen levels is recommended. Once-daily dosing may be advantageous. • Macrolide antibiotics, especially erythromycin, may cause enterocolitis (potentially fatal).

ALTERNATIVE DRUGS

Trimethoprim-sulfonamide (enteral or parenteral); potentiated penicillins (amoxicillin/sulbactam) may be useful.

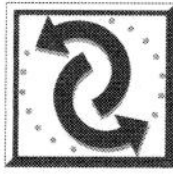

FOLLOW-UP

PATIENT MONITORING

Periodic peritoneal fluid analysis (every 2–3 days or if the patient does not show any improvement). Improvement may also be noted with normalization of blood parameters (white blood cell count, protein level, fibrinogen level).

POSSIBLE COMPLICATIONS

Laminitis and thrombophlebitis. Abscess formation and adhesion formation may also occur, resulting in a failure to thrive and colic, respectively.

MISCELLANEOUS

AGE-RELATED FACTORS

Immunodeficiency in the neonate

PREGNANCY

Peritonitis in a pregnant animal may cause loss of the fetus.

SEE ALSO

Colic

Suggested Reading

Davis JL. Treatment of peritonitis. Vet Clin North Am Equine Pract 2003;19:765-778.

Van Hoogmoed. Evaluation of peritoneal fluid pH, glucose concentration, and lactate dehydrogenase activity for detection of septic peritonitis in horses. JAVMA 1999;214:1032-1036.

Author Daniel G. Kenney
Consulting Editors Henry Stämpfli and Olimpo Oliver-Espinosa

PETECHIAE, ECCHYMOSES AND HEMATOMAS

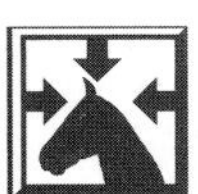

BASICS

OVERVIEW

• An increased hemorrhagic tendency may result in petechiae, ecchymoses and/or hematomas. • Petechiae are tiny, flat, round hemorrhages visible in the skin, mucous membranes, or serosal surfaces; ecchymoses are larger hemorrhages (1–2 cm), and a hematoma is a large, localized collection of clotted/ partially clotted blood. • A bruise is an ecchymosis/hematoma where hemoglobin is converted into bilirubin and hemosiderin, resulting in blue/green discoloration. • Bleeding disorders may result from blood vessel damage or impaired hemostasis. • Large blood vessel damage results from trauma, invasion, aneurism or other anomalies and usually results in hematomas. • Small blood vessel damage is commonly due to vasculitides causing petechial hemorrhages. • Impaired hemostasis may be primary (e.g., thrombocytopenia, von Willebrand's disease), secondary (e.g., hereditary or acquired defects in coagulation), or due to excessive fibrinolysis (e.g., DIC). • The pattern of bleeding may reflect the cause such that petechiae and/or ecchymoses should prompt consideration of severe thrombocytopenia, vasculitis or defects in secondary hemostasis. • Subcutaneous hematomas or hemorrhage into body cavities may result from trauma, platelet defects or defects in secondary hemostasis.

SIGNALMENT

• Acquired hemostatic abnormalities have no age, sex, or breed disposition. • Inherited coagulation disorders occur in young purebred horses, following an autosomal recessive pattern (see Coagulation Defects, Inherited).

SIGNS

Historical

Inappropriate hemorrhage or sudden onset of dark discolorations of skin or mucous membranes.

Physical Examination

• There may be variably sized, focal, flat, red areas within the skin, mucous membranes and/or serosal surfaces of internal organs. • Larger areas of hemorrhage are often associated with pressure points of skin and mucous membranes. • Additional signs may include pale mucous membranes, serosanguinous discharge or even frank hemorrhage from nose or rectum, red discoloration of feces or urine, melena, anorexia, tachypnea, tachycardia, respiratory distress, increased rectal temperature, ventral/peripheral edema, splenomegaly, ascites, colic, and pleural effusion.

CAUSES

Blood Vessel Damage

• Immune-mediated vasculitis (e.g., purpura hemorrhagica) • Vasculitis directly caused by infectious agents • Septicemia/bacteremia • Trauma

Platelet Abnormalities

• Decreased platelet production (e.g., myelophthisis, aplastic anemia, megakaryocytic and myeloid hypoplasia in Standarbreds) • Increased platelet destruction (e.g., primary IMTP, secondary IMPT, snake evenomation, toxin/drug induced direct platelet damage, neonatal alloimmune thrombocytopenia) • Increased platelet consumption (e.g., DIC, localized intravascular coagulation, excessive hemorrhage, severe trauma, vasculitis) • Platelet sequestration (e.g., splenomegaly, vascular neoplasms) • Platelet dysfunction (e.g., Glanzmann's thrombasthenia)

Defects in Coagulation

• Acquired coagulation defects (e.g., vitamin K deficiency) • Inherited coagulation defects (e.g., von Willebrand's disease, hemophilia A, prekallikrein deficiency) • Liver disease • Neoplasia • DIC

Multifactorial (Complex Vascular/Platelet/Coagulation Abnormalities)

• Infections (e.g., equine infectious anemia, equine granulocytic ehrlichiosis, equine monocytic ehrlichiosis, equine viral arteritis, Venezuelan equine encephalitis, African horse sickness, equine herpesvirus, equine influenza, babesiosis, trypanosomiasis) • Septicemia/endotoxemia/DIC • Neoplasia

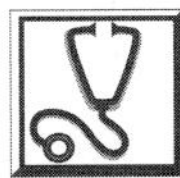

DIAGNOSIS

DIFFERENTIAL DIAGNOSIS

Petechiae, ecchymoses, and hematomas may be associated with a wide variety of disease processes.

CBC/BIOCHEMISTRY/URINALYSIS

• Highly variable depending on underlying cause of hemostatic abnormality • May include anemia, thrombocytopenia, and abnormal liver enzymes or function assays

OTHER LABORATORY TESTS

• Platelet count, ACT, PT, aPTT, fibrinogen, plasma D-dimer, antithrombin III, and protein C concentrations—to identify coagulation defects and DIC • Quantification of specific clotting factors (e.g., VIII), platelet aggregation tests/clot retraction time, and platelet function tests to help characterize platelet defects. • Serology (including Coggins test), blood smears and cultures may identify infectious agents. • Flow cytometry for detection of platelet bound antibody. • Platelet factor 3 test as an indirect test for IMTP

IMAGING

Ultrasonography of the thorax, abdomen, or soft tissues may be helpful for identifying a cause or may be used for ultrasound-guided centesis to help establish a definitive diagnosis.

OTHER DIAGNOSTIC PROCEDURES

• Avoid invasive procedures in patients at risk of bleeding. • Bone marrow aspirate/biopsy, centesis of abdomen/thorax to investigate cause and extent of bleeding tendency

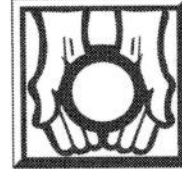

TREATMENT

AIMS OF TREATMENT

• Treatment of underlying disease is essential. • Supportive care may include: ○ Isotonic fluids for blood volume expansion and fluid balance maintenance ○ Whole blood, plasma, or platelet transfusions

MEDICATIONS

DRUG(S) OF CHOICE

These may include:

• Appropriate antimicrobials or antiparasitics for infectious causes • Immunomodulators (e.g., corticosteroids) for immune-mediated disease; dexamethasone is superior to short-acting corticosteroids • Cytotoxic drugs (e.g., azothioprine, vincristine) for refractory IMTP or neoplasia • Vitamin K_1 in cases of vitamin K deficiencies • Low-dose flunixin meglumine and antithrombotics (e.g., heparin) in cases of endotoxemia

CONTRAINDICATIONS

• Identification of the cause of the bleeding disorder is indicated before onset of therapy as drugs used to treat some causes are contraindicated in others. • Corticosteroids are contraindicated with preexistent laminitis or most infectious diseases. • Aspirin and other NSAIDs may impair platelet function. • Treatments that affect platelet function (e.g., colloids) or coagulation system function (e.g., heparin) may exacerbate bleeding.

PRECAUTIONS

Minimize activity to decrease risk of trauma.

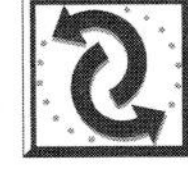

FOLLOW-UP

PATIENT MONITORING

Daily platelet counts to assess response to medications.

POSSIBLE COMPLICATIONS

Hypovolemic shock and/or sudden death due to internal hemorrhage

MISCELLANEOUS

SEE ALSO

• Coagulation defects, inherited • Coagulation defects, acquired • DIC • Purpura hemorrhagica • Thrombocytopenia

ABBREVIATIONS

• ACT = activated clotting time • aPTT = activated partial thromboplastin time • DIC = disseminated intravascular coagulation • IMTP = immune-mediated thrombocytopenia • PT = prothrombin time

Suggested Reading

Sellon DC. Disorders of the hematopoietic system. In: Reed SM, et al., eds. Equine Internal Medicine, ed 2. St Louis: Saunders, 2004;721–768.

Author Jennifer Hodgson
Consulting Editors David Hodgson and Jennifer Hodgson

PHEOCHROMOCYTOMA

BASICS

OVERVIEW

- PCC is a tumor of the catecholamine-producing cells of the adrenal medulla.
- Most reported equine PCCs have been unilateral, well-encapsulated, benign neoplasms, and almost half have been incidental findings at necropsy.
- Can be functional and release catecholamines, which include epinephrine and norepinephrine
- Clinical signs result from excessive catecholamine production or tumor growth. The most commonly reported signs in horses are sweating, tachycardia, tachypnea, abdominal pain, mydriasis, muscle tremors, and hyperglycemia.

SYSTEMS AFFECTED

- Endocrine
- Cardiovascular

SIGNALMENT

- Reported mainly in horses 12 years and older. However, one malignant PCC involving both adrenal glands has been reported in a 6-mo-old foal.
- No breed or sex predilection is apparent.

SIGNS

Many clinical signs associated with functional PCC are nonspecific and can be caused by other diseases. This explains why most cases are diagnosed postmortem.

Historical

- Horses may have a history of lethargy, anorexia, abdominal pain, sweating, tachycardia, diarrhea, or neurologic signs of ataxia.
- Pregnant mares may abort.
- One foal with a malignant PCC had a 4-mo history of poor growth and a 5-day history of progressive ataxia.

Physical Examination

- Sweating, tachycardia, tachypnea, abdominal pain, mydriasis, muscle tremors, ileus, and diarrhea are reported and attributable to excessive catecholamine production.
- A mass may be palpated per rectum medially to the left kidney.
- Signs of ataxia and paresis have been described in one case and resulted from compression of the spinal cord by the tumor's metastasis.

CAUSES AND RISK FACTORS

- PCC is a benign or malignant tumor of the chromaffin cells of the adrenal medulla.
- No risk factors have yet been identified.

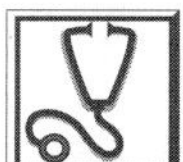

DIAGNOSIS

DIFFERENTIAL DIAGNOSIS

- Causes of abdominal pain and ileus (e.g., colic) should be considered.
- Clinical signs and biochemical abnormalities similar to those reported with PCC may be observed with renal disease, enteritis, colitis, hypoadrenocorticism, or other causes of cardiovascular, pulmonary, and neurologic diseases.
- Causes of hyperglycemia including stress, hyperadrenocorticism, or diabetes mellitus should be considered.

CBC/BIOCHEMISTRY/URINALYSIS

- Laboratory findings are variable and nonspecific.
- Hemoconcentration and inflammatory leukogram are common.
- Hyponatremia, hyperkalemia, metabolic acidosis, hypocalcemia, hyperphosphatemia, azotemia, hyperglycemia, glucosuria, and occult hematuria are common.

OTHER LABORATORY TESTS

Assays for catecholamines and their metabolites in plasma or urine are technically difficult and few laboratories perform these tests. Interpretation of the results may be complicated further by the intermittent nature of catecholamine release in horses with PCC and the fact that high catecholamine levels can be detected in stressed but otherwise normal horses.

IMAGING

Ultrasonography may reveal a mass medial to the kidney, along the aorta, or in the posterior vena cava.

DIAGNOSTIC PROCEDURES

Direct or indirect arterial blood pressure measurements may document hypertension.

PATHOLOGICAL FINDINGS

- Usually unilateral and infrequently bilateral.
- Unique or multiple nodular masses within the adrenal gland may vary in size from a few millimeters to >10 cm.
- A large PCC may invade the posterior vena cava and result in extensive hemorrhage. This can lead to numerous blood clots in the perirenal and retroperitoneal spaces in addition to the hemoperitoneum.
- Histologically, PCCs often are necrotic and hemorrhagic, which also may result in adrenocortical hemorrhage and necrosis.

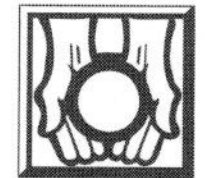

TREATMENT

- Suspected cases should be treated on an inpatient basis.
- Medical care should be aimed at controlling pain, using fluid therapy to normalize renal function and electrolyte abnormalities, and stabilizing the cardiovascular function.
- Complete rest is recommended.
- Avoid feed intake as long as intestinal motility is impaired.
- Consider surgical resection in cases of localized nodular tumors. This procedure is difficult technically and the risk of a fatal complication is high (hemorrhage, cardiac arrhythmia, or rhabdomyolysis).

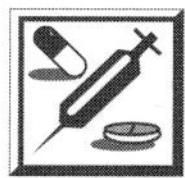

MEDICATIONS

DRUGS

In humans, small animals, α- and β-adrenergic blocking agents can control the effects of excessive catecholamine secretion.

FOLLOW-UP

PATIENT MONITORING

Monitor renal and cardiovascular function, electrolytes, and acid-base status.

POSSIBLE COMPLICATIONS

- Renal failure
- Hemorrhage
- Cardiac arrhythmia
- Hypotension may follow adrenalectomy.

EXPECTED COURSE AND PROGNOSIS

- There are no reports of successful treatment of functional PCC in horses.
- All reported cases involved death or euthanasia within a few hours to a few days of the onset of clinical signs.

MISCELLANEOUS

PREGNANCY

Abortion during late gestation and fatal hemorrhage during parturition have been reported.

ABBREVIATION

- PCC = Pheochromocytoma

Suggested Reading

Johnson PJ, Goetz TE, Foreman JH, Zachary JF. Pheochromocytoma in two horses. JAVMA 1995;206:837–841.

Author Laurent Couëtil
Consulting Editor Michel Lévy

BASICS

DEFINITION

The inability to protrude the penis from the prepuce

PATHOPHYSIOLOGY

Constriction of either the external preputial orifice or the preputial ring can result in phimosis.

SYSTEM AFFECTED

Reproductive

SIGNALMENT

Stallions or geldings of any age

SIGNS

Historical

Urination within the preputial cavity and/or dysuria

Physical Examination

- Visible or palpable thickening of the external preputial orifice or the preputial ring. Excoriations due to urine scalding may be apparent.

CAUSES

Congenital

- Stenosis of the preputial orifice
- Hermaphroditism
- Penile dysgenesis

Acquired

- Trauma—breeding injury, postsurgical edema, chronic posthitis
- Neoplasia—sarcoid, SCC, papilloma, melanoma, hemagioma
- Parasitism—habronemiasis
- Viral infections—EHV-3

RISK FACTORS

- Poor hygiene; accumulation of excessive smegma can lead to posthitis and subsequent phimosis from the formation of scar tissue.
- Light-colored skin is associated with an increased incidence of squamous cell carcinoma.
- Gray horses are more commonly diagnosed with melanomas.

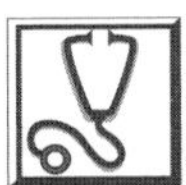

DIAGNOSIS

DIFFERENTIAL DIAGNOSIS

Differentiating Similar Signs

Phimosis during the first 30 days of life is normal due to fusion of the internal preputial lamina to the free portion of the penis.

CBC/BIOCHEMISTRY/URINALYSIS

N/A

OTHER LABORATORY TESTS

Virus isolation using fluid from vesicular lesions may be diagnostic for EHV-3.

IMAGING N/A

DIAGNOSTIC PROCEDURES

Cytology or biopsy (histopathology) may distinguish and/or provide a definitive diagnosis for neoplastic, granulomatous, or herpesvirus lesions.

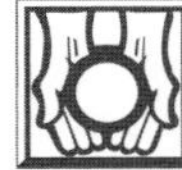

TREATMENT

If phimosis is due to:

- Postsurgical edema—Hydrotherapy, massage, exercise, and diuretics are indicated. Cleansing and application of topical emollients or antibiotics may be indicated.
- Neoplastic or granulomatous lesions—surgical excision, cryosurgery, chemotherapy, or radiation, as indicated by type, location, and size
- A stricture of the external preputial orifice—surgical removal of a triangular section of the external preputial lamina
- A stricture at the preputial ring—Incise the internal preputial fold (preputiotomy). Circumcision (reefing) may be necessary to remove the constricting tissue in its entirety.

MEDICATIONS

DRUG(S) OF CHOICE

- NSAIDs, including phenylbutazone (2–4 g/450 kg/day PO) or flunixin meglumine (1.1 mg/kg/day IV, IM, or PO), for symptomatic relief or to decrease inflammation
- Systemic or local antibiotics if indicated to treat local infections or prevent septicemia
- Diuretics—Furosemide (1–2 mg/kg IV q6–12h) may be indicated in the acute phase to reduce edema.
- Specific topical or systemic treatments for parasitic, fungal, or neoplastic conditions as indicated by test results

CONTRAINDICATIONS N/A

PRECAUTIONS

Phenothiazine tranquilizers should be avoided/used with caution (see Priapism).

POSSIBLE INTERACTIONS N/A

ALTERNATIVE DRUGS N/A

FOLLOW-UP

PATIENT MONITORING

- Initially, daily evaluations—Ensure that secondary posthitis, balanitis, balanoposthitis, urine scald, or penile/preputial excoriations are not complicating the phimosis.
- As the initial problem is effectively treated, less frequent examinations will be necessary.

POSSIBLE COMPLICATIONS

- Urination within the preputial cavity may cause inflammation of the epithelium, leading to a more extensive inflammation (posthitis, balanoposthitis) and scarring.
- Infertility or impotence can result if scarring becomes extensive.

MISCELLANEOUS

ASSOCIATED CONDITIONS

N/A

AGE-RELATED FACTORS

- Papillomas are more frequently diagnosed in young animals.
- Squamous cell carcinomas and melanomas are more frequently diagnosed in middle-age to aged horses.

ZOONOTIC POTENTIAL

N/A

PREGNANCY

N/A

SYNONYMS

N/A

SEE ALSO

- Paraphimosis
- Penile vesicles/erosions

ABBREVIATIONS

- EHV = equine herpesvirus

Suggested Reading

Blanchard TL, Varner DD, Schumacher J, Love CC, Brinsko SP, Rigby SL. Manual of Equine Reproduction, ed 2. St. Louis: Mosby, 2003:193–218.

Schumacher J, Varner DD. Surgical correction of abnormalities affecting the reproductive organs of stallions. In: Youngquist RS, Threlfall WR, eds. Current Therapy in Large Animal Theriogenology. St. Louis: Saunders Elsevier, 2007:23–36.

Schumacher J, Vaughan JT. Surgery of the penis and prepuce. Vet Clin North Am Equine Practice 1988;4;473–491.

Vaughan JT. Surgery of the penis and prepuce. In: Walker DF, Vaughan JT, eds. Bovine and Equine Urogenital Surgery. Philadelphia: Lea & Febiger, 1980:125–144.

Author Carole C. Miller

Consulting Editor Carla L. Carleton

PHOSPHORUS, HYPERPHOSPHATEMIA

BASICS

DEFINITION

Serum phosphate concentration greater than the reference interval (e.g., >4.5 mg/L)

PATHOPHYSIOLOGY

• Kidneys, small intestine, and skeleton are involved in phosphate homeostasis in conjunction with parathyroid hormone, calcitonin, vitamin D, and diet. • Decreased glomerular filtration or renal excretion, excessive intestinal absorption or dietary supplementation, or excessive bone resorption can result in hyperphosphatemia.

SYSTEMS AFFECTED

General

• Phosphorus and calcium metabolism and homeostatic mechanisms are closely linked.
• Hyperphosphatemia frequently occurs with hypocalcemia in many disorders; in these cases, effects of hyperphosphatemia on organ systems often are indirect and relate more to hypocalcemia.

Skeletal

• Skeletal effects result from concurrent secondary hypocalcemia due to excessive dietary intake or phosphorus imbalance. • In response to hypocalcemia, calcium is mobilized from bone to maintain other metabolic functions; consequences include too little or abnormal bone formation, bone demineralization, and a skeleton more prone to injury.

Endocrine

• Hyperphosphatemia stimulates PTH secretion. • Effects of PTH—increased resorption of calcium from bone, kidneys, and intestine; increased renal excretion of phosphorus; the net effect decreases plasma phosphorus and increases plasma calcium levels.

SIGNALMENT

• Varies with underlying disease or condition.
• Neonates and young, growing animals have increased serum phosphorus levels—often 4.5–9.0 mg/dL.

SIGNS

General Comments

Signs of hyperphosphatemia are associated with hypocalcemia: lameness, abnormal bone and cartilage development, or fractures.

Historical Findings

History varies with the underlying cause of hyperphosphatemia, and may reflect disorders associated with hypocalcemia or hypercalcemia.

Physical Examination Findings

• Dietary phosphorus excess or imbalance—clinical signs manifest in the skeletal system; early signs include intermittent shifting leg lameness, generalized joint tenderness, or stilted gait; as the disease progresses, abnormal bone formation and enlarged facial bones (e.g., bighead in NHP) occur. • Hypervitaminosis D—horses may exhibit limb stiffness, with painful flexor tendons and suspensory ligaments.

CAUSES

• Neonates and young, growing animals—hyperphosphatemia commonly is seen because of rapid bone turnover. • Endurance exercise—transient hyperphosphatemia may be seen after long-distance endurance activity.
• Decreased glomerular filtration—common cause of hyperphosphatemia associated with prerenal, renal, or postrenal azotemia; hyperphosphatemia may be seen in some cases of acute renal failure, but equine chronic renal failure usually is accompanied by hypophosphatemia. • Hypervitaminosis D—hyperphosphatemia and hypercalcemia result from excessive dietary supplementation with vitamin D–containing products; ingestion of plants (e.g., *Cestrum diurnum,* wild jasmine, *Solanum* sp., Hawaii) containing a vitamin D–like substance usually do not cause abnormalities in plasma phosphorus levels.
• Excessive dietary phosphorus or phosphorus imbalance—excessive phosphorus intake, dietary calcium:phosphorus imbalance, or excessive supplementation with bran, which is high in phosphorus content, inhibits absorption of calcium, thus altering calcium homeostatic mechanisms and the rate of bone turnover. This can result in calcium deficiency that may go undetected for weeks to months.
• In young animals, skeletal mass does not keep up with increasing body size; thus, the skeleton is more injury prone. NHP (e.g., bighead disease) occurs from excess phosphorus and low or marginal calcium intake. Secretion of PTH increases as a compensatory mechanism to correct the disturbance in mineral homeostasis induced by nutritional imbalance.

RISK FACTORS

Increased potential for soft-tissue mineralization with concurrent hyperphosphatemia and hypercalcemia

PHOSPHORUS, HYPERPHOSPHATEMIA

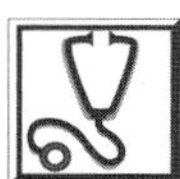

DIAGNOSIS

DIFFERENTIAL DIAGNOSIS

History is useful in determining if diet contains phosphorus excess or imbalances.

LABORATORY FINDINGS

Drugs That May Alter Lab Results

Citrate, oxalate, and EDTA anticoagulants interfere with biochemical methodology and should not be used.

Disorders That May Alter Lab Results

• Lipemia, hemolysis, and icterus may falsely elevate serum phosphorus concentrations because of interference with biochemical methodology. • Serum is the preferred specimen. Heparinized plasma can be used, but phosphate levels may be minimally lower than serum reference ranges. • Delayed separation of cells from the clot can result in leakage of phosphorus from cells and falsely elevate serum phosphorus concentration.

Valid If Run in Human Lab?

Yes

CBC/BIOCHEMISTRY/URINALYSIS

• NHP—normal renal function and, depending on stage of disease, hypocalcemia, hyperphosphatemia, and elevated ALP • Renal failure—azotemia; isosthenuria

OTHER LABORATORY TESTS

• Dietary deficiency or imbalance—review dietary history; inspect feed, and analyze chemically for calcium and phosphorus content. • NHP—increased urinary phosphorus fractional excretion

IMAGING

Conventional radiology has little benefit in detecting loss of skeletal mineralization until such losses exceed 30%.

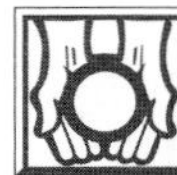

TREATMENT

• NHP—Correct dietary deficiency or imbalance by supplying the deficient nutrient; dietary calcium:phosphorus ratio must not exceed 1.5–2:1. • Removal of vitamin D sources and time may result in recovery; however, if soft-tissue mineralization in the heart or kidney occurs, prognosis is poor. • With suspected acute renal failure, fluid replacement and correction of electrolyte imbalances

MEDICATIONS

DRUG(S) OF CHOICE

Hypervitaminosis D—removal of source, fluid diuresis, corticosteroid administration, and low-calcium and -phosphorus feeds; in severe cases, treatment generally is unrewarding because of extensive soft-tissue mineralization.

MISCELLANEOUS

ASSOCIATED CONDITIONS

Hypocalcemia

AGE-RELATED FACTORS

• Hyperphosphatemia and elevated ALP levels are common in healthy, young, growing animals. Both parameters decrease with age. • Young animals are more prone to skeletal abnormalities resulting from dietary excess or imbalances.

SYNONYMS

NHP—bighead disease, bran disease, osteodystrophia fibrosa, Miller's disease

SEE ALSO

• Hypercalcemia • Hypocalcemia

ABBREVIATIONS

• ALP = alkaline phosphatase
• NHP = nutritional secondary hyperparathyroidism
• PTH = parathyroid hormone

Suggested Reading

Bertone JJ. Nutritional secondary hyperparathyroidism. In Robinson NE, ed. Current Therapy in Equine Medicine, ed 3. Philadelphia: WB Saunders, 1992:119–122.

Author Karen E. Russell
Consulting Editor Kenneth W. Hinchcliff

PHOSPHORUS, HYPOPHOSPHATEMIA

BASICS

DEFINITION

Serum phosphate concentration less than reference interval (<2.0 mg/dL)

PATHOPHYSIOLOGY

• Phosphorus is one of the most abundant elements in the body, with >80% occurring in bone and complexed with calcium in the form of hydroxyapatite. • Phosphorus is an important component of nucleic acids, phospholipids, and phosphoproteins. • Maintenance of cellular integrity and metabolism depends on phosphate-containing, high-energy compounds (e.g., ATP) and many enzyme systems that require phosphorus. • Skeletal-associated abnormalities (e.g., demineralization, deformation, poor growth) are potential consequences of hypophosphatemia. • Depletion of ATP can affect any cell with high-energy requirements; erythrocytes, skeletal muscle cells, and brain cells are especially susceptible.

SYSTEMS AFFECTED

• Skeletal—too little or abnormal bone formation, bone demineralization, and a skeleton more prone to injury • Reproductive—anestrus, irregular estrus, or reduced conception rates
• Hematologic—Severe deficiency may predispose to erythrocyte hemolysis.

SIGNALMENT

Varies with the cause

SIGNS

General Comments

• History and clinical signs reflect the underlying disorder rather than the serum abnormality.
• Pica and developmental orthopedic disease may be seen with phosphorus deficiency.

Historical

• Chronic renal failure—poor performance
• Dietary phosphorus deficiency—poor growth, poor reproductive history, anestrus, irregular estrus, and reduced conception rates

Physical Examination

• Chronic renal failure—weight loss • Dietary phosphorus deficiency—lameness, stiff painful gait, or pica

CAUSES

Renal Failure

Serum phosphorus in horses with chronic renal failure may be normal or low, depending on the presence and degree of hypercalcemia.

Dietary Phosphorus Deficiency

The condition is common in states of phosphate deficiency or starvation.

Primary Hyperparathyroidism

• Potential causes—parathyroid adenoma, parathyroid hyperplasia, or carcinoma • In case reports of horses with primary hyperparathyroidism, hypercalcemia, hypophosphatemia or low-normal phosphorus concentration, and increased fractional phosphorus excretion were common findings. Vitamin D_3 concentration was not elevated.
• This condition is rare in horses but should be considered if all other causes of hypercalcemia have been excluded.

Rickets

• Young, growing animals with vitamin D deficiency may be hypophosphatemic, hypocalcemic, and have elevated ALP levels.
• Vitamin D deficiency causes defective mineralization of new bone, resulting in painful swelling of the physis and metaphysis of the long bones and costochondral junctions, bowed limbs, and stiff gait. • Natural cases of rickets in foals probably are quite rare.

Halothane Anesthesia

• In one report, a few horses subjected to prolonged halothane anesthesia (>12 hr) were observed to have mild hyperphosphatemia initially, but developed hypophosphatemia persisting for a few days. • The pathogenesis is not known.

RISK FACTORS

• Severe hypophosphatemia has been associated with intravascular hemolysis and altered erythrocyte function in other species—bovine, human, and canine. • With horses in chronic renal failure that are hypercalcemic, do not feed legume hays (e.g., alfalfa, clover) or high-calcium rations, and do not treat with calcium-containing fluids.

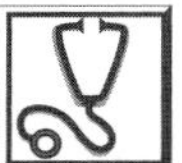

DIAGNOSIS

DIFFERENTIAL DIAGNOSIS

• Chronic renal failure—azotemia, isosthenuria, hypercalcemia, and exposure to nephrotoxins
• History—useful in determining dietary deficiency of phosphorus or calcium. • Primary hyperparathryoidism–hypercalcemia, hyperphosphatemia, increased serum PTH concentration, increased fractional phosphorus excretion, and low to normal concentrations of vitamin D_3

LABORATORY FINDINGS

Drugs That May Alter Lab Results

• Serum is the preferred specimen for phosphate determination. • Heparinized plasma can be used, but phosphorus levels may be minimally lower than serum reference ranges. • Citrate, oxalate, and EDTA anticoagulants interfere with biochemical methodology and should not be used.

Disorders That May Alter Lab Results

• Lipemia, hemolysis, and icterus may falsely elevate serum phosphorus concentrations.
• Delayed separation of cells from the clot can result in leakage of phosphorus from cells and falsely elevate serum phosphorus concentrations.

Valid If Run in Human Lab?

Yes

CBC/BIOCHEMISTRY/URINALYSIS

• Chronic renal failure—azotemia, hypercalcemia, isosthenuria are common findings; hypophosphatemia, mild hyponatremia and hypochloridemia, and normo- or hyperkalemia also may be present. • Moderate to marked proteinuria is common in cases of glomerulonephritis. • Suspect urinary tract infection with the finding of moderate to many leukocytes in urine sediment. • Primary hyperparathryoidism—renal function should be normal. • Severe calcium or phosphorus deficiency—elevated serum ALP level

OTHER LABORATORY TESTS

With suspected hypoparathyroidism, fractional phosphorus excretion and immunoreactive C-terminal PTH concentration help to confirm the diagnosis.

IMAGING

Conventional radiology has little benefit in detecting loss of skeletal mineralization until such losses exceed 30%.

DIAGNOSTIC PROCEDURES

With suspected dietary phosphorus and calcium deficiencies, thorough review of dietary history, inspection of feeds, and chemical evaluation of calcium and phosphorus content in feeds are necessary.

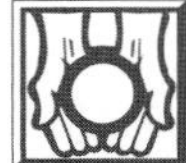

TREATMENT

• Supplementation with appropriate mineral sources to correct deficiency or imbalance in a particular diet • Common mineral supplements for phosphorus—defluorinated phosphate, bonemeal, dicalcium phosphate, monocalcium phosphate, or monosodium phosphate

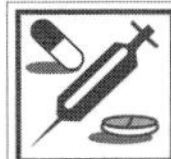

MEDICATIONS

PRECAUTIONS

Dietary calcium:phosphorus ratio must not exceed 1.5–2:1.

AGE-RELATED FACTORS

Young animals may be more prone to skeletal abnormalities resulting from dietary deficiency or imbalances.

SEE ALSO

• Hypercalcemia, chronic renal failure
• Hypocalcemia

ABBREVIATIONS

• ALP = alkaline phosphatase
• PTH = parathyroid hormone

Suggested Reading

Fleming SA, Yates DJ. Disorders of phosphorus metabolism: chronic phosphorus deficiency/hypophosphatemia. In: Smith BP, ed. Large Animal Internal Medicine, ed 2. St. Louis: Mosby–Year Book, 1996:1471–1474.

Freestone JF, Melrose PA. Endocrine diseases. In: Kobluk CN, Ames TR, Geor RJ, eds. The Horse: Diseases and Clinical Management. Philadelphia: WB Saunders, 1995:1137–164.

Schryver HF, Hintz HF. Minerals. In: Robinson NE, ed. Current Therapy in Equine Medicine, ed 2. Philadelphia: WB Saunders, 1987:393–405.

Author Karen E. Russell
Consulting Editor Kenneth W. Hinchcliff

PHOTIC HEAD SHAKING

BASICS

OVERVIEW

• Otherwise known as head tossing behavior, photic head shaking is a condition where, in the absence of any external stimuli other than light, a horse vigorously and violently shakes its head in horizontal, vertical, or rotary directions.
• This disorder is probably a form of optic-trigeminal nerve summation, where retina and optic nerve stimulation produces referred sensation to the nasal cavity. The irritability in the nasal cavity causes the horse to shake its head.
• Eye, CNS, and upper respiratory tract can be involved.

SIGNALMENT

• Hunter-type horses are most commonly affected.
• Affected horses are 7 years old with mean duration of signs prior to referral of 8 months.
• Heritability is unknown.
• Geldings are overrepresented.

SIGNS

Excessive and occasionally violent rubbing, sneezing, and flipping of the nose and head at rest or during exercise

CAUSES AND RISK FACTORS

Sunlight may stimulate parasympathetic activity in the infraorbital nerve resulting in irritating nasal sensations and head tossing; most horses are asymptomatic in winter.

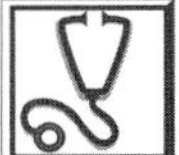

DIAGNOSIS

DIFFERENTIAL DIAGNOSES

Otitis media/interna from mites, premaxillary bone cysts, maxillary osteomas, guttural pouch disease, upper respiratory tract disease, bit and tack problems, and dental as well as ocular diseases such as iris cysts must also be ruled out as a cause.

CBC/BIOCHEMISTRY/URINALYSIS

Usually normal

OTHER LABORATORY TESTS

None

IMAGING

Radiography of skull and cervical spine to identify changes associated with otitis media and interna

DIAGNOSTIC PROCEDURES

• Blindfolding horse or placing in dark environments (improvement noted in head shakers)
• Upper respiratory tract examination
• Endoscopy of the guttural pouches
• Tympanocentesis under general anesthesia (may be helpful to rule out ear disease that lacks radiologic evidence)
• Thorough otic, oral, nasal, and ophthalmic examination
• Bilateral infraorbital nerve blocks

GROSS AND HISTOPATHOLOGIC FINDINGS

N/A

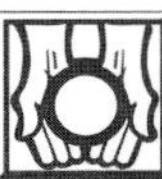

TREATMENT

• The complete workup may require overnight hospitalization. The medical management can be done by the trainer/owner.
• Head shaking can occur at rest or during exercise. Because most head shakers show signs shortly after the onset of activity, there may be unforeseen risks in working an uncontrolled photic head shaker.
• Medical therapy controls, but does not cure, the condition. If effective, medical treatment may only be needed during the season in which the horses exhibit head shaking behavior. Surgical infraorbital neurectomies are a salvage procedure.
• If a horse does not respond to medical therapy and infraorbital nerve blocks are successful, the horse may be a candidate for bilateral infraorbital neurectomy.

MEDICATIONS

DRUG(S) OF CHOICE

Cyproheptadine (H_1 blocker), a serotonin antagonist that alters POMC metabolism, has the potential to alleviate the clinical signs at a dose of 0.3 mg/kg PO BID for 7 days initially, then continued as needed. Some horses may require a dose up to 0.6 mg/kg PO BID. The antiepileptic drug carbamazepine can help others (10 mg/kg PO q6h, or 29 mg/kg PO q12h).

CONTRAINDICATIONS
Avoid in hypersensitive patients.

PRECAUTIONS
- Treatment of performance horses should comply with the rules of the governing organization.
- Mild lethargy, anorexia, and depression have been reported in horses treated with cyproheptadine.
- Drug eruptions have also been reported with cyproheptadine.

POSSIBLE INTERACTIONS
Additive CNS depression may be seen if combined with barbiturates or tranquilizers. Cyproheptadine has anticholinergic effects, which may be intensified by monoamine oxidase inhibitors (e. g., furazolidone).

ALTERNATE DRUGS
To mimic winter conditions physiologically, melatonin therapy at a dose of 12 mg PO on a sugar cube once between 17:00 and 18:00 daily may also be beneficial.

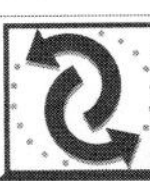

FOLLOW-UP
- A 7-day trial of cyproheptadine should determine whether the patient will respond favorably to medical management. Therapy can be stopped periodically and reinstated if the behavior recurs and there are no side effects.
- Horses kept in a dark environment may not show severe clinical head shaking. Light blocking protectors or a "nose net" may also help controlling the clinical signs for some horses. This type of management, however, may not be practical for the horse or its owner and trainer.
- A horse with uncontrolled head shaking may develop unwanted head trauma and the owner or trainer may find it difficult for the horse to optimally work or perform.
- Long-term, seasonal medical therapy can control, but not cure, this disease. Infraoribital nerve blocks relieved clinical signs in some horses. Posterior ethmoidal nerve (caudal nasal branch of the maxillary division of the trigeminal nerve) blocks were more effective in abolishing clinical signs.

MISCELLANEOUS

ASSOCIATED CONDITIONS
Photic sneezing in humans

PREGNANCY
No studies are available in the horse on safety of cyproheptadine in pregnant mares. It should be used with caution.

SYNONYMS
- Head tossing

ABBREVIATIONS
- CNS = central nervous system
- POMC = proopiomelanocortin

Suggested Reading

Brooks DE: Ophthalmology for the Equine Practitioner. Jackson, WY: Teton NewMedia, 2002.

Brooks DE, Matthews AG: Equine ophthalmology. In: Gelatt KN (ed). Veterinary Ophthalmology, ed 4. Philadelphia: Lippincott Williams and Wilkins, 2007.

Gilger BC (ed): Equine Ophthalmology. Philadelphia: WB Saunders, 2005.

Author Dennis E. Brooks

Consulting Editor Dennis E. Brooks

PHOTOSENSITIZATION

BASICS

OVERVIEW

• Photosensitization is defined as UVL-induced dermatitis caused by the presence of a photodynamic agent in the skin which increases the sensitivity of the skin to sunlight.
• Decreased skin pigmentation and hair cover facilitate cutaneous penetration of UVL.

PATHOPHYSIOLOGY

• Upon exposure to UVL, molecules of the photodynamic agent enter an excited or high energy state. These excited molecules may cause skin damage directly but damage occurs mostly through the production of reactive oxygen metabolites and free radicals.
• Photosensitization in horses generally fits into one of two categories: (1) *primary photosensitization,* which is caused when a preformed or metabolically derived photodynamic agent (e.g., plant or fungal products or chemicals) reaches the skin by ingestion, injection, or contact; and (2) *secondary (hepatogenous) photosensitization,* which occurs in cases of liver disease when phylloerythrin acts as a photodynamic agent. Phylloerythrin, a porphyrin compound formed by microbial degeneration of chlorophyll in the intestine, is normally conjugated in the liver and excreted in the bile. Liver dysfunction and/or biliary stasis may result in the accumulation of phylloerythrin in the blood and body tissues, including the skin. Some toxins derived from grasses are directly phototoxic and hepatotoxic, which makes the above classification of photosensitization less clear.

SYSTEMS AFFECTED

• Skin/exocrine system—lesions usually restricted to light-skinned, sparsely haired areas such as the coronary band, muzzle, ears, eyelids, tail, and vulva
• Hepatobiliary system—Secondary photosensitization can be associated with any cause of hepatic insufficiency. However, it appears to be more commonly associated with hepatic insufficiency caused by the ingestion of hepatotoxic plants.

SIGNALMENT

• All ages and breeds are susceptible.
• Light-skinned horses will have the most severe lesions.

SIGNS

Historical

• Initial signs noted are restlessness and scratching and rubbing of the ears, eyelids, and muzzle.
• Affected animals may be observed to seek out shade.
• Demarcated skin lesions characterized by redness, blister formation, weeping, and crusting may be reported.
• In cases of *secondary photosensitization* owners may notice signs suggestive of liver failure (e.g., altered mentation, weight loss, abdominal pain, diarrhea, etc.).

Physical Examination

Cutaneous Lesions (Primary and Secondary Photosensitization)

• Usually restricted to sparsely-haired, light-skinned areas on the dorsal aspects of the body (e.g., face, muzzle, eyelids, ears, coronary bands, vulva, and tail) but in severe cases, can extend to surrounding dark-skinned areas.
• Demarcation between lesions and normal skin is quite clear, particularly in multicolored animals.
• Acute signs include erythema followed by edema, serous exudation, and crust formation. Lesions are sensitive to touch.
• As lesions become more chronic, crust formation and sloughing of the skin is noted.
• Variable degrees of pruritus and pain may be present.
• Conjunctivitis, keratitis, and corneal edema may be seen in some cases.

Liver Failure Signs (May Accompany Cutaneous Lesions in Cases of Secondary Photosensitization)

• Icterus
• Pruritus
• Weight loss
• Diarrhea
• Abdominal pain
• Altered mentation

CAUSES AND RISK FACTORS

Causes of Primary Photosensitization

Associated with ingestion, injection, or contact with a photodynamic agent
• Photodynamic plants (e.g., St. John's wort [*Hypericum perforatum*], buckwheat [*Fagopyrum esculentum*], perennial ryegrass [*Lolium perenne*], burr trefoil [*Medicago denticulata*], spring parsley [*Cymopterus watsoni*], bishop's weed [*Amni majus*], oat grass [*Avena fatua*], rape [*Brassica* spp.], dutchman's breeches [*Thamnosma texana*], alsike clover [*Trifolium hibridum*], alfalfa [*Medicago* spp.], vetches [*Vichia* spp.], etc.)
• Chemicals (e.g., phenothiazines, thiazides, acriflavines, methylene blue, sulfonamides, tetracyclines, coal tar derivatives, furosemide, promazine, chlorpromazine, quinidine, etc.)
• Mycotoxins (e.g., phycocyanin produced by blue-green algae and phytoalexins produced by celery and parsnip).

Causes of Secondary Photosensitization

Associated most often with chronic liver failure or conditions that result in biliary obstruction
• Chronic active hepatitis
• Hepatic abscessation
• Neoplasia (cholangiocellular carcinoma, lymphosarcoma)
• Chronic megalocytic hepatopathy (*Senecio* spp., *Crotolaria* spp., *Heliotropium* spp.)
• Burning bush, fireweed (*Kochia scoparia*)
• Mycotoxicoses (blue-green algae [*Microcystis* spp.], *Phomopsis leptostromiformis* [on lupins])
• Cholelithiasis/cholangitis

RISK FACTORS

• Exposure to plants and chemicals that cause primary photosensitization
• Chronic liver failure or biliary obstruction
• Lack of skin pigment and/or sparse hair cover
• Exposure to sunlight

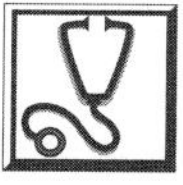

DIAGNOSIS

DIFFERENTIAL DIAGNOSES

The clinical signs in cases of photosensitization are identical regardless of the etiology. History and clinical findings can aid in the differentiation of primary vs. secondary photosensitization.

Primary Photosensitization

A history of exposure to plants (e.g., St. John's wort, buckwheat) or chemicals (phenothiazines, tetracyclines) known to cause primary photosensitization, and absence of liver failure signs, will support a tentative diagnosis of primary photosensitization.

Secondary Photosensitization

Photodermatitis accompanied by liver failure signs (e.g., icterus, weight loss, diarrhea, abdominal pain, neurologic lesions) should prompt the clinician to consider secondary photosensitization.

CBC/BIOCHEMISTRY/URINALYSIS

Primary Photosensitization

Liver enzyme activities (SDH, GGT, AST, ALP), bilirubin, and bile acid concentration are usually normal.

Secondary Photosensitization

Increased liver enzyme activities (SDH, GGT, AST, ALP), hyperbilirubinemia, and/or bilirubinuria will support a diagnosis of secondary or hepatogenous photosensitization.

OTHER LABORATORY TESTS

Increased serum bile acid concentration, prolonged clearance of foreign dyes such as BSP, and abnormal findings on a liver biopsy indicate a diagnosis of secondary photosensitization.

IMAGING

Ultrasonography

Can be used to demonstrate changes in liver size and abnormalities in the hepatic parenchyma (e.g., abscesses, neoplastic masses, dilated bile ducts, choleliths) in cases of secondary photosensitization

DIAGNOSTIC PROCEDURES

Liver Biopsy

May yield diagnostic, prognostic, and therapeutic information in cases of secondary photosensitization

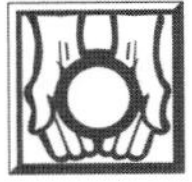

TREATMENT

- Varies depending on the underlying cause of photosensitization
- Identify and eliminate source of photodynamic agent.
- Restrict activity and avoid exposure to sunlight.
- Administer laxatives (mineral oil) and/or adsorbents (activated charcoal) to prevent further toxin absorption from the gastrointestinal tract.
- For secondary photosensitization, a diet that provides 40–50 kcal/kg body weight in the form of a low-protein, high-energy feed is recommended (e.g., milo, sorghum, beet pulp).

MEDICATIONS

DRUG(S) OF CHOICE

Medications for Cutaneous Lesions

- Use anti-inflammatory drugs (1.1 mg/kg of prednisolone or prednisone PO q24 h or 1.1 mg/kg flunixin meglumine PO IM, IV q8–12h) to decrease severity of inflammation in early stages.
- Topical antibiotic–corticosteroid creams may be applied to affected areas.
- Systemic antibiotics are indicated to manage secondary bacterial infections.
- Intravenous fluids may be required in severely affected animals.
- Surgical debridement is indicated to manage skin necrosis.

Treatment for Hepatic and Extracutaneous Disorders

Treat underlying liver disease as described in Liver Failure.

CONTRAINDICATIONS/POSSIBLE INTERACTIONS

Primary Photosensitization

Avoid use of drugs that may promote further photosensitization (e.g., tetracyclines, sulfonamides, or phenothiazines).

Secondary Photosensitization

- Avoid use of drugs metabolized primarily by the liver (e.g., anesthetics, barbiturates, or chloramphenicol).
- Sedatives metabolized by the liver (e.g., xylazine or diazepam) may have to be used at reduced dosages.

FOLLOW-UP

PATIENT MONITORING

Primary Photosensitization

Evaluate skin lesions every few days and debride necrotic lesions as required.

Secondary Photosensitization

- Monitor liver enzyme activities and bilirubin concentration weekly until improvement is noted.
- Repeat liver biopsy in 4–6 weeks to monitor disease progression.

PREVENTION/AVOIDANCE

Identify and eliminate photodynamic agent from environment.

POSSIBLE COMPLICATIONS

- Patients with secondary photosensitization often succumb to underlying liver disease.
- Rubbing and biting of affected areas may cause secondary self-trauma and bacterial infections.

EXPECTED COURSE AND PROGNOSIS

In general, prognosis is favorable for primary photosensitization and poor for secondary photosensitization.

MISCELLANEOUS

ASSOCIATED CONDITIONS

- Local edema of nostrils, lips, and eyelids can cause dyspnea, abnormal feed prehension, or lacrimation.
- Mares with teat lesions may not allow their foals to nurse, causing starvation.
- Secondary septicemia may develop in severe cases.

SEE ALSO

Liver disease topics

ABBREVIATIONS

- ALP = alkaline phosphatase
- AST = aspartate aminotransferase
- BSP = bromosulphotalein
- GGT = γ-glutamyltransferase
- SDH = sorbitol dehydrogenase
- UVL = ultraviolet light

Suggested Reading

Peterson AD, Schott AC. Cutaneous markers of disorders affecting adult horses. Clin Tech Equine Pract 2005;4:234–388.

Scott DW, Miller W. Equine dermatology. In Scott DW, Miller W, eds. Scott DW, Miller W. Environmental Skin Diseases. Philadelphia: Saunders, 2003:600.

Stegelmeier BL. Equine photosensitization. Clin Tech Equine Pract 2002;1:81–88.

Author Jeanne Lofstedt

Consulting Editor Michel Lévy

PICA

BASICS

OVERVIEW

Pica is an abnormal appetite for consumption of nonfood items, including substances such as dirt, sand, gravel, paint, tail hairs, feces, or other inanimate objects. The pathophysiology of pica is not completely understood. It has been associated with such conditions as obesity, parasitism, malnutrition, and deficiencies in fiber, electrolytes (sodium, chloride, or phosphorus), protein, or trace mineral imbalances (copper and zinc). It may also be due to a lack of oral stimulus or boredom. Decreased roughage in the diet has been associated with wood chewing, although it is considered normal for pastured horses to eat trees and shrubs. Wood chewing has been noted to be increased in cold, wet climates. Behavior-altering diseases, such as rabies, may result in pica; stereotypies can also lead to pica. Consumption of feces by foals is considered normal behavior.

SIGNALMENT

Miniature horses and foals appear to be more prone to pica, although no clear association with a particular signalment has been made. There is an association between stabled horses with limited pasture time, low-roughage/ high-concentrate diets, and wood chewing.

SIGNS

- History of eating nonfood items
- Colic, choke, or diarrhea may be secondary to consumption of inappropriate substances.

CAUSES AND RISK FACTORS

Pica is frequently associated with stereotypic behavior but may be secondary to deficiencies in the diet or parasitism. Inadequate housing, exercise, stimulus, or nutrition can be associated with pica. Foals appear to be more prone to pica due to their natural coprophagic behavior and inquisitive nature. Coprophagia is considered normal behavior in young foals.

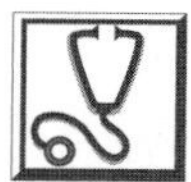

DIAGNOSIS

DIFFERENTIAL DIAGNOSIS

Deficiencies in the diet should be investigated before determining if the pica is behavioral. This disorder is usually associated with behavioral abnormalities, but may also be secondary to behavior-altering diseases, such as certain neurologic disorders (e.g., rabies), or malnutrition.

CBC/BIOCHEMISTRY/URINALYSIS

No consistent abnormalities are usually found, but should be evaluated to identify possible primary causes of pica. If no significant abnormalities are found and a complete neurological examination reveals no abnormalities, then the problem is likely behavioral.

OTHER LABORATORY TESTS

Fecal examination for parasites and any other tests indicated by prior testing; feed evaluations, especially for trace minerals such as copper, cobalt, phosphorus, and zinc, are diagnostic.

IMAGING

N/A

DIAGNOSTIC PROCEDURES

N/A

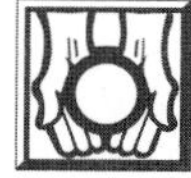

TREATMENT

- Treatment should be directed at any primary diseases or deficiencies identified (see section on specific diseases for treatment recommendations).

Once primary disease processes are eliminated, treatment should aim at redirecting the behavior. This can be accomplished through:

- Limiting exposure to the items of concern
- Providing an appropriate substitute
- Increasing roughage in the diet, especially if wood chewing
- Altering the environmental condition causing the stereotypy (see section on behavioral abnormalities)
- Altering the desirability of the nonfood item through application of repellents with an objectionable taste
- Increasing level of exercise
- If behavioral in origin, once established, the behavior is difficult to discourage; therefore, prevention is recommended.

MEDICATIONS

DRUG(S) OF CHOICE, CONTRAINDICATIONS, PRECAUTIONS, POSSIBLE INTERACTIONS, ALTERNATIVE DRUGS

N/A

FOLLOW-UP

- The amount of follow-up required depends on the primary disease. If no primary condition is evident, contact with the owners should be made within 2 weeks of any recommended treatment to determine if it has decreased the pica and if there is owner compliance. If the horse has made no improvements after a 2-week period, alternative recommendations should be given.
- Gastrointestinal disorders such as intestinal obstruction may occur. In addition, there may be abnormal wear to the teeth, which may in turn lead to further gastrointestinal disorders.

MISCELLANEOUS

ASSOCIATED CONDITIONS, AGE-RELATED FACTORS, ZOONOTIC POTENTIAL, PREGNANCY

N/A

SEE ALSO

See specific section.

Suggested Reading

Houpt KA. Stable vices and trailer problems. Vet Clin North Am Equine 1986;2:623–633.

Mass J. Pica. In: Smith BP, ed. Large Animal Internal Medicine. St. Louis: Mosby, 1996:193–195.

McGreevy P. Ingestive behavior. In: McGreevy P, ed. Equine Behavior. A Guide for Veterinarians and Equine Scientists. Edinburgh: Saunders, 2004:200–206.

McGreevy PD, et al Geophagia in horses: a short note on 13 cases. Appl Anim Behav Sci 2001;71:119–215.

Ralston SL. Feeding behavior. Vet Clin North Am Equine 1986;2:609–621.

Author Deborah A. Parsons

Consulting Editors Henry Stämpfli and Olimpo Oliver-Espinosa

PIGMENTURIA (HEMATURIA, HEMOGLOBINURIA, AND MYOGLOBINURIA)

BASICS

DEFINITION

- Discoloration of urine, red to brown in color, from increased excretion of RBCs (hematuria), hemoglobin (hemoglobinuria), or myoglobin (myoglobinuria)
- Factitious pigmenturia occurs when dehydrated horses pass concentrated urine that is dark or when porphyrins in urine are oxidized after being voided (red to brown discoloration of snow, wood shavings, or with storage of urine over time).
- Observed as a side effect of medication (e.g., orange with rifampin or pyridium and dark brown to black with doxycycline)

PATHOPHYSIOLOGY

Hematuria

- Normal urine contains ≅5000 RBCs/mL or <5 RBCs/hpf on sediment examination.
- Microscopic hematuria (10,000–2,500,000 RBCs/mL) can be detected as 10–20 RBCs/hpf on sediment examination or traced to +++ reaction on a reagent strip.
- Macroscopic or gross hematuria can be observed with >2,500,000–5,000,000 RBCs/mL (≅0.5 mL of blood per 1 L of urine).
- Hemorrhage from the kidneys, ureters, or bladder leads to hematuria during the entire urination. Hematuria at the beginning of urination indicates lesions of the distal urethra and at the end of urination indicates lesions in the proximal urethra or bladder neck.

Hemoglobinuria

Hemolysis and hemoglobinuria may be the result of immune-mediated diseases or secondary to infectious disease, neoplasia, or drug administration and may develop with liver disease or exposure to toxins (e.g., red maple leaves, onions, phenothiazines) that cause oxidant injury and Heinz body anemia.

Myoglobinuria

- Myoglobinuria can result from rhabdomyolysis, e,g., polysaccharide storage myopathy, recurrent exertional rhabdomyolysis, postanesthetic myopathy, or infectious diseases (e.g., *Streptococcus equi* myositis, clostridial myonecrosis).
- "Atypical myoglobinuria" has been used to describe a highly fatal syndrome of nonexertional rhabdomyolysis that has affected those on poor-quality pasture.

SYSTEMS AFFECTED

- Renal/urologic—pigmenturia, especially hematuria
- Hemic/lymphatic/immune—hemolysis; hemoglobinuria
- Hepatobiliary—hemolysis; hemoglobinuria
- Musculoskeletal—rhabdomyolysis

GENETICS

Polysaccharide storage myopathy is a genetic disease of Quarter Horse breeds and recurrent exertional rhabdomyolysis may be a genetic disease of thoroughbred horses.

INCIDENCE/PREVALENCE

Incidence of polysaccharide storage myopathy and other myopathies are common, yet clinical rhabdomyolysis is less common.

GEOGRAPHIC DISTRIBUTION

N/A

SIGNALMENT

Breed Predilections

- Proximal urethral defects most commonly are observed in QHs.
- Arabians appear predisposed to IRH.
- Polysaccharide storage myopathy is most common in QHs but may also affect draft breeds.
- Recurrent exertional rhabdomyolysis appears more common in TBs.

Mean Age and Range

- NI affects neonatal foals and mule foals.
- Vascular malformations more commonly occur in foals.
- Neoplasia affects old horses.

Predominant Sex

- Proximal urethral defects, habronemiasis, and neoplasia of the penis and distal urethra occur in geldings and stallions.
- Recurrent exertional rhabdomyolysis is a more significant problem in young, female racehorses.

SIGNS

General Comments

- Clinical signs in horses with pigmenturia vary with the primary disease, from severe muscle cramping with ER to lethargy, inappetence, and possible colic with signs with red maple toxicosis.
- However, with other disorders (e.g., neoplasia, proximal urethral defects, urolithiasis, or IRH), pigmenturia may be the primary complaint.

Historical

- Horses with pigmenturia often have obvious historical evidence of a primary problem—"tying-up," toxin ingestion, dysuria from lower UTI, or penile neoplasia.
- Observation of pigmenturia may be the presenting complaint for problems—vascular anomalies, cystolithiasis, proximal urethral defects, renal or bladder neoplasia, IRH, or exercise-associated hematuria.

Physical Examination

- Findings with hematuria are consistent with the underlying disease processes (e.g., ARF, urolithiasis, UTI, neoplasia, toxin ingestion) or may be normal (e.g., vascular malformations, proximal urethral defects, exercise-associated hematuria, IRH).
- Findings in horses with hemoglobinuria or myoglobinuria reflect the underlying disease processes—pale membranes, weakness, and anorexia with hemolytic anemia; dark-brown membranes with methemoglobinemia; icteric membranes and hepatoencephalopathy with liver disease; firm muscles and a stiff reluctant gait with rhabdomyolysis.

CAUSES

Hematuria

- ARF—microscopic hematuria is common due to glomerular and tubular damage.
- Urolithiasis—Stones anywhere in the urinary tract may lead to hematuria; postexercise hematuria is common with large cystoliths.
- UTI—Infection anywhere in the urinary tract, including habronemiasis of the prepuce and distal penis, may result in hematuria.
- Neoplasia—nephroblastoma, renal adenocarcinoma, hemangiosarcoma, squamous cell carcinoma of the lower urinary tract, transitional cell carcinoma, and other bladder tumors (e.g., leiomyoma, lymphosarcoma)
- Renal vascular anomalies—arteriovenous and arterioureteral malformations
- Proximal urethral defects—consistently found at the dorsocaudal aspect of the urethra near the ischial arch; likely from a "blowout" of the corpus spongiosum penis into the urethral lumen during contraction of the bulbospongiosus and urethralis muscles. It can produce hemospermia or hematuria at the end of urination.
- Exercise-associated hematuria—microscopic hematuria seems a normal physiological response to exercise due to increased blood pressure and extravasation of RBCs across glomerular capillaries; magnitude of hematuria increases with exercise intensity; gross hematuria after exercise may develop, when the bladder mucosa becomes "bruised" by trauma against the brim of the pelvis; urination prior to exercise increases risk, as urine in the bladder cushions against mucosal injury.
- Blister beetle (cantharidin toxicity) can lead to inflammation and bleeding of the urinary tract.
- IRH—syndrome of recurrent, potentially life-threatening hematuria of renal origin; unknown cause

Hemoglobinuria

- Primary immune-mediated hemolytic anemia —NI; incompatible blood transfusions
- Secondary immune-mediated hemolytic anemia—hemolysis with infectious diseases (e.g., equine infectious anemia, piroplasmosis, *Clostridium perfringens,* chronic infection), neoplasia, or drug administration (e.g., penicillins)
- Exposure to toxins—red maple leaves; onions; phenothiazines; ionophores
- Secondary to reabsorption of RBCs from previous hemorrhage into a body cavity
- Liver disease

Myoglobinuria

- Rhabdomyolysis—associated with exercise or other metabolic (e.g., polysaccharide

PIGMENTURIA (HEMATURIA, HEMOGLOBINURIA, AND MYOGLOBINURIA)

storage myopathy) and infectious (e.g., *Streptococcus equi*) diseases
• Nutritional myopathy—selenium deficiency
• Postanesthetic myopathy—due to crush injury of muscle during anesthesia and other factors, especially hypotension
• "Atypical myoglobinuria"—Ingestion of a toxic substance is a suspected cause.

RISK FACTORS

• Similar to those for ARF, urolithiasis, or UTI
• See Causes.

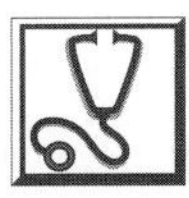

DIAGNOSIS

DIFFERENTIAL DIAGNOSES

• Blood accumulation at the vulvar margins in pregnant mares may be due to hemorrhage from varicosities in the vagina rather than bleeding from the urinary tract.
• Stallions with proximal urethral defects may present for hemospermia rather than hematuria.

CBC/BIOCHEMISTRY/URINALYSIS

Changes characteristic for ARF (see Acute Renal Failure), urolithiasis (see Urolithiasis), UTI (see Urinary Tract Infection), Liver Disease (see Acute Hepatitis, Cholelithiasis, Hepatic Abscess, and Toxic Hepatopathy) when these cause hematuria.

CBC

• Normal laboratory values—renal vascular anomalies with mild hematuria
• Anemia tends to have evidence of regeneration with increased MCV and RDW, and anisocytosis.
• Mild to moderate anemia—neoplasia, proximal urethral defects, IRH, primary or secondary immune-mediated hemolytic anemia
• Moderate to severe anemia—any disease causing severe hematuria, vascular anomalies, or IRH
• Hypoproteinemia—severe hemorrhage secondary to hematuria (IRH, vascular anomalies)
• Hemoglobinemia (red discoloration of plasma after centrifugation) and hemoglobinuria—primary or secondary immune-mediated hemolytic anemia

CHEMISTRY

• Hypergammaglobulinemia—neoplasia, chronic infection
• Prerenal azotemia—all related conditions
• Hyperbilirubinemia—primary or secondary immune-mediated hemolytic anemia (mostly indirect), liver disease (direct or indirect)
• Increased CK and AST—rhabdomyolysis
• Methemoglobinemia (oxidant injury)—red maple leaf toxicity, onions
• Increased liver enzymes (AST, GGT, SDH, ALP), serum bile acids, and coagulation times, hypoglycemia—liver disease

URINALYSIS

• See definitions in Pathophysiology.
• Proteinuria accompanies any hemorrhage into the urine.
• Abnormal cytology—neoplasia, UTI

OTHER LABORATORY TESTS

• Centrifugation of urine—RBCs form a red to brown pellet with clear supernatant (hematuria), whereas urine remains discolored with hemoglobinuria or myoglobinuria.
• Urine reagent strips impregnated with orthotoluidine—react with hemoglobin and myoglobin; RBCs produce scattered red spots as long as hematuria is <250,000 RBCs/mL.
• Blondheim test—Differential precipitation of hemoglobin and myoglobin with ammonium sulfate is a simple but sometimes inaccurate test.
• Hemoglobin—can be differentiated from myoglobin in urine by protein electrophoresis or specific tests (e.g., radioimmunoassays, enzyme-linked immunosorbent assays).
• Quantitative urine culture—perform in all cases of suspected hematuria to assess for concurrent UTI.

IMAGING

• Transabdominal and transrectal ultrasonography—size and echogenicity of the kidney, ureters, bladder, and proximal urethra
• Urethroscopy/cystoscopy—to confirm source of hematuria; diagnostic of choice for proximal urethral defects

DIAGNOSTIC PROCEDURES

• Liver biopsy—further evaluation of liver disease
• Muscle biopsy—for further evaluation of rhabdomyolysis and other myopathies
• Biopsy of abnormal tissue in bladder or distal urinary tract

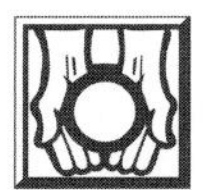

TREATMENT

This discussion is limited to hematuria; see other sections for treatment of disorders causing hemoglobinuria and myoglobinuria.

AIMS OF TREATMENT

Address underlying disease process, stabilize patient, ensure adequate circulating blood volume, and halt further hemorrhage.

APPROPRIATE HEALTH CARE

• ARF—see Acute Renal Failure.
• Urolithiasis—see Urolithiasis.
• UTI—see Urinary Tract Infection.
• Neoplasia—complete surgical excision (rarely possible) combined with topical, intralesional or systemic antineoplastic agents for bladder and urethral cancer
• Renal vascular anomalies—proper diagnosis and when hematuria persists, appropriate surgical intervention
• Proximal urethral defects—Because ≅50% of lesions heal spontaneously, no treatment is initially indicated; surgery is recommended for hematuria causing anemia or lasting for >1 mo.
• Exercise-associated hematuria—Bladder mucosal lesions in the rare horse with gross hematuria heal without treatment, but a few days of rest may be advised.
• IRH—supportive care for hemorrhagic shock, including repeated blood transfusions

SURGICAL CONSIDERATIONS

• Renal Neoplasia—Unilateral nephrectomy may correct hematuria but rarely produces long-term success; most neoplasms, especially renal adenocarcinoma, have metastasized prior to diagnosis.
• Renal vascular malformation—Nephrectomy, or renal arteriolar embolization (in foals), may be indicated with persistent hematuria; in other foals, hematuria may be self-limiting if a thrombus forms in the malformation.
• Proximal urethral defect—A perineal urethrotomy approach into the corpus spongiosum penis, but not extending into the urethral lumen. The procedure creates a "pressure relief valve" for the corpus spongiosum penis, allowing the urethral defect to heal.
• IRH—Nephrectomy in select cases that maintain normal renal function but continue to bleed from the affected kidney; repeat cystoscopies to confirm unilateral renal hemorrhage (because bilateral, episodic renal bleeding may occur) before nephrectomy is pursued.

NURSING CARE

• Although a straightforward procedure, surgical treatment of proximal urethral defects should be performed on an inpatient basis, with 1–3 days of postoperative hospitalization—bleeding from the surgical site can be substantial for a few days, and frequent washing of the perineum and limbs is necessary.
• Horses with IRH require frequent monitoring and supportive care and possibly a blood transfusion both before and after nephrectomy.

ACTIVITY

If moderate to severe anemia only, free choice exercise. Mild exercise restriction for horses with exercise-induced hematuria.

DIET

See Acute Renal Failure, Urolithiasis, and Urinary Tract Infection.

CLIENT EDUCATION

• Patients with neoplasia have a poor prognosis, but current treatments and supportive care may prolong life.
• Horses with vascular malformations may have other developmental anomalies that may not be apparent until later in life. Vascular malformations that resolve by spontaneous formation of a thrombus may redevelop.

PIGMENTURIA (HEMATURIA, HEMOGLOBINURIA, AND MYOGLOBINURIA)

- Counsel patience to owners of horses with proximal urethral defects with a short duration of hematuria and exercise-associated bladder mucosal damage, because spontaneous resolution may occur.
- The cause of hematuria in horses with IRH is unknown, so owners of affected horses must receive considerable education before nephrectomy is considered.

MEDICATIONS

DRUGS OF CHOICE

- 5-Fluorouracil and triethylenethiophosphoramide are antineoplastic agents that may be used topically (at weekly or more frequent intervals) for bladder or penile neoplasms.
- Piroxicam, a COX-2 inhibitor (80 mg PO q24–72 h), for transitional cell carcinomas
- Prophylactic antibiotics are recommended for horses undergoing nephrectomy (e.g., penicillin/gentamicin) or a perineal urethrotomy approach for correction of a proximal urethral defect (e.g., trimethoprim-sulfonamide combination).
- α-Aminocaproic acid (10 mg/kg IV q6 h) to enhance blood clot stabilization may be used in horses with renal hematuria from neoplasia or IRH, but success has not been reported.

CONTRAINDICATIONS

Do not perform nephrectomy in patients with azotemia.

PRECAUTIONS

Approach nephrectomy with caution, and consider it a last-resort procedure for control of refractory unilateral IRH.

POSSIBLE INTERACTIONS

N/A

ALTERNATIVE DRUGS

N/A

FOLLOW-UP

PATIENT MONITORING

- See Acute Renal Failure, Urolithiasis, and Urinary Tract Infection.
- Assess clinical status of patients with nephrectomy of perineal urethrotomy at least twice daily, and monitor urine production and PCV once daily, during the initial 2–4 days after surgery.

POSSIBLE COMPLICATIONS

- Dissemination of neoplasia
- IRH from the contralateral kidney after nephrectomy

EXPECTED COURSE AND PROGNOSIS

- Prognosis for recovery after surgical correction of a proximal urethral defect generally is favorable, but the problem may recur.
- Recurrent bouts of hematuria over several years may occur with IRH. Resolution may happen however, some may suffer acute, fatal renal hemorrhage.
- Guarded long-term prognosis for patients with renal hematuria initially treated successfully by unilateral nephrectomy due to the loss of renal functional reserve and potential for bleeding from the remaining kidney

MISCELLANEOUS

ASSOCIATED CONDITIONS

- ARF
- Urolithiasis
- UTI
- Immune-mediated hemolytic anemia—primary and secondary
- Intoxication with agents causing hemolysis and hemoglobinuria
- Liver disease
- Rhabdomyolysis

ZOONOTIC POTENTIAL

Leptospirosis, which may cause hematuria and ARF, has zoonotic potential; avoid direct contact with infective urine.

PREGNANCY

- Multiparous mares are at greater risk of producing alloantibodies that may lead to NI in their foals.
- Vulvar hemorrhage from varicosities can be confused with hematuria.

SYNONYMS

Azoturia (for ER)

SEE ALSO

- ARF
- UTI
- Urolithiasis

ABBREVIATIONS

- ARF = acute renal failure
- hpf = high-power field
- ER = Exertional Rhabdomyolysis
- IRH = idiopathic renal hematuria
- NI = neonatal isoerythrolysis
- PCV = packed cell volume
- RBC = red blood cell
- TB = Thoroughbred
- UTI = urinary tract infection

Suggested Reading

Fischer AT, Spier S, Carlson GP, et al. Neoplasia of the equine urinary bladder as a cause of hematuria. J Am Vet Med Assoc 1985;186:1294–1296.

Schott HC. Hematuria. In: Reed SM, Bayly WM, Sellon DC, eds. Equine Internal Medicine, ed 2. Philadelphia: WB Saunders, 2004:1270–1276.

Schott HC, Hodgson DR, Bayly WM. Haematuria, pigmenturia and proteinuria in exercising horses. Equine Vet J 1995;27:67–72.

Schumacher J, Varner DD, Schmitz DG, et al. Urethral defects in geldings with hematuria and stallions with hemospermia. Vet Surg 1995;24:250–254.

Schumacher J. Hematuria and pigmenturia of horses. Vet Clin North Am Equine Pract 2007;23:655–676.

Author Harold C. Schott II

Consulting Editors Gillian A. Perkins and Dominic Dawson

PLACENTAL BASICS

BASICS

DEFINITIONS/OVERVIEW

- Placental classification is by five major criteria:
  - Shape
  - Origin of tissues
  - Degree of invasion
  - Vascular structure
  - Degree of attachment
- Shape—diffuse in mares; normal placenta covers the entire endometrial surface; for normal avillous sites, see locations/exceptions below.
- Origin of tissues—allantochorionic; tissues derived from fusion of fetal-derived allantois and chorion
- Degree of invasion—epitheliochorial; fetal-derived tissue directly apposes maternal endometrium.
- Vascular structure—microcotyledonary/villous; unit of exchange is villous-like; maternal and placental vessels are in near apposition.
- Degree of attachment—adeciduate; no loss of maternal tissue in placenta formation or at time of expulsion

CHRONOLOGY

- Equine conceptus is mobile (i.e., transuterine migration) within the uterus to day 16 after conception (day 0).
- Conceptus is spherical until ≈day 35 and thereafter ellipsoid.
- Endometrial cup formation by day 36–38
- Pregnancy maintenance by allantochorionic placentation alone has been reported experimentally from 70 days' gestation.
- Placenta contacts the entire endometrial surface by ≈day 77.
- Placental development complete by day 150

ENDOMETRIAL CUPS

- Fetal trophoblast invasion of maternal endometrium—formation begins at ≈day 36–38; peak function of endometrial cups is at ≈day 70 of gestation.
- Cups undergo necrosis by day 120–150.
- Cups are sloughed and become allantochorionic pouches.
- Cups produce eCG and are responsible for formation and function of accessory CL.

EXAMINATION

- At parturition, fetus and fluid pressures rupture the placenta at the cervical star; allantochorion is usually passed inside out, with fetal surface (i.e., allantois) exteriorized.
- A complete placental examination requires also observing the chorionic surface (turn inside out), the amnion, and the umbilical cord.
- Identify the body and both uterine horns; lay out in the shape of the capital letter "F."
  - To ensure none of the placenta has been retained, confirm horn tips are present.
  - If areas are torn, match blood vessels on the exposed allantoic surface.
- The tip of the nonpregnant horn is the most likely part of the membranes to be retained and must be identified in all examinations.
- Cervical star is the site of fetal exit; its remnants require special attention.
  - Any allantochorionic thickening or exudates should be sampled.
- Assess amnion for uniform thickness, color, and presence of fecal staining.
- Assess umbilical cord length, degree of twisting, and for the presence of any vascular compromise.
- In healthy Thoroughbred mares, the placenta weighs ≈11% of the foal's birth weight.

VILLI

- There are potentially *5 normal avillous areas* on the chorionic side of the allantochorion.
  - Location of endometrial cups (may no longer be evident by term pregnancy)
  - Cervical star
  - Ostium (at tips of horns)
  - Site of umbilical attachment
  - Invaginated/redundant folds resulting from umbilical cord traction; appear longitudinal and symmetric
- *Pathological avillous areas*
  - Apposition of placentae in a twin pregnancy
  - Placentitits
  - Endometrial fibrosis
  - Endometrial cysts

ALLANTOCHORION

Normal

- Chorion appears as "red velvet" because of the diffuse microvilli over its entire surface.
- Tip of the pregnant horn usually is thicker and edematous compared to nonpregnant horn; unknown significance

Abnormal

- Any area of the placenta is abnormal if it is:
  - Grossly thickened
  - Covered with exudate
- Ascending placentitits
  - May involve cervical star and adjacent placental body
- Nocardioform placentitits
  - Prominent localized changes involving placental body and horn base
- Line of demarcation between affected and normal area may be prominent.
- Other causes may lead to more diffuse inflammatory changes.
- If grossly edematous or thickened, may indicate vascular disturbance or fescue toxicosis

AMNION

Normal

- Equine amnion is completely separate from allantochorion.
- White; translucent
- Focal proliferative areas may occur.

Abnormal

- Discolored or edematous—fetal distress (e. g., fetal diarrhea)
- Thickened—amnionitis
- Widespread edema and thickening may indicate fetal compromise because of decreased nutrient and gaseous exchange.
- Extension of allantochorionitis

UMBILICAL CORD

Normal

- Distinct allantoic and amniotic portions (60–83 cm in length)
- Normal twists in equine cord

Abnormal

- Length >100 cm increases risk of fetal strangulation and torsion.
- Umbilical cord torsion may also result in hypoperfusion; congestion, thrombosis, and mineralization of the allantochorion.
- If pregnancy is lost, examine for autolysis, vascular damage, thrombi (e. g., evidence of abnormal, excessive twisting), and urachal tearing.
- Neonate may have a patent urachus and elongated navel stump.

ALLANTOIC FLUID

- Clear to amber—hypotonic urine and fetal excretory products
- Within the allantoic fluid—hippomane, i.e., allantoic calculus; composed of concentric layers of cellular debris
  - Consistency—rubbery
  - Color—dark brown, green, or tan

AMNIOTIC FLUID

Opaque—respiratory, and buccal secretions of the fetus

SEE ALSO

Placentitis—bacterial, viral, fungal
Placental insufficiency
Retained fetal membranes

ABBREVIATIONS

- CL = corpus luteum
- eCG = equine chorionic gonadotropin

Suggested Reading

Bucca S, Fogarty U, Collins A, Small V. Assessment of feto-placental well-being in the mare from mid-gestation to term: transrectal and transabdominal ultrasonographic features. Therio 2005;64:542–557.

Morresey PR. How to perform a field assessment of the equine placenta. Proc AAEP 2004;409–414.

Author Peter R. Morresey
Consulting Editor Carla L. Carleton

PLACENTAL INSUFFICIENCY

BASICS

DEFINITION/OVERVIEW

• Placental exchange unit cannot meet fetal demands, results in fetal malnutrition • May result in intrauterine growth retardation, prolonged gestation, preterm delivery, or pregnancy loss

ETIOLOGY/PATHOPHYSIOLOGY

• Physical constrictions to placental development—body pregnancy; intraluminal adhesions, endometrial cyst formation with lymphatic stasis, endometrial fibrosis and glandular degeneration (endometrosis)
• Placentitis • Whether caused by failure to form or separation of microcotyledonary attachments, the area available for placental exchange between the endometrium and fetus is decreased.
• Histiotrophe, i.e., uterine milk, exchange occurs between the microcotyledonary attachments.
  ○ Production increases during pregnancy.
  ○ Sufficient production depends on the health and number of endometrial glands.

SYSTEM AFFECTED

Reproductive

SIGNALMENT

• Pregnant female, usually aged or multiparous
• May be a history of endometritis, reproductive failure
• Mares bearing twins—highlights a mare's inability to sustain two placentas and two fetuses

SIGNS

General Comments

• Preterm delivery of small, emaciated fetus or fetuses
• Prolonged gestation or term delivery of a small fetus for gestational age, dysmature fetus; underweight; silky haircoat; behavioral abnormalities; major organ system dysfunction; increased risk for sepsis

Historical

• May have previously delivered similar, compromised fetus • Endometrial changes are irreversible. Endometrial biopsy commonly reveals loss of endometrial epithelial layer, fibrosis, glandular nesting, or decreased number of glands.

Physical Examination

• Gross uterine abnormalities—intraluminal adhesions; segmental aplasia; cystic endometrial structures • Gross placental abnormalities—localized avillous areas or generalized poorly villous chorionic surface
• Histopathologic findings—See Pathologic Findings.

CAUSES

• Placentitis • Degenerative endometrial changes—endometritis, endometrosis; histologic biopsy diagnosis

RISK FACTORS

• Age • Increased parity • Chronic endometritis
• Poor vulvar conformation • Uterine infection
• Endometrial biopsy displays fibrosis, endometrosis.

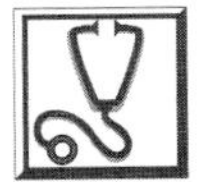

DIAGNOSIS

DIFFERENTIAL DIAGNOSIS

• Infectious causes of abortion—bacterial, viral, fungal
• Noninfectious causes of abortion—endotoxemia caused by systemic illness, uterine torsion, developmental anomalies, spontaneous fetal death
• Other causes of prolonged gestation—fescue toxicosis; fetal endocrine abnormalities • Other causes of fetal malnutrition—twinning; maternal disease

CBC/BIOCHEMISTRY/URINALYSIS

• Abnormalities reflect systemic pathologic process, if any, in mare. • No systemic changes are directly attributable to placental insufficiency.

IMAGING

Transabdominal U/S

• Small for gestational age fetus—crown–rump length; fetal orbit • Intrauterine growth retardation—more pronounced later in gestation.
• Asymmetrically affected fetal/neonatal development—long head, thin body, little body fat

Transrectal US

Thickness or detachment of placenta cranial to cervix—late gestation

PATHOLOGICAL FINDINGS

Gross

• Placental exam—avillous areas other than those previously described as normal. Classic placental lesion at site of apposition of the two placentas prevents attachment to the endometrium.
  ○ Grossly—avillous (pale) area at which no exchange can occur.
  ○ Usual outcome—abortion of both fetuses or one dead and/or mummified.
  ○ If pregnancy reaches term, remaining twin is small for gestational age.
• Thickened, edematous, or discolored areas
• Small placenta relative to size of neonatal foal
• Evidence of multiple pregnancies

Histopathologic

• Placenta—decreased microcotyledonary formation
• Endometrial biopsy—pronounced fibrosis, glandular nesting, lymphatic stasis of the endometrium, varying degrees of inflammation

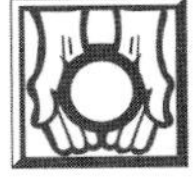

TREATMENT

• Placental insufficiency—a postpartum diagnosis • If suspected in periparturient mare, oxygen supplementation can be administered in an effort to raise fetal oxygen tension.

MEDICATIONS

DRUG(S) OF CHOICE

• Progestagen supplementation may be helpful to boost endometrial histiotrophe production.
• Progesterone in oil • Altrenogest

CONTRAINDICATIONS

Establish fetal viability before treating—transabdominal fetal U/S; fetal heart rate

FOLLOW-UP

PATIENT MONITORING

• U/S • Fetus—viability and fetal heart rate
• Placenta—for thickness and detachment

PREVENTION/AVOIDANCE

• Establish reproductive competence of mare when she is not pregnant (i.e., BSE). • Detect and repair anatomical defects—vulvar conformation, cervical competence.
• Endometrial biopsy to evaluate density of endometrial glands, presence of inflammation (e.g., acute—neutrophilia; chronic—plasmacytic, lymphocytic), and degenerative changes (e.g., periglandular fibrosis, diffuse; lymphatic, dilation, stasis)
• Endometrial cytology for eosinophilia; association with pneumovagina • Early detection by assessment of placental thickness and areas of detachment

POSSIBLE COMPLICATIONS

• Abortion • Birth of undersized, weak neonate
• Premature placental separation at parturition with risk for neonatal hypoxia

MISCELLANEOUS

ASSOCIATED CONDITIONS

• Placentitis • Premature placental separation
• Neonatal maladjustment/hypoxic ischemic encephalopathy • Fetal sepsis—bacterial, fungal

AGE-RELATED FACTORS

Endometrial competence declines with increasing age and parity of mares.

PREGNANCY

Abortion

SEE ALSO

• Placental basics • Placentitis

ABBREVIATION

• BSE = breeding soundness examination
• U/S = ultrasound/ultrasonography

Suggested Reading

Adams R. Identification of the mare and foal at high risk for perinatal problems. In: McKinnon AO, Voss JL, eds. Equine Reproduction. Philadelphia: Lea & Febiger, 1993:988–989.

Bucca S, Fogarty U, Collins A, Small V. Assessment of feto-placental well-being in the mare from mid-gestation to term: transrectal and transabdominal ultrasonographic features. Therio 2005;64:542–557.

Collins MH. Placentas and foetal health. Eq Vet J Suppl 1993;14:8–11.

Giles RC, Donahue JM, Hong CB, et al. Causes of abortion, stillbirth, and perinatal death in horses: 3,527 cases (1986–1991). J Am Vet Med Assoc 1993;203:1170–1175.

Rossdale PD. The maladjusted foal: influences of intrauterine growth retardation and birth trauma. Proc AAEP 2004;75–126.

Wilsher S, Allen WR. The effects of maternal age and parity on placental and fetal development in the mare. Eq Vet J 2003;35:476–483.

Author Peter R. Morresey
Consulting Editor Carla L. Carleton

PLACENTITIS

BASICS

DEFINITION/OVERVIEW

Inflammation of the placenta. Single most important cause of late-term abortion, stillbirth, and premature delivery in the mare

ETIOLOGY/PATHOPHYSIOLOGY

- An infectious agent (e.g., bacterial, viral, mycotic) invades the placenta, leading to an inflammatory response.
- Typically, initial location is in the area of the cervical star, when cause is ascending.
- Placental detachment and thickening—may be localized or widespread.
- Uterine motility is altered in response to local inflammation.
- Modes of entry
  - Ascending via cervix (most common)
  - Hematogenous, as part of systemic illness
  - Inoculation
  - Recrudescence of pre-existing focus of infection

SYSTEM AFFECTED

Reproductive

GENETICS

N/A

INCIDENCE/PREVALENCE

Common if any of modes of entry are in play or if VC is less than ideal (ascending route of infection)

SIGNALMENT

Pregnant mare typically during late gestation

SIGNS

- Vulvar discharge—purulent; hemorrhagic
- Cervical incompetence—discharge; inflammation
- Mammary—swelling; discharge; prepartum lactation
- Relaxation of pelvic musculature—vulva; sacrosciatic ligament
- Restlessness; premonitory foaling behavior
- Placenta—thickening; edema; increased weight; discoloration; discharge; adenomatous hyperplasia; plaque formation, especially centered on cervical star

CAUSES AND RISK FACTORS

Bacterial

- Throughout gestation
- Two presentations
  - Acute, focal or diffuse
  - Chronic, focal or extensive
- Acute, focal or diffuse
  - Neutrophil infiltration
  - Necrosis of chorionic villi
  - Primarily early to mid-gestation
- Chronic, focal or extensive
  - Centered around area of cervical star
  - Eosinophilic chorionic material
  - Necrosis of villi
  - Adenomatous hyperplasia
  - Mononuclear cell infiltration
  - Primarily mid- to late gestation
- Common pathogens
  - *Streptococcus equi* subsp. *zooepidemicus*
  - *Streptococcus equisimilis*
  - *Escherichia coli*
  - *Pseudomonas aeruginosa*
  - *Klebsiella pneumoniae*
- *Leptospira* spp.
  - Diffuse, spirochete invasion
  - Hematogenous spread only
- *Crossiella equi*
  - Other actinomycete species also occur; base of horns and body.
  - Gram-positive filamentous bacillus infiltration.
  - Chronic nature

Viral

- EVA
  - Thickening of allantochorion attributable to a longer incubation time before abortion
  - Compare/contrast with EHV-1, with which there are either no or nonspecific placental changes.

Fungal

- Usually 300 days of gestation or later
- *Aspergillus* spp.—chronic, focal placentitis at cervical star similar to chronic bacterial cases
- *Candida* spp.—diffuse; necrotizing; proliferative
- *Histoplasma* spp.—multifocal; granulomatous

Anatomic

- Cervical incompetence—laceration; age-induced degeneration. Bacterial invasion resulting in placentitis.
- Vulvar and vestibular incompetence—aspiration of external irritants and debris
- Production of $PGF_{2\alpha}$ by endotoxin release, leading to cervical relaxation

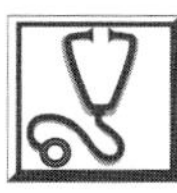

DIAGNOSIS

DIFFERENTIAL DIAGNOSIS

- Impending parturition
- Fescue toxicosis—placental edema; delayed parturition; decreased lactation
- Other causes of vulvar discharge
  - Vaginitis (speculum examination to assess cervical integrity/discharge)
  - Endometritis
  - Pyometra
  - Metritis
  - Vaginal varicosities
- Uterine trauma or hemorrhage
- Urinary tract infection
- Urine pooling
- Uterine or vaginal neoplasia
- Other causes of lactation—endocrine, seasonal
- Other causes of relaxation—impending parturition

CBC/BIOCHEMISTRY/URINALYSIS

- CBC may remain normal even with significant placental pathology.
- Leukocytosis with neutrophilia
- Hyperfibrinogenemia
- Biochemistry usually normal
- Urinalysis, normal

OTHER LABORATORY TESTS

- Mares with placentitis have been demonstrated experimentally to have increased concentrations of either pregnenolone (P5) and/or progesterone (P4) along with a number of metabolites.
  - This suggests increased fetal production of P5 and/or P4 and increased uteroplacental metabolism in response to chronic stress.

IMAGING

U/S

- Transrectal; transabdominal
- Marked increase in the CTUP measured by U/S, especially in the cervical region of the uteroplacental unit
  - Good indicator of ascending placentitis
- Normal ranges for the area immediately cranial to the cervix have been established from 4 mo of gestation to term in normal pregnant mares using transrectal U/S.
- Mean CTUP is:
  - Approximately 4 mm between the 4th and 9th months of pregnancy
  - After which time it increases 1.5–2 mm each month until the end of gestation
  - Alternately, CTUP of up to 7 mm prior to day 300 has been considered normal.
  - Obtain measurements from a consistent area on the ventral body of the uteroplacental unit.
  - Areas of placental folding or detachment from endometrium
- Allantoic fluid debris

OTHER DIAGNOSTIC PROCEDURES

- Microbial culture of discharge from cervix
- Cytology—neutrophils, with or without intracellular bacteria; fungal elements

PATHOLOGICAL FINDINGS

Examination of the allantochorion

Gross

- Thickened; discolored
- Bright red chorion becomes gray/brown, with plaques; avillous areas; exudative
- Examine umbilical cord, fetus for inflammatory changes.

Histopathologic

- Necessary to differentiate bacterial from mycotic
- Inflammatory infiltrate, fibrosis, thrombosis, edema; causative agent—bacteria or fungal elements

Microbiological Examination

Bacterial/fungal/viral isolation

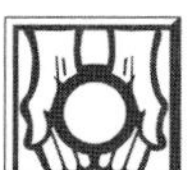

TREATMENT

APPROPRIATE HEALTH CARE

- Remove inciting cause—control infectious agent (bacterial, fungal).

- Control placental, endometrial inflammation, e.g., Caslick's vulvoplasty, progesterone supplementation.
- Clinical trials indicate that long-term treatment improves pregnancy outcome.
- Maintain fetoplacental function.
- Prevent fetal expulsion.
  - If mare carries to 300 days, chance of fetal survival increases.
  - Stress of intrauterine environment accelerates fetal maturity.
- Maintain maternal health.

NURSING CARE

Minimize maternal and fetal stress.

ACTIVITY

Stall rest the mare.

DIET

N/A

CLIENT EDUCATION

Monitor subsequent pregnancies.

SURGICAL CONSIDERATIONS

Repair of cervical and conformational defects, if present

MEDICATIONS

DRUG(S) OF CHOICE

Antibiotics

- Penicillin G; gentamicin
- Trimethoprim-sulfa
- Selection based on sensitivities of most likely pathogen

Anti-inflammatories

- NSAIDs decrease endotoxin production.
- Decrease luteolytic potential
- Decrease myometrial contractility
- Decrease incidence of laminitis

Anti-cytokine Therapies

- Pentoxifylline 8.5 mg/kg BID PO
- Decreases production of inflammatory mediators
- Has led to pregnancy maintenance in mouse endotoxemia model

Progestagen Supplementation

- Altrenogest (Regu-Mate) 0.44 mg/kg orally once daily for routine administration may be given at 0.088 mg/kg daily for the last 20 +/− 5 days of pregnancy; helps to decrease uterine excitability
- Maintains production of histiotrophe, fetal nutrition
- Aids cervical competency

CONTRAINDICATIONS

If fetal death occurs:
  - Discontinue progestagens.
  - Allow abortion to occur.
  - Avoid in utero fetal decomposition.
  - Continue antimicrobial and anti-inflammatory treatment of mare.
  - Monitor for laminitic changes.

PRECAUTIONS

N/A

POSSIBLE INTERACTIONS

N/A

ALTERNATIVE DRUGS

N/A

FOLLOW-UP

PATIENT MONITORING

Mare

- Transrectal U/S of cervix and caudal uterine body to evaluate thickness and detachment of placenta
- Transabdominal U/S to monitor placental integrity, fetal viability
- Attend parturition
  - Increased incidence of premature placental separation, and/or
  - Decreased likelihood of thickened allantochorion to rupture readily at cervical star during delivery
  - Either circumstance can lead to neonatal asphyxiation.
- Preterm mammary development (especially if >30 days before parturition)
- Premature lactation—loss of colostral antibodies; potential FPT
- Placental examination—to ensure no RFM
- Diagnostic samples—microbiological and histological from placenta, fetus
- Vaginal speculum examination to monitor cervix—closure, relaxation, and discharge
  - Use with caution.
  - This procedure disrupts existing vulvar and vestibular barriers to ascending uterine infection.

Neonate

- Increased potential for sepsis
- Increased potential for neurological compromise
- Possible IUGR
- Prepartum lactation may have depleted colostral antibodies.
- Fetal ECG in late gestation (final trimester)

PREVENTION/AVOIDANCE

- BSE of the mare when not pregnant; include examination of cervical competence
  - Best if in diestrus at time of examination
- Prebreeding preparation of mare and stallion—hygiene
- Keep environment and housing of pregnant mares as clean as possible.

POSSIBLE COMPLICATIONS

- Abortion
- Dystocia
- Sick, weak neonate

EXPECTED COURSE AND PROGNOSIS

N/A

MISCELLANEOUS

ASSOCIATED CONDITIONS

- Premature placental separation
- Laminitis
- Fetal sepsis—bacterial; fungal
- Neonatal sepsis and compromise

AGE-RELATED FACTORS

Endometrial health and cervical competence decline with age and increasing parity of mares.

ZOONOTIC POTENTIAL

N/A

PREGNANCY

Abortion

SEE ALSO

- Placental basics
- Placental insufficiency

ABBREVIATIONS

- BSE = breeding soundness examination
- CTUP = combined thickness of the uterus and placenta
- ECG/EKG = echocardiogram
- EHV = equineherpes virus
- EVA = equine viral arteritis
- FPT = failure of passive transfer
- IUGR = intrauterine growth retardation
- RFM = retained fetal membranes
- U/S = ultrasound, ultrasonography
- VC = vulvar conformation

Suggested Reading

Bucca S, Fogarty U, Collins A, Small V. Assessment of feto-placental well-being in the mare from mid-gestation to term: transrectal and transabdominal ultrasonographic features. Therio 2005;64:542–557.

Macpherson ML. Treatment strategies for mares with placentitis. Therio 2005;64:528–534.

Ousey JC, Houghton E, Grainger L, et al. Progestagen profiles during the last trimester of gestation in Thoroughbred mares with normal or compromised pregnancies. Therio 2005;63:1844–1856.

Renaudin CD, Troedsson MH, Gillis CL, et al. Ultrasonographic evaluation of the equine placenta by transrectal and transabdominal approach in the normal pregnant mare. Therio 1997;47:559–573.

Author Peter R. Morresey

Consulting Editor Carla L. Carleton

PLEURAL FLUID CYTOLOGY

BASICS

OVERVIEW

• Fluid is collected from the pleural space by aspiration between the intercostal spaces. • Fluid usually is taken from both the right and left sides of the chest. • Samples are collected aseptically into a sterile clot tube for bacterial culture and into EDTA for cell count, cytology, and protein determination. • Normal equine pleural fluid is clear to yellow, with no detectable odor.
• Protein content, as measured by refractometry, usually is <2.5 g/dL in samples from normal horses. Total nucleated cell count in fluid from normal horses is reportedly 800–12,000 cells/μL, with most samples containing <8000 cells/μL. • Nondegenerative neutrophils (low numbers) and large mononuclear cells, including mesothelial cells and macrophages, comprise most of the cells in normal pleural fluid. A few small lymphocytes occasionally, and eosinophils rarely, are seen. • Small numbers of RBCs commonly are present, presumably because of minor hemorrhage secondary to sampling.

PATHOPHYSIOLOGY

• Pleural fluid normally is a dialysate of the plasma, present in a small volume, and drained from the pleural cavity via lymphatic vessels.
• An increased volume of this fluid constitutes an effusion, the character of which reflects the process initiating the increased volume—inflammation, neoplasia, decreased oncotic pressure, or hemorrhage.

SYSTEMS AFFECTED

• Respiratory • Cardiovascular • Hemic/lymphatic/immune • Hepatobiliary

SIGNALMENT

Any breed, age, or sex

SIGNS

• Dyspnea • Depression • Weight loss • Fever
• Cough • Nasal discharge • Reduced lung sounds • Exercise intolerance • Ventral edema

CAUSES AND RISK FACTORS

• Pleuritis—inflammation caused by pleuropneumonia, ruptured abscess, external trauma, foreign bodies, or primary pleuritis; may be bacterial, viral, or fungal
• Neoplasia—lymphoma, metastatic squamous cell carcinoma, metastatic adenocarcinoma, melanoma or mesothelioma
• Hemorrhage
• Decreased oncotic pressure—hypoalbuminemia
• Increased hydrostatic pressure—congestive heart failure
• Chylothorax

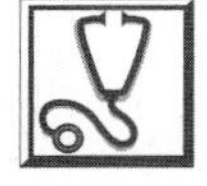

DIAGNOSIS

DIFFERENTIAL DIAGNOSIS

Pleuritis

• Inflammation causes an exudate or fluid with an increased cell count and protein content. This most commonly is associated with pneumonia or lung abscess and often is bacterial in origin.
• A predominantly neutrophilic response is seen in acute inflammation.
• If bacteria are present, neutrophils may appear degenerative (with pale, swollen nuclei), and bacteria may be seen, either intracellularly or free. Some bacteria cause fewer degenerative-type changes, however, so culture is suggested when neutrophil numbers are increased, even when the morphology appears normal.
• As inflammation becomes more chronic, the proportion of large mononuclear cells increases compared to neutrophils, and these cells may appear vacuolated or actively phagocytic.
• Lymphocytes and eosinophils may be present in very small numbers in exudates.

Neoplasia

• If cells from an intrathoracic tumor are shed into the pleural fluid, a diagnosis of neoplasia may be established on the basis of cytologic examination of the fluid.
• The most common tumor causing pleural effusions is lymphoma, sometimes characterized by large lymphocytes with large nuclei, prominent nucleoli, and scant, deeply basophilic cytoplasm. Lymphoma that is not lymphoblastic is harder to diagnose cytologically, because neoplastic lymphocytes may appear morphologically normal.
• Primary mesothelioma, metastatic gastric squamous cell carcinoma, melanoma and adenocarcinoma also may exfoliate cells into the pleural fluid.
• Intrathoracic tumors not uncommonly incite inflammation, which may make establishing the diagnosis more difficult. In addition, effusions typically cause exfoliation of reactive mesothelial cells, which have some cytologic features of malignancy.

Hemorrhage

• Most hemorrhage in fluid samples is mild, iatrogenic, and occurs at the time of sampling.
• Very recent hemorrhage may be associated with platelets in the sample.
• Hemorrhage into the thorax before sampling may cause a sample to appear hemolyzed, and phagocytosis of RBCs or erythrocyte breakdown products may be seen cytologically.

Decreased Oncotic Pressure

• Hypoalbuminemia may cause accumulation of a very low-protein, low-cellularity fluid in the pleural cavity because of reduced oncotic pressure in the plasma. This fluid is cytologically unremarkable, with low numbers of nondegenerative neutrophils, large mononuclear cells, and few lymphocytes.
• Mesothelial cells may appear reactive because of increased fluid volume.

Increased Hydrostatic Pressure

• Effusions that result from congestive heart failure or other causes of increased venous or lymphatic pressure usually have higher cell counts (5000–15,000 cells/ μL) and protein content (2.0–5.0 g/L) than a pure transudate.
• These modified transudates have a normal distribution of cells, including neutrophils and large mononuclear cells.

Chylothorax

This rare condition in horses has been associated with pleural fluid that is white and opaque grossly, with a predominance of small lymphocytes cytologically.

CBC/BIOCHEMISTRY/URINALYSIS

• Inflammatory conditions of the pleura may be associated with leukocytosis, left shift, toxic changes in neutrophils, and hyperfibrinogenemia. These changes are not always present, however, and are not specific for pleural inflammation.
• Hypoalbuminemia on a serum biochemical panel is helpful in establishing the diagnosis of a transudate.

OTHER LABORATORY TESTS

• Culture fluid with increased numbers of neutrophils both aerobically and anaerobically.
• Bronchoalveolar lavage or tracheal aspiration may help in establishing the diagnosis of pleuropneumonia or lung abscess.

IMAGING

Radiology and ultrasonography may help to localize pleural fluid and to characterize pathological processes—abscesses, masses, and pneumonias.

OTHER DIAGNOSTIC PROCEDURES

N/A

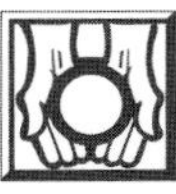

TREATMENT

Directed at the underlying cause

MEDICATIONS

DRUG(S) OF CHOIE N/A

CONTRAINDICATIONS/POSSIBLE INTERACTIONS N/A

FOLLOW-UP

PATIENT MONITORING N/A

POSSIBLE COMPLICATIONS N/A

MISCELLANEOUS

ASSOCIATED CONDITIONS, AGE-RELATED FACTORS, ZOONOTIC POTENTIAL, PREGNANCY

N/A

Suggested Reading

Parry BW. Pleural fluid. In: Cowell RL, Tyler RD, eds. Cytology and Hematology of the Horse. Goleta, CA: American Veterinary Publications, 1992:107–120.

Author Susan J. Tornquist
Consulting Editor Kenneth W. Hinchcliff

PLEUROPNEUMONIA

BASICS

OVERVIEW

The development of an inflammatory response in the lung parenchyma to bacterial pathogens, with extension to the pleural space and subsequent pleural effusion

SIGNALMENT

There is no breed or sex predilection. All ages can be affected but pleuritis with pneumonia is much less common in the foal than in the adult.

SIGNS

• Acute—fever, lethargy, anorexia, tachypnea, dyspnea, decreased bronchovesicular sounds ventrally, radiating heart sounds, pleural friction rubs, serous, serosanguinous or mucopurulent nasal discharge, pleural pain (pleurodynia), soft cough, ventral and/or limb edema • Subacute or chronic—fever (may be intermittent), weight loss, exercise intolerance, persistent ventral or limb edema, intermittent colic, tachypnea and dyspnea relative to the volume of pleural effusion. Cough, nasal discharge, and pleurodynia minimal to absent.

CAUSES AND RISK FACTORS

• Mixed infections are common. *Streptococcus zooepidemicus* is the primary gram-positive pathogen. *Escherichia coli* and *Klebsiella pneumoniae* are the most common gram-negative, enteric pathogens. *Actinobacillus* spp. and *Pasteurella* spp. are the most common gram-negative, nonenteric pathogens. Anaerobic bacteria are isolated in many cases of pleuropneumonia. Mycoplasma has been isolated from the pleural fluid in rare cases.
• Stress, transport, exercise-induced pulmonary hemorrhage, viral disease, esophageal obstruction (choke), dysphagia, thoracic trauma, general anesthesia

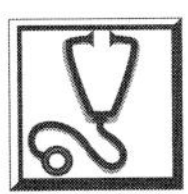

DIAGNOSIS

DIFFERENTIAL DIAGNOSIS

• Viral pneumonia (influenza, rhinopneumonitis, EVA), fungal pneumonia (coccidioidomycosis), neoplasia (lymphosarcoma, gastric squamous cell carcinoma), hemothorax, cardiac disease (congestive heart failure, pericarditis), equine infectious anemia, diaphragmatic hernia
• Thoracic auscultation, ultrasound, and radiography will indicate the presence of pleural fluid and cranioventral pulmonary consolidation. Serologic testing can be done to rule out coccidioidomycosis and equine infectious anemia. Hemothorax or diaphragmatic hernia should be considered if there is historical or physical evidence of thoracic trauma. Jugular venous distention or pulsation combined with cardiac murmur or arrhythmia suggests cardiac disease. Cytologic evaluation of pleural fluid is important in the differentiation of neoplasia.

CBC/BIOCHEMISTRY/URINALYSIS

• CBC—inflammatory leukogram (neutrophilic leukocytosis, hyperfibrinogenemia) or toxic leukogram, anemia (subacute or chronic).
• Biochemistry—hypergammaglobulinemia (subacute or chronic)

OTHER LABORATORY TESTS

Arterial blood gases will help to evaluate the severity of hypoxemia, hypercapnia, and respiratory compromise.

IMAGING

• Thoracic ultrasound—hypoechoic or anechoic fluid present between the thoracic wall and the lung parenchyma. Fluid may be loculated if there is significant fibrin deposition. Pulmonary consolidation or atelectasis can be detected. The presence of a pulmonary abscess can be detected if it is surrounded by nonaerated lung, or if it is in a subpleural location. Small hyperechoic images within the pleural fluid are suggestive of anaerobic infection. • Thoracic radiography—less useful than ultrasound for the accurate detection of pleural fluid. May be helpful after thoracocentesis and drainage of the pleural fluid to reveal the extent of the pneumonia.

OTHER DIAGNOSTIC PROCEDURES

The definitive diagnosis is established through the cytologic and microbiologic evaluation of aspirates. TTA and pleural fluid sample for cytology and culture. TTA is often more rewarding than thoracocentesis for the positive identification of pulmonary pathogens. Pleural fluid glucose concentration of <40 mg/dL, pH < 7.2, or lactate level higher than venous blood all suggest septic effusion.

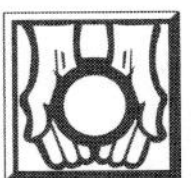

TREATMENT

• Mild cases with minimal fluid accumulation and respiratory compromise can be treated on an outpatient basis. Treatment as an inpatient is recommended for patients with significant fluid accumulation due to the need for frequent reevaluation by ultrasound, repeated thoracocentesis, or indwelling thoracic drainage.
• Fluids—oral or intravenous polyionic fluids should be used to correct dehydration and electrolyte or acid-base disturbances. • To stabilize patients in respiratory distress, nasal insufflation with oxygen and therapeutic thoracocentesis may be required.

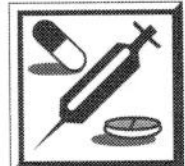

MEDICATIONS

• Optimally, antimicrobial therapy should be based on identification of the bacterial pathogens and results of in vitro sensitivity testing. If antimicrobial therapy is begun without culture results, then broad-spectrum drugs should be used due to the high number of mixed infections. Choose agents effective against both gram-positive and gram-negative, as well as aerobic and anaerobic, organisms. Penicillin is effective against the great majority of anaerobes but *Bacteroides fragilis*, a common anaerobic isolate, is often resistant to penicillin. A common treatment choice would be penicillin or ampicillin, gentamicin or amikacin, and metronidazole. • NSAIDs—phenylbutazone or flunixin meglumine may be used to reduce inflammation and endotoxemia, and provide analgesia. • Antithrombotic drugs—Heparin and aspirin have been used in endotoxic animals that may be at increased risk of DIC but their use is controversial.

CONTRAINDICATIONS/POSSIBLE INTERACTIONS

The nephrotoxicity of aminoglycoside antibiotics may be potentiated in the dehydrated patient or by concurrent administration of NSAIDs.

FOLLOW-UP

PATIENT MONITORING

Frequent auscultation and follow-up thoracic ultrasound examinations are the most sensitive indicators of patient progress. Repeated thoracic drainage or placement of an indwelling thoracic drain may be necessary in cases where pleural fluid continues to build up.

PREVENTION/AVOIDANCE

• Avoid or minimize risk factors. • Vaccination against upper respiratory viruses

POSSIBLE COMPLICATIONS

• Pulmonary or subpleural abscesses are not uncommon. • Bronchopleural fistulas, pleural adhesions, pericarditis, and laminitis are other serious sequelae.

EXPECTED COURSE AND PROGNOSIS

Guarded to good prognosis with early diagnosis and aggressive antibacterial and supportive treatment. Prognosis is guarded to poor in cases of pleuropneumonia, which reach the subacute to chronic stage prior to accurate diagnosis.

MISCELLANEOUS

ABBREVIATIONS

DIC = disseminated intravascular coagulation
EVA = equine viral arteritis
NSAID = nonsteroidal anti-inflammatory drug
TTA = Transtracheal aspirate

Suggested Reading

Chaffin MK, Carter GK. Bacterial pleuropneumonia. In: Robinson NE, ed. Current Therapy in Equine Medicine, ed 4. Philadelphia: WB Saunders, 1997:449–452.

Sweeney CR. Pleuropneumonia. In: Smith, BP, ed. Large Animal Internal Medicine. St. Louis: Mosby, 2002:500–504.

Author Joie Watson
Consulting Editor Daniel Jean

PNEUMONIA, NEONATAL

BASICS

DEFINITION

• Inflammation of pulmonary parenchyma occurring in foals less than 4 weeks of age
• One of the most common sites of infectious disease in neonatal foals

PATHOPHYSIOLOGY

Bacterial Septicemia

• Foals frequently develop septic pneumonia as a sequel to bacterial septicemia.
  ○ Most common cause of neonatal pneumonia
• Bacteria are borne hematogenously to the pulmonary parenchyma and cause infection.
• Pattern of affected lung is diffuse, consistent with a blood-borne infection. • Immune status of foal at time of exposure to pathogens is very important in pathogenesis.
  ○ Amount of colostrum ingested and serum IgG concentration highly correlated with incidence of disease, with foals ingesting an adequate quantity of good-quality colostrum less frequently affected
• Pathogens implicated in neonatal septicemia are most frequently isolated.
  ○ *Escherichia coli* ○ *Klebsiella pneumoniae* ○ *Actinobacillus equuli* ○ *Salmonella* spp. ○ *Streptococcus* spp.

Viral Infection

• Can cause severe, refractory pneumonia in neonatal period
  ○ Foals may be infected in utero or shortly after birth.
• Most foals affected with viral pneumonia succumb quickly (almost always fatal). • Foals may be born pre-term or aborted as consequence of maternal viral infection. • Most commonly associated with the following viruses:
  ○ Equine herpesvirus-1 (less frequently EHV-4) ○ Equine arteritis virus ○ Equine influenza virus ○ Equine adenovirus may cause pneumonia in Arabian foals with SCID.

Aspiration Pneumonia

• Aspiration of milk, oral secretions occurs as a result of neonatal pharyngeal dysfunction and/or weakness (any cause). • Pneumonia displays characteristic cranioventral/caudoventral distribution.
  ○ Cleft palate ○ Botulism ○ Sepsis ○ Iatrogenic (syringe, bottle feeding of colostrum/milk) ○ Perinatal asphyxia

SYSTEMS AFFECTED

• Respiratory system • In foals with septicemic disease, other systems (most notably the musculoskeletal and gastrointestinal systems) may be concurrently affected.

GENETICS

• No genetic predisposition • Exception is Arabian foals affected by SCID

INCIDENCE/PREVALENCE

• Up to 50% of neonatal foals examined and treated at referral institutions have pneumonia.
• Case-fatality rate is unknown but likely depends on timeliness of therapeutic intervention, etiologic agent, and immune status of foal, among other factors.

GEOGRAPHIC DISTRIBUTION

No geographic distribution in incidence of disease; however, there may be geographic differences in bacterial isolates.

SIGNALMENT

Breed Predilections

• No breed predisposition • Exception is Arabian foals with SCID.

Mean Age and Range

• Neonatal foals (<14 days of age) • Most cases are <7 days of age at the time of presentation.

Predominant Sex

No sex predisposition identified

SIGNS

General Comments

• Foals may have severe pulmonary disease without overt clinical signs referable to the respiratory tract. • Foals with pneumonia often display nonspecific signs of disease.

Historical

• See Risk Factors. • History of maternal disease
• Prematurity • History of inadequate colostral ingestion (any reason) common • Lethargy, depression, decreased nursing behavior

Physical Examination

• Often vague, nonlocalizing clinical signs
• Weak, often increasingly recumbent
• Decreased frequency of nursing • Fever, although affected foals may have increased, normal, or decreased body temperatures
• Tachypnea is a frequent finding, and affected foals may be dyspneic with an increased abdominal component to their respiratory pattern. • Pulmonary auscultation may reveal increased bronchovesicular sounds or absence of auscultable sounds over regions of consolidated/atalectatic lung, or may be normal (even in severely affected foals). • Cyanosis not common, and might not be noted in anemic foals (requires at least 5 g/dL unsaturated hemoglobin to be visible); occurs when Pao_2 less than 50 mm Hg (severe hypoxemia) • Cough and/or nasal discharge are not common findings in early disease.

RISK FACTORS

Failure of transfer of passive immunity is likely the single most important risk factor.
• Maternal risk factors
  ○ Maternal illness (colic, respiratory disease, etc.) ○ Dystocia ○ Running colostrum/milk prior to parturition ○ Ascending cervicitis/placentitis ○ Maternal rejection of neonate ○ Agalactia/hypogalactia (e.g., fescue exposure within final 4 weeks of gestation)
  ○ Maternal age (very young or old mares produce less colostrum of lower quality)
• Neonatal risk factors
  ○ Dystocia ○ Hypoxic-ischemic encephalopathy ○ Musculoskeletal disease preventing rising, nursing in timely fashion
• Unhygienic environment in immediate neonatal period— ingested or inhaled pathogens. Prolonged lateral recumbency—vascular congestion of dependent lung may predispose to infection.

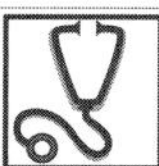

DIAGNOSIS

DIFFERENTIAL DIAGNOSIS

• Anemia (e.g., neonatal isoerythrolysis)—Weakness is similar, but hematocrit measurement will differentiate. • Cardiac disease (e.g., congenital cardiac anomaly)—tachypnea and lethargy may be seen; presence of heart murmur and diagnosis with echocardiography.
• Hyperthermia—tachypnea may be seen.
• Idiopathic tachypnea • Trauma (rib fracture, pulmonary contusion) • Neurologic disease (including PAS)—abnormal respiratory patterns may develop, potentially resulting in blood gas derangements. • Botulism—fatigue of ventilatory muscles can result in abdominal breathing and respiratory failure; other muscular weakness is seen with botulism. • Segmented neutrophil count may be increased, normal, or decreased. • Toxic granulation, vacuolation may be evident associated with sepsis. • Viral infection may induce profound lymphopenia, but this is inconsistent. • Elevated lymphocyte counts (greater than neutrophil count) may be noted in premature foals and may indicate a poor prognosis. • Plasma fibrinogen level often increases with pulmonary inflammation.

OTHER LABORATORY TESTS

Arterial Blood Gas Analysis

• Ideal method to determine adequacy of gas exchange and pulmonary function • Best sampling sites include dorsal metatarsal artery, brachial artery, femoral artery, or transverse facial artery. • Patient should be standing or sternally recumbent for ≈5–10 min prior to sampling.
• Useful for monitoring response to therapy and assessing changes in patient's status • Pao_2
  ○ Should be >80 mm Hg
  ○ Values between 60 and 80 mm Hg may be associated with pulmonary disease but also may be noted in foals that are laterally recumbent at time of sampling. ○ Values <60 mm Hg indicate hypoxemia and poor pulmonary function.
• $Paco_2$
  ○ Values >60 mm Hg with concurrent hypoxemia indicate respiratory failure.
  ○ Indication for mechanical ventilation

Blood Culture

• Likely to be helpful in identification of etiologic agent in septicemic cases
• Antimicrobial sensitivity helpful to guide therapy

Culture and Cytology of Samples of Respiratory Tract Secretions

• Important for establishing diagnosis, identifying etiologic agent • Not recommended in dyspneic patients—patient should be stabilized first. • Bacteria readily cultured, antimicrobial sensitivity helpful to guide therapy
• Viral isolation may be performed on respiratory tract samples.
  ○ Serology less helpful in neonate (interference by dam's colostral antibodies, assuming colostral ingestion)

PNEUMONIA, NEONATAL

Serum IgG Levels

• Serum IgG level often <400 mg/dL in affected neonates

IMAGING

• Thoracic radiography
  ○ Useful for documenting extent and severity of disease ○ Hematogenous bacterial pneumonia—diffuse disease with an alveolar or interstitial/alveolar pattern ○ Aspiration pneumonia—cranioventral/caudoventral pulmonary fields (alveolar pattern) ○ Useful for monitoring response to therapy, resolution of disease (radiographic disease will lag behind clinical status of patient)
• Thoracic ultrasonography
  ○ Can visualize parietal abscessation, pulmonary consolidation, pleural effusion ○ Also useful for monitoring response to therapy

OTHER DIAGNOSTIC PROCEDURES

• Endoscopy of the upper respiratory tract
  ○ May be useful for identifying cause in patients with aspiration pneumonia ○ Pharyngeal, laryngeal abnormalities may be noted.
• Pulse oximetry may be useful as a continuous, noninvasive estimate of Pa_{O_2}, although results should be periodically confirmed by arterial blood gas measurements.

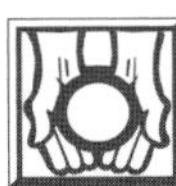

TREATMENT

AIMS OF TREATMENT

• Sterilize pulmonary parenchyma • Promote efficient gas exchange • Minimize inflammatory changes that may promote ARDS, SIRS, and subsequent death of the patient

APPROPRIATE HEALTH CARE

Best examined and treated as inpatients at referral facility; however, this depends somewhat on the severity of the disease. Emergency referral for intensive medical therapy, especially in dyspneic patients, is imperative for best possible outcome.

NURSING CARE

• Oxygen—Humidified oxygen should be administered via nasal cannula(s) inserted to the level of the nasopharynx at a rate of 5–10 L/min.
• Thoracic coupage may be peformed to mobilize secretions by striking the chest wall gently with a cupped hand; patients should be examined carefully for thoracic trauma (e.g., rib fractures) prior to instituting this therapy. • Foals should be maintained in sternal recumbency to minimize dependent lung atalectasis.
• Mechanical ventilation should be provided for foals in respiratory failure (hypoxemia with concurrent hypercapnia); this may only be required for a short period (12–24 hr) in foals with respiratory failure secondary to ventilatory muscle fatigue. • Judicious suctioning of respiratory secretions (use care—may cause pulmonary collapse and exacerbate hypoxemia); suction only as needed and for short periods (<2 seconds). • Fluid therapy
  ○ Isotonic polyionic electrolyte solutions should be administered to address dehydration and electrolyte and acid-base abnormalities.
  ○ Adequate hydration may also help moisten and mobilize pulmonary secretions, promote function of mucociliary apparatus.
• Pulmonary edema may result from overhydration, particularly dangerous in patients with already compromised pulmonary function.

ACTIVITY

Should be minimized to decrease metabolic oxygen demands, especially in hypoxemic patients

DIET

• Enteral nutrition should be provided via an indwelling nasogastric feeding tube, particularly in patients with pharyngeal dysfunction or weakness, which has resulted in aspiration.
• Parenteral nutrition may be required for foals that do not tolerate enteral feeding (colic, ileus, diarrhea).

MEDICATIONS

DRUG(S)

Antimicrobials

• Broad-spectrum bactericidal drugs should be administered prior to results of culture and sensitivity testing. • Aminoglycoside/beta-lactam combinations are good choices for empiric therapy.
  ○ Amikacin (25 mg/kg IV daily) or gentamicin (6.6 mg/kg IV daily) and penicillin (22,000 IU/kg IV q6h) or ampicillin (15–30 mg/kg IV q6h)
• Third-generation cephalosporins are also good empiric choices, particularly if patient has renal compromise (aminoglycosides contraindicated).
  ○ Ceftiofur (4–10 mg/kg IV q6h–q12h).
  ○ Ceftazidime (50 mg/kg IV q6h)
  ○ Ceftriaxone (25 mg/kg IV q12h)
  ○ Cefotaxime (40 mg/kg IV q12h)
• Therapy may be adjusted based on culture and sensitivity results. • Therapy should continue for 2–5 weeks (see comments on monitoring below).
• Antiviral therapy (acyclovir) has been used for viral pneumonia; unlikely to affect clinical course

Nonsteroidal Anti-inflammatory Medications

• Useful to minimize fever, inflammation
• Ketoprofen (2.2 mg/kg IV q12h) • Flunixin meglumine (1.1 mg/kg IV q12h)

Gastroprotectants

• May be useful in foals receiving nonsteroidal medications • See Gastric Ulcers, Neonate.

CONTRAINDICATIONS

Aminoglycosides should not be used in azotemic patients.

PRECAUTIONS

• Oxygen therapy may cause hypoventilation in hypercapnic patients. • Mechanical ventilation strategies should be lung-protective (lower tidal volumes, peak airway pressures) to minimize trauma.

ALTERNATIVE DRUGS

Depending on results of bacterial culture/sensitivity, alternative antimicrobial drugs may be needed.

FOLLOW-UP

PATIENT MONITORING

• Physical examination—Attitude, respiratory rate, and pattern should be observed frequently until stabilized. • Arterial blood gas analysis should be performed daily, or when status of patient changes (especially mechanically ventilated patients). • CBC, fibrinogen every 3–5 days; when status of patient changes; prior to discontinuation of antimicrobial therapy
• Thoracic radiography—weekly; when change in patient status; prior to discontinuation of antimicrobial therapy • Thoracic ultrasonography may be performed daily or every other day.

PREVENTION/AVOIDANCE

Ensure adequate transfer of passive immunity within the first 18–24 hr of life.

POSSIBLE COMPLICATIONS

• Pulmonary abscessation • Pleural adhesions
• Other septic foci (e.g., septic polyarthritis)

EXPECTED COURSE AND PROGNOSIS

• Approximately two-thirds of foals with pneumonia survive to hospital discharge.
• Effects on future athletic performance unknown

MISCELLANEOUS

ASSOCIATED CONDITIONS

• Septicemia • Prematurity

SEE ALSO

• Septicemia, neonatal • Failure of transfer of passive immunity

ABBREVIATIONS

• ARDS = acute respiratory distress syndrome
• PAS = perinatal asphyxia syndrome • SCID = severe combined immunodeficiency • SIRS = systemic inflammatory response syndrome

Suggested Reading

Benedice D. Manifestations of septicemia: foal with septic pneumonia. In: Paradis MR, ed. Equine Neonatal Medicine: A Case-Based Approach. Philadelphia: Saunders, 2006.

Dunkel B. Acute lung injury and acute respiratory distress syndrome in foals. Clin Tech Equine Pract 2006;5:127–133.

Koterba AM, Paradis MR. Specific respiratory conditions. In: Koterba AM, Drummond WH, Kosch PC, eds. Equine Clinical Neonatology. Philadelphia: Lea & Febiger, 1990.

Wilkins P. Lower respiratory problems of the neonate. Vet Clin North Am Equine Pract 2003;19:19–33.

Author Teresa A. Burns
Consulting Editor Margaret C. Mudge

PNEUMOTHORAX

BASICS

OVERVIEW

• PTX—presence of air within the pleural space, resulting in varying degrees of lung collapse and inadequate ventilation • Rarely encountered, but most commonly following penetrating thoracic wounds or birth trauma • One or both hemithoraces may be involved. • Open PTX—when air freely enters and leaves the pleural cavity through a chest wound • Closed PTX—when air freely enters and leaves the pleural cavity through a breach in the visceral pleura or mediastinum • Tension PTX—when air accumulates in the pleural space with each breath and cannot escape. Usually a flap of tissue in a wound acts as a one-way valve, causing a buildup of pressure in the pleural cavity. A rare but life-threatening condition.

SIGNS

Historical

• History of thoracic trauma or recent transtracheal wash, bone marrow aspiration
• Neonates from primiparous mares or dystocias are predisposed.

Physical Examination

• If PTX is not severe, no clinical signs may be evident at rest. • Tachypnea, nasal flaring, and superficial breathing may be evident. • Dyspnea may occur in more severe and bilateral cases and can progress to severe respiratory distress, tachycardia, and cyanosis. • Absence of lung sounds dorsally on thoracic auscultation, and increased resonance on percussion • Inspection and palpation of the thoracic cage and axillary area may reveal a penetrating wound. Localized thoracic pain, subcutaneous emphysema, and instability of the thoracic wall is compatible with fractured rib(s).

CAUSES AND RISK FACTORS

• Collision with an object (fences) • Birth trauma (primiparous mares or dystocia)
• Bronchopleural fistula from pleuropneumonia, distal tracheal or esophageal lacerations
• Transtracheal wash, bone marrow aspiration, or lung biopsy

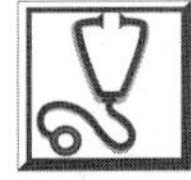

DIAGNOSIS

DIFFERENTIAL DIAGNOSIS

• Pain can cause rapid, shallow breathing.
• Diaphragmatic hernia • Pleural effusion—hemothorax or pyothorax

CBC/BIOCHEMISTRY/URINALYSIS

Stress leukogram and leukocytosis with secondary bacterial infection

OTHER LABORATORY TESTS

Arterial blood gas analysis may reveal hypercapnia and hypoxemia due to hypoventilation.

IMAGING

Thoracic Ultrasonography

• Air in the presence PTX accumulates dorsally in standing horse or laterally in a recumbent foal. • The pleural line appears (3.5 MHz) as a hyperechoic line in the intercostal space (below the intercostal muscles) which dynamically twinkles with normal lung movement ("sliding lung sign"). Absence of the "sliding lung sign" is strong, but not absolute, evidence for the presence of PTX on 2D mode. • In horses breathing rapidly, confirmation of the diagnosis of PTX can be made on M-mode ultrasonography, which permits assessment of tissue movements temporally. A normal lung appears diffusely grainy, like sand, below the visceral pleura and the superficially generated horizontal lines above the lung ("seashore sign"). In the presence of PTX, because of the complete absence of tissue movements, horizontal lines alone are visible throughout the image ("stratosphere sign").

Thoracic Radiography

Retraction of lung margins from the thoracic wall

OTHER DIAGNOSTIC PROCEDURES

Complete ultrasonographic examination of thorax and abdomen for horses with a history of trauma

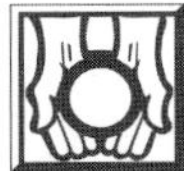

TREATMENT

• These animals may suffer from polytrauma; a clinical approach consisting of a first look, shock treatment, and frequent rechecks is suitable.
• Control of external hemorrhage and shock treatment with IV fluids are essential during the acute period. Remember, the contused lung in cases of trauma is extremely sensitive to fluid overload; therefore, use sparingly. • In cases with minimal clinical signs at rest, PTX will resorb without treatment in a couple of weeks if the animal is confined. • Administer oxygen by nasopharyngeal insufflation (5–10 L/min for foals; 10–15 L/min for adults) for dyspneic and hypoxemic patients. • Open PTX—Temporarily close the wound using sterile gauze impregnated with antibiotic ointment. Suture it whenever possible to rapidly achieve an air-tight seal. For wounds that are not amenable to primary closure, apply a thin film dressing to the skin to provide an airtight seal. • Thoracocentesis—Indicated when clinical signs of respiratory distress are present. The site for air evacuation is the dorsal thoracic cavity just in front of the 12th through 15th ribs. Avoid intercostal vessels which run along the caudal border of the ribs. • Perform thoracocentesis using a 14-gauge over-the-needle catheter, a teat cannula or a large-gauge needle attached to a three-way stop cock, extension set, and 60-mL syringe. • If severe or active PTX is present, a thoracostomy tube may be placed dorsally in the pleural cavity and attached to a Heimlich valve or, in the case of rapid reaccumulation of air, a continuous suction apparatus could be used. When PTX has persisted for some time it should be aspirated slowly to avoid reexpension pulmonrary edema.
• Uncontrolled PTX or recurrence is an indication for thoracoscopy. Also useful to evaluate pulmonary pathology and to diagnose a radiolucent foreign body.
• Intercostal nerve blocks can be used to control pain associated with fractured ribs.

MEDICATIONS

DRUG(S)

Broad-spectrum antibiotics (penicillin, gentamicin, and metronidazole), NSAIDs (flunixin or phenylbutazone), and tetanus prophylaxis

CONTRAINDICATIONS/POSSIBLE INTERACTIONS

Avoid drugs such as xylazine or opioids, because they may reduce PaO_2.

FOLLOW-UP

PATIENT MONITORING

• Monitor hourly the respiratory rate and character, mucous membrane color, and heart rate for the first 24–48 hours. • Serial ultrasonography or radiography and blood gas analyses reveal the effectiveness of pleural air evacuation and reexpansion of the lungs.
• Thoracostomy tubes may be removed if $\leq$50 mL of air are aspirated in 12 hours. • Full recovery is expected if the injury is not massive and the recognition and treatment of PTX is prompt.

POSSIBLE COMPLICATIONS

• Recurrence of PTX • Pyothorax with open PTX

EXPECTED COURSE AND PROGNOSIS

• Tension PTX is a serious life-threatening condition if left untreated. • Full recovery is expected if the injury is not severe and does not involve other thoracic structures.

MISCELLANEOUS

ASSOCIATED CONDITIONS

• Thoracic trauma • Fractured ribs
• Diaphragmatic hernia • Ruptured trachea
• Thoracic and abdominal organ lacerations
• Other complications of trauma

SEE ALSO

• Diaphragmatic hernia • Expiratory dyspnea
• Inspiratory dyspnea • Pleuropneumonia
• Thoracic trauma

ABBREVIATION

• NSAID = nonsteroidal anti-inflammatory drug • PTX = pneumothorax

Suggested Reading

Hassel MH. Thoracic trauma in horses. Vet Clin North Am Equine Pract 2007;23:67–80.

Jean D, Laverty S, Halley J, et al. Thoracic trauma in newborn foals. Equine Vet J 1999;31:149–152.

Laverty S, Lavoie JP, Pascoe JR, Ducharme N. Penetrating wounds of the thorax in 15 horses. Equine Vet J 1996;220–224.

Authors Florent David and Sheila Laverty
Consulting Editor Daniel Jean

PNEUMOVAGINA/PNEUMOUTERUS

BASICS

DEFINITION/OVERVIEW

• Air in the vagina or uterus • Usually results from vulvar conformational defect

ETIOLOGY/PATHOPHYSIOLOGY

• Air accumulates subsequent to poor vulvar conformation and relaxation of the vestibular sphincter. • The negative pressure within the lumen of the genital tract aids in movement of air into the vestibule, vagina, and uterus; elicits a "wind-sucking" sound. • With motion (e. g., running, rolling), air is forced back out, resulting in a characteristic expulsive sound.

SYSTEM AFFECTED

Reproductive

GENETICS

Possible genetic influence for less-than-ideal vulvar conformation

INCIDENCE/PREVALENCE

No statistics available regarding incidence. Condition is common and one of the major causes of equine infertility.

SIGNALMENT

• All breeds, but breeds/individuals with less perineal muscle are more severely affected. • All of breeding age • Older pluripara mares most commonly affected

SIGNS

General Comments

• Described as potential reproductive problem as early as 1937. • Condition remains a major cause of subfertility/infertility.

Historical

• May exhibit signs of chronic pneumovagina, including vaginal flatus, abnormal redness of the vaginal mucosa and accumulation of air in the uterus, coupled with abnormal vulvar conformation.
• Subfertility/infertility linked with uterine infections and/or inflammation – also common.

Physical Examination

• Determine if vulvar conformation is normal:
  ○ Assess relationship of dorsal vulvar commissure to the pubis; should lie at or below the floor of the pubis.
• Effect of poor vulvar conformation on fertility confirmed by the presence of vaginitis, pneumovagina, or pneumouterus.
• As age/parity increases:
  ○ Anus is pulled cranially and thus attached soft-tissue structures move forward with it.
  ○ The vulva is pulled in a cranial slant, up over the posterior brim of the pubis.

CAUSES

Predisposing Factors:

• Changes in general conformation, e. g., sway back • Loss of body condition and/or vaginal fat • Age, genetics, trauma-related changes of vulvar conformation • Weakness or stretching of the supporting soft-tissue structures in the perineal area

RISK FACTORS

• Diminishes protective barrier of a normal vulva by age, parity, genetic predisposition • Vulvar conformation also influenced by pregnancy—additional stretching of the perineal soft tissues • Poor nutritional condition may contribute to decreased vulvar conformation. • Normal estrual tissue relaxation may slightly affect vulvar conformation.

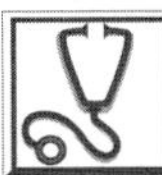

DIAGNOSIS

IMAGING

U/S—not necessary, unless to confirm pneumouterus

PATHOLOGICAL FINDINGS

• Evidence of vaginitis and endometritis:
  ○ Indicators of pneumovagina and/or pneumouterus
  ○ Other possible causes exist, but with poor vulvar conformation, the diagnosis is conclusive.
• This condition may result not only in subfertility and infertility, but also cause abortion in pregnant mares after vaginitis and cervicitis have developed.

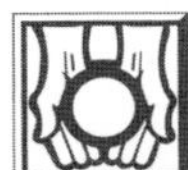

TREATMENT

APPROPRIATE HEALTH CARE

Little justification to treat a mare for uterine infection or inflammation if poor vulvar conformation is not corrected.

CLIENT EDUCATION

• Advise clients to evaluate the vulvar conformation of all mares. • If vulvar conformation is less than ideal, a Caslick's vulvoplasty surgery is needed.

SURGICAL CONSIDERATIONS

• Surgical correction for poor vulvar conformation (vulvoplasty or episioplasty) was first described by Dr. Caslick in 1937.
• First, wrap and tie the mare's tail away from the field of surgery, and thoroughly clean the perineal area with cotton and soap. • Carbocaine or other local anesthetic is infiltrated into the mucocutaneous junction of the vulva; ≅10–12 mL typically used to infiltrate both sides of the vulva. • The tissue edges are *freshened* before suturing, either by:
  ○ *Strip removal*: very narrow strip of tissue is cut away from the edge of the each vulvar lip, or by
  ○ *Split-thickness technique*: incising at the mucocutaneous junction along the line dilated with local anesthetic; i.e. no tissue is removed.
  ○ The latter is *tissue-sparing* and preferred for the long-term reproductive welfare of the mare.
  ○ Over the reproductive life of a mare, the split-thickness technique helps to retain the normal elasticity of vulvae during labor by minimizing prior, annual damage.
  ○ Both described techniques are in common use and considered acceptable.
• Use nonabsorbable suture material or staples, with removal in ≅10 days.
  ○ At the time of suture/staple removal, evaluate surgical site for presence of small fistulae through which contamination may continue.
• *Pouret technique*: in cases of severe/extremely poor vulvar conformation, it may be necessary to dissect the perineal body in a caudal (widest) to cranial (point), pie-shaped wedge, that permits the genital tract, ventral to the rectum, to slide caudally and away from fecal contamination, as well as aspiration of air; only the skin is closed, i.e., no deep reconstruction of dissected tissue.
• Check mare's tetanus toxoid vaccination status.

MEDICATIONS

DRUG(S) OF CHOICE

• No antibiotics are indicated. • Selection of local anesthetic is at the discretion of the surgeon.

FOLLOW-UP

PATIENT MONITORING

Remove sutures 10 days after surgery to prevent the possibility of stitch abscess forming at the suture site.

PREVENTION/AVOIDANCE

Select broodmares with excellent vulvar conformation.

POSSIBLE COMPLICATIONS

• Primary contraindication to vulvoplasty: necessity to reopen the vulvar commissure ≅5–10 days before parturition to prevent tearing of the perineum at delivery. • It should be replaced, i.e., incised and sutured, immediately after foaling or breeding and confirmation of ovulation in the next season, depending on severity of vulvar conformation abnormality, confirmed.
• Place the Caslick vulvoplasty following breeding as soon as ovulation has been confirmed:
  ○ Ensures the best uterine environment for the newly arriving embryo 6 days post-ovulation. ○ Do not wait until after the first pregnancy check. The unsutured vulva allows endometrial contamination to continue unabated and the embryo arrives into a more hostile uterine environment.

EXPECTED COURSE AND PROGNOSIS

Without surgical correction, mares may remain infertile or abort during pregnancy.

MISCELLANEOUS

AGE-RELATED FACTORS

High probability of vulvar conformation becoming worse with age

PREGNANCY

Surgery may be necessary to obtain a pregnancy.

SYNONYMS

• Windsucker • Windsucking

SEE ALSO

• Dystocia • Endometrial biopsy • Endometritis
• Perineal lacerations • Vulvar conformation

Suggested Reading

Caslick EA. The vulva and vulvo-vaginal orifice and its relationship to genital health of the thoroughbred mare. Cornell Vet 1937;27:178–186.

Colbern GT, Aanes WA, Stashak TS. Surgical management of perineal lacerations and recto-vestibular fistulae in the mare: a retrospective study of 47 cases. J Am Vet Med Assoc 1985;186:265–269.

Shipley WD, Bergin WC. Genital health in the mare. III. Pneumovagina. VM/SAC 1968;63:699–702.

Author Walter R. Threlfall
Consulting Editor Carla L. Carleton

POISONING (INTOXICATION) – GENERAL PRINCIPLES

BASICS

DEFINITION

• A *poison* or *toxicant* is a natural or synthetic substance causing disease via its own inherent qualities.
• A *toxin* is a type of toxicant with a biologic origin—plants, bacteria, or animals.
• *Toxicosis* refers to the disease caused by a poison.
• *Toxicity* refers to the amount of a poison that causes disease; substances with high toxicity require a lower dose to cause disease than do substances with low toxicity.

PATHOPHYSIOLOGY

Mechanisms of action vary with the different toxicants and are discussed in the specific chapters dealing with those toxicants.

SYSTEMS AFFECTED

• All systems have the potential to be affected by toxicants. The ones most commonly affected include the GI, hepatic, nervous, renal, hemic, and cardiovascular systems.
• The system affected depends on the type of toxicant and may also depend on other factors such as the dose or the route of exposure.
• Some toxicants affect more than one system. The effects can occur concurrently, sequentially, or independently of each other.

GENETICS

Genetics rarely plays a significant factor in the occurrence of clinical toxicosis in domestic animals.

INCIDENCE/PREVALENCE

The incidence, prevalence, case-fatality rate, and mortality rate vary with each specific toxicant.

GEOGRAPHIC DISTRIBUTION

The occurrence of specific toxicoses can vary depending on geographic location and weather conditions, as well as agricultural and management practices.

SIGNALMENT

• Some toxicants can have an age predilection, most often related to eating habits (and, therefore, dose ingestion) or to management practices.
• Very few toxicoses are related to breed or gender.

SIGNS

General Comments

• Establishing the diagnosis of poisoning often is difficult and the importance of a complete history and physical examination cannot be overstated.
• Thorough record keeping is necessary because of the possibility of legal action, especially if a poisoning results from a faulty product or the negligence of others.

Historical

• Establishing the history of the problem may be difficult and can require finesse by the veterinarian.
• The client may already be convinced that poisoning has occurred, even though the onset of clinical signs is only coincidental with exposure of the animal to a particular substance.
• Clients may not be forthcoming with complete information if they feel guilty because poisoning resulted from their own mistakes. Conversely, clients may give biased information if they believe poisoning resulted from a faulty product, the negligence of others, or suspected malicious intent.
• The clinician should determine how many animals are at risk of poisoning and how many are actually affected.
• Current or past health problems and treatments may reveal factors that can affect toxicity and influence therapeutic recommendations.
• Collect detailed information regarding the current poisoning situation—clinical signs, date of onset, time of onset, and treatments given by the owner.
• Determine how and when the animal was exposed to the toxicant.
• Record the full label name of the product, the manufacturer, the lot number, and the active ingredients, including their concentrations. If the product is a pesticide, record the EPA registration number.
• If a potential adverse reaction to a therapeutic agent is involved, record the lot or batch number, determine if the product was used according to the manufacturer's recommendations, and determine the amount of exposure to the product.

Physical Examination

• Clinical signs vary with the different toxicants.
• Not all potential signs are seen in every animal.

CAUSES

Substances that cause poisoning are discussed in the specific chapter regarding that toxicant.

RISK FACTORS

• The risk of developing toxicosis depends on the toxicity of the substance, exposure dose, exposure type (e.g., acute, multiple, chronic), and exposure route (e.g., dermal, oral, inhaled, injected).
• Individual risk factors may include age, breed, sex, reproductive status, body condition, weight, previous health status, and current treatments.

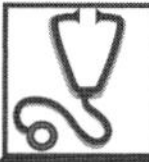

DIAGNOSIS

DIFFERENTIAL DIAGNOSIS

• First, attempt to determine if the illness actually resulted from a poisoning rather than from a medical or surgical disease. The diagnosis may be obvious from a quick history and physical examination but usually requires more thorough investigation by the clinician.
• The foremost consideration in confirming a diagnosis of poisoning is to establish that clinical signs or lesions are compatible with a toxic exposure to a specific toxicant.
• The list of differential diagnoses varies with different toxicants. Resources to assist veterinarians in diagnosing toxicoses include diagnostic laboratories and the ASPCA National Animal Poison Control Center.

CBC/BIOCHEMISTRY/URINALYSIS

These tests are often helpful in defining the cause of the problem and in determining the course of treatment.

OTHER LABORATORY TESTS

• Laboratory confirmation can be made for many toxicants via sample submission to diagnostic laboratories.
• Collect whole blood, serum, and urine from live animals and liver, kidney, brain, fat, urine, and GI contents from dead animals.
• Toxicologic testing can rarely be performed on samples preserved in formalin; thus, samples for toxicology testing (except whole blood) should be frozen. However, routine post-mortem samples should be collected and put in formalin for histologic examination to help narrow the differential list.
• Collect samples of feed, water, and any suspected source material; other samples also may be necessary to confirm a diagnosis, depending on the toxicant.
• Always contact the laboratory for specific information regarding submission protocols, because incorrect samples, inadequate sample size, and improper sample storage are common causes of diagnostic testing failures.

IMAGING

N/A

OTHER DIAGNOSTIC PROCEDURES

N/A

PATHOLOGICAL FINDINGS

• Gross and histopathological findings vary depending on the specific toxicant.
• Some toxicants cause nonspecific lesions.

POISONING (INTOXICATION) – GENERAL PRINCIPLES

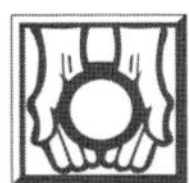

TREATMENT

AIMS OF TREATMENT

- With a life-threatening situation, immediately provide life support by maintaining respiratory and cardiac function. Control seizures if they occur.
- Once the animal is stabilized, institute symptomatic and supportive care.
- Decontaminate the animal as appropriate. Remove the animal from the toxic source so that further exposure does not occur.

APPROPRIATE HEALTH CARE

The type, the duration, and the intensity of medical management vary with each toxic incident.

NURSING CARE

- Maintain adequate hydration if necessary. Control acid-base imbalances if they occur.
- Maintain proper body temperature. Seizures or tremors can result in elevated temperatures. Conversely, severely depressed or comatose animals may have low body temperatures.
- With a dermal route of exposure, bathe the animal with mild dishwashing detergent. People who are washing and handling the animal should take measures (e.g., wearing gloves) to prevent self-exposure.
- With an ocular route of exposure, lavage the eye with copious amounts of water or normal saline.

ACTIVITY

The amount of activity to be allowed or encouraged varies with each toxic incident.

DIET

Dietary restrictions or additions vary with each toxic incident.

CLIENT EDUCATION

Client discussions will vary with each toxic incident.

SURGICAL CONSIDERATIONS

N/A

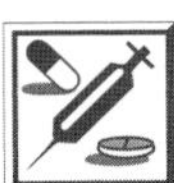

MEDICATIONS

DRUG(S) OF CHOICE

- Few poisons have specific antidotes.
- Relevant medications and antidotes are discussed in those sections dealing with the specific toxicants.
- Many toxicants are adsorbed by AC, thereby reducing the amount of toxicant absorbed from the GI tract. AC binds many organic compounds but is relatively ineffective against inorganic compounds (e.g., heavy metals). Mix the AC (1–4 g/kg) with warm water to form a slurry. Follow the AC with a laxative to hasten removal of the toxicant from the intestinal tract. The efficacy of mineral oil for treating intoxicated patients has not been established and its use is discouraged for routine GI decontamination.
- Some toxicants are eliminated primarily by the fecal route or undergo enterohepatic recirculation. AC followed by a laxative is the most effective means for increasing elimination of these toxicants.
- Many toxicants are eliminated by the kidneys, and in some cases, renal excretion can be enhanced by increasing urine output via fluid administration. Diuretics can be used to increase urine flow—furosemide (1 mg/kg IV); mannitol (0.25–2.0 g/kg as 20% solution by slow IV infusion).
- Manipulating the urine pH also can increase the excretion of some toxicants in the urine via ion trapping. Weak acids are ionized in alkaline urine, whereas weak bases are ionized in acidic urine. The normal range of urine pH in adult herbivores is alkaline, ranging from 7 to 9.

CONTRAINDICATIONS

N/A

PRECAUTIONS

- Toxicants typically are metabolized and/or excreted by the liver, GI tract, and/or kidneys. Select medications that will minimally affect these systems.
- Before administering oral products, determine that the horse is not exhibiting gastric reflux.
- Cathartics can result in significant diarrhea; therefore, ensure that the horse is adequately hydrated.

POSSIBLE INTERACTIONS

N/A

ALTERNATIVE DRUGS

- Magnesium sulfate (Epsom salts) is an osmotic laxative that draws water into the intestines. The recommended dose is 250–500 mg/kg mixed in several liters of water.
- Sorbitol 70% (3 mL/kg) or sodium sulfate (250–500 mg/kg mixed in several liters of water) is an alternative cathartic.

FOLLOW-UP

PATIENT MONITORING

Potential sequelae vary with the toxicant and severity of the poisoning and are discussed in those sections dealing with specific toxicants.

PREVENTION/AVOIDANCE

Minimize the risk of intoxication by using medications and pesticides according to the label directions, storing all chemicals safely, and identifying and removing all potentially toxic plants in the animal's environment.

POSSIBLE COMPLICATIONS

The type and severity of complications as well as potential sequelae will vary with each toxic incident.

EXPECTED COURSE AND PROGNOSIS

Prognosis will vary with the type of toxicant, dose received, and onset of treatment, as well as individual and environmental factors.

MISCELLANEOUS

ASSOCIATED CONDITIONS

Laminitis is a possible secondary condition to any severe disease in horses.

AGE-RELATED FACTORS

The effect of age will vary with the specific toxicant.

ZOONOTIC POTENTIAL

N/A

PREGNANCY

- Abortion or teratogenic disease may be a concern in pregnant mares depending on the toxicant and stage of pregnancy at the time of exposure.
- Some poisons can affect the fertility of mares or stallions.

SYNONYMS

Discussed in those chapters dealing with specific toxicants

SEE ALSO

Chapters dealing with specific toxicants

ABBREVIATIONS

- AC = activated charcoal
- GI = gastrointestinal

Suggested Reading

Galey FD. Diagnostic toxicology. In: Plumlee KH, ed. Clinical Veterinary Toxicology. St. Louis: Mosby, 2004.

Oehme FW. General principles in treatment of poisoning. In: Robinson NE, ed. Current Therapy in Equine Medicine, ed 2. Philadelphia: WB Saunders, 1987.

Poppenga RH. Treatment. In: Plumlee KH, ed. Clinical Veterinary Toxicology. St. Louis: Mosby, 2004.

Author Konnie H. Plumlee

Consulting Editor Robert H. Poppenga

POLYCYTHEMIA

BASICS

DEFINITION

• An increase in the circulating RBC (erythrocyte) mass, reflected by increases in RBCs and hemoglobin and PCV greater than the upper limits of laboratory reference values
• Increase in circulating RBC mass may be relative or absolute.

PATHOPHYSIOLOGY

Relative Polycythemia

• May be caused by hemoconcentration or splenic contraction
• Hemoconcentration results from a reduction in the plasma volume without a concomitant reduction in circulating RBC numbers. It is associated with either dehydration or fluid shifts between fluid compartments of the body.
• Common causes of hemoconcentration include dehydration association with reduced water intake, diarrhea, renal failure, diuresis or excessive sweating. Endotoxemia is a common cause of a shift in water from the plasma space to the interstitium.
• Splenic contraction (e.g., excitement, exercise) results in a transient polycythemia due to release of stored RBCs into the circulation. The spleen can store up to one third of the mature RBC volume and contraction may increase the PCV by up to 50% for several hours dependent on the stimulus.

Absolute Polycythemia

• An increase in circulating RBC mass without change in the plasma volume
• Increased erythropoiesis causes an increase in RBC count, hemoglobin concentration and PCV.
• May be primary or secondary
• Primary absolute polycythemia is an increase in the RBC mass associated with normal PO_2 and a normal or reduced EPO concentration. It is due to a myeloproliferative disorder of the bone marrow.
• Secondary absolute polycythemia results from increased erythropoiesis due to an increased synthesis of EPO that may be appropriate (response to tissue hypoxia; low PO_2) or inappropriate (excessive EPO or other hormone production and normal PO_2).

SYSTEMS AFFECTED

• Cardiovascular
• Hemic
• Pulmonary
• Hepatobiliary
• Nervous
• Renal
• Gastrointestinal

INCIDENCE/PREVALENCE

• Relative polycythemia is common in animals with cardiovascular/hemodynamic compromise and when blood is collected from horses that have been exercised or are excited.
• Absolute polycythemia is uncommon/rare.

GEOGRAPHIC DISTRIBUTION

• Horses kept at altitudes >2200 m (7200 feet) are likely to have appropriate secondary absolute polycythemia.

SIGNALMENT

Breed Predilections

• There are no breed predilections.
• Reference values for RBC count, hemoglobin concentration and PCV vary with breed; values are greater for light horse (i.e., hot-blooded) breeds (Thoroughbreds, Standardbreds, Arabians, and Quarter Horses) than draft (i.e., cold-blooded), pony and miniature breeds and donkeys.

Mean Age and Range

• Animals of any age can develop polycythemia.
• Reference values for RBC count, hemoglobin concentration and PCV of newborn foals are similar to adults, however values decrease rapidly after birth and take several months to increase.

SIGNS

General Comments

• Signs of relative polycythemia are associated with the primary disease process including signs of dehydration and impaired tissue perfusion.
• Signs of absolute polycythemia vary dependent on the degree of increase in RBC mass and any underlying condition.

Historical

• Relative polycythemia from splenic contraction may include a history of excitement, exercise, administration of catecholamines.
• Relative polycythemia from fluid shifts is dependent on underlying disease process.
• Absolute polycythemia may include a history of hemorrhagic diathesis, weight loss, lethargy, and inappetence.

Physical Examination

• Prolonged CRT, dry mucous membranes, cool extremities, reduced skin turgor, and reduced mentation may be observed in horses with relative polycythemia from fluid shifts.
• Mucosal hyperemia (dark red to purple in color), prolonged CRT, lethargy, epistaxis, melena, and laminitis may be observed in horses with absolute polycythemia.
• Abnormal mentation, tachycardia and tachypnea may be observed when PCV >60% as increased blood viscosity impairs tissue oxygenation.
• Cardiac murmur, tachycardia and other signs of cardiac disease may be observed if a congenital cardiac defect is present.
• Tachypnea, abnormal brochovesicular sounds, dyspnea may be observed if chronic pulmonary disease is present.

CAUSES

Relative Polycythemia

• Inadequate water consumption may be caused by dysphagia (altered prehension or swallowing—many causes), restricted access, or altered mentation.
• Increased fluid losses may be caused by diarrhea, diuretic therapy, polyuric renal failure, diabetes inspidus, excessive sweating, anterior enteritis, peritoneal or pleural effusion, metritis, ileus, or endotoxemia.
• Internal fluid shifts may be caused by endotoxemia, SIRS, musculoskeletal trauma, hyponatremia.
• Splenic contraction may be caused by exercise, excitement, administration of α_1-adrenegic agonists (epinephrine, phenylephrine).

Absolute Polycythemia

• Primary absolute polycythemia is an exceptionally rare myeloproliferative disorder that may occur as a single cell disorder or as a component of polycythemia vera (concurrent thrombocytosis and leukocytosis).
• Appropriate secondary absolute polycythemia is associated with congenital cardiac defects with right to left shunting (e.g., tetralogy of Fallot, pulmonary atresia with VSD, persistent truncus arteriosus, tricuspid atresia), chronic pulmonary disease and residence at high altitude.
• Inappropriate secondary absolute polycythemia is an exceptionally rare syndrome from inappropriate EPO, EPO-like protein or androgenic hormone secretion (associated with hepatocellular carcinoma, hepatoblastoma, metostatic carcinoma, or lymphoma) or administration of exogenous androgens. In other species, chronic nephropathies (tumors, cysts, or hydronephrosis) may result in increased EPO production.

Miscellaneous

• Administration of exogenous EPO
• Syndrome of red cell hypervolemia in Swedish Standardbred trotters has been reported.

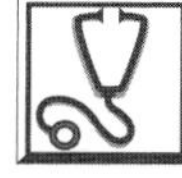

DIAGNOSIS

DIFFERENTIAL DIAGNOSIS

• Primary polycythemia is diagnosed on the exclusion of relative or secondary polycythemia.
• Laboratory error—insufficient centrifugation of a blood sample can result in an artificially high PCV.

CBC/BIOCHEMISTRY/URINALYSIS

• RBC count, hemoglobin concentration, and PCV values are greater than upper limit of laboratory reference ranges.
• Hyperproteinemia usually accompanies relative polycythemia from hemoconcentration unless protein loss occurs concurrently (e.g., diarrhea, glomerulonephritis, peritonitis, or pleuritis) whereby normal or reduced protein concentrations may be present.
• Mild thrombocytosis may accompany relative polycythemia from splenic contraction.
• Neutropenia, left shift, and toxic changes in neutrophils also may be reported in response to endotoxemia/SIRS.
• Increased hepatic enzymes may be present in cases of inappropriate secondary absolute polycythemia associated with hepatic neoplasia.

OTHER LABORATORY TESTS

• PaO_2 to differentiate between appropriate and inappropriate secondary absolute polycythemia
• Blood concentrations of EPO may assist in the diagnosis of inappropriate secondary absolute polycythemia.

• Detection of α-fetoprotein in blood is consistent with hepatic neoplasia (heptocellular carcinoma or hepatoblastoma).

IMAGING

• Echocardiography for detection of congenital cardiac defects
• Tracheal aspiration, bronchoalveolar lavage, thoracic ultrasonography and radiography, and pulmonary function testing to detect lung disease
• Renal and hepatic ultrasonography

OTHER DIAGNOSTIC PROCEDURES

• Liver biopsy if evidence of hepatic disease
• Renal biopsy if evidence of renal disease
• Bone marrow aspirate/biopsy for detection of myeloproliferative disorders

PATHOLOGICAL FINDINGS

Dependent on cause of polycythemia

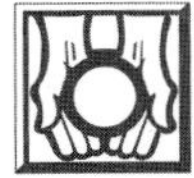

TREATMENT

AIMS OF TREATMENT

• Treatment of underlying disorder
• Reduction of RBC parameters to within normal laboratory range

APPROPRIATE HEALTH CARE

• Relative polycythemia from splenic contraction requires no treatment.
• Relative polycythemia from dehydration requires inpatient medical management. Once condition is stabilized, outpatient medical management can be recommended.
• Absolute polycythemia requires inpatient medical management.

NURSING CARE

• Relative polycythemia from dehydration requires IV fluid therapy. If protein loss is concurrent, colloid therapy may be necessary.
• Appropriate secondary absolute polycythemia requires oxygen therapy. If chronic pulmonary disease is present, corticosteroids and bronchodilators may be of benefit.
• Absolute polycythemia may require phlebotomy if PCV remains >50%, where 10–20 mL of blood/kg is removed and replaced by equivalent volume of polyionic crystalloid solution. Phlebotomy is repeated every 2–3 days until PCV <50% and then as required.
• Phlebotomy is contraindicated in relative polycythemia.
• Phlebotomy should be used with caution in polycythemia associated with hypoxia as the increased RBC mass is a compensatory mechanism for tissue hypoxia. If performed, phlebotomy should be less pronounced and the PCV necessary to satisfy tissue oxygen without complications is determined by careful monitoring.

ACTIVITY

In cases of absolute polycythemia, activity should be restricted as persistent polycythemia can result in hypertension, tissue hypoxia, thrombosis, and hemorrhage.

CLIENT EDUCATION

Response to treatment is dependent on the underlying cause. Most cases of absolute polycythemia have a poor to hopeless prognosis.

SURGICAL CONSIDERATIONS

Increased blood viscosity associated with marked absolute polycythemia may result in sludging of blood cells in small vessels and hypoxia, increasing the risk of anesthesia associated complications.

MEDICATIONS

DRUG(S) OF CHOICE

• Hydroxyurea causes reversible bone marrow suppression including reduced erythropoiesis and has been used successfully to treat polycythemia is humans and dogs.
• The use of hydroxyurea in horses has not been reported and appropriate dosage is unknown.
• A suggested protocol for dogs is 30 mg/kg PO once daily for 7–10 days, then a maintenance dose of 15 mg/kg PO once daily.

PRECAUTIONS

There are no reports of use of hydroxyurea in horses.

FOLLOW-UP

PATIENT MONITORING

• Monitor PCV, total plasma protein and clinical parameters of hydration status 3–4 times daily in dehydrated animals to monitor response to fluid therapy. If possible monitor bodyweight also as this reflects total body fluid balance.
• In cases of absolute polycythemia, PCV should be monitored initially every 2–3 days, particularly if phlebotomy is performed. Thereafter, measure PCV as required.

POSSIBLE COMPLICATIONS

Absolute polycythemia can increase viscosity of blood with an increased risk of tissue hypoxia, thrombosis, hemorrhage, and hypertension.

EXPECTED COURSE AND PROGNOSIS

• Relative polycythemia from splenic contraction resolves within hours.
• Most cases of relative polycythemia associated with fluid shifts resolve with appropriate IV fluid therapy; however, cardiovascular shock may be more refractory to treatment.
• Primary absolute polycythemia has a hopeless prognosis.
• Most cases of secondary absolute polycythemia have a poor to grave prognosis, except compensation to residency at high altitude.
• Syndrome of red cell hypervolemia in Swedish Standardbred trotters is associated with poor performance; however, horses are otherwise healthy.

MISCELLANEOUS

AGE-RELATED FACTORS

RBC count, hemoglobin concentration, and PCV in foals decrease rapidly after birth.

PREGNANCY

RBC count, hemoglobin concentration, and PCV tend to increase during pregnancy.

SYNONYMS

Erythrocytosis

SEE ALSO

• Congenital heart disease
• Endotoxemia
• Myeloproliferative disorders

ABBREVIATIONS

• CRT = capillary refill time
• EPO = erythropoietin
• PaO_2 = partial pressure of oxygen in arterial blood
• PCV = packed cell volume (hematocrit)
• PO_2 = partial pressure of oxygen in tissues
• RBC = red blood cell
• SIRS = systemic inflammatory response syndrome

Suggested Reading

Collatos C. Polycythemia. In Robinson NE, ed. Current Therapy in Equine Medicine, ed 5. St. Louis: Saunders, 2003:358.

Funkquist P, Sandhagen B, Persson SG et al. Effects of phlebotomy on haemodynamic characteristics during exercise in standardbred trotters with red cell hypervolaemia. Equine Vet J 2001;33:417–424.

Koch TG, Wen X, Bienzle D. Lymphoma, erythrocytosis and tumor erythropoietin gene expression in a horse, J Vet Intern Med 2006;20:1251–1255.

Lennox TJ, Wilson JH, Hayden DW, et al. Hepatoblastoma with erythrocytosis in a young female horse. J Am Vet Med Assoc 2000;216:718–721.

Sellon DC. Disorders of the hematopoietic system. In: Reed SM, et al., eds. Equine Internal Medicine, ed 2. St Louis: Saunders, 2004;721–768.

Author Kristopher Hughes
Consulting Editors Jennifer Hodgson and David Hodgson

POLYNEURITIS EQUI

BASICS

OVERVIEW

- Granulomatous inflammatory condition involving the extradural nerve roots of the cauda equina and often cranial nerves, which in at least some conditions may be immune mediated.
- Used to be known as "cauda equina neuritis" because it can present with only cranial nerve signs

SIGNALMENT

No age or sex predilection; not usually seen in the very young or very old

SIGNS

- Clinical signs usually include retention of feces, urine retention or incontinence, loss of tone of tail and anus, and analgesia of the tail and perineum.
- Abnormalities in the pelvic limb gait and muscle wasting are less often seen.
- Analgesia of the perianal skin may be surrounded by a zone of hyperaesthesia.
- The cranial nerves most often affected include VIII (head tilt), XII (tongue weakness), V (masseter atrophy and weakness), IX and X (difficulty swallowing), and III (depressed pupillary light reflex).
- Clinical signs generally progress more slowly than in typical EHV-1 cases and only rarely are horses ataxic.
- Lesions may progress to involve lumbar plexus, leading to pelvic limb weakness (initially subtle and asymmetric).

CAUSES AND RISK FACTORS

The cause is unknown, but it is thought to be predominantly an immune-mediated event that may be initiated by viral and/or bacterial infections.

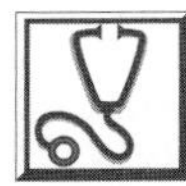

DIAGNOSIS

DIFFERENTIAL DIAGNOSIS

- Sacral fractures—far more common than PNE—Rule out using rectal palpation, radiography, and scintigraphy.
- EHV-1 myelopathy—tends have a more acute onset, stabilizes more rapidly, and responds well to treatment. May need CSF tap cytology and viral titers to differentiate.
- Equine protozoal myeloencephalitis—serum and CSF Western blot analysis, IFAT or ELISA

CBC/BIOCHEMISTRY/URINALYSIS

Most often normal—may be reflective of any secondary disease or complications that may have occurred, such as dehydration due to impaction colic or urinary tract infection due to urinary retention.

OTHER LABORATORY TESTS

Lumbosacral CSF tap to rule out EPM. CSF may be difficult to obtain from the lumbosacral area due to the space-occupying nature of the lesions.

IMAGING

Scintigraphy and radiography to help rule out sacral fractures

PATHOLOGIC FINDINGS

- Necropsy is the only way to reach a definitive diagnosis.
- Cauda equina and cranial nerves become thickened and covered with fibrous material.
- Granulomatous inflammation includes infiltrates of inflammatory cells, including neutrophils, lymphocytes, and macrophages. Axonal degeneration and myelin degeneration in the cauda equina and cranial nerves. Inflammation classically stops abruptly at the CNS/PNS border.

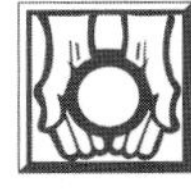

TREATMENT

- Supportive
- If cranial nerve signs are present and animals are having difficulty eating, may have to feed mash—bran mash if fecal retention is a problem; otherwise, can use complete feed or other feed for mash
- May have to evacuate feces manually
- Some horses can be maintained for a long time with supportive care, but the disease is relentlessly progressive.

MEDICATIONS

- Antibiotics for secondary urinary tract infections
- Anti-inflammatory drugs are ineffective in the long term.

FOLLOW-UP

Follow progress of hypalgesia in tail region.

PATIENT MONITORING

- Monitor for choke, impaction colic, fecal and urinary incontinence

EXPECTED COURSE AND PROGNOSIS

Disease usually progresses, and long-term prognosis is poor.

MISCELLANEOUS

ASSOCIATED CONDITIONS

- None

AGE-RELATED FACTORS

- Adult horses

ZOONOTIC POTENTIAL

- None

PREGNANCY

- N/A

SEE ALSO

- EHV-1
- Protozoal myeloencephalitis

ABBREVIATIONS

- CNS = central nervous system
- CSF = cerebrospinal fluid
- EHV-1 = equine herpesvirus 1
- ELISA = enzyme-linked immunosorbent assay
- EPM = equine protozoal myeloencephalitis
- IFAT = immunofluorescence antibody test
- PNE = polyneuritis equi
- PNS = peripheral nervous system

Suggested Reading

Divers TJ, Mayhew IG. Neurology. Clin Tech Equine Pract 2006;5(1).

Hahn CN, Mayhew IG, MacKay RJ, The nervous system. In: Collahan PT, Mayhew IG, Merritt AM, Moore JN, eds. Equine Medicine and Surgery, ed 5. St. Louis: Mosby, 1999.

The author and editors wish to acknowledge the contribution of S. G. Witonsky, author of this chapter in the previous edition.

Author Caroline N. Hahn

Consulting Editor Caroline N. Hahn

POLYSACCHARIDE STORAGE MYOPATHY

BASICS

OVERVIEW

• PSSM is one form of chronic exertional rhabdomyolysis most often found in Quarter Horse–related breeds. • It is an inherited metabolic myopathy characterized by increased glycogen concentrations and abnormal polysaccharide inclusions in skeletal muscle. • Affected horses have increased insulin sensitivity, increased glycogen synthesis, and enhanced uptake of glucose by muscle.

SYSTEMS AFFECTED

• Endocrine/metabolic • Neuromuscular • Renal

SIGNALMENT

• 2- to 4-year-old Quarter Horses • Can affect foals • PSSM has been reported in other breeds, common in Draft Horses and Warmbloods

SIGNS

In Quarter Horses

• Episodes of "tying-up" occur shortly after the onset of exercise characterized by muscle stiffness, sweating, and reluctance to move. • Excessive sweating, tachypnea, tachycardia, muscle fasciculations, tucked-up abdomen, camped-out stance, firm painful lumbar and gluteal muscles, gait asymmetry, and hindlimb stiffness • Episodes may be subclinical to severe with recumbency and renal failure. • Numerous episodes and poor performance • +/− Pawing or rolling, may resemble colic • +/− Rapid muscle atrophy after concurrent respiratory disease in some Quarter Horses

In Draft Horses

• Variable clinical signs from normal to weakness and recumbency • Muscle soreness • Generalize muscle atrophy • Exertional rhabdomyolysis • Hindlimb weakness, difficulty rising, reluctance to back up • Gait abnormalities such as shivers

CAUSES

Hereditary basis +/− environmental influence (e.g., high-starch diet, lack of exercise)

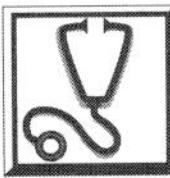

DIAGNOSIS

DIFFERENTIAL DIAGNOSIS

• Clinical signs of PSSM are not specific for the disease. Confirmation is achieved by elimination of other differentials and muscle biopsy.
• Differentials:
  ○ Sporadic or chronic exertional rhabdomyolysis
  ○ Non–exercise-associated rhabdomyolysis, e.g., infectious and immune-mediated myopathies (*Clostridium* sp., influenza, *Streptococcus equi,* sarcocystis), nutritional myodegeneration, traumatic myopathy, idiopathic pasture myopathy and toxic muscle damage, e.g., monensin, white snake root ingestion
  ○ Colic
  ○ Laminitis—Rule out with radiography.
  ○ Lameness
  ○ Pleuropneumonia—Rule out with imaging
  ○ Aorto-iliac thrombosis—Rule out with imaging.
  ○ Tetanus
  ○ HYPP—Rule out with DNA analysis.
  ○ Neurologic diseases resulting in recumbency or reluctance to move

CBC/BIOCHEMISTRY/URINALYSIS

• CK, LDH, AST elevations (usually >10,000 U/L) after exercise • Persistently elevated CK • Myoglobinuria • +/− Azotemia • In severe disease, high potassium and low sodium and chloride serum concentrations • +/− CK, AST, LDH elevation in Drafts

OTHER LABORATORY TESTS

• Serum vitamin E and whole blood selenium to rule out deficiency • Fractional excretion of urine electrolytes

OTHER DIAGNOSTIC PROCEDURES

• Muscle (semimembranosus/tendinosus) biopsy—detection of abnormal polysaccharide inclusions • Submaximal exercise test—Measure serum CK before 15 min of walk and trot and 4–6 hr after exercise. Abnormal response is indicated by >3- to 4-fold increase in CK.

PATHOLOGICAL FINDINGS

Muscle biopsy histopathology— subsarcolemmal vacuoles, dark periodic acid-Schiff staining for glycogen, and amylase-resistant (abnormal) polysaccharide accumulation

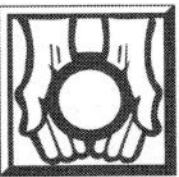

TREATMENT

• In acute episodes, oral and/or intravenous balanced polyionic fluids +/− electrolytes, analgesia, and rest • Daily turnout, gradual return to consistent exercise • Dietary management—Forage at 1.5% to 2% of body weight, limiting starch to <10% of daily digestible energy by eliminating grain and replacing it with a fat supplement. Caloric needs should be assessed to prevent obesity. Corn or soy oil may be added to alfalfa pellets, rice bran, or other commercial pelleted rations developed for exertional rhabdomyolysis with a low-starch, high-fat content.

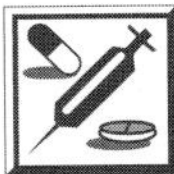

MEDICATIONS

DRUGS

• NSAIDs—phenylbutazone (4.4 mg/kg IV or PO q12 h for 1 day followed by 2.2 mg/kg PO q12 h) or flunixin meglumine (0.5–1.1 mg/kg IV or PO q12–24h) • Acepromazine (0.04–0.11 mg/kg IV or IM q8–12 h) • +/− Detomidine (0.005–0.02 mg/kg IV or IM) • +/− Methocarbamol (40–60 mg/kg PO daily) • +/− Intravenous dimethyl sulfoxide (<10% solution)

CONTRAINDICATIONS/POSSIBLE INTERACTIONS

• NSAIDs are contraindicated in dehydration or myoglobinuria. • Acepromazine is contraindicated in dehydration.

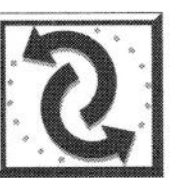

FOLLOW-UP

PATIENT MONITORING

• Effectiveness of treatment is judged by improvement in signs. • Frequent monitoring of clinical signs, especially during abrupt exercise/training changes • Serum CK activity (resting or 4 hours postexercise) can be measured prior to restarting exercise and during reintroduction of exercise. • If myoglobinuria is present, renal parameters should be monitored for evidence of renal dysfunction. • If the patient appears depressed or inappetent after an acute episode, acute renal failure should be suspected and treated promptly to reduce the potential for chronic renal compromise.

PREVENTION/AVOIDANCE

Strict adherence to a low-starch, fat-supplemented diet and provision of regular daily exercise and turnout appear to be the best way to avoid exertional rhabdomyolysis associated with PSSM.

POSSIBLE COMPLICATIONS

• The disease has a genetic basis (probable dominant expression with incomplete penetrance) in Quarter Horses, and therefore owners should be counseled regarding the breeding of animals affected with PSSM.

EXPECTED COURSE AND PROGNOSIS

• In acute severe disease, renal failure, recumbency, and death are possible. • With proper dietary and exercise management, prognosis is good to excellent for athletic endeavors.

MISCELLANEOUS

ASSOCIATED CONDITIONS

• Severe rapid muscle atrophy after concurrent respiratory disease in Quarter Horses • Severe rhabdomyolysis not associated with exercise in Quarter Horse foals

AGE-RELATED FACTORS

Clinical signs and rhabdomyolysis may be observed in foals at 1 day of age; however, muscle biopsy analysis may not reveal abnormal histological characteristics until 12 months of age or later.

SEE ALSO

• Exertional rhabdomyolysis syndrome • HYPP • Colic in foals

ABBREVIATIONS

• AST = aspartate aminotranferase • CK = creatine phosphokinase • HYPP = hyperkalemic periodic paralysis • LDH = lactate dehydrogenase • PSSM = polysaccharide storage myopathy

Suggested Reading

Valberg SJ, Hodgson DR. Diseases of muscle. In: Smith BP, ed. Large Animal Internal Medicine, ed 3. St. Louis: Mosby, 2002:1266–1291.

Author Anna M. Firshman
Consulting Editor Elizabeth J. Davidson

POLYURIA (PU) AND POLYDIPSIA (PD)

BASICS

DEFINITION

• PU—urine output >50 mL/kg per day
• PD—fluid intake >100 mL/kg per day

PATHOPHYSIOLOGY

• Production of concentrated or dilute urine requires generation of the interstitial concentration gradient from the renal cortex to the inner medulla, dilution of tubular fluid in the thick ascending limp of the loop of Henle and distal tubule (diluting segment of the nephron that has low water permeability), and presence or absence of water channels in the collecting ducts (controlled by ADH activity).
• Modest increases in plasma tonicity (≅3 mOsm/kg) stimulate production and release of ADH by the posterior pituitary gland and insertion of aquaporins (water channels) in the luminal membrane of collecting duct epithelial cells leading to increased water permeability and reabsorption. • Decreases in plasma tonicity inhibit ADH release and insertion of aquaporins. As a result, collecting ducts become less permeable to water, and dilute urine is produced. • Transient PU may be an effect of fluid or drug administration (e.g., furosemide and other diuretic agents) or a consequence of loss of the medullary concentration gradient—medullary washout • Persistent PU is generally associated with a number of disease processes—CRF, Cushing's disease, DI, diabetes mellitus, and endotoxemia. • There are two important stimuli for thirst—an increase in plasma tonicity and hypovolemia. • PD may be a physiologic response to PU (to prevent dehydration), a consequence of drug administration (e.g., corticosteroids), or a primary problem of excessive water intake. In horses, the latter problem usually is behavioral in origin (primary PD) but may also accompany excessive salt intake. • Urine production and water consumption vary with age, diet, workload, environmental temperature, and GI water absorption.

SYSTEMS AFFECTED

• Renal/urologic—excessive urine production
• Endocrine/metabolic—CD; diabetes mellitus
• Nervous—central DI

GENETICS

Unknown—familial nephrogenic DI in TB colts

INCIDENCE/PREVALENCE

CD may affect up to 15% of horses >20 years of age.

SIGNALMENT

Breed Predilections

CD appears more common in Morgan horses and ponies.

Mean Age and Range

• Foals consuming a predominantly milk diet (<2 mo of age) normally are polyuric. Daily fluid intake may approach 250 mL/kg per day (5-fold greater than adults), and a USG <1.008 is normal. • CD occurs in older horses and ponies.

Predominant Sex

Familial nephrogenic DI in TB colts

SIGNS

General Comments

PU/PD is often a primary complaint by owners. Affected horses may appear otherwise healthy or have other clinical signs of CD or mild to moderate weight loss with CRF.

Historical

• Horses with mild to moderate PU/PD often go undetected by owners, or the horse may stop to urinate while being ridden or have excessive thirst after exercise. • With more substantial PU/PD (e.g., with primary PD), the magnitude of PU typically is dramatic, with owners reporting that horses drink 2- to 3-fold more water and that stalls can be flooded with urine.
• Horses with acquired DI may have a recent history of medical problems or treatment with a potentially nephrotoxic medication.

Physical Examination

Consistent with the underlying disease processes (e.g., CRF, Cushing's disease) or normal (e.g., primary PD, excessive salt ingestion)

CAUSES

Primary PD

• Primary or "psychogenic" PD probably is the most common cause of PU/PD in adults. • The cause is unknown; however, in some horses it appears to be a stable vice, while in others it may develop after a change in management (e.g., stabling, diet, interaction with other horses, or medication administration).

Excessive Salt Consumption

"Psychogenic salt eaters" appear to be less common than primary PD; salt intake may have to exceed 5%–10% of dry matter intake before PU/PD becomes apparent.

Drug Administration

Administration of enteral or IV fluids, diuretics, α_2-agonists, and corticosteroids

CRF

• These horses cannot concentrate urine beyond the isosthenuric range (specific gravity, 1.008–1.014). • The degree of PU is modest compared to primary PD or DI, so it is a client complaint only in ≅ 50% of affected horses.

CD

• An osmotic diuresis when plasma glucose concentration exceeds the renal threshold, leading to glucosuria • Antagonism of the action of ADH on collecting ducts by cortisol • A primary dipsogenic effect of excessive cortisol
• Compression of the posterior pituitary by growth of an adenoma leading to central DI

DI

• May occur because of inadequate secretion of ADH (neurogenic or central DI) or decreased sensitivity of the epithelial cells of the collecting ducts to circulating ADH (nephrogenic DI).
• An acquired form of central DI has been described in horses and is idiopathic or secondary to encephalitis or other diseases accompanied by dehydration, endotoxemia, or administration of potentially nephrotoxic medications. • Nephrogenic DI has been described in sibling TB colts, suggesting an inherited form may occur.

Diabetes Mellitus

A state of chronic hyperglycemia accompanied by glucosuria resulting in an osmotic diuresis.

Sepsis/Endotoxemia

• PU/PD occasionally is observed in horses with sepsis or endotoxemia. • The mechanism is unclear but may result from endotoxin-induced prostaglandin production. Prostaglandin E_2 is a potent renal vasodilating agent that also can antagonize the effects of ADH.

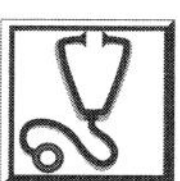

DIAGNOSIS

DIFFERENTIAL DIAGNOSIS

N/A

CBC/BIOCHEMISTRY/URINALYSIS

• CRF—mild anemia, azotemia, isosthenuria, and electrolyte and acid-base alterations in more advanced cases; see Chronic Renal Failure.
• CD—Mild anemia and a stress leukogram are characteristic CBC findings. Hyperglycemia and mild increases in hepatic enzyme activity may be found in more advanced cases. Glucosuria may be present. • Primary PD and DI—CBC and serum chemistry results are normal, but USG typically is <1.005. Fractional sodium clearance is increased (>1%) when excessive salt intake is the cause. • Diabetes mellitus—Hyperglycemia and glucosuria are present.
• Sepsis/endotoxemia—CBC and serum chemistry abnormalities reflect the underlying disease process.

OTHER LABORATORY TESTS

• Appropriate diagnostic tests for CD (see Cushing's disease) • Measurement of fractional sodium clearance (fractional excretion of sodium) in horses with primary PD
• Measurement of plasma ADH concentration would be useful in cases of DI to differentiate neurogenic (low ADH) from nephrogenic (high ADH when dehydrated) forms, but this assay is not commercially available.

IMAGING

Transabdominal/transrectal ultrasonography—to assess kidney size and echogenicity (should be normal, except with CRF)

OTHER DIAGNOSTIC PROCEDURES

• Overnight water deprivation is the most useful test to determine ability to concentrate urine. Horses with primary PD should concentrate urine to a specific gravity of 1.020–1.025; horses with CRF and DI fail to concentrate urine.
• Approach water deprivation cautiously in horses with suspected DI, and do not perform when azotemia is detected (with CRF). Measure body weight before water deprivation; extending the test beyond the time needed to lose 5% of body weight (may be <12 hr in horses with DI) has no benefit. • Horses were suspected to have DI because they failed to concentrate urine during water deprivation. Administration of desmopressin acetate (DDAVP, 0.1 mg/mL solution can be diluted in sterile water and 0.05 mg/kg can be administered intravenously for this

purpose) can be used to differentiate neurogenic DI (will concentrate urine to >1.020) from nephrogenic DI (will not concentrate urine).

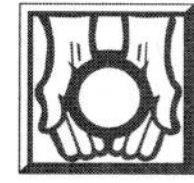

TREATMENT

AIMS OF TREATMENT

• Address underlying condition (CD, CRF).
• Provide appropriate availability of salt and water.

APPROPRIATE HEALTH CARE

• CRF—See Chronic Renal Failure. • CD—medical treatment (pergolide) with other necessary supportive care (nutrition, hoof care and analgesia for laminitis, antibiotics for secondary infections, etc.) • Primary PD—gradual restriction of water intake (initially to 100 mL/kg per day, which is approximately twice maintenance needs in a temperate climate, followed by a decrease to 75 mL/kg per day after several days) with careful monitoring of body weight and hydration status along with "trial and error" management changes; removal of supplemental salt when excessive consumption is the cause of PD • DI—mild water restriction (to 100 mL/kg per day with careful monitoring of body weight and hydration status) and use of medications may help in limiting PU/PD; discontinue water restriction if dehydration or >5% loss of body weight occurs. • Diabetes mellitus—exogenous insulin replacement therapy • Sepsis/endotoxemia—appropriate antibiotic treatment and supportive care (including judicious fluid therapy) for the underlying disease process

NURSING CARE

Long-term survival of horses with CD likely improves with close monitoring, prompt recognition, and appropriate treatment of complications—flare-ups of laminitis and secondary infections.

ACTIVITY

May increase activity to modify behavior of horses with psychogenic PD; otherwise normal activity

DIET

• See Chronic Renal Failure for dietary recommendations in horses with CRF. • Horses with CD usually are aged and may have dental disorders, requiring feeding of complete pelleted senior rations. • Increasing the amount of forage in the diet may help to decrease excessive water intake by horses with primary PD. • Limit availability of supplemental salt to horses with excessive salt consumption as the cause of primary PD.

CLIENT EDUCATION

• Inform clients that provision of adequate fresh water at all times is imperative to prevent dehydration with all pathological causes of PU/PD. • Horses with primary PD may need "trial and error" management changes (e.g., increasing turn-out time, increasing exercise, provision of a stablemate or other diversions in the stall) along with gradual water restriction. • When excessive salt consumption is the cause of PD, removing salt availability usually is corrective. • The magnitude of PU/PD with inherited forms of DI may be reduced with mild salt and water restriction and medical therapy. With acquired forms of DI, especially nephrogenic DI from reversible renal disease or drug treatment, PU/PD may last for weeks to months but often may resolve over time. • Some horses with diabetes mellitus are managed successfully with insulin replacement therapy, but most have a guarded to poor prognosis for long-term survival. Inform owners of the indications for euthanasia—loss of appetite and body condition; progressive weakness

SURGICAL CONSIDERATIONS

None

MEDICATIONS

DRUG(S) OF CHOICE

CD

The dopamine agonist pergolide (2–6 μg/kg PO q24 h) is the drug of choice.

DI

• With neurogenic DI, hormone replacement therapy with desmopressin (a potent ADH analogue administered as eye drops) has been successful in small-animal patients but has not been described in horses and may be cost prohibitive. • With nephrogenic DI, replacement hormone therapy is ineffective; the only practical treatment is to restrict sodium and water intake and to administer thiazide diuretics.

Diabetes Mellitus

Insulin replacement therapy in horses with low serum insulin concentrations (type 1 diabetes mellitus)

CONTRAINDICATIONS

Gradual water restriction is contraindicated in horses with CRF, CD, diabetes mellitus, or sepsis/endotoxemia.

PRECAUTIONS

• Perform water restriction with caution in horses with primary PD and DI to avoid significant dehydration. • Insulin therapy in diabetes mellitus could result in hypoglycemia.

FOLLOW-UP

PATIENT MONITORING

• Closely monitor water intake, urine output, USG in all patients with PU/PD to minimize the risk of dehydration; horses with DI are at greatest risk of developing significant dehydration, even during short periods (hours) of water deprivation. • See Chronic Renal Failure for specific follow-up recommendations in horses with CRF. • See Cushing's Disease for specific follow-up recommendations in horses with this condition.

POSSIBLE COMPLICATIONS

Moderate to severe dehydration may develop when horses with CRF, DI, or diabetes mellitus are unintentionally deprived of water for short periods.

EXPECTED COURSE AND PROGNOSIS

The course and prognosis for horses with PU/PD depend on the underlying cause. Horses with primary PD or excessive salt consumption generally respond rapidly and favorably with management changes. In contrast, horses with CRF, DI, and diabetes mellitus have a more guarded to poor long-term prognosis, while horses with CD can be effectively managed for years with appropriate treatment and management.

MISCELLANEOUS

ASSOCIATED CONDITIONS

• CRF • Cushing's disease • Diabetes mellitus

AGE-RELATED FACTORS

• During the first 2 mo of life, foals consuming a predominantly milk diet normally are polyuric.
• CD occurs in older horses and ponies.

SEE ALSO

• CRF • Cushing's syndrome

ABBREVIATIONS

• ADH = antidiuretic hormone
• CD = Cushing's disease
• CRF = chronic renal failure
• DI = diabetes insipidus
• PU = polyuria
• PD = polydipsia
• USG = urine specific gravity
• TB = Thoroughbred

Suggested Reading

Browning AP. Polydipsia and polyuria in two horses caused by psychogenic polydipsia. Equine Vet Educ/AE 2000;2:231–236.

Genetzky RM, Loparco FV, Ledet AE. Clinical pathological alterations in horses during a water deprivation test. Am J Vet Res 1987;48:1007–1011.

McKenzie EC. Polyuria and polydipsia in horses. Vet Clin North Am Equine Pract 2007;23:641–654.

Schott HC, Bayly WM, Reed SM, Brobst DF. Nephrogenic diabetes insipidus in sibling colts. J Vet Intern Med 1993;7:68–72.

Schott HC. Polyuria and polydipsia. In: Reed SM, Bayly WM, Sellon DC, eds. Equine Internal Medicine, ed 2. Philadelphia: WB Saunders, 2004:1276–1283.

Author Harold C. Schott II
Consulting Editor Gillian A. Perkins

POSTPARTUM METRITIS

BASICS

DEFINITION/OVERVIEW

- Acute metritis resulting from retained fetal membranes or contamination of the uterus after parturition or dystocia
- Marked by concurrent septicemia/endotoxemia and, possibly, laminitis

ETIOLOGY/PATHOPHYSIOLOGY

- Because of difficult foaling, retained fetal membranes, or heavy bacterial contamination of the uterus during foaling, coupled with septicemia/endotoxemia, the uterus is flaccid and thin walled compared with the normal involuting uterus (thick walls and longitudinal rugae are present as it rapidly involutes postpartum).
- Accumulated fluid and debris provide favorable conditions for bacterial growth, inflammation, and toxin release.
- Toxins are easily absorbed into the maternal circulation (i.e., endotoxemia) because of the highly vascularized and thin-walled postpartum uterus.

SYSTEMS AFFECTED

- Reproductive
- Hemic/lymphatic/immune
- Musculoskeletal

GENETICS

N/A

INCIDENCE/PREVALENCE

N/A

SIGNALMENT

- Postpartum mare
- Signs of abdominal pain or depression after dystocia, retained fetal membranes, or extensive intrapartum uterine contamination
- Also can occur after normal delivery if a mare does not exercise
  - Exercise aides in the clearance of postpartum debris and fluid accumulation.
  - A mare's need to exercise is often compromised if she has a foal with a limb deformity that necessitates restriction of exercise for the foal.

SIGNS

- Metritis may become evident by 12–24 hr post-partum, characterized by depression, abdominal pain, and anorexia.
- Depression is suggestive of shock or endotoxemia.
- Fever, elevated pulse and respiratory rate, and congested or toxic mucous membranes
- Uterus is enlarged, flaccid, and baggy from accumulation of fetid, dark-red to chocolate-colored fluid. The fetid odor can be striking in its severity.
- Attachment of retained fetal membranes usually at/in the previously nongravid horn. The retained fetal membranes may either be composed of a large portion of the total placenta and be seen hanging through the vulvae or be limited to only a small piece of the remaining placenta.
- Signs of laminitis (e.g., bounding digital pulses, lameness) may appear 12 hr to 5 days postpartum.

CAUSES AND RISK FACTORS

- Mares with a history of placentitis, retained fetal membranes, dystocia, abortion, prolonged or assisted delivery, fetotomy, or cesarean section are at greater risk of postpartum metritis.
- Postpartum complications depend on the amount and type of bacteria in the reproductive tract. Postpartum metritis is often associated with a dirty foaling environment or excessive manipulation at parturition.
- Aerobic gram-negative and gram-positive bacteria such as *Streptococcus zooepidemicus* and other β-hemolytic streptococci, *Staphylococcus* sp., *Escherichia coli, Pseudomonas aeruginosa,* and *Klebsiella pneumoniae* are frequently involved.
- The gram-positive anaerobe *Bacteroides fragilis* resides in the external genitalia of mares and stallions and is periodically introduced into the uterus by coitus or genital pathologies such as pneumovagina and vagino/cervical damage. Spontaneous or iatrogenic (i.e., excess manipulation) mucosal breakdown and necrotic tissue create favorable conditions for this bacterium's overgrowth.
- Autolytic retained fetal membranes, in concert with bacterial contamination, initially result in endometritis which progresses to the deeper layers; the end result is metritis.
- Metritis, left untreated, can lead to systemic illness—septicemia, endotoxemia, and laminitis.

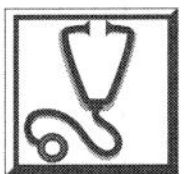

DIAGNOSIS

DIFFERENTIAL DIAGNOSIS

Other Causes of Postpartum Abdominal Pain/Depression

- Normal uterine involution and placental expulsion
- Uterine artery rupture, with or without internal hemorrhage—A clot forms between the myometrium and serosa; the uterus/broad ligament usually is enlarged and painful at palpation. The hematocrit may be normal or decreased. If the clot is not contained within the broad ligament (rupture of the broad ligament), abdominocentesis may reveal increased RBCs, PMNs, and some bacteria.
- Uterine torsion
- Uterine rupture may be difficult to identify at TRP. Abdominocentesis reveals PMN, bacteria, and elevated protein.
- Rupture of cecum or right ventral colon; strong abdominal contractions during parturition can rupture or bruise the large bowel if it is distended by gas or ingesta or if it becomes trapped between the uterus and the pelvis. Abdominocentesis reveals ingesta in the peritoneal cavity.

Other Causes of Postpartum Vaginal Discharge

Normal postpartum (≤6 days postpartum) lochia—odorless, dark red-brown vaginal discharge associated with a palpable, normally involuting uterus, with thickening and corrugation (i.e., TRP description) of uterine wall

CBC/BIOCHEMISTRY/URINALYSIS

- Marked leukopenia (≤2000 cells/μL) with toxic PMNs and left shift. Response to treatment is evaluated by the return of WBCs to normal values (5000–12,000 cells/μL).
- Fibrinogen may increase to ≥500 mg/dL during the acute phase but usually returns to normal values (≤400 mg/dL) 2–3 days after WBC count returns to the normal range.

OTHER LABORATORY TESTS

- Bacterial identification—Obtain a sample of uterine contents using a guarded swab. Plate the sample on blood and McConkey's agar. Blood agar will support growth of gram-positive, select gram-negative, and some yeasts, whereas McConkey's will only support growth of gram-negative organisms. Incubate plates at 37° C and examine at 24 and 48 hr.
- For anaerobes, streak swabs onto two Wilkins-Chalgren anaerobe agar plates and incubate in an atmosphere of 10% hydrogen, 10% CO_2, and 80% N_2 at 37° C and examine at 24 and 48 hr.
- Since diagnosis of *Bacteroides fragilis* is difficult, when conditions are present that support its growth (i.e., necrotic tissue, lacerations), assume it may be contributory.
- The presence of large numbers of mixed flora is expected from a uterine swab taken from normal postpartum mares.
- Collect a uterine culture before instituting antibiotic therapy, if possible, but do not wait for culture results before beginning treatment. Initiate treatment immediately with broad-spectrum antibiotics, metronidazole, IV fluids, and anti-endotoxic doses of anti-inflammatory drugs if metritis is suspected based on clinical signs, CBC, history of dystocia, retained fetal membranes (≥8–12 hr), or contamination/trauma has occurred. Adjust therapy when the culture and sensitivity results are available, switching to other, more appropriate antibiotics, if indicated.

IMAGING

U/S

- Large amounts of fluid may accumulate in the uterus 24–48 hr postpartum.
- Degree of echogenicity generally relates to the amount of debris or inflammatory cells in the fluid, but "clear" fluid can be misleading.
- Uterine wall appears thick and edematous.

OTHER DIAGNOSTIC PROCEDURES

N/A

PATHOLOGICAL FINDINGS

Postpartum acute inflammatory response extending from the endometrium to the deeper regions (i.e., stratum compactum, stratum spongiosum, to and including the myometrium [full-thickness, uterine wall disease]); contrast with endometritis and routine uterine infections/reaction in the mare, which are limited to the endometrium and luminal infections.

POSTPARTUM METRITIS

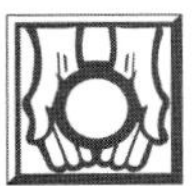

TREATMENT

APPROPRIATE HEALTH CARE

- Endotoxemia is prevented/treated by IV fluids for circulatory support and anti-endotoxic doses of flunixin meglumine. Polymyxin-B is used to neutralize circulating endotoxins.
- Administer systemic, broad-spectrum antibiotics and metronidazole to control uterine bacterial overgrowth and to prevent endotoxemia.
- Only after the mare is medically stable should removal of the source of infection (i.e., retained placenta, infected uterine fluid) be addressed; a critical point in the management of this condition. Uterine manipulation in the face of acute postpartum metritis (fever, systemic illness) may guarantee absorption of endotoxins from the uterus; and increase the likelihood of death by endotoxemia.
- Once medically stable, evacuate bacteria and inflammatory debris from the uterine lumen by uterine lavage with large volumes of warm saline solution. Three to 6 L is infused at each treatment period through a sterile nasogastric tube; uterine contents then are siphoned off, and the lavage is repeated until the recovered fluid is clear. Repeat 1–3 times daily based on TRP and U/S findings. Administer oxytocin routinely to aid uterine evacuation or if fluid remains after lavage.
- Finding a thickened, corrugated uterine wall at palpation indicates a positive response to treatment and stimulation of uterine involution.
- Unresponsive mares have flaccid, thin uterine walls and accumulate large amounts of fluid between treatments. Treatment is discontinued when intrauterine fluid is clear or slightly cloudy.
- Begin with a smaller volume (1 L) if a uterine tear is suspected. Finding fluid accumulation ventrally within the uterine lumen is one indicator that a tear is not present on the ventral aspect of the uterus.
- See Laminitis.

NURSING CARE

N/A

ACTIVITY

Exercise—turn out twice a day.

DIET

N/A

CLIENT EDUCATION

N/A

SURGICAL CONSIDERATIONS

N/A

MEDICATIONS

DRUG(S)OF CHOICE

Fluids

- Use polyionic solutions, e.g., Normosol.
- Estimate dehydration based on clinical signs (e.g., skin turgor), hematocrit (normal, 32%–53%), and total protein (normal, 5.7– 7.9 g/dL).
- Calcium gluconate (125 mL of 23% solution) and oxytocin (40 IU) may be added to every other 5-L bag of Normosol.
- Mild colic or discomfort will result from uterine contractions stimulated by treatment.
- Discontinue or slow the rate of administration if signs of severe colic occur.

Systemic Antibiotics

- Potassium penicillin for gram-positive organisms—loading dose of 44,000 IU IV, followed by 22,000 IU IV QID
- Combine with gentamicin for gram-negative organisms—2.2 mg/kg IV QID or 6.6 mg/kg IV daily
- For oral administration, use 15 mg/kg of trimethoprim sulfa (broad-spectrum) BID.
- Metronidazole, for anaerobes, should always be combined with IV or PO therapy—loading dose of 15 mg/kg PO, followed by 7.5 mg/kg PO QID or 15 to 25 mg/kg PO BID.

Uterotonic Drugs

- Oxytocin—Multiple protocols have been proposed and used.
  - 10 IU IV or 20 IU IM after uterine lavage
  - 40 IU added to IV fluids
  - 10 IU IV QID

NSAIDs

- Flunixin meglumine (Banamine)—anti-endotoxic dose, 0.25 mg/kg IV or IM TID; anti-inflammatory dose, 1.1 mg/kg IV or IM BID
- Phenylbutazone—4.4 mg/kg IV or PO BID; at the onset of laminitis, recommended loading dose is 8.8 mg/kg IV.
- Polymyxin B—administer 6000 U/kg IV in 1 L of sterile saline over 30–60 min; recommended BID for 1–2 days

CONTRAINDICATIONS

N/A

PRECAUTIONS

- NSAIDs may cause bone marrow dyscrasia and GI ulceration.
- Aminoglycosides can be nephrotoxic and ototoxic; ensure good hydration during treatment.
- Polymyxin B—potentially nephrotoxic at therapeutic doses
- Dehydration and NSAID administration may potentiate the nephrotoxicity associated with aminoglycosides and polymixin B.
- Metronidazole can decrease appetite in a number of circumstances. If it decreases appetite, then milk production in postpartum mares could be affected.

POSSIBLE INTERACTIONS

N/A

ALTERNATIVE DRUGS

See Laminitis.

FOLLOW-UP

PATIENT MONITORING

- Monitor CBC every 48–72 hr for signs of endotoxemia or response to treatment.
- See Laminitis.
- Monitor for signs of laminitis by early and repeated evaluation of digital pulses, signs of weight shift, and radiographs of the distal phalanx, rotation or sinking of P3.
- Monitor for postpartum constipation or post-surgical/dystocia ileus. Mineral oil (0.5–1.0 gallon) or bran mash may be used to prevent or treat ileus; fluid therapy also is helpful.

PREVENTION/AVOIDANCE N/A

POSSIBLE COMPLICATIONS

- Delayed uterine involution
- Mare will often be recumbent—to keep sternal support with bales; adjust positioning multiple times per day to avoid developing pressure sores.
- Septicemia/endotoxemia
- Laminitis
- Death

EXPECTED COURSE AND PROGNOSIS

- Prognosis depends on severity, duration, and secondary complications caused by metritis.
- Rapid response to therapy indicates a favorable prognosis.
- Laminitis after endotoxemia carries a guarded to grave prognosis.

MISCELLANEOUS

ASSOCIATED CONDITIONS, AGE-RELATED FACTORS, ZOONOTIC POTENTIAL, PREGNANCY N/A

SYNONYMS

- Metritis/laminitis/septicemia complex
- Toxic metritis

SEE ALSO

Delayed uterine clearance
Dystocia
Endometritis
Laminitis
Retained fetal membranes
Uterine torsion

ABBREVIATIONS

- CBC = complete blood count
- P3 = third phalanx
- PMN = polymorphonuclear leukocyte/WBC
- RBC = red blood cell
- TRP = transrectal palpation
- US = ultrasound/ultrasonography
- WBC = white blood cell

Suggested Reading

Asbury AC. Care of the mare after foaling. In: MacKinnon AO, Voss JL, eds. Equine Reproduction. Philadelphia: Lea & Febiger, 1993:976–980.

Ricketts SW, Mackintosh ME. Role of anaerobic bacteria in equine endometritis. J Reprod Fertil Suppl 1987;35:345–351.

Threlfall WR, Carleton CL. Treatment of uterine infections in the mare. In: Morrow DA, ed. Current Therapy in Theriogenology. Philadelphia: WB Saunders, 1986:730–737.

Author Maria E. Cadario
Consulting Editor Carla L. Carleton

POTASSIUM, HYPERKALEMIA

BASICS

OVERVIEW

• Potassium is the major intracellular cation in biological systems. • It plays a major role in determining the resting membrane potential of excitable tissue. • It is readily absorbed by the gastrointestinal tract in health (typically in excess of body need), and the average equine diet is potassium-rich. • Excretion of excess potassium from dietary intake is performed by the kidney, preventing potentially toxic hyperkalemia in health. • The quantity of potassium in the ECF is less than 2% of the total body potassium; as such, plasma potassium evaluation is a poor assessment of bodywide potassium status.
• However, since the ratio of ICF-to-ECF potassium concentration is critical in determining the resting membrane potential, changes in plasma potassium concentration can have marked effects on excitable tissue (muscle and nervous tissue). • *Hyperkalemia* is defined as an elevated concentration of potassium in the plasma. Precise numerical values defining hyperkalemia depend on the reference laboratory performing the assay. In general, values greater than 5.0 mmol/L are considered elevated. • The two largest clinically significant body potassium stores are erythrocytes and skeletal muscle; disorders of these tissues may perturb plasma potassium levels.

SYSTEMS AFFECTED

• Musculoskeletal • Cardiovascular

SIGNALMENT

• No sex predisposition • Certain common causes of hyperkalemia show age and/or breed predisposition.
  ○ Uroperitoneum in young foals
  ○ Hyperkalemic periodic paralysis (HYPP) in stock breeds (American Quarter Horse, American Paint Horse, Appaloosa)

SIGNS

• Skeletal muscle weakness
  ○ Fasciculations ○ Stiffness, myotonia ○ Staggering gait ○ "Dog-sitting" ○ Collapse
• Bradycardia, other cardiac dysrhythmias
• Sweating, anxiety • Sudden death

CAUSES AND RISK FACTORS

• Strenuous exercise—causes transient hyperkalemia, usually resolves shortly post work
• Likely reflects lactic academia that develops during exercise, but myocytes also leak potassium • Potassium may be responsible for peripheral vasodilation during exercise, increasing blood flow to skeletal muscle.
• Rhabdomyolysis (or any condition which results in severe, diffuse cellular injury/necrosis, resulting in leakage of large amounts of intracellular potassium)
• Intravascular hemolysis (severe)
• Hyperkalemic periodic paralysis—major cause of intermittent hyperkalemia in horses of stock breeds descended from the sire Impressive
• Laboratory error/poor sample handling—"pseudohyperkalemia" caused by leakage of intracellular potassium from erythrocytes and/or platelets; samples should be spun and removed from clot as soon as possible after collection to avoid this problem.
• Acidemia—intracellular translocation of interstitial fluid hydrogen ion in exchange for intracellular potassium results in elevation of plasma potassium concentration.
  ○ Usually mild to moderate elevation in plasma potassium ○ Affected horses likely to have total-body potassium *depletion* due to primary disease
• Renal insufficiency/failure
  ○ Inconsistent finding, as affected animals may be hypokalemic, eukalemic, or hyperkalemic ○ Anuria/oliguria more likely to produce clinically significant hyperkalemia.
• Iatrogenic—aggressive parenteral supplementation may cause dangerous hyperkalemia.
• Uroperitoneum—postrenal obstruction, decreased potassium clearance
• Hyperosmolality • Renal tubular acidosis

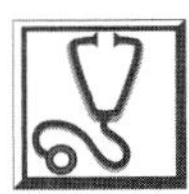

DIAGNOSIS

CBC/BIOCHEMISTRY/URINALYSIS

Biochemistry = increased potassium concentration (>5.0 mmol/L)

OTHER LABORATORY TESTS

• Arterial blood gas analysis may reveal acidemia.

IMAGING

May be useful in diagnosis of underlying cause

OTHER DIAGNOSTIC PROCEDURES

• Electrocardiography
  ○ Peaked, tented T waves ○ Decreased Q-T interval ○ Decreased amplitude of P waves, may progress to atrial standstill ○ Widened QRS complexes ○ Sinus bradycardia ○ Changes may be seen when plasma potassium level exceeds 6 mEq/L. ○ Changes are marked with plasma potassium level greater than 8 mEq/L. ○ Plasma potassium level >9–10 mEq/L often fatal
    • Ventricular fibrillation • Asystole

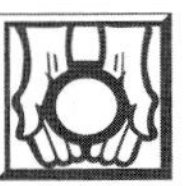

TREATMENT

• Definitive treatment depends on the underlying cause, which should be pursued diagnostically.
• Hyperkalemia should be addressed as an emergency; however, the necessity of hospitalization depends somewhat on the underlying cause. • Diuresis with potassium-free polyionic fluid may be helpful (e.g., 0.9% NaCl).
  ○ In mild cases, this may be all that is required to resolve the hyperkalemia. ○ More severe cases require additional emergency medical treatment (see below).
  ○ Use caution in anuric/oliguric patients with renal disease underlying the hyperkalemia.
• Hyperkalemia should be treated and the patient stabilized prior to induction of general anesthesia to minimize cardiovascular and musculoskeletal complications (especially regarding neonates with vesicular rupture).
○ Hyperkalemic patients should be offered potassium-poor diets; alfalfa hay, and concentrate feeds containing molasses should be avoided.

MEDICATIONS

DRUG(S)

• Calcium gluconate
  ○ Can use 0.2–0.4 mL/kg of 23% solution diluted in 1–2 L 5% dextrose, administered slowly
  ○ Calcium is cardioprotective and may be life-saving in cases with signs or evidence of cardiac effects (e.g., ECG changes).
• Dextrose/insulin
  ○ Insulin causes rapid intracellular translocation of potassium. ○ Dextrose induces endogenous insulin release, and is much safer and more convenient for field use than insulin. ○ Oral source may be given in emergency (oats, light corn syrup) but is not appropriate alone for severe cases. ○ Intravenous dextrose preferred (5%, 4.4–6.6 mL/kg; 1–2 L for 450-kg horse)
• Sodium bicarbonate
  ○ Use care—rapid alkalinization of patients with metabolic academia may result in acute, profound hypokalemia. ○ 1–2 mEq/kg IV as isotonic solution
• Diuretics
  ○ Acetazolamide (2–4 mg/kg PO q12h) is a potassium-wasting, carbonic anhydrase inhibitor diuretic that may be effective for managing horses with HYPP.

CONTRAINDICATIONS/POSSIBLE INTERACTIONS

Do not administer sodium bicarbonate with calcium-containing fluids.

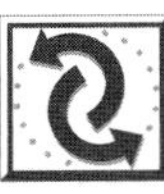

FOLLOW-UP

PATIENT MONITORING

• ECG monitoring (until normalized) ○ Serial evaluation of serum potassium concentration

PREVENTION/AVOIDANCE

• Depends on underlying cause • Preventive measures are described for horses with HYPP (see "HYPP" in this volume)

POSSIBLE COMPLICATIONS

• Cardiac dysrhythmias with resultant hemodynamic compromise • Sudden death

EXPECTED COURSE AND PROGNOSIS

Highly dependent on underlying cause

MISCELLANEOUS

SEE ALSO

• Hypokalemia • HYPP • Uroperitoneum

ABBREVIATIONS

• ECF = extracellular fluid • ECG = electrocardiography • ICF = intracellular fluid • HYPP = hyperkalemic periodic paralysis

Suggested Reading

Johnson PJ. Electrolyte and acid-base disturbances in the horse. Vet Clin North Am Equine Pract 1995;11:491–514.

Author Teresa A. Burns
Consulting Editor Kenneth W. Hinchcliff

POTASSIUM, HYPOKALEMIA

BASICS

OVERVIEW

• Potassium is the major intracellular cation in biological systems. • It plays a major role in determining the resting membrane potential of excitable tissue. • Readily absorbed by the gastrointestinal tract in health (typically in excess of body need); the average equine diet is potassium-rich, easily providing the daily requirement of 23 g for an adult horse.
  ○ Alfalfa hay—13 lb. provides 145 g potassium
  ○ Grass hay (average)—16 lb. provides 121 g potassium
  ○ Trace mineral salt—2 oz. provides 145 g potassium
• Excretion of excess potassium from dietary intake is performed by the kidney, preventing potentially toxic hyperkalemia in health.
• Renal conservation of potassium is nonspecific and inefficient, developing over the course of several days in horses with decreased dietary potassium intake and/or excessive potassium losses. This aspect of potassium physiology increases risk of clinically significant hypokalemia in horses with inappetence or potassium-wasting diseases. • Disorders involving this cation are relatively common in hospitalized horses.
• The quantity of potassium in the ECF is less than 2% of the total body potassium; as such, plasma potassium evaluation is a poor assessment of *body-wide* potassium status.
• However, since the *ratio* of ICF-to-ECF potassium concentration is critical to determining the resting membrane potential, changes in plasma potassium concentration can have marked effects on excitable tissue (muscle and nervous tissue). • *Hypokalemia* is defined as a decreased potassium concentration in serum, usually less than 2.5 mEq/L (depends on reference values of laboratory performing the assay). • May be due to total body potassium deficit, or, more likely, may reflect a shift in potassium distribution between ECF and ICF
• Hypokalemia is uncommon in horses with normal feed intake.

SIGNS

• Usually noted when serum potassium concentration falls below 1.8 mEq/L
• Musculoskeletal weakness • Collapse
• Arrhythmia (ventricular premature beats, ventricular tachycardia) • Sudden death (malignant ventricular arrhythmia)
• Gastrointestinal ileus

CAUSES AND RISK FACTORS

• Alkalemia (any cause)—extracellular potassium is exchanged for intracellular hydrogen ion in an attempt to restore acid-base equilibrium. • Profuse sweating (equine sweat contains high concentration of potassium)
• Polyuric renal failure (uncommon) • Renal tubular acidosis (types 1 and 2) • Decreased dietary intake (inappetence for any reason)
• Gastrointestinal loss
  ○ Diarrhea
  ○ Nasogastric reflux (persistent small intestinal functional or mechanical obstruction)
• Iatrogenic (administration of certain medications)
  ○ Sodium bicarbonate
  ○ Dextrose-containing fluids
  ○ Insulin
  ○ Prolonged parenteral nutrition

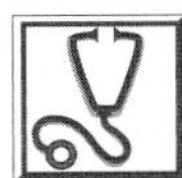

DIAGNOSIS

DIFFERENTIAL DIAGNOSIS

• Muscular weakness—underlying myopathy, other electrolyte, acid-base abnormalities (such as hypocalcemia, hypomagnesemia)
• Cardiac arrhythmia—underlying cardiomyopathy (rare), other electrolyte, acid-base abnormalities

CBC/BIOCHEMISTRY/URINALYSIS

• CBC—may be helpful for identification of underlying disease (e.g., neutropenia with toxic changes in patients with enterocolitis)
• Serum biochemistry—evidence of underlying disease may be present; other electrolyte abnormalities, such as hypomagnesemia and hypocalcemia, may be noted concurrently and may exacerbate clinical signs of hypokalemia. • Urinalysis—fractional clearance of potassium is variably affected; depends somewhat on primary disease

OTHER LABORATORY TESTS

Arterial blood gas analysis may reveal alkalemia.

OTHER DIAGNOSTIC PROCEDURES

• Electrocardiography
  ○ Peaked P waves
  ○ Decreased amplitude of T waves
  ○ Increased QRS duration
  ○ Ventricular ectopic rhythms (VPCs, ventricular tachycardia)

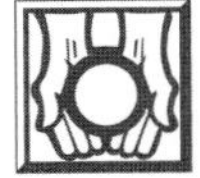

TREATMENT

• Definitive treatment of underlying cause is required. • A potassium-rich diet should be offered (e.g., alfalfa hay). • Oral supplementation with potassium chloride is typically sufficient in mild cases (trace mineral supplement, oral electrolyte pastes, etc.).
  ○ 25–40 g/day via nasogastric tube in divided doses
• Parenteral supplementation is required for severe cases, particularly if the patient is inappetent.
  ○ Potassium chloride supplementation of intravenous fluids (20–40 mEq/L; no more than 0.5 mEq/kg/hour to avoid potentially dangerous hyperkalemia)

MEDICATIONS

DRUG(S) OF CHOICE

Potassium chloride (see above)

CONTRAINDICATIONS/POSSIBLE INTERACTIONS

• Supplemental potassium should be given with caution in patients with known renal insufficiency; careful monitoring of serum potassium concentration should be performed in these horses. • Medications that may exacerbate hypokalemia should be avoided.
  ○ Sodium bicarbonate
  ○ Glucose/dextrose and insulin
  ○ Diuretics (acetazolamide, furosemide)

FOLLOW-UP

PATIENT MONITORING

• Serial assessment of serum potassium concentration • ECG monitoring should be continued until the trace normalizes.

PREVENTION/AVOIDANCE

• Assess serum potassium concentration in patients with diseases commonly associated with hypokalemia; supplement as necessary.
  ○ Enterocolitis
  ○ Renal insufficiency
  ○ Exhaustion/profuse sweating
  ○ Prolonged anorexia

POSSIBLE COMPLICATIONS

• Cardiac arrhythmias (especially idioventricular rhythms) • Sudden death
• Gastrointestinal ileus, colic • Predisposition to exertional rhabdomyolysis/myopathy

EXPECTED COURSE AND PROGNOSIS

Referable to underlying disease

MISCELLANEOUS

SEE ALSO

• Renal failure • Duodenitis/proximal jejunitis • Alkalosis

ABBREVIATIONS

• ECF = extracellular fluid
• ECG = electrocardiography
• ICF = intracellular fluid

Suggested Reading

Johnson PJ. Electrolyte and acid-base disturbances in the horse. Vet Clin North Am Equine Pract 1995;11:491–514.

Johnson PJ, Goetz TE, Foreman JH, Vogel RS, Hoffmann WE, Baker GJ. Effect of whole-body potassium depletion on plasma, erythrocyte, and middle gluteal muscle potassium concentration of healthy, adult horses. Am J Vet Res 1991;52:1676–1683.

Author Teresa A. Burns

Consulting Editor Kenneth W. Hinchcliff

POTOMAC HORSE FEVER (PHF)

BASICS

DEFINITION

PHF is an acute and potentially fatal enterotyphlocolitis of horses caused by infection with the monocytotropic rickettsia *Neorickettsia risticii* (formerly known as *Ehrlichia risticii*).

PATHOPHYSIOLOGY

- The pathophysiology of PHF is poorly understood. *N. risticii* is an obligate intracellular, gram-negative bacteria with a predilection for blood monocytes and tissue macrophages. Within days of infection, *N. risticii* can be found in blood monocytes. *N. risticii* survives within phagosomes in macrophages by inhibiting phagosome–lysosome fusion. The neoricketsemia persists throughout the disease.
- The pathogen has a predilection for the cecum and large colon, but is occasionally found in the jejunum and small colon. Colonic and small intestinal epithelial cells, colonic mast cells, and macrophages are the targets of infection. Mild cases of PHF without diarrhea have evidence of colitis. It is possible that many pathophysiologic changes observed in horses with PHF are secondary to effects of altered colonic flora.

SYSTEMS AFFECTED

- Gastrointestinal—predominantly cecum and large colon
- Cardiovascular—dehydration and shock may develop in severe cases.
- Reproductive—occasional cause of abortion

GENETCS

N/A

INCIDENCE/PREVALENCE

In Ohio, 13%–20% of horses on racetracks had serologic evidence of exposure to *N. risticii,* although only 10%–20% of the seropositive horses had clinical signs of the disease.

Geographic Distribution

PHF has been reported from 43 states in the United States, three provinces in Canada (Alberta, Nova Scotia, Ontario), South America (Brazil, Uruguay), Europe (France, The Netherlands), and India.

SIGNALMENT

All breeds and all ages may be affected. Horses younger than 1 year rarely develop PHF. Clinical cases of PHF occur sporadically, with rarely more than 5% of horses on any one affected farm. Only in a significant epizootic infection does the attack rate on individual farms become high (20%–50%).

SIGNS

There is a considerable variation in the severity of the clinical manifestations of PHF. The majority of clinical disease appears to be mild or subclinical. In overt clinical illness, the manifestation of colitis is common in all cases. Not all cases show colic or diarrhea.

- Depression (90%)
- Anorexia (80%)
- Fever (70%)—initially a transient fever of 39.4°–41.1° C (103°–106° F) followed in 3–7 days by a second, more persistent febrile episode
- Ileus (70%)—decreased intestinal sounds. Signs of ileus are one of the most consistent clinical findings.
- Mild to severe GI signs, ranging from mild colic and soft manure to profuse diarrhea
- Diarrhea (≈60%)—mild to severe, watery, pipe-stream diarrhea present in 45%–60% of cases. Course of diarrhea ranges from 1 to 10 days.
- Mild colic (30%) often accompanies diarrhea.
- Congested mucous membranes (70%)
- Dehydration
- Laminitis develops in about 20%–25% of PHF cases.
- Mortality rate from PHF—5%–30%
- Some horses show only mild signs of anorexia, depression, and fever.
- Clinical course is usually 5–10 days without treatment.
- Infrequent abortion may occur.

CAUSES AND RISK FACTORS

Causes

- Infection with *N. risticii*, an obligate intracellular gram-negative bacteria. Different strains of *N. risticii* have been identified; not all appear to be pathogenic.
- *N. risticii* DNA has been found in trematodes (virgulate cercariae) that parasitize freshwater snails in endemic areas (confirmed in northern California, central Ohio, and central Pennsylvania). In northern California, the number of snails harboring the trematode stages varied from 3% to 93%.
- During periods of warm water temperatures, cercariae infected with *N. risticii* are released from the snails, infecting and developing into metacercariae in the second intermediate host, aquatic insects, such as caddis flies, mayflies, damselflies, dragonflies, and stoneflies. Aquatic insects may represent a major source of infection because of their abundance in the natural environment and the mass hatches regularly observed during the summer and fall. Experimentally one horse fed adult caddis flies developed PHF.
- Under natural conditions, horses grazing near rivers or creeks could conceivably be exposed to *N. risticii* through skin penetration by infected cercariae in water, or ingest metacercariae in a second intermediate host such as an aquatic insect along with grass, consume adult insects trapped on the water surface, or consume adult insects that are attracted by stable lights or accumulate in feed and water. DNA of *N. risticii* has been found in adult trematodes, which infect the intestines of bats, birds, and amphibians.
- There is no evidence for the spread of PHF by arthropod vectors.

Risk Factors

Endemic areas have been identified. *N. risticii* infection has been strongly associated with rivers or other aquatic habitats. Increased risk of PHF is associated with horses grazing pastures bordering waterways (freshwater rivers, streams, irrigation ditches, etc.); horses coming from an area with a high PHF prevalence or a farm with history of PHF; or travel to an area with a high incidence of PHF.

Season

There is a seasonal pattern in temperate climates. Most clinical cases of PHF occur in mid to late summer. In the Northern Hemisphere, the majority of clinical PHF cases occur between July and September.

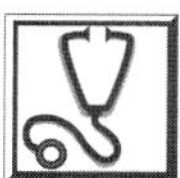

DIAGNOSIS

DIFFERENTIAL DIAGNOSIS

Differential diagnoses include all other causes of enterocolitis—acute salmonellosis, clostridial colitis, cyathostomes (small strongyles), antibiotic-induced colitis, intestinal ileus secondary to displacement or obstruction, NSAID toxicity, cantharidin toxicity; peritonitis; and dietary changes.

CBC/BIOCHEMISTRY/URINALYSIS

- Hematology is highly variable.
- The most consistent abnormalities are an elevated PCV and TPP. Hypoproteinemia may also be present in severe cases.
- Leukopenia with a neutropenia and lymphopenia may be initially present in some cases, and within a few days a marked leukocytosis may occur.
- Hyponatremia
- Hypochloremia
- Hypokalemia
- Metabolic acidosis
- Prerenal azotemia may be present.

OTHER LABORATORY TESTS

N/A

IMAGING

N/A

OTHER DIAGNOSTIC PROCEDURES

- A definitive diagnosis should be based on the isolation of *N. risticii* from blood culture or detection of the DNA of *N. risticii* from the blood or feces of an infected horse. Isolation of the organism requires collecting 100–400 mL heparinized blood and harvesting buffy coat for cell culture. It may take from several days to several weeks.
- The development of *N. risticii*–specific PCR assays that detect the partial 16 S rRNA gene of *N. risticii* has facilitated PHF diagnosis. In naturally infected horses, PCR on peripheral blood and feces is more sensitive than blood culture. PCR may also be used in the detection of *N. risticii* DNA in fresh or formalin-fixed and paraffin-embedded colon tissue.
- Serological tests using the IFA test or ELISA tests are of limited diagnostic value in a clinical case. The IFA test has been the most widely used diagnostic test for PHF; however, results interpretation can be difficult. PHF is diagnosed by demonstrating a ≥4-fold increase or decrease in titers between acute and convalescent serum samples. The acute sample should be collected as soon as first clinical signs are observed; the convalescent sample should be collected 5–7 days later. This is necessary because PHF-infected horses have a rapid rise in antibody titer that usually begins before the onset of clinical signs. Clinical signs of PHF may be delayed as long as 14 days after infection. As a

consequence, paired titers may demonstrate a rise, a decline, or no change. The IFA test produces >30% false-positives.

- Failure to seroconvert does not rule out PHF. The expected antibody titer of naturally affected horses is >1:80. Persistence of high antibody titers (1:2560) for more than 1 year has been noted in clinical and subclinical cases after natural infection.

PATHOLOGICAL FINDINGS

- Gross distention of the cecum and large colon with fluid contents
- Histologically the lesions are mild, with no inflammatory response or necrosis in the wall of the affected bowel. This is in marked contrast to the other causes of acute enterotyphylocolitis seen in the horse (e.g., enteric salmonellosis and clostridiosis).
- There may be mucus depletion of the goblet cells of the colon, with shortening and basophilia of the mucosal epithelial cells.

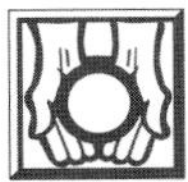

TREATMENT

APPROPRIATE HEALTH CARE

Mild cases can be managed on the farm, but severely affected animals may require intensive care. As other causes of some of the clinical signs are potentially highly infectious (e.g., salmonellosis), animals should be managed in isolation. The clinical signs of PHF are not sufficient to make a definitive diagnosis, and serologic confirmation is available only 7–10 days after the onset of clinical signs. However, early, appropriate treatment gives the best chance for a successful outcome. Failure to respond to therapy is often a diagnostic clue that the horse does not have PHF.

ACTIVITY

Stall rest during the course of therapy is recommended.

DIET

A grass hay diet is recommended until fecal consistency is normal.

CLIENT EDUCATION N/A

SURGICAL CONSIDERATIONS N/A

MEDICATIONS

DRUGS

- Oxytetracycline 6.6 mg/kg IV q 24 h for 5 days is the treatment of choice. A rapid recovery and dramatic decrease in fatality rate is observed when oxytetracycline therapy is commenced within 24 hr after the development of fever. Delaying oxytetracycline treatment may lessen the therapeutic value of the antibiotic.
- NSAIDs, such as flunixin meglumine, may be useful to treat endotoxemia.

FLUIDS

IV fluid and electrolyte replacement therapy is extremely important in the treatment of hypovolemia and shock.

CONTRAINDICATIONS

N/A

PRECAUTIONS

Diarrhea may occur in horses receiving parenteral antibiotics.

POSSIBLE INTERACTIONS

N/A

ALTERNATIVE DRUGS

N/A

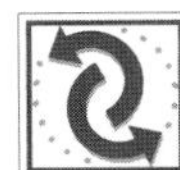

FOLLOW-UP

PATIENT MONITORING

Relapses rarely occur following the cessation of IV oxytetracycline therapy. If relapse occurs, administer a second course of IV oxytetracycline.

PREVENTION/AVOIDANCE

- Contact with recovered or currently ill animals is not associated with the development of PHF.
- Natural infection with PHF induces a protective immunity for as long as 20 mo.
- Horses do not remain chronic carriers.
- In endemic areas, access to freshwater streams and ponds should be limited, especially during the months of peak incidence.
- Methods to reduce snail numbers in adjacent creeks, ditches, or other bodies of water should be considered.
- Horses in endemic areas may be vaccinated with an inactivated, partially purified cell vaccine between early spring and early summer. They require 2-dose primary series 3–4 weeks apart. Revaccination at 6- to 12-mo intervals is dependent on whether in highly endemic area. Vaccination should occur 1 mo before the first cases of PHF are expected. Vaccine failure (89%) has been reported in endemic areas. There have been anecdotal reports of reduced severity of clinical signs in vaccinated horses.

POSSIBLE COMPLICATIONS

- Acute or chronic laminitis in 20–25% of PHF cases
- Thrombophlebitis
- Disseminated intravascular coagulopathy

EXPECTED COURSE AND PROGNOSIS

Horses with mild signs and that are treated aggressively and early in the course of the disease show a dramatic response to therapy and can be clinically normal in 3–5 days. Horses with more severe and long-standing problems require a longer period of therapy, and if secondary problems are present, then the clinical course may be much longer and the outcome less favorable.

MISCELLANEOUS

SYNONYMS

- Equine monocytic ehrlichiosis
- Equine ehrlichial colitis
- Acute equine diarrheal syndrome
- "Shasta River Crud" (northern California)

ABBREVIATIONS

- ELISA = enzyme-limited immunosorbent assay
- IFA = indirect fluorescent antibody
- PCR = polymerase chain reaction
- PCV = packed cell volume
- PHF = Potomac horse fever
- TPP = total plasma protein

Suggested Reading

Barlough JE, Reubel GH, Madigan JE, Vredevoe LK, Miller PE, Rikihisa Y. Detection of *Ehrlichia risticii*, the agent of Potomac horse fever, in freshwater stream snails (Pleuroceridae: *Juga* spp.) from northern California. Appl Environ Microbiol 1998;64:2888–2893.

Gibson KE, Rikihisa Y, Zhang C, Martin C. *Neorickettsia risticii* is vertically transmitted in the trematode *Acanthatrium oregonense* and horizontally transmitted to bats. Environ Microbiol 2005;7:203–212.

Madigan JE, Pusterla N, Johnson E, Chae JS, Pusterla JB, Derock E, Lawler SP. Transmission of *Ehrlichia risticii*, the agent of Potomac Horse fever, using naturally infected aquatic insects and helminth vectors: preliminary report. Equine Vet J 2000;32:275–279.

Madigan JE, Pusterla N. Life cycle of Potomac horse fever—implications for diagnosis, treatment, and control: a review. Proc Am Assoc Equine Pract 2005;51:158–162.

Mott J, Muramatsu Y, Seaton E, Martin C, Reed S, Rikihisa Y. Molecular analysis of *Neorickettsia risticii* in adult aquatic insects in Pennsylvania, in horses infected by ingestion of insects, and isolated in cell culture. J Clin Microbiol 2002;40:690–693.

Pusterla N, Johnson EM, Chae JS, Madigan JE. Digenetic trematodes, *Acanthatrium* sp. and *Lecithodendrium* sp., as vectors of *Neorickettsia risticii*, the agent of Potomac horse fever. J Helminthol 2003;77:335–339.

Pusterla N, Leutenegger CM, Sigrist B, Chae JS, Lutz H, Madigan JE. Detection and quantitation of *Ehrlichia risticii* genomic DNA by real-time PCR in infected horses and snails. Vet Parasitol 2000;90:129–135.

Rikihisa Y. New findings on members of the family Anaplasmataceae of veterinary importance. Ann N Y Acad Sci 2006;1078:438–445.

Wilson JH, Pusterla N, Bengfort JM, Arney L. Incrimination of mayflies as a vector of Potomac horse fever in an outbreak in Minnesota. Proc Am Assoc Equine Pract 2006;52:324–328.

Author John D. Baird

Consulting Editors Henry Stämpfli and Olimpo Oliver-Espinosa

PREGNANCY DIAGNOSIS

BASICS

DEFINITION/OVERVIEW

• *Pregnancy*—the condition post-fertilization of an embryo or fetus developing and maturing in utero • *Pregnancy diagnosis*—determination of a pregnant state based on clinical signs and laboratory and physical findings, including TRP and U/S

ETIOLOGY/PATHOPHYSIOLOGY

N/A

SYSTEMS AFFECTED

• Reproductive • Other systems may be affected in abnormal pregnancy.

GENETICS

N/A

INCIDENCE/PREVALENCE

N/A

SIGNALMENT

Nonspecific; puberty occurs between 12 and 24 mo in equine females. Pregnancy may occur anytime after puberty until advanced age in mares.

SIGNS

Historical

Failure of a mare that has been bred to return to estrus 16–19 days post-ovulation.

Physical Examination

• Early in pregnancy, little physical change may be noted. • As pregnancy advances, most mares will develop recognizable abdominal distention and weight gain. • In the final 2–4 weeks prior to parturition, most mares will have increased development of the mammary gland with secretion of fluid from the nipples ranging from thin and straw-colored to sticky and creamy.

CAUSES

Mating

RISK FACTORS

N/A

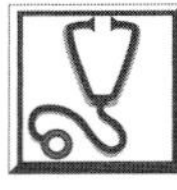

DIAGNOSIS

DIFFERENTIAL DIAGNOSIS

Other Causes of Failure to Cycle

• *Seasonal anestrus*—TRP and U/S reveal little ovarian activity; uterine and cervical tone is flaccid. • *Behavioral anestrus*—serial TRP and/or u/s will distinguish mares in estrus from those in diestrus or pregnancy. • *Prolonged luteal life span*—evidence of a CL detected by U/S examination of the ovary or progesterone assay. Responds to $PGF_{2\alpha}$ treatment.
• *Granulosa–theca cell tumor*—abnormally enlarged, multi-cystic ovary and small contralateral ovary. Confirm with elevated serum inhibin concentrations. • *Chromosomal abnormalities* (gonadal dysgenesis, testicular feminization)—confirm by karyotype determination.

Other US Findings Resembling Early Pregnancy

• *Uterine/lymphatic cysts*—U/S examination of the mare prior to breeding and pregnancy can aid in determining presence, number, size and shape of uterine cysts; a small *uterine map* (uterine horns and body) is drawn on each mare's TRP record and easily referenced at the time of the early pregnancy examinations. • This permanent record of cystic structures can be beneficial in distinguishing uterine cysts from early embryonic vesicles. • Update at the start of each breeding season to note the changing appearance and number of cysts as a mare ages.

CBC/BIOCHEMISTRY/URINALYSIS

N/A

OTHER LABORATORY TESTS

Progesterone Assay

• ELISA and RIA for serum or milk progesterone concentrations
  ○ Elevated concentrations of progesterone at 18–21 days post-ovulation imply that functional luteal tissue is present.
  ○ This is a presumptive, but not diagnostic, test for pregnancy.
• Progesterone assay may be a useful adjunct to other methods of early pregnancy diagnosis (i.e., TRP without U/S). • Confirmation of pregnancy, using an assay such as estrone sulfate or total estrogens, is advisable if early pregnancy was diagnosed solely by a progesterone assay.

eCG Assay

• eCG is a hormone secreted by endometrial cups in the pregnant mare uterus.
• Endometrial cups form between ≈36 and 37 days' gestation, when chorionic girdle cells (fetal trophoblasts) actively invade the endometrial epithelium.
  ○ The cups attain maximum size and hormone output between 55–70 days' gestation.
  ○ Endometrial cups regress between 80 and 120 days' gestation; secretion of eCG ceases at that time.
• eCG is measured using an ELISA.
• *False positives* occur if fetal death occurs after endometrial cups have formed.
  ○ The cups can persist up to 3–4 mo after a mare has lost a pregnancy, either a nonviable fetus in utero or fetal loss (early abortions often not noted).
• *False negatives* occur in samples evaluated:
  ○ Before the formation of endometrial cups (<36 days of gestation).
  ○ After the regression of the cups (>120 days of gestation)

Estrogen Assay

• Estrogens are secreted by the fetoplacental unit. • Total estrogens or estrone sulfate (conjugated estrogen) can be measured from plasma or urine to diagnose pregnancy after day 60 using RIA. • Estrone sulfate concentrations in milk are diagnostic for pregnancy after day 90 in the mare. • Fetal death, and subsequent compromise to the fetoplacental unit, results in an immediate decline in estrogen concentrations.

IMAGING

Transrectal US

• Pregnancy diagnosis can be determined as early as 9 days after ovulation, with a 5-MHz transducer and a high quality U/S scanner.
• *Days 13–15 days post-ovulation*
  ○ The optimal time to scan for early pregnancy. The embryonic vesicle is an anechoic, spherical yolk sac that averages between 12 and 20 mm in height.
  ○ Not only is the detection of an embryonic vesicle more reliable during this period, but twin embryonic vesicles can consistently be located at this time.
  ○ Early diagnosis of twin pregnancies increases the probability of successfully reducing twins to a singleton pregnancy using the manual reduction technique.
• *Days 18–24 post-ovulation*
  ○ The u/s appearance of the vesicle becomes more triangular by day 18 when the embryonic vesicle becomes less turgid.
  ○ The embryo proper often can be visualized by day 20–21 and a heartbeat can be seen as early as 24 days, and certainly should be evident on most u/s machines by 25 days.
  ○ The allantoic sac is visible ventral to the embryo by day 24.
• *Days 25–48 post-ovulation*
  ○ As the allantois develops and the yolk sac regresses, the embryo appears (during u/s exams) to be lifted from the ventral aspect of the vesicle to a dorsal location.
  ○ The embryo is visualized mid-vesicle by 28–30 days and is in the dorsal aspect of the vesicle by day 35.
  ○ The umbilical cord forms and attaches at the dorsal aspect of the vesicle around day 40.
  ○ As the cord elongates, the fetus migrates toward the ventral aspect of the allantoic sac.
  ○ Descent to the ventral wall is normally complete by day 48.

Fetal Sexing

Determination of fetal gender is best accomplished between 60 and 70 days of gestation. The technique is very useful in both horses and cattle, but high-resolution ultrasound equipment and experience are necessary for accurate identification of fetal gender.
• Fetal sex is determined by locating the position of the genital tubercle during its developmental migration. • The genital tubercle is the precursor to the clitoris in females and the penis in males.
• The structure is located on the ventral midline and is imaged as a hyperechoic, bilobed structure that is approximately 2 mm in diameter. • The tubercle migrates from between the rear legs caudally toward the tail in female fetuses and cranially toward the umbilicus in male fetuses. The location and orientation of the fetus must be determined. • Fetal position can be determined by locating the mandible, which points ventrally and caudally. • The heart is imaged on the ventral midline of the thorax.
• Examining the fetus cranially to caudally, the abdominal attachment of the umbilicus is located. • Immediately caudal to the umbilical attachment is the male genital tubercle. • The female tubercle is best visualized at the caudal most aspect of the fetus under the tailhead. The optimal image of the female tubercle appears

within a triangle formed by the tailhead and the distal tibias or hocks.

US findings from day 70–130 days

- Days 70–75, the fetus can be visualized using transrectal U/S. There will be some variation depending on the mare's age and parity. At this time, the weight of the developing pregnancy pulls the uterus over the brim of the pelvis.
- At 95 days' gestation, the fetus may move more dorsally within the pregnant uterus and can be imaged to determine fetal gender.
- From 95 to 130 days' gestation, gender can be determined by locating external genital structures:
  - Mammary gland, teats, and clitoris in the female
  - Penis, prepuce, and scrotum in the male

OTHER DIAGNOSTIC PROCEDURES

Behavioral Assessment

A mare teased to a stallion should begin to show signs of behavioral estrus 16–18 days after ovulation if not pregnant. Response of a mare to a stallion is a nonspecific indicator of pregnancy. This method should be used only as an adjunct to more reliable means such as TRP and U/S.

False Positive

• Failure to show estrus even as she returns to heat • Pregnancy loss occurs after formation of endometrial cups. • Prolonged luteal activity but not pregnant

False Negative

Mare continues to exhibit signs of behavioral estrus when pregnant.

Vaginal Speculum Examination

• Under the influence of progesterone, the cervix is tightly closed, pale, and dry. • This test is not diagnostic for pregnancy, as a functional CL in a cycling mare has the same effect on the cervix.

• Often, a speculum examination is used as an adjunct to TRP of the reproductive tract.

TRP of the Reproductive Tract

15–18 Days Post-ovulation

• Tubular tract becomes toned, and the "v" shape of the uterine bifurcation is often distinctly palpable. • Palpation of a vesicular bulge in the uterine horn has been reported as early as day 15; however, palpation of a true bulge at this stage is difficult in all but maiden mares with small uterine horns.

- The cervix is generally tightly closed, narrow and elongated.
- Both ovaries are often actively producing follicles during early pregnancy.
- False diagnosis of pregnancy, based on TRP findings, may occur at this stage due to EED or persistent/prolonged luteal activity.

25–30 Days of Gestation

- Uterine tone is very distinct (elevated) and the cervix is narrow and elongated.
- Follicular activity is present.
- A bulge the size of a small hen's egg can be appreciated at the caudoventral aspect of a uterine horn, adjacent to the uterine bifurcation.
- The uterine wall is slightly thinner over the fluid-filled, resilient vesicle.

35–40 Days of Gestation

- Uterus still demonstrates increased tone, the cervix is closed and elongated and the ovaries active.
- A tennis ball–sized bulge can be noted at the base of the uterine horn.
- Uterine tone begins to drop at/around the enlarging bulge.
- Greatly increased uterine tone is still present in the nonpregnant horn.

45–50 Days of Gestation

- Palpable bulge increases to softball size.

60–65 Days of Gestation

- Vesicle begins to expand into the uterine body, and the palpable bulge resembles the shape of a child-sized football.
- Wall of the uterine horn is distinctly thinner at this stage and the pregnancy begins to lose some of its resiliency.
- Good uterine tone is often maintained in the nongravid horn and the tip of the gravid horn.
- The increasing size of the pregnancy begins to pull the uterus ventrally.

To term

- Pregnancy occupies more of the uterus and uterine tone diminishes. It expands dorsally and resembles the size of a basketball.
- The pregnant uterus can be confused with a full urinary bladder.
- To distinguish the two, the fluid-filled uterus can be traced back to the closed cervix at the caudal aspect of the uterine body.
- Additionally, as the uterus continues to drop deeper into the abdomen, the ovaries are drawn ventrally and toward the midline.
- Occasionally the fetus may be visible during the latter aspect of this time period; however, it may not be possible or noticeable.

150–210 Days of Gestation

- Uterine descent into the ventral abdomen is complete; ovaries are often found at the midline.
- The fetus may consistently be ballotted within the fluid-filled uterus.

To term

- Tremendous fetal growth occurs from approximately to term.
- Ratio of the fluid volume of the pregnancy to the fetus decreases.
- Fetal growth is rapid and it occupies a greater percentage of the uterus late in gestation.

PATHOLOGICAL FINDINGS

N/A

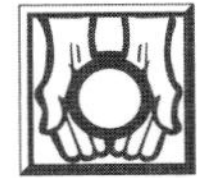

TREATMENT

APPROPRIATE HEALTH CARE, NURSING CARE, ACTIVITY, DIET, CLIENT EDUCATION, SURGICAL CONSIDERATIONS

N/A

MEDICATIONS

DRUG(S) OF CHOICE, CONTRAINDICATIONS, PRECAUTIONS, POSSIBLE INTERACTIONS, ALTERNATIVE DRUGS

N/A

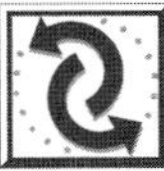

FOLLOW-UP

PATIENT MONITORING

- Pregnant mares are routinely examined in the last trimester of gestation to verify fetal viability.
- The most common method of pregnancy diagnosis as this stage is TRP with ballottement of the fetus.
- Transabdominal U/S may be used to measure fetal parameters such as fetal HR, aortic diameter, fetal activity, and fetal fluid quality.

PREVENTION/AVOIDANCE

N/A

POSSIBLE COMPLICATIONS

Embryonic or fetal loss, twins, placentitis, abortion, ruptured prepubic tendon, abdominal wall herniation, hydrallantois, hydramnion, uterine torsion, uterine rupture, prolonged gestation, dystocia

EXPECTED COURSE AND PROGNOSIS

A normal, viable fetus born at term gestation

MISCELLANEOUS

ASSOCIATED CONDITIONS, AGE-RELATED FACTORS, ZOONOTIC POTENTIAL, PREGNANCY

N/A

SEE ALSO

- Abortion
- Conception failure
- Early embryonic death
- Dystocia
- Placental basics
- Twinning
- Fetal sexing

ABBREVIATIONS

- CL = corpus luteum
- eCG = equine chorionic gonadotropin
- EED = early embryonic death
- ELISA = enzyme-linked immunosorbent assay
- HR = heart rate
- $PGF_{2\alpha}$ = natural prostaglandin
- RIA = radioimmunoassay
- TRP = transrectal palpation
- U/S = ultrasound, ultrasonography

Suggested Reading

Ginther OJ. Reproductive Biology of the Mare, ed 2. Cross Plains: Equiservices, 1992.

Ginther OJ. Ultrasonic Imaging and Reproductive Events in the Mare. Cross Plains: Equiservices, 1986.

McKinnon AO. Diagnosis of pregnancy. In: McKinnon AO, Voss JL, eds. Equine Reproduction. Philadelphia: Lea & Febiger, 1993.

Author Margo L. Macpherson

Consulting Editor Carla L. Carleton

PREMATURE PLACENTAL SEPARATION

BASICS

DEFINITION/OVERVIEW

- Premature disassociation (detachment) of the chorioallantoic membrane from the endometrium before delivery of the term fetus.
- The chorioallantoic is responsible for supplying the fetus with oxygen and nutrients and for removing its waste products; with premature detachment (e.g., late stage 1, early stage 2), the fetus dies from hypoxia if immediate assistance is unavailable to aid in delivery.

ETIOLOGY/PATHOPHYSIOLOGY

- Proposed origins—alterations in the chorioallantoic membrane in the area of the internal os of the cervix or abnormal attachment of the chorioallantoic membrane to the endometrium, which predisposes to premature separation.
- Occurs secondary to cervical relaxation (hormonal, ascending infection, cervical incompetency) and development of low-grade placentitis, which compromises the normal relationship of the chorioallantoic and the endometrium.

GENETICS

N/A

INCIDENCE/PREVALENCE

- Incidence increases significantly with induction of parturition.
- Incidence of <1% in medium-size to large breeds of horses, but higher in miniature horses

SIGNALMENT

- All breeds, with increased occurrence in miniature horses
- All females of breeding age

SIGNS

- This is an emergency.
- Because of the abrupt reduction in oxygen delivery to the fetus, immediate delivery assistance is essential as soon as the chorioallantoic membrane protrudes through the vulvar lips.
- Although it may happen for the first time at any parity, a history of premature placental separation is often found.
- Closely observe any mare with a history of premature placental separation.
- Physical examination findings are normal.
- Chorioallantoic membrane, when presented at the vulva, may appear to be characteristically velvety and roughened.

CAUSES AND RISK FACTORS

- Miniature horses
- Induction of parturition
- Older mares

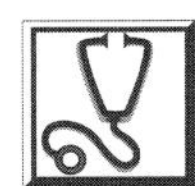

DIAGNOSIS

DIFFERENTIAL DIAGNOSIS

- Evagination of the vaginal wall
- Eversion of the urinary bladder
- Prolapse of the vaginal wall
- Lacerations of the vaginal wall and prolapse of the intestines

CBC/BIOCHEMISTRY/URINALYSIS

N/A

OTHER LABORATORY TESTS N/A

IMAGING

U/S:

- Prepartum examination may reveal an area of detachment cranial to the cervix, which also may indicate a mare at risk for placentitis.
- Intrapartum appearance of the chorioallantoic membrane protruding through the vulvar lips (i.e., "red velvet" or "red bagging") is diagnostic in itself.

OTHER DIAGNOSTIC PROCEDURES

Best diagnostic method—visual examination of the exposed tissue

PATHOLOGICAL FINDINGS N/A

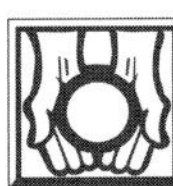

TREATMENT

When premature placental seperation is observed, tear chorioallantoic and assist in delivery.

APPROPRIATE HEALTH CARE N/A

NURSING CARE N/A

ACTIVITY N/A

DIET

N/A

CLIENT EDUCATION

- Knowledge regarding the normal appearance of placenta at parturition
- With normal parturition, the first membrane observed at the vulvae should be smooth and white, opaque, or pale pink.
- Any reddish or roughened protruding membrane indicates a problem requiring immediate action.
- This is a true emergency. Because of fetal hypoxia, insufficient time is available to seek outside assistance and still deliver a live foal.
- A normal placenta examined when freshly delivered serves as an excellent teaching tool to educate clients regarding what is normal and abnormal.
- If premature placental separation is observed and client cannot/will not tear chorioallantoic and assist in delivery, instruct the client to walk the mare until the veterinarian arrives
    - May reduce further/full abdominal contractions and thus decrease further/full separation (still only partial usefulness) for a few minutes

PREMATURE PLACENTAL SEPARATION

MEDICATIONS

DRUG(S) OF CHOICE
N/A

CONTRAINDICATIONS
Oxytocin is contraindicated before fetus has been delivered.

PRECAUTIONS
Oxytocin is contraindicated.

POSSIBLE INTERACTIONS
Oxytocin is contraindicated.

FOLLOW-UP

PATIENT MONITORING
- Mares do well after delivery.
- The potential problem is with the fetus and its inability to exchange oxygen upon placental separation.
  - The neonate, if alive when delivered, can suffer permanent damage from oxygen deprivation that occurred during delivery.

PREVENTION/AVOIDANCE
- No known method to prevent this condition
- Observe parturition for any mare with a history of a previous delivery involving premature placental separation.

POSSIBLE COMPLICATIONS
- Mare—none
- Fetus—death caused by lack of oxygenation; dummy foal post-partum

EXPECTED COURSE AND PROGNOSIS
Delayed delivery results in fetal death.

MISCELLANEOUS

ASSOCIATED CONDITIONS
N/A

AGE-RELATED FACTORS
N/A

ZOONOTIC POTENTIAL
N/A

PREGNANCY
Only occurs at the end of gestation

SYNONYMS
- Red bag
- Red bagging

SEE ALSO
- Dystocia
- Prolonged pregnancy

ABBREVIATION
- U/S = ultrasound, ultrasonography

Suggested Reading

Asbury AC, LeBlanc MM. The placenta. In: McKinnon AO, Voss JL, eds. Equine Reproduction. Philadelphia: Lea & Febiger, 1993:513.

Roberts SJ. In: Veterinary Obstetrics and Genital Diseases (Theriogenology). Woodstock, VT: published by the author, 1986:251–252.

Whitwell KE, Jeffcott LB. Morphological studies on the fetal membranes of the normal singleton foal at term. Res Vet Sci 1975;19:44–55.

Author Walter R. Threlfall

Consulting Editor Carla L. Carleton

PREPUBIC TENDON RUPTURE

BASICS

DEFINITION/OVERVIEW

Prepubic tendon separates from its attachment to the pubis.

ETIOLOGY/PATHOPHYSIOLOGY

• Weight of the mare's abdomen, plus the enlarging fetus, increasing quantity of fetal fluids and membranes, and the accumulation of ventral abdominal edema place pressure on the prepubic tendon's pelvic attachment that surpasses the tendon's load limit. • Separation occurs (partial tear, half, or full rupture).
• Abdominal wall falls ventrally as the tendon tears away from the pubis.

SYSTEMS AFFECTED

• Muscular • Reproductive

GENETICS

N/A

INCIDENCE/PREVALENCE

Extremely low

SIGNALMENT

• All breeds; all of breeding age • Older mares at increased risk • Females (predominant)
• Rupture occurs in the late/near-term pregnant mare due to excess weight of the fetus, uterine fluid and membranes and ventral edema. • The male's prepubic tendon may rupture after severe trauma.

SIGNS

General Comments

• Mares usually in advanced pregnancy with twins, hydrops, or other causes for a uterus to be enlarged beyond normal limits. • Prepubic tendon rupture may occur after severe trauma, e.g., being struck by a car.

Historical

• Mares usually present with an abdomen that has slowly enlarged, excessive size is quite noticeable. • Discomfort is associated with abdominal size; difficulty breathing—short shallow respirations, or reluctance to lie recumbent.

Physical Examination

• Dependent edema of ventral abdomen may extend to/involve the mare's legs.
• Characteristic appearance of the ventral abdomen after rupture:
  ○ Distinct profile viewed from the side
  ○ Ventral abdominal line appears flat, no rise in the flank region by the udder.
  ○ Udder loses its normal orientation—its anterior aspect slants steeply down and lies at a lower point than its posterior aspect.
  ○ Normal definition between udder and abdominal wall is absent.
• Transrectal palpation of the rupture may not be possible while the mare is pregnant. • Identify intestines immediately below the skin, i.e., outside the abdominal musculature; indicates rupture of the tendon or abdominal wall.

CAUSES

Excessive pressure and weight on the abdominal wall, usually from excessive uterine size, exceeds the physiologic limit that the attachment can withstand.

RISK FACTORS

• Pregnant with twins or triplets • Predisposed are individuals with excessive fluid accumulation:
  ○ Extra-abdominally from edema
  ○ Intra-abdominally with conditions such as hydrops

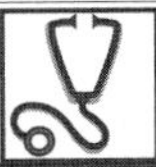

DIAGNOSIS

• Physical examination usually reveals dependant edema of ventral abdomen, may involve the legs.
• Side profile is flat from the front limbs to, and including, the udder. • Definition between the udder and abdominal wall is absent. • Intestines may be palpated immediately underlying the skin in the absence of the abdominal wall.

DIFFERENTIAL DIAGNOSIS

• Abdominal wall rupture • Tearing of the muscles near the prepubic tendon; may be impossible to distinguish from actual tendon rupture

IMAGING

Abdominal U/S examination may confirm abdominal viscera immediately under the skin near the udder.

PATHOLOGICAL FINDINGS

Tearing or rupture of the prepubic tendon

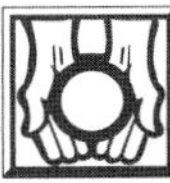

TREATMENT

APPROPRIATE HEALTH CARE

• With complete rupture, the mare cannot expel the fetus at term due to loss of abdominal musculature. • Precludes a normal abdominal press necessary for active labor • Once assisted delivery is complete, a better assessment can be made to determine if there are any realistic surgical options.

NURSING CARE

• Keep mare off surfaces that could lead to falling and/or further damage—slippery, angled, uneven. • Prevent rolling, if possible. • Close observation for intestinal obstruction or parturition, dystocia • Consider use of trusses or supportive devices, but:

- Problems may result from transferring all the abdominal weight and its contents onto the mare's back, plus pressure increases on the ventral abdomen and its contents as they have lost their normal orientation.

ACTIVITY

Restrict exercise to hand walking, prevent additional tearing of the ruptured tendon.

DIET

Changes in diet may be indicated; reduce additional abdominal cavity bulk.

CLIENT EDUCATION

• Because this occurs primarily late in gestation, discuss the mare's impaired ability to participate in active labor absent an intact abdominal wall. • Advise owners to seek veterinary help if a mare's abdominal size exceeds that of a normal pregnancy.

SURGICAL CONSIDERATIONS

• Dependent on degree of tissue damage as determined postpartum and mare's value • Reproductive life of the mare will be limited to embryo transfer, if repair is possible. • The mare is not a candidate to carry subsequent pregnancies.

MEDICATIONS

DRUG(S) OF CHOICE

• Diuretics (e.g., furosemide) may reduce edema in dependent areas. • Phenylbutazone, but only if the possibility of ulcer induction in the foal has been considered

CONTRAINDICATIONS

Avoid any medications with detrimental fetal effects.

PRECAUTIONS

• Goal of mare care—medical stabilization • Prepare and observe mare for an induced parturition.

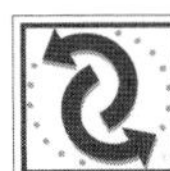

FOLLOW-UP

PATIENT MONITORING

• Close observation is essential. • Ensure assistance will be available at parturition.

PREVENTION/AVOIDANCE

Terminate pregnancy in seriously at-risk mares before prepubic tendon ruptures, especially if excessive abdominal size and/or ventral dependent edema is present late in gestation.

POSSIBLE COMPLICATIONS

Mares may die prepartum or postpartum from GI complications or rupture of the uterine or middle uterine arteries.

EXPECTED COURSE AND PROGNOSIS

• Mares have a high probability of survival, if managed properly. • Many do well after delivery without surgical repair, if they are not rebred. • Do not rebreed any mare with a partial prepubic tendon rupture; it will worsen with additional pregnancies.

MISCELLANEOUS

ASSOCIATED CONDITIONS

• Multiple pregnancies—twins; triplets; hydrops pregnancy • Any other condition that increases size and weight of the pregnant uterus.

AGE-RELATED FACTORS

• Increasing age • Old multiparous mares

PREGNANCY

• Usually associated with the late-pregnant mare • May occur in any horse that has suffered a severe, traumatic abdominal injury

SEE ALSO

• Dystocia • Prolonged pregnancy

ABBREVIATION

• GI = gastrointestinal

Suggested Reading

Löfstedt R: Miscellaneous diseases of pregnancy and parturition. In: McKinnon AO, Voss JL, eds. Equine Reproduction. Philadelphia: Lea and Febiger, 1993:596–603.

Roberts SJ: Veterinary Obstetrics and Genital Diseases (Theriogenology). Woodstock, VT: published by the author, 1986:229–230, 347–352.

Tulleners E, Fretz P. Prosthetic repair of large abdominal wall defects in horses and food animals. JAVMA 1983;192:258–262.

Author Walter R. Threlfall
Consulting Editor Carla L. Carleton

PRIAPISM

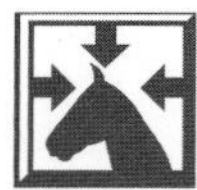

BASICS

DEFINITION/OVERVIEW

Persistent erection with engorgement of the CCP, in the absence of sexual arousal

ETIOLOGY/PATHOPHYSIOLOGY

- The pudendal nerves control the smooth muscles of the arteries that supply, and the veins that drain, the CCP.
- *Parasympathetic* stimulation of the pudendal nerves:
  - Stimulation of the pudendal nerves causes arterial dilation and venous constriction to/from the CCP to promote erection. ○ Allows relaxation of the retractor penis muscles (causing penile prolapse) and the smooth muscle cells located in the walls of the CCP (allows CCP to fill with blood).
- *Detumescence*—less well understood, thought to be under sympathetic control
  - With adrenergic stimulation, arterial blood flow to the CCP decreases, and smooth muscles lining the CCP constrict. ○ Agents/conditions interfering with sympathetic stimulation are thought to directly or indirectly block detumescence ○ When detumescence fails—CO_2 tension in the CCP increases, causing increased blood viscosity and RBC sludging, and further occlusion of venous outflow from the CCP. ○ Prolonged erection may lead to secondary problems—paraphimosis or penile paralysis due to injury to the retractor penis muscles and/or the pudendal nerves

SYSTEM AFFECTED

Reproductive

SIGNALMENT

- Predominantly in stallions. Geldings can be affected.
  - Serum testosterone may contribute to development of priapism. ○ Gelding's lack of testosterone may cause atrophy of the smooth muscles of the CCP, decreasing size of cavernous spaces available for filling with blood during the process of erection.

SIGNS

- The protruded, erect penis is usually evident.
- If the penis is only partially erect, the distended CCP can be detected by digital palpation.

CAUSES

- Phenothiazine-derivative TQ
  - Propiopromazine HCl, chlorpromazine HCl, acepromazine maleate
- Spinal cord injury or disease • Other causes are rare and include general anesthesia, neoplasia, infectious diseases (i.e., purpura hemorrhagica), postsurgical complications (castration), severe debilitation or starvation.

RISK FACTORS

Most cases of priapism occur subsequent to phenothiazine TQ to stallions. Do not use this class of drugs in stallions.

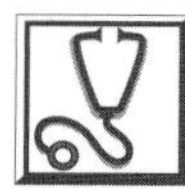

DIAGNOSIS

DIFFERENTIAL DIAGNOSIS

Differentiating Similar Signs

- Paraphimosis is the prolapse of the penis and prepuce, with extensive edema of those tissues. Paraphimosis may occur secondary to priapism:
- It is significant if history includes phenothiazine TQ or the presence of erection prior to edema formation.
- Penile paralysis is differentiated by a *flaccid* prolapsed penis, not erect or partially erect, as is seen in priapism.

Differentiating Causes

- History of phenothiazine TQ given to intact stallion
- With evidence of debilitation, starvation, systemic illness—merits further investigation and can contribute to the development of priapism
- A complete neurologic examination is indicated to rule out spinal cord injury or disease as the inciting cause of priapism.

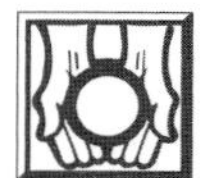

TREATMENT

- Penile support, as with paraphimosis, in the form of slings, massage, application of emollient dressings to the penis and prepuce, and hydrotherapy—prevents accumulation of edema and further penile injury
- With the horse under anesthesia, manual compression of the erect penis, physically replacing it in the prepuce—successful in some acute cases
- Flushing the CCP with heparinized saline (10 IU sodium heparin/mL 0.9% saline) using 12-gauge needles:
  - Proximal to the glans penis (ingress) and ○ At the level of the ischium (egress) ○ Has been used in cases of priapism unresponsive to cholinergic blocking or α-adrenergic agent administration
- Vascular shunt created between the CCP and CSP:
  - Surgical procedure successfully used in men, advocated for use in horses
- Chronic cases that ultimately undergo detumescence may need surgery:
  - Circumcision (reefing) ○ Retraction (Bolz technique) to retain the penis within the prepuce ○ Penile amputation has been necessary in some cases.

SURGICAL CONSIDERATIONS

Refer to Treatment.

MEDICATIONS

DRUG(S) OF CHOICE

- A cholinergic blocker (benztropine mesylate 8 mg IV slow administration) has been successful in treating priapism caused by the administration of α-adrenergic blocking agents (e.g., phenothiazine TQ).
  - Must be administered during the acute phase
- Injection of 10 mg of 1% phenylephrine HCl (an α-adrenergic agent) directly into the CCP during the acute phase
  - Advocated in cases unresponsive to cholinergic blocking agents
- Topical or systemic antibiotics—for superficial or deep lacerations, secondary to prolonged prolapse
- Anti-inflammatory medication (phenylbutazone at 2–4 g/450 kg/day PO)
  - Indicated if secondary paraphimosis or intractable inflammation exists

CONTRAINDICATIONS

- Phenothiazine TQ are absolutely contraindicated.
- Avoid benztropine mesylate and phenylephrine HCl in patients with tachycardia or hypertension.

ALTERNATIVE DRUGS

Although its effectiveness remains unproven, the β_2-agonist clenbuterol has been used (0.8–3.2 mg/kg PO) to treat priapism.

FOLLOW-UP

PATIENT MONITORING

- Hospitalization may be needed for frequent reevaluation; initial intensive management
- Pain and discomfort are managed with PT (massage, hydrotherapy, support) or pharmacologics.
- Successful reduction of the erection and return of the penis to the prepuce are considered good prognostic indicators.

POSSIBLE COMPLICATIONS

- Chronic priapism may cause inflammation of the pudendal nerve where it passes over the ischium. The pudendal nerve innervates the retractor penis muscle.
  - Pudendal nerve damage can cause malfunction of the retractor penis muscles and permanent penile paralysis.
- Secondary paraphimosis may develop as dependent edema accumulates.
- Impotence can occur as a result of desensitization of the glans penis (nerve damage) or fibrosis of the CCP (nerve damage) of fibrosis or the CCP.

MISCELLANEOUS

ASSOCIATED CONDITIONS

- Paraphimosis
- Penile paralysis

SEE ALSO

- Paraphimosis
- Penile paralysis

ABBREVIATIONS

- CCP = corpus cavernosum penis
- CSP = corpus spongiosum penis
- PT = physical therapy
- RBC = red blood cell
- TQ = tranquilizer

Suggested Reading

Pauwels F, Schumacher J, Varner D. Priapism in horses. Compend Cont Educ Pract 2005;27:311–315.

Pearson H, Weaver BMQ. Priapism after sedation, neuroleptanalgesia and anaesthesia in the horse. Equine Vet J 1978;10:85–90.

Rochat MC. Priapism: a review. Therio 2001;56:713–722.

Author Carole C. Miller

Consulting Editor Carla L. Carleton

PRIMARY HYPERPARATHYROIDISM

BASICS

OVERVIEW

- Caused by excessive PTH secretion by hyperplastic or neoplastic parathyroid cells. This results in increased calcium resorption from bones leading to hypercalcemia and clinical signs of fibrous osteodystrophy.
- Hypophosphatemia and hyperphosphaturia result from low renal tubular reabsorption of phosphate secondary to increased PTH secretion.
- Excessive PTH may originate from parathyroid hyperplasia, adenoma, or adenocarcinoma.

SYSTEMS AFFECTED

- Endocrine
- Musculoskeletal

SIGNALMENT

- Any sex or breed
- Reported only in old equids

SIGNS

- Intermittent weakness
- Weight loss
- Anorexia
- Enlargement of facial bones
- Shifting-leg lameness
- Difficult mastication

CAUSES AND RISK FACTORS

Excessive, uncontrolled secretion of PTH by chief cells of one or more parathyroid glands

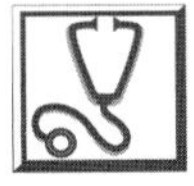

DIAGNOSIS

DIFFERENTIAL DIAGNOSIS

- Fibrous osteodystrophy may result from nutritional secondary HP in horses fed diets with low concentrations of calcium and high concentrations of phosphorus. However, hypocalcemia (or normocalcemia) and hyperphosphatemia characterize nutritional HP.
- Other causes of hypercalcemia—chronic renal failure, hypervitaminosis D, and neoplastic disease.
- Normal serum BUN, creatinine concentration, and urine specific gravity rule out chronic renal failure.
- Ingestion of oxalate-containing plants and vitamin D toxicosis can be eliminated based on history. In addition, vitamin D toxicosis is characterized by hyperphosphatemia.
- Certain neoplastic tissues produce a PTH-related protein with identical biologic properties to PTH that results in pseudo-HP, but ruling out neoplastic disease in live horses may be difficult. Measurements of intact PTH, using an immunoradiometric assay that does not cross-react with PTH-related protein, may help in differentiation.

CBC/BIOCHEMISTRY/URINALYSIS

- Hypercalcemia, hypophosphatemia, and hyperphosphaturia are characteristic.
- Hyperchloremic metabolic acidosis has been associated.

OTHER LABORATORY TESTS

- Fractional excretion of phosphorus (reference range, 0.04%–0.16%) and serum PTH are abnormally elevated.
- PTH may be measured by immunoradiometric assay for immunoreactive PTH (detects C-terminal portion) or for intact PTH (detects both C- and N-terminal portions). However, the latter assay does not measure PTH-related protein, which is often elevated in cases of pseudo-HP.

IMAGING

- Skull radiography may reveal osseous proliferation of the facial bones and loss of the lamina dura surrounding the premolars and molars.
- Detection of parathyroid neoplasia may be attempted with nuclear scintigraphy using ^{99m}Tc sestamibi.

DIAGNOSTIC PROCEDURES

Horses have two pairs of parathyroid glands: one cranial pair adjacent to the cranial pole of the thyroid gland and one caudal pair variably located along the neck anywhere from the thoracic inlet to the cranial third of the trachea. Therefore, if a mass is identified in that part of the neck, biopsy may be attempted.

PATHOLOGIC FINDINGS

- Parathyroid gland hyperplasia, adenoma, or adenocarcinoma
- Equine parathyroid glands may be difficult to distinguish from surrounding tissues.
- With parathyroid neoplasia, atrophy of the nonaffected parathyroid tissue is expected.
- Single or multiple glands may be affected.

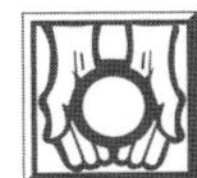

TREATMENT

- Removal of the affected parathyroid gland and medical treatment for hypercalcemia
- Eliminate exogenous sources of vitamin D and calcium.
- Successful surgical removal of a parathyroid adenoma has been reported in a pony.
- Disease progression may be slow: one pony has been reported to still be clinically normal 2 years after diagnosis.

MEDICATIONS

DRUG(S) OF CHOICE

IV fluid therapy, diuretics, and corticosteroids may promote calcium excretion.

CONTRAINDICATIONS/POSSIBLE INTERACTIONS

N/A

FOLLOW-UP

- Monitor electrolytes, acid-base status, and bone ossification.
- Possible complications—difficulty chewing because of loosening teeth and lameness secondary to osteopenia

MISCELLANEOUS

ASSOCIATED CONDITIONS, AGE-RELATED FACTORS, ZOONOTIC POTENTIAL, PREGNANCY

N/A

ABBREVIATIONS

- HP = hyperparathyroidism
- PTH = parathyroid hormone

Suggested Reading

Frank N, Hawkins JF, Couëtil LL, Raymond JT. Primary hyperparathyroidism with osteodystrophia fibrosa of the facial bones in a pony. JAVMA 1998;212:84–86.

Wong D, Sponseller B, Miles K, et al. Failure of technetium Tc99m sestamibi scanning to detect abnormal parathyroid tissue in a horse and a mule with primary hyperparathyroidism. J Vet Intern Med 2004;18:589–593.

Author Laurent Couëtil

Consulting Editor Michel Lévy

PROGRESSIVE ETHMOIDAL HEMATOMA

BASICS

OVERVIEW

• A PEH is an uncommonly encountered, slowly expanding, non-neoplastic mass originating in the submucosa of one of the ethmoturbinates that causes signs of disease referable to the respiratory system. • Lesions may arise from the nasal or sinusal portion of the ethmoidal labyrinth. • The mass expands slowly into the nasal cavity, paranasal sinuses, or nasopharynx, destroying adjacent tissue by compression.
• Occasionally bilateral

SIGNALMENT

• Any age, but rare in horses <3 years (median age, ≅10 years) • Occurs in most breeds, but predilection for Arabians and Thoroughbreds. Standardbreds appear to be spared. • No difference in prevalence between males and females or between geldings and stallions

SIGNS

• Most common—intermittent, scanty, serosanguineous nasal discharge from the affected side. • Other signs—halitosis, abnormal respiratory noise, dyspnea, coughing, head shaking, and facial deformity. • The mass may be visible at the nostril. • Small lesions may cause no clinical signs.

CAUSES AND RISK FACTORS

Cause unknown. The lesion may originate from a congenital or acquired hemangiomatous lesion that hemorrhages into the submucosa of the ethmoidal labyrinth.

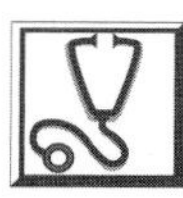

DIAGNOSIS

DIFFERENTIAL DIAGNOSIS

• Other conditions that may cause sanguineous nasal discharge—mycosis of the guttural pouch, paranasal sinuses, or nasal cavity; facial trauma; neoplasia of any region of the respiratory tract; exercise-induced pulmonary hemorrhage; respiratory amyloidosis; septic pneumonia; conidiobolomycosis; and infection of a nasolacrimal duct. • Lesions of the nasal cavities that resemble PEH endoscopically—polyps, fungal masses, and neoplasms

CBC/BIOCHEMISTRY/URINALYSIS

Usually normal but may reveal anemia

IMAGING

• If confined to the nasal cavity, the mass appears radiographically as an abnormal opacity of soft-tissue density with smooth margins ventral to the eye and rostral to the ethmoidal labyrinth. • A mass within the paranasal sinuses may result in fluid lines within the compartments of the sinuses. • Positive-contrast sinusography or CT may allow more complete evaluation of the lesion's extent.

OTHER DIAGNOSTIC PROCEDURES

• Endoscopic exam of the nasal cavity or paranasal sinuses reveals a yellow-red-green mass that appears to originate from the ethmoidal labyrinth. • White colonies of *Aspergillus* spp. may be present on the lesion. • The size of the mass may obscure its origin. • A nasal mass may protrude caudally around the nasal septum into the contralateral nasal cavity, obscuring the contralateral ethmoidal labyrinth and giving the impression of two masses; a mass that originates from the sinusal portion of the ethmoidal labyrinth is not seen during endoscopy of the nasal passage unless it protrudes into the nasal cavity through the nasomaxillary aperture. • A mass within the paranasal sinuses may distort the nasal cavity. • Always examine both nasal cavities because the lesion can occur bilaterally. • The diagnosis is established on the basis of clinical signs, the location and endoscopic appearance of the lesion, but biopsy of the lesion is confirmatory.

PATHOLOGIC FINDINGS

• The lesion is covered by respiratory epithelium, which overlies submucosal fibrous tissue as well as old and recent hemorrhage.
• The hemorrhage contains hemosiderin-filled macrophages and multinucleated giant cells.

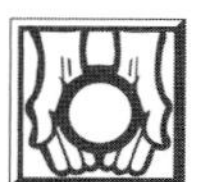

TREATMENT

• Affected horses can be treated by excising the lesion, by ablating the lesion using a cryogen or laser, or by injecting 10% formalin into the lesion. • Surgical ablation is performed through an osteoplastic frontonasal flap, usually with the horse anesthetized. A lesion on the nasal portion of the ethmoidal labyrinth is exposed by perforating the floor of the dorsoconchal sinus. The lesion and diseased portion of the ethmoidal labyrinth are excised. • Application of a cryogen (e.g., liquid nitrogen) to ablate the mass causes minimal hemorrhage and can be performed with the horse sedated. This method is useful only if the lesion is small. • A small mass can be ablated transendoscopically using a laser with the horse sedated. Laser therapy requires multiple treatments, and the cost of the equipment may limit its availability.

MEDICATIONS

DRUG(S) OF CHOICE

• The lesion can be ablated by injecting 10% formalin into it transendoscopically with the horse sedated. A lesion in the paranasal sinuses is accessed through a trephine hole in the caudal maxillary or conchofrontal sinus. • Lesions are injected until they distend and begin to leak formalin. • Horses are retreated at 3- to 4-week intervals until the lesion is eliminated or so small and deep within the ethmoidal recess that injection no longer is possible; small lesions deep within the ethmoidal recess may cause no clinical signs of disease.

CONTRAINDICATIONS/POSSIBLE INTERACTIONS

Formalin should not be injected into a lesion if the lesion has eroded the cribriform plate. Determining if the cribriform plate has been eroded requires CT or MRI imaging. Erosion of the cribriform plate is rare.

FOLLOW-UP

PATIENT MONITORING

Even when the condition appears to have resolved, the horse's nasal cavities should be endoscopically examined every 3–6 months indefinitely to determine if the lesion has reappeared at the same or other sites. Always examine both nasal cavities. Reappearance of a lesion in the paranasal sinuses is unlikely to be detected until the horse develops clinical signs of disease. Lesions may reappear years after apparent resolution.
0

POSSIBLE COMPLICATIONS

• Complications of surgical ablation include severe hemorrhage, especially if the dorsoconchal sinus must be perforated into the nasal cavity; encephalitis, if the mass has eroded the cribriform plate; dehiscence of the wound, and suture periostitis. • Laminitis may be a rare complication of injection with formalin.
• Injecting formalin into a lesion that has eroded the cribriform plate may result in death.

EXPECTED COURSE AND PROGNOSIS

• Regardless of the type of treatment, prognosis for long-term cure is guarded to poor. • The incidence of recurrence has been reported to range from 14%–45% but may be even higher.
• The incidence of recurrence seems to be much higher in bilaterally affected horses.

MISCELLANEOUS

SEE ALSO

• Exercise-induced pulmonary hemorrhage
• Guttural pouch mycosis • Hemorrhagic nasal discharge

ABBREVIATION

• PEH = progressive ethmoidal hematoma.

Suggested Reading

Schumacher J, Dixon P. Progressive ethmoidal haematoma. In: McGorum B, Dixon P, Robinson E, Schumacher J, eds. Equine Respiratory Medicine and Surgery. Oxford: Elsevier Science, 2006.

Author Jim Schumacher
Consulting Editor Daniel Jean

PROLIFERATIVE OPTIC NEUROPATHY

BASICS

OVERVIEW

A slowly enlarging white mass protruding from the optic disc into the vitreous. The lesion is generally "fixed" (i.e., it does not move when the eye moves). Can be associated with small hemorrhages.

SYSTEM AFFECTED

Ophthalmic

SIGNALMENT

Primarily horses older than 15 years

SIGNS

- None, or minimal effect on vision
- Pupillary light reflex is normal.
- Generally unilateral
- No signs of pain

CAUSE AND RISK FACTORS

Unknown

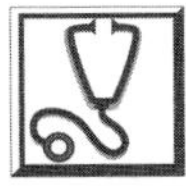

DIAGNOSIS

DIFFERENTIAL DIAGNOSIS

- Ischemic optic neuropathy
- Exudative optic neuritis
- Tumors—astrocytoma, medulloepithelioma, and neuroepithelioma
- Granuloma
- Abscesses

CBC/BIOCHEMISTRY/URINALYSIS, OTHER LABORATORY TESTS, IMAGING, DIAGNOSTIC PROCEDURES

N/A

PATHOLOGIC FINDINGS

- Histologically it resembles a schwannoma in many cases but may also be similar to an astrocytoma or xanthoma.
- Schwannomas are well-circumscribed masses attached to peripheral nerves, cranial nerves, or spinal nerve roots. They contain areas of densely packed spindle cells intermixed with looser, myxoid regions.

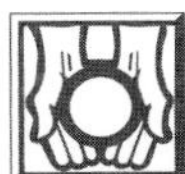

TREATMENT

There is no therapy for this condition.

MEDICATIONS

N/A

FOLLOW-UP

PATIENT MONITORING

Observe for vision changes.

POSSIBLE COMPLICATIONS

None

EXPECTED COURSE AND PROGNOSIS

No effect on vision; slowly progressive in size

MISCELLANEOUS

N/A

ASSOCIATED CONDITIONS

N/A

AGE-RELATED FACTORS

Primarily horses older than 15 years

SEE ALSO

- Exudative optic neuritis
- Traumatic optic neuropathy
- Ischemic optic neuropathy

Suggested Reading

Brooks .DE Ophthalmology for the Equine Practitioner. Jackson, WY; Teton NewMedia, 2002.

Brooks DE, Matthews AG. Equine ophthalmology. In: Gelatt KN, ed. Veterinary Ophthalmology, ed 4. Philadelphia; Lippincott Williams and Wilkins, 2007.

Gilger BC, ed. Equine Ophthalmology. Philadelphia; WB Saunders, 2005.

Authors Maria Källberg and Dennis E. Brooks

Consulting Editor Dennis E. Brooks

PROLONGED DIESTRUS

BASICS

DEFINITION/OVERVIEW

Persistence of a corpus luteum post-ovulation such that the normal return to estrus is delayed

ETIOLOGY/PATHOPHYSIOLOGY

- Post-ovulation, the corpus luteum forms and begins progesterone production. In the mare, a corpus luteum is unresponsive to $PGF_{2\alpha}$-induced luteolysis for 4–5 days after ovulation, due to immaturity of luteinization.
- Endogenous $PGF_{2\alpha}$, produced by the endometrium, is released approximately 14–15 days post-ovulation to initiate luteolysis in the nonpregnant mare.
- The life span of the corpus luteum is prolonged when $PGF_{2\alpha}$ release is inhibited or when it fails to respond to $PGF_{2\alpha}$ that is released.

SYSTEM AFFECTED

Reproductive

GENETICS N/A

SIGNALMENT

Mares of any age and breed

SIGNS

Historical

Failure to return to estrus at the expected time interval in the cycling mare

Physical Examination

- The general physical examination is usually normal.
- Transrectal palpation may reveal some ovarian activity (complete inactivity could indicate anestrus and is addressed elsewhere), a normal or enlarged uterus, and a closed cervix.
- Transrectal U/S may allow a corpus luteum to be visualized. If a mare is prone to multiple ovulations, more than one corpus luteum may be identified. A mature corpus luteum appears as a round or teardrop-shaped, uniformly hyperechoic area within the ovary. The periphery of a recent ovulation may appear as described, but the center of the corpus hemorrhagicum/corpus luteum is often hypoechoic or mottled. Transrectal U/S should also be used to evaluate the uterus for cysts, luminal fluid accumulations, or pregnancy.
- Vaginoscopy can confirm transrectal palpation findings regarding the degree of cervical relaxation and/or the presence of uterine or cervical discharge.

CAUSES

Idiopathic/Spontaneous Persistence of the Corpus Luteum

Associated with normal *diestrus* ovulations (after day 10 of the cycle), resulting in an immature corpus luteum being present at the time of normal luteolysis (day 14–15). Persistent corpus lutea have also been related to ingestion of fescue-contaminated feed.

Pregnancy

Corpus luteum function continues in the presence of a conceptus.

Early Embryonic Death

Maternal recognition of pregnancy occurs by day 14 post-ovulation. Embryonic death after this time results in a delayed return to estrus, i.e., a longer than expected interestrus interval. If embryonic death occurs after the formation of endometrial cups (35–40 days post-ovulation), the mare will not return to estrus until the endometrial cups regress and production of eCG by the cups ceases (120–150 days post-ovulation).

Uterine Infections/Endometrial Degeneration

Because endogenous $PGF_{2\alpha}$ is of endometrial origin, endometritis, pyometra, or other causes of declining uterine health can result in ineffective prostaglandin formation and/or release.

Iatrogenic/Pharmaceutical

- Parenteral administration of progestin compounds to suppress behavioral estrus
- NSAIDs can potentially interfere with endometrial $PGF_{2\alpha}$ release and result in prolonged luteal activity. There is no evidence that chronic administration at recommended therapeutic dosages inhibits the spontaneous formation and release of $PGF_{2\alpha}$ from the endometrium.
- GnRH agonist (deslorelin) implants used to stimulate ovulation have been associated with prolonged interovulatory intervals. The effect is more profound if $PGF_{2\alpha}$ is used during the diestrus period in an attempt to "short-cycle" the mare. The implant format is not currently sold in the United States, but the injectable product remains available.

Lactation

A corpus luteum may persist following the first, or *foal heat,* ovulation. This may be more likely in mares that are in less than optimal body condition (in caloric deficit).

RISK FACTORS

N/A

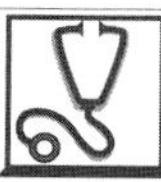

DIAGNOSIS

DIFFERENTIAL DIAGNOSIS

Differentiating Similar Signs

Diagnosis is based on finding a normal, nonpregnant, diestrus reproductive tract coupled with a history of failing to show estrus behavior >2 weeks post-ovulation and a serum progesterone concentration of >4 ng/mL. This assumes some ovarian activity has previously been observed and therefore is not being mistaken for anestrus. Regular teasing, serial transrectal palpation, and U/S are the cornerstones to proper interpretation of the reproductive cycle of an individual mare.

Differentiating Causes

- Pregnancy and/or early embryonic death can occur without any history of a scheduled breeding, if access to any stallion/colt is remotely possible in the mare's environment. Therefore, it is essential to palpate a mare before doing any invasive vaginal procedures (uterine culture or biopsy) or administering prostaglandin to short-cycle a mare experiencing a prolonged diestrus.
- Pyometra and endometritis are typically diagnosed on the basis of transrectal palpation, U/S, uterine culture, and biopsy. See Endometritis, Pyometra.
- History of a normal foal heat followed by reproductive quiescence can be due to either prolonged diestrus or lactational anestrus. Ovarian activity and serum progesterone concentration assays allow differentiation.

CBC/BIOCHEMISTRY/URINALYSIS

N/A

OTHER LABORATORY TESTS

- Serum progesterone concentrations—Basal levels of <1 ng/mL indicate no mature luteal tissue is present. Mature corpus luteum function is associated with levels of >4 ng/mL.
- Serum eCG levels—may be useful in cases of suspected early embryonic death after endometrial cup formation, especially if there is no evidence of pregnancy at the time of the examination. See Pregnancy Diagnosis.

IMAGING

N/A

DIAGNOSTIC PROCEDURES

Uterine cytology, culture, and endometrial biopsy are useful to diagnose and treat pyometra and endometritis. See Endometritis, Pyometra.

PATHOLOGICAL FINDINGS

N/A

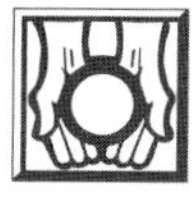

TREATMENT

- If deslorelin was used to stimulate ovulation, consider removing the implant 48 hr after administration (post-ovulation) on subsequent cycles. The implant format is not currently sold in the United States, but the injectable product remains available.
- Prolonged diestrus, if the presence of a corpus luteum is confirmed, is treated with $PGF_{2\alpha}$.
- Pregnancy should be definitively ruled out.
- Luteolysis is the goal of treatment, whether the release of endogenous $PGF_{2\alpha}$ is accomplished with uterine manipulation or exogenous $PGF_{2\alpha}$ is administered to the mare.
- Endogenous $PGF_{2\alpha}$ release can be stimulated by intrauterine infusion of sterile saline at ambient temperature or warmed to ≤120° F/48° C. Maintain aseptic technique; use a 500- to 1000-mL volume of flush solution.

- Endometrial biopsy or uterine culture may infrequently stimulate endogenous $PGF_{2\alpha}$ release.

APPROPRIATE HEALTH CARE, NURSING CARE, ACTIVITY, DIET, CLIENT EDUCATION, SURGICAL CONSIDERATIONS

N/A

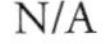

MEDICATIONS

DRUG(S) OF CHOICE

- $PGF_{2\alpha}$ (Lutalyse [Pfizer] 10 mg IM) or its analogs are used to stimulate luteolysis. Mares with a functional corpus luteum typically exhibit estrus 2–4 days post-injection and ovulate 6–12 days after treatment.
- Two doses of $PGF_{2\alpha}$ given 14–15 days apart are useful, if transrectal palpation cannot easily or safely be accomplished. This regimen ensures that immature/nonresponsive luteal tissue present at the time of the first injection has ample time to mature and be able to respond to the second $PGF_{2\alpha}$ injection.

CONTRAINDICATIONS

$PGF_{2\alpha}$ and its analogs are contraindicated in mares with heaves or other bronchoconstrictive disease.

PRECAUTIONS

- Horses
  - $PGF_{2\alpha}$ causes sweating and colic-like symptoms due to its stimulatory effect on smooth muscle cells. If cramping has not subsided within 1–2 hr, symptomatic treatment should be instituted.
  - $PGF_{2\alpha}$ should not be used in horses intended for food.
- Humans
  - $PGF_{2\alpha}$ and its analogs should not be handled by pregnant women, or persons with asthma or bronchial disease. Any accidental exposure to skin should be washed off immediately.

POSSIBLE INTERACTIONS

N/A

ALTERNATIVE DRUGS

Cloprostenol sodium (Estrumate [Schering-Plough Animal Health] 250 µg/mL IM) is a prostaglandin analog. This product is used in similar fashion as the natural prostaglandin but has been associated with fewer side effects. While it is not currently approved for use in horses, it is an analog in broad use in the absence of an alternative.

FOLLOW-UP

N/A

PATIENT MONITORING

- Serial (three times weekly) teasing, transrectal palpation, and U/S are recommended to evaluate the mare's reproductive tract for evidence of estrus.
- Serum progesterone concentrations, measured twice weekly for 2 weeks post-$PGF_{2\alpha}$ administration, can be used to determine the effectiveness of treatment and/or persistence of functional luteal tissue.

PREVENTION/AVOIDANCE

N/A

POSSIBLE COMPLICATIONS

Prolonged nonpregnant periods and/or infertility

EXPECTED COURSE AND PROGNOSIS

N/A

MISCELLANEOUS

ASSOCIATED CONDITIONS

N/A

AGE-RELATED FACTORS

N/A

ZOONOTIC POTENTIAL

N/A

PREGNANCY

Prostaglandin administration to pregnant mares can cause corpus luteum lysis and abortion. Carefully and absolutely rule out pregnancy before administering this drug or its analogs.

SYNONYMS

- Equine chorionic gonadotropin (eCG)
- Pregnant mare serum gonadotropin (PMSG)

SEE ALSO

- Abnormal estrus intervals
- Anestrus
- Early embryonic death
- Endometritis
- Abnormal estrus intervals
- Pseudopregnancy
- Pyometra

ABBREVIATIONS

- eCG = equine chorionic gonadotropin
- GnRH = gonadotropin releasing hormone
- $PGF_{2\alpha}$ = PGF, natural prostaglandin
- U/S = ultrasound, ultrasonography

Suggested Reading

Daels PF, Hughes JP. The abnormal estrous cycle. In: McKinnon AO, Voss JL, eds. Equine Reproduction. Philadelphia: Lea & Febiger, 1993:144–160.

Hinrichs K. Irregularities of the estrous cycle and ovulation in mares (including seasonal transition). In: Youngquist RS, Threlfall WR, eds. Current Therapy in Large Animal Theriogenology. St. Louis, MO: Saunders Elsevier, 2007:144–152.

Löfstedt RM. Some aspects of manipulative and diagnostic endocrinology of the broodmare. Proc Soc Therio 1986;67–93.

McCue PM, Farquhar VJ, Carnevale EM, Squires EL. Removal of deslorelin (Ovuplant™) implant 48 h after administration results in normal interovulatory intervals in mares. Therio 2002;58:865–870.

Sharp DC. Early pregnancy in mares: uncoupling the luteolytic cascade. Proc Soc Therio 1996;236–242.

Van Camp SD. Prolonged diestrus. In: Robinson NE, ed. Current Therapy in Equine Medicine. Philadelphia: WB Saunders, 1983:401–402.

Author Carole C. Miller

Consulting Editor Carla L. Carleton

PROLONGED PREGNANCY

BASICS

DEFINITION/OVERVIEW

• Gestation exceeding the normal range for the mare; gestation that appears to be lengthened by abnormal characteristics of the fetus
• Normal range of gestation is 320–355 days, but it is not rare for gestational length to fall outside this range.

ETIOLOGY/PATHOPHYSIOLOGY

• Multifactorial—individual variation, placental function or dysfunction, and hormonal changes; may also involve damage to the endometrium, thus reducing the nutrient supply to the fetus; still able to sustain life, but resulting in fetal growth retardation

SYSTEM AFFECTED

Reproductive

GENETICS

N/A

INCIDENCE/PREVALENCE

• No statistics are available regarding incidence.
• It is not a major reproductive problem.

SIGNALMENT

• Females
• All breeds
• All of breeding age

SIGNS

General Comments

• Differs from other domestic species, in which prolonged pregnancy is linked with iodine deficiency, increased progesterone, and inheritance
• May be caused by abnormal fetal pituitary and adrenal development or by lack of hypothalamic maturity at term

Historical

Usually appears to be a fetal problem, so historical information may have limited value

Physical Examination

• Mare—no abnormalities of the mare unless excessive uterine fluid has accumulated
• Fetus—postpartum examination usually reveals a dead or very weak fetus; smaller than normal; may appear undernourished

CAUSES AND RISK FACTORS

• Hormonal—Most commonly, the pituitary or adrenal glands are involved.
• Not a mare problem; mares can be bred again with little concern for recurrence.

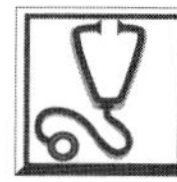

DIAGNOSIS

• Accurate history combined with transrectal palpation
• Outward gross appearance of the mare
• Appearance of the fetus—pre-partum, post-partum, and/or necropsy

DIFFERENTIAL DIAGNOSIS

Hydrops

• Prolonged pregnancy with a hydrops is invariably shorter than the lengthened gestation associated with a fetus having a higher center defect.
• Known breeding and ovulation dates facilitate differentiation.

CBC/BIOCHEMISTRY/URINALYSIS

N/A

OTHER LABORATORY TESTS

Peritoneal tap:
• To determine the location of excessive fluid accumulation
• To differentiate prolonged pregnancy from hydrops
• *Hydrops amnii*—due to a fetal defect; excessive fluid is amniotic.
• *Hydrops allantois*—due to a uteroplacental defect; excessive fluid is allantoic.

IMAGING

U/S imaging, to determine if
• Excessive fluid is present.
• The endometrium is thickened.
• Fetal extremities are smaller than normal.

OTHER DIAGNOSTIC PROCEDURES

• When >30 days postpartum, perform an endometrial biopsy of the mare to determine the endometrial status before prebreeding.

PATHOLOGIC FINDINGS

• The uterus may or may not be larger than normal.
• If the fetus is dead or dies postpartum, a necropsy should be done to determine if its adrenal and pituitary glands and hypothalamus are normal.

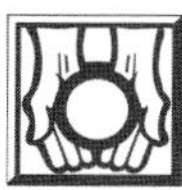

TREATMENT

• Parturition induction is an option. However, it is essential that the breeding date is accurate, and that records can confirm its validity, to avoid inducing a preterm, nonviable foal.
• Remind owners that fetal survival after a prolonged gestation is in question. The actual circumstances of survival may not be known until after delivery.
• Routine care for the mare during the postpartum period
• Emphasize to owners that prolonged pregnancies can occur and that most affected mares have normal foals.
• Remind owners that gestational length may fall outside the normal range and still be normal for that individual.

APPROPRIATE HEALTH CARE, NURSING CARE, ACTIVITY, DIET, CLIENT EDUCATION, SURGICAL CONSIDERATIONS

N/A

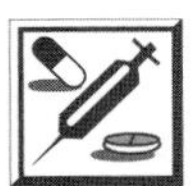

MEDICATIONS

DRUG(S) OF CHOICE

None required or indicated

CONTRAINDICATIONS

N/A

PRECAUTIONS

N/A

POSSIBLE INTERACTIONS

N/A

ALTERNATIVE DRUGS

N/A

FOLLOW-UP

PATIENT MONITORING

- Monitor mares once they are suspected to be "overdue."
- Take no action unless pregnancy goes beyond the expected due date in the absence of external evidence of advancing gestation and approaching parturition.
- A pluriparous mare should be close to a previous "term gestation" length in which she delivered a normal foal before considering inducing parturition.

PREVENTION/AVOIDANCE

Unknown, because the major causes involve abnormal fetal pituitary, adrenals, or hypothalamus

POSSIBLE COMPLICATIONS

- Prolonged pregnancy could result in dystocia.
- Because the fetus usually is smaller than normal and has no ankylosis of joints, dystocia usually is not a problem.

EXPECTED COURSE AND PROGNOSIS

Postpartum

- Normal postpartum examination of the mare
- The fetus is expected to be smaller than normal and has a low probability of survival.

MISCELLANEOUS

ASSOCIATED CONDITIONS

N/A

AGE-RELATED FACTORS

N/A

ZOONOTIC POTENTIAL

N/A

PREGNANCY

Occurs only during gestation

SEE ALSO

- Parturition induction
- Postpartum care

Suggested Reading

Vandeplassche M. Obstetrician's view of the physiology of equine parturition and dystocia. Equine Vet J 1980;12:45–49.

Author Walter R. Threlfall

Consulting Editor Carla L. Carleton

PROTEIN, HYPERFIBRINOGENEMIA

BASICS

DEFINITION

- A plasma fibrinogen concentration greater than the upper limit of the laboratory reference range—usually >400 mg/dL (4.0 g/L)
- Increased fibrinogen concentrations can be associated with a wide variety of inflammatory diseases and may be the only indicator of inflammation if the accompanying leukogram is normal.
- Concentrations usually peak 72–96 hours after the onset of inflammation and can exceed 1000 mg/dL (10.0 g/L). The normal half-life for plasma fibrinogen is ≅3 days. As inflammation subsides, concentrations return to normal and may be used to indicate resolution of inflammation.
- Plasma fibrinogen may also be increased with hemoconcentration and may be decreased with severe hepatic disease because of decreased production, or with DIC because of increased utilization, which may mask the hyperfibrinogenemia associated with inflammation.

PATHOPHYSIOLOGY

- Fibrinogen is a glycoprotein produced solely in the liver in response to inflammation.
- Cytokines (e.g., interleukins-1β and -6, tumor necrosis factor), released early in an inflammatory process, reduce hepatic synthesis of negative acute phase proteins (e.g., albumin, prealbumin, and transferrin) and increase synthesis of positive acute phase proteins (e.g., fibrinogen, complement, haptoglobin, C-reactive protein, serum amyloid A, ceruloplasmin, and α-acid glycoprotein). Subsequent exudation of these proteins into sites of inflammation allows conversion of fibrinogen to fibrin, where fibrin monomers provide the scaffolding for fibroblasts to wall off the inflammatory process and initiate tissue healing.
- The conversion of fibrinogen to fibrin also is an essential component of the clotting cascade.

SIGNALMENT

Fibrinogen concentrations may be increased in foals up to 6 mo of age and during pregnancy in mares (see Age-Related Factors and Pregnancy).

SIGNS

- There are no clinical signs specifically referable to hyperfibrinogenemia; signs observed usually relate to the underlying disease process or are nonspecific indicators of inflammation (e.g., fever, inappetence, weight loss).
- History varies with the underlying primary disease or may nonspecifically reflect inflammation.
- Establishing the etiology of the primary inflammatory condition is warranted.

CAUSES AND RISK FACTORS

- There are two primary causes of hyperfibrinogenemia; inflammation (inflammatory, infectious and neoplastic disorders) and dehydration (relative increase).
- The inflammatory process may be acute or chronic and occur in a wide variety of body systems.
- GI tract—e.g., colitis, enteritis, peritonitis, parasitism, endotoxemia, mesenteric abscessation, large colon torsion, ruptured esophagus, intussusception, tooth root abscess, neoplasia, and surgery.
- Respiratory tract—e.g., pneumonia (aspiration, broncho-, pleuro-, abscessation/*Rhodococcus equi*), guttural pouch empyema, sinusitis, and pyothorax.
- Hemic/lymphatic/immune systems—e.g., septicemia, endocarditis, pericarditis, thrombophlebitis, omphalophlebitis, lymph node abscessation (*Streptococcus equi*, *Corynebacterium pseudotuberculosis*), lymphangitis, immune-mediated vasculitis (purpura hemorrhagica), systemic viral infections (e.g., equine infectious anemia, equine viral arteritis), and leukemia.
- Urologic system—e.g., cystitis, urinary calculi, glomerulonephritis, pyelonephritis, canathardin poisoning, and neoplasia.
- Reproductive tract—e.g., pregnancy (see below), placentitis, endometritis, and orchitis.
- Musculoskeletal system—e.g., wound infections, cellulitis and abscesses, septic arthritis or osteomyelitis (e.g., fistulous withers), trauma and fractures, exertional rhabdomyolysis, myositis (e.g., infectious, postanesthetic) and neoplasia.
- Nervous system—e.g., bacterial meningitis and abscess.
- Hepatobiliary system—e.g., acute hepatic failure (i.e., Theiler's disease), cholangitis, hepatitis, and neoplasia
- Ophthalmic system—e.g., uveitis, trauma or injury to eye, and neoplasia
- Skin—e.g., pemphigus foliaceus, dermatophilosis, and chronic dermatitis

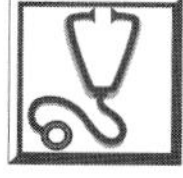

DIAGNOSIS

DIFFERENTIAL DIAGNOSIS

- Hyperfibrinogenemia should prompt a thorough, systematic physical examination and possibly further diagnostic testing to establish the origin of the inflammatory stimulus. Any area of heat, pain, or swelling is a likely source of the inflammatory stimulus and should be evaluated. The challenge lies in identifying the primary cause of hyperfibrinogenemia in a patient with no overt clinical signs of disease.
- Historical or physical examination findings may help localize the site of inflammation; colic, abdominal mass, diarrhea, or weight loss should prompt closer investigation of the GI tract; tachycardia, dyspnea, abnormal nasal discharge, or malodorous breath should prompt closer investigation of the respiratory tract; weight loss and lymph node enlargement might indicate *S. equi* or *C. pseudotuberculosis* infection, or lymphosarcoma/other neoplasms.

LABORATORY FINDINGS

- A number of analytical techniques may be used to determine fibrinogen concentrations and the sample type submitted for analysis must be consistent with the technique.
- Blood collected in standard EDTA tubes is suitable for analysis by the heat precipitation method. Human laboratories commonly use a thrombin clotting time (or Clauss modification of thrombin time) to determine fibrinogen concentration. In this test, fibrinogen quantification is based on the rate of clot formation in dilute, citrated plasma after addition to thrombin. For this assay, blood must be submitted in sodium citrate. Immunological assays for quantification of fibrinogen in human plasma may also be used on equine samples in human laboratories due to the high degree of immunologic cross-reactivity for fibrinogen between species. However, this assay has not been validated for use with equine plasma.
- Fibrinogen concentrations may be falsely lowered if the blood has clotted before analysis. Analytical error may also occur with hemolyzed, icteric, or lipemic samples; heparin contamination; over- or under-filling of citrated collection tubes; and methods dependent on normal clotting if submitted in EDTA tubes.
- Hyperproteinemia caused by dehydration, or hypoproteinemia caused by marked protein loss, can falsely increase or decrease plasma fibrinogen concentrations, respectively.
- The plasma protein:fibrinogen (PP:F) ratio can help interpretation of fibrinogen concentrations if hyperproteinemia is present. This ratio is calculated as:

$$\text{PP:F ratio} = \frac{[\text{plasmaTP mg/dL}]/[\text{fibrinogen mg/dL}]}{[\text{fibrinogen mg/dL}]}$$

- Ratios between 15 and 20 are considered normal. Elevated ratios (>20) are consistent with dehydration. Decreased ratios (<15) demonstrate a relative increase in plasma fibrinogen and indicate inflammation. If ratios are between 10 and 15, clinical impression and other diagnostic aids should be employed in these cases to determine if the ratio is significant. Ratios <10 are abnormal and indicate active inflammation.
- PP:F ratios should not be used in foals or mature horses with concurrent diseases causing hypoproteinemia. Increased fibrinogen consumption in the pathological state or concurrent dehydration and inflammation may also confound the interpretation.

CBC/BIOCHEMISTRY/URINALYSIS

- White blood cell count and the number of band (i.e., immature) neutrophils may be concurrently increased in horses with hyperfibrinogenemia.
- In cases where there are no overt clinical signs of inflammation, a CBC, chemistry panel, and urinalysis should be performed to screen specific organ systems for abnormalities.

OTHER LABORATORY TESTS

- A number of other acute phase proteins (e.g., serum amyloid A, haptoglobin, C-reactive protein) as well as plasma iron concentrations have been evaluated in horses as alternate indicators of systemic inflammatory disease.
- Of these analytes, plasma iron appears to be most sensitive. One study found decreases in plasma iron better reflected acute inflammation than did plasma fibrinogen concentration. Therefore, plasma iron concentrations may be a useful alternate or co-analyte for evaluation of inflammation in horses.

IMAGING

Radiography or ultrasonography may help localize and possibly allow quantitative assessment of involvement of a specific organ system.

OTHER DIAGNOSTIC PROCEDURES

- Ancillary diagnostic tests (e.g., tracheal wash, peritoneal or pleural fluid analysis, specific organ biopsies) may help localize an inflammatory focus.
- Bacteriology and serology may identify specific pathogens.

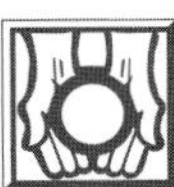

TREATMENT

AIMS OF TREATMENT

- Treatment should be aimed at the underlying primary disease process.
- Hyperfibrinogenemia is highly correlated with septic inflammatory processes; thus, empiric antibiotic treatment may be useful in some circumstances while awaiting results or while a more extensive diagnostic workup is being pursued.
- The degree of hyperfibrinogenemia may approximate the severity of disease and can be used, together with other clinical and laboratory findings (e.g., plasma iron concentrations), for determining the level of care, length of treatment and possibly prognosis for the primary disease process.

MEDICATIONS

DRUG(S)

- Therapeutic choices should be based on a tentative or definitive diagnosis of the primary underlying disease process.
- Broad-spectrum, bactericidal antimicrobial or anti-inflammatory agents often are indicated.

FOLLOW-UP

PATIENT MONITORING

- Treatment efficacy may be monitored by serial evaluation of CBC and plasma fibrinogen concentrations at 2–3-day intervals.
- Fibrinogen concentrations alone may be used to identify resolution of an inflammatory process, especially when the leukocyte count is unchanged or has returned to normal values.
- Fibrinogen concentrations peak within 72–96 hr after the onset of inflammation, although resolution of hyperfibrinogenemia may be lengthy if the inflammatory focus persists. In one study, fibrinogen concentrations had not returned to normal 15 days after surgical trauma.

POSSIBLE COMPLICATIONS

Increasing plasma fibrinogen concentrations positively correlate with mortality from the associated disease process.

MISCELLANEOUS

AGE-RELATED FACTORS

Fibrinogen increases in normal foals during the first 5 mo of age and can exceed normal adult concentrations. Ranges of 260 +/− 60 mg/dL (2.6 g/L) in 1-day-old foals to 460 +/− 70mg/dL (4.6 g/L) in 1- to 3-mo-old foals have been reported. The cause has been attributed to maturing hepatic function and is not associated with subclinical disease.

PREGNANCY

- In one study, fibrinogen concentrations showed a dramatic increase (>40%) in prepartum mares.
- These concentrations can further increase by another ≈10% between 12 and 36 hr postpartum, but return to prepartum concentrations by 14 days after foaling.

ABBREVIATION

- GI = gastrointestinal

Suggested Reading

Allen BV, Kold SE. Fibrinogen response to surgical tissue trauma in the horse. Equine Vet J 1988;20:441–443.

Andrews DA, Reagan WJ, DeNicola DB. Plasma fibrinogen in recognizing equine inflammatory disease. Compend Cont Educ 1994;16:1349–1356.

Borges AS, Divers TJ, Stokol T, Mohammed OH. Serum iron and plasma fibrinogen concentrations as indicators of systemic inflammatory disease in horses. J Vet Intern Med 2007;21:489–494.

Gentry PA, Feldman BF, O'Neill SL, Madigan JE, Zinkl JG. Evaluation of the haemostatic profile in the pre- and post-parturient mare, with particular focus on the perinatal period. Equine Vet J 1992;24:33–36.

Murata H, Shimada N, Yoshioka M. Current research on acute phase proteins in veterinary diagnosis: an overview. Vet J 2004;168:28–40.

The author and editors wish to acknowledge the contributions of Dina A. Andrews, author of this topic in the previous edition.

Author Jennifer Hodgson

Consulting Editors David Hodgson and Jennifer Hodgson

PROTEIN, HYPERPROTEINEMIA

BASICS

DEFINITION

- Dysproteinemia is the presence of normal protein at abnormal concentrations in blood or the presence of abnormal protein. Hyperproteinemia occurs when the protein concentration in peripheral blood is greater than the upper limit of the laboratory reference interval—usually >7.9 g/dL (>79 g/L) in serum.
- The increase in protein may be nonselective, due to higher than normal concentrations of all plasma proteins (i.e., panhyperproteinemia), or may be selective where some protein concentrations (e.g., globulins) are increased more than others.
- The predominant proteins present in blood include albumin, globulins, and fibrinogen. Globulins and albumin can be separated and quantified by serum electrophoresis. Using this technique, globulin proteins can be further divided into α_1, α_2, β_1, β_2, and γ globulins. Immunoglobulins are located in the β and γ regions of the serum electrophoretogram.
- Paraproteins are immunoglobulins produced by neoplastic immune cells, such as plasma cells in cases of multiple myeloma.

PATHOPHYSIOLOGY

- Collectively, plasma proteins perform a nutritive function, exert colloidal osmotic pressure, and aid in the maintenance of acid-base balance. Individual proteins serve as enzymes, antibodies, coagulation factors, hormones, and transport carriers.
- The major sites of plasma protein production are the liver, then the immune system.
- Filtration between intravascular and extravascular space, metabolic demands, hormonal balance, nutritional status, and water balance determine the plasma protein concentration of an individual.
- Plasma protein concentration in neonates is significantly influenced by passive transfer of immunoglobulins (see Age-Related Factors), while in adults the protein concentration remains relatively stable unless influenced by pathological processes.

Panhyperproteinemia

- Results from a relative water loss (dehydration), which concentrates all plasma proteins proportionally.
- Dehydration initially causes a shift of tissue fluid into the intravascular space as the body attempts to maintain adequate blood volume. As dehydration persists, intravascular fluid is lost, resulting in hemoconcentration with a relative increase in TP. If renal function is adequate, urine output decreases to compensate for the fluid loss, and urine concentration increases (see CBC/Biochemistry/Urinalysis).
- The water loss may be due to decreased fluid intake or excessive fluid losses (see Causes).
- There is usually an associated increase in PCV, though a hemoconcentrated patient that is concurrently anemic has hyperproteinemia with a normal or decreased PCV.

Hyperalbuminemia

Hyperalbuminemia represents a relative increase in albumin concentration secondary to dehydration. Concurrent hyperglobulinemia is usually also present.

Hyperglobulinemia

- Increases in globulin concentrations may be relative (i.e., secondary to hemoconcentration) or absolute.
- Absolute increases occur in horses with inflammatory disease and immunostimulation resulting in hepatic synthesis of acute-phase proteins and lymphocyte (plasma cell) synthesis of immunoglobulins.
- There are 3 major changes of plasma proteins in an inflammatory dysproteinemia:
    - Increased hepatic production of *positive acute phase proteins* (e.g., α_1 globulins, α_2 globulins, fibrinogen, serum amyloid A, and C-reactive protein) during acute inflammation. Production of these proteins may increase within hours of inflammatory stimulus and persist for the duration of the process, but increased plasma or serum concentrations are usually detectable ≈2 days after onset of inflammation.
    - Decreased hepatic production of *negative acute phase proteins* (e.g., albumin, transferrin) during acute and chronic inflammation. Due to the life span of these proteins, decreased concentrations may not be noted until inflammation has continued for at least 1 week, but will persist for the duration of the inflammatory response.
    - Increased production of *delayed response proteins* (e.g., immunoglobulins, and complement) during acute or chronic inflammation, which can be detected 1 to 3 weeks after onset of inflammation. Globulins produced are predominantly IgG (γ globulins) but also IgM and IgA (β globulins). Increased synthesis of a variety of immunoglobulins by many different lymphocytes produces a polyclonal gammopathy.
- Increased production of acute-phase proteins may cause mild increases in globulin concentration, whereas production of chronic phase proteins (e.g., immunoglobulins) can cause moderate to marked hyperglobulinemia/hyperproteineia.

Hyperfibrinogenemia

See related topic—Hyperfibrinogenemia.

Neoplastic Diseases

- An absolute increase in globulins also may be caused by B-lymphocyte neoplasia.
- A neoplastic (clonal) expansion of one type of B lymphocyte may result in production of large quantities of a single immunoglobulin type, with the resulting dysproteinemia being called a monoclonal gammopathy.
- The neoplastic cells may produce intact immunoglobulins, free light chains (Bence Jones proteins), only heavy chains or abnormal fragments.
- Monoclonal gammopathies can be caused by multiple myeloma (plasma cell neoplasia), lymphocytic leukemia, and lymphosarcoma. Polyclonal gammopathies may also be detected with lymphosarcoma or other tumors.
- The pattern of protein changes associated with monoclonal gammopathies includes a mild to marked hyperproteinemia, due to hyperglobulinemia that contains a monoclonal gammopathy. The monoclonal protein may migrate in the β or γ fraction. Concentrations of immunoglobulins, other than the monoclonal protein, frequently are decreased and there is a mild to moderate hypoalbuminemia.

SIGNALMENT

Hyperglobulinemia associated with a monoclonal gammopathy secondary to neoplasia is more likely in older animals.

SIGNS

General Comments

- There are no pathognomonic signs of hyperproteinemia.
- Nonspecific physical findings associated with dehydration, inflammation, or neoplasia warrant hematologic and serum chemistry evaluation, which may demonstrate hyperproteinemia.

Historical

Fever, decreased appetite, cough, nasal discharge, respiratory distress, exercise intolerance, poor performance, GI dysfunction, and weight loss may be observed.

Physical Examination

- In addition to the physical findings discussed above, signs of dehydration may include decreased capillary perfusion as demonstrated by increased CRT, decreased pulse pressure, tachycardia, decreased skin elasticity, sunken eyes, and decreased urine output.

CAUSES

Panhyperproteinemia

- Panhyperproteinemia is associated with dehydration, which may be due to decreased fluid intake or excessive fluid losses.
- Decreased fluid intake may be due to:
    - Dysphagia associated with pain (e.g., pharyngeal abscess, trauma), obstruction (e.g., esophageal obstruction/choke, nasal mass) or neurological dysfunction (e.g., botulism, guttural pouch mycosis, yellow star thistle/Russian knapweed poisoning, lead toxicity, rabies idiopathic),
    - Lack of thirst, e.g., toxemia
- Excessive fluid losses may be due to:
    - GI disorders e.g., diarrhea associated with acute colitis, salmonellosis, Potomac horse fever, intestinal clostridiosis, intestinal strangulating obstruction, proximal enteritis
    - Fluid sequestration subsequent to intestinal obstruction
    - Polyuria associated with chronic renal failure
    - Increased vascular permeability (e.g., purpura hemorrhagica, gram-negative sepsis, endotoxemia)
    - Loss from the vascular space via excessive sweating
    - Exudation from extensive skin wounds (e.g., burns)

Hyperglobulinemia

- Globulin concentrations may increase due to dehydration (relative increase), inflammation (infectious, inflammatory, and neoplastic disorders), in late stages of pregnancy, or due to

B-lymphocyte neoplasia (e.g., multiple myeloma).

- The inflammatory process is usually chronic and may occur in a wide variety of body systems:
  - GI tract—e.g., peritonitis, parasitism, mesenteric abscessation, tooth root abscess,
  - Respiratory tract—e.g., pulmonary abscessation (*Rhodococcus equi*), guttural pouch empyema, pyothorax,
  - Hemic/lymphatic/immune systems—e.g., endocarditis, pericarditis, lymph node abscessation (*Streptococcus equi*, *Corynebacterium pseudotuberculosis*), immune-mediated vasculitis (purpura hemorrhagica),
  - Urologic system—e.g., glomerulonephritis, pyelonephritis,
  - Reproductive tract—e.g., pregnancy (*see below*), endometritis,
  - Musculoskeletal system—e.g., abscesses, septic arthritis, osteomyelitis (e.g., fistulous withers),
  - Nervous system—e.g., bacterial meningitis and abscess,
  - Hepatobiliary system—e.g., cholangitis, chronic active hepatitis,
  - Skin—e.g., pemphigus foliaceus, chronic dermatitis, dermatophilosis.
- Specific neoplastic disorders causing hyperglobulinemia include multiple myeloma, lymphocytic leukemia, and lymphosarcoma. Other forms of neoplasia may also result in increased globulin concentrations via inflammation.

Hyperalbuminemia

- Dehydration

Hyperfibrinogenemia

- See related topic Hyperfibrinogenemia.

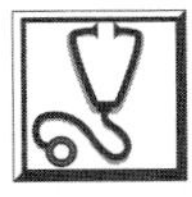

DIAGNOSIS

DIFFERENTIAL DIAGNOSIS

- Selective versus nonselective hyperproteinemia should first be determined. Evidence of dehydration supports nonselective (relative) hyperproteinemia.
- If selective hyperproteinemia is occurring—Infectious, inflammatory, and lymphoproliferative disorders should be differentiated and the site and cause of infectious/inflammatory/neoplastic processes should be determined.

CBC/BIOCHEMISTRY/URINALYSIS

- Total serum or plasma protein is most commonly measured by refractometry, which is influenced by the concentration of solids within a sample. Therefore, high concentrations of lipids, urea, Na^+, Cl^-, etc., may increase refractive index and cause spurious effects on TP values.
- Increased PCV, albumin concentration, and urine specific gravity and prerenal azotemia support dehydration.
- Laboratory findings associated with inflammation may include anemia of chronic disease, neutrophilia or neutropenia, lymphocytosis or lymphopenia, monocytosis, and hypoalbuminemia.
- Normal or decreased PCV with hyperproteinemia may indicate concomitant anemia with dehydration or infectious/inflammatory disease.

OTHER LABORATORY TESTS

- Calculation of the albumin:globulin (A/G) ratio may help interpretation of TP values.
- The A/G ratio will remain within the reference interval if both fractions are increased uniformly such as with dehydration,
- The A/G ratio may be abnormal if an alteration of one fraction predominates; e.g., decreased A/G ratio with renal proteinuria and/or immunoglobulin production following antigenic stimulation; increased A/G ratio from lack of immunoglobulin production in adults or lack of colostrum absorption in foals.
- Serum protein electrophoresis can be used to quantitate individual protein fractions encountered in hyperglobulinemic patients and to differentiate polyclonal from monoclonal gammopathies. Alternatively, immunochemical and radio-immunological methods allow specific identification and quantitation of individual proteins.
- Additional tests for infectious (e.g., serology) or other inflammatory diseases as indicated to establish a definitive diagnosis.

IMAGING

Ultrasonography and radiography of the thorax, abdomen, or relevant soft tissues may help identify the cause of the hyperglobulinemia.

OTHER DIAGNOSTIC PROCEDURES

Abdominocentesis, thoracocentesis, tracheal aspiration or bronchoalveolar lavage, endoscopy, laparoscopy, bone marrow aspiration, biopsy, and histopathology may be indicated to determine location and etiology of infectious, inflammatory or lymphoproliferative disorders.

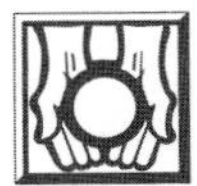

TREATMENT

AIMS OF TREATMENT

- If dehydration is cause of hyperproteinemia, the severity of dehydration and electrolyte imbalances will help determine route, volume and composition of fluids to be administered.
- Specific causes of dehydration, inflammation, or infection may require additional medical or surgical treatments.

FOLLOW-UP

PATIENT MONITORING

- Evaluation of hydration status using clinical (mucous membrane color, heart rate, and CRT) and laboratory (PCV/TP, creatinine) parameters
- Frequency of monitoring will depend on severity of the case and clinical response to therapy.

MISCELLANEOUS

AGE-RELATED FACTORS

- Plasma and serum protein concentrations are low at birth, increase after absorption of colostrum, decline over 1–5 weeks as antibodies in colostrum are metabolized, and then increase to adult concentrations within 6 mo to 1 year.
- Adult protein concentrations remain relatively stable, although albumin decreases slightly over time, while globulins, particularly immunoglobulins and acute phase proteins, progressively increase in old age.

PREGNANCY

- Fetal development stresses the maternal protein reserve, resulting in an increased globulin concentration with a concomitant decrease in albumin concentration.
- Serum immunoglobulin concentrations increase in the dam until ≈1 mo before term, at which time they are secreted into the mammary gland during colostrums production.
- Both albumin and TP concentrations decrease during lactation.

SYNONYMS

Gammopathy

SEE ALSO

- Hyperfibrinogenemia
- Multiple myeloma
- Lymphosarcoma

ABBREVIATIONS

- CRT = capillary refill time
- GI = gastrointestinal
- PCV = packed cell volume
- TP = total protein

Suggested Reading

Latimer KS, Maheffey EA, Prasse KW. Duncan & Prasse's Veterinary Laboratory Medicine. Clinical Pathology, ed 4. Ames, IA: Iowa State University Press, 2003.

Smith BP. Large Animal Internal Medicine, ed 3. St. Louis: CV Mosby, 2002.

Stockham SL, Scott MA. Fundamentals of Veterinary Clinical Pathology. Ames, IA: Iowa State University Press, 2002.

Author Jennifer Hodgson

Consulting Editors David Hodgson and Jennifer Hodgson

PROTEIN, HYPOPROTEINEMIA

BASICS

DEFINITION

• Dysproteinemia is the presence of normal protein at abnormal concentrations in blood or the presence of abnormal protein. Hypoproteinemia occurs when the TPP is <5.2g/dL (<52g/L). This may vary with age, sex, and physiologic state.
• The decrease in protein may be nonselective, due to lower than normal concentrations of the major plasma proteins (i.e., panhypoproteinemia), or may be selective where some protein concentrations (e.g., albumin, globulins) are decreased.
• Deficiencies in individual proteins can result in specific diseases including immune deficiency and defective hemostasis. These are discussed elsewhere. This topic is an overview of hypoproteinemia.

PATHOPHYSIOLOGY

• Plasma contains hundreds of proteins that, collectively, perform a nutritive function, maintain oncotic pressure, regulate immune function, aid in the maintenance of acid-base balance, and affect hemostasis/fibrinolysis.
• Major sites of production are the liver, then the immune system.
• TPP within an individual is determined by filtration between the intravascular and extravascular spaces, metabolic demands, hormonal balance, nutritional status, and water balance.
• TPP concentration in neonates is significantly influenced by passive transfer of immunoglobulins (see Age-Related Factors), while in adults, protein concentrations remain relatively stable unless influenced by pathological processes.
• Dysproteinemias associated with low concentrations of plasma proteins include:
  ○ Hypoproteinemia with decreased concentrations of albumin and globulin (nonselective or panhypoproteinemia),
  ○ Hypoproteinemia with hypoalbuminemia or hypoglobulinemia (selective hypoproteinemia).
  ○ Normal TPP concentrations with hypoalbuminemia and hyperglobulinemia,
  ○ Normal TPP concentrations with hyperalbuminemia and hypoglobulinemia (rare).

Panhypoproteinemia

• Panhypoproteinemia may be relative or absolute.
• A relative decrease occurs when TPP concentrations are lower than normal but the absolute content of protein in the vascular space is normal, e.g., dilution of plasma protein by overzealous fluid therapy.
• An absolute decrease occurs when there is a reduction in the amount of plasma proteins in the vascular space with normal plasma volume. This can be the result of impaired production or accelerated loss:
  ○ Reduced production of all plasma proteins occurs primarily as a result of malnutrition and starvation. Liver disease rarely causes hypoproteinemia,
  ○ Loss of protein is a common cause of panhypoproteinemia. The loss can be from either the vascular space into the extravascular compartment due to increased capillary permeability (e.g., endotoxemia, vasculitis) or from the body (e.g., compensated hemorrhage, protein-losing glomerulopathy/enteropathy). These may cause hypoalbuminemia/globulinemia or a selective loss of protein. In most protein-losing diseases, hypoalbuminemia occurs first, due to its small size and low MW. However, if the disease is severe or chronic, globulins also may be decreased.
• Severe, acute hemorrhage results in hypoproteinemia through a direct loss of protein followed by a dilution effect by movement of fluid into the vascular space to maintain circulatory volume. This is exacerbated by excess water intake—common after acute blood loss.
• Persistent, low-grade hemorrhage results in normovolemic anemia and hypoproteinemia. Hypoproteinemia persists as long as the rate of loss exceeds the rate of protein production.

Hypoalbuminemia

• Albumin is produced in the liver, has the lowest MW of the plasma proteins, and contributes 75% of the osmotic pressure.
• Hypoalbuminemia may be accompanied by decreased or normal total plasma protein concentrations, and normal, elevated, or decreased globulin concentrations. In many diseases, hypoalbuminemia precedes hypoglobulinemia due to the preferential loss of albumin or due to preferential synthesis of globulins when substrates are scarce.
• Hypoalbuminemia usually results from increased loss (primarily GI/renal), but decreased production and increased catabolism may occur.
• Decreased production is rarely due to liver disease, but may occur with starvation, malnutrition, and GI disorders. Albumin is a negative acute phase protein, with decreased production associated with inflammatory processes and increased globulin production. The $t^1/_2$ for albumin is ≈18 days; therefore, when decreased synthesis causes hypoalbuminemia, the underlying disease is usually chronic with globulins increased, resulting in normal or increased TPP concentrations.
• Catabolism of albumin may occur with increased metabolic demands and negative nitrogen balance (e.g., fever, trauma, surgery, neoplasia). Chronic antigenic stimulation also increases albumin catabolism to provide necessary amino acids for immunoglobulin production. The resulting hypoalbuminemia is usually offset by hyperglobulinemia with concurrent normal TPP concentration.
• Increased loss of albumin occurs with:
  ○ Protein-losing nephropathy—It is readily filtered through defects in the glomerular basement membrane and glomerulopathies result in albuminuria/hypoalbuminemia. Azotemia, dilute urine—Electrolyte abnormalities may reflect the extent of renal disease.
  ○ Protein-losing enteropathy—causes include ulceration, defective lymphatic drainage, increased mucosal permeability, and exudation due to inflammation.
  ○ Congestive heart failure—Retention of sodium and water forces fluid into the extravascular spaces (e.g., interstitial spaces, ascitic fluid, and GI tract) with concomitant loss of protein. Reduced food intake, inadequate protein absorption, and inadequate hepatic synthesis in severe heart failure also contribute to hypoalbuminemia.
  ○ Chronic inflammation—Albumin is lost through exudation (e.g., into the thoracic and abdominal cavities).
• Hypoalbuminemia causes low plasma oncotic pressure, allowing fluid movement from the vascular space into the extravascular space causing reduced plasma volume. This may be manifest as edema, decreased blood flow to tissues and organ dysfunction. Hypoalbuminemia also reduces transportation of molecules within plasma (e.g., hormones and Ca^{++}).

Hypoglobulinemia

• Hypoglobulinemia with normal plasma albumin concentration occurs rarely, except in FPT.
• Hypoglobulinemia also may occur with specific immunodeficiencies resulting in decreased production of gammaglobulins (e.g., SCID) and lymphoid hypoplasia/aplasia.
• A compensatory increase in albumin often occurs with hypoglobulinemia.

Hypofibrinogenemia

• It is rare and may result from increased consumption or decreased synthesis, but alone will not cause hypoproteinemia.
• Severe, diffuse liver damage may cause decreased fibrinogen production.
• Increased fibrinolysis is associated with DIC, but hypofibrinogenemia is rare as inflammation is often the initiating cause and this will mask the increased consumption.

SYSTEMS AFFECTED

Hypoproteinemia is most often associated with GI/renal disorders, hemorrhage, and chronic hepatic disease.

SIGNALMENT

Neonates with hypoproteinemia, particularly hypoglobulinemia, should be investigated for FPT.

SIGNS

General Comments

There are no pathognomonic signs for hypoproteinemia.

Historical

Fever, lethargy, edema, weight loss, GI dysfunction, dysuria, hemorrhage, or a history of prolonged NSAID administration warrants further diagnostic evaluation for hypoproteinemia.

Physical Examination

• May reflect the underlying cause (e.g., diarrhea, melena, polyuria)
• Hypoproteinemia/hypoalbuminemia may be indicated by symmetrical edema of the distal extremities, ventral body wall and head. Usually

PROTEIN, HYPOPROTEINEMIA

TPP must be <5 g/dL (50 g/L) and albumin <1.5 g/dL (15 g/L).
• Pulmonary edema can occur in hypoalbuminemic patients undergoing intravascular fluid therapy.

CAUSES

Panhypoproteinemia

• May be caused by relative dilution (excessive fluid therapy/water intake), decreased production or increased loss. • Reduced production occurs primarily as result of:
  ○ Malnutrition, starvation
  ○ Liver disease
• Increased loss can be due to:
  ○ Endotoxemia, vasculitis—e.g., purpura hemorrhagica, African horse sickness
  ○ Acute or chronic hemorrhage—e.g., trauma, epistaxis, internal vascular rupture, coagulation disorders such as immune-mediated thrombocytopenia, and all causes of chronic blood loss
  ○ Protein-losing nephropathy—e.g., glomerulonephritis, amyloidosis, pyelonephritis
  ○ Protein-losing enteropathy—e.g., intestinal parasitism, salmonellosis, clostridiosis, Potomac horse fever, *Lawsonia intracellularis*, gastric ulceration, granulomatous enteritis, eosinophilis enteritis, lymphosarcoma, NSAID toxicosis, exposure to caustic chemicals, strangulating GI obstructions/infarction
  ○ Peritonitis or pleuritis
  ○ Chronic heart failure

Hypoalbuminemia

• May occur initially in many diseases, causing panhypoproteinemia
• Chronic antigenic stimulation/infections
• Chronic, diffuse or severe liver disease—e.g., chronic hepatitis/fibrosis/neoplasia

Hypoglobulinemia

• FPT
• Specific immunodeficiencies—e.g., SCID, selective IgM deficiency, agammaglobulinemia, Fell Pony immunodeficiency syndrome
• Adult acquired immunodeficiency

Hypofibrinogenemia

• Impaired hepatic synthesis
• DIC
• Primary hyperfibrinolysis
• Uncompensated loss during massive hemorrhage

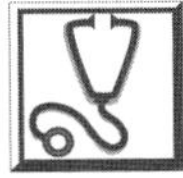

DIAGNOSIS

DIFFERENTIAL DIAGNOSIS

• The underlying cause should be determined.
• Clinical signs referable to specific body systems (e.g., diarrhea, polyuria, dyspnea) may help localize source of protein loss.

CBC/BIOCHEMISTRY/URINALYSIS

• If testing occurs in a human laboratory, albumin may not be accurate and fibrinogen not measured. Hypofibrinogenemia is best measured by thrombin clotting time. Falsely decreased fibrinogen concentrations will occur in samples containing clotted blood.
• PCV and TPP values should be interpreted simultaneously to determine if hemoconcentration or concurrent anemia is present.
• The albumin:globulin (A/G) ratio may help interpretation of hypoproteinemia.
• Hypoproteinemia with a normal A/G ratio reflects hemorrhage, starvation/malnutrition or chronic disease.
• A decreased A/G ratio occurs with inflammatory disease, B-lymphocyte neoplasia, and in early selective hypoproteinemias due to hypoalbumemia (e.g., protein-losing nephropathies, some protein-losing enteropathies, some liver diseases).
• An increased A/G ratio is rare and reflects erroneous albumin measurement or decreased synthesis of gammaglobulins (lymphoid hypoplasia or aplasia).
• Urine should contain little protein, but transient slight proteinuria occurs with exercise and stress, and in neonates.
• Proteinuria is an abnormal finding and warrants further investigation.

OTHER LABORATORY TESTS

• Selective protein deficiencies may be characterized by protein electrophoresis or measurement of specific proteins (e.g., immunoglobulins).
• Characterization of immune system function is indicated in cases of hypoglobulinemia (see FPT, Selective Immunoglobulin Deficiencies, SCID)
• Appropriate tests for infectious or inflammatory diseases may be indicated.

IMAGING

Ultrasonography and radiography of the thorax, abdomen, or soft tissue may help characterize the cause of protein loss.

OTHER DIAGNOSTIC PROCEDURES

Abdominocentesis, thoracocentesis, tracheal aspiration or bronchoalveolar lavage, endoscopy, laparoscopy, bone marrow aspiration, CSF evaluation, biopsy, and histopathology may be indicated.

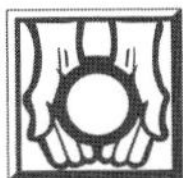

TREATMENT

• Principles include treatment of the inciting disease and correction of hypoproteinemia.
• Relative panhypoproteinemia will resolve within hours of discontinuation of excessive fluid therapy or restriction of water intake.
• Therapy for immunodeficient patients is supportive, because no specific treatment is available.

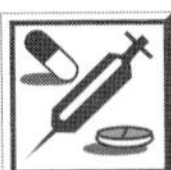

MEDICATIONS

DRUG(S)

• FPT requires oral administration of colostrum or IV adminstation of plasma depending on age. If equine colostrum is unavailable, bovine colostrum, equine plasma, or lyophilized equine IgG can be administered PO.
• Plasma administered IV may be warranted in adult horses with marked hypoproteinemia. Plasma transfusion is preferred over blood transfusion unless anemia is also present.
• Plasma should be transfused to increase albumin concentrations to >2.0 g/dL (20 g/L).
• Plasma oncotic pressure can be increased by IV administration of hydroxyethyl starch or high MW dextrans (8–10 mL/kg or 6% solution IV over 6–12 hr).

PRECAUTIONS

Anaphylactic reactions can occur during IV plasma administration; monitor closely during treatment.

FOLLOW-UP

PATIENT MONITORING

• Evaluate laboratory variables (TPP, albumin, globulins) and hydration status.
• Frequency of monitoring will depend on severity and response to therapy.

POSSIBLE COMPLICATIONS

• Complications depend on the cause of hypoproteinemia.
• Dependent and pulmonary edema are possible.
• Upper airway obstruction may develop due to pharyngeal and laryngeal edema and require a tracheotomy.

EXPECTED COURSE AND PROGNOSIS

Depend on the underlying cause

MISCELLANEOUS

AGE-RELATED FACTORS

Reference intervals for TPP, albumin and globulin concentrations for foals are lower than those for mature horses.

SEE ALSO

• Anemia
• Failure of passive transfer
• Selective immunoglobulin deficiencies
• SCID
• Hyperfibrinogenemia

ABBREVIATIONS

• DIC = disseminated intravascular coagulopathy
• GI = gastrointestinal
• MW = molecular weight
• PCV = packed cell volume
• SCID = severe combined immunodeficiency
• TPP = total plasma protein

Suggested Reading

Diseases of the hemolymphatic and immune systems. In: Radostits O, Gay C, Hinchcliff K, Constable P, eds. Veterinary Medicine, ed 10. Philadelphia: WB Saunders, 2007:439–469.

Smith BP. Large Animal Internal Medicine, ed 3. St. Louis: CV Mosby, 2002.

Author Jennifer Hodgson
Consulting Editors David Hodgson and Jennifer Hodgson

PROTEIN-LOSING ENTEROPATHY (PLE)

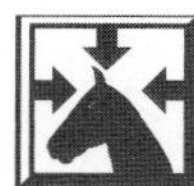

BASICS

OVERVIEW

• Normally, the intestinal capillary endothelium allows a small amount of protein to enter the mucosal interstitium; however, the movement of protein and fluid into the intestinal lumen is restricted by the tight intercellular bridges. Plasma proteins such as albumin are present in low concentrations in normal gastrointestinal secretions, and protein usually undergoes complete degradation within the intestinal lumen. • GI protein loss may result from mucosal ulceration and plasma exudation, lymphatic obstruction with leakage and rupture of dilated lacteals, passive diffusion through intracellular spaces, active secretion by mucosal cells, intracellular loss, increased permeability of capillaries and venules, and disordered cell metabolism. • The excessive loss of proteins into the GI tract causes hypoproteinemia. The early intestinal protein loss in PLE involves relatively larger quantities of albumin than globulins. If severe, hypoalbuminemia may result in the development of subcutaneous edema. In the later stages of the disease, all protein fractions may be lost. Feces are frequently normal in consistency, if large colon function is not impaired. • PLE is usually a progressive condition; however, accelerated protein leakage can occur in acute GI diseases such as salmonellosis.

SIGNALMENT

• GE and eosinophilic gastroenteritis are most common in young adult horses (range, 1–5 years). Standardbreds are more frequently affected with GE. • Intestinal lymphosarcoma and intestinal parasitism may occur in horses of all ages. • Gastric squamous cell carcinoma affects mainly older horses. • Ponies and young animals are reportedly more susceptible to NSAID toxicity. • *Lawsonia intracellularis* in weanling foals (3–12 months) • Severe gastric ulceration in young (1–3 years) racehorses

SIGNS

Affected animals show some of the following signs:

• Chronic, progressive weight loss • Edema (dependent edema involving ventral thorax, ventral body wall, distal extremities)
• Depression • Anorexia • Reduced performance
• Lethargy • Intermittent or chronic colic
• Diarrhea is not present in PLE cases with lesions primarily in the small intestine because the colon can effectively absorb electrolytes and water. • Skin lesions (focal or patchy alopecia, thin or rough hair coat) may be present.
• Enlarged peripheral lymph nodes in some cases
• Acute colic and signs of endotoxemia may occur in horses with intestinal parasitism or NSAID toxicity. • On per-rectal examination, may be able to palpate enlarged mesenteric lymph nodes (lymphoma) and thickened bowel wall in some PLE cases • Occasionally, pharyngeal and laryngeal edema may develop in severely hypoproteinemic animals and may produce an upper airway obstruction. • Pain after eating may be observed in some horses with gastric squamous cell carcinoma.

CAUSES AND RISK FACTORS

Diseases that have been most commonly associated with PLE include chronic inflammatory bowel diseases (GE, idiopathic eosinophilic enterocolitis, multisystemic eosinophilic epitheliotropic disease, lymphocytic–plasmacytic enterocolitis), GI neoplasia (lymphosarcoma, squamous cell carcinoma), parasitic thrombosis of the cranial mesenteric artery (*Strongylus vulgaris*), cyathostomiasis, NSAID toxicity, acute salmonellosis, other causes of acute enterocolitis, proliferative enteropathy due to *L. intracellularis*, congestive heart failure, and amyloidosis.

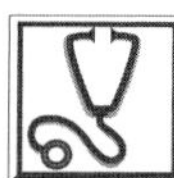

DIAGNOSIS

DIFFERENTIAL DIAGNOSIS

The diagnosis of PLE is usually made after protein loss through other routes (e.g. urine, into body cavities such as thorax and abdomen) and inability to synthesize protein (liver disease) are ruled out.

CBC/BIOCHEMISTRY/URINALYSIS

• Hypoalbuminemia
• Decreased, normal, or increased plasma globulin concentrations

- Serum protein electrophoresis is the preferred test for quantifying protein fractions.
- Panhypoproteinemia
- Hypocalcemia may occur in conjunction with hypoalbuminemia because a large portion of serum calcium is protein bound.
- Anemia

OTHER LABORATORY TESTS

- Coprology for parasitic ova and larvae
- Fecal occult blood test may be positive in horses with GI blood loss from gastric squamous cell carcinoma, intestinal parasitism, or iatrogenic following per-rectal examination.
- Fecal PCR test for *L. intracellularis* in young foals and weanlings
- Ultrasonography to determine thickness of intestinal wall
- Oral D-xylose absorption test is preferable to the oral glucose tolerance test as an indicator of small intestine absorptive function.
- Abdominocentesis—cytology to detect neoplasia. A normal abdominal fluid does not rule out neoplasia.

OTHER DIAGNOSTIC PROCEDURES

- Immunoelectrophoresis (elevated serum IgA; lower serum IgM [lymphoma])
- Gastroduodenoscopy to visualize stomach and duodenum
- Rectal mucosal biopsy—histopathological examination may be useful in the diagnosis of GE, eosinophilic enterocolitis, or alimentary lymphoma.
- Exploratory laparotomy and intestinal biopsy often necessary for definitive diagnosis
- Increased fecal radioactivity following [^{51}Cr]albumin documents gastrointestinal protein loss.

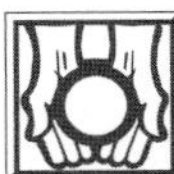

TREATMENT

Because the condition is usually well advanced when the first clinical signs are recognized, the prognosis for recovery is generally guarded to very poor and treatment is frequently unrewarding.

MEDICATIONS

Treatment depends on the primary disease causing PLE or treating the hypoproteinemia.

DRUG(S) OF CHOICE

- Plasma transfusion is usually indicated when total plasma protein concentration is or falls below 40 g/L (4 g/dL). The effect may be minimal due to the continued protein losses.
- If horse is receiving NSAIDs, therapy should be discontinued.
- When internal parasites are suspected as the cause, administer larvicidal anthelmintics (moxidectin 0.4 mg/kg PO, ivermectin 0.2 mg/kg PO, or fenbendazole 10 mg/kg daily PO for 5 days).
- For *L. intracellularis* proliferative enteropathy—erythromycin phosphate (37.5 mg/kg PO q12h) and rifampin (10 mg/kg PO q24h) for a minimum of 21 days.
- Total parenteral nutrition may be indicated in valuable horses.
- Corticosteroid therapy is often ineffective in treating chronic inflammatory bowel disease. Prolonged courses are required.

DIET

Dietary management—feed pelleted feed and restrict roughage. Provide palatable, easily assimilated, high-energy and -protein sources supplying electrolyte mixtures to include calcium, magnesium, and to a lesser extent, zinc, copper, and iron, and supplementing fat- and water-soluble vitamins.

FOLLOW-UP

- Monitor total serum protein and albumin concentrations.
- Monitor body weight.

MISCELLANEOUS

ABBREVIATIONS

- GE = granulomatous enteritis
- GI = gastrointestinal
- PLE = protein-losing enteropathy

Suggested Reading

Roberts MC. Protein-losing enteropathy in the horse. Compend Cont Educ Pract Vet 1983;5:S550–S556.

Author John D. Baird
Consulting Editors Henry Stämpfli and Olimpo Oliver-Espinosa

PROTOZOAL MYELOENCEPHALITIS (EPM)

BASICS

DEFINITION

Multifocal neurologic disease of horses caused by *Sarcocystis neurona* and possibly *Neospora hughesi*.

PATHOPHYSIOLOGY

• Infection results from ingestion of sporocysts of *S. neurona* in feed and water contaminated with feces of opossums, the definitive host. • Sporocysts can be transmitted by vectors such as birds, rodents, and insects. • Sporocysts excyst in the horse's small intestine, releasing sporozoites that penetrate the enterocytes and enter the bloodstream. • Two rounds of replication (i.e., merogony) occur, and *S. neurona* invade the entire organism before forming sarcocysts in the muscles of intermediate hosts, including horses. • Parasites appear to gain access to the CNS either by direct penetration of the blood-brain barrier or through infected WBCs. Merozoites multiply within neurons and leukocytes, resulting in cell death. • Clinical signs are caused by neuronal loss and inflammation and swelling, which disrupt normal CNS architecture, compromise blood flow, and reduce oxygen delivery.
• Incubation time can be as short as 10 days but latent infections can persist for months. • Life cycle of *N. hughesi* and its importance as a causative agent of EPM are not well understood.

SYSTEMS AFFECTED

• Nervous—multifocal CNS infection results in variable sensory, motor, and cognitive dysfunction; cranial nerve deficits can occur
• Neuromuscular—discrete, neurogenic muscle atrophy and weakness are common
• Musculoskeletal—occasional secondary injuries and soreness from ataxia; asymmetric muscle weakness/atrophy
• Gastrointestinal—cranial nerve signs associated with prehension, mastication, and swallowing; loss of anal tone
• Skin—hyporeflexia, discrete areas of sensory loss and hyperhidrosis
• Respiratory—laryngeal hemiplegia and pneumonia secondary to dysphagia
• Ophthalmic—loss of ocular reflexes and blindness • Renal/urologic—urinary incontinence

GENETICS

No apparent genetic predisposition

INCIDENCE/PREVALENCE

• Seroprevalence of *S. neurona* reaches approximately 50% in many parts of the United States, 70% in Brazil, and 35% in Argentina.
• Incidence of the disease is low, with 0.014% of the population of horses affected in the United States. • Seroprevalence of *Neospora* spp. in North and South America is very low—3.4% and 2.5%, respectively.

GEOGRAPHIC DISTRIBUTION

• The geographic range of EPM cases is defined by the distribution of the opossum. • Native cases of EPM have only been reported in the Western hemisphere. • Cases of neosporosis have been described in the United States and in France.

SIGNALMENT

Breed Predilections

Thoroughbreds, Standardbreds, and Quarter Horses are most frequently affected.

Mean Age and Range

Horses may be affected at any age.
Most cases confirmed at post mortem have involved horses 3 months to 30 years old; the average age is 6 years.

Predominant Sex

No sex predilection

SIGNS

General Comments

• There is a great variation in clinical signs due to the multifocal localization of the parasites in the CNS. • The onset of the disease may be acute or insidious and can progress rapidly or remain stable for a long period of time.

Historical Findings

• Apparent lameness from asymmetrical ataxia and muscle weakness is the most common clinical complaint. • Muscle atrophy, sore back, and cranial nerve deficits also may be reported.

PHYSICAL EXAMINATION FINDINGS

• Affected horses are usually bright and alert.
• Clinical signs suggestive of spinal cord lesions, with variable degrees of ataxia and weakness in one or more limbs, are the most frequent finding. • Localized muscle atrophy, head tilt, facial paralysis, diminished ocular reflexes, poor prehension, mastication or dysphagia, laryngeal hemiplegia, urinary incontinence, localized sweating, seizure, and head shaking are also common.

CAUSES

• *Sarcocystis neurona* • Possibly *Neospora hughesi*

RISK FACTORS

• Presence of opossums or previous diagnosis of EPM on the premises • Stress or adverse health event less than
90 days before presentation

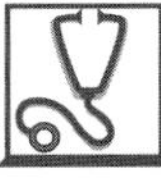

DIAGNOSIS

DIFFERENTIAL DIAGNOSIS

• Ataxia and paresis often confused with lameness • CSM—has similar breed predilection and usually produces symmetric ataxia
• Trauma—History, external evidence of injury, and anatomic localization to a single area of the CNS are common. • EDM—progressive, symmetrical ataxia, and weakness in horses younger than 2 years • EHV-1 myeloencephalopathy—Typically affects more than one horse in a group and often follows respiratory disease. Is commonly associated with symmetric, posterior ataxia and weakness, bladder dysfunction, and loss of tail and anal tone. • West Nile virus infection—depression and fever • Any conditions causing central and peripheral nervous system dysfunctions

CBC/BIOCHEMISTRY/URINALYSIS

CBC and serum biochemistry are usually unremarkable.

OTHER LABORATORY TESTS

• Gold standard remains post-mortem identification of characteristic lesions and parasites within the CNS. Immunohistology can help identify the parasites on fixed tissues.
• WBT—Positive serology is only indicative of exposure to the parasite. Negative tests indicate a high probability that the horse is not infected with *S. neurona*. • In a study on 234 horses, sensitivity of WBT on CSF was 87%–88% regardless of whether the horses showed signs of neurologic diseases. Specificity reported on CSF varies from 44% to 60% depending on the presence or absence of neurologic signs, respectively. • False-positive results on CSF samples may occur due to blood contamination of the CSF, subclinical infection with other concurrent neurologic disease, cross-reactivity with other *Sarcocystis* or *Neospora* spp., or natural passage of antibody from the blood to the CSF after vaccination or colostrum ingestion.
• IFAT—Sensitivity and specificity using serum samples of horses naturally infected with *S. neurona* are 83.3% and 96.9%, respectively. Using CSF, sensitivity is 100% and specificity is 99%. • An ELISA to detect *S. neurona*–specific IgG has been described. Sensitivity and specificity are 95.5% and 92.9%, respectively.
• PCR detection of *S. neurona* DNA on the CSF has a high specificity but poor sensitivity. • IFAT is more accurate to diagnose *N. hughesi*–infected horses than ELISA and direct agglutination test. Sensitivity is 100% and specificity varies from 71.5% to 100% depending of the cutoff value.

IMAGING

Lesions localized in the brain, brainstem, and cervical spinal cord can be visualized using CT/MRI.

OTHER DIAGNOSTIC PROCEDURES

• CSF is usually within normal limits, although its analysis may help rule out other diseases.
• Cytology on the CSF—more than 50 RBC/μL indicates blood contamination and prevents interpretation of a positive WBT.

PATHOLOGIC FINDINGS

• Gross lesions not always visible at necropsy
• CNS lesions due to *S. neurona* are commonly multifocal characterized by hemorrhage and necrosis in the brain, brainstem, and spinal cord. Infective organisms are found primarily in neurons but also occasionally in leukocytes and vascular endothelium. • *N. hughesi* causes multifocal granulomas in the CNS.

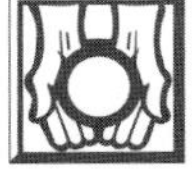

TREATMENT

AIMS OF TREATMENT

• Stopping progression of the disease
• Improving the neurologic status of the horse
• Preventing lesions from self-trauma
• Preventing relapse when possible

Protozoal Myeloencephalitis (EPM)

APPROPRIATE HEALTH CARE

General supportive care in horses with severe neurologic dysfunction primarily aimed at avoiding self-traumatic injuries (deep bedding, sling support, and protective gear)

ACTIVITY

• Prolonged inactivity does not enhance recovery. • However, premature return to heavy work may prolong the time to recovery and promote relapse.

DIET

• Use of folate inhibitors may result in bone marrow suppression and anemia. If life-threatening anemia develops, discontinue medication for 2–3 weeks to allow recovery or switch to an alternative medication.
High-quality pasture and alfalfa hay are excellent sources of folinic acid and highly recommended during treatment. Folic acid is poorly absorbed by the horse and has been associated with toxicity. • Supplementation with vitamin E 6,000–10,000 IU PO daily has been recommended during therapy and rehabilitation.

NURSING CARE

• Severely ataxic horses should be confined in a heavily bedded box stall. • Turning of the recumbent horse must be attempted every 2–6 hours. • Legs should be bandaged to avoid traumatic injuries. • Adequate nutritional support must be provided. Diets and routes of administration must be adapted to each patient.

MEDICATIONS

DRUG(S) OF CHOICE

• Ponazuril (Marquis, Bayer) is administered orally at 5 mg/kg daily for 28 days and is well tolerated in horses. Few adverse effects have been described at recommended dosages. • Oral administration of nitazoxanide (Navigator; Idexx Pharmaceuticals) starts at 25 mg/kg daily for 5 days and then 50 mg/kg daily for a total of 28 days. • Folate inhibitors are still widely used at 20 mg/kg sulfadiazine and 1.0 mg/kg pyrimethamine orally daily for 4–6 months or at least 1 month after the horse stops showing further improvement. Many veterinarians now recommend 1.5- to 2.0-fold the standard dose of pyrimethamine for the initial treatment or after 30 days without satisfactory progress. The combination should be given on an empty stomach to prevent interference with absorption from the gut. • Administration of flunixin meglumine (1.1 mg/kg BID) or phenylbutazone (2.2 mg/kg BID) the first 1–2 weeks of treatment and anytime the condition appears to worsen may help minimizing further damage due to parasite death and the host response.
• DMSO (1.0 g/kg in 10% saline IV daily for 3 days) may be beneficial. • Use of dexamethasone (0.05 mg/kg IV daily or BID) in severely affected horses may help reducing CNS inflammation but remains controversial. • Treatment of *N. hughesi* remains a challenge. In one report, the parasite was not affected by treatment with folate inhibitors and nitazoxanide, while in vitro studies indicate their susceptibility to those compounds.

CONTRAINDICATIONS

Known sensitivity to one of the drugs

PRECAUTIONS

• Corticosteroids should be used with caution because they can suppress the immune response to the parasite. Their use should not exceed 1–3 days to avoid exacerbating the disease. • Fatal enterocolitis, anorexia, weight loss, depression, colic, discoloration of the urine, fever, peripheral edema, and laminitis have been described in horses treated with nitazoxanide. • Stallions may be at increased risks of developing laminitis while treated with nitazoxanide. • Folic acid supplementation in horses treated with folate inhibitors may paradoxically exacerbate the deficiency. • Abortion and decreased stallion fertility may occur using folate inhibitors.

POSSIBLE INTERACTIONS

Use of potentiated sulfas and pyrimethamine may increase the side effects of folic acid depletion.

ALTERNATIVE DRUGS

• Diclazuril and toltrazuril (5–10 mg/kg PO daily for 28 days) have been used in the treatment of EPM in the horse. Their efficacy appears to be comparable to folate inhibitors.
• Immunostimulants such as levamisol, killed *Propionobacterium acnes*, and mycobacterial cell wall extract have been recommended, but their efficacy has not been documented.

FOLLOW-UP

PATIENT MONITORING

• Neurologic examination of affected horses is recommended at regular intervals during treatment. • Relapse may occur in 10%–25% of horses. • To reduce the relapse rate, medication should not be discontinued until CSF became negative, but some horses remain CSF positive for an extended period after full recovery or stabilization. • The relapse rate among horses with negative CSF at the time treatment is stopped has been extremely low. • When using folate inhibitors, monthly CBCs are recommended to monitor anemia.

PREVENTION/AVOIDANCE

• Ataxic horses represent a risk for themselves and their handlers. • Management should aim at preventing physical stress from injury and bacterial infection. Long trailer rides are stressful and commonly mentioned in clinical histories of affected horses. • Prevention should aim at limiting the access of opossums and other wildlife to the horse's environment, feed, and water supply.

POSSIBLE COMPLICATIONS

Secondary injuries may occur from ataxia. Keep performance animals out of training during therapy.

EXPECTED COURSE AND PROGNOSIS

• Regardless of treatment used, improvement usually varies between 60% and 75%. • Full recovery rate are <25%. Mildly affected horses treated early in the course of infection have better prognosis. Improvement often is observed during the first week of therapy and frequently progresses steadily for several weeks. The rate of improvement typically slows as the horse gradually improves over many weeks, until a plateau is reached. Chronic signs of CNS damage (e. g., muscle atrophy) rarely improve.

MISCELLANEOUS

ASSOCIATED CONDITIONS

Secondary injuries

ZOONOTIC POTENTIAL

N/A

PREGNANCY

• Transplacental transmission of *S. neurona* is unlikely, with infected mares producing normal foals. Abortion and death of foals born from mares treated with folate inhibitors and supplemented with folic acid and vitamin E are reported.

ABBREVIATIONS

- CNS = central nervous system
- CSF = cerebrospinal fluid
- CSM = cervical stenotic myelopathy
- EDM = equine degenerative myeloencephalopathy
- EHV-1 = equine herpesvirus 1
- EMND = equine motor neuron disease
- EPM = equine protozoal myeloencephalitis
- IFAT = immunofluorescence antibody test
- IgG = immunoglobulin G
- PCR = polymerase chain reaction
- WBT = Western blot test

Suggested Reading

Furr M, MacKay R, Granstorm D. Clinical diagnosis of equine protozoal myeloencephalitis (EPM). J Vet Intern Med 2002;16:618–621.

Packham AE, Conrad PA, Wilson WD, et al. Qualitative evaluation of selective tests for detection of *Neospora hughesi* antibodies in serum and cerebrospinal fluid of experimentally infected horses. J Parasitol 2002;88:1239–1246.

Sellon DC, Dubey JP. Equine protozoal myeloencephalitis. In: Sellon DC, ed. Equine Infectious Diseases. St. Louis: Saunders, 2007:453–464.

The author and editor wish to acknowledge the contribution of David E. Granstrom, author of this topic in the previous edition.

Author Laureline Lecoq
Consulting Editor Caroline N. Hahn

PTYALISM

BASICS

OVERVIEW

• Excessive salivation (ptyalism) arises either through excessive production of saliva or saliva that cannot be swallowed. Saliva is produced continuously from the salivary glands and is secreted into the oral cavity. Any condition that causes dysphagia may produce ptyalism through inhibiting swallowing of saliva [see causes of dysphagia (e.g., oral pain), neurologic conditions, obstruction of the esophagus]. • Increased production of saliva may occur following the ingestion of forage or hay contaminated with *Rhizoctonia leguminicola.* This produces a mycotoxin, slaframine, that has parasympathomimetic properties. It is an indole alkaloid that requires hepatic activation. The active compound is thought to either cause the release of histamine or have direct histaminergic effects. Heavy-metal toxicity, parasympathomimetic poisoning, neurologic disease, and stomatitis (e.g., vesicular stomatitis) may also increase saliva production. Gastroesophageal reflux secondary to gastroduodenal ulceration is also associated with ptyalism, particularly in foals. • Primary diseases of the salivary glands are uncommon and can include sialoadenitis, salivary calculi, salivary mucocele, trauma, neoplasia (adenocarcinomas, acinar cell tumors, melanomas), or infection (e.g., *Streptococcus equi,* rabies). Some of these may also be associated with increased production of saliva. • Horses have relatively high levels of salivary chloride and low levels of bicarbonate. Therefore, loss of saliva causes a transient metabolic alkalosis due to loss of the chloride.

SIGNALMENT

Depends on the primary problem

Foals

• Esophageal disorders due to dysmaturity, septicemia, botulism, and congenital disorders
• Increased risk of gastroduodenal ulceration

Young Horses

Esophageal disorders due to improper chewing during tooth eruption

Aged Horses

• Esophageal disorders due to neoplasia or improper chewing of feed due to poor teeth
• Feeding practices and pica can increase likelihood of foreign body obstruction or choke with feed material. • Feeding/grazing mold-infected legumes such as red clover increase likelihood of slaframine toxicity.

SIGNS

Increased saliva from the mouth. Other signs are associated with the primary disease and include:
• Enlargement of the esophageal area with cervical esophageal obstruction • Signs of dysphagia include coughing during swallowing, frequent swallowing motions, extension of the neck, and regurgitation of feed material out the nostrils; differentiate choke by the mixture of feed material with the saliva. • Salivation following slaframine ingestion usually occurs within 30–60 min and may persist for 24 hr. May also be accompanied by diarrhea, anorexia, polyuria, or abortion. Clinical signs resolve within 48–96 hr of removing the infected feed.
• Gastroduodenal ulceration frequently accompanied by bruxism, colic, and decreased appetite, especially for grain.

CAUSES AND RISK FACTORS

• Secondary to stomatitis—vesicular stomatitis, irritants, caustic chemicals, yellow bristle grass, foxtails, NSAID toxicity, erosions secondary to point on teeth • Decreased ability to swallow the saliva produced may be secondary to esophageal disorders such as obstruction or disorders in motility or structure secondary to obstructions.
• Secondary to botulism or sepsis • Secondary to pharyngeal trauma as a result of improper administration of bolus medication • Secondary to other causes of dysphagia; neurogenic, obstructive • Toxin ingestion • NSAID administration leading to gastroduodenal ulceration • Grass sickness

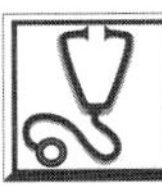

DIAGNOSIS

DIFFERENTIAL DIAGNOSIS

Determine the primary conditions resulting in ptyalism:
• Neurogenic dysphagia • Pharyngeal obstruction • Esophageal disorders • Gastric /gastroduodenal ulceration • Toxin ingestion

CBC/BIOCHEMISTRY/URINALYSIS

• Results of the CBC are often normal, but may reflect the primary disease (neonatal septicemia, *S. equi* infection) • Stress leukogram
• Biochemical analysis may be normal or may reflect changes consistent with the primary disease. After prolonged ptyalism, horse may develop metabolic alkalosis due to loss of chloride in the saliva.

OTHER LABORATORY TESTS

HYPP testing if dysphagia is also present along with suspect lineage

IMAGING

• Radiographs of the skull if trauma is suspected, or to localize foreign bodies, temporomandibular joint disease, or retropharyngeal masses
• Ultrasound examination if primary salivary gland disease is suspected

DIAGNOSTIC PROCEDURES

Oral Examination

Rabies is a possible cause, and therefore care should be taken to wear gloves when examining the mouth and limit exposure of nonvaccinated individuals/animals.

Nasogastric Intubation

• Endoscopy—pharynx, guttural pouches, esophagus, stomach, duodenum • Postmortem immunofluorescent antibody testing on brain tissue for rabies, if suspected • Examination of hay source or pasture

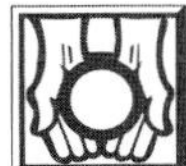

TREATMENT

• Treat the primary condition (see section on specific conditions). • Symptomatic treatment rarely attempted • Treat any fluid and acid-base disorders that may have resulted from chronic loss of saliva • Remove any feed material that may contain *R. leguminicola.*

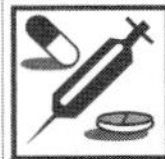

MEDICATIONS

DRUGS AND FLUIDS

The appropriate crystalloid fluid should be given intravenously to treat any existing dehydration or acid-base disorders that may have developed.

FOLLOW-UP

• Monitor for signs of aspiration pneumonia or rupture of the esophagus. • Possible complications include aspiration pneumonia, dermatitis, and dehydration and electrolyte disorders.

MISCELLANEOUS

SEE ALSO

• Stomatitis • Esophageal disorders
• Gastroduodenal ulceration • Dental eruptions and disorders • Dysphagia • Rabies
• Mycotoxicosis • Fracture of the mandible or maxilla • Extramedullary plasmocytoma

ABBREVIATIONS

• CBC = complete blood count • HYPP = hyperkalemic periodic paralysis

Suggested Reading

Baker SJ, Johnson PJ, David A, Cook CR. Idiopathic gastroesophageal reflux disease in an adult horse. JAVMA 2004;224:1967–1970.

Easley KJ. Salivary glands and ducts. In: Smith BP, ed. Large Animal Internal Medicine. St. Louis: Mosby, 1996:697.

Jones SL. Oral diseases. In: Reed SM, Bayly WM, Sellon DC, eds. Equine Internal Medicine. Philadelphia: WB Saunders, 2004: 854.

Laryngospasm, dysphagia, and emaciation associated with hyperkalemic periodic paralysis in a horse. JAMA 1996;209:115–117.

McConkey S, Lopez A, Pringle J. Extramedullary plasmacytoma in a horse with ptyalism and dysphagia. JAVMA 2000;12:282–284.

Schmitz DG. Toxicological problems. In: Reed SM, Bayly WM, Sellon DC, eds. Equine Internal Medicine. Philadelphia: WB Saunders, 2004:1450.

Author Deborah A. Parsons

Consulting Editors Henry Stämpfli and Olimpo Oliver-Espinosa

PURPURA HEMORRHAGICA

BASICS

DEFINITION

• An acute disease of horses characterized by an immune-mediated vasculitis, extensive edema of the head and limbs, petechial and ecchymotic hemorrhages in mucosae, musculature and viscera, and sometimes glomerulonephritis.
• The vasculitis is aseptic and the disease noncontagious.
• PH is most common secondary to *Streptococcus equi* ss *equi* infection, although may be associated with other infectious agents and/or vaccination.

PATHOPHYSIOLOGY

• PH is believed to be an immune-mediated vasculitis associated with a type III hypersensitivity reaction.
• Soluble immune complexes, formed in moderate antigen excess, become deposited in the walls of small blood vessels with subsequent fixation and activation of complement to C5a, a potent chemotactic factor for neutrophils.
• Release of proteolytic enzymes from localized neutrophils directly damages vessel walls causing leakage and luminal compromise. The net effect is edema, hemorrhage, thrombosis, and ischemic changes in supplied tissues.
• The circulating immune complexes are most commonly composed of IgA and *S. equi* ss *equi* M protein.
• Blood vessels of the skin are predominantly affected due to the size and physicochemical properties of the immune complexes and blood flow turbulence. Hydrostatic pressures within vessels in dependent areas of the body result in distribution of lesions in lower limbs and ventral abdomen.

SYSTEMS AFFECTED

• Hemic/lymphatic/immune
• Cardiovascular system
• Skin

INCIDENCE/PREVALENCE

• Sporadic disease
• Reported incidence subsequent to *S. equi* ss *equi* infection varies from 0.5% to 5%.
• Highest incidence reported in extensive outbreaks of strangles, possibly because of reinfection of horses already sensitized by previous infection(s)

SIGNS

Historical Findings

• Exposure to, or infection with, respiratory pathogens frequently reported within previous 2–4 weeks.
• Vaccination may precede disease.

Physical Examination Findings

• Clinical signs associated with PH vary and range from a mild transient reaction to a severe and fatal disease.
• Horses with PH frequently have signs of depression, are febrile with tachycardia and tachypnea, are reluctant to move, and have reduced or absent appetite.
• Dermal or subcutaneous edema is a common early sign, with swelling beginning around the nostrils and muzzle then progressing to the whole head, distal limbs, and ventral abdomen.
• The edema initially appears as well-demarcated areas of hot, sensitive swellings, which become cold and painless over time and merge gradually into normal tissue without a line of demarcation. The swellings can develop suddenly or gradually over several days, are usually asymmetric and nonpruritic, and pit with gentle pressure.
• Hyperemia and petechial and ecchymotic hemorrhages (purpura) may be observed in light-skinned areas and on mucous membranes.
• The edema and hemorrhage may progress to skin infarction, necrosis, and exudation with large, distended areas oozing red-tinged serum. The skin of the distal limbs is most commonly and severely affected. These sites may eventually slough and leave granulating wounds.
• Mucosal surfaces may also ulcerate and slough.
• If the larynx is involved, dysphagia and dyspnea may be observed due to swelling and pain.
• Edema, hemorrhage, and necrosis also can occur in other body systems—lameness, colic, dyspnea, and ataxia may be observed.
• Subclinical renal disease is common.
• Secondary complications such as laminitis, thrombophlebitis, and localized infections are common.
• Death may ensue as a result of pneumonia, cardiac arrhythmias, renal failure, or GIT disorders.
• An uncommon, although more severe, manifestation of PH (infarctive PH), is characterized by infarction of multiple tissues including the GIT and muscle. Affected horses have colic and muscle swelling. The course of disease is ≈3–5 days, with death a common outcome due to severe colic and rapidly deteriorating metabolic status.

CAUSES

• Antigens involved in PH can be derived from infectious agents (bacteria, viruses) or drugs.
• In 1 study, approximately 32% of horses had been infected with, or exposed to, *S. equi* ss *equi*; 9% had been vaccinated with *S equi* ss *equi* M protein; 17% had been infected with *Corynebacterium pseudotuberculosis*; and 9% had a history of apparently infectious respiratory disease of unknown cause. A further 28% of horses had no history of recent infectious diseases.
• Equine influenza virus, equine herpeviruses, *S. equi* ss *zooepidemicus*, *Rhodococcus equi*, and prolonged drug administration also have been implicated in some cases.
• Horses vaccinated excessively with either modified live, killed whole cell, or M protein–based *S. equi* ss *equi* vaccines may also develop PH due to high concentrations of antibody and antigen.
• No inciting cause may be found in some cases (idiopathic vasculitis)

RISK FACTORS

• The role of vaccination in development of PH is currently contentious.
• Streptococcal vaccines have not definitively been shown to be a risk factor for development of PH. However, some authors recommend that horses with high serum antibody titers to streptococcal M protein not be vaccinated for strangles.
• It is also not clear whether infected horses should be vaccinated during an outbreak of strangles due to the potential association with development of PH.

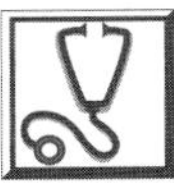

DIAGNOSIS

DIFFERENTIAL DIAGNOSIS

• Immune-mediated vasculitis must be differentiated from vasculitis directly caused by infectious agents (e.g., EVAV, EIAV, and *Anaplasma phagocytophilum* [EGE]), IMTP, and other causes of edema or petechial and ecchymotic hemorrhages.
• Serological testing for EVAV, EGE, and EIAV (Coggins).
• Blood smears may demonstrate cytoplasmic inclusions within neutrophils in EGE.
• Congestive heart failure can be readily differentiated on physical examination.
• Angioneurotic edema is not associated with petechiation.
• Horses with IMTP will have decreased platelet counts.
• Horses with warfarin toxicity and moldy sweet clover toxicity have increases in PT and, ultimately, aPTT.
• Stachybotryotoxicosis can be diagnosed by identification of mold on straw (may appear blackened as if with soot).

CBC/BIOCHEMISTRY/URINALYSIS

• No characteristic abnormalities are associated with PH and length of illness, organ involvement, and secondary complications will influence changes observed.
• Neutrophilic leukocytosis, hyperfibrinogenemia, hyperglobulinemia, and mild anemia are commonly observed due to chronic inflammation. Moderate anemia may be observed in some cases due to increased RBC destruction.
• The platelet count is usually normal.
• Creatinine may be elevated, and urinalysis may show traces of hematuria and/or proteinuria if there is glomerulonephritis.
• Elevations in CK and AST activities may be present due to muscle lesions.
• Horses with infarctive PH have marked elevations in serum CK and AST and neutrophilia, and in severely affected horses there is evidence of a concomitant consumptive coagulopathy, which will result in thrombocytopenia and decreased PT and aPTT.

OTHER LABORATORY TESTS

Serology for infectious agents associated with immune-mediated vasculitis should include demonstration of elevated IgA titers to *S equi* ss *equi*.

IMAGING

• Endoscopy of upper airways for *S. equi* ss *equi* lymphadenopathy
• Thoracic radiography for evidence of lower respiratory tract infection

OTHER DIAGNOSTIC PROCEDURES

- Diagnosis of PH is often based on history, clinical signs, and response to therapy.
- Documentation of leukoclastic vasculitis and/or presence of immune complexes add support to the diagnosis.
- Full-thickness punch biopsies (at least 6 mm in diameter) of skin on affected sites should be obtained and preserved in 10% formalin (for histopathology) and Michel's transport medium (for IFA testing).
- Multiple biopsies of early lesions (8–24 hr of age) are required as distribution of lesions is patchy. Lesions >24 hr may be nondiagnostic.
- IFA may reveal the presence of immune complexes in the walls of small blood vessels.

PATHOLOGICAL FINDINGS

- Subcutaneous edema and numerous, discrete, petechial, and ecchymotic hemorrhages throughout the skin, submucosa, musculature, kidney, respiratory, and GIT tracts are seen on PM.
- Leucoclastic vasculitis (neutrophilic infiltration of small blood vessels with nuclear debris in and around involved vessels and fibrinoid necrosis) may be observed in scattered blood vessels, particularly in the skin, lung, muscle, and GIT.
- Horses with infarctive PH have dark red to black, multifocal coalescing hemorrhages in skeletal muscles, hemorrhages in the lungs, and GIT. Histologic examination reveals coagulative necrosis of muscle and other tissues.

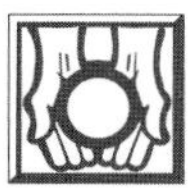

TREATMENT

AIMS OF TREATMENT

- Treatment of PH involves removal of the inciting cause, reduction of inflammation within blood vessels, reduction of the immune response, and provision of supportive care.
- Identification of the underlying infection/disease is required to remove the source of antigenic stimulation. Although the sensitizing infection has often resolved by the time signs of PH occur, ongoing antigen production may prolong the immune-mediated vasculitis.
- Administration of any drugs should be discontinued as PH could be caused by an adverse drug reaction.

NURSING CARE

- Horses with PH usually require aggressive nursing care, which should be instituted immediately.
- Hydrotherapy can minimize edema, and pressure wraps are used to decrease swelling of limbs.
- Isotonic fluid administration (IV or via a nasogastric tube) may be required to maintain hydration in animals with severe depression or dysphagia.
- Sloughed areas of skin should receive topical wound therapy.

ACTIVITY

Limited—Hand walking may be useful to increase peripheral circulation, especially in cases with significant edema of the limbs.

DIET

Swelling of the head and pharynx may necessitate placement of a nasogastric feeding tube to permit enteral feeding of dysphagic horses.

SURGICAL CONSIDERATIONS

- Any accessible, mature abscesses should be drained.
- Emergency tracheostomy may be required to relieve respiratory distress and prevent asphyxiation.

MEDICATIONS

DRUG(S)

- The use of corticosteroids remains controversial and mild cases of PH may resolve without immunosuppressive therapy. However, horses with life-threatening edema or organ dysfunction require early, aggressive corticosteroid treatment.
- Dexamethasone (0.05–0.2 mg/kg IV or IM q12–24h) or prednisolone (0.5–1.0 mg/kg IM or PO q12h) should be administered at the dosage and rate necessary to effect reduction in edema. Dexamethasone may be more effective than prednisolone.
- Once edema starts to resolve, the dosage of corticosteroids can be gradually reduced (10%–15% every 1–2 days) over 7–21 days while carefully monitoring for recurrence. Some cases require more than 4–6 weeks of corticosteroid therapy, and relapse may occur if therapy is truncated or if dexamethasone is switched to prednisolone too early (<10 days).
- For horses suffering a relapse, the corticosteroid dose may need to be increased over the previously efficacious concentrations. In these instances use of flunixin meglumine may enhance steroid efficacy.
- Antimicrobials should be used in conjunction with corticosteroids to help reduce the occurrence and severity of cellulites or other septic sequelae. In addition, when streptococcal infection is suspected, horses should be treated with penicillin (procaine penicillin 22,000 IU/kg IM q12 h or potassium penicillin 22,000 IU/kg IV q6 h) for at least 2 weeks or until clinical signs resolve.
- NSAIDs (e.g., flunixin meglumine 1.1 mg/kg PO or IV q12h or phenylbutazone 2.2 mg/kg PO or IV q12h) may help reduce vascular inflammation and edema and provide analgesia.

PRECAUTIONS

High-dose corticosteroid therapy may be associated with laminitis or secondary infections.

FOLLOW-UP

PATIENT MONITORING

Glomerulonephritis can progress to chronic renal failure. Creatinine and urine protein should be monitored weekly.

PREVENTION/AVOIDANCE

- Control of upper respiratory tract infections, e.g., strangles, will reduce the incidence.
- Careful consideration should be given to the use of streptococcal vaccines in horses at low risk of developing strangles.
- Measurement of serum antibodies to M protein may help determine the need for vaccination in endemic areas or when risk is high. Horses with antibody titers >1:32,000 should not be vaccinated.

POSSIBLE COMPLICATIONS

- Skin sloughing may be followed by exuberant granulation tissue and require excision followed by skin grafting.
- Laminitis and various infections such as cellulitis, pneumonia, colitis, and thrombophlebitis may occur due to long-term corticosteroid therapy.

EXPECTED COURSE AND PROGNOSIS

- Most horses recover with early aggressive therapy and supportive care within 2–4 weeks, although sequelae may prolong convalescence.
- Prognosis depends on severity and extent of disease—Extensive skin sloughing, evidence of internal organ involvement, development of secondary septic processes or laminitis are poor prognostic indicators.

MISCELLANEOUS

SEE ALSO

Streptococcus equi ss *equi* (strangles)

ABBREVIATIONS

- aPTT = activated partial thromboplastin time
- AST = aspartate aminotransferase
- CK = creatine kinase
- EGE = equine granulocytic ehrlichiosis
- EIAV = equine infectious anemia virus
- EVAV = equine viral arteritis virus
- IFA = immunofluorescence assay
- IMPT = immune-mediated thrombocytopenia
- PH = purpura hemorrhagica
- PT = prothrombin time

Suggested Reading

Kaese HJ, Valberg SJ, Hayden DW, et al. Infarctive purpura hemorrhagica in five horses. J Am Vet Med Assoc 2005;226:1893–1898.

Pusterla N, Watson JL, Affolter VK, et al. Purpura hemorrhagica in 53 horses. Vet Rec 2003;153:118–121.

Sellon DC. Disorders of the hematopoietic system. In: Reed et al., eds. Equine Internal Medicine, ed 2. St Louis: Saunders, 2004;721–768.

Author Jennifer Hodgson

Consulting Editors David Hodgson and Jennifer Hodgson

PURULENT NASAL DISCHARGE

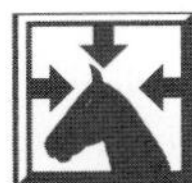

BASICS

DEFINITION

Fluid discharge of varying turbidity, color, amount, frequency, and odor from one or both nostrils

PATHOPHYSIOLOGY

• Composed of combinations of leukocytes and varying amounts of fluid and/or mucus from any location in the respiratory tract.
• Production originates from an inflammatory process incited by traumatic, immune, allergic, infectious, or noxious stimuli.
• Discharge can be septic or nonseptic.
• Color varies—white, yellow, green, reddish, or brown depending on the presence of bacteria, ingesta, blood or necrotic tissue.
• Unilateral discharge is most likely associated with a condition of the ipsilateral nasal cavity or paranasal sinus. • Bilateral discharge more likely originates caudal to the nasal septum, especially the lower airways. • Nasal discharge from the guttural pouches can be unilateral or bilateral depending on the volume of discharge • Malodorous discharge is associated with anaerobic infections, foreign bodies, necrotic bone, and tooth root abscesses.

SYSTEMS AFFECTED

• Respiratory—lower tract, consisting of alveoli, bronchioles, bronchi, and trachea; upper tract, consisting of nasopharynx, guttural pouches, larynx, turbinates, conchae, nasal passages, paranasal sinuses, and false nostrils. • Gastrointestinal—oropharynx and esophagus

GENETICS

N/A

INCIDENCE/PREVALENCE

Variable depending on underlying cause

GEOGRAPHIC DISTRIBUTION

Variable depending on underlying cause

SIGNALMENT

• Foals and young horses or any immunocompromised animal more prone to infections. • Neonates with milk in the discharge may have cleft palate or selenium deficiency and resulting aspiration pneumonia. • Older horses—(heaves), tooth infections, sinusitis, and neoplasia • Any age horse can have trauma, IAD, or bacterial infection.

SIGNS

Historical

• Nasal discharge accompanied by coughing, fever, reluctance to eat, dyspnea, respiratory noise, or odor
• Discharge that is continuous or intermittent, spontaneous, and/or associated with exercise or eating. • Discharge may be copious or scant, unilateral or bilateral.
• Previous signs of respiratory disease or exposure to other animals with disease
• Previous treatments and management changes and responses • Seasonal correlation with worsening or alleviation may indicate allergic disease. • Exercise intolerance • Facial swelling or bony remodeling is indicative of a chronic sinus problem and/or tooth disease.

Physical Examination

• Ongoing discharge or dried material at nares
• Normal or decreased airflow at the nares with airway compromise • Fever—consistent with infectious agent • Chronic dyspnea, tachypnea, nostril flaring, increased abdominal respiratory effort, and "heave line" are suggestive of heaves • Lymphadenopathy with swelling and inflammation of retropharyngeal and/or submandibular lymph nodes with *Streptococcus equi* (strangles) or *S. zooepidemicus* infection • Guttural pouch distention with empyema tympany or chondroids
• Dull areas on percussion and auscultation of paranasal sinuses indicate exudate or cystic structure • Evidence of dental disease associated with sinusitis • Odor occurs with tooth root infection, bony necrosis (i.e., neoplasia), foreign body, gram-negative lung abscessation, or necrotizing pneumonia
• Abnormal lung sounds consistent with pneumonia, pleuropneumonia, or heaves; may be exacerbated or elicited with use of a rebreathing bag • Percussion of lung field—dull areas are indicative of pleural fluid, abscess, or consolidated lung • Auscultation of fluid in trachea with exudate in pneumonia, IAD, or heaves • Dysphagia with esophageal obstruction, guttural pouch disease (resulting neuropathy), or episodes of hyperkalemic periodic paralysis • Milk in discharge with cleft plate in neonates, severe depression, botulism, or nutritional myopathy (selenium deficiency) • Depression—severe illness with severe pneumonia or pleuropneumonia • Plaque of edema between the front legs in cases of pleuropneumonia

CAUSES

• Common causes are bacterial infections, bacterial infections following initial viral infections and heaves. • Bacterial infections—*S. equi* lymphadenitis, guttural pouch empyema, sinusitis, lung abscessation, pneumonia, and pleuropneumonia
• Mycotic rhinitis, mycotic guttural pouch infection • Foreign bodies or trauma with subsequent inflammation/infection
• Esophageal obstruction or pharyngeal dysfunction resulting in dysphagia and aspiration

RISK FACTORS

• Viral infections—influenza and equine herpesvirus especially with young animals and congregated housing • Exposure to animals infected with upper respiratory virus or strangles • Lack of vaccination against respiratory pathogens • Poor deworming history, migrating ascarids predispose foals and yearlings to secondary bacterial pneumonia • Immunodeficiency—FPT, SCIDS, and steroid therapy
• Immunosuppression associated with PPID
• Environmental—indoors, dust, molds, air pollutants, and smoke inhalation
• Transport—subsequent pleuropneumonia
• Ethmoid hematoma, EIPH • Dental disease/sinusitis • Dysphagia and aspiration associated with esophageal choke, cranial nerve damage, guttural pouch disease (mycosis), botulism, hyperkalemic periodic paralysis episodes affecting pharyngeal muscles • Orphan foal aspirating milk
• Selenium deficiency in foals resulting in dysphagia and aspiration

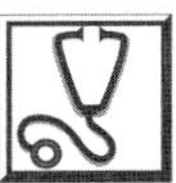

DIAGNOSIS

DIFFERENTIAL DIAGNOSES

• Unilateral discharge suggests a problem affecting the upper airways; bilateral discharge may originate from either the upper (caudal to nasal septum) or the lower airway
• Presence of food may indicate esophageal obstruction or pharyngeal dysfunction
• Infectious—bacterial, viral, and fungal
• Immune-mediated—allergic, airway hypersensitivity • Trauma—foreign body
• Congenital cleft palate or sinus cyst
• Nutritional (selenium) deficiency in foals
• Neuromuscular problem such as botulism or cranial nerve damage due to guttural pouch disease • Abscessation • Inflammation
• Neoplasia

CBC/BIOCHEMISTRY/URINALYSIS

• May or may not have an inflammatory leukogram with neutrophilia and hyperfibrinogenemia if localized or extensive
• Leukogram may be degenerative, with left shift and toxic cells depending on severity (especially with pneumonia). • Anemia may be a feature if there is chronic hemorrhage or chronic inflammation.

OTHER LABORATORY TESTS

• Serum immunoglobulin levels for FPT or immunodeficiency in neonates
• Serum/plasma *S. equi* titers and upper respiratory virus titers • PCR detection of bacterial pathogens such as *Rhodococcus equi* and *Streptococcus equi* • Arterial blood gases—PaO_2 for lower airway disease or pneumonia

IMAGING

• Endoscopy—nasal passages, sinuses, pharynx, guttural pouches and trachea bronchi • Radiography—sinuses, teeth, guttural pouches, pharynx, and lungs
• Ultrasonography—thorax • Scintigraphy, MRI, or CT scan may be available for further detailed imaging if the source of the discharge is ellusive.

OTHER DIAGNOSTIC PROCEDURES

• Culture and sensitivity of nasopharynx or guttural pouch to detect strangles • Bronchoalveolar lavage—cytology in diffuse lower airway disorders • Transtracheal wash—culture and cytology • Lymph node (if affected) aspiration—culture and cytology
• Sinus aspiration/trephination—culture and cytology • Thoracocentesis—culture and cytology • Respiratory function testing for airway disease

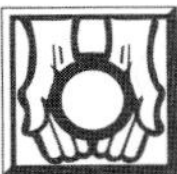

TREATMENT

• Environmental management for IAD and heaves • Institute isolation measures if strangles suspected/confirmed • Removal of foreign body • Trephination, drainage, flushing of the sinuses • Surgical tooth expulsion • Flushing of guttural pouches
• Drainage of abscesses • Chest drainage may be indicated in pleuropneumonia
• Appropriate intensive care, nursing care, oxygen administration, rest for pneumonia and pleuropneumonia patients

AIMS OF TREATMENT

• Eliminate underlying infection. • Prevent spread of infectious agents to susceptible animals. • Manage heaves through environmental modification, anti-inflammatories, and bronchodilators.

APPROPRIATE HEALTH CARE

• Routine vaccination of susceptible animals against infectious respiratory diseases
• Minimize dust and mold exposure.
• Routine dental examinations

NURSING CARE

Variable depending on underlying disease

ACTIVITY

Most respiratory infections require a period of rest to allow recovery. Insult to the airway mucociliary apparatus may take up to 7 weeks to repair.

DIET

• Appropriate for change in activity.
• Decreased plane of nutrition for athletic animals during recovery period. • Adequate plane of nutrition for serious respiratory disease such as pleuropneumonia where animals may be in catabolic disease state

CLIENT EDUCATION

Contingent on the diagnosis. Infectious disease control, and environmental management control if appropriate

SURGICAL CONSIDERATION

• May be required for sinus, guttural pouch, or dental conditions • Hemorrhage may be an issue. Remember tetanus prophylaxis.

MEDICATIONS

DRUG(S) OF CHOICE

• Antimicrobial regimen based on culture and sensitivity results for bacterial infections
• NSAIDs such as flunixin meglumine
• Inhalant or systemic steroids for IAD and heaves patients • Bronchodilators

CONTRAINDICATIONS

• Clenbuterol bronchodilator should *not* be administered to horses being slaughtered for human consumption. • Clenbuterol is *not* recommended for use in horses with cardiovascular disease.

PRECAUTIONS

• Aminoglycoside antibiotics such as gentamicin and amikacin should be monitored closely to avoid renal toxicosis.
• Expectorants such as Na and K iodide if used for long periods can cause iodinism. This will resolve when the expectorant is discontinued. • Do not use steroids alone in the face of an infection. • NSAIDs can exacerbate gastrointestinal ulceration, especially in foals. • Methylxanthine bronchodilator (aminophylline) has a narrow therapeutic index and can cause seizures and death in sick foals.

POSSIBLE INTERACTIONS

Methylxanthine bronchodilator (aminophylline) and cimetidine

ALTERNATIVE DRUGS

• Expectorants • Interferon alpha immune stimulant for IAD in young horses

FOLLOW-UP

Contingent on diagnosis

PATIENT MONITORING

Contingent on diagnosis

PREVENTION/AVOIDANCE

Contingent on diagnosis

POSSIBLE COMPLICATIONS

• Aspiration pneumonia if dysphagia
• Recurrence if sinus infections • Fatal hemorrhage if ethmoid hematoma or guttural pouch mycosis • Purpura hemorrhagica if strangles

EXPECTED COURSE AND PROGNOSIS

Contingent on diagnosis

MISCELLANEOUS

ASSOCIATED CONDITIONS

N/A

AGE-RELATED FACTORS

• Foals and young horses at risk to respiratory infections • Foals with congenital cleft palate, selenium deficiency • Young horses with congenital sinus cysts • Older horses with PPID prone to recurring infections

ZOONOTIC POTENTIALS

N/A

PREGNANCY

Clenbuterol should be discontinued in pregnant mares near term as it is a tocolytic.

SEE ALSO

• Aspiration pneumonia • Esophageal choke
• Guttural pouch empyema • Heaves (RAO)
• Paranasal sinusitis • Pleuropneumonia
• Pneumonia • *Streptococcus equi* infection

ABBREVIATIONS

• EIPH = exercise-induced pulmonary hemorrhage
• FPT = failure of passive transfer of immunity
• IAD = inflammatory airway disease
• PCR = polymerase chain reaction
• PPID = pars pituitary intermedia dysfunction or equine Cushing's disease.
• SCIDS = severe combined immunodeficiency syndrome

Suggested Reading

Colahan PT. Nasal discharge. In: Colahan PT, Merritt AM, Moore JN, Mayhew IG, eds. Equine Medicine and Surgery, ed 5. St. Louis: Mosby, 1999:30–31.

McGorum BC, Dixon PM, Robinson NE, Schumacher J. eds. Equine Respiratory Medicine and Surgery. Philadelphia: WB Saunders, 2007.

Rush B, Mair T. eds. Equine Respiratory Disease. Ames, Iowa: Blackwell Publishing, 2004.

Author Wendy Duckett
Consulting Editor Daniel Jean

PYOMETRA

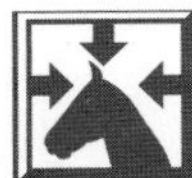

BASICS

DEFINITION

Accumulation of a large volume of purulent exudate within the uterine lumen

ETIOLOGY/PATHOPHYSIOLOGY

- Impaired drainage of uterine fluids
- Frequently a sequel to metritis, cervicitis, or cervical adhesions/trauma
- Associated with severe endometrial inflammatory changes, loss of epithelium, and permanent gland atrophy
- Signs of systemic disease, e.g., anorexia, weight loss, and depression, are rare.

SYSTEM AFFECTED

Reproductive

GENETICS

N/A

INCIDENCE/PREVALENCE

No geographic distribution

SIGNALMENT

Aged pluriparous mares are predisposed to recurrent uterine infections because of anatomic defects and failing mechanical uterine defense mechanisms.

- Poor vulvar conformation
- Pendulous uterus
- Aging
- Cervical/uterine trauma or adhesions

SIGNS

General Comments

- The mare may cycle regularly or remain in a prolonged diestrus.
- Prolonged diestrus is associated with decreased ability of the uterus to secrete endogenous $PGF_{2\alpha}$ because of extensive endometrial destruction.

Historical

- Watery, milky, or purulent vaginal discharge may be continuous, intermittent (i.e., open pyometra), or absent (i.e., closed pyometra) depending on cervical patency and stage of the estrous cycle.
- Contact dermatitis and alopecia of the inner thighs and hocks may be evident.
- Can be an incidental finding on routine examination

Physical Examination

- External conformation may be normal.
- Chronic or intermittent purulent vaginal discharge
- TRP reveals an enlarged, fluid-filled uterus that may be further described with U/S. A large fluid volume (0.5–60 L) may accumulate within the uterine lumen.
- Digital cervical examination often reveals adhesions, constrictions, or other abnormalities.
- Culture and cytology results show bacteria and fungi similar to those associated with infectious endometritis. Bacterial isolation ranges from a mixed population of organisms to no bacterial growth.
- Presence of different amounts of PMNs is consistent.

CAUSES AND RISK FACTORS

Infectious

- Bacteria do not cause pyometra in the mare, they are opportunists.
- Most common isolates—*Streptococcus zooepidemicus*, *Escherichia coli*, *Actinomyces* sp., *Pasteurella* sp., and *Pseudomonas* sp.
- Chronic infection with *P. aeruginosa* or fungi may predispose the mare to developing a pyometra.

Noninfectious

- Mechanical impairment preventing normal uterine drainage
- Physical obstruction of the cervical canal that inhibits uterine evacuation, e.g., trauma, cervical fibrosis/induration that prevents either complete closure or dilation, and obstruction of the cervical lumen by adhesions
- Extrauterine impairment caused by abdominal adhesions to the uterus may prevent the uterus from involuting or evacuating completely.
- Chronic uterine distention also impairs ability of the uterus to contract and evacuate its contents.
- Age and parity—multiparous; >14 years of age
- Conformational abnormalities—history of postpartum metritis/cervicitis; history of cervical laceration, trauma, or incomplete cervical dilation

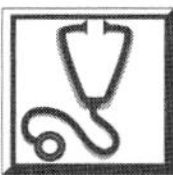

DIAGNOSIS

DIFFERENTIAL DIAGNOSIS

Pregnancy

- The uterine walls of a pregnant mare demonstrate a characteristic tone and responsiveness.
- The uterine walls of a mare with a pyometra may become thickened. The purulent exudate causes the uterus to feel "doughy."
- U/S findings provide additional differentiating characteristics. Uterine fluid with a pyometra has a characteristic appearance/characteristics—hyperechoic, flocculent, echo-dense.

Pneumouterus

- Associated with abnormal vulvar conformation and poor uterine tone, resulting in wind-sucking and pneumovagina
- Poor tone of the vestibulovaginal sphincter allows air to pass through the cervix and into the uterus. This most commonly occurs during estrus because of vulvar/cervical relaxation and also after administration of sedatives, e.g., acepromazine.

Mucometra

Mucoid exudate accumulation associated with hormonally induced cystic endometrial hyperplasia in old mares is a very rare condition.

Placentitis

- May be characterized by a purulent vaginal discharge in a pregnant mare
- Ascending placentitis occurs late in gestation and is localized at the cervical star.
- Premature mammary development also may be present.

Distended Bladder

Distinguish the uterus from the bladder by the ability to locate ovaries and/or trace along either the uterine horns or the cervix during TRP.

OTHER CAUSES OF VAGINAL DISCHARGE

See Endometritis.

CBC/BIOCHEMISTRY/URINALYSIS

Mild normocytic, normochromic anemia, and/or neutropenia in some mares

OTHER LABORATORY TESTS—FOR INFECTIOUS CAUSES

Bacteria

- Endometrial cells and intraluminal contents may be obtained by scraping the endometrial surface with the swab tip or cap (if using a Kalayjian culture swab). The sample is then stained with Diff-Quik. The presence of neutrophils indicates active inflammation.
- Evaluation of the endometrial contents for bacteria is obtained using a guarded swab.
    - The sample should be cultured in blood agar and McConkey's at 37° C and examined at 24 and 48 hr.
    - Blood agar will support growth of gram-positive, select gram-negative organisms, and some yeasts.
    - McConkey's will support only the growth of gram-negative organisms.
    - Both should be used.

Yeasts

- Samples obtained for bacterial culture can also be used to isolate *Candida* and *Aspergillus* sp., because these organisms grow in blood agar.
- Branching hyphae can be identified in stained smears or wet mounts.
- For fungal-specific culture, the sample is inoculated in Sabouraud agar and incubated for 4 days at 37° C.

IMAGING

U/S

- Intrauterine fluid can be categorized by its presence, quantity, and quality.
- Depending on the amount of accumulated debris and inflammatory cells, the exudate may be moderately to highly hyperechoic.

OTHER DIAGNOSTIC PROCEDURES

Endometrial Biopsy

- An important prognostic tool
- Collect the initial sample before treatment.
- Evacuate uterine content before performing the biopsy to lessen what is a slight likelihood of rupturing/penetrating the uterine wall during the procedure.

Endoscopy

- May reveal intrauterine adhesions that are precluding effective uterine drainage
- Purulent exudate may be attached to the walls and/or found free in the lumen.

PATHOLOGICAL FINDINGS

- Wide range of findings, depending on the severity and duration of the condition
- Especially pronounced in old mares—severe endometrial inflammatory changes; glandular atrophy
- Atrophy may be permanent and confers an extremely poor prognosis for the mare's reproductive life.

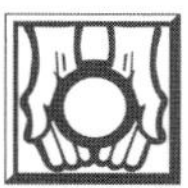

TREATMENT

APPROPRIATE HEALTH CARE

- Mechanical evacuation of purulent contents by repeated uterine lavage (daily or alternate days) using a nasogastric tube and large volumes of warm saline
- Follow lavage with administration of an ecbolic drug (oxytocin or $PGF_{2\alpha}$).
- The uterus is then infused with antibiotics based on culture and sensitivity results.
- Note: Antibiotics should be infused 45–60 min after oxytocin administration to avoid their premature evacuation.
- Administer a luteolytic dose of $PGF_{2\alpha}$ if a persistent corpus luteum is suspected.

NURSING CARE

N/A

ACTIVITY

N/A

DIET

N/A

CLIENT EDUCATION

N/A

SURGICAL CONSIDERATIONS

- If the option is to forego further breeding or there is chronic pyometra, treatment may be left undone, or hysterectomy, although not often used, is an option.
- If hysterectomy is performed, the uterus must be emptied as completely as possible before surgery.
- Life-threatening complications after hysterectomy have decreased significantly due to improved techniques.

MEDICATIONS

DRUGS OF CHOICE

- See Endometritis.
- $PGF_{2\alpha}$, dinoprost tromethamine (Lutalyse; 5–10 mg total IM)

CONTRAINDICATIONS

See Endometritis.

PRECAUTIONS

Infuse fluid for uterine lavage carefully into the distended and friable uterus, beginning with relatively low volumes to avoid rupture.

POSSIBLE INTERACTIONS

N/A

ALTERNATIVE DRUGS

N/A

FOLLOW-UP

PATIENT MONITORING

- TRP and U/S to evaluate response to treatment—uterine size and tone; amount of intrauterine fluid
- Endometrial biopsy and/or endoscopy after treatment for endometrial visualization, evaluation of response to treatment, and prognosis

PREVENTION/AVOIDANCE

N/A

POSSIBLE COMPLICATIONS

Contamination of abdomen during surgery can cause peritonitis.

EXPECTED COURSE AND PROGNOSIS

- Recurrence is common.
- Prognosis for fertility is poor.
- The prognosis for fertility is grave in cases with severe uterine or cervical adhesions.

MISCELLANEOUS

ASSOCIATED CONDITIONS

Cervical adhesions may obliterate the cervical lumen and keep it from opening and closing properly.

AGE-RELATED FACTORS

Repeated uterine stretching associated with pregnancy results in a uterus suspended low in the abdomen, predisposing to fluid accumulation and increased risk for pyometra.

ZOONOTIC POTENTIAL

N/A

PREGNANCY

- Pregnancy can be achieved in few of the treated mares.
- Mares with chronic uterine inflammation or anatomical problems may require the use of assisted reproductive techniques to obtain a pregnancy (e.g., oocyte transfer, in vitro fertilization, intracytoplasmatic sperm injection).

SEE ALSO

- Cervical lesions
- Endometritis/delayed uterine clearance
- Postpartum metritis
- Vulvar conformation

ABBREVIATIONS

- TRP = transrectal palpation
- U/S = ultrasonography

Suggested Reading

Hughes JP, Stabenfeldt GH, Kindahl H, et al. Pyometra in the mare. J Reprod Fertil Suppl 1979;27:321–329.

Murray WJ. Uterine defense mechanisms and pyometra in mares. Compend Contin Educ Pract Vet 1991;13:659–663.

Rotting AK, Freeman DE, Doyle AJ, Lock T, Sauberli D. Total and partial ovariohysterectomy in seven mares. Equine Vet J 2004;36:29–33.

Author Maria E. Cadario

Consulting Editor Carla L. Carleton

PYRROLIZIDINE ALKALOID TOXICOSIS

BASICS

DEFINITION

• A disease associated with chronic ingestion of PA-containing plants; PAs are a distinct group of structurally similar molecules found in approximately 6000 plant species worldwide. • Hundreds of different alkaloids, defined as saturated or unsaturated, exist, along with their corresponding *N*-oxide forms. • Some PAs are hepatotoxic; some are not. • Alkaloid composition and concentration, as well as toxicity, vary tremendously among plants. The alkaloid concentration varies within different parts of the plant, along with stage of plant maturity. • Three plant families (i.e., Compositae, Leguminosae, and Boraginaceae) account for most PA-containing plants. The most common plant responsible for clinical disease in the United States is probably *Senecio* spp.; *Amsinckia, Cynoglossum,* and *Crotalaria* can cause disease but are less commonly implicated. • Economic losses caused by these plants once were estimated at ≈$20 million per year in the Pacific Northwest alone. Because of widespread recognition of the problem and effective livestock management and biologic control measures (particularly with *S. jacobaea*), intoxications resulting from these plants are much less common. • Intoxications usually occur when horses graze paddocks or pastures heavily contaminated with these plants or consume contaminated hay during a period of several weeks to months. • Acute intoxications are rare, primarily because of the large amount of plant material a horse would need to ingest at any one feeding or several feedings.

PATHOPHYSIOLOGY

• PAs are rapidly absorbed from the GI tract and undergo extensive hepatic metabolism by mixed-function oxidases. • Some are detoxified to harmless metabolites, primarily by ester hydrolysis and conversion to *N*-oxides, which then are eliminated via the urine or bile. Others are activated by conversion to toxic metabolites, primarily by dehydrogenation, yielding highly toxic pyrrole derivatives. • Pyrroles alkylate double-stranded DNA, thus inhibiting cell mitosis. Nuclear and cytoplasmic cell masses expand because of the impaired ability to divide, thus forming megalocytes. As megalocytes die, they are replaced by fibrous connective tissue. • Pyrroles also bind to cellular constituents in lung and kidney tissues, either because of systemic distribution of reactive pyrroles from the liver or in situ metabolism of the parent PA.

SYSTEMS AFFECTED

• Hepatobiliary—Interference with cell replication leads to hepatocytomegaly and necrosis with bile duct proliferation and fibrosis; endothelial proliferation in centrilobular and hepatic veins occurs. • Renal/Urologic—Pyrrole-bound molecules can lead to megalocytosis of the proximal convoluted tubules, atrophy of glomeruli, and tubular necrosis; this has not been described in horses. • Respiratory—Pyrrole-bound molecules can lead to alveolar hemorrhage and edema, progressive proliferation of alveolar walls, pulmonary arteritis and hypertension; this is not commonly reported in horses. • Cardiovascular—Right ventricular hypertrophy and cor pulmonale have been documented experimentally, most likely secondary to PA-induced lung damage.

GENETICS N/A

INCIDENCE/PREVALENCE

Most intoxications occur during late spring, summer, and early fall, when there is access to the growing plant; however, intoxications can occur at any time because of the persistent toxicity of these alkaloids in baled hay.

SIGNALMENT N/A

SIGNS

General Comments

• Most affected horses suffer chronic weight loss and debilitation associated with hepatic insufficiency, which can be subtle in nature; this is referred to as the chronic-delayed form. • In the chronic-delayed form, clinical signs can appear quite suddenly, despite exposure and liver lesions having been chronic and progressive. • The extent of hepatic damage depends greatly on the daily amount of alkaloid consumption, degree of pyrrole conversion, age of the animal, and metabolic and mitotic status of the target cells. • Food intake and nutritional status also can modify the effects of PAs. • Most affected patients, particularly those suffering from the chronic-delayed form, exhibit neurologic signs.

Physical Examination

• Loss of appetite • Weight loss • Weakness and sluggishness • Photodermatitis • Icterus • Behavioral abnormalities—mania, derangement, yawning, aimless walking, head pressing, drowsiness, blindness, and ataxia • Inspiratory dyspnea—related to paralysis of the pharynx and larynx • Gastric impaction • Ascites • Diarrhea with tenesmus

CAUSES

• Plants incriminated in the United States—*Senecio jacobaea* (tansy ragwort), *S. vulgaris* (common groundsel), *S. douglasii* var *longiilobus* (threadleaf groundsel), *S. riddelli* (Riddell's groundsel), and *Cynoglossum officinale* (hound's-tongue)
• Depending on the species, stage of maturity, environmental conditions, and age of the horse, most animals must ingest 1%–5% of body weight in plant material daily before effects are observed. Sometimes as much as 50% is required before clinical signs become apparent.
• With tansy ragwort, some authors suggest a chronic lethal dose for horses of 0.05–0.20 kg/kg. Thus, for a 500-kg horse, ingestion of one dried hound's-tongue plant per day for 2 weeks can cause clinical disease.
• *Amsinckia* and *Crotalaria* spp. rarely cause problems, because the highest percentage of alkaloid is presumably present in the seed. Most intoxications result from ingestion of contaminated grain or cakes; however, horses have been poisoned after chronic ingestion of *Amsinckia* spp.–contaminated hay.

RISK FACTORS

Intoxication occurs from grazing heavy stands of the plants or eating contaminated hay for extended periods of time (2–4 weeks to several months).

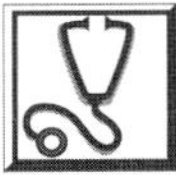

DIAGNOSIS

DIFFERENTIAL DIAGNOSIS

• Alsike clover (*Trifolium hybridum*) or red clover (*Trifolium pratense*) intoxication
• Acute hepatitis—Theiler's disease
• Cholangiohepatitis
• Liver abscess
• Cholelithiasis
• Viral encephalitis
• Nigropallidal encephalomalacia
• Leukoencephalomalacia
• Equine protozoal encephalomyelitis
• Miscellaneous hepatotoxic chemicals—more acute in nature; causing more necrosis (e. g., carbon tetrachloride, chlorinated hydrocarbons, pentachlorophenols, coal-tar pitch, phenol, iron, phosphorus)
• Aflatoxin poisoning—rare

CBC/BIOCHEMISTRY/URINALYSIS

• Elevations in GGT and ALP
• Hyperbilirubinemia
• Hypoalbuminemia
• Hypoproteinemia
• Inflammatory leukogram
• Hyperammonemia

OTHER LABORATORY TESTS

• Prolonged BSP clearance time
• Elevated bile acids
• Abnormal liver biopsy

IMAGING

Ultrasonography may detect extensive liver fibrosis.

DIAGNOSTIC PROCEDURES

• Detection of pyrrole metabolites in blood or hepatic tissue can be performed by some laboratories. This is more successful in the acute stages of the disease.
• Identification of PA-containing plants on premise or in feed (less commonly stomach contents) is the preferred method of confirming exposure.
• Identification and quantification of the active PA in feed or stomach contents can be performed by some laboratories, but this is not routinely done.

• Liver biopsy to detect characteristic lesions is critical to the diagnosis.

PATHOLOGICAL FINDINGS

• Poor body condition; loss of body fat
• Jaundice
• Ascites and generalized edema
• Small, pale, firm liver with a mottled, cut surface
• Megalocytosis, with mild necrosis
• Fibrosis—centrilobular and periportal
• Veno-occlusive lesions
• Biliary hyperplasia
• Pulmonary edema
• Interstitial pneumonia
• Brain status spongiosus
• Other, less-recognized lesions—myocardial necrosis, cecal and colonic edema and hemorrhage, and adrenal cortical hypertrophy

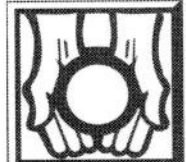

TREATMENT

APPROPRIATE HEALTH CARE

• No specific treatment
• Primary goal—to provide supportive therapy until enough liver tissue can regenerate and function adequately for the intended use of the horse
• Most PA-poisoned patients respond poorly to treatment, because by the time the disease is diagnosed, adequate liver regeneration is no longer possible.

NURSING CARE

• IV fluids to correct dehydration often are necessary.
• Photodermatitis can be treated with an appropriate combination of cleansing, hydrotherapy and debridement, along with restricting exposure to sunlight.

ACTIVITY

Plenty of rest, with reduction of stress, is important.

DIET

• Replace contaminated feed with a high nutrient diet (i.e., highly digestible, high in calories, low in protein) divided into 4–6 daily feedings.
• One suggested diet includes 1–2 parts beet pulp and 0.25, 0.50, or 1 part cracked corn mixed with molasses and fed at a rate of 2.5 kg per 100 lb. Sorghum or milo can be substituted for beet pulp.
• Oat or grass hay is a good source of roughage.
• Avoid alfalfa and other legumes because of their high protein content.
• Oral pastes and IV preparations containing high concentrations of branched-chain amino acids and antioxidants have been used, but with questionable success.
• Consider weekly vitamin B_1, folic acid, and vitamin K_1 supplementation.

CLIENT EDUCATION

• Recognize PA-containing plants of concern in the geographic area, and prevent access by the horse.
• Provide adequate forage and prevent overgrazing to limit ingestion of toxic plants.

SURGICAL CONSIDERATIONS

N/A

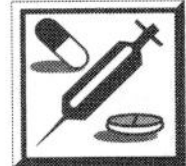

MEDICATIONS

DRUG(S) OF CHOICE

• Horses with neurological signs may require diazepam (foals: 0.05–0.4 mg/kg IV; adults: 25–50 mg IV; may be necessary to repeat) or xylazine (1.1 mg/kg IV or 2.2 mg/kg IM).
• With septic photodermatitis, consider oral, broad-spectrum antibiotics—e.g., cephalosporins.
• With low blood glucose, a continual 5% dextrose drip may be administered IV at a rate of 2 mL/kg/hr. Dilute the 5% dextrose in normal saline or LRS if the infusion will last longer than 24–48 hr.
• Oral neomycin (50–100 mg/kg q6h for 1 day), lactulose (0.3 mL/kg q6h), or mineral oil has been used to decrease blood ammonia concentrations, but with varying results.

CONTRAINDICATIONS

N/A

PRECAUTIONS

• Diarrhea is a common sequela after neomycin or lactulose therapy.
• Neomycin can predispose to salmonellosis.
• Exercise care when administering any medication that undergoes extensive hepatic metabolism.

POSSIBLE INTERACTIONS

N/A

ALTERNATIVE DRUGS

N/A

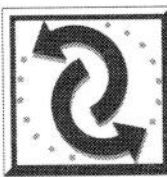

FOLLOW-UP

PATIENT MONITORING

• Monitor appetite, weight, serum liver enzymes and bile acids every 2–4 weeks.
• Magnitude of the elevation of serum hepatic enzymes does not always correlate with degree of hepatic impairment.

PREVENTION/AVOIDANCE

• Recognize PA-containing plants, both in the field and in feeds.
• Use good management practices and appropriate herbicide control to avoid overexposure of horses to these plants.
• Sheep and goats are relatively resistant and have been used to graze heavily contaminated land.

POSSIBLE COMPLICATIONS

Pneumonia and chronic wasting are the most common sequelae.

EXPECTED COURSE AND PROGNOSIS

• Most affected horses are given a poor prognosis and are euthanized because of severe debilitation or nonresponsive neurologic signs.
• Some animals can recover after several months of care but generally cannot regain their former fitness or activity level.

MISCELLANEOUS

ASSOCIATED CONDITIONS

N/A

AGE-RELATED FACTORS

Although not documented, foals or young ponies may be at slightly greater risk because of their smaller body mass, less discriminating eating habits, higher metabolic activity, and higher susceptibility of tissues in which cells are rapidly dividing.

ZOONOTIC POTENTIAL

N/A

PREGNANCY

• PAs have been detected in milk collected from PA-exposed cattle and goats, but the levels have been considered clinically insignificant.
• PAs cross the placenta in other species, causing various fetotoxic effects.

SYNONYMS

• Walking disease
• Yawning disease

SEE ALSO

N/A

ABBREVIATIONS

• ALP = alkaline phosphatase
• BSP = bromosulfophthalein
• GGT = γ-glutamyltransferase
• GI = gastrointestinal
• LRS = lactated Ringer's solution
• PA = pyrrolizidine alkaloid

Suggested Reading

Craig AM, Pearson EG, Meyer C, Schmitz JA. Clinicopathologic studies of tansy ragwort toxicosis in ponies: sequential serum and histopathological changes. Equine Vet Sci 1991;11:261.

Mendel VE, Witt MR, Gitchell BS, et al. Pyrrolizidine alkaloid-induced liver disease in horses: an early diagnosis. Am J Vet Res 1988;49:572.

Pearson EG. Liver failure attributable to pyrrolizidine alkaloid toxicosis and associated with inspiratory dyspnea in ponies: three cases (1982–1988). J Am Vet Med Assoc 1991;198:1651.

Author Patricia A. Talcott

Consulting Editor Robert H. Poppenga

QUERCUS SPP. (OAK) TOXICOSIS

BASICS

OVERVIEW

- This genus of plants contains a variety species, including trees and shrubs.
- Species more commonly associated with poisoning include Gambel's oak (*Q. gambelii*), Havard or shinnery oak (*Q. havardii*), and white shin oak (*Q. durandii* var. *brevilobata*). Other species implicated in poisonings include wavyleaf oak (*Q. undulata*), Emory oak (*Q. emoryi*), shrub live oak (*Q. turbinella*), and silverleaf oak (*Q. hypoeucoides*).
- All *Quercus* spp. should be considered toxic. Ingestion of large quantities of leaves, leaf buds, or acorns results in a severe gastroenteritis/nephrotoxic syndrome.
- Poisoning is most commonly associated with ingestion of new leaf buds, hence the common name "oak-bud poisoning."
- Gallotannins are the toxic principals. Ingested tannins react with dietary and tissue proteins rendering them nonfunctional. Toxicosis generally occurs when oak is >50% of the diet.
- Poisonings most commonly occur in early spring with ingestion of new leaf buds or in late fall with ingestion of acorns.

SIGNALMENT

- Poisoning is rare in horses.
- It can occur at any age.
- Male and female equids are equally susceptible.

SIGNS

- Abdominal pain, depression, anorexia, constipation (early) followed by hemorrhagic diarrhea
- Peripheral edema, diphtheritic membranes in feces
- Weakness, polydipsia, and polyuria
- Tachycardia
- Prostration and death

CAUSES AND RISK FACTORS

- Intoxication is often associated with a lack of available forage or dietary supplementation.
- Drought or conditions that inhibit other forages from growing predisposes to ingestion of oak.
- Most common in the early spring when leaf buds are developing or late fall when acorns are dropping

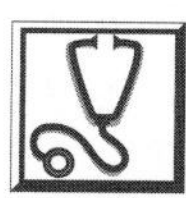

DIAGNOSIS

CBC/BIOCHEMISTRY/URINALYSIS

Increased serum BUN and creatinine, hyposthenuria, proteinuria, hematuria, hyperphosphatemia, hypocalcemia, increased AST

OTHER LABORATORY TESTS

N/A

IMAGING

N/A

DIAGNOSTIC PROCEDURES

N/A

PATHOLOGICAL FINDINGS

Gross

- Subcutaneous edema, mucoid and/or hemorrhagic enteritis, pseudomembranous enteritis, edema of mesenteric lymph nodes, hydropericardium, perirenal edema, swollen and pale kidneys, ascites, petechial hemorrhage of kidneys, and hepatic congestion

Histopathological

- Kidneys—numerous pink to brown casts in the proximal tubules, proximal tubular necrosis, medullary congestion
- Gastrointestinal—pseudomembranous, necrotizing enteritis with hemorrhage and ulceration
- Other—vascular congestion of the liver and lungs, generalized tissue congestion

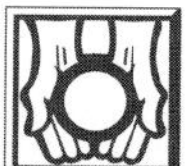

TREATMENT

- Prevent further exposure by removing horses from access to oaks.
- Minimize further gastrointestinal and renal damage with general decontamination and supportive care.
- Decontamination may decrease the duration and severity of signs. Activated charcoal binds tannins in GI tract, rendering them unabsorbable, but this has not been proved.
- Decrease GI transit time with mineral oil or cathartics such as magnesium sulfate (Epsom salt). Use gastric demulcents or sucralfate for severe GI damage.
- Administer intravenous normal saline to keep the horse hydrated and maintain urine flow.

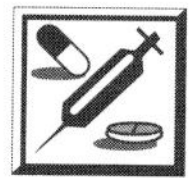

MEDICATIONS

DRUG(S) OF CHOICE

AC (1–4 g/kg PO once in a water slurry), magnesium sulfate (250–500 mg/kg as a 20% solution PO once), sucralfate (2 mg/kg PO TID)

CONTRAINDICATIONS/POSSIBLE INTERACTIONS

Do not give AC with mineral oil as the oil prevents binding of compounds to the charcoal. Do not give AC if there is evidence of severe GI mucosal damage, as the charcoal can imbed in mucosal erosions.

FOLLOW-UP

PATIENT MONITORING

Monitor renal function daily. Maintenance of renal function is a good indicator of treatment efficacy.

PREVENTION/AVOIDANCE

Avoid pasturing horses in areas containing oaks unless other adequate forage is available. Supplementation with calcium hydroxide (15% pellet) to inactivate tannins has been beneficial in other species, but its effectiveness in horses is unknown.

POSSIBLE COMPLICATIONS

With severe GI ulceration and necrosis, scarring and strictures are possible.

EXPECTED COURSE AND PROGNOSIS

Recovery may require 2–3 weeks of intense care.

MISCELLANEOUS

ASSOCIATED CONDITIONS, AGE-RELATED FACTORS, ZOONOTIC POTENTIAL, PREGNANCY

N/A

ABBREVIATIONS

- AC = activated charcoal
- AST = aspartate aminotransferase
- GI = gastrointestinal

Suggested Reading

Harper KT, Ruyle GB, Rittenhouse LR. Toxicity problems associated with the grazing of oak in the intermountain and southwestern U.S.A. In: James LF, Ralphs MH, Nielsen DB, eds. The Ecology and Economic Impact of Poisonous Plants on Livestock Production. Boulder, CO: Westview Press, 1988:197–206.

Author Jeffery O. Hall

Consulting Editor Robert H. Poppenga

BASICS

DEFINITION

A lethal encephalitis caused by a neurotropic, single-stranded RNA virus in the family Rhabdoviridae, genus *Lyssavirus*

PATHOPHYSIOLOGY

• Rabies is usually transmitted via salivary contamination of a bite wound. Historically, an animal may have been bitten by a dog, racoon, skunk, fox, or bat several months prior to the onset of signs, although most rabies cases have no such evidence and usually bite wounds are healed by the onset of neurologic signs.
• The virus may amplify in muscle tissue before invading the peripheral nervous system. It is not known how the virus enters the peripheral nerves.
• The virus moves to the CNS by axoplasmic flow and passes along neurons within the nervous system.
• Initially, there may be hyperactivity of affected neurons with signs such as hyperesthesia, tremor, straining, and salivation.
• Ultimately, the neurons die, and signs such as flaccid paralysis, dysphagia, and anesthesia then can be expected.

SYSTEM AFFECTED

CNS

SIGNALMENT

Any breed, sex, and age

SIGNS

Historical

Horses may be in areas where rabies is more common.

Physical Examination

• The presenting signs and progressive syndromes that can result from rabies virus infection are extremely varied.
• Classically, the syndromes are divided into a cerebral or furious form, the brainstem or dumb form, and the spinal cord or paralytic form. Almost certainly, these partly relate to the site of inoculation into the body and subsequent neuronal spread of the virus and the body's response to it.
• Forebrain signs often include aggressive behavior, hyperesthesia, vocalization, sialosis, tenesmus, and convulsions.
• In the brainstem, or dumb form, somnolence, dementia, stupor, opisthotonus, facial hypalgesia, pharyngeal paralysis, excessive drooling, and ataxia occur.
• The spinal cord, or paralytic, form is characterized by progressive, ascending paralysis; monoparesis/plegia; truncal, limb, and perineal hyporeflexia and hypalgesia; priapism; and altered frequency of miction; and urinary incontinence.
• Self-mutilation can be associated with any form.
• Once signs start, the untreated clinical course is less than 14 days, but usually less than 5 days, and the animal dies in a mean period of 3 days.
• Prodromal colic, lameness, listlessness, anorexia, and, rarely, hydrophobia may be recalled by owners in large animal cases.
• Fever may occur independent of seizure activity.

CAUSE

• The disease is caused by serotype 1 rabies virus. This is a bullet-shaped, neurotropic, single-stranded RNA virus of the genus *Lyssavirus* and family Rhabdoviridae. There are approximately 25 viruses in this family, but only serotype 1 is pathogenic.
• Rabies has two cycles, which include canine (urban) and wildlife (sylvatic) rabies. Most wildlife vectors are small omnivores, like skunks, raccoons, or foxes.
• There is extension into domestic animals, which are essentially dead-end hosts.

RISK FACTORS

Horses in enzootic areas

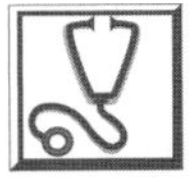

DIAGNOSIS

DIAGNOSIS/PATHOLOGY

The patient can be evaluated for 10 days and, if it needs to be destroyed or dies, the head or $\frac{1}{2}$ fresh and $\frac{1}{2}$ formalin-fixed brain and fresh salivary gland should be sent to a veterinary diagnostic laboratory equipped to handle rabies virus–infected tissue. Direct and indirect immunofluorescent antibody testing for rabies virus may be done there, as well as mouse inoculation studies if indicated.

DIFFERENTIAL DIAGNOSIS

• Any disease associated with progressive gray matter disruption should be considered.
• Togaviral encephalitides, heavy metal toxicity, neuritis of the cauda equina, acute protozoal myeloencephalitis, sorghum-sudan grass poisoning, hepatoencephalopathy, CNS trauma, moldy corn poisoning, and probably many other disorders

CBC/BIOCHEMISTRY/URINALYSIS

No specific abnormalities

OTHER LABORATORY TESTS

CSF is often normal but may show moderate elevations in protein and mononuclear cell numbers.

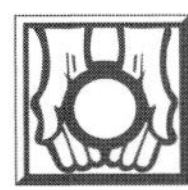

TREATMENT

• Only palliative treatment can be offered.
• Anti-inflammatory therapy for other diseases may delay progression of signs.

PREVENTION

Horses in enzootic areas may be immunized with annual vaccination beginning at 6 months of age with commercial inactivated vaccine. Horses previously immunized and bitten by suspect rabid animals can be given a three-booster immunization series over 7 days. They should be quarantined for a minimum of 90 days.

MEDICATIONS

N/A

FOLLOW-UP

N/A

MISCELLANEOUS

ZOONOTIC POTENTIAL

Horse-to-human transmission appears to be very rare. Nevertheless, exposure to nervous and other tissues from horses suspected to be rabid should be avoided and documented if occurred.

ABBREVIATION

• CNS = central nervous system
• CSF = cerebrospinal fluid

Suggested Reading

Green SL. Rabies. Vet Clin North Am Equine Pract 1997;13:1–11.

The author and editor wish to acknowledge the contribution of Joseph J. Bertone and Pamela Wilkins, authors of this chapter in the previous edition.

Author Caroline N. Hahn
Consulting Editor Caroline N. Hahn

RECTAL PROLAPSE

BASICS

OVERVIEW

With rectal prolapse, tissue is protruding through the anus, and depending on the layers involved, it can be categorized in four types:

- Type 1 = rectal mucosa and submucosa protrude
- Type 2 = complete prolapse of all layers of the rectal ampulla
- Type 3 = complete prolapse of the rectal ampulla and invagination of the terminal small colon into the rectum
- Type 4 = intussusception of the peritoneal rectum and varying lengths of the small colon through the anus

PATHOPHYSIOLOGY

Rectal prolapse results from an increase in pressure gradient between the abdominal cavity and the anus (i.e., tenesmus), which causes the rectal mucosa and submucosa to glide backward over the muscularis layer. Unreduced prolapses become edematous and cyanotic due to compromise of venous outflow. With type 3 and 4 prolapses, the entire rectum disengages from the perirectal tissues, resulting in complete displacement of the rectum as well as the distal small colon. Because the mesocolon of the distal small colon is relatively short, caudal displacement and tearing of the mesocolon during prolapse often result in avulsion of the colonic blood supply. If the blood supply to the small colon is disrupted, ischemic necrosis ensues.

SYSTEMS AFFECTED

- Gastrointestinal—rectal impaction, small colon necrosis, or peritonitis
- Behavioral—tenesmus or mild to moderate abdominal pain
- Cardiovascular—circulatory shock may be evident in horses with thrombosis or rupture of the small colonic vasculature or due to endotoxemia caused by small colon necrosis.

SIGNALMENT

More common in adult horses and mares. Type 4 rectal prolapse is seen with dystocia in mares.

SIGNS

Historical

Prolonged tenesmus due to diarrhea or colic; dystocia

Physical Examination

Palpation and inspection are simple means of differentiating between the four types of rectal prolapses. Types 1, 2, and 3 are continuous with the mucocutaneous junction of the anus. Characteristic findings include:

- Type 1—a circular, doughnut-shaped, edematous swelling at the anus that is usually most prominent ventrally
- Type 2—a larger, cauliflower-shaped swelling that is often thicker ventrally than dorsally
- Type 3—appears similar to type 2, but is firmer due to the presence of invaginated peritoneal rectum or small colon within the mass.
- Type 4—a palpable trench exists between the prolapse and the anus, and can be appreciated by sliding a finger underneath the prolapse and past the normal mucocutaneous junction. Usually has tube-like appearance.

CAUSES

Rectal prolapse is most often associated with tenesmus secondary to a variety of conditions:

- Parturition
- Dystocia
- Uterine prolapse
- Diarrhea
- Constipation
- Colitis
- Proctitis
- Rectal masses—neoplasms (leiomyoma, lipoma), foreign bodies, abscesses, polyps, hematomas
- Grade 2 rectal tears
- Intestinal parasitism
- Urethral obstruction—urolithiasis

In many cases, however, a cause cannot be identified.

RISK FACTORS

Any condition that induces tenesmus. Poor body condition due to loss of tone in the anal sphincter or decreased elasticity of the connective tissue may increase risk. Type 1 rectal prolapses are often seen in horses with severe diarrhea, and type 4 rectal prolapses are most often associated with dystocia in broodmares.

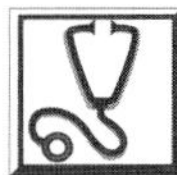

DIAGNOSIS

DIFFERENTIAL DIAGNOSIS

Prolapsed tissues may be mistaken for a neoplastic mass. Visual inspection and palpation can differentiate between the two conditions. Evaginated rectal tissues are obvious with a prolapse, whereas a neoplasm arises from a localized aspect of the rectal or perirectal tissues.

CBC/BIOCHEMISTRY/URINALYSIS

Systemic abnormalities corresponding to the inciting cause may be identified. Early in the course of type 3 and 4 prolapses, leukocytosis and neutrophilia with a left shift may be observed, as well as increases in PCV, fibrinogen, TP, sodium, and potassium levels. With longer duration, leukopenia and neutropenia ensue. Chronicity may lead to decreases in potassium, sodium, and chloride levels and increases in BUN, creatinine, and bilirubin.

OTHER LABORATORY TESTS

Abdominocentesis to assess if compromise to the small colon has occurred. Peritoneal fluid in horses with type 3 or 4 prolapse may have an increase in WBC count or TP level.

IMAGING

Transabdominal ultrasound may be used to identify possible free fluid in the abdomen and evaluate motility of the intestine.

OTHER DIAGNOSTIC PROCEDURES

A flank laparotomy, ventral midline celiotomy, or laparoscopy can be used to assess the degree of compromise to the mesocolon and small colon in type 3 and 4 prolapse; however, access to the terminal small colon can be challenging with a flank or ventral midline laparotomy. In the standing horse, laparoscopy provides superior visualization and selection of the most appropriate surgical procedure in a minimally invasive manner.

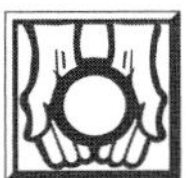

TREATMENT

- The first step in the treatment of rectal prolapse is to prevent tenesmus. The specific cause of the prolapse should therefore be identified and addressed. Epidural anesthesia is an effective means of alleviating tenesmus. Alternatively, heavy sedation, use of lidocaine gel, a lidocaine enema, or infiltration of the inflamed tissues with local anesthetic may provide some relief.
- Early type 1 and 2 rectal prolapses without extensive edema, trauma, or contamination usually respond to conservative therapy aimed at reduction of tissue edema, manual reduction of the prolapse, and placement of a purse-string suture in the anus to prevent recurrence, and treatment of the primary cause for the prolapse.
    - Reduction of edema—application of topical glycerin, or mannitol, or magnesium sulfate
    - Purse-string suture—use of a large (size 1–3), nonabsorbable (nylon, polypropylene, umbilical tape, caprolactam) material; placed using four wide bites located 1–2 cm from the anus. Following placement, the external anal sphincter should be dilatable to a diameter of 4–6 cm to permit defecation. Epidural anesthesia/analgesia should be maintained to prevent straining against the suture. The suture should be removed within 24–48 hr to minimize complications.

- The horse should be taken off feed for the first 24 hr.
- Mineral oil or other laxatives should be administered and a laxative diet maintained for at least 1 week.
- Horse should be kept cross tied in a box stall for the first week to prevent recumbency (increased abdominal pressure when recumbent).

• Type 1 and 2 prolapses that are chronic in nature or that have failed to respond to conservative therapy can be treated successfully by submucosal resection or by rectal amputation. Both procedures can be performed in the standing, sedated horse using epidural anesthesia. Submucosal resection is preferred over rectal amputation because the rectal vasculature and muscular layers are preserved, an aseptic peritoneal environment is maintained, there is decreased risk of postoperative perirectal abscess formation or of rectal stricture, and postoperative tenesmus is decreased.

• Types 3 and 4 rectal prolapses require referral to a surgical facility. Balanced polyionic intravenous fluid therapy may be required by horses with type 3 or 4 prolapses for treatment of hypovolemia or endotoxemic shock. The fluid rate should be based on the horse's hydration status and clinical condition.

CLIENT EDUCATION

Horses with type 4 rectal prolapse have a serious condition carrying a guarded to poor prognosis for survival. Depending on the length of intussuscepted tissues, chronicity of the prolapse, the horse's medical status and value, and the owner's intentions for the horse, euthanasia may be warranted. If the owner wishes to pursue treatment, factors that require discussion include cost, the need for extensive postoperative care, and multiple possible complications following resection/anastomosis or colostomy. Horses undergoing colostomy require a second procedure for revision; the second procedure necessitates general anesthesia, incurs additional costs, and provides additional opportunities for complications to arise.

SURGICAL CONSIDERATIONS

Notable hemorrhage may occur during submucosal resection or rectal amputation, but can be controlled with electrocautery or ligation.

MEDICATIONS

DRUGS OF CHOICE

• Sedation may be achieved with xylazine (0.2–1.1 mg/kg IV) or detomidine (0.005–0.02 mg/kg IV). Both duration and quality of sedation may be enhanced by the co-administration of butorphanol tartrate (0.1 mg/kg IV).

• Epidural administration of a variety of agents may provide anesthesia for initial evaluation and treatment, as well as analgesia for prevention of postoperative tenesmus (for details and dosages, see Rectal Tear).

PATIENT MONITORING

Following treatment, the patient should be observed regularly for evidence of tenesmus, rectal impaction, or relapse. Purse-string sutures should be removed within 24–48 hr to minimize complications.

PREVENTION/AVOIDANCE

Prompt recognition and treatment of factors predisposing to tenesmus reduce the likelihood of rectal prolapse.

POSSIBLE COMPLICATIONS

• Rectal impaction
• Reprolapse
• Dehiscence of suture lines
• Perirectal abscess formation
• Rectal stricture
• Ischemic necrosis of the small colon
• Complications associated with colostomy, celiotomy, or resection/anastomosis procedures

EXPECTED COURSE AND PROGNOSIS

The prognosis for type 1 and 2 rectal prolapses is favorable, whereas the prognosis for type 3 and 4 prolapses is guarded to poor.

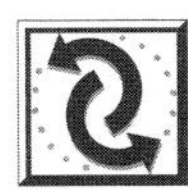

FOLLOW-UP

N/A

MISCELLANEOUS

ASSOCIATED CONDITIONS

• Endotoxemia
• Laminitis
• Uterine prolapse

SEE ALSO

• See individual factors listed under Causes.

ABBREVIATIONS

• BUN = blood urea nitrogen
• CBC = complete blood count
• PCV = packed cell volume
• TP = total protein
• WBC = white blood cell

Suggested Reading

Freeman DE. Rectum and anus. In: Auer JA, Stick JA eds. Equine Surgery, ed 3. St. Louis: Saunders Elsevier, 2006.

Authors Judith B. Koenig and Annette M. Sysel

Consulting Editors Henry Stämpfli and Olimpo Oliver-Espinosa

RECTAL TEAR

BASICS

DEFINITION

A partial- to full-thickness tear in the wall of the retroperitoneal or peritoneal rectum

PATHOPHYSIOLOGY

Rectal tears are usually iatrogenic, occurring most commonly as a complication of manual palpation per rectum. Less commonly, they occur as complication of enema administration, especially in foals, dystocia, and breeding accidents. Most tears involve the dorsal aspect of the rectum and are located 15–55 cm from the anus; they are usually located parallel to the longitudinal axis of the rectum. Based on severity, they are divided into the following four grades:

- Grade 1—Tearing of the rectal mucosa and submucosa.
- Grade 2—The muscular layer of the rectum is torn, and the mucosa and submucosa prolapse through the defect to create a diverticulum, which may act as a pocket for fecal impaction.
- Grade 3(a)—Disruption of the rectal mucosa, submucosa, and muscularis layers, resulting in a palpable void in the rectal wall that exposes the serosa.
- Grade 3(b)—Disruption of the rectal mucosa, submucosa, and muscularis layers, without involvement of the mesorectum. This tear is palpable as a defect in the rectal wall that exposes the fat-filled mesorectum. Grade 3 tears can cause formation of a retroperitoneal space within the pelvic cavity that can become impacted, then rupture and convert to a grade 4 tear. The presence of intact serosa or mesorectum prevents contamination of the abdominal cavity with fecal material; however, movement of bacteria through these tissues may induce local peritonitis.
- Grade 4—Tearing of all layers of the rectum; as a result, direct communication exists between the rectum and the abdominal cavity, resulting in septic peritonitis, which may result in development of endotoxemia and circulatory shock.

SYSTEM AFFECTED

Gastrointestinal

Local and diffuse peritonitis may develop within 2 hr of a rectal tear. Ileus secondary to diffusion of bacteria and toxins may follow. Abdominal discomfort and straining may accompany rectal impactions, especially in horses with grade 2 rectal tears.

Behavioral

Signs of colic secondary to peritonitis and ileus may be present initially, but progress to signs of depression and endotoxic shock.

Cardiovascular

Vascular collapse secondary to endotoxemic shock may be evident within 2 hr following a rectal tear.

GENETICS

None

INCIDENCE/PREVALENCE

N/A

GEOGRAPHIC DISTRIBUTION

None

SIGNALMENT

Breed Predilections

- Arabians
- Miniature horses and other small breeds
- Ponies

Mean Age and Range

Rectal tears can occur in horses of any age. Young horses that have a small rectal diameter or those that are unaccustomed to rectal examination may be predisposed.

Predominant Sex

May occur more often in males than in females

SIGNS

General Comments

Tearing of the rectum during a palpation per rectum may not be felt by the examiner, but should be suspected if a significant amount of blood is evident on the rectal sleeve or in the feces following rectal examination.

Historical

Horses with grades 1 or 2 rectal tears rarely demonstrate signs relative to the tear. Grade 2 tears are often not identified until signs of rectal impaction develop; frequently, these tears are identified during an unassociated rectal examination. Grade 3 or 4 rectal tears are often associated with signs of sweating, pawing, a splinted abdomen, or tachycardia within 2 hr following breeding or rectal palpation.

Physical Examination

Rectal findings are summarized under Pathophysiology.

CAUSES

- Rectal palpation of the gastrointestinal or urogenital system
- Misdirected intromission of a stallion's penis during breeding
- Enema administration
- Meconium extraction with forceps
- Dystocia
- External trauma
- Fractures of the pelvis or vertebrae
- Sodomy
- Displaced granulosa cell tumors
- Ruptured small colon hematomas
- Spontaneous

RISK FACTORS

Any condition that necessitates repeated rectal examination

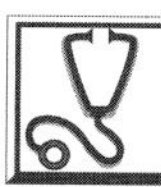

DIAGNOSIS

DIFFERENTIAL DIAGNOSIS

Mild mucosal irritation may result in a few flecks of blood or blood-tinged fluid on the palpation sleeve following rectal examination. Colitis or conditions that compromise the vascular supply of the small colon, with or without compromise to its lumen, may produce bloody or malodorous brown fluid on rectal examination.

CBC/BIOCHEMISTRY/URINALYSIS

Leukocytosis and neutrophilia with a left shift, as well as increases in PCV, fibrinogen, TP, sodium, and potassium occur early in the course of grades 3 and 4 rectal tears, as well as leukopenia and neutropenia; decreases in potassium, sodium, and chloride levels; and increases in BUN, creatinine, and bilirubin may occur later.

OTHER LABORATORY TESTS

An increase in peritoneal fluid, WBC count, or TP level is consistent with a diagnosis of peritonitis. The presence of degenerate neutrophils, bacteria, or plant material on cytologic examination is indicative of septic peritonitis and is associated with a poor prognosis.

IMAGING

Abdominal ultrasound may be useful in assessment of quantity and quality of peritoneal fluid.

DIAGNOSTIC PROCEDURES

- After administration of epidural lidocaine, bare-armed evaluation of the rectum is useful in ruling out the presence of a rectal tear. The veterinarian's arm should be lubricated copiously with a water-soluble gel and the feces gently removed from the rectum. Rectal tears can be identified through circumferential palpation of the rectum cranially from the anus in 3- to 4-inch (6- to 10-cm) increments. The rectal tear should be assessed for depth of penetration, size, position, and distance from the anus.
- A vaginal speculum may be used for visualization of the tear, but infolding of the mucosa around the end of the speculum often hampers adequate assessment.
- The severity of damage to the rectal wall can be assessed endoscopically.
- Laparoscopy may be performed in horses with severe grade 3 or 4 tears to determine presence and degree of fecal contamination of the abdominal cavity. Laparoscopy may also permit direct visualization and assessment of tears of the peritoneal rectum.

PATHOLOGICAL FINDINGS

See Pathophysiology.

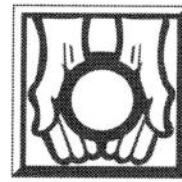

TREATMENT

AIMS OF TREATMENT

- Reduce straining.
- Reduce motility.
- Decrease fecal contamination.
- Prevent infection.
- Prevent shock.

APPROPRIATE HEALTH CARE

If a rectal tear is suspected, straining and rectal peristalsis should be reduced by sedation, epidural anesthesia, and/or parasympatholytic drugs. A lidocaine enema (12–25 mL of 2% lidocaine in 50 mL water) or lidocaine jelly may be used. Fecal softeners and a laxative diet are valuable in the management of all rectal tear cases. Grade 1 rectal tears usually respond well to a 3- to 5-day course of anti-inflammatory and broad-spectrum antibiotic therapy. Periodic cleaning and delicate debridement with gauze squares may be needed to hasten healing and prevent abscess formation, a permanent diverticulum, or a rectal stricture. In addition to the above, grade 2 rectal tears may be treated with a combination of flushing and drainage of the diverticulum. Horses with grade 3(a), 3(b), or grade 4 rectal tears should be considered emergencies that require referral to a surgical facility. Prior to transport, the rectal tear should be packed with 3-inch (7.5-cm) stockinette filled with moistened roll cotton. This should be sprayed with povidone–iodine and lubricated with surgical gel and inserted to a point 10 cm proximal to the tear. The tear should not be overpacked. The packing may be secured by closing the anus with towel clamps or a purse-string suture. Epidural anesthesia should be maintained to prevent straining during transport. Parenteral anti-inflammatory and broad-spectrum antibiotic therapy should be initiated, and intravenous fluids should be administered to horses in shock. Feed should be withheld, and fecal softeners should be administered via nasogastric tube.

NURSING CARE
See appropriate health care.

ACTIVITY
Horses that have undergone surgical treatment should be confined to a stall for appropriate postoperative monitoring and management.

DIET
All horses with rectal tears should be fed a low-bulk laxative diet, such as green grass, a complete pelleted ration, or alfalfa pellets soaked in water.

CLIENT EDUCATION
The owner should be informed of the presence of a rectal tear or a suspected tear immediately. If treatment is pursued, the owner should be advised of the cost, extensive postoperative care, and multiple complications that can be associated with surgical treatment.

SURGICAL CONSIDERATIONS
A grade 3 or 4 rectal tear may require placement of a rectal liner, may be sutured directly or under laparoscopic guidance, or may require a loop colostomy.

MEDICATIONS

DRUG(S) OF CHOICE
- Parasympatholytic agents such as propantheline bromide 0.014 mg/kg IV or IM or atropine 0.44–0.1 mg/kg IM or SC decrease rectal peristalsis and prevent straining during transport.
- Sedation may be achieved with xylazine 0.2–1.1 mg/kg IV or detomidine 0.005–0.02 mg/kg IV. Both duration and quality of sedation may be enhanced by the co-administration of butorphanol tartrate 0.1 mg/kg IV.
- Epidural administration of a variety of agents (e. g., lidocaine, xylazine, detomidine) may provide anesthesia for initial evaluation and treatment as well as analgesia for prevention of postoperative tenesmus. A caudal epidural catheter allows repeated administration of agents to alleviate straining and provide analgesia/anesthesia to the perineal region.
- Broad-spectrum antibiotic therapy is recommended for 3–10 days with grades 1 and 2 rectal tears. Extensive broad-spectrum antibiotic therapy is required for grades 3 and 4 tears.
- Tetanus prophylaxis should be considered.
- Flunixin meglumine therapy is recommended in horses with endotoxemia.

CONTRAINDICATIONS
- Acepromazine is contraindicated for sedation of hypovolemic horses.
- Indiscriminate use of atropine can result in gastrointestinal complications, such as prolonged ileus with tympanic distention of the bowel, mild to moderate abdominal pain, and tachycardia.

PRECAUTIONS
Administration of epidural lidocaine may be associated with ataxia.

POSSIBLE INTERACTIONS
If sedatives have been administered by the intramuscular or intravenous route, the epidural dosage of xylazine or detomidine should be adjusted to avoid excessive cumulative sedation.

ALTERNATIVE DRUGS
N/A

FOLLOW-UP

PATIENT MONITORING
- Horses with grade 1 rectal tears should be monitored closely for 4–8 days, with serial CBCs, fibrinogen levels, and peritoneal fluid analyses.
- Rectal palpation should be avoided for 30 days. Most grades 1 and 2 tears heal within 7–14 days.
- Horses with grades 3 and 4 rectal tears should be monitored for complications associated with the surgical procedure(s) performed. These horses should be assessed with serial CBCs, fibrinogen levels, and peritoneal fluid analyses.

PREVENTION/AVOIDANCE
- Rectal examination of horses should be reserved for veterinarians. Rectal examinations should be done only when necessary, and the history of the problem as well as the size and temperament of the patient should be considered.
- Appropriate restraint and careful technique should be used.
- Appropriate supervision during breeding may reduce the likelihood of inadvertent tearing by the stallion.

POSSIBLE COMPLICATIONS
- Progression of the tear
- Fecal contamination of the tear or of the abdomen
- Peritonitis
- Extensive cellulitis
- Abscess formation
- Rectoperitoneal fistula formation
- Rectal impaction or stricture
- Ileus
- Abdominal adhesions
- Complications associated with primary closure—excessive tissue trauma; incomplete closure; inadvertent suturing of mucosal folds leading to stricture
- Complications associated with temporary liner placement—tearing of the liner; retraction of the liner into the rectum to uncover the tear; premature sloughing
- Complications associated with colostomy—dehiscence; adhesions; abscessation; herniation/prolapse; rupture of mesenteric vessels; infarction; spontaneous closure

EXPECTED COURSE AND PROGNOSIS
Chances for survival improve with adequate and immediate first aid. Grades 1 and 2 rectal tears have a good prognosis; grade 3(a) tears have a fair to guarded prognosis; grade 3(b) tears have a guarded to poor prognosis because of the likelihood of greater tissue damage and undermining; and grade 4 tears have a poor to grave prognosis because gross fecal contamination of the abdomen predisposes to massive adhesion formation and fatal peritonitis.

MISCELLANEOUS

ASSOCIATED CONDITIONS
- Peritonitis
- Endotoxemia
- Laminitis
- Abdominal adhesions

AGE-RELATED FACTORS
None

ZOONOTIC POTENTIAL
None

PREGNANCY
Broodmares left with permanent colostomies are prone to intestinal herniation in advanced pregnancy and at parturition due to unusual abdominal pressures placed against the colonic stoma.

SYNONYMS
None

SEE ALSO
- None

ABBREVIATIONS
- BUN = blood urea nitrogen
- PCV = packed cell volume
- TP = total protein

Suggested Reading

Freeman DE. Rectum and anus. In: Auer JA, Stick JA, eds. Equine Surgery, ed 3. St. Louis: Saunders Elsevier, 2006.

Mair TS. The medical management of eight horses with grade 3 rectal tears. Equine Vet J Suppl 2000;32:104–107.

Meagher DA. Rectal surgery. In: White NA, Moore JN, eds. Current Practice of Equine Surgery. Philadelphia: JB Lippincott, 1990.

Rick MC. Management of rectal injuries. Vet Clin North Am Equine Pract 1989;5:407–428.

Watkins JP, Taylor TS, Schumacher J, et al. Rectal tears in the horse: an analysis of 35 cases. Equine Vet J 1989;21:186–188.

Authors Judith B. Koenig and Annette M. Sysel

Consulting Editors Henry Stämpfli and Olimpo Oliver-Espinosa

RECUMBENT HORSE

BASICS

DEFINITION

Down horse that is unable to get up without assistance

PATHOPHYSIOLOGY

Recumbency may occur secondary to pain, weakness, and/or incoordination produced by an underlying primary condition of such severity that the horse can no longer get up. Some horses are able to rise with assistance (tail assistance, sling assistance). Organ systems that are commonly associated with the primary disease include:
• Respiratory • Metabolic • Musculoskeletal
• Cardiovascular • Gastrointestinal
• Neurologic

SYSTEMS AFFECTED

It is crucial to find the cause of recumbency in order to plan on a therapy and give prognostic information. In recumbent horses, it may be hard to assess all body systems, but it is important to be thorough and complete. Safety measures should be considered while working on down horses, in particular, when the cause of recumbency is unclear. Secondary to recumbency the following systems may become affected:
• Cardiovascular—hydration status
• Respiratory—atelectasis underperfused lung areas • Gastrointestinal—impaction or diarrhea (depending on disease), hydration status, and diet • Musculoskeletal—muscle disease • Skin—decubital ulcers

GENETICS

Some breeds of horses are more prone to developing initiating disease. For example, young Thoroughbreds are more likely to develop grade 4–5/5 neurologic deficits and subsequent recumbency due to cervical vertebral stenotic myelopathy.

INCIDENCE/PREVALENCE

Incidence of recumbency is higher in certain diseases such as botulism and laminitis. Some diseases have a higher prevalence in certain geographic areas.

GEOGRAPHIC DISTRIBUTION

Some diseases that may lead to recumbency are more prevalent in certain geographic areas, such as botulism in the northeastern United States.

SIGNALMENT

None specific

SIGNS

General Comments

Down horse that cannot get up on its own. The horse may be quiet, restless, or violently thrashing.

Historical

Consider whether the change in status has occurred acutely or whether a more chronic disease process has deteriorated over time. Are there more animals affected? Consider trauma. Consider infectious disease.

Physical Examination

Monitor respiration, heart rate, temperature, pain, gastrointestinal system, musculoskeletal system, and neurologic status.

CAUSES

• Trauma • Respiratory—severe hypoxemia may lead to collapse and recumbency. Treatment and prognosis depend on the origin of hypoxemia. Causes include upper airway obstructions, *Streptococcus equi* abscesses, HYPP, and severe pulmonary disease. Emergency tracheostomy may be required for stabilization of the horse in cases of upper airway disease. • Cardiovascular—hemorrhagic, (endo)toxic and hypovolemic shock, sepsis, cardiac arrhythmias that lead to syncope and collapse, and cardiac failure can result in recumbency. The cause of recumbency in these situations is inadequate tissue perfusion and oxygenation. Generally these pathologic conditions are recognized through signalment, history, and physical examination. Treatment depends on the primary disease process and prognosis depends on cause and treatment options.
• Musculoskeletal disease—Tractures, rhabdomyolysis, and laminitis are the main musculoskeletal causes of recumbency. Laminitis is perhaps the most common cause of (excessive) recumbency in the horse. Although most horses will have a positive response to hoof testers placed over the sole, this disease may be difficult to recognize in a recumbent animal. Encouraging a recumbent horse to stand may facilitate the diagnosis of laminitis. However, it may be contraindicated to force a horse with limb fractures to stand up. Lower limb fractures are generally easily detectible, but upper limb fractures, pelvic fractures, and vertebral fractures may be more difficult to diagnose and may only be suspected by assessing the horse's ability to stand in the sling or through the use of ancillary diagnostics. Severe exertional rhabdomyolysis may lead to recumbency and is diagnosed by an accurate signalment, history, and physical and laboratory examinations. Other types of myositis, such as clostridial myonecrosis and post-anesthetic muscle compartment injury may lead to (post-anesthetic) recumbency. Multiple joint lameness and severe degenerative joint disease in young and geriatric horses are other potential causes of recumbency. White muscle disease can cause recumbency. • Metabolic disease—Derangements that lead to hypoglycemia, hyponatremia, or hypocalcemia may be causes of recumbency. Horses that develop an episode of HYPP may become recumbent. Liver disease, through the development of hepatoencephalopathy, may lead to abnormal behavior and subsequent recumbency. Weakness due to chronic disease, anorexia, and/or old age may become a cause of recumbency and inability to rise. Further, various toxicoses or administration of drugs can lead to recumbency. • Neurologic disease—Cervical vertebral stenotic myelopathy, equine protozoal myeloencephalitis, equine degenerative myelopathy, equine motor neuron disease, equine herpes myeloencephalitis, other encephalitis (West Nile virus, EEE, VEE, WEE), meningitis, leukoencephalomalacia, cholesterol granuloma, peripheral nerve injury, rabies, botulism, tetanus

RISK FACTORS

Cervical vertebral stenotic myelopathy, HYPP positive, unvaccinated for infectious diseases, laminitis

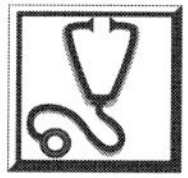

DIAGNOSIS

CBC/BIOCHEMISTRY/URINALYSIS

Depending on initiating disease

OTHER LABORATORY TESTS

Serology/polymerase chain reaction for infectious diseases

IMAGING

Radiology, ultrasound, myelography, magnetic resonance imaging, computed tomography

OTHER DIAGNOSTIC PROCEDURES

Electromyelography, endoscopy, rectal examination, nasogastric intubation

PATHOLOGICAL FINDINGS

Specific for underlying disease

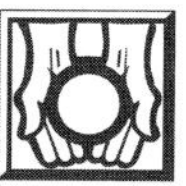

TREATMENT

AIMS OF TREATMENT

Management of a recumbent horse is a combination of intensive supportive care and specific treatment aimed at the underlying or secondary complicating disease processes. Supportive care is directed at protection of the animal and maintenance of adequate hydration and nutritional status. In addition to supportive care, many recumbent horses will need specific treatments for their primary disease and for treatment of conditions associated with the recumbent state.

NURSING CARE

• Transportation—Minimize self-trauma. An empty trailer without supporting bars and a wide door (stock trailer) should be used and the horse may need to be heavily sedated or anesthetized. Legs and head should be bandaged to minimize trauma to extremities. Deep bedding or padding is optimal, particularly for longer duration of transport.
• Bedding—Prolonged recumbency of horses may lead to the development of pressure sores, muscle compartment injury, and compressive neuropathies. The prevention and care of muscle compartmental injury, peripheral

nerve injury, and decubital ulcers are important aspects in the management of a recumbent animal. Bedding should be absorbent, nonabrasive, and conformable. The type of bedding may need to be adjusted when the horse makes (successful) attempts to stand or is standing in the sling. Then it is very important that the bedding provides adequate footing. Deep bedding in those situations may hinder the horse's attempts to stand or to ambulate and straw may be slippery. • Turning—Regular turning of the recumbent horse (every 2–6 hr) is necessary to provide adequate perfusion of the skin and musculature of the down side. Also, it will improve perfusion and ventilation of the down lung. If the horse is able to maintain a sternal position, this should be encouraged and, if necessary, assisted with the placement of straw bales or other materials. If a horse is in a comfortable sternal position, turning of the hindlimbs is still necessary. • Hydration—Unless horses can maintain itself standing or in sternal recumbency long enough to drink, the water intake will not be sufficient to meet the maintenance requirement (60 mL/kg/day). Fluid therapy can be provided intravenously or intragastrically via frequent nasogastric intubation at which 8–10 L can be administered in an adult horse (500 kg) or by indwelling nasogastric feeding tube through which gavage feeding can be administered. Depending on the dietary protocol, electrolytes and glucose may be added to the fluids. • Bladder/rectum emptying may be required.

DIET

• Regular diet or, if not possible, gruel through nasogastric tube, or PPN intravenously
• Some horses are able to ingest a sufficient amount of roughage (+/−2% of body weight) with or without grain while they are in sternal recumbency or standing with sling assistance.
• Pellet gruel—A large nasogastric tube can accommodate a diet consisting of soaked pellets such as alfalfa pellets or a soaked complete pelleted feed. Depending on the energy density of the pellet, 4–8 kg of pellets should be fed. Corn oil and electrolytes can be added to this diet to increase calories and maintain electrolyte balance.
• Liquid diet—Complete liquid diets are available for use in horses. For example, Osmolite (Ross Products Division, Abbott Laboratories, Columbus, OH, USA), contains approximately 1 cal/ml, so an adult horse would need 15 L of Osmolite in order to fulfill the caloric requirements. It is generally not possible to feed this amount to a horse because it is very costly and there is a risk of inducing colitis. This diet would be suitable for use in smaller horses or to meet only part of the nutritional requirements. Critical Care Meals (MD's Choice Inc., Louisville, TN, USA) provides a diet for horses that consists of 4 parts. Parts 1 and 4 can be diluted in approximately 8 L of water and parts 2 (vitamins and minerals) and 3 (glutamine, salt, yeast, arginine, carnitine) can be added to that. According to the directions, an adult horse should receive 2 feedings of 8 L and that would provide approximately 10 Mcal per day. This diet does not contain sufficient fiber, so it could be supplemented with pellet gruel if it is used for a longer period of time; however, a larger-bore tube is then required. Both of these diets should be started at approximately 25% of the total nutritional demand and should be gradually increased (3–4 days). The typical maintenance requirement is 30 kcal/kg and dietary intake should be started at 25% of this amount and gradually increased (3–4 days).
• Parenteral nutrition—Continuous intravenous access is required. Similar to the enteral diets, parenteral nutrition should be started at 25% of the nutritional demand (30 kcal/kg) and gradually increased. Disadvantages are the expense of the diet and expense of close monitoring of blood glucose concentrations. Provision of sufficient calories is important, particularly in animals with chronic disabling disease.

MEDICATIONS

DRUG(S) OF CHOICE

• Sedative/anesthetic/analgesics—xylazine, detomidine, medetomidine, acepromazine, diazepam, midazolam, phenobarbital, potassium bromide, pentobarbital, morphine, butorphanol
• Anti-inflammatory and edema-reducing agents—NSAIDs, corticosteroids, dimethylsulfoxide, mannitol, glycerol, hypertonic saline
• Antimicrobials—trimethoprim-sulfamethoxazole, penicillin-aminoglycoside
• Others as indicated for specific disease

FOLLOW-UP

PATIENT MONITORING

Gastrointestinal Tract/Urinary Tract

Down horses are prone to developing impactions of the cecum or large or small colon. Reduced fecal output may be a preliminary sign of impaction formation and the administration of laxatives such as magnesium or sodium sulfate, or polyethylene glycol containing solutions is then indicated. Some horses may develop ileus.

Respiratory Tract

Adequate ventilation, maintaining a clean stall environment, and preventing aspiration of food are important factors in reducing the chance of respiratory tract disease. Regular turning of the horse may minimize development of lung disease. In addition to decubital ulcers, the development of aspiration pneumonia is the most common complication seen in horses with botulism.

Ophthalmic Disease

Protection of the head is often required in recumbent horses primarily to protect the eyes. Protection may be accomplished by use of adequate padding or of helmets or bandages. The most common ophthalmic disorders seen in recumbent horses are corneal ulcers and (fungal) keratitis. Eyes need to be examined daily and treated carefully.

Physiotherapy

Physiotherapy is an important aspect of supportive care and the rehabilitative process of injured horses. Physiotherapy can be provided in the recumbent animal by manipulating limbs or by assisting the horse to stand with a sling.

Sling

When a horse is unable to rise but otherwise appears to have a normal mentation, it may be helpful in the examination to assist the horse to stand with a sling. Using the sling to assist a horse to stand may provide information for short-term management purposes. Deterioration or improvement of disease may be determined by daily sling-assistance. The sling is a valuable in the long-term management of recumbent animals. Depending on the horse's primary disease and compliance, horses can be comfortably managed in the sling until they have regained sufficient control to ambulate freely.

MISCELLANEOUS

ZOONOTIC POTENTIAL

• Due to the risk of diseases such as rabies, precautions should be taken in neurologic cases of unknown origin.

ABBREVIATIONS

• EEE, WEE, VEE = Eastern, Western, and Venezuelan encephalitides
• HYPP = hyperkalemic periodic paralysis
• PPN = partial parenteral nutrition

Suggested Reading

McConnico, R. S.; Clem, M. F. *et al*. (1991) Supportive medical care of recumbent horses. Compend. Contin. Educ. Pract. Vet. 13, 1287–1295.

Nout, Y. S. and Reed, S.M. (2005) Examination and treatment of the recumbent horse. Equine Veterinary Education 7 (6) 416—432. December 2005.

Radostitis OM, Gay CC, Hinchcliff KW, Constable PD. Diagnosis and care of the recumbent horse. In: Veterinary Medicine; a textbook of the diseases of cattle, horses, sheep, goats, and pigs. 10th ed. 2007:120–124.

Author Yvette S. Nout

Consulting Editor Michel Lévy

RECURRENT UVEITIS

BASICS

DEFINITION

ERU is a common cause of blindness in horses. It is a group of immune-mediated diseases of multiple origins. Recurrent attacks of uveitis are the hallmark of ERU.

PATHOPHYSIOLOGY

ERU appears to have characteristics of an infection-mediated autoimmune disease. The triggers for ERU are not completely understood. ERU can occur as a late sequela to systemic infection with ocular signs developing months postexposure. Hypersensitivity to infectious agents such as *Leptospira interrogans* is possible.

SYSTEM AFFECTED

Ophthalmic

GENETICS

Unknown but some genetic predisposition has been shown in German Warmblood and Appaloosa horses

INCIDENCE/PREVALENCE

Up to 8% affected in the United States

SIGNALMENT

- Breed predilection—*L. interrogans*–seropositive Appaloosas were 8.3 times as likely to develop uveitis as other breeds, and 3.8 times more likely as other breeds to lose vision following development of uveitis.
- Mean age and range—All ages can be affected.
- Predominant sex—none

SIGNS

- Horses experiencing classic, acute inflammatory ERU episodes display increased lacrimation, blepharospasm, and photophobia. Subtle amounts of corneal edema, conjunctival hyperemia, and ciliary injection will be present initially, and can become prominent as the condition progresses. Aqueous flare, hyphema, intraocular fibrin, and hypopyon may be observed. Miosis can result in a misshapen pupil and posterior synechiae. Inability to achieve pharmacologic mydriasis is common when uveitis is active. IOP is generally low, but ERU may be associated with intermittent elevations in IOP. Cataract formation may occur.
- In some horses, especially Appaloosas, the uveitis may be insidious without any overt signs of ocular discomfort.
- There can be evidence of active or inactive chorioretinitis. Choroiditis may result in focal or diffuse retinal detachments. The vitreous may develop haziness due to leakage of proteins and cells from retinal vessels. The optic nerve head can appear congested.
- In chronic cases, corneal vascularization, permanent corneal edema, calcific band keratopathy, synechiation, cataract formation, and iris color changes can result. Secondary glaucoma and phthisis bulbi can occur. Irreversible blindness is a common sequela to ERU.

CAUSES

- While the pathogenesis is clearly immune mediated, the causes are often unknown.
- Hypersensitivity to infectious agents such as *L. interrogans* serovar *pomona* is commonly implicated as a possible cause.
- Toxoplasmosis, salmonellosis, *Streptococcus*, *Escherichia coli*, *Rhodococcus equi*, borreliosis, strongyles, onchocerciasis, parasites, and viral infections have also been implicated as causes of ERU.

RISK FACTORS

Leptospira infections increase the risk for ERU.

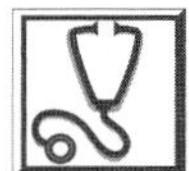

DIAGNOSIS

DIFFERENTIAL DIAGNOSIS

It is imperative to immediately differentiate a painful eye in a horse as a result of ulcerative keratitis from ERU, by using a fluorescein dye test. While corticosteroids are the treatment of choice for ERU, they are detrimental to an eye with a corneal ulcer.

CBC/BIOCHEMISTRY/URINALYSIS

None

OTHER LABORATORY TESTS

- Conjunctival biopsies for examination for *Onchocerca* microfilaria may be performed.
- Detection of *Leptospira* organisms by culture or PCR in aqueous or vitreous humor samples may be considered, as well as serologic evaluation. Results of serology can be difficult to interpret as many horses have positive titers with no evidence of ocular or systemic diseases. Leptospiral titers for *Pomona*, *Bratislava,* and *Autumnalis* should be requested in the United States. Positive titers for serovars of 1:400 or greater are of importance.

IMAGING

N/A

DIAGNOSTIC PROCEDURES

N/A

PATHOLOGIC FINDINGS

- In acute stages, lymphocytic infiltration with neutrophils can be found in the uveal tract, resulting in edema and plasmoid vitreous.
- In addition, fibrin and leukocytes are present in the anterior chamber.
- The vessels of the iris, ciliary body, choroid, and retina can be cuffed by lymphocytes and plasma cells.
- The chronic stages manifest by corneal scarring, cataract formation, and peripapillary chorioretinitis with retinal degeneration.

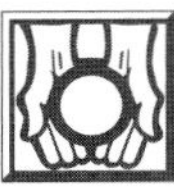

TREATMENT

APPROPRIATE HEALTH CARE

- The major goals of treatment of ERU are to preserve vision, decrease pain, and prevent or minimize the recurrence of attacks of uveitis.
- Specific prevention and therapy are often difficult as the etiology is not identified in each case.
- Treatment should be aggressive and prompt in order to maintain the transparency of the ocular structures.
- Therapy can last for weeks or months and should not be stopped abruptly or recurrence may occur.

NURSING CARE

N/A

ACTIVITY

Activity should be reduced pending resolution of clinical signs.

DIET

Diet should be appropriate for the degree of activity.

CLIENT EDUCATION

A complete cure is not possible in most affected horses. Treatment of the disease can be both time consuming and expensive. The owner should be educated immediately about the potential recurrence and the blinding nature of this disease.

SURGICAL CONSIDERATIONS

- Pars plana vitrectomy in horses with ERU has been used successfully to remove vitreal debris and infectious organisms in order to improve vision and delay the progression of the clinical signs in horses with ERU.
- A slow-release implant of cyclosporine A in the suprachoroidal space can suppress the intensity of the uveitis in many eyes with ERU. The drug can last 5–9 years.

MEDICATIONS

DRUGS OF CHOICE

- Prednisolone acetate (1%) or dexamethasone (0.1%) should be applied a minimum of 4–6 times per day initially. When the frequent application of topical steroids is not practical, the use of subconjunctival corticosteroids may be used. Methylprednisolone acetate (40 mg every 1–3 weeks) and triamcinolone acetonide (4 mg every 1–3 weeks) are commonly used subconjunctivally in the horse.

- Systemic corticosteroids may be beneficial in severe, refractory cases of ERU but should be used with caution.
- The NSAIDs such as topical flurbiprofen, indomethacin, diclofenamic acid, and suprofen (BID to TID) can provide additive anti-inflammatory effects to the corticosteroids, and are effective at reducing the intraocular inflammation when a corneal ulcer is present.
- Flunixin meglumine (0.25–1.0 mg/kg PO BID), phenylbutazone (1 g IV or PO BID), or aspirin (15 mg/kg/day) is frequently used systemically to control intraocular inflammation.
- Mydriatic and cycloplegic medications minimize synechiae formation by inducing mydriasis, and alleviate some of the pain of ERU by relieving spasm of ciliary body muscles (cycloplegia). These drugs also narrow the capillary interendothelial cell junctions to reduce capillary plasma leakage. A combination of topically administered phenylephrine (2.5%) and atropine (1%) can also be used to attempt to obtain maximum dilation in the inflamed ERU eye.
- The use of systemically or topically administered antibiotics is often recommended for ERU. Topical antibiotics are indicated in cases of uveitis due to penetrating ocular trauma, or ulcerative keratitis. Antibiotic treatment for horses with positive titers for *Leptospira* remains speculative but streptomycin (11 mg/kg IM BID) may be a good choice for horses at acute and chronic stages of the disease. Penicillin G sodium (10,000 U/kg IV or IM QID) and tetracycline (6.6–11 mg/kg IV BID) at high dosages may be beneficial during acute leptospiral infections. Oral doxycycline at 10 mg/kg BID does not enter the aqueous or vitreous of normal horse eyes at therapeutic levels high enough to affect *Leptospira* but might reach higher levels in inflamed eyes.
- Intravitreal gentamicin prevented episodes of uveitic attacks in one study. A majority (17/18) of eyes had no episodes of uveitis and vision was maintained in 30%. One dose of 4 mg was injected into the vitreous at the 12 o'clock position 8 mm from the limbus.

CONTRAINDICATIONS

N/A

PRECAUTIONS

- A complete ophthalmic examination should be performed to determine if the uveitis is associated with a corneal ulcer or stromal abscess.
- Gut motility should be strictly monitored by abdominal auscultation and observation of signs of abdominal pain when using topically administered atropine in adult horses and foals, as gut motility can be markedly reduced by atropine in some horses. Should gut motility decrease during treatment with topically administered atropine, one can either discontinue the drug or change to the shorter-acting tropicamide.

ALTERNATIVE DRUGS

- Homeopathic remedies (e.g., poultices of chamomile and oral methylsulfonylmethane) for ERU have been discussed.
- Acupuncture at ST1 (stomach 1, intersection of the nasal and middle third of the lower eyelid) and BL1 (bladder 2, at the supraorbital foramen) every 3 days has been used to treat active ERU.

FOLLOW-UP

PATIENT MONITORING

Repeated examination of the anterior and (if possible) the posterior eye segment should be performed to monitor effect of treatment.

PREVENTION/AVOIDANCE

In horses where the disease tends to flare up after routine vaccination or deworming, prophylactic treatment of the eye may be beneficial.

POSSIBLE COMPLICATIONS

ERU can potentially blind the horse.

EXPECTED COURSE AND PROGNOSIS

Recurrence of anterior uveitis due to immunologic mechanisms is the hallmark of ERU. Overall, the prognosis for ERU is usually poor for a cure to preserve vision, but the disease can be controlled.

MISCELLANEOUS

ASSOCIATED CONDITIONS

Systemic infection by the ERU-causing organism

AGE-RELATED FACTORS

N/A

ZOONOTIC POTENTIAL

Infectious agents such as *Leptospira* can be a health risk for people, especially if basic hygienic principles are disregarded.

PREGNANCY

Leptospira infection may lead to abortion. The potential side effects of the medications (especially glucocorticoids and NSAIDs) have to be considered.

SYNONYMS

- Periodic ophthalmia
- Moon blindness
- Iridocyclitis

SEE ALSO

- Corneal/scleral ulcerations
- Corneal stromal abscesses
- Stationary night blindness
- Chorioretinitis
- Systemic infectious diseases
- Calcific band keratopathy
- Glaucoma

ABBREVIATIONS

- ERU = equine recurrent uveitis
- IOP = intraocular pressure

Suggested Reading

Brooks DE. Ophthalmology for the Equine Practitioner. Jackson, WY; Teton NewMedia, 2002.

Brooks DE, Matthews AG. Equine ophthalmology. In: Gelatt KN, ed. Veterinary Ophthalmology, ed 4. Philadelphia; Lippincott Williams and Wilkins, 2007.

Gilger BC, ed. Equine Ophthalmology. Philadelphia; WB Saunders, 2005.

Authors Andras M. Komaromy and Dennis E. Brooks

Consulting Editor Dennis E. Brooks

REGURGITATION/ VOMITING/DYSPHAGIA

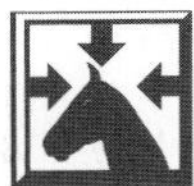

BASICS

DEFINITION

Regurgitation is defined as the retrograde flow of esophageal or gastric contents through the nares or, rarely, mouth. Vomiting is the forceful expulsion of gastric contents. Regurgitation and vomiting indicate an immediate and severe threat to horses' life. Dysphagia is defined as difficult prehension, mastication, or swallowing.

PATHOPHYSIOLOGY

- Regurgitation and vomiting in horses occur from the nose rather than from the mouth, because of the specific anatomy of the soft palate. Anatomical esophageal barriers such as the cranial esophageal sphincter, esophageal motor function, and the caudal (lower) esophageal sphincter (cardia) must be breached to allow food to travel retrograde from the stomach. Partial or complete physical obstruction (choke) at any of these levels may result in regurgitation. Esophageal barriers may be compromised by congenital anatomical malformations involving esophagus or surrounding tissues, central or peripheral neurologic disorders, and extreme intragastric pressure.
- Dental problems as well as other problems in the oral cavity and anatomical parts of the head and neck that support prehension, mastication, and swallowing predispose to dysphagia. Dysphagia does not always lead to regurgitation.

SYSTEMS AFFECTED

- The gastrointestinal system is primarily affected, which includes small intestine, stomach, esophagus, pharynx/larynx, and oral cavity. Infectious or noninfectious diseases of the central or peripheral nervous system can affect normal function of the gastrointestinal system.
- Involvement of the cardiovascular system is possible in cases where the regurgitation is secondary to a persistent right aortic arch. Development of aspiration pneumonia should always be considered in cases of regurgitation/vomiting, particularly in foals.

SIGNALMENT

Predispositions are variable and dependent on primary disease.

SIGNS

Historical

Dehydrated, exhausted, chronically debilitated horses, and horses with dental abnormalities are more prone to regurgitation/vomiting. The owner should be questioned about horse's age and diet, and possible exposures to poisonous plants, snakes, or other toxins. Health status of other horses on the premises should be inquired. Information about the time of regurgitation in relation to feeding may further localize the anomaly. Usually, regurgitation immediately following feeding is due to an obstruction of the oral cavity or pharynx. A prolongation in the time between feeding and regurgitation indicates an obstruction of the esophagus or stomach.

Physical Examination

- Adult horses have bilateral nasal discharge consisting of feed and saliva. Horses may cough and express odynophagia (painful swallowing) and ptyalism (excessive flow of saliva). Depending on the severity and duration of clinical signs, dehydration may be evident. Nursing foals have a nasal discharge consisting of milk. All foals should be examined for the presence of a cleft palate or signs of septicemia. Horses may show signs of respiratory disease, including tachypnea, coughing, and increased lung sounds. Other clinical signs are specific to the primary cause of regurgitation/vomiting/dysphagia.
- Dysphagia is often associated with dropping feed from the mouth while attempting to chew. In some cases, signs of aspiration pneumonia can be present.

CAUSES

Causes may be congenital or acquired in nature. The location of the defect may be oral, pharyngeal, esophageal, or gastroduodenal/jejunal. The physical defects may be caused by a physical obstruction (i.e., an intraluminal mass or a cleft palate), whereas the functional defects may involve a disruption in the nervous or muscular control of swallowing (i.e., tetanus, botulism).

RISK FACTORS

Specific risk factors exist depending on the primary underlying condition. Please refer to specific chapters for details.

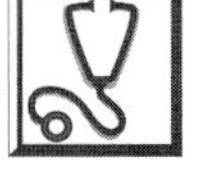

DIAGNOSIS

DIFFERENTIAL DIAGNOSIS

Differential diagnoses include:

- Esophageal obstruction
- Choke
- Atresia, agenesis
- Stenosis
- Persistent right aortic arch
- Tetanus
- Botulism
- Rabies
- Equine protozoal myeloencephalitis
- Head trauma
- Bacterial meningitis
- Hydrocephalus
- Gastric rupture
- Gastric ulceration
- Cleft palate
- Guttural pouch tympany or mycosis
- Weakness in neonatal foals with a poor suckle reflex (transient)
- Foreign body or mass of the oral cavity, pharynx, esophagus, or stomach
- Diaphragmatic hernia
- Megaesophagus
- Subepiglottic or pharyngeal cysts
- Dorsal displacement of the soft palate
- Rostral displacement of the palatopharyngeal arch
- Severe inflammatory condition of the oral cavity, pharynx, esophagus, or stomach
- Various plant toxins (including oleander)
- Various other toxins (including snake bite venom, lead, arsenic)

CBC/BIOCHEMISTRY/URINALYSIS

The CBC and serum biochemistry profile may be normal or show evidence of dehydration (elevated PCV, TP, BUN, and creatinine). The profile may also reveal hypochloremia and metabolic alkalosis secondary to loss of saliva.

OTHER LABORATORY TESTS

These are variable, depending on the primary condition. Please refer to specific chapters for details.

CLINICAL EXAMINATION SPECIFICS

Thorough physical examination of oral cavity is essential (observation, palpation, smelling).

IMAGING

Cranial Gastrointestinal Radiography

- Radiography of the oral cavity, pharynx, esophagus, and/or stomach may be performed to further localize and define the cause of regurgitation.
- Disorders such as a mass, foreign body, guttural pouch tympany, esophageal impaction, or diaphragmatic hernia may be diagnosed using plain radiography.
- Fluoroscopy is a valuable diagnostic modality in which barium is administered orally followed by fluoroscopic examination. Abnormalities in transit and clearance times may be estimated. In foals, normal emptying of contrast from the stomach occurs in <2 hr and reaches the large intestine within 3 hr. Irregularities, including luminal obstructions

or esophageal dilatation, can be identified. Extraluminal masses may be discovered due to displacement of the esophagus from its normal anatomic position. An "hour-glass" appearance of the dilated esophagus has been described. In this case, the esophagus is constricted, either by fibrous tissue at the level of the thoracic inlet or by vasculature.

DIAGNOSTIC PROCEDURES

Passage of a Stomach Tube

A stomach tube assesses the patency of the pharynx and esophagus and indicates the presence of fluid or gas under pressure in the stomach. Care must be taken not to injure or perforate esophagus during intubation.

Endoscopy

Endoscopic evaluation of the pharynx, esophagus, trachea, and guttural pouches may be performed. Cleft palate, gastric and esophageal ulcerations, intraluminal masses or foreign bodies, and guttural pouch disorders may be identified. The integrity of the gastrointestinal tract should be determined, as any ulceration or rupture will worsen prognosis.

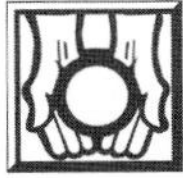

TREATMENT

Patients with regurgitation should be treated as an intensive-care medical inpatient in most cases. Balanced polyionic fluids with or without chloride supplementation should be considered. Total (in foals) or partial parenteral nutrition may be considered. The patient should be stall rested until it is stabilized. In most cases, the horse should be held off feed to prevent further regurgitation and possible aspiration. The owner should be aware of the severe complication of aspiration pneumonia. Surgical options exist for certain primary conditions that cause regurgitation; please refer to specific chapters for details.

MEDICATIONS

DRUG(S) OF CHOICE

Drugs prescribed are variable depending on the primary condition.

CONTRAINDICATIONS

N/A

PRECAUTIONS

N/A

POSSIBLE INTERACTIONS

N/A

ALTERNATIVE DRUGS

N/A

FOLLOW-UP

PATIENT MONITORING

Monitoring is variable depending on the primary condition.

POSSIBLE COMPLICATIONS

Common complications include aspiration pneumonia, dehydration, electrolyte abnormalities, and malnutrition.

MISCELLANEOUS

ASSOCIATED CONDITIONS

- Aspiration pneumonia
- Dehydration
- Colonic impaction
- Malnutrition
- Septicemia (in young animals)
- Depression

AGE-RELATED FACTORS

The most likely differential diagnosis for an adult horse with regurgitation is an esophageal obstruction or neurologic disorder, whereas congenital defects such as cleft palate or persistent right aortic arch are seen only in foals.

ZOONOTIC POTENTIAL

Some differential diagnoses, especially neurologic disorders such as rabies, must be ruled out. The necessary precautions should be undertaken during handling and management of these cases.

PREGNANCY

The most significant consideration in a pregnant animal with regurgitation is the often poor prognosis for survival of the mare. Under special circumstances, cesarian section may be considered in order to attempt salvage of a near-term fetus.

SYNONYMS

- Pharyngeal dysphagia
- Esophageal dysphagia
- Gastroesophageal reflux

SEE ALSO

- Esophageal obstruction (choke)
- Cleft palate
- Dysphagia
- Gastric ulceration
- Specific neurologic disorders (tetanus, EPM)
- Specific toxins (lead, oleander)

ABBREVIATIONS

- BUN = blood urea nitrogen
- CBC = complete blood count
- PCV = packed cell volume
- TP = total protein

Suggested Reading

Barton MH. Nasal regurgitation of milk in foals. Compend Cont Educ Vet Pract 1993;15:81–91, 93.

Campbell NB. Esophageal obstruction (choke). In Robinson NE, ed. Current Therapy in Equine Medicine. Philadelphia: WB Saunders, 2003:90–94.

Greet TRC. Observations on the potential role of oesophageal radiography in the horse. Equine Vet J 1982;14:73–79.

Milne E. Differential diagnosis of dysphagia. In Robinson NE, ed. Current Therapy in Equine Medicine. Philadelphia: WB Saunders, 1997:141–143.

Smith BP. Regurgitation/vomiting. In Smith BP, ed, Large Animal Internal Medicine. St. Louis: Mosby, 2002:114–116.

Smith BP. Dysphagia. In Smith BP, ed. Large Animal Internal Medicine. St. Louis: Mosby, 2002:116–118.

Authors Modest Vengust

Consulting Editors Henry Stämpfli and Olimpo Oliver-Espinosa

RETAINED DECIDUOUS TEETH

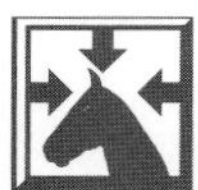

BASICS

OVERVIEW

• Between the ages of 2.5 and 4 years, deciduous incisors and the first three cheek teeth (premolars 2, 3, and 4) are replaced with permanent dentition in the horse. The permanent teeth erupt under the roots of the deciduous teeth, depriving them of their blood supply and force them to be shed into the mouth.
• Abnormal retention of deciduous cheek teeth (termed *caps*) may lead to oral discomfort as a result of gingivitis, periodontal disease, or lingual and buccal laceration. Furthermore, retained deciduous cheek teeth or incisors may cause maleruption of the permanent hypodontic teeth and distortion of their bony sockets.
• Entrapment (impaction) of the deciduous premolars may lead to delayed eruption of the permanent teeth and the formation of enlarged eruption cysts (characterized by progressive lysis of the alveolar bone and symmetrical bony swelling. These swellings, beneath the developing apices of the permanent cheek teeth, occur more commonly on the mandible (termed *3- or 4-year-old bumps*) than maxilla and may increase the susceptibility of the tooth root to hematogenous bacterial colonization termed *anachoretic pulpitis*. This may progress to a periapical abscess and a draining fistulous tract to the mandible or maxilla.
• Lingual displacement of the permanent incisors and premolars is also recognized as a common sequel to prolonged retention of the deciduous teeth.

SIGNALMENT

The deciduous teeth of the second, third, and fourth premolars are shed at approximately 2.5, 3, and 4 years of age, respectively. The first, second, and third incisors erupt according to a similar schedule. Although there can be much individual variation in the timing of deciduous tooth shedding, these defined eruption times determine the age of affected horses. Breed and sex predilections have not been reported, although horses with smaller heads and relative overcrowding of the teeth may be predisposed.

SIGNS

Pain associated with laceration of gums from caps can be associated with head-shy behavior and resistance to the bit. In addition, maleruption and tooth impaction can cause oral discomfort with head shaking while eating, quidding, hemorrhage from the oral cavity, and rubbing of incisors against fixed objects. Retained caps may also cause abnormal mastication, uneven dental wear, and weight loss.

CAUSES AND RISK FACTORS

Retained deciduous teeth are relatively common and may be caused by abnormalities of mastication either as a result of inadequate roughage in the diet or other causes of abnormal dental wear. Overcrowding of the dental arcades can also cause retention of deciduous teeth. Hooks or ramps in young animals may cause a displacement of the opposing dental arcade with a resultant overcrowding of the premolars. An excessively large first premolar (wolf tooth) or supernumerary teeth (polyodontia) may also lead to relative overcrowding.

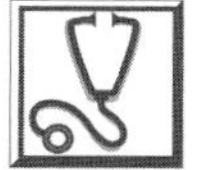

DIAGNOSIS

DIFFERENTIAL DIAGNOSIS

There are few differential diagnoses, as the characteristic age and the presence of dental caps or malerupted teeth are pathognomonic. However, periapical abscess formation may need to be differentiated from sepsis caused by trauma, infundibular necrosis, or (less commonly) neoplasia. Any painful condition of the mouth resulting from trauma (e.g., tongue laceration), infection (e.g., vesicular stomatitis), or neurologic dysfunction can cause some of the signs seen with retained deciduous teeth.

CBC/BIOCHEMISTRY/URINALYSIS

N/A

OTHER LABORATORY TESTS

N/A

IMAGING

Radiographic projections of the cheek teeth may assist in the diagnosis of retained premolars. The characteristic findings of an eruption cyst include a cystic extension of the periodontal ligament (lamina dura) with a regular outline and the absence of sclerosis and periosteal reaction. Eruption cysts are also associated with an erupting tooth.

DIAGNOSTIC PROCEDURES

A thorough oral examination should reveal the presence of caps, which are also palpable when the border between the permanent and deciduous tooth extends above the gingiva. An oral examination should also reveal malerupted teeth in the premolar or incisor arcades. Radiographs are also useful as outlined above.

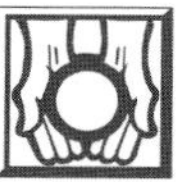

TREATMENT

• Removal of loose incisor and cheek teeth caps should be undertaken after their identification; specialized "cap extractors" are available, but any long slim-bladed instrument may be used for the purpose.
• Wolf tooth extraction forceps work well for the removal of premolars 3 and 4—rolling the cap toward the lingual surface will reduce the breakage of the buccal roots, which can leave slivers of cap behind that may cause soft tissue damage and subsequent irritation. If one cap has been shed, some authors recommend all other caps in that corresponding quadruplet be removed. This should only be done provided that the permanent teeth concerned have erupted through the gingiva. The practice of methodically removing deciduous teeth at set ages in an attempt to prevent the problem of retained caps will result in the premature removal of deciduous teeth in some horses and may predispose to infundibular caries later in life. Occasionally, caps may extend above the occlusal surface of the adjacent teeth but extraction is not possible without the use of excessive force. These caps should be floated down with the adjacent occlusal surface and evaluated for extraction 6–8 weeks later.

MEDICATION

DRUG(S) OF CHOICE

Antimicrobial therapy may be useful in cases of impacted teeth to prevent formation of anachoretic pulpitis. Antimicrobials used early in the course of a periapical infection in young horses have been reported to be successful. However, resolution of the infection commonly requires extraction of the affected tooth.

CONTRAINDICATIONS/POSSIBLE INTERACTIONS

N/A

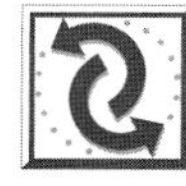

FOLLOW-UP

PREVENTION/AVOIDANCE

Adequate dental care for younger horses may decrease abnormal dental wear and resultant overcrowding of the dental arcades. Regular dental care should also identify retained deciduous teeth prior to their causing significant problems.

EXPECTED COURSE AND PROGNOSIS

Removal of retained deciduous teeth usually results in the normal alignment and development of the permanent teeth. When abnormal conformation of the arcades remains, this should be corrected.

MISCELLANEOUS

ASSOCIATED CONDITIONS

Associated conditions include abnormal dental wear and periapical abscessation.

AGE-RELATED FACTORS

The ages at which the permanent teeth erupt (between 2.5 and 4 years) are the times at which deciduous teeth become retained. The actual age of eruption is variable, and the deciduous teeth of the lower arcade are usually shed before the upper arcade. One report suggests that 2 years 8 mo, 2 years 10 mo, and 3 years 8 mo may be a more accurate eruption schedule for premolars 2, 3, and 4, repsectively, than outlined previously.

Suggested Reading

Dixon PM, Dacre I. A review of equine dental disorders. Vet J 2005;169:165–187.

Authors Hugo Hilton
Consulting Editors Henry Stämpfli and Olimpo Oliver-Espinosa

RETAINED FETAL MEMBRANES

BASICS

DEFINITION/OVERVIEW

Fetal membranes are defined as retained if they have not been passed within 3 hr postpartum.

ETIOLOGY/PATHOPHYSIOLOGY

Suggested Causes

• Pathological sites of adherence between the endometrium and chorion with the first occurrence that may recur during future pregnancies • Infections between the endometrium and chorion • Any debilitating condition—excessive fatigue, poor conditioning, unhygienic environment, or advanced age

SYSTEM AFFECTED

Reproductive

INCIDENCE/PREVALENCE

• The most common postpartum condition in mares, with an incidence of 2%–10%
• Incidence is reported to increase after dystocia or cesarean section, in draft mares, with a hydrops pregnancy, and after prolonged pregnancy.

SIGNALMENT

• All breeds • All females of breeding age

SIGNS

General Comments

• The portion of retained fetal membranes visible at the vulvar lips is not a reliable indicator of the proportion that may yet be attached (i.e., retained) within the uterus. • As mares move about immediately postpartum, portions of the membranes may be torn or break free. • A careful look through stall bedding may yield the balance of the placental membranes and decrease concern regarding a retained portion.

Historical

• Previous history of partial or complete failure to pass the fetal membranes. • Higher occurrence after dystocia, prolonged pregnancy, or abortion. • Incidence increases in mares of >15 years. • No effect of previous reproductive status (maiden, barren, or foaling) the previous year • No effect attributed to breeding by artificial insemination versus natural (i.e., live) cover the previous year. • No effect from sex of foal or birth of a weak or dead fetus.

PHYSICAL EXAMINATION

• TRP examination to determine size and tone of the uterus and to gauge amount of fluid in the uterine lumen. • Vaginal examination may be necessary, but is not always essential, depending on condition of the placenta and the uterus.

CAUSES

See Etiology/Pathophysiology.

RISK FACTORS

See Historical.

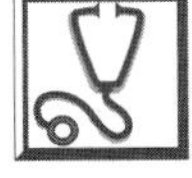

DIAGNOSIS

DIFFERENTIAL DIAGNOSIS

• Uterine infection • Delay or failure of postpartum involution

PATHOLOGIC FINDINGS

See Etiology/Pathophysiology.

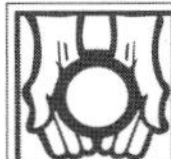

TREATMENT

APPROPRIATE HEALTH CARE

• Treat primarily with oxytocin, best results. • Initiate oxytocin treatment <3 hr postpartum if membranes have not passed.
  ○ Repeat q60–120 min for the first 12–18 hr postpartum.
• Once >12–18 hr, if membranes still retained, may treat intrauterine with irritants or antibiotics or systemically with antibiotics. Prostaglandin therapy should also be considered. • Use of systemic antibiotics is not necessary unless systemic disease develops subsequent to the retained fetal membranes. • Flushing the uterus can have great value if a portion of the placenta is retained. • Insufflation—If the membranes are by-in-large intact, place fluid (preferably isotonic saline solution; alternatively LRS or water) to dilate the uterine lumen within the innermost aspect of the fetal membranes, sufficient to expand the uterus and stimulate uterine activity.
  ○ Gather the exposed (external to the vulvae) portion of placental membrane; tie around it outside of the vulvae to maintain fluid within the uterus and placenta for a brief time.
  ○ This maintains the uterine expansion, stretching the myometrium/endometrium to facilitate release of the microvilli.
  ○ Cost of this larger-volume treatment may be more expensive, but it yields a modest increase in benefit.

NURSING CARE

• Administer oxytocin postpartum to all mares with a history of retained fetal membranes. Such mares are at higher risk for recurrence.
• Examine in its entirety after passage to determine that all portions of the placenta are present.

ACTIVITY

Affected mares should have normal exercise.

DIET

No changes are indicated.

CLIENT EDUCATION

• Retained fetal membranes is relatively common and should be treated if not passed within 3 hr postpartum, regardless of the time at which foaling occurred.
• Advise owners to maintain a supply of oxytocin, with administration beginning only after 3 hr have passed.

MEDICATIONS

DRUG(S) OF CHOICE

• Oxytocin (≤20 IU per injection), with injections repeated at 60- to 120-min intervals.
• After 18–24 hr—$PGF_{2\alpha}$ or analogues can be administered and antibiotics can be infused into the uterus.

CONTRAINDICATIONS

Higher doses of oxytocin may lead to uterine prolapse.

PRECAUTIONS

• Oxytocin may induce uterine cramping. • The mare may go down, with potential to cause harm to the foal.

ALTERNATIVE DRUGS

None as effective as oxytocin

FOLLOW-UP

PATIENT MONITORING

• Examine the mare to determine if placenta has been expelled. • Evaluate uterine size and tone to determine if they are normal relative to the number of days postpartum.

PREVENTION/AVOIDANCE

• Exercise and dietary supplementation with selenium may have value. • Avoid pasturing mares on fescue near term.

POSSIBLE COMPLICATIONS

• Septic metritis • Laminitis

EXPECTED COURSE AND PROGNOSIS

• Of mares treated with oxytocin, >90% pass the retained fetal membranes without any other problem, and the prognosis is excellent.
• Retained fetal membranes passed without secondary involvement have no effect on foal heat breeding conceptions. • Affected mares treated with intrauterine antibiotics have higher rates of conception and higher rates of pregnancy termination.

MISCELLANEOUS

ASSOCIATED CONDITIONS

See Historical.

AGE-RELATED FACTORS

Old mares have a higher incidence on some farms.

PREGNANCY

• Follows parturition • May increase with induction of parturition

SYNONYMS

• Retained afterbirth

ABBREVIATION

• TRP = transrectal palpation

Suggested Reading

Alexander RW. Excessive retainment of the placenta in the mare. Vet Rec 1971;89:175–176.

Burns SJ, Judge NG, Martin JE, Adams LG. Management of retained placenta in mares. Proc Am Assoc Equine Pract 1977;381–390.

Provencher R, Threlfall WR, Murdick PW, Wearly WK. Retained fetal membranes in the mare. A retrospective study. Can Vet J 1988;29:903–910.

Threlfall WR. Retained placenta. In: McKinnon AO, Voss JL, eds. Equine Reproduction. Philadelphia: Lea & Febiger, 1993:614–621.

Threlfall WR, Carleton CL. Treatment of uterine infections in the mare. In: Morrow DA, ed. Current Therapy in Theriogenology, ed 2. Philadelphia: WB Saunders, 1986:730–737.

White TE. Retained placenta. Mod Vet Pract 1980;61:87–88.

Author Walter R. Threlfall
Consulting Editor Carla L. Carleton

RHODOCOCCUS EQUI

BASICS

DEFINITION

Rhodococcus equi is an important cause of pneumonia in foals less than 6 months of age. Infection with *R. equi* may also result in diarrhea, joint sepsis, intra-abdominal abscessation, and multifocal abscesses throughout the body.

PATHOPHYSIOLOGY

R. equi is a gram-positive pleomorphic intracellular facultative organism that normally inhabits soil. Inhalation of dust containing the organism is thought to be the primary route of exposure for both the horse and humans. *R. equi* then resides within the alveolar macrophages, replicates, and can produce a severe, potentially life-threatening pyogranulomatous bronchopneumonia as necrosis and destruction of lung parenchyma occur. Intestinal forms of the disease include ulcerative colitis and abdominal lymphadenitis. Associated gastrointestinal infections likely arise from infected foals swallowing sputum containing the organism. Peyer's patches become infected and ulcerated and, with time, significant mesenteric lymphadenitis can occur. *R. equi* may disseminate to other body sites and produce septic arthritis, serositis, vertebral body abscesses, and cutaneous ulcerative lymphangitis. Other extrathoracic manifestations of the disease include immune-mediated polysynovitis, uveitis/keratouveitis, immune-mediated hemolytic anemia, immune-mediated thrombocytopenia, hyperthermia associated with erythromycin-rifampin, hyperlipemia, and telogen effluvium.

SYSTEMS AFFECTED

- Respiratory
- Gastrointestinal
- Musculoskeletal
- Hemic/lymphatic/immune
- Ophthalmic
- Renal
- Skin
- Hepatobiliary
- Nervous

SIGNALMENT

Foals 1–6 months of age. Most foals show clinical signs before 4 months of age. *R. equi* infection has been reported in immunocompromised adults or adults with concurrent illness.

SIGNS

Fever, cough, lethargy, depression, anorexia, poor weight gain, exercise intolerance, diarrhea, respiratory distress, joint distention, and sudden death. Foals may have abnormal thoracic auscultation and percussion findings, although severely affected foals may not have auscultable abnormalities.

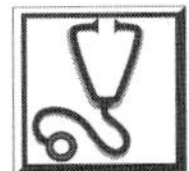

DIAGNOSIS

DIFFERENTIAL DIAGNOSIS

Primary differentials are other causes of pneumonia in foals, including *Streptococcus equi* var *equi, S. equi* var *zooepidemicus,* parasite migration, and viral respiratory infections. There has been a suggestion that EHV-2 infection may predispose foals to *R. equi.* Definitive diagnosis is based on culture of *R. equi.*

CBC/BIOCHEMISTRY/URINALYSIS

CBC is characterized by leukocytosis with a mature neutrophilia. Fibrinogen concentration is increased. Serum protein may be increased. Foals with severe disease may have anemia and thrombocytopenia. Foals with diarrhea may have electrolyte abnormalities, including hyponatremia and hypochloremia. Creatinine and BUN concentration may be increased in foals with dehydration secondary to diarrhea or respiratory distress. Urinalysis is usually normal, excepting cases with renal and/or urinary tract involvement.

OTHER LABORATORY TESTS

- AGID serology for detection of precipitating antibody for equifactors and exoenzymes produced by *R. equi*
- ELISA serology for detection of antibody to cell surface *R. equi* antigen. PCR testing of tracheal fluid, bronchoalveolar lavage fluid, aspirates from other sites

DIAGNOSTIC PROCEDURES

Transtracheal Aspirate

Cytology reveals gram-positive to gram-variable pleomorphic ("Chinese character") intracellular rods. Culture is positive for *R. equi.*

Bronchoalveolar Lavage

- Results similar to TTA
- May recognize concurrent infection with *Pneumocystis carinii,* and requires specialized stain (silver stain)
- *Caution:* Either TTA or bronchoalveolar lavage may be detrimental to a foal with significant respiratory disease.

PATHOLOGIC FINDINGS

- Findings are related to the organ system involved. Characteristic finding at necropsy is bilateral bronchopneumonia with severe coalescing abscess formation. Ventral lung field involvement is generally more severe. Abscesses may range in size from a few millimeters to more than 10 cm. Generalized miliary abscess formation is also common. Pulmonary parenchyma surrounding pulmonary abscesses is usually congested or consolidated. Bronchial and mediastinal lymphadenopathy with abscessation is common. Pleural empyema can occur. Pleural inflammation is unusual unless empyema secondary to abscess rupture has occurred.
- Gastrointestinal lesions are variable and may involve the entire gastrointestinal tract. Lesions include mucosal villous atrophy, mucosal necrosis, diphtheritic membrane formation, ulcerative enterocolitis, and mesenteric lymphadenopathy with abscess formation. Pulmonary histology abnormalities are predominately pyogranulomatous. Abscesses have a necrotic central core with surrounding degenerate neutrophils. Adjacent areas are infiltrated with macrophages, lymphocytes, and occasional giant cells. There is congestion, edema, and alveolar infiltration by macrophages and neutrophils, acute suppurative bronchitis, and peribronchitis. Organisms may be identified using hematoxylin eosin stain (H&E) and/or Gram stains. Some organisms demonstrate acid-fast characteristics. There are reports of concurrent infection with *Pneumocystis carinii.* Identification of concurrent infection is facilitated by the use of silver stains.
- Gastrointestinal histology abnormalities are characterized by infiltration of phagocytic cells into the lamina propria. Necrosis of the villi and submucosa and mucosal ulceration are prominent. Peyer's patches are frequently involved.

IMAGING

Ultrasonography

Consolidation of lung parenchyma; pulmonary and intra-abdominal abscessation. Lesions deep within pulmonary parenchyma and not in contact with pleura will not be recognized.

Radiography

Abnormalities range from increased interstitial density to dense patchy areas of alveolar pattern to areas of consolidation and abscessation in the thorax. Radiographs may be useful in monitoring response to therapy and determining the severity of pulmonary involvement.

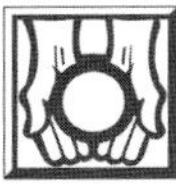

TREATMENT

APPROPRIATE HEALTH CARE

Affected foals may be treated at the farm. Severely affected foals may benefit from treatment at a referral facility with climate-controlled environments. Foals being sent to such facilities should be transported during cool times of the day and stress should be minimized. Foals with *R. equi* infection should not be transferred from an endemic farm to a farm with no previous history of *R. equi* infection.

NURSING CARE

The most important aspect of nursing care is minimizing stress. Provision of climate-controlled environments, air conditioning, and good ventilation may improve the short-term prognosis with severely affected foals.

ACTIVITY

Exercise should be restricted. Stall confinement is not necessary as long as turnout is in a small area only. Affected foals should be completely restricted from exercise during the hot periods of the day.

DIET

There are no specific dietary considerations. Severely affected foals experiencing weight loss and anorexia may benefit from parenteral nutrition.

CLIENT EDUCATION

R. equi probably infects all horse farms to some degree. The difference in disease appearance is related to differences in environments, management techniques, and virulence of the isolate. On enzootic farms, *R. equi* infections result in huge economic losses associated with costs of prevention, treatment, and the death of some foals.

Most foals treated for *R. equi* infection recover. Severely affected foals are less likely to survive.

Severely immunocompromised humans have been diagnosed with *R. equi* infection. It then becomes important to inform people with diseases resulting in immunodeficiency that *R. equi* is endemic on certain farms, and that they may be at risk of developing this disease if they either reside or work at these farms.

SURGICAL CONSIDERATIONS

Surgical drainage of easily accessible abscesses may be reasonable. However, surgical removal of abdominal abscesses is unlikely to be rewarding.

MEDICATIONS

DRUG(S) OF CHOICE

Erythromycin (10–37.5mg/kg BID to QID PO) or rifampin (5–10mg/kg SID to BID PO) is the traditional standard therapy. Newer macrolide antimicrobials azithromycin (10mg/kg PO SID) and clarithromycin (7.5mg/kg PO BID) have been efficacious and may have reduced side effects. Treatment continues until CBC, fibrinogen, and clinical presentation are normal. If possible, pneumonia should be resolved radiographically.

CONTRAINDICATIONS/PRECAUTIONS/ POSSIBLE INTERACTIONS/ ALTERNATIVE DRUGS

- Some foals receiving the above-mentioned drug combinations may develop severe diarrhea. Decreasing the erythromycin dose may resolve the problem.
- Mares housed with foals receiving the combination have developed severe fatal colitis, thought to be associated with *Clostridium difficile* infection secondary to ingestion of small amounts of erythromycin from the foal.
- Idiosyncratic hyperthermia and tachypnea have been reported in foals receiving erythromycin. Use of the estolate form of the drug may decrease this adverse response.
- Aminophylline should not be used in combination with erythromycin due to potential toxicity.
- Foals diagnosed very early in the clinical course of infection may respond to trimethoprim-sulfa combinations.
- Rifampin-resistant strains of *R. equi* have been identified. Rifampin should never be used alone due to the rapidity of development of resistance.

FOLLOW-UP

PATIENT MONITORING

Response to therapy can be monitored by resolution of clinical signs, normalization of CBC and fibrinogen, and radiographic improvement. Treatment should be continued until all recognized abnormalities have resolved.

PREVENTION/AVOIDANCE

- Several strategies for prevention of *R. equi* infection exist. Decreasing the size of infective challenge by good housing and management practices and isolation of affected foals is important.
- Early recognition of infection is important. This can be facilitated by serologic (AGID and/or ELISA) monitoring, daily temperature monitoring of foals, frequent routine physical examinations, and frequent thoracic ultrasound examinations.
- Passive immunization by the intravenous administration of *R. equi* hyperimmune plasma has been used as a preventative technique, but its efficacy has recently been questioned. Timing of this treatment, if effective, is purportedly important and depends on expected exposure; it is typically administered during the first month of life.
- To date, no active immunization protocol has been effective.

EXPECTED COURSE AND PROGNOSIS

In well-established pulmonary cases, therapy may extend over 3–5 weeks.

MISCELLANEOUS

ABBREVIATIONS

- AGID = agar gel immunodiffusion
- EHV = equine herpesvirus
- ELISA = enzyme-linked immunosorbent assay
- TTA = transtracheal aspirate

Suggested Reading

Davis JL, Gardner SY, Jones SL, et al. Pharmacokinetics of azithromycin in foals after i.v. and oral dose and disposition into phagocytes.J Vet Pharmacol Ther 2002;25:99–104.

Giguere S, Gaskin JM, Miller C, et al. Evaluation of a commercially available hyperimmune plasma product for prevention of naturally acquired pneumonia caused by *Rhodococcus equi* in foals. J Am Vet Med Assoc 2002;220:59–63.

Giguere S, Jacks S, Roberts GD, et al. Retrospective comparison of azithromycin, clarithromycin, and erythromycin for the treatment of foals with *Rhodococcus equi* pneumonia. J Vet Intern Med 2004;18:568–573.

Jacks S, Giguere S, Gronwall PR, et al. Pharmacokinetics of azithromycin and concentration in body fluids and bronchoalveolar cells in foals. Am J Vet Res 2001;62:1870–1875.

Jacks S, Giguere S, Gronwall PR, et al. Disposition of oral clarithromycin in foals. J Vet Pharmacol Ther 2002;25:359–362.

Wilkins PA, Lesser FR, Gaskin JM. *Rhodococcus equi* infection in foals: Comparison of AGID and ELISA serology on a commercial Thoroughbred breeding farm. AAEP Proc 1992:289.

Author Pamela A. Wilkins

Consulting Editors Ashley G. Boyle and Corinne R. Sweeney

RIB FRACTURES IN FOALS

BASICS

OVERVIEW

• Rib fracture is a significant contributor to morbidity and mortality in affected neonates and is the most commonly diagnosed fracture occurring within the first 24 hr of life, most typically due to trauma sustained during foaling. • Foals may present primarily with respiratory compromise secondary to the rib fracture or, more commonly, for signs relating to sepsis or neonatal maladjustment syndrome with the rib fractures diagnosed as an additional finding. Early recognition of life-threatening injury is necessary to implement appropriate therapeutic intervention.

SIGNALMENT

• Neonatal foals are most commonly affected as the injury is most often as a result of a dystocia. Foals born to maiden mares and multiparous mares are thought to be equally affected. • In one retrospective report, colts were affected 3 times as frequently as fillies. It remains undetermined whether there is a breed disposition to the problem.

SIGNS

• Plaques of subcutaneous edema overlying injured ribs, especially caudal to the elbows or along the ventrum. Subcutaneous emphysema is occasionally present but when noted should alert the clinician to the high potential for rib fracture. • Audible or palpable crepitation when the examiner's hand is gently pressed over the fracture. The foal may groan or grunt when moving and flinch when the affected rib is palpated. • Tachypnea or dyspnea frequently present • Abnormal thoracic auscultation may indicate the presence of hemothorax or pneumothorax. • Patients that have significant hemothorax may present in hemorrhagic shock due to intracavitary blood loss.

CAUSE AND RISK FACTORS

• Dystocia has been well documented as a significant risk factor for neonatal rib fractures. • Neither fetal thoracic diameter nor birth weight has been shown to play a role in occurrence of birth trauma.

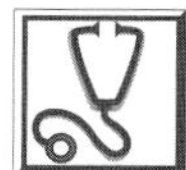

DIAGNOSIS

DIFFERENTIAL DIAGNOSIS

• Pleuropneumonia— Thoracic radiography and ultrasonography will help to rule out primary or concurrent pneumonia. • Sepsis—Rib fractures may be found incidentally in septicemic foals, although both the sepsis and rib fracture can be clinically important. • Perinatal asphyxia syndrome—may be a concurrent condition in neonatal foals with rib fractures

CBC/BIOCHEMISTRY/URINALYSIS

• Anemia secondary to hemorrhage
• Septicemic foals may have abnormalities on CBC—Leukopenia or leukocytosis are most common.

OTHER LABORATORY TESTS

• IgG—Pain or debilitation from rib fractures may prevent the foal from ingesting adequate colostrum. • Blood culture to identify concurrent septicemia

IMAGING

Thoracic ultrasonography is the superior imaging modality in detection and characterization of thoracic soft tissue abnormalities.

• Thoracic ultrasonography—Nondisplaced fractures may be identified, requiring less manipulation and positioning than radiography. The degree of fracture displacement and proximity of fragment ends to the heart should be assessed. Ultrasonographic changes of the pleural surface may reveal pleural effusion/ hemothorax, pulmonary contusion, thickened pleura, or pneumonia. Pneumothorax may be identified dorsally. • Thoracic radiography—Although a less sensitive imaging modality for this particular lesion, pneumothorax, hemothorax, and pulmonary contusion can be readily identified. Radiography is also useful to rule out pneumonia.

OTHER DIAGNOSTIC PROCEDURES

• Palpation of the thoracic wall will reveal firm, focal swelling of one or more ribs, most typically at, or 2–3 inches dorsal, to the costochondral junction. Visibility of the thoracic wall contour may be improved by wetting the hair with alcohol to allow chest wall indentation or soft tissue swelling to be seen. • Thoracocentesis to evaluate for hemothorax

PATHOLOGICAL FINDINGS

• Pulmonary contusions, hemothorax, pneumothorax, diaphragmatic hernia, and hemopericardium are significant consequences of rib fracture. • Sudden death can result from fracture fragments lacerating the myocardium, pleural vessels, and pleura.

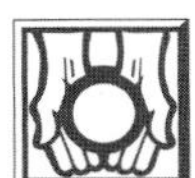

TREATMENT

• In patients with single nondisplaced rib fractures with minimal respiratory compromise, conservative management comprising severely restricted exercise for 4–6 weeks with weekly reevaluation is sufficient. • Foals that do not have dyspnea evident or concomitant pneumonia should be managed by encouraging lateral recumbency with the affected side down to minimize ventilatory embarrassment to the undamaged lung. • Foals with pneumonia associated with sepsis should be managed in sternal recumbency for optimal gas exchange. In foals with dyspnea and hemothorax evident on physical examination and ultrasonography, thoracocentesis to drain the excess fluid is indicated. If hemothorax is diagnosed in the absence of any ventilatory compromise to the foal, the chest may not be drained to allow for autotransfusion and the hemostatic effect of positive pressure to help minimize continued bleeding. • Patients with hemorrhagic shock should be referred for fluid therapy, possible blood transfusion and intranasal oxygen therapy. • Multiple (3 or more) displaced fractured ribs, a single displaced fragment in the vicinity of the heart, or a patient with flail chest warrants evaluation for internal fixation of the fracture fragments, and immediate referral is recommended.

MEDICATION

For Pain Management

• NSAIDs—ketoprofen (1.1 mg/kg IV q12–24h) or flunixin meglumine (0.5–1.1 mg/kg q12h) • Butorphanol (0.04–1.0 mg/kg IV q8–24h)

Prevention of Secondary Infections

Broad-spectrum antibiotics including potassium penicillin (22,000 IU/kg IV q6h) and amikacin (25 mg/kg IV q24h)

CONTRAINDICATIONS

• Analgesia should be used judiciously as any sudden movement can cause rib fragments to lacerate internal vascular structures or the heart. • NSAIDs and aminoglycosides can have adverse renal affects—they should be used with caution in dehydrated or debilitated foals. • NSAIDs can contribute to gastrointestinal ulceration—ulcer prophylaxis may be indicated in some cases.

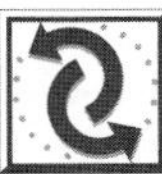

FOLLOW-UP

• Sequential thoracic ultrasonography should be performed to assess fracture and pulmonary healing. • Six weeks is considered necessary for stabilization is most circumstances. • The clients should be warned that sudden death is not an uncommon feature of this condition.

MISCELLANEOUS

• The patient must be carefully evaluated for other common neonatal ailments associated with dystocia, including bladder rupture in colt foals. • As with any case, sepsis and failure of transfer of passive immunity must be ruled out.

Suggested Reading

Sprayberry KA, Bain FT, Seahorn TL, et al. 56 cases of rib fractures in neonatal foals hospitalized in a referral center intensive care unit from 1997–2001. AAEP Proc 2001;47:395–399.

Author Katie J.Smith
Consulting Editor Margaret C. Mudge

RIGHT AND LEFT DORSAL DISPLACEMENT OF THE COLON

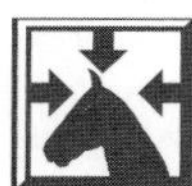

BASICS

DEFINITION

Right Dorsal Displacement

• An anatomic relocation of the colon due to migration of the pelvic flexure cranially followed by migration to the right abdominal quadrant until it is located between the cecum and the body wall.
• Rotation along the long axis (either clockwise or counterclockwise) of the colon can also occur.

Left Dorsal Displacement

An anatomic relocation of the colon such that it travels dorsally between the body wall and the spleen until it becomes entrapped in the nephrosplenic (i.e., renosplenic) space.

PATHOPHYSIOLOGY

• Speculative, as with other intestinal displacements
• Lack of mesenteric attachment of the large colon to the body wall makes it very mobile and more prone to displacements.
• Microbial fermentation takes place in the large colon; excess soluble carbohydrate diet may result in increased fermentation leading to increased gas production and possibly displacements.
• Alteration of normal colonic motility patterns could also lead to displacements.

Right Dorsal Displacement

• Can occur in two directions—clockwise and counterclockwise
• Clockwise (as viewed from above) displacement occurs more frequently than counterclockwise displacement and consists of the pelvic flexure being displaced between the cecum and the body wall in a cranial-to-caudal direction. The pelvic flexure then often continues in a clockwise direction and is located near the diaphragm.
• Counterclockwise displacement consists of the pelvic flexure being displaced lateral to the cecum in a caudal-to-cranial direction.

Left Dorsal Displacement

• A result of the pelvic flexure passing through the nephrosplenic space in a cranial-to-caudal direction or of the left dorsal and ventral colon passing lateral to the spleen in a ventral-to-dorsal direction.
• The colon ascends dorsally between the spleen and the body wall. The dorsal colon is proposed to fall into the nephrosplenic space first, followed by the ventral colon.
• The entrapped colon often is rotated 180° in the nephrosplenic space, lending credence to the theory of ventral-to-dorsal mechanism for left dorsal displacement.
• The left colon can be palpated between the spleen and the body wall in resolving left dorsal displacements, suggesting this route is important in the pathogenesis of the condition.

Vascular Compromise

Vascular compromise is usually minor. It is associated with torsion of the colon at the root of the mesentery for right dorsal displacements and with torsion at the site of entrapment over the nephrosplenic ligament in left dorsal displacements.

SYSTEMS AFFECTED

GI

• The colon is displaced, and other sections of the abdominal GI tract can be displaced as a result—especially the cecum, but also the small colon and small intestine.
• Mechanical traction on the mesentery can result in considerable pain.
• Vascular obstruction results in compromise of the colon, resulting in colonic necrosis.

Cardiovascular

With long duration or vascular compromise, dehydration and fluid shifts may lead to circulatory compromise.

GENETICS

N/A

INCIDENCE/PREVALENCE

• In one study of exploratory celiotomies, 14% of cases were diagnosed as nonstrangulating colonic displacements.
• In another study, 23% of all colic cases presented to a referral practice were large colon displacements.

SIGNALMENT

No particular signalment. Mares, particularly following parturition, may be predisposed to displacement of the ascending colon.

SIGNS

• Referable to the amount of colonic distention and any vascular compromise
• Mild to moderate abdominal discomfort after 12–24 hr
• Colic usually responds to analgesia initially but returns when the analgesic efficacy decreases.
• Acute escalation of signs is associated with increased colon distention or bowel compromise.
• Gastric reflux is inconsistent and usually caused by mechanical obstruction of the proximal small intestine.
• Heart rate often is less than might be expected from the degree of pain displayed (left dorsal displacement).

CAUSES

• Possible causes include alteration to the intestinal motility and changes in the weight of the colon because of excess gas formation or mild impactions.
• Changes in intra-abdominal volume and GI activity after parturition may predispose postpartum mares to colonic displacement.
• Left dorsal displacement—in addition to the above, gastric distention resulting in displacement of the spleen from the body wall, splenic contraction, and displacement of the spleen because of adhesions between the spleen and previous ventral midline celiotomy incisions.

RISK FACTORS

• Adhesions of the spleen to midline because of previous celiotomies, previous colonic displacements, and other forms of colic may cause a horse to roll.
• Sudden dietary changes

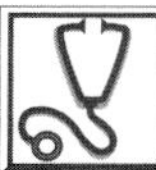

DIAGNOSIS

DIFFERENTIAL DIAGNOSIS

• Colonic/cecal tympany
• Retroflexion of the pelvic flexure
• Colonic impaction
• Colonic volvulus
• Enterolithiasis
• A diagnosis of left dorsal displacement may be established on the basis of rectal examination by identifying the colon running across the dorsal aspect of the nephrosplenic ligament in conjunction with characteristic ultrasound images.
• Right dorsal displacement is more problematic, because excessive distention of the colon may preclude a thorough rectal examination of the caudal abdomen; however, the need for surgery is based on the degree of colon distention, tight bands, edematous bowel wall, and the lack of response to analgesia.

CBC/BIOCHEMISTRY/URINALYSIS

• CBC and biochemistry may be normal, with mild alkalosis to mild acidosis in cases of nonstrangulating displacements.
• Decreased hematocrit may result from sequestration of RBCs in the spleen.
• If strangulation of the colon occurs, significant dehydration, with a relatively decreased protein and metabolic acidosis, is common.

OTHER LABORATORY TESTS

• Peritoneal fluid usually is normal, unless the bowel is compromised.
• Abdominocentesis may result in perforation of the spleen in patients with left dorsal displacement, because the spleen is forced medially and ventrally.

IMAGING

• Ultrasound of right dorsal displacement may reveal large intestine distended with gas and fluid. Ultrasonography of a left dorsal displacement is characterized by failure to visualize the left kidney because of gas in the large colon and a flat, horizontal border of the dorsal spleen, which is displaced ventrally.
• A false-positive diagnosis can result from a gas-distended viscus near the left kidney, obstructing visualization of the kidney.
• A false-negative diagnosis can result from lack of gas in the entrapped colon.
• One study reported a correct diagnosis in 89% of cases of nephrosplenic entrapment, with no false-positive results.

DIAGNOSTIC PROCEDURES

• Abnormal findings on rectal examination for right dorsal displacement—transverse tight bands in the caudal abdomen, gas distention of the large intestine, and inability to palpate the cranially displaced cecum. If the cecum is palpable, it may be distended, and the colon may be palpable between the cecum and the right body wall. Sections of impacted colon may be palpable as well.
• Abnormal findings on rectal examination for left dorsal displacement—distended large bowel on the left, with tight bands coursing

RIGHT AND LEFT DORSAL DISPLACEMENT OF THE COLON

craniodorsally toward the nephrosplenic space; medial or caudal displacement of the spleen; and gas distention of the cecum. The colon above the nephrosplenic ligament may be clearly palpable in some horses. Correct rectal diagnosis of left dorsal displacement varies, with one report claiming a definitive diagnosis in 32% of cases and another that nephrosplenic entrapment was correctly diagnosed in 61% of cases (false-positive results not included).

PATHOLOGICAL FINDINGS

Left dorsal displacement—sometimes a focal area of bowel necrosis can be associated with the site of entrapment.

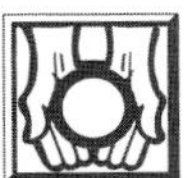

TREATMENT

APPROPRIATE HEALTH CARE

- Right dorsal displacement—surgical correction is often required; correction of nonstrangulating colonic displacements may occur with conservative therapy, but these cases need to be monitored carefully and delay may worsen the prognosis.
- Left dorsal displacement—surgical correction, rolling the horse under general anesthesia, administration of phenylephrine (with or without controlled exercise) and conservative management as for right dorsal displacement—7.5% of horses were reported to have another concurrent lesion (i.e., small intestinal obstruction, 360-degree colon torsion, etc.).
- Choice of treatment depends on several factors—certainty of the diagnosis, degree of colonic distention, and financial limitations of the client.
- If the diagnosis is not certain or colonic distention is marked, rolling and controlled exercise may be contraindicated.
- Reported success rates for conservative regimens vary widely and may relate to the accuracy of the original diagnosis.

NURSING CARE

- Vital
- Exploratory celiotomy—large deficits in fluid volume need to be addressed before surgery, as do acid-base and electrolyte imbalances.
- Abdominal distention restricting respiratory tidal volume—supplemental oxygen therapy may be required. In addition, deflation of a markedly distended large intestine via percutaneous trocarization may be beneficial but may cause leakage of intestinal contents; therefore, administer prophylactic antibiotics if performed.
- Passage of a nasogastric tube and decompression of the stomach are vital when a mechanical obstruction of the small intestine results in gastric distention.

ACTIVITY

- Controlled exercise may assist resolution of left dorsal displacement of the colon.
- Uncontrolled rolling may convert a nonstrangulating to a strangulating displacement.

DIET

No food should be administered.

CLIENT EDUCATION

- Counsel owners on the decision of whether to treat left dorsal displacement conservatively, either by close monitoring alone, rolling, or with controlled exercise or phenylephrine.
- Stress that treatment without surgery has obvious benefits, but that risks are associated with conservative treatment—rupture or further strangulation of a markedly distended viscus.

SURGICAL CONSIDERATIONS

When the colon is not strangulated, the condition usually is straightforward to correct.

MEDICATIONS

DRUG(S) OF CHOICE

- Administer standard analgesia for colic—see Acute Abdominal Pain. Drug use and dosage vary depending on the nature of the colic and the therapy to be instituted.
- Left dorsal displacement—phenylephrine. The rationale is that phenylephrine causes splenic contraction and may facilitate conservative therapy aimed at dislodging the colon from the nephrosplenic space. Commonly used dosages include 3–5 μg/kg/min infused over 15 min or a bolus of 45 μg/kg injected slowly.

FOLLOW-UP

PATIENT MONITORING

- Routine postoperative monitoring after surgery or conservative therapy
- Recurrence of displacement is well recorded for some horses, but data regarding the frequency of recurrence are difficult to find.

PREVENTION/AVOIDANCE

- The cause of displacement is poorly understood; therefore, avoidance is difficult.
- Management that may alter colonic activity, production of excess gas, and formation of impactions should be minimized; therefore, institute nutritional changes gradually.
- Prevent horses from rolling when showing signs of mild colic.

POSSIBLE COMPLICATIONS

Displacement can progress such that the colon becomes strangulated; at this stage, horses can rapidly succumb to cardiovascular shock from endotoxemia and hypovolemia or to colonic rupture from devitalization of the colon.

EXPECTED COURSE AND PROGNOSIS

- The prognosis is good, provided there has been no volvulus or significant vascular insult to the colon.
- In one study, long-term survival of horses with nonstrangulating displacements was >70%.

MISCELLANEOUS

ASSOCIATED CONDITIONS

- Cholestasis
- Colonic volvulus
- GI impaction

PREGNANCY

- The colon is held in place largely by its association with surrounding organs, and the gravid uterus, as well as the empty abdomen in postpartum mares, may predispose to displacement.
- Volvulus rather than dorsal displacement is more commonly associated with the postpartum mares.

SYNONYM

Left dorsal displacement is also called nephrosplenic ligament entrapment.

SEE ALSO

- Impaction
- Large colon torsion

ABBREVIATIONS

- CBC = complete blood count
- GI = gastrointestinal
- RBC = red blood cell

Suggested Reading

Hackett RP. Nonstrangulating colonic displacement in horses. JAVMA 1983;182:235–240.

Hardy J, Minton M, Robertson JT, *et al.* Nephrosplenic entrapment in the horse: a retrospective study of 174 cases. Equine Vet J Suppl 2000;32:95–97.

Johnston JK, Freeman DE. Diseases and surgery of the large colon. Vet Clin North Am Equine Pract 1997;13:317–340.

Santschi EM, Slone DE Jr, Frank WM. Use of ultrasound in horses for diagnosis of left dorsal displacement of the large colon and monitoring its nonsurgical correction. Vet Surg 1993;22:281–284.

Authors Judith B. Koenig and Simon G. Pearce
Consulting Editors Henry R. Stämpfli and Olimpo Oliver-Espinosa

RIGHT DORSAL COLITIS

BASICS

DEFINITION

Localized ulcerative inflammation of the right dorsal colon associated with administration of NSAIDs, particularly phenylbutazone, in the presence of hypovolemia or deprivation of water

PATHOPHYSIOLOGY

• Phenylbutazone, like any NSAID, inhibits cyclooxygenase (COX) activity. This drug is a competitive antagonist for both constitutive COX-1, responsible for the production of prostaglandins involved in physiologic functions, and for inducible COX-2, involved in inflammation pathway. Intestinal mucosal cell production of prostaglandin E_2 and prostaglandin $F_{2\alpha}$ is decreased by the inhibition of COX-1 activity. This inhibition results in the loss of the prostaglandin-mediated protective effect on the intestinal mucosa. When the intestinal mucosa integrity is sufficiently compromised, local bacterial invasion of the mucosa, luminal endotoxin absorption, and plasma protein leakage into the intestinal lumen may occur.
• Phenylbutazone toxicity is potentiated in hypovolemic or water-deprived horses because the normal protective vascular changes guarding against ischemic injury and intestinal mucosal cell atrophy from reduced blood flow are inhibited.

SYSTEM AFFECTED

Gastrointestinal Tract

• The right dorsal colon is the only portion of the gastrointestinal tract to be affected by this condition.
• Histologically, the lesions are characterized by multifocal to coalescing ulcerations in the wall of the right dorsal colon. Islands of mucosal regeneration may be observed.
• Lesions can be subacute or chronic. Subacute lesions are characterized by a fibrinonecrotic ulcerative colitis.
• In chronic cases, fibrous connective tissue is present in the lamina propria underlying the ulcerated mucosa.
• In chronic severe cases, colonic stenosis with ingesta impaction and subsequent necrosis and rupture of the colon can be observed.

GENETICS

N/A

INCIDENCE/PREVALENCE

Initially, RDC was thought to be associated with the administration of high dosage of phenylbutazone (> 10 mg/kg PO q24 h for 7–10 days). More recently, RDC has been observed in horses receiving lower doses of phenylbutazone (4.4–8.8 mg/kg PO q24 h for 5–30 days). The variable occurrence of the toxic side effects of phenylbutazone at the manufacturer's recommended daily dose (4.4–8.8 mg/kg PO q24h) have been attributed to individual variation in response to NSAID, duration of treatment, diet composition, health status, age, and hydration status.

GEOGRAPHIC DISTRIBUTION

N/A

SIGNALEMENT

Reported to be more frequently in ponies and in young performing horses

SIGNS

General Comments

All cases have a common history of administration of oral or parenteral phenylbutazone. Phenylbutazone is usually administrated for a problem not related to the gastrointestinal tract, most frequently for a painful musculoskeletal condition.

Historical

• All cases have also a history of systemic dehydration due to either a systemic illness or an inability to maintain proper hydration.
• Horses with acute disease may have clinical signs that include depression, lethargy, partial or complete anorexia, fever, colic, and, shortly thereafter, diarrhea.
• Horses with more chronic disease may have clinical signs that include intermittent colic, soft unformed feces, weight loss, and ventral edema.

Physical Examination

• In horses with acute disease, profuse watery diarrhea, severe dehydration, and deterioration of mucous membranes are observed.
• In horses with more chronic disease, the feces can be normal in amount but with the consistency of "cow patty" feces.

CAUSES

The exact cause of this condition is not known. It is not understood why the lesions are localized only in the right dorsal colon.

RISK FACTORS

A degree of hypovolemia and exposure to NSAIDs such as phenylbutazone are prerequisites for the development of this condition.

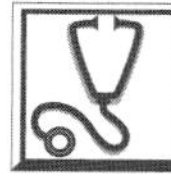

DIAGNOSIS

DIFFERENTIAL DIAGNOSES

• Other causes of colitis, such as salmonellosis, *Clostridium difficile* infection, and Potomac horse fever, should be included in the differential diagnoses. However, negative serology (Potomac horse fever), fecal cultures (salmonellosis), and fecal ELISA testing (*Clostridium difficile*) would help to rule out these conditions.
• For the chronic form of the disease, all disorders resulting in chronic abdominal pain, chronic diarrhea, or weight lost in the horse should be included in the differential diagnosis. These disorders include sand enteropathy, cyathostomiasis, chronic inflammatory bowel disease, alimentary lymphosarcoma, gastric ulcer disease, and chronic salmonellosis. Making a definitive diagnosis depends on the history of the case, a complete physical examination, and appropriate ancillary testing.

CBC/BIOCHEMISTRY/URINALYSIS

Complete Blood Count

Hematologic abnormalities include the presence of mild to moderate toxic neutrophils with either a regenerative or a degenerative left shift. Neutropenia is occasionally observed. Polycythemia (hemocontrentation), characterized by an increased PCV, is frequently observed.

Biochemistry Profile

Biochemistry abnormalities include hypoproteinemia, hypochloremia, azotemia, and metabolic acidosis. Hypoproteinemia may be observed despite hemoconcentration. Hypoalbuminemia is common, but when total protein concentration is <4.5 g/dL (45 g/L), panhypoproteinemia is observed.

OTHER LABORATORY TESTS

Abdominal Paracentesis

Elevation of total solids concentration and nucleated cell count may be observed.

Fecal Occult Blood Test

May be positive

IMAGING

• Transabdominal ultrasonography—Transabdominal ultrasonography at the right 10th, 11th, 12th and 13th intercostal spaces can be used in standing horses to image the right dorsal colon. Horses with RDC have an ultrasonographic mural thickness significantly greater than that of healthy horses (0.9–1.8 cm versus 0.3–0.4 cm in healthy horses). The right dorsal colon of affected horses also has a prominent hypoechoic layer associated with submucosal edema and inflammatory infiltrates.
• Nuclear scintigraphy with technetium-99 m hexamethylpropyleneamine oxime (^{99m}Tc-HMPAO)–labeled white blood cells—The application of ^{99m}Tc-HMPAO–labeled white blood cells can be used in specialized referral centers for imaging inflammatory bowel disease in horses. This technique is not specific of RDC but supports its diagnosis and facilitates prompt and appropriate management of affected horses.
• Gastroscopy—To rule out gastric and duodenal ulcers

OTHER DIAGNOSTIC PROCEDURES

Exploratory Celiotomy/Laparoscopy

Rarely necessary. A tentative diagnosis of this condition can be made when gross findings of marked edema or thickening or reduction in diameter of the intestinal tract are restricted to the right dorsal colon.

Intestinal Biopsy

The definitive diagnosis of the condition is made by histopathological examination of a biopsy of the right dorsal colon collected during celiotomy or at necropsy.

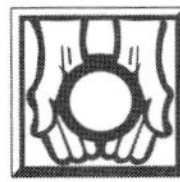

TREATMENT

AIMS OF TREATMENT

The treatment consists primarily of withdrawal of phenylbutazone and supportive therapy and care.

APPROPRIATE HEALTH CARE

Most patients with RDC require hospitalization to receive medical supportive therapy.

NURSING CARE

Acute Right Dorsal Colitis

Horses with acute disease are treated with supportive treatment, including intravenous fluids (lactated Ringer's solution), systemic broad-spectrum antibiotics, and analgesics. All NSAIDs should be used with extreme caution. When hypoproteinemia is severe (<4 g/dL; 40 g/L), plasma transfusion should be instituted.

Chronic Right Dorsal Colitis

- Horses with chronic disease can be managed with feeding and environmental adjustments and avoidance of treatment with NSAIDs.
- Dietary management consists of frequent feeding of a complete pelleted concentrate that contains 30% dietary fiber and 14% protein. Pelleted feed is advocated because it decreases the mechanical and physiologic load of the large colon. Roughage is eliminated or restricted to small amounts of fresh grass for at least 3 mo. The concentrate is fed according to the manufacturer's recommendations. The diet change is gradually completed over a period of 8 days. On the first day, 25% of the recommended amount of pelleted feed is offered, then the amount is increased by 25% every other day. Once on the new diet, the recommended amount of pelleted feed is divided in 4–6 equal aliquots and the horse is fed every 4–6 hr.

ACTIVITY

Managements to decrease stress include discontinuing or decreasing workloads such as strenuous exercise

SURGICAL CONSIDERATION

The surgical treatment is advocated when the RDC cannot be controlled with medical treatment. It consists of either bypassing or resecting the diseased RDC. Side-to-side colo-colostomy, between the proximal intact part of the RDC and the small colon, can be performed to bypass the diseased part of the RDC. End-to-end colo-colostomy after resection of the diseased RDC can also be performed. The prognosis for horses that undergo surgery is guarded.

DRUGS

Supportive treatment for horses with acute disease includes:

- Lactated Ringer's solution (6–12 mL/kg/hr IV) as a fluid volume replacement
- Broad-spectrum systemic antibiotics (sodium penicillin G 20,000 IU/kg IV QID and gentamicin sulfate 6.6 mg/kg IV daily or ceftiofur 2.2 mg/kg IV BID or trimethoprim-sulfamethoxazole 5–25 mg/kg IV BID)
- Analgesics such as xylazine (0.2–0.5 mg/kg IV) alone or in combination with butorphanol (0.02 mg/kg IV) can be administered.

PRECAUTION

- NSAIDs such as flunixin meglumine should be used with caution because they may also be involved in the pathogenesis of the disease.
- Aminoglycoside as well as flunixin meglumine should be used with caution when clinical signs of severe dehydration (prerenal azotemia) and hypoproteinemia are present.

PATIENT MONITORING

Hematocrit and plasmatic protein concentration should be monitored when intravenous fluid therapy is administered. If plasma protein concentrations decrease below 4 g/dL (40 g/L) during fluid therapy, plasma transfusion should be instituted.

POSSIBLE COMPLICATION

- Horses with acute disease can develop a persistent diarrhea with progressive edema, laminitis, or renal disease.
- The chronic disease can be associated with progressive weight loss, hypoproteinemia, colic, and loose feces.

MEDICATIONS

N/A

FOLLOW-UP

N/A

MISCELLANEOUS

ABBREVIATION

- RDC = right dorsal colon

Suggested Reading

East LM, Trumble TN, Steyn PF, Savage CJ, Dickinson CE, Traub-Dargatz JL. The application of technetium-99 m hexamethylpropyleneamine oxime (99mTc-HMPAO) labeled white blood cells for the diagnosis of right dorsal ulcerative colitis in two horses. Vet Radiol Ultrasound 2000;41:360–364.

Jones SL, Davis J, Rowlingson K. Ultrasonographic findings in horses with right dorsal colitis: five cases (2000–2001). JAVMA 2003;222:1248–1251.

Karcher LF, Dill SG, Anderson WI, King JM. Right dorsal colitis. J Vet Int Med 1990;4:247–253.

Author Ludovic Bouré
Consulting Editors Henry Stämpfli and Olimpo Oliver-Espinosa

ROBINIA PSEUDOACACIA (BLACK LOCUST) TOXICOSIS

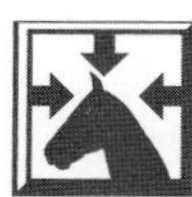

BASICS

OVERVIEW

• *Robinia pseudoacacia* (black locust) toxicosis results from an unknown toxin found in all portions of the plant except the flowers.
• A glycoprotein called robin is the putative toxin.
• The tree is widely distributed east of the Mississippi River.
• Signs relate to GI and cardiovascular effects of the toxin.
• Among domestic livestock species, horses may be the most susceptible.
• Most cases involve horses eating the bark of the tree.

SIGNALMENT

No known breed, age, or genetic susceptibilities

SIGNS

• Depression
• Colic
• Diarrhea or constipation
• Decreased intestinal peristalsis
• Weakness
• Cardiac dysrhythmias
• Hyperexcitability
• Dyspnea
• Laminitis

CAUSES AND RISK FACTORS

• Leaves are palatable and will be eaten if other forage is of poor quality or unavailable.
• Clinical signs have been reported in horses ingesting as little as 70 g of bark.
• Boredom and hunger predispose to ingestion.

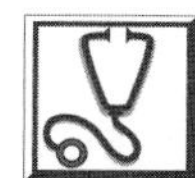

DIAGNOSIS

DIFFERENTIAL DIAGNOSIS

• Ionophore intoxication—differentiated by detection of an ionophore in feed
• *Eupatorium rugosum* (white snakeroot) intoxication—evidence of plant consumption
• Other causes of colic—appropriate physical examination and imaging (e.g., ultrasonography; radiography)

CBC/BIOCHEMISTRY/URINALYSIS

• Hypocalcemia was noted in two ill horses after leaf ingestion.
• Recumbent horses have increased serum CK concentrations.

OTHER LABORATORY TESTS

N/A

IMAGING

N/A

DIAGNOSTIC PROCEDURES

ECG may demonstrate cardiac dysrhythmias, but the types of dysrhythmias are not well documented.

PATHOLOGICAL FINDINGS

Gross

• Plant material (e.g., bark, leaves, pods) in stomach contents
• Watery and hemorrhagic intestinal contents

Histopathological

Enteritis characterized by diffuse villus-tip necrosis and hemorrhage

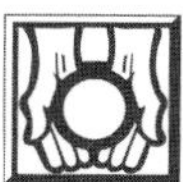

TREATMENT

• Decontamination with AC and saline cathartic or mineral oil
• Balanced electrolyte fluids

ROBINIA PSEUDOACACIA (BLACK LOCUST) TOXICOSIS

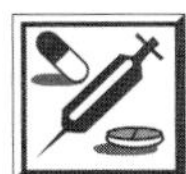

MEDICATIONS

DRUG(S) OF CHOICE

- AC (1–4 g/kg PO in water slurry [1 g of AC in 5 mL of water])
- One dose of cathartic PO with AC if no diarrhea or ileus—70% sorbitol (3 mL/kg) or sodium or magnesium sulfate (250 mg/kg), with the latter two in a water slurry
- Treat cardiac dysrhythmias as appropriate; although dysrhythmias are reported to occur they are not well described.
- Analgesics for abdominal discomfort—flunixin meglumine (1.1 mg/kg IV or IM as necessary)

CONTRAINDICATIONS/POSSIBLE INTERACTIONS

- Use NSAIDs with caution in dehydrated patients.
- Do not give mineral oil concurrently with AC because of impaired binding ability of AC.

FOLLOW-UP

PATIENT MONITORING

N/A

PREVENTION/AVOIDANCE

Prevent access to black locust; if not practical, provide good-quality diet in adequate amounts.

POSSIBLE COMPLICATIONS

N/A

EXPECTED COURSE AND PROGNOSIS

- Guarded prognosis in symptomatic animals
- No long-term sequelae are expected in recovered animals.

MISCELLANEOUS

ASSOCIATED CONDITIONS, AGE-RELATED FACTORS, ZOONOTIC POTENTIAL, PREGNANCY

N/A

ABBREVIATIONS

- AC = activated charcoal
- CK = creatine kinase

Suggested Reading

Burrows GE, Tyrl RJ. Toxic Plants of North America. Ames, IA: Iowa State University Press, 2001: 602.

Author Robert H. Poppenga

Consulting Editor Robert H. Poppenga

SALMONELLOSIS

BASICS

DEFINITION

Salmonellosis refers to clinical disease resulting from infection with various serovars of *Salmonella enterica* ssp. *enterica.* Shedding refers to detection of *Salmonella* spp. in a fecal sample whether or not the animal is demonstrating clinical signs of disease.

PATHOPHYSIOLOGY

Exposure to *Salmonella* spp. usually occurs through the alimentary tract. *Salmonella* spp. can invade pharyngeal, intestinal, and colonic mucosa. Bacteria attach to mucosa, invade epithelial cells, and spread through mucosa to lymphoid tissue and into bloodstream. Virulence factors may promote the ability of bacteria to invade host tissues; the production of toxins damaging host cells or stimulating fluid secretion in the GI tract or causing severe cardiovascular impairment; and stimulate the host's inflammatory response, which can cause further signs of toxemia. The infective dose can vary by type of *Salmonella* spp. as well as with host factors.

SYSTEMS AFFECTED

The GI tract is the principal system affected. *Salmonella* bacteria can enter the blood and disseminate to other organs, including bone, lung, liver, and kidneys.

INCIDENCE/PREVALENCE

- Outbreaks of salmonellosis have been recognized on farms, stables, sales facilities, and veterinary hospitals.
- Prevalence of *Salmonella* varies according to whether clinical disease or fecal shedding is being studied, the equine population being tested (hospitalized versus general population), the test method used to detect organism, sampling method (e.g., fecal swabs versus at least 1 g of feces), and season of year. Prevalence of fecal shedding by clinically normal horses has been reported to be as low as 0.8% and as high as 20% using fecal culture and PCR methods, respectively. The prevalence of fecal shedding among horses with a GI disorder is higher than in clinically normal horses.

SIGNALMENT

No breed or sex predilection has been reported.

SIGNS

- Fever, lethargy, diarrhea, and abdominal discomfort are common.
- Cardiovascular function can be severely compromised because of dehydration that accompanies diarrhea and the systemic effects of endotoxemia and proinflammatory cytokines.
- Tachycardia, injected mucous membranes, delayed capillary refill time, hypoproteinemia, and peripheral edema typically accompany severe intestinal inflammation.
- Adult horses may have fever and colic signs, without diarrhea.
- The role of *Salmonella* spp. infection in chronic diarrhea in horses is not clear.
- Neonatal foals may be septicemic and thus clinical signs may vary according to the organ system being involved. Young foals may be lame from primary musculoskeletal involvement or develop pneumonia caused by *Salmonella* spp.

CAUSES

Frequency of serovars isolated varies, but *Salmonella* Typhimurium, Newport, Anatum, and Agona are the most frequent isolates from clinical cases in United States. In Canada, common serovars isolated in the past 2 years were *Salmonella* Typhimurium and Heidelberg.

RISK FACTORS

- Ingestion of contaminated feed or water or contact with the bacteria through exposure to feces containing the organism or direct exposure to shedding animals, e.g., patient hospitalized during a noscomial salmonellosis outbreak.
- Several factors can predispose to salmonellosis, including transportation, sudden feed changes or spoiled feedstuffs, other illnesses, and surgical interventions, that can disrupt normal GI bacterial flora, reduce GI motility, or reduce the stomach acid or other natural barriers to colonization. Antimicrobial treatment has been reported to increase risk of salmonellosis.

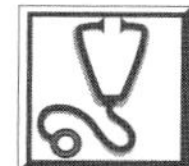

DIAGNOSIS

DIFFERENTIAL DIAGNOSIS

- Other causes of diarrhea, including PHF, intestinal clostridiosis, small strongyle infestation, and idiopathic colitis.
- Signs of endotoxemia occur with other GI disorders and in mares with placental retention.
- Signs of colic may be referable to many other disorders.
- Peripheral edema may result from other causes of hypoproteinemia, congestive heart failure, and vasculitis.

CBC/BIOCHEMISTRY/URINALYSIS

CBC

- Hemoconcentration
- Decreased to normal (with dehydration) total solids
- Leucopenia due to neutropenia
- Leukocytosis can occur in horses with colitis of several days' duration and with septic thrombophlebitis.
- White blood cells can have a highly reactive appearance.
- +/− hyperfibrinogenemia

Serum Chemistries

- Azotemia
- Hypoalbuminemia
- Hyponatremia, hypochloremia, hypokalemia, hypocalcemia
- Metabolic acidosis
- Hyperglycemia

Urine Analysis

Hyposthenuria may result from renal insult from toxemia or be due to toxicity of NSAIDs given to dehydrated animals.

OTHER LABORATORY TESTS

- Fecal culture or PCR testing for *Salmonella*
- Serotyping of isolated *Salmonella* bacteria
- Antibiogram of isolated *Salmonella* bacteria
- Abdominocentesis for animals with signs of colic

IMAGING

Transabdominal or transrectal ultrasonography may be used to determine whether there is bowel wall thickening (infiltrative disease, edema) or excessive peritoneal fluid accumulation.

DIAGNOSTIC PROCEDURES

- Rectal palpation with colic
- Exploratory laparotomy may be indicated to rule out causes of colic; when performed, intestinal biopsy for bacterial culture may be done to confirm a suspected case of salmonellosis. The risk versus benefit of such a biopsy must be considered on a case-by-case basis.

PATHOLOGICAL FINDINGS

Lesions at necropsy include congested, purple cecal and colonic serosal surfaces. Mucosa may be thickened, sometimes markedly. Colon infarction and perforation occur infrequently. Gross renal lesions, such as infarctions, may be found in severe cases. In severe cases, disseminated bacterial or fungal infection in multiple organs, particularly the lungs, may be found.

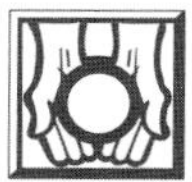

TREATMENT

NURSING CARE

Isolation of suspect or confirmed cases along with optimal biosecurity and biocontainment precautions is indicated. Control of insects and regular cleaning of bedding are indicated to minimize the spread of bacteria. Regular cleaning of soiled areas on the patient to reduce skin damage from fecal material is also indicated.

ACTIVITY

Horses recovering from salmonellosis should have their activity restricted proportionate to severity of illness, and biosecurity precautions should be considered regarding where horse could be walked or turned out.

DIET

Depends on severity of intestinal disease. Concentrate feed, particularly in large amounts, is withheld in acute cases of salmonellosis because of possible adverse effects on perturbed intestinal microflora. Hay and pellets are likely to be poorly digested in horses with colitis because of changes in the microflora, but acetic acid produced by fermentation of cellulose may be beneficial in cecal and colonic mucosal healing. Feeding small amounts of palatable feed frequently may improve food consumption. Fresh water should always be available. Some horses will consume electrolyte-containing fluids orally, which can reduce need for supplementation of intravenous electrolytes. Patients with prolonged anorexia benefit from parenteral nutrition.

CLIENT EDUCATION

- It is optimal to isolate *Salmonella* shedding horses from other horses. The risk that the shedding horses pose to normal herd mates is really unknown. It is likely that normal horses are less likely to become diseased if exposed compared to hospital patients.
- Clients should be informed about potential for fecal shedding of *Salmonella* bacteria into

environment. The number of *Salmonella* spp. per gram of feces may vary based on horse's clinical status, with potentially fewer organisms in feces from horses with formed manure that are convalescing compared to acutely ill horses with diarrhea.
• Also, formed feces are likely to contaminate a smaller area and be removed more easily than are watery feces.
• Specific isolation procedures should be developed for any diarrheic horse.
• It is important to limit contact of personnel and other animals, including dogs. Dogs may have a habit of consuming horse manure, if given contact with a shedding horse.
• The zoonotic potential of salmonellosis should also be discussed with clients.

SURGICAL CONSIDERATION

If shedding or suspect horses are taken into surgery, optimal biosecurity procedures should be used.

MEDICATIONS

DRUG(S) OF CHOICE

• Restoration and maintenance of fluid volume are critical for salmonellosis patients with severe diarrhea. Polyionic fluids should be used for replacement and maintenance. Electrolyte deficits should be corrected with supplemental solutions.
• Opinions differ as to whether antimicrobial drugs should be given to adult horses with salmonellosis. Foals with salmonellosis, particularly with concurrent septicemia, are routinely treated with antimicrobial drugs.
• Antimicrobials used in salmonellosis include combinations of penicillin and gentamicin; ceftiofur and gentamicin; and fluoroquinolones such as enrofloxacin and orbifloxicin.
• Flunixin meglumine and ketoprofen have been shown to ameliorate effects of endotoxemia and are often used in salmonellosis patients.
• Dimethylsulfoxide and products that contain antibody to LPS or that neutralize circulating LPS, such as polymyxin B, have been used with variable results.
• Plasma, with or without heparin, if severe hypoproteinemia and edema
• Gastric ulcer prophylaxis may be indicated. Use of products to absorb bacterial toxins in digestive tract from di-tri-octahedral smectite and/or bismuth subsalicylate and those that may benefit enterocyte recovery such as psyllium may be indicated if the horse's GI motility is such that these products are likely to be well tolerated.

CONTRAINDICATIONS

• Use of NSAIDs, aminoglycosides, and polymixin B in azotemic or moderately or severely dehydrated patients without ensuring rehydration and adequate urine production
• Use of various medications via nasogastric tube in patients with gastric reflux or severe ileus.

PRECAUTIONS

If glomerular filtration is impaired, administering drugs that depend on renal clearance, particularly aminoglycosides or NSAIDs, should be done judiciously.

POSSIBLE INTERACTIONS

Concurrent use of NSAIDs along with aminoglycosides particularly in dehydrated or azotemic patients can potentiate nephrotoxicity of each drug given alone.

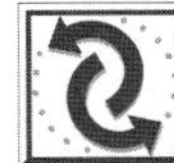

FOLLOW-UP

PATIENT MONITORING

• Heart rate—should progressively decrease toward normal (32–40 bpm)
• Rectal temperature should decrease to normal.
• Peripheral leukocyte count should increase toward normal but not become elevated.
• Leukocyte morphology—should progressively change from highly reactive appearance ("toxic") to normal
• Attitude, appetite should improve toward normal.
• Fecal *Salmonella* culture should eventually become negative.
• Weight loss should gradually resolve.
• Serum protein concentration, if low, should increase to normal.
• Serum creatinine, if elevated, should decrease with fluid treatment.

PREVENTION/AVOIDANCE

• Thorough cleaning followed by disinfection of areas where fecal contamination is likely (stalls, including water buckets or automatic waterers; drains and cracks in the floors and wall); equipment used needs to be cleaned and disinfected.
• Prompt detection of illness of any diarrheic horse followed by isolation away from any contact with other horses
• Biocontainment protocols that address prevention of spread of *Salmonella* spp. by personnel and equipment need to be developed and enforced.

POSSIBLE COMPLICATIONS

• Laminitis
• Thrombophlebitis
• Colon infarction
• Disseminated bacterial infection
• Chronic diarrhea
• Chronic or recurrent colic
• Persistent poor body condition
• Persistent fecal shedding of *Salmonella* spp.

EXPECTED COURSE AND PROGNOSIS

Horses with profuse diarrhea and toxemia require intensive care; prognosis for survival is approximately 50%. Horses that survive typically show substantial improvement within 7 days, and horses that do not substantially improve in 7–10 days have a very poor prognosis for survival.

MISCELLANEOUS

ASSOCIATED CONDITIONS

• Dehydration
• Hypoproteinemia
• Toxemia
• Laminitis
• Venous thrombophlebitis
• Weight loss

AGE-RELATED FACTORS

Foals predisposed to developing extraintestinal sites of infection such as joint and bone infections

ZOONOTIC POTENTIAL

Salmonellosis has a high zoonotic potential that should be communicated to all personnel. Personnel on antimicrobial treatment, on immunosuppressive treatment, or who have immunocompromising illnesses should advised to avoid contact with salmonellosis patients.

PREGNANCY

Abortion caused by *Salmonella* bacteria is rare as *Salmonella* Abortusequi is no longer recognized in the United States; however, pregnancy may be affected by any severe illness of a mare.

SEE ALSO

• PHF
• Intestinal clostridiosis
• Small strongyle infestation

ABBREVIATIONS

• GI = gastrointestinal
• LPS = lipopolysaccharide
• PCR = polymerase chain reaction
• PHF = Potomac horse fever

Suggested Reading

Dwyer RM: Environmental disinfection to control equine infectious diseases. Vet Clin North Am Infect Control 2004;20: 531–543.

Hyatt DR, Weese JS: Salmonella culture: sampling procedures and laboratory techniques. Vet Clin North Am Infect Control 2004;20:577–587.

Schott HC, Ewart SL, Walker RD, et al: An outbreak of salmonellosis among horses at a veterinary teaching hospital. JAVMA 2001;218;1152–1159.

Tillotson K, Savage CJ, Salman MD, Gentry-Weeks CR, Rice D, Fedorka-Cray PJ, Hendrickson DA, Jones RL, Nelson AW, Traub-Dargatz JL: Outbreak of *Salmonella infantis* infection in a large animal veterinary teaching hospital. JAVMA 1997;211;1554–1557.

Traub-Dargatz JL, Besser TE: Salmonellosis. In: Sellon DC, Long MT, eds. Equine Infectious Diseases. St. Louis: Saunders Elsevier, 2007:331–345.

Author Josie Traub-Dargatz

Consulting Editors Henry Stämpfli and Olimpo Oliver-Espinosa

SAND IMPACTION AND ENTEROPATHY

BASICS

DEFINITION

Gravitational sedimentation of ingested sand in the large intestine causing colonic impaction and mucosal irritation

PATHOPHYSIOLOGY

Horses ingest sand while grazing on loose sandy soil or while eating from the ground in sandy stalls or paddocks. Some horses, particularly foals, develop pica and intentionally eat sand or fine grit contained in decomposed granite used for stall or paddock floors. Ingested sand sediments and accumulates in the large colon until impaction and partial or complete obstruction may occur. The intestinal contents become dehydrated, the sand may dry out and take on a concrete-like consistency. Fine sand tends to accumulate in the ventral colon, whereas coarse sand or grit may also accumulate in the dorsal and transverse colons. Colonic displacement and/or volvulus is found in up to 54% of horses treated surgically for sand accumulation. The amount of accumulated sand required to induce clinical signs is not known and some horses may tolerate more sand than others. Abdominal pain is caused by colonic distention from the impaction or from ingesta and gas accumulating proximally due to partial or complete obstruction, and by reflex intestinal spasms stimulated by distention. Chronic irritation of the bowel wall and reduction in the absorptive surface area by accumulated sand may interfere with normal water absorption in the colon and give rise to diarrhea.

SYSTEM AFFECTED

Gastrointestinal

INCIDENCE/PREVALENCE

- Worldwide distribution, but more common in geographic locations with loose sandy soil or where horses are kept in sandy paddocks or stalls and fed on the ground
- Underfed horses, horses being fed a diet of insufficient or poor-quality roughage, and horses on closely grazed overstocked pastures appear to be at greatest risk.

SIGNALMENT

There is no breed and age predilection. Miniature horses may be predisposed due to behavioral, environmental, and management issues.

SIGNS

Historical

- Feeding hay and/or grain on the ground or grazing on pastures with sandy soil
- Recurrent or chronic colic of mild to moderate severity, intermittent or chronic diarrhea, weight loss, and ill thrift despite a good appetite

Physical Examination

- Typical signs reflect mild to moderate colic unless a concurrent large colon displacement or torsion is present.
- Scant or absent feces are typical, although watery to "cow pie" diarrhea may accompany or precede the onset of colic and may be the major presenting sign.
- Other signs include anorexia, lethargy, depression, abdominal distention, prolonged capillary refill time, and tachypnea.
- Auscultation of the colon over the most dependent portion of the abdomen for 1–5 min reveals typical "sand sounds" from sand/sand and mucosal/sand friction. These occur at a rate of 2–5 per min and last for 2–5 seconds.
- Sounds also arise from propulsive–retropulsive contractions at intervals of 2–3 min and last for 15–30 seconds and sound like the sound generated by slowly rotating sand in a partially filled paper bag. Sand sounds are sensitive and reliable indicators of sand accumulation.
- In thin horses with massive accumulations of sand in the colon, external palpation and ballottement of the ventral and ventrolateral abdomen may reveal a firm, heavy viscus. Rectal examination usually reveals distinct distention of the large colon and/or cecum. Definitive diagnosis of sand impaction by rectal palpation alone is achieved in only about 15% of cases. Fecal sand may be detected as a "gritty" feeling during rectal examination and sand may sediment on the floor of the rectum in horses with concomitant diarrhea.

CAUSES

See Pathophysiology.

RISK FACTORS

See Pathophysiology.

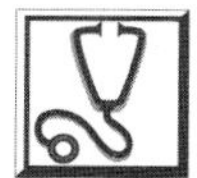

DIAGNOSIS

DIFFERENTIAL DIAGNOSIS

- Large colon feed impaction, unless a concurrent large colon displacement or torsion is present.
- All other causes of colic, but particularly those that are recurrent, including enterolithiasis, internal abdominal abscess, gastric ulcer, thromboembolic colic, peritonitis, abdominal neoplasia, cholelithiasis, and nephrolithiasis.
- Chronic diarrhea and ill thrift due to parasitism, inflammatory bowel disease with malabsorption, intestinal neoplasia, and abnormal fermentation associated with noninflammatory bowel disease or antibiotic use.

CBC/BIOCHEMISTRY/URINALYSIS

Changes are nonspecific for sand impaction or enteropathy.

OTHER LABORATORY TESTS

- Feces may contain frank or occult blood.
- Abdominocentesis should be performed with great care so as not to perforate the colon. If the colon is penetrated, sand in the abdominal fluid sample is diagnostic. Abdominal fluid may be normal in horses with sand accumulation, but if the colon is compromised, the total protein concentration and white blood cell count may be elevated.

IMAGING

- Abdominal radiography is frequently diagnostic for presence of accumulated sand and serves to monitor the disappearance of sand with medical treatment, particularly in small horses, ponies, and foals. Sand may appear as a homogeneous or granular radiodense accumulation with a horizontal dorsal margin in one or more dependent portions of viscera in the cranioventral abdomen.
- Ultrasonographic evidence of sand is less specific. Signs suggesting sand accumulation include increased contact of the large colon with the ventral abdominal wall, decreased gut motility, and hyperechoic acoustic shadowing.

DIAGNOSTIC PROCEDURES

- Observation of sand in the feces, abdominal auscultation, rectal palpation, abdominal radiography, abdominal ultrasound, or sand palpated or obtained during abdominocentesis
- The sand sedimentation test is performed by breaking up three or four fecal balls in a rectal sleeve and mixing them with water to form a slurry. The sleeve is tied off and suspended to allow the sand to settle inside the fingertips. A sediment of more than 0.6 cm (0.25 inch) in the fingertips indicates that the horse is passing excessive quantities of sand in feces. In a more quantitative test, the finding of more than a teaspoon (5 g) of sand in the bottom of a bucket after suspending six fecal balls in water and allowing organic matter to float out is considered abnormal. The appearance of sand on sedimentation is considered a sign of clearance of sand. Horses with sand impaction may not necessarily have sand in their feces at the time of examination.

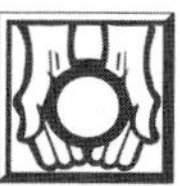

TREATMENT

- Horses with well-formed impactions or profuse diarrhea benefit from intragastric administration of water and electrolytes or intravenous administration of balanced electrolyte solutions. The choice of analgesics and the frequency of administration are dictated by the degree of pain.
- Withholding of food for ≥24 hr and intragastric administration of mineral oil and water promote lubrication and dissolution of the feed impaction that frequently complicates sand impaction. Resuspension and removal of sand are best accomplished by intragastric administration of lubricating, motility-stimulating bulk laxatives containing *Psyllium hydrophila* mucilloid (0.25–0.5 kg/500 kg). Because psyllium gels quickly when mixed with water and may occlude the nasogastric tube, it is best administered mixed with 2 L of mineral oil, followed by 4 L of water. Continued daily administration of 0.25–0.5 kg of psyllium orally mixed with grain or sweet feed or administered by nasogastric tube for 10–14 consecutive days is recommended. Thereafter, further treatment is based on whether all of the accumulated sand has been removed from the large colon. Medical treatment is most likely to be successful in horses with good intestinal motility, modest accumulations of sand, low levels of abdominal pain, and pain that is easily controlled.

APPROPRIATE HEALTH CARE

Initial evaluation and treatment of horses with sand colic are handled appropriately on an outpatient basis. Transportation to a referral center is usually necessary for radiographic confirmation of the diagnosis and surgical management of horses that do not respond to medical therapy.

NURSING CARE

- Prevention of rolling and self-induced trauma, provision of analgesia, and maintenance of hydration
- Placement of an indwelling nasogastric tube and fluid therapy are recommended before referral and during transportation for horses that may need surgical treatment.

ACTIVITY

Stall-rested and hand-walked as necessary until the sand impaction has resolved

DIET

Feed should be withheld during medical treatment for sand colic until the impaction has broken down, significant quantities of feces have been passed, and signs of abdominal pain have abated.

CLIENT EDUCATION

Feeding practices must be modified to prevent further accidental or intentional ingestion of sand.

SURGICAL CONSIDERATION

Affected horses with reduced or absent intestinal motility, with large accumulations of sand, and horses that fail to respond to medical treatment within 48–72 hr, have uncontrollable pain, abdominal distention, gaseous distention of the bowel palpable on rectal examination, repeated gastric reflux, bowel displacement, a rising white cell count in peritoneal fluid, or sudden worsening of clinical signs. Prognosis for long-term survival is favorable if successful evacuation of the colon is achieved. Intraoperative complications include the inability to remove all of the sand, rupture of the intestine, and contamination of the abdomen leading to peritonitis. The most common postoperative complication is diarrhea.

MEDICATION

CONTRAINDICATIONS

Acepromazine is contraindicated in affected horses showing evidence of shock.

PRECAUTIONS

Repeated use of potent analgesics such as flunixin meglumine, ketoprofen, or phenylbutazone to control colic pain should be avoided unless appropriate diagnostic and therapeutic intervention are also pursued.

FOLLOW-UP

PATIENT MONITORING

Repeat physical examinations including abdominal auscultation and sand sedimentation—testing of feces at weekly intervals for 2–4 weeks. Abdominal radiographs can also be performed to confirm the clearance of sand. Thereafter, abdominal auscultation and sand sedimentation tests should be performed at intervals of 3–6 mo during routine health examinations.

PREVENTION/AVOIDANCE

- Identification and evacuation of accumulated sand from the large colon and modification of feeding and management practices to minimize further ingestion of significant quantities of sand
- Auscultation of the ventral abdomen frequently identifies horses with significant accumulations of sand before overt clinical signs become apparent.
- The source of sand and causes of pica should be identified, horses should not be fed on the ground, and pastures should not be grazed too short.
- Feeders should be placed above a solid, sand-free surface such as rubber mats or provided with a solid bottom. Feeders made from two tractor tires bolted on top of each other and to a plywood base have proved to be very effective for feeding horses in dry paddocks when feeders cannot be placed on a solid base.
- Sufficient feeder space should be provided for all horses in order to discourage them from pulling hay out of the feeder and eating it from the ground. Horses should receive appropriate quantities of feed, including good-quality roughage, on a regular schedule, and fresh water should be freely available.
- Overgrazed bare pastures should be rested, fertilized, irrigated, and, when necessary, reseeded to promote lush growth before reintroducing horses.
- Avoiding sand as the flooring material for stalls and paddocks for horses that habitually eat sand or dirt may also be necessary.
- If management practices cannot be modified to prevent ingestion of sand, intermittent "purge" treatments with psyllium-containing products is recommended. Daily oral administration of 0.25 kg of psyllium for 7 consecutive days each month has proved to be effective.

POSSIBLE COMPLICATIONS

Chronic diarrhea, bowel perforation, peritonitis, and bowel displacement, with or without strangulation

EXPECTED COURSE AND PROGNOSIS

- Medical therapy is usually successful in resolving sand impaction and relieving signs of colic within 1–4 days; however, complete removal of accumulated sand often takes several weeks.
- Prognosis is good for sand impactions diagnosed at an early stage.
- A guarded prognosis is given in more chronic, high-volume sand impactions, which are more likely to require surgical intervention, although survival after surgery is reported to be 75%–90%.
- The long-term prognosis depends on preventing sand ingestion and on the degree of mucosal injury and scarring resulting from the original episode of sand impaction.
- Some horses, presumably those with extensive mucosal injury, may show diarrhea and ill thrift for extended periods after evacuation of the offending sand.

MISCELLANEOUS

ASSOCIATED CONDITIONS

Chronic diarrhea, ill thrift, colonic displacement, colonic rupture, septic peritonitis, endotoxemia, and the other postoperative complications listed above have been recognized in association with sand impaction.

AGE-RELATED FACTORS

Sand impaction can occur in horses of any age, including foals as young as a few weeks.

PREGNANCY

- Pregnant mares requiring surgical treatment for sand colic are likely at increased risk for abortion.
- Prophylactic use of NSAIDs (flunixin meglumine) and progestogens such as altrenogest are indicated in pregnant mares.

SYNONYMS

- Sand impaction
- Sand colic
- Sand enteritis
- Sand enteropathy

SEE ALSO

- Colic

Suggested Reading

Ragle CA, Meagher DM, Schrader JL, Honnas CM. Abdominal auscultation in the detection of experimentally induced gastrointestinal sand accumulation. J Vet Int Med 1989;3:12–14.

Ragle CA, Meagher DM, Lacroix CA, Honnas CM. Surgical treatment of sand colic: results in 40 horses. Vet Surg 1989;8:48–51.

Ruohoniemi M, Kaikkonen R, Raekallio M *et al.* Abdominal radiography in monitoring the resolution of sand accumulations from the large colon of horses treated medically. Equine Vet J 2001;33:59–64.

Authors W. David Wilson and Sarah S. le Jeune
Consulting Editors Henry Stämpfli and Olimpo Oliver-Espinosa

SARCOID

BASICS

DEFINITION

Benign, locally aggressive, fibroblastic cutaneous neoplasm that has variable clinical manifestations

PATHOPHYSIOLOGY

- Not completely understood
- There is cumulative evidence that BPV types 1 and 2 are the principal causative agents of sarcoid.
- Most sarcoids appear to contain detectable viral DNA and mRNA and express the major BPV transforming protein E5, but papilloma viral particles have not been isolated.
- There may be a strong association between risk of sarcoid development and certain MHC class II genes.
- BPV may be transmitted via flies, stable management practices, or the contact of wounds with an environment that has been contaminated with the virus.

SYSTEM AFFECTED

Skin

GENETICS

A genetic predisposition involving specific equine MHC haplotypes (W13 and A5) has been demonstrated; however, the underlying mechanisms are not clear.

INCIDENCE/PREVALENCE

- The most commonly reported neoplasm of horses worldwide, representing up to 90% of the skin tumors and 20% of all tumors
- The proportional morbidity rate of sarcoids among the veterinary colleges ranges between 0 and 14 per 1000 cases, with an average of 6 per 1000.

GEOGRAPHIC DISTRIBUTION

None reported

SIGNALMENT

Breed Predilections

- Higher risk—Appaloosas, Arabians, and Quarter Horses
- Lower risk—Standardbreds

Mean Age and Range

- Mean age—3–6 years
- Range—1–15+ years

Predominant Sex

Geldings appear to be predisposed.

SIGNS

General Comments

Sarcoids do not metastasize.

Historical

- Single or multiple skin tumors that can be present in different areas of the body
- Frequently occur at sites of previous injury or scarring
- Variable clinical presentations and growth rates
- High propensity for recurrence and become more aggressive if subject to accidental or iatrogenic interference
- Spontaneous regression is rare.

Physical Examination

A large majority of affected horses have more than one lesion, most often detected on the paragenital regions, thorax, abdomen, limbs, neck, head, and periocular areas.
Six distinct clinical types of sarcoids can be recognized.

1. Occult—one or more small cutaneous nodules or roughened areas with a mild thickened appearance. Predilection sites include periocular area, neck, and other relatively hairless areas of the body.
2. Verrucous (warty)—warty appearance with variable flaking and scaling. Predilection sites include face, body, and groin.
3. Nodular—firm, well-defined dermal or subcutaneous nodules of variable sizes. Predilection sites include groin, sheath, and eyelid areas.
4. Fibroblastic—most aggressive type, "proud flesh" appearance, pedunculated or extensive sessile tumors with prominent ulceration and exudation. Predilection sites include groin, eyelid, lower limbs, and coronet. This tumor type often shows secondary bacterial infections.
5. Mixed—progressive/transient state between 2 or more types of sarcoids.
6. Malevolent sarcoid—may show extensive infiltration of lymphatics with numerous ulcerative nodules and surface involvement as well as possible extension to local lymph nodes. Predilection sites include jaw, face, elbow, and medial thigh.

CAUSES

Likely caused by an association between BPV types 1 and 2, the environment, and the inheritable traits of the horse

RISK FACTORS

- Possible genetic predisposition
- Flies as potential vectors, stable management practices, or the introduction of the BPV into a wound from a contaminated environment

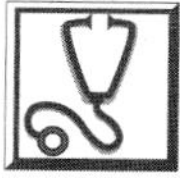

DIAGNOSIS

DIFFERENTIAL DIAGNOSIS

- Occult—dermatophytosis, skin excoriations, ectoparasites
- Verrucous—papillomatosis, hyperkeratosis, sarcoidosis, molluscum contagiosum, horsepox, SCC
- Nodular—fibroma, neurofibroma, hypodermyasis, dermoid cysts, allergic/axillary collagen necrosis, melanoma
- Fibroblastic—exuberant granulation tissue, botryomycosis, fibrosarcoma, neurofribroma/fibrosarcoma, SCC
- Mixed—varies with clinical appearance.
- Malevolent—lymphangitis, chronic skin infections (e. g., glanders, epizootic, and histoplasmosis)

CBC/BIOCHEMISTRY/URINALYSIS

No specific findings

OTHER LABORATORY TESTS

N/A

IMAGING

Radiography may be needed if suspect orbital or bone involvement.

OTHER DIAGNOSTIC PROCEDURES

- Skin biopsy is needed for definitive diagnosis.
- Anecdotal reports suggest that biopsy of occult, nodular, or small verrucous sarcoids may transform these tumors into more aggressive types; however, such reports should not prevent pursuing a biopsy as a mean of appropriate diagnostic testing.

PATHOLOGICAL FINDINGS

- The gross appearance of a sarcoid can be quite variable; however, six broad categories are recognized—occult, verrucous, nodular, fibroblastic, mixed, and malevolent. All types may have smaller satellite lesions surrounding the main tumor.
- Histologically, sarcoids are characterized by dermal proliferation of fibroblastic cells. Neoplastic cells are spindle-shaped or fusiform with pointed nuclei and large, irregular, pleomorphic nuclei. The mitotic rate is variable, but it is usually low. The dermis shows variable amounts of fibroblasts and collagen fibers that form whorls, interlacing bundles, and disorganized arrays. Fibroblastic cells are frequently oriented perpendicular to the overlying basement membrane, in a so-called "picket-fence" pattern. The overlying epidermis is usually hyperplastic and hyperkeratotic with rete ridges often attenuated and pointed.

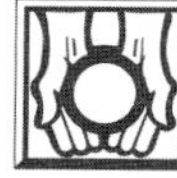

TREATMENT

AIMS OF TREATMENT

- Observation without treatment may be indicated for small tumors that do not cause harm.
- Surgical excision and/or medical therapy is recommended for large tumors or tumors that impede the horse's use.

APPROPRIATE HEALTH CARE

The appropriate health care will depend on elected therapy. For surgical procedures of small tumors and intralesional drug administration, the horse may be standing with sedation and local anesthesia. Surgical excision of larger and/or more invasive tumors may require general anesthesia and hospitalization. Combination of different treatment modalities and repeated treatments are usually necessary.

NURSING CARE

Specific nursing/supportive care is dictated from selected treatment modality.

ACTIVITY

Activity may need to be altered depending upon the treatment modality chosen, e.g., restricted activity is recommended during postoperative period.

DIET

N/A

CLIENT EDUCATION

High propensity for recurrence of tumor(s) at treated or new site(s).

SURGICAL CONSIDERATIONS

- The propensity for regrowth at the site of the lesion is a significant problem associated with surgical removal of sarcoid. Regrowth is closely dependent on the invasiveness, type and location of the tumor, and the ability to obtain clean surgical margins. Regrowth can occur within days of incomplete excision and is followed by rapid wound dehiscence and subsequent failure to heal.
- The use of various adjunctive therapies (cryosurgery, immunotherapy, hyperthermia, carbon dioxide, laser therapy, topical and intralesional chemotherapy and radiotherapy) appears to improve the overall success rate.
- The reported curative success rate for conventional surgical excision alone is approximately 82% compared to CO_2 laser (71%), cryosurgery (79%), interstitial brachytherapy using Ir (87%–94%), radium 226 and Co (>60%), gold 198 and Rn (92%), and intralesional administration of interleukin-2 and cisplatin (80%).

MEDICATIONS

DRUG(S) OF CHOICE

- Immunotherapy with intratumoral injections of mycobacterial products such as bCG (1 mL of bCG/cm^2 of tumor surface injected up to 6 times at 2- to 4-week intervals). This modality is mostly indicated for periocular sarcoids.
- Intratumoral therapy with chemotherapeutic drugs may be useful in some cases. These drugs include bleomycin (5 mg/20 mL sterile water; 1 mm solution/10-mm-diameter lesion injected 1–5 times at 1- to 2-week intervals) and cisplatin (1 mg/cm^3 tissue injected 4 times at 2-week intervals). Cisplatin can be combined with interleukin-2. Additionally, intratumoral administration of 5-FU (50 mg/mm^3 tissue injected up to 7 times at 2-week intervals) was reported to have a long-term resolution rate of 61.5%.
- Topical application of cytotoxic agents may be effective with daily applications; however, results are anecdotal and inconsistent. These drugs include AW-3-LUDES (5-FU/thiorouracil/heavy metal salts), 50% podophyllin in alcohol, 1% arsenic pentoxide in DMSO, 50% podophyllin and 5% 5-FU, XTERRA (Eastern bloodroot and zinc chloride), and Animex (blood root extract that contains *Sanguinaria canadensis*, puccoon, gromwell, distilled water, and trace minerals).
- Topical application of imiquimod 5%, an immune response modifier, was recently shown to be of benefit for different types of sarcoids with at least 75% reduction in tumor size in 80% of the sarcoids treated. Treatment involves once-daily 3-times-a-week applications until cure is achieved or for up to 16 weeks. Cleaning the tumor area prior to treatment is advised to remove dry exudate and allow better drug absorption through the affected skin. Information regarding the recurrence rate associated with imiquimod therapy is not available.
- Other therapies reported to have anecdotal benefits include intravenous and intralesional administration of heat-killed *Propionibacterium acnes* (EqStim); intratumoral administration of xanthates; autogenous sarcoid vaccines; and homeopathic drugs.
- Topical and/or systemic antibiotics may be required to manage secondary bacterial skin infections and to prevent infections after certain treatment modalities such as surgical excision.
- Analgesic/anti-inflammatory drugs such as the NSAID flunixin meglumine may be needed after surgical excision or adjunctive therapy.

CONTRAINDICATIONS

N/A

PRECAUTIONS

- A severe inflammatory reaction and discomfort may develop at the application sites(s) with use of some of the topical therapies, mainly with imiquimod therapy. Temporary treatment interruption or reduction in the frequency of application is needed in these circumstances.
- Anaphylaxis may occur with use of intralesional immunotherapy; however, pretreatment with flunixin meglumine and corticosteroids or diphenhydramine may minimize risk.

POSSIBLE INTERACTIONS

None reported

ALTERNATIVE DRUGS

N/A

FOLLOW-UP

PATIENT MONITORING

- Monitor for anaphylaxis after intralesional immunotherapy.
- Monitor for long-term, potential recurrence of tumor(s).

PREVENTION/AVOIDANCE

Fly control/avoidance is anecdotally reported to reduce incidence in herds with affected horses.

POSSIBLE COMPLICATIONS

- Tumor progression, depending on location, may lead to dysfunction (e.g., eyelid deformation, altered locomotion).
- Secondary bacterial or fungal infections, and rarely septicemia, may occur.
- Myiasis may occur at tumor sites, mainly on unsupervised horses.

EXPECTED COURSE AND PROGNOSIS

- Several factors affect prognosis of sarcoids, including tumor type and size, location, number of tumors, and invasiveness.
- Malevolent and fibroblastic sarcoids tend to have a poor prognosis.
- Horses with a single sarcoid carry a better prognosis than do horses with multiple sarcoids.
- Post therapy recurrence rates are usually high and vary according to the therapy used.

MISCELLANEOUS

ASSOCIATED CONDITIONS

N/A

AGE-RELATED FACTORS

N/A

ZOONOTIC POTENTIAL

Not reported

PREGNANCY

N/A

SYNONYMS

N/A

SEE ALSO

- Aural plaques
- Papillomatosis
- Melanoma
- Mast cell tumor

ABBREVIATIONS

- bCG = bacillus Calmette-Guérin
- BPV = bovine papilloma virus
- 5-FU = 5-fluorouracil
- MHC = major histocompatibility complex
- SCC = squamous cell carcinoma

Suggested Reading

Bogaert L, et al. Bovine papillomavirus load and mRNA expression, cell proliferation and p53 expression in four clinical types of equine sarcoid. J Gen Virol 2007;88:2155–2161.

Nogueira SAF, et al. Efficacy of imiquimod 5% cream in the treatment of equine sarcoids: a pilot study. Vet Dermatol 2006;17:259–265.

Scott DW, Miller WH Jr. Equine Dermatology. St. Louis: Saunders, 2003:719.

Author Sandra Nogueira Koch

Consulting Editor Gwendolen Lorch

SCRAMBLING IN TRAILERS

BASICS

OVERVIEW

- A horse that leans its shoulder, hip, or barrel against the side wall of the trailer or against an interior partition and moves its feet rapidly in a treading motion as if it were attempting to regain normal standing posture and balance; the treading motion can be any locomotor pattern and usually involves the feet slipping across the contact surface.
- Severe scrambling may involve the horse leaning against one wall of a trailer and moving its feet against the opposite wall, rather than on the floor, and may result in the fall of the horse.
- Can occur while the trailer is stationary or in motion
- Most cases are not caused by disease. However, impaired vision or balance may contribute.
- The horse may be unfamiliar with the confinement of a trailer or van or may have had an unpleasant experience or injury involving a trailer.

SIGNALMENT

Any age, sex, or breed

SIGNS

- Behavioral signs range from mild anxiety with locomotor involvement to severe fear responses with the corresponding involvement of organ systems.
- Signs of anxiety, active escape, and/or aggressive behaviors are seen in some cases.
- Physiologic signs may be consistent with sympathetic stimulation (e.g., tachycardia and vasodilation), increases in ACTH and cortisol concentrations, perspiration, defecation.
- Respiratory rate may be increased.

Physical Examination

Findings unremarkable, unless the horse has been injured by falling or hitting the sides of the trailer or pathophysiology is suspected.

CAUSES AND RISK FACTORS

- Innately, horses are claustrophobic.
- They desire to remain standing during stress-producing situations and initiate flight responses in an effort to maintain their balance.
- Scrambling involves a vicious cycle in which the horse perceives it is slipping, or actually slips, then rapidly moves its feet to regain its balance causing more slipping and more frantic attempts to regain an upright posture.
- Unpleasant experiences and injuries involving trailering can create anxiety about confinement in the trailer or van.
- Trailers that are too small, have slippery flooring, or are poorly designed and drivers with poor trailer driving skills (e.g., sudden starts and stops or sharp turns) can contribute to the problem.

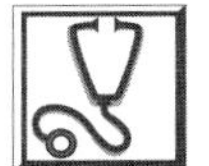

DIAGNOSIS

DIFFERENTIAL DIAGNOSIS

- Scrambling is usually behavioral in nature.
- Evaluate for normal vision, balance, and kinesis (ruling out confounding conditions, e.g., spinal ataxia, vestibular diseases, equine protozoal myelitis, myositis, lameness, etc.). If no abnormalities are found, the problem probably is behavioral.

CBC/BIOCHEMISTRY/URINALYSIS

If suspect a pathophysiology

OTHER LABORATORY TESTS

If suspect a pathophysiology

IMAGING

If suspect a pathophysiology

OTHER DIAGNOSTIC PROCEDURES

If suspect a pathophysiology

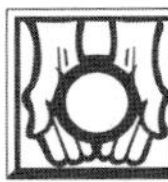

TREATMENT

Adjust the trailering situation so that the horse experiences less anxiety and is better able to maintain its balance.

Mild Problems

- Modify the trailer to make it easier for the horse to maintain its balance; generally, a horse that can spread its legs apart and brace against the movement of the trailer will not scramble.
- Rubber mats to make the floors nonslip
- Reduce the vertical width of the interior partitions so that the trailer is open from the horse' s stifle to the floor, allowing room for a wide stance, or either remove the interior partition or swing it to one side and secure it.

- Use a trailer with larger interior dimensions.
- Use a trailer in which individual stalls are situated diagonally to the direction of travel.
- Tie the horse's head so that it has enough range of head motion to help it maintain its balance but so that it cannot turn its neck around completely.
- The driver of the towing vehicle must execute slow, smooth turns as well as controlled accelerations and decelerations.

Severe Problems

- Problems in which the horse becomes self-injurious may require major modifications.
- The best treatment is to use an open stock trailer and turn the horse loose in the trailer; generally the more freedom the horse has, the less anxiety and the less scrambling.
- Most horses hauled loose in an open trailer quickly assume a position with their body diagonal to the long axis of the trailer and facing the rear; horses traveling facing the rear generally show less anxiety and maintain their balance more easily than horses facing forward.
- A trailer that has a center of gravity close to the coupling with the tow vehicle reduces the amount of sway, which would reduce occurrences of the horse losing its balance laterally.
- A tow vehicle and braking system designed to support and control the weight of the trailer also reduces lateral sway.

MEDICATIONS

DRUG(S) OF CHOICE

Tranquilizers may alleviate anxiety, but generally are contraindicated due to their influence on the muscle-skeletal system.

CONTRAINDICATIONS/POSSIBLE INTERACTIONS

N/A

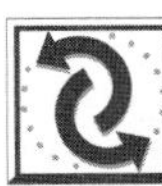

FOLLOW-UP

PATIENT MONITORING

N/A

PREVENTION/AVOIDANCE

- Ensure trailers are large enough to accommodate the horse comfortably.
- Use good trailer driving practices.
- Use leg protection (wraps, boots) on horses to reduce injury. Make sure trailer side walls are smooth and/or padded.
- Incorporate trailer loading in basic training procedures.
- Acclimate horses to trailer rides gradually. Initially, try very short and slow trips, on straight roads, and in safe, comfortable trailers.

POSSIBLE COMPLICATIONS

Injury caused by the behavior

EXPECTED COURSE AND PROGNOSIS

Depends on severity of problem and compliance with management changes

MISCELLANEOUS

ASSOCIATED CONDITIONS

Aversion to loading and enclosed spaces

SEE ALSO

- Fears and phobias
- Trailer loading/unloading problems
- Training and learning problems

Suggested Reading

Clark DK, Friend TH, Dellmeier G. The effect of orientation during trailer transport on heart rate, cortisol and balance in horses. Appl Anim Behav Sci 1993;38:179–189.

Creiger SE. Reducing equine hauling stress: a review. Equine Vet Sci 1982;2:187–198.

Author Cynthia A. McCall

Consulting Editors Victoria L. Voith and Daniel Q. Estep

SEIZURE DISORDERS

DEFINITION

Seizures are paroxysmal, transient electrical disturbances of brain function that have a sudden onset, cease spontaneously, and have a tendency to recur.

PATHOPHYSIOLOGY

- Disease processes that alter cortical brain function can result in clinical signs that include behavioral changes, altered states of consciousness, central blindness, and seizures.
- Seizures are caused by excessive neuronal excitation or loss of neuronal inhibition.
- Seizures in horses almost always have a focal onset that may secondarily generalize. In horses, this is generally secondary to trauma (which can have occurred a long time previously) or diseases or toxins that have an effect on neuronal function.
- Classic idiopathic epilepsy as seen in humans and dogs has not been reported in this species.

SYSTEMS AFFECTED

Central nervous system, trauma to other systems from seizure, systems affected by the initiating disease

GENETICS

Juvenile epilepsy in Arabian foals is likely to have a genetic basis.

INCIDENCE/PREVALENCE

Low prevalence

GEOGRAPHIC DISTRIBUTION

N/A

SIGNALMENT

There is no associated signalment for seizures in general. A benign form of juvenile epilepsy can occur in young growing Arabian foals of Egyptian lineage up to 12 months old.

SIGNS

Historical

A history of trauma or toxin exposure can be present, but often no historical associations can be made.

Physical Examination

- Seizures are classified as generalized, focal, or focal with secondary generalization. The type of seizure is often associated with the extent of the lesion.
- Diffuse cortical disturbances are often associated with generalized disease processes. The onset of a generalized seizure is often preceded by a short period of restlessness and disorientation (preictal period). Inappropriate chewing, teeth grinding, and other bizarre behavior may occur during this period. Subsequently, generalized muscular rigidity, recumbency, and unconsciousness can occur. Dorsocaudal positioning of the pupils (rolled back eyes), tonic/clonic paddling movements, and signs of autonomic activity, such as salivation, urination, and defecation are common. Between seizures, other localizing neurologic deficits may be evident.
- Signs of a focal seizure depend on the portion of the cerebral cortex that is discharging and the site of the seizure focus (the origin of the abnormal electrical activity): in horses, the most common expression of a focal seizure is involuntary movement of facial muscles. If the electrical discharge spreads through the entire cerebral cortex, a partial seizure may progress to a generalized form.

CAUSES

- Many disease processes can be associated with seizures. Trauma, neoplasm, cholesterol granuloma, hydrocephalus, cerebral abscess, thromboembolism, intracarotid injection, neonatal maladjustment syndrome, hypoxemia, moldy corn poisoning, hepatoencephalopathy, hypoglycemia, hyposmolality, hyperosmolality, and bacterial, viral, verminous, and protozoal encephalitides have all been associated with seizures.
- In juvenile epilepsy, no other disease process is evident.

RISK FACTORS

Exposure to infectious diseases and toxins, etc., associated with seizure

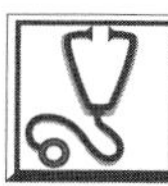

DIAGNOSIS

- Neuroanatomic diagnostic examination may help localize the site of a seizure focus.
- CSF analysis may be useful as well.
- Disease-specific tests may be useful.
- Magnetic resonance imaging may be useful to identify structural lesions.

DIFFERENTIAL DIAGNOSIS

- Any disease causing abnormal movements and loss of consciousness such as syncope (e. g., heart blocks), and sleep disorders
- HYPP and blood electrolyte abnormalities such as hypocalcemia may result in tremors and recumbency but are not associated with loss of consciousness.

CBC/BIOCHEMISTRY/URINALYSIS

No pathognomonic abnormalities

OTHER LABORATORY TESTS

- Dependent on associated disease
- CSF may reveal evidence of infection or neoplasia.

IMAGING

Skull radiographs or preferably computed tomography or magnetic resonance imaging if post-trauma.

PATHOLOGIC FINDINGS

Dependent on associated disease. Some CNS changes such as hippocampal sclerosis or ischemic neurons may be secondary to the seizures rather than due to the primary disease.

TREATMENT

AIMS OF TREATMENT

The goals of treatment should be to reduce harm to the patient and to protect those surrounding the animal.

APPROPRIATE HEALTH CARE

Horses may require supportive care until the seizures are controlled. Drug therapies will depend on the initiating disease.

Treatment of Status Epilepticus

- Diazepam—adults 25–200 mg IV as needed; foals 5–15 mg IV as needed
- Pentobarbitone—adults loading dose 12–20 mg/kg IV, maintenance 6–12 mg/kg PO BID; foals 2–3 mg/kg IV to effect

Blood concentrations should be performed initially after 3 weeks. Once effective plasma concentrations (8–12 μg/mL) have been reached, then assessment may occur after longer intervals dependent on the patient.

NURSING CARE

Treat any lesions secondary to trauma that occurred during seizure episodes.

ACTIVITY

A horse in anticonvulsant treatment is not safe to be ridden, and a useful guide is that a horse that has had seizures should only be ridden once it has been off medication and seizure free for 6 months.

CLIENT EDUCATION

Severity and frequency of seizure episodes may increase with time. Horse is a danger to himself and his handler during seizuring.

MEDICATIONS

DRUG(S)

- See above

CONTRAINDICATIONS

- Drugs that reduce seizure threshold (e.g., acetylpromazine)

PRECAUTIONS

Any drugs that may lower seizure thresholds

FOLLOW-UP

PREVENTION/AVOIDANCE

Dependent on the initiating disease process

POSSIBLE COMPLICATIONS

Trauma associated with the seizure episode and complications associated with other diseases

EXPECTED COURSE AND PROGNOSIS

- For most seizure conditions, the prognosis is fair for long-term management.
- Most juvenile epilepsy foals have a reduction in frequency to cessation of seizures.

MISCELLANEOUS

ASSOCIATED CONDITIONS

See above.

AGE-RELATED FACTORS

Seizures can occur at any age; juvenile epilepsy occurs in foals often less than 5 months.

ZOONOTIC POTENTIAL

See specific related diseases.

ABBREVIATIONS

- CSF = cerebrospinal fluid
- HYPP = hyperkalemic periodic paralysis

Suggested Reading

Chang BS, Lowenstein DH. Epilepsy. N Engl J Med 2003;349:1257–1266.

Hahn CN, Mayhew IG, MacKay RJ, The nervous system. In: Collahan PT, Mayhew IG, Merritt AM, Moore, JN, eds. Equine Medicine and Surgery, ed 5. St. Louis: Mosby, 1999.

Author Caroline N. Hahn

Consulting Editor Caroline N. Hahn

SEIZURES IN FOALS

BASICS

DEFINITION

• Abnormal movement or loss of consciousness associated with abnormal electrical activity of the brain • Partial seizures involve a focal area of the cerebral cortex, with clinical signs such as facial or limb twitching. • Generalized seizures involve the entire cerebral cortex, and result in generalized tonic-clonic activity and loss of consciousness. • Status epilepticus is rarely seen, but appears as multiple generalized seizures in succession.

PATHOPHYSIOLOGY

• Mechanisms of abnormal electrical activity in the brain include increased excitatory neurotransmitters and decreased inhibitory neurotransmitters. Firing of neurons under these conditions can lead to the spread of electrical activity over the entire cerebral cortex, leading to a generalized seizure. • Electrolyte abnormalities, such as derangements in sodium and potassium, can cause abnormal electrical activity, leading to seizures. Alterations in intracellular potassium and calcium concentrations can lead to neuronal firing. Rapid influx of sodium can cause rapid firing of neurons. Unlike in dogs, hypoglycemia is a rare cause of seizures in foals. • Perinatal asphyxia is the most common cause of seizures in neonatal foals. It is proposed that periods of asphyxia may be associated with cerebral edema and necrosis. Hypoxia leads to a breakdown of cerebral energy metabolism, causing dysfunction of the Na^+/K^+ pump, and subsequent leakage of calcium into the cell. Hypoxic injury also stimulates release of glutamate due to cellular depolarization. Glutamate binds to NMDA receptors, opening calcium channels, and this inflow of calcium causes neuronal injury through activation of proteases, lipases, and endonucleases. Glutamate also activates receptors that regulate intracellular G-protein signal cascades, leading to a further increase in intracellular calcium.

SYSTEM AFFECTED

Nervous—primary system involved

GENETICS

• Idiopathic epilepsy affects Arabians. A genetic link is suspected. • Lavender foal syndrome also affects the Arabians of pure Egyptian lineage—thought to be genetic, although the specific gene has not been identified.

GEOGRAPHIC DISTRIBUTION

Locoweed is most commonly found in the Midwest and Rockies. This is a very uncommon cause of seizures in foals.

SIGNALMENT

Breed Predilections

• Idiopathic epilepsy in the Arabian breed
• Persistent seizures in foals of Egyptian Arabian breeding affected by lavender foal syndrome

Mean Age and Range

• Foals with hypoxic brain injury and secondary seizures generally present when they are less than 2 days of age. • Trauma can affect foals of any age. • Foals with bacterial meningitis and systemic sepsis are generally less than 2 weeks of age. • Seizures secondary to congenital abnormalities usually occur within the first few days of birth.

Predominant Sex

None

SIGNS

General Comments

Generalized seizures are the most common form of seizure in foals, although focal seizure activity may be seen. Status epilepticus is seen uncommonly.

Historical

A history of dystocia, placental insufficiency or placentitis, and maternal illness should raise the suspicion of perinatal asphyxia as a cause of seizures.

Physical Examination

• Partial seizures can appear as facial twitches, rapid eye movements, or compulsive chewing or suckling. • Generalized seizures result in tonic-clonic muscle contractions. Paddling of the limbs, jaw movements, extensor rigidity, and opisthotonus are common. Depression is seen after the seizure (postictal). • Foals with hepatoencephalopathy or kernicterus will have icteric mucous membranes. • Signs of sepsis combined with seizure activity are suggestive of bacterial meningitis. • Abrasions and corneal ulcers may indicate a previous seizure.

CAUSES

Perinatal Asphyxia

• Dystocia • Premature placental separation
• Maternal illness (colic, endotoxemia)

Congenital Neurologic Abnormalities

• Hydrocephalus • Hydraencephaly • Idiopathic epilepsy of Arabians

Traumatic

Brain trauma

Metabolic

• Electrolyte abnormalities—hyponatremia, hyperkalemia, hypocalcemia, hypomagnesemia
• Hypoglycemia • Hepatoencephalopathy
• Kernicterus (secondary to neonatal isoerythrolysis)

Infectious

• Septicemia • Bacterial meningitis • Cerebral abscesses • Viral meningitis (EHV-1)

Toxic

• Moldy corn • Locoweed • Organophosphates
• Strychnine • Metaldehyde • Moxidectin

RISK FACTORS

• Dystocia, placental insufficiency, and maternal illness are associated with PAS. • Failure of transfer of passive immunity, poor environmental hygiene, and early infections (omphalophlebitis, pneumonia) are associated with systemic sepsis, which can lead to septic meningitis.

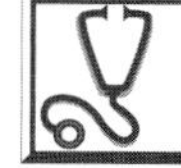

DIAGNOSIS

DIFFERENTIAL DIAGNOSIS

• Septicemia—Depression and weakness are often seen with septicemia. Septic meningitis can occur with generalized septicemia, and may result in seizure activity. • Colic/pain—Muscle contractions and paddling/flailing may been seen, but the tonic-clonic contractions typical of seizures are not seen. Gastrointestinal signs such as abdominal distention and straining are more typical of colic. Despite pain, overall mentation is generally normal during episodes of colic or pain. • Hyperkalemic periodic paralysis—Muscle fasciculations and prolapsed nictitating membrane are typical but do not progress to tonic-clonic movements or loss of consciousness. Occurs in Quarter Horse and Quarter Horse cross breeds—signs are not commonly seen in young foals. High serum potassium levels are often noted early in an episode of HYPP. • Syncope—Cardiac abnormalities (congenital defects or arrhythmias) can lead to episodes of syncope. ECG and echocardiography can help to rule out cardiac abnormalities causing syncope.
• Tetanus—Muscular rigidity may appear similar to seizure activity, but contractions are progressive and not "tonic-clonic" as with seizures. Usually occurs in foals >7 days

CBC/BIOCHEMISTRY/URINALYSIS

• Foals with septic meningitis may have neutrophilia and hyperfibrinogenemia on CBC. Septicemic foals may also present with neutropenia. • Kernicterus—Bilirubin levels are generally >20 mg/dL before neurologic signs are seen. • Hypoglycemic seizures are generally not seen until blood glucose concentrations are below 40 mg/dL. • Hepatoencephalopathy may be suspected if there are marked elevations in GGT, ALP, AST, and SDH.

OTHER LABORATORY TESTS

• IgG should be checked since neonatal foals with neurologic deficits may not have ingested adequate colostrum. • Blood culture should be performed to confirm septicemia in cases of septic meningitis.

IMAGING

• Skull radiographs to rule out fracture • MRI or CT of brain/skull to rule out skull fracture, subdural hematoma, intracranial abscess, and cerebral edema

OTHER DIAGNOSTIC PROCEDURES

• CSF analysis—collection from cisterna magna—increased protein and white blood cell count can be indicative of meningitis. Increase in red blood cells may indicate trauma or disruption of the blood-brain barrier.
• Electroencephalography can document abnormal electrical activity from the cerebral cortex.

PATHOLOGICAL FINDINGS

Post-mortem examination of the brain may reveal edema, necrosis, or abscessation. There are no specific pathological findings associated with seizures due to metabolic or hypoxic disorders.

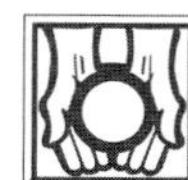

TREATMENT

AIMS OF TREATMENT

• Control seizure activity—Anticonvulsant therapy should be initiated immediately with status epilepticus or when there are multiple seizures in a short period of time. • Prevent additional seizures. • Prevent or decrease hypoxic-ischemic damage. • Antimicrobial coverage—Treat underlying septic meningitis, or provide broad-spectrum coverage for neonates at risk of septicemia.

APPROPRIATE HEALTH CARE

• Any foal with signs of seizure activity should have further evaluation to address any underlying cause. Initial treatment and monitoring require emergency inpatient intensive care management.

NURSING CARE

• Pressure sores or decubital ulcers are common in foals that are recumbent and paddling for long periods of time. Soft bedding, careful attention to keeping the foal clean and dry, and immediate treatment of any developing sores are important. • Eyes should be lubricated with Artificial Tears and examined for self-trauma/corneal ulcers. Head pads and helmets may be used for further protection.
• Plasma should be given intravenously if the foal's serum IgG is <800 mg/dL. • Global hypotension will lead to decreased cerebral perfusion and possible worsening of neurologic function. Intravenous fluids and pressors may be needed to maintain adequate blood pressure and perfusion. • If hypoglycemia is suspected as the cause of the seizure activity, dextrose should be administered immediately and the blood glucose levels should be monitored closely. • Respiratory function should be monitored carefully, and oxygen supplementation and ventilation started, if indicated by increasing arterial Co_2 and decreasing Pao_2. Elevated $Paco_2$ can worsen cerebral edema.

ACTIVITY

Foals may need to be restrained to prevent trauma during seizure activity.

DIET

• Foals with active seizures should not be fed. Normal mentation, suckle reflex, and swallowing reflex should be confirmed before nursing from the mare is permitted. If the foal is unable to nurse but is able to sit sternally it may be fed via nasogastric feeding tube. • If the foal is minimally responsive or if intestinal function is uncertain, parenteral nutrition should be instituted.

CLIENT EDUCATION

If a genetic or heritable condition (lavender foal syndrome and idiopathic juvenile epilepsy of Arabians) is suspected, owners should be informed of the possible genetic link.

SURGICAL CONSIDERATIONS

Craniotomy for abscess drainage has been described in horses.

MEDICATIONS

DRUG(S) OF CHOICE

For Seizure Control

• Diazepam—0.1–0.4 mg/kg IV
• Midazolam—0.1–0.4 mg/kg IV or IM, or CRI of 1–3 mg/hr in a 50-kg foal for recurrent seizures • Phenobarbital—5–20 mg/kg IV (maintenance, 2–10 mg/kg PO q12h). Start with the lowest dosage and increase until desired effect is achieved. Phenobarbital has a long half-life in foals and therefore increases in dosing should be done with caution.
• Phenytoin—1–5 mg/kg IV or PO

Antimicrobial Coverage

• Trimethoprim sulfa—20–30 mg/kg PO q12h; broad-spectrum coverage with good CNS penetration, but not the most appropriate if septic meningitis is suspected, due to risk of resistant organisms. • Cefotaxmine (40 mg/kg IV q6h) or ceftazidime (50 mg/kg IV q6h—third- generation cephalosporins with good CNS penetration; good choices for septic meningitis) • If septic meningitis is not present, but treatment of septicemia is needed, penicillin (22,000 IU/kg IV q6h) and amikacin (25 mg/kg IV q24h) may be used for broad-spectrum coverage.

Prevent Further Neurologic Damage

• Magnesium sulfate—50 mg/kg/hr as a 1% solution for 1hr, then decrease to maintenance dose of 25 mg/kg/hr • DMSO—0.5–1.0 g/kg as a 10% solution IV q12h • Mannitol—0.25–1.0 g/kg as a 20% solution IV, up to q12h to decrease cerebral edema
• Corticosteroids—dexamethasone sodium phosphate 0.4 mg/kg IV q12h has been used for early treatment of septic meningitis and CNS trauma, although the use of corticosteroids is controversial. • Thiamine and antioxidants have also been used for prevention of further neurologic damage, without empiric evidence of effect.

CONTRAINDICATIONS

• Acetylpromazine—may lower the seizure threshold • Xylazine—in foals with sepsis or PAS, may increase intracranial pressure and decrease cerebral blood flow enough to cause further cerebral hypoxia • Ketamine—increases intracranial pressure • Corticosteroids—High doses are contraindicated with septicemia.

PRECAUTIONS

• Higher or repeated doses of phenobarbital can cause hypotension, hypothermia, and decreased respiratory drive. • Mannitol should not be used if intracranial bleeding is suspected. • The use of corticosteroids with cerebral inflammation or trauma is controversial, and steroids should be used with caution if underlying septicemia is suspected.

POSSIBLE INTERACTIONS

N/A

ALTERNATIVE DRUGS

N/A

FOLLOW-UP

PATIENT MONITORING

• The foal should have 24-hr monitoring to detect further seizure activity and to prevent self-trauma during seizures or struggling. • Daily assessments of neurologic status help aid in making adjustments to the treatment plan and in formulating a more accurate prognosis.

POSSIBLE COMPLICATIONS

• Head trauma during seizure activity • Pressure sores • Corneal ulceration

EXPECTED COURSE AND PROGNOSIS

• Survival of foals with uncomplicated PAS is 70%–80%. Concurrent septicemia will decrease the prognosis. • Foals with head trauma have variable prognosis, largely dependent on the severity and extent of injury. • Foals with septic meningitis have a guarded to poor prognosis.
• Arabian foals affected by lavender foal syndrome have a grave prognosis. Arabian foals with idiopathic juvenile epilepsy will generally outgrow the seizure activity by 12 mo of age.

MISCELLANEOUS

ASSOCIATED CONDITIONS

• Perinatal asphyxia syndrome • Septicemia

SYNONYMS

• Epilepsy • Convulsions

SEE ALSO

• Perinatal asphyxia syndrome • Bacterial meningitis • Lavender foal syndrome

ABBREVIATIONS

• ALP = alkaline phosphatatse • AST = aspartate aminotransferase • CSF = cerebrospinal fluid • CT = computed tomography • GGT = γ-glutamyl transferase
• HYPP = hyperkalemic periodic paralysis
• MRI = magnetic resonance imaging • PAS = perinatal asphyxia syndrome • SDH = sorbitol dehydrogenase

Suggested Reading

Cornelisse CJ, Schott HC, Lowrie CT, Rosenstein DS. Successful treatment of intracranial abscesses in 2 horses. J Vet Intern Med 2001;15:494–500.

MacKay RJ. Neurologic disorders of neonatal foals. Vet Clin North Am Equine Pract 2005;21:387–406.

Wilkins PA. How to use midazolam to control equine neonatal seizures. Proc AAEP 2005.

Author Margaret C. Mudge
Consulting Editor Margaret C. Mudge

SELENIUM INTOXICATION

BASICS

OVERVIEW

• Acute selenosis almost invariably results from oversupplementation, via either treated feedstuffs or parenteral medications. • Plant species that accumulate sufficient selenium to be acutely toxic are so unpalatable that horses will usually starve rather than eat them. • Clinical signs involve the respiratory, cardiovascular, hematologic, and GI systems. • Chronic selenosis is most often associated with naturally contaminated forages or hay; the most obvious clinical signs involve the epithelium (hair, hoof).
• Research during the last two decades indicates that the condition described as "blind staggers" is, in fact, a potpourri of other maladies mistakenly ascribed to selenium toxicosis.

SIGNALMENT

• No known breed, age, or sex predilections
• Horses are somewhat more sensitive to chronic selenosis than ruminants and, thus, may be poisoned on pastures that do not affect cattle.

SIGNS

Acute Selenosis

• Can present as sudden death with few, if any, clinical signs • When clinical signs do occur, they progress rapidly. • Affected horses exhibit lassitude, muscular weakness, anorexia, and progressively worsening dyspnea beginning 1–24 hr after exposure. • Colic and diarrhea may occur. • Heart rate and respiration are elevated, pulse is weak, and animals frequently are cyanotic. • Fever, polyuria, and hemolytic anemia have been reported in some cases.
• Lethally poisoned animals usually become comatose and die with 12–48 hr.

Chronic Selenosis

• Sometimes called alkali disease • It usually requires chronic (30–90 days) exposure to seleniferous forages or pastures. • In rare cases, the condition may result from shorter exposures but still requires approximately 30 days to manifest clinical signs. • The most obvious clinical manifestations are bilaterally symmetric alopecia and dystrophic hoof growth. • Alopecia typically involves the mane and tail but, in severe cases, may involve other parts of the body.
• Lameness, erythema, and swelling of the coronary bands follow in a few days to weeks by a circumferential crack parallel to and just distal to the coronet and subsequent hoof separation. The damaged claw is displaced from underneath by new growth and subsequently sloughs or the damaged claw is not shed but remains attached, resulting in an extended, upwardly curled toe that places abnormal stresses on the appendicular skeleton. Affected animals become so lame that they cannot eat or drink and, thus, starve.

CAUSES AND RISK FACTORS

• Selenium- or vitamin E–deficient animals are more susceptible to acute selenosis.
• Chronic selenosis usually is associated with naturally seleniferous vegetation; as such, specific geographic localities are high risk.

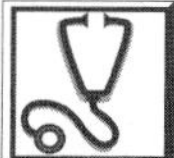

DIAGNOSIS

DIFFERENTIAL DIAGNOSIS

• Acute—heavy metal (e.g., arsenic) intoxication (clinical signs, lesions, metal detection in blood, urine, or tissues), endotoxemia (clinical signs and pathology, detection of endotoxin, presence of septic process), and blister beetle intoxication (detection of beetles in forage, clinical signs, lesions, detection of cantharidin in feed, GI contents, or urine) • Chronic—*Leucaena leucocephala* intoxication (clinical signs, detection of plant in environment, evidence of plant consumption), ergotism (clinical signs, detection of ergot bodies in feed, measurement of ergot alkaloids), laminitis (history, clinical signs, and physical examination), and thallium intoxication (clinical signs, detection of thallium in blood, urine, or hair).

CBC/BIOCHEMISTRY/URINALYSIS

• Hematology and serum enzymes in horses with acute selenosis suggest nonspecific damage to the heart, liver, and GI tract.
• Uncomplicated chronic selenosis is not generally associated with abnormalities.

OTHER LABORATORY TESTS

• Tissue selenium concentrations are less reliably predictive of damage than with other toxic elements. Consideration must be given to the form of Se ingested (organic selenium forms in forage versus inorganic selenium salts) when interpreting results. • Blood and liver concentrations <1.0 ppm usually rule out selenosis; the only exception might be a chronic case in which the first samples are not taken until several weeks after the onset of signs. • Higher concentrations may indicate excessive exposure but, by themselves, do not prove selenosis.

IMAGING N/A

OTHER DIAGNOSTIC PROCEDURES

N/A

PATHOLOGICAL FINDINGS

Acute Selenosis

• The most obvious gross lesions occur in the thorax and GI tract. • The heart may be pale or mottled and flaccid. • Petechial or ecchymotic hemorrhages are found within the myocardium and throughout the thoracic viscera. • The lungs are wet, heavy, and congested, with prominent septal edema and froth in the airways.
• Congestive heart failure is manifested as hydrothorax and ascites. • The intestinal tract may be hyperemic or hemorrhagic, especially after oral exposure, and usually is edematous.
• Hepatic centrilobular necrosis and renal proximal tubular necrosis often occur but seldom are recognizable grossly.

Chronic Selenosis

• Alopecia of the mane and tail and separation of the hoof wall • Histologically, hoof damage begins as ballooning degeneration and necrosis of keratinocytes near the tips of the primary laminae. Neutrophils and dyskeratotic debris accumulate around the tips of the epidermal papillae and in the lumen of keratin tubules.
• Alopecia results from atrophy of the primary hair follicles. Accessory follicular structures (e.g., sebaceous glands and erector pili muscles) are unaffected.

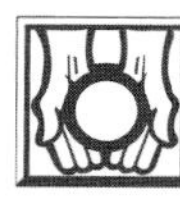

TREATMENT

• There are no proved therapies for acute selenosis. Supportive care for shock and antioxidants (vitamin E) may be helpful.
• Uncomplicated chronic selenosis has been successfully treated with palliative measures (e.g., heart-bar shoes, therapeutic trimming, analgesics and intensive nursing care).

MEDICATIONS

DRUG(S) OF CHOICE

• No specific drugs for treating acute selenosis
• Analgesics and NSAIDs are essential in keeping a horse with chronic selenosis both mobile and eating.

CONTRAINDICATIONS/POSSIBLE INTERACTIONS N/A

FOLLOW-UP

PATIENT MONITORING

N/A

PREVENTION/AVOIDANCE

• Prevention consists of avoiding excess selenium exposure. • Total dietary concentrations as low as 5 ppm of dry matter are potentially, but not always, toxic. • Avoid selenium-containing mineral supplements if possible in seleniferous areas. • Low dietary protein levels potentiate selenium toxicity, but it is doubtful that extremely high protein levels are protective.

POSSIBLE COMPLICATIONS N/A

EXPECTED COURSE AND PROGNOSIS

• Poor prognosis with acute selenosis
• Prolonged recovery with chronic selenosis

PREGNANCY

Most research seems to indicate that selenium is not teratogenic in mammals; the author has seen several normal foals born to mares recovering from chronic selenosis.

MISCELLANEOUS

ABBREVIATIONS

• GI = gastrointestinal
• ppm = parts per million

Suggested Reading

Raisbeck MF. Selenosis. Vet Clin North Am Food Anim Pract 2000;16:465–481.

Author Merl F. Raisbeck
Consulting Editor Robert H. Poppenga

SELF-MUTILATION

BASICS

OVERVIEW

- Biting at the flank, stifle, or chest
- The cause is unknown.
- Generally thought to be behavioral in origin
- In mild cases, only the hair is bitten; in more severe cases, the skin is torn.

SIGNALMENT

- Almost always a male, usually an intact male. Arabians are most apt to be affected.
- The median age of onset is 18 mo. Arabians and American Saddlebreds are overrepresented.

SIGNS

- Biting at the flank or, more rarely, the pectoral area, forelimbs, prepuce, or stifle. The biting may not break the skin, especially if the affected animal is a colt or a gelding, but a stallion may produce severe injuries to his skin or even underlying tissue.
- Geldings and mares are more apt to rub, roll, and spin than stallions.
- Most horses self-mutilate on both sides, but those who have a side bias turn to the right significantly more often. The horses frequently vocalize and kick out.
- The behavior may occur many times a day or as rarely as monthly. Bouts range from seconds to hours. The median duration is 1–10 min.

CAUSES AND RISK FACTORS

- The cause is unknown, but it usually occurs in isolated stallions and geldings in social groups with mares. It may be more common in males in contact with their dams. Almost all free-living male horses leave their mother's band, so it would be very unusual for them to have contact with their dam.
- Aggression may be a displacement behavior and that could lead to aggression re-directed to self.
- A stallion may see another stallion walk past his stall and, when unable to aggress against that stallion, aggresses against himself. The risk factors are male sex, sexually intact, in visual and olfactory contact with other stallions or the dam, but isolated from direct contact with mares.
- Horses aroused by the presence of other horses or, in severe cases, by any environment stimulation may self-mutilate.
- Seasonal changes, excitement, and/or anticipation of food can lead to an increase in frequency.

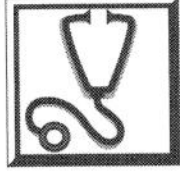

DIAGNOSIS

DIFFERENTIAL DIAGNOSIS

- Any pain-producing condition such as injury, internal parasites, or colic must be ruled out.
- Any pruritic condition such as external parasites or dermatitis must also be ruled out.

CBC/BIOCHEMISTRY/URINALYSIS

If physical examination warrants

OTHER LABORATORY TESTS

If physical examination warrants

IMAGING

If physical examination warrants

OTHER DIAGNOSTIC PROCEDURES

- A rectal examination and a neurologic examination should be done.
- A skin scraping should be taken.

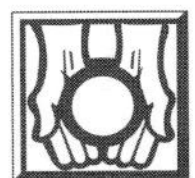

TREATMENT

- Castration of 10 horses was reported as curative in 3, substantially improve in 2, and slightly improved in 2.
- Change in the social environment. Allowing a stallion to live with a mare and away from other stallions will usually resolve the problem. Unfortunately, owners of valuable stallions are reluctant to allow a stallion to live on pasture with a mare because of the risk of injury.
- Donkeys or goats have been used as stall companions.
- A mirror might help, although the stallion may attack it first. The minor should be polished metal or some other unbreakable material.
- Removing mares, particularly his dam, from a gelding's environment may be helpful.
- Modifications to the diet and increased exercise can help. In one case reported, the stallion's ration was reduced from 3.6 kg of sweet feed and 3.6 kg of oats to 0.25 kg of sweet feed. Also, 4.5 kg of alfalfa was omitted from his diet and replaced with ad libitum coastal hay. He was hand-walked for 25 min per day. The self-mutilation stopped and, when the horse returned to the owners, round pen training for 20 min four times a week and a companion goat were enough, with the dietary changes, to resolve the self-mutilation.
- Applying a cradle may prevent the horse from injuring himself but does not change his motivation. In addition, he will still be able to kick out, which can be dangerous to humans. Blanketing the horse can reduce hair coat and skin damage.

MEDICATION

- An opioid antagonist, nalmefene, has been reported to reduce self-mutilation in a dose-related manner when given IM at doses of from 100 mg to 800 mg over a 4-day period to an Arabian stallion.
- Amitriptyline, a tricylic antidepressant, has been used successfully at a dose of 250 mg/day/horse orally to reduce self-mutilation. The author has treated several geldings successfully using chronic amitriptyline treatment. Tricyclic antidepressants have anticholinergic and antihistaminic properties. Their use would be contraindicated in patients with cardiac conduction abnormalities, glaucoma, seizures, and urinary and fecal retention problems.
- A wide variety of drugs have been tried therapeutically with mixed results. The sample size of horses treated in reports on the efficacy of medical therapy is small (1–12). Generally, the drugs are used in conjunction with other techniques, and if there is a response to drug therapy, it is transitory. Medications reported to have some effect on the behavior are topical applications (antiseptics, shampoos, parasiticides, anti-inflammatory agents, and taste repellents), ulcer medication, antihistamines, steroids, phenylbutazone, flunixin meglumine, synthetic progesterone, acepromazine, and fluphenazine decanoate.

FOLLOW-UP

- Environmental changes should reduce the self-mutilation within 2 weeks.
- Drug therapy may take up to 3 weeks. If there is no improvement in one month, another treatment should be tried.

Suggested Reading

Dodman NH, Normile JA, Shuster L, Rand W. Equine self-mutilation syndrome (57 cases). J Am Vet Med Assoc 1994;204:1219–1223.

Dodman NH, Shuster L, Court MH, Patel J. Use of a narcotic antagonist (nalmefene) to suppress self-mutilative behavior in a stallion. J Am Vet Med Assoc 1988;192:1585–1587.

Dodman NH, Shuster L, Patronek GJ, Kinney L. Pharmacologic treatment of equine self-mutilation syndrome. Intern J Appl Res Vet Med 2004;2:90–98.

McClure SR, Chaffin MK, Beaver BV. Nonpharmacologic management of stereotypic self-mutilative behavior in a stallion. J Am Vet Med Assoc 1992;200:1975–1977.

Author Katherine Albro Houpt

Consulting Editors Victoria L Voith and Daniel Q. Estep

SEPTIC ARTHRITIS, NEONATAL

BASICS

DEFINITION

Septic arthritis is infection of the articular structures, usually bacterial in origin, resulting in inflammation, pain, and effusion.

PATHOPHYSIOLOGY

• Foals are most commonly affected by hematogenous seeding of the synovium and subsequent joint infection. Growing foals have increased blood flow through the transphyseal vessels and to the joint capsule.
• Organisms involved are similar to those seen with systemic sepsis. *Enterobacter, Escherichia coli, Klebsiella, Salmonella, Pseudomonas, Acinetobacter*, and *Actinobaclillus* are common gram-negative isolates. *Streptococcus* spp. and *Staphylococcus* spp. are common gram-positive isolates. • Increased production of cytokines and migration of neutrophils result in a painful, effusive joint. Synovial fluid has increased protein and white blood cells, and the inflammatory and degradative enzymes in this fluid can eventually cause articular cartilage damage. • Traumatic joint penetration (wounds, lacerations, punctures) can also lead to joint sepsis, although this etiology is more common in adult horses than in neonates.

SYSTEMS AFFECTED

• Musculoskeletal—synovium, cartilage, bone, and surrounding soft tissues can all be affected.
• Neonates can have multiple systems (e.g., gastrointestinal, pulmonary, ocular) affected if systemic sepsis is present.

GENETICS N/A

INCIDENCE/PREVALENCE

Approximately 25% of septic foals are affected with septic arthritis.

GEOGRAPHIC DISTRIBUTION N/A

SIGNALMENT

Breed Predilections N/A

Mean Age and Range

Septic arthritis secondary to hematogenous spread is most common in foals less than 1 month of age. Foals can be affected as early as 1 day of age and foals with other systemic bacterial disease (e.g., pneumonia) may be affected at several months of age.

Predominant Sex N/A

SIGNS

Historical

• Frequent recumbency or reluctance to rise
• Inadequate ingestion of colostrum—mare leaking colostrum prior to foaling; delayed ingestion of colostrum • Prematurity or dysmaturity

Physical Examination

• Stilted gait or lameness; lameness may not be noted if the foal is mostly recumbent (as with severe septicemia) or if the lameness is bilateral.
• Joint effusion +/− heat, pain on manipulation
• Tarsocrural, stifle, and carpal and fetlock joints are most commonly affected. • Periarticular edema • Fever
• Decubital ulcers due to frequent or prolonged recumbency

CAUSES

• Septicemia (see Pathophysiology above)
• Penetrating wounds • Iatrogenic—joint injections (uncommon in foals)

RISK FACTORS

• Systemic sepsis is the most important risk factor in neonates. Pneumonia, enteritis, and omphalophlebitis are often associated with septic arthritis. • Low serum IgG concentration (failure of transfer of passive immunity)
• Premature/dysmature foals can maintain increased blood flow through the transphyseal vessels for longer periods of time, keeping the physis and joint at higher risk of sepsis.

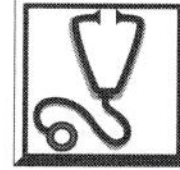

DIAGNOSIS

DIFFERENTIAL DIAGNOSIS

• Septic physitis—can occur concurrently with septic arthritis; radiographs can identify septic physitis. • Osteomyelitis—can occur concurrently with septic arthritis; radiographic changes may not be evident for 10–14 days.
• Trauma—fracture and/or soft tissue damage. Radiographs, ultrasound, and arthrocentesis can differentiate. • Foot abscess—sensitive to pressure or hooftesters. Abscess may be found during paring of the sole.

CBC/BIOCHEMISTRY/URINALYSIS

Hyperfibrinogenemia is consistently seen. Leukocytosis or leukopenia may be found on CBC, but these changes are not specific for septic arthritis.

OTHER LABORATORY TESTS

Serum IgG concentration—often low (<800 mg/dL)

IMAGING

• Radiography—Bony abnormalities are often not seen in the early stages of septic arthritis. Radiographic changes associated with osteomyelitis may not been seen for 1–2 weeks. Initial radiographs are useful for determining prognosis and as a baseline for identifying changes on follow-up radiographs.
• Computed tomography—likely to show osteomyelitis and/or physitis or bony abscesses earlier than would be seen on radiographs
• Magnetic resonance imaging—Cartilage and early bone defects will be detected earlier; it requires general anesthesia, and availability is limited to referral centers. • Nuclear scintigraphy—rarely needed for identification of septic arthritis but may be useful when the site of sepsis is difficult to localize. Radiolabeled leukocyte scintigraphy may more specifically detect areas of infection or significant inflammation. • Ultrasound of joints—Joint effusions and bony irregularity can help to identify likely septic joints or areas of abscessation. • Ultrasound of the umbilicus should be performed in neonates to rule out concurrent omphalophlebitis.

OTHER DIAGNOSTIC PROCEDURES

• Joint aspirates—cytology. Increases in WBCs (>30,000/μL and often >100,000/μL, with 80%–90% neutrophils) and total protein (>4 g/dL) are typical of septic arthritis. Protein will rise first in the early stages of infection, but elevations can also be seen with severe inflammation. Low pH is also found in the synovial fluid of septic structures. Normal synovial fluid has total protein <2 g/dL and WBC <300/μL with <10% neutrophils.
• Joint aspirates—culture and sensitivity. Sample should ideally be taken before the foal is started on antibiotics. Do not discontinue antimicrobial therapy in order to obtain a culture if the foal is septicemic or has a septic synovial structure. Treatment with antimicrobials should begin immediately after culture is taken, but culture results can help to guide therapy if there is poor response to the initial treatment.
• Blood culture can be very useful for identifying the cause of septicemia. • If septic physitis is suspected, needle aspirate of the abnormal physeal area can be performed.

PATHOLOGICAL FINDINGS

Early in the course of septic arthritis, there may not be significant gross lesions of bone or cartilage. Advanced septic arthritis can result in significant cartilage degradation and osteomyelitis/septic physitis.

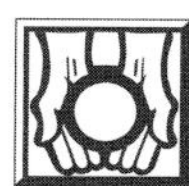

TREATMENT

AIMS OF TREATMENT

Joint Drainage and Lavage

• Primary treatment for any septic synovial structure • Via 14-gauge needles or teat cannulas—through-and-through lavage with several liters of balanced electrolyte solution (volume depends on severity of sepsis and size of synovial structure). Multiple lavages (usually 48 hr apart) are often needed.

Local Antimicrobial Delivery

• Intra-articular injection—delivers the highest concentration of antibiotics to the joint. Aminoglycosides such as amikacin (250–500 mg) or gentamicin are commonly used. Continuous infusion catheters have also been used successfully to deliver high concentrations of antibiotics to septic synovial structutes. • Regional limb perfusion—a regional vein is used for delivery of diluted antibiotic (commonly amikacin, for example, 500 mg diluted to 30 mL with saline or lactated Ringer's) with a tourniquet above (and sometimes also below) the septic structure. The tourniquet is left in place for 20–30 min. Regional limb perfusion may also be performed through the medullary cavity (intraosseous perfusion) in a similar manner.

Systemic Antimicrobial Treatment

• Broad-spectrum, parenteral, bactericidal antimicrobials are initiated immediately after fluid is sampled for culture. The combination of beta-lactams and aminoglycosides provides good coverage in most cases. • When culture and susceptibility results are available, antimicrobial coverage can be altered. If clinical response is not adequate, antimicrobials may need to be changed empirically. • Systemic antimicrobials are generally continued for approximately 2 weeks after resolution of the infection.

Pain Management

• It is important for foal to be comfortable enough to willingly rise and nurse. • NSAIDs are used for pain management, control of fever, and control of inflammation related to the septic structure. • Opioids may be used if additional analgesia is needed or if there are contraindications to using NSAIDs.

APPROPRIATE HEALTH CARE

Inpatient medical and surgical therapy

NURSING CARE

• Stall should be deeply bedded to prevent decubital ulcers. • Foals are often reluctant to rise and should therefore be encouraged or assisted to rise in order to nurse, ideally every hour. • Immunologic support—plasma transfusion if IgG < 800 mg/dL

ACTIVITY

Stall rest is necessary until the joint inflammation has resolved. Concurrent systemic disease may be the limiting factor in the foal's activity.

DIET

Foals should be encouraged or assisted to rise and nurse frequently (at least every 1–2 hr). Debilitated foals or those unable to stand for long periods of time require supplemental feedings via nasogastric feeding tube.

CLIENT EDUCATION

Management practices of good hygiene and ensuring adequate colostrum intake should be emphasized.

SURGICAL CONSIDERATIONS

• Joint drainage and lavage: Through-and-through needle lavage may be successful in the early treatment of septic arthritis. If there is significant fibrin or long-standing infection, arthroscopic lavage and visualization or arthrotomy should be performed. • Umbilical resection should be performed in cases of septic omphalophlebitis.

MEDICATIONS

DRUG(S)

Antimicrobials

• Initial broad-spectrum coverage often includes penicillin and amikacin, although third-generation cephalosporins may also be used. • Penicillin—22,000–44,000 IU/kg IV q6h • Amikacin—25 mg/kg IV q24h
• Ceftiofur—10 mg/kg IV q6h
• Ceftazidime—50 mg/kg IV q6h
• Cefotaxime—40 mg/kg IV q6h

NSAIDs

• Ketoprofen (1.1–2.2 mg/kg IV q12h)
• Flunixin meglumine (0.5–1.1 mg. kg IV or PO up to q12h) • Phenylbutazone (1.1–2.2 mg/kg IV or PO q12h)

Antiulcer Medication

• Ranitidine 6.6 mg/kg PO q8h or omprazole 4 mg/kg PO q24h • May be needed for foals under stress, especially if treated with NSAIDs. Septicemic foals may actually have alkaline gastric pH, so antiulcer medications may not be indicated in this group.

CONTRAINDICATIONS

Enrofloxacin should not be used as part of the antimicrobial regimen in foals.

PRECAUTIONS

• Aminoglycosides can cause renal compromise, especially in dehydrated or debilitated foals.
• All NSAIDs can cause renal and gastrointestinal damage, although ketoprofen is less ulcerogenic and has more renal safety than phenybutazone. • Chloramphenicol can cause aplastic anemia in humans.

POSSIBLE INTERACTIONS N/A

ALTERNATIVE DRUGS

• Gentamicin (6.6 mg/kg IV q24h) may be used in place of amikacin, however, there may be more bacterial resistance to this drug, and there may be more risk of renal damage.
• Chloramphenicol 50 mg/kg PO q6–8h or cefpedoxime 10 mg/kg PO q8–12h—useful for longer term therapy when an oral antimicrobial is needed • Imipenem (10 mg/kg IV q6h)—should only be used if guided by culture results.

FOLLOW-UP

PATIENT MONITORING

• Foals should be monitored twice daily for development of additional sites of sepsis (palpation of joints and umbilicus; monitoring for diarrhea, pneumonia). • If lameness and joint effusion persist, repeat radiographs (at 7–10 days) are indicated to determine presence of septic physitis or osteomyelitis. • Repeat joint aspiration to help assess response to therapy.

PREVENTION/AVOIDANCE

• Consumption of adequate amounts of high-quality colostrum • Good hygiene in foaling area • Routine measurement of IgG levels

POSSIBLE COMPLICATIONS

• Degenerative joint disease • Osteomyelitis

EXPECTED COURSE AND PROGNOSIS

• Response to therapy depends upon the severity of infection and the presence of concurrent systemic disease. Prognosis appears to be improved if therapy is initiated early in the course of sepsis. • Reported prognosis for survival ranges from approximately 40% to 86%. • Septic arthritis decreases the likelihood of racing for Thoroughbreds, and appears to prolong the period of time needed to start in their first race. • Multisystem disease decreases the prognosis for discharge from the hospital to approximately 50%. • Multiple joint involvement and infection with *Salmonella* spp. appear to further decrease the prognosis. Presence of concurrent osteomyelitis also decreases the prognosis (guarded).

MISCELLANEOUS

ASSOCIATED CONDITIONS

• Septic physitis • Septicemia • Diarrhea
• Omphalophlebitis • Pneumonia

AGE-RELATED FACTORS

Physeal infections appear to be more common in older foals, whereas synovial sepsis alone is more common in younger foals.

ZOONOTIC POTENTIAL N/A

PREGNANCY N/A

SYNONYMS

• Septic joint • Joint ill

SEE ALSO

• Septicemia, neonatal
• Failure of transfer of passive immunity

ABBREVIATION

• WBC = white blood cell

Suggested Reading

Smith LJ, Marr CM, Payne RJ, Stoneham SJ, Reid SW. What is the likelihood that Thoroughbred foals treated for septic arthritis will race? Equine Vet J 2004;36:452–456.

Steel CM, Hunt AR, Adams PL, Robertson ID, et al. Factors associated with prognosis for survival and athletic use in foals with septic arthritis: 93 cases (1987–1994). J Am Vet Assoc 1999;215:973–977.

Trumble TN. Orthopedic disorders in neonatal foals. Vet Clin North Am Equine Pract 2005;21:357–385.

Author Margaret C. Mudge
Consulting Editor Margaret C. Mudge

SEPTIC MENINGOENCEPHALOMYELITIS

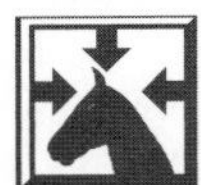

BASICS

DEFINITION

Septic meningoencephalomyelitis is defined as bacteria-associated inflammation of the CNS.

PATHOPHYSIOLOGY

Histologic meningoventriculitis often occurs with neonatal septicemia in foals, with overt neurologic signs being unseen. It is possible that the meningeal tissues become involved by infected mononuclear cells migrating to the CNS.

SYSTEMS AFFECTED

CNS

SIGNALMENT

Most often, young foals, but adult horses may (rarely) be affected.

SIGNS

Historical

Reasons for inadequate passive transfer of maternal immunoglobulin are important historical factors, as is a history of or current evidence of prematurity and other illnesses such as enteritis and omphalophlebitis.

Physical Examination

- Fever (not always present in neonates), lethargy, behavioral changes (e. g., aimless walking, somnolence, abnormal vocalization lack of affinity for the mare), etc., characterize the prodromal period of septic meningitis.
- Later, tactile and auditory hyperaesthesia over the entire body and a stiff and extended neck posture may be noted.
- CNS pain is often manifested by reluctance to move the head or neck and trismus (spasms of the muscles of mastication).
- Signs progress rapidly to loss of the suckling reflex, cranial nerve abnormalities, ataxia, paresis, and blindness.
- Recumbency, coma, seizures, and death quickly follow.

CAUSES

- Bacterial meningoencephalomyelitis is most commonly associated with hematogenous extension of a suppurative process or results from traumatic penetration of the CNS.
- The bacteria involved are those most commonly associated with neonatal sepsis.
- Organisms that commonly affect foals include coliforms, *Salmonella* spp., and *Actinobacillus equuli.*
- Adult horse meningitis has been associated with *Streptococcus equi* and *Actinomyces* spp.
- On only rare circumstances has disease related to *Listeria monocytogenes* been identified.

RISK FACTORS

Risk factors include those that are associated with septic conditions of foals—Maternal uterine infection, premature placental separation, poor hygiene during parturition, failure of passive transfer of maternal immunoglobulins, adverse environmental conditions in early life, etc., have all been associated with this condition.

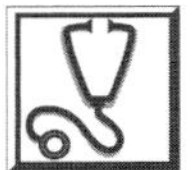

DIAGNOSIS

- Early diagnosis and aggressive treatment are essential for these animals to survive.
- Clinical signs alone obligate the initiation of aggressive therapy.
- A complete blood count may reveal a neutrophilic leukocytosis, but neonatal animals, especially foals, frequently have neutropenia with sepsis.
- In acute cases, CSF contains increased numbers of neutrophils and an increased protein content and in protracted and treated cases mononuclear cells often are prominent. Glucose content of CSF measured on a urinary reagent strip can be negative and is a good field test that is consistent with the presence of inflammatory cells and microbes, although hypoglycemia must be considered as a cause of this.
- Blood cultures are often positive and antimicrobial therapy should be guided by this and CSF Gram stain results and cultures.

DIFFERENTIAL DIAGNOSIS

Viral encephalitis, intoxication

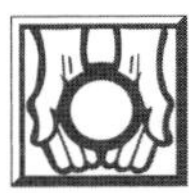

TREATMENT

N/A

MEDICATIONS

DRUGS

- In meningitis, the blood-brain barrier is damaged and most antibiotics are likely to get into the CSF and brain parenchyma. However, the organisms are often extremely pathogenic and resistant to many antibiotics.
- Third-generation cephalosporins, such as cefotaxime and moxalactam, may be worth using, although they are expensive. Ceftiofur is a third-generation–like cephalosporin that is inexpensive. Fluphenicol also appears to be a useful choice for meningitis due to its antimicrobial spectrum and penetration into CSF.
- The fluroquinolone antibiotics are probably quite efficacious but risk of induction of antimicrobial resistance in animal and human pathogens and the adverse effects on cartilage metabolism must be weighed with the use of fluoroquinolone antibiotics in foals.

• Antimicrobial administration cannot wait for sensitivity testing. Penicillin (22,000 IU/kg IV q6h), ceftiofur (2.2 mg/kg IV q8h), or cephazolin (15 mg/kg IV q8h) plus amikacin (21 mg/kg IV q24h) or gentamicin (6.6 mg/kg IV q24h) provides a good initial spectrum.
• Antimicrobial therapy should be continued for at least 7 days after resolution of clinical signs. Supportive treatment is essential as in any foal that is impaired. Caloric, fluid, electrolyte, respiratory, and thermic support may be required for a successful outcome.
• Seizures may be managed with diazepam, 5 to 20 mg IV, and repeated as necessary in 50-kg foals. Intractable seizures may require phenobarbital (10–20 mg/kg diluted in saline and administered slowly over 15 minutes IV q12h). The time to peak effect is 15–30 minutes. Pentobarbital and xylazine can be used when other drugs are not available. However, cardiovascular and respiratory depression is likely to occur with these formulations.
• Corticosteroids (dexamethasone 0.05–0.1 mg/kg or equivalent) should be considered when progression is rapid.
• Drugs to resolve secondary problems should be considered (e. g., antiulcer medications, ocular preparations, etc).

FOLLOW-UP

PATIENT MONITORING

Foals will need to be continuously monitored and supported. See Septicemia.

POSSIBLE COMPLICATIONS

The prognosis for foals with septic meningitis is poor. Even with appropriate intensive treatment, greater than 50% of affected foals die.

AGE-RELATED FACTORS

Young foals are most often affected.

SEE ALSO

Seizure disorders

ABBREVIATIONS

• CNS = central nervous system
• CSF = cerebrospinal fluid

Suggested Reading

Cherubin CE, et al. Treatment of gram-negative bacillary meningitis: Role of the new cephalosporin antibiotics. Rev Infect Dis 1982;4:S453–S464.
Hahn CN, Mayhew IG, MacKay RJ, The nervous system. In: Collahan PT, Mayhew IG, Merritt AM, Moore JN, eds. Equine Medicine and Surgery, ed 5. St. Louis: Mosby, 1999.
Smith JJ, Provost PJ, Paradis MR. Bacterial meningitis and brain abscesses secondary to infectious disease processes involving the head in horses: Seven cases (1980–2001). J Am Vet Med Assoc 2004;224:739–742.

The author and editor wish to acknowledge the contribution of Joseph J. Bertone, author of this chapter in the previous edition.

Author Caroline N. Hahn
Consulting Editor Caroline N. Hahn

SEPTICEMIA, NEONATAL

BASICS

DEFINITION

• SIRS—Systemic inflammatory response syndrome with at least 2 of the 4 following clinical abnormalities: (1) fever or hypothermia, (2) tachycardia, (3) tachypnea of hypocapnia, and (4) leukopenia, leukocytosis or left shift.
• Sepsis—SIRS with a source of confirmed or suspected infection • Septic shock—sepsis with hypotension and reduced perfusion refractory to fluid resuscitation • Bacteremia—presence of viable bacteria in the bloodstream
• Septicemia—Bacterial invasion into the bloodstream with systemic inflammatory response; bacteria may not remain in the bloodstream, but the persistence of bacterial toxins perpetuates systemic disease.

PATHOPHYSIOLOGY

• In utero infection and postnatal infection within the first week of life are the most common causes of neonatal septicemia. Bacteria can gain entry via placental infection, ingestion of organisms at birth, open umbilical structures or wounds, or the respiratory tract.
• Overwhelming bacterial infection or inappropriate response to invading pathogens can lead to sepsis. Gram-negative bacteria are most commonly involved, although the incidence of gram-positive septicemia is high in some recent reports. *Escherichia coli, Enterobacter* spp., *Actinobacillus* spp., *Klebsiella* spp., and *Streptococcus* spp. are common isolates. Anaerobes are an infrequent cause.

SYSTEMS AFFECTED

• Cardiovascular—Early "hyperdynamic" sepsis causes an increase in cardiac output, but this can rapidly progress to decompensated or "hypodynamic" sepsis, in which there is a decrease in cardiac output, blood pressure, and vascular tone.
• Endocrine/metabolic—Commonly disregulated with severe sepsis—relative adrenal insufficiency may occur.
• Gastrointestinal—The intestinal tract may be the primary site of infection (as with colitis and enteritis) or secondary ileus.
• Hemic/lymphatic/immune—Neutropenia and immune compromise are common.
• Hepatobiliary—Inflammatory cytokines can impair hepatocellular function.
• Musculoskeletal—Septic arthritis and septic physitis are common sequelae of septicemia.
• Nervous/depression—Infection can localize as meningitis (rare). • Ophthalmic—uveitis
• Renal/urologic—renal insufficiency secondary to hypoperfusion or direct damage by inflammatory cytokines. Nephritis has been reported secondary to *Actinobacillus* infections.
• Respiratory—Bacterial pneumonia secondary to sepsis occurs most often via hematogenous spread.

GENETICS

There does not appear to be a genetic predisposition to sepsis, although it is possible that there may be genetic polymorphisms that help determine the response to bacterial and inflammatory insults, as is seen in humans.

INCIDENCE/PREVALENCE

Sepsis is one of the most common reasons for neonatal foals to present to referral centers. It is reported as the cause of death in approximately 25%–30% of neonatal deaths.

GEOGRAPHIC DISTRIBUTION

Incidence of septicemia does not appear to have specific geographic distribution, although bacterial isolates may vary by geographic location.

SIGNALMENT

Mean Age and Range

In utero infection can occur; it is most common within the first week of life.

Predominant Sex

None

SIGNS

Historical

• Illness or stress in mare prior to parturition
• Placentitis, vulvar discharge, milk leakage prior to parturition • Premature delivery or prolonged gestation • Dystocia • Foal has never nursed or was slow to stand and nurse.

Physical Examination

• Lethargy/depression • Decreased nursing; loss of suckle reflex • Fever or hypothermia
• Tachycardia and tachypnea—not always present in septic foals; in late (decompensation) stages, bradycardia may be present. • Injected mucous membranes; petechiation
• Late/decompensated sepsis—obtunded, cold extremities, cyanotic, weak pulses, hypoothermia
• Localizing signs—diarrhea, joint effusion, respiratory distress, uveitis, omphalophlebitis

CAUSES

• In utero infection • Bacterial inoculation via the gastrointestinal tract or respiratory tract
• Entry of bacteria via umbilical structures or wounds

RISK FACTORS

• Inadequate colostral intake or poor quality colostrum • Environmental contamination/poor hygiene • Maternal (prenatal) risk factors—systemic illness, placentitis, dystocia, premature placental separation • Prematurity and dysmaturity/prolonged gestation
• Immunosuppression due to viral infection or SCID

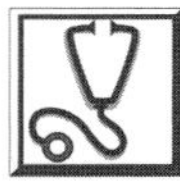

DIAGNOSIS

DIFFERENTIAL DIAGNOSIS

• PAS—fever, leukopenia, and localized infection are not seen with uncomplicated PAS.
• Prematurity/dysmaturity—Foaling dates and appearance (domed head, silky haircoat) help to differentiate from sepsis; there may be concurrent sepsis. • White muscle disease—recumbent with weak or absent suckle; muscle enzymes are significantly elevated; fever and neutropenia are not usually present.
• Congenital neurologic or cardiac abnormalities—may present with primary complaints of lethargy, depression, and lack of suckle

CBC/BIOCHEMISTRY/URINALYSIS

• WBC—most commonly leukopenia (usually neutropenia +/− left shift and toxicity), although can present with normal WBC count or leukocytosis. Older septicemic foals more commonly have a leukocytosis.
• Hyperfibrinogenemia shortly after birth is suggestive of in utero infection. • Hypoglycemia is common, although hyperglycemia can also occur. • Azotemia and elevated liver and muscle enzymes may be present depending on the severity of hypoperfusion and organ dysfunction.

OTHER LABORATORY TESTS

• Serum IgG levels—Some degree of failure of transfer of passive immunity is common in septic foals. • Blood cultures (aerobic and anaerobic) —aseptic collection; can confirm sepsis and help direct antimicrobial therapy
• Blood lactate—Normal foals <12 hr old have lactate concentrations up to 4 mmol/L, but this decreases to <2.5 mmol/L by 24 hr of age. Severely elevated lactate concentration on admission and at 18–36 hr appears to be a poor prognostic indicator. • Blood gas—Mixed metabolic and respiratory acidosis is common.
• Arthrocentesis with cytology and culture if septic arthritis suspected • CSF aspirate with cytology and culture if bacterial meningitis suspected

IMAGING

Radiography

• Musculoskeletal radiography if septic arthritis/physitis suspected • Thoracic radiography—Pneumonia may be seen; it can be normal in the very early stages of disease.

Ultrasonography

• Abdominal ultrasonography—detects signs of ileus and enterocolitis. • Ultrasound of umbilical remnants— Umbilicus may appear normal externally, but internal structures are commonly affected. • Thoracic ultrasound—detects pleural effusion, abscessation, or pleural roughening.

OTHER DIAGNOSTIC PROCEDURES

Sepsis score—historical data, clinical examination, CBC, and other laboratory data are scored to give a prediction of sepsis. If in doubt, treat the foal for septicemia pending results of blood culture.

PATHOLOGICAL FINDINGS

• Localized infection (pneumonia, septic arthritis, enterocolitis, etc.) is confirmed.
• Generalized petechiation and adrenal hemorrhage are consistent with, but not specific to, neonatal septicemia.

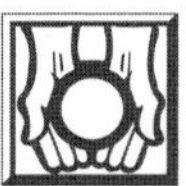

TREATMENT

AIMS OF TREATMENT

• Elimination of infection—treatment with antimicrobials should begin immediately and can be altered based on culture results and response to treatment. • Provide adequate immunogloblins. • Anti-inflammatory therapy—control inflammation, fever, pain, and effects of endotoxemia. • Antiendotoxin therapy in cases of gram-negative bacterial infection • Supportive care—Maintain perfusion, oxygenation; correct acid-base and electrolyte abnormalities.

APPROPRIATE HEALTH CARE

Inpatient medical management, and often emergency inpatient intensive care management

NURSING CARE

• Fluid therapy—needed to maintain hydration and perfusion, especially in hypotensive foals. See Fluid Therapy, Neonate. • Dextrose supplementation for hypoglycemic foals • Immunoglobulin therapy—transfusion with hyperimmune plasma for foals with IgG <800 mg/dL. IgG levels should be rechecked in septic foals as they often consume large amounts of immunoglobulin. If the foal is <12 hr of age, also supplement with colostrum orally or via feeding tube. • Oxygen therapy—if Pa_{O_2} is low. Mechanical ventilation may be needed if significant hypoxemia and hypercapnea are present. If oxygen therapy does not improve oxygen delivery, fluid therapy, use of pressors and inotropes, and blood transfusion to correct anemia should be considered. • Prevention of pressure sores—good padding; a "foal sitter" or frequent nursing care is needed to keep the debilitated foal clean, dry, comfortable, and in sternal recumbency. Eye lubrication is usually indicated in very debilitated foals due to the risk of corneal ulceration.

ACTIVITY

Activity is restricted (stall rest) in weak foals and those with musculoskeletal involvement.

DIET

• Enteral feeding via nasogastric feeding tube is usually needed initially in foals with a weak suckle reflex or an inability to stand and nurse adequately. • Use parenteral feeding for foals that are unable to remain standing or in sternal recumbency, or in foals with gastrointestinal ileus or enterocolitis.

CLIENT EDUCATION

Sepsis with multisystem involvement can be very expensive to treat and has a guarded prognosis. Clients should be aware of the costs and potential complications.

SURGICAL CONSIDERATIONS

• Joint lavage, arthroscopic exploration, and/or arthrotomy may be needed for treatment of septic arthritis. • Omphalophlebitis that does not respond to medical therapy may require umbilical resection.

MEDICATIONS

DRUG(S)

Antimicrobials

• Broad-spectrum parenteral antimicrobial treatment is initiated immediately and guided by culture results if there is not adequate response to the initial therapy. • A penicillin (22,000–44,000 IU/kg q6h) and aminoglycoside (amikacin 25 mg/kg IV q24h) combination is a common initial choice. • A third-generation cephalosporin with or without an aminoglycoside is another common choice. • Metronidazole (15 mg/kg PO q6–8h) if anaerobic infection is suspected

Anti-inflammatories

• Flunixin meglumine (0.5–1.1 mg/kg IV q12h) • Ketoprofen (1.1–2.2 mg/kg IV q12h) • Corticosteroids—Low-dose hydrocortisone has been advocated for human patients with relative adrenal insufficiency or for refractory septic shock. There is no clear evidence in favor of the use of steroids for treatment of septic foals. High-dose corticosteroid treatment is contraindicated in septic patients.

Antiendotoxin Therapy

Polymyxin B (3000–5000 IU/kg IV q8–12h)

Vasopressors/Inotropes

• Dobutamine (1–5 μg/kg/min IV CRI) for inotropic effects • Norepinephrine (0.1–1.0 μg/kg/min IV CRI) for vasopressor effects

Gastroprotectants

Sucralfate, omeprazole, and ranitidine may be used to treat gastric ulcers. Routine use of acid-suppressors to raise the gastric pH is discouraged in septic foals, as these foals already tend to have an alkaline gastric pH, and further alkalinization may encourage bacterial overgrowth and translocation.

PRECAUTIONS

• Aminoglycosides, NSAIDs, and polymyxin B should be used with caution in hypotensive and hypovolemic foals due to the risk of renal damage. Therapeutic drug monitoring of aminoglycosides can be very useful. • NSAIDs may contribute to development of gastric ulcers.

ALTERNATIVE DRUGS

Dopamine and vasopressin may also be used for treatment of septic shock.

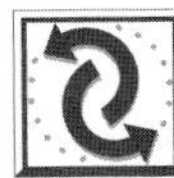

FOLLOW-UP

PATIENT MONITORING

• Intensive monitoring with frequent checks of vital parameters (q1–4h; may be required more often) is essential in the early stages of sepsis and septic shock. Foals with septic shock or organ failure may require more advanced monitoring, including blood pressure, urine output, and cardiac output measurements. • Lactate, blood glucose, renal parameters, electrolytes, and CBC should be monitored frequently to assess the need for changes in therapy and to help determine an accurate prognosis. Localized infections (septic arthritis, pneumonia, etc.) may develop during hospitalization.

PREVENTION/AVOIDANCE

• Clean foaling environment; reduce contamination of mare's udder and limbs. • Ensure adequate colostrum intake; administer intravenous plasma if IgG is not adequate or foal is at high risk of sepsis. • Umbilical dipping with dilute chlorhexidine or povidone-iodine (Betadine) may reduce the risk of bacterial entry or umbilical infection.

POSSIBLE COMPLICATIONS

• Organ failure (renal, respiratory) • Decreased athletic performance after septic arthritis

EXPECTED COURSE AND PROGNOSIS

Short-term survival is approximately 50%, although reported survival ranges from ≈30% to 70%. Gram-negative septicemia has been shown to have a worse prognosis than gram-positive septicemia. Multisystem disease and high sepsis score have also been correlated with higher mortality. The ability of the foal to stand and normal lactate concentration on admission are positively correlated with survival.

MISCELLANEOUS

ASSOCIATED CONDITIONS

• Septic arthritis • Omphalophlebitis • Diarrhea

AGE-RELATED FACTORS

Foals are most commonly affected in the first week of life.

SYNONYMS

• Bacteremia • Sepsis

SEE ALSO

• Bacterial meningitis, neonate • Diarrhea, neonatal • Gastric ulcers, neonate • Omphalophlebitis • Pneumonia, neonatal • Septic arthritis, neonatal

ABBREVIATIONS

• PAS = perinatal asyphyxia syndrome • SCID = severe combined immunodeficiency syndrome • SIRS = systemic inflammatory response syndrome

Suggested Reading

Corley KT, Donaldson LL, Furr MO. Arterial lactate concentration, hospital survival, sepsis, and SIRS in critically ill neonatal foals. Equine Vet J 2005;37:53–59.

Roy MF. Sepsis in adults and foals. Vet Clin North Am Equine Pract 2004;20:41–61.

Sanchez LC. Equine neonatal sepsis. Vet Clin North Am Equine Pract 2005;21:273–293.

Author Margaret C. Mudge
Consulting Editor Margaret C. Mudge

SEVERE COMBINED IMMUNODEFICIENCY

BASICS

OVERVIEW

• SCID is a lethal disease of Arabian or Arabian cross foals characterized by a complete absence of functional B and T lymphocytes. • The disease is inherited as an autosomal recessive trait—affected (homozygous) foals fail to produce antigen-specific immune responses, whereas heterozygous foals show no abnormalities. • Foals with SCID are unable to resist or recover from infections due to the absence of a functional immune system.

SIGNALMENT

• Only Arabian or Arabian cross foals are affected. • Clinical signs develop by 2–3 mo of age; most foals die by 5 mo. • No apparent sex predilection

SIGNS

• Affected foals appear physically normal at birth. • Onset of clinical signs is determined by the extent of maternal antibody transfer and the degree to which affected foals are isolated from other horses carrying equine pathogens; commonly occurs around 4–8 weeks of age. • As protective antibodies acquired from the dams' colostrum are catabolically eliminated, SCID foals become more susceptible to infectious agents. • The most common presenting signs involve the respiratory tract and may include nasal discharge, cough and increased respiratory sounds. • Additional clinical signs reflect alternate locations of infection and may include recurrent pyrexia (bacteremia), diarrhea (enteritis), lameness (arthritis), and colic (peritonitis). • Infection of the pancreas may result in proliferation of pancreatic duct cells, loss of endocrine and exocrine pancreatic tissue and an increase in connective tissue contributing to impaired growth and weight loss in foals with SCID. • Equine adenovirus is the most common pathogen isolated from affected foals and is found in up to two-thirds of affected animals. • *Cryptosporidium parvum* may also be involved initially and some foals present with severe diarrhea. • A range of infectious agents can be isolated from foals including those that rarely cause disease in immunocompetent foals (e.g., adenovirus, *Pneumocystis carinii*, *C. parvum*) and also more common equine pathogens (e.g., *Rhodococcus equi*). • Herpesvirus infections are rare in foals with SCID, although they are highly susceptible to most other pathogens. This may be a result of the natural killer cell function detected in SCID foals.

CAUSES AND RISK FACTORS

• SCID is due to a mutation in the gene encoding the catalytic subunit of the enzyme DNA-dependent protein kinase. • Loss of functional enzyme causes failure of V(D)J recombination and thus absence of mature, functional T and B lymphocytes. • About 16%–25% of Arabian horses are carriers and 2%–3% of Arabian foals are affected. • Reported in Arabian foals from Australia, Canada, the United Kingdom, Europe, and the United States

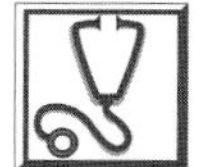

DIAGNOSIS

DIFFERENTIAL DIAGNOSIS

• A major challenge when diagnosing foals with severe infectious diseases is determining if it is a primary problem in an immunonaïve animal, or is secondary to an immunodeficient state.
• There are a number of primary, inherited disorders of the immune system in horses that must be differentiated from SCID. • Foals with selective IgM deficiency have persistently low serum IgM and a normal lymphocyte count and usually develop infections at an older age.
• Agammaglobulinemia is characterized by a complete lack of immunoglobulins but lymphocyte counts are often normal due to the presence of T lymphocytes. This disease has not been reported in Arabian foals. • Foals with failure of passive transfer (a secondary disorder) will also present in a transient immunodeficient state. This syndrome is characterized by the lack of transfer of maternal antibodies, which results in low serum IgG concentrations in foals >24 hr of age; lymphocyte counts will mostly be normal. In contrast, most foals with SCID have normal serum IgG concentrations after birth until >3 weeks of age due to successful passive transfer of antibodies.

CBC/BIOCHEMISTRY/URINALYSIS

• Immature or severely ill foals can be transiently lymphopenic; therefore, profound, *persistent* lymphopenia (<1000 lymphocytes/μL) in multiple absolute lymphocyte counts over 1–2 weeks should be observed for a presumptive diagnosis of SCID. • Total WBC and neutrophil counts can be low, normal, or high depending on secondary infections. • Many foals with SCID develop anemia late in the clinical course of disease. • Biochemistry and urinalysis usually are normal or reflect the organ system involved in infection.

OTHER LABORATORY TESTS

• The presumptive diagnosis can be aided by quantitation of serum IgM, which is absent before colostrum consumption or after ≈26 days in affected foals due to catabolism of maternally derived antibodies. • A PHA intradermal test is negative in affected foals, indicating an absence of cell-mediated immune responses. • Definitive diagnosis of SCID in an Arabian foal can be made by demonstrating the foal is homozygous for the defective SCID gene. • Blood or cheek swabs may be submitted for genetic testing (VetGen LLC, Ann Arbor, MI) to determine if the foal is free of, heterozygous (carrier), or homozygous for the defective gene.

PATHOLOGICAL FINDINGS

• On postmortem examination, small or grossly undetectable thymus and lymph nodes are suggestive of SCID. • Histopathological examination of these tissues reveals severe cellular hypoplasia.

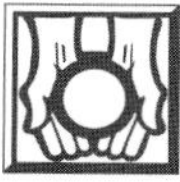

TREATMENT

• Medical management of foals with SCID is unrewarding, as death is inevitable. • Therapy is supportive and directed at acquired secondary infections. • SCID can be corrected by transplanting histocompatible stem cells from a genetically matched donor, but this technique is rarely practical.

MEDICATIONS

DRUG(S) OF CHOICE

Antimicrobials for treatment of acquired secondary infections

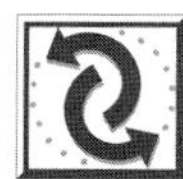

FOLLOW-UP

PATIENT MONITORING

Affected animals may be monitored for development of infection.

PREVENTION/AVOIDANCE

• The solution to equine SCID is to avoid the production of affected foals. • Prevention can be accomplished by DNA testing both the stallion and mare before breeding and only breeding those free of the SCID gene.
• Breeding two SCID gene carriers (heterozygous) will result in 25% of offspring with SCID, 50% as carriers, and 25% that are normal. • Breeding a SCID gene carrier with an SCID gene–negative horse will produce nonaffected foals, but with a 50% chance of being a carrier. If such a breeding occurs, the owners should be advised to have all offspring tested and heterozygous animals used for nonreproductive pursuits.

POSSIBLE COMPLICATIONS

Ongoing infections

EXPECTED COURSE AND PROGNOSIS

• Prognosis is grave, even with intensive conventional therapy. • Most foals die from acquired infections by 5 mo of age.

MISCELLANEOUS

ASSOCIATED CONDITIONS

Bacterial infections

AGE-RELATED FACTORS

Only observed in young animals

SEE ALSO

Immunoglobulin deficiencies

ABBREVIATIONS

• PHA = phytohemagglutinin • SCID = severe combined immunodeficiency

Suggested Reading

Perryman LE. Primary immunodeficiencies of horses. Vet Clin North Am Equine Pract 2000;16:105.

Author Jennifer Hodgson
Consulting Editors David Hodgson and Jennifer Hodgson

SHIVERS (SHIVERING)

BASICS

OVERVIEW

Classic shivering is a neurologic or neuromuscular disease characterized by involuntary jerky flexion of the pelvic limb and testicles as well as extension of the tail. In some syndromes, shivering is an expression of generalized hypertonia also affecting the thoracic limbs.

SIGNALMENT

Classic shivering is most often seen in draft horses, but other breeds may be affected.

SIGNS

Mild cases may be difficult to detect due to clinical signs occurring at irregular intervals. However, in most cases the clinical signs are characteristic. Clinical signs are usually noticed when an attempt is made to back or turn the affected horse or when the affected horse is forced to step over an object. The affected limb is held off the ground in a flexed and abducted manner while muscles of the upper limb and tail may quiver. After a short time, the quivering ceases and the affected limb and tail return to a normal position. The horse then appears normal, but clinical signs reappear if attempts are made to turn or back the affected horse. The difficulties backing into traces made this a disease of significant morbidity when draft horses were historically used.

CAUSE AND RISK FACTORS

The etiology is unknown but is likely to involve an alteration in the feedback loop between α-afferent and γ-efferent fibers. Some other diseases that include shivering as a clinical sign are equine polysaccharide storage myopathy and "stiff-horse syndrome."

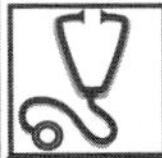

DIAGNOSIS

DIFFERENTIAL DIAGNOSIS

- Shivering should be distinguished from stringhalt, which also results in increased flexion but occurs during forward motion in which a degree of delayed protraction is also seen.
- Equine polysaccharide storage myopathy should have other clinical signs including generalized weakness, mild to moderately increased serum creatine kinase, and abnormal polysaccharide accumulations in muscle fibers.
- "Stiff-horse syndrome" is a recently recognized syndrome that is associated with generalized myotonia with severe muscle cramps. It appears to be related to a deficiency in the inhibitory neurotransmitter glutamic acid decarboxylase.

CBC/BIOCHEMISTRY/URINALYSIS

N/A

OTHER LABORATORY TESTS

N/A

IMAGING

- N/A

OTHER DIAGNOSTIC PROCEDURES

Muscle biopsy to rule out equine polysaccharide storage disorder

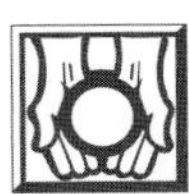

TREATMENT

No effective treatment is presently available.

MEDICATIONS

DRUG(S) OF CHOICE

None

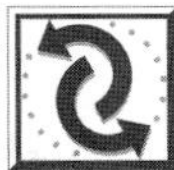

FOLLOW-UP

PATIENT MONITORING

Follow severity of clinical signs.

PREVENTION/AVOIDANCE

None known

POSSIBLE COMPLICATIONS

N/A

EXPECTED COURSE AND PROGNOSIS

Classic shivering is slowly progressive, and the prognosis for affected horses is poor. Polysaccharide storage myopathy may be reasonably well controlled with a consistent exercise program and a low-carbohydrate/high-fat diet. Too little is currently known about stiff-horse syndrome to offer good treatment advice.

MISCELLANEOUS

ASSOCIATED CONDITIONS

None

AGE-RELATED FACTORS

Adult horses

ZOONOTIC POTENTIAL

None

PREGNANCY

N/A

SEE ALSO

Polysaccharide storage myopathy

Suggested Reading

Nollet H, Vanderstraeten G, Sustronck B, et al. Suspected case of stiff-horse syndrome. Vet Rec 2000;146:282–284.

Valentine BA. Equine polysaccharide storage myopathy. Equine Vet Educ 2003;15:254–262.

The author and editors wish to acknowledge the contribution of Steven T. Grubbs, author of this chapter in the previous edition.

Author Caroline N. Hahn

Consulting Editor Caroline N. Hahn

SINUSITIS (PARANASAL)

BASICS

DEFINITION

Paranasal sinusitis is inflammation of the paranasal sinuses usually caused by primary or secondary bacterial or mycotic infection.

PATHOPHYSIOLOGY

- Infection of the paranasal sinuses may be primary, following transient, systemic bacterial infection (often streptococcal). Sinusitis commonly occurs secondary to periradicular infection of one of the four most caudal maxillary cheek teeth (Triadan 08–011); the tooth most commonly affected is the first molar (Triadan 09). Periradicular infection can be blood-borne, or it can result from idiopathic dental fracture, infundibular caries, or periodontal disease.
- Bacterial sinusitis less commonly occurs secondary to facial fracture or tissue necrosis caused by an expanding mass within the sinuses, such as a cyst, neoplasm, osteoma, or progressive ethmoidal hematoma.
- Generally accompanied by empyema that, regardless of its cause, may become inspissated. Inspissated exudate is found most commonly in the VCS.
- Mycosis of the paranasal sinuses is caused most commonly by *Aspergillus fumigatus* and less commonly by *Pseudallescheria boydii*, both of which are saprophytic fungi.
- All compartments communicate directly or indirectly with each other, so all may be involved.

SYSTEMS AFFECTED

Respiratory

GENETICS

None

INCIDENCE/PREVALENCE

- Worldwide
- Primary and secondary bacterial sinusitis is common. Mycotic infection of the sinuses is uncommon.

GEOGRAPHIC DISTRIBUTION

- None for bacterial paranasal sinusitis
- Mycosis of the paranasal sinuses is most common in warm, humid climates and is more common in Europe than in North America.

SIGNALMENT

No age, sex, or breed predilections

SIGNS

- The most common clinical sign, regardless of the cause, is persistent, unilateral, mucoid, purulent, or mucopurulent nasal discharge from the affected side. Mycotic infection frequently causes a sanguineous discharge.
- Horse may uncommonly be bilaterally affected.
- Flow of exudate from the naris may increase when the head is lowered.
- Malodorous nasal exudate is characteristically associated with dental sinusitis, an expanding mass, or mycotic sinusitis, whereas odorless exudate is more characteristic of primary bacterial sinusitis; malodorous nasal discharge can also occur, however, with primary bacterial sinusitis, especially if exudate becomes inspissated.

Historical

Commonly a complication of strangles (*Streptococcus equi* var *equi* infection) or may accompany signs of dental disease.

Physical Examination

- Common signs include epiphora, conjunctivitis, and enlargement of the submandibular lymph nodes on the affected side.
- Facial distortion and obstructed airflow are features of horses with expanding masses, such as inspissated exudate, within the sinuses.
- Oral examination may reveal evidence of sepsis of one of the caudal maxillary cheek teeth, such as infundibular caries or fracture, or a diastema between two of the caudal cheek teeth.

CAUSES

Unknown

RISK FACTORS

- Horses 1–5 years old are most susceptible to *Streptococcus equi* var *equi* infection and, therefore, are most susceptible to primary bacterial sinusitis.
- The incidence of infundibular caries and periodontal disease, both of which are causes of periradicular dental disease, increases with age, as does the incidence of neoplasia.
- Horses that are confined to a stable or have recently undergone surgery of the paranasal sinuses are most at risk of developing mycotic infection of the paranasal sinuses.

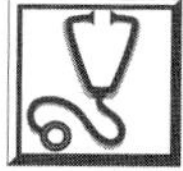

DIAGNOSIS

DIFFERENTIAL DIAGNOSIS

- Other sources of purulent exudate at the nares are the nasal cavities, guttural pouches, nasopharynx, and lungs.
- Nasal discharge caused by disease caudal to the caudal edge of the nasal septum is usually bilateral.
- Inspissated exudate in the VCS may cause clinical signs characteristic of those caused by any mass in the paranasal sinuses.

CBC/BIOCHEMISTRY/URINALYSIS

Usually normal

OTHER LABORATORY TESTS

N/A

IMAGING

- The different radiodensities of teeth and paranasal sinuses necessitate multiple radiographs with different factors of exposure and positions of the tube head to clearly demonstrate detail of the paranasal sinuses and dental structures. The cassette should be positioned on the affected side of the skull.
- Lateral and dorsoventral radiographs usually show increased opacity of the affected sinuses. Horizontal fluid lines in the sinuses generally are visible during examination of lateral radiographs of the skull taken with the horse standing. Obtaining radiographs after exudate is lavaged from the sinuses may be necessary to demonstrate masses.
- The VCS is the usual site of inspissated exudate. Identification of a soft-tissue density dorsal to the maxillary molars on a lateral radiograph and medial to those teeth on a dorsoventral radiograph is evidence of a mass, usually inspissated exudate, in the VCS. Dorsoventral radiographs may demonstrate medial deviation of the ventral concha by insipissated exudate.
- To examine the roots of the maxillary teeth, the cassette is positioned on the affected side. The tube is placed dorsally, angled 30° ventrally, and centered on the rostral end of the facial crest.
- Periradicular disease of teeth whose roots reside within the paranasal sinuses can be recognized radiographically with confidence in only half of the cases.
- The presence of apical infection can sometime be confirmed by gamma scintigraphy, computed tomography, or magnetic resonance imaging.

OTHER DIAGNOSTIC PROCEDURES

- Percussion may identify loss of resonance within the sinuses, especially if sinuses are completely filled with fluid or tissue.
- The oral cavity should be examined for dental abnormalities.
- Nasal endoscopy may reveal exudate discharging from the middle meatus at the drainage angle or distortion of one or both conchae caused by an expanding mass, such as inspissated exudate, within the sinuses.
- The sinuses can be examined endoscopically for the presence of exudate or mycotic plaques through trephine holes. The VCS can be examined through a portal in the conchofrontal or caudal maxillary sinus, but only after the maxillary septum has been perforated with an instrument.

PATHOLOGIC FINDINGS

- Cytological examination and culture of exudate obtained by sinocentesis may help to determine whether sinusitis is caused by primary infection or is secondary to other disease. If infection is caused by periradicular dental disease, plant material sometimes can be identified and multiple bacterial colonies cultured. Identification of a single bacterial organism, usually a β-hemolytic *Streptococcus* sp., during cytological examination or culture is a good indication that the infection is primary, but a mixed bacterial population is sometimes cultured, obscuring the etiological agent responsible for initiating the primary infection.

• The cause of sinusitis is determined to be mycotic based on histological observation of fungal hyphae and conidiophores in the plaques removed from the sinuses and culture of a heavy and pure growth of potentially pathogenic fungi from these plaques.

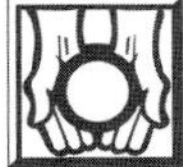

TREATMENT

AIMS OF TREATMENT

The aim of treatment for primary sinusitis is to resolve infection by appropriate antimicrobial therapy and by evacuation of exudate. The aim of treatment for secondary sinusitis is to resolve the cause of infection.

APPROPRIATE HEALTH CARE

• For noninspissated empyema of the paranasal sinuses caused by primary bacterial infection, lavage of the sinuses and parenteral administration of an antimicrobial drug are indicated. Bacterial organisms commonly isolated are frequently sensitive to penicillin.
• The paranasal sinuses are usually lavaged through an ingress portal created in the conchofrontal or caudal maxillary sinus; the rostral maxillary and VCS are most effectively lavaged, however, through a portal created in the rostral maxillary sinus. The nasomaxillary aperture provides egress of the lavage solution.
• Inspissated purulent exudate in the VCS should be suspected when primary bacterial sinusitis does not resolve with lavage and parenteral administration of an antimicrobial drug; horses with inspissated exudate in the VCS require surgical removal of exudate.
• For primary mycotic sinusitis, lavage of the affected sinuses with an antifungal agent (e.g., itraconazole, fluconazole, enilconazole, miconazole, ketoconazole, natamycin, and clotrimazole) for one to two weeks is indicated.
• For bacterial or mycotic sinusitis secondary to other diseases (e.g., periradicular dental disease or a mass in the sinuses), eliminating the cause of the sinusitis, often by surgical intervention, is indicated. Resolution of sinusitis secondary to periradicular dental infection usually necessitates removal of the infected tooth.

NURSING CARE

NSAIDs, such as phenylbutazone or flunixin meglumine, may be required to reduce discomfort.

ACTIVITY

Exercise should be restricted for at least several weeks after clinical signs of disease have resolved.

DIET

No change required.

CLIENT EDUCATION

N/A

SURGICAL CONSIDERATIONS

• Inspissated exudate is most easily removed from the VCS through a frontonasal osteoplastic flap, which often can be created with the horse standing. The maxillary septum must be perforated to expose the VCS.
• An infected cheek tooth can be removed by extraction performed per os, by repulsion or by lateral buccotomy. Lateral buccotomy cannot be performed on the last three cheek teeth. Endodontic therapy is often ineffective in resolving dental infection.
• Extracting an infected tooth per os is usually accompanied by few complications and can be accomplished with the horse standing, whereas repelling a tooth is often accompanied by serious complications and is best accomplished with the horse anesthetized.

MEDICATIONS

DRUG(S) OF CHOICE

• Primary bacterial empyema—parenteral administration of an antimicrobial drug to which streptococci are susceptible, usually a β-lactam antibiotic (e.g., procaine penicillin 20,000–50,000 IU/kg IM q12h) in conjunction with lavage of the sinuses.
• Sinusitis secondary to other disease—antimicrobial drugs, either broad spectrum or based on culture and sensitivity results.
• Ancillary treatment for mycotic infection includes systemic administration of sodium iodide (67 mg/kg IV once daily) for 2–5 days and then oral administration of organic iodide (ethylenediamine dihydroiodide) (40 mg/kg PO once daily) indefinitely.

CONTRAINDICATIONS

Sodium iodide and organic iodide should not be administered to pregnant mares.

PRECAUTIONS

Side effects of systemic treatment with sodium iodide or organic iodide include excessive lacrimation, nonpruritic generalized alopecia, a nonproductive cough, abortion, or birth of a hypothyroid foal.

POSSIBLE INTERACTIONS

None

ALTERNATIVE DRUGS

None

FOLLOW-UP

PATIENT MONITORING

• Resolution of abnormal nasal discharge, especially after antimicrobial therapy has been discontinued, indicates resolution of infection.
• Distortion of the turbinates into the nasal passage caused by an expanding mass gradually resolves over several weeks after removal of the mass.
• Increased opacity of the sinuses may be observed radiographically long after the disease has resolved.

PREVENTION/AVOIDANCE

• Vaccination of susceptible horses against *Streptococcus equi* on farms where strangles is endemic may decrease the incidence of primary paranasal sinusitis.
• Routine dental care may decrease the incidence of dental disease that leads to periradicular infection and associated dental sinusitis.

POSSIBLE COMPLICATIONS

• Unsuccessful treatment for primary paranasal sinusitis can usually be attributed to retention of inspissated exudate, usually in the VCS.
• Unsuccessful treatment for dental sinusitis can usually be attributed to persistent alveolar infection caused by retention of osseous or dental sequestra within the alveolus or less commonly, from retention of inspissated exudate in the VCS.

EXPECTED COURSE AND PROGNOSIS

The long-term prognosis for horses affected by primary or secondary dental sinusitis is good, provided that the horse receives proper treatment.

MISCELLANEOUS

ASSOCIATED CONDITIONS

Horses affected by primary sinusitis caused by *S. equi* infection may also have additional sites of infection, including the guttural pouch.

AGE-RELATED FACTORS

N/A

ZOONOTIC POTENTIAL

N/A

PREGNANCY

N/A

SEE ALSO

• Guttural pouch empyema
• Purulent nasal discharge

ABBREVIATION

• VCS = ventral conchal sinus

Suggested Reading

Tremaine H, Freeman DE. In: McGorum B, Dixon P, Robinson E, Schumacher J, eds. Equine Respiratory Medicine and Surgery. Oxford: Elsevier Science, 2006:393–407.

Author Jim Schumacher
Consulting Editor Daniel Jean

SLAFRAMINE TOXICOSIS

BASICS

OVERVIEW

• Slaframine, or slobber factor as it is commonly called, is a mycotoxin produced by *Rhizoctonia leguminicola*.
• As the name indicates, this fungus is a pathogen of legumes, usually red clover (*Trifolium pratense*).
Other less likely substrates include alfalfa (*Medicago sativa*) and ladino or white clover (*Trifolium repens*). Slaframine has a high affinity for the muscarinic receptor subtype responsible for regulation of secretory glands. It has been suggested that the slobbers syndrome involves other physiologically active compounds, such as swainsonine, that are also produced by *R. leguminicola*.

SIGNALMENT

All horses are susceptible. There are no breed, age, or sex predispositions.

SIGNS

• Onset of hypersalivation within hours of ingestion is the hallmark of this condition. Polydipsia is a consequence of fluid loss.
• Less commonly reported signs include anorexia, excessive lacrimation, polyuria, and diarrhea.

CAUSES AND RISK FACTORS

• Black patch is the fungal disease of clover associated with slaframine production. The plant pathogen, *R. leguminicola*, is most likely to grow on clover during wet, humid weather.
• A moist, humid environment with a temperature range of 25°–29° C and a substrate pH of 5.9–7.5 is needed to support growth. The fungus appears as dark spots or concentric rings on diseased leaves and stems. Contaminated seed spreads the fungus. Consumption of infected pastures or second-cutting forage is usually associated with intoxication.

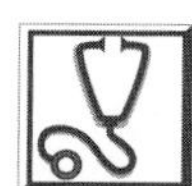

DIAGNOSIS

DIFFERENTIAL DIAGNOSIS

• Excessive salivation can be induced by dental disease, stomatitis, or foreign objects lodged in the pharynx.
• Ptyalism may result from inflammation of the oral mucosa or salivary glands by penetrating wounds or plant awns such as foxtail.
• Hypersalivation seen in organophosphate and carbamate poisoning is associated with more life-threatening signs of dyspnea, colic, and diarrhea.

CBC/BIOCHEMISTRY/URINALYSIS

N/A

OTHER LABORATORY TESTS

• Diagnosis is based on rapid onset of profuse salivation associated with consumption of legume forage infected with *R. leguminicola*.
• Chemical analysis of suspect forage will confirm the presence of slaframine.
• Plant pathologists can confirm black patch disease on suspect forages.

IMAGING

N/A

DIAGNOSTIC PROCEDURES

N/A

PATHOLOGICAL FINDINGS

N/A

TREATMENT

Although specific antidotes are not available or in most cases necessary, introduction of uncontaminated forage will resolve the condition in 1–3 days.

MEDICATIONS

DRUGS

Response to atropine is questionable. Empirical evidence suggests that atropine given prior to exposure will prevent hypersalivation, although administration after the onset of hypersalivation is not particularly effective. Atropine should be used cautiously in horses.

CONTRAINDICATIONS/POSSIBLE INTERACTIONS

N/A

FOLLOW-UP

Resolution of the problem occurs when horses are provided uncontaminated forage.

PATIENT MONITORING

N/A

PREVENTION/ AVOIDANCE

Storage of contaminated hay for several months results in significant reduction in toxicity. Red clover hay containing 50–100 ppm slaframine contained about 7 ppm after 10 mo of storage. Reseeding with newer clover varieties that are resistant to *Rhizoctonia* infection can solve persistent problems.

POSSIBLE COMPLICATIONS

N/A

COURSE AND PROGNOSIS

Removal of contaminated forage results in uncomplicated recovery in 1–3 days.

MISCELLANEOUS

ASSOCIATED CONDITIONS, AGE-RELATED FACTORS, ZOONOTIC POTENTIAL, PREGNANCY

N/A

ABBREVIATION

• ppm = parts per million

Suggested Reading

Croom WJ, Hagler WM, Froetschel MA, Johnson AD. The involvement of slaframine and swainsonine in slobbers syndrome: a review. J Anim Sci 1995;73:1499–1508.

Author Stan W. Casteel
Consulting Editor Robert H. Poppenga

SMALL STRONGYLE INFESTATION

BASICS

OVERVIEW

Cyathostomes are acquired by horses on pasture and the larvae undergo a period of weeks to months of arrested development in the mucosa and/or submucosa of the large intestine and cecum. The clinical manifestation of disease is primarily due to the simultaneous emergence of large numbers (millions) of previously "encysted" (hypobiotic) larvae. Adults within the intestinal lumen may also cause some damage by digesting small plugs of mucosa, resulting in pinpoint or coalescing ulcer formation. Seasonal patterns of severe clinical disease associated with larval emergence have been reported in Europe and North America. In Europe, most cases occur in late winter and early spring, whereas in Canada, most cases have been seen in the fall and early winter.

PATHOPHYSIOLOGY

Cyathostome eggs passed in the feces hatch and develop on pasture to the L_3 stage in 1–3 weeks. Ingested L_3 and L_4 larvae penetrate the intestinal mucosa of the cecum and large colon, with eventual intramural "encapsulation. "Larvae may remain in a hypobiotic state for varying periods of time before emerging to mature into adults in the intestinal lumen. The prepatent period may vary between 5 weeks and 20 mo. The initial host inflammatory response to encysted larvae includes a granulomatous reaction. Additional lesions include inflammation, edema, and pinpoint ulcerations or regional areas of denuded mucosa in the cecum and large colon. There may be catarrhal, hemorrhagic, or fibrinous enteritis with multiple nodules on the mucosal surface from larval cysts or visible larvae beneath the mucosal wall. Adult parasites (6–20 mm) may be present in large numbers within the intestinal lumen.

SIGNALMENT

All ages can be infested, although young (6 mo to 3 years of age) and naïve animals or geriatric horses are more susceptible.

SIGNS

• Diarrhea, anorexia, and dramatic weight loss—might be seasonal, continuous, acute, chronic, and in varying degrees and combinations • Recurrent colic, transient fever of unknown origin, episodic diarrhea, ventral abdominal edema, anemia, and generalized slow debilitation may also occur.

CAUSES AND RISK FACTORS

• High stocking density and overgrazing of pastures lead to an extremely high level of contamination with larvae. • Infective-stage larvae and eggs can remain viable in the environment for extended periods of time. Dry, hot weather often destroys hatched larvae. Adult horses may shed high numbers of cyathostome eggs.

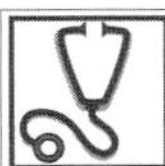

DIAGNOSIS

DIFFERENTIAL DIAGNOSIS

Differential diagnoses includes other causes of diarrhea. For ill thrift, include other GI parasites as well as chronic infection, abscessation, dental disease, or protein-caloric malnutrition. Colic is a nonspecific clinical sign associated with multiple causes.

BIOCHEMISTRY/CBC

Hypoalbuminemia and microcytic anemia are often present. Transient systemic eosinophilia is rare.

OTHER LABORATORY TESTS

Abdominocentesis and fecal culture are generally unrewarding but might be of value to evaluate other differential diagnoses.

IMAGING

Abdominal ultrasound may be useful to differentiate thickening of small intestine due to other reasons.

DIAGNOSTIC PROCEDURES

Fecal flotation for specific egg count per gram of feces

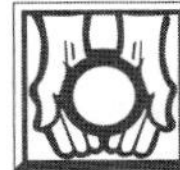

TREATMENT

Treatment is indicated for fecal egg cell counts >200 eggs per gram. Treatment relies on anthelmintic treatment and symptomatic treatment of dehydration, intestinal inflammation, serum hypoproteinemia, peripheral edema, and complications such as laminitis.

MEDICATIONS

DRUG(S) OF CHOICE

• Moxidectin 0.4 mg/kg PO is effective against encysted cyathostome larvae in addition to benzimidazole-resistant intraluminal forms of the parasite. This drug provides protection against cyathostomiasis for up to 3 mo following treatment. • Ivermectin 0.2 mg/kg PO does not eliminate encysted larvae reliably. • Oxfendazole 10 mg/kg PO or fenbendazole 30–60 mg/kg PO once or 7.5–10 mg/kg PO daily for 5 consecutive days may be used against adult cyathostomes, although benzimidazole resistance has been identified. • Pyrantel tartrate 2.2 mg/kg/day PO kills ingested larvae, preventing subsequent infection. • In acute severe diarrhea due to larval cyathostominosis, treatment with either a single dose of moxidectin 0.4 mg/kg PO or fenbendazole daily for 5 consecutive days is indicated.

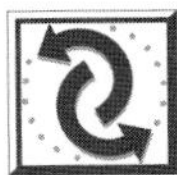

FOLLOW-UP

PATIENT MONITORING

Monitoring of high-risk patient is indicated after anthelmintic treatment since severe protein-losing enteropathy is possible. Treatment efficacy should be monitored by fecal flotation on the day of treatment and 10 days after treatment. Retreatment with an anthelmintica from a different drug group is indicated if the fecal egg count is reduced by <90%.

PREVENTION/AVOIDANCE

• Anthelmintic therapy is *only* an adjunct to proper pasture management and hygiene; negligence on selected farms might lead to parasite resistance. Continuous removal of feces from pastures and paddocks is paramount in reducing pasture parasite burden. Stocking density on pastures or turnout facilities should ideally provide 2–3 acres per horse. Harrowing, pasture rotation, or grazing horse pastures with cattle or small ruminants assist in reducing herbage contamination with infective larvae. One anthelmintic drug class should be used for one full year before rotating to another drug class.

• A fecal egg count should be performed minimum once a year in the late summer when the extent of larval hypobiosis is at the lowest level. This annual evaluation should be used to evaluate the success of the previous year's anthelmintic control program, to identify horses in need of treatment (>200 EPG) and to identify potential carriers.

POSSIBLE COMPLICATIONS

• Acute colitis may result in severe dehydration, dramatic weight loss, thrombophlebitis, laminitis and death due to hypovolemic shock.

• Anthelminthic therapy may cause clinical deterioration due to the abrupt killing of high numbers of larvae. Administration of NSAIDs or prednisolone is controversial but might be reasonable if severe intestinal mucosal inflammation is suspected.

EXPECTED COURSE AND PROGNOSIS

Approximately 40% of horses affected with acute diarrhea from larval cyathostomiasis survive if treated with appropriate anthelmintic and supportive therapy. Return to normal intestinal function may be slow.

MISCELLANEOUS

AGE-RELATED FACTORS

Horses 6 mo to 3 years are most at risk of clinical disease.

Suggested Reading

Peregrine AS, McEwen B, Bienzle D, Koch TG, Weese JS. Larval cyathostominosis in horses in Ontario: an emerging disease? Can Vet J 2006;47:80–82.

Steinbach T, Bauer C, Sasse H, Baumgärtner W, Rey-Moreno C, Hermosilla C, Damriyasa IM, Zahner H. Small strongyle infection: consequences of larvicidal treatment of horses with fenbendazole and moxidectin. Vet Parasitol 2006;139:115–131.

Authors Thomas G. Koch

Consulting Editors Henry Stämpfli and Olimpo Oliver-Espinosa

SMALL INTESTINAL OBSTRUCTION

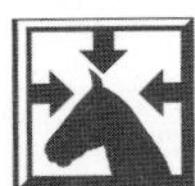

BASICS

DEFINITION

Impaired aboral transit of ingesta between the stomach and cecum

PATHOPHYSIOLOGY

• Can be a result of either a nonstrangulating (simple or functional) or a strangulating obstruction. Intestinal obstruction causes prestenotic distention with gas, fluid, and ingesta that can compress intestinal veins, which increases venous and capillary pressure and results in edema of the intestinal wall. Once a certain threshold is reached (intraluminal hydrostatic pressure rises above 15 cm H_2O), fluid will be sequestered into the bowel lumen, further exacerbating distention, and resulting in hypovolemia. Experimental distention of equine jejunum for 2 hr results in significant damage to the intestinal wall, which may contribute to adhesion formation. Intestinal distention results in local stretching of the bowel wall and activation of pain receptors. In cases of strangulating obstruction, simultaneous occlusion of the intestinal lumen and its blood supply occurs, which leads to ischemic injury and possibly necrosis of the affected intestinal segment. • Concurrent distention, inflammation, and sympathetic stimulation result in ileus.

SYSTEMS AFFECTED

• Gastrointestinal
• Behavioral—Activation of pain receptors is associated with clinical signs of abdominal pain; with progressive distention, depression may ensue. • Cardiovascular—Shock occurs secondary to hypovolemia, endotoxemia, and altered electrolyte status; with gastric distention, pressure on the vena cava decreases cardiac return. • Respiratory—Decreased pulmonary function may be secondary to pressure on the diaphragm from gastric distention or diaphragmatic herniation. • Endocrine/ metabolic—Affected patients frequently demonstrate metabolic alkalosis secondary to loss of hydrochloric acid in gastric reflux; as the condition progresses and hypovolemia ensues, metabolic acidosis develops.
• Hemic/lymphatic/immune—Once tissue pressures exceed venous portal pressures, the small veins, venules, and lymphatics that drain the affected intestine collapse, and net fluid movement into the bowel is potentiated.
• Renal/urologic—Hypovolemia is associated with decreased glomerular filtration rate.

SIGNALMENT

• Any age, sex, or breed • Ascarid impactions frequently are seen in foals/weanlings/yearlings.
• Small intestinal intussusception and volvulus occur most often in horses <3 years old. • Small intestinal volvulus is most common in foals between 2 and 4 mo. • Abdominal tumors usually are identified in horses >5 years.
• 47%—71% of horses with epiploic foramen entrapment are <11 years old. • Incidence of strangulating lipoma is 5 times higher in horses >15 years old. • Scrotal hernias are observed in stallions. • Proximal enteritis may occur more commonly in stallions. • Gastrosplenic ligament incarceration of the small intestine has been described most often in male horses.
• Mesoduodenal rents and diaphragmatic hernias can be seen in mares during late gestation.
• Warmbloods, Standardbreds, Tennessee Walking Horses, and American Saddlebreds appear to be predisposed to inguinal herniation.

SIGNS

Historical

• Horses with partial obstruction may display subacute, intermittent signs of abdominal pain or vague signs of lethargy, weakness, or weight loss. Transient episodes of abdominal pain may recur over a period of weeks to months and may progress in severity with time. • Complete small intestinal obstruction is associated with signs of severe, persistent abdominal pain and ileus. Horses may display a dog-sitting posture with distention of the stomach. • Recent abdominal surgery may indicate abdominal adhesions.
• Recent antihelmintic treatment contributes to ascarid impaction. • Prolonged or high-dose NSAID therapy may indicate duodenal ulceration. • Previous infection with *Streptococcus equi* can result in abscessation within the small intestinal mesentery.

Physical Examination

• Clinical signs depend on the lesion present and the location, duration, and severity of that lesion. • Most common signs—abdominal discomfort, tachycardia, discolored mucous membranes, prolonged capillary refill time, clinical dehydration, decreased to absent small intestinal borborygmi, reflux from the small intestine (yellow-brown, fetid odor, pH 6–8), and distended loops of small intestine and/or dehydrated colon contents contained within prominent colon haustra on rectal examination.

CAUSES

Nonstrangulating, Intraluminal Obstruction

• Impaction—feed, trichobezoar, ascarids, or tapeworms • Foreign body • Healed duodenal ulcer, with scarring and stricture
• Granulomatous enteritis

Nonstrangulating, Extraluminal Obstruction

• Tension on duodenocolic ligament secondary to distention or displacement of the large colon
• Adhesions—ischemic bowel, peritonitis, prolonged distention, excessive or traumatic surgical manipulation, anastomotic leakage, tissue dehydration, and inappropriate suture or technique
• Ileal muscular hypertrophy
• Ileal neurogenic stenosis
• Ileocecal valve edema or infarction secondary to migrating strongyle larvae
• Diverticula—traction, pulsion, or Meckel's
• Mesenteric abscess
• Neoplasia—pedunculated lipoma, lymphosarcoma, leiomyosarcoma, or carcinoid
• Intramural hematoma

Strangulating Obstruction

• Volvulus
• Herniation—inguinal/scrotal, umbilical, diaphragmatic, epiploic foramen, gastrosplenic, nephrosplenic, or tears in mesentery/omentum/ligaments/fibrous bands/adhesions
• Intussusceptions
• Vaginal evisceration

Functional (Ileus)

• Intestinal distention
• Intestinal ischemia
• Intestinal inflammation—duodenitis/proximal jejunitis, enterocolitis, surgical manipulation, or resection/ anastomosis
• Endotoxemia
• Peritonitis
• Pain—GI, musculoskeletal, etc.
• Drugs—α-adrenergic agonists, opioids, etc.
• General anesthesia
• Hypovolemia/hypotension
• Electrolyte imbalances—hypocalcemia secondary to massive sweat loss
• Parasitism

RISK FACTORS

Diet

• Sudden changes in feed or feeding practices
• Moldy hay or grain
• Poor-quality or low-grade roughage
• Decreased roughage intake over 24 hr
• Coastal Bermuda hay—ileal impaction
• Pelleted feed—impaction
• Decreased water intake or availability—impaction

Management

Poor deworming program—ascarid/tapeworm impaction, large strongyle migration, and infarction

Body Condition

Obesity—pedunculated lipoma

Geographic Location

Southeastern United States—ileal impaction and proximal enteritis

Genetic

Inflammatory bowel disease—granulomatous enteritis and eosinophilic gastroenteritis

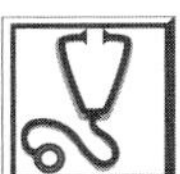

DIAGNOSIS

DIFFERENTIAL DIAGNOSIS

Differentiating Similar Signs

GI reflux usually is pathognomonic for small intestinal lesions but may be present secondary to large colon lesions that compress the small intestine or place tension on the duodenocolic ligament.

Differentiating Causes

The ability to differentiate between causes depends on the severity of clinical findings, which may be influenced by location of the lesion, length of intestine involved, and stage of disease.

Clinical Findings

• Intestinal involvement in an umbilical hernia usually is evident on palpation—pain on palpation of the hernia may indicate a strangulating hernia.
• Scrotal hernias may be accompanied by mild to severe scrotal swelling, palpable loops of intestine

within the scrotum, and decreased scrotal temperature because of vascular obstruction.

Palpation per Rectum

- Only the caudal 30%–40% of the abdomen is palpable on rectal evaluation, but distention usually pushes affected intestinal segments into reach.
- Any distended loops should be evaluated for position, degree of distention, wall thickness, gas versus fluid content, and pain on palpation.
- In cases of small intestinal strangulation, distended loops of small intestine were palpated in 50%–98% of horses.
- A thick, tubular structure palpable in the center of the abdomen may indicate ileal impaction, jejunal intussusception, or ileal intussusception.
- Resentment to palpation of the ileocecal region often accompanies ileocecal intussusception.
- Asymmetric inguinal rings, intestine or mesentery extending into an inguinal ring, or inability to identify one inguinal ring represent palpation findings in horses with inguinal herniation.
- If ileum is involved in inguinal herniation, the edematous antimesenteric ileocecal band may be palpable entering the ring on the affected side.

CBC/BIOCHEMISTRY/ URINALYSIS

- Leukocytosis/neutrophilia with a left shift may be observed with peritonitis, proximal enteritis, or mesenteric abscessation.
- Leukopenia/neutropenia may develop secondary to intestinal necrosis or endotoxemia.
- Often increased PCV and TP because of fluid sequestration within the bowel.
- Hypoproteinemia may develop as the disease progresses.
- Hypoalbuminemia may be observed with proximal enteritis or mesenteric abscessation.
- Hypergammaglobulinemia may be found with mesenteric abscessation or lymphosarcoma.
- Decreased potassium and chloride levels occur with loss into the bowel, and decreased sodium and calcium levels occur secondary to extracellular fluid shifts.
- Loss of hydrochloric acid with gastric reflux results in metabolic alkalosis.
- Acute strangulating obstructions associated with release of endotoxin, increased production of lactic acid, and hypoperfusion result in metabolic acidosis.
- If small intestinal obstruction occurs in the region of the hepatopancreatic ampulla, increases in total bilirubin, ALP, and GGT may be observed.

IMAGING

- Abdominal ultrasonography to assess small intestinal wall thickness and movement
- Edema of the wall of the small intestine (>3-mm wall thickness), distention, and absence of motility are suggestive of strangulating obstruction.
- Intestinal intussusception may display a characteristic concentric ring or "bull's eye" appearance.
- Abdominal radiography may be useful in distinguishing small from large intestinal problems in foals.
- Contrast radiography in foals may be used to demonstrate gastrointestinal obstruction.

DIAGNOSTIC PROCEDURES

Abdominocentesis

- Normal nucleated cell count for adults ranges from 5000 to 10,000 cells/µL; however, in foals, cell count >1500 cells/µL is considered elevated.
- As peritonitis and intestinal ischemia progress, the fluid becomes increasingly serosanguineous and cloudy as the cellularity and protein levels increase.
- WBC:TP ratios <3 and RBC:TP ratios <15 represent nonstrangulating obstructions or proximal enteritis; ratios >3 or <15 indicate strangulating lesions.
- Peritoneal fluid may be evaluated cytologically for neoplastic cells.

Endoscopy

- May be used to identify duodenal ulcers
- A 2.5–3.0-m endoscope is needed to visualize this region in adults.

Laparoscopy and Celiotomy

May be performed to diagnose and correct the cause of obstruction or for intestinal biopsy.

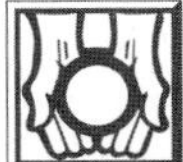

TREATMENT

- Most affected horses require referral to a hospital facility for further evaluation and treatment.
- Horses with strangulating lesions are candidates for surgery.
- Before transport, nasogastric decompression is vital. Horses may be transported with nasogastric tubes left in place.
- Surgical intervention is necessary if a surgical lesion can be identified at examination per rectum or abdominocentesis, if abdominal pain becomes uncontrollable, or if there is a lack of response to medical therapy.
- IV fluid therapy is important to maintain hydration and tissue perfusion and to correct electrolyte and acid-base abnormalities. Balanced polyionic IV solutions (e.g., lactated Ringer's solution) are ideal; rate and quantity depend on the horse's status.
- The decision whether to administer IV fluids before transport depends on horse's condition. Often, rehydration increases the volume of gastric reflux, so gastric decompression may need to be performed more frequently.
- Hyperimmune serum may benefit horses with endotoxemia.

MEDICATIONS

DRUG(S) OF CHOICE

- Sedation and analgesia may be achieved with xylazine 0.2–1.1 mg/kg IV or detomidine 0.005–0.02 mg/kg IV; both duration and quality of sedation or analgesia may be enhanced by coadministration of butorphanol tartrate (0.1 mg/kg IV).
- NSAIDs such as flunixin meglumine 1.1 mg/kg IM or IV BID or phenylbutazone 2.2–4.4 mg/kg PO or IV BID may be used for analgesic and anti-inflammatory effects as well as to mediate the effects of endotoxin.
- Endotoxemia also may be mediated with polymixin B 6000 U/kg diluted in 0.5–1.0 L of saline IV BID or pentoxifylline 8.5 mg/kg PO BID.
- Specific therapies for ileus, sepsis, gastric ulcers, and laminitis are discussed elsewhere.

CONTRAINDICATIONS

Acepromazine for sedation in hypovolemic horses

PRECAUTIONS

- Continued monitoring after administration of analgesics is important to ensure the drug is not masking signs of pain while the disease process progresses.
- Certain drugs (e.g., xylazine, detomidine) decrease GI motility.
- Gentamicin, amikacin, and polymixin B are nephrotoxic drugs.

FOLLOW-UP

PATIENT MONITORING

Depends on cause of obstruction and method of treatment

POSSIBLE COMPLICATIONS

- Gastric rupture
- Intestinal necrosis
- Abdominal adhesions
- Thrombophlebitis
- Laminitis

MISCELLANEOUS

ASSOCIATED CONDITIONS

- Endotoxemia
- Ileus
- Impaction of the large or small colon secondary to dehydration
- Laminitis

PREGNANCY

Outcome of pregnancy is determined more by cardiovascular and metabolic status of the mare and fetus than by the specific cause of the condition.

SEE ALSO

- Endotoxemia
- Ileus
- Proximal enteritis

ABBREVIATIONS

- ALP = alkaline phosphatase
- GGT = γ-glutamyltransferase
- GI = gastrointestinal
- PCV = packed cell volume
- TP = total protein

Suggested Reading

Freeman DE. Small intestine. In: Auer JA, Stick JA eds. Equine Surgery, ed 3. St. Louis; Saunders Elsevier, 2006.

Authors Judith B. Koenig and Annette M. Sysel
Consulting Editors Henry R. Stämpfli and Olimpo Oliver-Espinosa

SMOKE INHALATION

BASICS

OVERVIEW

- A mixture of hot air, solid particulates, gases, fumes, and vapors
- Composition depends on burning material(s) and fire environment.
- Two principal mechanisms lead to respiratory and systemic dysfunction—direct thermal injury and injury by asphyxiants and irritating combustion products.
- Heat/flame causes laryngotracheitis.
- Irritants and asphyxiants cause both local and systemic effects. Carbon dioxide, carbon monoxide, and cyanide are common asphyxiants.
- Water-soluble irritants like ammonia cause irritation in the URT leading to epithelial necrosis and edema.
- There are three clinical phases of a severe smoke inhalation event: early phase (within 24 hr), intermediate phase (12 hr to 5 days), and late phase (>5–7 days).
- Clinical signs of early phase are caused by carbon monoxide and cyanide.
- Clinical signs of the intermediate phase are caused by pulmonary edema.
- Late phase is caused by bronchopneumonia—impaired mucociliary clearance and alveolar macrophage function, together with the effects of smoke inhalation, to predispose patients to gram-negative bacterial infection.
- Other systems affected include skin, cardiovascular, nervous, and renal systems.

SIGNALMENT

N/A

SIGNS

- Depend on the composition of inhaled smoke, duration of exposure, and presence or absence of predisposing medical conditions
- Singed hair, URT inflammation, soot-stained nasal discharge, and the smell of smoke suggest smoke exposure; observe asymptomatic patients closely for 1 week after exposure.
- In the early phase, clinical signs may reflect carbon monoxide and/or cyanide poisoning. Affected horses may show signs of severe hypoxemia, depression, irritable behavior or be moribund to comatose. Horses may exhibit tachypnea and tachycardia.
- Heat and chemical injuries may cause tarchypnea, dyspnea, cough, drooling, or nasal discharge.
- Cyanosis and dehydration may be observed.
- Severe respiratory distress and signs of shock may be evident in the intermediate phase.
- Upper airway edema may be progressive and lead to airway obstruction.
- Thoracic auscultation may reveal decreased lung sounds, crackles, or wheezes.
- Signs of multiple organ failure may be present in severe cases—acute renal failure, cardiac failure, and CNS effects like ataxia, seizures, and coma.
- In the late phase, clinical findings may be similar to bronchopneumonia.
- In case of secondary bacterial infection, fever will be present.
- Worsening of clinical signs after initial improvement suggests secondary bacterial bronchopneumonia.

CAUSES AND RISK FACTORS

- Confined/enclosed spaces
- Preexisting conditions like asthma, chronic obstructive pulmonary disease, and cardiovascular or renal disease increase risk of a severe outcome.

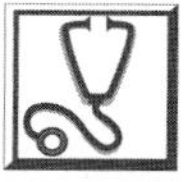

DIAGNOSIS

DIFFERENTIAL DIAGNOSIS

- Allergic airway diseases—endoscopy, physical examination, tracheobronchial aspirates or lavage, clinical pathology
- Acute respiratory distress syndrome—physical examination, history, radiographs, arterial blood gases
- Pneumonia (bacterial or fungal)—clinical signs, physical examination, clinical pathology, endoscopy, radiography, tracheobronchial aspirates or lavage, ultrasound
- Chronic obstructive pulmonary disease—seasonal disorder associated with environmental changes, physical examination, endoscopy, radiography, bronchoalveolar lavage
- Exposure to poisonous gases or vapors—history of exposure, possible environmental gas measurement
- Pulmonary neoplasia—endoscopic examination, tracheobronchial aspirates or lavage, radiography, ultrasound, biopsy

CBC/BIOCHEMISTRY/URINALYSIS

- Leukocytosis and hyperfibrinogenemia indicate an inflammatory process.
- Severe cases may reveal increased creatinine and BUN, suggesting prerenal or renal failure.
- Decreased oxygen saturation using pulse oximetry
- Carboxyhemoglobinemia
- Measurable blood cyanide
- Methemoglobinemia
- Lactic acidosis

OTHER LABORATORY TESTS

- Cytology of tracheal fluid may reveal carbon particles in phagocytic cells.
- Bacterial culture and antibiotic sensitivity testing of transtracheal fluid to document bronchopneumonia and to determine appropriate antibiotic therapy

IMAGING

Thoracic Radiography

- Chest radiographs are a very important diagnostic aid.
- Because the disease is progressive, take serial chest radiographs to monitor presence or lack of disease progression. Expect diffuse bronchial and peribronchial lesions or diffuse, patchy interstitial infiltration, which are suggestive of edema.
- Radiographic lesions may not correlate with the severity of pulmonary dysfunction.
- Radiographic findings indicative of pneumothorax, pneumomediastinum, and emphysema may be found in severe cases.

DIAGNOSTIC PROCEDURES

- Endoscopy may reveal airway edema and inflammation, mucosal necrosis, and soot deposits.
- Electrocardiograms are recommended for animals with pre-existing cardiovascular disease.

TREATMENT

• Remove animals from further exposure.
• General supportive care should be aimed at providing a patent airway, reversing bronchospasms and hypoxemia, decreasing pulmonary inflammation and edema, and providing ventilatory support.
• Specific treatment for carbon monoxide and cyanide poisoning if indicated
• Supplemental humidified 100% oxygen may be needed if hypoxemia is severe.
• Suction the upper respiratory tract to clear mucus and fluid, soot, and cell debris.
• Perform a tracheotomy if signs suggest upper airway obstruction; patients maintained with tracheal tubes require careful and frequent nursing care to prevent obstruction of the tube by secretions.
• IV fluid administration is indicated in most horses, because dehydration and renal failure often are present. Administer with caution, however, to prevent exacerbation of pulmonary edema and overhydration. Fluid selection is based on serum electrolyte disturbances and acid-base status.

MEDICATIONS

DRUG(S) OF CHOICE

• Early use of bronchodilators to control bronchospasm and airway obstruction—β_2-adrenergic agonists (e.g., clenbuterol 0.8–3.2 μg/kg PO q12h, terbutaline sulfate 0.02–0.06 mg/kg PO q12h, or albuterol 1–2 μg/kg) may be administered safely to most horses; aminophylline (5–10 mg/kg PO or IV q12h) may be associated with toxic side effects (e.g., tachycardia, hyperesthesia, and excitement).
• Furosemide (1–2 mg/kg IM or IV) may be given for treatment of upper airway or pulmonary tract edema.
• Dimethyl sulfoxide (1.0 g/kg in a 20% solution IV [slowly] q24h or q12h) may be potentially effective.
• Antibiotic prophylaxis in affected horses is controversial because it may lead to development of bacterial resistance. In severe cases, however, early antibiotic treatment with broad-spectrum activity may be justified. In case of confirmed secondary bacterial infection, use specific antibiotics as determined by culture and sensitivity tests.
• NSAIDs (e.g., phenylbutazone 4.4 mg/kg PO or IV daily) may be beneficial in decreasing mediator release and controlling fever.

CONTRAINDICATIONS/POSSIBLE INTERACTIONS

• Concurrent treatment with aminophylline may potentiate the diuretic effect of furosemide.
• Corticosteroid therapy is controversial and associated with increased septic complications (e.g., bacterial bronchopneumonia); avoid such therapy if possible.

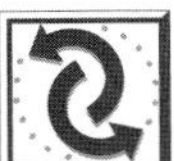

FOLLOW-UP

• Horses with no or minimal respiratory tract edema have a favorable prognosis and those with bronchopneumonia have a guarded prognosis.
• Horses should preferably be hospitalized for at least 12 hr post exposure and monitored closely for 1 week. Sudden deterioration can occur.
• The time required for complete recovery varies with the severity of the injury; several months may be needed before the animal can return to work.
• Modify the environment to reduce dust, molds, and other irritants to avoid development of airway hypersensitivity.
• Serial chest radiographs over several days or weeks should be helpful in assessing recovery.
• Possible complications are chronic pulmonary obstructive disease, bronchopneumonia, or permanent neural complications (e.g., seizures).

MISCELLANEOUS

ASSOCIATED CONDITIONS, AGE-RELATED FACTORS, ZOONOTIC POTENTIAL, PREGNANCY

N/A

SEE ALSO

• Inspiratory dyspnea
• Pleuropneumonia
• Pneumothorax

ABBREVIATION

• URT = upper respiratory tract

Suggested Reading

Geor RJ, Ames TR. Smoke inhalation injury in horses. Compend Cont Educ Pract Vet 1991:13;1162–1169.

Kemper T, Spiers S, Barratt-Boyes SM, Hoffman R. Treatment of smoke inhalation in five horses. J Am Vet Med Assoc 1993:202;91–94.

Author Wilson K. Rumbeiha
Consulting Editor Robert Poppenga

SNAKE ENVENOMATION

BASICS

DEFINITION

• Disease associated with bites from two families of venomous snakes in the U. S.—Elapidae, which includes the eastern coral snake (*Micrurus fulvius fulvius*) and Texas coral snake (*M. fulvius tenere*); and Crotalidae (pit viper), which includes the genera *Agkistrodon* (copperheads and cottonmouth water moccasins), *Crotalus* (rattlesnakes) and *Sistrurus* (pygmy and massasauga rattlesnakes). • Coral snakes have a relatively small head, black snout and round pupils. Their color pattern consists of fully encircling bands of red, yellow and black. Coral snakes are not only shy and nocturnal but have fixed front fangs of the upper jaw, which makes them less of a threat to large livestock. • Pit vipers have bilateral pits between the nostril and eye, elliptical pupils, well-developed and retractable maxillary fangs, and an undivided row of ventral scales caudal to the cloaca. The hollow, hinged front fangs rotate forward for striking and delivering the venom.
• Copperheads are stout and orange/brown; their head typically is a solid copper tone. Cottonmouths are brown to black, thick-bodied, aggressive snakes with a white oral mucosa they display when agitated. • There are numerouse subspecies and color variations of rattlesnakes; however, they are typically identified by the special keratin rattles on the ends of their tails.

PATHOPHYSIOLOGY

• Pit viper venom is a complex mixture of enzymes including myotoxins, proteases, hyaluronidase, bradykinin-releasing enzyme, and phospholipase A_2; the toxins are primarily responsible for causing significant local tissue destruction—myonecrosis, edema, hemorrhage and inflammation at the bite site. • These enzymes, in addition to other nonenzymatic proteins, cause an increase in capillary permeability, with subsequent loss of plasma volume and peripheral pooling of blood. The sequelae of these events are decreased cardiac output, hypoproteinemia, hypotension, and a metabolic acidosis that, if not corrected, can lead to complete respiratory and circulatory collapse.
• Other toxins are associated with hemolysis, thrombocytopenia and alterations in the coagulation cascade. • Hemorrhagins are responsible for hemorrhage observed either at the bite wound or systemically. • Coral snake venom consists mostly of neurotoxins; phospholipase A causing hemolysis can also be present.

SYSTEMS AFFECTED

• Cardiovascular—interference with vascular endothelial intercellular cement substance, RBC lysis, vasodilation, enhanced degradation of fibrinogen to fibrin, enhanced activation of factor X to Xa, enhanced production of degradation products, enhanced platelet aggregation and hypoxia.
• Skin/exocrine/musculoskeletal—dilatation of the sarcoplasmic reticulum; inhibition of the calcium ion pump; hydrolysis of peptide linkages of amino groups of aliphatic, hydrophobic amino acids; disruption of connective tissue viscosity by depolymerizing hyaluronic acid; hydrolysis of the ester bond at C-2 of lecithin, which results in release of histamine, serotonin, bradykinin and prostaglandins. • Respiratory—direct damage to alveolar membranes; hemorrhage of the pulmonary capillary bed.
• Neuromuscular—neurotransmitter decrease, resulting in neuromuscular junction dysfunction and respiratory center paralysis.
• Renal/urologic—nephrotoxic effects of myoglobinuria, hemoglobinuria, defibrination syndrome, DIC-like syndrome, direct toxic effect and hypovolemic shock. • Nine rattlesnake species have subpopulations with venom containing Mojave toxin, a potent neurotoxin that interrupts neurotransmission at the neuromuscular junction. This can lead to loss of control of skeletal musculature resulting in flaccid paralysis and respiratory failure.
• Coral snake venom also contains a potent neurotoxin that causes an irreversible decrease of acetylcholine release at the neuromuscular junction. Possible sequelae include bulbar paralysis and respiratory collapse from paralysis of the diaphragm. Other systemic effects from coral snake venom include RBC lysis and rhabdomyolysis.

INCIDENCE/PREVALENCE

• Most snakebites occur from April to October and result from accidental encounters. • Several hundred horses are bitten each year by pit vipers, mostly rattlesnakes in the western U.S. • Coral snakes are small and shy, and bites from these snakes are infrequent.

SIGNS

General Comments

• Most horses are bitten on or near the muzzle, which results in severe local tissue destruction often leading to acute head swelling and airway obstruction. • A smaller percentage of horses receive bites on the limbs below the carpus or tarsus; bites to the trunk are not common. • Less than half of bitten horses develop multiple or severe manifestations of envenomation. • In addition to airway obstruction, hemolytic anemia or coagulopathies can be acute, life-threatening problems. • Determining the species of pit viper involved is not necessarily important, but determining whether the snake delivered sufficient venom is important. • Most envenomations elicit local signs of swelling within 60 minutes. • Onset of systemic signs may be delayed for up to 6 hours; monitor the patient for at least this time period. • Lack of local signs does not preclude life-threatening problems from occurring, particularly with bites from a pit viper, whose venom contains neurotoxins. • Coral snake venom is primarily neurotoxic, and envenomations that elicit neurologic signs in the victim carry a poor prognosis. • Horses bitten by coral snakes may show a lag phase of up to 18 hours between the bite and onset of clinical signs; once neurologic signs appear, they are difficult to reverse.

Physical Examination Findings

Pit Vipers:
• Painful soft-tissue swelling with hemorrhage at the bite marks; possible ecchymosis and petechiation • Dyspnea and tachypnea caused by upper airway obstruction, pulmonary edema or hemorrhage • Cardiac abnormalities—tachycardia, dysrhythmias
• Fever • Epistaxis • Other signs—lethargy, diarrhea, salivation caused by dysphagia, flaccid paralysis, incontinence, tremors, clotting abnormalities, laminitis, colic, coma and shock

Coral Snakes:
• Puncture wounds—usually small and without hemorrhage • Salivation caused by dysphagia
• Bulbar paralysis—flaccid paralysis
• Respiratory arrest

CAUSES AND RISK FACTORS

• Primary factors determine severity of a venomous snake bite—species of snake, circumstances of the bite, age of the snake and venom composition. • The snake controls the degree of envenomation—defensive bites tend to be less severe than offensive and agonistic bites.
• Decapitated heads can reflexively bite for up to 1 hour. • Venom from young snakes tends to contain a high peptide fraction, so although tissue slough may not be as severe, systemic effects may be worse. • Peptide fractions have been reported by some to have higher concentrations in venoms during the spring, thus causing more serious problems. • Bite site location can affect the speed of systemic uptake of the venom. • Size of the victim and their activity level after envenomation influence the extent of venom systemic circulation and severity of the toxicosis. • Time from bite to medical intervention can significantly alter the prognosis.

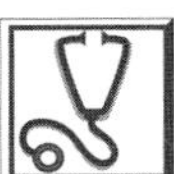

DIAGNOSIS

DIFFERENTIAL DIAGNOSIS

• Angioedema secondary to insect sting/bite
• Trauma • Foreign body/abscess • Botulism—no evidence of bite wound, detection of toxin using mouse bioassay. • *Centaurea solstitialis* (yellow star thistle) or *Acroptilon repens* (Russian knapweed) poisoning—evidence of plant consumption, postmortem brain lesion.
• Purpura hemorrhagica—recent history of strangles or equine influenza.

CBC/BIOCHEMISTRY/URINALYSIS

• Elevated CPK, AST, and SDH and immediate hemoconcentration, followed by a hemolytic or coagulopathy-induced anemia, leukocytosis with an inflammatory leukogram, hyper- or hypofibrinogenemia, hypoproteinemia, thrombocytopenia, hyperglobulinemia, azotemia, and nonspecific abnormal renal changes.

OTHER LABORATORY TESTS

• Prolonged clotting times—ACT, PT and PTT
• High FDP • Metabolic acidosis

IMAGING

Echocardiography to assess cardiac dysfunction

DIAGNOSTIC PROCEDURES

Electrocardiography to assess cardiac dysfunction

PATHOLOGIC FINDINGS

• Extensive soft-tissue edema, hemorrhage and myonecrosis at and around the bite site
• Generalized congestion, with petechiation of major organs • Hepatocellular necrosis • Possible

myocardial inflammation and fibrosis with pleural and pericardial effusions • Laminitis, pneumonia and chronic changes associated with wound complications; osteomyelitis
• Secondary opportunistic infections

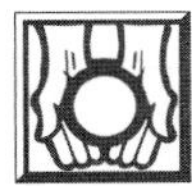

TREATMENT

APPROPRIATE HEALTH CARE

• First-aid measures—calm the patient, and immediately transport to a veterinary facility for appropriate monitoring. • Inpatient medical management may last for several days; short-term goals include preventing or controlling shock, neutralizing the venom, minimizing tissue necrosis and preventing secondary bacterial infections (especially clostridial infections).
• Establishing a patent airway is essential; horses with bites on the head and accompanying head and neck swelling may require tracheotomy.
• Some form of rigid tubing can be sutured into the nostrils to keep the nasal passages patent.

NURSING CARE

• IV crystalloid fluids to combat shock and hypotension and to increase tissue perfusion and maintain hydration; alternatively, whole blood or blood products to correct anemias, thrombocytopenias and clotting abnormalities
• Local wound management—continuous cleansing, hydrotherapy, and debridement
• Administer tetanus toxoid or antitoxin as appropriate.

ACTIVITY

Calm the patient to decrease distribution of the venom.

CLIENT EDUCATION

• Size and condition of the wound site may not correlate with severity of the systemic signs.
• Avoid first-aid techniques such as tourniquets, cryotherapy, lancing, suction and electroshock.
• Systemic signs may be delayed by several hours, so immediate treatment is essential.

SURGICAL CONSIDERATIONS

Fasciotomies are not indicated, except for extremely rare circumstances with documented, elevated compartmental pressures.

MEDICATIONS

DRUGS OF CHOICE

• Specific antivenin against pit viper or coral snake envenomations—*M. fulvius* (equine origin, for coral snakes, Wyeth); antivenin (Crotalidae) polyvalent, equine origin (Wyeth)
• Consider antivenin for bites in foals and ponies because of their smaller body mass.
• Adult horses have some innate protection from envenomations because of their large body mass, but fatalities do occur. • Antivenin is most effective shortly after envenomation has occurred. This is especially true in combating local tissue necrosis and neurologic sequela.
• Initial dose of antivenin should be 5 vials IV. The total number of vials used depends on the clinical signs, progression of the syndrome, degree of hypotension and the bite site. Do not administer antivenin IM or into the bite site itself. • All animals should receive a broad-spectrum antibiotic (e.g., cephalosporin) for at least 7–10 days. • NSAIDs (e.g., flunixin meglumine) can be used 24 hours after the bite for control of pain and swelling. • Approach use of pain-control medications conservatively, and take care using compounds that interfere with platelet function.

CONTRAINDICATIONS

• Heparin • Dimethyl sulfoxide

PRECAUTIONS

• Use of corticosteroids (e.g., dexamethasone) is debatable. Avoid long-term, high dose of corticosteroids, which may depress the immune response to the venom and alter clinically relevant laboratory parameters that are useful in monitoring progression of the syndrome. Corticosteroids also may interfere with effectiveness of the antivenin and may have little effect on local tissue response to snake venom.
• Antihistamines are of little benefit.

FOLLOW-UP

PATIENT MONITORING

• Assess CBC, serum chemistry panel, clotting panel, and fibrinogen every 12–24 hours at a minimum and more often if the patient is deteriorating. • Close observation of vital signs along with the respiratory and cardiovascular systems is recommended.

POSSIBLE COMPLICATIONS

Common chronic problems after rattlesnake bites include cardiac dysfunction, liver disease, pneumonia, colitis, laminitis, pharyngeal paralysis and various wound complications.

EXPECTED COURSE AND PROGNOSIS

• Clinical signs can last as long as 2 weeks, with close inpatient monitoring. • Poor prognosis after coral snake bites results from the neuromuscular effects of the venom, leading to respiratory collapse as the most common cause of death. • Estimated mortality rate after rattlesnake bites is ~10–30%.

MISCELLANEOUS

AGE-RELATED FACTORS

Young foals or ponies are at greatest risk because of their small body mass.

ABBREVIATIONS

• ACT = activated clotting time • AST = aspartate aminotransferase • CPK = creatine phosphokinase • DIC = disseminated intravascular coagulation • FDP = fibrin degradation products • SDH = sorbitol dehydrogenase • PT = prothrombin time
• PTT = partial thromboplastin time

Suggested Reading

Dickinson CE, et al. Rattlesnake venom poisoning in horses: 32 cases (1973–1993). J Am Vet Med Assoc 1996;208:1866–1871.

Hudelson S, Hudelson P. Pathophysiology of snake envenomation and evaluation of treatments—part I. Compend Contin Educ Pract Vet 1995;17:889–898.

Hudelson S, Hudelson P. Pathophysiology of snake envenomation and evaluation of treatments—part II. Compend Contin Educ Pract Vet 1995;17:1035–1041.

Hudelson S, Hudelson P. Pathophysiology of snake envenomation and evaluation of treatments—part III. Compend Contin Educ Pract Vet 1995;17:1385–1396.

Authors Patricia A. Talcott and Michael Peterson

Consulting Editor Robert H. Poppenga

SODIUM, HYPERNATREMIA

BASICS

DEFINITION

A serum sodium concentration greater than the upper limit of normal horses—generally >144 mEq/L

PATHOPHYSIOLOGY

- Sodium is the major extracellular cation in the body and therefore is critical for maintenance of the extracellular space.
- Serum sodium concentration reflects the ratio of total-body sodium to total-body water; therefore, knowledge of the hydration state is important for accurate interpretation of serum sodium concentrations.
- Hypernatremia usually reflects an absolute or relative water deficiency.

SYSTEM AFFECTED

Nervous—hypernatremia may lead to hyperosmolality and intracellular water loss from neurons, in turn leading to CNS shrinkage.

SIGNALMENT

No breed, sex, or age predilections

SIGNS

- Lethargy
- Weakness
- Seizures
- Coma
- Death
- Severity of signs depends on the duration and degree of hypernatremia.
- Other signs depend on the underlying cause.

CAUSES

- Normal total-body sodium with pure water loss—water deprivation because of unavailable water source or physical abnormality causing decreased ingestion (e.g., botulism or dysphagia); prolonged hyperventilation; central and nephrogenic diabetes insipidus (DI); evaporative loss from extensive burns; exhausted horse syndrome
- Low total-body sodium with hypotonic fluid loss—urinary loss (osmotic diuresis; i.e., osmotic diuretic administration such as mannitol); GI loss (early stages of diarrhea, before the point of compensatory water intake occurs)
- High total-body sodium—excessive intake of sodium chloride (i.e., salt poisoning) with water restriction; IV or oral administration of hypertonic saline or sodium bicarbonate solutions

RISK FACTOR

Inadequate water intake

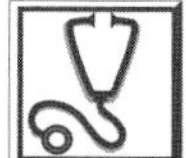

DIAGNOSIS

DIFFERENTIAL DIAGNOSIS

- History or physical examination to detect decreased water intake or excessive water loss resulting in (hypertonic) dehydration
- See other causes.

LABORATORY FINDINGS

Drugs That May Alter Lab Results

Sodium salts of EDTA, fluoride, and heparin can result in pseudohypernatremia.

Problems That May Alter Lab Results

Sample dehydration or evaporation can result in pseudohypernatremia.

Valid If Run in Human Lab?

Yes

CBC/BIOCHEMISTRY/URINALYSIS

- High serum sodium concentration
- Hyposthenuria—consider diabetes insipidus
- Decreased potassium, chloride, calcium, and magnesium; stress neutrophilia and lymphopenia, occasionally leukopenia—consider exhausted horse syndrome

OTHER LABORATORY TESTS

- Urinary fractional excretion of sodium (FE_{Na})—a single urine sample can be used for sodium and creatinine measurements, which are compared with serum sodium and creatinine concentrations determined at the same time ($[Na^+{}_u/Na^+{}_s]/[Cr_u/Cr_s]$; normal <1%); suspect extrarenal water loss if urine volume with FE_{Na} <1% and clinical signs of dehydration; suspect osmotic diuresis if urine volume is increased with FE_{Na} >1% and clinical signs of dehydration.
- Plasma osmolality—should be high with hypernatremia.
- Other laboratory tests depend on the underlying cause (i.e., vasopressin concentration in conjunction with water deprivation—nephrogenic DI if vasopressin ≥3 normal and neurogenic DI if vasopressin normal; ADH response test with vasopressin administered IV and urine osmolality measured at 2-hr intervals—neurogenic DI if urine osmolality increases to ≥1.025).

IMAGING

N/A

OTHER DIAGNOSTIC PROCEDURES

N/A

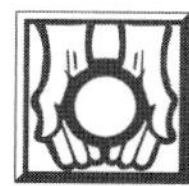

TREATMENT

- Treatment depends on the severity of hypernatremia and the underlying disorder.
- If increases in sodium and chloride are proportional, assure adequate water availability.
- If hypernatremia and hyperchloremia are long-standing, correction should be gradual.
- If chloride is increased disproportionately compared with sodium, evaluate and treat the acid-base imbalance.

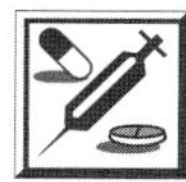

MEDICATIONS

DRUG(S) OF CHOICE

Treat the underlying disorder.

CONTRAINDICATIONS

N/A

PRECAUTIONS

The combination of hypernatremia and dehydration is a therapeutic dilemma, because rapid reduction of serum sodium concentrations can lead to cerebral and pulmonary edema.

POSSIBLE INTERACTIONS

N/A

ALTERNATIVE DRUGS

N/A

FOLLOW-UP

PATIENT MONITORING

Electrolytes, acid-base status, urine output, water intake, and body weight

POSSIBLE COMPLICATIONS

Seizures, convulsions, and probable permanent neurological damage in severe, long-standing cases

MISCELLANEOUS

ASSOCIATED CONDITIONS, AGE-RELATED FACTORS, ZOONOTIC POTENTIAL, PREGNANCY, SYNONYMS

N/A

SEE ALSO

- Hyperchloremia

ABBREVIATION

- ADH = antidiuretic hormone
- DI = diabetes insipidus

Suggested Reading

Carlson GP. Clinical chemistry tests. In: Smith BP, ed. Large Animal Internal Medicine, ed 3. St. Louis: Mosby, 2002.

Authors Wendy S. Sprague and Martin David
Consulting Editor Kenneth W. Hinchcliff

SODIUM, HYPONATREMIA

BASICS

DEFINITION

A serum sodium concentration less than the lower limit of normal horses—generally <132 mEq/L

PATHOPHYSIOLOGY

• Sodium is the major extracellular cation in the body and, therefore, is critical for maintenance of the extracellular space. • Serum sodium concentration reflects the ratio of the total-body sodium to total-body water; therefore, knowledge of the hydration state is important for accurate interpretation of serum sodium concentrations. • Hyponatremia usually results from relative water excess and usually is not clinically significant until serum sodium concentrations are <122 mEq/L.

SYSTEMS AFFECTED

• Nervous—cerebral edema (also seen with rapid correction of severe hyponatremia) • Renal/urologic—medullary washout • Hemic/lymphatic/immune intravascular hemolysis

SIGNALMENT

No breed, sex, or age predilections

SIGNS

• Lethargy • Tremors • Abnormal gait • Central blindness • Seizures • Severity of signs depends on the rapidity and degree of hyponatremia.
• Other signs depend on the underlying cause.

CAUSES

• Loss of sodium-containing fluid—diarrhea, pronounced sweating, hemorrhage, excessive GI fluid drainage by nasogastric intubation, excessive pleural fluid drainage, saliva loss, sustained exercise, protein-losing gastroenteropathies, chronic/subacute colitis, and acute renal disease (usually in foals)
• Adrenal insufficiency (i.e., iatrogenic) or adrenal exhaustion • Sequestration of fluid (third spacing)—peritonitis, ascites, uroperitoneum (usually in foals), and gut torsion, volvulus, obstruction or ileus • Iatrogenic—oral administration of hypotonic fluids, and inappropriate fluid therapy (i.e., excessive IV administration of 5% dextrose solution to horse with renal disease) • Inappropriate water retention—psychogenic polydipsia, renal disease, inappropriate ADH secretion, congestive heart failure, hepatic fibrosis, and severe hypoalbuminemia • Prolonged diuresis secondary to hyperglycemia and glucosuria may result in medullary washout and subsequent hyponatremia and hypochloremia.

RISK FACTORS

• Heavy sweating • Colic or other GI disorders
• Furosemide treatment

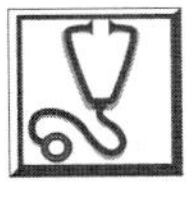

DIAGNOSIS

DIFFERENTIAL DIAGNOSIS

• Azotemia and hyperkalemia in foals—consider renal disease and uroperitoneum. • Other clinical signs can help to differentiate causes—diarrhea, abdominal pain, ascites, polyuria/polydipsia, etc.

LABORATORY FINDINGS

Drugs That May Alter Lab Results

Mannitol can cause pseudohyponatremia.

Disorders That May Alter Lab Results

• Hyperlipidemia and hyperproteinemia can cause pseudohyponatremia unless an ion-specific electrode is used for measurement.
• Marked hyperglycemia causes dilution of circulating sodium concentration by osmotic water movement.

Valid If Run in Human Lab?

Yes

CBC/BIOCHEMISTRY/URINALYSIS

• Low serum sodium concentration • Other abnormalities depend on the underlying cause.

OTHER LABORATORY TESTS

• Urinary fractional excretion of sodium (FE_{Na})—a single urine sample can be used for sodium and creatinine measurements, which are compared with serum sodium and creatinine concentrations determined at the same time. ($[Na^+{}_u/Na^+{}_s]/[Cr_u/Cr_s]$; normal <1%); suspect renal disease if FE_{Na} >1%.
• Plasma osmolality—should be low with hyponatremia; if in the normal or high range, rule out renal failure and causes of pseudohyponatremia.
• Other laboratory tests depend on the underlying cause (i.e., abdominal fluid cytology and creatinine concentration determination in foals with uroperitoneum, etc.).

IMAGING

N/A

OTHER DIAGNOSTIC PROCEDURES

N/A

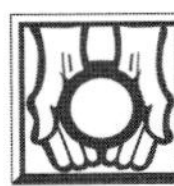

TREATMENT

• Treatment depends on the severity of hyponatremia and the underlying disorder.
• Correct acute hyponatremia rapidly and chronic hyponatremia (≅48 hr) gradually.
• Moderate hyponatremia (122–132 mEq/L)—treatment probably not critical, but depends on clinical signs
• Treat severe hyponatremia; therapy depends on the acuteness of the disorder.
• Acute hyponatremia—elevate serum sodium to 125 mEq/L over 6 hr, then gradually increase to normal. The amount of Na^+ needed to elevate serum Na^+ to a concentration of 125 mEq/L = (125 – measured serum Na^+ [mEq/L] × 0.67 × BW [kg]). Isotonic or hypertonic (3%) saline is suggested for states of volume contraction.
• Chronic hyponatremia—not well defined in horses; appropriate fluid would be 0.45% NaCl in 2.5% dextrose; use the formula above to calculate the amount of Na^+ needed.
• If chloride is decreased disproportionately compared with sodium, evaluate and treat the acid-base imbalance.

MEDICATIONS

DRUG(S) OF CHOICE

• Sodium bicarbonate—if indicated for concurrent, severe metabolic acidosis; calculate the dosage carefully to avoid correcting serum sodium too rapidly.
• DMSO and NSAIDs (i.e., phenylbutazone, flunixin meglumine) can be used for treatment of cerebral ischemia and inflammation.
• Corticosteroids may be used with caution for cerebral edema.
• Mannitol can be used to reduce cerebral edema in cases of acute hyponatremia if serum sodium concentrations are concurrently normalized, but it is not recommended with suspected cerebral hemorrhage or chronic hyponatremia.

CONTRAINDICATIONS N/A

PRECAUTIONS

Rapid correction of serum sodium in cases of chronic hyponatremia has led to osmotic cerebral demyelination in humans, but this has not been reported in horses.

POSSIBLE INTERACTIONS N/A

ALTERNATIVE DRUGS

N/A

FOLLOW-UP

HORSE MONITORING

Electrolytes, acid-base status, urine output, and body weight

POSSIBLE COMPLICATIONS

Depend on the underlying disorder

MISCELLANEOUS

ASSOCIATED CONDITIONS

Other acid-base and electrolyte abnormalities

AGE-RELATED FACTORS

N/A

ZOONOTIC POTENTIAL

N/A

PREGNANCY

N/A

SYNONYMS

N/A

SEE ALSO

Hypochloremia

ABBREVIATIONS

• ADH = antidiuretic hormone
• BW = body weight
• DMSO = dimethylsulfoxide

Suggested Reading

Carlson GP. Clinical chemistry tests. In: Smith BP, ed. Large Animal Internal Medicine, ed 3. St. Louis: Mosby, 2002.

Authors Wendy S. Sprague and Martin David
Consulting Editor Kenneth W. Hinchcliff

SOLANUM SPP. (NIGHTSHADE) TOXICOSIS

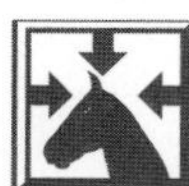

BASICS

OVERVIEW

- Numerous *Solanum* spp. (nightshade family) are potentially toxic to animals—*S. nigrum* (black nightshade), *S. dulcamera* (bittersweet nightshade), *S. carolinense* (horse nettle), *S. rostratum* (buffalo burr), *S. tuberosum* (potato), and others.
- Plants in this genus are widely distributed.
- Toxicity is attributed primarily to tropane alkaloids and steroidal glycoalkaloids (e.g., solanine), but few equine data are available.
- Anticholinergic, muscarinic, and GI irritant effects have been described in intoxicated animals.
- Muscarinic effects may result from cholinesterase inhibition, but this has not been verified clinically.
- GI irritation is believed to result from a saponin-like effect of the steroidal glycoalkaloids.
- Toxicity varies with environment, plant part ingested, and time of year.
- Unripe berries contain the highest glycoalkaloid concentration, which declines with maturity.
- Green portions of potato contain the highest toxin concentration.
- Documented cases of equine intoxication are rare, and those in the literature do not provide significant information concerning pathophysiologic effects.

SIGNALMENT

No known breed, age, or sex predispositions

SIGNS

- GI signs predominate—anorexia, nausea, salivation, colic, and diarrhea with or without blood.
- Nervous system signs—apathy, drowsiness, trembling, progressive weakness or paralysis, recumbency, and coma

CAUSES AND RISK FACTORS

- Contamination of hay with *Solanum* spp.
- Unavailability of alternative desirable forage
- Access to old potatoes or potato refuse

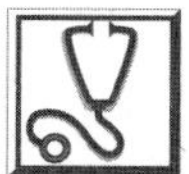

DIAGNOSIS

DIFFERENTIAL DIAGNOSIS

- Establishing the diagnosis relies on evidence of consumption of *Solanum* spp.
- Detection of alkaloids in GI contents is possible but not commonly performed.
- Other causes of colic—physical examination, lack of exposure to *Solanum* spp.

CBC/BIOCHEMISTRY/URINALYSIS

N/A

OTHER LABORATORY TESTS

N/A

IMAGING

N/A

DIAGNOSTIC PROCEDURES

N/A

PATHOLOGICAL FINDINGS

- Evidence of plant in the stomach
- Grossly, there may be evidence of GI irritation and diarrhea with or without hemorrhage.
- Histopathologically, there is congestion, inflammation, hemorrhage, and ulceration of the GI mucosa.

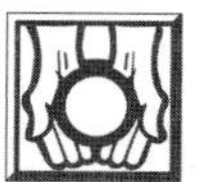

TREATMENT

- Remove animal from source of exposure.
- If soon after ingestion, consider GI decontamination.
- Symptomatic and supportive care

MEDICATIONS

DRUGS

- AC (1–4 g/kg PO in water slurry [1 g of AC in 5 mL or water])
- One dose of cathartic (70% sorbitol at 3 mL/kg PO or sodium or magnesium sulfate at 250 mg/kg PO, the latter two being administered in a water slurry) with AC if no diarrhea or ileus
- NSAIDs—flunixin meglumine (0.1 mg/kg IV or IM as necessary)

CONTRAINDICATIONS/POSSIBLE INTERACTIONS

N/A

FOLLOW-UP

PATIENT MONITORING

N/A

PREVENTION/AVOIDANCE

- Limit or prevent access to *Solanum* spp.
- Do not feed potatoes or potato refuse.

POSSIBLE COMPLICATIONS

N/A

EXPECTED COURSE AND PROGNOSIS

- With early intervention and appropriate symptomatic and supportive care, prospects for recovery are good.
- With severe clinical signs, prognosis is guarded.

MISCELLANEOUS

ASSOCIATED CONDITIONS

N/A

AGE-RELATED FACTORS

N/A

ZOONOTIC POTENTIAL

N/A

PREGNANCY

Congenital craniofacial malformations have been induced in fetuses of pregnant laboratory animals fed *Solanum* spp. glycoalkaloids. The significance of this finding for horses is unknown, but do prevent pregnant mares from ingesting any *Solanum* spp.

ABBREVIATIONS

- AC = activated charcoal
- GI = gastrointestinal

Suggested Reading

Burrows GE, Tyrl RJ. Toxic Plants of North America. Ames, IA: Iowa State University Press, 2001:1127.

Dalvi RR, Bowie WC. Toxicology of solanine: an overview. Vet Hum Toxicol 1983; 25:13–15.

Author Robert H. Poppenga

Consulting Editor Robert H. Poppenga

BASICS

OVERVIEW

- Infection in the superficial subsolar tissues of the foot due to penetration of the sole with a sharp object followed by premature closure of the entrance hole resulting in abscess formation
- Subsolar hematoma in severely bruised foot may become secondarily infected through small cracks allowing bacterial penetration.

SYSTEM AFFECTED

Musculoskeletal—foot

SIGNALMENT

No breed, sex, age, or sport predilection

SIGNS

- Sudden acute severe lameness and pointing of the toe of the affected foot
- Heat in the hoof capsule and pounding digital pulses
- Swelling of the heel bulb or at the coronary band may indicate proximal migration of infection. Just before drainage, a soft painful focal area may be appreciated.
- Focal sensitivity to hoof tester application or generalized solar pain
- Distal limb swelling may be noted especially with deep or severe infections.
- Gray or black malodorous fluid leaks from the tract once the abscess breaks open.

CAUSES AND RISK FACTORS

- Penetration of the bottom of the foot with a sharp object (e.g., horseshoe nail, rock*)
- Risk factors include laminitis, thin soles, and Cushing's disease.

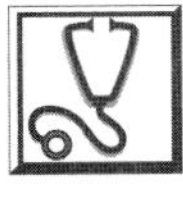

DIAGNOSIS

DIFFERENTIAL DIAGNOSIS

- Severe solar bruising—no drainage will rule out
- Close horseshoe nail or nail prick ("quickening")—injury location at nail entrance and pain soon after shoeing
- Laminitis—Rule out with radiography.
- Deep penetrating wound through the sole—Rule out with contrast radiography.
- Coffin bone fracture—Rule out with radiography.
- Navicular bone fracture—Rule out with radiography.

CBC/CHEMISTRY/URINALYSIS

Usually normal; may have hyperfibrinogenemia in severe or extensive disease

OTHER LABORATORY TESTS

None

IMAGING

- Radiography—Radiolucent gas or fluid may be appreciated within the sole. Radiology is also useful to rule out other causes of foot lameness and identify possible complications.
- Radiographic evaluation should be repeated in 2–3 weeks if complications such as infectious osteitis are suspected. Radiographic signs include bone lysis, irregular margins, increased vascular size, and bone sequestrum formation.

OTHER DIAGNOSTIC PROCEDURES

- Hoof tester application to the sole
- Paring of the sole and frog with a hoof knife. Care should be taken not to remove normal tissue.
- Application of foot poultice or foot soaks often helps to localize the affected sole.
- Microbial culture and sensitivity of exudate is not necessary.

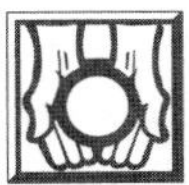

TREATMENT

- The object of treatment is to open and drain the abscess, remove diseased tissue, and protect the site from contamination.
- Drainage is established by paring the sole with a sharp hoof knife or hoof groover. The hole should be just large enough for adequate drainage. Aggressive or overzealous debridement is discouraged.
- For superficial, localized infection, antiseptic dressing and foot protection are all that is needed.
- For deep infection, perineural analgesia of the foot may be necessary to facilitate extensive debridement.
- The affected foot may be periodically soaked in hot or warm Epsom salt and povidone-iodine solutions until drainage and infection subside.
- Foot protection is accomplished with bandages, bandages with duct tape, waterproof foot boot, and, in some cases, a shoe with a hospital treatment plate.
- Horses are stall confined or limited to small paddock turnout. Bedding should be dry and clean.
- Long term, horses may be shod with pads until the solar defect fills in.

MEDICATIONS

DRUG(S) OF CHOICE

- Tetanus toxoid and antitoxin
- NSAIDs—phenylbutazone 2.2–4.4 mg/kg daily to BID as needed
- Tincture of iodine can be applied to the wound.
- Systemic broad-spectrum antimicrobials are indicated for horses with infectious osteitis and severe infections.
- Regional limb antimicrobial perfusion is rarely necessary.

CONTRAINDICATIONS/POSSIBLE INTERACTIONS

Systemic broad-spectrum antimicrobials may be contraindicated in mild cases since they prolong the clinical signs.

FOLLOW-UP

PATIENT MONITORING

Significant improvement in lameness and other clinical signs is apparent once drainage is established.

PREVENTION/AVOIDANCE

Horseshoes with pads are indicated in flat-soled horses and in horses ridden on rocky or uneven terrain.

POSSIBLE COMPLICATIONS

- Infectious osteitis and bone sequestrum formation
- Contralateral limb laminitis in horses with prolonged non–weight-bearing lameness

EXPECTED COURSE AND PROGNOSIS

- For horses with superficial uncomplicated infections, disease course is short and prognosis is excellent.
- Horses with complicated infections require longer and aggressive treatment. Prognosis is fair to good.

MISCELLANEOUS

ASSOCIATED CONDITIONS

- Laminitis
- Older horses with Cushing's disease

AGE-RELATED FACTORS

None

ZOONOTIC POTENTIALS

None

PREGNANCY

N/A

SEE ALSO

- Penetrating injuries to the foot
- Laminitis
- Cushing's disease

Suggested Reading

Stashak TS. Penetrating wounds of the foot. In: Stashak TS, ed. Adam's Lameness in Horses, ed 5. Baltimore: Lippincott Williams & Wilkins, 2002:703–710.

Author Elizabeth J. Davidson
Consulting Editor Elizabeth J. Davidson

SOLUBLE OXALATE TOXICOSIS

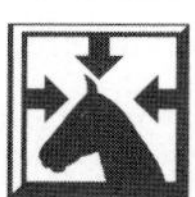

BASICS

OVERVIEW

• Disease follows ingestion of plants containing oxalic acid or soluble sodium and potassium oxalates.
• Oxalate concentrations in plant material vary widely between different parts of the plant, along with seasonal, environmental, and geographical factors.
• Green leaves and fruiting structures tend to contain higher oxalate concentrations.
• *Halogeton* spp. are an exception—Concentrations may increase as the plant matures and are often highest when the plant is dead and dry.
• Plants potentially containing dangerous amounts of soluble oxalates include—*Agave americana*, *Amaranthus* spp., *Anagallis arvensis*, *Beta vulgaris*, some *Brassica* spp., *Chenopodium* spp., *Galenias* spp., *Halogeton glomeratus, Kochia scoparia*, *Mesembryanthemum* spp., *Oxalis* spp., *Phytolacca americana*, *Portulaca oleracea, Rheum rhaponticum, Rumex* spp., *Salsola* spp., *Sarcobatus vermiculatus*, *Setaria* spp., *Tetragonia* spp., and *Trianthema* spp.; most of these plants are considered unpalatable when the oxalate content is high.
• Cases of poisoning are seen more commonly in the summer and fall months, when other forage is unavailable and large amounts of plant material are ingested over a short period of time.
• Ingestion of excess soluble oxalates causes GI discomfort along with muscular weakness and paralysis due to hypocalcemia. Ultimately, the disease can lead to acute renal damage.
• Nephrosclerosis and osteodystrophia fibrosa have been recorded in horses after chronic ingestion of oxalates, but these changes are uncommon.

SIGNALMENT

Equine intoxication with these plants is reportedly uncommon; horses appear relatively resistant to acute oxalate-induced nephrosis.

SIGNS

• Acute signs relate predominantly to hypocalcemia.
• Within 2–6 hr of ingestion, signs observed include depression, mild to moderate colic, and muscular weakness.
• Weakness may lead to recumbency, convulsions, unconsciousness, and death.
• Chronic signs may relate to renal disease, including polydipsia, polyuria, and generalized weight loss.

CAUSES AND RISK FACTORS

• Overgrazing areas highly contaminated with oxalate-containing plants
• Inadequate supplemental feed
• Hungry animals are more likely to ingest potentially toxic amounts.
• Low-calcium diets enhance soluble oxalate absorption; calcium binds oxalate in the GI tract to form insoluble calcium oxalate.

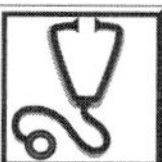

DIAGNOSIS

DIFFERENTIAL DIAGNOSIS

• Oxalate-induced hypocalcemic syndrome must be differentiated from hypocalcemia caused by poor diet and starvation, forced exercise, transit tetany (i.e., hypocalcemia during and after transportation), and lactation tetany (occurs 10 days after foaling or 1–2 days after weaning).
• Causes of equine acute renal disease—ischemia, vitamin K_3, NSAIDs, vitamin D, heavy metal (e.g., arsenic, mercury, lead), aminoglycoside, and acorn toxicoses
• Causes of equine chronic renal failure—proliferative glomerulonephritis, renal glomerular hypoplasia, chronic interstitial nephritis, pyelonephritis, amyloidosis, and neoplasia
• Known access to oxalate-containing plants is critical in helping to differentiate this disease from all others.

CBC/BIOCHEMISTRY/URINALYSIS

• Hypocalcemia is the most consistent finding.
• Other findings in cattle and sheep—modest elevations in liver enzymes (e.g., AST, ALT), proteinuria, albuminuria, hematuria, hyperglycemia, azotemia, hyperphosphatemia, and hyperkalemia

OTHER LABORATORY TESTS

Oxalate content of suspect plant material can be assayed by some laboratories.

IMAGING
N/A

DIAGNOSTIC PROCEDURES
N/A

PATHOLOGICAL FINDINGS
- Erythema and edema of the GI mucosa are most commonly seen.
- Other findings—necrosis of the proximal renal tubules and collecting ducts, with birefringent crystals; crystals also may be seen within vascular spaces.

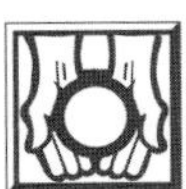

TREATMENT

- Hospitalize patients for initial medical workup and management.
- Fluid replacement therapy for any volume deficits and correction of any electrolyte and acid-base abnormalities are critical in patients with GI distress or possible renal failure.
- Fluid therapy also tends to slow precipitation of calcium oxalate crystals within the renal tubule lumen.

MEDICATIONS

DRUG(S) OF CHOICE
- Hypocalcemic patient should receive a slow IV infusion of calcium gluconate (e.g., 250–500 mL of 23% calcium gluconate diluted in fluids; alternatively, 150–250 mg/kg calcium gluconate IV slowly to effect).
- Rare patients exhibiting acute or chronic renal failure should be treated accordingly; treatment options vary depending on whether oliguria or polyuria is present.

CONTRAINDICATIONS/POSSIBLE INTERACTIONS
N/A

FOLLOW-UP

PATIENT MONITORING
- Monitor respiration and cardiac rate and rhythm during administration of calcium gluconate.
- Monitor serum concentrations of calcium, sodium, chloride, potassium, bicarbonate, urea nitrogen, creatinine, PCV, total protein, phosphorus, and central venous pressure in patients with severe GI distress or impaired renal function.

PREVENTION/AVOIDANCE
- Prevent access to soluble oxalate–containing plants through pasture management—animal rotation; herbicide treatment.
- Do not allow hungry animals access to highly contaminated areas.
- Make adequate supplemental forage available to animals grazing contaminated areas.
- Oral dicalcium phosphate prevents this disease in cattle and sheep.

EXPECTED COURSE AND PROGNOSIS
- Many clinically affected horses may not recover.
- Animals that survive acute intoxication often suffer renal failure, which carries a poor prognosis.
- Horses, being relatively resistant to the renal effects of soluble oxalates, may have a somewhat better prognosis than do affected cattle and sheep.

MISCELLANEOUS

ASSOCIATED CONDITIONS, AGE-RELATED FACTORS, ZOONOTIC POTENTIAL, PREGNANCY
N/A

ABBREVIATIONS
- ALT = alanine aminotransferase
- AST = aspartate aminotransferase
- GI = gastrointestinal
- PCV = packed cell volume

Suggested Reading

Radostits OM, Gay CC, Blood DC, Hinchcliff KW. Veterinary Medicine, ed 9. London: WB Saunders, 2000:1636–1639.

Author Patricia A. Talcott
Consulting Editor Robert H. Poppenga

SORBITOL DEHYDROGENASE (SD)/IDITOL DEHYDROGENASE (IDH)

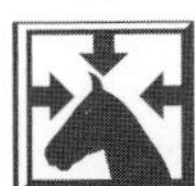

BASICS

DEFINITION

- SD catalyzes the reversible oxidation of D-sorbitol to D-fructose with the help of NAD.
- Although present at high concentration in hepatocytes, kidneys, and testes, SD is a liver-specific enzyme, with essentially all serum activity attributed to hepatocytes.
- Because of low ALT activity in hepatocytes of horses and other large animals, SD is the enzyme of choice for detection of hepatocellular injury/necrosis.
- Reported normal SD activity for horses ranges from 1.9–18.3 U/L.

PATHOPHYSIOLOGY

- Increases in SD activity are indicative of hepatocellular injury.
- SD is a specific indicator of acute and ongoing hepatocellular injury because of its short half-life (a few hours) and tissue specificity.
- The magnitude of the elevation generally is proportional to the number of hepatocytes affected, not to the severity of a particular insult. For example, injury to many hepatocytes (e.g., diffuse hepatitis) may cause higher serum SD activity than injury to fewer hepatocytes (e.g., small localized abscess).
- Activity of SD may increase within 4 hr of a single episode of hepatocellular injury and return to the reference range within 2–3 days. In contrast, AST (also an "injury" enzyme) takes longer to peak after injury and has a half-life of several days.
- After hepatocellular injury, SD increases quickly, before AST. Elevated SD, with normal or increased AST, indicates acute or ongoing hepatocellular injury.
- If serial serum chemistries reveal continuously or progressively elevated SD activity, ongoing hepatocellular injury is likely.
- During treatment of hepatic disease, the enzymes can be used to monitor cessation of the insult. If, after documenting recent hepatocellular injury, serial serum chemistries reveal elevated AST and progressively decreasing or normal SD activity, cessation of the original insult is likely.

SYSTEM AFFECTED

Hepatobiliary

GENETICS

Depends on the primary disease process and secondary complications

INCIDENCE/PREVELANCE

Depends on the primary disease process and secondary complications

GEOGRAPHIC DISTRIBUTION

Depends on the primary disease process and secondary complications

SIGNALMENT

Depends on the primary disease process and secondary complications

SIGNS

- Vary according to the primary cause
- Typically, horses with liver disorders may exhibit jaundice, discolored urine, neurologic deficits, and many other nonspecific signs—anorexia, abdominal pain, weight loss, and fever.
- Horses also may present with no significant clinical signs.
- Clinical signs of hepatic failure generally do not appear until 75% of the hepatic functional mass is lost.

CAUSES

- Degenerative conditions—cirrhosis; cholelithiasis
- Anomaly, congenital diseases— portal-vascular shunts, biliary atresia
- Metabolic diseases—shock, hypovolemia, hypoxia caused by severe anemia or during anesthesia, and severe GI disease
- Neoplastic or nutritional diseases—primary neoplasia, metastatic neoplasia, leukemia, and hepatic lipidosis
- Infectious and immune-mediated disease—hepatitis of various causes (e.g., viral, bacterial, protozoal, fungal, parasitic), serum sickness, amyloidosis, endotoxemia, and chronic active hepatitis.
- Toxic or trauma—pyrrolizidine alkaloid–containing plants, ferrous fumarate in newborn foals, cottonseed, castor, oaks, alsike clover, fungal toxins (e.g., aflatoxins, cyclopiazonic acid, fumonisin, phalloidin [mushrooms], rubratoxins), blue-green algae, and chemical compounds/elements (e.g., ethanol, chlorinated hydrocarbons, carbon tetrachloride, monensin, copper, iron, petroleum and its products, phosphorus)

RISK FACTORS

- Familial disease, exposure to infected animals, overweight and miniature ponies with hyperlipidemia, poor nutrition, or exposure to toxic compound or plants; these vary according to the specific disease.
- Halothane anesthesia, particularly of prolonged duration, may result in hepatic injury in horses.

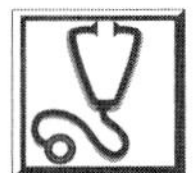

DIAGNOSIS

DIFFERENTIAL DIAGNOSIS

See Causes.

CBC/BIOCHEMISTRY/URINALYSIS

CBC

- Erythrocytes—Liver disease may cause nonregenerative anemia and morphologic changes (e.g., acanthocytes, target cells, nonspecific poikilocytosis, normochromic microcytosis in portosystemic vascular shunts); severe anemia of any cause may cause cellular injury due to tissue hypoxia.
- Leukocytes—Leukocytosis or leukopenia may be seen with inflammatory diseases and leukemia; morphologic changes in leukocytes may be seen (e.g., neutrophil toxicity in inflammation; neoplastic cells).
- Platelets—Quantitative decreases and increases may be seen with a variety of systemic diseases that affect the liver.

SERUM/PLASMA BIOCHEMISTRY PROFILE

- Various parameters may be abnormal, with the direction and magnitude of the change depending on the primary causes, severity of the disease, and other concurrent diseases or factors.
- Glucose—increased in diabetes mellitus and glucocorticoid influence (e.g., exogenous, endogenous); decreased in end-stage liver disease and sepsis/endotoxemia
- BUN—decreased in liver insufficiency and end-stage liver disease because of decreased conversion of ammonia to urea
- Albumin—decreased in end-stage liver disease because of decreased production; minimally to mildly decreased in inflammation
- Globulins—generally increased in end-stage liver disease and/or chronic antigenic stimulation
- AST—increased with injury to striated muscle and/or hepatocytes
- ALP—increased with concurrent cholestatic disease
- GGT—increased with cholestatic disease or hepatocellular injury
- Conjugated bilirubin—increased in cholestatic disease
- Unconjugated bilirubin—increased with anorexia and prehepatic cholestasis (i.e., massive in vivo hemolysis)
- Cholesterol—may be increased with cholestasis and lipid disorders, and decreased with hepatic insufficiency.
- Triglycerides—may be increased in association with hepatic lipidosis.
- Unlike other enzymes (e.g., AST), SDH is unstable at room temperature or when refrigerated and may lose as much as 25% of its activity during freezing after 1 week.
- If the serum or plasma sample is not analyzed within 8–12 hr, storage in a freezer is recommended.

Urinalysis

Bilirubinuria—conjugated bilirubin, detected by the commonly used "dipstick" and the diazo tablet methods, indicates cholestatic disease and should not be elevated if only hepatocellular injury is present.

OTHER LABORATORY TESTS

SBAs

- Sensitive test for hepatobiliary disease but not specific for the type of hepatobiliary disease
- May be increased with cell injury, cholestasis, or hepatic insufficiency/decreased functional mass. Specificity for the latter condition is greatly increased when SBAs are elevated with normal or minimally elevated markers for hepatocellular injury (i.e., SD, AST, GGT) and cholestasis (i.e., ALP, GGT, conjugated bilirubin).
- The main advantage of SBAs compared with plasma ammonia (i.e., a more specific test for hepatic insufficiency/decreased functional mass) is that immediate analysis of the sample is not necessary.

Plasma Ammonia Concentration

- Hepatic insufficiency/decreased functional mass is indicated by increased fasting or challenged concentration of ammonia.
- A sensitive and specific test, because it is not affected by other factors (e.g., cholestasis);

SORBITOL DEHYDROGENASE (SD)/IDITOL DEHYDROGENASE (IDH)

however, ammonia measurement requires special handling, which limits its general availability.
• Consult the reference laboratory for specific sample submission requirements.

Coagulation Tests and Fibrinogen

• The liver synthesizes many coagulation factors, and significant decreases in liver function may lead to deficiencies in these factors and to coagulation abnormalities.
• APTT and PT— decreases in these parameters occur when approximately 30% of the activity of the factors is present.

Serologic Tests

May help in detecting an infectious cause

Toxicology

• Analysis of tissue biopsy material, feed, ingesta, serum/plasma, or other body fluids may indicate presence of a toxin.
• Contact a reference laboratory regarding sample selection and submission.

Bacterial, Fungal, or Viral Culture

• May establish a definitive diagnosis regarding the infectious agent involved and help to guide treatment
• Request bacterial antibiotic sensitivity to determine appropriate antibiotic therapy.
• Contact a reference laboratory regarding sample selection and submission.

Sulfobromophthalein and Indocyanine Green Dye Clearance for Evaluation of Hepatic Function

These tests have been replaced by serum ammonia and SBAs.

IMAGING

Abdominal Ultrasonography

• Limited by the position and size of the liver
• Evaluate size, echogenicity, shape, and position.
• Useful in obtaining biopsy material for cytology, histopathology, and microbiology
• Findings depend on the primary disease condition.
• Other diagnostic imaging modalities such as radionucleotide imaging are expensive and available only at selected institutions.

OTHER DIAGNOSTIC PROCEDURES

• Aspiration cytology and histopathology of formalin-fixed tissue
• Cytology has the advantages of simplicity, quicker turnaround, better individual cellular detail, and better recognition of individual infectious organisms.
• Histopathology has the advantage of permitting examination of the tissue architecture and distribution of the lesion.
• The success of these procedures depends on the quality of the sample submitted, the area sampled, and the disease process itself—some hepatic diseases do not have significant microscopic alterations.

PATHOLOGICAL FINDINGS

Pathological findings depend on the primary disease and complications.

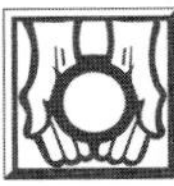

TREATMENT

AIMS OF TREATMENT

Depend on the primary disease process and secondary complications

APPROPRIATE HEALTH CARE

Depends on the primary disease process and secondary complications

NURSING CARE

Depends on the primary disease process and secondary complications

ACTIVITY

Depends on the primary disease process and secondary complications

DIET

Depends on the primary disease process and secondary complications

CLIENT EDUCATION

Depends on the primary disease process and secondary complications

SURGICAL CONSIDERATIONS

Depends on the primary disease process and secondary complications

MEDICATIONS

DRUG(S) OF CHOICE

Depend on the primary disease process and secondary complications

CONTRAINDICATIONS

N/A

PRECAUTIONS

With suspected hepatic insufficiency, assess the relative safety/risk of performing invasive procedures (e.g., fine-needle aspiration, tissue biopsy, laparoscopy, surgery) in light of the coagulation panel results.

POSSIBLE INTERACTIONS

Depend on the primary disease process and secondary complications

ALTERNATIVE DRUGS

Depend on the primary disease process and secondary complications

FOLLOW-UP

PATIENT MONITORING

Serial serum biochemical analyses to monitor progression or improvement of the disease process (see Pathophysiology)

PREVENTION/AVOIDANCE

Depends on the primary disease process and secondary complications

POSSIBLE COMPLICATIONS

Depend on the primary disease process and secondary complications

EXPECTED COURSE AND PROGNOSIS

Depend on the primary disease process and secondary complications

MISCELLANEOUS

ASSOCIATED CONDITIONS

Depend on the primary disease process and secondary complications

AGE-RELATED FACTORS

See Signalment.

ZOONOTIC POTENTIAL

Possible with some infectious diseases such as salmonellosis

PREGNANCY

See Signalment.

SYNONYMS

• IDH
• SDH

SEE ALSO

See Causes.

ABBREVIATIONS

• GI = gastrointestinal
• SBA = serum bile acids

Suggested Reading

Pearson EG. Diseases of the hepatobiliary system. In: Smith BP, ed. Large Animal Internal Medicine, ed 3. St. Louis: Mosby, 2002.

Kramer JW, Hoffmann WE. Clinical enzymology. In: Kaneko JJ, Harvey JW, Bruss ML, eds. Clinical Biochemistry of Domestic Animals, ed 5. San Diego: Academic Press, 1997.

Tennant BD. Hepatic function. In: Kaneko JJ, Harvey JW, Bruss ML, eds. Clinical Biochemistry of Domestic Animals, ed 5. San Diego: Academic Press, 1997.

Bain PJ. Liver. In: Latimer KS, Mahaffey EA, Prasse KW, eds. Duncan and Prasse's Veterinary Laboratory Medicine Clinical Pathology, ed 4. Ames, IA: Iowa State University Press, 2003.

Peek SF. Liver disease. In: Robinson NE. Current Therapy in Equine Medicine, ed 5. Philadelphia: Saunders, 2003.

The author and editor wish to acknowledge the contribution to this chapter of John A. Christian, co-author in the previous edition.

Author Armando R. Irizarry-Rovira
Consulting Editor Kenneth W. Hinchcliff

SORGHUM SPP. TOXICOSIS

BASICS

OVERVIEW

• *Sorghum vulgare* var. sudanense (sudangrass or hybrid sudangrass) causes cystitis, ataxia and teratogenesis in horses. The sorghum cystitis – ataxia syndrome is also referred to as cauda equine syndrome. Grazing of sudan pastures and ingestion of freshly cut hay are associated with the syndrome but feeding of cured hay is not.
• Generally, intoxication occurs during periods of high rainfall and rapid plant growth. Fertilization has no effect on toxicity.
• The toxin is believed to be a lathyrogenic agent, β-cyanoalanine. Onset of clinical signs is after weeks to months (average of 8 weeks) of grazing a sudangrass pasture.
• Geographically, sudangrass is most commonly used as a forage in the southwestern and central United States. Ingestion of *Sorghum* spp. is also associated with cyanide and nitrate toxicoses (see Cyanide Toxicosis and Nitrate Toxicosis for more in-depth discussion of these intoxications).

SIGNALMENT

Sorghum cystitis – ataxia is more common in mares but can occur in geldings or studs. All ages are susceptible.

SIGNS

• Posterior ataxia and incoordination
• Forced movement enhances ataxia
• Falling when backed up
• Recumbency
• Constant urine dribbling from a full bladder
• Urine scalding
• Cystitis
• Frequent opening and closing of vulva (winking)
• Mares may appear to be in constant estrus.
• Fetal malformations (extreme flexion of joint or ankylosis) when mares graze sudangrass between days 20–50 of gestation

CAUSES AND RISK FACTORS

Grazing sudangrass is the primary risk.

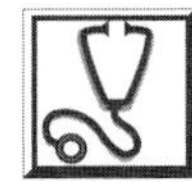

DIAGNOSIS

DIFFERENTIAL DIAGNOSIS

• Trauma
• Abscess
• neoplasia
• EHV-1 myeloencephalitis
• EPM
• rabies

CBC/BIOCHEMISTRY/URINALYSIS

• Leukocytosis
• Lymphocytosis
• Sediment—large numbers of RBCs, WBCs, epithelial cells, bacteria, hyaline casts, and granular casts
• Normal pH and specific gravity
• Proteinuria

OTHER LABORATORY TESTS

Urine bacterial cultures generally isolate opportunistic bacteria such as *Escherichia coli*, *Proteus vulgaris*, *Staphylococcus* spp., *Pseudomonas aeruginosa,* or *Corynebacterium* spp.

IMAGING

N/A

DIAGNOSTIC PROCEDURES

N/A

PATHOLOGICAL FINDINGS

• Gross pathology—cystitis with marked thickening of the bladder wall
• Full bladder
• Hyperemic ureters
• Hyperemic urethra
• Vaginal hyperemia
• Ulcerations of the bladder mucosa
• External abrasions from falling
• Areas of urine-scalded skin
• Pyelonephritis
• Histopathology—necrotizing cystitis
• Pyelonephritis
• Inflammation of the ureters, urethra, bladder, and vagina
• Axonal degeneration of the spinal cord and cerebellum
• Myelomalacia of the spinal cord and cerebellum

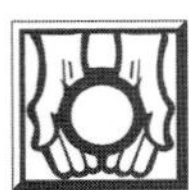

TREATMENT

- Treatment can be managed on an outpatient basis.
- Generally, treatment is unsuccessful in horses that exhibit incoordination and/or urine dribbling.
- Temporary cure of cystitis/pyelonephritis can be achieved but recurrence 2–3 weeks after therapy is stopped is common.
- Prevent further exposure by removing horses from access to sudangrass.
- Treat urine-scalded areas.
- Antimicrobial treatment of cystitis/pyelonephritis should be based upon culture and sensitivity tests.

NURSING CARE

N/A

MEDICATIONS

DRUGS

Antibiotics should be chosen based on culture and sensitivity tests.

CONTRAINDICATIONS/POSSIBLE INTERACTIONS

Avoid use of potentially nephrotoxic antibiotics.

FOLLOW-UP

PATIENT MONITORING

Monitor urine for evidence of bacteria/cystitis twice weekly during and after antibiotic therapy.

PREVENTION/AVOIDANCE

Avoid exposure to sudangrass pastures.

POSSIBLE COMPLICATIONS

With severe ulceration and necrosis, scarring and strictures are possible.

EXPECTED COURSE AND PROGNOSIS

- Recovery of clinically effected horses is extremely rare.
- Horses that do not continue to have recurrent cystitis should not be used for work or riding due to residual nervous system damage.
- Horses may still be used for breeding, but cystitis, vaginitis, or urethritis can complicate breeding efforts.

MISCELLANEOUS

ASSOCIATED CONDITIONS

N/A

AGE-RELATED FACTORS

N/A

ZOONOTIC POTENTIAL

N/A

PREGNANCY

Fetal malformations (extreme flexion of joints or ankylosis) occur when mares graze sudangrass between days 20–50 of gestation.

SEE ALSO

Nitrate toxicosis
Cyanide toxicosis

Suggested Reading

Burrows GE, Tyrl RJ. Toxic Plants of North America. Ames, IA: Iowa State University Press, 2001:929.

Van Kampen KR. Sudan grass and sorghum poisoning of horses: a possible lathyrogenic disease. J Am Vet Med Assoc 1970;156:629–630.

Author Jeffery O. Hall
Consulting Editor Robert H. Poppenga

SPERMATOGENESIS AND FACTORS AFFECTING SPERM PRODUCTION

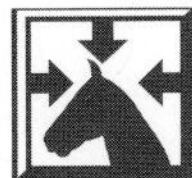

BASICS

DEFINITION/OVERVIEW

• *Spermatogenesis*—occurs in testicular seminiferous tubules and is the process of:
 ○ Mitotic proliferation of spermatogonia ○ Meiotic divisions of primary (first meiotic division) and secondary spermatocytes (second meiotic division) to form spermatids ○ Maturation of spermatids into spermatozoa capable of motility and fertilization.
 ○ In the horse, this sequence takes 55–57 days.
• *Spermiogenesis*—portion of spermatogenesis that involves the maturation of round spermatids into spermatozoa • *Epididymal maturation*—In many animals, including the horse, passage through the epididymis is thought to be a necessary for spermatozoa to achieve normal motility and fertilizing ability.
 ○ Passage through the epididymis takes 9 days in the horse.

ETIOLOGY/PATHOPHYSIOLOGY

Normal Physiology

Endocrine Considerations

• Testosterone tissue concentrations in the testis seem to be positively associated with spermatogenic activity.
 ○ Tissue concentrations of testosterone are related to blood concentrations. ○ It is difficult to assess testosterone activity in the testis or circulating levels with a single blood sample.
• Modulation of spermatogenesis involves LH, FSH, GnRH, testosterone, estrogen, inhibin, and other paracrine/autocrine factors not yet completely characterized.

Seasonal Patterns

• Some studies report a higher testicular concentration of testosterone in stallions during the breeding season.
○ Sperm production during the winter short-daylight months may be half of the level observed during months of maximum photoperiod. ○ Normal stallions produce spermatozoa year-round (and are potentially fertile year-round).
 ○ Sperm motility and percent normal morphology vary little throughout the year. ○ There are seasonal variations in sperm production and output.

SIGNS—AZOOSPERMIA AND OLIGOSPERMIA

• Small testes • Softening or reduction in size of the testes • Poor semen characteristics of reduced motility, increased morphological defects, and reduced total sperm numbers per ejaculate or DSO
• Azoospermia—There are *no* spermatozoa.
• Oligospermia or oligozoospermia—few spermatozoa present

CAUSES OF ARRESTED OR DISRUPTED SPERMATOGENESIS

Congenital

• Testicular hypoplasia due to hypogonadotropic hypogonadism
 ○ Abnormally low GnRH, LH, and FSH result in low testosterone. ○ Probably rare
• Primary testicular degeneration
 ○ Unknown if this is part of a congenital lesion or acquired
• Chromosomal anomalies such as XXY
• Intersex conditions • Cryptorchidism

Acquired

• Testicular neoplasia is rare. • Testicular heating due to infection, fever, environment, and scrotal insulation
 ○ *Heating* could result from a hydrocele, ventral edema, inflammation, and trauma.
• Testicular degeneration associated with testicular metabolic changes is incompletely characterized at present but might be associated with either of the following:
 ○ Anabolic steroid treatment, or treatment with steroids or medications with steroid-like effects, i.e., androgens, estrogens, or progestins, administered for behavioral or medical conditions ○ Interference with normal metabolism by nutritional deficiencies, or exposure to toxic substances, of which there are many (see Table). Diagnosis is challenging and few cases have specifically been documented in the stallion.

RISK FACTORS—OLIGOSPERMIA AND AZOOSPERMIA

• Toxins • Metabolic disorders • Testicular heating
• Trauma • Neoplasia • Inflammation

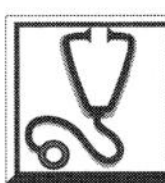

DIAGNOSIS

• Semen evaluation—a set of *two ejaculates* collected at a 1-hr interval
 ○ The minimum sample size to assess fertility and/or sperm production ability
• DSO—arrived at by collecting daily until sperm numbers stabilize • Rule out:
 ○ Bilateral blockage of the excurrent duct system
 ○ Ejaculatory disturbances ○ Behavioral abnormalities that cause failure of normal ejaculation

DIFFERENTIAL DIAGNOSIS

Refer to Causes and Age-Related Factors.

IMAGING

U/S

• Assess testicular dimensions and volume, and presence of fluid within space between the parietal and visceral vaginal tunics. • Assess testicular texture and presence of abnormal masses in testis or epididymis.
• Evaluate ampullae if blockage or sperm accumulation is suspected.

OTHER DIAGNOSTIC PROCEDURES

• Measurement of serum/plasma concentrations of FSH, LH, estrogen, inhibin, and testosterone.
 ○ Daily blood samples for 3 days recommended by some labs.
• GnRH stimulation test—single dose of 25 μg GnRH given IV at 9 AM
 ○ Blood collected at 30 (pre-GnRH treatment), 0, 30, 60, 90, and 120 min ○ Serum/plasma assayed for LH and testosterone
• Triple pulse GnRH stimulation test (given in nonbreeding season)
 ○ Three IV doses of 5 μg given 1 hr apart ○ Samples taken 1 hr before and 6 hr after GnRH ○ Assayed for LH
• hCG stimulation test—give 10,000 units hCG IV
 ○ Collect blood samples 1 hr before and 6 hr after hCG. ○ Assay for testosterone and estrogen.
• Testicular biopsy—three tissue samples recommended
 ○ One biopsy sample fixed in Bouin's fluid or modified Davidson's solution for histopathological evaluation ○ Two tissue samples placed in PBS and snap-frozen for assay of paracrine/autocrine factors
• Flow cytometric procedures such as the SCSA or SUTI
 ○ Detect alterations in sperm integrity. ○ May be available in some specialized university and/or research settings

PATHOLOGICAL FINDINGS (CONDITIONS)

Azoospermia—Absence of Spermatozoa in the Ejaculate

• *Causes*—absence of germ cells in the seminiferous tubules (rare), arrested spermatogenesis, bilateral blockage of the epididymis or ductus deferens, and abnormal ejaculation • Typically, stallions with congenital absence of spermatogenesis or arrested spermatogenesis will have smaller testes than normal.

Oligospermia—Fewer Spermatozoa in the Ejaculate Than Considered Normal

• *Causes*—small testicular volume with reduced sperm-producing tissue, congenital disorders, partial blockage of the duct system, ejaculatory disturbances, and disruption of spermatogenesis due to toxins, metabolic disorders, testicular heating, trauma, neoplasia, and inflammation
• Typically, stallions with chronic oligospermia due to reduced testicular production of spermatozoa will have smaller than normal testes.

Poor Fertility Following Cryopreservation and/or Cooling

• The sperm's ability to tolerate these special procedures varies by stallion. • The causes of increased susceptibility of some stallion's sperm to damage during cryopreservation and/or cooling are best described as "idiopathic."
 ○ Subtle disruptions in spermatogenesis may not have been identified and cannot be ruled out.

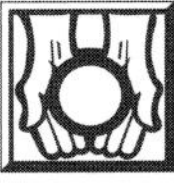

TREATMENT

• Resolve underlying condition, if it can be identified.
• Hemicastration may be indicated if one testis in a valuable breeding animal has been affected by trauma, inflammation, infection, or neoplasia. • Treatments of infertility due to abnormal spermatogenesis are speculative at best if the etiology and underlying pathological process remain unidentified.

CLIENT EDUCATION

• An understanding of the length of the spermatogenic cycle and the need for patience are critical. • Minimum recheck interval or BSE of an injured or affected stallion—two months from date of recovery, e. g., body temperature has returned to normal (post-fever), following episode of frost-bite affecting the scrotum, following a hemicastration of a testicular tumor, etc.

FOLLOW-UP

• Semen evaluation following treatment or resolution of underlying condition • Depending on what aspects of spermatogenesis are affected, the period of recovery might be as long as 60–70 days (the duration of spermatogenesis and epididymal maturation and transport)

MISCELLANEOUS

AGE-RELATED FACTORS

• At puberty, testis weight is positively correlated with:
 ○ Potential DSO based on histologic evaluation of seminiferous tubules
 ○ Quantitative measures of spermatogenesis
• In 1- to 3-year-old horses, spermatogenic efficiency does not reach normal adult levels of 14–18 million spermatozoa per gram of testicular tissue per day until

SPERMATOGENESIS AND FACTORS AFFECTING SPERM PRODUCTION

the individual testis weight reaches 70–80 g, or a combined testicular volume of 133 to 152 mL (or cm^3).
  - Some 3-year-olds may reach this testicular volume without producing sufficient spermatozoa to rank them as *satisfactory* during a BSE. ○ From puberty on, sperm production may continue to increase for years. Some studies have found sperm production continues to increase past 12 years of age. Full maturity of the stallion with regard to sperm production is often considered to be 6 years.
- Intratesticular testosterone (testosterone produced per gram of testicular tissue) increases with age and is related to sperm production.
  - Differences in intratesticular testosterone between stallions may explain differences in sperm production.
- In general
  - Testicular size increases with age. ○ Sperm production and sperm output increase with testicular size.

SYNONYMS

• Oligospermia • Oligozoospermia

SEE ALSO

• Abnormal testicular size • Castration, routine and Henderson technique • Cryptorchidism • Disorders of sexual development • Inquinal hernias • Spermatogenesis

ABBREVIATIONS

• BSE = breeding soundness examination • DSO = daily sperm output • FSH = follicle-stimulating hormone • GnRH = gonadotrophin-releasing hormone • hCG = human chorionic gonadotropin • LH = luteinizing hormone • PBS = phosphate-buffered saline • SCSA = sperm chromatin structure assay • SUTI = sperm ubiquitin tag immunoassay • US = ultrasound, ultrasonography

Suggested Reading

Card C. Cellular associations and the differential spermiogram: making sense of stallion spermatozoal morphology. Theriogenology 2005;64:558–567.

Proceedings of the 4th International Symposium on Stallion Reproduction, Hannover, Germany, October2005. Anim Reprod Sci 2005;89:1–321.

Roser J. Endocrine Diagnostics for Stallion Infertility. In: Recent Advances in Equine Reproduction, B. A. Ball(ed.), International Veterinary Information Service (www.ivis.org), Ithaca, New York (2001)

Samper JC, et al., eds. Current Therapy in Equine Reproduction. St. Louis: Elsevier, 2007.

Authors Rolf E. Larsen and Tim J. Evans

Consulting Editor Carla L. Carleton

Table 1

Toxicants and Physiological Factors That Adversely Affect Spermatogenesis

Toxicant/Factor	Potential Adverse Effect(s) on Stallions*
Antimicrobials	
Metronidazole	High doses: ↓ sperm number and ↑ abnormal morphology
Tetracycline	Very high doses: ↓ sperm number; ↓ sperm capacitation; testis atrophy
Trimethoprim	One-month course: ↓ sperm number by 7%–88%
Exogenous Hormones	
Androgens	↓ Sperm number; testicular degeneration
Anabolic steroids	↓ Sperm number, motility and normal morphology
Estrogens	↓ Sperm number; behavioral feminization
Progestins	↓ Sperm number and normal morphology; ↓ aggression
Antihistamines	
Chlorpheniramine	In vitro experiments: ↓ sperm motility
Gastrointestinal Tract Drugs	
Cimetidine	↓ Sperm number
Anti-inflammatory Medications	
Phenylbutazone	Inhibition of sperm acrosome reaction; unknown effect on fertility
Prednisone	↓ sperm number and motility; ↓ testosterone
Insecticides	
Pyrethrins	In vitro: 40%–60% ↓ in testosterone binding to androgen receptor
Heavy Metals	
Lead	↓ Testosterone; ↓ sperm number; ↓ fertilization rates
Physiologic Factors	
Stress	↓ Sperm motility
Fever (hyperthermia)	Damaged sperm chromatin and quality

* Note:
• These potential toxicants (many of them are medications commonly used in equine practice) and physiologic factors have adversely affected spermatogenesis in one or several animal species (including horses in some instances).
• It is assumed that high enough or long enough exposures to any of these could potentially have similar effects in stallions, despite few or no reported cases.
• Depending on the stage of sexual development at the time of exposure, adverse effects can vary in their severity and reversibility.

Adapted, with permission, from Ellington JE, Wilker CE. In: Peterson ME,Talcott PA, eds. Small Animal Toxicology, ed 2. St. Louis: Elsevier Saunders, 2006.

SPIDER ENVENOMATION

BASICS

OVERVIEW

- Spider bites are not common.
- Diagnosis is often difficult because the spider is usually not present when treatment is needed.
- The two most common poisonous spiders in the United States are the fiddleback, *Loxosceles reclusa,* and the black widow, *Latrodectus* spp.
- Fiddleback spiders, also known as brown recluse, are brown with a dark brown violin shape on their back. They have delicate legs that span 1–2 inches in diameter as adults. They are nocturnal and are often found in closets and attics.
- Black widow spiders are black with a red hourglass or other red shape on the ventral abdomen of the female. Females consume their mate. They prefer to be outside, under old woodpiles or in dark places. Their adult leg span is approximately 1 inch in diameter.
- Fiddleback venom contains hyaluronidase, esterases, alkaline phosphatases, and 32-kDa sphingomyelinase and causes localized necrosis.
- Black widow venom contains neuroactive proteins and proteolytic enzymes and is neurotoxic. The principal toxin is α-latrotoxin, which causes an initial large release of acetylcholine and norepinephrine at postganglionic sympathetic synapses followed by depletion of the neurotransmitters.
- Horses are reportedly very sensitive to black widow (*Lactrodectus mactans* or *hesperus*) spider bites, with resultant hypertension, pain, and muscle spasms 15 min to 6 hr after envenomation.

SIGNALMENT

N/A

SIGNS

Black Widow

- Subcutaneous edema and pain at the bite site are the main clinical signs.
- Generalized hypertension and pain associated with regional lymph nodes and extremities as it spreads
- Muscle fasciculations and rigidity
- Abdominal pain (colic)
- Ataxia
- Flaccid paralysis progressing to ascending paralysis
- Dyspnea if respiratory muscles are involved
- Most black widow spider bites produce symptoms that peak in 2–4 hr.

Fiddleback

- Local and systemic signs
- Little or no pain from initial bite
- It starts as a central vesicle that becomes an ulcer with tissue around the site becoming red, swollen and painful.
- Tissue will slough over a period of weeks. Severity depends on site of bite (e. g., near veins or arteries).
- Systemic signs are less common but can include (in humans): hemolysis, nausea, vomiting, fever, and malaise.

CAUSES AND RISK FACTORS

- All mammalian species are susceptible to the venom of fiddleback and black widow spiders.
- Garbage, sheds, old tarpaulins, and discarded furniture or farm equipment are good black widow spider habitats.
- Old buildings, clothes, old newspapers, attics, and undisturbed places are good fiddleback habitats.
- Many modern houses and barns have problems with fiddleback spider infestation.

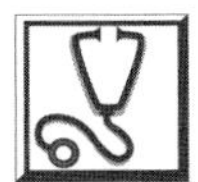

DIAGNOSIS

DIFFERENTIAL DIAGNOSIS

- Actually observing a spider on a horse is probably the only way to associate a bite wound with a spider.
- Colic resulting from other causes can be confused with *Lactrodectus* spp. envenomation.
- Ataxia, pain, stiffness, and muscle fasciculation may resemble ionophore toxicosis: detection of ionophore in feed sample, post-mortem lesions associated with cardiotoxicity of ionophores
- Ascending paralysis is also a symptom of botulism—detection of botulinum toxin in environmental (feed) or biological samples
- Nonhealing ulcerative lesions could resemble *Loxosceles* spp. envenomation.

CBC/BIOCHEMISTRY/URINALYSIS

- A serum chemistry and CBC may show evidence of a Coomb's negative hemolytic anemia.
- Elevation of enzymes indicating skeletal muscle damage (creatine kinase, aspartate transaminase) may occur after a black widow bite.

OTHER LABORATORY TESTS

N/A

IMAGING

N/A

OTHER DIAGNOSTIC PROCEDURES

N/A

PATHOLOGICAL FINDINGS

- Swelling and erythema around the bite may be the only pathology noted with a black widow spider bite.
- Tissue necrosis is the primary lesion with fiddleback spider bites.

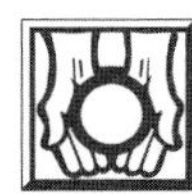

TREATMENT

- Depends on the type of spider
- Supportive and symptomatic
- Both types should be treated as emergencies, but usually time of bite is not known.

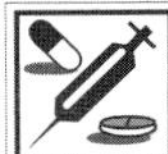

MEDICATIONS

DRUG(S) OF CHOICE

Black Widow

- Diazepam for muscle rigidity
- Methocarbamol for muscle rigidity
- Opioids for pain
- A black widow antivenin exists but should be used only if necessary, because it is of equine origin and can result in anaphylaxis. If used, give undiluted (one vial/horse) and administer IV.

Fiddleback

- There is no antidote.
- Chlorhexadine diacetate topical 1% q6h
- Dapsone at 1 mg/kg q12h for 10 days (human treatment); efficacy questionable
- Analgesics such as flunixin at 0.5–1.1 mg/kg IV, IM, or PO q8–12h
- Antibiotics

CONTRAINDICATIONS/POSSIBLE INTERACTIONS

Watch the animal closely for signs of anaphylaxis if antivenin is administered.

FOLLOW-UP

PATIENT MONITORING

- The course of a black widow bite will generally occur much faster than a fiddleback bite unless systemic signs occur.
- Fiddleback spider bites must be monitored at least twice a day to determine severity and secondary complications.

PREVENTION/AVOIDANCE

Clean up potential spider habitats.

POSSIBLE COMPLICATIONS

Areas that slough from fiddleback bites should be monitored, particularly if the blood supply is affected.

EXPECTED COURSE AND PROGNOSIS

Recovery from a spider bite generally is within 7–14 days.

Suggested Reading

Gwaltney-Brant SM, Dunayer EK, Youssef HY. Terrestrial zootoxins. In: Gupta RC, ed. Veterinary Toxicology: Basic and Clinical Principles. New York: Elsevier, 2007:785.

Roder JD. Spiders. In: Plumblee KH, ed. Clinical Veterinary Toxicology. St. Louis: Mosby, 2004:111.

Author Sandra E. Morgan

Consulting Editor Robert H. Poppenga

SPLENOMEGALY

BASICS

OVERVIEW

• The spleen serves a number of functions in the horse—storage for blood cells, a source of extramedullary erythropoiesis, a major component of the RES, and an important component of the immune system.
• Splenomegaly is a diffuse enlargement of the spleen and is usually secondary to other disease processes. • Splenomegaly can be caused by increased workload (hypersplenism), inflammation of the spleen (splenitis), infiltration by neoplastic cells, venous congestion, splenic infarction, or hematoma.

SIGNS

• Complete destruction of splenic function associated with splenomegaly is virtually free of signs, especially if loss of function occurs gradually. • In most cases clinical signs are restricted to those caused by the enlarged spleen impinging on other organs—for example, colic due to displacement of the bowel. • Splenic abscesses may be associated with systemic signs of depression, fever, anorexia, weight loss, tachycardia, and tachypnea if the abscess is extensive and/or acute. Pain may be evident on palpation over the area of the spleen.
• Peritonitis is often coexistent with splenic abscess and produces signs of mild, recurrent abdominal pain with arching of the back and disinclination to move. • Acute hematoma or splenic rupture results in pooling of blood within the splenic capsule and abdomen. Clinical signs may include colic, tachycardia, cold extremities, and pallor of the mucous membranes, all suggestive of hemorrhagic shock.

CAUSES AND RISK FACTORS

Hypersplenism

• Hypersplenism is caused by destruction of abnormal blood cells in the spleen and may be associated with disseminated intravascular coagulation, immune-mediated hemolytic anemia, immune-mediated thrombocytopenia, and purpura hemorrhagica. • Hypersplenism can be associated with hyperplasia of the RES (increase in number and size of macrophages), giant cell formation, and marked hemosiderin accumulation.

Infectious

• Acute splenitis or splenic abscess(es) results from infections with blood-borne pathogens and may result when a septic embolus lodges in the spleen (metastatic spread) or, more commonly, is due to extension of infection from a neighboring organ (e. g., gastric penetration by sharp metal or perforation of a gastric ulcer).
• The cellular infiltrates vary from neutrophilic, pyogranulomatous to granulomatous depending on the infectious agent. • Splenic abscesses due to metastatic spread has been reported for a number of agents including *Streptococcus equi* ss *equi, Corynebacterium pseudotuberculosis,* and *Rhodococcus equi.* • Moderate degrees of splenomegaly occur in many systemic infectious diseases, especially salmonellosis, anthrax, babesiosis, equine infectious anemia, equine anaplasmosis (formerly ehrlichiosis), and, more rarely, trypansomiasis and echinococcosis.

Infiltrative

• Accumulations of neoplastic cells, or intracellular accumulations of abnormal lipid, result in infiltrative disease and cause an increase in splenic mass and size. • Primary neoplasia of the spleen is rare in horses but disseminated disease such as lymphoma and hemangiosarcoma often involves the spleen. Splenomegaly will also occur with leukemia (e. g., myelocytic) or metastic neoplasia (e. g., melanoma).

Congestive States

• Right-sided heart failure or, more rarely, portal hypertension may cause splenomegaly due to poor venous drainage, congestion of hepatic or splenic veins and venous overload. • Portal or splenic vascular occlusion may also occur secondary to parasites. • Lightning strike, electrocution, and euthanasia with barbiturates may be associated with moderate splenomegaly, but enlargement is less than that observed with congestive heart failure, portal obstruction, or neoplastic change.

Miscellaneous

Splenic hematoma or, in more severe cases, splenic rupture usually results from trauma, e. g., falling on a stirrup or blunt trauma to the left side of the rib cage.

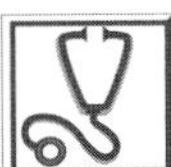

DIAGNOSIS

DIFFERENTIAL DIAGNOSIS

• To differentiate from primary intestinal lesions associated with colic, a complete workup for abdominal pain is indicated. • Left dorsal displacement of the colon and nephrosplenic entrapment cause splenic displacement medially and may give the impression that the organ is enlarged. Rectal examination and ultrasonography will detect the position of the colon. • Hepatomegaly may be differentiated by evaluation of liver enzymes, abdominal ultrasound, or liver biopsy. • Abdominal abscesses in other organs can be differentiated from splenic abscess with rectal examination and ultrasonography to locate the abdominal mass.
• Abdominal tumor—similar to that for abdominal abscess.

CBC/BIOCHEMISTRY/URINALYSIS

• Highly variable depending on underlying cause • Changes associated with hypersplenism may include anemia, thrombocytopenia, leukopenia, neutropenia, lymphopenia, hyperfibrinogenemia, increased hepatic enzyme activity, and hematuria. • Changes associated with chronic splenic abscesses may include leucocytosis with neutrophilia, hyperglobulinemia, hyperfibrinogenemia, and anemia—marked leukocytosis with a distinct left shift may occur in acute cases.

OTHER LABORATORY TESTS

Blood culture and serology for infectious agents

IMAGING

• Transadominal ultrasonography may be performed over the left 13th to 17th intercostal spaces to assess splenic size, detect infiltrative disease, alterations in echogenicity (hyperechoic or hypoechoic masses), and homogeneity and allow for guided biopsy. • The echogenicity of the left kidney should be concurrently evaluated for comparison and should be less echogenic.

OTHER DIAGNOSTIC PROCEDURES

• An enlarged spleen may be palpable per rectum, but this is not a consistent finding due to marked variations in size. • Abdominocentesis may provide evidence of chronic peritonitis (septic exudates) in cases of splenic abscess.
• Splenic aspiration or biopsy, then cytology and histopathology to determine underlying disease process

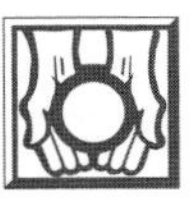

TREATMENT

• Level of care and specific treatment will depend on cause and severity of the primary underlying disease. • Splenic abscess may be treated with splenectomy if adhesions and associated peritonitis are absent, but is often unrewarding due to the extensive nature of the lesion before clinical signs appear.

MEDICATIONS

DRUG(S) OF CHOICE

Appropriate antimicrobials and antiparasitics depending on the causative agent

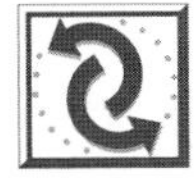

FOLLOW-UP

PATIENT MONITORING

• Monitor primary disease process.
• Monitor splenic size by rectal palpation or sonography.

POSSIBLE COMPLICATIONS

Splenic rupture of a grossly enlarged spleen may cause sudden death due to internal hemorrhage.

MISCELLANEOUS

SEE ALSO

• Anemia
• Babesiosis
• EIAV

ABBREVIATION

• RES = reticuloendothelial system

Suggested Reading

Diseases of the hemolymphatic and immune systems. In: Radostits O, Gay C, Hinchcliff K, Constable P, eds. Veterinary Medicine, ed 10. Philadelphia: WB Saunders, 2007;439–469.

Author Jennifer Hodgson
Consulting Editors David Hodgson and Jennifer Hodgson

STALLION SEXUAL BEHAVIOR PROBLEMS

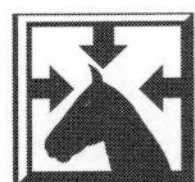

BASICS

DEFINITION

- Includes slow or variably inadequate precopulatory behavior, sexual arousal, erection, or copulatory behavior
- Particular preferences and aversions for mares, handlers, breeding locations, procedures, or equipment have also been demonstrated; can also be general or specific to certain conditions
- In stallions, can be chronic or intermittent and can include certain aberrant precopulatory or copulatory behaviors—excessive biting or licking, savaging the mare or handler, or premature dismount

PATHOPHYSIOLOGY

In stallions, can be the result of single or multiple factors—genetic predisposition, inadequate social maturation, simple inexperience, suboptimal breeding stimuli, or aversive experience associated with sexual behavior, breeding, or general handling

SYSTEMS AFFECTED

- Behavior—other behavior problems, including aggression stereotypies, can follow unresolved or ill-handled sexual behavior dysfunction; it is not uncommon for managers to physically abuse stallions for failure to perform sexually.
- Reproduction—subfertility or infertility

SIGNALMENT

Novice and experienced breeders of any age, breed, or performance type

SIGNS

Historical

- Current and past general health, attitude, and temperament? Early socialization experience?
- Training and performance history?
- What is the stallion fed, including supplements?
- Any current medications?
- Current work and performance schedule?
- How is the stallion housed?
- Breeding experience?
- Age of first use?
- Libido and temperament?
- General behavior in stall and at pasture?
- Step-by-step details of behavior in sexual situation?
- Past and current breeding schedules and results?
- Natural cover or collection of semen?
- Stimulus and mount mares used?
- How is the stallion handled for breeding?
- Experience of personnel?
- Behavior of any other stallions at same facility?

Physical Examination

Usually normal, but take care to identify any evidence of possible past sources of discomfort (e.g., stallion ring, other scars).

CAUSES

- Inexperience
- Pain associated with breeding—legs, feet, chest, shoulder, stifle, back, penis, testicles, cord torsion, or inguinal testicle
- Punishment associated with sexual behavior
- Antimasturbatory devices or practices
- Injudicious punishment or rough or inconsistent handling during breeding, particularly intolerance of normal sexual behavior or overhandling of the head
- Breeding accidents—slipping during breeding, hitting the head on a low ceiling when mounting, or being kicked by a mare
- Overuse as a breeding stallion or overwork in performance
- Abuse
- Suboptimal stimulus mare
- Innate mare preferences
- Suboptimal breeding environment—poor footing, low ceilings, or noise and distractions
- Suboptimal artificial vagina or dummy mount conditions or techniques
- Too rigid or too flexible breeding organization

RISK FACTORS

- Age <2 years
- Novice breeders >5 years
- Sire with low or temperamental libido
- Heavy training or work
- Exposure to anabolic steroids and other performance-enhancing medications and feed supplements
- Discipline for showing normal sexual behavior
- Heavy breeding schedule
- Poor general health
- Physical abuse
- Handrearing, particularly if isolated from other horses during development
- Housing conditions—deliberate or inadvertent sensory, exercise, and social deprivation
- Injudicious, rough, or inconsistent handling during breeding
- Any musculoskeletal or genital pain, discomfort, or instability
- Fear of people or a particular person
- Obesity
- Severely underweight
- Extreme hot or cold environmental temperatures
- Change in environment, housing conditions, or management, which can suppress sexual response
- Self-serve dummy mounts

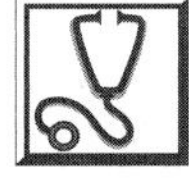

DIAGNOSIS

DIFFERENTIAL DIAGNOSIS

Medical differentials must be ruled out before a primary psychogenic diagnosis can be established.

CBC/BIOCHEMISTRY/URINALYSIS

Should be normal

OTHER LABORATORY TESTS

- Endocrinology—stallion panel (i.e., testosterone, estradiol, LH, FSH, T_3, T_4, insulin, and cortisol) should be normal. For old stallions or those with suspected testicular degeneration, hCG and GnRH challenge tests may be useful. Use challenge and sampling protocols of an equine endocrine laboratory with a large stallion database and knowledge regarding interpretation of their protocol results.
- Semen—can be evaluated for signs of infection or hemospermia that might suggest urogenital lesions causing discomfort

IMAGING

Radiography, scintigraphy, ultrasonography, and endoscopy to identify or rule out any sources of present or past musculoskeletal or urogenital pain.

DIAGNOSTIC PROCEDURES

- Cardiovascular examination to rule out aortic iliac disease that may affect breeding ability
- Musculoskeletal and neurologic examinations on the ground and during breeding
- Video surveillance in the stall to observe erection and penile movement during normal, spontaneous erections
- Video surveillance of the stallion in the stall next to a mare or turned out at liberty with or near a mare to determine stallion-like behavior under less-controlled conditions
- Video or direct observation of breeding procedures and stallion handling

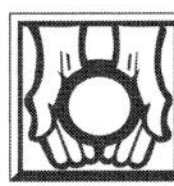

TREATMENT

MANAGEMENT AND ENVIRONMENT

- To the extent possible, correct obvious housing, handling, and breeding environment deficiencies, providing optimal stimulus mares and physical facilities for breeding—excellent footing, ample head room, and plenty of space
- Establish a feeding and exercise program to maximize fitness for breeding and to minimize fatigue and pain.
- Establish a breeding schedule to maximize libido and breeding performance; for stallions with low or variable libido, a breeding schedule of two or three times weekly usually maximizes arousal and performance.
- To the extent possible, identify and abide any specific preferences or aversions of the animal.

BEHAVIOR MODIFICATION

- Provide as much uncontrolled access to mares as possible; this likely will increase endogenous male hormones and build confidence in responding to mares.

- For slow-starting, novice breeders, continue daily exposure to breeding, with patient and gentle handling and a variety of stimulus mares; pasture breeding opportunities can build confidence and naturally train a stallion to breed.
- When people are present, they can encourage and positively reinforce sexual arousal and response.
- Educate handlers to use positive reinforcement–based stallion handling procedures to encourage spontaneous erection and masturbation.

MEDICATIONS

DRUGS OF CHOICE

- Analgesics, acupuncture, and related therapies for management of any potential sources of physical discomfort or instability during breeding
- Anxiolytics as a training aid to overcome past, negative breeding experiences—diazepam (0.05 mg/kg [to maximum of 20 mg] slow IV 5–7 min before breeding; extralabel use)
- Unless androgen levels are greater than the normal range, administer GnRH (50 μg SC 2 hr and again 1 hr before breeding; extralabel use) to boost endogenous androgens, which often increases sexual interest and arousal and appears to make genital tissues more sensitive to stimulation.
- If quick results are needed, short-term treatment with aqueous testosterone (50–80 mg SC every other day for at least 1 week; extralabel use) can effectively increase circulating testosterone and boost libido; the greatest improvement in libido typically occurs after 4–7 days of treatment.
- Imipramine hydrochloride (500–800 mg for each 1000 lb PO 2–3 hr before breeding; extralabel use) to lower the ejaculatory threshold and reduce the amount of work needed to breed
- Drug-induced ejaculation regimens (extralabel use) are available as substitutes for in copula breeding or collection of semen.

PRECAUTIONS

- Benzodiazepine anxiolytics release innate aggressive as well as sexual behavior. Caution handlers to expect and to prepare for possibly increased aggressive behavior before or during the increased sexual behavior. Similarly, increasing male hormone levels with GnRH or androgens also likely increases aggressive behavior. If the aggression is not skillfully directed or abided, mare or handler interaction with the stallion can be counterproductive. Increasing the dose of testosterone often is tempting, but possible adverse side effects on pituitary gonadal function are a concern.
- At certain levels, imipramine hydrochloride can inhibit rather than enhance ejaculation, disturb bladder neck function, and cause premature flaring of the glans penis. Should these occur, a lower dose usually is more effective at enhancing ejaculation without these side effects.

POSSIBLE INTERACTIONS

N/A

ALTERNATIVE DRUGS

N/A

FOLLOW-UP

PATIENT MONITORING

- Once- to twice-weekly follow-up for at least 1 mo, with monthly follow-up thereafter during the current breeding season to monitor and fine-tune improvements and medications
- Reexamination near the end of the current breeding season and near the beginning of the next breeding season, or with change in environment or health status

POSSIBLE COMPLICATIONS

- Best results occur if everyone involved with the care and handling of the horse communicates positively among each other and with the clinician toward a positive outcome for the stallion.
- Counterproductive blaming or failure of all to cooperate or comply with the treatment plan

MISCELLANEOUS

ASSOCIATED CONDITIONS

- Some stallions become "sour" if continually failing at breeding and may develop self-mutilation or tendencies to savage the mare or handlers.
- Many stallions with low libido actually began high-energy, unruly stallions that, in association with discipline, became uninterested or slow to respond.
- Subclinical lameness, neurologic disease, or aortic iliac disease that may specifically disturb pelvic circulation or cause hindlimb pain or weakness during copulation

AGE-RELATED FACTORS

- Inadequate sexual interest and response in young novice stallions more likely is primarily psychogenic than a libido problem in old experienced stallion that has been breeding successfully for years.
- Most healthy, sound stallions maintain stable libido through their mature years and into old age. However, with advancing age and accumulated minor physical deterioration, once tolerable musculoskeletal discomfort or disabilities may become more problematic for breeding stallions.
- Cardiac pathology, particularly with advancing age, often is associated with reduced libido, apparent anxiety on exertion during breeding, and delayed or urgent dismount.

ZOONOTIC POTENTIAL

N/A

PREGNANCY

N/A

SYNONYMS

- Libido problem
- Erection dysfunction
- Breeding dysfunction
- Sexual behavior dysfunction
- Poor breeding performance

SEE ALSO

- Aggression
- Fears and phobias
- Self-mutilation

ABBREVIATIONS

- FSH = follicle-stimulating hormone
- GnRH = gonadotropin-releasing hormone
- hCG = human chorionic gonadotropin
- LH = luteinizing hormone
- T_3 = triiodothyronine
- T_4 = thyroxine

Suggested Reading

Martin BB, McDonnell SM, Love CC. Effects of musculoskeletal and neurologic disease on breeding performance in stallions. Compend Cont Educ Pract Vet 1998;20:1159–1169.

McDonnell SM. Ejaculation: physiology and dysfunction. Equine Pract 1992;8:57–70.

McDonnell SM. Normal and abnormal behavior. Equine Pract 1992;8:71–89.

McDonnell SM. Sexual behavior dysfunction of stallions. In: Robinson NO, ed. Current Therapy in Equine Medicine, ed 3. 1992;3:633–637.

McDonnell SM. Libido, erection, and ejaculatory dysfunction in stallions. Compend Cont Educ Pract Vet 1999;21:263–266.

McGreevy P. Equine Behaviour: A Guide for Veterinarians and Equine Scientists. Philadelphia: WB Saunders, 2005.

Mills DS, McDonnell S. Domestic Horse: The Origins, Development, and Management of its Behaviour. New York: Cambridge University Press, 2005.

Waring GH. Horse Behavior, ed 2. Norwich, NJ: Noyes Publications/William Andrew Publishing, 2003.

Author Sue M. McDonnell

Consulting Editors Victoria L Voith and Daniel Q. Estep

STAPHYLOCOCCAL INFECTIONS

BASICS

DEFINITION

Infections caused by staphylococci, gram-positive, facultatively anaerobic bacteria

PATHOPHYSIOLOGY

Staphylococcus spp. can be found worldwide in mammals as well as the environment. At least 30 species of *Staphylococcus* spp. occur as commensals on the skin of domestic animals and humans. They can also be found on mucous membranes of the upper respiratory tract and lower urogenital tract and transiently in the gastrointestinal tract.

Staphylococcal bacteria are divided into CPS and CNS groups based on the ability to coagulate plasma. The CNS species were once considered normal skin flora but are now recognized as opportunistic pathogens responsible for infections related to the use of invasive medical procedures, medical implants, and intravenous catheterization.

Three species of CPS are important pathogens of domestic animals: *S. aureus* (SA), *S. intermedius*, and *S. hyicus*. All three species have been isolated from the skin of horses. SA is the most virulent species, although asymptomatic humans and animals can serve as carriers and reservoirs for sources of infection. The most frequent carrier sites in humans are the anterior nares and perineum. Asymptomatic equine carriers have been demonstrated with nasal swab cultures. SA possesses many characteristics and virulence factors that contribute to its pathogenicity. A variety of extracellular enzymes and toxins allow the organism to invade tissues and escape normal host defenses.

SA also has a significant ability to acquire or develop resistance to antimicrobials and antiseptics. Methicillin-resistant *Staphylococcus aureus* (MRSA) has become an increasing concern in veterinary medicine. MRSA strains are frequently resistant to many other classes of antimicrobials including the aminoglycosides, macrolides, chloramphenicol, tetracyclines, fluoroquinolones, and the beta-lactams. Many veterinary teaching hospitals have now identified MRSA strains in equine patients.

SYSTEMS AFFECTED

Integument

- Folliculitis/furunculosis
- Pseudomycetoma (granulomatous masses)
- Secondary infections
  - Traumatic wounds
  - Postoperative surgical incisions
- Cellulitis
- Musculoskeletal
  - Septic arthritis/osteomyelitis
- Hemic
  - Thrombophlebitis
  - Omphalophlebitis
- Urogenital
  - Scirrhous cord (infections of stump of the spermatic cord)
  - Metritis
- Respiratory
  - Pneumonia

INCIDENCE/PREVALENCE

Incidence of staphylococcal folliculitis usually increases in spring and summer months when humidity is high and horses are still shedding winter hair coats. Nosocomial infection with MRSA has now been identified in equine patients of multiple veterinary teaching hospitals. MRSA comprised 22% of all SA isolates from horses in one multicenter study. Horses have also been identified as carriers on horse farms, and 70% of MRSA carrier horses identified were less than 1 year old.

SIGNALMENT

No breed, sex, or age is predisposed to infection with staphylococci, although 70% of MRSA-positive carriers in one study were less than 1 year of age.

SIGNS

Historical

Weather changes and some seasons or climates may be associated with some dermatoses. Previous antimicrobial or other therapies may have been given with skin and wound infections. Occasionally, there is no history of a wound, or a penetrating injury can be very difficult to find in some cases of cellulitis.

Physical Examination

• Clinical signs will depend on the organ systems involved. • Earliest signs of staphylococcal folliculitis include small, raised tufts of hair that are easily epilated. These lesions may be more easily palpated than visualized. Papules develop with central ulceration, serosanguinous to purulent exudate and crust formation. Lesions range in diameter from 2–3 mm up to 1 cm. Pain may be present as lesions progress and areas of alopecia and scald develop. Pruritis is uncommon. Development of nodular lesions and draining tracts is suggestive of furunculosis. • Tail pyoderma and pastern dermatitis are cases of folliculitis/furunculosis specific to these areas. Pseudomycetomas are masses composed of firm nodules with purulent cores containing white granules. • Acute swelling of a limb with severe lameness is seen with cellulitis. The affected limb is typically warm and painful on palpation. The patient may be depressed, tachycardic, and febrile. Abscessation may develop with ulceration and skin sloughing. Concurrent infectious osteitis or osteomyelitis may also be present. • Signs of postoperative or wound infection include heat, pain, swelling, redness, and serous to purulent drainage. Local cellulitis, abscessation, and dissemination to other organs can follow.

CAUSES AND RISK FACTORS

• Dermatoses develop when the protective barriers of the skin or mucous membranes are disrupted. Minor abrasive trauma from harness or tack, maceration from water and sweat, abrasions, cuts, punctures, rubbing and scratching, or insect bites may be involved. Poor grooming habits and poor sanitation appear to increase risk, as well as exposure to excessively damp environments or contaminated fomites. • Lack of aseptic technique during surgical procedures and wound treatment provides exposure for wounds and surgical incisions. Immunosuppression, antimicrobial therapy or exposure to asymptomatic carriers and contaminated environments with MRSA may predispose to infection with resistant strains. • Transmission from humans to horses and horses to humans has been demonstrated in veterinary teaching hospitals. • Asymptomatic carriers of MRSA have been identified in horses and horse care personnel by nasal swab cultures. Farm size was the only demonstrable risk factor with all colonized horses living on a farm with a population of more than 20 horses.

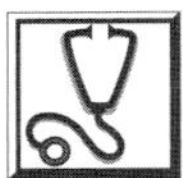

DIAGNOSIS

DIFFERENTIAL DIAGNOSIS

Dermatoses

• Dermatophilosis • Corynebacterial abscessation/folliculitis • Allergic dermatitis • Dermatomycosis • Pemphigus foliaceous

Pseudomycetoma

• Eosinophilic granuloma • Pythiosis • Habronemiasis • Sarcoid

Cellulitis

• Vasculitides • Lymphangitis

CBC/BIOCHEMISTRY/URINALYSIS

Bloodwork may be normal or show leukocytosis and hyperfibrinogenemia. Anemia can occur with chronic infection. Other changes will depend on organ system affected.

OTHER LABORATORY TESTS

N/A

DIAGNOSTIC PROCEDURES

Impression smears of crusts or exudates may aid in diagnosis of dermatophilosis. Gram stained smears may reveal typical gram-positive clusters of cocci with staphylococcal infections. Skin scrapings and fungal cultures are useful in cases of dermatophytosis. Histopathology can be helpful for severe acute or chronic skin conditions and mass lesions. Culture of exudates or tissue should be performed if bacterial infection is suspected and species identified for all staphylococci isolated. Antimicrobial sensitivity testing can aid in treatment planning and identify local trends. Methicillin or oxacillin should be included to rule in/out MRSA. Strain typing may be applicable in epidemiological studies such as nosocomial outbreaks.

Other tests may be useful depending on organ system involved (e.g., ultrasound and blood culture for thrombophlebitis).

IMAGING

Ultrasound and radiographs of areas with wounds or cellulitis may identify a primary lesion, foreign bodies, or damage to deeper tissue and bone such as concurrent osteomyelitis.

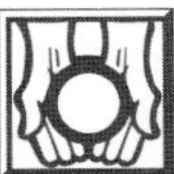

TREATMENT

- Treatment of folliculitis is highly dependent on removal of any underlying predisposing factors such as poorly fitting tack or inadequate hygiene. Shelter with dry, clean bedding is necessary for healing of pastern dermatitis. An adequate grooming routine should be implemented and all tack and grooming equipment regularly cleaned. Medicated baths with a dilute antiseptic such as povidone-iodine or chlorhexidine can be effective at eliminating bacteria. Occasionally, systemic therapy may be necessary in severe, unresponsive cases. The trimethoprim-sulfas are the antimicrobial of choice, although antimicrobial selection should be based on culture and sensitivity whenever possible. With more severe cases of pastern dermatitis, initial cleaning followed by generous application of antibiotic-corticosteroid ointment under a soft bandage for several days may soften the area and allow more thorough removal of crusts and exudates. Mupirocin ointment has been reported to be efficacious against staphylococcal infections with pastern dermatitis.
- Pseudomycetomas require surgical removal followed by systemic antimicrobial therapy for several weeks.
- Cases of infectious cellulitis typically respond well to systemic broad-spectrum antimicrobial therapy. Surgical debridement and lavage may be necessary early on in treatment. Daily cold hydrotherapy and bandaging along with administration of NSAIDs can help reduce swelling and increase comfort.
- Drainage must be established with wound and incisional infections and abscesses. Debridement and lavage should be performed as necessary.

MEDICATIONS

DRUG(S) OF CHOICE

- Staphylococci found in skin infections may be sensitive to a wide range of antimicrobials. When found in wounds and other invasive infections, staphylococci are usually resistant to penicillins, tetracyclines, and occasionally other antimicrobials. Broad-spectrum antimicrobial therapy such as penicillin and an aminoglycoside or trimethoprim-sulfonamide should be instituted initially in severe dermatoses, pseudomycetoma, cellulitis, and wound infections. Results of culture and sensitivity should guide further therapy.
- Antimicrobial resistance of SA is a growing concern with sensitivity to trimethoprim-sulfonamides, erythromycin, ceftiofur, and gentamicin variable. Many are sensitive to amikacin, enrofloxacin, and chloramphenicol.
- Vancomycin may be effective against MRSA, but its use in animals is controversial due to emergence of resistant organisms in human medicine. The use of vancomycin should be reserved for cases in which there are no other alternatives and antimicrobial sensitivity testing indicates vancomycin will be effective. Rifampin has been shown to have synergistic properties in treating MRSA but cannot be used alone as resistance develops quickly. Gentamicin has also been reported to be synergistic will vancomycin.

CONTRAINDICATIONS/POSSIBLE INTERACTIONS

- Rifampin is a potent inducer of microsomal enzymes of the liver, whereas erythromycin inhibits these systems. Serum levels of other drugs given concurrently may be affected.
- Fluoroquinolones have been associated with cartilage damage in young foals. Exposure to fluoroquinolones has also been linked to MRSA isolation or infection in humans although no evidence for this has been demonstrated in horses.
- Renal function should be monitored in patients receiving aminoglycosides. Some horses may demonstrate allergic hypersensitivity to topical therapies.

FOLLOW-UP

PATIENT MONITORING

Rectal temperature should be monitored daily in patients with wound or invasive infections or cellulitis. Persistent fever or fever spikes are indicative of inadequate response to therapy or further dissemination of infection. Patients with severe lameness caused by cellulitis should be monitored closely for development of laminitis in the contralateral limb. Skin biopsy may be indicated if dermatoses are unresponsive to treatment.

POSSIBLE COMPLICATIONS

Complications following invasive infection with MRSA depend on sites affected. Thrombophlebitis has been associated with bacteremia and dissemination to other sites including the lung, spinal cord and meninges, and liver. Osteomyelitis and sequestra may be seen with extensive cellulitis. Infection around orthopedic implants can lead to bony lysis and failure of fixations.

PREVENTION/AVOIDANCE

Adequate hygiene and environmental management can prevent some dermatoses. Horses should have access to dry, clean housing. Stalls or sheds should be cleaned frequently to help prevent pastern dermatitis. Masks and gloves may be necessary for horse care personnel of horses colonized with MRSA. Control measures such as isolation of colonized horses and associated equipment from noncolonized horses can reduce or eliminate carriers; however, this is labor intensive and may be cost prohibitive. Thorough hand washing has been shown to prevent transmission of staphylococci in humans.

EXPECTED COURSE AND PROGNOSIS

Prognosis is good for dermatoses and superficial wound infections but guarded for more invasive infections, especially if MRSA is present.

MISCELLANEOUS

ZOONOTIC POTENTIAL

Humans are susceptible to colonization with staphylococcal organisms from contact with horses. Horses are also susceptible to colonization from contact with humans. Colonization will not necessarily result in infection.

ABBREVIATIONS

- CNS = coagulase-negative staphylococci
- CPS = coagulase-positive staphylococci
- MRSA = methicillin-resistant *Staphylococcus aureus*
- SA = *Staphylococcus aureus*

Suggested Reading

Outerbridge CA, Ihrke PJ. Folliculitis: Staphylococcal pyoderma, dermatophilosis and dermatophytosis. In: Robinson NE, ed. Current Therapy in Equine Medicine, ed 5. St. Louis: Elsevier Science, 2003:197–200.

Middleton JR, Fales WH, et al. Surveillance of *Staphylococcus aureus* in veterinary teaching hospitals. J Clin Microbiol 2005;2916–2919.

Rosenkrantz WS. Systemic/topical therapy. In: Fadok VA, ed. Vet Clin N Am Equine Pract Dermatol 1995;11:127–146.

Weese JS, Archambault M, et al. Methicillin-resistant *Staphylococcus aureus* in horses and horse personnel, 2000–2002. Emerg Infect Dis 2005;11:430–435.

Weese JS, Rousseau J. Attempted eradication of methicillin-resistant *Staphylococcus aureus* colonization in horses on two farms. Equine Vet J 2005;37:510–514.

Author Christopher Ryan

Consulting Editors Ashley G. Boyle and Corinne R. Sweeney

STATIONARY NIGHT BLINDNESS

BASICS

OVERVIEW

Equine stationary night blindness is a disease of the outer and/or middle retina that is present at birth and persists throughout the horse's life. The rod photoreceptors, which are responsible for vision at low light levels (i.e., scotopic vision), are more severely affected than the cone photoreceptors, which allow the animal to see in daylight with higher light levels (i.e., photopic vision).

SYSTEM AFFECTED

Ophthalmic

SIGNALMENT

- Appaloosas are affected, but also Quarter Horses, Thoroughbreds, Paso Finos, and Standardbreds.
- No sex predilection is known.
- Disease is present at birth and persists throughout life.

SIGNS

- There is visual impairment in dim light with generally normal vision in daylight, behavioral uneasiness and unpredictability occurring at night, despite normal ophthalmoscopic examination.
- Foals may appear disoriented and stare off into space, and may have a bilateral dorsomedial strabismus.
- Owners may report repeated injuries to the horses during the evening hours.
- Poor day or photopic vision can also occur in a few cases.
- In mild cases, the disease is not observable until weaning, when the mare's guidance is no longer available. Some foals appear clumsy and a vision problem is not suspected until 1 year of age.
- If visual disturbance is not obvious in normal lighting, the horse should be observed in a dark area.

CAUSES AND RISK FACTORS

- There appears to be a defect in the neural transmission between photoreceptors and cells of the inner retina.
- It is a congenital, recessive trait in Appaloosas. It was once believed to be sex linked, but this may not be true. The prevalence was 25% in one study in Appaloosas. A single dominant allele, *Lp* (Leopard complex), is responsible for the color dilute white spotting patterns of coat color in Appaloosas and other horse breeds may be involved.

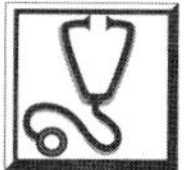

DIAGNOSIS

DIFFERENTIAL DIAGNOSIS

Other congenital and acquired blinding disorders of the retina, optic nerve, and brain have to be ruled out, such as colobomas, retinal detachments, and chorioretinitis. In the latter diseases, the visual impairment is not strictly limited to dim light.

Stationary Night Blindness

CBC/BIOCHEMISTRY/URINALYSIS
N/A

OTHER LABORATORY TESTS
N/A

IMAGING
N/A

DIAGNOSTIC PROCEDURES
Ophthalmoscopically, the ocular fundi appear normal. Electroretinography is required for definitive diagnosis. Decreased b-wave amplitude and a large negative, monotonic a-wave potential in the scotopic flash ERG confirm the presence of night blindness. The photopic flash ERG shows reduced amplitude and increased implicit time of the b-wave.

PATHOLOGIC FINDINGS
Histologic examination of the affected retinas is normal; subtle microphthalmos may occur.

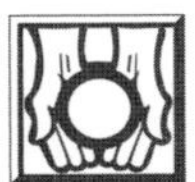

TREATMENT
None

MEDICATIONS
N/A

FOLLOW-UP

PREVENTION/AVOIDANCE
Affected horses should not be used for breeding.

POSSIBLE COMPLICATIONS
The disease may, in a very few cases, progress to poor photopic or day vision.

EXPECTED COURSE AND PROGNOSIS
Horses can undergo training and perform well during the day.

MISCELLANEOUS

SEE ALSO
- Ocular problems in the neonate
- Chorioretinitis
- Optic nerve atrophy

ABBREVIATION
- ERG = electroretinogram

Suggested Reading

Brooks DE. Ophthalmology for the Equine Practitioner. Jackson, WY; Teton NewMedia, 2002.

Brooks DE, Matthews AG. Equine ophthalmology. In: Gelatt KN, ed. Veterinary Ophthalmology, ed 4. Philadelphia; Lippincott Williams and Wilkins, 2007.

Gilger BC, ed. Equine Ophthalmology. Philadelphia; WB Saunders, 2005.

Sandmeyer LS, Breaux CB, Archer S, Grahn BH. Clinical and electroretinographic characteristics of congenital stationary night blindness in the Appaloosa and the association with the kopard complex. Vet Othalmol 2007;10:368–375.

Witzcl DA, Smith EL, Wilson RD, Aguirre GD. Congenital stationary night blindness: an animal model. Invest Ophthmol Vis Sci 1978;17:788–795.

Authors Andras M. Komaromy and Dennis E. Brooks

Consulting Editor Dennis E. Brooks

STREPTOCOCCUS EQUI INFECTION

BASICS

DEFINITION

Streptococcus equi subsp *equi* infection (strangles) is an acute upper respiratory infection characterized by fever, lethargy, purulent rhinitis, and regional lymph node abscessation.

PATHOPHYSIOLOGY

S. equi is inhaled or ingested after direct contact with mucopurulent discharge from infected horses or contaminated equipment. It adheres to the epithelial cells of the buccal and nasal mucosa. Eventually it spreads to the regional lymph nodes, such as the submandibular, submaxillary, and retropharyngeal lymph nodes. The M-protein is important for adherence of the organism to the epithelium and also protects the bacteria from ingestion by polymorphonuclear leukocytes. The hyaluronic acid capsule is important in the pathogenicity by repelling phagocytic cells due to its strong negative charge. Fever occurs 3–14 days after exposure. Nasal shedding occurs 2–3 days after the onset of fever, persisting for 2–3 weeks. Seventy-five percent of horses develop immunity after natural infection that can last up to 5 years. Older horses may develop a mild form of strangles. Carrier horses are responsible for maintaining the infection in affected herds. These carriers are asymptomatic, and the organism is often isolated from their guttural pouches.

SYSTEMS AFFECTED

• Respiratory • Hemic/lymphatic/immune

INCIDENCE/PREVALENCE

Disease occurs sporadically on farms, but once present, morbidity rates will depend on age of the animals (ranging from 32% to 100%). Mortality rates are considered low in uncomplicated cases (<2%) but higher for cases of bastard strangles.

GEOGRAPHIC DISTRIBUTION

S. equi occurs worldwide.

SIGNALMENT

S. equi can occur in any age group, although those between the ages of 1 and 5 years are predisposed. There is no breed or sex predilection.

SIGNS

• Fever of >103° F (>39.5°) • Depression and listlessness • Lymphadenopathy and abscessation of retropharyngeal and submandibular lymph nodes (rarely parotid and cranial cervical lymph nodes) • Bilateral mucopurulent nasal discharge • Guttural pouch empyema • Respiratory stridor • Dysphagia, anorexia, cough, and neck extension • Ocular discharge

CAUSES

S. equi subsp. *equi*, a gram-positive cocci

RISK FACTORS

The immunologically naïve, young equine population housed in highly concentrated and transient populations

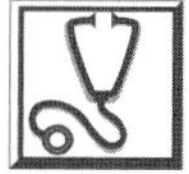

DIAGNOSIS

DIFFERENTIAL DIAGNOSIS

For Nasal Discharge

• Influenza • EHV-1 and EHV-4 • Rhinovirus • Adenovirus • Reovirus • EHV-2 • Pharyngitis • Chronic pharyngeal lymphoid hyperplasia • Nasal/paranasal sinus infection/cysts/polyps/tumors • Early bacterial pneumonia/pleuritis • Guttural pouch infection/mycosis • Overflow of nasolacrimal ducts • Heaves

For Fever

Any disease that causes inflammation

For Lymphadenopathy and Abscessation

• Lymphoma • Upper respiratory tract infection • *C. pseudotuberculosis* lymphadenitis • Bacterial endocarditis • Ulcerative/epizootic/sporadic lymphadenitis • Glanders • Plasma cell myeloma • Tuberculosis • Hemolytic/uremic–like syndrome

CBC/BIOCHEMISTRY/URINALYSIS

Hyperfibrinogenemia, leukocytosis characterized by a neutrophilia, and possibly anemia of chronic disease are commonly seen. Serum biochemistry and urinalysis are normal. Any abnormalities may indicate complications.

OTHER LABORATORY TESTS

Suspicion of disease can be supported, but not confirmed with cytologic evaluation revealing gram-positive extracellular cocci in long chains. Definitive diagnosis via cultures from nasal swabs, nasal washes, guttural pouch washes, or pus aspirated from abscesses remains the gold standard. PCR can be used in conjunction with culturing. This detects both dead and alive DNA in nasal washes, guttural pouches, etc. Serology via the specific ezyme-linked immunosorbent assay for SeM protein is useful for detecting recent but not current infection, need for vaccination, diagnosis of purpura hemorrhagica. and metastatic abscessation. Antibody titers peak 5 weeks after infection and remain high for at least 6 months. Responses to commercial extract vaccines peak at 2 weeks post vaccination and remain high for 6 months. Recommendations include not vaccinating if titer is greater than 1:1600 due to possible higher risk of developing purpura hemorrhagica.

IMAGING

Imaging is typically not performed in uncomplicated cases of strangles. Swellings of the upper respiratory tract can occlude the trachea, which can be seen on radiographs. Intra-abdominal abscessation can be detected on abdominal ultrasound using a 2.5-MHz probe or per rectum using a 5-MHz probe depending on the location of the abdominal mass.

OTHER DIAGNOSTIC PROCEDURES

Endoscopy and radiographs of the guttural pouches aid in the diagnosis of guttural pouch empyema with or without chondroids.

PATHOLOGIC FINDINGS

Hyperplastic lymph nodes are found with increased numbers of neutrophils, monocytes, and macrophages, all due to antigenic stimulation. Also, gram-positive cocci are present. Nasal lesions are characterized by edematous, hyperemic, and occasionally ulcerated mucosa with a variable amount of creamy yellow exudate. In cases of complicated strangles, the pathologic findings are variable, depending on the organ system involved.

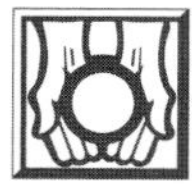

TREATMENT

AIMS OF TREATMENT

To control transmission of *S. equi* and to eliminate infection while providing future, effective immunity to the disease

APPROPRIATE HEALTH CARE

A dry and isolated stall, rest, and soft, moist, palatable food may be all that are necessary while letting the disease run its course. Care depends on the stage of the disease. Acute phase of the fever and depression can be treated with antibiotics but this will prevent protective immunity for the future. It can prevent the formation of abscessation. This practice is considered controversial for it has been argued that this will make the animal more susceptible to septicemia and metastatic abscessation. Horses with lymph node abscessation require hot packing or topical treatment with 20% icthamol to encourage maturation of the abscess and drainage, followed by flushing with 3%–5% povidone-iodine solution once opened. Judicious use of nonsteriodals can decrease swelling and promote eating. Horses with complications benefit from systemic antibiotic therapy (dose: 22,000–44,000 IU/kg IM q12h of procaine penicillin or IV q6h of aqueous potassium penicillin). Horses with chondroids within their guttural pouches require copious lavage with or without 20% acetylcysteine solution.

NURSING CARE

Minimal unless respiratory obstruction or complications occur

ACTIVITY

Horses and stables should be quarantined until there are no clinical signs and three negative nasopharyngeal swab or guttural pouch cultures (1 week apart) are negative for *S. equi.*

DIET

Soft, moist, palatable food.

CLIENT EDUCATION

Appropriate measures should be taken for segregation and preventing cross-contamination. Stables that housed infected animals should be rested for 4 weeks after cleaning and disinfecting.

SURGICAL CONSIDERATIONS

Tracheostomy may need to be performed for horses in severe respiratory distress. Surgical removal of chondroids from the guttural pouch is sometimes necessary in horses for which copious lavage is not successful.

MEDICATIONS

DRUG(S) OF CHOICE

See Appropriate Health Care.

ALTERNATIVE DRUGS

Most antimicrobials that provide good gram-positive coverage could theoretically be administered.

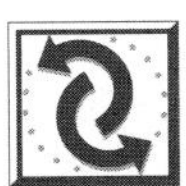

FOLLOW-UP

PATIENT MONITORING

• In cases of uncomplicated strangles, response to therapy can be noted by resolution of clinical signs.

• Temperature, attitude, and appetite must be noted several times a day.

• In cases of complicated strangles, patient monitoring depends on the severity of the disease and the system affected.

PREVENTION/AVOIDANCE

Nonimmunologic strategies of control include the following recommendations:

• Isolation of new horses for 3 weeks, with close observation for signs of strangles or any disease.

• Temperature should be monitored twice daily.

• Affected horses or horses suspected of being affected should be quarantined immediately, with isolation of all equipment and tools that were in contact with these animals.

• People who care for the infected horses should avoid any contact with healthy horses.

• Those horses that were in contact with the affected horses should be observed closely for signs of disease and have their temperatures monitored.

• The appropriate disinfectants, including phenols, iodophores, and chlorhexidine compounds, should be used to destroy the *S. equi* organism.

• Exposure to air is essential for disinfection. Several vaccines are available but do not guarantee the prevention of strangles. The level of immunity stimulated by these vaccines is lower than that produced during recovery from the disease because of failure to provide local protection. Natural infection causes a rise in both systemic and local antibodies, whereas vaccine only causes a rise in systemic antibodies. Currently, the following systemic vaccines are available: Strepvax II (concentrated M-protein extract of *S. equi*) and Strepquard (purified M-protein extract of *S. equi*). These intramuscular vaccines tend to cause injection-site reactions; therefore, routine administration is not performed unless there is a persistent endemic problem on the farm. An intranasal vaccine (Pinnacle, -IN) contains an attenuated live strain of *S. equi* that is antigenic but has low pathogenicity. Live vaccine should be administered only to healthy animals with no known exposure to infected animals during an outbreak.

Persistent carriers of *S. equi* with the guttural pouch are a potential source of new infections on a farm. Shedding can persist intermittently for years. Some farms require culture and/or PCR of the guttural pouch prior to entering the resident population. Persistent carriers have been cleared of infection via repeated infusion of gelatin-pencillin mixtures into the guttural pouch via a chambers catheter under endoscopic guidance +/− systemic pencillin treatment.

POSSIBLE COMPLICATIONS

In the majority of the horses with strangles, the disease runs its course and the horse recovers uneventfully. Complications have been reported in about 20% of the cases.

• Atypical or bastard strangles results when *S. equi* metastasize to other lymph nodes or body systems. Most common sites include the lungs, mesentery, liver, spleen, kidney, and brain. This occurrence is usually fairly low but was reported as high as 28% in a recent study of a strangles outbreak.

• Horses may present in respiratory distress due to upper respiratory tract obstruction from retopharyngeal lymph node abscessation. Suppurative necrotic bronchopneumonia can result from either aspiration of pus from the upper respiratory tract or metastatic spread to the lungs. Guttural pouch empyema is a result of pus from an abscessed lymph node draining into the guttural pouch. Other clinical signs include laryngeal hemiplegia, facial nerve palsy, and Horner's syndrome.

• Myocarditis can result from myocardial abscesses and endocarditis.

• Purpura hemorrhagica is an aseptic vasculitis reported in mature horses after second natural exposure to infection or after vaccination of animals that previously had strangles. Clinical signs vary from mild to life-threatening. Typical signs include pitting edema of dependent areas of the head, trunk, and extremities and petechiation and ecchymoses of mucous membranes. Therapy consists of antimicrobials, corticosteroids, and supportive care. Septicemia and the development of infectious arthritis, pneumonia, and encephalitis are also possible sequelae.

EXPECTED COURSE AND PROGNOSIS

Prognosis is good for full recovery in cases of uncomplicated strangles. The course of the disease depends on the phase of the infection.

MISCELLANEOUS

AGE-RELATED FACTORS

Horses between the ages of 1 and 5 years are immunologically naïve; therefore, they are most prone to developing the disease. Older horses have probably been exposed to the disease.

ZOONOTIC POTENTIAL

Cases in debilitated humans and a dog have been reported.

PREGNANCY

As with any other infectious disease, avoiding infection in a pregnant mare is preferable. Newborn foals have more resistance to disease when dams recovered from infection while pregnant or when vaccinated with an intramuscular extract vaccine. No data are available on colostral antibody levels when broodmares are vaccinated with the modified live intranasal vaccine.

SYNONYMS

Strangles, distemper

ABBREVIATION

• EHV = equine herpesvirus
• PCR = polymerase chain reaction

Suggested Reading

Ladlow J, Scase T, Waller A. Canine strangles case reveals a new host susceptible to infection with *Streptococcus equi*. J Clin Microsc 2006;44:2664–2665.

Smith PA. How to eliminate strangles infections caused by silent carriers. AAEP Proc 2006;52:101–103.

Sweeney CR, Timoney JF, Newton RJ, Hines MT. *Streptococcus equi* infections in horses: Guidelines for treatment, control, and prevention of strangles. J Vet Intern Med 2005;19:123–134.

Verheyen K, Newton JR, Talbot NC, et al. Elimination of guttural pouch infection and inflammation in asymptomatic carriers of *Streptococcus equi*. Equine Vet J 2000;32:527–532.

Waller AS, Jolley KA. Getting a grip on strangles: Recent progress towards improved diagnostics and vaccines. Vet J 2007;173:492–501.

Author Ashley G. Boyle

Consulting Editors Ashley G. Boyle and Corinne R. Sweeney

STRESS FRACTURES

BASICS

DEFINITION

Repetitive overuse bone injury

PATHOPHYSIOLOGY

• Repetitive mechanical loading of bone secondary to physical activity that stimulates incomplete remodeling response • Bone changes shape and structure in response to use (Wolff's law). Under normal stress, there is balance between bone resorption and replacement. Cortical bone responds to stress by forming new bone (modeling), demonstrated by periosteal callus and remodeling of existing bone. Subchondral bone responds to stress by remodeling with sclerosis and lysis. • With excessive or intense training, bone resorption may exceed replacement resulting in a transient period of weakness. With continued stress, focal weakness can function like a stress riser and allow stress or fatigue fracture to occur under otherwise physiologic conditions. • Catastrophic fracture and fatal injuries are severe manifestations of milder stress related injury. Complete fractures of the pelvis, scapula, humerus, and tibia commonly have evidence of unrecognized preexisting stress-related bony remodeling.

SYSTEMS AFFECTED

Musculoskeletal—long bones (MCIII/MTIII, humerus, scapula, tibia), C3, pelvis (ilium), distal phalanx

INCIDENCE/PREVALENCE

• Exact incidence is unknown. • 53%–68% of racehorses unable to train due to lameness. • Musculoskeletal injuries prevent 45%–63% of Thoroughbreds from racing; incidence is 3.3 to 7.3 per 1000 race starts. • Prevalence of catastrophic musculoskeletal injuries (end result of unrecognized stress related bone injury) resulting in death is 1.1 to 1.8 injuries per 1000 starts. • Type of racing largely determines the location and type (cortical or subchondral) injury. • Thoroughbreds are 8.6 times more likely to develop dorsal metacarpal bone disease than are Standardbreds.

GEOGRAPHIC DISTRIBUTION

Regions where racing is prevalent (North America, England, Japan, Australia)

SIGNALMENT

Breed Predilections

• Racehorses (Thoroughbreds, Standardbreds, Quarter Horses, Arabians) • Site-specific breed predilections:

- Distal phalanx—Standardbred overrepresented, Thoroughbred
- Dorsal aspect of MCIII—Thoroughbred, Quarter Horse
- Distal palmar/plantar aspect of MCPJ/MTPJ—Thoroughbred (forelimb), Standardbred (hindlimb)
- Subchondral injury of C3— Standardbred, Thoroughbred
- Humerus—Thoroughbred
- Scapula—Thoroughbred
- Tibia—Thoroughbred, also Standardbred, Quarter Horse
- Pelvis (ilium)—Thoroughbred

Mean Age and Range

• Young, naïve 2- to 5-year-old racehorses
• Mean age as determined by IRU is 3.1 years for Standardbreds and 3.3 years for Thoroughbreds.

SIGNS

General Comments

• Clinical recognition is challenging. • Lameness is variable and physical examination findings are often subtle or absent.

Historical Findings

• Acute lameness after racing or training that responds quickly to rest • Poor performance
• Intermittent unilateral lameness or lameness in numerous limbs

Physical Exam Findings

• Variable lameness in duration and severity
• Cortical bone stress fractures—+/− periosteal thickening, variable pain during palpation and manipulation • Subchondral bone stress injury—+/− joint effusion, pain during flexion with chronic injury • Examination findings specific to site:

- Distal phalanx—unilateral lameness, distal interphalangeal joint distension, variable response to hoof tester application
- Palmar/plantar aspect of MCPJ/MTPJ—short chopping shifting limb lameness, MCPJ/MTPJ distension, painful flexion in chronic disease
- Dorsal cortex of MCIII—"bucked shins": periosteal thickening of the dorsal MCIII, pain on palpation; "saucer fracture": focal bony bump of the dorsal MCIII, focal pain
- Proximal palmar aspect of MCIII—pain, heat or swelling is absent or subtle.
- Subchondral injury of C3—joint effusion, +/− pain during carpal flexion, limb abduction and swinging wide when trotting
- Humerus—+/− pain during upper forelimb manipulation
- Scapula—equivocal findings
- Tibia—pain elicited when applying firm pressure or percussion to medial diaphysis, pain during upper hindlimb flexion or tibial torsion
- Pelvis (ilium)—plaiting or poor hindlimb action, painful to palpation of affected tuber sacrale

CAUSES

• Repetitive, intense high-speed exercise*
• Maladaptive or nonadaptive bone remodeling*

RISK FACTORS

• First introduction to race training • Race training after lay-ups (periods of rest without race or timed work) for illness • Racing and/or race training • Inconsistent racetrack surfaces
• Poor hoof conformation—long toe, underrun heel • Horseshoe with toe grab • Previous injury and/or prerace physical exam abnormality

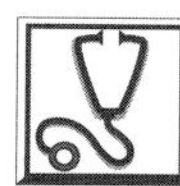

DIAGNOSIS

DIFFERENTIAL DIAGNOSES

• Complete bone fracture at common sites of stress injury (i.e., condylar fracture of distal MCIII/MTIII, slab fracture of C3)—affected horses have severe or non–weight-bearing lameness, joint distension. Rule out with imaging. • Osteoarthritis—chronic subchondral bone disease may result in cartilage injury and synovitis. Joint effusion and pain during joint flexion may be present in both types of injury. Nuclear scintigraphic and radiographic abnormalities assist in differentiation.
• Suspensory desmitis—Rule out with ultrasonography.

IMAGING

• Nuclear scintigraphic findings—Focal, moderate to intense areas of IRU is the hallmark of stress fracture. Specific sites of IRU associated with stress fracture/reaction include:

- Distal phalanx—lateral aspect of left front, medial aspect of right front
- Palmar/plantar aspect of MCPJ/MTPJ—distal palmar/plantar aspect of MCIII/MTIII, respectively. Flexed lateral images differentiate IRU of proximal sesamoid bones.
- Dorsal cortex of MCIII—"bucked shins": diffuse IRU of dorsal MCIII; "saucer fracture": focal IRU of dorsal cortex
- Palmar proximal aspect of MCIII—palmar proximal MCIII
- Subchondral injury of C3—medial aspect of middle carpal joint or C3. Flexed dorsal images differentiate IRU of radiocarpal bone.
- Humerus—caudoproximal and craniodistal humerus, medial diaphysis
- Scapula—caudal distal aspect
- Tibia—caudolateral aspect of the middle third of tibia
- Pelvis (ilium)—ilial wing, 10–15 cm lateral to tuber sacrale. Dorsal oblique views enhance identification.

• Radiographic findings—often normal; periosteal reaction, callus formation, unicortical incomplete fracture; subchondral sclerosis and/or lysis with subchondral injury; +/− supplement views. Specific sites of stress fracture and potential radiographic findings include:

- Distal phalanx—oblique incomplete fracture line through the lateral or medial wing, usually nonarticular
- Palmar/plantar aspect of MCPJ/MTPJ—subchondral lucency and/or sclerosis of distal palmar/plantar aspect of MCIII/MTIII; down-angled oblique views of the MCPJ/MTPJ enhance identification.
- Dorsal cortex of MCIII—"bucked shins": periosteal roughening and/or thickening; "saucer fracture": cortical fracture in the middle third
- Proximal palmar aspect of MCIII—crescent-shaped radiolucent defect (avulsion fracture), incomplete longitudinal fracture, subchondral sclerosis
- Subchondral injury of C3—subchondral sclerosis of radial facet; dorsoproximal-dorsodistal (skyline) view is recommended.
- Humerus—callus formation, +/− distinct fracture line
- Scapula—equivocal, difficult to obtain radiographic evaluation
- Tibia—cortical thickening, callus formation, unicortical oblique fracture line
- Pelvis (ilium)—limited pelvic radiography in the standing horse

- Ultrasonographic findings
  - Proximal palmar aspect of MCIII—bony irregularity or avulsion fracture at the origin of suspensory ligament, accompanying suspensory desmitis
  - Pelvis (ilium)—irregular bony surface or clear discontinuity of the bone contour, hematoma in acute injury

DIAGNOSTIC PROCEDURES

- Diagnostic analgesia—response is variable. Upper limb stress fracture is suspected when lameness does not "block out" with distal limb analgesia. Intra-articular analgesia often incompletely or poorly alleviates pain from subchondral bone injury. Specific sites of stress fracture and diagnostic analgesia procedures:
  - Distal phalanx—abaxial analgesia, intra-articular distal interphalangeal analgesia
  - Palmar/plantar aspect of MCPJ/MTPJ—low palmar/plantar or lateral palmar/plantar metacarpal/metatarsal analgesia, incomplete analgesia with intra-articular MCPJ/MTPJ
  - Dorsal cortex of MCIII—high palmar and dorsal ring block
  - Proximal palmar aspect of MCIII—high palmar or lateral palmar analgesia, intra-articular middle carpal analgesia
  - Subchondral injury of C3—intra-articular middle carpal analgesia
  - Humerus—pain not alleviated with distal forelimb analgesia
  - Scapula—pain not alleviated with distal forelimb analgesia
  - Tibia—pain not alleviated with distal hindlimb analgesia
  - Pelvis (ilium)—pain not alleviated with distal hindlimb analgesia
- Rectal examination (ilium)—+/− crepitus or hematoma

PATHOLOGICAL FINDINGS

Periosteal callus, cortical remodeling, microfractures, subchondral sclerosis, and lysis

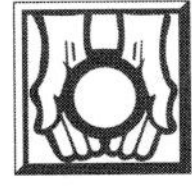

TREATMENT

AIMS OF TREATMENT

- Halt or alter the continuum of stress placed on a bone when weakened or fatigued. • Prevent cortical bone injury becoming catastrophic fracture. • Prevent subchondral bone injury progressing to osteoarthritis and/or osteochondral fragmentation.

APPROPIATE HEATLH CARE

- Early recognition via nuclear scintigraphic and/or radiographic evaluation • Once identified most injuries respond favorably to conservative management. • +/− Extracorporeal shockwave therapy (single treatment, 2000 shocks)
- Restore or improve hoof balance, flat shoe
- Bar shoe for distal phalanx stress fracture

ACTIVITY

- For cortical stress fractures (distal phalanx, MCIII, humerus, tibia, ilium)—4 weeks stall rest, then 4 weeks stall rest with hand walking, then 2 mo of small paddock turnout • For subchondral bone–related injury (distal palmar/plantar MCIII/MTIII, proximal palmar MCIII, C3)—controlled exercise program and gradual return to exercise, i.e., 3 weeks of hand walking, then 3 weeks of walking under saddle, then 3 weeks of trotting. For severe injury, 3–4 mo of rest. Intra-articular medications are indicated with subsequent osteoarthritis.

DIET

Mild to moderate caloric reduction of intake while stall confined or resting

CLIENT EDUCATION

The most important concept to understand is that stress related bone injuries are a continuum. If unrecognized, not treated or treated inappropriately, catastrophic fracture (cortical bone stress) or osteoarthritis (subchondral bone stress) will be the end result.

SURGICAL CONSIDERATIONS

- "Saucer fracture"—osteostixis (fenestration), screw fixation, or a combination of both. • For subchondral bone injures, arthroscopy allows global visualization and assessment of joint health. Debridement of subchondral bone injury is often unrewarding.

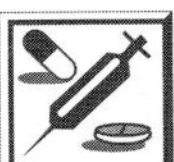

MEDICATIONS

DRUG(S) OF CHOICE

- For subchondral bone injury:
  - NSAIDs—phenylbutazone (2.2–4.4 mg/kg BID)
  - Systemic chondroprotective drugs—polysulfated glycosaminoglycan (500 mg IM q4days for 7 treatments) or sodium hyaluronate (40 mg IV q7days for 3 treatments)
  - Isoxsuprine hydrochloride (1 mg/kg PO BID)
  - Intrasynovial corticosteroids—methylprednisolone acetate (20–40 mg) or triamcinolone (3–6 mg)
  - Intrasynovial sodium hyaluronate (10–20 mg)
  - Combination of intrasynovial corticosteroids and sodium hyaluronate

CONTRAINDICATIONS

Long-term NSAID use is contraindicated due to their ability to impair bone healing and risk of catastrophic fracture.

FOLLOW-UP

PATIENT MONITORING

- Ideally, nuclear scintigraphic reassessment (dramatic decrease in or absence of IRU) should be obtained prior to resuming race training.
- With early subchondral bone disease, lameness examination after each exercise increment

PREVENTION/AVOIDANCE

- Bone should be given time to adapt before progressing to the next speed or gait. Strict conditioning recommendations cannot be defined since bony remodeling is an ongoing slow process. In general, 1-mo increments for any increase in gait or speed may be advantageous. • Any signs of lameness in young racehorses should be investigated fully. The full range of imaging, especially nuclear scintigraphy, is vital for accurate diagnosis.

POSSIBLE COMPLICATIONS

- Catastrophic long bone fracture • Reduced or poor performance • Osteoarthritis in chronic subchondral sclerosis and/or lysis

EXPECTED COURSE AND PROGNOSIS

- After recognition and conservative treatment, cortical stress fractures have an excellent prognosis for return to previous athletic function. • Subchondral bone injuries are frequently chronic and insidious in nature. Even with early recognition and treatment, horses may be chronically lame or drop in class. • If unrecognized, stress-related bone injuries may result in fatal long bone fracture or career ending osteoarthritis.

MISCELLANEOUS

AGE-RELATED FACTORS

Stress-related injuries occur in young naïve racehorses.

SYNONYMS

- Fatigue fracture • Incomplete fracture • Stress related bone injury • Stress reaction
- Maladaptive or nonadaptive bone disease

SEE ALSO

- Dorsal metacarpal bone disease
- Osteoarthritis • Suspensory desmitis

ABBREVIATIONS

- C3 = third carpal bone • IRU = increased radiopharmaceutical uptake • MCIII = third metacarpus • MTIII = third metatarsus
- MCPJ = metacarpophalangeal joint
- MTPJ = metatarsophalangeal joint

Suggested Reading

Davidson EJ, Moss MW. Clinical recognition of stress-related bone injury in racehorses. Clin Techn Equine Pract 2003;2:296–311.

Stover SM. The epidemiology of Thoroughbred racehorse injuries. Clin Techn Equine Pract 2003;2:312–322.

Hill T. On-track catastrophe in the Thoroughbred racehorse. In: Ross MW, Dyson SJ, eds. Diagnosis and Management of Lameness in the Horse. St. Louis: Saunders, 2003:854–861.

Author Elizabeth J. Davidson
Consulting Editor Elizabeth J. Davidson

SUMMER PASTURE-ASSOCIATED OBSTRUCTIVE PULMONARY DISEASE

BASICS

OVERVIEW

• Seasonal, reversible, inflammatory condition of lower airways characterized by airway obstruction resulting from bronchoconstriction, mucus hypersecretion, neutrophilic exudates, and pathologic changes of the bronchiolar epithelia • Shares many similarities with heaves, but occurs while horses are pastured rather than stabled

PATHOPHYSIOLOGY

• Exposure to inhaled particulates present in pasture during warm months of the year leads to inflammation and obstruction of lower airways. Mold spores and grass pollen grains are suspected. • Affected horses have excessive production of mucus secretion and decreased mucociliary clearance. • Airway obstruction leads to ventilation- perfusion inequalities and hypoxemia.

SYSTEM AFFECTED

Respiratory

GENETIC

Unknown

INCIDENCE/PREVALENCE

Unknown; unpublished survey in 1970s reported prevalence of 5% in Louisiana

GEOGRAPHIC DISTRIBUTION

• First described in southeastern United States • More recently described in England and Scotland • Anecdotal reports in other places

SIGNALMENT

• Overrepresentation of horses of Quarter Horse–type breeds (e.g., Quarter Horse, Appaloosa, Paint) and ponies • Mature horses, average age 12 +/− 6 years • No sex predilection

SIGNS

• Clinical exacerbation occurs during warm months of the year. • Initial signs limited to exercise intolerance and occasional cough, but these are often missed by owners. • Most prominent signs are labored expiratory effort, flared nostrils and coughing. • Affected horses are alert, and appear anxious because of respiratory difficulty. • Vital signs may be increased, especially respiratory rate. Mildly increased body temperature is common.
• Severity and frequency of coughing episodes worsen, often become paroxysmal. • In severe cases, affected horses stand with the head and neck extended forward, increased respiratory rate, flared nostrils, and end-expiratory effort. These horses are dehydrated, anorexic, undergo weight loss, and may become emaciated.
• Affected horses develop a "heave line" (hypertrophy of the external abdominal oblique muscles). • Appearance of clinical signs is seasonal and very predictable based on time of the year, if the animal is kept in the same environment. • In mild cases, thoracic auscultation reveals increased bronchovesicular sounds at rest, wheezes and expiratory crackles are evident during forced breathing (rebreathing bag or exercise).
• Thoracic auscultation of severely affected horses reveals wheezes, generally expiratory (sometimes inspiratory too) and expiratory crackles at rest. Wheezes may be audible without stethoscope.

CAUSES

Exposure to pasture environment for extended periods of time, especially during warm months of the year.

RISK FACTORS

• In southeastern United States, horses performing their primary activity in grassy areas are at higher risk. • Airborne particulates inhaled during grazing are incriminated as the inciting agents.

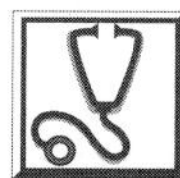

DIAGNOSIS

DIFFERENTIAL DIAGNOSIS

• Lower RT infections of viral, bacterial or fungal etiology may lead to increased respiratory effort and coughing. Diagnostic workup reveals evidence of infectious process. • Anhydrosis, although not a respiratory condition, often occurs in horses exposed to the similar environmental conditions (hot and humid). Affected horses are tachypneic and anxious, and it may be mistakenly interpreted as a respiratory condition. • Pharyngeal disease may cause chronic coughing and increased respiratory effort. Clinical examination reveals normal lung sounds and absence of typical increased end-expiratory effort.

CBC/BIOCHEMISTRY/URINALYSIS

• Mildly increased WBC associated with mild mature neutrophilia is common. • Mildly increased fibrinogen may occur.

OTHER LABORATORY TESTS

• Tracheal wash yield mucopurulent material, consisting mostly of nondegenerate neutrophils (<90%); presence of bacteria and fungal elements are common, and may reflect impaired mucociliary clearance rather than pulmonary infection. • Bacterial culture of tracheal secretions may yield bacterial growth, and it may represent colonization of the lower airways because of impaired mucociliary clearance.
• Cytology of BALF (preferred diagnostic test) is representative of small airways; consistent finding is increased percentage of nondegenerate neutrophils (>25%). • Arterial blood gases: PaO_2 values often <80 mm Hg and may be as low as 40 mm Hg in horses with labored breathing; $PaCO_2$ values may be slightly elevated. • The diagnostic value of lung biopsy in SPAOPD may be outweighed by the risk of rare, but possibly fatal, bleeding.

IMAGING

• Endoscopy usually reveals copious mucopurulent exudate in trachea, accumulating at the carina. • Thoracic radiography may reveal no abnormalities or increased bronchointerstitial pattern.

OTHER DIAGNOSTIC PROCEDURES

• Tentative diagnosis is established on the basis of history of seasonal onset of signs associated with exposure to pasture, signalment and clinical findings; diagnosis is confirmed by >25% neutrophils in BALF. • Exclusion of other diseases affecting the RT; favorable response to environmental changes and therapy.

PATHOLOGIC FINDINGS

• Histology reveals bronchiolitis with accumulation of mucus and neutrophils in the small airways, epithelial hyperplasia with goblet cell hyper- and metaplasia. • Airway smooth muscle hyperplasia/ hyperthrophy, peribronchiolar mononuclear inflammatory infiltrate and areas of alveolar overinflation due to air trapping are common. • Peribronchial fibrosis and emphysema are rare.

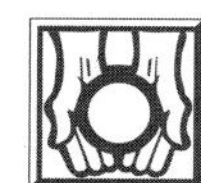

TREATMENT

AIM OF TREATMENT

Control airway inflammation and decrease airway obstruction

APPROPRIATE HEALTH CARE

In- or outpatient medical management

NURSING CARE

• Disease is reversible with proper control of environmental exposure, which is best achieved by keeping horses in a dust-free indoor environment, avoiding pasture during warm months of the year. • If animal not severely affected, it may be kept on pasture. The pasture should be cut very short and the horse should be offered a complete diet to decrease grazing and inhalation of particulates. • Severely affected horses must be removed from pasture and kept in dust-free indoor environment, preferably in a stall with rubber mats and no bedding; and they should be fed a complete diet. Signs of airway obstruction may subside with just environmental changes. • Respiratory signs usually recur within days of reexposure to pasture during warm months of the year. • Although clinical remission occurs during the cooler months, it is recommended that the pasture be kept relatively short (only a few inches high), and the horses fed a complete diet. • In some cases, the response to appropriate environmental control is striking and no drug therapy is required. In other cases, despite strict environmental management, the horse may take a long time to shown clinical improvement and drug therapy is recommended. • In horses with profound hypoxemia (PaO_2 <60 mm Hg), inhaled oxygen supplementation is recommended.

ACTIVITY

• Horses with signs of clinical exacerbation and severely compromised respiratory function should be rested. • Horses in clinical remission may be exercised normally.

DIET

• It is preferable to keep affected horses on the same complete diet throughout the year.
• Complete feed, cubed forage, or haylage are preferred over hay, even at times of clinical remission. • Round hay bales should not be offered to affected horses, even during clinical remission.

SUMMER PASTURE–ASSOCIATED OBSTRUCTIVE PULMONARY DISEASE

CLIENT EDUCATION

• Maintain affected horses away from pasture during the warm month of the year. • With clinical exacerbation, horses must be kept in dust-free indoor environment. • As affected horses appear to have a poor pulmonary clearance, the susceptible horse should be kept in a low-dust environment when stabled even during clinical remission. Follow recommendations to minimize exposure to dust.

SURGICAL CONSIDERATIONS

N/A

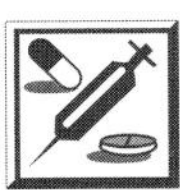

MEDICATIONS

DRUG(S) OF CHOICE

The medications recommended for the treatment of heaves are usually also efficacious for the treatment of SPAOPD.

Corticosteroids

• Systemic corticosteroids allow effective control of the airway inflammation. • In severe cases, use dexamethasone (0.05 mg/kg q24h), then decrease dose and increase interval. • Inhaled corticosteroids allow maximal concentration of drug in the RT, minimizing systemic side effects. • Inhaled drugs can be delivered using nebulization, MDIs, and dry-powder inhalers. • Inhaled corticosteroids: beclomethasone diproprionate (5–7 μg/kg q12h) and fluticasone propionate (4 μg/kg q12h) are efficacious and have minimal residual effects. • The response to inhaled corticosteroids takes longer than that to systemic steroids. Combination of inhaled bronchodilators and corticosteroids are recommended.

Bronchiodilators

• Affected horses may develop hypoxic vasoconstriction; bronchodilators may be life-saving. • Long-term administration of bronchodilators should be combined with strict environmental control and corticosteroid, because inflammation of the lower RT may progress despite the improvement of clinical signs. • β_2-Adrenergic agonist bronchodilators are used to relieve small airway obstruction caused by the airway smooth muscle contraction. • Oral β_2-adrenergic agonist bronchodilators: clenbuterol syrup (0.8–3.2 μg/kg q12h) is commonly used; albuterol oral syrup and tablets (0.8 μg/kg q8h) may be used; terbutaline sulfate has poor bioavailability when given orally and is not recommended. • Several inhaled β_2-adrenergic agonist bronchodilators are effective for horses. Fast-acting and short-lasting: albuterol MDI (1–2 μg/kg); Fast-acting and long-lasting: pirbuterol MDI (1–1.5 μg/kg) and fenoterol MDI (1–2 μg/kg); Slow-acting and long-lasting: salmeterol MDI (1 μg/kg). Appropriate delivery devices must be used. • Long-term use of β_2-adrenergic agonist may result in tachyphylaxis. • Parasympatholytic (anticholinergic) bronchodilators given systemically (atropine and glycopyrrolate) are not recommended because of their adverse effects on the gastrointestinal tract and risk in precipitating colic in horses. • Inhaled muscarinic receptor antagonist bronchodilator, ipratropium bromide MDI (2–3 μg/kg), is effective in horses and has minimal adverse systemic effects. Other muscarinic antagonists (oxitropium and tiotropium) are not currently used in horses.

Expectorant, Mucolytic, and Mucokinetic Agents

• Efficacy of mucolytic, expectorants and mukokinetic agents (such as acetylcysteine, dornase, guaifenesin, and iodides) in improving clinical signs of SPAOPD are limited to anecdotal reports. • β_2-Adrenergic agonists, in addition to their bronchodilatory effect, improve mucociliary clearance by decreasing the viscosity of the respiratory secretions and increasing mucociliary beating; these mucokinetic properties are helpful for the management of clinical exacerbation of airway obstruction.

Contraindications/Possible Interactions

• Corticosteroid administration is contraindicated in the face of infectious process. • Administration of bronchodilators may exacerbate ventilation-perfusion inequalities, temporarily worsening hypoxemia; in severe cases oxygen therapy is recommended in conjunction with bronchodilators. • Oral mucokinetic agents that stimulate the gastropulmonary mucokinetic vagal reflex such as the iodides can induce or exacerbate bronchospasm.

ALTERNATIVE DRUGS

• The use of chloride channel blockers as mast cell stabilizers (sodium cromoglycate 80–200 mg q12–24h or nedocromil sodium 24 mg q12h) in horses in clinical remission may be helpful as adjunctive in the prevention of seasonal exacerbation. • It is important to remember that no drug therapy can replace appropriate environmental management.

FOLLOW-UP

PATIENT MONITORING

• Monitoring of expiratory effort and pulmonary adventitious sounds following appropriate environmental changes • Severely affected horses that are hypoxemic during clinical exacerbation should be monitored by serial PaO_2 determination to evaluate response to therapy.

PREVENTION/AVOIDANCE

Dust-free environment, away from pasture during the warm months of the year.

POSSIBLE COMPLICATIONS

• SPAOPD is a debilitating disease that can lead to death in severe cases, especially if proper environmental control and effective medical treatment are not provided. • In severe cases, hypoxic vasoconstriction associated with severe hypoxemia can lead to pulmonary hypertension and right heart failure.

EXPECTED COURSE AND PROGNOSIS

• The condition is reversible with adequate environmental control and medical therapy. • As the onset of clinical exacerbation is fairly predictable from year to year, environmental control and prevention are critical. • Inadequate environmental control is associated with worsening of the condition (increase severity of signs and shorten length of clinical remission) from year to year. • Pulmonary neutrophilia may persist even if the horse is asymptomatic. • Affected horses may be at risk to develop airway obstruction associated with indoor dusty environment and moldy hay.

MISCELLANEOUS

AGE-RELATED FACTORS

• Rare in horses <6 years • Incidence increases with age

PREGNANCY

Fetal growth retardation and death may occur in hypoxic mares with severely compromised respiratory function.

SYNONYMS

• Summer pasture heaves • Summer pasture–associated recurrent airway obstruction

SEE ALSO

• Heaves • Cough • Expiratory dyspnea

ABBREVIATIONS

• BALF = bronchoalveolar lavage fluid • MDI = metered dose inhaler • RT = respiratory tract • SPAOPD = summer pasture–associated obstructive pulmonary disease

Suggested Reading

Beadle RE. Summer pasture-associated obstructive pulmonary disease In: Robinson NE, ed. Current Therapy in Equine Medicine. Philadelphia: Saunders, 1983:512–516.

Author Lais R. R. Costa
Consulting Editor Daniel Jean

SUPERFICIAL NONHEALING ULCERS WITH ANTERIOR STROMAL SEQUESTRATION

BASICS

OVERVIEW
Superficial nonhealing ulcers are injuries of the corneal epithelium that do not penetrate the basement membrane. These ulcers can progress to deeper ulcers once the basement membrane is injured. In the horse, superficial ulcers are commonly seen associated with protein deposits in the anterior stroma.

SYSTEM AFFECTED
Ophthalmic

SIGNALMENT
All ages and breeds affected

SIGNS
- Chronic superficial corneal erosions have an opalescent grayish color, display faint retention of fluorescein dye, and have thin, undulating, acellular, stromal surface membranes.
- Erosions are surrounded by loose lip of migrating, nonattached epithelium, corneal vascularization, and crystalline stromal deposits.
- Slight uveitis is noted.

CAUSES AND RISK FACTORS
Unknown; possible primary corneal disease with chronic secondary irritation. For example, this may be secondary to acute corneal ulceration from rubbing of a silicone subpalpebral lavage system.

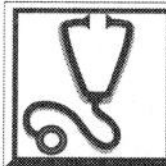

DIAGNOSIS

DIFFERENTIAL DIAGNOSIS
- Lid abnormalities such as distichiasis, trichiasis, and entropion; neuroparalytic and neurotrophic keratitis; keratoconjunctivitis sicca; corneal dystrophies; and corneal foreign bodies
- Inappropriate topical corticosteroid therapy causing delayed corneal healing.

CBC/BIOCHEMISTRY/URINALYSIS
N/A

OTHER LABORATORY TESTS
Rule out infectious causes (bacterial or fungal) with corneal scrapings for cytology and culture.

IMAGING
N/A

DIAGNOSTIC PROCEDURES
N/A

PATHOLOGIC FINDINGS
- Histologically, ulceration with a thin membrane of altered corneal stroma, representing corneal stromal sequestration
- Lack of epithelial migration and/or attachment onto the ulcerated surface is present.

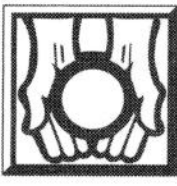

TREATMENT
- Epithelial debridement of the loose lip of epithelium.
- Superficial grid keratotomy for debridement of ulcers and disruption of the superficial membrane.
- Superficial keratectomy.
- Postoperatively, temporary partial tarsorraphy prevents trauma to ulcers from blepharospasm.
- Contact lenses act as bandages.

MEDICATIONS

DRUGS
- Topical broad-spectrum antibiotics (e.g., chloramphenicol, bacitracin-neomycin-polymyxin)
- Topical serum every 4 hours or topical polysulfated glycosaminoglycans TID (Adequan, diluted with artificial tears solution to 50mg/mL) may be beneficial.

SUPERFICIAL NONHEALING ULCERS WITH ANTERIOR STROMAL SEQUESTRATION

CONTRAINDICATIONS/POSSIBLE INTERACTIONS

- Gentamicin topically may slow corneal healing. If an infection of the corneal defect is not ruled out first by culture and/or cytology, a grid keratotomy can potentially lead to an infection of the deep corneal stroma with loss of vision or globe.
- Use solutions, not ointments.

FOLLOW-UP

EXPECTED COURSE AND PROGNOSIS

- Lavage system induced ulcers are notoriously slow to heal.
- Infection is a risk due to epithelial loss.
- Scarring of the cornea may result.

MISCELLANEOUS

ASSOCIATED CONDITIONS

- Infection
- Uveitis

SEE ALSO

- Corneal ulceration
- Corneal/scheral lacerations
- Ulcerative keratomycosis
- Corneal stromal abscesses
- Recurrent uveitis
- Glaucoma
- Nonulcerative keratouveitis
- Eosinophilic keratitis
- Viral and herpes keratitis
- Burdock pappus bristle keratopathy
- Calcific band keratopathy
- Limbal keratopathy

Suggested Reading

Brooks DE. Ophthalmology for the Equine Practitioner. Jackson, WY; Teton NewMedia, 2002.

Brooks DE, Matthews AG. Equine ophthalmology. In: Gelatt KN, ed. Veterinary Ophthalmology, ed 4. Philadelphia; Lippincott Williams and Wilkins, 2007.

Gilger BC, ed. Equine Ophthalmology. Philadelphia; WB Saunders, 2005.

Authors Andras M. Komaromy and Dennis E. Brooks

Consulting Editor Dennis E. Brooks

SUPRAVENTRICULAR ARRHYTHMIAS

BASICS

DEFINITION

• Supraventricular arrhythmias originate from an ectopic focus in the atria or the AV junction that is overdriving the sinus pacemaker. • The term *supraventricular premature depolarization* (SVPD) refers to isolated ectopic complexes. More than four SVPDs in succession is SVT, and this can be either paroxysmal or sustained. • Atrial fibrillation is also a supraventricular arrhythmia but is described in a separate section of this textbook.

PATHOPHYSIOLOGY

• A number of different electrophysiologic mechanisms are responsible for the development of ventricular arrhythmias, including reentry, enhanced automaticity, and accelerated conduction. • Primary myocardial disease is an infrequent cause. • Horses are often able to block conduction of SVPD into the ventricles at the level of the atrioventricular node, under the influence of the vagus, and consequently there is rarely a rapid ventricular rate in the presence of supraventricular ectopy.

SYSTEMS AFFECTED

Cardiovascular

SIGNALMENT

There are no specific age, breed, or sex predilections.

SIGNS

General Comments

• SVPDs are common but often are detected incidentally during routine examinations.
• SVPDs occurring during the warm-up and cool-off periods of exercise are rarely of any immediate clinical significance, although they may represent a risk factor for atrial fibrillation.
• SVT is uncommon, but when it occurs, it may be associated with poor performance.

Historical

Poor performance

Physical Examination

Individual premature beats or runs of rapid rhythm, usually with a rapid onset and offset

CAUSES

• Hypoxia • Sepsis • Toxemia • Drugs such quinidine sulfate • Autonomic imbalance
• Metabolic and electrolyte imbalance
• Primary myocardial disease

RISK FACTORS

• Atrioventricular valvular disease leading to atrial enlargement • Infective endocarditis
• Treatment with quinidine sulfate

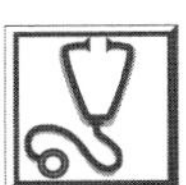

DIAGNOSIS

DIFFERENTIAL DIAGNOSIS

• Ventricular premature depolarizations—differentiate electrocardiographically. • Sinus tachycardia—The heart rate usually speeds up and slows down more subtly with sinus tachycardia than with SVT; differentiate electrocardiographically.

CBC/BIOCHEMISTRY/URINALYSIS

Electrolyte or metabolic abnormalities may be present.

OTHER LABORATORY TESTS

• Elevated cardiac isoenzymes (CK-MB, HBDH, or LDH-1 and LDH-2) or cardiac troponin I may be present. • Blood culture and viral serology may be indicated in some cases.

IMAGING

Electrocardiography

• SVPD are represented by a premature p wave which may (conducted) or may not (unconducted) be followed by a QRS-T complex. • The shape of the premature p wave may be different from those of sinus origin, but the configurations of the premature QRS complex and T wave are the same as those of sinus origin as conduction through the ventricle is not affected. • The premature p wave may not be visible if it occurs sufficiently early that it is buried in the preceding T wave. • Junctional complexes do not have a p wave but do have the same QRS configuration as those of sinus origin. • Occasionally, SVPD have QRS complexes that are of slightly larger similar duration and morphology compared to the sinus QRS complexes. • It can be helpful to examine multiple leads to differentiate premature p waves and confirm that all premature QRS complexes have a configuration that is identical to those of sinus origin.

Echocardiography

• The echocardiogram is most often normal, or there may be a slightly low shortening fraction, particularly with SVT. • With primary myocardial disease, there are more profound decreases in fractional shortening and abnormalities of myocardial wall motion (dyskinesis or akinesis) and mitral and aortic valve motion. • Foci of increased or decreased echogenicity are occasionally seen within the myocardium. • Echocardiography may reveal evidence of other cardiac diseases such as infective endocarditis or severe valvular disease.

Thoracic Radiology

Pulmonary edema may be present in rare cases of sustained, prolonged SVT.

OTHER DIAGNOSTIC PROCEDURES

Continuous 24-Hour Holter Moitoring

This is particularly helpful in identifying intermittent or paroxysmal supraventricular arrhythmias, in quantifying numbers of isolated SVPDs and assessing response to therapy.

Exercise Electrocardiography

Characterization of the effect of exercise on supraventricular arrhythmias is important in assessing their clinical significance.

PATHOLOGIC FINDINGS

• The heart may be normal, grossly and histopathologically, in horses with no underlying cardiac disease. • Focal or diffuse myocardial necrosis, inflammation, or fibrosis may be present. • Atrial enlargement and concurrent valvular pathology may be identified.

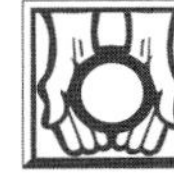

TREATMENT

AIMS OF TREATMENT

• Address any predisposing causes.
• Antiarrhythmic therapy in selected cases

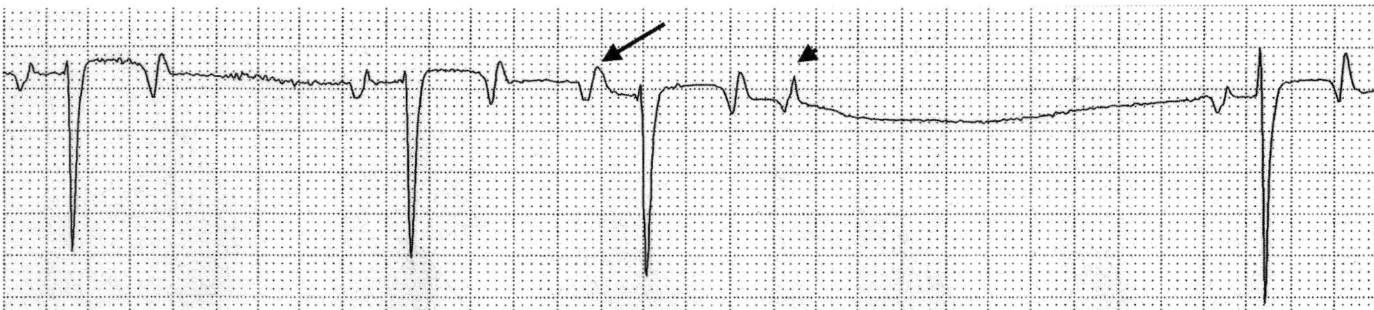

Figure 1.

Conducted (arrow) and unconducted (arrowhead) SVPD: the premature p waves differ slightly from those of sinus origin whereas all QRS are the same—base apex lead, 25 mm/sec, 5 mm = 1 mV.

APPROPRIATE HEALTH CARE

• Emergency antiarrhythmic therapy is restricted to cases in which the rhythm is unstable and life-threatening. This is very rarely necessary except in cases in which the rapid SVT is due to drug treatment such as quinidine sulfate. • Oral antiarrhythmic therapy is occasionally used when frequent SVPDs are present, particularly if these are associated with episodes of atrial fibrillation and/or SVT.

NURSING CARE

• Continuous electrocardiographic monitoring should be performed during antiarrhythmic therapy. • Horses should be kept quiet and not moved during the antiarrhythmic therapy.

ACTIVITY

• SVPDs are not thought to be an important cause of collapse during exercise; and if there is no poor performance, horses with SVPDs can usually be exercised normally. • Horses with poor performance associated with SVPDs may benefit from a period of rest. • Horses with SVT during maximal exercise should not be exercised.

DIET

N/A

CLIENT EDUCATION

Clients should be counseled that the main risk associated with SVPD is that it may predispose the horse to developing atrial fibrillation in the future. Normal exercise can be performed in most horses with SVPD providing there is no poor performance.

SURGICAL CONSIDERATIONS

Surgical ablation techniques that are used to treat supraventricular arrhythmias in human beings have not been performed in horses and are unlikely to be relevant.

MEDICATIONS

DRUG(S)

• In the absence of any predisposing causes precluding their use, such as infective endocarditis, corticosteroids are often used in horses with SVPD. Either prednisolone 1 mg/kg PO every other day or dexamethasone 0.05–0.1 mg/kg IV, or 0.1 mg/kg PO once a day for 3 or 4 days and then continued every 3–4 days in decreasing dosages is recommended. • Phenytoin given orally at doses of 5–15 mg/kg BID may be effective in suppressing SVPD, but the arrhythmia may recur on discontinuation of therapy. • Digoxin is given intravenously at 0.0022 mg/kg for emergency treatment of rapid SVT, particularly where it is associated with quinidine administration. For less rapid SVT during quinidine therapy, digoxin can be given at 0.011 mg/kg PO BID. Digoxin is less likely to be effective against SVPD, although occasionally favorable responses have been observed when it is used orally. • Propanolol given intravenously at 0.03–2 mg/kg can be used for emergency treatment of rapid SVT, particularly if digoxin is unsuccessful. • Quinidine sulfate (single dose of up to 22 mg/kg PO) and quinidine gluconate (0.5–2.2 mg/kg IV boluses to a maximum of 12 mg/kg) are indicated for treating rare cases of rapid SVT where it is not associated with quinidine administration.

CONTRAINDICATIONS

Corticosteroids should *not* be used in horses with concurrent pituitary pars intermedia dysfunction or active laminitis.

PRECAUTIONS

• Horses should be monitored for signs of laminitis if receiving corticosteroid therapy.
• Adverse effects of digoxin include anorexia, depression, abdominal pain, and ventricular arrhythmias. Ideally, therapeutic drug monitoring should be used to ensure that plasma digoxin concentrations remain at therapeutic levels (1–2 μg/mL). • Adverse effects of phenytoin include excitement, sedation, and other neurological signs. Ideally, therapeutic drug monitoring should be used to ensure that plasma phenytoin concentrations remain at therapeutic levels (5–10 mg/mL). • Adverse effects of quinidine include myocardial depression, colic, diarrhea, and ventricular arrhythmias. Ideally, therapeutic drug monitoring should be used to ensure that plasma phenytoin concentrations remain at therapeutic levels (3–5 μg/mL)

POSSIBLE INTERACTIONS

There is interaction between quinidine and digoxin.

ALTERNATIVE DRUGS

Other drugs used in human beings for treatment of SVT may be beneficial in horses, but protocols for their use have yet to be defined.

FOLLOW-UP

PATIENT MONITORING

24-hour Holter monitoring and exercise electrocardiography are the most useful tools to assess the success of therapy and, where no treatment has been recommended, to monitor for any progression of the supraventricular arrhythmia.

POSSIBLE COMPLICATIONS

• The main risk associated with SVPD is that it may predispose the horse to developing atrial fibrillation in the future. However, the magnitude of this risk in horses that have not previously had paroxysmal or sustained atrial fibrillation has not been quantified. Horses that have previously had atrial fibrillation are more likely to have recurrences if SVPDs are detected after treatment of the atrial fibrillation or SVT occurs during treatment. Atrial fibrillation is also more likely to develop if there is underlying heart disease such as severe atrioventricular valvular insufficiency.
• Horses that develop SVPDs in association with atrial enlargement and severe underlying cardiac disease are at particular risk of developing atrial fibrillation and this often marks the onset of declining clinical status and congestive heart failure. In these cases, the SVPDs can be regarded as a complication of the underlying condition rather than a cause of atrial fibrillation.

EXPECTED COURSE AND PROGNOSIS

Horses in which SVPDs are detected as an incidental finding may frequently remain asymptomatic in work for prolonged periods.

MISCELLANEOUS

ASSOCIATED CONDITIONS

• Atrioventricular valvular disease (tricuspid and mitral regurgitation) • Atrial septal defect
• Infective endocarditis
Supraventricular premature beats

SEE ALSO

• Atrial septal defect • Myocardial disease
• Atrial fibrillation • Ventricular arrhythmias
• Infective endocarditis • Ionophore toxicosis

ABBREVIATIONS

• CK-MB = MB isoenzyme of creatine kinase
• HBDH = α-hydroxybutyrate dehydrogenase
• LDH = lactate dehydrogenase • SVT = supraventricular tachycardia • SVPD = supraventricular premature depolarization

Suggested Reading

Bowen IM, Marr CM, Elliott JE. Cardiovascular pharmacology. In Bertone J, Horspool LJI, eds. Clinical Pharmacology of the Horse. Philadelphia: WB Saunders, 2004:193–216.
Guthrie AJ, Nichas E, Viljoen FV, Hartmann AM, Killeen VM. Sustained supraventricular tachycardia in a horse. J S Afr Vet Assoc 1989;60:46–47.
Reef VB. Arrhythmias. In Marr CM, ed. Cardiology of the Horse. Philadelphia; WB Saunders, 1999:179–209.

Author Celia M. Marr
Consulting Editor Celia M. Marr

SUSPENSORY DESMITIS

BASICS

OVERVIEW

• SLD is inflammation of the proximal portion, body, and/or branches of the ligament. • DSLD is a progressive, debilitating disorder of the suspensory ligament resulting in continuous enlargement of the ligament due to ineffective collagen fiber repair and generalized interstitial and periligamentous fibrosis.

SYSTEM AFFECTED

Musculoskeletal—palmar/plantar MCIII/MTIII

SIGNALMENT

SLD

• Performance horses of all ages and breeds
• Standardbred racehorses and upper-level dressage horses have highest incidence of hindlimb SLD.
• Suspensory ligament rupture is part of catastrophic breakdown injury in Thoroughbred flat racers.

DSLD

• Most common in Peruvian Paso • Recognized in other breeds (Arabian, American Saddlebred, Quarter Horse, Thoroughbred) • Heritability is not yet established but appears to run in families.

SIGNS

SLD

• Acute or insidious onset of mild to moderate lameness • Lameness resolves with rest and recurs with exercise. • In forelimb, lameness may be exacerbated when trotting in a circle with the affected limb on the outside. • In hindlimb, lameness subtle in early disease, worse when ridden • In acute disease, localized heat, swelling, and pain • In chronic disease, palpable thickening and pain • +/− Positive to lower limb flexion and upper limb flexion (hindlimb) • +/− Fetlock joint distention with branch injuries
• Dropped fetlock and severe lameness with complete rupture

DSLD

• Early signs include generalized stiffness, changes in attitude, reluctance to work, and back pain. • Subtle, chronic intermittent or persistent unilateral to quadrilateral lameness • End-stage cases become reluctant to move and frequently lie down. • Palpable thickening and pain of the suspensory ligament
• Positive fetlock flexion
• Progressive fetlock drop

CAUSES AND RISK FACTORS

SLD

• Foot imbalance, long pasterns, fetlock hyperextension • Back at the knee or tied-in below the knee, straight hock • Axial periosteal proliferation on splint bones ("blind splint")

DSLD

• Peruvian Paso heritage • Abnormal proteoglycan deposition between collagen and elastin fibers in connective tissues

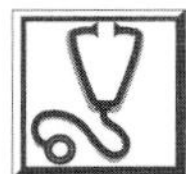

DIAGNOSIS

DIFFERENTIAL DIAGNOSIS

SLD

• Proximal forelimb SLD—middle carpal or carpometacarpal joint pain, palmar proximal cortical stress or avulsion fracture of MCIII, carpal sheath or retinaculum pain • Proximal hindlimb SLD—tarsometatarsal joint pain, avulsion or stress fracture of MTIII

DSLD

• Injury mediated SLD

IMAGING

Ultrasonography

• High-quality images in both transverse and longitudinal planes and cross-sectional measurements are necessary. Comparison to the contralateral limb distinguishes variations in normal from pathology. • In acute injury, focal isoechoic or anechoic core lesions
• In chronic injury, decreased echogenicity and abnormal fiber pattern • Increased cross-sectional area
• Periligamentous thickening and adhesion formation
• Dystrophic calcification
• Associated bony abnormalities
• DSLD—progressive enlargement, loss of echogenicity and fiber pattern, primarily in the branches

Radiography

• Often normal • Subchondral sclerosis and/or avulsion fracture of proximal MCIII/MTIII
• Sesamoiditis, proximal sesamoid fracture
• Splint bone exostosis or fracture

Nuclear Scintigraphy

• Generalized increased radiopharmaceutical uptake of the proximal palmar/plantar aspect of MCIII/MTIII is uncommon but strongly suggestive for desmitis when present. • Focal increased radiopharmaceutical uptake in the proximal palmar/plantar aspect of MCIII/MTIII with avulsion fracture

OTHER DIAGNOSTIC PROCEDURES

SLD

• Diagnostic analgesia—High palmar/plantar, lateral palmar (forelimb), subtarsal (hindlimb) and local infiltration of the suspensory ligament. Intra-articular middle carpal and tarsometatarsal analgesia may diffuse into proximal suspensory ligament.

DSLD

• Diagnostic analgesia as for SLD • Nuchal ligament biopsy is under investigation.

PATHOLOGICAL FINDINGS

DSLD—Histopathological examination reveals large accumulations of proteoglycans between collagen and elastin fibers in suspensory ligament(s) and other connective tissues.

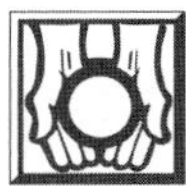

TREATMENT

SLD

• Local and/or systemic analgesic and anti-inflammatory therapy if acute • Controlled exercise program—stall rest and hand walking for weeks to months followed by gradual return to exercise. Duration determined by sonographic findings and lameness assessment. • Hoof balance, caudal heel support, eggbar shoes
• Ancillary therapies:
  ○ Extracorporeal shockwave therapy
  ○ Percutaneous ligament splitting (desmoplasty)
  ○ Fasciotomy of deep palmar/plantar metacarpal/metatarsal fascia
  ○ Tibial or deep branch of the lateral plantar neurectomy
  ○ Intralesional injections (bone marrow, adipose-derived stem cells, bioscaffold material)

DSLD

• Local and/or systemic analgesic anti-inflammatory therapy • Controlled exercise program • Stall confinement in chronic or severe disease • Extended caudal heel support, eggbar shoes

MEDICATIONS

DRUG(S)

• NSAIDs—phenylbutazone 2.2–4.4 mg/kg daily to BID for a few days • Systemic chondroprotective drugs—polysulfated glycosaminoglycan (500 mg IM q4days for 7 treatments) or sodium hyaluronate (40 mg IV q7days for 3 treatments) • Oral chondroprotective medications—glucosamine/chondrotin sulfate powder (1 scoop [3.3 g] BID)

CONTRAINDICATIONS/POSSIBLE INTERACTIONS

Intralesional corticosteroids

FOLLOW-UP

PATIENT MONITORING

• Sonographic and lameness reevaluation every 8 weeks • Recurrence of lameness, heat, or swelling during rehabilitation prompts discontinuation of exercise and sonographic reevaluation.

POSSIBLE COMPLICATIONS

Chronic lameness despite treatment

EXPECTED COURSE AND PROGNOSIS

• Lameness resolves within 2–5 days of discontinuing exercise. • Total convalescence ranges from 6 to 12 mo depending on severity of lesion. • Prognosis depends on location of the lesion, forelimb versus hindlimb, and presence of associated conditions. • Prognosis is good for return to full work in forelimb proximal SLD and poor for hindlimb proximal SLD. • Recurrence is high in horses that are inadequately rested. • DSLD—poor prognosis

MISCELLANEOUS

ASSOCIATED CONDITIONS

SLD

• Avulsion fracture of MCIII/MTIII at the origin of suspensory ligament • Splint bone fracture and exostosis • Proximal sesamoid bone fractures and sesamoiditis

SEE ALSO

Tendonitis

ABBREVIATIONS

• DSLD = degenerative suspensory ligament disease
• MCIII = third metacarpus • MTIII = third metatarsus • SLD = suspensory ligament desmitis

Suggested Reading

Dyson SJ. The suspensory apparatus. In: Ross M, Dyson S, eds. Diagnosis and Management of Lameness in the Horse. St. Louis: Saunders, 2003:654–666.

Author JoAnn Slack
Consulting Editor Elizabeth J. Davidson

SYNCHRONOUS DIAPHRAGMATIC FLUTTER

BASICS

OVERVIEW

- A contraction of the diaphragm that is synchronous with the heartbeat
- Also known as "thumps"
- Results from hyperexcitability of the phrenic nerve usually secondary to fluid and electrolyte imbalance; the electric impulse generated from atrial depolarization stimulates the phrenic nerve and causes diaphragmatic contraction.
- Commonly observed in endurance horses exercising in hot, humid conditions. Also noted in Thoroughbred and Standardbred race horses, and severely ill horses

SIGNALMENT

Any breed, age, or sex

SIGNS

Historical

- Often a recent history of prolonged exercise accompanied by intense sweating
- Also associated with GI disease, blister beetle toxicosis, lactation tetany, transportation, and trauma

Physical Examination

- Pathognomonic sign—a spasmodic contraction of the flank that is synchronous with the first heart sound.
- Flank movements are associated with diaphragmatic contractions and are independent of the normal respiratory cycle.
- Flank twitching may not occur with every heartbeat, but when it does, it is always associated with atrial depolarization.
- Strong contractions may produce a thumping noise, which has led to the name "thumps."

CAUSES AND RISK FACTORS

- Electrolyte and acid-base imbalances may increase phrenic nerve excitability. The equine phrenic nerve runs over the right atrium, allowing it to produce an action potential when stimulated by atrial depolarization. In addition, physical irritation of the nerve through the pericardium may induce SDF.
- Hypocalcemia, hypokalemia, and alkalosis, either individually or in combination, have been associated with SDF. Excessive sweating, GI disturbances, transportation, lactation tetany, furosemide therapy, urethral obstruction, and hypoparathyroidism may cause these electrolytic abnormalities. Equine sweat is hypertonic and may lead to substantial loss of electrolytes, particularly sodium, chloride, potassium, and calcium.
- Hypocalcemia increases the excitability of nerve and muscle cells by lowering the depolarization threshold.
- Hypokalemia increases the resting membrane potential of cells and results in increased nerve excitability. Alkalosis, which is often accompanied by hypokalemia, increases albumin binding of calcium and results in decreased ionized calcium concentration.

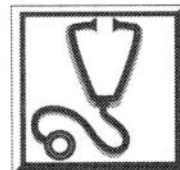

DIAGNOSIS

DIFFERENTIAL DIAGNOSIS

- Rather than a disease, SDF is a clinical manifestation of deranged electrolyte levels and acid-base status; therefore, many diseases may be associated with this condition.
- Hiccups and nonsynchronous diaphragmatic flutter have been observed. However, in these cases, diaphragmatic twitching is not synchronous with cardiac contraction.
- Forceful contractions of the abdominal muscles may accompany severe respiratory disease (e.g., recurrent airway obstruction, pneumonia). Affected horses present with obvious signs of respiratory disease, however, and each abdominal contraction is associated with expiration, not with a heartbeat.

CBC/BIOCHEMISTRY/URINALYSIS

- Hypocalcemia, hypokalemia, and alkalosis (metabolic or respiratory) are the most common metabolic abnormalities.
- Serum ionized calcium concentration is more accurate than total calcium concentration to diagnose hypocalcemia.

OTHER LABORATORY TESTS

Blood gas analysis is useful to assess acid-base status.

DIAGNOSTIC PROCEDURES

The diagnosis can be confirmed by simultaneously recording the electrocardiogram and the diaphragmatic contractions, either manually or with electromyography or phonocardiography.

PATHOLOGICAL FINDINGS

Lesions relate to the primary associated disease, not to SDF itself.

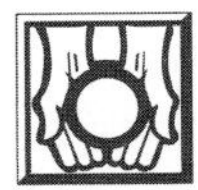

TREATMENT

Correction of the underlying condition and restoring electrolyte homeostasis

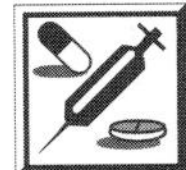

MEDICATIONS

DRUG(S) OF CHOICE

- Oral or parenteral administration of balanced electrolyte solutions is beneficial and often sufficient to correct electrolytic abnormalities.
- Hypocalcemia may be corrected by IV infusion of 20% calcium-borogluconate solution (contains 21.4 mg/mL of elemental calcium). Estimate calcium deficit according to the following formula:
- Ca deficit in mg = [(normal total Ca) – (measured total Ca) in mg/dl] × 6 [body weight in kg]
- Administration of isotonic-saline solution helps to correct metabolic alkalosis and hypokalemia.
- Horses with excessive sweating may be treated with oral or parenteral administration of solutions containing sodium, chloride, potassium, and calcium.

CONTRAINDICATIONS/POSSIBLE INTERACTIONS

Excessive administration of alkalinizing solutions (e.g., bicarbonate) may worsen clinical signs by decreasing available free calcium.

FOLLOW-UP

PATIENT MONITORING

Monitor electrolytes, acid-base status, and clinical signs.

PREVENTION/AVOIDANCE

- When large electrolyte losses are anticipated (e.g., endurance ride), administer electrolytes before, during, and after losses occur.
- Avoid excessive calcium supplementation as a prophylactic measure, because it reduces parathyroid hormone secretion and may impair rapid mobilization of calcium from bone when needed.

POSSIBLE COMPLICATIONS

Electrolyte abnormalities may lead to ileus, muscle weakness, and cardiac arrhythmia.

EXPECTED COURSE AND PROGNOSIS

SDF is not life-threatening; in most cases; it is a transient condition that resolves either spontaneously or in response to treatment of the underlying problem.

MISCELLANEOUS

ASSOCIATED CONDITIONS

- Prolonged exercise in hot, humid conditions
- Lactation
- GI disturbances

AGE-RELATED FACTORS N/A

ZOONOTIC POTENTIAL N/A

PREGNANCY N/A

SEE ALSO

Hypocalcemia

ABBREVIATION

- GI = gastrointestinal

Suggested Reading

Toribio RE. Calcium Disorders in the Horse. In: Reed SM, Bayly WM & Sellon DC, ed. Equine Internal Medicine, ed 2. St. Louis: Saunders, 2004:1312–1315.

Author Laurent Couëtil
Consulting Editor Michel Lévy

SYNOVIAL FLUID

BASICS

DEFINITION

• A dialysate of plasma with the addition of hyaluronan and certain glycoproteins
• Normal synovial fluid is light yellow, clear, and free of particulate material and viscous, producing a strand ≅2.5 cm in length. It is found in joints, tendons sheaths, and bursae.
• Leukocyte counts usually may be done manually using a hemocytometer or using electronic cell counters.
• Smears from normal synovial fluid have low cellularity <1000 cells/μL (1×10^9/mL), consisting primarily of a mixture of small lymphocytes, macrophages, and synovial lining cells. The ratio of lymphocytes, macrophages, and synovial lining cells is variable and generally not of diagnostic significance. Many labs report all these cells collectively as mononuclear cells.
• One consistent feature of normal synovial fluid is that neutrophils should comprise <10% of the cells present. Few (if any) erythrocytes should be present.
• Normal values for equine synovial fluid protein vary between author and method. Upper limits of normal, as reported by various authors, generally range from 1–3g/dL, usually about 25–35% of the plasma protein level of the same animal.
• Synovial fluid functions as a biological lubricant and as a media for transfer of nutrients and cytokines to avascular cartilage.

PATHOPHYSIOLOGY

• Synovial fluid evaluation alone generally does not establish a specific diagnosis, but it reflects the degree and type of inflammation of the synovial lining—synovitis.
• Damage to articular cartilage often is not reflected in routine synovial fluid analysis.
• Synovial fluid analysis is most useful in the diagnosis of sepsis in synovial structures and has little value in differentiating the many causes of degenerative and traumatic joint conditions.
• Gross appearance is insensitive and should not be used alone.

SYSTEM AFFECTED

Musculoskeletal

SIGNALMENT

Any horse

SIGNS

Historical

Lameness

Physical Examination

• Lameness
• Swollen joints or synovial structures
• Pain

CAUSES

Septic Arthritis/Synovitis

• A clinical emergency that causes marked changes in synovial fluid.
• Routine synovial fluid examination usually provides sufficient information to establish a presumptive diagnosis.
• Depending on the cell count, fluid color may range from a slightly cloudy, dark yellow to an opaque cream. Red to red-brown is common with inflammation-induced hemorrhage.
• Flocculent material may be apparent.
• Fluid viscosity is markedly reduced.
• Cytology usually shows >90% neutrophils.
• Total nucleated cell counts usually >10,000 cells/μLl (10×10^9 /L), often much higher.
• Total protein concentrations also are markedly elevated, typically >4.0g/dL.
• In many, if not most, cases bacteria are not seen on cytological examination. Lack of identifiable bacteria, however, should not diminish consideration of sepsis in fluids with markedly elevated neutrophil counts.
• Culture of bacteria from the synovial fluid from septic joints can be expected to be positive in only about 50% of cases.
• Many times, neutrophils do not show marked degenerative changes with septic arthritis.
• As a general rule, synovial fluid should be considered infected if total nucleated cell counts are >30,000 cells/μL (30×10^9 /L), differentials indicate >80% neutrophils and/or total protein >40g/L.

Resolving Synovial Disease or Chronic Synovitis

• Synovial disease that is resolving, especially from previous joint sepsis, may appear similar to traumatic or degenerative joint disease.
• There often is a mononuclear component with very vacuolated macrophages and variable numbers of synovial cells and lymphocytes.
• Neutrophils usually are <10% of the cell component.
• Cell counts are within normal limits to slightly increased.
• Chronic synovitis may have a predominance of macrophages/monocytes or lymphocytes.
• Lymphocytic synovial fluid reflects lymphocytic inflammation within the synovial membrane and, rarely, may have plasma cells.
• Lymphocytic synovitis has been attributed to proliferative synovitis and infectious agents.

Degenerative/Traumatic Joint Disease

• Many conditions result in traumatic or degenerative joint injury. Associated inflammation is variable and often mild.
• Synovial fluid usually is clear, unless there is associated hemorrhage, in which case it may be red tinged.
• Viscosity may be decreased proportionately to the amount of effusion.
• Cell counts vary from normal to moderately increased, usually being <10,000 cells/μL (10×10^9/L) and consisting of >90% mononuclear cells.
• Macrophages may be large and vacuolated, sometimes containing phagocytosed debris.
• Low-grade degenerative changes may have normal synovial fluid characteristics.
• An increased percentage of neutrophils (>10%) may occur in some cases of acute trauma or with hemorrhage into the joint that adds peripheral blood neutrophils to the joint fluid. The total nucleated cell count (and absolute number of neutrophils) generally is much less than typically seen with septic arthritis.
• Traumatic injury usually is associated with a mild <5000 cells/μL (5×10^9/L), predominantly mononuclear cell response, but neutrophilic responses with cell counts up to 30,000 cells/μL (30×10^9/L) have been reported. These can be difficult to differentiate from septic responses, but cell counts in untreated cases of sepsis are usually much higher and the cell count with traumatic injury generally declines rapidly.
• Cartilage fragments may be seen in synovial fluid associated with trauma or degenerative joint disease, but this finding is uncommon.

RISK FACTORS

• Septic arthritis—failure of passive transfer in neonates
• Penetrating injuries or wounds near synovial structures
• Performance horses

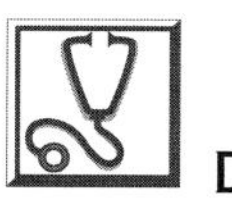

DIAGNOSIS

DIFFERENTIAL DIAGNOSIS

See Causes.

LABORATORY FINDINGS

General

• Place samples in an EDTA tube for the most important parameters—cell counts, cytology, and protein concentration.
• If only a small amount (<0.25mL) of fluid can be retrieved, make and submit air-dried direct smears.
• Placing extremely small quantities of fluid in an EDTA tube results in excessive dilution of the sample and, possibly, in a falsely increased total protein concentration (if determined by refractometry) resulting from EDTA as a solute.

Physical Characteristics

• Color, clarity, and an estimate of viscosity are noted.
• Viscosity may be estimated by placing a drop of synovial fluid between the thumb and forefinger, slowly pulling the fingers apart, and evaluating the strand length before breaking. Alternatively, strand length before breaking can be noted as synovial fluid is expelled through the tip of a needle.
• Normal synovial fluid may gel on standing, appearing to have clotted, but will return to a liquid state on warming and agitation.

Leukocyte Count (WBC)

• Cell counts often are too low to be accurately determined with an electronic cell counter.
• Leukocyte counts are subject to sources of analytic error and must not be interpreted too strictly when comparing serial counts.
• Markedly exudative samples (e.g., from septic joints) with dramatically elevated leukocyte counts >50,000 cells/μL (50×10^9/L) often contain numerous cell clumps that preclude an accurate cell count.
• Samples of low cellularity are subject to a different source of error. In samples with normal viscosity, cell counts may be falsely low, because the sample fails to mix evenly with the diluent. Despite these difficulties, samples with normal,

mildly elevated, and markedly elevated cells counts can be reliably differentiated.

- If a diluent system is used (e.g., Unopette system) along with a hemocytometer, avoid use of a product containing acetic acid as a diluent, because acetic acid causes precipitation of the mucin in synovial fluid.

Erythrocyte Count

- Erythrocyte counts are obtained from electronic cells counters or hemocytometers if a diluent that does not lyse erythrocytes is used.
- Erythrocytes indicate contamination during sample collection or hemorrhage secondary to hemostatic abnormalities, traumatic injury, or inflammatory disease. This is best differentiated at sample collection because hemorrhage during collection is usually apparent as a nonuniformly red-discolored fluid.
- Marked blood contamination increases the nucleated cell count and alters the differential leukocyte count, usually increasing the percentage of neutrophils.

Cytology

- Along with nucleated cell count, probably the most diagnostically important parameter of synovial fluid evaluation
- With a limited sample, direct smears, from which the cell count could be estimated, should be made first.
- Blood contamination, in additional to adding RBCs, can add various leukocytes in proportions typical of peripheral blood (i.e., predominantly neutrophils).
- Predominance of neutrophils, rather than of mononuclear cells, indicates inflammation of the synovial lining.
- In most species, neutrophilic inflammation is seen with septic and immune-mediated joint diseases.
- Because immune-mediated arthritis has not been well documented in horses, the main consideration for neutrophilic inflammation is septic arthritis, but traumatic injury and chemical synovitis should be considered.
- Gram stain may demonstrate bacteria, although often bacteria are not seen even with sepsis. If bacteria are seen, it may be useful to direct antibiotic choice.
- Erythrocytes indicate blood contamination during sample collection or hemorrhage from hemostatic defects, trauma, or inflammatory disease. Differentiating these conditions based on cytology is difficult. Macrophages containing phagocytized RBCs (i.e., erythrophagocytosis) indicate intra-articular hemorrhage if the slides were made soon after collection. Phagocytosis of erythrocytes by macrophages can occur in vitro during prolonged transport (i.e., several hours). Platelets or platelet clumps suggest blood contamination during sample collection.

Mucin Clot Test

- Provides a crude estimate of hyaluronate concentration
- May be reduced in both septic and nonseptic synovitis so is of little clinical use

Total Protein Concentration

- Some laboratories measure protein concentration using a dye-binding method; others use refractometric readings as estimates of protein concentrations.
- Protein measurements may help to indicate the presence of inflammation but are not useful in differentiating between types of inflammation.
- Increased protein concentrations are seen with synovial inflammation. Concentrations of >2.5g/dL probably are abnormal.
- Nonseptic inflammatory conditions usually result in protein levels of <4.0g/dL.

Drugs That May Alter Lab Results

- Previous therapeutic procedures must be considered.
- Intra-articular injections can produce high leukocyte counts and neutrophil percentages, but the magnitude generally is lower than that seen with septic arthritis.
- Injection of sterile saline produces cell counts of up to 30,000 cells/μL (30×10^9/L), with neutrophils being the predominant cell type (≅70%).
- Injection of chemicals irritating to the synovial membrane can result in higher counts.
- Intra-articular corticosteroid injections can cause a neutrophilia (up to 98% neutrophils), with cell counts near 20,000 cells/μL (20×10^9/L).
- With inflammation caused by intra-articular injection, cell counts and neutrophil percentages decline significantly by 3–4 days after the injection.
- Previous intra-articular injections of corticosteroids may delay the onset of changes in synovial fluid with septic arthritis; however, the typical changes still occur.

Disorders That May Alter Lab Results

N/A

Valid If Run in Human Lab?

Yes, if familiar with synovial fluid analysis

CBC/BIOCHEMISTRY/URINALYSIS

Dependent on the underlying disease

OTHER LABORATORY TESTS

- Evaluation of hyaluronan content, serum enzymes and isoenzymes (i.e., creatine kinase, lactate dehydrogenase), glucose, and cartilage fragments have been suggested, but none has gained wide use.
- With further research, direct and indirect biomarkers may become important in the diagnosis and monitoring of joint disease.
- Polymerase chain reaction may provide rapid sensitive diagnosis of bacterial sepsis in the presence of antibiotics but gives no information on antibiotic sensitivities.
- Bacterial culture and sensitivity of purulent samples

IMAGING

Radiography, ultrasonography, and nuclear scintigraphy may be useful for establishing a diagnosis.

DIAGNOSTIC PROCEDURES

Arthroscopy

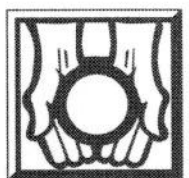

TREATMENT

Directed at the underlying cause

MEDICATIONS

DRUGS OF CHOICE

Specific for the underlying cause

PRECAUTIONS

Samples must be collected aseptically.

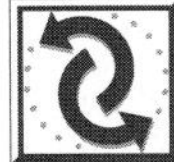

FOLLOW-UP

Serial monitoring of synovial fluid often useful diagnostically and to monitor response to treatment

PATIENT MONITORING

Dependent on the underlying disease

ASSOCIATED CONDITIONS

Laminitis

AGE-RELATED FACTORS

Neonates with failure of passive transfer can develop sepsis and septic joints.

SYNONYMS

Joint fluid

SEE ALSO

Related musculoskeletal topics

Suggested Reading

Madison JB, Sommer M, Spencer PA. Relations among synovial membrane histopathologic findings, synovial fluid cytologic findings, and bacterial culture results in horses with suspected infectious arthritis: 64 cases (1979–1987). JAVMA 1991;198:1655–1661.

McIwraith CW. Use of synovial fluid and serum biomarkers in equine bone and joint disease: a review. Equine Vet J 2005;37:473–482.

Steel CM. Equine synovial fluid analysis. Vet Clin North Am Equine Pract 2008;24(2).

Trotter GW, McIlwraith CW. Clinical features and diagnosis of equine joint disease. In: McIlwraith CW, Trotter GW, eds. Joint Disease of the Horse. Philadelphia: WB Saunders, 1996:137–141.

Tulamo R, Bramlage L, Gabel A. Sequential clinical and synovial fluid changes associated with acute infectious arthritis in the horse. Equine Vet J 1989;21:325–331.

The author and editor wish to acknowledge the contribution to this chapter of James Meinkoth and Rick L. Crowell, the authors in the previous edition.

Author Mattias A. Muurlink

Consulting Editor Kenneth W. Hinchcliff

TEMPOROHYOID OSTEOARTHROPATHY

BASICS

DEFINITION

THO can cause ankylosis between the hyoid bone and the petrous temporal bone. The condition can result in a number of clinical signs and, if fractured, acute vestibular disease and/or facial nerve paresis.

PATHOPHYSIOLOGY

The cause of THO is unknown. Initial publications indicated that the bone reaction is secondary to chronic middle ear infection or guttural pouch disease; however, only rarely has an infectious process been shown histologically. Another scenario may be that osteochondroarthrosis of the temporohyoid joint precedes other changes, and that involvement of the osseous bulla and proximal stylohyoid bone occurs by extension of the degenerative joint disease. The fused joint may then suddenly fracture during normal movements of mastication and phonation, leading to fracture of the petrous temporal bone, and impingement of the facial and vestibular nerve, respectively, in the middle and inner ear.

SYSTEMS AFFECTED

Peripheral nervous system

SIGNALMENT

The disease is most common in middle-aged horses.

CLINICAL SIGNS

Clinical signs include difficulty chewing, pain on external palpation of the temporohyoid joint area, head shaking, and behavior problems, particularly when ridden.

Acute signs of vestibular disease are common with or without facial nerve paresis and involve a head tilt and sometimes nystagmus with the fast phase away from the side of the lesion. Horses with a severe case can circle toward the lesion or end up recumbent with the affected side down. All branches of the facial nerve are usually affected, leading to ptosis, muzzle deviation away from the side of the lesion, and a dropped lower lip and ear on the side of the lesion. Chronic facial nerve paresis can result in exposure keratitis.

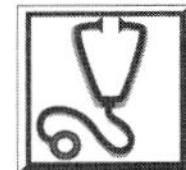

DIAGNOSIS

- Endoscopic and radiographic changes of temporohyoid bone ankylosis and enlargement of the proximal stylohyoid bone are usually extensive by the time neurologic abnormalities are evident.
- Radiographs are not as sensitive a diagnostic tool as endoscopy unless a ventrodorsal view can be obtained (usually under anesthesia).
- Computed tomography provides an excellent assessment of the bony abnormalities.

DIFFERENTIAL DIAGNOSIS

Trauma, equine protozoal myeloencephalitis in affected regions

CBC/BIOCHEMISTRY/URINALYSIS

No specific abnormalities

OTHER LABORATORY TESTS

Atlanto-occipital cerebrospinal fluid—Most cases have xanthochromia with elevated protein and nondegenerate inflammatory cells.

IMAGING

Radiographic changes and endoscopy are consistent. See Pathophysiology.

PATHOLOGIC FINDINGS

See Pathophysiology.

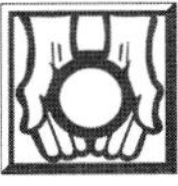

TREATMENT

- As with most peripheral vestibular syndromes, signs of vestibular dysfunction will improve regardless of therapy.
- Supportive care is essential.

• Antibiotics with a good spectrum against *Staphylococcus aureus* have been recommended for 2–4 weeks (e. g., trimethoprim-sulfa and enrofloxacin).
• Horses with severe vestibular disease are sometimes treated with a tapering course of corticosteroids (beginning with 0.04–0.08 mg/kg dexamethasone) to try to more rapidly decrease the inflammatory response and improve the horse's balance.
• Removal of a section of the stylohyoid bone and a ceratohyoidectomy have been described to reduce stresses on the temporohyoid joint.
• A partial tarsorrhaphy may be necessary to manage palpebral dysfunction.
• Vestibular function will improve with time, but even with surgery, facial and other cranial nerve disorders often remain constant with only slight improvement over time.
• In addition, the acute nature of the fracture and subsequent vestibular disease can make these horses dangerous to riders!

MEDICATIONS

PRECAUTIONS

The acute nature of the fracture and subsequent vestibular disease can make these horses dangerous to riders. Even horses that appear to have no residual signs can look profoundly worse when blindfolded. Brainstem auditory evoked potentials have been used in referral institutions to document the integrity of the vestibulocochlear nerve.

FOLLOW-UP

POSSIBLE COMPLICATIONS

• Uveitis and ocular rupture have been seen in a few horses.
• Weight loss and aspiration pneumonia can be seen when dysphagia is evident.

PROGNOSIS

Fair for long-term resolution even with surgery

MISCELLANEOUS

ABBREVIATION

• THO = temporohyoid osteoarthropathy

Suggested Reading

Divers, TJ, Mayhew IG. Neurology. Clin Tech Equine Pract 2006;5(1).
Pease AP, et al. Complication of partial stylohyoidectomy for treatment of temporohyoid osteoarthropathy and alternative surgical technique in three cases. Eq Vet I, 2004,36:546–550.

The author and editors wish to acknowledge the contribution of Joseph J. Bertone, author of this chapter in the previous edition.

Author Caroline N. Hahn
Consulting Editor Caroline N. Hahn

TENDONITIS

BASICS

DEFINITION

Inflammation of a tendon and/or musculotendinous junction; most commonly refers to inflammation of the SDFT and DDFT

PATHOPHYSIOLOGY

• The normal SDFT of a galloping Thoroughbred can elongate up to 16% of its original length. SDFT failure occurs with percentage elongations (strains) of approximately 20%. This small safety margin is probably a major factor in the high incidence of SDFT injury in Thoroughbred racehorses. • Excessive loading of the digital flexor tendons results in disruption of the collagen fibrils and extracellular matrix. Intratendinous hemorrhage and hematoma formation occur. Fibrin and inflammatory cells are released in proportion to the size of the injury. • Scar formation begins with the production of type III collagen, which provides early stability but little tensile strength. Type III collagen predominates for the first 6–8 weeks of healing. • Remodeling begins after 6–8 weeks. Type I collagen slowly replaces type III collagen. The tendon is resized and reshaped. Collagen fibers become aligned in the direction of stress and tendon tensile strength improves. Remodeling continues for many months.
• Abnormal quantities of type III collagen, small collagen fibrils, and lack of linear fiber arrangement can persist for up to 14 mo. This slow rate of healing contributes to the high rate of reinjury.

SYSTEMS AFFECTED

Musculoskeletal—tendons, musculotendinous junctions, areas of tendon insertion, tendon sheaths

GENETICS

Unknown

INCIDENCE/PREVALENCE

• Incidence of SDFT injury in all Thoroughbred racehorses is between 8% and 43%. • Incidence of SDFT injury in the event horse is higher in those competing in Concours Complet International (CCI) competitions than in those competing in 1-day events. • Injury to the SDFT is unusual in show jumpers except in those competing at the international level or older than 15 years. • SDFT injuries occur more frequently in the forelimb than in the hindlimb. Bilateral lesions are common. • Injury to the DDFT occurs most commonly in the hindlimb of dressage horses and show jumpers.

SIGNALMENT

• Thoroughbred racehorses (flat and steeplechase) are most likely to sustain an injury to the SDFT followed by upper-level event horses then Grand Prix level show jumpers.
• Standardbred racehorses, racing Arabians and Quarter Horses, polo ponies, fox hunters, cutting horses, and barrel racers experience SDFT injury infrequently. • DDFT injuries occur most commonly in jumpers and dressage horses older than 10 years.

SIGNS

Historical

• Acute unilateral lameness that responds to rest
• Swelling, focal sensitivity, and/or heat along the palmar/plantar aspect of the metacarpus/metatarsus • Tendon enlargement with chronic injury

Physical Examination—SDF Tendonitis

• Bowed (convex) tendon profile when weight bearing • Distension of the digital sheath much less common than with DDFT injury • "Curb" if injury to tarsal region • Variable lameness depending on the severity, location, and chronicity • Mild and/or chronic injuries tend not to cause lameness. • Moderate or moderately severe injuries tend to be transiently lame in the acute phase. • Lesions in the carpal canal region cause mild distention of the carpal sheath and consistent lameness that is accentuated by carpal flexion; horse may stand with the knee slightly flexed. • Pastern branch lesions frequently but not always cause lameness. • Complete rupture causes severe lameness and a dropped fetlock.

Physical Examination—DDF Tendonitis

• Subtle bowed tendon profile • Mild to moderate lameness that may worsen with distal limb flexion • +/− Distention of the digital tendon sheath • In distal injury (within the foot), unilateral lameness with no physical examination abnormalities

CAUSES

• Excessive biomechanical load • Direct blunt or penetrating trauma • Sepsis secondary to a wound that penetrates the tendon sheath
• Secondary to encircling bandages; "bandage bow"

RISK FACTORS

• Performing at speed • Performing over fences
• Increasing age with tendon matrix deterioration • Abnormal conformation—long pasterns, tied in behind the knee, long toe/low heel, medial-to-lateral hoof imbalance • Rough uneven ground, wet slippery surfaces, and deep footing • Palmar digital neurectomy may be a predisposing factor for rupture of the distal DDFT.

DIAGNOSIS

DIFFERENTIAL DIAGNOSIS

• Suspensory desmitis • Inferior check desmitis
• Long plantar desmitis or other causes of curb
• Primary/noninfectious tenosynovitis • Tears of the manica flexoria • Palmar/plantar annular ligament syndrome • All of the above differential diagnoses can be ruled out with ultrasonography.

IMAGING

• Ultrasonography—The tendon should be evaluated in both transverse and longitudinal planes. Size, shape, echogenicity, and fiber pattern should be evaluated. Length of the lesion and cross-sectional measurements of both the tendon and the lesion should be obtained in each zone. These measurements are used to determine severity of lesion—
mild = <15%, moderate = 15%–25%, severe = >25% of total cross-sectional area.
• Sonographic abnormalities include:
  ○ In acute injury, focal anechoic core lesions completely lacking in fibers, +/− hematoma formation
  ○ In chronic injury, areas of decreased echogenicity and abnormal fiber pattern, +/− hyperechoic areas that cast strong acoustic shadows (dystrophic calcification)
  ○ Increased tendon cross-sectional area
  ○ Adhesions between tendon and surrounding tissues can be identified by performing a dynamic scan. (The vinculum of the SDFT and the mesotendon of the DDFT are normal structures often mistaken for adhesions.)
  ○ Increased fluid, +/− fibrin within the carpal/tarsal or digital sheath
  ○ The lateral margins of the DDFT should be carefully scanned as lateral lesions are common and easily missed.
• MRI (for DDFT injury within the foot)—core lesions, sagittal tears, dorsal border lesions, insertional injuries, and combination injuries
• Radiography—dystrophic mineralization within a tendon, bony irregularity at tendon insertion, osteochondroma of the distal radius

OTHER DIAGNOSTIC PROCEDURES

• Diagnostic analgesia—High palmar/plantar analgesia, intrathecal digital sheath analgesia are diagnostic especially with subtle or absent abnormal physical examination findings.
• Tenoscopic exploration of the tendon sheath—identification of marginal tears of the DDFT

PATHOLOGICAL FINDINGS

• Lesions < 2 weeks—fragmented collagen fibers surrounded by strands of fibrin and edema, polymorphonuclear cells and macrophages; intratendinous and peritendinous hemorrhage • Lesions 1–5 mo duration—large numbers of fibroblasts, granulation tissue and immature fibrous tissue; proliferation of paratenon and endotenon • Lesions of ≥6 mo duration—various degrees of fibrosis characterized by irregular collagen arrangement, widespread scar formation and prominent endotendinous tissue; fibrosis of the paratenon
• After 14 mo—scar still hypercellular with little subdivision into bundles

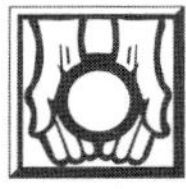

TREATMENT

AIMS OF TREATMENT

• Limit inflammatory process, control pain, and prevent further injury. • Optimize the quality of the tendon repair in order to have the best chance of returning the horse to a similar level of performance with the lowest risk of reinjury.

APPROPRIATE HEALTH CARE

• Rest and controlled exercise program are essential. • Resuming athletic work is based on lameness and sonographic reevaluations every 6–8 weeks.

NURSING CARE

• Cold water hydrotherapy • Poultice • Support wrap

ACTIVITY

- Controlled exercise program (rest, confinement, and gradual reintroduction of exercise) is the mainstay of tendonitis treatment.
- Duration is determined by the location, severity, and response to treatment. • Stall rest initially • Turnout should be limited to small paddock initially and occur no sooner than 4 mo following mild injury; no sooner than 6 mo if moderate to severe injury.
- Controlled exercise program for horses recovering from SDF tendonitis (example):
  - Level 1—walking 30 min/day for 4 weeks followed by 45 min/day for an additional 4 weeks
  - Level 2—jogging 5 min/day for 4 weeks followed by 10 min/day for 4 weeks
  - Level 3—jogging 15 min/day for 4 weeks followed by 20 min/day for 4 weeks
  - Level 4 (for horses with moderate to severe injuries; horses with mild injuries can go on to level 5) —continued jogging exercise 25 min/day for 4 weeks followed by 30 min/day for 4 weeks
  - Level 5—canter or slow gallop 1 mile/day for 4 weeks followed by 2 miles/day for 4 weeks
  - Level 6—breeze 4 weeks
  - Level 7—race
- Walking exercise can be performed in hand, on a walker, or with rider up. • Ultrasound and lameness evaluations should be repeated between each level of exercise. If appropriate sonographic improvement does not occur at any level, exercise should not be increased and in some cases may need to be decreased.

DIET

Mild to moderate caloric reduction of intake while stall confined or resting

CLIENT EDUCATION

- Early recognition and strict adherence to controlled exercise program are essential to tendon healing and return to athletic performance.
- Risk of reinjury is high, especially during early phases of healing and inappropriate exercise.

SURGICAL CONSIDERATIONS

- Superior check desmotomy—for SDF tendonitis, improved outcome in Standardbreds, recommended for moderate to severe lesions, +/− suspensory desmitis after surgery
- Percutaneous tendon splitting—for tendon core lesions during the acute stage of injury to decompress areas of hemorrhage and maybe promote vascularization • Fetlock palmar/plantar annular desmotomy—for treatment of distal metacarpal/metatarsal tendonitis where normal gliding of the tendon is impaired • Proximal metacarpal fasciotomy and carpal retinacular release—for treatment of proximal SDF tendonitis, especially injuries within the carpal canal region • Tenoscopy of the digital flexor tendon sheath—Therapeutic value consists of debridement of the injured digital flexor tendon, breakdown of adhesions, and removal of foreign material in the case of penetrating injury; procedure may result in further adhesion formation and therefore should be used judiciously.

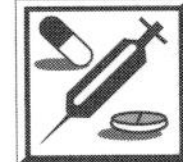

MEDICATIONS

DRUG(S)

- Systemic NSAIDs—phenylbutazone (4.4 mg/kg per day) for 7–10 days • Intrathecal sodium hyaluronan (10–20 mg) • Intrathecal corticosteroids— methylprednisolone acetate (40 mg) or triamcinolone (6 mg)

CONTRAINDICATIONS

Intralesional or perilesional corticosteroids

ALTERNATIVE DRUGS/THERAPIES

- Intralesional β-aminoproprionitrile fumarate (BAPTN) 1 mL (0.7 mg) per 3% total lesion area, up to 10 mL • Intralesional stem cells derived from fat or bone marrow • Intralesional platelet-rich plasma • Extracorporeal shock wave therapy • Appropriate hoof care and shoeing
- Therapeutic ultrasound • Counterirritation (iodine-based liniments, internal peritendinous injection of 2% iodine in almond oil, pin firing)

FOLLOW-UP

PATIENT MONITORING

- The quality of healing as judged by ultrasound should be used to determine the level of exercise.
- Lameness and sonographic evaluations every 8 weeks until adequate tendon healing in the face of exercise
- Lameness, heat, or swelling over the tendon should prompt discontinuation of exercise and sonographic reevaluation.

PREVENTION/AVOIDANCE

- Prevention is limited to addressing risk factors that can be avoided such as inappropriate hoof balance and dangerous work surfaces. • Once an injury occurs, limiting reinjury becomes the focus. Appropriate rest period with controlled exercise and sonographic monitoring is critical for preventing reinjury.

POSSIBLE COMPLICATIONS

- Adhesion between the tendon and peritendinous tissue or digital sheath • Tendon rupture with severe tendonitis and continued exercise

EXPECTED COURSE AND PROGNOSIS

- Rehabilitation takes 8–12 mo on average, regardless of treatment. • SDF tendonitis carries a guarded prognosis for return to previous level of athletic performance in any horse that is required to work at speed. • Rate of recurrence of SDF tendonitis is high. • Prognosis for SDF tendonitis is better for Standardbred racehorses than for Thoroughbred racehorses.
- Approximately 50% of event horses and most show jumpers with SDFT injury will return to full athletic function. • Prognosis for return to previous level of athletic activity is guarded for DDF tendonitis.

MISCELLANEOUS

ASSOCIATED CONDITIONS

- Tenosynovitis of the digital sheath • Navicular syndrome • Desmitis of the accessory ligament of the DDFT • Annular ligament constriction
- Osteochondroma of the distal radius

AGE-RELATED FACTORS

- Older horses tend to heal more slowly and require longer rehabilitation. • Older horses may develop injuries to SDFT without significant athletic activity. • Injuries to the SDFT in the carpal canal region occur more frequently in older horses.

SYNONYMS

Bowed tendon

SEE ALSO

- Suspensory desmitis • Navicular syndrome

ABBREVIATIONS

- CCI = Concours Complet International
- DDFT = deep digital flexor tendon
- MRI = magnetic resonance imaging
- SDFT = superficial digital flexor tendon

Suggested Reading

Dyson SJ. The deep digital flexor tendon. In: Ross M, Dyson S, eds. Diagnosis and Management of Lameness in the Horse. St Louis: Saunders, 2003:644–650.

Jorgensen JS, Genovese RL. Superficial digital flexor tendinitis. In: Ross M, Dyson S, eds. Diagnosis and Management of Lameness in the Horse. St. Louis: Saunders, 2003:628–643.

Author JoAnn Slack
Consulting Editor Elizabeth J. Davidson

TENESMUS

BASICS

OVERVIEW

• An involuntary straining to evacuate the rectum or bladder, with passage of little fecal matter or urine • Constant stimulation of the sacral nerves by inflammation or physical pressure gives the horse a continual sensation of the need to defecate or urinate, which leads to repeated attempts to evacuate the bowel or bladder as long as the stimulation remains unrelieved by the attempts. • Stimulation may result from intrinsic disease of the organ involved (e.g., rectal inflammation); therefore, tenesmus may be seen with diarrhea.
• Stimulation also may result from physical pressure on the organ from within (e.g., rectal stimulation by constipated feces) or from without (e.g., rectal stimulation by a pararectal abscess). • May lead to rectal or uterine/bladder prolapse (in females only)

SIGNALMENT

More common in females

SIGNS

• Repeated attempts to defecate or urinate
• Prolapse of the penis • Sometimes a visibly prolapsed rectum, uterus, or bladder (mares) secondary to tenesmus

CAUSES AND RISK FACTORS

• Internal pressure of the rectum—constipation or foreign body (meconium impaction in foals)
• External pressure on the rectum—pararectal abscess or neoplasm • Inflammation of the rectum—proctitis/ diarrhea or rectal tear
• Inflammation of the urethra—lower urinary tract infection • Urinary tract obstruction—cystic/urethral calculi
• Inflammation of the vagina—vaginitis
• Direct stimulation of the nervous system—hepatic encephalopathy or damaged nerves caused by rabies • Parturition/dystocia

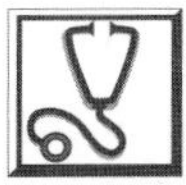

DIAGNOSIS

DIFFERENTIAL DIAGNOSIS

• Inflammation of the colon or rectum • Rectal tears, strictures, polyps, neoplasms, or small colon intussusceptions • Pararectal abscess or anorectal lymphadenopathy • Meconium impaction or uroperitoneum (i.e., ruptured bladder or urachus) in foals • Vaginitis or retained placenta • Urolithiasis or lower urinary tract infection and uroperitoneum • Neurologic disorders involving sacral nerves or CNS disorder—hepatic encephalopathy, rabies, or others • Oak (acorn) poisoning, *Psilocybe* (magic mushroom) poisoning, or lolitrem B toxicity

CBC/BIOCHEMISTRY/URINALYSIS

• Urinalysis may be abnormal with urinary tract involvement. • CBC may show neutropenia and thrombocytopenia with a rectal tear, retained placenta, or intussusception. • CBC may show neutrophilia in cases of inflammation.
• Eosinophilia was reported in one case of eosinophilic proctitis. • Elevated serum globulins with pararectal abscess • Biochemistry may demonstrate liver failure in cases of hepatic encephalopathy; bile salts and blood ammonia also may be elevated. • Hyponatremia and hypochloremia may occur with uroperitoneum and in foals with meconium impaction if repeated enemas with water have been administered previously. • Hyperkalemia occurs in cases of uroperitoneum.

OTHER LABORATORY TESTS

• Abdominocentesis for uroperitoneum and rectal tears • Urinary gallic acid equivalent concentration in acorn poisoning

IMAGING

• Abdominal radiography for meconium impaction • Abdominal ultrasonography for uroperitoneum, intussusception, and pararectal abscess, or lymphadenopathy • Bladder ultrasonography for urolithiasis or neoplasia

DIAGNOSTIC PROCEDURES

• Manual vaginal and rectal examination
• Rectal endoscopy for tears, polyps, neoplasia, strictures, or intussusception • Vaginoscopy or endoscopy for vaginitis • Endoscopy of the urethra and bladder for lower urinary tract problems • Rectal biopsy for proctitis, polyps, or neoplasia

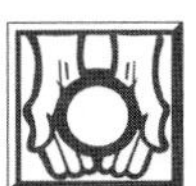

TREATMENT

• Depends on the inciting cause; eliminating the cause relieves the symptom of tenesmus. • Rectal or uterine/bladder prolapse— reduction of the prolapse is required. Temporary relief from tenesmus can be obtained with caudal epidural (i.e., regional) anesthetic. A caudal epidural also is required before attempting to reduce a prolapse or for surgery of the perineal area. Addition of xylazine in the epidural injection can reduce the dose of local anesthetic required to avoid postepidural hindlimb ataxia. • Rectal stricture or narrowing due to a pararectal mass—add laxatives and stool softeners to the diet. • If rectal prolapse has occurred, prevent recumbency until the prolapse has been reduced to minimize tissue trauma. • Surgical management by permanent colostomy if untreatable neoplasia of perianal region
• Retention enema in meconium impaction

MEDICATIONS

DRUGS

No specific medication; treatment depends on the inciting cause.

FOLLOW-UP

PATIENT MONITORING

• Depends on the inciting cause • Rectal prolapse can recur.

POSSIBLE COMPLICATIONS

• Repeated attempts to evacuate the bowel or bladder may lead to rectal or uterine/bladder prolapse (in females only). • Rectal prolapse may recur after correction if feces are not softened enough.

EXPECTED COURSE AND PROGNOSIS

Prognosis depends on the cause.

MISCELLANEOUS

ASSOCIATED CONDITIONS

• Rectal prolapse • Uterine or bladder prolapse (in females only)

AGE RELATED FACTORS

• Meconium impaction in neonatal foals
• Ruptured bladder in neonatal foals and parturient mares • Hamartomatous polyp in neonatal foal • Urolithiasis in young adults
• Bladder neoplasia in old individuals

PREGNANCY

Dystocia

SYNONYMS

• Urgency (human) • Straining to defecate; dyschezia (although commonly meant to convey pain) • Straining to urinate; strangury; dysuria (although commonly meant to convey pain)

SEE ALSO

• Dystocia • Hepatic encephalopathy
• Inflammation of the colon or rectum; colitis; proctitis • Intussusception • Meconium impaction • Rabies • Rectal prolapse • Rectal tears or strictures • Retained placenta
• Ruptured bladder; uroperitoneum
• Urolithiasis or lower urinary tract infection
• Vaginitis • Other neurologic disorder involving sacral nerves

ABBREVIATIONS

• CBC = complete blood count
• CNS = central nervous system

Suggested Reading

Colbourne CM, Bolton JB, Yovich JV, Genovese L. Hamartomatous polyp causing intestinal obstruction and tenesmus in a neonatal foal. Aust Equine Vet 1996;14:78–80.

Frazer GS. Post partum complications in the mare. Part 2: fetal membrane retention and conditions of the gastrointestinal tract, bladder and vagina. Equine Vet Educ (Am Ed) 2003;5:118–128.

Jones J. 'Magic mushroom' (Psilocybe) poisoning in a colt. Vet Rec 1990;127:603.

Laverty S, Pascoe JR, Ling GV, Lavoie JP, Ruby AL. Urolithiasis in 68 horses. Vet Surg 1992;21:56–62.

Munday BL, Monkhouse IM, Gallagher RT. Intoxication of horses by lolitrem B in ryegrass seed cleanings. Aust Vet J 1985;62:207.

Author Gail Abells Sutton

Consulting Editors Henry Stämpfli and Olimpo Oliver-Espinosa

TERATOMA

BASICS

DEFINITION/OVERVIEW

- Germ cell tumor of the gonad
- Generally benign, but can become malignant and metastasize into the abdominal cavity
- Contains mixture of mature and poorly differentiated structures
- Other types—dysgerminoma (female); seminoma (male)
- Characterized by multiple tissue types within the tumor
- Contains somatic structures derived from all embryonic germ cell layers arranged randomly throughout tumor—
  - Ectoderm (hair, teeth)
  - Neuroectoderm (nerves, melanocytes)
  - Endoderm (salivary gland, lung)
  - Mesoderm (fibrous, adipose, bone, muscle)
  - Nervous and adipose tissue (nearly always present)

ETIOLOGY/PATHOPHYSIOLOGY

- Generally a benign, incidental finding
- Hormonally inactive, does not preclude pregnancy or normal cyclicity in female

SYSTEMS AFFECTED

- Reproductive
- Gonad, placenta also reported
- Rarely a systemic effect, unless metastasis occurs

GENETICS

See Causes.

INCIDENCE/PREVALENCE

Rare, although second most common ovarian neoplasm following granulosa thecal cell tumor

SIGNALMENT

- Horses of any age may display signs because of teratoma, colic.
- Young males—usual presenting age, 1–2 years
- Cryptorchid testes—Presence of a teratoma in the fetus can prevent testicular descent.
- Females—discovered during routine reproductive examination

SIGNS

- Effects from physical presence of a teratoma if it is of high mass/weight
  - May lead to discomfort and extramural intestinal obstruction.
- Has been associated with small colon torsion in a foal, colic in mares, and testicular cyst formation
- Females—palpably abnormal ovarian mass, altered consistency of ovarian tissue
  - Generally unilateral
  - Solid and cystic areas, replacing normal tissue
- Males—scrotal mass
  - Most often a cryptorchid testicle
  - May decrease spermatogenesis or induce tubular atrophy of adjacent testicular tissue

CAUSE

Congenital

RISK FACTORS

May be concurrent with other gonadal neoplasia—carcinoma; granulosa thecal cell tumor

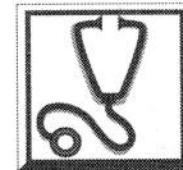

DIAGNOSIS

DIFFERENTIAL DIAGNOSIS

- Females—ovarian hematoma; granulosa thecal cell tumor; dysgerminoma; carcinoma; fibroma; abscess, lymphosarcoma, cystadenoma
- Males—seminoma; Sertoli cell tumor; interstitial cell tumor; carcinoma; testicular hematoma; fibroma, abscess

CBC/BIOCHEMISTRY/URINALYSIS

N/A

OTHER LABORATORY TESTS

Lack of endocrinological abnormality consistent with other causes of ovarian enlargement

IMAGING

U/S

- Couple with transrectal palpation.
- Abnormal paraovarian mass—solid; multilocular
- May have hyperechoic structures present (mineralized bone, teeth)

OTHER DIAGNOSTIC PROCEDURES

N/A

PATHOLOGICAL FINDINGS

- Histopathological findings—Multiple tissue types may be present within neoplasm (adipose, bone, cartilage, hair, nervous elements, and teeth).
- Gross findings—solid, cystic multilocular form; yellow-white

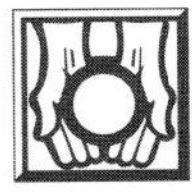

TREATMENT

APPROPRIATE HEALTH CARE

Surgical removal

NURSING CARE

N/A

ACTIVITY

N/A

DIET

N/A

CLIENT EDUCATION

N/A

SURGICAL CONSIDERATIONS

May necessitate concurrent gonadectomy

MEDICATIONS

DRUG(S) OF CHOICE, CONTRAINDICATIONS, PRECAUTIONS, POSSIBLE INTERACTIONS, ALTERNATIVE DRUGS

N/A

FOLLOW-UP

PATIENT MONITORING, PREVENTION/AVOIDANCE, POSSIBLE COMPLICATIONS, EXPECTED COURSE AND PROGNOSIS

N/A

MISCELLANEOUS

ASSOCIATED CONDITIONS, AGE-RELATED FACTORS, ZOONOTIC POTENTIAL, PREGNANCY, SYNONYMS

N/A

SEE ALSO

- Large ovary syndrome

ABBREVIATION

- U/S = ultrasound, ultrasonography

Suggested Reading

Allison N, Moeller RB Jr, Duncan R. Placental teratocarcinoma in a mare with possible metastasis to the foal. J Vet Diagn Invest 2004;2:160–163.

Buergelt CD. Color Atlas of Reproductive Pathology of the Domestic Animals. St. Louis: Mosby–Year Book, 1997:55–56,106–107.

Catone G, Marino G, Mancuso R, Zanghi A. Clinicopathological features of an equine ovarian teratoma. Reprod Domest Anim 2004;39:65–69.

Gurfield N, Benirschke K. Equine placental teratoma. Vet Pathol 2003;40:586–588.

Jubb KVC, Kennedy PC, Palmer N. Pathology of the Domestic Animals, ed 4. San Diego: Academic Press, 1993:368, 510.

Lefebvre R, Theoret C, Dore M, Girard C, Laverty S, Vaillancourt D. Ovarian teratoma and endometritis in a mare. Can Vet J 2005;46:1029–1033.

Author Peter R. Morresey

Consulting Editor Carla L. Carleton

TETANUS

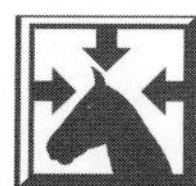

BASICS

DEFINITION

Tetanus is a disease characterized by muscular spasm, caused by a neurotoxin produced by *Clostridium tetani*.

PATHOPHYSIOLOGY

C. tetani is a gram-positive, spore-forming bacillus. The spores are widespread in the environment, particularly in soil and mammalian feces. They typically gain access to the animal via a wound. The oxygen tension within the wound must be low to allow germination. Concurrent infection with other bacteria and the presence of foreign bodies or necrosis within the wound can help produce a favorable anaerobic tissue environment. Under such conditions, *C. tetani* organisms proliferate locally. Death and lysis of the organisms within the wound result in liberation of tetanospasmin, a neurotoxin responsible for the characteristic clinical signs. Tetanospasmin travels to the central nervous system via the hemolymphatic system and via peripheral motor nerves. The toxin exerts its effect on presynaptic inhibitory interneurons in the ventral horn of the spinal cord. There it cleaves synaptobrevin, a vesicle-associated membrane protein necessary for release of the neurotransmitters glycine and GABA. This results in a loss of motor neuron inhibition, and the subsequent hypertonia and muscular spasm. Two other exotoxins are produced by *C. tetani*. Tetanolysin is thought to increase local tissue necrosis, promoting proliferation within the wound. Another nonspasmogenic toxin may have a sympathomimetic effect.

The incubation period is highly variable, but it is usually 1–3 weeks. The spores can survive in tissue and germinate after wound healing if conditions then become favorable. Castration wounds and injection sites have also been associated with the development of tetanus.

SYSTEMS AFFECTED

- Neuromuscular
- Secondary effects on other systems (respiratory, skeletal, etc.) depending on the presence of complications

GENETICS

N/A

INICIDENCE/PREVALENCE

- Horses are exquisitely sensitive to the toxin, and the disease has a worldwide distribution.
- A higher incidence may be associated with poor husbandry.
- There may be a higher incidence in warmer areas.

SIGNALMENT

No sex, age, or breed predilections

CLINICAL SIGNS

- There is usually a history of a wound 1–4 weeks earlier.
- There may be lack of vaccination, although tetanus may occur in the face of vaccination.
- The first signs may be vague (local stiffness, lameness, colic).
- The progression of signs depends on the extent of the infection, the vaccination status, and the age and size of the horse.
- Generally, the signs progress within 24 hours, with the horse beginning to exhibit a stiff/spastic gait.
- Trembling, a raised tail head, flared nostrils, and erect ears are seen.
- Preferential effects on postural muscles result in the characteristic "sawhorse stance."
- Retraction of the eyes and protrusion of the third eyelids occur following a stimulus (noise or menace).
- Spasm of the masseter muscles can cause inability to open the mouth ("lockjaw").
- Dysphagia results in accumulation of saliva in the mouth and aspiration of feed material.
- Pyrexia and profuse sweating occur in response to prolonged muscular spasm.
- All signs are exacerbated by stimulation and excitement.
- Recumbency, with difficulty or inability to rise, occurs as the disease progresses. This can be accompanied by severe extensor rigidity,
- Horses may exhibit difficulty urinating and defecating,
- Respiratory failure occurs in fulminant cases.

CAUSES

Infection of a necrotic wound with *C. tetani*.

RISK FACTORS

Unvaccinated horses that have sustained a contaminated soft tissue wound or penetrating wound to the foot are most at risk.

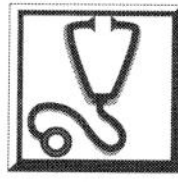

DIAGNOSIS

DIFFERENTIAL DIAGNOSIS

- Laminitis
- Hypocalcemia
- Rhabdomyolysis
- Rabies
- Myotonia

CBC/BIOCHEMISTRY/URINALYSIS

- Nonspecific
- Hemoconcentration and a stress leukogram may present.
- May see hyperfibrinogenemia and leukocytosis with secondary aspiration pneumonia

OTHER LABORATORY TESTS

Anaerobic culture of *C. tetani* may be attempted from a wound.

IMAGIING

- No specific diagnostic indications
- Thoracic radiography or ultrasonography if aspiration pneumonia is suspected
- Ultrasonography of wound sites may help confirm anaerobic infection.

DIAGNOSTIC PPROCEDURES

No specific diagnostic procedures—Diagnosis is made based on clinical signs coupled with the history of a recent wound.

PATHOLOGIC FINDINGS

- Nonspecific
- May demonstrate a *C. tetani*–infected wound
- Secondary traumatic injury or aspiration pneumonia may be present.

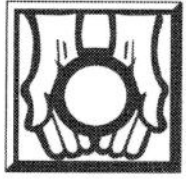

TREATMENT

APPROPRIATE HEALTH CARE

- Initial treatment is aimed at neutralizing unbound toxin and preventing further release by eliminating the infection.
- Appropriate nursing care, particularly if the horse is recumbent, is vital to maximize the chances of a successful outcome.
- Intravenous fluids may be necessary to maintain hydration.

NURSING CARE

- Confine to a quiet, dark stall with deep bedding.
- Minimize auditory stimulation with ear plugs.
- Padded walls and/or a padded helmet to minimize injury
- Frequent turning of recumbent horses (every 2–4 hours)
- Recumbent horses that are unable to rise may benefit from slinging.
- Manual rectal evacuation and/or urinary catheterization may be necessary.

ACTIVITY

Restrict activity as much as possible through confinement and sedation.

DIET

- High-quality feed and free choice water should be made easily accessible.
- If the horse is dysphagic, a nasogastric tube can be placed for the administration of feed, water and electrolytes. The tube can be left in place to avoid the stress of repeated passage.
- Parenteral nutrition may be required if caloric needs cannot be met by nasogastric administration.

CLIENT EDUCATION

Appropriate tetanus prophylaxis should be discussed.

SURGICAL CONSIDERATIONS

Debride the wound and maximize exposure to air.

MEDICATIONS

DRUG(S) OF CHOICE

- Tetanus antitoxin—100–200 U/kg IV or IM (single dose) will bind circulating toxin.
- Acepromazine—0.05–0.08 mg/kg IV or IM q3–6h or as required
- Phenobarbital 6–12 mg/kg slow IV followed by 6–12 mg/kg PO q12h alone or in combination with acepromazine
- Penicillin G (potassium or sodium)—22,000–44,000 IU/kg IV q6h for 7–10 days
- Consider intrathecal administration of 50 mL TAT (20–30 mL in foals) after removal of an equal amount of CSF from the atlanto-occipital space (requires general anesthesia). This is thought to be most beneficial early in the disease process.
- Local infiltration of the wound with procaine penicillin and/or tetanus antitoxin (3,000–9,000 IU). This may help eliminate the infection and neutralize toxin present at the site.
- Vaccination with tetanus toxoid—Clinical disease does not result in a sufficient immune response. Use separate injection site for antitoxin.

CONTRAINDICATIONS

N/A

PRECAUTIONS

- TAT has been associated with the development of Theiler's disease (serum hepatitis).
- General anesthesia and intrathecal TAT administration can result in significant complications (meningitis, seizures). A significant improvement in outcome has not been definitively demonstrated with this procedure.

POSSIBLE INTERACTIONS

TAT will bind tetanus toxoid. These agents should be administered at different sites.

ALTERNATE DRUGS

- Haloperidol 0.01 mg/kg IM every 7 days for long-acting sedation
- Diazepam 0.01–0.4 mg/kg IV q2–4h

FOLLOW-UP

PATIENT MONITORING

Regular physical examination

PREVENTATION/AVOIDANCE

- Initial vaccination with 2 doses of tetanus toxoid 3–4 weeks apart
- Annual toxoid booster thereafter
- Tetanus toxoid should be administered in the case of a wound if there has not been vaccination within the past 6 months.
- Pregnant mares should be given a toxoid booster 4–6 weeks prior to expected parturition.

POSSIBLE COMPLICATIONS

- Myopathy
- Aspiration pneumonia
- Trauma (fractures, decubital ulcers) .

EXPECTED COURSE AND PROGNOSIS

- Horses that are recumbent and unable to rise have a grave prognosis, particularly if progression has been rapid.
- Horses that retain the ability to stand and ambulate have a fair prognosis.
- The clinical signs may persist for weeks; however, survivors will generally stabilize after 7 days and begin to show improvement after 2 weeks.
- Recovery may take as long as 6 weeks but is usually complete.
- The attitude of the individual horse and the ability to provide ideal nursing care are important factors affecting outcome.
- The overall mortality rate in horses is reported to be 50%–80%.

MISCELLANEOUS

ASSOCIATED CONDITIONS, AGE-RELATED FACTORS, ZOONOTIC POTENTIAL, PREGNANCY

N/A

SYNONYMS

Lockjaw

ABBREVIATIONS

- CSF = cerebrospinal fluid
- GABA = γ-aminobutyric acid
- TAT = tetanus antitoxin

Suggested Reading

George LW, Smith MO. Tetanus. In: Smith BP, ed. Large Animal Internal Medicine, ed 3. St. Louis, Mosby, 2002, pp. 995–998.

Green SL, et al. Tetanus in the horse: A review of 20 cases (1970–1990). J Vet Intern Med 1994;8:128–132.

Steinman A, et al. Intrathecal administration of tetanus antitoxin in three cases of tetanus in horses. Equine Vet Educ 2000;12: 237–240.

Author Andrew W. van Eps

Consulting Editors Ashley G. Boyle and Corinne R. Sweeney

TETRALOGY OF FALLOT

BASICS

DEFINITION

A complex of congenital defects that includes a ventricular septal defect, overriding aorta, right ventricular outflow tract obstruction, and right ventricular hypertrophy

PATHOPHYSIOLOGY

- Blood shunts from right to left in affected horses.
- The overriding aorta, right ventricular outflow tract obstruction, and ventricular septal defect result in blood from the right ventricle shunting out the aorta during systole, creating the right-to-left shunt.
- Some shunting of blood between the right and left ventricle also occurs during systole and diastole.
- A pressure overload of the right ventricle occurs secondary to the right ventricular outflow tract obstruction, resulting in right ventricular hypertrophy.
- The size of the ventricular septal defect and severity of the right ventricular outflow tract obstruction are the primary determinants for the severity of clinical signs.
- Horses with severe right ventricular outflow tract obstruction have marked resting arterial hypoxemia caused by the large right-to-left shunt.

SYSTEM AFFECTED

Cardiovascular

GENETICS

Not yet determined in horses

INCIDENCE/PREVALENCE

- Low prevalence in the equine population
- Reported in <5% of congenital cardiac disease in horses

SIGNALMENT

- Murmurs are detectable at birth.
- Diagnosed most frequently in neonates, foals, and young horses

SIGNS

General Comments

Tetralogy of Fallot is usually detected in very young foals during routine auscultation postpartum or because the foal is unthrifty.

HISTORICAL

- Unthrifty youngster that has grown poorly
- Exercise intolerance
- Congestive heart failure

Physical Examination

- Grade 3–6/6 coarse, band- or crescendo-decrescendo–shaped, pansystolic murmur with its point of maximal intensity in the pulmonic valve area (left third intercostal space)
- Grade 3–6/6 coarse, band-shaped, pansystolic murmur with its point of maximal intensity in the tricuspid valve area (right fourth intercostal space); this murmur usually is 1 grade softer than that found in the pulmonic valve area.
- Tachycardia
- Cyanotic mucous membranes—occurs in some but not all affected foals at rest; more likely after exercise

CAUSES

Congenital malformation of the interventricular septum, aorta and right ventricular outflow tract, pulmonic valve, or pulmonary artery

RISK FACTORS

N/A

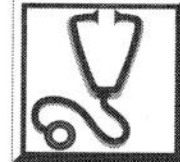

DIAGNOSIS

DIFFERENTIAL DIAGNOSIS

- Ventricular septal defect with pulmonic stenosis or bicuspid pulmonic valve—Murmurs are similar; differentiate echocardiographically.
- Ventricular septal defect with overriding aorta—Loudest murmur is usually located on the right hemithorax; differentiate echocardiographically.
- Outflow tract ventricular septal defect—no cyanosis; differentiate echocardiographically.
- Pulmonic stenosis—rare; differentiate echocardiographically.
- Tricuspid regurgitation—Murmur has point of maximal intensity over the tricuspid valve area; foal not stunted; no cyanosis present; differentiate echocardiographically.
- Mitral regurgitation—Murmur has point of maximal intensity over the mitral valve area; foal not stunted; no cyanosis present; differentiate echocardiographically.

CBC/BIOCHEMISTRY/URINALYSIS

Polycythemia may be present but rarely is reported.

OTHER LABORATORY TESTS

Arterial blood gas analysis, at rest and during exercise, will reveal peripheral arterial hypoxemia.

IMAGING

Electrocardiography

A right-axis shift may be detected associated with right ventricular hypertrophy.

Echocardiography

- Ventricular septal defect usually is in the membranous and perimembranous portion of the interventricular septum, immediately beneath the septal leaflet of the tricuspid valve and right or noncoronary leaflet of the aortic valve.
- The aorta overrides the interventricular septum and may appear dextraposed.
- The pulmonary artery and pulmonic valves usually are hypoplastic, but valvular pulmonic stenosis also occurs.
- Poststenotic dilatation of the pulmonary artery may be present.
- The right ventricle is enlarged, and the right ventricular free wall and moderator band are thickened.
- Contrast echocardiography reveals shunting of blood from the right ventricle to the aorta; some blood flow from the right to the left ventricle also may be detected.
- Continuous-wave Doppler echocardiography confirms the right ventricular outflow tract obstruction by the presence of a high-velocity turbulent jet in the pulmonary artery and right outflow tract.
- Pulsed-wave or color-flow Doppler echocardiography demonstrates shunting of blood from the right ventricle out the aorta. The pressures between the two ventricles are similar; thus, there may be relatively little shunting through the ventricular septal defect.

Thoracic Radiography

- Decreased pulmonary vascularity may be detected.
- Cardiac enlargement may be confirmed by observation of elevation of the trachea and increase in the size of the cardiac silhouette.

DIAGNOSTIC PROCEDURES

- Right-sided cardiac catheterization can be performed to directly measure right atrial, right ventricular, and pulmonary arterial and aortic pressures and to sample blood for oxygen content.
- Elevated right ventricular pressure and decreased oxygen saturation of blood obtained from the left ventricle, aorta, and peripheral arteries in affected horses
- The catheter also may be guided through the ventricular septal defect to sample blood from the left ventricle and to measure left ventricular pressure.

PATHOLOGIC FINDINGS

- Ventricular septal defect overriding aorta and cause of the right ventricular outflow tract obstruction are detected.
- In most horses, the pulmonary artery and pulmonic valve are hypoplastic.
- Poststenotic dilatation may be detected in the main pulmonary artery.
- Jet lesions may be detected along the ventricular septal defect margins and around the outflow tract obstruction.
- The right ventricular free wall and moderator band are thicker than normal and hypertrophied.
- Congestive heart failure—Ventral and peripheral edema, pleural effusion, pericardial effusion, and chronic hepatic congestion may be detected.

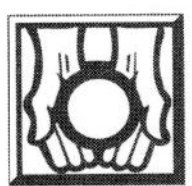

TREATMENT

AIMS OF TREATMENT

Palliative therapy for congestive heart failure aimed at reducing congestion and improving cardiac output may be appropriate in the short term, but euthanasia on humane grounds is inevitable.

APPROPRIATE HEALTH CARE

- Affected horses usually develop congestive heart failure by 2 years of age.
- Ultimately, the prognosis is hopeless and affected horses should be humanely destroyed once clinical signs of severe congestive heart failure develop or at diagnosis.

NURSING CARE

N/A

ACTIVITY

Affected horses are not safe to use for athletic performance and should not be broken to ride or drive.

DIET

N/A

CLIENT EDUCATION

- Do not use affected horses for any type of athletic work.
- Do not breed affected horses.
- If humane destruction is not chosen at diagnosis, closely monitor the horse for exercise intolerance, respiratory distress, tachycardia, venous distention, jugular pulsations, ventral edema or deteriorating body condition that, if detected, should prompt euthanasia.

SURGICAL CONSIDERATIONS

Surgical repair of the defect is not practical and does not result in an equine athlete.

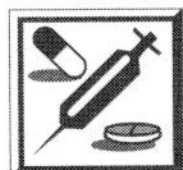

MEDICATIONS

DRUG(S) OF CHOICE

N/A

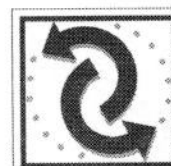

FOLLOW-UP

PATIENT MONITORING

Monitor clinical findings including heart rate, venous distension, jugular pulsations. body condition, peripheral edema, and exercise tolerance to assess the quality of life and onset of congestive heart failure in affected foals.

PREVENTION/AVOIDANCE

N/A

POSSIBLE COMPLICATIONS

N/A.

EXPECTED COURSE AND PROGNOSIS

- All affected horses have a grave prognosis for life.
- Foals with large ventricular septal defects (>4 cm) and severe right ventricular outflow tract obstruction are likely to develop congestive heart failure during the first year of life; foals with less severe right ventricular outflow tract obstruction may survive slightly longer.
- The oldest reported horse with the tetralogy of Fallot was 3 years old.

MISCELLANEOUS

ASSOCIATED CONDITIONS

- Tricuspid regurgitation can develop in horses with significant right ventricular volume and pressure overload secondary to stretching of the tricuspid annulus.
- Aortic regurgitation can develop in horses with large aortic roots and aortic valve prolapse. The aortic valve leaflet lacks the support from the interventricular septum and prolapses into the defect, resulting in aortic regurgitation.
- Patent ductus arteriosus also may be present in some horses, which is a condition known as pentalogy of Fallot.
- Foals with congenital cardiac disease consisting of ventricular septal defect with bicuspid pulmonic valve leading to obstruction of the right ventricular outflow tract and right ventricular hypertrophy without overriding aorta or ventricular septal defect with overriding aorta but no obstruction to the right ventricular outflow tract have also been reported. Affected foals present similarly, although usually with milder signs. These variations can be distinguished echocardiographically.

AGE-RELATED FACTORS

Young horses are more likely to be diagnosed.

PREGNANCY

Do not breed affected horses.

SEE ALSO

Ventricular septal defect

Suggested Reading

Cargile J, Lombard C, Wilson JH, Buergelt CD. Tetralogy of Fallot and segmental uterine aplasia in a three-year-old Morgan filly. Cornell Vet 1991;81:411–418.

Marr CM. Cardiac murmurs: congenital heart disease. In: Marr CM, ed. Cardiology of the Horse. Philadelphia: WB Saunders, 1999:210–232.

Reef VB. Cardiovascular ultrasonography. In: Reef VB, ed. Equine Diagnostic Ultrasound. Philadelphia: WB Saunders, 1998:215–272.

Reef VB. Echocardiographic findings in horses with congenital cardiac disease. Compend Contin Educ Pract Vet 1991;13:109–117.

Author Virginia B. Reef

Consulting Editor Celia M. Marr

THORACIC TRAUMA

BASICS

DEFINITION

• May be penetrating or blunt • Penetrating trauma usually results from collision with an object • Blunt trauma occurs in neonatal foals at parturition

PATHOPHYSIOLOGY

• Fracture of bones of the thoracic cage, lung injury, air in the pleural space and mediastinum, diaphragmatic injury and heart or large vessel injury may occur. Concurrent trauma to the abdomen is also possible. • Axillary laceration—Often result of a horse running into a fence or barbed wire. Can be accompanied by severe subcutaneous emphysema, pneumomediastinum, or PTX. • Pulmonary contusion—Occurs when the chest wall is compressed against the lung parenchyma, or by rib fractures. May cause hemorrhage into the alveolar spaces and induce respiratory distress and pneumonia. • Pulmonary laceration—A traumatic disruption of the lung that causes PTX or HTX. Caused by a sudden compression of the thoracic wall or direct puncture of the lung by a fractured rib. Complications such as pulmonary abscess or bronchopleural fistula may arise.
• PTX causes varying degrees of lung collapse, mechanical inability to inflate the lung, and inadequate ventilation. • Fractured ribs cause pain and may lead to hypoventilation. When combined with pulmonary contusions, they can lead to pneumonia. • Large vessel or cardiac laceration can cause HTX, hemopericardium, and cardiac tamponade. • HTX displaces the pulmonary lobes and may reduce ventilatory capacity. A penetrating injury combined with HTX carries a risk of septic pleuritis.
• Transdiaphragmatic perforation can cause viscus rupture and septic peritonitis.

SYSTEMS AFFECTED

• Respiratory—PTX, rib fracture, and pulmonary contusions or lacerations
• Cardiovascular—cardiac tamponade or laceration, great vessel, and intercostal artery or pulmonary parenchymal vessel injury
• Gastrointestinal—foreign body penetration of the abdominal cavity, causing intestinal or abdominal organ injury

INCIDENCE/PREVALENCE

• Penetrating trauma is rare. • Blunt trauma occurs in 20% of newborn foals (primiparous and dystocic) at birth. However, related clinical signs are rare. • In foals referred to neonatal intensive care units, fractured ribs were identified in 65% of foals; mortality attributable to rib fractures may be as high as 25%.

GEOGRAPHIC DISTRIBUTION

None

SIGNALMENT

• Neonatal foals are predisposed to rib fracture and costochondral fracture/dislocation. • No sex or breed predilections

SIGNS

Historical

• History of penetrating or blunt trauma
• Tachypnea or increased respiratory effort
• Colic • History of dystocia or birth from a primiparous mare. Affected foals may be lethargic, grunt, or lie in a sternal position.

Physical Examination

• Cyanotic or pale mucous membranes
• Absence of lung sounds dorsally on thoracic auscultation and increased resonance on percussion—indicative of PTX • Reduced lung sounds ventrally and decreased resonance on percussion— suggestive of HTX • Inspection and palpation of the thoracic cage and axillary area may permit detection of penetrating wound, edema, fractured ribs or thoracic wall instability. • Subcutaneous emphysema is usually palpated with penetrating thoracic wounds.
• Thoracic cage asymmetry, caused by fractured rib displacement or costochondral dislocation.

CAUSES

• Collision with an object, particularly fences, is the most common cause of penetrating thoracic wounds. • Birth trauma in foals most likely results from compression of the thorax during passage through the dam's pelvic canal. Fractured ribs may lacerate the lungs, causing PTX; the heart, causing sudden death or HTX; or the diaphragm, causing diaphragmatic hernia.

RISK FACTORS

• Horses at pasture • Newborn foals from primiparous mares • Dystocia

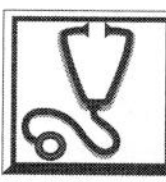

DIAGNOSIS

As these horses may suffer from polytrauma, an approach consisting of a first look, shock and emergency treatment, recheck, and then diagnosis is suitable.

DIFFERENTIAL DIAGNOSIS

• Pain can cause rapid shallow breathing.
• Diaphragmatic hernia • Pneumonia
• HTX—pleural septic effusion or hydrothorax

CBC/BIOCHEMISTRY/URINALYSIS

• CBC—stress leukogram may be observed. Leukocytosis and hyperfibrinogenemia are common if secondary bacterial infection is present; anemia caused by blood loss. • Serum chemistry—hypoproteinemia indicating early blood loss.

OTHER LABORATORY TESTS

Arterial blood gas analysis anomalies depending on the magnitude of pulmonary contusion, PTX and HTX and the ability of the animal to compensate.

IMAGING

Thoracic Ultrasonography

• A thorough thoracic examination is recommended in an emergency situation and unstable patients. This permits immediate identification of specific problems. • Air resulting from PTX accumulates dorsally in the standing horse or laterally in a recumbent foal. Blood (hemothorax) accumulates ventrally in the standing horse. • A 3.5- to 5-MHz probe is mandatory. • Absence of the "sliding lung sign" is strong evidence for the presence of PTX (see PTX). • HTX may be identified by the presence of fluid located ventrally in the pleural space.
• The presence of fluid located in the pericardial space may result from hemopericardium, septic pericarditis or hydropericardium. Cardiac tamponade is a form of obstructive shock that is associated with a large pericardial accumulation of fluid that interferes with the mechanical function of the heart. • Ribs (5- to 7.5-MHz probe) and diaphragm evaluation may reveal the presence of fractured ribs or diaphragmatic hernia. • Foreign bodies or lung contusion (alveolar consolidation emanating from the visceral pleura) may also be identified.
• Abdominal fluid may indicate hemoperitoneum caused by diaphragmatic perforation and abdominal organ damage or peritonitis caused by viscus trauma.

Thoracic Radiography

• Performed when the horse is stabilized. However, radiographs are less sensitive than ultrasonography for the detection of rib fractures. • Retraction of lung margins from the thoracic wall, with varying degrees of lung collapse is characteristic of PTX; radiopaque foreign objects, fluid in the thorax, fractured ribs, or diaphragmatic hernia also may be seen.

OTHER DIAGNOSTIC PROCEDURES

• Thoracocentesis confirms a diagnosis of tension PTX or HTX and should be performed as a therapeutic measure in dyspneic animals.
• Thoracoscopy to evaluate pulmonary pathology and to detect nonradiopaque foreign bodies. • Abdominal paracentesis when abdominal cavity perforation is suspected.

PATHOLOGIC FINDINGS

• Hemothorax • Rib fracture and flail chest
• Pulmonary contusion or laceration • Large vessel injury, hemopericardium and cardiac laceration • Diaphragmatic laceration
• Intestinal or abdominal organ injury • Septic pleuritis or peritonitis • Extrathoracic trauma

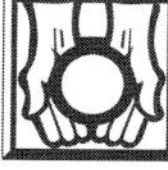

TREATMENT

AIMS OF TREATMENT

• Support and restore respiratory function
• Treat shock if necessary • Close wound whenever possible • Administer broad spectrum antibiotics, anti-inflammatory and analgesic drugs.

APPROPRIATE HEALTH CARE

• Emergency care and continuous monitoring for severe cases • Inpatient care until stabilized

NURSING CARE

• Administer oxygen by nasopharyngeal insufflation to dyspneic and hypoxemic patients (10–15 L/min for adults;

5–10 L/min for foals). • Control of external hemorrhage and shock treatment with IV fluids (hypertonic/isotonic) during in the acute period. Blood or plasma transfusions should be considered if hemorrhage has caused severe blood loss. Remember that contused lungs in cases of trauma are extremely sensitive to crystalloid fluid overload. • Temporarily close penetrating wounds with sterile antibiotic ointment and gauze; minimal debridement and closure once the patient is stabilized.
• Decision to decompress the pleural cavity (air or blood) should be based on:
  ○ Apparition or exacerbation of clinical signs at rest when the wound is sealed.
  ○ Presence of a tension PTX or an increase in PTX size.
  ○ Presence of a large accumulation of blood in the pleural space (improves respiratory function and prevents development of a fibrinous layer around the lung, which could impede pulmonary expansion).
  ○ Presence of HTX combined with the presence of a penetrating thoracic wound.
• The site for air evacuation is the dorsal thoracic cavity just in front of the 12th to 15th ribs. The site for fluid evacuation is the ventral thoracic cavity and is best evaluated by ultrasonography (usually, the 5th–8th intercostal spaces). Avoid intercostal vessels which run along the caudal border of the ribs. • Perform thoracocentesis using a 14-gauge over-the-needle catheter, a teat cannula, or a large-gauge needle attached to a three-way stop cock, extension set, and 60-mL syringe. • For severe or active PTX or HTX, place a thoracostomy tube in the pleural cavity, and attach to a "home made tip-truncated unlubricated condom," a Heimlich valve, or continuous-suction apparatus in cases of rapid reaccumulation. Evacuation pressures $\leq$20 cm H_2O should be used, and the air or fluid should be removed from the thorax slowly. • Drain pericardial effusions when cardiac tamponade is detected. Ideally, a 14-gauge over-the-needle catheter is inserted through the pericardium under ultrasonographic guidance. ECG monitoring is recommended both during and after the procedure. • Fractured ribs are usually not stabilized, but rough edges may be rongeured and fragments removed in cases of open fracture. Indications for internal fixation are:
  ○ Foals with existing extensive internal thoracic trauma or potential for such a trauma (fractured rib(s) with large displacement, sharp edges close from the heart or diaphragm).
  ○ Presence of flail chest (three or more consecutive ribs that are each fractured in at least two sites, resulting in a free-floating segment of the chest wall and paradoxical associated respiration) with severe respiratory dysfunction not responding to intensive medical support.

ACTIVITY

• Box stall rest until all associated problems resolve. • When clinical signs caused by PTX are minimal at rest, the PTX should gradually resorb if the animal is confined. • Confine foals with fractured ribs for 2–3 weeks, and if possible, avoid manipulation of these foals to prevent exacerbating injuries by the fractured ribs.

CLIENT EDUCATION

• Discuss clinical signs of PTX, and advise immediate return with recurrence. • Rib and sternal fistula are potential complications of open thoracic wounds (bone sequestrum, osteomyelitis, foreign body). Reevaluation is recommended if wound drainage occurs.

SURGICAL CONSIDERATIONS

• Stabilization of the patient, decompression of PTX and positive-pressure ventilation are mandatory for surgery. • Suture wounds whenever possible to rapidly achieve an air-tight seal. Conservative debridement is advised to permit primary closure. If impossible, apply an occlusive bandage. • Consider thoracoscopy for severe or recurrent PTX or when a foreign body is suspected. • Certain types of rib fractures may be successfully reduced and stabilized in foals using reconstruction plates, self-tapping screws and cerclage wire, or nylon strand suture.
• Wound and/or thoracic exploration is indicated for uncontrolled hemorrhage.

MEDICATIONS

DRUG(S) OF CHOICE

• Broad-spectrum antibiotics for patients with wounds. Combination of penicillin sodium (22,000 UI/kg IV QID), gentamicin (6.6 mg/kg IV SID), and metronidazole (25 mg/kg PO QID) is particularly appropriate for cases with penetrating wounds and associated HTX. • NSAIDs for first line pain management to avoid splinting and hypoventilation because of pain from fractured ribs. If pain is not controlled, long lasting intercostal blocks (bupivacaine) or opioid analgesics may be indicated.

PRECAUTIONS

Drugs such as xylazine or opioids should be used sparingly, because they may reduce PaO_2.

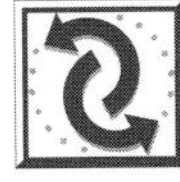

FOLLOW-UP

PATIENT MONITORING

• Respiratory rate and effort, mucous membrane color, heart rate and pulse quality, auscultation, and measurement of PCV and total solids during the first 24–48 hours. • Serial blood gas analyses reveal effectiveness of ventilation. Check for signs of hypoventilation—increased $PaCO_2$, decreased PaO_2. • Thoracic ultrasonography and radiography can be repeated every 24–48 hours until the condition is stable.

POSSIBLE COMPLICATIONS

• Recurrence of PTX or hemothorax
• Pyothorax • Bacterial pneumonia in young foals • Septic peritonitis and shock when intestinal viscus penetration has occurred • Rib and sternal fistulas • Diaphragmatic hernia

EXPECTED COURSE AND PROGNOSIS

• Tension PTX and cardiac tamponade are serious life-threatening conditions if left untreated. • Cardiac or great vessel laceration carries a poor prognosis. • Full recovery is expected if the injury is not severe and does not involve the great vessels, heart or abdominal cavity.

MISCELLANEOUS

ASSOCIATED CONDITIONS

• Fractured ribs • Diaphragmatic hernia
• Ruptured trachea • Thoracic and abdominal organ lacerations • Other complications of trauma

SEE ALSO

• Diaphragmatic hernia • Expiratory dyspnea
• Inspiratory dyspnea • Pleuropneumonia
• Pneumothorax

ABBREVIATIONS

• HTX = hemothorax • PTX = pneumothorax

Suggested Reading

Bellezzo F, Hunt RJ, Provost R, et al. Surgical repair of rib fractures in 14 neonatal foals: case selection, surgical technique and results. Equine Vet J 2004;36:557–562.

Hassel DM. Thoracic trauma in horses. Vet Clin Equine 2007;23:67–80.

Jean D, Picandet V, Macieira S, et al. Detection of rib trauma in newborn foals in an equine critical care unit: A comparison of ultrasonography, radiography and physical examination. Equine Vet J 2007;39: 158–163.

Schambourg MA, Laverty S, Mullim S, et al. Thoracic trauma in foals: post mortem findings. Equine Vet J 2003;35:78–81.

Authors Florent David and Sheila Laverty
Consulting Editor Daniel Jean

THROMBOCYTOPENIA

BASICS

DEFINITION

A platelet (thrombocyte) count in the peripheral circulation less than the lower limit of the reference range; usually <100,000/μL (<100 × 10^9/L)

PATHOPHYSIOLOGY

• Platelets are anucleate fragments derived from megakaryocytes in the bone marrow and are the smallest cellular particles in blood. • Play a pivotal role in primary hemostasis through interactions with the endothelium and other platelets, and also contribute to secondary hemostasis • Have a short life span in circulation (≈3–5 days), and in health, numbers are balanced between removal from the circulation and replacement by the bone marrow
• Thrombopoeisis is stimulated by interleukin 3 (IL-3), IL-6, GM-CSF, and thrombopoeitin.
• From 30% to 50% of mature platelets can be stored in the spleen. • Thrombocytopenia can arise from decreased production, increased consumption, increased destruction, or increased sequestration. • In addition, platelet dysfunction can occur, leading to impaired primary hemostasis.

Decreased Platelet Production

• Usually results from myelophthisis or aplastic anemia (intrinsic stem cell failure or disruption of their interactions with other cells in the microenvironment). Circulating granulocyte, monocyte, and erythrocyte counts are usually reduced concurrently. Lymphocyte counts may be normal due to continued production in extramedullary sites.

Increased Platelet Destruction

• Usually results from immune-mediated mechanisms—primary autoimmune IMTP, neonatal alloimmune thrombocytopenia, or secondary IMTP (secondary to various antigens derived from neoplasms, drugs, or infections)
• Primary IMTP is associated with production of autoantibodies directed against normal platelet surface antigens or against novel platelet antigens that develop in response to a primary disease process. • Neonatal alloimmune thrombocytopenia develops when a foal inherits a platelet alloantigen from the sire that is not present on the dam's platelets; the dam produces alloantibodies against this antigen, and they are secreted into colostrum that the foal ingests after birth. • Secondary IMTP occurs when either circulating immune complexes attach to platelets nonspecifically, antibodies are directed against antigens that attach to the platelets, or via molecular mimicry. • Irrespective of the source of antibody, platelets coated with antibody are removed from circulation by cells of the reticuloendothelial system. • Non–immune-mediated destruction may occur in response to infections and after exposure to various toxins and drugs.

Increased Platelet Consumption

• Usually occurs in DIC • Can also occur with localized activation of coagulation, trauma, and severe hemorrhage • DIC is the most common cause of thrombocytopenia in the horse.

Platelet Sequestration

Can occur in splenomegaly and in vascular neoplasms

Other

Pseudothrombocytopenia can occur with collection of blood into EDTA or, less commonly, heparin.

SYSTEMS AFFECTED

• Hemic/lymphatic/immune • Hemorrhage can occur when the platelet count in <30,000/μL (<30.0 × 10^9/L) where lesions in the skin, renal/urologic, gastrointestinal, and respiratory systems are most common.

GENETICS

• There is a genetic basis to neonatal alloimmune thrombocytopenia due to inheritance of platelet alloantigens by the foal from the sire that are not present on the dam's platelets. • A genetic basis of familial megakaryocytic and myeloid hypoplasia in Standardbreds is suspected.

INCIDENCE/PREVALENCE

Unknown, although at one veterinary teaching hospital, 1.49% of horses that had a CBC performed were thrombocytopenic.

SIGNALMENT

Breed Predilections

Standardbred horses may be at increased risk.

Mean Age and Range

• Neonatal alloimmune thrombocytopenia occurs in foals <7 days of age and is more common in mules. • Animals of any age can be affected by thrombocytopenia.

Predominant Sex

N/A

SIGNS

General Comments

• Signs of spontaneous hemorrhage are most commonly observed in animals with platelet counts <10,000/μL (<10.0 × 10^9/L) or after trauma/surgery/venipuncture if platelet count is <30,000/μL (<30.0 × 10^9/L). • Hemorrhagic diatheses are consistent with dysfunction of primary hemostasis. • Signs of underlying disease may be observed.

Historical

• Spontaneous or post-traumatic hemorrhage involving mucous membranes, skin, nasal cavity, GIT, and urogenital tract may be reported.
• Weight loss, lethargy, and inappetence may be reported if an underlying condition is present.

Physical Examination

• Petechiation and ecchymotic hemorrhages of oral, ocular, vaginal, and nasal mucous membranes • Epistaxis • Prolonged hemorrhage from venipuncture or surgical sites • Hyphema
• Hematuria • Melena

CAUSES

Decreased Platelet Production

• Myelophthisis—including myelofibrosis, myelodysplasia, leukoproliferative disorders (myeloproliferative disorders [monocytic, myelomonocytic, eosinophilic, or myelogenous leukemia] or lymphoproliferative disorders [multiple myeloma or lymphoid leukemia])
• Aplastic anemia due to idiopathic pancytopenia, drugs (e.g., phenylbutazone, estrogens, chloramphenicol), infectious or immune-mediated disease • Megakaryocytic and myeloid hypoplasia in related Standardbreds

Increased Platelet Destruction

• Primary IMTP—can be autoimmune or idiopathic • Neonatal alloimmune thrombocytopenia • Secondary IMTP due to neoplasia (e.g., lymphosarcoma), bacterial infection (sepsis), viral infection (e.g., EIA), drugs (e.g., heparin), or concurrent immune-mediated hemolysis • Snake envenomation • Toxin- or drug-induced platelet damage

Increased Platelet Consumption

• DIC • Localized intravascular coagulation due to hemangioma/hemangiosarcoma, hemolytic uremic syndrome, thrombosis • Excessive hemorrhage • Severe trauma • Vasculitis

Platelet Sequestration

• Splenomegaly • Vascular neoplasms

Pseudothrombocytopenia

Collection of blood into EDTA

Miscellaneous with Complex Mechanisms

• EIA • EGE (*Anaplasma phagocytophilum*)
• Equine monocytic ehrlichiosis (*Neorickettsia risticii*) • Viral—including EHV, EVA, VEE, EVA, African horse sickness • Bacterial infections—neonatal septicemia
• Neoplasia—lymphosarcoma • Endotoxemia
• Fell Pony syndrome

RISK FACTORS

• Any drug may potentially precipitate IMTP. Most common with heparin and myelosuppressive drugs • Certain viral and bacterial infections (see Causes) • Neoplasia (see Causes) • Immune-mediated diseases

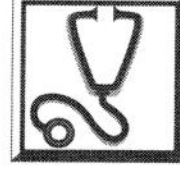

DIAGNOSIS

DIFFERENTIAL DIAGNOSIS

• Other causes of petechial/ecchymotic hemorrhages or spontaneous hemorrhage must be differentiated. • Heparin therapy due to disruption of secondary hemostasis and platelet dysfunction. History of heparin administration.
• Vitamin K antagonism (e.g., warfarin toxicity). Evaluate hemostasis. • Hepatopathy due to impaired production of clotting factors. Elevated liver enzymes or products • Hemophilia A (factor VIII deficiency). Only occurs in males.
• von Willebrand's disease. Evaluate for quantitative or qualitative defects in vWF.
• Platelet dysfunction (e.g., Glanzmann's thrombasthenia). Evaluate hemostasis.
• Vasculitis—histopathological evaluation of biopsies

CBC/BIOCHEMISTRY/URINALYSIS

• Platelet count <100,000/μL (<100 × 10^9/L)
• Equine platelets are smaller than human platelets and laboratory equipment must be calibrated accordingly. • Neutropenia and left shift may indicate endotoxemia/DIC.

THROMBOCYTOPENIA

Derangements of hemostasis and fibrinolysis parameters also may be present and include prolonged PT and aPTT, decreased ATIII, and increased FDPs. • Concurrent anemia may occur with chronic disease, EIA, immune-mediated hemolysis, and hemorrhage. • Concurrent anemia and leukopenia reflects decreased production. • Hyperfibrinogenemia suggests chronic inflammation. • Inclusions may be observed in neutrophils in EGE. • Poor venipuncture or collection of blood into EDTA may result in platelet clumping and pseudothrombocytopenia—Examine feathered edge of blood smear for evidence of clumping. Repeat platelet count on blood sample collected into lithium heparin. • Various biochemical derangements may be present with underlying conditions.

OTHER LABORATORY TESTS

• Coggins test for EIA • Serology for *Anaplasma phagocytophilum, Neorickettsia risticii,* and various viral agents • aPTT, PT for assessment of secondary hemostasis • ATIII • FDPs for assessment of fibrinolysis • Quantification of specific clotting factors (e.g., VIII) • Clot retraction time and in vitro testing of platelet aggregation • Blood culture for septicemia • Immunophenotypic techniques for classification of leukemia • Flow cytometry for detection of platelet-bound antibody • Platelet factor 3 test as indirect test for IMTP

IMAGING

• Abdominal and thoracic ultrasonography for detection of space-occupying lesions and effusions • Thoracic radiography for detection of neoplasia, abscess, pneumonia

OTHER DIAGNOSTIC PROCEDURES

• Abdominocentesis • Thoracocentesis • Bone marrow biopsy to determine megakaryocyte numbers and evidence of myelophthisis or bone marrow hypoplasia • Fine needle aspirate/biopsy of internal/external space-occupying lesion

PATHOLOGICAL FINDINGS

• Petechial and ecchymotic hemorrhages in various tissues • Other findings dependent on specific underlying disease

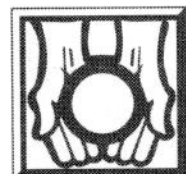

TREATMENT

AIMS OF TREATMENT

• Improvement/increase in platelet count
• Treatment of underlying disease • Prevention of recurrence of thrombocytopenia

APPROPRIATE HEALTH CARE

Severe thrombocytopenia (<30,000/μL [<30.0 × 10^9/L]) necessitates hospitalization for treatment; once condition and platelet count are stabilized, treat on an outpatient basis.

NURSING CARE

• Minimize the number of invasive procedures performed to limit potential for hemorrhage.
• Apply prolonged pressure to venipuncture sites. • Prevent trauma. • Discontinue any medications if IMTP is suspected. • Life-threatening hemorrhage may require transfusions with whole blood or platelet-rich plasma.

ACTIVITY

Restrict to minimize trauma and spontaneous hemorrhage.

CLIENT EDUCATION

Thrombocytopenia indicates the presence of an underlying disease that is the focus of diagnostic assessment and treatment.

SURGICAL CONSIDERATIONS

• Elective surgery should be avoided until platelet counts are normal. • Emergency surgery may require concomitant administration of whole blood or platelet-rich plasma.

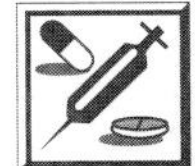

MEDICATIONS

DRUG(S) OF CHOICE

• For IMTP, corticosteroids are recommended. Initially dexamethasone (0.1 mg/kg IV or IM once daily, then reduce dose by 0.01 mg/kg/day when platelet count is >100,000/μL [>100 × 10^9/L]). Longer-term therapy can be provided with oral prednisolone (1–2 mg/kg PO or IM once daily). • EGE and equine monocytic ehrlichiosis—oxytetracycline (7 mg/kg IV once or twice daily for 7 days) • Bacterial infection—antimicrobial therapy based on culture and sensitivity testing. • DIC, heparin, NSAIDs

CONTRAINDICATIONS

• Corticosteroids—preexistent laminitis or infectious disease • NSAIDs (especially aspirin) in most circumstances due to impairment of platelet function

POSSIBLE INTERACTIONS

Avoid concurrent use of corticosteroids and NSAIDs due to possible increased risk of GIT damage.

ALTERNATIVE DRUGS

• For refractory IMTP, use azothiaprine (3 mg/kg PO once daily) or vincristine (0.01–0.025 mg/kg IV weekly). • In other species, danazol and gammaglobulin infusions have been used.

FOLLOW-UP

PATIENT MONITORING

• Monitor for hemorrhagic diathesis. • Daily platelet count until stabilized, thereafter weekly until >100,000/μL (>100 × 10^9/L)
• Appropriate use of laboratory, imaging, and diagnostic procedures if underlying disease is being treated

PREVENTION/AVOIDANCE

Avoid use of any drugs suspected in development of IMTP.

POSSIBLE COMPLICATIONS

Excessive hemorrhage

EXPECTED COURSE AND PROGNOSIS

• Variable, dependent on cause
• Most cases of IMTP secondary to drugs or infection respond with withdrawal of the drug or successful treatment of the underlying infection.
• Many cases of IMTP recover in 3–4 weeks.
• Myeloproliferative disorders have a grave prognosis.
• EIA and neoplasia have a poor to grave prognosis.
• Some cases of IMTP are recurrent and require intermittent corticosteroid therapy.
• Response to therapy is a useful prognostic indicator in the majority of cases.

MISCELLANEOUS

ASSOCIATED CONDITIONS

• Immune-mediated hemolysis
• Bacterial, vira, or fungal infection
• Neoplasia
• Endotoxemia/DIC

AGE-RELATED FACTORS

Platelet counts in young animals (<3 years) are often higher than older animals.

ZOONOTIC POTENTIAL

VEE

SEE ALSO

• Anemia, immune-mediated
• Aplastic anemia
• Coagulation defects, acquired
• Coagulation defects, inherited
• Disseminated intravascular coagulation
• Equine granulocytic erlichiosis
• Hemangiosarcoma
• Lymphosarcoma
• Myeloproliferative diseases
• Pancytopenia
• Petechiae, ecchymoses, and hematomas
• Thrombocytosis

ABBREVIATIONS

• aPTT = activated partial thromboplastin time
• ATIII = antithrombin III
• EGE = equine granulocytic ehrlichiosis
• EHV = equine herpesvirus
• EIA = equine infectious anemia
• EVA = equine viral arteritis
• FDP = fibrin degradation product
• GIT = gastrointestinal tract
• IMTP = immune-mediated thrombocytopenia
• PT = prothrombin time
• VEE = Venezuelan equine encephalomyelitis

Suggested Reading

Davis E, Wilkerson MJ. Thrombocytopenia. In Robinson NE, ed. Current Therapy in Equine Medicine, ed 5. St Louis: Saunders, 2003:349–350.

Perkins GA, Miller WH, Divers TJ, et al. Ulcerative dermatitis, thrombocytopenia and neutropenia in neonatal foals. J Vet Intern Med 2005;19:211–216.

Sellon DC. Disorders of the hematopoietic system. In: Reed et al., eds. Equine Internal Medicine, ed 2. St Louis: Saunders, 2004;721–768.

Author Kristopher Hughes
Consulting Editors Jennifer Hodgson and David Hodgson

THROMBOCYTOSIS

BASICS

OVERVIEW

• A platelet (thrombocyte) count in the peripheral circulation greater than the upper limit of the laboratory reference interval—usually >350,000/μL (>350× 10^9/L) • Most commonly occurs due to increased production of platelets in horses with chronic inflammatory or infectious diseases (secondary reactive thrombocytosis). Cytokines produced during an inflammatory response (e.g., IL-3, IL-6, and GM-CSF) may stimulate megakaryopoiesis and release of increased numbers of platelets into the circulation.
• Increased production of platelets can occur due to a myeloproliferative disorder (primary thrombocytosis). • Physiologic causes are possible, also.

SIGNALMENT

• Stallions have higher platelet counts than geldings or mares. • Young horses have a higher count than older horses (>3 years old).

SIGNS

Signs specific to thrombocytosis are seldom observed.

Historical

May relate to a primary underlying inflammatory, infectious or neoplastic disease process (e.g., inappetence, lethargy)

Physical Examination

• Signs reflective of an underlying disease process may be present. • Hemostatic function is usually normal; however, hemorrhagic diathesis can occur if platelet function is abnormal and thrombosis may occur with platelet counts >1,000,000/μL (>1000 × 10^9/L).

CAUSES AND RISK FACTORS

Primary Thrombocytosis

• Occurs as a primary myeloproliferative disorder (essential thrombocytemia) or associated with polycythemia vera • Yet to be diagnosed definitively in horses

Secondary (Reactive) Thrombocytosis

• Physiologic causes can include exercise and excitement (release of splenic platelet reserves).
• Rebound phenomenon occurs after thrombocytopenia or hemorrhage.
• Immune-mediated hemolysis, including neonatal isoerythrolysis • Iron deficiency anemia (associated thrombocytosis more prevalent in humans) • Corticosteroid therapy • Chronic inflammatory/infectious conditions, e.g., pneumonia, peritonitis, septic arthritis, polyarthritis, bacterial abscess, colitis, IBD, and hepatitis • Neoplasia • Musculoskeletal trauma
• Splenectomy

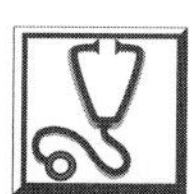

DIAGNOSIS

DIFFERENTIAL DIAGNOSIS

• Underlying cause of thrombocytosis must be determined. • If pyrexia is observed, consider inflammatory, infectious, immune-mediated, or neoplastic disease or trauma. • If inflammation is present, site and cause of inflammatory process should be determined. • If colic or diarrhea observed, consider colitis, IBD. • If anemia present, consider hemorrhage, hemolysis, or bone marrow disease. • If hyperfibrinogenemia reported, consider chronic inflammation. • If leukocytosis present, consider infectious, inflammatory, or neoplastic disorder. • If excitement or post-exercise, consider splenic contraction. • If lameness observed, consider skeletal or soft-tissue trauma, septic, or immune-mediated arthritis. • If pleural or peritoneal effusion observed, consider neoplasia or inflammatory/infectious disorder. • If thoracic or abdominal space-occupying lesion identified, consider abscess or neoplasia.

CBC/BIOCHEMISTRY/URINALYSIS

• Platelet count > upper limit of laboratory reference interval. Counts of 401,000 to >1,000,000/μL (401–1000 × 10^9/L) have been recorded. • Hyperfibrinogenemia, leukocytosis, neutrophilia, and/or a left shift indicate inflammatory or infectious disease.
• Normocytic, normochromic anemia may be present in chronic disease. • Microcytic, hypochromic anemia may be present with iron deficiency. • Macrocytic anemia and hemoglobinemia/hemoglobinuria may be present with hemolytic anemia. • Polycythemia may be present with splenic contraction, hemoconcentration, organ disease, or polycythemia vera. • Mature neutrophilia, eosinopenia, and lymphopenia may be present with exogenous corticosteroid administration.
• Blast or poorly differentiated cells may be observed in leukoproliferative disorder.
• Increased AST and CK activities in serum are associated with skeletal muscle trauma.
• Increased hepatic enzymes, bile acids, and bilirubin are consistent with presence of a hepatopathy.
• Hypoproteinemia/hypoalbuminemia may be associated with protein-losing enteropathy/nephropathy or effusive disorder into body cavities.

OTHER LABORATORY TESTS

• Coombs test • Decreased iron, ferritin, and percentage saturation of transferrin in serum, decreased iron in bone marrow, and increased total iron-binding capacity are typical of iron deficiency. • Immunophenotypic techniques for classification of leukemia

IMAGING

• Abdominal ultrasonography for detection of effusion and space-occupying lesions • Thoracic ultrasonography and radiography for detection of space-occupying lesions and pneumonia
• Musculoskeletal ultrasonography and radiography for detection of trauma or joint disease

OTHER DIAGNOSTIC PROCEDURES

• Abdominocentesis to detect peritonitis or neoplasia • Thoracocentesis to detect pleuritis or neoplasia • Arthrocentesis to detect septic or immune-mediated arthritis • Bone marrow aspirate/biopsy to detect leukoproliferative disorder • Endoscopy of the lower airways
• Tracheal aspirate for detection of pneumonia
• Liver biopsy • Fine needle aspirate/biopsy of internal/external space-occupying lesion • Oral glucose absorption test to detect small intestinal malabsorption • Rectal biopsy to detect IBD or neoplasia • Laparascopy/thoracoscopy
• Mucosal bleeding time and clot retraction test to assess primary hemostasis

PATHOLOGICAL FINDINGS

Dependent on the underlying disorder

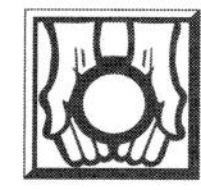

TREATMENT

• Specific treatment to reduce platelet count is seldom indicated. • Any underlying disease process should be treated.

MEDICATIONS

DRUG(S) OF CHOICE

• Treatment of any underlying disease process
• Aspirin therapy if an increased tendency of thrombosis is suspected or platelet counts are increased markedly

CONTRAINDICATIONS/POSSIBLE INTERACTIONS

Avoid use of NSAIDs, especially aspirin, if there is evidence of platelet dysfunction.

FOLLOW-UP

PATIENT MONITORING

• Hematologic monitoring as needed • Monitor response of underlying disease to treatment; resolution of thrombocytosis suggests improvement.

POSSIBLE COMPLICATIONS

• Hemorrhagic diathesis with platelet dysfunction • Thrombosis and possible ischemic tissue damage (e.g., laminitis, organ dysfunction)

EXPECTED COURSE AND PROGNOSIS

Dependent on successful treatment of underlying condition

MISCELLANEOUS

AGE-RELATED FACTORS

Young horses are at increased risk.

SEE ALSO

• Thrombocytopenia • Coagulation defects

ABBREVIATIONS

• GM-CSF = granulocyte-macrophage colony-stimulating factor • IBD = inflammatory bowel disease • IL = interleukin

Suggested Reading

Sellon DC, Levine JF, Plamer K, et al. Thrombocytosis in 24 horses (1989–1994). J Vet Intern Med 1997;11:24–29.

Author Kristopher Hughes
Consulting Editors Jennifer Hodgson and David Hodgson

THYROID TUMORS

BASICS

OVERVIEW

- Thyroid adenomas, adenocarcinoma, and C-cell (parafollicular) tumors have been reported in horses.
- Adenomatous change is quite common in older horses. In a postmortem survey of 100 horses, 34 had normal thyroids, 20 had hyperplastic changes, 9 colloid tumors, and 37 had adenomas.
- Tumors are usually incidental findings not associated with clinical signs.

SIGNALMENT

- Common in older horses—over 10 years of age. There are no reported sex or breed predilections.
- There is no known genetic basis for thyroid tumors.

SIGNS

- Typically, there are no clinical signs associated with thyroid tumors. They are detected on physical examination by palpation of an enlarged thyroid gland.
- Signs are more commonly associated with adenocarcinoma and C-cell tumors. These signs may be associated with either hypothyroidism or hyperthyroidism. The most frequently reported physical sign is weight loss. Other signs associated with thyroid tumors include nervousness, work intolerance, respiratory embarrassment, and cold intolerance. Behavioral disturbances include pacing and difficulty when being handled. Tachypnea and tachycardia may also be present.
- Alterations in blood calcium, both total calcium and ionized calcium levels can occur with C-cell tumors. Although calcium levels outside the normal range may be detected on chemistry panels, clinical signs associated with alterations in blood calcium are not typically observed.

CAUSES AND RISK FACTORS

No known risk factors for development of thyroid tumors

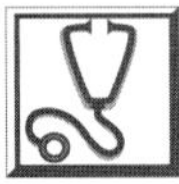

DIAGNOSIS

- Diagnosis is usually made by a combination of physical examination and diagnostic tests.
- Thyroid adenoma should be suspected in any old horse with an enlarged thyroid gland.

DIFFERENTIAL DIAGNOSIS

- Goiter without neoplasia
- Retropharyngeal lymph node enlargement
- Hematoma
- Guttural pouch distention

CBC/BIOCHEMISTRY/URINALYSIS

Generally normal in horses with thyroid tumors

OTHER LABORATORY TESTS

Serum T_4 and T_3 levels may be increased or decreased if the tumor lead to either hypothyroidism or hyperthyroidism. In the one horse described with hyperthyroidism due to an adenocarcinoma, free T_4 concentrations were quite elevated above the normal range. The total T_4 levels were not increased. In horses with hypothyroidism, T_3 and T_4 serum concentrations will be below reference ranges.

IMAGING

A thyroid tumor can be imaged via ultrasound examination as one or more nodules within the thyroid gland. If it is so large that the entire gland is enlarged, this may be seen on radiographs of the cervical region as a soft tissue density.

DIAGNOSTIC PROCEDURES

- A fine needle aspirate will allow one to identify the tumor as being thyroid in origin but will not often allow one to differentiate between an adenoma and adenocarcinoma.
- A biopsy of the thyroid gland mass will provide the definitive diagnosis, though results are often equivocal

PATHOLOGICAL FINDINGS

Most tumors are adenomas. Other tumor types occur infrequently but have been reported.

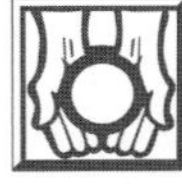

TREATMENT

If a discrete noninvasive thyroid tumor is found, surgical removal of the affected thyroid lobe should be curative. If metastatic disease has occurred, prognosis is poor. Even C-cell tumors and adenocarcinoma spread slowly, however, and surgical removal is generally curative.

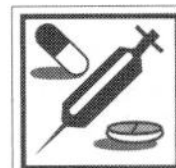

MEDICATIONS

DRUG(S) OF CHOICE

Propylthiouracil has been used to induce hypothyroidism experimentally, but has not been reported as a treatment for clinical cases. Its use could be considered if local invasion or metastasis precludes complete surgical removal. If bilateral tumors occur and the complete gland is removed, then thyroxine supplement (20 μg/kg per day) is indicated. Calcium supplementation is not necessary as horses have parathyroid tissue spread diffusely in the cervical area.

CONTRAINDICATIONS/POSSIBLE INTERACTIONS

N/A

FOLLOW-UP

Anesthetic complications have been reported following the removal of thyroid tumors. For this reason, surgery on hyperthyroid horses should be done in a controlled setting where monitoring equipment and emergency treatments are available. Once the tumor is removed, any clinical signs should gradually resolve.

MISCELLANEOUS

ASSOCIATED CONDITIONS

N/A

AGE-RELATED FACTORS

Horses with thyroid tumors tend to be older, above 10 years of age.

ZOONOTIC POTENTIAL

N/A

PREGNANCY

N/A

SEE ALSO

- Hypothyroidism
- Hyperthyroidism

ABBREVIATIONS

- T_3 = triiodothyronine
- T_4 = thyroxine

Suggested Reading

Held JP, Shaftoe S, Rose ML *et al*. Work intolerance in a horse with thyroid carcinoma. JAVMA 1985;197:1187–1189.

Author Janice Sojka
Consulting Editor Michel Lévy

TOXIC HEPATOPATHY

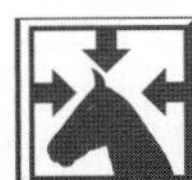

BASICS

OVERVIEW

- Many toxins can cause liver disease (i.e., toxic hepatopathy) in horses.
- Fortunately, most toxins do not cause liver failure and, therefore, likely go unnoticed unless a chemistry panel is performed.
- The pathophysiology of the hepatic disease will vary depending upon the specific toxin. Pyrrolizidine alkaloids are known to inhibit mitosis and to cause fibrosis. Some plant hepatotoxins may cause mostly periportal inflammation/apoptosis and fibrosis while other toxins such as iron may cause zonal hepatic necrosis/apoptosis and fibrosis. Regardless of the initial site and mechanism of disease, prolonged injury and activation of hepatic stellate cells will often result in hepatic fibrosis. Proliferation of hepatocytes, beginning in the periportal region and moving in toward perivenous zones, will occur in many toxic hepatopathies as an attempt to repair the injury. Once severe hepatic fibrosis and/or prolonged attempts of proliferative repair are established microscopic examination of the liver may be of little help in identifying the initial type of injury or specific toxin.

SIGNALMENT

- Any age, breed, or sex
- Acute iron (i.e., ferrous fumarate) poisoning was common when a previously available product was administered PO to foals before colostrum nursing. A hepatopathy will sometimes occur in foals recovering from neonatal isoerythrolysis but etiology is unknown.
- Adult horses in the western United States and eastern Canada often are fed alfalfa hay containing pyrrolizidine alkaloid–containing plants.
- Outbreaks may occur in horses grazing toxic pastures (i.e., alsike clover) or in horses fed toxic hays containing pyrrolizidine alkaloids or saponin.

SIGNS

- Mostly those of hepatoencephalopathy—head pressing, circling, blindness, maniacal behavior or depression, and excessive yawning
- Photosensitization may occur on white-haired parts of the body or mucous membranes. A more generalized dermatitis may occur in association with liver disease. This more generalized disease may be caused by the adverse dermatologic effects of elevated serum bile acids, nutrient deficiencies caused by intestinal malabsorption or from immune-mediated dermatitis. Uveitis may also occur from immune mechanisms.
- Icterus and discolored urine may be noted.
- Colic may occur because of gastric impaction.
- Weight loss has occurred in a few cases of chronic poisoning.

CAUSES AND RISK FACTORS

Numerous, but the most common include the following:

Pyrrolizidine Alkaloid–Containing Plants

- Usually ingested when mixed in "first cutting" alfalfa hay
- *Senecio* sp. (i.e., groundsel and ragwort) and *Amsinckia intermedia* (i.e., fiddleneck) are common in parts of North America.

Panicum Hay

- Fall panicum hay may cause outbreaks of liver disease and failure.
- The toxic principal is thought to be saponin.

Iron Toxicosis

- Generally a result of overzealous oral iron administration
- In newborn foals, even small amounts of iron given orally before colostrum may be fatal.
- In adult horses, very large amounts of iron given orally are necessary to produce toxicity.

Mycotoxins

- May cause hepatic failure in horses
- *Fusarium moniliformis* in horses fed moldy corn
- *Aspergillus flavus* (rarely) in horses fed peanuts or other sources
- Most horses with *Fusarium* sp. poisoning have clinical signs associated with leukoencephalomalacia rather than hepatic failure.

Pasture-Associated Hepatopathy

- May occur in horses grazing on alsike clover (northeastern United States and Canada) or kleingrass (southwestern United States)
- Incidence will vary from year to year, suggesting environmental factors play a role in toxin concentration. This is also true for panicum hay.

Drug-Induced Hepatopathy

This appears to be rare in the horse. Fortunately, horses appear to be very resistant to NSAIDs (currently available ones, at least). Foals being treated with a variety of antibiotics (most commonly for enteritis) and gastric ulcer medications have occasionally had marked increases in liver enzymes in spite of clinical improvement for their primary condition. The enzymes decreased as medication was withdrawn.

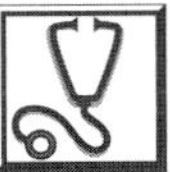

DIAGNOSIS

DIFFERENTIAL DIAGNOSIS

- The differential for hepatoencephalopathy includes primary hyperammonemia seen in adult horses with intestinal disease, Morgan foals, and foals with portosystemic shunts and encephalitis, CNS trauma, and selected metabolic disorders (e.g., severe acidosis).
- These disorders generally involve no increase in hepatic enzymes and, even more rarely, abnormalities in liver function tests (e.g., direct bilirubin, bile acids).
- Morgan foals with hyperammonemia will have mild elevations in some liver enzymes, and foals with portosystemic shunts will have elevated plasma bile acids. Horses with intestinal disease or severe ileus may have mild elevations in conjugated bilirubin without other evidence of liver dysfunction.

CBC/BIOCHEMISTRY/URINALYSIS

- CBC abnormalities most often involve neutrophilia and sometimes erythrocytosis.
- Liver enzymes, both hepatocellular (i.e., AST, SDH) and biliary (i.e., GGT), are markedly elevated in acute toxic hepatopathy. In chronic toxicities (e.g., pyrrolizidine alkaloid poisoning), enzymes may not be markedly elevated, although GGT remains elevated in most cases, even with chronic fibrosis.
- Serum bile acids will be elevated in most cases if there is moderate loss of liver function.
- BUN and fibrinogen generally are abnormally low.
- Albumin, because of its long half-life, may remain normal or slightly low.
- Both conjugated and unconjugated bilirubin levels are increased with liver failure. In most cases, the greatest increase involves unconjugated bilirubin. With severe cholestasis the conjugated bilirubin concentration may be $\geq$25% of the total bilirubin.
- Urine may be discolored (dark brown to orange), and when shaken, the foam may appear green.
- Urine dipstick examination usually is positive for bilirubin.

OTHER LABORATORY TESTS

- Prothrombin and partial thromboplastin times are prolonged.
- Blood ammonia may be high or normal.
- Urinary and/or hepatic concentrations of specific toxins may be found.
- Serum ferritin and measurement of hepatic iron may help to confirm the diagnosis of iron

hepatopathy. Serum iron is frequently and secondarily elevated with a variety of liver diseases in the horse.

IMAGING

Ultrasonography is the procedure of choice.

DIAGNOSTIC PROCEDURES

- Liver biopsy is most commonly performed for microscopic diagnosis of either hepatocellular necrosis (e.g., acute iron poisoning), periportal or diffuse fibrosis from chronic toxicosis, and/or megalocytosis (e.g., pyrrolizidine alkaloids).

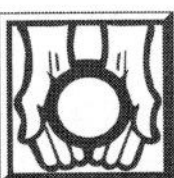

TREATMENT

- In some cases, such as with hepatoencephalopathy, horses may need hospitalization to control abnormal behavior and supply supportive therapy (see Icterus).
- Avoid activity, sunlight, and high-protein feeds.

MEDICATIONS

DRUGS

- Detomidine (5–30 μg/kg IV) may be required to control maniacal behavior.
- For horses with hepatic failure, anorexia, and neurologic signs, IV fluids should be used — acetated Ringer's solution supplemented with 20–40 mEq KCl/L and dextrose (50 g/L).
- In cases of hepatoencephalopathy, neomycin (10 g/500 kg) should be given PO mixed in molasses via syringe q8 h for 2 days. Prebiotics or probiotics can also be given.
- Pentoxifylline (8.4 mg/kg BID), *S*-adenosylmethionine (10 mg/kg daily), and colchicine (0.03 mg/kg daily) may be administered PO in hopes of decreasing fibrosis.

CONTRAINDICATIONS/POSSIBLE INTERACTIONS

- Colchicine should not be used to treat pyrrolizidine alkaloid toxicosis.
- Although PT and aPTT are often prolonged with liver failure, liver biopsy has a low risk of serious hemorrhage. This is most likely because platelet numbers and function remain normal.

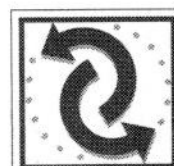

FOLLOW-UP

- Prevent toxin exposure to all horses in the future.
- Feed a moderate-protein/high-energy feed, protect from sunlight.
- Avoid stress.
- Monitor serum enzymes and bile acids for progression of hepatic disease.
- Prognosis depends on toxin, degree of fibrosis, and progression of disease.
- All cases with moderate to extreme fibrosis have a guarded to poor prognosis for life >1 year.

MISCELLANEOUS

ASSOCIATED CONDITIONS

N/A

AGE-RELATED FACTORS

N/A

ZOONOTIC POTENTIAL

N/A

PREGNANCY

N/A

SEE ALSO

- Icterus
- Photosensitization

ABBREVIATIONS

- AST = aspartate aminotransferase
- GGT = γ-glutamyltransferase
- SDH = sorbitol dehydrogenase

Suggested Reading

Durham AE, Newton JR, Smith KC, Hilyer MH, Hilyer LL, Smith MR, Mar CM. Retrospective analysis of historical, clinical, ultrasonographic, serum biochemical and haematological data in prognostic evaluation of equine liver disease. Equine Vet J 2003;35:542–547.

Durham AE, Smith KC, Newton JR, Hillyer MH, Hillyer LL, Smith MR, Marr CM. Development and application of a scoring system for prognostic evaluation of equine liver biopsies. Equine Vet J 2003;35:534–540.

Johnson AL, Divers TJ, Freckleton ML, McKenzie HC, Mitchell E, Cullen JM, McDonough SP. Fall panicum (Panicum dichotomiflorum) hepatotoxicosis in horses and sheep. J Vet Intern Med 2006;20:1414–1421.

Smith MR, Stevens KB, Durham AE, Marr CM. Equine hepatic disease: the effect of patient- and case-specific variables on risk and prognosis. Equine Vet J 2003;35:549–552.

Author Thomas J. Divers

Consulting Editor Michel Lévy

TRAILER LOADING/UNLOADING PROBLEMS

BASICS

OVERVIEW

• The most common problem is hesitating or refusing to enter or exit a trailer or van. The problem can range from mild hesitation in which the horse takes more than 60 seconds to begin to enter or exit the trailer, to complete refusal to approach or exit the trailer. In some horses this refusal includes fearful, active escape and/or aggressive behaviors. • The other extreme is the horse that enters or exits the trailer too rapidly, creating a safety problem for itself and its handlers. • Most cases are not caused by disease; however, impaired vision, impaired balance, or musculoskeletal pain in the back or hindquarters may contribute aversion to the trailer or van. • Behavioral signs range from balking to severe fear responses, with the corresponding involvement of other organ systems consistent with sympathetic stimulation (e.g., tachycardia and vasodilation, increases in ACTH and cortisol concentrations, sweating, defecation, increased respiration rate).

SIGNALMENT

Any age, sex, or breed

SIGNS

Behaviors indicative of fear

CAUSES AND RISK FACTORS

• Horses are innately claustrophobic about small, dark, enclosed areas. • Unpleasant experiences and injuries involving trailering • Trailers that are too small or poorly designed. Inexperienced handlers and drivers can contribute to the problem.

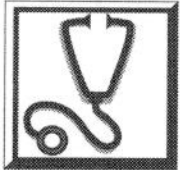

DIAGNOSIS

DIFFERENTIAL DIAGNOSIS

• Trailer loading/unloading problems usually are behavioral in nature. • Evaluated for normal vision, balance and kinesis (ruling out confounding conditions, e.g., spinal ataxia, equine protozoal myelitis, myositis, lameness, etc.); if no abnormalities are found, the problem is probably behavioral.

CBC/BIOCHEMISTRY/URINALYSIS

If pathophysiology is suspected

OTHER LABORATORY TESTS

If pathophysiology is suspected

IMAGING

If pathophysiology is suspected

OTHER DIAGNOSTIC PROCEDURES

If pathophysiology is suspected

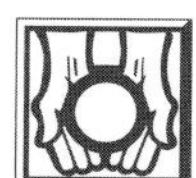

TREATMENT

MILD PROBLEMS

• Modify the trailer to make it appear more open and less threatening. • Use rubber mats to make the trailer floors nonslip and less noisy. • Bedding is not recommended because it contributes to dust and airborne irritants in the trailer. Some bedding materials are inherently slippery (e.g., straw) and may contribute to poor loading/hauling behavior. • Open doors and windows; use interior lights and/or place the trailer where the interior is illuminated.
• Remove the interior partition or swing it to one side and secure it. • Change to a step-up or to a ramp type trailer depending on the horse's preference. It may be helpful to utilize a natural fiber mat on a ramp to muffle ramp "noise."
• Use a trailer with larger interior dimensions, or try an open stock trailer. • Use an existing fence or alleyway to limit the horse's movement away from the trailer • Make sure the footing in the loading area is nonslip (grass or packed soil is preferable to pavement) and that the ramp, if used, is covered with a nonslip surface. • Keep the loading ramp level or minimize the step-up height by parking the trailer on a slight hill.
• Load a quiet horse on the trailer before the reluctant horse. • Load the horse frequently as part of its normal training/handling routine.
• Be patient and allow the horse time to investigate the trailer and make several attempts at loading.

SEVERE PROBLEMS

Unless the practitioner is an expert in solving trailering problems and has the time to adequately instruct the owner, owners should be instructed to consult a qualified, competent individual.

SAFETY ISSUES

- Never stand in front of the horse and pull on the lead or try to pulley the horse into the trailer; the horse may pull back and fall over backwards or leap on top of the handler.
- Never tie the horse in the trailer until it is fully loaded and the trailer doors are securely shut. A tied horse that tries to back out of a trailer usually panics, hits its head on the trailer, and may break its legs if they slip under the back of the trailer. Teach the horse to stand quietly while tied before trailering it, or trailer it loose in a stock trailer.
- Always untie the horse and remove butt bars or chains before opening the trailer doors.
- Never get between the horse and the trailer. The handler should always have an escape route. The escape door should be closed during loading or unloading to prevent a frightened horse from using it.
- Never allow the lead rope to become wrapped around the handler.
- Use protective equipment for the handler (e.g., boots, gloves) and for the horse (e.g., leg wraps, bell boots, head bumper). Accustom the horse to protective gear prior to loading.
- Never load a horse in a lightweight trailer that is not coupled to the tow vehicle because the trailer could tip or roll with the horse.
- Young foals should be trailered loose in a stock trailer with their dam tied in the trailer. Never turn a foal loose in a trailer with an open half-door as they may panic and jump out.
- When loading mares with young foals, catch and hold the foal while the dam is loaded so that the foal does not run away from the trailer if startled by the noise associated with the loading process.

MEDICATIONS

DRUGS

Tranquilizers may alleviate loading and unloading problems temporarily but are not an effective, permanent therapy. They can also impair a horse's balance.

CONTRAINDICATIONS

N/A

FOLLOW-UP

PATIENT MONITORING

If the horse continues to exhibit problems, advise the owner to consult a highly qualified individual for assistance.

PREVENTION/AVOIDANCE

- Encourage owners to practice loading/unloading horses prior to travel.
- Horses should not be unloaded during rest stops unless the stop has a specific facility dedicated to livestock handling.

MISCELLANEOUS

Check compliance with federal and state regulations regarding transport of horses.

ASSOCIATED CONDITIONS

- Poor hauling behavior such as scrambling, kicking, or excessive movement in trailers or vans leading to anxiety and possible injury
- Respiratory irritation/disease. Long distance travel should have frequent rest stops in which the horse is allowed to lower its head to clear nasal passages. Bedding materials (e.g., wood shavings) produce more dust than nonslip rubber mats. Trailers should be well ventilated. Most horses will not consume feed while the trailer is in motion and hay blowing around the trailer increases the chance of lung and eye irritation. Hay or forage should be offered at rest stops.
- Dehydration can be reduced by frequent rest stops in which the horse is offered water and by ensuring the trailer is well ventilated.
- Frequent rest stops give the horse an opportunity to urinate.
- Eye irritation/injury may occur if horse is allowed to put its head out the trailer window.
- Trailer type and weather conditions determine the necessity of blanketing the horse during travel. Horses expend significant energy while traveling, so overheating is generally a greater concern than cold stress.

SEE ALSO

- Fears and phobias
- Training and learning problems

Author Cynthia A. McCall
Consulting Editors Victoria L. Voith and Daniel Q. Estep

TRAINING AND LEARNING PROBLEMS

BASICS

DEFINITION

• *Training* is a term used to describe the process of teaching an animal to perform a new behavior or exhibit a species-typical behavior in designated circumstances. Acquisition of trained behaviors is based on learning.
• Learning influences everything a horse does throughout its life. It is a consequence of the animal's experience with the environment and is one of the basic mechanisms of survival.
• The term *behavior modification,* historically, refers to the treatment of observable, undesirable behaviors by applying principles of learning to substitute desirable responses for undesirable ones. Over the years, parallel and overlapping terminology has evolved within diverse groups of people engaged in similar activities with animals.
• Training and behavior modification often require a delicate balance of modifying a specific segment in a sequence of behaviors without interfering with other components of the behavior pattern and without introducing new behavior problems.
• Familiarity with species-typical behaviors and principles of learning are fundamental to recognizing when a behavior is affected by pathophysiologic states, experience, or learning.
• Undesirable behaviors exhibited by a horse can be a normal species-typical behavior or a consequence of pathophysiology, a learned behavior, or combinations thereof. For example, bucking under saddle could be a predator response, play, due to pain or anticipation of pain.

PATHOPHYSIOLOGY

• Pain, anxiety, and fear are common causes of training and other behavior problems.
• Numerous physiologic states and pathologies can affect learning.
• Common pathophysiological conditions that can induce training or learning problems are:
  ○ Dental problems—sharp edges on molars, caps on molars, or normal wolf-teeth. Contact of the bit or pressure from the halter on these tooth structures can result in bridling and haltering avoidance, bit chomping, head tossing, rearing, and sometimes, bucking. If the pathology is unilateral, the horse's response may be very specific to how the bit or halter is manipulated (e.g., the horse only reacts when asked to take the left lead or only tosses his head when the halter is used to turn the head in one direction).
  ○ Skeletal and muscular problems—pain in the spinal column, back, hip, or stifle, but can occur in anywhere
  ○ Infection, parasites, or foreign body in ears can result in head shyness, pinning ears when the head is reached for, and resistance of bridling and/or haltering
  ○ Vision problems—shying (also when not in training situations; more likely to occur in unfamiliar environments), stopping at jumps, or refusing to traverse obstacles that were previously traversed
  ○ Endocrine states can affect temperament, motivation, and species-typical behaviors, which in turn can result in training and behavior problems.
• Perinatal experiences have been shown in several species to affect development of the nervous system and consequently influence the animal's temperament and reaction to environmental changes.

SYSTEMS AFFECTED

• Training and learned behavior problems are often either precipitated by fear or result in fear. Fear, anxiety, and pain can affect almost all physiologic systems.
• Behavior modification and training procedures can change the physiologic state of the horse, by reducing or alleviating fear, and consequently can change numerous physiologic systems.

GENETICS

• Training and other learned behaviors are constrained by temperament and physical ability to perform specific behaviors. Often the most practical way to gauge the influence of genetics on the behavior of an individual is to determine if siblings, parents, and other closely related individuals (under different management) exhibit the same problems.
• Training and behavior modification are genetically constrained by how and what an animal can learn.

INCIDENCE/PREVALENCE

Unknown

GEOGRAPHIC DISTRIBUTION

Regional training practices may influence the type and frequency of specific training and learning problems.

SIGNALMENT

Breed Predilections

Breeds vary in temperament and physical abilities, which can influence performance and learning.

Mean Age and Range

Any age

Predominant Sex

Any sex. Intact males may pose more problems for handlers and thereby result in more training problems.

SIGNS

General Comments

• Behavioral signs may be the same or similar whether the cause is pathophysiologic, learned, or a species-typical behavior.
• Analysis of training and learning problems requires excellent observational skills and understanding of principles of learning.

Historical

• Objective, detailed descriptions and history are critical. Observation by the clinician is often necessary. Sometimes the horse will exhibit the behavior when brought to the clinician. Sometimes video recordings will suffice. Often a personal visit to where the horse exhibits the behavior is required. This allows observation of the horse's environment and provides details the owner may have overlooked in the history or when obtaining a video recording.
• History of punitive training techniques or traumatic incidents
• Expectations of owner exceed ability of horse.
• Common signs of discomfort—wringing or whipping of the tail, champing or fussing with the bit, tossing the head, bucking, head shyness, pinning back of ears, aggression, and evasive behaviors
• Common signs of conflict and "frustration"—pawing, yawning, closing the eyes, and repetitive compulsive behaviors
• Common signs of fear or anxiety—pacing or attempts to escape, defecation, neighing, "rolling of the eyes" defense responses, and behaviors associated with sympathetic arousal such as tachycardia, sweating, etc.

Physical Examination

• Should be unremarkable unless an underlying pathology is present
• Signs indicative of pain or fear.
• Evidence of trauma
• Observe horse in a different environment or circumstance, e.g., different rider, different tack, not being ridden, different handler, different location, etc. This may help determine if the problem is related to the environment as opposed to a medical problem, but be aware that an aroused animal can override physical signs of pain.

CAUSES

• Normal, species-typical behaviors that interfere with management or training, such as defensive responses; play; social behaviors (e.g., greeting behaviors, separation distress responses, courtship behaviors, intermale aggression or displays).
• Fear
• Pain
• Common inappropriate training and handling techniques: inconsistency, not allowing the horse to distinguish between training cues, inadvertently rewarding the wrong behaviors, and/or inappropriately applied aversive stimuli. Training problems frequently arise from the trainer/rider giving a signal the horse does not understand; punishment can further compound the problem.

• A handler's response to a problem behavior can profoundly affect the horse not only in the context of the problem but also in other situations. For example, a punitive technique to discourage a stallion from neighing at another horse or having an erection may stop the unwanted behaviors at the time. However, later the horse may not maintain an erection during a desired breeding situation and, even, become aggressive toward people who approach him. Use of a whip to teach a horse in a stall to always face a person, never presenting the side or rear, may interfere with training a horse to move away from a person using a whip with lunge lines or driving lines.

RISK FACTORS

• Trainers, handlers, and owners who base their training philosophies on "showing the horse who is the boss" and "teaching the horse a lesson" and believe that horses "are trying to get away with something" or are "willfully disobedient." Rider/trainers with such philosophies are less likely to analyze situations critically for the precise stimuli and conditions eliciting the undesirable behaviors and are more likely to be punitive.
• Sometimes it is not possible for a horse to perform specific tasks at the level an owner expects. A mismatch of expectations and ability can lead to welfare problems for the horse and frustration for the owner.
• Neonatal and young animals are especially susceptible to experiences. Isolation, barren environments, and lack of exposure to novel environments and novel stimuli can alter the structure of the nervous and endocrine systems. In turn, these changes affect the animal's subsequent responses to the environment and learning processes. Some types of neonatal handling have been shown to result in beneficial effects on the development of the nervous, endocrine, and immune systems and subsequent learning.

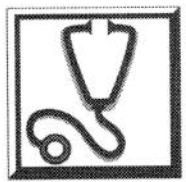

DIAGNOSIS

DIFFERENTIAL DIAGNOSIS

• Identification of the precise stimuli and conditions associated with the behavior problem. If necessary, brief exposure to the stimuli, or reduced intensity of the stimulus, can confirm the eliciting stimuli.
• If unwanted behaviors arise only during training sessions, the training methods should be carefully examined. If those methods adhere to sound principles of learning and the horse is not subject to abusive techniques, pathophysiological conditions are more likely.
• Pathophysiological conditions can exist concurrently with inappropriate training and riding techniques.
• Addressing learning and training problems can be complex and requires the cooperation of open-minded, competent, and experienced rider/trainer/owners.
• The clinician should determine if fear is a motivation for the behavior problems. Many fears can be treated with behavior modification techniques.

CBC/BIOCHEMISTRY/URINALYSIS

• Usually normal; possible stress leukogram
• Dependent on presenting signs
• Abnormalities may suggest metabolic or endocrine explanations.

OTHER LABORATORY TESTS

Dependent on presenting signs; may be indicated to rule out medical explanations.

IMAGING

Dependent on presenting signs

OTHER DIAGNOSTIC PROCEDURES

Dependent on presenting signs

PATHOLOGICAL FINDINGS

Usually not found, although central nervous system and endocrine abnormalities are a possibility

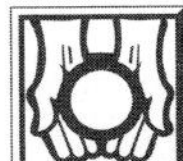

TREATMENT

AIMS OF TREATMENT

• Identify and treat physical problems.
• It is extremely important to remember that after physical problems are successfully treated, behavior problems may persist due to conditioned responses that have been acquired. Retraining or behavior modification may still be required.
• Recognize species-typical behaviors and implement management to alleviate, minimize, or accommodate these behaviors.
• Treat or refer to appropriate expert for treatment of learned aspects of the problems.
• Educate, refer, or supply sources of information to owners, handlers, and trainers pertaining to learning principles and normal behaviors of the horse.

PRINCIPLES OF LEARNING

• Even if a clinician does not assume responsibility for treating a behavior problem, knowledge of some learning principles is helpful in making a differential diagnosis, assisting the owner, and assessing experts to whom to refer the owner. Basic psychology, learning, and behavior modification textbooks are generally good sources for detailed information.
• Learning influences everything a horse does throughout its life. It is a consequence of the animal's experience with the environment and is one of the basic mechanisms of survival.
• Animals learn in many ways. Learning can occur as a consequence of exposure to environmental situations or by direct interaction with stimuli in the environment. It may not be immediately apparent by the animal's behavior that it has learned something.
• *Conditioning* is a term that refers to learning associations between stimuli or between a stimulus and a response. Conditioning processes allow the horse to anticipate, predict, and/or prepare for subsequent stimuli. Conditioning also provides the horse with responses for coping with the occurrence of specific stimuli.
• It is almost intuitive that people know that horses can associate pain with stimuli in the environment, such as a white coat, a syringe, a specific saddle, a specific rider, a specific location. Identifying the relevant stimuli, however, can sometimes be difficult.
• What is not so obvious is that a horse with a problem during training may also associate several environmental stimuli with the acquired problem. If these stimuli are removed or changed, the problem behavior is often altered. For example, changing type equipment or location of training may decrease the intensity of the problem behavior and make it easier to teach new, desired behaviors.
• Operant or instrumental conditioning is a process by which the frequency of a behavior is modified by the consequences of the behavior. Reinforcers (stimuli or events that increase the occurrence of a behavior) can be positive (usually pleasant) or negative (usually aversive).
• Positive reinforcers are essentially rewards that increase the probability that an animal will repeat a behavior. Owners can unintentionally reward unwanted behaviors. It often takes a knowledgeable observer to notice this happening.
• Behaviors acquired by intermittent positive reinforcement may persist for a prolonged time after reinforcement stops (call to mind the persistence with which people gamble without reinforcement).
• Behaviors previously positively reinforced may temporarily intensify when reinforcement ceases. The behavior often gets worse before it begins to wane.
• Negative reinforcers also increase the occurrence of behaviors. Horses perform behaviors to avoid or escape aversive stimuli. If appropriately used, aversive stimuli are not always contraindicated. However, such stimuli must be of the appropriate intensity and applied appropriately. For example, many behaviors under saddle are acquired via negative reinforcement with use of bits, reins, and leg pressure. The horse engages in a specific response to escape from a specific stimulus and thus the response is reinforced (the aversive stimulus goes away). If a signal (light touch, shift of weight, voice) precedes the aversive stimulus (pressure), the horse can learn to completely avoid the aversive stimulus.
• Horses also learn to avoid aversive stimuli by throwing their heads back, bucking, fleeing, and other evasive maneuvers.

TRAINING AND LEARNING PROBLEMS

- Successful escape and avoidance of an aversive stimulus are highly reinforcing and difficult to extinguish by only withholding the aversive reinforcer. A counterconditioning program is usually required to remedy these behaviors.
- Punishment is the use of aversive stimuli to stop a behavior and reduce/prevent the future occurrence of a behavior. Considerable judgment and timing are required to appropriately implement punishment. A correctly used punisher (the aversive stimulus) should be of high enough intensity to interrupt a behavior but not so high as to cause side effects—such as anxiety, fear, and aggression. A punisher should be applied immediately at the onset of the behavior and used every time the unwanted behavior is initiated. It helps many people to think of punishing the behavior, not punishing the horse. An effective punisher should work within a few applications. Attempts to use an aversive stimulus as a punisher without adhering to these guidelines are, at best, harassment and, at worse, abuse.
- The intensity, timing, and consistently of use of any aversive technique are critical. Use of aversive stimuli often backfires. Even if use of an aversive stimulus achieves a specific result, the horse may also acquire undesirable, detrimental, and dangerous behaviors as a consequence.
- The wave of acceptance and success of "natural horsemanship" techniques attests to the value of positive reinforcement and nonpunitive techniques in training and management of horses.
- Aversive stimuli ALWAYS carry the potential of inducing anxiety, fear, and defensive aggression. Aversive stimuli are almost always contraindicated if fear is a component of an undesirable behavior.

APPROPRIATE HEALTH CARE

Adequate exercise and social interaction are integral parts of maintaining health.

NURSING CARE

N/A

ACTIVITY

Meet the species-typical behavioral needs of the horse. e.g., exercise, opportunity play, etc.

DIET

Investigation of the role of diet in learning and behavior is continuously ongoing.

CLIENT EDUCATION

Educate, refer, or supply sources of information regarding learning principles and normal behaviors of the horse.

SURGICAL CONSIDERATIONS

Castration or ovariectomy may be indicated.

MEDICATIONS

DRUGS OF CHOICE

There are many verbal and written recommendations regarding the use of drugs and across-the-counter remedies to treat fears, phobias, and facilitate training of horses. However, there are no drugs approved for these uses in horses. To date, there are no substantial safety and efficacy data for the use of any of these drugs or remedies for these purposes.

CONTRAINDICATIONS

Off-label use of tranquilizers or sedatives may alter the visual perception, balance, proprioception, and musculoskeletal coordination of horses. These effects could be detrimental to horse, handler, bystanders, riders, and drivers.

PRECAUTIONS

Although use of medications may reduce excitability or fear and minimize or suppress unwanted behaviors, there is no guarantee that a horse will learn the desired behaviors while under the influence of the medications. Anxiolytics, sedatives, and tranquilizers can have animistic properties.

POSSIBLE INTERACTIONS N/A

ALTERNATIVE DRUGS

Modipher EQ is a commercially available synthetic pheromone reported to prevent/reduce anxiety and fearful reactions if administered before exposure to the anxiety/fear-eliciting situations.

FOLLOW-UP

PATIENT MONITORING

- Behavior modification programs frequently need to be adjusted.
- If veterinarians assume partial or full responsibility for treatment of a learning problem or fear/phobic response, they should instruct the client to contact them immediately if the behavior gets worse and otherwise within 2 weeks of initiating treatment procedures. Thereafter, frequency of contact depends on the individual problem and treatment.
- If medical problems have been ruled out or successfully treated and the horse continues to exhibit the problem behavior, the client should be advised to consult with a person qualified to deal with that specific problem.
- If the veterinarian refers the client to a nonveterinarian, it is still beneficial to periodically contact the owner. Signs of a previously subclinical medical problem may become apparent. Follow-up information is also helpful in assessing the success of the treatment program that the owner is implementing.

PREVENTION/AVOIDANCE

- Gradually introduce horses to novel environments and new tasks.
- Be cognizant of inadvertently reinforcing unwanted behaviors.
- Do not inappropriately use aversive stimuli in attempts to change behavior.
- Horses that have been successfully treated for fear-based behavior problems should periodically be exposed to the fear-eliciting stimuli to prevent "spontaneous recovery" of the fearful behaviors.

POSSIBLE COMPLICATIONS

- Undetected underlying medical cause of the problem
- Persistence of behavior after successful treatment of initial medical cause

EXPECTED COURSE AND PROGNOSIS

Highly variable dependent on recognition of underlying medical problems, diagnosis of the behavior problem, temperament of the horse, management strategies, and abilities of owner, handler, trainer, and behavior expert.

MISCELLANEOUS

ASSOCIATED CONDITIONS

- Medical problems, especially those causing pain
- Fearful behavior

AGE-RELATED FACTORS N/A

ZOONOTIC POTENTIAL N/A

PREGNANCY

Pregnancy is sometimes associated with a "calmer" disposition, perhaps related to progesterone.

SYNONYMS N/A

SEE ALSO

- Fears and phobias
- Trailer loading/unloading problems
- Stallion sexual behavior problems

Suggested Reading

Borchelt PL, Voith VL. Punishment. In: Voith VL, Borchelt PL, eds. Readings in Companion Animal Behavior. Trenton, NJ: Veterinary Learning Systems, 1996:72–80.

Domjan M. The Principles of Learning and Behavior: Active Learning Edition. Belmont, CA: Thomson/Wadsworth, 2006.

McGreevy P. Equine Behaviour: A Guide for Veterinarians and Equine Scientists. Philadelphia: WB Saunders, 2005.

Mills DS, McDonnell S. Domestic Horse: The Origins, Development, and Management of Its Behaviour. New York: Cambridge University Press, 2005.

Waring GH. Horse Behavior, ed 2. Norwich, NJ: Noyes Publications/William Andrew Publishing, 2003.

Author Victoria L. Voith

Consulting Editors Victoria L. Voith and Daniel Q. Estep

TREMORGENIC MYCOTOXIN TOXICOSES

BASICS

OVERVIEW

• Several mycotoxins cause equine neurologic disease—fumonisins, swainsonine, slaframine, lolitrems, and paspalitrems. • Those considered to be "tremorgens" are the lolitrems (lolitrems A, B, C, and D) produced by *Neotyphodium lolii* and causing perennial ryegrass (*Lolium perenne*) staggers and paspalitrems (paspalinine, paspalitrem A and B) produced by *Claviceps paspali* and causing dallis grass or paspalum staggers (associated with dallis grass [*Paspalum dilatatum*] and bahia grass [*Bahia oppositifolia*]). • A tremorgenic disease associated with ingestion of bermuda grass (*Cynodon dactylon*) is believed to result from a mycotoxin, but a specific tremorgen has not been isolated. • *N. lolii* is an endophytic fungus of ryegrass and propagates via seed. • *C. paspali* is a soil fungus that invades dallis and bahia grass under favorable environmental conditions. • Tremorgens are believed to competitively inhibit CNS postsynaptic GABA receptors and, therefore, chloride influx; GABA-receptor antagonism leads to increased nerve discharge and neurologic signs. • Annual ryegrass toxicosis, whose clinical presentation is similar to that of tremorgenic mycotoxins, can result when the bacterium *Clavibacter toxicus* is carried into annual ryegrass seedheads by the nematode *Anguina funesta. C. toxicus* produces the neurotoxin corynetoxin, a glycolipid that inhibits the synthesis of lipid-linked oligosaccharides and blocks protein glycosylation.

SIGNALMENT

No breed, sex, or age predispositions

SIGNS

Perennial Ryegrass Staggers

• Signs can occur 5–10 days after grazing highly toxic pastures. • Initial signs include head tremors and muscle fasciculations of the neck and legs, which progress to head nodding and swaying while standing. • Animals that are excited or forced to move develop dysmetria and leg stiffening, leading to collapse and tetanic spasms; if left alone, animals recover in a few minutes and walk away with a relatively normal gait. • Affected animals rarely die unless they injure or entrap themselves during a tetanic spasm. • Affected animals may lose weight and are difficult to handle or move because of inducible spasms..

Paspalum Staggers

Signs are identical to those of perennial ryegrass staggers but often less severe.

Annual Ryegrass Staggers

Signs are similar to those of perennial ryegrass staggers.

CAUSES AND RISK FACTORS

Perennial Ryegrass Staggers

• Pastures must be predominantly perennial ryegrass for toxicosis to occur. • Incidence is greater during the late summer and fall and on ryegrass pastures that have been heavily grazed. • Environmental temperatures are generally >23° C. • Frequency of intoxication relates to the degree of fungal infection of the ryegrass. Infection rates <25% are associated with sporadic outbreaks, whereas rates >90% are associated with large outbreaks.

Paspalum Staggers

Toxin production is greatest during a wet period following seedhead formation.

Annual Ryegrass Staggers

• Toxin concentration increases in seedheads during the summer and is greatest as the plant dries and seeds ripen. • Annual ryegrass occurs in patches, and alterations in grazing patterns may predispose to ingestion. • Newly introduced animals may ingest more ryegrass.

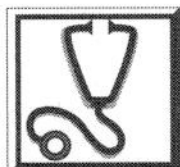

DIAGNOSIS

DIFFERENTIAL DIAGNOSIS

Other plant intoxications such as locoism (*Astragalus* spp.) and white snakeroot (*Eupatorium rugosum*)—evidence of plant consumption, characteristic histopathological lesions, detection of tremetol in white snakeroot toxicosis

CBC/BIOCHEMISTRY/URINALYSIS

N/A

OTHER LABORATORY TESTS

Perennial Ryegrass Staggers

• Positive identification of perennial ryegrass
• Microscopic detection of fungus in ryegrass
• Mouse bioassay of methanol extracts from ryegrass to produce characteristic clinical signs
• Detection of lolitrems in ryegrass—concentrations of lolitrem B >2 ppm are associated with effects in sheep and cattle.

Paspalum Staggers

• Positive identification of dallis or bahia grass and associated fungal sclerotia on grass seedheads
• Detection of tremorgen

Annual Ryegrass Staggers

• Positive identification of annual ryegrass
• Identification of galls associated with nematode infestation • ELISA for detection of corynetoxin

IMAGING

N/A

DIAGNOSTIC PROCEDURES

N/A

PATHOLOGICAL FINDINGS

• Gross and histopathological lesions generally are absent. • Animals with chronic ryegrass staggers may have loss of Purkinje cells in the cerebellum, which is believed to be secondary to hypoxia and hypoglycemia. • Histopathological changes associated with annual ryegrass staggers include cerebellar, hepatic, and splenic hemorrhages that may be secondary to endothelial cell damage.

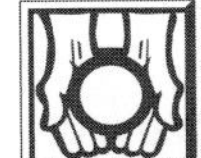

TREATMENT

Remove animals from affected grass pastures.

MEDICATIONS

DRUGS

N/A

CONTRAINDICATIONS/POSSIBLE INTERACTIONS

N/A

FOLLOW-UP

PATIENT MONITORING

Attempt to prevent self-injury during tetanic spasms

PREVENTION/AVOIDANCE

Perennial Ryegrass Staggers

• Reduce overgrazing of pastures. • Remove animals from pastures during critical periods—late summer and fall for endophyte-infested ryegrass pastures. • Use endophyte-free ryegrass seed. • Use fungicides—reduces seed viability.

Paspalum Staggers

Mow pastures to remove toxic seedheads.

Annual Ryegrass Staggers

• Break nematode life cycle by killing ryegrass for two or three growing seasons. • Integrated control measures—herbicide use in the spring, seeding pastures with legumes, burning infested pastures in the early autumn, applying herbicides to selectively kill ryegrass during the summer, and heavy winter grazing.

POSSIBLE COMPLICATIONS

• Traumatic injury • Bloating or drowning during tetanic spasm.

EXPECTED COURSE AND PROGNOSIS

• Once removed from affected pastures, animals generally recover within several weeks without treatment. • Degenerative CNS lesions associated with chronic perennial ryegrass staggers likely prevent full recovery.

MISCELLANEOUS

ASSOCIATED CONDITIONS, AGE-RELATED FACTORS, ZOONOTIC POTENTIAL, PREGNANCY

N/A

ABBREVIATIONS

• CNS = central nervous system
• ELISA = enzyme-linked immunosorbent assay
• GABA = γ-aminobutyric acid

Suggested Reading

Plumlee KH, Galey FD. Neurotoxic mycotoxins: a review of fungal toxins that cause neurologic disease in large animals. J Vet Intern Med 1994;8:49–54.

Author Robert H. Poppenga
Consulting Editor Robert H. Poppenga

THYROID-RELEASING HORMONE (TRH) AND THYROID-STIMULATING HORMONE (TSH) STIMULATION TESTS

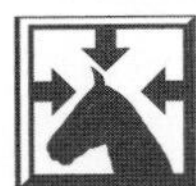

BASICS

DEFINITION

• TRH and TSH stimulation tests are performed to evaluate the ability of the thyroid gland to secrete T_3 and T_4. No increase in blood T_3 and T_4 levels after TRH or TSH administration indicates hypothyroidism. TRH also may be used as a screening test in horses with suspected pituitary tumors; increased cortisol or MSH after administration of TRH indicates a pars intermedia tumor of the pituitary gland (i.e., equine Cushing's syndrome).
• TRH test to evaluate thyroid function: Give TRH (1 mg IV) and measure T_3 and T_4 levels at 0, 2, and 4 hr. Normally, the baseline T_3 and T_4 are in the reference range with the T_3 concentration doubling at 2 hr, and the T_4 concentration doubling at 4 hr.
• The TSH test (5 IU IV) is performed in the same manner, with the same expected end points.
• TRH test to evaluate pituitary function: Give TRH (1 mg IV), and measure blood cortisol or MSH at 0, 15, 30, 60, 120, and 180 min. Normally, the hormone concentrations do not change; however, an increased concentration over 1.5 times baseline suggests the presence of a pars intermedia dysfunction.

PATHOPHYSIOLOGY

• Thyroid hormone levels in blood are regulated by the thyroid-pituitary-hypothalamic axis. Endogenous TRH is released from the hypothalamus and travels to the pituitary gland. The pituitary gland then secretes TSH into the circulation, which stimulates release of T_4 and T_3 from the thyroid gland.
• When exogenous TSH is given, the thyroid gland's ability to secrete hormone is tested.
• When TRH is given, the pituitary gland's ability to respond to this by secreting TSH and then the thyroid gland's ability to respond to the endogenous TSH are tested.
• In equine medicine, test selection is based primarily on availability of the reagents. Presently, TSH is not available for clinical use. However, TRH can be obtained, although quite expensive.
• Why pituitary tumor cells respond inappropriately to TRH while normal cells do not is not completely understood. Tumor cells are hypothesized to have an alteration in the receptor/adenylate cyclase system that allows for a paradoxic response to specific and nonspecific challenges.

SYSTEM AFFECTED

• The endocrine system is primarily affected by abnormal results of the TSH or TRH stimulation tests—decreased thyroid hormone response to the stimulation test is diagnostic of hypothyroidism while increased cortisol in response to TRH is suggestive, although not diagnostic, of pituitary pars intermedia dysfunction.

SIGNALMENT

• No sex or breed predilections
• Hypothyroidism can occur at any age.
• Pars intermedia dysfunction occurs in older horses (>13 years)

SIGNS

• Signs associated with an abnormal TRH/TSH stimulation test are those of hypothyroidism or equine pituitary pars intermedia dysfunction.
• Clinical signs of congenital hypothyroidism in foals—prognathism, ruptured common digital extensor tendon, forelimb contracture, retarded ossification, crushing of the carpal and tarsal bones, weakness, and poor suckle reflex.
• Less common signs of congenital hypothyroidism in foals—goiter, angular limb deformities, respiratory distress, abdominal hernia, poor muscle development, and osteoporosis.
• Hypothermia and bradycardia are consistent findings in adults with hypothyroidism. Other signs include myositis, anhydrosis, laminitis, infertility, agalactia, poor hair coat, and poor growth.
• Clinical signs of pituitary pars intermedia dysfunction include hirsutism and failure to shed a winter coat. Also common are abnormal fat distribution, pendulous abdomen, weight loss, polyuria and polydipsia, laminitis, and chronic infections.

CAUSES

• The primary cause for lack of response in a TSH/TRH stimulation test is primary hypothyroidism. Many factors can cause low resting T_3 and T_4 levels in blood; however, unless the horse is truly hypothyroid, the gland responds normally to exogenous stimulating hormones. When it does not, hypothyroidism is diagnosed.
• The primary cause for increased cortisol after TRH administration is stress response. Increased cortisol and MSH may result from an inappropriate response of a pituitary tumor to TRH.

RISK FACTORS

• Known risk factors for thyroid abnormalities are primarily dietary. Intake of excess or inadequate iodine or ingestion of other goitrogens can lead to hypothyroidism.
• In old populations, thyroid tumor is a risk factor for development of thyroid abnormalities.
• Pituitary tumor is a risk factor for development of abnormal cortisol secretion in response to TRH.

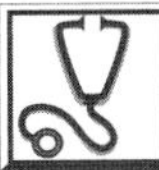

DIAGNOSIS

DIFFERENTIAL DIAGNOSIS

• The primary differential diagnosis for increased cortisol after TRH administration is stress response. Psychic stress from handling, receiving injections, and blood sample collections result in increased blood cortisol.
• Stress response can be differentiated from pituitary tumor by more specific tests for that condition—endogenous ACTH assay or dexamethasone suppression test.

LABORATORY FINDINGS

Drugs That May Alter Lab Results

N/A

Disorders That May Alter Lab Results

N/A

Valid If Run in a Human Lab?

Laboratory determination of T_3, free T_3, T_4, and free T_4 is valid if run in a human laboratory. Human thyroid hormone values are commonly higher than equine; therefore, use equine reference ranges to interpret results. Free T_3 and T_4 should be determined by equilibrium dialysis method.

CBC/BIOCHEMISTRY/URINALYSIS

• Hypothyroidism—anemia, leukopenia, and hypercholesterolemia
• Pituitary pars intermedia dysfunction—stress response with a mature neutrophilia, lymphopenia, and eosinopenia; possibly increased blood glucose and glucosuria

OTHER LABORATORY TESTS

Pituitary function—endogenous ACTH determination, dexamethasone suppression testing, and insulin response test; if results are consistent with equine Cushing's syndrome, this would support a positive TRH test.

IMAGING

• Ultrasonography—rarely useful in hypothyroidism, but an enlarged thyroid gland caused by tumor or goiter could be visualized.
• Radiography—An enlarged thyroid gland caused by tumor or goiter might be seen as an increased soft-tissue density in the throat-latch area.
• Increased pituitary gland size may be visualized with specialized modalities—CT or venous contrast.

DIAGNOSTIC PROCEDURES

Fine-needle aspiration or biopsy may assist in assessing the thyroid gland.

THYROID-RELEASING HORMONE (TRH) AND THYROID-STIMULATING HORMONE (TSH) STIMULATION TESTS

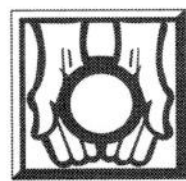

TREATMENT

APPROPRIATE HEALTH CARE

- Foals with congenital hypothyroidism may require inpatient medical management with severe disease.
- All other horses with abnormal TRH/TSH tests can be treated as outpatients.

NURSING CARE

- Foals may need assistance standing and milk administered via nasogastric tube if they are too weak to suckle.
- Foals may need mechanical ventilation if they cannot breathe on their own.
- Animals with poor hair coat may need blanketing.
- Horses with laminitis need corrective hoof trimming and shoeing.

ACTIVITY

- Limit activity of foals with musculoskeletal deformities—incomplete ossification of the carpal or tarsal bones
- Limit activity of horses with laminitis.

DIET

- Examine the diet of any horse with hypothyroidism and of dams with foals born having hypothyroidism to ensure that the proper amount of iodine is being fed.
- Pregnant mares should not receive endophyte-infected fescue hay or iodine supplementation, particularly during the last months of gestation.
- Horses with laminitis generally benefit from a low-carbohydrate, high-fiber diet.

CLIENT EDUCATION

- The prognosis for soundness is poor in most foals with congenital hypothyroidism and, thus, should be discussed with owners before expensive treatments begin.
- Adult horses with hypothyroidism respond well to exogenous replacement hormone. Their prognosis generally is good.
- Horses with pituitary pars intermedia dysfunction may be managed via medication (pergolide) and nursing care, but their prognosis is quite variable. Some do well for several years; others are refractory to treatment. Owners need to understand that treatment is palliative and required for life.

SURGICAL CONSIDERATIONS

If the abnormal TRH/TSH response test results from a tumor of the thyroid gland, surgical removal of the affected thyroid lobe should be curative.

MEDICATIONS

DRUG(S) OF CHOICE

- For decreased T_3 and T_4 caused by hypothyroidism, replacement therapy with T_4 is the drug of choice—20 μg/mL maintains T_4 and T_3 levels in the normal range for 24 hr; this constitutes a dose of 10 mg in a 1000-lb horse.
- The agent most commonly used to alter symptoms of pituitary pars intermedia dysfunction is pergolide (0.75–2 mg/day).

CONTRAINDICATIONS

If the horse has low resting T_3 and T_4 values because of some other severe disease (e. g., euthyroid sick syndrome), thyroid replacement therapies may cause further deterioration. Perform provocative testing before administering medication in any horse with suspected hypothyroidism that is debilitated or exhibits signs of any other disease.

PRECAUTIONS

- Exogenous thyroid hormone causes down-regulation and, potentially, atrophy of the thyroid gland. Discontinue the supplement gradually over the course of several weeks.
- Horses that receive overdoses of pergolide may exhibit anorexia, lethargy, and ataxia.

POSSIBLE INTERACTIONS

N/A

ALTERNATIVE DRUGS

Other sources of thyroid hormone supplement are iodinated casein (5.0 g/day) and concentrated bovine thyroid extract (10 g/day).

FOLLOW-UP

PATIENT MONITORING

- Monitor horses on thyroid supplement by retesting serum T_4 and T_3 levels every 30–60 days. If the serum level is low, increase the dosage until the normal range is achieved. If the serum level is too high or on the higher end of the normal range, decrease the dosage and retest the horse.
- Failure to respond clinically after 6 weeks of therapy should prompt reconsideration of the original diagnosis of thyroid disease.
- Retest horses with pituitary pars intermedia dysfunction every 12–20 weeks by endogenous ACTH determination or dexamethasone response test. Abnormal results indicate the need for an increased dose or a change in medication.

MISCELLANEOUS

ASSOCIATED CONDITIONS

- Angular limb deformities, hypognathism, weakness, and respiratory distress often are associated with congenital hypothyroidism.
- Infertility, skin problems, and myositis have been associated with hypothyroidism in adults.
- Hirsutism, chronic infections, and laminitis are commonly associated with equine Cushing's syndrome.

AGE-RELATED FACTORS

On the first day of life, foals have little T_3 response to TRH/TSH administration. Only a T_4 response should be evaluated in neonatal foals.

ZOONOTIC POTENTIAL

N/A

PREGNANCY

N/A

SEE ALSO

- ACTH
- Hypothyroidism
- Pituitary tumors
- T_3
- T_4

ABBREVIATIONS

- ACTH = adrenocorticotrophic hormone
- MSH = melanocyte-stimulating hormone
- TRH = thyroid-releasing hormone
- TSH = thyroid-stimulating hormone
- T_3 = triiodothyronine
- T_4 = thyroxine

Suggested Reading

Frank N, Sojka J. Equine thyroid dysfunction. Vet. Clin. North Am. 2002;18:305–319.

Author Janice Sojka
Consulting Editor Michel Lévy

TRICUSPID REGURGITATION

BASICS

DEFINITION

• Occurs when the tricuspid (right atrioventricular) valve allows blood to leak backward into the right atrium during systole and creates a systolic murmur with its point of maximal intensity in the tricuspid valve area
• The murmur radiates toward the right heart base dorsally or cranially.
• Occasionally, the murmur can be auscultated in the left second to third intercostal space.

PATHOPHYSIOLOGY

• Tricuspid leaflets do not form a seal between the right atrium and ventricle.
• During systole, blood regurgitates into the right atrium, and if severe, this causes increased right atrial pressure and right atrial and ventricular volume overload.
• As the regurgitation becomes more severe, further increases in right atrial pressure produce increased central venous pressure, hepatic congestion, and right-sided congestive heart failure.

SYSTEM AFFECTED

Cardiovascular

GENETICS

N/A

INCIDENCE/PREVALENCE

Reported more frequently in Thoroughbreds, particularly National Hunt racehorses, and in Standardbred racehorses.

SIGNALMENT

N/A

SIGNS

General Comments

Usually an incidental finding during routine auscultation unless the horse is in congestive heart failure. Tricuspid regurgitation can develop as a physiological adaptation to athletic training and in these horses there is no effect on performance. The severity of signs is dependent on the nature and severity of any valvular pathology.

Historical Findings

• Sometimes poor performance
• Sometimes congestive heart failure

Physical Examination Findings

• Grade 2–6/6, band-shaped to crescendo or crescendo-decrescendo holosystolic murmur with its point of maximal intensity in the tricuspid valve area (right fourth intercostal space) radiating to the right heart base.
• Approximately 30% of horses with infective endocarditis affecting the tricuspid valve do not have cardiac murmurs.
• Other, less common findings—atrial fibrillation, accentuated third heart sound, jugular pulsations, generalized venous distention, and ventral edema

CAUSES

• Physiological tricuspid regurgitation, often related to cardiac adaptation in response to athletic training
• Degenerative changes of the tricuspid leaflets
• Pulmonary hypertension
• Nonvegetative valvulitis
• Ruptured chordae tendineae
• Infective endocarditis
• Congenital malformation

RISK FACTORS

N/A

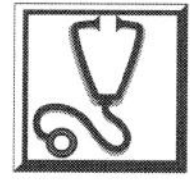

DIAGNOSIS

DIFFERENTIAL DIAGNOSIS

Ventricular septal defect—this causes a loud murmur over the right hemithorax but is also accompanied by the murmur of relative pulmonic stenosis murmur over the pulmonic valve area (left third intercostal space); differentiate echocardiographically.

CBC/BIOCHEMISTRY/URINALYSIS

Possible neutrophilic leukocytosis and hyperfibrinogenemia with infectivel endocarditis

OTHER LABORATORY TESTS

• Elevated cardiac isoenzymes may be present (e.g., cardiac troponin I, CK-MB, HBDH, LDH 1 and 2) with concurrent myocarditis or other myocardial disease.
• Positive blood culture may be obtained in horses with infective endocarditis.

IMAGING

Electrocardiography

• Atrial premature depolarizations may be present in horses with right atrial enlargement.
• Atrial fibrillation may be present in horses with tricuspid regurgitation leading to significant right atrial enlargement.

Echocardiography

• Most affected horses have normal tricuspid valve leaflets.
• Prolapse of a tricuspid leaflet into the right atrium frequently is detected in affected horses.
• Thickening of the valve leaflets is not seen often but diffuse thickening of the free edge of the leaflets is more common than nodular thickening of the leaflets' free edge.
• Ruptured chordae tendineae, flail tricuspid leaflets, or vegetations associated with infective endocarditis infrequently are detected.
• Right atrium—enlarged and dilated, with a rounded appearance.
• Right ventricle—enlarged and dilated, with a rounded apex and thinning of the right ventricular free wall and interventricular septum.
• A pattern of right ventricular volume overload, including paradoxic septal motion, in severe cases.
• Dilatation of the cranial and caudal vena cava and hepatic veins in severe cases.
• Pulsed-wave or color-flow Doppler reveals a jet (or jets) of tricuspid regurgitation in the right atrium. In most horses with mild to moderate regurgitation, the jet is directed toward the aortic root. The size and extent of the jet are a good method of semiquantitating severity, as is the strength of the regurgitation signal.

Thoracic Radiography

Cardiac enlargement may be detected, with increased contact between the heart and the sternum.

DIAGNOSTIC PROCEDURES

Cardiac Catheterization

Right-sided catheterization may reveal elevated right atrial and central venous pressures, with normal oxygen saturation of the blood from the right atrium and central veins.

Continuous 24-Hour Holter Monitoring

Useful in horses with suspected atrial or ventricular premature depolarizations

Ultrasonography

• Perform in cases with a thrombosed jugular vein; note the absence of a cardiac murmur does not rule of infective endocarditis of the tricusid valve or other right-sided structures.
• Detection of a cavitated thrombus is consistent with septic jugular vein thrombophlebitis.

PATHOLOGIC FINDINGS

• Where the regurgitation relates to physiological adaptation to athletic training, no pathological findings are expected.
• Most horses have relatively normal-appearing tricuspid valve leaflets at postmortem examination.
• Focal or diffuse thickening or distortion of one or more tricuspid leaflets may be present.
• Ruptured chordae tendineae, flail tricuspid leaflets, vegetations due to infective endocarditis, or congenital malformations of the tricuspid valve are infrequent.
• Jet lesions may be detected in the right atrium.
• Right atrial enlargement and thinning of the atrial myocardium in cases with significant regurgitation.
• Right ventricular enlargement and thinning of the right ventricular free wall and interventricular septum in horses with significant regurgitation
• Dilatation of the cranial and caudal vena cava and hepatic veins in horses with severe regurgitation.
• Pale areas may be seen in the atrial myocardium, with areas of atrial fibrosis detected histopathologically.
• Inflammatory cell infiltrate has been documented in affected horses with myocarditis.
• Myocardial necrosis occasionally is detected in affected horses with primary myocardial disease.

• In horses with congestive heart failure, ventral and peripheral edema, pleural effusion, pericardial effusion, chronic hepatic congestion, and occasionally, ascites may be detected.

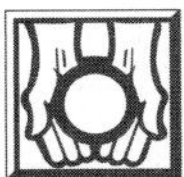

TREATMENT

AIMS OF TREATMENT

• Management by intermittent monitoring in horses with tricusid regurgitation that is mild or moderate in severity
• Palliative care in horses with severe tricuspid regurgitation and signs of right-sided or congestive heart failure

APPROPRIATE HEALTH CARE

• Most affected horses require no treatment and can be monitored on an outpatient basis.
• Treat horses with severe regurgitation and congestive heart failure for congestive heart failure with positive inotropic drugs, vasodilators, and diuretics on an inpatient basis, if possible, and monitor response to therapy.

NAURSING CARE

N/A

ACTIVITY

• Affected horses with tricuspid regurgitation are safe to continue in full athletic work unless the regurgitation is severe or the horse develops exercise intolerance or congestive heart failure.
• Horses with significant right ventricular dysfunction and exercise intolerance are no longer safe to ride.

DIET

N/A

CLIENT EDUCATION

• Monitor the cardiac rhythm regularly; any irregularities other than second-degree atrioventricular block should prompt ECG.
• Carefully monitor for exercise intolerance, jugular or generalized venous distention, jugular pulses, ventral edema, prolonged recovery after exercise, or increased resting heart rate; if detected, perform a cardiac re-examination.

SURGICAL CONSIDERATIONS

N/A

MEDICATIONS

DRUG(S) OF CHOICE

Treat affected horses in congestive heart failure with digoxin, furosemide, and vasodilators.

CONTRAINDICATIONS

N/A

PRECAUTIONS

N/A

POSSIBLE INTERACTIONS

N/A

ALTERNATIVE DRUGS

N/A

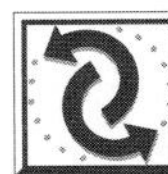

FOLLOW-UP

PATIENT MONITORING

• Frequently monitor cardiac rhythm and respiratory system.
• Annual echocardiographic re-examinations are recommended in moderate to severe cases.

PREVENTION/AVOIDANCE

N/A

POSSIBLE COMPLICATIONS

Chronic cases—atrial fibrillation; congestive heart failure

EXPECTED COURSE AND PROGNOSIS

• Many affected horses have normal performance and life expectancy.
• Prognosis for horses with tricuspid valve prolapse and mild regurgitation is excellent, and in many, the amount of regurgitation remains unchanged for years.
• Progression of regurgitation associated with degenerative valve disease usually is slow. If regurgitation is mild, these horses have a good to excellent prognosis.
• Horses with ruptured chordae tendineae, flail tricuspid valve leaflets, or infective endocarditis have a more guarded prognosis, because the regurgitation usually becomes more severe and may result in a shortened performance and life expectancy.
• Affected horses with congestive heart failure usually have severe underlying valvular heart and myocardial disease and a guarded to grave prognosis for life.
• Most affected horses being treated for congestive heart failure respond to supportive therapy and improve. Such improvement usually is short lived, however. Most of these horses are euthanized within 2–6 mo of initiation of treatment.

MISCELLANEOUS

ASSOCIATED CONDITIONS

Mitral regurgitation

AGE-RELATED FACTORS

• Physiologic regurgitation due to cardiac adaptation to athletic training is the most common form and is usually diagnosed in horses of racing age.
• Old horses are more likely to be affected with severe tricuspid regurgitation.

ZOONOTIC POTENTIAL

N/A

PREGNANCY

• Affected mares should not experience any problems with the pregnancy unless regurgitation is severe.
• The volume expansion of late pregnancy places an additional load on the already volume-loaded heart, which may precipitate congestive heart failure in mares with severe regurgitation.
• Pregnant mares with congestive heart failure should be treated for the underlying cardiac disease with positive inotropic drugs and diuretics.
• ACE inhibitors are contraindicated because of potential adverse effects on the fetus.

SYNONYMS

Tricuspid insufficiency

SEE ALSO

• Atrial fibrillation
• Infective endocarditis
• Mitral regurgitation

ABBREVIATIONS

• ACE = angiotensin-converting enzyme
• CK-MB = MB isoenzyme of creatine kinase
• HBDH = α-hydroxybutyrate dehydrogenase
• LDH = lactate dehydrogenase

Suggested Reading

Gardner SY, Reef VB, Spencer PA. Ultrasonographic evaluation of 46 horses with jugular vein thrombophlebitis: 1985–1988. J Am Vet Med Assoc 1991;199:370–373.
Patteson MW, Cripps PJ. A survey of cardiac auscultatory findings in horses. Equine Vet J 1993;25:409–416.
Reef VB. Heart murmurs in horses: determining their significance with echocardiography. Equine Vet J 1995;19(suppl):71–80.
Reef VB. Cardiovascular ultrasonography. In: Reef VB, ed. Equine Diagnostic Ultrasound. Philadelphia: WB Saunders, 1998:215–272.
Young LE, Wood JL. Effect of age and training on murmurs of atrioventricular valvular regurgitation in young thoroughbreds. Equine Vet J. 2000;32:195–199.

Author Virginia B. Reef
Consulting Editor Celia M. Marr

TRIFOLIUM HYBRIDIUM (ALSIKE CLOVER) TOXICOSIS

BASICS

OVERVIEW

• *Trifolium hybridum* (alsike clover) has been implicated as the cause of equine hepatic failure and neurologic impairment. • Clinical manifestations of intoxication are acute and neurologic or chronic and cachectic.
• Postmortem histopathological lesions consistently are found in the liver and include biliary fibrosis and marked bile duct proliferation. • Occurrence of the two syndromes is associated with ingestion of alsike clover, but a specific toxin has not been identified. • Photosensitization can occur in conjunction with both syndromes but is uncommon. • Morbidity varies, but mortality is high. • A reversible, alsike clover–induced photosensitization has been described and is considered by some to be unrelated to the other two syndromes.

SIGNALMENT

• When both syndromes are considered together, there are no apparent breed, age, or sex predispositions; however, a retrospective study of alsike clover–associated disease suggested the nervous form occurs more commonly in old, female horses. • Not all horses in an exposed group develop clinical signs.

SIGNS

• Acute and neurologic—alternating depression and excitement, head pressing, aimless walking, incoordination, yawning and bruxism, coma, and death • Chronic and cachectic—variable appetite, progressive loss of body condition, weakness, sluggishness, dry and rough haircoat, icterus, yawning, head pressing, and periodic excitement preceding sudden death
• Photosensitization—skin erythema and swelling, pruritus, exudation of serum, hair matting, skin exfoliation, lacrimation, conjunctivitis, photophobia, and keratitis

CAUSES AND RISK FACTORS

• The disease is associated with ingestion of alsike clover–containing pasture or hay.
• Alsike clover is believed to be less palatable than other forages and horses on pasture may eat less if alternative plants are available.
• The ability of horses to avoid alsike clover in hay is less than those on pasture; thus, horses fed alsike clover–containing hay may ingest more of the plant.

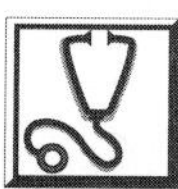

DIAGNOSIS

DIFFERENTIAL DIAGNOSIS

• Ingestion of plants containing pyrrolizidine alkaloids—evidence of consumption; characteristic histopathologic lesions
• Locoism (*Astragalus* spp.)—evidence of consumption; characteristic histopathological lesions • *Equisetum arvense* (horsetail) or *Pteridium aquilinum* (bracken fern)—evidence of consumption; response to thiamine administration
• Fumonisin mycotoxins—detection in feed; characteristic gross and histopathological brain lesions
• Rabies—fluorescent antibody test on brain tissue
• EPM—CSF evaluation; characteristic histopathologic lesions; response to treatment
• Viral encephalitides—CSF evaluation; serology; histologic evaluation of brain
• Brain abscesses or meningitis—clinical signs; CSF evaluation; gross or histopathological examination
• Narcolepsy—EEG; response to drug administration
• Other causes of liver disease, with or without hepatoencephalopathy

CBC/BIOCHEMISTRY/URINALYSIS

Clinicopathological changes have not been described in most suspected cases, but one had elevated serum SD and AP and blood ammonia concentrations.

OTHER LABORATORY TESTS

• CSF—normal
• Serology—normal

IMAGING

Ultrasonography—enlarged and irregular liver

DIAGNOSTIC PROCEDURES

Liver biopsy can be useful in differentiating alsike clover toxicosis from other liver diseases.

PATHOLOGICAL FINDINGS

Gross

• Enlarged and irregular liver
• Some fibrosis may be evident.
• Icterus is variable.

Histopathological

• Hepatic lesions include fibrosis of portal triads and around proliferating biliary epithelium.
• Inflammatory changes—uncommon

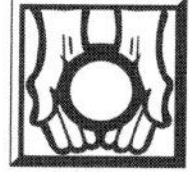

TREATMENT

• Treat photosensitivity by preventing sun exposure.
• Remove animal from the source of exposure to the plant.
• Treatment of the hepatic and nervous syndromes commonly is unrewarding.
• Symptomatic and supportive care including sedation for nervous syndrome, balanced electrolyte fluid administration, correction of hypoglycemia if present, and treatment of liver failure and hyperammonemia
• If the animal is eating, small meals given frequently are suggested.
• Diet should provide adequate energy and limited protein, primarily as branched-chain amino acids.

MEDICATIONS

DRUGS

• Sedation—xylazine (0.3–0.5 mg/kg IV as needed)
• Hyperammonemia—neomycin (20–30 mg/kg PO q6h) or lactulose (90–120 mL PO q6h–q8h)
• Energy provision—continuous 5% or 10% dextrose drip (2 or 1 mL/kg/hr IV, respectively)

CONTRAINDICATIONS/POSSIBLE INTERACTIONS

• Diazepam is contraindicated in hepatoencephalopathy.
• Use care when administering drugs requiring hepatic metabolism for activity or elimination.

FOLLOW-UP

PATIENT MONITORING

Monitor hepatic function.

PREVENTION/AVOIDANCE

Because the conditions under which animals are intoxicated are poorly defined, the only specific recommendation is to prevent horses from ingesting alsike clover.

POSSIBLE COMPLICATIONS

N/A

EXPECTED COURSE AND PROGNOSIS

• Recovery from hepatic and neurologic syndromes is unlikely.
• Recovery from uncomplicated photosensitization is expected with appropriate treatment.

MISCELLANEOUS

ASSOCIATED CONDITIONS, AGE-RELATED FACTORS, ZOONOTIC POTENTIAL, PREGNANCY

N/A

SEE ALSO

N/A

ABBREVIATIONS

• AP = alkaline phosphatase
• CSF = cerebrospinal fluid
• EEG = electroencephalography
• EPM = equine protozoal myelitis
• SD = sorbitol dehydrogenase

Suggested Reading

Nation PN. Hepatic disease in Alberta horses: a retrospective study of "alsike clover poisoning" (1973–1988). Can Vet J 1991;32:602–607.

Author Robert H. Poppenga
Consulting Editor Robert H. Poppenga

TROPANE ALKALOIDS

BASICS

OVERVIEW

- Tropane alkaloids include hyoscyamine, hyoscine, atropine, and scopolamine.
- Tropane alkaloids act as competitive antagonists to acetylcholine at the muscarinic receptors (antimuscarinic).
- Tropane alkaloid-containing plants include *Datura stramonium* (jimsonweed), *Atropa belladonna* (belladonna), and *Hyoscyamus niger* (henbane).
- All parts of the plant should be considered toxic, especially the seeds that accumulate higher amounts of the toxins.
- Horses have been poisoned through ingestion of *Datura* seeds or *Datura*-contaminated hay.
- Due to the plant's particular odor and taste, animals seldom are poisoned by direct consumption of the fresh plant.
- The toxic effects include gastrointestinal signs, neurological signs, teratogenic effects, and death.

SIGNALMENT

No known breed, age or sex predispositions

SIGNS

- Mildly elevated rectal temperature
- Tachypnea (shallow breathing, nostrils wide open)
- Tachycardia (may have a weak pulse) due to removal of the parasympathetic tone
- Mydriasis and diffusely reddened conjunctiva
- Anorexia, lack of thirst, defecation, and urination
- Dry mucosae (oral, nasal, vaginal, and rectal)
- Hyperesthesia and/or ataxia
- Colic, with signs of abdominal pain, anxiety, and increased borborygmi
- Intestinal gas accumulation due to ileus

In more severe cases:

- Lateral recumbency accompanied by kicking
- Sweating
- Bruxism
- Seizures
- Respiratory failure
- Death

CAUSES AND RISK FACTORS

- There is a lack of information about the toxic levels of *Datura* in horses.
- Toxic dose is estimated to be about 0.75 mg seeds/kg body weight, equivalent to 0·5% of *Datura* seeds in the feed, over a period of 10 days.
- Contamination of feed with about 25% by volume of *Datura* can to be sufficient to induce peracute signs of poisoning and death in horses.

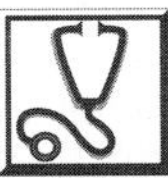

DIAGNOSIS

DIFFERENTIAL DIAGNOSIS

Causes of colic

CBC/BIOCHEMISTRY/URINALYSIS

N/A

OTHER LABORATORY TESTS

N/A

IMAGING

N/A

OTHER DIAGNOSTIC PROCEDURES

Analysis of GI contents or urine for tropane alkaloids

PATHOLOGICAL FINDINGS

Gross

- Gastrointestinal irritation and diarrhea with or without hemorrhages
- Ruptured diaphragm
- Intestinal and gastric gas accumulation
- Plant parts in stomach

Microscopic

- Hyperemic mesenteric blood vessels
- Petecial hemorrhages on mesenteric and intestinal serosa

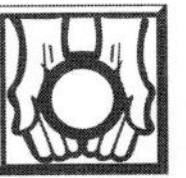

TREATMENT

- Remove the source of exposure.
- Gastric lavage in cases of acute exposure
- Activated charcoal through nasogastric intubation
- Symptomatic and supportive care

MEDICATIONS

DRUG(S)

- Activated charcoal 1–4 g/kg PO in water slurry (1 g of activated charcoal in 5 mL of water)
- If no diarrhea or ileus, then 1 dose of cathartic should be given orally (70% sorbitol at 3 mL/kg or sodium or magnesium sulfate at 250–500 mg/kg as a 20% solution in water).
- NDAIDs—flunixin meglumine (0.1 mg/kg IV or IM as necessary)
- Diazepam (0.05–0.4 mg/kg IV for foals; 25–50 mg IV for adult horses) for controlling seizures. Repeat in 30 min if necessary.

CONTRAINDICATIONS/POSSIBLE INTERACTIONS

- Avoid stressing or stimulating the horse.
- Do not give activated charcoal with mineral oil because oil can potentially prevent binding of the alkaloids to the activated charcoal.

FOLLOW-UP

PATIENT MONITORING

Monitor hydration status and behavior.

PREVENTION/AVOIDANCE

Avoid exposure of the horses to tropane alkaloid–containing plants.

POSSIBLE COMPLICATIONS

- Colic
- Intestinal or diaphragmatic rupture

EXPECTED COURSE AND PROGNOSIS

- Course of the disease may be as short as minutes or hours and is usually less than 2–5 days (unless there is continuing exposure).
- The prognosis is favorable if, during the recovery from intoxication, polydipsia, polyuria, and frequent defecation are observed.
- With severe clinical signs, the prognosis is guarded.

MISCELLANEOUS

ASSOCIATED CONDITIONS

N/A

AGE-RELATED FACTORS

N/A

ZOONOTIC POTENTIAL

N/A

PREGNANCY

Plants containing high amounts of scopolamine can be potentially teratogenic; risk of teratogenesis is unclear.

SEE ALSO

N/A

Suggested Reading

Burrows GE, Tyrl RJ. Toxic Plants of North America. Ames, IA: Iowa State University Press, 2001:1113.

Author Asheesh K. Tiwary
Consulting Editor Robert H. Poppenga

TRYPANOSOMIASIS

BASICS

OVERVIEW

• Blood-borne parasitic disease, subtropical and tropical climates. • Several species of trypanosomes, differentiated by clinical disease, morphology, and country of origin. • Genetic techniques will likely re-organize these parasites. • *Trypanosoma congolense, T. evansi, T. vivax*, and *T. brucei brucei* all infect horses. • Disease organized into New (South and Central America) or Old World animal trypanosomiasis (Africa and Asia), by disease presentation (surra, dourine, and African animal trypanosomiasis), or by parasite-vector relationships. • *T. evansi, T. equinum*: surra, mal de caderas • *T. congolense, T. vivax, T. brucei brucei*: tsetse fly disease, African animal trypanosomiasis, nagana, sleeping sickness • *T. equiperdum*: dourine, quite possibly a strain or subspecies of either *T. evansi* or *T. brucei brucei* • Hallmark: hemic/lymphatic/immune system disease and secondary effect on hepatobiliary, nervous, ophthalmic, renal, reproductive systems • Some species directly infect reproductive tract

SIGNALMENT

• No known sex, age, or breed predilection
• Horses, mules, and donkey • More severe disease in horses • For venereal disease: donkeys are likely reservoir
  ○ Light breeds more susceptible and develop more severe disease ○ Indigenous breeds less susceptible
• Females have less mortality than males

SIGNS

General Signs

• Icterus, mucous membrane pallor, lymphadenopathy, splenomegaly • Direct ocular infection: edema, hyperemia, and petechiation of conjunctiva • Clinical signs are cyclical

Surra (mal de caderas)

• Variable: inapparent to overt clinical signs
• Onset varies from acute to chronic and insidious
• Primarily fever, progressive anemia, weight loss, despite good appetite • Urticaria with edematous plaques on ventral abdomen, distal limb edema and petechial hemorrhages
• Neurological signs: weakness and ataxia
• Reproductive signs: stillbirth and abortion

African Animal Trypanosomiasis

• Initial infection of skin with chancre
• Anemia, intermittent fever, edema, weight loss
• Neurologic signs: common with *T. brucei*
• Reproductive signs: Abortion infertility

CAUSES AND RISK FACTORS

Surra

• *Trypanosoma evansi*: host adapted with acute to chronic forms • Disease present in horses and camels, but also seen in cattle, buffalo, llamas, dogs, cats, sheep, goats, pigs, and elephants.
• Found in South America, northern Africa, Middle East, Asia, Indonesia, Philippines
• Transmitted mechanically by biting flies (*Tabanus* and *Stomoxys*) • Likely transmitted by vampire bats (*Desmodus rotundus, Diphylla ecaudata, Diaemus youngi*) • New emergence has high mortality • *T. equiperdum* (dourine): indistinguishable by diagnostic testing from *T. evansi*

African Animal Trypanosomiasis

• *T. vivax*—moderate to severe disease • *T. congolense*—mild, peripheral edema • *T. brucei*—peripheral and scrotal edema; relapse with CNS infection common despite treatment
• Risk: range of the tsetse fly infected areas of Africa extending from the southern edge of the Sahara to Angola, Zimbabwe, and Mozambique.
• Disease in horses severe, disease in donkeys chronic • Cattle likely reservoir • Etiologic agents: *T. congolense, T. vivax, T. brucei*
• Transmitted by the biological vector *Glossina* spp. (tsetse fly) • Other mechanical vectors: *Tabanus, Haematopota, Liperosia, Stomoxys, Chrysops* • Hippobosid flies implicated in spread of *T. brucei* beyond African tsetse fly range • Incubation varies between species but generally 4 to 14 days. • Transmitted transplacentally but not colostrally • Foals seropositive after suckling, but seronegative by 4–5 months of age if not infected

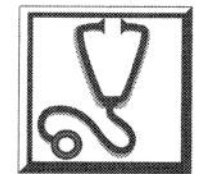

DIAGNOSIS

DIFFERENTIAL DIAGNOSES

Trypanosomiasis, Anemia, Vasculitis, Edema

• Equine infectious anemia virus: cyclical fevers, anemia, thrombocytopenia • Equine viral arteritis: edema, vasculitis, fever • African horse sickness • *Babesia caballi, Babesia equi* (equine piroplasmosis): cyclical fever, anemia, thrombocytopenia • *Leptospira interrogans*: mostly in young animals, although adult disease occurs sporadically • *Anaplasma phagocytophila*
• Systemic clostridial infections • Immune medicate hemolytic anemia (extravascular): usually not febrile, edema limited • Heinz body anemia • Purpura hemorrhagica: vasculitis, fever

CNS Disease

• Flaviviral encephalitis
  ○ West Nile virus ○ Japanese encephalitis virus
• Alphaviral encephalitis
  ○ Eastern, Western, Venezuelan equine encephalitis virus ○ Ross River virus ○ Getah virus

Dourine

• Vesicular exanthema • Equine herpesvirus 3

CBC/BIOCHEMISTRY/URINALYSIS

• Decreased PCV • Decreased erythrocyte count
• Decreased hemoglobin • Leukopenia, neutropenia, lymphocytosis, monocytosis
• Thrombocytopenia • Metabolic acidosis
• Hyperbilirubinemia • Hyperglobulinemia
• Hypoalbuminemia • Increased BUN

OTHER LABORATORY TESTS

• Antibody and antigen detection methods for other infectious diseases • Crystal violet or new methylene blue stain for Heinz bodies • Clotting profile

DIAGNOSTIC PROCEDURES

• Thick/thin smears of Giemsa or Leish-stained blood smears or lymph nodes aspirates
• Hematocrit centrifuge technique for detection of trypanosomes—better for chronic infection. Mouse inoculation—parasitemia detected within 48–72 hours. • Organism detected within tissues
• Antigen and antibody based ELISA's, card agglutination, IFA, CFT are available in a variety of laboratories • For many tests, sensitivity and specificity for equine infection not established
• CFT can not differentiate *T. equiperdum* from *T. evansi, T. gambiense*, or *T. brucei*.

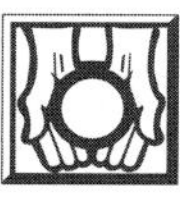

TREATMENT

• Supportive care • Blood transfusion
• Intravenous fluids

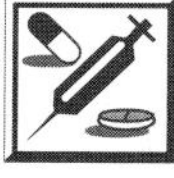

MEDICATIONS

• Suramin (Germanin®): polysulphonated naphthylurea receptor antagonist with antiparasitic and antitumor activities.
• Quinapyramine sulfate: acute and chronic infections, but many adverse local reactions
• Isometamidium chloride • Melarsen oxide: CNS infection • Diminazene: side effects common

FOLLOW-UP

• Re-infection common; limited long term immunity • Monitor PCV, appetite/weight loss, rectal temperature

PREVENTION/AVOIDANCE

• Prevention only with continuous chemotherapy
  ○ Quinapyramine salt ○ Combination suramine and diminazene
• Segregation, quarantine, vector control

MISCELLANEOUS

ZOONOTIC POTENTIAL

None known for animal trypanosomiasis

PREGNANCY

Abortion

SEE ALSO

• African horse sickness • Infectious anemia
• Erhlichiosis, Equine granulocytic • Babesiosis
• Clostridal myositis • Dourine • Eastern/Western equine encephalitis virus
• Equine infectious anemia virus • Equine viral arteritis • Heinz body anemia • Immune mediated hemolytic anemia • Leptospirosis
• Purpura hemorrhagica • West Nile virus

ABBREVIATIONS

• ELISA = enzyme-linked immunosorbent assay
• CFT = complement fixation test
• IFA = immunofluorescent assay

Suggested Reading

http://www.oie.int/fr/normes/mmanual/a_00066.htm

Author: Maureen T. Long
Consulting Editors: Ashley Boyle and Corinne Sweeney

TUBERCULOSIS

BASICS

OVERVIEW

Tuberculosis is a rare infection in the horse. Most cases are related to infection with *Mycobacterium bovis,* although some reported cases have been caused by *M. avium-* complex. No specific syndromes have been described.

SIGNALMENT

There is no apparent age or breed predilection.

SIGNS

Signs are variable, and relate to the system or systems involved. The infections are chronic and slowly progressive. An intermittent fever may be recorded. Weight loss is a common feature. In primary pulmonary cases varying degrees of dyspnea may be present, and in some cases cough and nasal discharge may also be observed. Infection of cervical vertebrae and neurologic signs consistent with a cervical spinal cord lesion have been described. In some horses with granulomatous enteritis, *M. avium* has been identified in the feces or the intestinal tissues. These latter horses have clinical signs of malabsorption or protein-losing enteropathy or both.

CAUSES AND RISK FACTORS

No specific risk factors have been identified. Cases are too rare and sporadic to establish any particular pattern.

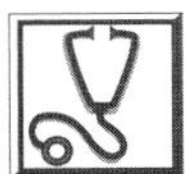

DIAGNOSIS

DIFFERENTIAL DIAGNOSIS

As the infection can occur at almost any site, tuberculosis can be considered as a differential diagnosis in almost any chronic progressive disease of the horse. It is, however, rare, and therefore should be low on the list for most of these syndromes.

CBC/BIOCHEMISRY/URINALYSIS

There are no specific clinical pathology data typical for this disease in horses. Hematology may be consistent with a chronic inflammatory process, (i.e., neutrophilia, hyperfibrinogenemia, and anemia). Other laboratory abnormalities may be observed depending on the organ system(s) involved.

OTHER LABORATORY TESTS

Results of tuberculin testing in horses are variable and the tests are considered to be unreliable for diagnostic purposes. Many false positives occur, and the tuberculin may induce an anaphylactic response. Identification of the organisms in aspirates or biopsies using acid-fast staining is strongly supportive of a diagnosis of equine tuberculosis.

IMAGING

Depending on the region of the body affected, radiography or ultrasonography or both may demonstrate the nature and extent of the infection. For example, miliary lesions have been described in the lung, and these provide a very suggestive radiographic image.

DIAGNOSTIC PROCEDURES

Biopsies of affected organs may be indicated to determine the nature of the lesions, and collection of exudate (e.g., by transtracheal aspiration or bronchoalveolar lavage) is indicated in specific cases.

PATHOLOGIC FINDINGS

Multiple lesions are often present in a variety of organs, particularly in lymph nodes and spleen. Involvement of bone is said to be more frequent in horses than cattle. Lesions tend to be firm in all tissues, and may appear to be neoplastic. Histopathologic evaluation is needed to confirm the diagnosis.

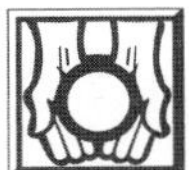

TREATMENT

There is no effective treatment for equine tuberculosis.

MEDICATIONS

DRUG(S) OF CHOICE

There does not appear to be any reports of successful treatment of confirmed cases of equine tuberculosis. Drugs used in other species (isoniazid, rifampin, streptomycin, etc.) could be considered, but there are no guidelines for their use in the horse for this condition. Based on experiences in human medicine it would be expected that therapy, if attempted in an equine case, would have to be given for several months or even a year or more.

CONTRAINDICATIONS/POSSIBLE INTERACTIONS

N/A

FOLLOW-UP

N/A

EXPECTED COURSE AND PROGNOSIS

As therapy is not usually a viable option, the prognosis for established cases is hopeless, and a recommendation for euthanasia would be appropriate.

MISCELLANEOUS

ZOONOTIC POTENTIAL

This is a potential zoonosis, particularly to immunocompromised persons. If a confirmed case is to be kept alive, either to attempt treatment or for other reasons (e.g., for an affected mare to foal), then specific cautions should be issued to the owner and handlers. It would be prudent to seek permission to advise appropriate health-care workers of the situation.

Suggested Reading

No review of the subject is available.

Author Christopher M. Brown

Consulting Editors Ashley Boyle and Corinne R. Sweeney

TUMORS OF RESPIRATORY SYSTEM

BASICS

OVERVIEW

• Tumors of the respiratory system are most commonly located in the thoracic or sinusal/parasinusal structures. Nonrespiratory thoracic tumors (mediastinal lymphosarcomas and tumors of the thymus for example) are not included in this section. • Incidence is very low—Neoplasia involving thoracic cavity in a necropsy study: 35 of 5629 (0.62%). Primary lung tumors are even less common: an abattoir survey reported 2 of 1308 horses. • Although rare, the most frequent primary lung tumor is the granular cell tumor (or myoblastoma). They may be accompanied by osteoproliferative abnormalities of carpal, tarsal, and fetlock joints. • Lung is a relative frequent site for secondary metastases from lymphosarcoma, adenocarcinoma, squamous cell carcinoma and hemangiosarcoma from other organs. • From 50% to 68% of the nasal passage tumors are malignant with squamous cell carcinoma being the most frequent. Squamous cell carcinoma originates from mucosal or alveolar teeth epithelium and start invading locally before metastasizing regionally (larynx, ocular, oral cavity).

SIGNALMENT

• Nasal/paranasal tumors—Squamous cell carcinoma (most frequent): usually mature adults, more frequent in aged horses, but also found in young animals. Mean age 8–12.4 years. • Primary pulmonary tumors—older than 7 years. Pulmonary granular cell tumor (most frequent): mean age 13 years, range 8–22 years • Lung metastases from distant primary tumors—mean age 8 years, range 3 months to 14 years • Sex predilection—Majority of cases reported for pulmonary granular cell tumor are females. Majority of males for intrathoracic metastatic adenocarcinoma. • No breed predilection • No genetic basis reported

SIGNS

Historical

• Weight loss • Dullness • Exercise intolerance
• Intermittent fever

Physical Examination

- Thoracic respiratory tumors
  - Underweight
  - Signs of pleural effusion and ventral edema
  - Tachypnea
  - Coughing
  - Dyspnea
  - Hemoptysis
  - Abnormal lung auscultation sounds (wheezes, decreased breath sounds)
  - Pallor, icterus and epistaxis in cases of hemangiosarcoma.
  - Squamous cell carcinoma of the stomach with thoracic metastases does not necessary cause respiratory manifestations.
  - Proliferative osteopathy of carpal, tarsal, fetlock joints rarely seen
- Nasal/parasinusal tumors
  - Nasal discharge (frequent). May be foul smelling
  - Facial deformity for large tumors

CAUSES AND RISK FACTORS

Undetermined

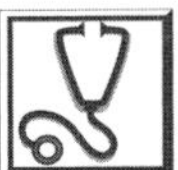

DIAGNOSIS

DIFFERENTIAL DIAGNOSIS

- Thoracic respiratory tumors
  - Chronic inflammatory diseases
  - Heaves
  - Granulomatous pneumonia
  - Squamous cell carcinoma
  - Lymphosarcoma
  - Multisystemic eosinophilic epitheliotropic disease
  - Idiopathic pleuritis
  - Mycotic pneumonia and cryptococcosis
  - Cardiac neoplasia
- Nasal/paranasal tumors
  - Primary sinusitis
  - Nasal inflammatory polyps
  - Progressive ethmoidal hematoma

CBC/BIOCHEMISTRY/URINALYSIS

• CBC—Results depend on the invasiveness of the primary tumor—CBC can be normal, but often inflammatory hemogram (anemia, mature neutrophilia, hyperfibrinogenenaemia).
• Chemistry—No particular abnormalities unless a specific organ is showing functional insufficiency.

OTHER LABORATORY TESTS

• Thoracocentesis—Neoplastic cells can be observed on cytology of the pleural fluid (adenocarcinoma, fibrosarcoma, metastatic squamous cell carcinoma). • Lung biopsy—Preferentially ultrasound-guided to sample a mass. Biopsies can also be performed through an endoscope if a mass is visible in the large airways. • Cytological examination of a transtracheal aspiration may reveal neoplastic cells. • For nasal/paranasal tumors—Biopsy samples obtained deep within the mass is preferable. Superficial samples obtained through the endoscope are often nondiagnostic.

IMAGING

• Head radiography—Nasal/paranasal squamous cell carcinoma: Primarily maxillary and frontal sinuses. Opaque soft tissue. A dorso-ventral view is useful. • Thorax radiography—Pulmonary tumors: Mass of soft tissues density in the lung (single large mass or several smaller nodules). Some cases reported with hypertrophic osteopathy of carpal, tarsal, fetlock joints.
• Thorax ultrasound—Pleural effusion, masses in the lung parenchyma with irregular surface.
• Upper and lower airway endoscopy—Nasal paranasal squamous cell carcinoma: Often ulcerated, and mottled. Pulmonary tumor: Masses in the main bronchi or carina (for granular cell tumor) are occasionally seen.

OTHER DIAGNOSTIC PROCEDURES

Thoracoscopy—To visualize and biopsy masses affecting the pleura or the lung surface

PATHOLOGIC FINDINGS

• Nasal/paranasal squamous cell carcinoma—Classified as well, moderately or poorly differentiated. Degrees of differentiation not correlated with the presence of metastasis. • Lung tumor—Neoplastic cells (large cells with small nucleus and granular cytoplasm) seen at a needle aspiration • Pulmonary granular cell tumor—Most frequent primary pulmonary tumor. Usually affecting one lung side. Local metastases frequently reported • Pulmonary carcinoma—Usually unilateral, caudal lung. Pleomorphic epithelial cells. Rarely metastasize. • Metastatic hemangiosarcoma—Primary tumor more frequently in skeletal muscle or skin
• Metastatic squamous cell carcinoma—Primary tumor more frequently in the stomach, but also on the penis, vulva, and eye.

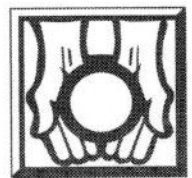

TREATMENT

• Lung neoplasm—lung mass and lung resection have been attempted. • Nasal/paranasal mass removal—Often malignant with risks of recurrence and metastasis

MEDICATIONS

None

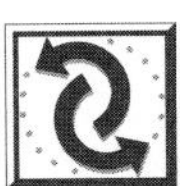

FOLLOW-UP

PATIENT MONITORING

Improvement in attitude, clinical signs (e.g. breathing effort, nasal discharge), and weight gain can be observed when nasal/paranasal mass is removed successfully.

EXPECTED COURSE AND PROGNOSIS

Grave for lung tumors and malignant nasal passage tumors with a short life expectancy after diagnosis.

MISCELLANEOUS

ASSOCIATED CONDITIONS

• Primary neoplasms when lung metastases are present • Some cases of proliferative osteopathy of carpal, tarsal, fetlock joints

Suggested Reading

Facemire PR, Chilcoat CD, et al. Treatment of granular cell tumor via complete right lung resection in a horse. JAVMA 2000;217:1522–1525.
Heinola T, Heikkila M, et al. Hypertrophic pulmonary osteopathy associated with granular cell tumour in a mare. Vet Rec 2001;149:307–308.
Ohnesorge B, Gehlen H, et al. Transendoscopic electrosurgery of an equine pulmonary granular cell tumor. Vet Surg 2002;31:375–378.
Pusterla N, Norris AJ, et al. Granular cell tumours in the lungs of three horses. Vet Rec 2003;153:530–532.
Scarratt KW, Crisman MV. Neoplasia of the respiratory tract. Vet Clin North Am Equine Pract 1998;143:451–473.

Author Renaud Leguillette
Consulting Editor Daniel Jean

TWIN PREGNANCY

BASICS

DEFINITION/OVERVIEW

The simultaneous intrauterine production of two or more embryos/fetuses

ETIOLOGY/PATHOPHYSIOLOGY

- The majority of multiple pregnancies in the mare are twins.
  - Most twins are dizygotic and result from double ovulations.
  - Early twin vesicles behave similarly to a singleton conceptus.
  - The vesicles undergo transuterine migration until 15 days of gestation, when fixation occurs in one or both uterine horns at approximately day 16–17 of gestation.
  - Approximately 75% of twin vesicles fix in the same horn (unicornual).
- Approximately 75% of *unicornual* twin pregnancies <40 days of age undergo natural reduction to one embryo.
  - The remaining embryo develops normally to term as a singleton.
  - If natural reduction of one embryo fails to occur by 40 days of gestation, there is a strong probability that the twins will continue to develop, only to abort later in gestation.
- *Bicornual* twins do not undergo natural reduction. Instead, the twins usually develop through the last trimester of gestation, at which time abortion is common.

SYSTEM AFFECTED

Reproductive

GENETICS

Higher incidence of double ovulations in some breeds of horses

INCIDENCE/PREVALENCE

- The incidence of twin pregnancy is related to age, breed, and reproductive status.
- Twin pregnancy occurs more frequently in older mares, barren mares, Thoroughbreds, and draft breeds.
- Arabians, Quarter Horses, ponies, and primitive breeds are reported to have a lower incidence of twin pregnancy.

SIGNALMENT

Mares that develop twin pregnancies tend to have twins in subsequent pregnancies.

SIGNS

N/A

CAUSES

- Ovulation and fertilization of multiple ova, in most cases
- Rare incidences of monozygotic multiple pregnancies have been reported.

RISK FACTORS

Breed, age, and reproductive status

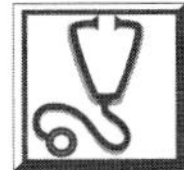

DIAGNOSIS

DIFFERENTIAL DIAGNOSIS

Differentiating Similar Signs

- Uterine cysts can be confused with developing embryonic vesicles causing an improper diagnosis of twin pregnancy.
- Differentiation of uterine cysts from embryonic vesicles may be simplified by recording the location, size, and shape of uterine cysts prior to pregnancy.
- If records are unavailable from a prior season, reexamine the mare in 2 days. The vesicle of pregnancy will demonstrate a noticeable increase in diameter by U/S; the uterine/lymphatic cyst will not increase in that limited period of time.
- Differentiation of an embryonic vesicle from a uterine cyst may also be made with the observation of an embryonic heartbeat present at 24+ days of gestation.

CBC/BIOCHEMISTRY/URINALYSIS

N/A

OTHER LABORATORY TESTS

N/A

OTHER DIAGNOSTIC PROCEDURES

TRP of the Reproductive Tract

- Pregnancy diagnosis by TRP at 25–30 days of gestation is characterized by distinct uterine tone and a narrow, elongated cervix.
- A bulge the size of a small hen's egg can be appreciated at the caudoventral aspect of a uterine horn, adjacent to the uterine bifurcation.
- If twin vesicles of pregnancy are bicornual in location, it may be possible to diagnose twin pregnancies at this time.
- If the vesicles of pregnancy are unicornual in location, it is impossible to determine the presence of twin pregnancy using TRP alone, but an experienced practitioner may note the bulge of pregnancy seems to be larger than anticipated.

IMAGING

Transrectal U/S

- U/S examination of the reproductive tract early in gestation allows for prompt diagnosis and treatment of twin pregnancies.
- Pregnancies may be detected as early as day 9 of gestation; however, twin pregnancies may differ in age by as much as 2 days.
- Due to the possible differences in age and size of twin pregnancies, U/S diagnosis of twins is recommended between 13 and 15 days of gestation.
- The embryonic vesicle(s) at this time is an anechoic, spherical yolk sac that averages between 12 and 20 mm in height.
- Twin vesicles are highly mobile for the first 15–16 days and can be located adjacent to one another or in different locations within the uterus.
- To properly determine if twin vesicles are present, it is critical to scan both uterine horns and the uterine body to the cervix, sequentially, with at least two full sweeps across the tract.

Transabdominal U/S

- Transabdominal U/S is useful for diagnosing twin pregnancies at >75 to 100 days of gestation.
- Diagnosis is generally made by identification of two fetal heartbeats.

PATHOLOGICAL FINDINGS

N/A

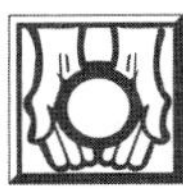

TREATMENT

Management of Twins prior to Day 40 of Gestation

- Twins detected during transuterine migration of the conceptus (days 9–15) are best managed by crushing one embryonic vesicle. One vesicle is manipulated, transrectally, to the tip of a uterine horn. Pressure is placed on the vesicle, and it is crushed.
- The remaining vesicle survives in approximately 90% of the cases.
- The crush technique is useful for twins in the mobility phase and bilateral twins prior to 30 days of gestation.
- After 30 days of gestation, fluid released from the crushed vesicle tends to disrupt the remaining pregnancy.
- Unicornual twins are usually both destroyed when crushing of one vesicle is attempted.

Management of Twins after Day 40 of Gestation

- Management of twin pregnancies in the fetal period (≥day 40) is further complicated by the formation of endometrial cups.
- Pregnancy loss once endometrial cups have formed has been shown to cause irregular estrous cycles and/or delay a return to fertile cycles.
- Consequently, maintenance of a singleton pregnancy following a reduction procedure is critical to the reproductive success of the mare if reduction is done later than day 40.

Alternate Methods of Twin Management That Have Been Attempted Include:

- *Dietary restriction*—In one study, mares with twin pregnancies (diagnosed by TRP) were limited to poor-quality grass hay early in gestation (day 21–49 of gestation).
  - One viable foal (reduction had occurred) was delivered in 56% (23 of 41) of the cases examined.
- *Surgical removal of one twin*—Surgical removal of one twin was attempted in 7 unicornual and 8 bicornual twins at 41–62 days of gestation.
  - None of the unicornual twins survived.
  - Five of eight bicornual twin pregnancies were successfully reduced to a singleton.
- *Intracardiac injection of potassium chloride (KCl)*—Using transcutaneous u/s, one fetal heart is located and fetal death is caused by intracardiac injection of KCl.
  - The technique has been successful in approximately 50% of the cases attempted.
  - This procedure is most useful from 115 to 130 days of gestation.
- *Transvaginal allantocentesis*—Transvaginal U/S has been used to aid in identification of the allantoic sac in one twin fetus, pass a needle into the allantois, and aspirate the allantoic fluid.
  - Aspiration of the fluid causes collapse of the vesicle and fetal death.
  - To date, this technique has been successful in approximately 30% of the attempted cases.
  - The technique is most applicable for bicornual twins.

APPROPRIATE HEALTH CARE
N/A

NURSING CARE
N/A

ACTIVITY
N/A

DIET
See Alternate Methods, above.

CLIENT EDUCATION
- Importance of TRP in the periovulatory period (before and after breeding and insemination), and noting >1 ovulation during an estrus.
- Emphasis of early (latest 16 days following ovulation), serial evaluations of a high-risk mare:
  - Multiple ovulations
  - Prior history of twinning
  - Breeds with higher incidence of twinning
  - Suspicious appearance of vesicle of pregnancy at initial examination warrants follow-up U/S within 2–4 days.
- Earlier reduction of twins (<16 days, prior to fixation) increases likelihood of success—continuation of remaining embryo/fetus to term.

SURGICAL CONSIDERATIONS
N/A

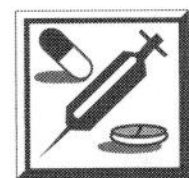

MEDICATIONS

- Flunixin meglumine 1 mg/kg IV is often administered at the time of attempted twin reduction to prevent prostaglandin release from the uterus and subsequent lysis of the CL.
- Exogenous progestins (Altrenogest 1 mL/50 kg body weight [0.044 mg Altrenogest/kg body weight] PO daily) at double the recommended dose (2 mL/50 kg) may be administered when twin reduction is attempted to maintain uterine and cervical tone following uterine manipulation and to counter the effects of possible fetal fluid release into the uterine lumen.

DRUG(S) OF CHOICE
N/A

CONTRAINDICATIONS
Twinning is undesirable in the mare and routinely ends in abortion.

PRECAUTIONS
N/A

POSSIBLE INTERACTIONS
N/A

ALTERNATIVE DRUGS
N/A

FOLLOW-UP

PATIENT MONITORING
- After any method of twin reduction is performed, it is useful to monitor the progress and viability of the remaining embryo/fetus using U/S.
- It is critical to monitor the mare for embryo/fetal death if the mare is being treated with exogenous progestins.
- Once-weekly U/S examinations are warranted for the first 3 weeks following the procedure.
- Less frequent examinations, i.e., once monthly, after the initial examinations, would be useful to monitor fetal progress.
- The mare can also be monitored for signs of abortion such as mammary development, vulvar discharge, or fetal expulsion.

PREVENTION/AVOIDANCE
- Serial, complete TRP and maintenance of individual records for broodmares
- Record sizes of all follicles >30 mm on both ovaries during estrus (average growth is 5–6 mm/day) to account for ovulation or regression.
- Double ovulation—the earliest indicator of mares at higher risk for developing twins
- Early diagnosis of pregnancy in mares from families with a history of twinning, or one known to have twinned in a prior pregnancy (same season or prior years)
- Earlier reduction is associated with greater success in achieving a singleton pregnancy.

POSSIBLE COMPLICATIONS
Embryonic or fetal loss, abortion, dystocia

EXPECTED COURSE AND PROGNOSIS

Success Association with Each Reduction Technique
- 90% success with early crush of a bicornual twin
- 50% with KCl intracardiac injection between days 115–130 of gestation
- 20%–30% with transvaginal aspiration of allantoic fluid from one of bicornual twins

MISCELLANEOUS

ASSOCIATED CONDITIONS, AGE-RELATED FACTORS, ZOONOTIC POTENTIAL, PREGNANCY
N/A

SEE ALSO
- Abortion
- Early embryonic death
- Dystocia and parturient complications
- Placental basics, placentitis

ABBREVIATIONS
- TRP = transrectal palpation
- U/S = ultrasound, ultrasonography

Suggested Reading

Ginther OJ. Reproductive Biology of the Mare, ed 2. Cross Plains: Equiservices, 1992.

Ginther OJ. Ultrasonic Imaging and Reproductive Events in the Mare. Cross Plains: Equiservices, 1986.

Author Margo L. Macpherson
Consulting Editor Carla L. Carleton

TYZZER'S DISEASE (CLOSTRIDIUM PILIFORMIS)

BASICS

OVERVIEW

- A rapidly progressive, highly fatal disease of foals caused by *Clostridium piliformis* (previously *Bacillus piliformis*) characterized by peracute progressive hepatitis
- Worldwide distribution

SIGNALMENT

- Can be sporadic or occur in outbreaks
- Foals of any breed and sex are affected.
- Typically 1–6 weeks old

SIGNS

- Affected foals are usually normal at birth and then develop rapidly progressive signs including nonspecific findings such as lethargy, loss of suckle reflex, diarrhea, and dehydration.
- Tachycardia and tachypnea are common.
- Icterus—mucous membranes may vary from red and injected to profoundly icteric.
- Fever is a common feature, although hypothermia may also be seen.
- Seizure activity is followed by rapid-onset recumbency, weakness, coma, and death.
- Foals are usually found dead without significant premonitory signs.

CAUSES AND RISK FACTORS

- Infectious disease of foals thought to be caused by the ingestion of spore-containing feces from carrier horses with subsequent colonization of the intestine and liver via the portal circulation. This has also been supported with experimental replication of disease in horses.
- The causative agent is *C. piliformis*, a gram-negative, spore-forming, obligate intracellular bacterium found in soil and feces.
- Foals born to nonresident mares and/or mares <6 years old are more likely to develop disease. This is thought to be due to differences in colostral quality and specific protective immunoglobulin.

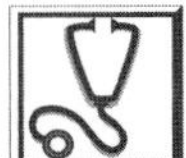

DIAGNOSIS

- Ante-mortem diagnosis is difficult. Presumptive diagnosis may be made on history, physical examination, diagnostic imaging and clinicopathologic data. Definitive ante-mortem diagnosis requires demonstration of *C. piliformis* on liver biopsy.

DIFFERENTIAL DIAGNOSIS

- Neonatal septicemia—usually does not have marked icterus; clinicopathologic features include low IgG and neutropenia.
- Neonatal isoerythrolysis—icterus, but foals have moderate to severe anemia; positive Coomb's test.
- Viral hepatitis (EHV-1)—icterus due to hepatic necrosis is similar; marked leukopenia
- Toxic hepatopathy (rare)—iron toxicity, mycotoxin/leukoencephaolomalacia

CBC/BIOCHEMISTRY/URINALYSIS

- CBC—Many foals will have evidence of hemoconcentration (elevation in PCV), hyperfibrinogenemia and normal to low numbers of blood leukocytes.
- Biochemistry—Hypoglycemia is common. Serum liver enzyme activities are markedly elevated with increases in SDH, GGT, ALP. Serum total, indirect, and direct bilirubin concentrations are also elevated.
- Acid-base—Metabolic acidosis is characterized by low pH, base deficit, and low Tco_2 (or bicarbonate) on venous blood analysis.

OTHER LABORATORY TESTS

- PCR testing has been reported as a diagnostic tool but not commercially available at this time.
- Serologic testing detecting specific antibody using a monoclonal inhibition assay has been described in horses but is also not commercially available.
- Coagulation profiles—Many foals will have prolonged PT and aPTT, increases in fibrin degradation products, and decreases in antithrombin.

IMAGING

- Abdominal radiography may reveal hepatomegaly.
- Transabdominal ultrasound may reveal hepatomegaly with diffuse hyperechogenicity.

OTHER DIAGNOSTIC PROCEDURES

- Percutaneous liver biopsy and demonstration of characteristic histopathologic findings (see later)
- *Clostridium piliformis* is extremely difficult to culture in vitro.

PATHOLOGIC FINDINGS (OPTIONAL)

- Gross pathologic findings include hepatomegaly with multifocal regions of light discoloration and petechiation. Necrotic splenic foci and myocarditis may also be evident.
- These areas represent multifocal to confluent central coagulative necrosis surrounded by degenerate hepatocytes and neutrophilic (suppurative) inflammatory cell migration.
- Confirmation of Tyzzer's disease is achieved by histologic demonstration of intrahepatocellular filamentous bacteria (*C. piliformis*) at the periphery of the lesions within the liver.
- Special staining of histologic sections of liver with Warthin-Starry (a silver stain) will facilitate the visualization of bacteria.

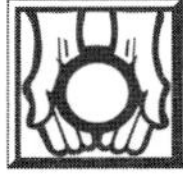

TREATMENT

- There is only a single paper that described the successful confirmation and treatment of this condition in a foal (Borchers 2006).
- Fluid therapy is essential in these cases. Volume resuscitation, glucose provision and electrolytes to assist in correcting metabolic acidosis are indicated.
- Lactated Ringer's solution, Plasmalyte-148 replacement solutions
- Plasmalyte-56, 0.45% sodium chloride maintenance solutions

• Dextrose (2.5%–5% solutions) should be added.
• Sodium bicarbonate supplementation is indicated with acidosis.
• Total or partial parenteral nutrition with vitamin supplementation should be considered for nutritional support.
• If colloid support or immunoglobulin and coagulation factors are needed, plasma transfusion may be given.

MEDICATIONS

DRUG(S) OF CHOICE

• Broad-spectrum antimicrobials are indicated, including gram-negative anaerobic coverage such as penicillin (22,000 IU/kg IV q6h), tetracycline (10 mg/kg IV q12h), erythromycin (25 mg/kg PO q6h), and metronidazole (10 mg/kg PO q2h).
• Seizure management using diazepam (0.1–0.4 mg/kg IV) or midazolam (0.02–0.06 mg/kg/hr CRI) is indicated.
• Ulcer prophylaxis is indicated including omeprazole (4 mg/kg PO q24h) and/or H_2 receptor antagonists (ranitidine 6.6 mg/kg PO q8h). Sucralfate (10 mg/kg PO q6h) may also be used.
• Anti-inflammatory drugs such as ketoprofen (1.1–2.2 mg/kg IV q12h) are indicated.
• Supportive therapies such as vitamin E and selenium can be given.
• Lactulose (0.1–0.25 mL/kg PO q6–8h) may be given to help reduce intestinal ammonia production.

CONTRAINDICATIONS/POSSIBLE INTERACTIONS

• Barbiturates should be given with caution for seizure management given their extensive hepatic metabolism. Benzodiazepines have the potential to worsen hepatoencephalopathy due to potentiation of GABA-induced sedation.
• Metronidazole is given at a lower dose due to reduced hepatic metabolism.

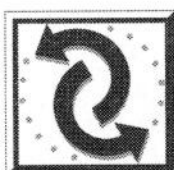

FOLLOW-UP

PATIENT MONITORING

• The average time from the onset of disease to death in nonsurvivors is reported to be 35hr (1–2 days).
• Monitor plasma ammonia, acid-base status, and glucose frequently during therapy.
• Consider decreasing doses of any medication that undergoes hepatic metabolism.

PREVENTION/AVOIDANCE

• None specific. Ensure adequate transfer of passive immunity at birth with an appropriate serum IgG concentration.

POSSIBLE COMPLICATIONS

N/A

EXPECTED COURSE AND PROGNOSIS

• Grave prognosis. Most foals die within 24hr from the onset of clinical signs. Early recognition, referral to an intensive care institution, and therapeutic intervention are required to have any chance of clinical resolution.

MISCELLANEOUS

ASSOCIATED CONDITIONS

N/A

AGE-RELATED FACTORS

N/A

ZOONOTIC POTENTIAL

Unknown zoonotic potential

PREGNANCY

N/A

ABBREVIATIONS

• ALP = alkaline phosphatase
• aPTT = activated partial thromboplastin time
• GABA = γ-aminobutyric acid
• GGT = γ-glutamyl transferase
• PCR = polymerase chain reaction
• PT = prothrombin time
• SDH = serum sorbitol dehydrogenase

Suggested Reading

Borchers A, Magdesian KG, Halland S, Pusterla N, Wilson WD. Successful treatment and polymerase chain reaction (PCR) confirmation of Tyzzer's disease in a foal and clinical and pathologic characteristics of 6 additional foals (1986–2005). J Vet Intern Med 2006;20:1212–1218.

Fosgate GT, Hird DW, Read DH, et al. Risk factors for *Clostridium piliforme* infection in foals. J Am Vet Assoc 2002;220:785–590.

Author Samuel D. A. Hurcombe
Consulting Editor Margaret C. Mudge

ULCERATIVE KERATOMYCOSIS

BASICS

DEFINITION

Keratomycosis is manifest clinically in the horse as ulcerative keratitis, stromal abscessation, and iris prolapse. Ulcerative keratitis refers to a disruption of the corneal epithelium with varying amounts of stromal loss, which may have concurrent bacterial and/or fungal infection. Ulcers infected with fungi range from minor corneal epithelial abrasions/erosions, to superficial plaques, to extremely deep and severe, interstitial keratitis.

PATHOPHYSIOLOGY

- Fungi are normal inhabitants of the equine conjunctival microflora, but can become pathogenic following corneal injury. Fungal organisms are ubiquitous in the equine environment, although regional geographic differences undoubtedly exist to account for variation in the presence of particular fungal species to specific regions. Exposure to vegetative material (hay, grasses, shavings, straw) and dust in the horse environment may influence exposure to fungi.
- The pathogenesis of ulcerative fungal keratitis commonly begins with corneal trauma resulting in an epithelial defect and stromal invasion by the commensal fungal organism or seeding of fungi from a foreign body of plant origin. Tear film instability also predisposes to fungal keratitis or is induced by the fungi prior to fungal attachment and invasion. Stromal destruction results from the release of proteases and other enzymes from the fungi, leukocytes, and keratocytes. Fungi appear to have an affinity for Descemet's membrane, with hyphae frequently found deep in the equine cornea. Deeper corneal invasion by the fungi can lead to sterile or infectious endophthalmitis.

SYSTEM AFFECTED

Ophthalmic

GENETICS

NA

INCIDENCE/PREVALENCE

Keratomycosis is much more common and the diseases are more aggressive in warm climates.

SIGNALMENT

All ages and breeds of horses may be affected.

SIGNS

- Clinical signs associated with equine ulcerative keratomycosis include miosis, blepharospasm, epiphora, and photophobia.
- Slight droopiness of the eyelashes of the upper eyelid may be a subtle sign of corneal ulceration.
- The cornea can be dry in appearance, or display cellular invasion with varying amounts of vascularization.

CAUSES

Septate filamentous fungi associated with ulcerative keratomycosis include several species common to the equine eye (*Fusarium, Aspergillus, Penicillium*).

RISK FACTORS

- Horses may be more susceptible to fungal corneal invasion and infection due to the large surface area and prominence of the equine eye and some weakness in the corneal immune system.
- Topical antibiotic and/or corticosteroid therapy of a noninfected corneal ulcer may predispose to fungal colony invasion and colonization.

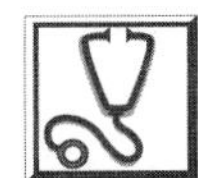

DIAGNOSIS

DIFFERENTIAL DIAGNOSIS

Ocular pain may also be found with bacterial corneal ulcers, uveitis, conjunctivitis, glaucoma, blepharitis, and dacryocystitis.

CBC/BIOCHEMISTRY/URINALYSIS

N/A

OTHER LABORATORY TESTS

N/A

IMAGING

N/A

DIAGNOSTIC PROCEDURES

The diagnosis of keratomycosis is based on finding fungal hyphae, mold, or yeast on at least one of the following: (1) cytologic examination of a corneal scraping, (2) culture of the corneal lesion, (3) polymerase chain reaction of corneal cytologic specimens, or (4) surgical histopathologic examination of a keratectomy specimen.

PATHOLOGIC FINDINGS

- Fungi show marked affinity for the deep corneal stroma and Descemet's membrane.
- Hyphae are often found with neutrophils in the stroma and are rarely found free in the anterior chamber.

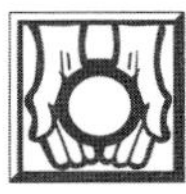

TREATMENT

ACTIVITY

- Horses with keratomycosis and secondary uveitis should be stall-rested until the condition is healed.
- Intraocular hemorrhage and increased severity of uveitis are sequelae to overexertion.

DIET

Diet should be consistent with the training level of the horse.

CLIENT EDUCATION

- Ulcerative keratomycosis is a serious, sight-threatening disease in the horse.
- Long duration of antifungal drug exposure is required for complete fungal destruction and resolution of the clinical signs.

SURGICAL CONSIDERATIONS

- Combined medical and surgical therapy is indicated if ulcers are extremely deep, if they are not responding to medical treatment, or if they worsen despite medical treatment.
- Surgeries for keratomycosis include conjunctival pedicle grafts, bridge grafts, hood grafts, island grafts, and full- and split-thickness penetrating keratoplasty. While surgical treatment may leave the horse with a larger scar, bulbar conjunctival grafts usually prevent corneal rupture and allow for physical support, a regional blood supply, and a supply of endogenous antiproteases to the ulcer site.

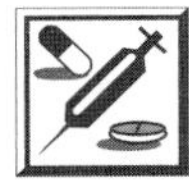

MEDICATIONS

DRUG(S) OF CHOICE

- Treatment must be directed against the fungi, as well as against the corneal and intraocular inflammatory responses that occur following fungal replication and hyphal death.
- Miconazole (1%) has been used successfully and frequently as a topical antifungal agent. The intravenous form is preferred, but the vaginal product may be used.
- Natamycin is employed topically in horses and is very effective against *Fusarium* and *Aspergillus*.
- Amphotericin B (1.5 mg/mL) may be administered topically.
- Silver sulfadiazine is a topical antimicrobial agent with both antifungal and antibacterial activity that is believed to be fungicidal and is used in horses' eyes. It is not effective in some geographic areas.
- Dilute (1:50) povidone-iodine is effective topically against *Fusarium* isolates.
- Itraconazole, voriconazole, and fluconazole are being used successfully topically for keratomycosis in horses.
- Topically administered antifungal therapy for equine keratomycosis is administered 3–4 times per day the first few days. This treatment frequency was determined empirically as the intensity of the iridocyclitis was often noted to be dramatically magnified the day following topical antifungal drug administration at drug treatment frequencies higher than this. Sudden death of stromal fungi due to initiation of antifungal drug therapy can result in acute iridocyclitis. Topical antifungal medications are then increased to 6 times per day on subsequent days.

• Corneal ulcerations result in massive increases in tear film protease activity. Topical serum and topical EDTA are critical to speed healing. They should be administered as many times a day as possible.
• Iridocyclitis is present any time a horse has a corneal ulcer, and can escalate in intensity following hyphal death after antifungal therapy is initiated. Flunixin meglumine (1 mg/kg BID IV, IM, PO) is the most frequently used NSAID in horses for systemic treatment of iridocyclitis. It may also reduce the speed of corneal vascularization.
• One percent atropine sulfate, a parasympatholytic agent, is used in all cases for its mydriatic and cycloplegic effects to dilate the pupil and diminish ciliary body muscle spasms associated with the axon reflex uveitis that occurs with corneal ulceration in the horse. It may be administered q4h until the pupil is dilated, and then the frequency of administration reduced.

CONTRAINDICATIONS, PRECAUTIONS, POSSIBLE INTERACTIONS, ALTERNATIVE DRUGS

N/A

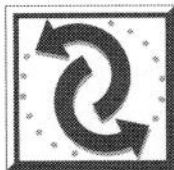

FOLLOW-UP

PATIENT MONITORING

• The horse should be protected from self-trauma with hard- or soft-cup hoods.
• Patients should be monitored for colic and persistent signs of eye pain.

PREVENTION/AVOIDANCE

N/A

POSSIBLE COMPLICATIONS

• Persistent pain, uveitis, endophthalmitis, and blindness are complications.
• Topically administered atropine must be used cautiously in horses as it may predispose some horses to colic.

EXPECTED COURSE AND PROGNOSIS

• Vision following keratomycosis in horses may be retained in as few as 50% of the eyes if treatment is not aggressive.
• Aggressive medical and surgical therapy for ulcerative keratomycosis in horses should, however, result in a positive visual outcome and ocular survival in over 90% of the eyes. Despite this success, therapy is quite prolonged and scarring of the cornea may be prominent.
• Enucleation may be necessary in horses that become blind and continue to experience ocular pain.

MISCELLANEOUS

ASSOCIATED CONDITIONS

Severe uveitis

AGE-RELATED FACTORS, ZOONOTIC POTENTIAL, PREGNANCY, SYNONYMS

N/A

SEE ALSO

Corneal ulceration

Suggested Reading

Brooks DE. Ophthalmology for the Equine Practitioner. Jackson, WY; Teton NewMedia, 2002.
Brooks DE, Matthews AG. Equine ophthalmology. In: Gelatt KN, ed. Veterinary Ophthalmology, ed 4. Philadelphia; Lippincott Williams and Wilkins, 2007.
Gilger BC, ed. Equine Ophthalmology. Philadelphia; WB Saunders, 2005.

Author Dennis E. Brooks
Consulting Editor Dennis E. Brooks

UPWARD FIXATION OF THE PATELLA

BASICS

OVERVIEW

• Gait abnormality characterized by the hindlimb locked in extension, dragging the toe • The patella is fixed medially by the medial patellar ligament hooking over the medial trochlear ridge of the femur effectively locking the reciprocal apparatus. When the patella becomes fixed in this position or its release is delayed, the condition is referred to as upward fixation of the patella.

SYSTEM AFFECTED

Musculoskeletal—stifle

SIGNALMENT

• More common in young horses and ponies
• Shetland ponies are most commonly affected. • May also be noted in an older unfit horse or in a horse taken abruptly out of work and confined to a stall

SIGNS

• In mild cases, delayed patellar release, "catching" of the stifle, is noted. The leg may snap or jerk into flexion. Horses may stumble or knuckle over in the affected hindlimb. The gait is more pronounced during downward transitions or going down hill. • In severe cases, the affected hindlimb is locked in extreme extension, pointing backward and dragging the toe. • Femoropatellar joint distention is common in chronic or severely affected horses. • Low-grade lameness may be noted in chronic intermittent cases.

CAUSES AND RISK FACTOR

• Straight hindlimb conformation* • Poor muscle mass • The gait is frequently manifested in horses that are confined to a stall or abruptly decreased fitness level.

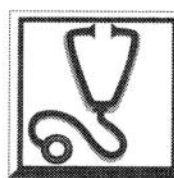

DIAGNOSIS

DIFFERENTIAL DIAGNOSIS

• Coxofemoral joint luxation—Affected limb may be fixed in extension. Differentiating signs include outward rotation of the stifle and foot, inward rotation of the tarsus, and shortening of the affected hindlimb; the affected hindlimb will not be extended caudally. • Luxation or lateral luxation of the patella—Although this term has been used to describe upward fixation of the patella, this is a misnomer. True luxation of the patella is a separate entity occurring primarily in foals and is most common in miniature horses. Severely affected horses stand in a crouched position and are unable to extend the stifle. Less severely affected horses will be reluctant to flex the stifle and have a stiff gait. Hypoplasia of the lateral trochlear ridge is often present.
• Stringhalt—Exaggerated upward hindlimb flexion with every walk stride and absent or less apparent when trotting are classic signs.
• Shivers—Early or mild disease may resemble stringhalt or intermittent upward fixation of the patella. Episodic hindlimb hyperflexion and limb abduction prior to hoof placement are differentiating characteristics.

CBC/CHEMISTRY/URINALYSIS

None

OTHER LABORATORY TESTS

None

IMAGING

• Radiography—Osteochondral fragmentation or osteophyte formation along the distal aspect of the patella may be noted in chronically affected horses. Evaluation for osteochondrosis is important for prognosis.
• Ultrasonography—Evaluate the periarticular and articular soft tissue structures for potential concurrent injury.

OTHER DIAGNOSTIC PROCEDURES

• Diagnostic analgesia—Intra-articular analgesia of the femoropatellar joint for confirmation of disease in horses with intermittent clinical signs. • Diagnostic testing for neuromuscular diseases such as polysaccharide storage disease, equine protozoal myelitis, shivers, or equine lower motor neuron disease may be warranted.

UPWARD FIXATION OF THE PATELLA

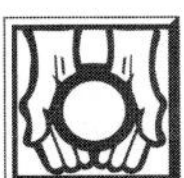

TREATMENT

• For mildly affected horses, a conditioning program to improve muscle strength of the quadriceps is indicated. Consistent daily exercise in good footing and uphill work should be encouraged. Stall confinement is contradicted. • Wedged heel pads or eggbar shoes may be beneficial. • For horses with a locked patella, manually push the patella medially and distally while backing the horse. • Transection of the medial patellar ligament or ultrasound guided percutaneous splitting of the medial patellar ligament is advocated for horses that do not respond to conservative management and for severely affected horses. After surgery, the horse is confined to a stall and handwalked for 6–8 weeks.

MEDICATIONS

DRUG(S)

• Counterirritant (2% iodine, volatile salts, Serapin) injections along the medial and middle patellar ligaments; 2 mL of counterirritant is injected along the medial and lateral borders of the ligaments close to their insertion on the tibia. • Intramuscular estrogen compounds (20 mg weekly for 3–4 weeks, then decreased by 5-mg increments weekly to 10 mg, treatment duration 6–8 weeks)

CONTRAINDICATIONS/POSSIBLE INTERACTIONS

Swelling after counterirritant injection is expected.

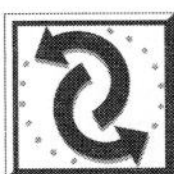

FOLLOW-UP

PATIENT MONITERING

• Immediate resolution of the abnormal gait with successful treatment in horses with a locked patella. • Gradational elimination of clinical signs is noted after treatment in horses affected with mild, intermittent disease. • Immature horses tend to outgrow the problem. • Recurrence in ponies is not uncommon.

PREVENTION/AVOIDANCE

• Stall confinement or abrupt changes in exercise regimen should be avoided if possible. • Consistent exercise program of adequate rigor

POSSIBLE COMPLICATIONS

• Fibrous thickening at the surgical site • Severe complications after medial patellar desmotomy include osteoarthritis, distal patellar fragmentation, chondromalacia of the patella, and patella fracture.

EXPECTED COURSE AND PROGNOSIS

• Most horses respond favorably to conservative management. • Horses with concurrent stifle osteochondrosis or soft tissue injury are more likely to be lame. • Surgical treatment is reserved for severely affected horses and horses in which the patella remains locked despite manipulation. Approximately 30% of horses will develop patellar lesions after medial patellar desmotomy. Arthroscopic removal of minor patella fragmentation is often successful.

MISCELLANEOUS

ASSOCIATED CONDITIONS

None

AGE-RELATED FACTORS

Gait abnormality is commonly seen in young horses and ponies.

ZOONOTIC POTENTIAL

None

PREGANANCY

N/A

Suggested Reading

Miller SM, Swanson TD. Upward fixation of the patella. In: Robinson NE, ed. Current Therapy in Equine Medicine, ed 5. St. Louis: Saunders, 2003:536–537.

Author Elizabeth J. Davidson

Consulting Editor Elizabeth J. Davidson

URINALYSIS

BASICS

DEFINITION

• Analysis of urine as an aid in the diagnosis of disease via visual inspection, dipstick analysis, refractometry or osmometry, and microscopy of sediment • Urine is collected by free catch during voiding or via urethral catheterization. Cystocentesis is not a method of urine collection in horses. Voided urine samples are easily contaminated. Catheterization is preferred for bacteriologic examination.
• Urine appearance changes during urination especially toward the end of micturition (more crystals voided). • Urine volume and composition influenced by feed and water intake, salt supplementation, environmental factors, exercise, stress, systemic disease, and drug administration

Normal Adult Urine

• Visual inspection—Color ranges from pale yellow to dark tan (may turn brown/red color after prolonged storage or exposure to air). Cloudy/turbid from large quantities of calcium carbonate (some calcium oxalate and phosphate). Viscous from the presence of mucus. Urine often appears red on snow or shavings. • Dipstick—Alkaline, pH typically >7.5 (7.0–9.0). Negative glucose. Negative blood. Negative/trace protein. Negative ketones. Negative bilirubin. Positive urobilinogen. • Osmometry—Osmolality the most accurate determinate of solute concentration of urine; typically 1500 mOsm/kg • Refractometry—Urine specific gravity (SG), measured with a refractometer, estimates solute concentration of urine (presence of larger molecules [e. g., glucose, protein]) leads to overestimation of urine concentration, but this is an appropriate test; typically >1.025 (1.008–1.040). • Urine concentration classified as hyposthenuric (SG <1.008; osmolality <269 mOsm/kg); isosthenuric (SG 1.008–1.012; osmolality 260–300 mOsm/kg); hypersthenuric (SG >1.012; osmolality >300 mOsm/kg).
• Microscopy of sediment—Refrigerate sample. Must evaluate within an hour, contents of urine not stable, cells/casts deteriorate, crystals dissolve/form. Method of collection can affect analysis—Catheterization may result in mild trauma, increasing urine protein and RCB. Due to large quantities of calcium salts some samples require addition of 10% acetic acid or hydrogen chloride to dissolve crystals. Normally abundant calcium carbonate crystals, small numbers of triple phosphate and calcium oxalate. No casts. RBCs <5/hpf. WBCs <5/hpf. Epithelial cells. Small numbers of bacteria in voided sample (surface contamination)

Normal Foal Urine

• Visual inspection—Color typically clear. More calcium oxalate crystals than in adults.
• Dipstick—acidic (5.0–7.0) • Refractometry or osmometry—Typically SG <1.008; osmolality <250 mOsm/kg. This reflects normal high-volume milk diet. May be elevated in healthy foals in the first 24 hr.

PATHOPHYSIOLOGY

• Kidneys are responsible for fine tuning body water content and ion composition.
• Important components of this regulation include renal blood flow, glomerular filtration, tubular modification of glomerular filtrate.
• Blood is filtered by the glomeruli in the kidneys. Small solutes are freely filtered at the glomerulus. The renal tubules then extensively modified ultrafiltrate by reabsorbing or secreting solutes to produce the final product.
• Urinary bladder stores urine for elimination through the urethra.
• Feed and water intake, salt supplementation, environmental factors, exercise, stress, systemic disease, and drug administration can produced changes in urinary parameters.
• Abnormalities in various organ systems can produce changes in urinary parameters.
• Abnormalities of the kidney, ureters, bladder, urethra, reproductive tract, or external urogenital structures are likely to change urinary parameters.

SYSTEM AFFECTED

Renal/urologic

CAUSES

See Disorders That May Alter Lab Results and Drugs That May Alter Lab Results.

VISUAL INSPECTION

• Change in color—pigmenturia, bacteruria, spermuria, excessive crystaluria. Dilute urine—polyuria. Pigmenturia throughout micturition—bladder or renal lesion. Pigmenturia at the beginning or end of micturition—urethral or accessory gland lesion.

Dipstick Analysis

• Decreased pH—vigorous exercise, high concentrate diet, dehydration, anorexia, metabolic acidosis, hypochloremic metabolic alkalosis, bacteriuria
• Positive protein—false-positive (alkaline or hemoglobinuria). More sensitive methods—sulfosalicylic acid precipitation test or by specific quantification with colormetric assay. Proteinuria and absence of WBCs, RBCs, bacteria, or casts—glomerulonephritis or amyloidosis. Bacteria, WBCs, and proteinuria—infection. Hemorrhage or inflammation associated with proteinuria. Transiently after exercise. Often detected in foals after colostrum ingestion (first 48 hr).
• Positive glucose—Severe hyperglycemia above renal threshold (serum glucose >150 mg/dL). Systemic disease such as equine metabolic syndrome, pituitary pars intermedia dysfunction. Elevated catecholamines or cortisol with corticosteroid therapy, intense exercise, pain, stress, or shock. Transiently after α_2-agonist. Glucosuria without hyperglycemia—renal tubular damage.
• Positive blood—false-positive (extremely alkaline urine). Dipstick cannot differentiate Hb, Mb, or RBC. Proteinuria generally present. Hematuria—hemorrhage in urogenital tract. Hemoglobinuria—intravascular hemolysis. Myoglobinuria—severe myopathy. Differentiate by centrifugation—RBCs from hemorrhage clear from supernatant, but Hb and Mb do not. Centrifugation of whole blood and examination of plasma—hemoglobinuria is accompanied by hemoglobinemia (red plasma); Mb not retained in blood and plasma is a normal color. Examination of sediment—intact RBCs present in urine with hemorrhage but not with hemoglobinuria or myoglobinuria.
• Positive ketones—horses rarely ketotic
• Positive bilirubin—Increased circulation of conjugated bilirubin; consider myopathy, hepatic disease, post hepatic obstruction.
• Positive urobilinogen—Presence indicates patent bile duct. Increases—hemolytic, hepatic, post hepatic disease

Specific gravity/Osmolality

• Do not measure SG with dipstick—poor correlation reported when compared to refractometry
• Random SG <1.025 is meaningless alone, without knowledge of water intake and other factors.
• SG >1.012 indicates ability to concentrated urine.
• SG <1.008 indicates ability to dilute urine.
• Azotemia and SG >1.020—prerenal cause
• SG <1.012 in the face of dehydration—altered renal function; primary renal disease, diabetes insipidus, medullary washout, or nephrogenic diabetes inspidus
• SG <1.012 and azotaemia—altered renal function
• SG 1.008–1.017 and azotaemia—CRF
• SG <1.008—diabetes inspidus, medullary washout, nephrogenic diabetes insipidus, psychogenic polydypsia, or chronic liver failure

Change in Sediment

• Casts—Indicate renal dysfunction particularly tubular abnormality. Can consist of RBCs, WBCs, or renal tubular cells
• Increased WBC (>5 cells/hpf)—Inflammatory process does not localize site unless WBC casts present—pyelonephritis. In association with bacteruira—infection in urinary tract. Primary cystitis is rare in horses.
• Increased RBCs (>5 cells/hpf)—hematuria—trauma, hemorrhage (including renal seen in renal tubular NSAID toxicity), urolithiasis, inflammation, infection, toxemia, neoplasia, coagulopathy, exercise, fulminate liver failure; count does not localize the site unless RBC casts are present.
• Bacteria—Contaminants in voided sample. Associated with pyuria—infection. Primary cystitis is rare in horses.
• Epithelial cells—normal unless numerous/bizarre or renal tubular cells

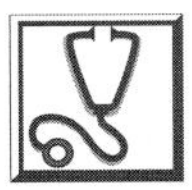

DIAGNOSIS

DIFFERENTIAL DIAGNOSIS

See Causes.

CBC/BIOCHEMISTRY/URINALYSIS

CBC

- Elevated WBC count, protein, fibrinogen—inflammatory or infectious process
- Mild anemia (packed cell volume 20%–30%)—decreased erythropoietin production and shortened RBC life in CRF

Biochemistry

- BUN and creatinine—do not increase until >75% nephrons nonfunctional
- Hyponatremia and hypochloremia—renal disease
- Potassium normal or elevated—ARF or CRF
- Hypocalcemia (variable) and hyperphosphatemia—ARF
- Hypercalcemia, hypermagnasemia, and hypophosphatemia—CRF
- Decreased albumin—protein losing glomeruopathy
- Hyperglycaemia (>150–175 mg/dL)—stress, exercise, sepsis, pituitary adenoma, diabetes mellitus—can result in glucosuria
- Elevated CK and AST—myopathy (differentiate myoglobinuria from hematuria or hemoglobinuria)

Drugs That May Alter Lab Results

- Xylazine—(diuretic effect) transient increase in urine volume, decrease in SG and glucosuria
- Diuretics, corticosteroids, and fluid therapy—increase urine volume, decrease SG, alter electrolyte excretion
- Sulphonamides—produce distinctive crystals
- Rifampin—urine discoloration (dark orange-red)

Disorders That May Alter Lab Results

- Feed and water intake, salt supplementation, environmental factors, exercise, stress, systemic disease, and drug administration can alter urinary parameters.
- Alkaline urine—falsely positive protein; verify with chemical methods (e. g., sulfosalicylic acid precipitation).
- Ascorbic acid, lactose, galactose, pentose, ascorbic acid, conjugated gluconates, and salicylates—alter glucose results
- Hyposthenuria—lysis of RBCs
- Discolored urine—affects interpretation of all dipstick color reactions
- Delayed analysis—affects ketones, bilirubin, urobilinogen, pH, and sediment examination
- Exposure to light—false-negative bilirubin
- Microbial peroxidase—false-positive blood

OTHER LABORATORY TESTS

- γ-Glutamyltransferase (GGT): creatinine ratio—GGT released into the urine from damaged proximal tubules. Normal range 0.1–2.3 IU/mmol. Most sensitive indicator of renal tubular damage (normal horse receiving phenylbutazone or gentamicin will have an elevated ratio). High sensitivity makes interpretation difficult.
- Fractional clearance/excretion—evaluates tubular function. Damaged renal tubules fail to adequately reabsorb electrolytes resulting in excessive loss in the urine. Collect urine and serum samples at similar time. FE of all electrolytes increased in RF. FE of sodium may help distinguish prerenal and renal azotemia. Dehydrated horse, FE should be low as body conserves sodium. Primary renal disease, FE increases (>1%).
- Distinguishing between hemoglobinuria and myoglobinuria—Ammonium sulfate precipitation method is imprecise and frequently fails to detect Mb. Accurate differentiation requires sophisticated methods. Assay is not commonly available, but diagnosis usually reached with hematology and biochemistry.
- Urinary protein–to–urinary creatinine ratio—determines significance of proteinuria; ratio >1:1 abnormal
- Indwelling bladder catheters—critically ill neonatal foals—quantify urine output to monitor fluid balance
- Culture and sensitivity—Sample aseptically collected via catheterization. Indication—significant WBCs and bacteria in urine sediment examination
- Water deprivation test—Evaluate patients with polydipsia and hyposthenuria polyuria when other causes excluded. Generally performed to determine if horse has psychogenic polydipsia or diabetes inspidus. Contraindicated in azotemic or dehydrated animals
- Enzymuria—Inflammation or necrosis of tubular epithelial cells—elevated urinary activity of enzymes—may provide evidence of early renal tubular damage and assist identifying segment of nephron affected

IMAGING

- Ultrasound of bladder and ureters—transrectally or transabdominally in adults and transabdominally in foals
- Ultrasound of kidneys—transcutaneously
- Abdominal ultrasound—if ruptured bladder and uroperitoneum suspected
- Excretory urography or intravenous pyelogram—identifies a nonfunctional or hypoplastic kidney or an ectopic or torn ureter
- Retrograde contrast studies—identify ectopic ureter or ruptured bladder
- Nuclear scintigraphy—provides qualitative information about renal function and is the only method currently available for assessing individual kidney function

OTHER DIAGNOSTIC PROCEDURES

- Rectal palpation of kidneys, ureters, and bladder
- Cystoscopy—if abnormal urination or hematuria. Allows examination of the urethra, bladder, and occasionally ureters. May sample urine from individual ureters to assess individual kidneys
- Biopsy—ultrasound guided

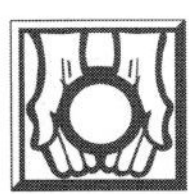

TREATMENT

- Urinalysis is an essential part of a complete diagnostic workup in many conditions, not just urinary tract disease, that complements history, clinical examination, hematology, biochemistry, but urinalysis should not be used alone. Therefore, urinalysis findings themselves generally do not require treatment.
- Exceptions include hemoglobinuria and myoglobinuria, which require immediate, aggressive fluid therapy because of their potential for causing permanent damage to the renal tubules.

POSSIBLE COMPLICATIONS

- Hemogloginuria and myoglobinuria can result in permanent renal tubular damage.
- Uncorrected dehydration can result in permanent renal compromise.
- Uroliths/cystoliths can result in urethral obstruction.

SEE ALSO

- BUN
- CK
- Creatinine
- Hemolysis
- Polyuria/polydipsia
- Renal failure
- Urine chemistry

ABBREVIATIONS

- ARF = acute renal failure
- AST = aspartate aminotransferase
- BUN = blood urea nitrogen
- CK = creatine kinase
- CRF = chronic renal failure
- GGT = γ-glutamyltransferase
- Hb = hemoglobin
- hpf = high-power field
- Mb = myoglobin

Suggested Reading

Carlson GP. Clinical chemistry test. In: Smith BP, ed. Large Animal Internal Medicine, ed 2. St Louis: Mosby, 1996.

Schott HD II. Examination of the urinary system. In: Equine Internal Medicine, ed 2. St. Louis: Saunders, 2004.

Toribio RE. Essentials of equine renal and urinary tract physiology. Vet Clin Equine 2007;23:533–561.

Wilson ME. Examination of the urinary tract in the horse. Vet Clin Equine 2007;23:563–575.

The author and editor wish to acknowledge the contribution to this chapter of Ellen W. Evans, the author in the previous edition.

Author Grace Forbes

Consulting Editor Kenneth W. Hinchcliff

URINARY INCONTINENCE

BASICS

DEFINITION

• Urinary incontinence is the inability to control urination with the involuntary passage of urine and in horses is manifested as scalding of the perineal area (mares) and inner aspect of the hindlimbs in both sexes.
• Bladder paralysis results from partial or complete loss of detrusor function. Incontinence develops when intravesicular pressure exceeds resting urethral sphincter pressure.

PATHOPHYSIOLOGY

• Bladder paralysis can be caused by a variety of disease processes and is typically separated into 3 types: (i) reflex or upper motor neuron (UMN) bladder (also known as spastic or autonomic bladder); (ii) paralytic or lower motor neuron (LMN) bladder; and (iii) myogenic or noneurogenic bladder.
  ○ Initially, a UMN bladder is characterized by increased urethral resistance, leading to increased intravesicular pressure before voiding can occur. Voiding may occur as short bursts of urine passage with incomplete bladder emptying, and rectal examination will reveal a turgid bladder that is small to increased in size.
  ○ In contrast, LMN and myogenic bladder paresis result in chronic bladder distension due to decreased or absent detrusor activity. Rectal palpation reveals a large, flaccid bladder and urine can usually be expressed by placing pressure on the bladder.
  ○ Although signs of a UMN bladder are initially different from those of the other two types, this type of problem is usually not recognized in horses until more significant incontinence develops in association with progressive loss of detrusor function.
  ○ Similarly, although LMN disease limited to the external urethral sphincter could result in incontinence with normal detrusor function, such a clinical syndrome has not been well documented in horses but may be related to hypoestrogenism in an occasional mare.
  ○ By the time incontinence develops into a clinically important problem in many horses, underlying pathology may be longstanding and the inciting cause can often not be determined.
• In both sexes, but perhaps more importantly in male horses, lower back pain has also been a suggested cause for development of bladder paresis/paralysis. Lumbar pain could make it difficult for horses to posture to urinate and completely empty the bladder. Incomplete bladder emptying would lead to accumulation of crystalline sludge in the ventral aspect of the bladder (termed sabulous urolithiasis), progressive bladder distension, loss of detrusor function, and paralysis (myogenic bladder).
• Trauma or malformation of the distal urinary tract could lead to urinary incontinence. In mares, trauma during natural breeding or during parturition is an additional mechanism by which direct injury to the urethral sphincter could occur and lead to a syndrome of urinary incontinence (and infertility).
• In young horses, incontinence due to ectopic ureter is the result of an anomaly of development; affected horses also posture and urinate normally when ectopic ureter is a unilateral problem.

SYSTEMS AFFECTED

• Renal/urologic
• Neurologic
• Musculoskeletal
• Reproductive

INCIDENCE/PREVALENCE

Low

SIGNALMENT

Breed Predilections

None documented

Mean Age and Range

Ectopic ureter is an anomaly of development and results in incontinence from birth.

Predominant Sex

• Bladder paralysis, accompanied by sabulous urolithiasis, appears to be more common in male horses due to the longer urethra.
• Postpartum mares may also be at greater risk for incontinence due to trauma sustained during parturition.
• An occasional mare may also develop incontinence consequent to hypoestrogenism.

SIGNS

• Urinary incontinence and scalding of the perineal area (mares) and inner aspect of the hindlimbs in both sexes
• Horses may appear painful while posturing to urinate or may not assume a normal voiding posture.
• Weakness, ataxia, etc., if bladder paralysis/incontinence is due to an underlying neurologic disease
• Fever, partial anorexia, weight loss may be observed if complicated by upper UTI (pyelonephritis).

CAUSES

• *Neurologic disease*—equine herpes myelitis, equine protozoal myeloencephalitis, spinal cord compression, cauda equine neuritis
• *Intoxication*—grazing *Sorghum* hybrids (Sudan grass and Johnson grass) that contain hydrocyanic acid
• *Trauma*—postbreeding or postpartum in mares
• *Hypoestrogenism*—a suspected cause of incontinence in an occasional mare
• *Ectopic ureter*—young horses
• *Idiopathic*—possibly a consequence of lumbar pain/orthopedic disease resulting in posturing difficulty and incomplete bladder emptying

RISK FACTORS

• Trauma to spinal cord or associated with breeding or parturition
• Other neurologic diseases
• Exposure to cyanogenic plants
• Musculoskeletal problems affecting posturing to urinate

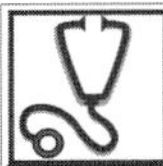

DIAGNOSIS

DIFFERENTIAL DIAGNOSIS

• Normal estrous behavior in mares can cause perineal staining with crystalloid material and can be confused with incontinence.
• Bladder paralysis/incontinence accompanying neurologic disease—equine herpes myelitis, equine protozoal myeloencephalitis, spinal cord compression, cauda equine neuritis

CBC/BIOCHEMISTRY/URINALYSIS

• CBC normal in most cases unless UTI extends to upper urinary tract leading to variable leukocytosis
• BUN and Cr normal unless complicated by moderate to severe bilateral pyelonephritis
• UA—Urine specific gravity usually normal (1.020–1.035) but increased numbers of RBCs, WBCs, and bacteria may be seen on sediment examination if complicated by UTI.

OTHER LABORATORY TESTS

Urine culture—Quantitative urine culture should be performed in all cases of bladder paralysis and incontinence.

IMAGING

• *Transabdominal ultrasonography*—renal parenchymal architecture may be abnormal (loss of detail of corticomedullary junction, cavitary lesions with abscess formation, and/or nephrolithiasis) if complicated by pyelonephritis
• *Transrectal ultrasonography*—confirms bladder size and may demonstrate accumulation of sabulous material in ventral aspect of bladder
• *Abdominal radiography*—intravenous pyelography may confirm ectopic ureter in foals with incontinence; intrarenal pyelography (contrast injected transabdominally directly into renal pelvis) has a greater likelihood of outlining the ectopia.
• *Urethroscopy/cystoscopy*— useful to assess bladder mucosa for inflammation, accumulation of sabulous material, and integrity of ureteral orifices (they may be wide open with chronic bladder paralysis supporting vesiculoureteral reflux and probable ascending pyelonephritis)
• *Lumbar radiographs +/− nuclear scintigraphy*—may be useful to evaluate possible thoracolumbar musculoskeletal disease

OTHER DIAGNOSTIC PROCEDURES

• *Bulbocavernosus reflex* (male horses)—When normal, contraction of the urethral sphincter can be palpated per rectum when the glans penis is gently squeezed by an assistant.
• *Cystometry*—continuous recording of intravesicular pressure during saline infusion to assess detrusor muscle function; threshold for onset of detrusor contraction in normal horses is 90 +/−20 cm H_2O.
• *Urethral pressure profile*—After passage of a balloon-tipped catheter into the bladder, the pressure in the balloon is continuously recorded as the catheter is withdrawn through the urethral sphincter to assess external sphincter muscle function; the pressure in normal horses typically exceeds 100 cm H_2O and waves of contractions can be appreciated on the tracing.

• *Neurologic examination*—document additional neurologic deficits.
• *Collection and analysis of cerebrospinal fluid*—cytologic analysis and appropriate testing for equine protozoal myeloencephalitis
• *Electromyography*—assess perineal and tail muscles for evidence of denervation (LMN disease).

PATHOLOGICAL FINDINGS

• The bladder often contains a concretion of chalky/sabulous material.
• The bladder mucosa may be thickened and hemorrhagic with a neutrophilic or lymphocytic infiltrate.
• The bladder contents can be culture positive.
• Attempts to investigate the neurologic component of the urinary incontinence are often unrewarding (no lesions identifiable).

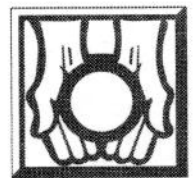

TREATMENT

AIMS OF TREATMENT

• Proper recognition and treatment of all underlying primary neurologic disease processes
• Removal from exposure to cyanogenic grasses
• Medications to improve detrusor function (bethanecol) or to enhance urethral sphincter tone (phenoxybenzamine or estradiol cypionate)
• Appropriate antimicrobial therapy for secondary UTIs
• In cases of myogenic bladder and sabulous urolithiasis, manual lavage of the bladder with saline may provide temporary relief of distension and can remove accumulated urine sediment.

NURSING CARE

• Nursing care including daily cleaning of perineum and hindlimbs to minimize skin irritation from incontinence, application of petrolatum to scalded areas

ACTIVITY

• In cases of neurologic disease, advise not to ride the horse until resolution of ataxia or other underlying conditions.
• If gait is normal and the horse is outwardly healthy, mild to moderate exercise

DIET

• Grass hay is preferable to alfalfa or other legumes (higher in calcium).
• Urine acidifying agents can be supplemented (NH_4Cl or NH_4SO_4) or an anionic diet can be fed in attempt to limit urine crystal formation; however, no currently available products are palatable enough to be efficacious.
• NaCl 1–2 oz. BID added to feed or mixed with water and administered as an oral slurry will increase urine flow and decrease sedimentation of crystalloid material in ventral aspect of bladder.

CLIENT EDUCATION

Urinary incontinence can be managed but requires dedication and repeated examinations and treatments for UTI.

SURGICAL CONSIDERATIONS

Surgical correction of ectopic ureter by unilateral nephrectomy or attachment of the distal ureter to the bladder neck

MEDICATIONS

DRUG(S) OF CHOICE

• Bethanecol (0.25–0.75 mg/kg SQ or PO q8 h)—parasympathomimetic agent that has a somewhat selective effect on smooth muscle of the gastrointestinal tract and bladder, stimulates postganglionic effector cells (detrusor myocytes) to improve detrusor muscle tone and strength of contraction; response to treatment is usually poor because of long-standing detrusor paresis/paralysis before problem is clinically recognized (except perhaps with acute herpes myelitis or equine protozoal myeloencephalitis). If no improvement is noted within 3–5 days of treatment, bethanecol therapy should be discontinued.
• Phenoxybenzamine 0.7 mg/kg PO q6 h—α-adrenergic blocker that can be used to decrease urethral sphincter tone in cases of UMN bladder; again, this condition has not been well documented in horses.
• Estradiol cypionate 4 μg/kg IM every other day)–estrogen appears to modulate the effect of norepinephrine on α-adrenergic receptor activity in the urethral sphincter and may improve urethral sphincter tone in mares with hypoestrogenism associated incontinence.
• Antimicrobials—Sulfamethoxazole-trimethoprim or sulfadiazine-trimethoprim (preferable due to less hepatic metabolism of sulfadiazine than sulfamethoxazole) combinations (20 mg/kg PO q12h or q24h) are the most practical long-term treatment; can be used prophylactically or therapeutically for established UTI; because these agents are concentrated nearly 100-fold in urine, they may achieve therapeutic minimum inhibitory concentrations in urine against pathogens that are reported to be resistant (see Urinary Tract Infection).

PRECAUTIONS

Bethanecol—must be used cautiously as may increase gastrointestinal motility and lead to colic signs

FOLLOW-UP

PATIENT MONITORING

• The prognosis for recovery of cases of bladder paresis/paralysis and associated incontinence due to neurologic disease is *guarded* and will depend on response to treatment of the underlying disease and duration of paresis/incontinence (generally more favorable if <2 weeks in duration); evidence of some detrusor function on cystometry and a normal urethral pressure profile improve the prognosis and such horses warrant aggressive treatment; patient monitoring should include regular repeat physical and neurologic examination, cystometry and urethral pressure profiles could be repeated at 2- to 4-week intervals if clinical improvement is uncertain.
• The prognosis for recovery of cases of long standing "idiopathic" bladder paralysis and associated incontinence is *poor;* management will require daily nursing care (cleaning the perineum and hindlimbs), prophylactic or therapeutic antimicrobial treatment, and possibly intermittent bladder lavage to remove sabulous material; patient monitoring should include regular (weekly or monthly) assessment of overall condition (attitude, appetite, body weight, etc.); owner frustration often leads to a decision for euthanasia within a few months after the problem is first recognized.

POSSIBLE COMPLICATIONS

• Moderate to severe dermatitis consequent to urine scald
• Sabulous urolithiasis
• UTI—cystitis, possibly complicated by ascending pyelonephritis

MISCELLANEOUS

ASSOCIATED CONDITIONS

• Equine herpes myelitis
• Equine protozoal myeloencephalitis
• Cauda equina neuritis
• Spinal cord trauma
• Thoracolumbar trauma/pain
• Hypoestrogenism
• Urine pooling and infertility (mares)

AGE-RELATED FACTORS

Hypoestrogenism would be more likely in older mares, and ectopic ureter is a problem recognized in young horses.

PREGNANCY

Increased risk of breeding and foaling trauma—induced incontinence

SYNONYMS

Enzootic ataxia and cystitis (herd outbreaks associated with intoxication)

SEE ALSO

• Urinary tract infection
• Sabulous urolithiasis
• Ectopic ureter

ABBREVIATIONS

• Cr = creatinine
• LMN = lower motor neuron
• UMN = upper motor neuron
• UTI = urinary tract infection

Suggested Reading

Bayly WM. Urinary incontinence and bladder dysfunction. In: Reed SM, Bayly WM, Sellon DC, eds. Equine Internal Medicine, ed 2. Philadelphia: WB Saunders, 2004:1290–1294.

Schott HC. Clinical Commentary: Urinary incontinence and sabulous urolithiasis–chicken or the egg? Equine Vet Educ 2006;8:17–19.

Author Harold C. Schott II

Consulting Editor Gillian A. Perkins

URINARY TRACT INFECTION (UTI)

BASICS

DEFINITION

• Two categories—those affecting the upper urinary tract (i.e., kidneys, ureters), and those affecting the lower urinary tract (i.e., bladder, urethra) • Bacterial infection is most common, but yeast (*Candida* spp.), protozoa (*Klossiella equi*), and other parasites (e.g., *Strongylus vulgaris, Halicephalobus gingivalis* [*deletrix*], and *Dioctophyma renale*) may also cause UTI.

PATHOPHYSIOLOGY

Bacterial Upper UTI

• Recognized infrequently • Most commonly develop as ascending infections secondary to stasis of urine flow (as with bladder paralysis) and vesiculoureteral reflux (retrograde flow of urine into ureters) or damage to renal parenchyma (i.e., polycystic disease and medullary crest necrosis) • Less commonly a result of neonatal septicemia (*Actinobacillus equuili*, etc.)

Bacterial Lower UTI

• Usually a consequence of abnormal urine flow (anatomic or functional) • Frequently accompanied by urolithiasis • Single large cystoliths predispose to UTI; however, it is difficult to determine if uroliths are a predisposing cause or a consequence of UTI.

Parasitic Infection

• *H. gingivalis* infection (rare) can be life threatening due to CNS involvement. Large granulomatous lesions full of rhabditiform nematodes usually are found in the kidneys. Renal involvement typically is inapparent.
• *D. renale* is a large (the female may reach up to 100 cm in length) bright-red nematode. Typical hosts are carnivorous species, but horses can ingest the intermediate host (i.e., annelid worm) while grazing or drinking from natural water sources. Once localized in the kidney, the parasite may live 1–3 years, shedding eggs in the urine. The renal parenchyma is completely destroyed, and death of the parasite leads to fibrosis of the kidney. • Occasionally, hydronephrosis or renal hemorrhage may be a serious complication of parasitic infection. • In contrast to infection with nematodes, infection with the coccidian parasite *K. equi* is common, but clinically benign, and thus an incidental finding.

Yeast Infection

Foals on broad-spectrum antibiotics may develop secondary *Candida* spp. cystitis.

SYSTEMS AFFECTED

• Renal/urologic—infection and failure (with bilateral upper UTI) • Nervous—with *H. gingivalis* infection • Dermatologic—urine scalding of hindlimbs

GENETICS

None documented

INCIDENCE/PREVALENCE

• Bacterial UTIs are uncommon. • "Outbreaks" of cystitis have been described in association with eating hybrids of *Sorghum* spp. (e.g., Johnson grass, Sudan grass) in the southwestern United States, but UTIs were likely a complication of sublethal intoxication that resulted in bladder paralysis. • Another outbreak of "cystitis," manifested by hematuria more than UTI or incontinence, was seen in horses on range pasture in Western Australia. A fungal toxin was suspected, because similar bladder lesions in sheep and cattle have been seen with sporidesmin, a toxin produced by the fungus *Pithomyces chartarum.* • Clinically significant renal nematode infections are rare, despite necropsy surveys revealing that up to 20% of equine kidneys have evidence of *Strongylus vulgaris* migration. • *K. equi* infection of equine kidneys occurs worldwide; one necropsy survey found the protozoa in 12% of horses examined.

GEOGRAPHIC DISTRIBUTION

Worldwide

SIGNALMENT

Breed Predilections

None documented

Mean Age and Range

• Foals <30 days of age are at greater risk for septic nephritis associated with septicemia.
• Critically ill neonates receiving broad-spectrum antibiotic treatment may develop ascending UTI with *Candida* spp.

Predominant Sex

• A shorter urethra increases risk of UTI in females; however, UTI is still rare in mares.
• Injury to the lower urinary tract during breeding and parturition increase risk of bladder paresis and UTI, especially after dystocia.

SIGNS

Historical

• Upper UTI—usually weight loss or fever of undetermined origin, less commonly, hematuria or pyuria. Occasionally, recurrent colic may be reported when obstruction with a urolith accompanies UTI. • Lower UTI—dysuria (e.g., pollakiuria, stranguria, hematuria) is common presenting complaint. Urinary incontinence and skin scalding may be observed with either bladder paresis or pollakiuria.

Physical Examination

Upper UTI

• Lethargy, fever, partial anorexia, intermittent colic, and mild dehydration • Rectal examination may reveal enlarged ureters and kidneys. • Occasionally, obstructing ureteroliths can be palpated.

Lower UTI

• Dysuria with or without urine scalding, but general health usually is good. • Rectal examination—thickened bladder wall; cystoliths or other bladder masses may be detected if bladder is not full. Assess for bladder paresis (i.e., large atonic bladder with incontinence produced by compressing bladder) versus the small bladder usually present with pollakiuria.

CAUSES

Upper UTI

• Bacterial ascending infections with bladder paralysis and vesiculoureteral reflux or obstructive disease— *Escherichia coli, Proteus mirabilis, Klebsiella* spp., *Staphylococcus* spp., *Enterobacter* spp., *Corynebacterium* spp., and *Pseudomonas aeruginosa.* Mixed infections may be seen. • Less commonly, a hematogenous infection with septicemia occurs—*Rhodococcus equi, Actinobacillus equuili,* and other gram-negative bacteria.

Lower UTI

• Ascending infections usually develop from abnormal urine flow (anatomic or functional), especially bladder paralysis. • Organisms are similar to those causing upper UTIs. • Chronic antibiotic treatment or instrumentation of the urinary tract (e.g., indwelling bladder catheters, ureteral stents) may cause UTI with *Enterococcus* spp. (formerly *Streptococcus faecalis*) or other antibiotic-resistant microbes. • Infection with *Candida* spp. may develop in recumbent neonatal foals receiving broad-spectrum antibacterial therapy.

RISK FACTORS

• Vesiculoureteral reflux, which may develop with bladder paresis or partial obstruction, is an important predisposing problem for ascending upper UTI. • Abnormal urine flow, especially with bladder paralysis, increases risk for lower UTI. • Use of indwelling catheters is a significant risk factor, but routine instrumentation of the urinary tract (e.g., bladder catheterization, cystoscopy) is relatively low risk. • Dystocia and subsequent trauma to the lower urinary tract may allow ascending infections.

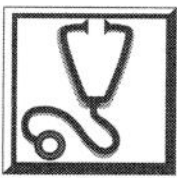

DIAGNOSIS

DIFFERENTIAL DIAGNOSIS

• Upper UTI—disease processes that may lead to lethargy, partial anorexia, weight loss, fever, recurrent colic, or hematuria • Lower UTI—normal estrus activity in mares, ectopic ureter, and other causes of dysuria (e.g., urolithiasis, neoplasia)

CBC/BIOCHEMISTRY/URINALYSIS

• Usually normal PCV, normal WBC, leukocytosis with upper UTI • Azotemia usually is not present unless bilateral pyelonephritis results in CRF. • USG—usually normal (>1.020) unless UTI is associated with CRF and isosthenuria (1.008–1.014) • Urinalysis generally reveals microscopic or macroscopic hematuria and pyuria; bacteria, yeast, and protozoa may be seen on sediment examination.

OTHER LABORATORY TESTS

• Perform quantitative urine culture and antimicrobial sensitivity testing in all suspected cases; recovery of >10,000 CFU/mL is diagnostic.
• Consider bacterial culture of the center of uroliths accompanying UTIs, because many have positive results despite negative urine culture results.

IMAGING

Transabdominal Ultrasonography

• Kidneys may be shrunken or enlarged, have loss of the corticomedullary junction or have areas of decreased echogenicity, particularly with pyelonephritis.
• Nephroliths (diameter >1 cm) should be readily detected.

Transrectal Ultrasonography

Useful for evaluation of the left kidney, ureters, and bladder

Urethroscopy/Cystoscopy

Useful to assess traumatic and anatomic defects of the lower urinary tract as well as uroepithelial damage and urine flow from the ureteral orifices

OTHER DIAGNOSTIC PROCEDURES

- Vaginal examination and vaginoscopy may reveal traumatic lesions resulting in abnormal passage of urine in the post-foaling mare
- Urethral pressure profile measurements to confirm inadequacy of the urethral sphincter
- Ureteral catheterization—during cystoscopy (or by a manual transurethral approach in mares) collect urine from each side of the upper urinary tract when unilateral pyelonephritis is suspected.

PATHOLOGICAL FINDINGS

- Pyelonephritis—mild to marked deformation of normal renal architecture, with complete loss in severe unilateral infection, nephroliths, ureteroliths, and ureteral dilation
- Lower UTI—diffusely thickened bladder wall, inflamed mucosa with areas of erosion/ulceration, adhesion of crystalloid material, and possible cystolithiasis

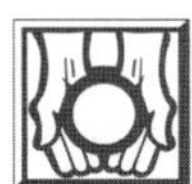

TREATMENT

AIMS OF TREATMENT

Eliminate infection and treat underlying predisposing cause.

APPROPRIATE HEALTH CARE

- Assess for predisposing causes; institute appropriate antimicrobial therapy.
- Surgical correction of anatomic defects or removal of uroliths that may accompany UTI

NURSING CARE

- Regular cleaning of perineum and hindlimbs to minimize skin irritation from incontinence
- Application of petrolatum to scalded areas

ACTIVITY

Normal, unless systemically ill from upper UTI

DIET

- Sodium chloride (1 oz. PO BID–QID) to increase urine flow
- Acidification diet to decrease infection or urolith formation; however, none seem adequate or palatable enough to be efficacious.

CLIENT EDUCATION

- Primary UTIs are rare; further diagnostics needed to rule out predisposing causes.
- With bladder paralysis, the prognosis for elimination of UTI is guarded to poor.

SURGICAL CONSIDERATIONS

- Nephrectomy to remove unilaterally infected kidney. Ensure appropriate renal function in contralateral kidney.
- Surgical removal of uroliths in the lower urinary tract
- Surgical repair of anatomic abnormalities of the lower urinary tract

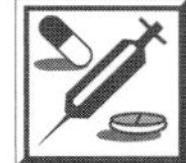

MEDICATIONS

DRUG(S) OF CHOICE

- Trimethoprim-sulfonamide combinations (20–40 mg/kg PO q12 h)—Sulfadiazine may be preferred over sulfamethoxazole, because the former is excreted largely unchanged in urine but the latter is largely inactivated before urinary excretion.
- Procaine penicillin G (22,000 IU/kg IM q12 h) and sodium ampicillin (10–20 mg/kg IV or IM q6–8 h) are effective for upper or lower UTI caused by susceptible *Corynebacterium* spp., *Streptococcus* spp., and some *Staphylococcus* spp. Many isolates of the Enterobacteriaceae family demonstrate resistance to ampicillin in vitro, but this drug is highly concentrated in urine. Thus, many organisms that are resistant in vitro may still be effectively treated with ampicillin.
- Ceftiofur (4.4 mg/kg IV or IM q12 h) or enrofloxacin (2.5 mg/kg PO q12 h) when other antibiotic resistance demonstrated
- Reserve gentamicin (6.6 mg/kg IV q24 h) and amikacin (15 mg/kg IV q24 h) for lower UTI caused by highly resistant organisms or acute, life-threatening upper UTI caused by gram-negative organisms
- NSAIDs—phenylbutazone (2.2 mg/kg PO q12–24 h) or flunixin meglumine (0.5–1.0 mg/kg PO q12–24 h) may be useful with pollakiuria or dysuria.

CONTRAINDICATIONS N/A

PRECAUTIONS

- Enrofloxacin—Consider potential cartilage damage in young horses.
- Administration of long-term antibiotics without correcting underlying cause (i.e., bladder paralysis) may lead to resistant bacterial growth.
- Aminoglycoside antibiotics and NSAIDs—Avoid or used sparingly in cases with renal compromise or azotemia.

POSSIBLE INTERACTIONS N/A

ALTERNATIVE DRUGS N/A

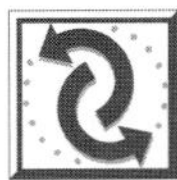

FOLLOW-UP

PATIENT MONITORING

- Institute antibiotic treatment for at least 1 week for simple (i.e., no apparent underlying cause) lower UTI; follow-up with another quantitative urine culture the week after treatment is discontinued.
- Institute antibiotic treatment for 4–6 weeks for upper UTI; follow-up with a quantitative urine culture the week after treatment is discontinued.
- Assess renal function of patients with azotemia at regular intervals (i.e., monthly or longer) during the early stages of CRF.
- Discontinuation of broad-spectrum antibiotics usually is sufficient for treating lower UTI caused by *Candida* spp. in neonates.

PREVENTION/AVOIDANCE

Salt supplementation may increase urine flow and decrease risk of recurrence.

POSSIBLE COMPLICATIONS

- Urolithiasis
- CRF

EXPECTED COURSE AND PROGNOSIS

- Favorable prognosis for simple lower UTI
- Guarded prognosis in patients with upper UTI and recurrent lower UTI where the underlying cause remains (e.g., bladder paralysis)
- Guarded prognosis in patients with bilateral pyelonephritis accompanied by azotemia; typically progresses to CRF

MISCELLANEOUS

ASSOCIATED CONDITIONS

- Urolithiasis
- Bladder paralysis
- CRF

AGE-RELATED FACTORS

- Foals <30 days of age are at greatest risk for septic nephritis associated with septicemia.
- Neonates on broad-spectrum antibiotic treatment are predisposed to ascending UTI with *Candida* spp.

ZOONOTIC POTENTIAL

N/A

PREGNANCY

Postpartum mares are at risk of urethral and bladder trauma leading to urethral sphincter incontinence and bladder paralysis.

SYNONYMS

- Cystitis
- Pyelonephritis

SEE ALSO

- CRF
- Urolithiasis
- Bladder paralysis and incontinence

ABBREVIATIONS

- CFU = colony-forming unit
- CRF = chronic renal failure
- PCV = packed cell volume
- USG = urinary specific gravity
- UTI = urinary tract infection

Suggested Reading

Frye MA. Pathophysiology, diagnosis and management of urinary tract infection in horses. Vet Clin North Am Equine Pract 2006;497–517.

Divers TJ. Urinary tract infections. In: Smith BP, ed. Large Animal Internal Medicine, ed 2. St. Louis: Mosby, 1995:962–965.

Divers TJ, Byars TD, Murch O, Sigel CW. Experimental induction of *Proteus mirabilis* cystitis in the pony and evaluation of therapy with trimethoprim-sulfadiazine. Am J Vet Res 1981;42:1203–1205.

Schott HC. Urinary tract infections. In: Reed SM, Bayly WM, Sellon DC, eds. Equine Internal Medicine, ed 2. Philadelphia: WB Saunders, 2004:1253–1258.

Author Harold C. Schott II

Consulting Editors Gillian Perkins and Dominic Dawson

URINE POOLING/UROVAGINA

BASICS

DEFINITION/OVERVIEW

• Reflux of urine from the urethral orifice into the vagina • Once in the vagina, urine may enter the uterus when the cervix relaxes during estrus or after irritation (and relaxation) of the cervix. • May cause infertility and permanent endometrial, cervical, or vaginal damage

ETIOLOGY/PATHOPHYSIOLOGY

• Caused by an altered position of the urethral orifice relative to the vulvar opening and vestibular sphincter that results in incomplete voiding and retention of urine within the vestibule and vagina

SYSTEMS AFFECTED

• Reproductive • Urinary

GENETICS

Inherited predisposition for vulvar conformation and, thus, the location of the urethral orifice

INCIDENCE/PREVALENCE

Incidence may increase with age, parity, and worsening vulvar conformation

SIGNALMENT

• All breeds • Most common in breeds with less muscle in the perineal area • Greater problem in old pluriparous mares • Females

SIGNS

• Few to no outward signs • Sole complaint may be infertility. • Mares bred multiple cycles that remain open/barren • On dismount, stallion may have urine evident on the glans and shaft of the penis. • Transrectal examination may disclose fluid within the uterus. • Vaginal examination may disclose urine in the vagina. • Speculum examination may reveal increased hyperemia and ulcers (from urine scalding) of the vaginal wall and external cervical os.

CAUSES AND RISK FACTORS

• With increasing age, vulvar conformation often worsens. • Frequently described as an elevation of the vulvar commissure. • Frequently coupled with relaxation of the vestibule, which elevates the caudal urethral opening and permits urine to reflux into the cranial vagina. • Inherited conformational traits • Multiparous mares

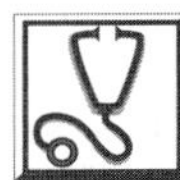

DIAGNOSIS

DIFFERENTIAL DIAGNOSIS

• Vaginitis • Pneumovagina

IMAGING

U/S imaging may demonstrate urine in the uterus.

PATHOLOGICAL FINDINGS

• Urine in the uterus and or vagina accompanied by severe inflammation of the uterus and vagina • Relative dorsal displacement of the external urethral os and downward slant (i.e., caudocranial) of the vagina to the cervix • Careful examination of the spatial relationship of the urethral opening to the ventral vulvar commissure, vestibular sphincter, and vagina

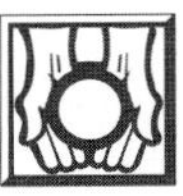

TREATMENT

SURGICAL CONSIDERATIONS

Surgical repair is the only permanent means of correction.

Pouret

• Correction of inadequate vulvar conformation by transection of the perineal body, allowing the vulva to lie more posterior and ventral, with subsequent movement of the urethral orifice posteriorly. • Decreases the possibility of urine pooling.

Urethral Extension

• Posterior relocation of the urethral orifice by undermining strips of the vaginal wall, folding the mucosa medially, and suturing it to extend the urethra to be longer than it initially was • Serves to move the external urethral opening closer to the vulvae, permitting urine to exit without reflux

Monin Vaginoplasty

• Ventral tissue dam of, or immediately cranial to, the vestibular sphincter; limited success • The dam is to reduce the likelihood of urine entering the vagina. • This procedure is usually torn at the time of delivery, and surgery must be performed again after delivery to again correct the urine pooling.

MEDICATIONS

None

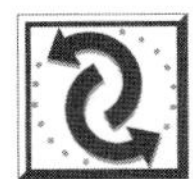

FOLLOW-UP

PATIENT MONITORING

Examine mares after treatment to determine success of the approach used.

PREVENTION/AVOIDANCE

- No specific way to prevent this condition
- Conformation of the perineal area is inherited.

POSSIBLE COMPLICATIONS

• Infertility • Vaginitis

EXPECTED COURSE AND PROGNOSIS

• Early recognition and treatment may assist in avoiding permanent damage to the vagina and endometrium. • Without surgical correction, mares continue to pool urine. • As the condition progresses, greater irritation and increase in urine accumulation in the vagina and uterus occur.

MISCELLANEOUS

• In the absence of systemic signs, no systemic therapy is justified and/or necessary. • Flushing the uterus and vagina before insemination may increase the likelihood of conception but does not prevent subsequent urine accumulation and pregnancy loss. • The condition (i.e., increasing angulation) becomes more extreme with increase of uterine weight later during gestation; pulls the vestibule further cranial and ventral. • If poor vulvar and vestibular conformations are secondary to loss of vaginal fat (e. g., mare that is cachectic, thin, poor conditioning), urine pooling may be a slight problem and may resolve as the mare gains weight.

- ○ Increasing fat within the pelvic cavity may elevate the vestibular floor in relationship to the ventral vulvar opening.
- ○ This is considered to be a temporary solution, however, because the condition most likely will recur with age, parity, or subsequent weight loss.

ASSOCIATED CONDITIONS

• Thin mares may be more predisposed to urine pooling. • Usually most severe when the mare is in estrus and vestibular tissues are relaxed
• Increased inflammation and fibrosis of the endometrium

AGE-RELATED FACTORS

• Possible tendency for soft-tissue supporting structures of the vestibule to decrease their tonicity with age • Old mares have a higher occurrence of this condition.

PREGNANCY

May observe infertility or loss of pregnancy because of urine pooling

SYNONYM

Vesicovaginal reflux

Suggested Reading

McKinnon AO, Beldon JO. Urethral extension technique to correct urine pooling (vesicovaginal reflux) in mares. J Am Vet Med Assoc 1988;192:647–650.

Shires GM, Kaneps AJ. A practical and simple surgical technique for repair of urine pooling in the mare. Proc AAEP 1986;51–56.

Author Walter R. Threlfall
Consulting Editor Carla L. Carleton

UROLITHIASIS

BASICS

DEFINITION

• Urolithiasis—macroscopic concretions of urine crystals (calculus or stone) in any portion of the urinary tract that may occur separately or together.
• Sabulous urolithiasis—accumulation of a large mass of urine sediment in the ventral aspect of the bladder as occurs with bladder paresis.

PATHOPHYSIOLOGY

• Despite the large amount of calcium carbonate crystals in normal equine urine, urolithiasis is rare compared to small animals, possibly due to protective lubricating mucus produced by glands in the renal pelvis and proximal ureter.
• The main component of equine uroliths is calcium carbonate along with inorganic elements (magnesium ammonium phosphate, calcium oxalate, or calcium sulfate) and organic matrix (mucoproteins).
• Urolith formation usually requires damage to the renal parenchyma or the uroepithelium of the ureters, bladder or urethra. Compromised uroepithelium allows for adherence of calcium carbonate crystals, which serve as a nidus for stone formation.
• Most spontaneously occurring bladder stones are disc-shaped, mildly spiculated, and porous.

SYSTEM AFFECTED

Renal/urologic—stone formation, infection, and occasionally, postrenal failure or bladder rupture (with obstructive disease)

GENETICS

None documented

INCIDENCE/PREVALENCE

• Urolithiasis is uncommon and reported to be responsible for 0.11% of equine admissions to 22 teaching hospitals, accounting for ≅8% of all urinary tract disorders.
• In the same study, cystoliths were most common (60% of all urinary stones) followed by urethroliths (24%), nephroliths (12%), and ureteroliths (4%); ≅10% of affected horses had multiple calculi at different sites.

SIGNALMENT

Breed Predilections

None documented

Mean Age and Range

Adult horses (mean age ≅10 years) with wide age range with horses <1 year also being possibly affected

Predominant Sex

• ≅75% of all reports are in males—stallions and geldings.
• A longer and less distensible urethra increases risk of cystolithiasis and urethrolithiasis in males, but calculi at other sites are similar in both sexes.

SIGNS

Historical

• Nephrolithiasis and ureterolithiasis—weight loss or fever of undetermined origin, with hematuria or pyuria less common. Occasionally, recurrent colic may be reported.
• Cystolithiasis—lower urinary tract signs (e.g., pollakiuria, stranguria, hematuria) predominate, and hematuria after exercise is common. Sometimes horses will exhibit behavior changes during exercise.
• Sabulous urolithiasis—urinary incontinence
• Urethrolithiasis—may cause severe renal colic signs (e.g., pollakiuria, stranguria, anuria) with partial to complete obstruction (e.g., pollakiuria, stranguria, anuria), and bladder rupture may occur

Physical Examination

• Nephrolithiasis and ureterolithiasis—lethargy, fever, partial anorexia, intermittent colic, and mild dehydration
• Cystolithiasis—dysuria and possibly urine scalding, but general health usually good
• Urethrolithiasis—A distended, sometimes pulsating urethra may be found below the anus, and careful palpation may allow location of the obstructing urolith.
• Rectal examination—Nephrolith—may palpate abnormal shaped left kidney due to hydronephrosis. Ureteroliths—enlarged, turgid ureters with focal concretions. Cystoliths—the calculi can be palpable in the neck of the bladder at the level of the pelvic canal (hand inserted to the wrist) if the bladder is not distended. The bladder wall is thickened. Sabulous urolithiasis—large atonic bladder with incontinence produced by compressing bladder indicates bladder paresis. Urethrolithiasis—markedly distended bladder when obstructed.

CAUSES

• Nephrolithiasis—developmental anomalies, ascending or hematogenous infection, acute tubular necrosis due to nephrotoxic or ischemic injury, and neoplasms can cause parenchymal damage that may serve as a nidus for nephrolithiasis. Ureterolithiasis most commonly is due to passage of small nephroliths into the ureters.
• Cystolithiasis—may develop from ascending infections, anatomic or functional causes of abnormal urine flow(or stasis), or with damage to the bladder uroepithelium.
• Sabulous urolithiasis—bladder paresis (caused by lumbosacral disease such as EPM, EHM, trauma, degenerative joint disease of the lumbosacral region) leading to incomplete voiding and sedimentation of normal urine crystals is a risk factor for developing sabulous urolithiasis in the ventral bladder. Unlike cystoliths, this urolith often indents with firm digital pressure (similar to clay).
• Urethrolithiasis—may develop at sites of damaged uroepithelium (e.g., site of previous perineal urethrotomy) but more commonly results from passage of small uroliths into the urethra.
• Repeated obstruction with urethroliths provides support for upper tract disease as a source of uroliths.

RISK FACTORS

• Although poorly documented, high-calcium diets (e.g., alfalfa and other legume hays) are likely risk factors for calculi along the entire urinary tract.
• An area of damaged uroepithelium usually serves as a nidus for initiation of stone formation.
• Renal medullary crest necrosis due to NSAID use is a risk factor for developing stones in and adjacent to the renal pelvis.

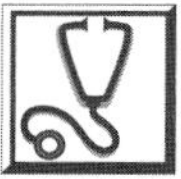

DIAGNOSIS

DIFFERENTIAL DIAGNOSIS

• Upper tract lithiasis—broad list of disease processes that may lead to lethargy, partial anorexia, weight loss, fever, recurrent colic, dysuria, or hematuria
• Lower tract lithiasis—normal estrus activity in mares and other causes of hematuria or dysuria (e.g., UTI, neoplasia)

CBC/BIOCHEMISTRY/URINALYSIS

• Normal to low PCV (with more severe hematuria), normal WBC count or leukocytosis (with concurrent upper tract infection), and normal to mildly decreased platelets (with hematuria)
• Azotemia—usually not present unless lower tract obstruction develops (i.e., postrenal azotemia) or bilateral nephrolithiasis/ureterolithiasis is associated with CRF
• USG—usually normal (>1.020) unless lithiasis is associated with CRF and isosthenuria (1.008–1.014)
• Urinalysis—generally reveals microscopic or macroscopic hematuria and pyuria; bacteria may be detected on sediment examination with concurrent UTI.

OTHER LABORATORY TESTS

• Perform quantitative urine culture along with antimicrobial sensitivity in all cases of suspected urolithiasis to assess for concurrent UTI.
• Consider bacterial culture of the urolith center after surgical removal, as many will culture positive despite negative urine culture results.

IMAGING

Transabdominal Ultrasonography

• Nephroliths (diameter >1 cm) should be readily detected as echogenic structures producing acoustic shadows, possible increased echogenicity in adjacent renal tissue.
• Dilation of the renal pelvis and proximal ureter (hydronephrosis) may be detected with obstructive ureterolithiasis.

Transrectal Ultrasonography

Useful in evaluating the left kidney, ureters, bladder, and proximal urethra. Calculi can be visualized, along with sabulous urolithiasis and a thickened bladder wall.

Urethroscopy/Cystoscopy

To assess uroepithelial damage and urine flow from each side of the upper urinary tract

PATHOLOGICAL FINDINGS

• Nephroliths and ureteroliths may be incidental findings at necropsy if bilateral obstructive disease was absent.
• Small, irregularly shaped kidneys are found with CRF, but nephroliths and ureteroliths occasionally may produce hydronephrosis when obstruction is complete.
• Cystolithiasis leads to bladder-wall thickening.
• Extensive mucosal damage accompanies cystolithiasis and urethrolithiasis.

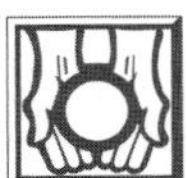

TREATMENT

APPROPRIATE HEALTH CARE

- Appropriate antimicrobial therapy for prophylaxis or treatment of UTI
- Dietary modification, salt supplementation, and medication with urinary acidifying agents may prevent recurrence.
- With sabulous urolithiasis, the underlying problem of bladder paralysis should be addressed.

NURSING CARE

- Regular cleaning of the perineum and hind-limbs to minimize skin irritation from incontinence or after perineal urethrotomy; application of petrolatum to scalded areas
- Horses with obstructive urethrolithiasis may benefit from temporary placement (1–3 days) of an indwelling bladder catheter after perineal urethrotomy if bladder distension was prolonged (>24 hr) or incomplete emptying is detected via rectal palpation.

ACTIVITY N/A

DIET

- Decrease dietary calcium intake by limiting legume hay.
- Oral electrolyte supplementation—sodium chloride (1 oz.) can be administered in concentrate feed or as an oral slurry/paste BID–QID to encourage increased drinking and urine output (to decrease risk of further urolith formation).
- Use of urinary acidifying agents may be considered.

CLIENT EDUCATION

- Urolithiasis may recur in as many as 40% of patients.
- Avoid use of NSAIDs in horses with upper tract lithiasis.
- With sabulous urolithiasis, prognosis for recovery is guarded to poor because of underlying bladder paralysis.

SURGICAL CONSIDERATIONS

- Nephrotomy for removal of obstructing nephroliths or possible unilateral nephrectomy for nephroliths accompanied by pyelonephritis and limited function of the affected kidney
- Elective surgical removal of cystoliths via cystotomy, parainguinal laparocystotomy, laparascopic cystotomy, or perineal urethrotomy; manual removal of small cystoliths may be accomplished in mares.
- High porosity, due to sedimentation of concentric layers of calcium carbonate crystal, makes cystoliths relatively easy to fragment during removal. Less commonly, increased phosphate content of precipitating material leads to more dense concretions and more difficult fragmentation.
- Possible emergency perineal urethrotomy for relief of urethral obstruction or repair of ruptured bladder —after initial stabilization of electrolyte (i.e., hyperkalemia with uroperitoneum) and acid–base alterations
- Fragmentation using electrohydraulic or laser lithotripsy is the treatment of choice for ureteroliths and may be the preferred treatment for cystoliths and urethroliths when equipment is available.
- Placement of a bladder catheter and aggressive lavage and rectal manipulation of the bladder may improve sabulous urolithiasis. There is a high risk for secondary UTI after catheterization of an atonic bladder.

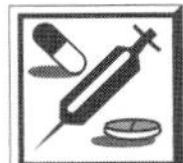

MEDICATIONS

DRUG(S) OF CHOICE

- Appropriate antibiotic agents for prophylaxis or treatment of urinary tract infection—see Urinary Tract Infection.
- Urinary acidifying agents—ammonium chloride (50–200 mg/kg per day PO) and ammonium sulfate (200–300 mg/kg per day PO)—may help decrease urine pH and, thereby, the amount of calcium carbonate crystals in urine; however, they are unpalatable.
- Developing an anionic diet (i.e., low cation–anion balance) will also reduce urine pH, however it requires testing of hay and addition of necessary supplements.
- Changing from alfalfa to grass hay likely will decrease the amount of calcium carbonate crystals more effectively than adding acidifying agents to a legume-based diet.

CONTRAINDICATIONS N/A

PRECAUTIONS

- Evaluate horses with recurrent urethral obstruction for upper tract lithiasis and infection.
- Passing a urinary catheter or performing cystoscopy can complicate UTI in horses with sabulous urolithiasis. UTI is difficult to eliminate when incomplete evacuation of the bladder continues due to bladder paresis.

POSSIBLE INTERACTIONS N/A

ALTERNATIVE DRUGS N/A

FOLLOW-UP

PATIENT MONITORING

- Surgical patients—Assess clinical status at least twice daily during the 2–4 days after surgery, emphasizing urine output and signs of dysuria.
- Nephrolithiasis or ureterolithiasis—Assess renal function at regular intervals (monthly or longer) during the early stages of CRF.
- Recurrent cystolithiasis or urethrolithiasis—Carefully examine the entire urinary tract for predisposing causes such as anatomic defects or pyelonephritis.

PREVENTION/AVOIDANCE

- Dietary modifications
- Use of urinary acidifying agents

POSSIBLE COMPLICATIONS

- Recurrent urolithiasis
- CRF
- Bladder rupture and uroperitoneum
- Urethral stricture
- UTI

EXPECTED COURSE AND PROGNOSIS

- Prognosis for recovery after surgical correction of cystolithiasis and urethrolithiasis generally is favorable, unless the problem is recurrent (guarded long-term prognosis). • Issue a guarded long-term prognosis for patients with nephrolithiasis or ureterolithiasis; these problems usually are accompanied by loss of renal function and, when lithiasis is bilateral, eventual progression to CRF. • Poor prognosis for sabulous urolithiasis where underlying cause of bladder paresis cannot be resolved.

MISCELLANEOUS

ASSOCIATED CONDITIONS

- Renal colic—with obstructive disease • UTI
- Bladder paralysis • CRF

AGE-RELATED FACTORS N/A

ZOONOTIC POTENTIAL N/A

PREGNANCY

Postpartum mares may be at greater risk of developing bladder paralysis or bladder rupture, especially after dystocia.

SYNONYMS

- Lithiasis
- Calculus formation
- Urinary tract stones

SEE ALSO

- CRF
- UTI
- Bladder paralysis and incontinence

ABBREVIATIONS

- CRF = chronic renal failure
- EPM = equine protozoal myelitis
- EHM = equine herpes myeloencephalitis
- PCV = packed cell volume
- USG = urine specific gravity
- UTI = urinary tract infection

Suggested Reading

Duesterdieck-Zellmer KF. Equine urolithiasis. Vet Clin North Amer: Eq Pract 2007:613–629.

Holt PE, Mair TS. Ten cases of bladder paralysis associated with sabulous urolithiasis in horses. Vet Rec 1990;127:108–110.

Laverty S, Pascoe JR, Ling GV, Lavoie JP, Ruby AL. Urolithiasis in 68 horses. Vet Surg 1992;21:56–62.

Mair TS, Holt PE. The etiology and treatment of equine urolithiasis. Equine Vet Educ 1994;6:189–192.

Neumann RD, Ruby AL, Ling GV, Schiffman P, Johnson DL. Ultrastructure and mineral composition of urinary calculi from horses. Am J Vet Res 1994;55:1357–1367.

Schott HC. Clinical Commentary: Urinary incontinence and sabulous urolithiasis – chicken or the egg? Equine Vet Educ 2006;8:17–19.

Author Harold C. Schott II

Consulting Editors Gillian Perkins and Dominic Dawson

UROPERITONEUM, NEONATAL

BASICS

DEFINITION

• Uroperitoneum is an accumulation of urine in the peritoneal cavity and is considered a medical emergency with a surgical cure. • Several known causes/situations can lead to uroperitoneum including congenital rupture of the bladder, bladder rupture associated with sepsis, rupture of the urachus, ureteral tear, or avulsion of the bladder from its urachal attachment from trauma or strenuous exercise.

PATHOPHYSIOLOGY

• Urine is composed of many solutes including a high concentration of potassium, low concentrations of sodium and chloride, and variable concentrations of urea, creatinine, and water. • With urine accumulation within the abdomen, urea, creatinine, and electrolytes move across the semipermeable peritoneal membrane to equilibrate with plasma, leading to azotemia (especially urea), hypochloremia, hyponatremia, and hyperkalemia. • These electrolyte derangements are further exacerbated by the diet of mare's milk, which has a high concentration of potassium (≈25 mEq/L) and low concentrations of sodium (≈12 mEq/L) and chloride. • Creatinine is less permeable than other solutes and may remain disproportionately elevated free within the abdomen. • Pathological abnormalities may not be apparent for several days following urine leakage. • Hyperkalemia is a MEDICAL EMERGENCY and represents the most serious of electrolyte derangement in these foals, where profound electrocardiographic dysfunction can occur. Bradycardia, atrial standstill, and cardiac arrest may occur with uncorrected hyperkalemia. • Restrictive respiratory failure and colic may be observed in foals with progressive abdominal distention, and ventilation may become impaired.

SYSTEMS AFFECTED

Urinary

• Rupture of one or more structures of the urinary tract; bladder most common • Septic foci may predispose to bladder rupture.

Gastrointestinal

• Colic and ileus associated with pain and progressive abdominal distention • Inappetence • Sterile peritonitis

Cardiovascular

Hyperkalemic dysrhythmias—atrial standstill, cardiac arrest, complete third-degree AV blockade, ventricular fibrillation

Respiratory

Tachypnea associated with progressive abdominal distention and restrictive lung expansion

Neurologic

Depression associated with hyponatremia, progressing to seizure activity

GENETICS N/A

INCIDENCE/PREVALENCE

Sporadic event; greatest incidence in newborn foals

GEOGRAPHIC DISTRIBUTION

Worldwide

SIGNALMENT

Breed Predilections

No known breed predilection

Mean Age and Range

• The age at the time of diagnosis varies between congenital and acquired uroperitoneum, as does the range. • Congenital uroperitoneum tends to occur during vigorous parturition and in the immediate post-partum period. Most cases are recognized within 3–5 days of age. Acquired or secondary uroperitoneum occurs in foals from 1 to 60 days, with most cases diagnosed within the first 2 weeks of life.

Predominant Sex

• Congenitally acquired uroperitoneum occurs more commonly in colt foals (>80%). Dorsal urinary bladder tears can occur during parturition. It is believed to occur more commonly in colts due to the relatively long urethra, high tone of the urethral sphincter, and high intraluminal hydrostatic pressures of the distended bladder contributing to an increased resistance to emptying. Also, increased intra-abdominal pressures during passage through the pelvic canal may contribute.
• Congenital ureteral defects occur more commonly in fillies. • Secondarily acquired uroperitoneum occurs equally among colts and fillies. Conditions such as neonatal septicemia, omphalophlebitis, omphaloarteritis, patent urachus, and umbilical abscessation are risk factors.

SIGNS

Historical

• Foals usually are born normal. • Foals may be observed to still void some urine. • Clinical signs are usually evident by 24–72 hr of age, yet can occur as late as 3–4 weeks.

Physical Examination

• Frequent attempts to urinate that may be partially successful and void a small stream. Often no urine is passed. • Progressive inappetence, dehydration, depression, lying down • Progressive abdominal distention and the development of colic and/or tachypnea. Fluid ballotment may be possible. • Ventral edema may be present. • As electrolytes become more deranged, weakness and recumbency become a prominent feature. • Bradycardia or tachycardia

CAUSES

• Congenital rupture during and/or shortly after parturition • Acquired urachal or bladder rupture associated with sepsis and/or local septic focus (e.g., omphalophlebitis) • Rarely, embryological failure of the halves of the bladder to unite (schistocystitis) or ureteral defects can cause uroperitoneum. • Iatrogenic rupture associated with catheters • Traumatic rupture

RISK FACTORS

• Males for congenital rupture • Age <4 days
• Septicemia • Prematurity • Abdominal trauma

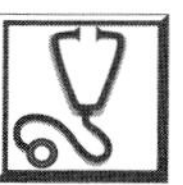

DIAGNOSIS

DIFFERENTIAL DIAGNOSIS

• Colic for various gastrointestinal reasons
• Meconium impaction should be differentiated from ruptured bladder. Generally, foals that strain to urinate adopt a base-wide stance with ventroflexion of the back whereas foals straining to defecate often show dorsoflexion in their back.

CBC/BIOCHEMISTRY/URINALYSIS

• Hematologic abnormalities may reflect concurrent disease such as septicemia.
• Electrolyte derangements include hyperkalemia, hyponatremia, hypochloremia.
• Acid-base evaluation often reveals metabolic acidosis (hypobicarbonatemia). • Azotemia

OTHER LABORATORY TESTS

Abdominocentesis may yield copious volumes of clear-yellow fluid of low cellularity with a uriniferous odor. Peritoneal fluid creatinine concentration is at least twice the serum creatinine concentration. Occasionally, calcium carbonate crystals may be present in peritoneal fluid.

IMAGING

Abdominal Ultrasonography

• Increased hypoechoic fluid with abdominal viscera floating within this fluid • A flaccid collapsed urinary bladder may be visualized.
• Urachal examination may show the margins of a tear. • *Note:* The thorax should be evaluated as pleural fluid often accumulates and detection is important when considering anesthesia for surgical repair.

Abdominal Radiography

• Loss of serosal detail of abdominal viscera
• Standing films may show obvious fluid line.
• Positive contrast cystography using water-soluble contrast agent (e.g., 10% iohexol) should be considered to evaluate the position of urogenital tear.

OTHER DIAGNOSTIC PROCEDURES

Electrocardiography is indicated to assess potassium related dysrhythmias, especially when potassium >6 mEq/L.

PATHOLOGIC FINDINGS

• Necropsy examination confirms the presence of uroperitoneum (high volume effusion) and the structural defect allowing leakage of urine into the abdomen. Bladder defects tend to be dorsal. Ureteral defects lead to an accumulation of retroperitoneal urine. • The urologic defect can have signs of healing, which can make it readily confused with a malformation, because affected foals can survive for days after the rupture occurs— sufficient time for partial healing of the defect.

UROPERITONEUM, NEONATAL

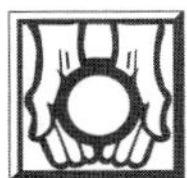

TREATMENT

AIMS OF TREATMENT

• Correct hypovolemia, electrolyte. and acid-base disturbances. • Effective abdominal drainage • Correct structural defects.

APPROPRIATE HEALTH CARE

• Immediate referral to a surgical facility is recommended. • Surgery should be performed after metabolic stabilization.

NURSING CARE

Stabilization

• Correction of hydration, electrolyte abnormalities and acid-base derangements should be initiated before surgery. Isotonic saline solutions (e.g., 0.9% NaCl) with or without dextrose (2.5%–5%) are often given. Occasionally hypertonic solutions are used (e.g., 1.8% NaCl). Half-strength saline (0.45% NaCl) should not be used as it may exacerbate hyponatremia. • Note that where profound hyponatremia exists, correction should be done slowly to avoid hyponatremic encephalopathy (≤1 mEq/L/hr). • Where profound metabolic acidosis exists, isotonic sodium bicarbonate solutions are indicated. • Plasma transfusion should be administered where failure of transfer of passive immunity is evident. • Abdominal drainage should be performed via placement of an abdominal catheter. A balloon-tip Foley catheter or peritoneal dialysis catheter is ideal and can be placed through a small (5 mm) incision under local anesthesia. A paramedian inguinal caudal abdominal approach is recommended to avoid contamination of a future surgical site and the omentum is least likely to cause drain blockage in this location. • Placement of a urinary catheter and bladder decompression should be done before surgery and may be useful for small defects in the bladder, where these may heal without surgery.

Hyperkalemia

• Isotonic saline solutions with dextrose (2.5%–5%) administered intravenously • For unresponsive hyperkalemia, regular (crystalline) insulin can be administered with a continuous infusion of dextrose. Regular assessment of serum glucose should be performed. • Calcium gluconate may be administered via slow intravenous injection. Caution: Do not mix with bicarbonate containing solutions as these will precipitate out.

ACTIVITY

• Restricted movement is recommended before and after surgery for at least 7–14 days.
• Limit walking or exercise until the abdominal sutures are removed and the abdominal incision is healed (usually 30–60 days).

DIET

• Allow the foal to continue to nurse until shortly before surgery. • Mare's milk after recovery from surgery and anesthesia

CLIENT EDUCATION

• Clients will need to know about correct care for the abdominal incision. • Careful observation for recurrence suggesting surgical failure

SURGICAL CONSIDERATIONS

• Emergency surgery is not indicated to repair the defect until the metabolic status of the patient is improved with medical therapy and abdominal drainage. • Before surgery, place a urethral catheter (e.g., Foley). • Constant ECG monitoring and acid-base assessment should be performed during surgery. • Ventral midline celiotomy and laparoscopic techniques are described. • Thorough inspection and assessment of structural defects should identify any necrotic/infected tissue. These should be resected, including the umbilical remnants.
• Conservative treatment is placement of urinary catheter (via urethra) for 3–5 days to allow constant drainage of bladder without surgical correction of tear. It is useful when surgical repair is not available (cost, expertise).

MEDICATIONS

DRUG(S)

• Broad-spectrum antimicrobial coverage, especially neonates with presumed sepsis and acquired rupture, e.g. sodium penicillin or ampicillin (25–40,000IU/kg IV q6 hr or 10 mg/kg IV q6hr, respectively) and amikacin sulfate (25 mg/kg IV q24hr) • NSAIDs may be given to control pain and inflammation related to surgery (ketoprofen 1–2 mg/kg q12–24h).
• Insulin (0.1–0.2 IU/kg SC or IV) may be given with dextrose infusions to help reduce the extracellular potassium concentration.

CONTRAINDICATIONS

Avoid potassium containing intravenous fluids or medications composed of potassium salts, e.g. potassium penicillin.

PRECAUTIONS

In hypovolemic patients, aminoglycosides and NSAIDs should be used with caution and at judicious dosages. Where possible, amikacin is the preferred aminoglycoside and ketoprofen is the preferred NSAID.

POSSIBLE INTERACTIONS N/A

ALTERNATIVE DRUGS

For broad-spectrum antimicrobial coverage, third-generation cephalosporins may be used.

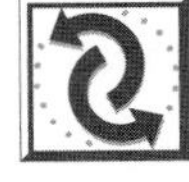

FOLLOW-UP

PATIENT MONITORING

• Serum electrolytes (especially potassium and sodium) and urea/creatinine concentrations should be performed every 2–4h to assess response to stabilization therapy and suitability for anesthesia and surgery. • Monitoring of urine output postoperatively is important. This should be at least 1 mL/kg/hr. • Postoperative indwelling urinary catheter use is controversial although effective at reducing distention on the surgical site, which is important particularly if there is friable tissue. The risk of ascending infection is increased with indwelling urinary catheters.

PREVENTION/AVOIDANCE N/A

POSSIBLE COMPLICATIONS

• Significant anesthetic risk occurs where electrolyte derangements exist. • Surgical dehiscence and re-rupture of the bladder
• Incisional complications include infection, dehiscence, hernia, although uncommon.
• Peritonitis

EXPECTED COURSE AND PROGNOSIS

• Congenital uroperitoneum associated with ruptured bladder carries a favorable prognosis, >80%, provided timely medical and surgical therapy is administered. • The prognosis for secondary uroperitoneum is considered less favorable, 50%–60%, largely influenced by the primary disease process, which in most cases is septicemia.

MISCELLANEOUS

ASSOCIATED CONDITIONS, AGE-RELATED FACTORS, ZOONOTIC POTENTIAL, PREGNANCY N/A

SYNONYMS

• Uroabdomen • Ruptured bladder

SEE ALSO

• Patent urachus • Meconium retention
• Colic in foals

ABBREVIATIONS

• AV = atrioventricular
• ECG = electrocardiograph

Suggested Reading

Bryant JE, Gaughan EM. Abdominal surgery in neonatal foals. Vet Clin North Am Equine Pract 2005;21:511–535.

Dunkel B, Palmer JE, Olson KN, Boston RC, Wilkins PA. Uroperitoneum in 32 foals: influence of intravenous fluid therapy, infection, and sepsis. J Vet Intern Med 2005;19:889–893.

Kablack KA, Embertson RM, Bernard WV, Bramlage LR, Hance S, Reimer JM, Barton MH. Uroperitoneum in the hospitalised equine neonate: retrospective study of 31 cases, 1988–1997. Equine Vet J 2000;32:505–508.

Richardson DW, Kohn CW. Uroperitoneum in the foal. J Am Vet Med Assoc 1983;182:267–271.

Author Samuel D. A. Hurcombe
Consulting Editor Margaret C. Mudge

URTICARIA

BASICS

DEFINITION

• Urticaria and angioedema are common inflammatory reaction patterns that result from mast cell and, to a lesser extent, basophil degranulation. Angioedema is a focal or diffuse excessive accumulation of tissue fluid within the interstitium, often at gravitative surfaces that presents as edematous swellings that may exhibit serum leakage or hemorrhage. Urticarial reactions may or may not be pruritic and vary in severity from inconsequential to systemic problems of a life-threatening nature.

PATHOPHYSIOLOGY

The release of cellular inflammatory mediators such as histamine, platelet-activating factor, and prostaglandins contributes to increased vascular smooth muscle relaxation and endothelial cell retraction, causing plasma to extravasate and cause turgid edematous wheals, or angioedema. Angioedema is due to increased capillary hydrostatic pressure and permeability, or low plasma colloid osmotic pressure. Stimuli for urticaria are classified as immunologic, immediate IgE-mediated (type I), immune complex-mediated (type III), or a delayed cell-mediated (type IV) hypersensitivities, or nonimmunologic.

SYSTEMS AFFECTED

• Skin/exocrine
• Respiratory

GENETICS

Genetic predisposition and heritability are unknown.

INCIDENCE/PREVALENCE

Urticaria is within the top 10 most common equine dermatoses, whereas angioedema is rare.

GEOGRAPHIC DISTRIBUTION

Worldwide; local environmental factors (temperature, humidity, and flora) can influence the seasonality, severity, and duration of signs if the urticaria has an underlying allergic etiology.

SIGNALMENT

Breed Predilections

Arabians, Thoroughbreds, Quarter Horses, and Warmbloods may be predisposed because of their propensity to develop allergic dermatitis.

Mean Age and Range

Mean age of onset is unknown; a range of 1–10 years has been documented.

Predominant Sex

Equal distribution exists between males and females.

SIGNS

General Comments

• Onset of lesions can be acute or peracute episodes occurring 15 min to hours post challenge. Chronic urticaria is a relapsing, remitting presentation that persists for at least 6–8 weeks. The characteristic lesion is a wheal—a flat-topped papule/nodule with steep-walled sides resulting from localized transient edema within the dermis. Pitting edema is a key clinical feature of urticaria or angioedema, although gyrate urticaria often does not pit. Clinical classification of urticaria relies on size and morphologic appearance.
• Conventional—Wheal size varies from 2–3 mm to 3–5 cm in diameter.
• Papular—Wheal size is uniform and small, ≈3–6 mm in diameter.
• Gyrate (polycyclic)—Wheals have unusual shapes such as annular, doughnut, serpignious, linear, curvilinear, arciform, and can persist for months.
• Giant—single or multiple wheals that range from 20 to 40 cm in diameter
• Exudative—Severe dermal edema oozes from the skin, mats the hair, and causes alopecia, often mistaken for pyoderma, dermatophytosis, and pemphigus foliaceus.
• Angioedema (angioneurotic edema)—diffuse subcutaneous edema, affecting head, thorax, ventral abdomen, and/or gravity-dependent extremities

CAUSES

Causes are either immunologic or nonimmunologic, with the former the most common.

• Immunologic causes include
  ○ Insect hypersensitivity (stinging and biting insects), atopic dermatitis (pollens, molds and epidermals), food allergy
  ○ Drugs (including vaccines, anthelmintics)
  ○ Various others such as penicillin, tetracycline, sulfonamides, neomycin, ciprofloxacin, streptomycin, aspirin, phenylbutazone, flunixin, phenothiazines, guaifenesin, ivermectin, moxidectin, iron, dextrans, hormones, and vitamin B complex
  ○ Infections—bacterial (e.g., strangles, salmonellosis, botulinum, tetanus), pyoderma, cellulitis, lymphangitis, abscess, dermatophytosis, parasitic protozoal, (e. g., *Trypanosoma equiperdum*), and viral (e.g., horsepox)
  ○ Vasculitis (immune-mediated or photo-activated)
  ○ Contact with substance (e.g., leather soaps, conditioners, or rubber tack)
  ○ Snakebite
  ○ Plants (e.g., nettle and buttercup)
  ○ Mast cell or lymphoreticular neoplasia
• Nonimmunologic factors include psychological stresses, genetic abnormalities, temperature (heat, cold or sunlight), physical (pressure or dermatographism), exercise, cholinergic, and administration of radiocontrast media and opiates.
• Idiopathic—the likelihood of documenting a specific etiology of chronic urticaria is low, thus the diagnosis of "idiopathic" is common.

RISK FACTORS

• Temperate environments with long allergy seasons
• Concurrent pruritic dermatoses, such as insect hypersensitivity (summation effect)
• Treatment by polypharmacy

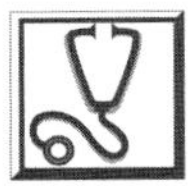

DIAGNOSIS

DIFFERENTIAL DIAGNOSIS

The differential diagnosis for urticaria varies with the morphologic presentation.

• Conventional—vasculitis
• Papular—infectious and sterile folliculitides, frequently associated with biting insects, in particular, mosquitoes and *Culicoides* spp.
• Giant—vasculitis
• Gyrate—erythema multiforme, drug reactions
• Lymphoreticular disease
• Amyloidosis

CBC/BIOCHEMISTRY/URINALYSIS

• Leukocytosis suggests inflammatory or infectious disease.
• Thrombocytopenia may be secondary to vasculitis.

OTHER LABORATORY TESTS

Relevance equated to etiology

IMAGING N/A

OTHER DIAGNOSTIC PROCEDURES

• Biopsy—used to differentiate urticaria, pyoderma, pemphigus, dermatophytosis, or vasculitis
• Dermatographism test—Scratch the skin with blunt object and observe for reaction within 10–15 min. A positive reaction is an edematous wheal that follows the path of the scratch.
• Heat- or cold-induced urticaria is confirmed by applying a reusable hand warmer or ice cube to the skin for a few minutes with the formation of a wheal within 15 min.
• Exercise-induced urticaria requires a period of active exercise to occur, whereas cholinergic urticaria results from an active (such as exercise) or a passive (hot bath) increase in core body temperature.
• An IDT is used to identify causative allergens (pollens, molds, epidermals) for inclusion into allergen-specific immunotherapy. The benefit of allergen-specific immunotherapy for treatment of insect hypersensitivity remains unknown. An IDT is performed in cases of chronic urticaria where the history and elimination of other differential diagnoses suggest atopic dermatitis.
• Horses with a suspected adverse reaction to food should undergo a food exclusion trial. Start with a 4- to 8-week trial of a novel food source such as single-source hay (alfalfa, orchard, timothy, or coastal Bermuda grass). Single-source grains include rolled oats, beet pulp, or barley. Commence food trial by

eliminating all grains, supplements, and drugs, and feed single-source hay. For horses in moderate to heavy work, consider both single-source hay and grain. After resolution of urticaria, confirm food allergy by rechallenging with the introduction of one item each week. Food allergy may be seasonal due to the seasonal variances in hay and supplements.
- A patch test is used to identify contact reactions. Clip a small area on the lateral aspect of the neck with a No. 40 blade. Place a small amount of the test substance on a piece of gauze and affix it so that the substance is in contact with the clipped area. Remove the gauze and observe for urticaria 24–48 hr after application.
- Skin scrapings, fungal and bacterial cultures, and impression smears should be performed if infectious causes are suspected.

PATHOLOGICAL FINDINGS

The histological description for allergic urticaria is superficial to mid-dermal, moderate to severe edema, and superficial vascular congestion. Perivascular to interstitial inflammation is often mild and extends from the superficial to the midfollicular dermis. Eosinophils, lymphocytes, histiocytes, and variable neutrophils are present. In more severe urticaria, prominent edema may expand the superficial dermis and result in secondary dermal-epidermal separation. Angioedema results in severe edema that extends to the subcutis.

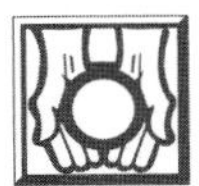

TREATMENT

AIMS OF TREATMENT

Identify and eliminate the primary cause.

APPROPRIATE HEALTH CARE

Depends on etiology

NURSING CARE

Frequent bathing using cool water (antimicrobial shampoos, sulfur/salicyclic acid, +/−colloidal oatmeal rinses or leave-on conditioners) removes allergens, crusts, bacteria, debris, controls secondary infections, hydrates skin, and counters pruritus.

ACTIVITY

Determined by severity and cause

DIET

Essential fatty acid supplementation may be beneficial.

CLIENT EDUCATION

Depends on etiology

SURGICAL CONSIDERATIONS

N/A

MEDICATIONS

DRUG(S)

- Anaphylaxis; see Anaphylaxis chapter.
- Glucocorticoids are indicated to reverse persistent bronchospasm and angioedema and to break the cycle of mediator-induced inflammation. Use a rapid-acting glucocorticoid such as prednisolone sodium succinate (0.25–10.0 mg/kg IV).
- If patient does not respond to antihistamine therapy, use prednisolone tablets or syrup (compounded) at 0.5–1.5 mg/kg q24h until control achieved; then reduce to lowest-dose alternate-day regimen, for example, 0.2–0.5 mg/kg q48h.
- For horses that do not respond to prednisolone (refractory cases), try dexamethasone powder or injectable. Initial loading oral or IV dose of 0.02–0.1 mg/kg q24h for 2–4 days followed by oral maintenance dose of 0.01–0.02 mg/kg q48–72h for maintenance
- Repository injectable corticosteroids should be avoided as withdrawal upon an adverse reaction is not possible.
- Antihistamines—hydroxyzine hydrochloride or pamonate at 1–1.5 mg/kg PO q12h or chlorpheniramine at 0.25–0.5 mg/kg PO q12h may be effective in controlling acute or chronic urticaria.

CONTRAINDICATIONS

- Diuretics generally aggravate edema of noncardiogenic origin.
- Steroids worsen edema secondary to infectious disease.
- Due to the anticholinergic properties of antihistamines and tricyclic antidepressants, do not use in patients with a history of cardiac arrhythmias, colic, glaucoma, or urinary retention disorders. Antihistamines may thicken mucus in the respiratory tract. Use extra caution in horses with respiratory problems due to excess mucus.
- Avoid corticosteroid use during pregnancy and lactation unless the benefits outweigh the risks.

PRECAUTIONS

- Epinephrine may cause excitement in horses; if administered SC, its potent vasoconstriction activity leads to poor absorption and local tissue necrosis.
- Adverse effects of epinephrine therapy are tachyarrhythmia and myocardial ischemia.
- The use of epinephrine should be avoided with the use of α_2-adrenoreceptor agonists such as xylazine or detomidine HCl as they potentate α_2-agonist effects.
- Taper patients on long-term steroid therapy so endogenous steroid production resumes.
- Transient sedation of several days may occur with antihistamines.

POSSIBLE INTERACTIONS

- Prednisolone interacts with phenytoin, phenobarbital, rifampin, erythromycin, neostigmine, and pyridostigmine.
- Antihistamines have an additive effect with other CNS-depressant drugs, such as tranquilizers.

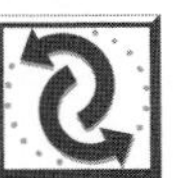

FOLLOW-UP

PATIENT MONITORING

Horses with respiratory and/or gastrointestinal involvement should be monitored at a facility with an intensive care unit.

PREVENTION/AVOIDANCE

Depends on the etiology

POSSIBLE COMPLICATIONS

- Most serious complication of angioedema is respiratory compromise.
- Angioedema may involve the gastro-intestinal tract, leading to intestinal wall edema and clinical signs of colic and/or diarrhea.
- Central nervous signs may occur secondary to focal cerebral edema.

EXPECTED COURSE AND PROGNOSIS

- Prognosis is generally good to excellent for control of urticaria, whereas the prognosis for angioedema depends on the cause and systemic manifestations.
- Linear urticaria may be more difficult to control or resolve.
- Spontaneous remission may occur.

MISCELLANEOUS

ASSOCIATED CONDITIONS

Angioedema—pleural or peritoneal effusion

AGE-RELATED FACTORS

Severity may worsen with age.

ZOONOTIC POTENTIAL

Certain fungal (*Sporothrix*) and bacterial (MRSA) organisms may transfer to people via direct contact.

PREGNANCY

- Corticosteroids—contraindicated during pregnancy
- Antihistamines—no information on teratogenicity is available for horses; consider this before treating pregnant mares.

SYNONYMS

Hives

SEE ALSO

- Vasculitits, systemic
- Insect hypersensitivity
- Atopic dermatitis
- Bacterial dermatitis

ABBREVIATIONS

- IDT = intradermal test
- MRSA = methicillin-resistant *Staphylococcus aureus*

Suggested Reading

Scott DW, Miller WH Jr. Equine Dermatology. St. Louis: Saunders, 2003:420.

Author Gwendolen Lorch
Consulting Editor Gwendolen Lorch

UTERINE INERTIA

BASICS

DEFINITION/OVERVIEW

Primary Uterine Inertia

- Lack of myometrial contractions
- May result in retained fetal membranes
- Associated/related conditions—lack of exercise, overconditioning, chronic illnesses, twinning, uterine disease, and aging

Secondary Uterine Inertia

- Usually follows prolonged labor without expulsion of the fetus and exhaustion of the myometrium
- More common than primary uterine inertia
- To increase the likelihood of delivering a live fetus, assist mares with uterine inertia, once the condition is diagnosed.

ETIOLOGY/PATHOPHYSIOLOGY

- *Primary inertia*—may result from failure of the myometrium to respond to hormonal stimulation; lack of hormonal release; or deficiency of hormonal receptors for oxytocin, estrogen, and/or $PGF_{2\alpha}$
- *Secondary inertia*—The exact mechanisms responsible for secondary uterine inertia are understandable, because exhaustion of the muscle fibers occurs with prolonged labor.

SYSTEM AFFECTED

Reproductive

GENETICS

N/A

INCIDENCE/PREVALENCE

Secondary inertia—<1% of foaling mares

SIGNALMENT

- All breeds
- All females of breeding age

SIGNS

- Mares in dystocia frequently are affected.
- Often a history of prolonged labor, then an absence of the signs of labor

CAUSES AND RISK FACTORS

- The major cause is dystocia.
- Lack of exercise has been incriminated repeatedly as a cause.
- Benefits observed in fit mares—less fatigue with/during delivery, shortened time for parturition, and improved body tone and abdominal strength
- Overconditioning—overweight
- Restricted exercise during pregnancy
- Old mares
- Mares in dystocia

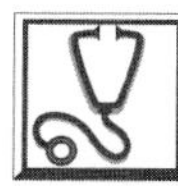

DIAGNOSIS

DIFFERENTIAL DIAGNOSIS

Dystocia from any cause

CBC/BIOCHEMISTRY/URINALYSIS

N/A

OTHER LABORATORY TESTS

N/A

IMAGING

N/A

OTHER DIAGNOSTIC PROCEDURES

Assess the effectiveness of uterine contractions—Observe the mare's expulsive efforts, and examine the uterus to determine if purposeful contractions are occurring.

PATHOLOGICAL FINDINGS

None specific

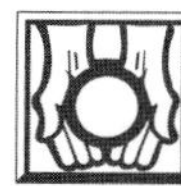

TREATMENT

- At the time when secondary uterine inertia is diagnosed, no correction is possible before the dystocia is resolved.
- With primary uterine inertia, first assist with the delivery of the fetus, then administer oxytocin.
    - If oxytocin is administered before fetal delivery, it will cause the uterus to contract around the fetus and compound delivery problems.
- Foaling mares need assistance if normal delivery times for stages 1 and 2 are exceeded.

The window of time for successful delivery (i.e., to deliver a live foal) is very short in the mare.

APPROPRIATE HEALTH CARE, NURSING CARE, ACTIVITY, DIET, CLIENT EDUCATION, SURGICAL CONSIDERATIONS

N/A

MEDICATIONS

DRUG(S) OF CHOICE

After removal of the fetus, oxytocin 10 IU IM is the hormone of choice.

CONTRAINDICATIONS

N/A

PRECAUTIONS

N/A

POSSIBLE INTERACTIONS

- Avoid high doses of oxytocin, which are unnecessary and may cause excessive contractions and the likelihood of uterine prolapse.
- $PGF_{2\alpha}$ enhances uterine contractions, but the clinical significance of these contractions has been questioned, but the author believes it to be beneficial.
- Do not attempt correction of uterine inertia before the fetus is delivered, and only then treat with low doses (10 IU IM) of oxytocin.

ALTERNATIVE DRUGS

N/A

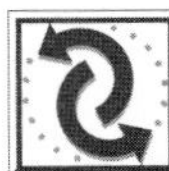

FOLLOW-UP

PATIENT MONITORING

Postpartum uterine examinations—Determine if involution is proceeding normally after oxytocin administration; determine if fetal membranes have all passed.

PREVENTION/AVOIDANCE

- Exercise and proper nutrition play important roles in preventing primary uterine inertia.
- Secondary uterine inertia occurs most often, but may be impossible to prevent unless parturition is observed and assistance is rendered as soon as dystocia is observed.

POSSIBLE COMPLICATIONS

- Retained fetal membranes
- Delayed uterine involution
- Both retained fetal membranes and delayed uterine involution may result in uterine infection and/or inflammation, which can delay rebreeding or result in infertility.

EXPECTED COURSE AND PROGNOSIS

- Excellent prognosis with proper treatment
- May be warranted to skip breeding on foal heat
- Reserve making the final decision regarding foal-heat breeding until examination of the uterus near/at the time of breeding, because some mares recover quickly.

MISCELLANEOUS

ASSOCIATED CONDITIONS

- Dystocia can cause secondary uterine inertia.
- Retained fetal membranes can occur after uterine inertia.

AGE-RELATED FACTORS

Incidence increases with age.

ZOONOTIC POTENTIAL

N/A

PREGNANCY

Occurs only at parturition and shortly thereafter

Suggested Reading

Roberts SJ. Veterinary Obstetrics and Genital Diseases (Theriogenology), ed 3. Woodstock, VT: published by the author, 1986:347–352.

Author Walter R. Threlfall

Consulting Editor Carla L. Carleton

UTERINE TORSION

BASICS

DEFINITION/OVERVIEW

Torsion or twisting of the uterus at its body less often extends caudally to involve the cervix in the mare.

ETIOLOGY/PATHOPHYSIOLOGY

- Lengthening of the broad ligament, which permits the uterus additional leeway to twist on itself, is of primary importance.
- This lengthening may result from repeated stretching during previous gestations, rapid movement of the fetus, or rolling or falling and turning of the mare, faster than the speed with which the fetus and uterus can rotate.

SYSTEM AFFECTED

Reproductive

GENETICS

- No hereditary predisposition is linked to uterine torsion.
- If the supporting tissue (i.e., broad ligament) is longer in some animals because of genetics, this would support the theory of hereditary predisposition.

INCIDENCE/PREVALENCE

- Infrequent occurrence; at anytime during the last 6 mo of pregnancy
- It is frequently found at 6–9 mo and should be corrected when diagnosed.
- The later in gestation that uterine torsion occurs, the more serious the consequences can be.

SIGNALMENT

- Females; all breeds
- Most affected are mares with deeper bodies or larger abdomens
- All mares of breeding age
- Increased occurrence in pluripara

SIGNS

General Comments

The mare exhibits a variety of clinical signs, depending on the stage of gestation when torsion occurs.

Historical

May present with signs of slight to mild colic, inappetence, depression, or general decrease or increase in activity, sweating, and increased urination

Physical Examination

- Depending on stage of gestation, the mare may exhibit tense abdomen, increased heart rate on auscultation, and increased respiratory rate.
- TRP reveals twisting of the broad ligament and body of the uterus and/or cervix.
- Vaginal examinations are less valuable in mares (compared with cows), because involvement of the vagina in the torsion is uncommon.
- At term, mares fail to show signs of labor, because the fetus is unable to enter the pelvic canal and cervix (i.e., absence of Ferguson reflex). Therefore, fetal death may occur from placental separation without the owner's knowledge.

CAUSES

- Cause unknown
- There appears to be a relationship to relaxation or decrease of the suspensory nature of the broad ligament.
- Fetal movement plus the possibility of the mare falling or rolling can add to the probability of developing uterine torsion.

RISK FACTORS

- Dam with a large abdomen
- Multiple pregnancies
- Primipara may be affected.

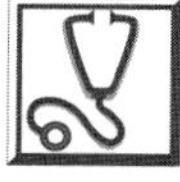

DIAGNOSIS

DIFFERENTIAL DIAGNOSIS

- Intestinal colic—Rule out by TRP to determine if the broad ligament twists to the left or right.
- Normal labor—Rule out by the absence of membrane rupture, release of chorioallantoic fluid, etc. suspensory nature.

CBC/BIOCHEMISTRY/URINALYSIS

N/A

OTHER LABORATORY TESTS

N/A

IMAGING

Transabdominal U/S examination if necessary determines viability of the fetus.

OTHER DIAGNOSTIC PROCEDURES

N/A

PATHOLOGICAL FINDINGS

- The uterus is turned clockwise or counterclockwise, with increased tension on the broad ligament, and the uterine wall may have increased tone.
- Counterclockwise torsion is more common than clockwise torsion.

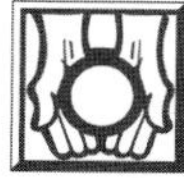

TREATMENT

APPROPRIATE HEALTH CARE

- Accurate diagnosis is important to correct torsion before the fetus dies.
- If left untreated, a torsion of >180° compromises the blood supply to the fetus and uterus, and fetal death may occur, especially if the mare is near term.

Rolling

- Usually not indicated, unless sufficient help is available and the mare is not near term (<9 mo of gestation)
- Mare must be anesthetized. Multiple people are necessary to rapidly roll the mare in the direction of the torsion.
  - Lay the mare down on the side toward which the torsion is turning.
  - Clockwise torsion, on the right side.
  - Counterclockwise torsion, on the left side.
  - Then roll the mare over on its back.
- Contraindications as the mare approaches term pregnancy: uterine artery rupture or uterine wall tears (more common than when this procedure is used to relieve torsion in cows)
- Assistance required after the procedure until the mare recovers from anesthesia and stands.

Laparotomy

- Excellent technique, because minimal assistance is necessary and repositioning is very successful, especially <9 mo of gestation.
- As the mare approaches term, additional help may be required, including the possibility of a second incision to allow a second surgeon to work from the opposite flank.
- If one incision is to be used:
  - Must be adequate to allow the surgeon to pull the ventral aspect of the uterus into proper position
  - It is easier to pull the uterus than it is to push the uterus and fetus.
- If an additional incision is necessary, the second surgeon can pull the dorsal aspect as the primary surgeon applies traction to the ventral aspect of the uterus.

Cesarean Section

- Can be performed in cases of uterine torsion, but correcting the torsion before incising the uterus makes it easier to extract the fetus and to suture the uterus
- Usually only necessary when the fetus is at term and delivery must be immediate, or if the fetus is dead and vaginal delivery is not possible
- Usually not necessary, because most torsions occur before the onset of labor

NURSING CARE

- Implement care by:
  - Bedding changes in the stall
  - Cross-tying, or
  - Other managerial options that may discourage the mare from rolling in the stall

ACTIVITY

- After correction of the torsion, stall rest the mare.
- Hand-walk the mare until parturition, if possible.
- Prevent the mare from running or having the opportunity to roll.

DIET

- Permit access to free-choice hay.
- Quality is not as important as quantity, keep the abdomen as full as possible.

CLIENT EDUCATION

Remind owners that as with any condition of pregnant mares, subtle changes in the mare's demeanor or behavior may indicate abnormal gestation and immediate assistance should be sought.

SURGICAL CONSIDERATIONS

- A grid incision usually fails to provide sufficient area for manipulation, and incision of the abdominal muscles is necessary.
- A hand is moved ventrally under the uterus, and a fetal hock or other extremity is grasped and then pulled toward the incision.
- At first, the uterus will be difficult to move, but as it begins returning to its normal position, movement will become easier.
- Once uterine detorsion passes the halfway point, it will easily move the remainder of the distance.
- If one person cannot return the uterus to its normal position, a second incision can be made on the opposite side of the mare, and both surgeons can pull the uterus to its normal position.

MEDICATIONS

DRUG(S) OF CHOICE

- Xylazine IV, followed 5–10 min later with IV morphine, detomidine, or drug of choice
- Infiltrate the area for incision with 2% carbocaine, to effect.

CONTRAINDICATIONS

N/A

PRECAUTIONS

- Confirm the diagnosis as rapidly as possible, especially if the mare is near term, to save the fetus.
- Administration of the previously mentioned agents should not be detrimental to fetal viability at any stage of gestation.

POSSIBLE INTERACTIONS

N/A

ALTERNATIVE DRUGS

N/A

FOLLOW-UP

PATIENT MONITORING

- Frequent after correction of uterine torsion
- Close, daily observation and TRP examination of the uterus at 1- to 2-week intervals until it appears that recurrence is not likely
- For mares at term and in labor, recurrence of this condition after delivery has not been reported.

PREVENTION/AVOIDANCE

- Limiting exercise is one possible method to reduce the likelihood of the mare falling or rolling, but rarely is indicated or warranted.
- Limited exercise also creates other problems: increase in difficult deliveries because of lack of exercise.
- Free-choice hay is advisable and also may reduce the occurrence of abdominal colic.

POSSIBLE COMPLICATIONS

Uterine torsion can result in prolonged delivery and fetal death.

EXPECTED COURSE AND PROGNOSIS

Correction before term requires follow-up examinations; recurrence is possible.

MISCELLANEOUS

N/A

ASSOCIATED CONDITIONS

N/A

AGE-RELATED FACTORS

Old mares may have increased occurrence because of previous broad ligament stretching.

ZOONOTIC POTENTIAL

N/A

PREGNANCY

Only occurs in pregnant animals

SYNONYMS

N/A

SEE ALSO

- Dystocia
- Premature placental separation
- Stages of normal parturition

ABBREVIATIONS

- TRP = transrectal palpation
- U/S = ultrasound, ultrasonography

Suggested Reading

Guthrie RG. Rolling for correction of uterine torsion in a mare. J Am Vet Med Assoc 1982;181:66–67.

Perkins NR, Robertson JT, Colon LA. Uterine torsion and uterine tear in a mare. J Am Vet Med Assoc 1992;201:92–94.

Vaughan JT. Equine urogenital systems. In: Morrow DA, ed. Current Therapy in Theriogenology, ed 2. Philadelphia: WB Saunders, 1986:756–775.

Wichtel JJ, Reinertson EL, Clark TL. Nonsurgical treatment of uterine torsion in seven mares. J Am Vet Med Assoc 1988; 193:337–338.

Youngquist RS. Equine obstetrics. In: Morrow DA, ed. Current Therapy in Theriogenology, ed 2. Philadelphia: WB Saunders, 1986:699.

Author Walter R. Threlfall

Consulting Editor Carla L. Carleton

VACCINATION PROTOCOLS

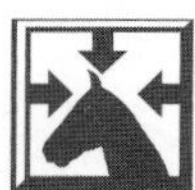

BASICS

Numerous factors must be considered when determining the need for vaccination of horses. The efficacy of the vaccine must be weighed against the risk and consequences of infection and the adverse effects and cost of the vaccine. The timing of the primary series may be influenced by the effect of passively acquired maternal antibodies on the foal's response to vaccination. The timing of subsequent vaccination is influenced by the duration of immunity provided by the vaccine and time of anticipated risk of exposure. The guidelines that follow have evolved with the consideration of these factors.

RABIES

Because rabies is a fatal zoonosis, all horses residing in endemic areas should be vaccinated. Foals from nonvaccinated mares should be vaccinated at 3 and 4 months of age. Initial vaccination of foals of vaccinated mares should occur at 6 months of age or older using two doses administered 4 weeks apart. These protocols are then followed by annual vaccination. Vaccination with the inactivated product is safe but has not been approved for use in pregnant mares. Broodmares should be vaccinated when not pregnant.

TETANUS

Due to the sensitivity of the horse to tetanus toxin and frequency of this pathogen in the environment, all horses should be vaccinated beginning at 6 months of age, with an initial series of three doses of toxoid 4 weeks apart. Thereafter, yearly boosters are adequate. Although vaccination confers long-lasting immunity, it is an accepted practice to booster horses that incur lacerations more than 6 months since the last vaccination. Tetanus toxoid should be given to broodmares 4–6 weeks prior to the anticipated foaling date.

Unvaccinated horses or horses with an uncertain vaccination history should receive tetanus antitoxin and tetanus toxoid if wounded. Vaccination should be given at separate sites. Foals born to unvaccinated mares should receive tetanus antitoxin and toxoid shortly after birth. Tetanus antitoxin is rarely associated with fatal acute hepatic necrosis.

ENCEPHALOMYELITIS

In North America, EEE is restricted to the eastern and southeastern United States, and although WEE occurs primarily in the western United States and western Canada, cases of WEE have been reported on the East Coast. All commercially available encephalomyelitis vaccines are inactivated and provide protection against both EEE and WEE. Because VEE has been reported in Mexico, horses residing in states on the Mexican border are frequently vaccinated.

The vaccines should be given in the spring prior to the emergence of the insect vector in cool climates. In warm climates, where the vector is present throughout the year, biannual vaccination is appropriate. Pregnant mares should be vaccinated 4–6 weeks prior to the anticipated foaling date. Foals that receive adequate colostral antibody are protected for the first 6 months of life and thus may not need to receive the primary immunization series of three doses until the following spring in climates without year-round vector exposure. There is debate about the effect of passive transfer of maternal antibodies on the efficacy of vaccination; therefore, in the southeastern United States where there is high risk year round, vaccination is recommended starting at 3–4 months of age.

RHINOPNEUMONITIS

Vaccination against EHV-1 and EHV-4 provides a short-lived and incomplete protection against abortion and respiratory disease. Both modified-live and inactivated vaccines are available. Vaccines are specifically labeled for protection against only respiratory disease or abortion. There is no vaccine licensed to protect against the neurologic strain of EHV-1. Foals should be vaccinated at 4–6 months of age with the inactivated vaccine 3–4 weeks apart and a third dose administered 8–12 weeks later. Vaccination against rhinopneumonitis depends on the risk of infection, need for protection, and use of the horse. For example, performance horses in which potential viral exposure is frequent should be vaccinated every 3 months to maintain protective immunity. Conversely, some owners may wish to accept the low risk of infection in horses that are not frequently exposed to other horses rather than perform frequent vaccinations.

To aid in the prevention of abortion, brood mares should be vaccinated during the 5th, 7th, and 9th months of gestation, with an optional dose at the 3rd month of gestation. Furthermore, vaccination against EHV-1 and EHV-4 at 4–6 weeks prior to foaling increases colostral antibodies that are necessary to protect the foal from these common respiratory diseases.

INFLUENZA

As with rhinopneumonitis, vaccination for influenza provides immunity that is short in duration and incomplete in protection. However, due to the ubiquitous nature of this pathogen and the explosive nature of outbreaks, regular vaccination is especially beneficial for horses entering high-risk environments, such as shows, training centers, and breeding farms.

Commercially available inactivated products are given by intramuscular injection. There are also commercially available modified live and killed intranasal vaccines available. Manufacturers generally recommend a primary series of two doses 3–6 weeks apart; however, a three-dose series may provide a higher antibody titer and longer immunity. Depending on the brand of vaccine, boosters are recommended every 3–6 months. Vaccination of brood mares 4–6 weeks prior to the anticipated foaling date enables passive transfer of colostral antibodies to the foal. Timing of foal vaccinations is controversial. Although some manufacturers suggest initiation of the primary series anytime after 3 months of age, there is evidence that maternal antibodies interfere with vaccination before 6 months of age. It is recommended that foals born to vaccinated mares receive their first dose at 9 months of age. Vaccination of foals born to seronegative, unvaccinated mares can be initiated at 3 months of age.

There have been no reports of the modified live vaccine causing problems in pregnant mares, but it is not recommended to be used in pregnant mares until more data are available.

BOTULISM

Clostridium botulinum produces several different toxins. In North America, horses are most frequently affected by type B. Types A and C also occur in the United States, but they are rare compared to type B. Although all three forms cause severe neuromuscular paralysis, the currently available toxoid only protects against type B. Ideally, horses in endemic areas should receive an initial series of three vaccinations 1 month apart and then an annual booster. Vaccination of brood mares is especially important due to the frequent occurrence of toxicoinfectious botulism in foals, with the third dose of the initial series given 4 weeks prior to the anticipated foaling date. Thereafter, a single yearly booster is given 4 weeks prior to foaling. Foals born to vaccinated mares should receive three vaccinations at monthly intervals beginning at 3 months of age. On farms where botulism is common, vaccination of foals may begin earlier because maternal antibodies do not appear to interfere with vaccination. Foals born to unvaccinated mares may benefit from vaccination at 2, 4, and 8 weeks of age. Vaccination is effective and is not associated with side effects; thus, it is highly recommended for horses in endemic areas.

POTOMAC HORSE FEVER

PHF is caused by *Neorickettsia risticii* and is characterized by fever, diarrhea, depression, anorexia, laminitis, colic, and death. Although the disease has been documented in most of the United States, risk factors include environments including access to water in the form of rivers, creeks, and irrigation ditches. *N. risticii* inhabits fluke-infested snails, and there has been recent documentation of caddisfly and mayfly involvement in the life cycle. Vaccination is generally limited to areas with a high prevalence. Unfortunately, there are several concerns about the efficacy of vaccination. First, the duration of immunity is short and protection is incomplete. The latter problem may be due to heterogeneity of the organism. Despite these shortcomings, the vaccine is safe and should be given prior to the disease season. In the eastern and midwestern United States, PHF occurs from mid-summer to fall, and in California it occurs from fall to spring. Due to the short duration of immunity, revaccination may be necessary 3–4 months later. Brood mares are vaccinated 4–6 weeks prior to the anticipated foaling date. It is recommended that foals in endemic areas receive three doses 1 month apart, beginning at 3–5 months of age.

STRANGLES

Strangles is a highly contagious disease caused by *Streptococcus equi* subspecies *equi.* Whole-cell bacteria, M-protein extract, and modified live intranasal vaccines are available in the United States. Two or three doses are given at 2- to 4-week intervals followed by semiannual or annual boosters for the whole-cell bacteria and M-protein extract vaccines. Mares should be vaccinated with an approved M-protein vaccine product 4–6 weeks prior to the anticipated foaling date because foals suckling these mares are frequently resistant to infection until weaned. Vaccination of foals should begin at 4–9 months of age with the intranasal live vaccine with the primary two-dose series and then annually thereafter. Foals may be safely initiated as early as 6 weeks of age if necessary, but a third dose should be administered prior to weaning, and the efficacy of this vaccine in young foals has not been adequately studied. The modified live vaccine has the advantage of promoting the mucosal secretory antibody that is important in preventing infection. Alternatively, vaccinate foals at 4–6 months of age with the IM M-protein vaccine using at least three does in the primary series and booster every 6 months. Vaccination is generally limited to horses at risk; horses residing on farms with previous outbreaks or horses entering these farms are candidates for vaccination. Although vaccination is not indicated for horses already infected, uninfected and unexposed horses may benefit from vaccination during an outbreak. Purpura hemorrhagica is a rare adverse reaction to vaccination.

EQUINE VIRAL ARTERITIS

EVA is characterized by abortion in mares and severe respiratory disease in neonates. In adult horses, clinical signs include fever, anorexia, limb and ventral edema, and nasal and ocular discharge. The virus is frequently spread by aerosolized respiratory secretions during outbreaks of respiratory disease. Chronically infected carrier stallions act as a reservoir for the virus and may infect mares by the venereal route.

A modified-live vaccine has been effective in controlling outbreaks of respiratory disease, protecting mares that are to be bred to infected stallions, and preventing stallions from becoming chronically infected. Some states have developed programs aimed at controlling spread of the virus, and state or U.S. Department of Agriculture officials and breed associations should be consulted prior to vaccination. Recommendations include vaccination of at-risk breeding stallions 4 weeks prior to the breeding season. Mares to be bred to infected stallions should be vaccinated not less than 3 weeks prior to breeding. Pregnant mares should not be vaccinated. Foals should not be vaccinated prior to 6 months of age as maternal antibodies may interfere with the development of an effective antibody response. Owners should be aware that seropositive horses may be ineligible for export to some countries; therefore, horses should be tested by a proficient laboratory for antibodies to this virus prior to vaccination to confirm that they are seronegative.

ROTAVIRUS

Rotavirus infection can cause outbreaks of infectious diarrhea in the majority of a foal crop on individual farms during the first few weeks of life. Older foals and adults are more resistant to infection. An inactivated rotavirus A vaccine containing the G3 (H-2) serotype is conditionally licensed in the United States for use in pregnant mares on endemic farms as an aid to preventing diarrhea in their foals caused by rotaviruses of serogroup A. The vaccine has been shown to be safe and there is evidence of partial efficacy. The recommended program includes vaccinating the mare during the 8th, 9th, and 10th months of pregnancy. This series should be repeated during each at risk pregnancy.

WEST NILE VIRUS

West Nile virus is transmitted by infected mosquitos and results in meningoencephalitis. Cases have been seen almost all year in the southeastern United States, but infection most commonly occurs from July to October. None of the available vaccines have a label for pregnant mares, but recent studies using the killed vaccine have shown no adverse effects on pregnant mares. Pregnant mares should be vaccinated 4–6 weeks prior to parturition. Foals from both vaccinated and unvaccinated mares should be vaccinated at 3–4 months of age with an initial series of three vaccines 1 month apart (maternal antibodies have been shown to not interfere with foal vaccination). Initial series for adult horses consists of two vaccines, 1 month apart. Annual to triannual boosters are recommended, prior to expected risk, depending on geographical location and duration of mosquito exposure.

ABBREVIATIONS

- EEE = Eastern equine encephalitis
- EHV = equine herpesvirus
- EVA = equine viral arteritis
- PHF = Potomac horse fever
- WEE = Western equine encephalitis
- VEE = Venezuelan equine encephalitis

Suggested Reading

American Association of Equine Practitioners Guidelines for Vaccination of Horses. 2001. Available at: www.myhorsematters.com/aaepOrg Vaccinations.html.

Horohov DW, Lunn DP, Townsend HGG, Wilson D. Equine vaccination. J Vet Intern Med. 2000;14:221–222.

West Nile virus vaccination guidelines. American Association of Equine Practitioners. Available at: www.aaep.org/pdfs/AAEP_WNV_Guidelines_2005.pdf-2005-01-10

Wilson WD. Strategies for vaccinating mares, foals, and weanlings. AAEP Proc 2005;51:421–438.

Author Kerry E. Beckman
Consulting Editors Ashley G. Boyle and Corinne R. Sweeney

VAGINAL PROLAPSE

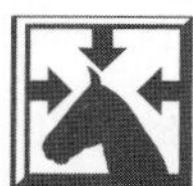

BASICS

DEFINITION/OVERVIEW

Displacement of all or part of the vaginal wall posteriorly through the vulva

ETIOLOGY/PATHOPHYSIOLOGY

Predisposing factors thought to be involved:

- Relaxation of the vaginal wall, such as occurs postpartum
- Relaxation of the vulvar lips, which permits protrusion of the vaginal wall
  - Secondary to increased abdominal pressure
  - Places additional pressure on the vaginal wall
  - A previous dystocia that may have damaged the perineal area, including the vagina and vulva

SYSTEMS AFFECTED

Reproductive

GENETICS

N/A

INCIDENCE/PREVALENCE

Low

SIGNALMENT

- All breeds
- All females of breeding age

SIGNS

- The vaginal wall protrudes through the vulva.
- The vaginal wall may become damaged and permit paravaginal fat to protrude through the prolapsed wall.
  - This protruded fat may cause additional straining and further prolapse.
- The protruding tissue has a characteristic pink to red color, depending on the length of time it has been outside the body.
- Differentiating the vagina from the bladder, intestines, uterus, cervix, and vestibule is essential before initiating treatment.

CAUSES AND RISK FACTORS

- Generally secondary to other abnormalities that initially predispose mares to everting part of the vaginal wall
- This may cause straining and additional tissue protrusion and injury.

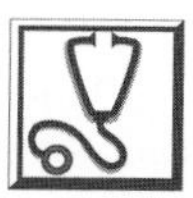

DIAGNOSIS

DIFFERENTIAL DIAGNOSIS

- Eversion of the bladder, uterus, or cervix
- Vaginal tears through which paravaginal fat or intestines may be protruding
- Eversion of the vestibular wall

CBC/BIOCHEMISTRY/URINALYSIS

N/A

OTHER LABORATORY TESTS

N/A

IMAGING

N/A

OTHER DIAGNOSTIC PROCEDURES

Careful visual and digital examination to differentiate the vaginal wall from other prolapsed tissues

PATHOLOGICAL FINDINGS

Protrusion of the vaginal wall through the vestibule and vulvar lips

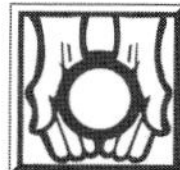

TREATMENT

- Reduce of prolapse (i.e., return tissues to their normal anatomic location) and terminate subsequent expulsive efforts; critical to permanent resolution
- Reduction of inflammation, if present, is advisable.
- No restriction of activity, unless the activity increases abdominal pressure
- Any protrusion of tissue through the vulvar lips requires immediate attention.
- Caslick's vulvoplasty may help prevent further vaginal irritation and, thus, decrease the likelihood of additional straining and tissue damage.
  - Vulvoplasty, however, does not prevent recurrent prolapse from straining.

APPROPRIATE HEALTH CARE, NURSING CARE, ACTIVITY, DIET, CLIENT EDUCATION, SURGICAL CONSIDERATIONS

N/A

MEDICATIONS

DRUG(S) OF CHOICE

- Epidural anesthetic may be indicated to reduce straining.
- Application of local, nonirritating antibiotics may aid in recovery.

CONTRAINDICATIONS

N/A

PRECAUTIONS

N/A

POSSIBLE INTERACTIONS

N/A

FOLLOW-UP

PATIENT MONITORING

At reexamination, careful and gentle assessment of previously affected tissues to prevent renewed irritation and reinitiation of straining

PREVENTION/AVOIDANCE

- Treat any conditions (e. g., vaginal damage or irritation) that may initiate straining and result in eventual prolapse of the vaginal wall.
- Once recognized, initiating treatment of prolapsed vaginal tissue as quickly as possible is critical to limit tissue trauma.

POSSIBLE COMPLICATIONS

Infections and abscessation of/within the vagina

EXPECTED COURSE AND PROGNOSIS

- Rapid recovery if the inciting cause is removed
- Satisfactory recovery if further damage can be avoided

MISCELLANEOUS

ASSOCIATED CONDITIONS

N/A

AGE-RELATED FACTORS

N/A

ZOONOTIC POTENTIAL

N/A

PREGNANCY

Usually occurs after parturition

SEE ALSO

- Dystocia
- Vaginitis

Suggested Reading

Cox JE. Surgery of the Reproductive Tract in Large Animals. Liverpool: Liverpool University Press, 1987:127–143.

Author Walter R. Threlfall

Consulting Editor Carla L. Carleton

VAGINITIS AND VAGINAL DISCHARGE

BASICS

DEFINITION/OVERVIEW

- Inflammation of the vagina
- Can be infectious or solely inflammatory in nature
- Vulvar discharge can occur, but only infrequently is discharge an obvious/external sign.

ETIOLOGY/PATHOPHYSIOLOGY

- Establish if discharge originates from the vagina, vestibule, or urethra.
- Pneumovagina—one of the major causes of vestibular and vaginal inflammation; caused by abnormal vulvar conformation
- Also may occur in fillies or mares in training or racing because of incomplete vulvar development
- Breed differences—increased incidence in mares with poor body condition (i.e., little fat) or less muscle around/in the perineal area (e. g., contrast Thoroughbreds and Standardbreds with Quarter Horses)

SYSTEM AFFECTED

Reproductive

GENETICS

Possible inheritance of poor vulvar conformation, which results in vaginitis

INCIDENCE/PREVALENCE

Increases with age, parity

SIGNALMENT

- All breeds
- All females of breeding age
- Occurs more often in old mares

SIGNS

Normal Discharge

- Urine, especially the characteristic appearance of calcium carbonate crystals that may accumulate at/on the ventral vulvar commissure during estrus
- This occurs secondary to frequent urination and evacuation of sediment common in equine urine, especially during estrus.

Abnormal Discharge

- Can be of mucoid or fluid consistency, and may be odiferous
- Color can range from white to yellow to brown.
- Note—Mares may have vaginitis without external discharge.

Historical

- Infertility or subfertility
- Periodic discharge throughout the cycle

Physical Examination

When secondary to infection or inflammation, there may be:

- Discharge on the tail and perineum
- Fluid in the vagina or uterus

CAUSES AND RISK FACTORS

- Poor vulvar conformation
- Trauma at parturition
- Vaginal breeding injury
- Pneumovagina
- Multiparous broodmares are highest risk
- Less frequent in young maidens (not broodmares)

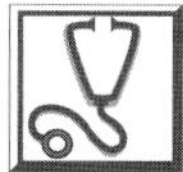

DIAGNOSIS

DIFFERENTIAL DIAGNOSIS

- Uterine disease/infection
- Urinary tract infection

CBC/BIOCHEMISTRY/URINALYSIS

N/A

OTHER LABORATORY TESTS

N/A

IMAGING

N/A

OTHER DIAGNOSTIC PROCEDURES

Careful speculum examination per vagina is the best means to establish a definitive diagnosis.

PATHOLOGICAL FINDINGS

- Hyperemia of the vaginal mucosa
- Fluid accumulation may be observed.
- Abrasions, ulcerations, and lacerations may be present:
  - Recent or chronic—adhesions or fibrin deposition
- Vulvar discharge does not always accompany vaginitis.
- Large amounts of discharge may be adhered to the tail or attract flies during summer months.
- Discharge may be evident only when the mare is more excitable, being ridden, or otherwise worked.

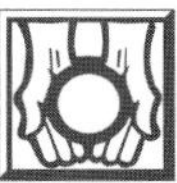

TREATMENT

- Exact cause must be determined before treatment is initiated.
- If only vaginitis (i.e., not secondary to injury), treatment need only halt additional contamination, and the inflammation should subside.
- Systemic antibiotics have no value.
- Local therapy if antibiotics are indicated and used
- Caslick's vulvoplasty to repair deficits in vulvar conformation, if present

APPROPRIATE HEALTH CARE, NURSING CARE, ACTIVITY, DIET, CLIENT EDUCATION, SURGICAL CONSIDERATIONS

N/A

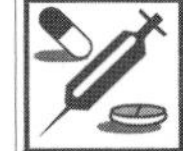

MEDICATIONS

DRUG(S) OF CHOICE

- If indicated after vulvoplasty, nonirritating, local application of antibiotics may reduce the mare's discomfort.
- This is usually unnecessary, as inflammation decreases rapidly once the source of irritation is resolved.

CONTRAINDICATIONS, PRECAUTIONS, POSSIBLE INTERACTIONS, ALTERNATIVE DRUGS

N/A

FOLLOW-UP

PATIENT MONITORING

Reexamination 1–2 weeks after vulvoplasty

PREVENTION/AVOIDANCE

Caslick's vulvoplasty or other cosmetic repair of vulvae:

- Mares born with poor vulvar conformation have an increased likelihood of vaginitis—breed or individual mare predisposition
- Postpartum, if injured at foaling

POSSIBLE COMPLICATIONS

If left untreated, may result in infertility, endometrial damage, and/or vaginal adhesions.

EXPECTED COURSE AND PROGNOSIS

If treated early in the course of disease, excellent resolution and normal fertility

MISCELLANEOUS

ASSOCIATED CONDITIONS

Linked with chronic vaginitis and uterine contamination:

- Metritis
- Endometritis
- Pyometra

AGE-RELATED FACTORS

- Prevalence increases with age.
- Conformation problems and/or damage to the caudal genital tract increase with age and parity.

ZOONOTIC POTENTIAL

N/A

PREGNANCY

May prevent pregnancy or cause abortion

SEE ALSO

- Dystocia
- Endometritis
- Metritis
- Pneumouterus
- Pneumovagina
- Vulvar conformation

Suggested Reading

Ricketts SW. Vaginal discharge in the mare. In: Boden E, ed. Equine Practice. Philadelphia: Bailliere Tindall, 1991:1–26.

Author Walter R. Threlfall
Consulting Editor Carla L. Carleton

VENTRICULAR ARRHYTHMIAS

BASICS

DEFINITION

Ventricular arrhythmias originate from an ectopic focus in the ventricle that is overdriving the sinus pacemaker. The term *ventricular premature depolarization* (VPD) refers to isolated ectopic complexes. More than four VPDs in succession is VT and can be either paroxysmal or sustained. Complexes that have a uniform appearance are termed monomorphic, whereas if there are more than two configurations, the VT is described as polymorphic.

PATHOPHYSIOLOGY

• A number of different electrophysiologic mechanisms are responsible for the development of ventricular arrhythmias, including reentry, enhanced automaticity, and accelerated conduction. • Ventricular arrhythmias often occur in association with other systemic illness. • Primary myocardial disease is an infrequent cause.

SYSTEM AFFECTED

Cardiovascular

SIGNS

General Comments

• VPDs may be found incidentally when they are infrequent. • VT is often associated with what is perceived to be abdominal pain.

Historical

• Acute onset • Poor performance • Weakness and collapse • Congestive heart failure

Physical Examination

• Individual premature beats or runs of rapid, regular or irregular rhythm • Loud booming heart sounds • Jugular pulses • Respiratory distress • Generalized venous distention and congestive heart failure

CAUSES

• Hypoxia • Sepsis • Toxemia • Drugs such as inhalation anesthetics, digoxin, and quinidine sulfate • Autonomic imbalance • Metabolic and electrolyte imbalance • Primary myocardial disease

RISK FACTORS

• Gastrointestinal and renal disease
• Endotoxemia • Left-sided infective endocarditis

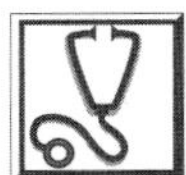

DIAGNOSIS

DIFFERENTIAL DIAGNOSIS

• Supraventricular arrhythmias— Differentiate electrocardiographically. • Sinus tachycardia—Differentiate electrocardiographically.

CBC/BIOCHEMISTRY/URINALYSIS

Electrolyte or metabolic abnormalities may be present.

OTHER LABORATORY TESTS

• Elevated activity in serum of cardiac isoenzymes (CK-MB, HBDH, or LDH-1 and LDH-2) or serum concentration of cardiac troponin I may be present. • Blood culture and viral serology may be indicated in some cases.

IMAGING

Electrocardiography

• VPDs are represented by a QRS-T complex that occurs prematurely and is different in configuration from those arising in the ventricle. The QRS complex usually appears widened and bizarre, with a T wave oriented in the opposite direction of the QRS complex. • With VT, there is a rapid ventricular rate with QRS and T complexes that are abnormal for the lead. P waves are present but occur less frequently than the ventricular depolarizations and are buried in the other complexes. The R-R interval may be regular or irregular. All ventricular QRS complexes and T waves may look identical (monomorphic) or vary in appearance (polymorphic).

Echocardiography

• With isolated VPD and monomorphic VT and no underlying cardiac disease, the echocardiogram is often normal or there may be a slightly low shortening fraction. • With polymorphic VT and primary myocardial disease, there are more profound decreases in fractional shortening and abnormalities of myocardial wall motion (dyskinesis or akinesis) and mitral and aortic valve motion. • Foci of increased or decreased echogenicity are occasionally seen within the myocardium. • Echocardiography may reveal evidence of other cardiac diseases such as infective endocarditis, severe valvular disease, pericarditis, or aortic root rupture.

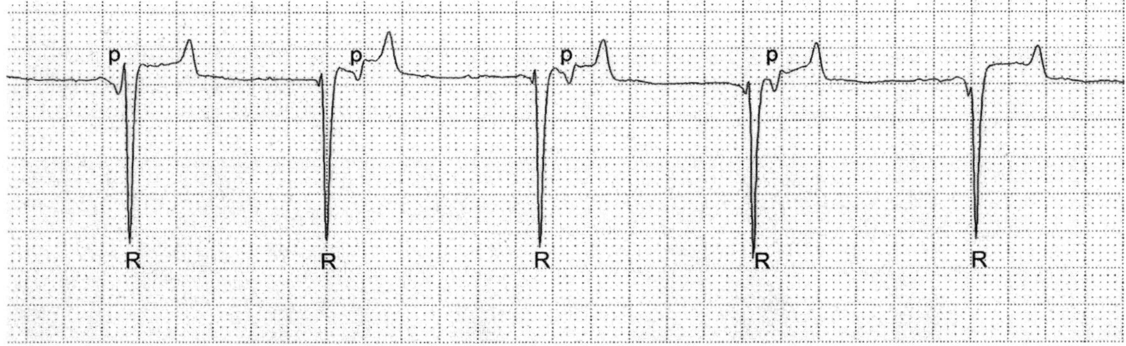

Figure 1.

Monomorphic ventricular tachycardia: the VPDs (R) have the same configuration and have no relationship to the p wave—base apex lead, 25 mm/sec, 5 mm = 1 mV.

Thoracic Radiology

Pulmonary edema is detected in horses with VT.

OTHER DIAGNOSTIC PROCEDURES

Continuous 24-Hour Holter Monitoring

This is particularly helpful in identifying intermittent or paroxysmal ventricular arrhythmias, in quantifying numbers of isolated VDP and in assessing response to therapy.

Exercise Electrocardiography

Characterization of the effect of exercise on ventricular arrhythmias is important in assessing their clinical significance.

PATHOLOGIC FINDINGS

• The heart may be normal, grossly and histopathologically, in horses with no underlying cardiac disease. • Focal or diffuse myocardial necrosis, inflammation, or fibrosis may be present.

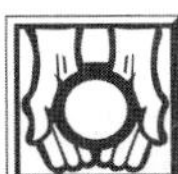

TREATMENT

AIMS OF TREATMENT

• Address any predisposing causes.
• Antiarrhythmic therapy is restricted to cases in which the rhythm is unstable and life-threatening.

APPROPRIATE HEALTH CARE

Antiarrhythmic therapy is considered if the horse shows signs of low cardiac output, the ventricular rate exceeds 100 bpm, R-on-T phenomenon is present (QRS complexes come immediately after the preceding T wave), and/or the VT is polymorphic.

NURSING CARE

• Continuous ECG monitoring should be performed during antiarrhythmic therapy.
• Horses should be kept quiet and not moved during the antiarrhythmic therapy.

ACTIVITY

Horses with VT or frequent isolated VPD during exercise should not be exercised.

CLIENT EDUCATION

The risks associated with the treatment need to be discussed with the owner (see Possible Complications).

MEDICATIONS

DRUG(S) OF CHOICE

• VPDs are not usually treated with antiarrhythmics but may respond to corticosteroids if due to primary myocarditis.
• Treatment of VT is usually an emergency and requires the use of intravenous preparations. The choice of the first drug used depends on the severity of the ventricular arrhythmia present and the onset of action of the drug selected, as well as the other side effects that the drug may have such as being a negative inotrope.
• Intravenous magnesium sulfate (25 g/450kg slowly IV over 20–30 min) is occasionally successful in correcting sustained ventricular tachycardia in both hypomagnesemic and normomagnesemic horses and has no negative inotropic effect. • Lidocaine hydrochloride is very rapidly acting but has central nervous system side effects that limit the dose that can be administered to an awake horse (0.25 mg/kg IV as a bolus). • Quinidine gluconate is one of the most successful antiarrhythmic drugs for horses with sustained ventricular tachycardia. Quinidine has a negative inotropic effect that is thought to be present only at high dosages but that may be a problem in horses with severe myocardial dysfunction. Quinidine gluconate is administered is small boluses of 0.5–1 mg/kg every 5–10 min up to a total dose of 10 mg/kg. Quinidine sulfate is rarely indicated in horses with sustained ventricular tachycardia because it has to be administered via nasogastric intubation.
• Procainamide 1 mg/kg/min to a total dose of 20 mg/kg IV has also been successful and its negative inotropic effect is thought to be less than that of quinidine.

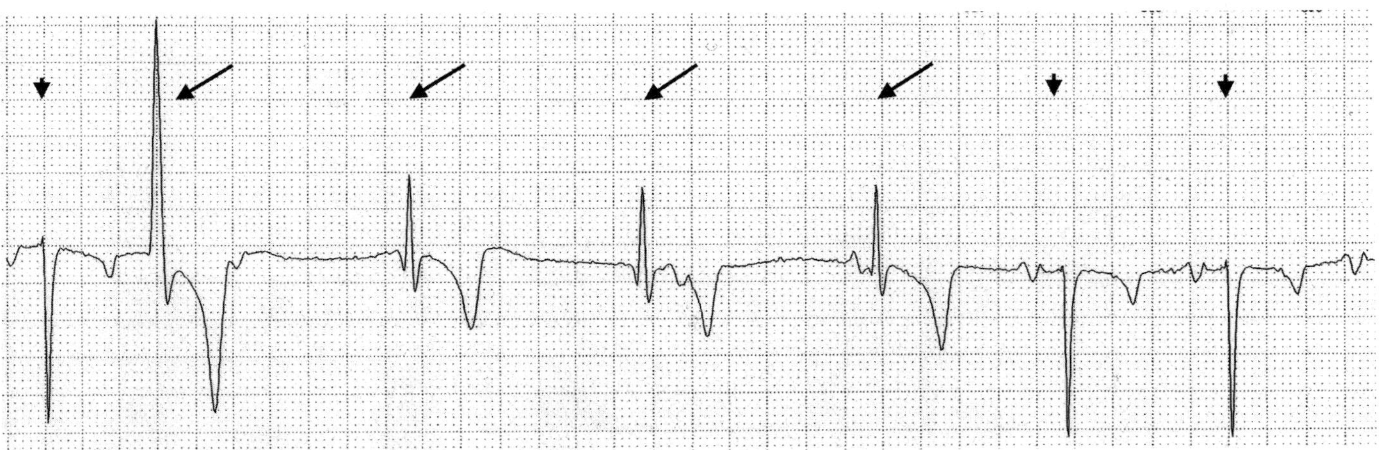

Figure 2.

Polymorphic ventricular tachycardia: four VPDs (arrows) with two configurations that differ from those of sinus origin (arrowheads)—base apex lead, 25 mm/sec, 5 mm = 1 mV.

VENTRICULAR ARRHYTHMIAS

CONTRAINDICATIONS

Quinidine gluconate should be administered carefully to horses with VT and severe myocardial dysfunction.

PRECAUTIONS (see Possible Complications)

• Intravenous lidocaine can cause seizures that may last for 5–10 min. • The QRS duration should be measured prior to each quinidine treatment. A prolongation of the QRS duration greater than 25% of the pretreatment duration should prompt discontinuation of quinidine treatment. The development of colic, ataxia, convulsions, or bizarre behavior is a sign of quinidine toxicity and should prompt discontinuation of treatment.

POSSIBLE INTERACTIONS

Antiarrhythmic drugs with different mechanisms of action can be used in combination, but specific guidelines are lacking and interactions are possible.

ALTERNATIVE DRUGS

• Most other drugs with efficacy against ventricular arrhythmias may be beneficial in converting horses with VT but have been less effective. • Phenytoin has been effective in VT refractory to other antiarrhythmias and is given orally at a starting dose of 20–22 mg/kg BID PO and then modified to keep drug in target range (usually 10–15 mg/kg). Side effects include excitement, sedation, and other neurologic signs.
• Digoxin at 0.011 mg/kg orally BID has been successful in converting two horses with VT.
• Intravenous propafenone at a dose of 0.5–1 mg/kg in 5% dextrose given slowly to effect over 5–8min has been successful in converting one horse with ventricular tachycardia but is not available in the United States in the IV formulation. Oral propafenone in conjunction with IV procainamide may have been helpful in achieving conversion in several horses.
• Propranolol can be tried at 0.03 mg/kg IV but is not as successful in correcting VT as many of the other antiarrhythmic drugs.

FOLLOW-UP

PATIENT MONITORING

• Continuous ECGmonitoring should be performed in all horses being treated for VT, as the antiarrhythmic drugs administered are also arrhythmogenic. • Following treatment of VT or VPD, continuous 24-hour Holter ECGs are useful in assessing whether complete resolution has occurred. Before returning to athletic activities, an exercise ECG should be obtained.
• Owners and trainers should regularly monitor their horse's cardiac rhythm before high-intensity exercise. Any irregularities in the cardiac rhythm or poor performance should prompt a cardiac reexamination.

PREVENTION/AVOIDANCE

The possibility of ventricular arrhythmias should be considered in horses with systemic illness, particularly if the heart rate is unexpectedly high.

POSSIBLE COMPLICATIONS

• With sustained VT, congestive heart failure or sudden death may ensure. • There are a myriad of complications that have been reported in horses treated for VT which can be broken down into the following categories:

Cardiovascular

• Other ventricular arrhythmias—may need to be treated with antiarrhythmic unless ventricular rhythm is slow (<100 bpm) and uniform and no R-on-T detected
• Hypotension—needs to be monitored and treated with intravenous polyionic fluids and if severe with intravenous phenylephrine at 0.1–0.2 μg/kg/min to effect • Congestive heart failure—Treat with digoxin at 0.0022 mg/kg IV and furosemide at 1–2 mg/kg IV, if needed.
• Sudden death—Try to prevent it with continuous ECG monitoring and treatment of arrhythmias that do occur.
• Neurologic—Indicative of quinidine, phenytoin or lidocaine toxicity

- Ataxia—Resolves upon return of plasma quinidine concentration to negligible levels
- Convulsions—Administer anticonvulsants.
- Sedation and bizarre behavior—resolves upon return of plasma drug concentrations to negligible levels
- Colic—Indicative of quinidine toxicity, treat with analgesics as needed; has also been seen in several horses with magnesium sulfate and severe multiform ventricular tachycardia and congestive heart failure

EXPECTED COURSE AND PROGNOSIS

- The majority of horses with monomorphic VT convert to sinus rhythm with antiarrhythmic therapy if there is little or no underlying cardiac disease. Recurrences of VT can occur as the antiarrhythmic medication wears off.
- Horses with sustained polymorphic VT are more difficult to convert and are more likely to have underlying myocardial disease.

MISCELLANEOUS

AGE-RELATED FACTORS

Older horses that develop ventricular tachycardia are more likely to have significant underlying cardiac disease.

PREGNANCY

VT leading to low cardiac output is likely to lead to fetal compromise.

SYNONYMS

VTach

SEE ALSO

- Aortic root rupture
- Infective endocarditis
- Mitral regurgitation
- Myocardial disease
- Ionophore toxicity
- Endotoxemia
- Septicemia

ABBREVIATIONS

- CK-MB = MB isoenzyme of creatine kinase
- HBDH = α-hydroxybutyrate dehydrogenase
- LDH = lactate dehydrogenase
- VPD = ventricular premature depolarization
- VT = ventricular tachycardia

Suggested Reading

Bowen IM, Marr CM, Elliott JE. Cardiovascular pharmacology. In: Bertone J, Horspool L, eds. Clinical Pharmacology of the Horse. Philadelphia; WB Saunders, 2004:193–216.

Ellis EJ, Ravis WR, Malloy M, et al. Pharmacokinetics and pharmacodynamics of procainamide in horses after intravenous administration. J Vet Pharmacol Ther 1994;17:265–270.

McGuirk SM, Muir WW, Sams RA. Pharmacokinetic analysis of intravenously and orally administered quinidine in horses. Am J Vet Res 1981;42:938–942.

Reimer JM, Reef VB, Sweeney RW. Ventricular arrhythmias in the horse: twenty-one cases (1984–1989). J Am Vet Med Assoc 1992; 201:1237–1243.

Wijnberg ID, Ververs FF. Phenytoin sodium as a treatment for ventricular dysrhythmia in horses. J Vet Intern Med 2004;18:350–353.

Author Virginia B. Reef
Consulting Editor Celia M. Marr

VENTRICULAR SEPTAL DEFECT (VSD)

BASICS

DEFINITION

• A congenital defect (i.e., hole) in the interventricular septum resulting in communication between the right and left ventricles
• Can be located in any portion of the interventricular septum—membranous (most common) or muscular

PATHOPHYSIOLOGY

• Blood shunts from the higher-pressure left ventricle to the lower-pressure right ventricle, the excessive volume then returns to the left ventricle via the lungs, creating primarily a left atrial and ventricular volume overload and, to a lesser degree, a right ventricular volume overload.
• The size and location of the VSD determine the severity of the volume overload and the degree of involvement by the right ventricle.
• With a large, membranous VSD, the left ventricular and atrial volume overload is severe. Over time, stretching of the mitral annulus occurs, and mitral regurgitation can develop. As the mitral regurgitation becomes more severe, increases in left atrial pressure cause increased pulmonary venous pressure, increased pulmonary capillary pressure, pulmonary edema, pulmonary hypertension, and clinical signs of left-sided congestive heart failure. As pulmonary hypertension becomes more severe, clinical signs of right-sided congestive heart failure appear.
• With a large, muscular VSD, the left atrial and ventricular volume overload and right ventricular volume overload are severe, and clinical signs of right-sided heart failure may predominate.
• When a large VSD is located immediately below the aortic valve, the valve may become incompetent which further exacerbates left ventricular volume overload.

SYSTEM AFFECTED

Cardiovascular

GENETICS

Not yet determined in horses, but likely to be heritable

INCIDENCE/PREVALENCE

• Welsh Mountain ponies are reported to be at significantly higher risk than Thoroughbreds.
• Standardbreds also appear to be more frequently affected than Thoroughbreds.

SIGNALMENT

• Murmurs are detectable at birth.
• Diagnosed most frequently in neonates, foals, and young horses but may be found at any age if careful auscultation has not been performed earlier in life

SIGNS

General Comments

Often detected as an incidental finding in mature horses if the VSD is small

Historical

• Medium to large VSDs—poor performance
• Large VSDs—congestive heart failure

Physical Examination

• Grade 3–6/6, coarse, band-shaped, pansystolic murmur with PMI in the tricuspid valve area (right fourth intercostal space); membranous defect has loudest murmur here.
• Grade 3–6/6, coarse, band- or crescendo-decrescendo, ejection shaped, holosystolic or pansystolic murmur with PMI in the pulmonic valve area (left third intercostal space); outflow defect has loudest murmur here. With membranous VSD, there is also a murmur in this location, usually 1 grade quieter than the right-sided murmur due to relative pulmonic stenosis (extra blood leaving the right ventricle through a structurally normal right ventricular outflow tract).
• Other, less common findings—accentuated third heart sound, grade 1–6/6 holodiastolic decrescendo murmur with PMI in aortic valve area (left fourth intercostal space), and atrial fibrillation.

CAUSES

Congenital malformation of the interventricular septum

RISK FACTORS

N/A

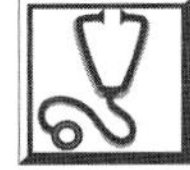

DIAGNOSIS

DIFFERENTIAL DIAGNOSIS

• Tricuspid regurgitation—no relative pulmonic stenosis murmur; differentiate echocardiographically.
• VSD with pulmonic stenosis or bicuspid pulmonic valve—loudest murmur usually in the pulmonic valve area; differentiate echocardiographically.
• Tetralogy of Fallot—Foals are often stunted and may be tachycardic and hypoxemic; loudest murmur usually in the pulmonic valve area; differentiate echocardiographically.

CBC/BIOCHEMISTRY/URINALYSIS

N/A

OTHER LABORATORY TESTS

N/A

IMAGING

Electrocardiography

Atrial premature depolarizations or atrial fibrillation may be present in horses with left atrial enlargement. Ventricular premature depolarizations also occur in some cases.

Echocardiography

• The most common location for a VSD is the membranous portion of the interventricular septum, immediately beneath the septal leaflet of the tricuspid valve and right or noncoronary leaflet of the aortic valve. Defects in this location that are <2.5 cm in two mutually perpendicular planes are generally restrictive with little hemodynamic impact. For smaller ponies, a ratio of the VSD to the aortic root of <1:3 suggests a restrictive defect.
• Outflow VSD is less common and more difficult to detect echocardiographically, because it is ventral to the aortic and pulmonic valves and difficult to detect on the long axis.
• Muscular VSD in other portions of the interventricular septum is less common, but if suspected, the entire ventricular septum should be examined.
• More than one defect may be present.
• Left atrium and ventricle—enlarged, dilated, and rounded in appearance
• Left ventricular free wall and interventricular septum—thinner than normal; pattern of left ventricular volume overload if the ventricle is coping well with the left-to-right shunt
• Normal or decreased fractional shortening in horses with left ventricular enlargement is consistent with myocardial dysfunction.
• Pulmonary artery dilatation in horses with a large shunt fraction
• Pulsed-wave or color-flow Doppler reveals the shunt from left to right through the VSD.
• Hemodynamic significance can be determined from the peak velocity of the shunt through the VSD—A peak velocity >4 m/sec is consistent with a restrictive defect and a shunt of lesser hemodynamic significance; a peak shunt velocity ≤3 m/sec indicates a very hemodynamically significant shunt and a large VSD.
• A jet of mitral regurgitation may be present with a large VSD and marked left atrial and ventricular volume overload.

Thoracic Radiography

• An enlarged cardiac silhouette, tracheal elevation, and increased pulmonary vascularity may be detected in horses with a large VSD.
• Pulmonary edema may be present in affected horses with congestive heart failure.

DIAGNOSTIC PROCEDURES

Cardiac Catheterization

• Right-sided catheterization can be performed to directly measure right atrial, right ventricular, and pulmonary arterial pressures and to sample blood for oxygen content.
• Elevated right ventricular pressure should be detected with an increased oxygen saturation of blood obtained from the right ventricle and pulmonary artery if the shunt is left to right.

Continuous 24-Hour Holter Monitoring
Useful in the diagnosis of suspected arrhythmias

PATHOLOGIC FINDINGS

- Most frequently found in the membranous septum underneath the septal leaflet of the tricuspid valve and the right or noncoronary leaflet of the aortic valve but also can be present in any portion of the interventricular septum
- Associated jet lesions along the margins of the defect and on the adjacent right ventricular endocardium
- Left atrial and ventricular enlargement and thinning of the left atrial and ventricular myocardium and interventricular septum in horses with a large shunt
- Right ventricular enlargement and thinning of the right ventricular free wall in horses with a VSD that is large or in a muscular location
- Pulmonary artery dilatation in horses with a large shunt fraction and in those with pulmonary hypertension

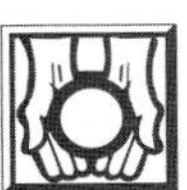

TREATMENT

AIMS OF TREATMENT

- Management by intermittent monitoring in horses with small membranous VSD
- Palliative care in horses with large membranous or muscular VSD and congestive heart failure

APPROPRIATE HEALTH CARE

- Most affected horses require no treatment and can be monitored on an outpatient basis.
- Monitor horses echocardiographically on an annual basis.
- Affected horses with congestive heart failure can be treated for congestive heart failure with positive inotropic drugs, vasodilators, and diuretics on an inpatient basis, if possible. Consider humane destruction if congestive heart failure progresses, however, because only short-term, symptomatic improvement can be expected.

NURSING CARE

N/A

ACTIVITY

- Horses with small VSD are safe to continue in athletic work provided there is no significant arrhythmias or pulmonary artery dilation.
- Horses with small VSDs can have unrestricted activity and may be able to compete reasonably successfully.
- Monitor horses with hemodynamically significant VSDs echocardiographically on an annual basis to ensure they are safe to ride and compete. These horses can be used for lower-level athletic work but are unlikely to compete successfully at upper levels.
- Horses with significant pulmonary artery dilatation are no longer safe to ride.
- Affected horses that develop significant arrhythmias often decompensate and are no longer safe to use for athletic performance.

DIET

N/A

CLIENT EDUCATION

- Regularly monitor cardiac rhythm; any irregularities other than second-degree AV block should prompt electrocardiography.
- Carefully monitor for exercise intolerance, respiratory distress, prolonged recovery after exercise, increased resting respiratory or heart rate, or cough; if detected, perform a cardiac reexamination.
- Because the defect most likely is heritable, do not breed affected horses.

SURGICAL CONSIDERATIONS

- Closure of the VSD would be possible with transvenous umbrella catheters if the umbrella diameter was large enough to close the defect. There are no published reports of this technique being successfully performed in horses to date.
- Surgical closure would require rib resection for the thoracotomy and cardiac bypass, however, which are not financially feasible or practical for obtaining an equine athlete.

MEDICATIONS

DRUGS OF CHOICE, CONTRAINDICATIONS, PRECAUTIONS, POSSIBLE INTERACTIONS, ALTERNATIVE DRUGS

N/A

FOLLOW-UP

PATIENT MONITORING

- Frequently monitor cardiac rate and rhythm and respiratory rate and effort.
- With defects >2.5 cm in two mutually perpendicular planes or peak shunt velocity <4 m/sec, echocardiographic reexaminations every 6–12 mo are recommended.

PREVENTION/AVOIDANCE

N/A

POSSIBLE COMPLICATIONS

Large VSD—atrial fibrillation; congestive heart failure

EXPECTED COURSE AND PROGNOSIS

- Horses with small, membranous VSDs (≤ 2.5 cm) that are restrictive (peak shunt velocity, >4 m/sec) should have normal performance and life expectancy. Horses with small VSDs can even race successfully, although not at the top levels.
- Progression of mitral regurgitation in horses with moderate VSDs usually is slow. These horses have normal life expectancy, but usually perform successfully only at lower levels of athletic competition.
- Horses with large VSDs (>4 cm) that are hemodynamically significant (peak flow velocity, ≤ 3 m/sec) have a guarded prognosis, because they usually have shortened performance and life expectancy.
- Affected horses with congestive heart failure and mitral regurgitation have a guarded to grave prognosis for life. Most affected horses being treated for congestive heart failure respond to supportive therapy and transiently improve, but once congestive heart failure develops, euthanasia of the horse is recommended.

MISCELLANEOUS

ASSOCIATED CONDITIONS

- Aortic regurgitation can develop in horses with VSDs and aortic valve prolapse. The aortic valve lacks the support normally provided by the interventricular septum and prolapses into the defect, resulting in aortic regurgitation.
- Mitral regurgitation can develop in horses with significant left atrial and ventricular volume overload secondary to stretching of the mitral annulus, further contributing to left atrial and ventricular volume overload.

AGE-RELATED FACTORS

Young horses are more likely to be diagnosed.

ZOONOTIC POTENTIAL

N/A

PREGNANCY

Do not breed affected horses because of the possibly heritable nature of these defects.

SYNONYMS

- Septal defect
- Interventricular septal defect

SEE ALSO

Aortic insufficiency

ABBREVIATIONS

- AV = atrioventricular
- PMI = point of maximal intensity
- VSD = ventricular septal defect

Suggested Reading

Pipers FS, Reef V, Wilson J. Echocardiographic detection of ventricular septal defects in large animals. J Am Vet Med Assoc 1985;19(suppl):86–95.

Reef VB. Echocardiographic findings in horses with congenital cardiac disease. Compend Contin Educ Pract Vet 1991;13:109–117.

Reef VB. Heart murmurs in horses: determining their significance with echocardiography. Equine Vet J 1995;19(suppl):71–80.

Author Virginia B. Reef
Consulting Editor Celia M. Marr

VERMINOUS MENINGOENCEPHALOMYELITIS

BASICS

DEFINITION

Meningoencephalomyelitis is most often associated with aberrant and unusual helminth and insect parasitic invasion of nervous tissues.

PATHOPHYSIOLOGY

- Aberrant migration of parasitic organisms of other species or organ systems.
- The clinical signs result from physical tissue destruction, hemorrhage and inflammation, or a space-occupying effect, depending on the parasite.
- An additional immune-associated inflammatory response may contribute to the pathophysiology.

SYSTEMS AFFECTED

CNS and other specific tissues associated with the more common parasitic migration pattern

GENETICS

N/A

INCIDENCE/PREVALENCE

Much decreased with the introduction of modern anthelmintics

GEOGRAPHIC DISTRIBUTION

None

SIGNALMENT

- Not specific
- No breed, sex, or age predisposition

SIGNS

- The history and physical examination signs are associated with the migratory pattern in each specific case.
- Signs often progress with further migration and inflammation.
- Any CNS defect(s) can occur.

CAUSES

Many parasites have been implicated and identified: *Strongylus vulgaris, Micronema deletrix, Hypoderma* spp., *Setaria* spp., and others.

RISK FACTORS

Horses may not be under good deworming management schemes.

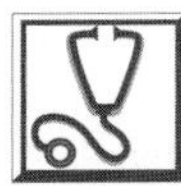

DIAGNOSIS

Most commonly, the diagnosis is made histologically on necropsy specimens.

Verminous involvement should be suspected in any case of acute CNS disease without a history of trauma or intracarotid injection.

DIFFERENTIAL DIAGNOSIS

Any central nervous system dysfunction

CBC/BIOCHEMISTRY/URINALYSIS

None specific to the disease

OTHER LABORATORY TESTS

Good diagnostic evidence of cerebrospinal helminthiasis and myiasis would be an eosinophilic or neutrophilic, aseptic pleocytosis in cerebrospinal fluid with varying numbers of macrophages and red blood cells. Inflammatory or hemorrhagic cytologic findings (e. g., xanthochromia, elevated protein concentration, red blood cells), however, are more common.

IMAGING

Cervical vertebral radiographs if horse is ataxic: cervical vertebral malformation is a far more common disease.

OTHER DIAGNOSITIC PROCEDURES

N/A

PATHOLOGIC FINDINGS

Parasitic lesions with typical eosinophilic and other inflammatory infiltrates

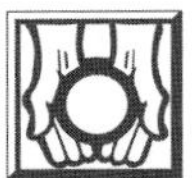

TREATMENT

APPROPRIATE HEALTH CARE, NURSING CARE, ACTIVITY, DIET

N/A

CLIENT EDUCATION

Appropriate anthelmintic schedule

SURGICAL CONSIDERATIONS

N/A

MEDICATIONS

DRUG(S) OF CHOICE

- Anti-inflammatory therapy (e. g., flunixin meglumine, 1.1 mg/kg q12–24h; dexamethasone 0.05–0.1 mg/kg q6–24h) may be useful.
- Suggested larvacidal doses of antiparasitic drugs should be administered.
- Treatment of suspect horses with fenbendazole (60 mg/kg) given once is justified.
- Avermectins may be useful.
- Others may become available.

CONTRAINDICATIONS

Avermectins function by GABA inhibition. A concern for safety is the distribution of these drugs across the blood-brain barrier and CNS GABA inhibition. However, a concern for efficacy is that for these drugs to be larvacidal in the CNS, they must reach concentrations that would induce GABA inhibition in the CNS.

PRECAUTIONS

Regular anthelmintic treatment

POSSIBLE INTERACTIONS

N/A

ALTERNATIVE DRUGS

N/A

FOLLOW-UP

Regular detailed neurologic examination to assess response to therapy

PREVENTION/AVOIDANCE

Regular anthelmintic treatment

POSSIBLE COMPLICATIONS

Trauma associated with the primary neurologic deficits

EXPECTED COURSE AND PROGNOSIS

Depends on severity of initial neurologic signs

MISCELLANEOUS

ASSOCIATED CONDITIONS, AGE-RELATED FACTORS, ZOONOTIC POTENTIAL, PREGNANCY

N/A

ABBREVIATIONS

- CNS = central nervous system
- GABA = γ-aminobutyric acid

Suggested Reading

Divers, TJ, Mayhew IG. Clinical techniques in equine practice. Neurology 2006;5(1).

Lester G. Parasitic encephalomyelitis in horses. Comp Cont Educ Pract Vet 1992;14:1624–1630.

Van Biervliet J, de Lahunta, A, Ennulat, D et al. Acquired cervical scoliosis in six horses associated with dorsal grey column chronic myelitis. Equine Vet J 2004;36:86–92.

The author and editor wish to acknowledge the contribution of Joseph J. Bertone, author of this chapter in the previous edition.

Author Caroline N. Hahn

Consulting Editor Caroline N. Hahn

VESICULAR STOMATITIS

BASICS

OVERVIEW

Vesicular stomatitis is a viral disease that primarily affects horses, cattle, and swine and occasionally sheep, goats, camelids, and wildlife. Rarely, humans may become infected by handling infected animals. The disease is caused by an RNA virus in the genus Vesiculovirus of the family Rhabdoviridae, of which two primary serotypes (New Jersey and Indiana) affect animals in North and Central America. Vesicular stomatitis may occur as an epidemic or involve only a few animals, and clinically resembles foot-and-mouth disease in cattle but is considerably milder.

SIGNALMENT

Any age, sex, or breed of animal can be affected.

SIGNS

• Vesicles or ulcers occur most often in the oral cavity, and less frequently on the nares, coronary bands, mammary glands, or external genitalia. • Transient fever • Ptyalism • Anorexia • Weight loss • Lameness and/or hoof wall deformation (secondary to coronitis) • Laminitis and hoof wall sloughing (occurs rarely, secondary to severe coronitis) • Epistaxis • Nasal edema, laryngitis, or pharyngitis • Drop in milk production if lactating

CAUSES AND RISK FACTORS

How vesicular stomatitis spreads is not fully known; insect vectors, mechanical transmission, and movement of animals are probably responsible. Animals housed where insect populations are greater than normal or near running water are at increased risk. Spread of the virus occurs via direct and indirect contact, and arthropod vectors (the biting midge, *Culicoides sonorensis*, has been shown to allow replication of the virus).

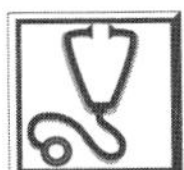

DIAGNOSIS

DIFFERENTIAL DIAGNOSIS

• Nonsteroidal anti-inflammatory drug toxicosis can be differentiated by a detailed history. Lesions are on the oral mucosa, but not necessarily at the mucocutaneous junction, and no skin lesions will be present. • Candidiasis can be differentiated by cytologic or histopathologic examination. • Blister beetle (cantharidin) toxicosis is usually accompanied by abdominal pain and hypocalcemia. Anamnesis typically includes ingestion of alfalfa hay. • Organophosphate paste dewormers (i.e. trichlorfon, dichlorvos) administered orally may result in oral ulcerations. • Plant awn stomatitis ulcerations (caused by foxtail, yellow bristle grass, etc) may occur at the mucocutaneous junction of the mouth or within the oral cavity, most commonly at the labial periodontal pocket of the incisors. Lesions are packed with fine awns. • Equine coital exanthema (equine herpesvirus 3) lesions are primarily found on the genitals, and are related to sexual contact. • Autoimmune diseases, such as bullous pemphigoid or paraneoplastic bullous stomatitis, may be differentiated by histopathologic examination. • Uremia can be differentiated by a serum biochemistry profile.

CBC/BIOCHEMISTRY/URINALYSIS

• Often within normal limits • Stress leukogram may be present. • Electrolyte abnormalities and hemoconcentration secondary to dysphagia or anorexia

OTHER LABORATORY TESTS

Complement fixation, virus neutralization, and ELISA (capture ELISA for IgM or competitive ELISA) tests provide a prompt diagnosis. Virus isolation may be performed on saliva, fluid from a recently ruptured vesicle, or epithelial tissue. Other diagnostic tests available are electron microscopy and fluorescent antibody tests on serum or tissues.

DIAGNOSTIC PROCEDURES

Cytologic and histopathologic examination of lesions may be useful in differentiating vesicular stomatitis from other diseases. Tissue samples may also be submitted for virus isolation.

PATHOLOGIC FINDINGS

Biopsy of acute lesions reveals nonspecific neutrophilic dermatitis, edema, epidermal necrosis, and reticular degeneration.

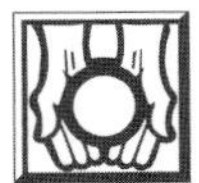

TREATMENT

Supportive care; no specific treatment is available. Providing softened feeds may decrease cachexia if oral discomfort leads to anorexia. Cleansing lesions with mild antiseptics may help avoid secondary bacterial infections.

MEDICATIONS

Oral or intravenous nonsteroidal anti-inflammatory drugs may be indicated to control painful lesions. Studies suggest recombinant equine interferon-β-1 given at a dose of 0.3–1.0 μg/kg IM every 2 days may be useful as a prophylactic treatment for animals at high risk, or animals showing the initial signs of the disease.

FOLLOW-UP

EXPECTED COURSE AND PROGNOSIS

The disease is self-limiting. Lesions often heal within two weeks, however two months may be required for complete regression. Scarring or depigmentation may occur at ulcerated sites. Prognosis is excellent for recovery, providing that complications such as laminitis or secondary bacterial infections are not present. Immunity to re-infection is hypothesized to be up to a few years, but may be as short as a few months. Immunity to one strain of vesicular stomatitis virus does not confer immunity to other strains.

EPIDEMIOLOGY/PREVENTION

Vesicular stomatitis is a disease of high morbidity and low mortality. The virus is endemic in northern South America, Central America, and southern North America, but sporadic outbreaks may occur in more temperate climates. Transmission from animal to animal occurs via aerosol or contact exposure to saliva or fluid from ruptured vesicles. Incubation period is typically 2 to 8 days, but may be as long as 21 days. Animals are highly contagious for the first 3 days of clinical signs, and should be quarantined from all other livestock until after lesions have healed. Premises should be disinfected with chlorine, iodine, or a quaternary ammonium compound. Insect control measures are indicated. There is not currently a commercially available vaccine in the United States. The inactivated vaccine developed for use in horses during the 1995 outbreak was not proven to be protective.

COMPLICATIONS

• Secondary bacterial infections • Laminitis
• Dehydration and weight loss secondary to anorexia

MISCELLANEOUS

ZOONOTIC POTENTIAL

Humans rarely contract vesicular stomatitis when handling infected animals, but can become infected. Vesicular stomatitis in humans results in an influenza-like illness. Most cases of human vesicular stomatitis have occurred under laboratory conditions, however protective measures such as gloves and eyewear should be utilized when working with infected animals to prevent transmission.

PUBLIC HEALTH

The Office Internationale des Epizooties classifies vesicular stomatitis as a "Class A" disease, which is defined as a communicable disease that has the potential to spread rapidly, is of serious socioeconomic or public health consequence, and is of major importance in the international trade of livestock. Rapid detection of this reportable disease is prudent, as it is clinically indistinguishable from hoof and mouth disease in ruminants and swine.

PREGNANCY

No known effects on pregnancy are documented.

ABBREVIATION

• ELISA = enzyme-linked immunosorbent assay

Suggested Reading

Kim L, Morley P, McCluskey B, et al. Oral vesicular lesions in horses without evidence of vesicular stomatitis virus infection. JAVMA, 2000;216(9):1399–1404.

Author Kerry Beckman
Consulting Editors Ashley G. Boyle and Corinne R. Sweeney

VICIA VILLOSA (HAIRY VETCH) TOXICOSIS

BASICS

OVERVIEW

- A systemic granulomatous disease described in horses grazing green *Vicia villosa* (hairy vetch) and hypothesized to result from an unknown immunogen
- Other *Vicia* spp. (e.g., *V. dasycarpa, V. benghelensis*) also have been implicated.
- *Vicia* spp. are legumes found throughout temperate regions of the U.S. and used as pasturage, hay, and silage.
- There are no reports of disease in animals fed hay or silage.
- Low morbidity, but high mortality in affected individuals

SIGNALMENT

No reported breed, age, or sex predispositions

SIGNS

- Listlessness
- Welts on the skin
- Alopecia
- Dermatitis
- Skin peeling around the nares
- Lymphadenomegaly
- Dependent-limb edema
- Low-grade, persistent fever
- Wasting
- Diarrhea

CAUSES AND RISK FACTORS

- The specific phytochemical responsible is unknown.
- The condition is hypothesized to be a type IV hypersensitivity reaction.
- Associated with ingestion of the green plant
- Outbreaks are more common at the peak of plant growth during the spring.
- Not all individuals grazing hairy vetch are affected, so unknown factors (e.g., growth stage of plant, dietary or environmental factors, or individual susceptibility) may be involved.

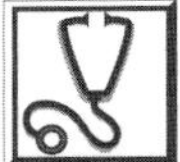

DIAGNOSIS

DIFFERENTIAL DIAGNOSIS

- Systemic granulomatous disease caused by other unidentified causes—no known exposure to *Vicia* spp.
- Dermatophytosis—negative fungal cultures
- Bacterial dermatitis—negative cultures for dermatopathogens
- Pemphigus foliaceus—skin biopsy
- Drug eruption—history of recent drug administration
- Chronic urticaria—skin lesions pit with pressure.

CBC/BIOCHEMISTRY/URINALYSIS

- Lymphocytosis
- Hyperproteinemia

OTHER LABORATORY TESTS

N/A

IMAGING

N/A

DIAGNOSTIC PROCEDURES

Skin biopsy

PATHOLOGICAL FINDINGS

Gross

- Thickened skin with scaling and alopecia
- Paleness of organs—heart, kidney, adrenal, and lymphoid tissues
- Lymphadenomegaly

Histopathological

- Cellular infiltrations of monocytes, lymphocytes, plasma cells, eosinophils, and multinucleated giant cells in multiple organs
- Lesions are especially prominent perivascularly.

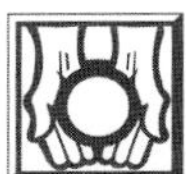

TREATMENT

Generally unrewarding

MEDICATIONS

DRUG(S) OF CHOICE

Glucocorticoids—prednisolone (0.2–4.4 mg/kg PO daily or BID) or dexamethasone (0.02–0.2 mg/kg PO daily)

CONTRAINDICATIONS/POSSIBLE INTERACTIONS

N/A

FOLLOW-UP

PATIENT MONITORING

N/A

PREVENTION/AVOIDANCE

Avoid reintroduction to pastures containing *Vicia* spp.

POSSIBLE COMPLICATIONS

N/A

EXPECTED COURSE AND PROGNOSIS

Mortality is high in affected animals.

MISCELLANEOUS

ASSOCIATED CONDITIONS, AGE-RELATED FACTORS, ZOONOTIC POTENTIAL, PREGNANCY

N/A

Suggested Reading

Woods LW, Johnson B, Hietala SK, Galey FD, Gillen D. Systemic granulomatous disease in a horse grazing pasture containing hairy vetch (*Vicia* sp.). J Vet Diagn Invest 1992;4:356–360.

Author Robert H. Poppenga
Consulting Editor Robert H. Poppenga

VIRAL AND HERPES KERATITIS

BASICS

OVERVIEW

Keratopathy with associated conjunctivitis and epiphora caused by equine herpesvirus type 2

SYSTEM AFFECTED

Ophthalmic

SIGNALMENT

All ages and breeds affected; may be seen in herds

SIGNS

- Multiple, superficial, white, punctuate, or linear opacities of the cornea, with or without fluorescein dye retention, varying amounts of ocular pain, conjunctivitis, corneal edema, epiphora, and iridocyclitis
- May stain with Rose Bengal dye
- Drooping of upper lid eyelashes is present.

CAUSES AND RISK FACTORS

EHV-2 is suspected agent, but equal prevalence of positive PCRs for EHV-2 has been found in normal control horses.

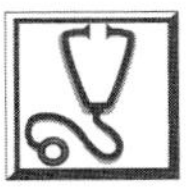

DIAGNOSIS

DIFFERENTIAL DIAGNOSIS

- Corneal ulcers
- Immune-mediated keratitis
- ERU
- Glaucoma
- Blepharitis
- Conjunctivitis
- Dacryocystitis

CBC/BIOCHEMISTRY/URINALYSIS

N/A

OTHER LABORATORY TESTS

- Rule out other infectious causes (bacterial or fungal) of keratitis with corneal scrapings for cytology and culture.
- Culturing virus from ocular specimens, and identification of viral isolates by use of PCR or electron microscopy

IMAGING, DIAGNOSTIC PROCEDURES, PATHOLOGIC FINDINGS

N/A

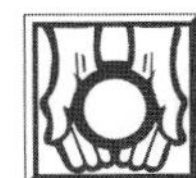

TREATMENT

N/A

MEDICATIONS

DRUG(S) OF CHOICE

- Topical idoxuridine or trifluorothymidine: initially every 2 hours, then 4–6 times per day.
- Topical NSAIDs (diclofenamic acid BID or flurbiprofen BID) may be beneficial.
- Topical antiproteases such as serum can also aid healing.

CONTRAINDICATIONS/POSSIBLE INTERACTIONS

N/A

FOLLOW-UP

EXPECTED COURSE AND PROGNOSIS

Treatment often successful, but recurrence common

MISCELLANEOUS

ASSOCIATED CONDITIONS

Secondary bacterial infection

AGE-RELATED FACTORS

Multiple foals in a herd may be affected.

SEE ALSO

- Corneal ulceration
- Corneal/scheral lacerations
- Ulcerative keratomycosis
- Corneal stromal abscessation
- Recurrent uveitis
- Glaucoma
- Nonulcerative keratouveitis
- Eosinophilic keratitis
- Burdock pappus bristle keratopathy
- Calcific band keratopathy
- Superficial nonhealing ulcers with anterior stromal sequestration

ABBREVIATIONS

- EHV-2 = equine herpesvirus type 2
- ERU = equine recurrent uveitis
- PCR = polymerase chain reaction

Suggested Reading

Brooks DE. Ophthalmology for the Equine Practitioner. Jackson, WY; Teton NewMedia, 2002.

Brooks DE, Matthews AG. Equine ophthalmology. In: Gelatt KN, ed. Veterinary Ophthalmology, ed 4. Philadelphia; Lippincott Williams and Wilkins, 2007.

Gilger BC, ed. Equine Ophthalmology. Philadelphia; WB Saunders, 2005.

Authors Andras M. Komaromy and Dennis E. Brooks

Consulting Editor Dennis E. Brooks

VIRAL ARTERITIS

BASICS

DEFINITION

EVA is a disease characterized by panvasculitis leading to edema, hemorrhage, and abortion in mares; respiratory disease and edema in other adults; and severe illness or death in the neonate.

PATHOPHYSIOLOGY

- EVA is an arterivirus. It is a small, enveloped, positive-stranded RNA virus. The virion is resistant to freezing, drying, and long storage at −70°C, although it is reliably destroyed by a 1:32 dilution of commercially available sodium hypochlorite solution. Virus can be isolated from the urine for up to 3 weeks postinfection. There is only one recognized serotype of EVA, the Bucyrus strain, although there is evidence of antigenic variation among different isolates and variation in the degree of clinical signs produced by various isolates.
- Infection with EVA can occur in horses of any age or use due to its highly contagious nature and its spread by direct contact with infected horses and their body secretions, including urine and milk. The disease classically has high morbidity and low mortality in adults. The mortality in known infected neonates is much greater than previously suspected. The incidence of infection, determined by seroconversion, varies considerably by population and geographic location. The chief mode of transmission among racehorse populations appears to be through nasal droplet spray. Transmission at breeding farms is generally via the venereal route.
- The carrier of the virus is the intact male. Seronegative mares bred to either short- or long-term carrier stallions, shedding the virus in their semen, serve as a primary source of virus spread. Carrier stallions harbor the virus in their accessory sex glands, and the carrier state is testosterone dependent. Virus may be present in frozen or cooled semen from carrier stallions.
- Seropositive mares bred to a carrier stallion may also shed virus for a short period of time. Abortion due to EVA infection is thought to occur secondary to myometrial necrosis and edema, resulting in failure to the uteroplacental unit, although there is evidence of direct infection of the placenta.
- Foals born to seropositive dams acquire passive immunity through the colostrum and become seronegative after passive immunity wanes. Foals may also acquire the virus through colostrum and milk; at least two foals are thought to have acquired a fatal form of the disease in this manner.
- Experimental inoculation of animals by nasal challenge has shown that the virus first replicates within bronchoalveolar macrophages of the lung and then appears in the bronchial lymph nodes. The virus is then spread throughout the body via the circulation. Vascular lesions develop associated with virus present in tunica media of myocytes and within the endothelium. Arterial damage may persist for weeks after infection. The kidney is a site of virus localization, as is the placenta, bronchiolar epithelium, thymic tissue, and enterocytes in foals.

SYSTEMS AFFECTED

- Whole body, except central nervous system
- Predominant systems affected by age group—respiratory system in young horses, foals, and urogenital system in pregnant broodmares and intact males

GENETICS

N/A

SIGNALMENT

- Horses of any age or breed can develop EVA, although Standardbreds have the highest seroconversion rates in the United States.
- Foals in the immediate perinatal period, young horses in race training, and broodmares at farms with a carrier stallion have the highest rates of incidence.

SIGNS

EVA infection can present a wide range of signs, from clinically silent and recognizable only by seroconversion to acute-onset severe disease resulting in abortion and neonatal death.

Historical

- In the case of abortion and neonatal death, the history will include possible exposure by residing on a farm where a carrier stallion is present.
- There may also be history of a seronegative mare returning to the farm after being bred by a carrier stallion.
- Young horses in training may have history of being associated with an outbreak of respiratory disease ranging from mild to severe.
- Neonates born to seronegative mares or that have failure of passive transfer of maternal antibody when born to seropositive mares seem to be at greatest risk.

Physical Examination

- Young adults and broodmares that develop clinical signs typically are febrile for 5–9 days.
- Distal limb edema, particularly of the hindlimbs, may be present, as may edema in other sites, including the conjunctiva, periorbital region, scrotum, and prepuce.
- Epiphora and nasal discharge associated with rhinitis and conjunctivitis may be observed.
- An urticarial skin rash may be present.
- Cough, lethargy, anorexia, lameness, and exercise intolerance have been reported during outbreaks.
- Abortion and stillbirth are seen in pregnant mares.
- Sudden death, although rarely reported in adults, may occur with particularly virulent isolates.
- Foals may be born normal or weak, and may also have edema and lethargy. They may present with sudden death or go through a period resembling hypoxic ischemic asphyxia syndrome before progressing to respiratory failure and death, although foals with EVA perinatal infection have been known to survive for more than 2 weeks prior to death.

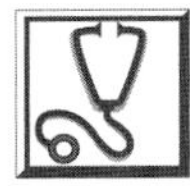

DIAGNOSIS

DIFFERENTIAL DIAGNOSIS

In young adults, differential diagnoses for EVA include all other infectious causes of respiratory disease, including, but not limited, to

- Equine influenza
- Equine herpesvirus, types 1 and 4
- Equine rhinovirus
- Equine infectious anemia
- Equine adenovirus
- Hendra virus

Differentials for edema due to vasculitis include:

- Equine infectious anemia
- Equine ehrlichiosis
- Purpura hemorrhagica

The primary differential in an abortion storm is equine herpesvirus type 1. Differentials for affected neonates include:

- Equine herpesvirus type 1
- Bacterial sepsis
- Severe hypoxic ischemic asphyxial or inflammatory perinatal insult

CBC/BIOCHEMISTRY/URINALYSIS

- CBC may demonstrate lymphopenia and thrombocytopenia, although these are variable and nonspecific findings.
- Serum biochemistry analysis is nondiagnostic.
- Urinalysis may reveal renal tubular inflammation with or without casts.

OTHER LABORATORY TESTS

Virus Isolation

Can be diagnostic antemortem. Acute cases have positive virus isolation from nasopharyngeal swabs or buffy coats from EDTA or citrated whole blood samples. Virus can be isolated from the urine in more chronic cases. EVA is isolated from the placenta or fetal tissues in the case of abortion, although maternal blood and urine may also be submitted.

Serology

CF and VN tests can be used. CF is best in acute cases and will show a rise in titer 2–4 weeks after infection. This titer becomes undetectable after about 8 months. VN titers develop along with CF titers, peak at 2–4 months, and remain increased for years.

DIAGNOSTIC PROCEDURES

Immunohistochemistry

Immunoperoxidase histochemistry performed on post-mortem or biopsy tissues can provide an accurate diagnosis in cases where EVA is suspected but has not been confirmed or as an adjunct to virus isolation and serology.

PATHOLOGIC FINDINGS

- Aborted and stillborn fetuses seldom have gross or histologic lesions, although EVA antigen may be identified in the fetus and/or placenta by immunoperoxidase histochemistry.
- Adults and foals that die of fulminant EVA infection have a bronchointerstitial pneumonia. The lungs are heavy, wet, and congested grossly. The pneumonia is characterized by hypertrophy and hyperplasia of type II pneumocytes and the presence of eosinophilic laminar to granular material scattered within the alveolar lumen. Histologically, the pneumonia may appear similar to morbillivirus (Hendra virus) infection in adults. Lymphocytic arteritis and periarteritis with varying degrees of tunica media fibrinoid necrosis may also be observed.
- Some infected foals are also reported to have pronounced gastrointestinal lesions.
- Renal tubular epithelial necrosis and interstitial nephritis are present in most chronic cases.
- Areas of edema are characterized by a lymphocytic vasculitis and perivasculitis.

IMAGING

Thoracic radiographs–possible increased bronchiolar and interstitial pattern with areas of consolidation

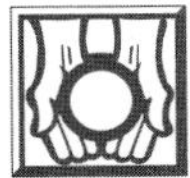

TREATMENT

APPROPRIATE HEALTH CARE

- Most horses with clinical disease recover with only supportive care. Horses may be best managed at home.
- In the case of an outbreak, all affected horses should be kept isolated for a period of 40 days following the appearance of the last case.
- Affected neonates need intensive medical management and should be hospitalized, although kept isolated from the rest of the hospital population, particularly pregnant mares.

NURSING CARE

- Nursing care is minimal for adults.
- Animals should be encouraged to eat and have stalls with good ventilation.
- Hydrotherapy and support wraps may benefit those patients with distal limb edema.
- Affected foals require intensive nursing, including intravenous fluid administration, frequent turning, feeding by nasogastric tube or by intravenous parenteral nutrition, and respiratory management, up to and including assisted ventilation.

ACTIVITY

- Activity should be minimal.
- Racehorses should be out of training until they are no longer shedding virus, a period of about 40 days.
- Handwalking is permissible, and may benefit those with edema, but contact with other horses should be minimal while the horse continues to shed virus.
- Acutely affected colts and stallions should have a prolonged period of sexual rest to decrease their chance of being chronic carriers.
- Affected foals are incapable of activity.

DIET

No dietary changes are required.

CLIENT EDUCATION

- Owners of affected foals should be informed of the poor prognosis for survival.
- Owners of affected colts and stallions should be informed of the risk of their horse becoming a carrier.
- All owners should be informed of the potential economic implications of seroconversion to EVA regarding import and export.

SURGICAL CONSIDERATIONS

N/A

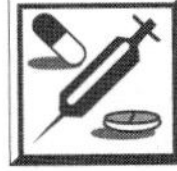

MEDICATIONS

DRUG(S) OF CHOICE

- There is no specific treatment for EVA.
- NSAIDs may be used to treat fever in adults.
- Affected neonates may be treated with broad-spectrum antimicrobial drugs to combat secondary bacterial infection. Anecdotally, treatment of foals with plasma harvested from a donor with high EVA titers has been attempted.

CONTRAINDICATIONS/PRECAUTIONS/ POSSIBLE INTERACTIONS/ ALTERNATIVE DRUGS

N/A

FOLLOW-UP

PATIENT MONITORING

Patients should be monitored for continued fever and potential secondary bacterial invaders.

CLIENT EDUCATION

It is important that clients be educated regarding control of EVA. Many states have regulations surrounding the use of EVA carrier stallions, notably New York and Kentucky. These programs have significant decreased the incidence of the disease in those states.

PREVENTION/AVOIDANCE

- Vaccination against EVA is available but is tightly controlled in some states. It is a modified-live vaccine and control programs usually involve vaccination of all noncarrier stallions and seronegative mares served by carrier stallions. Carrier stallions are evaluated periodically by breeding to seronegative mares and performing virus isolation on semen samples.
- Although international rules are loosening, seroconversion of a horse may result in problems regarding import and export to certain countries.

MISCELLANEOUS

ABBREVIATIONS

- CF = complement fixation
- EVA = equine viral arteritis
- NSAID = nonsteroidal anti-inflammatory drug
- VN = virus neutralization

Suggested Reading

Del Piero F, Wilkins PA, Lopez JW, et al. Equine viral arteritis in newborn foals: clinical, pathological, serological, microbiological and immunohistochemical observations. Equine Vet J 1997;29:178–185.

Doll ER, Knappenberger RE, Bryans JT. An outbreak of abortion caused by the equine arteritis virus. Cornell Vet 1957;47:69–75.

McCollum WH, Swerczek TW. Studies on an epizootic of equine viral arteritis in racehorses. Equine Vet J 1978;2:293–297.

McKenzie J. Equine viral arteritis and trade in horses from the USA. Surveillance 1990;16:17.

Timoney PJ, McCollum WH. Equine viral arteritis. Vet Clin North Am Equine Pract 1993;9:295–309.

Author Pamela A. Wilkins

Consulting Editors Ashley G. Boyle and Corinne R. Sweeney

VISION

BASICS

OVERVIEW

• The equine eye has developed a number of unique anatomic and physiologic features to suit its special visual needs. Adaptive influences include the horse's role as a prey species, its grazing habits, and the need for arrhythmic (diurnal and nocturnal) activity. Important adaptations to avoid predators are a large visual field and improved detection of motion. These adaptations, however, limit the ability to detect fine visual detail and color perception.

• The horse has a wide total visual field of about 350° due to the extreme lateral globe position, the nasal extension of the retina, and the horizontal shape of the pupil. It has narrow blind spots immediately below the nose and posterior to the tail.

• The visual fields of the two eyes overlap anteriorly and below the nose for 65°–70°. The binocular overlap is oriented down the nose in horses. A horse rotating its nose upward to better observe distant objects may be an attempt to exploit its improved binocular depth perception.

• Binocular depth thresholds are comparable to cats and indicate that horses possess stereopsis. Horses are also capable of utilizing monocular depth cues in judging distance. Nevertheless, the binocular threshold for depth perception in horses is five times better than the monocular threshold.

• The horse has 0.6 times the acuity of humans, 1.5 times that of dogs, and 3 times that of cats. That would mean a Snellen acuity of 20/33 (i.e., a horse viewing an object at a distance of 20 feet has approximately the visual acuity of a person viewing the object at 33 feet).

• Horses refractive errors range from +3 D to −3 D with most horses being emmetropic (normal).

• The aphakic equine globe is +9.9 D hyperopic (20/1200 Snellen equivalent). Despite this, aphakic horses after cataract surgery seem to perform well visually.

• The retina of the horse contains both rod and cone photoreceptors with rods outnumbering cones. Rods are most sensitive to dim light and are useful for motion detection. Cones are most sensitive to bright light, are responsible for color vision, and provide good visual resolution.

• Cone density in the retina of the horse is highest in the area centralis which provides the area of maximal visual acuity. The equine area centralis is divided into two areas: (1) area centralis rotunda—a small, circular region temporal and dorsal to the optic disc, and (2) the visual streak—a horizontal, narrow band above the optic nerve.
• Changes in head orientation, dynamic accommodation, and the presence of an area centralis aid near vision in horses.
• Horses have only two cone pigments and dichromatic color vision, whereas most humans typically have three cones and trichromatic vision. Each cone pigment responds to certain wavelengths better than others. Measurements of equine spectral sensitivity have shown a primary peak at 550 nm (greenish yellow), with a second peak at the far blue end of the color spectrum. The horse thus sees blue and yellow colors but may not see red. Since the cones are primarily located in the central retina, color vision is largely restricted to the central retina, and the ability of the peripheral retina to detect color is substantially reduced.
• The fibrous tapetum of the dorsal fundus enhances night vision but might, by scattering of light, degrade photoreceptor image resolution.
• The optic nerve of the horse is unique in that it contains a substantial proportion of axons of large diameter. Large retinal ganglion cells possess large-diameter axons and are involved in motion detection, stereopsis, and sensitivity to dim light, suggesting that the horse has strong retinal adaptations for these visual characteristics.
• The equine eye also show diurnal adaptations, such as the corpora nigra (protects the ventral retina during grazing), occludable pupils, and yellow pigment in the lens (limits transmittance of very short wavelengths which helps protect the photoreceptors in the retina).

ORGAN SYSTEM

Ophthalmic

ABBREVIATION

• D = Diopter

Suggested Reading

Brooks DE. Ophthalmology for the Equine Practitioner. Jackson, WY; Teton NewMedia, 2002.

Brooks DE, Matthews AG. Equine ophthalmology. In: Gelatt KN, ed. Veterinary Ophthalmology, ed 4. Philadelphia; Lippincott Williams and Wilkins, 2007.

Gilger BC, ed. Equine Ophthalmology. Philadelphia; WB Saunders, 2005.

Author Maria Källberg
Consulting Editor Dennis E. Brooks

VULVAR CONFORMATION

BASICS

DEFINITIONOVERVIEW

• The quality/grade of vulvar conformation is determined by the anatomic orientation of the anal sphincter to the vulva and pubis. This orientation impacts directly on the mare's reproductive health and affects her ability to maintain a healthy uterus and to carry pregnancies to term.

• *Good vulvar conformation* implies the dorsal commissure of the vulva is at or below the level of the pubis. This generally is coupled with vulvae that exhibit an effective side-to-side seal and are not slanted cranially, effectively protecting the genital tract from fecal contamination or aspiration of air.

• *Fair vulvar conformation* implies the dorsal vulvar commissure is elevated above the floor of the pubis and/or the vulva slope anteriorly, permitting pneumovagina or fecal contamination of the vestibule.

• *Poor vulvar conformation* implies the dorsal vulvar commissure is elevated above the pubis. This usually is accompanied by an obvious anterior slant of the vulva. Fecal contamination of the vestibule occurs frequently to continually.

• Problems with vulvar conformation account for a major portion of equine subfertility and infertility.

ETIOLOGY/PATHOPHYSIOLOGY

Factors predisposing mares to poor vulvar conformation—breeds/individuals with less muscle in the perineal area; perineal lacerations, and being underweight

SYSTEMS AFFECTED

Reproductive

GENETICS

• Influences vulvar conformation (mother/daughter) and should be considered when selecting broodmares. This is particularly important if farm-born fillies are to be the source of replacement stock.

• Mares with good vulvar conformation have fewer reproductive problems.

INCIDENCE/PREVALENCE

• Abnormal vulvar conformation is extremely common, especially in some breeds—Thoroughbreds, Standardbreds.

• More muscular breeds or certain families within breeds have less of a problem with less-than-ideal vulvar conformation.

SIGNALMENT

• Compromises of vulvar conformation can occur in all breeds and in any stock of breeding age.

• Incidence of poor vulvar conformation increases in old, pluriparous mares.

SIGNS

• The condition is fairly easy to evaluate. Assessment of each broodmare's vulvar conformation should be noted on her record at the start of each breeding season.

• Can worsen with age

Historical

• History of subfertility or infertility because of failure to conceive or termination of pregnancy

• In addition to endometritis, vaginitis or cervicitis may be present.

Physical Examination

• Less than ideal vulvar conformation may result in gross/histopathologic changes of the tubular genital tract.

• TRP—enlargement of uterine horns, increased uterine size, intraluminal fluid accumulation, and aspiration of air (e.g., pneumovagina, pneumouterus); if severe, echogenicities identified at U/S may be caused by fecal aspiration into the uterus.

• Vaginal examination using sterile lubricant and sterile vaginal speculum may reveal inflammation, discharge (e.g., endometritis, cervicitis, vaginitis), urine pooling, and/or adhesions (if chronic).

• Other physical parameters usually are normal.

CAUSES

• Inherited poor vulvar conformation

• Perineal laceration resulting from abnormal posture or fetal position at parturition

• Fetal extremities pushed dorsally, causing the fetus' feet to tear into the wall of the vagina or vestibule

RISK FACTORS

• Inherited

• No specific risk factors other than compromising the mare's ability to carry a healthy pregnancy to term

• Posterior presentation of a fetus might be linked with an increased incidence of perineal lacerations, but this has not been reported.

• Fetal posture and position can change within minutes of birth, so previous examinations for fetal position and posture have little predictive value.

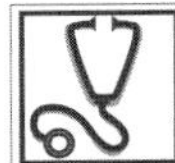

DIAGNOSIS

DIFFERENTIAL DIAGNOSIS

N/A

CBC/BIOCHEMISTRY/URINALYSIS

N/A

OTHER LABORATORY TESTS

N/A

IMAGING

N/A

OTHER DIAGNOSTIC PROCEDURES

• Determination of the location of the dorsal vulvar commissure in relation to the pubis

• Careful palpation of the vestibule, vagina, and rectum—to identify lacerations

• Rectovaginal fistulas may be small and not readily identified but result in sufficient contamination of the uterus to affect fertility.

PATHOLOGIC FINDINGS

• Partial- to full-thickness lacerations of the vestibule and/or vagina

• Aspiration of air into the vagina and/or uterus

• Fecal contamination of the vagina and vestibule, with resulting inflammation of the vestibule, vagina and cervix, and possibly, the endometrium

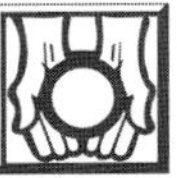

TREATMENT

APPROPRIATE HEALTH CARE

• Determine that a laceration does not extend into the perineal cavity—rare with perineal laceration or rectovaginal fistula.

• Systemic antibiotics seldom are indicated.

• Local medication is rarely indicated.

• Repair lacerations before attempting rebreeding.

• Boost tetanus toxoid vaccination, if status is not current or is unknown

NURSING CARE

N/A

ACTIVITY

Normal activity, no restrictions

DIET

Normal; no restrictions

CLIENT EDUCATION

• Review importance of closely observing foaling.
• Many lacerations occur before a foaling problem is noticed, even with trained attendants.

SURGICAL CONSIDERATIONS

General Comments

• Surgical correction for poor vulvar conformation (episioplasty) was first described by Caslick in 1937, i.e., Caslick's vulvoplasty.
• First, wrap and tie the mare's tail away from the field of surgery, and thoroughly clean the perineal area with cotton and soap.
• Carbocaine or another local anesthetic is infiltrated into the mucocutaneous junction on the vulva; ≅10–12 mL can be used to infiltrate both sides of the vulva.
• The tissue edges are freshened before suturing, either by removing a very narrow strip of tissue from the edge or by incising at the mucocutaneous junction along the line dilated with local anesthetic, the split-thickness technique; i.e., no tissue is removed.
• The split-thickness technique is tissue sparing, in that it helps to retain the normal elasticity of vulva during labor by minimizing damage with annual vulvoplasty. Both described techniques can be used, however, and are acceptable.
• Use nonabsorbable suture material or staples, with removal in ≅10 days.
• Check tetanus toxoid vaccination status.
• Pouret technique—In cases of severe/extremely poor vulvar conformation, it may be necessary to dissect the perineal body in a caudal (widest) to cranial (point), pie-shaped wedge, which permits the genital tract, ventral to the rectum, to slide caudally and away from fecal contamination as well as aspiration of air; only the skin is closed (i.e., no deep reconstruction of dissected tissue).

MEDICATIONS

N/A

DRUG(S) OF CHOICE

• No antibiotics are indicated.
• Selection of local anesthetic is at the discretion of the surgeon.

CONTRAINDICATIONS

N/A

PRECAUTIONS

N/A

POSSIBLE INTERACTIONS

N/A

ALTERNATIVE DRUGS

N/A

FOLLOW-UP

PATIENT MONITORING

Suture removal 10 days after surgery to prevent the possibility of stitch abscesses at the suture site

PREVENTION/AVOIDANCE

Select broodmares with excellent vulvar conformation.

POSSIBLE COMPLICATIONS

• Primary contraindication to vulvoplasty is the necessity to re-open the vulvar commissure ≅ 5 to 10 days before parturition to prevent perineum from tearing at delivery.
• Caslick's vulvoplasty should be replaced (i.e., incised and sutured) immediately after foaling or breeding and confirmation of ovulation in the next season, depending on severity of vulvar conformation abnormality.

EXPECTED COURSE AND PROGNOSIS

Without surgical correction, mares may remain infertile or abort during pregnancy.

MISCELLANEOUS

ASSOCIATED CONDITIONS

N/A

AGE-RELATED FACTORS

High probability of this condition becoming worse with age

ZOONOTIC POTENTIAL

N/A

PREGNANCY

Surgery may be necessary to obtain a pregnancy.

SYNONYM

Wind sucker

SEE ALSO

• Dystocia
• Endometrial biopsy
• Endometritis
• Perineal lacerations, fistulas
• Pneumovagina/pneumouterus
• Urine pooling

ABBREVIATIONS

• TRP = transrectal palpation
• U/S = ultrasound, ultrasonography

Suggested Reading

Aanes WA. Surgical repair of third degree perineal lacerations and recto-vaginal fistulas in the mare. JAVMA 1964;144:485–491.
Caslick EA. The vulva and vulvo-vaginal orifice and its relationship to genital health of the thoroughbred mare. Cornell Vet 1937;27:178–186.
Colbern GT, Aanes WA, Stashak TS. Surgical management of perineal lacerations and recto-vestibular fistulae in the mare: a retrospective study of 47 cases. JAVMA 1985;186:265–269.
Heinze CD, Allen AR. Repair of third-degree perineal lacerations in the mare. Vet Scope 1966;11:12–15.
Shipley WD, Bergin WC. Genital health in the mare. III. Pneumovagina. VM/SAC 1968;63:699–702.
Stickle RL, Fessler JF, Adams SB, et al. A single stage technique for repair of rectovestibular lacerations in the mare. J Vet Surg 1979;8:25–27.

Author Walter R. Threlfall
Consulting Editor Carla L. Carleton

WEANING SEPARATION STRESS

BASICS

DEFINITION

Weaning separation stress includes any of a number of reactions of the foal to separation from the dam and/or cessation of nutrition from the dam. Foals that are weaned naturally by the dam or that are weaned artificially but kept physically near or with the dam are rarely stressed as long as nutritional needs are met.

PATHOPHYSIOLOGY

- Under natural social conditions, cessation of nursing of foals occurs gradually over a period of months to years within the first 1–3 years of life. Significant nutrition from nursing at regular intervals usually ends at about 7–10 mo of age. Separation of the young from the dam typically does not occur until maturity. Long after nutritional dependence on regular nursing, offspring as old as 3 years or greater appear to gain social comfort by return to the dam and from nuzzling of the udder at moments of fear or threat, sometimes briefly latching on and apparently ingesting a small amount of milk.
- Under most traditional equine industry protocols, weaning is imposed at 2 to 6 mo of age by physical separation of the foal and dam. Abrupt separation from the nutritional and psychosocial support of the dam typically results in signs of physical and/or psychological stress reaction for the foal.

SYSTEMS AFFECTED

- Nervous system (behavior)—frantic locomotor activity, calling vocalizations, and interruption of foraging
- Gastrointestinal—frequent defecation; gastric ulcers are common.
- Immune—compromised immune function
- Musculoskeletal—Physical injuries may be incurred during panic, usually related to attempts to breech barriers; reduced rate of weight gain
- Respiratory—increased respiratory disease
- Skin—loss of coat and body condition

GENETICS

Inherited temperament likely affects maturational readiness and the behavioral and physical response to separation from the dam.

INCIDENCE/PREVALENCE

- Incidence of weaning separation stress varies in direct association with the methods and management.
- Abrupt permanent separation with re-location and without preweaning adaptation to alternative nutrition and hydration results in nearly all foals showing mild to moderate stress, loss of condition, and gastric ulcers.
- With gradual separation and careful nutritional preparation, the incidence of weaning and eventual separation stress or complications is very low.

GEOGRAPHIC DISTRIBUTION

May vary regionally with prevalent breeds and management practices, including weaning protocols, facilities

SIGNALMENT

Breed Predilection

More easily excitable breeds, such as Egyptian Arabians or Thoroughbreds, and lines within breeds appear to have greater separation stress response than less-excitable breeds and lines.

Mean Age and Range

Very early weaned foals 1–3 mo are believed to be at greater risk than more mature foals of 5–12 mo of age.

Predominant Sex

One study of 10 foals (6 females and 4 males) weaned at 6 mo of age resulted in the suggestion that female foals have greater locomotion response to weaning separation than males.

SIGNS

- Behaviors suggesting nonpathological stress of social separation include occasional whinny vocalization, increased level of alertness, calm walking, increased frequency of defecation, loose stool, mildly increased heart rate, and less recumbent rest but eating well.
- Signs of distress of social separation include frequent whinny vocalization, pawing, pacing, nervous walking or trotting, frequent defecation, watery stool, increased heart and respiratory rate, little standing or recumbent rest, and interrupted or poor eating.
- Signs of severe distress include reduced locomotion, depression, standing with lowered head, apathy, and not eating.

General Comments

- Locomotor and vocalization behavior of separation stress is adaptive for finding the dam or family group. In domestic confinement, it is the physical barriers and thwarted locomotion that typically lead to injuries.
- Groups of foals weaned and separated simultaneously often appear to suffer prolonged stress. Removal of only one or two dams at a time from a group of foals usually results in less stress for each foal than removing multiple or all dams at once. It is also useful to remove the dams of the most mature and behaviorally independent foals first.

Historical

Signs and observations often reported by the owner

CAUSES

N/A

RISK FACTORS

- Abrupt weaning
- Weaning less than 3 mo old
- Age at weaning
- Change of environment

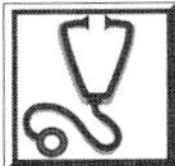

DIAGNOSIS

DIFFERENTIAL DIAGNOSIS

- Temporal association of behavioral distress responses and separation from the dam usually make the diagnosis clear.
- Weaning separation stress appears to be immediately evident.
- If a foal is calm within the minutes and hours after separation, a delayed onset is not expected without further social change, relocation, or other stressor.

CBC/BIOCHEMISTRY/URINALYSIS

As indicated to diagnose complications, e. g., gastric ulcers, dehydration, nutrition

OTHER LABORATORY TESTS

Cortisol will be elevated, as it is in many circumstances, so it is not diagnostic for separation stress.

IMAGING

Gastroscopy can be used to evaluate for gastric ulcers.

OTHER DIAGNOSTIC PROCEDURES

None

PATHOLOGICAL FINDINGS

Gastric ulcers

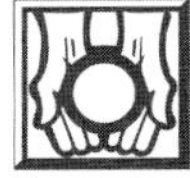

TREATMENT

AIMS OF TREATMENT

- Physical safety, social comfort, adequate nutrition, and distraction
- Diagnosis and treatment of related injuries or illnesses. Specifically, gastric ulcers should be addressed and treated.
- In cases of injury or frenetic distress, it may be advisable to re-unite the mare and foal and undertake separation at a much more mature age.

APPROPRIATE HEALTH CARE

Provide adequate nutrition, physical safety

NURSING CARE

- Ensure hydration and nutrition.
- If the dam is available, return foal to fence line—direct access to the dam may be considered.
- If the dam still has milk, udder covers are commercially available to block nursing.
- If return to the dam is not an option, companion horses, ponies, donkeys, goats, or chickens can provide social comfort and distraction. Also, human contact can be distracting and ameliorative.
- A simultaneously weaned foal may not be the best companion, due to a tendency for interfoal aggression, which appears to emerge in foals stressed by separation from the dam.

ACTIVITY

- Depending on the particular locomotor response, and the facilities, injuries may be greater with stall confinement than in a paddock.
- Foals that have been started in training or have had interactions with people before weaning/separation may be distracted and calmed from engaging in those activities.

DIET

- A preweaning diet high in fat and fiber compared to a high sugar and starch diet has been associated with less severe stress response to weaning separation.
- Milk from the dam (milked at the time or from a frozen bank) for 1 to a few days after separation can appear to provide some comfort.

CLIENT EDUCATION

See Patient Monitoring and Prevention/Avoidance.

SURGICAL CONSIDERATIONS

N/A

MEDICATIONS

DRUG(S) OF CHOICE

- Anxiolytics and other psychotropic medications have not been systematically evaluated for relieving weaning stress.
- For the frenetically active foal, tranquilization may be useful. Effectiveness varies with the level of panic.

CONTRAINDICATIONS

Some animals have paradoxical reactions to tranquilizers.

PRECAUTIONS

If tranquilizers are used, the foal should be watched carefully for at least an hour. Great care must be used to avoid incoordination, ataxia, or impaired judgment by the foal.

POSSIBLE INTERACTIONS

N/A

ALTERNATIVE DRUGS

A synthetic pheromone, Modipher EQ, is marketed as a calming agent for horses and specifically lists mare-foal separation as an indication for use. Apparently, the effectiveness has not been critically evaluated in controlled studies.

FOLLOW-UP

PATIENT MONITORING

- The foal should be observed for a return to a normal 24-hr time budget of behaviors. For a 4- to 6-mo-old foal, this would include at least 50% of time foraging, 25% standing or recumbent rest, minimal vocalization, at least 10% of time playing or playfully investigating environment and interacting socially, with no stereotypic pawing, cribbing, perimeter walking, or running.
- The activity pattern of a nonstressed foal includes alternating periods of foraging, play, and rest, with each foraging and rest period lasting ≈30 to 60 min.

PREVENTION/AVOIDANCE

Preventive measures to reduce weaning stress and associated injury and illness include:

- Introducing the independent diet high in fat and fiber well before separation from the dam, including a balanced mineral supplement and salt
- Separating/weaning only healthy, thriving foals of at least 4 mo of age
- Removing the dam from the established social group, rather than removing the foal to a new group
- Allowing the foal to establish play groups of foals and/or yearlings with which it can remain when the dam is removed
- Including in the foal group a familiar adult herd mate/s (e. g., mare or gelding) before weaning that can remain with the foal/s after separation from the dam as an adult guardian/s
- Employing gradual weaning/separation protocols versus abrupt separation
- In mare and foal groups, removing one mare at a time, leaving foals and remaining mares together and in familiar surroundings
- Separating/weaning older (4–6 mo) versus younger (2–4 mo) foals
- Observing behavior of foals to determine readiness for weaning
- Minimizing additional stress at the time of separation from the dam (e. g., new social groups, new location, transportation, immunization, deworming, intense human interaction or stressful handling or training)
- Ensuring a familiar, healthy, and safe environment for the foal at the time of separation (the most recent environment, good soft slip-free footing, safe fencing, free of obstacles, free of dust that can be stirred up with increased activity)

Evidence indicates that foals confined indoors in stalls at the time of separation, whether alone or in weanling pairs, are at greater risk of behavior and health problems related to weaning and separation stress than when kept at pasture. Respiratory complications are higher with the increased activity with greater dust and poorer ventilation in stalls. Injuries are greater in pair-stalled weanlings in association with interfoal aggression.

POSSIBLE COMPLICATIONS

In addition to long-term effects of injury and interference with weight gain, foals experiencing weaning separation stress are believed to be at greater risk of developing abnormal behavior, including separation anxiety, isolation panic, cribbing, and other stereotypies.

EXPECTED COURSE AND PROGNOSIS

Separation stress has a variable duration, usually from a few hours to several days.

Suggested Reading

Hoffman RM, Kronfeld DS, Holland JL, Greiwe-Crandell KM. Preweaning diet and stall weaning method influences on stress response in foals. J Anim Sci 1995;73:2922–2930.

Householder DD. Minimizing weaning stress in foals. Available at http://animalscience.tamu.edu/main/academics/equine/hrg018-weanfoals.pdf. Accessed September 30, 2007.

Malinowski K, Hallquist NA, Helyar L, Sherman AR, Scanes CG. Effect of different separation protocols between mares and foals on plasma cortisol and cell-mediated immune response. J Equine Vet Sci 1990;10:363–368.

McCall CA, Potter GD, Kreide JL. Locomotor, vocal and other behavioral responses to varying methods of weaning foals. Appl Anim Behav Sci 1985;14:27–35.

McCall CA, Potter GD, Kreider JL, Jenkins WL. Physiological responses in foals weaned by abrupt or gradual methods. J Equine Vet Sci 1987;7:368–374.

McGreevy P. Equine Behavior: A Guide for Veterinarians and Equine Scientists. Philadelphia: Saunders, 2004:279–282.

Moons C, Laughlin K, Zanella A. Effects of short-term maternal separations on weaning stress in foals. Appl Anim Behav Sci 2005;91(3–4):321–335.

Nicol CJ, Badnell-Waters AJ, Bice R, Kelland A, Wilson AD, Harris PA. The effects of diet and weaning method on the behaviour of young horses. Appl Anim Behav Sci 2005;95:205–221.

Author Sue M. McDonnell

Consulting Editors Victoria L. Voith and Daniel Q. Estep

WEST NILE VIRUS

BASICS

OVERVIEW

• West Nile virus (WNV) is a seasonal and potentially fatal neurotropic disease, introduced into the United States in 1999; WNV is now found in all 48 contiguous states; equine cases occur between May and January. • Outbreak peaked in 2002 with 15,257 equine WNV cases reported to U.S. Department of Agriculture; approximately 1000 cases were reported annually in 2004 and 2005. • Most infected horses are asymptomatic, but infection can present as neurologic disease. • WNV is carried and transmitted by mosquitoes. • Wild birds are the principal host for WNV; the virus is amplified in the bird population. • When the virus reaches high levels in the bird population, increasing number and species of mosquitoes are infected, thus increasing the risk to horses.
• WNV enters the body through the bite of an infected mosquito and then multiplies in the bloodstream. If it crosses the blood-brain barrier, it leads to meningoencephalitis and sometimes death.

SIGNALMENT

• Any age, breed, or sex • Species—horses, human, and birds (especially corvids); sporadic reports of titers and disease in other species

SIGNS

• Incubation period 5–15 days • Signs range from asymptomatic through acutely neurologic.
• Neurologic signs not pathognomonic—diagnosis cannot be based on clinical signs alone • Neurologic signs often include ataxia or incoordination, generalized weakness, lethargy/depression, muscle fasciculations, caudal paresis, and recumbency.
• Fever is not a common presenting sign.

CAUSES AND RISK FACTORS

• WNV is a member of the genus *Flavivirus,* family Flaviviridae. • Risk factor—exposure to infected mosquitoes

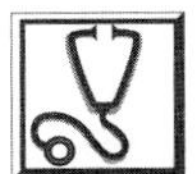

DIAGNOSIS

DIFFERENTIAL DIAGNOSIS

Other causes of equine neurologic disease include but are not limited to
• Eastern, Western, and venezuelan equine encephalitis • Rabies • EPM • EHV
• Poisoning—moldy corn; lead • Equine degenerative myelopathy • Aberrant strongyles migration • Wobbler's syndrome • Head trauma

CBC/BIOCHEMISTRY/URINALYSIS

Typical of viral infection

OTHER LABORATORY TESTS

Serum

• IgM-ELISA—the most reliable test available, particularly in horses previously vaccinated or of unknown vaccination status • Plaque reduction neutralization (PRN)—in horses never before vaccinated, a 4-fold rise in titer indicates infection; test is of no diagnostic value if the horse was previously vaccinated. • Brain tissue—hindbrain preferable • RT-PCR—virus load is low in horses; use a lab familiar with equine RT-PCR • Virus isolation useful if RT-PCR does not yield results

Notes

• Previous vaccination can significantly affect test results. • Check with local lab for preferred testing protocol. • When collecting brain samples, maintain brain tissue viability for rabies testing.

PATHOLOGIC FINDINGS

Lesions of the brain and spinal cord consistent with encephomyelitis

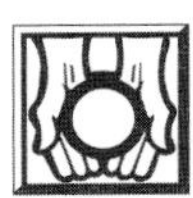

TREATMENT

• No specific treatment • Supportive care

FOLLOW-UP

PREVENTION/AVOIDANCE

Vaccination

• Four vaccines are currently licensed for horses and foals. • No vaccine is currently labeled for pregnant mares.

Avoidance

• Most important, minimize the standing water in which WNV-carrying mosquitoes breed. • To eliminate standing water: eliminate containers that collect water; keep watering devices, especially automatic waterers, clean; improve existing drainage; maintain basic sanitation.
• Potential mosquito-breeding sites: discarded tires; rain gutters and drainage ditches; water buckets and troughs; wash stall drains; wheelbarrows; bird baths; plastic wading pools; unused swimming pools; anything else that collects water.

POSSIBLE COMPLICATIONS

In one large study, 80% of horses who recovered did so fully; the remainder had residual effects such as weight or body condition loss, decreased stamina, ataxia, stumbling, and cranial nerve deficits.

EXPECTED COURSE AND PROGNOSIS

• Mortality rates range from 20% to 44%. • More severely affected horses have poorer prognoses. Horses are more likely to die if they develop caudal paresis or recumbency. • Severity of clinical signs tends to increase with age. • Vaccination appears to reduce severity of clinical signs and the risk of death from WNV. • Studies indicate vaccine protection is significantly increased if vaccination is completed prior to exposure to infected mosquitoes and according to manufacturer's instructions.

MISCELLANEOUS

AGE-RELATED FACTORS

Mortality increases with age among clinically ill infected horses.

ZOONOTIC POTENTIAL

• Humans are susceptible. • Infected mosquitoes transmit the virus. Horses do not seem to transmit WNV to other horses or humans, and humans do not seem to transmit the virus to other humans or horses. • Humans in areas with WNV-positive mosquitoes, birds, or horses should take measures to protect themselves from mosquitoes. • Humans exposed to potentially infected horse brain and spinal cord tissue should wear appropriate personal protective equipment.

PREGNANCY

• It is recommended that mares be fully vaccinated before breeding. • Studies of the safety of WNV vaccination in pregnant mares are ongoing.

ABBREVIATIONS

• EHV = equine herpesvirus • EPM = equine protozoal myeloencephalitis • PRN = plaque reduction neutralization • ELISA = enzyme-linked immunosorbent assay • RT-PCR = reverse transcription–polymerase chain reaction • WNV = West Nile virus

Suggested Reading

American Association of Equine Practitioners West Nile Virus Vaccination Guidelines. 2005. Available at: http://www.aaep.org/pdfs/AAEP_WNV_Guidelines_2005.pdf.

Center for Food Health and Public Safety. West Nile fever. January 2004. Available at: http://www.cfsph.iastate.edu/Factsheets/pdfs/west_nile_fever.pdf.

Long M. Flavivirus infections. In: Sellon DC, Long M, eds. Equine Infectious Diseases. Philadelphia: WB Saunders, 2006:198–206.

Salazar P, Traub-Dargatz JL, Morley PS, et al. Outcome of equids with clinical signs of West Nile virus infection and factors associated with death. J Am Vet Med Assoc 2004;225:267–274.

Schuler LA, Khaitsa ML, Dyer NW, et al. Evaluation of an outbreak of West Nile virus infection in horses: 569 Cases (2002). J Am Vet Med Assoc 2004;225:1084–1089.

USDA Animal and Plant Health Inspection Service (APHIS) Veterinary Services. West Nile virus monitoring and surveillance. Available at: http://www.aphis.usda.gov/vs/nahss/equine/wnv/; West Nile Virus Factsheet (October 2004).

Ward MP, Levy M, Thacker HL, et al. Investigation of an outbreak of encephalomyelitis caused by West Nile virus in 136 horses. J Am Vet Med Assoc 2004;225:84–89.

Authors Jennifer Jacobs Fowler, Susan C. Trock, and Brianne Gustafson
Consulting Editors Ashley G. Boyle and Corrine R. Sweeney

WHITE MUSCLE DISEASE

BASICS

OVERVIEW

• White muscle disease (nutritional muscular dystrophy, nutritional myodegeneration, dystrophic myodegeneration) is a noninflammatory degenerative disease of skeletal and cardiac muscle induced by a dietary deficiency of selenium (Se) and vitamin E.
• The regional distribution of cases corresponds to areas where Se-deficient soils predominate.
• Affected animals may be presented with acute fulminant disease with myocardial involvement or with subacute, insidious disease; in either case, mortality is high and animals often do not respond to treatment. Comorbidity is common and may mask the underlying primary problem.
• Prevention via monitoring of dietary and animal Se status and supplementation of pregnant mares is effective and recommended in Se-deficient areas or on farms where cases have been documented.

SIGNALMENT

• Young foals, with the majority of cases diagnosed within the first 60 days of life. Animals up to 1 year of age may be affected, and lesions have been noted in aborted fetuses.
• No breed or sex predisposition
• There does not appear to be a genetic component.

SIGNS

Acute Form

• Sudden death
• Circulatory collapse
• Cyanosis
• Tachycardia, arrhythmia, systolic cardiac murmur
• Respiratory distress (pulmonary edema, respiratory muscle failure)
• Inability to rise, often with violent struggling

Subacute Form

• *Profound muscular weakness = hallmark sign*
• Stiff, stilted gait
• Muscle fasciculation/trembling
• Inability to rise or stand unassisted
• Dysphagia and/or poor suckle reflex (milk at nares, ptyalism)
• Aspiration pneumonia
• Weight loss or failure to gain due to inadequate dietary intake
• Swollen, painful muscles—limbs, lumbar, cervical musculature

CAUSES AND RISK FACTORS

• Selenium deficiency—Selenium is an important component of GPx, an enzyme found in all animal tissue (high concentrations in liver and erythrocytes) that functions to reduce highly reactive oxygen metabolites that are produced during normal cellular metabolism. Deficiency of GPx increases membrane lipid peroxidation by these metabolites, resulting in membrane degradation and destruction of cells. Severe oxidative stress to myocytes and subsequent rhabdomyolysis underlie the pathogenesis of WMD in Se-deficient foals.
• While vitamin E deficiency may also play a role, deficiency of this nutrient alone is not sufficient to cause clinical disease in foals; vitamin E deficiency likely promotes disease in the setting of Se deficiency.
• Foals born to mares with dietary deficiency of Se are affected; not all Se-deficient foals display clinical signs of disease.

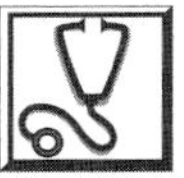

DIAGNOSIS

DIFFERENTIAL DIAGNOSIS

• Dysphagia
  ○ Cleft palate
  ○ Pharyngitis/pharyngeal malformation
  ○ Botulism
  ○ Weak foal for any reason (e.g., sepsis)
• Muscular weakness
  ○ Botulism
  ○ Tick paralysis
  ○ Neurologic/neuromuscular disease
• Stiff gait
  ○ Tetanus
  ○ Septic (poly)arthritis
  ○ Bacterial meningitis
  ○ Trauma
• Pneumonia
• Congenital cardiac anomaly
• Polysaccharide storage myopathy
• Glycogen branching enzyme deficiency
• Neonatal isoerythrolysis
• Sepsis

CBC/BIOCHEMISTRY/URINALYSIS

• CBC—hematocrit normal or increased (helpful to differentiate from neonatal isoerythrolysis, which may also cause pigmenturia)
• Biochemistry—hyponatremia, hypochloremia, hyperkalemia, hyperphosphatemia, azotemia (prerenal or postrenal), significant increases in CK, AST, and LDH; hypogammaglobulinemia
• Urinalysis—pigmenturia (myoglobinuria)

OTHER LABORATORY TESTS

• Whole blood Se concentration—documents recent Se deficiency; may be used to assess adequacy of supplementation; performed prior to supplementation
• Glutathione peroxidase concentration (erythrocyte)—documents Se deficiency in past weeks to months (Se incorporated during erythropoiesis); should be interpreted according to reference ranges of laboratory performing analysis

IMAGING

N/A

OTHER DIAGNOSTIC PROCEDURES

• Muscle biopsy—may be helpful to diagnose myopathy in animals with normal whole blood Se, GPx

PATHOLOGICAL FINDINGS

Pale streaking of major skeletal muscle groups and myocardium (especially left ventricle) seen at necropsy. Histologically, hyaline degeneration and myolysis are seen acutely; chronic cases may display fibrosis and calcification of lesions.

WHITE MUSCLE DISEASE

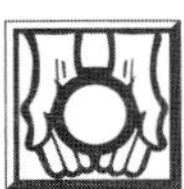

TREATMENT

- Affected foals should be strictly rested to avoid additional undue muscle damage.
- Supportive care in the form of supplemental nutrition (preferably via an indwelling nasogastric feeding tube to provide energy and avoid aspiration pneumonia)
- Fluid therapy (avoid potassium-containing fluids in hyperkalemic foals), and plasma are often required.

MEDICATIONS

DRUG(S) OF CHOICE

- Vitamin E/Se combination—2.5 mg Se/ml; recommended dose is 1 ml/45 kg deep IM divided into two sites (semimembranosus/semitendinosus recommended; do not use cervical, gluteal muscles); can be repeated at 5- to 10-day intervals if necessary
- Vitamin E (oral): 500 IU vitamin E/mL; recommended dose is 1–2 IU/kg PO daily.
- NSAIDs—flunixin meglumine (1 mg/kg IV BID) or ketoprofen (2.2 mg/kg IV BID) may be used to reduce muscle pain and swelling; may be ulcerogenic in neonates
- Broad-spectrum antimicrobials—Affected foals often have failure of transfer of passive immunity due to decreased colostral intake (recumbent/weak, dysphagic); concurrent aspiration pneumonia common (antimicrobial therapy best directed with results of bacterial culture of percutaneous transtracheal aspirate)

CONTRAINDICATIONS/POSSIBLE INTERACTIONS

Anaphylactoid reactions may occur with intravenous administration of commercial vitamin E/Se preparations; this is not recommended.

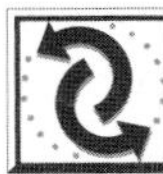

FOLLOW-UP

PATIENT MONITORING

- Rapid decreases (24–48 hours) in plasma CK concentration indicate cessation of muscle damage; AST and LDH decrease much more slowly (weeks).
- Monitoring of whole blood Se and GPx concentrations is recommended to gauge efficacy of supplementation.

PREVENTION/AVOIDANCE

Since WMD is associated with a high mortality rate, even with appropriate treatment, prevention of the disease is far preferred.

- Farms in known Se-deficient areas should practice routine feed analysis; all dietary components (forage and grain) should contain at least 0.10 ppm Se, preferably 0.30 ppm.
- Pregnant mares should be supplemented with dietary Se at the rate of 1 mg Se/mare/day through provision of a trace mineral salt (15–30 ppm) or in the ration at 0.50 ppm. Supplementation of mares in this fashion has been shown to prevent myopathy in foals and is more effective than supplementation of foals at birth (which may be born diseased). Alternatively, intramuscular administration of commercial vitamin E/Se preparations may be used for prevention.

POSSIBLE COMPLICATIONS

- Selenium toxicity may occur with over zealous supplementation; the toxic dose is 200 μg/kg in foals.
- Concurrent aspiration pneumonia and failure of transfer of passive immunity/septicemia are common.
- Fibrosis of severely affected muscle groups may result in permanent gait deficits in recovered animals.

EXPECTED COURSE AND PROGNOSIS

Guarded prognosis. Acute form, >90% mortality; subacute form, 50%–75%. Animals that do not respond to therapy within 2–5 days will likely not recover.

MISCELLANEOUS

ASSOCIATED CONDITIONS

- Septicemia
- Aspiration pneumonia

AGE-RELATED FACTORS

N/A

ZOONOTIC POTENTIAL

N/A

PREGNANCY

N/A (see Prevention/Avoidance)

SEE ALSO

- Septicemia
- Pneumonia, neonatal
- Glycogen branching enzyme deficiency
- Tetanus
- Botulism

ABBREVIATIONS

- AST = aspartate aminotransferase
- CK = creatine kinase
- GPx = glutathione peroxidase
- LDH = lactate dehydrogenase
- Se = selenium
- Ppm = parts per million
- WMD = white muscle disease

Suggested Reading

Moore RM, Kohn CW. Nutritional muscular dystrophy in foals. Comp Contin Educ Pract Vet 1991;13:476–490.

Author Teresa A. Burns
Consulting Editor Margaret C. Mudge

INDEX

Text in **boldface** denotes chapter discussions.

B

C

D

F

H

I

J

K

L

M

N

Q

T

V

W

X

Y

Z